Critical Heart Disease in Infants and Children

Second Edition

David G. Nichols, MD, MBA
Professor of Anesthesiology and Critical Care Medicine
  and Pediatrics
Vice Dean for Education
Mary Wallace Stanton Professor of Education
Johns Hopkins University School of Medicine
Baltimore, Maryland

Ross M. Ungerleider, MD
Professor and Chief, Cardiothoracic Surgery
Oregon Health and Sciences University
John C. Hursh Chair, Pediatric Cardiac Surgery
Doernbecher Children's Hospital
Portland, Oregon

Philip J. Spevak, MD
Associate Professor of Pediatrics and Medicine
Johns Hopkins University School of Medicine
Director of Pediatric Echocardiography
Johns Hopkins Hospital
Baltimore, Maryland

William J. Greeley, MD, MBA
Professor of Anesthesiology/Critical Care Medicine and
  Pediatrics
J.J. Downes Endowed Chair in Critical Care Medicine
University of Pennsylvania School of Medicine
Chair, Department of Anesthesiology and Critical Care
  Medicine
The Children's Hospital of Philadelphia
Philadelphia, Pennsylvania

Duke E. Cameron, MD
Professor of Surgery, The James T. Dresher Sr.
  Professor of Cardiac Surgery
Johns Hopkins University School of Medicine
Director of Pediatric Cardiac Surgery
Co-Director, The Dana and Albert "Cubby" Broccoli
  Center for Aortic Diseases
Johns Hopkins Hospital
Baltimore, Maryland

Dorothy G. Lappe, RN, MS, MBA
Baltimore, Maryland

Randall C. Wetzel, MBBS, MBA
Professor of Anesthesiology and Pediatrics
The Anne O'M. Wilson Professor of Critical Care
  Medicine
Keck School of Medicine of the University of Southern
  California
Chair, Department of Anesthesiology and Critical Care
  Medicine
Childrens Hospital Los Angeles
Los Angeles, California

MOSBY

ELSEVIER

MOSBY
ELSEVIER

1600 John F. Kennedy Blvd.
Ste 1800
Philadelphia, PA 19103-2899

CRITICAL HEART DISEASE IN INFANTS AND CHILDREN ISBN-13: 978-0-323-01281-2
Copyright © 2006, 1995 by Mosby, Inc., an affiliate of Elsevier Inc. ISBN-10: 0-323-01281-7

Notice

Knowledge and best practice in this field are constantly changing. As new research and experience broaden our knowledge, changes in practice, treatment, and drug therapy may become necessary or appropriate. Readers are advised to check the most current information provided (i) on procedures featured or (ii) by the manufacturer of each product to be administered, to verify the recommended dose or formula, the method and duration of administration, and contraindications. It is the responsibility of the practitioner, relying on their own experience and knowledge of the patient, to make diagnoses, to determine dosages and the best treatment for each individual patient, and to take all appropriate safety precautions. To the fullest extent of the law, neither the Publisher nor the Editors assume any liability for any injury and/or damage to persons or property arising out or related to any use of the material contained in this book.

The Publisher

Library of Congress Cataloging-in-Publication Data
Critical heart disease in infants and children / [edited by] David G. Nichols ... [et al.].—
  2nd ed.
    p. ; cm
  Includes bibliographical references and index.
  ISBN 978-0-323-01281-2
  1. Pediatric cardiology. 2. Pediatric intensive care. I. Nichols, David G. (David Gregory), 1951-
    [DLNM: 1. Heart Diseases—therapy—Child. 2. Heart Diseases—therapy—Infant. 3. Critical Care—Child. 4. Critical Care—Infant. WS 290 C934 2005
  RJ421.C75 2005
  618.92'12—dc22   2004053077

Acquisitions Editor: Natasha Andjelkovic
Project Manager: Mary Stermel
Marketing Manager: Emily Christie

Printed in the United States of America

Last digit is the print number: 9 8 7 6 5

*This book is dedicated to
children with critical heart disease
and to those adults who work together
to share their knowledge and skill
in the hope of restoring
these children to health.*

*This lifelong devotion to children
was exemplified throughout the career of*

Catherine A. Neill, M.D.

*In respect and with deep regard we dedicate
this book to the memory of this
dedicated physician,
consummate clinician,
devoted teacher.*

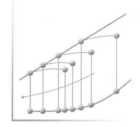

Contributors

Judith A. Ascenzi, RN, MSN

Nurse Clinician III/Unit Educator
Pediatric Intensive Care Unit
Johns Hopkins Hospital
Baltimore, Maryland

Robyn J. Barst, MD

Professor of Pediatrics in Medicine
Columbia University College of Physicians
    and Surgeons
Attending Pediatrician
Morgan Stanley Children's Hospital of
    New York-Presbyterian Medical Center
New York, New York

Robert D. Bart, MD

Assistant Professor of Pediatrics
Keck School of Medicine of the University of
    Southern California
Attending Physician, Department of Anesthesiology
    and Critical Care Medicine
Childrens Hospital Los Angeles
Los Angeles, California

Frank E. Berkowitz, MBBCh, MPH

Professor of Pediatrics
Emory University School of Medicine
Pediatrician
Hughes Spalding Children's Hospital
Atlanta, Georgia

Katherine Biagas, MD

Assistant Professor of Pediatrics
Columbia University College of Physicians
    and Surgeons
Director, Pediatric Critical Care Medicine Fellowship
Morgan Stanley Children's Hospital of
    New York-Presbyterian Medical Center
New York, New York

David P. Bichell, MD

Associate Professor of Surgery
University of Chicago School of Medicine
Director, Pediatric and Congenital Cardiac Surgery
University of Chicago Comer Children's Hospital
Chicago, Illinois

Ross Macrae Bremner, MD, PhD

Assistant Professor of Cardiothoracic Surgery
Keck School of Medicine of the University of
    Southern California
Chief of General Thoracic Surgery
St. Joseph's Hospital and Medical Center
Phoenix, Arizona

Duke E. Cameron, MD

Professor of Surgery
The James T. Dresher Sr. Professor of Cardiac Surgery
Johns Hopkins University School of Medicine
Director of Pediatric Cardiac Surgery
Co-Director of The Dana and Albert "Cubby" Broccoli
    Center for Aortic Diseases
Johns Hopkins Hospital
Baltimore, Maryland

Michael P. Carboni, MD

Assistant Clinical Professor in Pediatrics
Duke University School of Medicine
Division of Pediatric Cardiology
Duke Children's Hospital
Durham, North Carolina

Ira M. Cheifetz, MD

Associate Professor of Pediatrics
Division Chief, Pediatric Critical Care Medicine
Duke University School of Medicine
Medical Director, Pediatric Intensive Care Unit
Medical Director, Pediatric Respiratory Care and
    ECMO Programs
Duke Children's Hospital
Durham, North Carolina

Steve Davis, MD

Chair, Department of Pediatric Critical Care Medicine
Vice Chair, Department of Pediatrics
Cleveland Clinic Foundation
Cleveland, Ohio

Antonio DeMaio, PhD

Professor of Surgery
Vice Chairman of Research
University of California, San Diego
La Jolla, California

Jayant K. Deshpande, MD, MPH

Professor of Anesthesiology and Pediatrics
Vanderbilt University School of Medicine
Director, Division of Pediatric Critical Care Medicine
Medical Director, Performance Management and
    Improvement
Monroe Carell, Jr., Children's Hospital at Vanderbilt
Nashville, Tennessee

Scott M. Eleff, MD

Professor of Clinical Anesthesiology
Division of Neuro-Anesthesiology
University of Illinois at Chicago School of Medicine
Attending Anesthesiologist
University of Illinois Medical Center
Chicago, Illinois

David Epstein, MD

Assistant Clinical Professor of Pediatrics
University of California, Los Angeles
Pediatric Critical Care
Mattel's Children's Hospital at UCLA
Los Angeles, California

Thomas O. Erb, MD, MHS

Associate Professor of Anesthesia and Critical Care
University Basel, Medical Faculty
Division of Anesthesia
University Children's Hospital Beider Basel
Basel, Switzerland

Barbara A. Fivush, MD

Professor of Pediatrics
Johns Hopkins University School of Medicine
Chief of Pediatric Nephrology
Johns Hopkins Hospital
Baltimore, Maryland

Charles D. Fraser, MD

Professor of Surgery and Pediatrics
Baylor College of Medicine
Chief, Cardiac Surgery
Chief, Division of Congenital Heart Surgery
Donovan Chair in Congenital Heart Surgery
Texas Children's Hospital
Houston, Texas

J. William Gaynor, MD

Associate Professor of Surgery
University of Pennsylvania School of Medicine
Division of Cardiothoracic Surgery
The Children's Hospital of Philadelphia
Philadelphia, Pennsylvania

William J. Greeley, MD, MBA

Professor of Anesthesiology and Critical Care Medicine
    and Pediatrics
J. J. Downes Endowed Chair in Critical Care Medicine
University of Pennsylvania School of Medicine
Chair, Department of Anesthesiology and
    Critical Care Medicine
The Children's Hospital of Philadelphia
Philadelphia, Pennsylvania

Laura A. Hastings, MD

Assistant Professor of Anesthesiology and
    Pediatrics
Keck School of Medicine of the University of
    Southern California
Attending Physician, Cardiac Anesthesiology and
    Cardiac Intensive Care
Childrens Hospital Los Angeles
Los Angeles, California

Eugenie S. Heitmiller, MD

Associate Professor of Anesthesiology and
    Critical Care Medicine and
    Pediatrics
Johns Hopkins University School of
    Medicine
Vice Chairman for Clinical Affairs
Department of Anesthesiology and
    Critical Care Medicine
Johns Hopkins Hospital
Baltimore, Maryland

Mark A. Helfaer, MD

Professor of Anesthesiology and Critical
    Care Medicine and Pediatrics
University of Pennsylvania School of
    Medicine
Chief, Division of Critical
    Care Medicine
Department of Anesthesiology and
    Critical Care
The Children's Hospital of
    Philadelphia
Philadelphia, Pennsylvania

Allan J. Hordof, MD

Professor of Pediatrics
Columbia University College of Physicians
    and Surgeons
Interim Director, Division of Pediatric
    Cardiology
Morgan Stanley Children's Hospital of
    New York-Presbyterian Medical Center
New York, New York

Stephen B. Horton, PhD, CCP (Aus), CCP (USA)

Senior Fellow, Faculty of Medicine
Department of Paediatrics
The University of Melbourne
Director of Perfusion, Cardiac Surgery
Royal Children's Hospital
Victoria, Australia

Daphne T. Hsu, MD

Professor of Clinical Pediatrics
Columbia University College of Physicians
    and Surgeons
Attending Physician
Morgan Stanley Children's Hospital of
    New York-Presbyterian Medical Center
New York, New York

Elizabeth A. Hunt, MD, MPH

Assistant Professor of Anesthesiology and
  Critical Care Medicine
Director, Johns Hopkins Simulation Center
Johns Hopkins University School of Medicine
Pediatric Intensive Care Unit
Johns Hopkins Hospital
Baltimore, Maryland

Laura Ibsen, MD

Associate Professor of Pediatrics and
  Anesthesiology
Oregon Health and Sciences University
Medical Director, Pediatric Intensive Care Unit
Doernbecher Children's Hospital
Portland, Oregon

James Jaggers, MD

Associate Professor of Surgery
Duke University School of Medicine
Chief, Pediatric Cardiac Surgery
Duke Children's Hospital
Durham, North Carolina

David R. Jobes, MD

Professor of Anesthesiology and Critical
  Care Medicine
University of Pennsylvania School of Medicine
Senior Attending Anesthesiologist
The Children's Hospital of Philadelphia
Attending Anesthesiologist
The Hospital of the University of Pennsylvania
Philadelphia, Pennsylvania

James A. Johns, MD

Associate Professor of Pediatrics
Director, Pediatric Cardiology
  Training Program
Vanderbilt University
Monroe Carell, Jr., Children's Hospital
  at Vanderbilt
Nashville, Tennessee

Patricia A. Kane, MSN, CPNP

Pediatric Nurse Practitioner
Pediatric Cardiology and Cardiac Surgery
Johns Hopkins Hospital
Baltimore, Maryland

Ronald J. Kanter, MD

Associate Professor of Pediatrics
Duke University School of Medicine
Director of Pediatric Electrophysiology
Duke Children's Hospital
Durham, North Carolina

Tom R. Karl, MD, MS

Professor of Surgery and Pediatrics
University of California at San Francisco
  School of Medicine
Chief of Pediatric Cardiothoracic Surgery
UCSF Children's Hospital
San Francisco, California

Frank H. Kern, MD

Professor of Anesthesiology and Pediatrics
Duke University School of Medicine
Vice Chair, Department of
  Anesthesiology
Chief, Pediatric Anesthesia
Duke Children's Hospital
Durham, North Carolina

Paul M. Kirshbom, MD

Assistant Professor, Division of Cardiothoracic
  Surgery
Emory University School of Medicine
Cardiac Surgeon
Children's Healthcare of Atlanta and Emory
  University Hospital
Atlanta, Georgia

Dorothy G. Lappe, RN, MS, MBA

Baltimore, Maryland

Maureen A. Lefton-Greif, PhD

Assistant Professor of Pediatrics
Johns Hopkins University School
  of Medicine
Speech-Language Pathologist
Johns Hopkins Hospital
Baltimore, Maryland

Andrew J. Lodge, MD

Assistant Professor of Surgery
Duke University School of Medicine
Division of Cardiovascular and
  Thoracic Surgery
Duke Children's Hospital
Durham, North Carolina

Josephine M. Lok, MD

Instructor in Pediatrics
Harvard Medical School
Assistant in Pediatrics
Massachusetts General Hospital
Boston, Massachusetts

Bradley S. Marino, MD, MPP, MSCE

Assistant Professor of Anesthesiology and
  Critical Care Medicine and Pediatrics
University of Pennsylvania School
  of Medicine
Staff Intensivist and Cardiologist
Cardiac Intensive Care Unit
The Children's Hospital of Philadelphia
Philadelphia, Pennsylvania

Lynn D. Martin, MD

Professor of Anesthesiology
Professor of Pediatrics (Adjunct)
University of Washington School
  of Medicine
Director, Department of Anesthesiology
  and Pain Medicine
Children's Hospital Regional Medical Center
Seattle, Washington

Lynne G. Maxwell, MD

Associate Professor of Anesthesiology and
    Critical Care
University of Pennsylvania School of Medicine
Associate Director, General Anesthesia Division
Senior Anesthesiologist
The Children's Hospital of Philadelphia
Philadelphia, Pennsylvania

Brian W. McCrindle, MD, MPH, FRCP (C)

Professor of Pediatrics
University of Toronto
Staff Cardiologist
The Hospital for Sick Children
Toronto, Canada

Jon N. Meliones, MD, MS

Professor of Pediatrics and Anesthesiology
Duke University School of Medicine
Director, Pediatric Cardiovascular Intensive
    Care Unit
Duke Children's Hospital
Durham, North Carolina

Coleen Elizabeth Miller, RN, MS, PNP

Pediatric Nurse Practitioner
Pediatric Cardiac Surgery
Duke Children's Hospital
Durham, North Carolina

Anne M. Murphy, MD

Associate Professor of Pediatrics
Johns Hopkins University School of Medicine
Division of Pediatric Cardiology
Johns Hopkins Hospital
Baltimore, Maryland

Catherine A. Neill, MD*

Professor Emerita of Pediatrics
Johns Hopkins School of Medicine
Baltimore, Maryland

Alicia M. Neu, MD

Associate Professor of Pediatrics
Johns Hopkins University School of Medicine
Clinical Director, Pediatric Nephrology
Medical Director, Pediatric Dialysis and
    Kidney Transplantation
Johns Hopkins Hospital
Baltimore, Maryland

David G. Nichols, MD, MBA

Professor of Anesthesiology and Critical Care Medicine
    and Pediatrics
Vice Dean for Education
Mary Wallace Stanton Professor of Education
Johns Hopkins University School of Medicine
Attending Physician, Pediatric Intensive Care Unit
Johns Hopkins Hospital
Baltimore, Maryland

John J. Nigro, MS, MD

Director of Congenital Heart Center
St. Joseph's Hospital and Medical Center
Phoenix, Arizona

Daniel Nyhan, MD

Professor of Anesthesiology and Critical Care Medicine
Johns Hopkins University School of Medicine
Executive Vice Chairman, Department of
    Anesthesiology and Critical Care Medicine
Chief, Division of Cardiac Anesthesia
Department of Anesthesiology and Critical Care Medicine
Johns Hopkins Hospital
Baltimore, Maryland

Martin P. O'Laughlin, MD, PC

Pediatric Cardiologist
Kansas City, Missouri

Charles N. Paidas, MD, MBA

Professor of Surgery and Pediatrics
University of South Florida
Chief, Pediatric Surgery
Tampa General Hospital
Tampa, Florida

Rulan Parekh, MD, MS

Associate Professor of Pediatrics
Johns Hopkins University School of Medicine
Division of Pediatric Nephrology
Johns Hopkins Hospital
Baltimore, Maryland

F. Bennett Pearce, MD

Professor of Pediatrics
U.A.B. School of Medicine
L.M. Bargeron, Jr., Division of Pediatric
    Cardiology
Children's Health System
Birmingham, Alabama

Timothy Phelps, MS, FAMI

Associate Professor, Medical Illustrator
Art as Applied to Medicine
Assistant Director
Department of Art as Applied to Medicine
Johns Hopkins University School of Medicine
Baltimore, Maryland

Lorraine C. Racusen, MD

Professor of Pathology
Johns Hopkins University School of Medicine
Active Staff, Anatomic Pathology
Johns Hopkins Hospital
Baltimore, Maryland

J. Mark Redmond, MD, FRCSI

Professor of Surgery
Royal College of Surgeons
Consultant, Pediatric Cardiac Surgeon
Our Lady's Hospital for Sick Children
Dublin, Ireland

---

*Deceased

Richard E. Ringel, MD

Associate Professor of Pediatrics
Johns Hopkins University School of Medicine
Director, Pediatric Cardiac Catheterization Laboratory
Co-Director, Adult Congenital Heart Disease Program
Johns Hopkins Hospital
Baltimore, Maryland

James L. Robotham, MD

Chairman of the Department of Anesthesiology
Professor of Anesthesiology, Pediatrics, and Pharmacology
    & Physiology
University of Rochester School of Medicine and Dentistry
Director of Perioperative Services
Strong Health
Strong Memorial Hospital
Rochester, New York

Charles L. Schleien, MD

Professor of Pediatrics and Anesthesiology
Deputy Chairman for Finance
Columbia University College of Physicians and Surgeons
Medical Director, Pediatric Critical Care Medicine
Morgan Stanley Children's Hospital of New York-
    Presbyterian Medical Center
New York, New York

Scott R. Schulman, MD

Associate Professor of Anesthesiology and Pediatrics
Duke University School of Medicine
Attending Physician, Pediatric Intensive Care Unit
Duke Children's Hospital
Durham, North Carolina

Laureen M. Sena, MD

Instructor in Radiology
Harvard Medical School
Staff Radiologist
Children's Hospital Boston
Boston, Massachusetts

Shaun P. Setty, MD

Fellow in Cardiovascular and Thoracic Surgery
University of Minnesota School of Medicine
University of Minnesota Medical Center
Minneapolis, Minnesota

Donald H. Shaffner, Jr., MD

Associate Professor of Anesthesiology and
    Critical Care Medicine
Johns Hopkins University School of Medicine
Director, Division of Pediatric Anesthesiology
    and Critical Care Medicine
Johns Hopkins Hospital
Baltimore, Maryland

Irving Shen, MD

Associate Professor of Surgery
Oregon Health and Sciences University
Division of Cardiothoracic Surgery
Doernbecher Children's Hospital
Portland, Oregon

Michael J. Silka, MD

Professor of Pediatrics
Keck School of Medicine of the University of
    Southern California
Chief, Division of Pediatric Cardiology
Childrens Hospital Los Angeles
Los Angeles, California

Arthur J. Smerling, MD

Associate Clinical Professor of Pediatrics and
    Anesthesiology
Columbia University College of Physicians and
    Surgeons
Director of Cardiac Critical Care
Morgan Stanley Children's Hospital of New York-
    Presbyterian Medical Center
New York, New York

Philip J. Spevak, MD

Associate Professor of Pediatrics and Medicine
Johns Hopkins University School of Medicine
Director of Pediatric Echocardiography
Johns Hopkins Hospital
Baltimore, Maryland

Thomas L. Spray, MD

Professor of Surgery
Alice Langdon Warner Endowed Chair in Pediatric
    Cardiothoracic Surgery
University of Pennsylvania School of Medicine
Chief, Division of Cardiothoracic Surgery
Executive Director, The Cardiac Center
The Children's Hospital of Philadelphia
Philadelphia, Pennsylvania

Vaughn A. Starnes, MD

Hastings Distinguished Professor of Cardiothoracic
    Surgery
Keck School of Medicine of the University of
    Southern California
Head, Division of Cardiothoracic Surgery
Childrens Hospital Los Angeles
Los Angeles, California

James M. Steven, MD, MS

Associate Professor of Anesthesiology
    and Pediatrics
University of Pennsylvania School of
    Medicine
Senior Vice President for Medical Affairs
    and Chief Medical Officer
Senior Anesthesiologist
The Children's Hospital of Philadelphia
Philadelphia, Pennsylvania

Dylan Stewart, MD

Assistant Professor of Surgery
University of Maryland School of Medicine
Division of Pediatric Surgery
University of Maryland Medical Systems
Baltimore, Maryland

James D. St. Louis, MD

Assistant Professor of Surgery and Pediatrics
Medical College of Georgia
Director, Pediatric Cardiac Surgery
Children's Medical Center
Augusta, Georgia

Sarah Tabbutt, MD, PhD

Assistant Professor of Anesthesiology and
    Critical Care Medicine
Assistant Professor of Pediatrics
University of Pennsylvania School of Medicine
Director, Cardiac Intensive Care Unit
The Children's Hospital of Philadelphia
Philadelphia, Pennsylvania

Masao Takata, MD, PhD

Reader in Anaesthesia and Intensive Care
Head, Critical Care Research Group
Department of Anaesthetics, Pain Medicine and
    Intensive Care
Imperial College London
Chelsea and Westminster Hospital
London, UK

Robert Charles Tasker, MD, MBBS

Senior Lecturer in Paediatric Intensive Care
Cambridge University School of Clinical Medicine
Cambridge University
Consultant in Paediatric Intensive Care
Addenbrooke's Hospital, Hill's Road
Cambridge, UK

W. Reid Thompson, MD

Assistant Professor of Pediatrics
Johns Hopkins School of Medicine
Division of Pediatric Cardiology
Johns Hopkins Hospital
Baltimore, Maryland

Joseph D. Tobias, MD

Professor of Anesthesiology and Pediatrics
Russell and Mary Shelden Chair in Pediatric
    Critical Care
University of Missouri School of Medicine
Vice-Chairman, Department of Anesthesiology
Chief, Division of Pediatric Anesthesiology
University of Missouri Hospital
Columbia, Missouri

Peter Mark Trinkaus, MD

Clinical Associate Professor of Pediatrics
Division of Pediatric Intensive Care
Stanford University School of Medicine
Associate Attending Pediatrician
Lucile Packard Children's Hospital at Stanford
Palo Alto, California
Good Samaritan Hospital
San Jose, California

Ross M. Ungerleider, MD

Professor and Chief, Cardiothoracic Surgery
Oregon Health and Sciences University
John C. Hursh Chair, Pediatric Cardiac Surgery
Doernbecher Children's Hospital
Portland, Oregon

Gil Wernovsky, MD

Professor of Pediatrics
University of Pennsylvania School of Medicine
Director of Program Development, The Cardiac Center
Staff Cardiologist, Cardiac Intensive Care Unit
The Children's Hospital of Philadelphia
Philadelphia, Pennsylvania

Randall C. Wetzel, MBBS, MBA

Professor of Anesthesiology and Pediatrics
The Anne O'M. Wilson Professor of Critical Care Medicine
Keck School of Medicine of the University of
    Southern California
Chair, Department of Anesthesiology and
    Critical Care Medicine
Childrens Hospital Los Angeles
Los Angeles, California

Jeannette R.M. White, MD, PhD

Assistant Professor of Pediatrics
University of Maryland School of Medicine
Attending Physician, Pediatric Intensive Care Unit
University of Maryland Medical Systems
Baltimore, Maryland

Aaron L. Zuckerberg, MD

Assistant Professor of Pediatrics
University of Maryland School of Medicine
Director, Division of Pediatric Anesthesiology and
    Critical Care Medicine
Sinai Hospital
Baltimore, Maryland

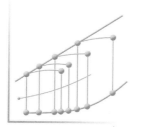

Preface

Enormous advances in care of the child with critical heart disease have marked the last decade. These have ranged from refinements in the staged management of the child with a univentricular heart to the explosion in diagnostic imaging capabilities to the understanding of the factors governing neurologic outcomes. The extreme rarity of intraoperative death has only heightened the focus on the peri-operative period for these children.

Within this changing environment, the objectives of this second edition of *Critical Heart Disease in Infants and Children* remain the same. Our goal is to offer a comprehensive understanding of critical heart disease based on scientific principles and best evidence combined with practical management plans. The care of these children is a multidisciplinary effort; therefore, the authors reflect the various disciplines that collaborate in the care of children with life-threatening heart disease. Their common language of pediatric cardiac intensive care is now more of a reality than it was when the first edition was published.

Since the disease processes for these children are often complex, we have approached the discussion from five interrelated perspectives that are represented by the five sections of the book. The first section on *basic principles* adopts a systems approach to elucidate the effects of critical heart disease on major integrated systems in the body. The second section on *special problems* provides an in-depth discussion of the major problems faced by this population such as dysrhythmias, CPR, and nutrition, to name a few. The huge role of technology in this field is discussed in the third section on *equipment and techniques*. The fourth and largest section of the book is devoted to the management of *congenital heart defects*. This section, like the rest of the book, is heavily illustrated to provide the non-surgeons a picture of what happens in the operating room. The fifth section discusses the diverse list of diseases that do not require or are not amenable to surgery (other than perhaps transplantation) but nevertheless may threaten the lives of these children.

On behalf of all the editors, I thank the authors and their staffs for their dedicated work; our principal artist, Tim Phelps, for beautiful illustrations; and our publisher, Natasha Andjelkovic, for her patient support. However, most of all, this book is dedicated to children with critical heart disease and to those adults who are willing to stand at their bedsides and apply their knowledge and skill in the hope of restoring these children to health.

David G. Nichols, MD

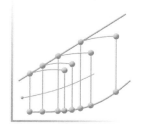

Contents

PART ONE

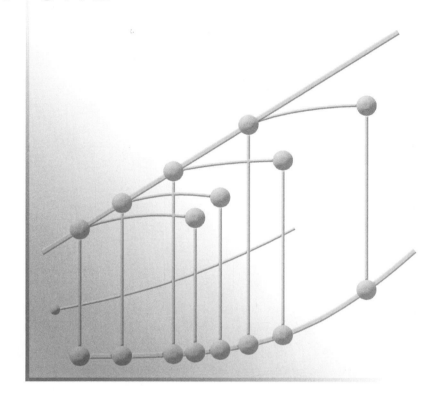

Basic Principles

Chapter 1

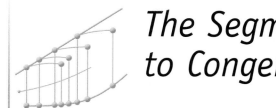

The Segmental Approach to Congenital Heart Disease

CATHERINE A. NEILL, MD, W. REID THOMPSON, MD,
and PHILIP J. SPEVAK, MD

INTRODUCTION

Given the potential complexity of congenital heart disease, an accurate and consistent nomenclature is a desirable if not an absolute necessity. Various anatomists and pathologists have proposed terminology and methods of description. At times, there has been inconsistency between the methods proposed so that a historical perspective of the development of nomenclature is useful to understanding the anatomic description of congenital heart disease.

The chambers of the heart have been called "right" and "left" from ancient times. William Harvey[13] in 1628 called them "dexter" (right) and "sinister"(left), (although he called the pulmonary artery the "vena arteriosa" or artery-like vein). This right-left labeling is based on relationships and imperfectly describes the situation, because the septa separating the two sides are not in the sagittal plane, and when considered in three-dimensional space are varyingly oblique.

Lev[30] in 1954 proposed that the chambers of the heart should be called by what they were, rather than by where they were; that each chamber had characteristics that identified it, no matter where it was in relation to the rest of the heart. This basis allowed Van Praagh[58] to propose a "segmental" approach to the heart, one in which the three major segments—atria, ventricles, and great arteries—were looked at in turn. Using an embryologic footing, he suggested that the two major determining features were the visceroatrial situs, which dictated where the atria were, and the bulboventricular loop, which did the same for the ventricles and the great arteries. This approach has withstood the test of time and is used by many.

Anderson and colleagues in the 1970s,[52] while supporting the segmental approach, thought that it focused too much on relationships, and that there was benefit in placing emphasis on how the blood moved through the heart. They directed attention to how the chambers are connected—or not connected—to one another. Thus, they teach that there are three separate facets to the make-up of the heart: the morphology of the chambers, their connections, and their relations. All three facets have their own terminology. Definitions of morphology require anatomic terms; in describing connections, terms such as concordant or discordant, absent or double are used; and spatial terms such as right and left are used to define relationships. The "sequence" of connections between segments is emphasized, leading to the sequential segmental approach.[2] More recently, Freedom[18,19] has sought to reconcile these really complementary approaches, and has underlined how they can be used to describe the malformed heart. He describes the three cardiac segments as the "building blocks" of the heart.

In this chapter, we will not attempt to duplicate all of the tables and diagrams used by the Van Praaghs, Anderson, and Freedom, who in their extensive writings have detailed almost all of the numerous segmental anomalies and variants.[5,59,63,64] Instead we will review how some of the terminology can be applied in clinical settings of varying complexity. Starting with the different positions of the heart and some of the embryologic considerations as they affect cardiac looping, we will then define the various segments and their connections, and how abnormalities can be diagnosed. The emphasis is on how essential it is to consider the segments and connections in every child with a cardiac malformation encountered in an intensive care setting.

POSITION OF THE HEART

The normal position of the heart in the left hemithorax, with the apex directed to the left, levocardia, is so usual that it is often left unstated. The term dextrocardia[6,24,42] is mostly used to describe a heart occupying the right hemithorax, although some authors prefer to distinguish dextrocardia from dextroversion. In that case, dextroversion means that the heart is in the right chest while dextrocardia means that the heart is in the right chest and that the apex is also pointed to the right. In mesocardia,[32] the heart is in the midline. Although dextrocardia can occur with a functionally normal heart, abnormalities of segmental relationships and connections are much more frequent than in the normally positioned heart.

EMBRYOLOGIC CONSIDERATIONS

The primitive heart tube is initially straight (Fig. 1-1), and the atrial portion receives venous blood from both the left and right sinus venosus. The straight heart tube begins to loop inside the pericardial sac when the embryo is about 11 somites, or 15 days.[9] The atrioventricular junction comes to lie to the left side of the pericardial cavity. In the primitive heart, there is a single atrium, single atrioventricular connection, and single ventricle communicating by an outflow (infundibulum or conus) to the undivided truncus arteriosus.

As the heart progresses from the straight tube stage, and with the proximal and distal ends more or less fixed, the tube grows and loops anteriorly (see Fig. 1-1). In normal hearts, the looping is anterior and to the right, termed by Van Praagh[58,60] a D-(dextro = right) loop. This usually results in the right ventricle being on the right with the aorta posterior and rightward of the pulmonary artery. The aorta is connected to the left ventricle and the main pulmonary artery to the right ventricle (Fig. 1-2, normally related great vessels).

In the most common form of transposition resulting in cyanosis, the aorta lies anteriorly and on the right and each great artery is connected to the "wrong" ventricle (i.e., aorta to the right ventricle and main pulmonary artery to the left ventricle) (see Fig. 1-2, D-TGA).[57] Pexieder[46] has recently recommended that transposition be considered an isolated defect of arterial looping, rather than being included with conotruncal malformations. This concept is compatible with clinical and epidemiologic data showing a much lower incidence of associated extracardiac anomalies in transposition than in tetralogy and other defects involving mesenchymal cell migration.[8,16]

If the heart loops anteriorly and to the left, a L-(levo = left) loop, then the ventricles are inverted. There is a form of transposition in this situation that is called physiologically corrected or congenitally corrected transposition. Again, the

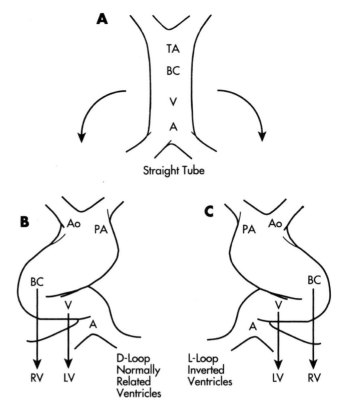

FIGURE 1-1 Cardiac looping. **A,** The heart initially develops as a straight tube (TA, truncus arteriosus, BC, bulbus cordis, V, ventricle, A, atrium). **B,** In normal cardiac looping, the bulbus cordis (future right ventricle) loops to the right (dextro or D-loop) and generally comes to lie to the right of the ventricle (future left ventricle). The truncus divides into the aorta (Ao) and the pulmonary artery (PA). **C,** An abnormal ventricular L-loop results in the developing right ventricle generally lying to the left of the anatomic left ventricle. (From Van Praagh R: The segmental approach to understanding complex cardiac lesions. In Eldredge WJ, Goldberg, Lemole GM [eds]: *Current Problems in Congenital Heart Disease.* New York: SP Medical and Scientific Books, 1979, pp 1–18.)

great arteries are connected to the "wrong" ventricles, but physiologically, the patient is not cyanotic (see Fig. 1-2, L-TGA). Rarely the viscera and atria are inverted and the ventricle and truncus are equally involved in a leftward (L) loop, resulting in dextrocardia with situs inversus and an otherwise normal heart. In this case the great vessels are connected with the appropriate ventricle (see Fig. 1-2, Inverted normally related great arteries).

The mechanisms underlying normal looping are still being studied, but they are under strong genetic control.[4,5,22] Recently, Overbeek and associates[68] have described a recessive mutation in a family of transgenic mice that resulted in situs inversus with dextrocardia in 95% of homozygotes studied. The mutation was mapped to chromosome 4. The authors observed that the direction of postimplantation body turning was reversed in the homozygotes. Although the clinical implications of this work are still pending, it suggests that situs inversus with dextrocardia and a normal heart is a basic abnormality of whole body polarity, under different control mechanisms from the more frequently encountered anomalies of cardiac looping. Failure of normal looping (i.e., looping of the heart tube to the left) is a very early embryologic defect,[29] and it is not surprising

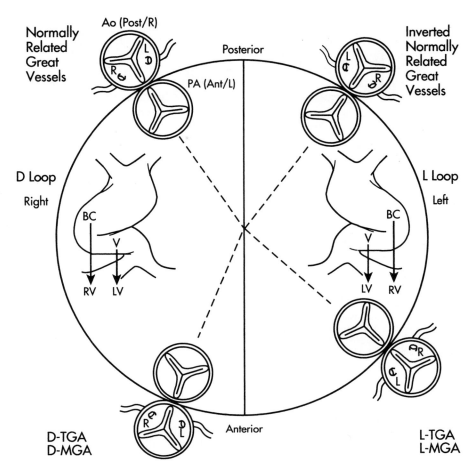

FIGURE 1-2 Arterial relationships. Orientation: Superior sagittal view of great arteries (Ao, PA). Frontal view of ventricular looping (BC, V, RV, LV). With normal ventricular looping to the right (D-loop), the arterial relationship may be normal, Ao posterior and to the right of the PA, which is anterior and to the left. Or there may be transposition (D-TGA) or malposition (D-MGA) in which the Ao is anterior and to the right. With abnormal ventricular looping to the left (L-loop), there may be inverted normally related great arteries, or levo-transposition L-TGA (corrected transposition), or malposition L-MGA. BC, bulbus cordis; V, ventricle; RV, right ventricle; LV, left ventricle; Ao, aorta; PA, pulmonary artery. (From Van Praagh R: The segmental approach to understanding complex cardiac lesions. In Eldredge WJ, Gberg H, Lemole GM [eds]: *Current Problems in Congenital Heart Disease*. New York: SP Medical and Scientific Books, 1979, pp 1–18.)

that associated defects of septation and valve formation are the rule rather than the exception.

With growth of the heart, the sinus venosus and paired superior and inferior cardinal veins become differentiated, resulting in persistence of the right-sided venous channels and atrophy of the left cardinal system except for the coronary sinus. The later development of the proximal part of the inferior vena cava is closely linked to the growth of the liver, so that the anatomic right atrium and the liver almost invariably develop on the same side of the body. This concept of visceroatrial situs is fundamental to the segmental approach. An important concept underlying the segmental approach is the recognition that the arrangement of the ventricles does not necessarily follow that of the visceroatrial situs. When the right atrium does not connect normally to the right ventricle, this results in a "discordant" atrioventricular connection.

The partitioning of the conotruncus results in the normal pulmonary artery and aorta. Recent work has shown that this normal partitioning involves migration of mesenchymal cells from the neural crest.[9] Unequal partitioning can result in tetralogy of Fallot and in some forms of abnormal connections between the great vessels and the ventricles.

The three segments of the heart can thus be distinguished in the very early embryo. The gradual development of the ventricular trabeculations, ventricular septum, and heart valves can be observed.[67] The segmental approach involves the sequential analysis of the three cardiac segments, atria, ventricles and great arteries, and knowledge of their connections.

THE ATRIA

The right atrium normally lies in the right hemithorax, and receives blood from the right-sided superior and inferior vena cava and, the coronary sinus. Identification of the right atrium as an anatomic structure in an abnormal heart is achieved by considering the visceroatrial situs, the great veins, and the atrial morphology.[2,3,18]

Visceroatrial Situs

The term "situs" means position, site, or location. In the overwhelming majority of patients seen in an intensive care unit, the visceral situs is "normal." This brief word summarizes a lot of expectations, namely that the stomach and spleen lie to the left, the right lobe of the liver is larger than the left, and the appendix is right-sided (Fig. 1-3). This normal asymmetry of the abdominal organs is accompanied by differences in lobulation between the right and left lung, with a trilobed right and a bilobed left lung. This arrangement is termed by different authors normal situs, or situs solitus, often abbreviated to "S" or sometimes "N," for normal. Van Praagh describes the segmental arrangement of the normal heart as {S,D,S}, indicating visceroatrial situs solitus (the first "S" referring to the atrial situs), a normal (D) ventricular loop to the right, and normal (S)olitus relationship of the semilunar valves.[71] Normally the inferior vena cava courses to the right of the descending aorta to enter the right atrium. The relationship of aorta and inferior vena cava can be recognized by echocardiography.[2,26,53,54]

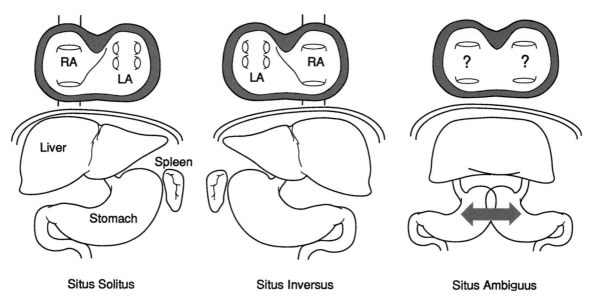

FIGURE 1-3 Visceroatrial situs. *Situs solitus* or normal situs, with right sided liver, superior vena cava, and right atrium. *Situs inversus,* with left sided liver, superior vena cava, and morphologic right atrium. *Situs ambiguous,* with midline liver, and ambiguity of venous connections and atrial morphology, shown as ?. Situs ambiguous with heterotaxy syndrome, also called Ivemark or asplenia/polysplenia syndrome, is discussed in Chapter 50. (From Van Praagh R: The segmental approach to understanding complex cardiac lesions. In Eldredge WJ, Gberg H, Lemole GM [eds]: *Current Problems in Congenital Heart Disease.* New York: SP Medical and Scientific Books, 1979, pp 1–18.)

In situs inversus, the position of the abdominal organs is reversed, with the stomach lying on the right, the dominant lobe of the liver on the left, and there is a left-sided appendix and left-sided inferior vena cava. The arrangement is a mirror image of the normal situs. The left lung is trilobed, and the right has two lobes. Pulmonary venous return is again to the left atrium but the left atrium is on the right side of the heart (i.e., inverted atria).

In the third type of situs, situs ambiguous (denoted as "A" in the Van Praagh method), the stomach may lie on either side of the epigastrium or in the midline, the liver is not clearly differentiated into unequal sized lobes, and there is frequently intestinal malrotation (see Fig. 1-3).

Another term related to situs is heterotaxy syndrome in which there is a loss of the normal order in organization.[40,41,65] Heterotaxy syndrome is sometimes also called cardiosplenic or Ivemark syndrome. There are two subtypes: asplenia and polysplenia syndrome. In asplenia there is an absence of a normal spleen. In polysplenia syndrome, multiple small spleens occur. In both cases, splenic function is usually abnormal. Anderson and colleagues[2,3,50] find the morphology of the atrial appendages a useful indication of the type of intracardiac defect and use the terms right and left atrial isomerism rather than asplenia or polysplenia. Two trilobed lungs (or in Anderson's terms right bronchial isomerism) may be seen in asplenia, and in polysplenia there may be left bronchial isomerism, with two bilobed lungs. There are exceptions to either method of classification. Both are useful methods for remembering the commonly associated features of each syndrome. In practice, each of the segments and connections needs to be ascertained, usually using echocardiography, before management can proceed.

Most infants and children with cardiac malformations have situs solitus that is, there is no derangement of the normal abdominal order. Approximately 1:10,000 individuals are born with situs inversus, dextrocardia, and with the cardiac segments arranged in the mirror image of normal (see Fig. 1-2). Mirror image dextrocardia with situs inversus was the first cardiac abnormality to be attributed to a single gene defect,[10] and a recessive mode of inheritance is usual. Such children may be otherwise entirely normal, though a few have ciliary dyskinesia, or Kartagener's syndrome.[1,12,23,28,39,45] If cardiac defects are present in the mirror image heart, they may be "mirror images" of those found in children with situs solitus, and often can be repaired with equal facility. Simple septal defects, tetralogy of Fallot,[27] and aortic atresia[47] have all been reported. Recently, coronary artery surgery and coronary angioplasty have been described in adults with mirror image arrangement and structurally normal hearts.[33] However, the majority of children seen in a cardiac center with dextrocardia and situs inversus do not have a mirror image of the normal heart but, have major abnormalities of cardiac septation, cardiac connections, and arterial relationships.

The Great Veins

The superior and inferior vena cavae are normally right-sided structures draining into the right atrium. A persistent additional left superior vena cava, draining into the coronary sinus, is present in 1% to 2% of the normal population, and is more frequent in those with malformed hearts. A wall normally separates the coronary sinus and left superior vena cava from the left atrium. If this wall is absent or fenestrated, the coronary sinus is described as "unroofed" and shunting in either direction can occur. In asplenia syndrome (called right atrial isomerism by Anderson), bilateral superior vena cavae are frequent, and the coronary sinus may be absent. In polysplenia (termed left atrial isomerism by Anderson), the suprarenal portion of the inferior vena cava is absent and the more inferior portion of the inferior vena cava drains via the azygous system. This is sometimes called an interrupted inferior vena cava. Abnormalities of pulmonary venous connections[34,43] are much more frequent in asplenia syndrome than in those with polysplenia syndrome.

Right and Left Atria

The right atrium normally receives the systemic venous return and flow from the coronary sinus. Distinguishing morphologic features include the presence of the terminal sulcus and crest, and the rim of the oval fossa. Anderson[2] has stressed the distinctive shape of the right atrial appendage (Fig. 1-4), "a blunt triangle with a broad junction to the

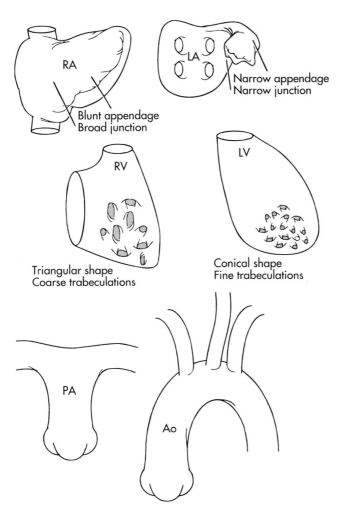

FIGURE 1-4 Morphologic features. Top, The right atrium (RA) has a blunt appendage with a broad junction to the body of the atrium; the left atrium (LA) has a narrower appendage with a crenellated edge and narrow junction to the left atrial body. Middle, The right ventricle (RV) has a characteristic triangular (or pyramidal) shape and coarse trabeculations. The left ventricle (LV) has a more conical (or bullet ellipsoid) shape and fine trabeculations. Bottom, The pulmonary artery (PA) is characterized by early bifurcation into two branches. The aorta (Ao) gives rise to coronary arteries (not shown) and systemic arteries. (From Van Praagh R, Weinberg PM, Smith SD, et al: Malpositions of the heart. In Adams FH, Emmanouilides GC, Riemenschneider TA [eds]: *Moss' Heart Disease in Infants, Children, and Adolescents.* Baltimore: Williams and Wilkins, 1989, pp 530–580.)

venous component of the atrium." He has found that two such appendages are common in right atrial isomerism[3,50] although echocardiographically, it is easier to identify atrial morphology by the venous connections than the morphology of appendages.

The left atrium contains the flap-valve aspect of the fossa ovalis. Again, Anderson finds the shape of the left atrial appendage a useful differentiating feature with the left-sided appendage narrower than the right-sided appendage[3] (see Fig. 1-4).

Noninvasive Clues to Visceroatrial Situs

While echocardiography is generally definitive in establishing atrial morphology and venous connections, the chest radiograph and electrocardiogram can be useful to the clinician in the intensive care unit in screening for abnormal visceroatrial situs. One can refer to Chapter 17 on noninvasive diagnosis for the details concerning evaluation using echocardiography and magnetic resonance imaging. Two-dimensional echocardiography should be able to define the intracardiac anatomy to avoid invasive diagnostic procedures in the majority of patients prior to initial surgical intervention.

On chest radiograph in normal situs or situs solitus, the stomach gas bubble is on the left and the liver on the right; in abdominal situs inversus, the stomach gas bubble is on the right, the liver on the left. In situs ambiguous, the liver is commonly in the midline and there is often discordance between the position of the stomach gas bubble and the direction of the cardiac apex.[56]

The electrocardiogram is often helpful. In normal situs solitus, the spread of electrical activation from the SA node over the atrial surface results in the normal inferior and leftward P-wave vector (Fig. 1-5). When the atria are inverted, the SA node is left sided and the major P-wave vector is left to right, resulting in inverted P waves in lead I and in the left precordial leads. In situs ambiguous, there may be no distinct SA node. Junctional rhythm or ectopic atrial rhythms with P-wave inversion in leads II and III are present in approximately 50% of patients. In asplenia, arrhythmias are less frequent, although bilateral SA nodes have been described.[55] The P-wave axis may be directed leftward and superiorly, particularly in polysplenia syndrome.[18]

VENTRICLES AND ATRIOVENTRICULAR CONNECTIONS

Once the visceral and atrial situs and venous connections are identified with echocardiography, attention is directed toward the atrioventricular connections and the spatial arrangements of the two ventricles. One cardinal rule is to realize that the normal situation, namely right atrium connects to right ventricle via a right-sided tricuspid valve, does not always apply in the presence of complex heart disease. Thus the function and connections of each atrioventricular valve must be established and the position and size of the ventricles carefully determined.

Atrioventricular Connections

Anderson[2] has emphasized that the atrial myocardium is connected to ventricular myocardium around the atrioventricular

Atria

1. **X-ray** - Position of stomach gas bubble & liver

2. **ECG** - P wave Axis

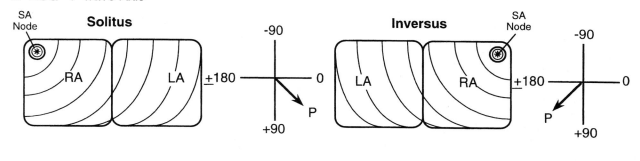

3. **Echo** - Relation of aorta to IVC
(also morphology of atrial appendages)

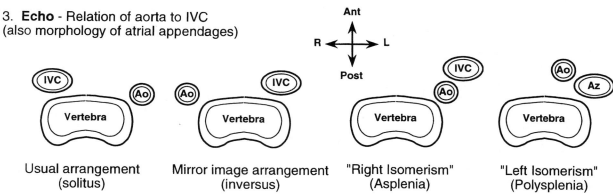

| Usual arrangement (solitus) | Mirror image arrangement (inversus) | "Right Isomerism" (Asplenia) | "Left Isomerism" (Polysplenia) |

Ventricles

1. **ECG** - Sequence of ventricular activation in precordial leads

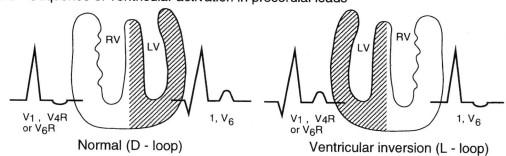

Normal (D - loop) Ventricular inversion (L - loop)

2. **Echo** - Ventricular Morphology

Characteristic	Right Ventricle	Left Ventricle
Shape	Triangular	Elipsoid
Trabeculation	Prominent	Minimal
Atrioventricular valve attachment	Septum	Free wall

Arteries

1. **Echo** - Ventriculoarterial connections/arterial relationships

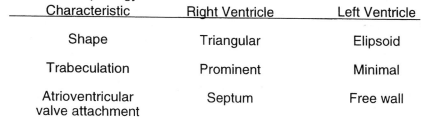

FIGURE 1-5 Noninvasive clinical signs. Atria, The chest x-ray, electrocardiogram (ECG), and echocardiogram provide information on visceroatrial situs. Ventricles, The ECG may help determine ventricular relationships from analysis of the sequence of ventricular activation in the precordial leads. Echocardiography can distinguish the different morphology of right and left ventricles. Arteries, Echocardiography can show ventriculoarterial connections and arterial relationships. (Adapted from Anderson RH: Terminology. In Anderson RH, Shinebourne EA, Macartney FJ, Tynan M [eds]: *Paediatric Cardiology*. Edinburgh: Churchill Livingstone, 1987, pp 65–82; and Park MK: Chamber localization and cardiac malposition. In Park MK [ed]: *Pediatric Cardiology for Practitioners*. Chicago: Year Book Medical, 1988, pp 201–205.)

junction, and these connections may be present even when there is an imperforate or atretic atrioventricular valve. The atrioventricular valves follow the ventricle, rather than the atrium. Thus, the tricuspid valve is related to the anatomic right ventricle and the mitral valve to the left ventricle. The tricuspid valve typically has attachments to the right ventricular septal surface (so-called "septophilic" valve) while the mitral valve is "septophobic" and typically only attaches to the free wall of the left ventricle.

When the ventricles are inverted, as in corrected transposition with a left-sided right ventricle, the tricuspid valve also lies on the left. Normally there are two patent atrioventricular valves but in malformed hearts, the atrioventricular valves may be atretic, straddle, or override. Straddling refers to abnormal attachment in the contralateral ventricle. Overriding means that the atrioventricular annulus is not positioned entirely over the appropriate ventricle (i.e., the tricuspid valve annulus is partially over the left ventricle or the mitral valve partially over the right ventricle).[20] Finally, there may be a single or common atrioventricular valve as in atrioventricular septal defect, or both atrioventricular valves may attach into the same ventricule (double inlet left or right ventricle).

Right and Left Ventricles

Ventricles are defined by their anatomic structure, not by their spatial relationships. Thus, the anatomic right ventricle is heavily trabeculated, while the anatomic left ventricle has a smoother lining with fine trabeculations. The right ventricle is a more triangular or pyramidal shape while the left ventricle is bullet ellipsoid (or conical) shape (see Fig. 1-4). Depending on the ventricular loop during development, the right ventricle may be located spatially on the right or left side of the heart. When the ventricles are inverted, the anatomic left ventricle generally lies to the right and the anatomic right ventricle lies to the left.

GREAT VESSELS AND VENTRICLES

Great Vessel Connections

There may or may not be normal connections of the great vessels. When the great vessels are abnormally connected or related they are termed malposed. There are four types of malposition: transposition of the great arteries, double outlet right ventricle, double outlet left ventricle, and anatomically corrected malposition. They are mutually exclusive from one another. Transposition means that the left ventricle gives rise to the main pulmonary artery and the right ventricle to the aorta. Double outlet right ventricle means that both great vessels arise predominantly from the right ventricle and double outlet left ventricle means that both vessels arise predominantly from the left ventricle. Anatomically corrected malposition means that the great vessels connect with the appropriate ventricle but in a manner different than normal. Anatomically corrected malposition is a rare condition and beyond the scope of this chapter. Let us review an example of how these terms are applied to patients.

Illustrative Case

An infant is scheduled for postoperative admission to the pediatric intensive care unit, with the diagnosis of "TGA {S,D,D} with IVS." What information is intended to be transferred by this succinct acronymic label, and what may the PICU team reasonably expect to arrive from the OR?

TGA stands for transposition of the great arteries and as noted previously, the aorta is connected to the right ventricle and the main pulmonary artery to the left ventricle. "{S,D,D}" means that there is atrial situs solitus, D-looped ventricles, and the final "D" means that the aorta is to the right of the main pulmonary artery. It is possible for the aorta in TGA {S,D,D} to be right and anterior, right and side-by-side, or right and posterior; however, a right and anterior relationship is most common. There are other forms of transposition in which the segments are {S,D,A} indicating that the aorta is anterior or {S,D,L}, indicating the aorta is left of the main pulmonary artery. "IVS" indicates that there is an intact ventricular septum (i.e., no ventricular septal defect is present). D-transposition of the great arteries is the most common form of transposition and cause of cardiac cyanosis.

The evolution of the nomenclature of transposition can be confusing. Transposition was the term originally introduced by von Rokitansky[66] in 1875 to describe hearts in which the aorta instead of being posterior to the pulmonary artery as in the normal heart was anterior to the pulmonary artery. Cardell,[7] Shaher,[51] and Goor and Edwards[21] advocated that the term transposition refer only to the anteroposterior relationship of the semilunar valves, regardless of their ventricular origin. Some cardiologists may use the terms double outlet right ventricle and transposition in the same patient when both great vessels arise from the right ventricle and the aorta is anterior. This can create confusion because the two diagnoses are conceptually mutually exclusive. Van Praagh[57,61] proposed a strict definition of transposition and that is what is used here, namely that transposition of the great arteries is present when the left ventricle connects with the main pulmonary artery and the right ventricle with the aorta. This definition is now generally accepted and other unusual relationships are termed "arterial malpositions" (see Fig. 1-2, D-MGA and L-MGA).

The connection between the ventricles and the great arteries is formed in the embryo from the bulbus cordis, which in the mature human heart is represented by the conus, or infundibulum. A conus is a "collar of muscle" separating a semilunar valve from the atrioventricular valve. In normally related great arteries, there is a well-developed conus proximal to the pulmonary valve, raising the valve, and allowing the pulmonary artery to connect with the right ventricle. In the most common form of D-transposition, subaortic conus is well developed, but subpulmonary conus is absent.

Continued

Illustrative Case—Cont'd

In transposition {S,D,D}, the ventricular looping is to the right. One can determine the ventricular loop from the echocardiographic imagining by imagining placing the palm of one's right hand on the right ventricular septal surface and the thumb of one's right hand in the tricuspid valve. The outstretched fingers extend into the outlet portion of the right ventricle. It is not possible to do this with the left hand in D-looped ventricles (Fig. 1-6).

Conversely, in physiologically corrected transposition {S,L,L}, the ventricular looping is to the left resulting usually in the right ventricle on the left side and the left ventricle usually located on the right side. Now one must use the left hand to imagine placing the thumb in the tricuspid valve, the palm on the right ventricular septal surface, and the outstretched fingers into the outflow (see Fig. 1-6).

To return to the infant with TGA {S,D,D}, the pediatric intensivist knows, from the segmental description, the key features of the heart disease. As importantly, by understanding the segmental basis and nomenclature, the intensivist can extend the concepts to understanding even more complex congenital heart disease. The ability to quickly and concisely refer to the orientation of each of the three main cardiac segments relative to the others facilitates description of complex anatomy and allows the clinician to better understand the physiologic implications of unusual segmental relationships (Fig. 1-7).

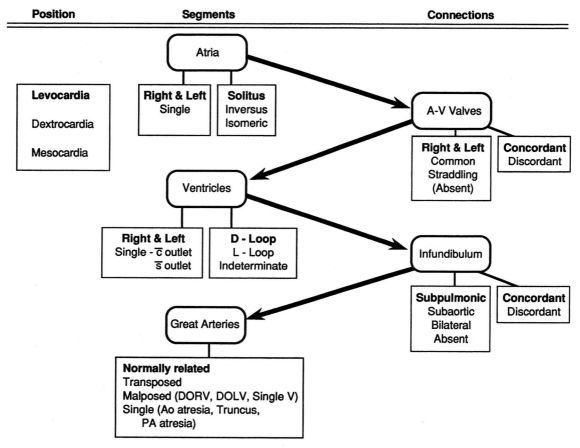

FIGURE 1-6   Transposition. *Complete transposition* (d-transposition, D-TGA). Although the arteries are transposed (discordant ventriculoarterial connection), the right ventricular organization is normal. The relationship of inlet, trabecular, and outlet portions is shown compared to the right hand. *Corrected transposition* (l-transposition, L-TGA) with inversion of the ventricles (discordant atrioventricular connection). The abnormal relationship of the right ventricular inlet, trabecular, and outflow portions of the right ventricle is shown compared to the left hand. (From Anderson RH: Terminology. In Anderson RH, Shinebourne EA, Macartney FJ, Tynan M [eds]: *Paediatric Cardiology.* Edinburgh: Churchill Livingstone, 1987, pp 65–82; and Van Praagh R, Weinberg PM, Smith SD, et al: Malpositions of the heart. In Adams FH, Emmanouilides GC, Riemenschneider TA [eds]: *Moss' Heart Disease in Infants, Children, and Adolescents.* Baltimore: Williams and Wilkins, 1989, pp 530–580.)

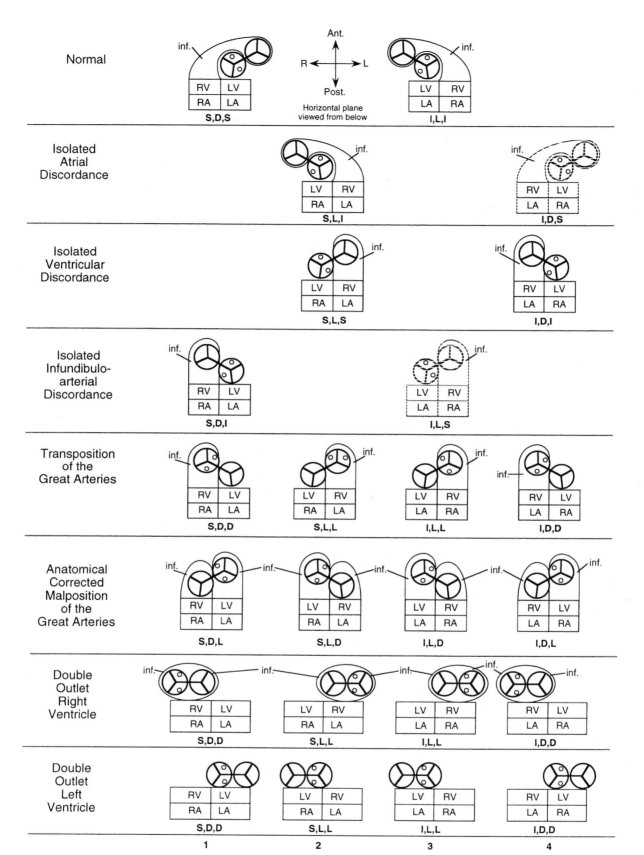

FIGURE 1-7 Types of human heart: segmental sets and alignments.[17] The diagrams depict the relationships of the three main cardiac segments to each other, as shown from below. Ant, anterior; Post, posterior; R, right; L, left; RA, morphologic right atrium; LA, morphologic left atrium; RV, morphologic right ventricle; LV, morphologic left ventricle; Inf, infundibulum. The aortic valve is designated by the coronary ostia. {} indicates "the set of." Each cardiac set has three segmental members, the atria, the ventricles, and the great arteries. Atrial situs may be solitus (usual) {S,-,-}, inversus {I,-,-}, or ambiguous {A,-,-} (not shown). Ventricular situs may be d-looped {-,D,-} or l-looped {-,L,-}. The great arterial situs may be solitus normal {-,-,S}, inverted normally related {-,-,I}, d-malposed {-,-,D}, l-malposed {-,-,L}, or ambiguously malposed {-,-,A} (not shown). Columns 1 and 3 have atrioventricular concordance; columns 2 and 4 atrioventricular discordance. Rows 1 to 4 have normal ventriculoarterial alignments; rows 5 to 8 have abnormal ventriculoarterial alignments. Sets depicted in broken lines have not yet been reported.

Double Inlet or Single Ventricle

So far, we have considered the segmental approach to hearts with two ventricular chambers. In double inlet ventricle, also called, although less precisely, single ventricle, there is typically one ventricle that receives the input of both atrioventricular valves. There may be a very small second ventricle or just an outflow chamber, but practically, the small chamber is not functionally useful. The same segmental method discussed previously can be applied with double inlet ventricle. There are many variants of double inlet ventricle and the reader is referred to Chapter 41 for a more complete discussion or to the discussion of Colvin.[11] Here, we outline only a brief summary of the major anatomic types, emphasizing how the segmental approach allows for accurate understanding of these defects.

Double inlet ventricle can be of a left ventricular, right ventricular, or indeterminate morphology. The atrioventricular connections also vary from a common atrioventricular valve, straddling right or left valve, or atresia of one of the atrioventricular valves. In reported series of double inlet ventricle, the dominant ventricle has had left ventricular morphology over 70% of the time. A notable though rare form of double inlet left ventricle is that with normally related great vessels, the so-called "Holmes heart."[11,49] In this heart, atrial situs is normal, the aorta arises from the left ventricle and the main pulmonary artery from a right sided outflow chamber. There is D-looping of the ventricles with the left ventricle in the normal position and the right ventricular outflow chamber rightward and anterior. The segmental description is double inlet left ventricle with normally related great arteries {S,D,S}.

The most common form of double inlet left ventricle has segmental description TGA {S,L,L}. The readers should now be able to deduce that there is atrial situs solitus, the ventricle loop is levo (i.e., there is ventricular inversion), and that the aorta is left of the main pulmonary artery. Because there is transposition, the main pulmonary artery arises from the single left ventricle and the aorta from the left-sided right ventricular outflow chamber.

Although most hearts with double inlet ventricle receive blood from both atria, in some cases there is atresia of one or other atrioventricular valves. Even in these cases, the valve apparatus of both atrioventricular valves relates to the "double inlet" single ventricle.

Double Outlet Ventricle

This term is used when both arteries arise from the same ventricle[31] and represents another form of malposition of the great vessels (see Chapter 34). The most common variant is double outlet right ventricle where both aorta and pulmonary artery connect with the right ventricle. The left ventricle receives blood through the mitral valve (which may be patent or atretic) and the only outlet is through a ventricular septal defect(s). The term double outlet right ventricle conveys that one artery arises entirely from the right ventricle, and the other overrides the ventricular septum by 50% or more.[35] Double outlet right ventricle results in a spectrum of clinical presentations. The newborn is cyanotic when there is significant pulmonary stenosis. If there is aortic stenosis, coarctation is common. Whether a two ventricle repair is possible (versus management towards a Fontan procedure like with single ventricle) depends primarily on the adequate size of each ventricle to pump a cardiac output, the potential to reliably connect each great vessel to a ventricle without obstruction, and finally, the ability to separate the two circulations.[62,69]

Illustrative Case

A 13-year-old child with heterotaxy, polysplenia, and dextrocardia had a Blalock-Taussig shunt as a newborn, followed by modified Fontan procedure at age 3 years (involving connection of each of bilateral superior vena cava to their ipsilateral branch pulmonary artery). The patient is admitted now because of atrial fibrillation. An echocardiogram shows double outlet right ventricle {A,D,D} with complete common atrioventricular canal defect and severe subvalvular and valvular pulmonary stenosis. The atrial situs is ambiguous (A). The inferior vena cava is interrupted with the infrahepatic portion of the inferior vena cava continuing posteriorly via a left-sided azygous vein to join the left superior vena cava. The coronary sinus is unroofed and the pulmonary veins drain ipsilaterally (right veins to right-sided atrium, left veins to left-sided atrium). The hepatic drains drain into the floor of the nearly common atrium.
The common atrioventricular valve is malaligned toward the right ventricle and there is severe left ventricular hypoplasia. There is severe atrioventricular valve regurgitation and atrial dilation. The ventricular loop is normal (D) with the morphologic right ventricle on the right side. There is double outlet right ventricle with the aortic valve positioned to the right of the pulmonary valve (D). There is moderate biventricular dysfunction. The caval connections are not well seen nor are the branch pulmonary arteries. The main pulmonary artery is tied off (performed at the time of the modified Fontan procedure). No intracardiac thrombus is seen. The systemic arterial oxygen saturation is 85% by pulse oximetry. Does a complete understanding of the anatomy assist in accurately assessing the acute problems? Does the longer-term management plan hinge on complete familiarity with these issues?

While the anatomy is extremely complex, the segmental method is very helpful in reaching an understanding of the anatomy and in creating a management plan. The patient required a Fontan procedure and single ventricle management because the left ventricle was severely hypoplastic and not able to pump a systemic output. As a newborn, cyanosis was due to the severe pulmonary stenosis and a Blalock-Taussig shunt was required. The Fontan procedure involved connecting the systemic venous circulation directly to the branch pulmonary arteries; in this case, bilateral caval-branch pulmonary artery connections were made. Note that the hepatic veins were left draining into the common atrium along with the pulmonary venous return, and that explains somewhat the arterial desaturation. Patients who have had a Fontan procedure have average oxygen saturation of approximately 93%. Because the hepatic veins continue to drain into the common atrium, all of the hepatic venous blood enters the systemic circulation and further reduces the systemic saturation. Furthermore, there is an increased frequency of pulmonary arteriovenous fistulae when the hepatic venous blood does not pass through the pulmonary circulation. In the more recent surgical era, the hepatic veins would be baffled to the pulmonary arteries to achieve more normal oxygen saturation and reduce the risk for the development of fistulae.

Continued

Illustrative Case—Cont'd

The atrial fibrillation is probably related to the marked atrial dilation from the atrioventricular regurgitation and the ventricular dysfunction. Afterload reduction may be helpful in this context. One would also want to document that the caval connections are unobstructed and that the branch pulmonary arteries are undistorted. After a Blalock-Taussig shunt, branch pulmonary artery distortion occurs in between 10% and 20% of patients. In the older child, the branch pulmonary arteries and Fontan connections may be better seen using magnetic resonance imaging rather than echocardiography.

Achievement of sinus rhythm would certainly improve the cardiac output and likely lessen the severity of atrioventricular regurgitation. Unfortunately, the ventricular dysfunction and atrioventricular regurgitation will likely remain or even worsen, increasing the chances for recurrent atrial arrhythmia.

THE UNUSUAL CASE: RELEVANCE IN THE INTENSIVE CARE SETTING

The logical sequential approach to the intracardiac arrangements is helpful when considering what special problems are likely to be encountered perioperatively in a specific child or adult.

Illustrative Case

A 9-month-old infant is to undergo a bidirectional Glenn procedure for tricuspid atresia with normally related great vessels, hypoplastic right ventricle, and pulmonary stenosis. What does this description convey of the cardiac segments, and what other anatomic problems are likely to be present?

The visceroatrial situs has not been described but is probably normal. It would be unusual in tricuspid atresia with normally related great arteries for the atrial situs to be abnormal and in such cases it is common to assume that it is normal if not described otherwise. The fact that the great vessels are normally related means that the aorta arises from the left ventricle and the pulmonary valve from the hypoplastic right ventricle. Given there is tricuspid atresia, blood reaches the pulmonary valve through the ventricular septal defect. Often there is subvalvular pulmonary stenosis because of narrowing at the ventricular septal defect or of the subpulmonary infundibulum. Aortic outflow obstruction or coarctation is unusual in tricuspid atresia with normally related great arteries.

Other information the intensivist caring for this patient in the postoperative period would want to know would be the preoperative hemodynamics including the pulmonary artery pressure and resistance, and whether there was branch pulmonary artery distortion. This should be determined on a preoperative catheterization. From the echocardiogram, one would want to know about ventricular and mitral valve function. All of these factors could affect postoperative hemodynamics and oxygen saturation.

SUMMARY

In summary, the basic concept of analyzing cardiac anatomy into segments is useful and indeed essential, and has, in Van Praagh's words, "withstood the test of time."[60] Newer diagnostic methodologies like magnetic resonance imaging,[69] fast computed tomography scanning, and three-dimensional echocardiography are increasingly being used to supplement two-dimensional echocardiography. Two-dimensional echocardiography remains the means whereby the anatomy is initially determined in the intensive care unit. Cardiac catheterization is less often used to clarify anatomy but is instead used to assess the hemodynamics and to intervene therapeutically.

Knowledge concerning laterality and cardiac looping is developing from the disciplines of genetics and embryology. Yost[70] in a recent review has stated that "the orientation of the cardiac tube looping is dependent on a cascade of genes in noncardiac embryonic cells … suggesting a linkage between complex cardiac defects and subtle midline defects in early embryos." Experimental studies in the chick embryo[36] also suggest an intricate linkage between the growth of the heart and the embryonic head flexures. In the next few years as part of the "genetic revolution," a nomenclature may appear separating more clearly defects of cardiac laterality (as in "mirror image dextrocardia") from the more complex defects of cardiac looping seen in "situs ambiguous" or isomerism.

For the present, the intensivist encountering a patient with a complex heart defect such as in heterotaxy syndrome should use all the information available to make his or her own diagram of the heart. Applying the principles of the segmental approach will allow the caretaker to more completely understand the anatomy and physiology with congenital heart disease.

References

1. Afzelius BA: A human syndrome caused by immotile cilia. *Science* 193:317–319, 1976.
2. Anderson RH: Terminology. In Anderson RH, Shinebourne EA, Macartney FJ, Tynan M (eds): *Paediatric Cardiology.* Edinburgh: Churchill Livingstone, 1987, pp 65–82.
3. Becker AE, Anderson RH: Isomerism of the atrial appendages - goodbye to asplenia and all that. In Clark EB, Takao A (eds): *Developmental Cardiology: Morphogenesis and Function.* Mount Kisco, NY: Futura, 1990, pp 659–670.
4. Brueckner M, D'Eustachio P, Horwich AL: Linkage mapping of a mouse gene, iv, that controls left-right asymmetry of the heart and viscera. *Proc Natl Acad Sci USA* 86:5035–5038, 1989.
5. Burn J: Disturbance of morphological laterality in humans. Ciba Foundation Symposium 282–300, 1992.
6. Calcaterra G, Anderson RH, Lau KC, Shinebourne EA: Dextrocardia—value of segmental analysis in its categorisation. *Br Heart J* 42:497–507, 1979.
7. Cardell BS: Corrected transposition of the great vessels. *Br Heart J* 18:186–192, 1956.

8. Clark EB: Growth, morphogenesis and function: The dynamics of cardiovascular development. In Moller JM, Neal WA, Lock JA (eds): *Fetal, Neonatal and Infant Heart Disease*. New York: Appleton–Century-Crofts, 1989, pp 1–14.

9. Clark EB, Van Mierop LHS: Development of the cardiovascular system. In Adams FH, Emmanouilides GC, Riemenschneider TA (eds): *Moss' Heart Disease in Infants, Children, and Adolescents*, Baltimore: Williams and Wilkins, 1989, pp 2–15.

10. Cockayne EA: The genetics of transposition of the viscera. *Q J Med* 7:479–493, 1938.

11. Colvin EV: Single ventricle. In Garson A Jr., Bricker JT, McNamara DG (eds): *The Science and Practice of Pediatric Cardiology*. Philadelphia: Lea and Febiger, 1990, pp 1246–1279.

12. Dietz R, Schanen G: CT in the preoperative clarification of Kartagener's syndrome. *Rontgenblatter* 43:463–464, 1990.

13. Dunseath R, Williams W, Patton D: A scintigraphic demonstration of dextrocardia and complete abdominal situs inversus. *Clin Nucl Med* 15:501–503, 1990.

14. Elliott LP: Complete transposition of the great vessels. I. An anatomic study of 60 cases. *Circulation* 27:1105–1117, 1963.

15. Ewing T: Genetic 'master switch' for left-right symmetry found. *Science* 260:624–625, 1993.

16. Ferencz C, Rubin JD, McCarter RJ, et al: Cardiac and noncardiac malformations: Observations in a population-based study. *Teratology* 35:367–378, 1987.

17. Foran RB, Belcourt C, Nanton MA, et al: Isolated infundiboarterial inversion {S,D,I}: A newly recognized form of congenital heart disease. *Am Heart J* 116:1337–1350, 1988.

18. Freedom RM: The "anthropology" of the segmental approach to the diagnosis of complex congenital heart disease. *Cardiovasc Intervent Radiol* 7:121–123, 1984.

19. Freedom RM: The application of a segmental nomenclature. In Freedom RM, Culham JAG, Moes CAF (eds): *Angiocardiography of Congenital Heart Disease*. New York: Macmillan, 1984, pp 17–45.

20. Geva T, Van Praagh S, Sanders SP, et al: Straddling mitral valve with hypoplastic right ventricle, crisscross atrioventricular relations, double outlet right ventricle and dextrocardia: Morphologic, diagnostic and surgical considerations. *J Am Coll Cardiol* 17:1603–1612, 1991.

21. Goor DA, Edwards JE: The spectrum of transposition of the great arteries: with specific reference to developmental anatomy of the conus. *Circulation* 48:406–415, 1973.

22. Hanzlik AJ, Binder M, Layton WM, et al: The murine situs inversus viscerum (iv) gene responsible for visceral asymmetry is linked tightly to the Igh-C cluster on chromosome 12. *Genomics* 7:389–393, 1990.

23. Ho AM, Friedland MJ: Kartagener's syndrome: Anesthetic considerations. *Anesthesiology* 77:386–388, 1992.

24. Huhta JC, Hagler DJ, Seward JB, et al: Two–dimensional echocardiographic assessment of dextrocardia: A segmental approach. *Am J Cardiol* 50:1351–1360, 1982.

25. Huhta JC, Smallhorn JF, Macartney FJ: Two dimensional echocardiographic diagnosis of situs. *Br Heart J* 48:97–108, 1982.

26. Huhta JC, Smallhorn JF, Macartney FJ, et al: Cross–sectional echocardiographic diagnosis of systemic venous return. *Br Heart J* 48:388–403, 1982.

27. Iga K, Hori K, Matsumura T, et al: A case of unusual longevity of tetralogy of Fallot confirmed by cardiac catheterization. *Jpn Circ J* 55:962–965, 1991.

28. Kartagener M, Strucki P: Bronchiectasis with situs inversus. *Arch Pediatr* 79:193–207, 1962.

29. Layton WM, Jr, Manasek FJ: Cardiac looping of early iv/iv mouse embryos. In Van Praagh R, Takao A (eds): *Etiology and Morphogenesis of Congenital Heart Disease*. Mount Kisco, NY: Futura, 1980, pp 109–126.

30. Lev M: Pathologic diagnosis of positional variations in cardiac chambers in congenital heart in congenital heart disease. *Lab Invest* 3:71–82, 1954.

31. Lev M, Bharati S, Meng CC, et al: A concept of double-outlet right ventricle. *J Thorac Cardiovasc Surg* 64:271–281, 1972.

32. Lev M, Liberthson RR, Gen JG, et al: The pathologic anatomy of mesocardia. *Am J Cardiol* 28:428–435, 1971.

33. Lewis BE: Successful directional coronary atherectomy in a patient with dextrocardia and situs inversus. *Cath Cardiovasc Diagn* 29:47–51, 1993.

34. Lucas RV, Krabill KA: Anomalous venous connections, pulmonary and systemic. In Adams FH, Emmanouilides GC, Riemenschneider TA (eds): *Moss' Heart Disease in Infants, Children, and Adolescents*. Baltimore: Williams and Wilkins, 1989, pp 580–617.

35. Macartney FJ, Rigby ML, Anderson RH, et al: Double outlet right ventricle: Cross sectional echocardiographic findings, their anatomical explanation, and surgical relevance. *Br Heart J* 52:164–177, 1984.

36. Manner J, Seidl W, Steding G: Correlation between the embryonic head flexures and cardiac development. *Anat Embryol* 188:269–285, 1993.

37. Marino B, Sanders SP, Pasquini L, et al: Two-dimensional echocardiographic anatomy in crisscross heart. *Am J Cardiol* 58:325–333, 1986.

38. Meyer RA, Schwartz DC, Covitz W, Kaplan S: Echocardiographic assessment of cardiac malposition. *Am J Cardiol* 33:896–903, 1974.

39. Miralles A, Muneretto C, Gandjbakhch I, et al: Heart-lung transplantation in situs inversus: A case report in a patient with Kartagener's syndrome. *J Thorac Cardiovasc Surg* 103:307–313, 1992.

40. Morishima M, Ando M, Takao A: Visceroatrial heterotaxy syndrome in the NOD mouse with special reference to atrial situs. *Teratology* 44:91–100, 1991.

41. Morishima M, Ando M, Takao A: Visceroatrial heterotaxy syndrome in the nonobese diabetic mouse. In Clark EB, Takao A (eds): *Developmental Cardiology*. Mount Kisco, NY: Futura, 1990, pp 431–441.

42. Nachlieli T, Gershoni-Baruch R: Dextrocardia, microphthalmia, cleft palate, choreoathetosis, and mental retardation in an infant born to consanguineous parents. *Am J Med Genet* 42:458–460, 1992.

43. Neill CA: Development of the pulmonary veins. With reference to the embryology of anomalies of pulmonary venous return. *Pediatrics* 18:880–887, 1956.

44. Park MK: Chamber localization and cardiac malposition. In Park MK (ed): *Pediatric Cardiology for Practitioners*. Chicago: Year Book Medical, 1988, pp 201–205.

45. Pedersen H, Mygind N: Absence of axonemal arms in nasal mucosa cilia in Kartagener's syndrome. *Nature* 262:494–495, 1976.

46. Pexieder T, Rousseil MP, Prados Frutos JC: Prenatal pathogenesis of transposition of the great arteries. In Vogel M, Buhlmeyer K (eds): *Transposition of the Great Arteries: 25 years after Rashkind balloon septostomy*. Darmstadt: Steinkopff Verlag, 1992, pp 11–27.

47. Raines KH, Armstrong BE: Aortic atresia with visceral situs inversus with mirror-image dextrocardia. *Pediatr Cardiol* 10:232–235, 1989.

48. Robinson PJ, Kumpeng V, Macartney FJ: Cross sectional echocardiographic and angiocardiographic correlation in criss cross hearts. *Br Heart J* 54:61–67, 1985.

49. Rosenquist G, Olney M, Roe BB: The Holmes heart: A variant of cor triloular biatritum. Report of a case in a child. *Circulation* 27:1143–1147, 1963.

50. Seo JW, Brown NA, Ho SY, Anderson RH: Abnormal laterality and congenital cardiac anomalies: Relations of visceral and cardiac morphologies in the iv/iv mouse. *Circulation* 86:642–650, 1992.

51. Shaher RM: *Complete Transposition of the Great Arteries*. New York: Academic Press, 1973.

52. Shinebourne EA, Macartney FJ, Anderson RH: Sequential chamber localization-logical approach to diagnosis in congenital heart disease. *Br Heart J* 38:327–340, 1976.

53. Silverman NH: An ultrasonic approach to the diagnosis of cardiac situs, connections, and malpositions. In Friedman WF, Higgins CB (eds): *Pediatric Cardiac Imaging*. Philadelphia: WB Saunders, 1984, pp 188–201.

54. Snider AR, Serwer GA: Diagnostic approach to complex congenital heart disease. In Snider AR, Serwer GA (eds): *Echocardiography in Pediatric Heart Disease*. St. Louis: Mosby-Year Book, 1992, pp 348–368.

55. Van Mierop LHS, Patterson PR, Reyns RW: Two cases of congenital asplenia with isomerism of the cardiac atria and the sinoatrial nodes. *Am J Cardiol* 13:407–414, 1964.

56. Van Mierop LH, Eisen S, Schiebler GL: The radiographic appearance of the tracheobronchial tree as an indicator of visceral situs. *Am J Cardiol* 26:432–435, 1970.

57. Van Praagh R: Transposition of the great arteries. II. Transposition clarified. *Am J Cardiol* 28:739–741, 1971.

58. Van Praagh R: The segmental approach to diagnosis in congenital heart disease. *Birth Defects*: Original Article Series 8:4–23, 1972.

59. Van Praagh R: The segmental approach to understanding complex cardiac lesions. In Eldredge WJ, Gberg H, Lemole GM (eds): *Current Problems in Congenital Heart Disease*. New York: SP Medical and Scientific Books, 1979, pp 1–18.

60. Van Praagh R: Diagnosis of complex congenital heart disease: morphologic-anatomic method and terminology. *Cardiovasc Intervent Radiol* 7:115–120, 1984.

61. Van Praagh R, Perez-Trevino C, Lopez-Cuellar M, et al: Transposition of the great arteries with posterior aorta, anterior pulmonary artery,

subpulmonary conus and fibrous continuity between aortic and atrioventricular valves. *Am J Cardiol* 28:621–631, 1971.

62. Van Praagh R, Chacko KA: Intraventricular anatomic correction of double outlet right ventricle: When is it anatomically feasible? In Crupi G, Parenzan L, Anderson RH (eds): *Perspectives in Pediatric Cardiology,* Vol. 2. *Pediatric Cardiac Surgery,* Part 2. Mount Kisco, NY: Futura, 1989, pp 62–64.

63. Van Praagh R, Vlad P: Dextrocardia, mesocardia, and levocardia: The segmental approach to diagnosis in congenital heart disease. In Keith JD, Rowe RD, Vlad P (eds): *Heart Disease in Infancy and Childhood.* New York: Macmillan, 1978, pp 638–695.

64. Van Praagh R, Weinberg PM, Smith SD, et al: Malpositions of the heart. In Adams FH, Emmanouilides GC, Riemenschneider TA (eds): *Moss' Heart Disease in Infants, Children, and Adolescents.* Baltimore: Williams and Wilkins, 1989, pp 530–580.

65. Van Praagh S, Kreutzer J, Alday L, Van Praagh R: Systemic and pulmonary venous connections in visceral heterotaxy, with emphasis on the diagnosis of the atrial situs: A study of 109 postmortem cases. In Clark EB, Takao A (eds): *Developmental Cardiology: Morphogenesis and Function.* Mount Kisco, NY: Futura, 1990, pp 671–727.

66. Von Rokitansky CF: *Die Defekte der Scheidewande des Herzens.* Vienna, Wilhelm Braumuller, 1875.

67. Wenink AC, Gittenberger-de Groot AC: Left and right ventricular trabecular patterns: Consequence of ventricular septation and valve development. *Br Heart J* 48:462–468, 1982.

68. Yokoyama T, Copeland NG, Jenkins NA, et al: Reversal of left-right asymmetry: A situs inversus mutation. *Science* 260:679–682, 1993.

69. Yoo SJ, Lim TH, Park IS, et al: MR anatomy of ventricular septal defect in double-outlet right ventricle with situs solitus and atrioventricular concordance. *Radiology* 181:501–505, 1991.

70. Yost HJ: The genetics of midline and cardiac laterality defects. *Curr Opin Cardiol* 13:185–189, 1998.

Chapter 2

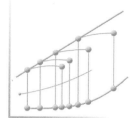

Cardiovascular Physiology and Shock

DAVID EPSTEIN, MD, and RANDALL C. WETZEL, MBBS, MBA

INTRODUCTION

The circulation, or cardiovasuclar system is a dynamic system responsible for the delivery of oxygen, nutrients, hormones, and host defense mechanisms throughout the body. It transports secretory products from tissues for action at distant sites (hormones) and by-products of cellular metabolism for excretion via the lungs, liver, skin, and kidneys. In addition to these transport functions, the cardiovascular system comprises dynamic metabolic tissue, synthesizing and modifying vasoactive compounds for regulation of vascular tone and myocardial function and self-repair after injury.

Cardiovascular regulatory mechanisms and their integration are severely affected by the stresses inherent in cardiovascular disease and cardiovascular surgery. An understanding of circulatory physiology forms the foundation of the critical care and surgical management of these children.

CONTRACTILE AND METABOLIC PROPERTIES OF THE CARDIOVASCULAR SYSTEM

The Heart

The prenatal heart develops a significant increase in contractile element expression, which continues after birth. However the newborn heart does not have as high a density of contractile elements as the adult heart.[102] Contractile force of the newborn myocardial sarcomere is equal to that in the adult; but with fewer sarcomeres per gram of tissue and other differences in control or modulation of sarcomere function, the newborn heart does not respond to stress as well as the adult heart.

With decreased density of contractile elements, the newborn has less cardiac reserve. The higher percentage of noncontractile elements results in decreased ventricular compliance and therefore less responsiveness to changes in vascular tone and preload than in adults.[237] Along with the incompletely developed contractile apparatus, the newborn heart has lower oxidative capability secondary to fewer mitochondria.[288]

In contrast, the newborn heart has a greater glycogen store than the adult heart and has an increased capacity for glycolytic pathway adenosine triphosphate (ATP) production.[236]

Sympathetic and parasympathetic innervation of the heart occurs at differing times. Although sympathetic innervation is extensive by 28 weeks gestation, it is still incomplete at birth, and development continues postnatally.[112] This may explain the increased sensitivity of the newborn heart to exogenous norepinephrine,[101] since less endogenous norepinephrine has been present to regulate the receptor-mediated response. Other inotropic agents may not be as potent in newborns.[91] Functionally, the newborn heart appears hypercontractile[284] and is capable of responding to at least a moderate degree of increased afterload.[22] In contrast, the parasympathetic vagal innervation of the heart is apparently complete at birth. This differential development may partially explain the tendency toward bradycardia during stress in the newborn; however, it seems likely that incomplete development of a mature central nervous system (CNS) control also contributes.

Vascular Development

Growth of the vasculature is a complex process. Mechanical forces of blood flow are clearly involved, but the primary mesodermal structures form before functional oxygen delivery and blood flow. It was theorized as early as 1896 by Thoma that "(1) increase in luminal size depends on the rate of blood flow, (2) growth in wall thickness is related to tension, and (3) length changes in vessels depend on the tension exerted by external tissues in the longitudinal direction."[285] These tenets underscore the intraluminal and extravascular forces that mediate development.

Endothelial cells lining the vessels grow in single layers, and vascular smooth muscle arises from mesodermal pericytes and fibroblasts. The vascular tree appears to be mature in structure at a young age in rats. Growth of the vascular tree occurs with increasing tension (blood pressure) and somatic growth of other body tissues. The vascular endothelium expresses different metabolic activity in youth from that in adulthood. These properties are discussed later in this chapter.

The aorta is an elastic artery composed of multiple lamellae of smooth muscle cells and elastic laminae. This structure empowers the aorta to act as a reservoir for blood delivered during ventricular systole. This blood is then distributed further during diastole, particularly to the heart. This elastic property of the aorta lessens left ventricular work, provides myocardial blood flow in diastole, and generates a continuous (albeit phasic) pressure gradient for blood flow into the arterial tree. The muscular arteries are primarily conduits for delivery of blood to the microcirculation. Nevertheless these vessels demonstrate dynamic responses to neural innervation, mechanical and chemical irritants, and pharmacologic vasoactive agents. These large vessels participate to different degrees in regional vascular tone and blood flow regulation. Arterioles (microvasculature proximal to capillaries) are the major circulatory resistance vessels. The largest resistance decrease occurs at this level, and local regulation of blood flow occurs primarily via changes in arteriolar radius and tone (Fig. 2-1). The arterioles as well as major conductance vessels are innervated by the autonomic nervous system and respond to changes in sympathetic tone and to pharmacologic

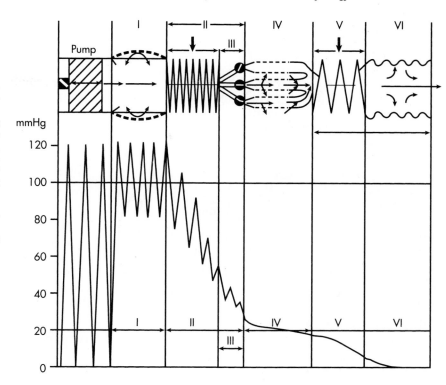

FIGURE 2-1 Schema for subdividing the circulation. The schematic along the top demonstrates various components of the circulation (from the heart pump to VI) and on the bottom shows an idealized systolic-diastolic pressure waveform for each of these components. The areas represented are the heart; I, the large arterial conduit vessels; II, the precapillary resistance vessels showing both the vessels and, III, the precapillary sphincters; IV, the capillary vessels where nutrient exchange occurs; V, the postcapillary resistance vessels; and VI, the veins, which consist of the venous capacitance and conduit vessels. As can be seen, the major fall in pressure occurs across the precapillary resistance vessels, which therefore represent the majority of the resistance in the circulation. (From Folkow B: The resistance vasculature: Functional importance in the circulation. In Bevan JA, Halpern W, Mulvany MJ (eds): *The Resistance Vasculature.* Totowa, NJ, Humana Press, pp 23–43, 1991; with permission.)

agents that act via receptors that evoke changes in contractile mechanisms in vascular smooth muscle.

The capillaries provide a large surface area for delivery of nutrients to all cells by diffusion and for passage of cellular secretory and waste products from tissues for transport. Capillary endothelium is not as well studied as large vessel or other microcirculatory endothelium. Although anatomic site of origin dependent heterogeneity is common, the capillary endothelium is undoubtedly metabolically active and dynamic and is mechanically active in providing a semipermeable barrier. This barrier function is altered in many states when the endothelium is injured. Migration of polymorphonuclear leukocytes and movement of macromolecules out of the circulation occur with inflammation, thermal injury, and hypoxic injury. Microvascular occlusion occurs at capillary, precapillary, and postcapillary vessel sites. The interaction of endothelium, leukocytes, and platelets occurs in each of these areas. Differences in receptor expression exist; for example, capillary endothelial cells express receptors for platelet-derived growth factor, whereas arterial endothelial cells do not.[241]

The venous component of the circulation is frequently considered merely a conduit that completes the cardiovascular system. However, the venous tree is critically important as a dynamic reservoir for blood. The venous circulation is innervated by the sympathetic nervous system, which promotes constriction. Also, venous vascular smooth muscle dilates in response to nitrovasodilators and loss of sympathetic tone. The venous limb tone is a major contributor to the dynamics of preload.

The Transitional Circulation

The fetus lives in an environment that is hypoxic by newborn or adult standards. Umbilical venous blood from the placenta is relatively highly saturated (80% to 85% saturation) with

a PO_2 of 30 to 35 mm Hg. This mixes with other venous (inferior vena cava) return to the right atrium and is shunted to the left atrium for left ventricular ejection to provide the highest oxygen delivery to the brain and myocardium via the ascending aorta (Fig. 2-2). Nevertheless the PO_2 of the preductal, ascending aortic blood, which supplies the coronary circulation, is even lower (25 to 28 mm Hg).[242] Any reduction in maternal oxygen tension can adversely affect the fetus because the oxygen tension is normally already low.

Fetal circulatory pressures are quite low when compared with adults. As the vascular system develops with growth of the fetus, the systemic pressure rises slightly, achieving 60/45 to 70/45 mm Hg by near term (see Fig. 2-2). Right and left ventricular pressures are nearly equal in utero, but right ventricular pressure falls at birth in response to dramatic changes in pulmonary vascular resistance (PVR). Systemic pressures, similar to late gestation pressures, are maintained in the newborn period. With loss of the low-resistance uteroplacental circuit and a large increase in pulmonary blood flow, a marked increase in left ventricular output and a smaller increase in right ventricular output occur.[11] This results in the high cardiac output necessary to provide support to the high metabolic requirements of the newborn.

The circulation abruptly changes at birth from a parallel system to one in series. In utero, the high PVR and low lung volumes direct most of the right ventricular output through the patent ductus arteriosus to combine with left ventricular output. Oxygenated blood from the placenta returns to the right heart via the ductus venosus (bypassing the liver to the suprahepatic inferior vena cava. Venous return from the inferior vena cava blood enters the right atrium and passes to the left atrium via the foramen ovale. Most superior vena cava return enters the right atrium and crosses the tricuspid valve to the right ventricle. The high PVR causes most right ventricular output to cross the patent ductus arteriosus, and both

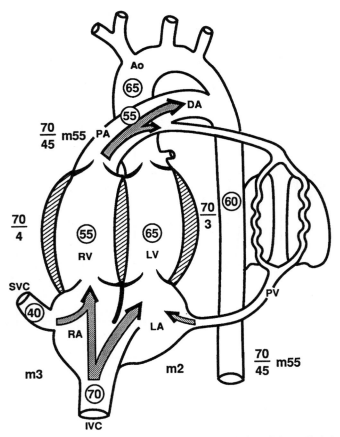

FIGURE 2-2 The in utero late gestational fetal circulation of sheep. Circled figures represent percentages of oxygen saturation; the other numbers represent the pressures in each chamber. The direction of flow is indicated by the arrows. (From Rudolph AM: The fetal circulation. In Rudolph AM (ed): *Congenital Diseases of the Heart.* Chicago, Mosby–Year Book, pp 1–16, 1974; with permission.)

ventricles combine output to provide systemic blood flow. With the multiple right-to-left connections and low-pressure requirements, the fetus can survive with major vascular anomalies without severe distress. At birth, many changes occur: (1) there is reduction in PVR attendant with the first breath; (2) there is loss of the low-resistance placenta and its gas exchange function; (3) there is increased systemic vascular resistance from loss of the placenta, and the left ventricular and left atrial pressures rise, which functionally closes the flap-valve foramen ovale; (4) the ductus venosus and ductus arteriosus become unnecessary; and (5) the lungs become the obligate organ of oxygen and carbon dioxide exchange. With these changes, the circulatory system is now in series pattern. In the immediate postnatal period, the only permanent anatomic change is the removal of the uteroplacental unit. Each of the other changes is dynamic in nature.

The cardiac output in relation to body weight is extremely high in the neonatal period compared with adults.[164] In the newborn, this reaches greater than 200 mL/kg/minute. The cardiac index (4.0 L/min/m² at 1 hour of age) diminishes slowly with age to achieve adult norms (2.5 to 3 L/min/m²) by adolescence (Fig. 2-3). The cardiac output is tightly coupled with oxygen consumption, which is also higher per unit mass in newborns than in adults. This increased oxygen consumption is secondary to thermogenesis as the infant responds to the stress of the extrauterine environment.[129,253] In the newborn,

oxygen consumption reaches 6 to 8 mL/kg/minute in comparison with the adult normal values of 4 to 5 mL/kg/minute. Some of this increased oxygen consumption is due to thermogenesis, but even when infants are placed in a neutral thermic environment, they demonstrate increased oxygen utilization. This is believed to be due to growth requirements, which are responsible for a large percentage of caloric utilization in young children.

Cardiovascular function depends on the intimate relationship and balance between the circulation and cardiac function. This is clear in the simple expression:

Blood Pressure = Cardiac Output
× Systemic Vascular Resistance

The regulation of cardiovascular function can be discussed from the viewpoint of regulation of cardiac output and control of vascular tone, but it must be realized that this is an artificial dichotomy. In reality the circulation is regulated by a highly complex crosstalk between all of its elements. For purposes of discussion, the cardiac output will be addressed first.

DETERMINANTS OF CARDIAC OUTPUT

Two relatively simple but crucial relationships are essential to an understanding of cardiovascular physiology. These can be stated as follows:

Cardiac Output = Stroke Volume × *Heart Rate*,
Stroke Volume ∝ *Preload, Afterload, and Contractility.*

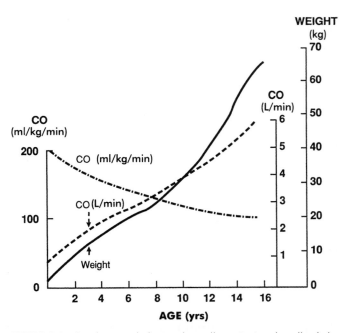

FIGURE 2-3 Developmental changes in cardiac output and cardiac index with regard to weight and age. As can be seen, although the cardiac output increases with increasing age and body weight, the cardiac output per kilogram falls. (From Rudolph AM: Changes in the circulation after birth. In Rudolph AM (ed): *Congenital Diseases of the Heart.* Chicago, Mosby–Year Book, pp 17–28, 1974, with permission.)

Circulatory function is determined by both cardiac and vascular function. Blood pressure provides a clinically useful, albeit insensitive and crude integrated indication of circulatory function. *Cardiac function* depends on the structure of the heart, its rhythmicity, and its contractile function. Cardiac output is an integrated indicator of overall cardiac function. *Myocardial function* is determined by the contractile state of the heart, which is influenced by the intrinsic inotropic state of the heart and the work it has to perform (preload and afterload). Stroke volume is a clinical indicator of myocardial function. Each of these primary determinants of cardiovascular function (previous italics) must be individually understood to comprehend the integrated function of the cardiovascular system.

The average heart rate for quiet, awake newborns in the first week of life is approximately 145 beats/minute, and 120 to 125 beats/minute during sleep. However, the range for heart rate is 70 to 220! Strong influences of the autonomic nervous system are apparent very early in life. Coordinated electric activity and automaticity of the conduction system in the newborn heart are essential to maximize the active phase of atrioventricular filling. The cardiac output is clearly dependent on a coordinated heart rate with conduction and adequate diastolic filling time. The newborn heart has a limited ability to increase stroke volume, whereas stroke volume can fall easily secondary to severe tachycardia.[25] Heart rate and the effect of irregularities in cardiac rate and rhythm in the critically ill child are further discussed in Chapter 8.

DETERMINANTS OF STROKE VOLUME

The Contractile Unit

The myocyte consists of multiple elements, including the basic contractile unit: the sarcomere. The sarcomere contains the myofibrillar contractile elements and is the functional unit of the myocardial myocyte. Other myocyte constituents are cytoplasm, mitochondria, sarcoplasmic reticulum, and the cell envelope, which is an excitable membrane. The myofibrillar contractile elements consist of actin, tropomyosin, troponin complexes (thin filaments), and myosin filaments (thick filaments) containing myosin crossbridge components (heads) (Fig. 2-4).

Excitation-Contraction Coupling

The spreading action potential in the myocardium leads to myocyte membrane depolarization along the T-tubule system. Extracellular calcium enters the cell through voltage-gated calcium channels. The increase in cytoplasmic calcium concentration leads to the release of intracellular calcium stores from the sarcoplasmic reticulum (SR) and a further rise in cytoplasmic calcium content. This process is called *calcium-induced calcium release*.

Free, intracellular calcium causes actin-myosin binding, which is the basis of myocyte contraction. In the resting state, actin and myosin binding is inhibited by troponin and tropomyosin. Tropomyosin is a filament that overlies the actin. Troponin is a complex of three subunits: troponin T attaches to the tropomyosin, troponin C is a high-affinity calcium-binding site, and troponin I inhibits the actin-myosin interaction. When intracellular calcium content rises, it binds to the troponin C subunit. This binding antagonizes troponin I and

causes a conformational change in tropomyosin and troponin that exposes the myosin-binding sites on the actin filaments. These actin-binding sites are then free to bind with the myosin heads forming cross-bridges. As this binding occurs, the actin and myosin filaments slide along each other and draw the myocyte Z-bands closer together, resulting in myocyte and ultimately myocardial contraction. The force and rapidity of contraction are directly proportional to the amount of free intracellular calcium. The myosin head contains the actin-myosin ATPase that is responsible for the hydrolysis of ATP and the release of energy that allows relaxation of the actin and myosin crossbridges. The mutual affinity of actin and myosin is so great that energy is required to separate them and allow further cross-bridging, which leads to contraction. The amount of ATP hydrolyzed determines the rapidity of this unbridging and relinking cycle, and thus the velocity of fiber shortening.[270]

Clearly, the intracellular calcium content is the crucial determinant of myocardial contraction. Intracellular calcium increases during contraction from 10^{-7} M during diastole to 10^{-5} M during systole.[256] Cyclic AMP (cAMP) plays an important role in regulating contractility by (1) enhancing inward calcium flow, (2) increased sarcoplasmic reticulum calcium release, (3) phosphorylation of troponin I to promote binding of myosin to actin, (4) phosphorylation of sarcoplasmic reticulum to decrease reuptake of calcium, and (5) possibly enhancing mitochondrial release of calcium. Thus, agents that stimulate adenylate cyclase will act as inotropes.[315] Most inotropic agents (including catecholamines) increase intracellular calcium, while negative inotropes (including calcium channel blockers and beta-antagonists) decrease intracellular calcium. Drugs such as phosphodiesterase inhibitors (amrinone, milrinone) that prevent the breakdown of cAMP to 5′-AMP will also have a positive inotropic effect.

The other elements of the myocyte also play a role in myocyte contraction. The cytoplasm contains the mitochondria, which provide energy for contraction and relaxation. During development, the mitochondria demonstrate increased cristae formation and become larger and plumper.[10] The neonatal myocyte is relatively deficient in mitochondria, which accounts for 35% to 40% of the muscle mass by adulthood. The cytoplasm also contains calmodulin, which regulates phosphorylation of the contractile proteins, and parvalbumin, which plays an important role in sequestration of intracellular calcium and may modulate muscle relaxation. Calmodulin's role is complex; it is involved as a calcium-binding protein and in activation of phosphorylation via protein kinases.[10] It functions in a balancing (both synergy and antagonism) fashion with cAMP-mediated effects.

In the fetus and neonate the tropomyosin isoforms are different from those in adults: The amount of actin and myosin per cell and the amount of ATPase activity are less, and the intracellular water content is greater.[162] In addition the cardiac myocyte shape and dimensions change with development. The cardiac myocyte progresses in shape from sphere-like in extreme immaturity to that of a blunt-ended rectangle in adulthood. The myocyte of the newborn heart typically is 40 μm long and 5 μm wide, whereas that of the adult heart may exceed 150 μm in length and 25 μm in width. When shortening of the neonatal and the adult myocyte are compared, the adult myocyte contracts more rapidly and by a proportionately larger amount, with shortening occurring in the long axis of the cell.[11] In addition, the myofibrils (consisting of actin and myosin) are

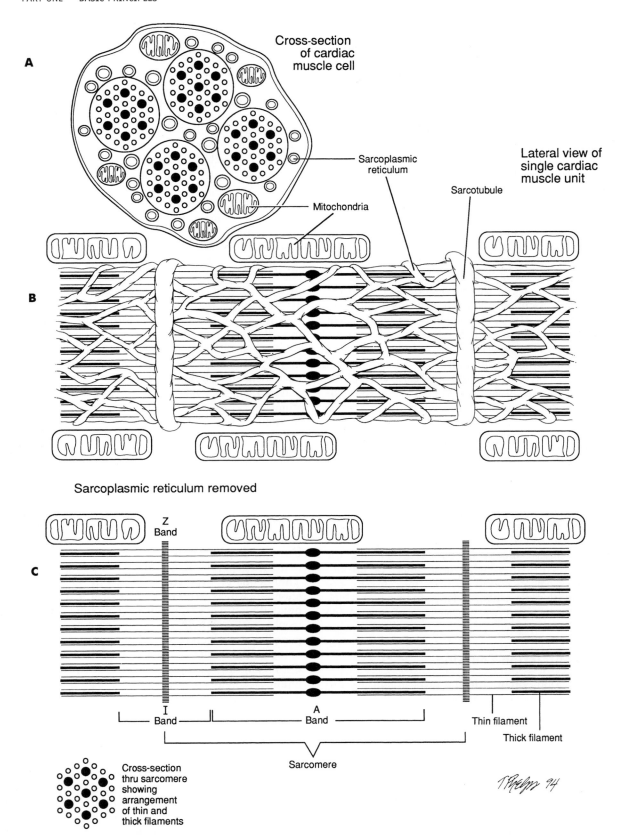

FIGURE 2-4   **A,** The myocyte (or fiber) consists of bundles (or fibrils) of aligned actin and myosin filaments surrounded by cytoplasm containing mitochondria. **B,** The fibrils with sarcoplasmic reticulum and T-tubule systems are responsible for conduction of ionic currents and electrical depolarization, which increases the intracellular calcium around the actin and myosin. **C,** Each fibril consists of sarcomeres connected in series and each sarcomere consists of bundles of actin and myosin connected at the Z plates. The muscle bundles consist of thick filaments (myosin) and thin filaments (actin) and multiple regulatory protein compounds (tropomyosin, troponin C complex). The myosin heads join to their actin-binding sites when the tropomyosin–troponin C complex exposes these binding sites in the presence of increasing calcium concentrations. This is the actual process of contraction.

in a less parallel array than in older children and adults.[198] This is analogous to the myocytes, which are also in a nonparallel array compared to the adult myocytes within the myocardium. These multiple factors contribute to the relative resistance of the neonatal heart to increasing the inotropic state.

Excitation-contraction coupling and factors that affect the rate of spread of depolarization through the myocardium (dromotropy) are the primary determinants of calcium entry into the myocytes. Myocyte contractility is also affected by myocyte receptors. Both beta$_1$ and beta$_2$ receptors are present in the fetus and increase in density with age.[45,184] Histamine, vasoactive intestinal peptide (VIP), acetylcholine M$_2$, adenosine, and somatostatin receptors are also present on myocytes.

Receptor-mediated signal transduction is linked to contractility by two major pathways. The first is the G protein-linked adenylate cyclase receptor.[95,161] Ligand-receptor binding leads to a conformational change in the G protein complex, which activates adenylate cyclase.[231] This in turn causes diverse activity of multiple protein kinases, activation of voltage-dependent calcium channels, troponin I inactivation, crossbridge formation, and ultimately contraction. Another signal transduction pathway is the phospholipase pathway. Phospholipase A activation leads to release of arachidonate (and thus eicosanoid metabolites) and a diacyl phospholipids, which are further metabolized by phospholipase C.[29] The products of phospholipase C are diacylglycerol (DAG) and inositol (1,4,5) triphosphate (IP$_3$). DAG, in conjunction with intracellular calcium, activates membrane-bound protein kinases to enhance enzyme phosphorylation and activate regulatory proteins. IP3 binds to the sarcoplasmic reticulum to cause release of intracellular calcium. These combined effects tend to interact with the effects of cAMP. This pathway, although critical in vascular smooth muscle, plays a minor role in the myocardial myocyte. The developmental aspects of these pathways are poorly understood. In heart failure, downregulation of beta receptors and vasoactive intestinal peptide receptors occurs and may play a role in the reduced contractility.[45,127]

Cell Mechanics

The sarcomere length-tension relationship has been inferred from studies of myocardial muscle strips. Starling's famous demonstration of the length-tension relationship, describing how preload and afterload affect contractility, underlies the concepts that continue to influence patient management in the intensive care unit (ICU). Increasing resting muscle strip length before excitation increases developed tension until a plateau is reached. This is then followed by a decrease in developed tension with increasing length. This is the Starling relationship. Increasing the weight against which the muscle contracts (afterload) decreases developed tension (Fig. 2-5). Resting sarcomere Z-Z distance is about 1.6 microns. Optimal overlap occurs around 2.2 microns, and distraction occurs around 3.5 microns.[267] Thus a muscle fiber must be stretched to twice its resting length before the descending limb of the Starling curve is reached. In reality this is a rare occurrence that has virtually no clinical correlate.

In the clinical setting, preload augmentation is most likely to increase resting fiber length and, if all else remains the same, to increase developed tension, which is associated with increased stroke volume. Clinically, excessive preload does not overdistract the myocyte (although it may overdistend

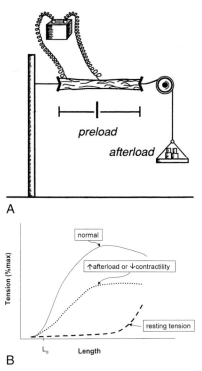

FIGURE 2-5 The classic Starling experiment. **A,** The muscle strip is suspended between two points at a given length that determine the preload. L_0 is the resting unstressed fiber length. After electrical stimulation, the muscle contracts against the weight (afterload). **B,** The length-tension curves for resting tension (dashed line), normally developed peak tension (solid line), and either increased afterload or decreased contractility (dotted line). The ordinate is expressed as percent of maximum tension developed. These are the classic length-tension relationships, which are by analogy extrapolated to our understanding of pressure-volume relationships.

the ventricle and lead to AV valve regurgitation and increased volume load on the heart), but rather alters myocardial perfusion and energy balance in such a fashion as to decrease contractile function. This system is best represented by a shift of the Starling curve downward to the right: that is, for the same preload, less tension is developed (if afterload is constant). Clinically, this is associated with decreased stroke volume, not on the basis of the "descending limb" but on the basis of decreased contractility.

Myocardial Structure

The myocytes exist in an array of connective tissue that binds the myocytes into bundles and maintains their alignment with each other and their capillaries. With maturation, most of this collagen changes from type III to type I.[183] The relationship of the myocyte cytoskeleton plays a crucial role in linking contraction of the sarcomeres to actual cell and then myocardial shortening.[198] Developmental differences exist, although their full implications are as yet poorly understood.[70] The capillary network of the myocardium is extremely dense, and the ratio of endothelial cells to myocytes is approximately 1:1. Thus, the coronary and endocardial endothelium are in a strategic location to affect myocyte function, just as the endothelium is in the vasculature. The organization of the myocardial framework varies. With increasing age, the bundles become more tightly packed and aligned in a highly organized parallel fashion. The neonatal myocardium is more chaotic, with less obvious structure and with more loose connective tissue.[198] This may account for the relatively greater "stiffness" of the neonatal myocardium and its decreased compliance characteristics. These factors may explain why preload limitation is more pronounced in the neonatal period.

The muscle fibers of the myocardium are arranged in a complex helical array.[275] Midwall circumferential fibers parallel to the AV groove are encased in a double figure-eight series of fibers twisting toward the surfaces of the heart, so that at the epicardium they lie at a 75° angle and at the endocardium at a 60° angle to the circumferential fibers. This gross anatomy accounts for the "bottom-up" squeezing-rotating action on the ventricles with contraction. In general the myocardium grows by hyperplasia before birth and hypertrophy postnatally. Increase in cell number ceases by early infancy. Although the right ventricular thickness (approximately 0.3 cm at the AV valve ring) increases little postnatally, left ventricular thickness doubles (to approximately 1.2 cm) and mass increases approximately 20-fold, completely by cellular hypertrophy. The right ventricular to left ventricular weight ratio shifts from 1 at birth to 0.5 in later childhood.[176]

Preload

For an isolated muscle strip, preload is readily conceptualized as the resting fiber length before contraction. In the intact heart, preload, by analogy, becomes resting or end-diastolic ventricular volume. Obviously, the structure of the heart, the alignment of the myocytes, and the organization of the myocardium convert the simple relationship between resting fiber length and developed tension into a complex relationship between end-diastolic volume (EDV) and myocardial function. This complex relationship is further modified by geometry and structural changes associated with congenital heart disease (CHD). Generally, in the isolated heart that is not allowed to eject, increased ventricular EDV, or pre-load, causes increased pressure generation during systole. This observation was made by Otto Frank. If the heart is permitted to eject against a constant afterload, a greater stroke volume (SV) results (Starling's law). Combined, this Frank-Starling law states that if preload is increased, SV and the capability for pressure generation are increased.

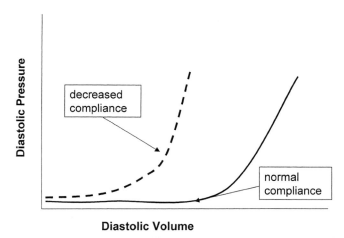

FIGURE 2-6 The diastolic compliance curve of the ventricle. Diastolic pressure is graphed against diastolic volume. In the normally compliant ventricle, volume may be increased with minimal increase in pressure initially. However, at the steep end of the curve, small increases in volume lead to steep increases in pressure. In a ventricle with decreased compliance, this curve is displaced to the left as shown.

In clinical practice preload is rarely measured as ventricular EDV. Instead we measure or infer (from wedge and atrial pressures) ventricular end-diastolic pressure (EDP).[226] The relationship between pressure and volume is described by compliance, which is the ratio of change in volume per unit change in pressure. For a given EDV, the EDP will depend on the compliance of the ventricle. Thus, for a given preload, hypertrophy, ischemia, infarction, or structural abnormality may decrease ventricular compliance and increase EDP (Fig. 2-6). The compliance curve of the heart is similar to that of other structures. Volume may be increased without an increase in pressure until a point of steep increase in pressure is reached. Although the relationship between EDV and SV is linear, the relationship between EDP and SV is curvilinear, owing to the nature of the compliance of the heart (Fig. 2-7).[266] Decreased compliance leads to higher EDP for a given preload, and this may limit ventricular filling by impeding venous return to the heart (see discussion following).

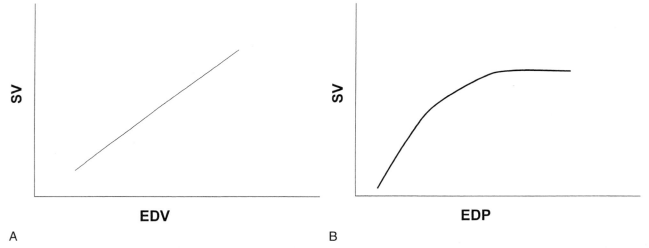

A   B

FIGURE 2-7   A, Linear increase in stroke volume (SV) with increasing end-diastolic volume (EDV). **B,** Curvilinear increase in SV with increasing end-diastolic pressure (EDP). Increased end-diastolic volume virtually always increases stroke volume. Note that as end-diastolic pressure increases, stroke volume plateaus, because of the nature of the compliance relationship of the ventricle.

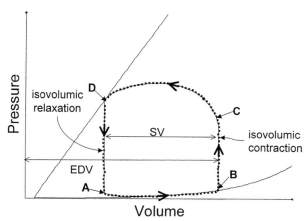

FIGURE 2-8 A prototypic pressure-volume loop of the left ventricle. At point A the mitral valve opens and diastole begins. At point B diastole ends (mitral valve closes) prior to ventricular contraction. Point C is the end of isovolumic contraction when the aortic valve opens prior to ejection. Point D is the end of ventricular ejection (systole) when the aortic valve closes before isovolumic relaxation. Line A-B thus represents ventricular filling during diastole. Line B-C represents the period of isovolumic contraction with rising ventricular pressure and no change in ventricular volume. Line C-D represents ventricular ejection. Line D-A is isovolumic relaxation. Stroke volume (SV) and end-diastolic volume (EDV) are also shown. The area encompassed by the loop represents cardiac work. (Figure generated by the Heart Simulator, courtesy of Marc Dickstein, MD, and Daniel Burkhoff, MD, Columbia University.)

The *ventricular pressure-volume loop* is a helpful concept for analyzing the relationship between preload and contractility (Fig. 2-8).[309] If ventricular pressure and volume are simultaneously recorded, the resultant loop provides useful information concerning ventricular function. The concept of *elastance* describes these pressure-volume relationships. Elastance is the change in pressure per unit change in volume (and is therefore the reciprocal of compliance).

Figure 2-8 represents the prototypic pressure-volume relationship.[245] Point A is the point at which left ventricular pressure falls below left atrial pressure, the mitral valve opens, and the ventricle begins to fill during diastole. Point B represents the pressure-volume relationship at end-diastole, just before ventricular contraction occurs. Point C is the point at which the aortic valve opens. Line BC is therefore the phase of isovolumic contraction, when ventricular pressure rises and volume (which is in fact EDV) does not change. From point C to point D (line CD) the ventricle is ejecting; ventricular volume falls and pressure changes relatively little. Point D represents closure of the aortic valve as ventricular pressure falls below aortic pressure. The final line (DA) represents isovolumic relaxation as ventricular pressure falls and volume remains constant at end-systolic volume (ESV). In this construct, SV is the difference between lines AD and BC. The ejection fraction (EF) is the ratio of SV:EDV. The external stroke work of the ventricle is the area enclosed within the loop. Pressure-volume loops can be normalized to body surface area to allow comparison among children. Pressure-volume loops in normal children and those with heart disease are shown in Figure 2-9.[114] It should be noted that this description of pump function of the heart is directly determined by the mechanical properties of the myocardium and the individual myocytes.

Now consider the changes that occur in the pressure-volume relationship with increased preload when contractility remains the same (Fig. 2-10). If aortic end-systolic pressure remains the same, a volume infusion will extend the loop to

the right. The constant end-systolic pressure in the face of volume infusion is mediated in part by the baroreceptor reflex (see the following), which results in vasodilation and bradycardia in response to increased stretch in the walls of the atria, aorta, and carotid sinus. Notice that EDV and EDP are increased (B to B_1) and SV is increased. Note that EF is also increased, although contractility is unchanged. Thus pure preload augmentation may increase EDV, SV, and apparent EF without changing contractility.

As long as contractility remains constant, preload augmentation will increase SV and therefore cardiac output. As mentioned previously, limitation in this Starling mechanism is uncommon. Nevertheless, preload augmentation does have limitations. The increase in EDV increases EDP. If this occurs on the steep portion of the ventricular compliance curve, the increase in left ventricular EDP (LVEDP) may be excessive. Because LVEDP is the downstream pressure for myocardial perfusion, excessively high EDPs (more than 15 to 20 mm Hg) may impair myocardial perfusion, with subsequent loss in function and deterioration in contractility. If preload augmentation decreases myocardial perfusion pressure (mean arterial blood pressure minus LVEDP) below 50 to 55 mm Hg, serious concern about myocardial ischemia is warranted. This mechanism underlies the so-called descending limb of the Starling or myocardial function curve. A further limitation to preload augmentation is excessive increase in venous pressure (pulmonary and systemic). This has two consequences: increased transcapillary fluid flux leading to edema (systemic and, more seriously, pulmonary) and possible decreased organ perfusion because venous pressures are the downstream pressures for perfusion. For example, if the mean arterial pressure is 60 mm Hg and the inferior vena cava pressure rises from 15 to 25 mm Hg with volume infusion, renal perfusion pressure will fall from 45 to 35 mm Hg, well below the autoregulatory threshold of the kidney; thus renal hypoperfusion will ensue. These sequelae of volume infusion make it clear that the danger in preload augmentation is not volume but rather the pressure generated by increased volume.

It is clear that the newborn heart responds to increased preload in a fashion similar to the adult heart. These relationships can be demonstrated in utero.[25] Although increased preload increases SV in neonates, there are developmental differences that are important. The compliance relationship of the newborn heart differs from that of the adult. The newborn heart is stiffer and maintains an equivalent volume at a higher EDP. In the neonate, normalized left ventricular EDV (LVEDV) is less than in children (42 ± 10 versus 73 ± 11 mL/m²) and diastolic pressures are similar. With less contractile structures per gram of tissue, the ventricles do not tolerate excessive preload as well as later in life.[237] Excessive increases in preload, which readily lead to increased EDP with elevated venous pressures, limit the effectiveness of volume infusion in neonates. Evidence in the fetal lamb indicates that when EDPs are greater than 10 to 12 mm Hg, further preload augmentation does not increase SV. With less compliant ventricles, heart failure may occur earlier in newborns. Therefore, with less tolerance of preload and maximized contractility, the stressed newborn augments cardiac output by increasing heart rate. This mechanism is in part responsible for the heart rate dependence of cardiac output in newborns and infants.

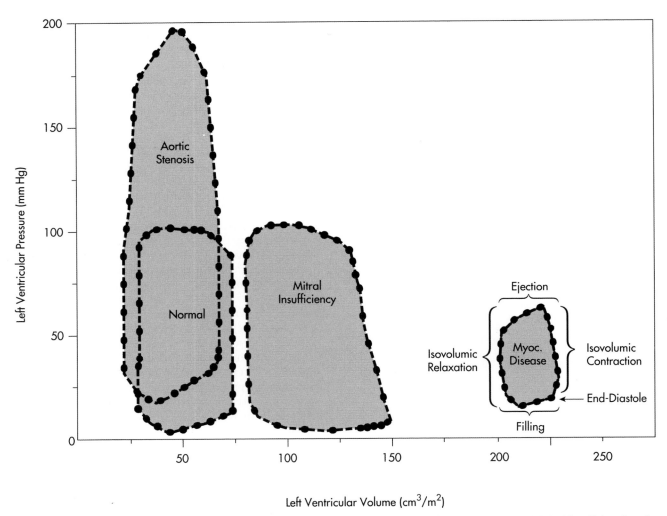

FIGURE 2-9   Pressure-volume loops for children with various congenital heart diseases. Myocardial disease, volume overload (mitral insufficiency), and pressure overload (aortic stenosis) are demonstrated. (From Graham TP Jr, Jarmakani MM: Evaluation of ventricular function in infants and children, *Pediatr Clin North Am* 18:1109–1132, 1971, with permission.)

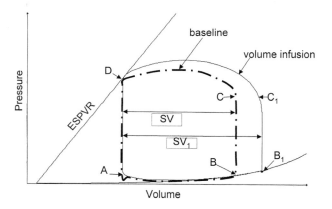

FIGURE 2-10   The effect of preload augmentation on the pressure-volume loop. The infused volume raises end-diastolic volume (B-B_1). Stroke volume is augmented by the difference between SV and SV_1. Note that end-systolic pressure (D) has not changed significantly in this example, because of the effects of baroreceptor reflexes and other regulatory responses. (Figure generated by the Heart Simulator, courtesy of Marc Dickstein, MD, and Daniel Burkhoff, MD, Columbia University.)

Contractility

To further understand the relationship between preload and contractility, consider the pressure-volume relationship of the ventricle in Figure 2-11. The example in Figure 2-10 assumed that ejection would occur to the same end-systolic pressure-volume point (D). In fact, the position of end-systolic pressure-volume point (D) may change with changes in preload. Figure 2-11 shows a series of pressure-volume loops (1...n). If intravascular and therefore ventricular volume is successively reduced, both end-diastolic and end-systolic ventricular volumes decrease. The entire pressure-volume loop moves downward and toward the left. SV is decreased (from SV_1 to SV_n). Hence, the end-systolic pressure point is also left-shifted. As successive amounts of volume are removed, that is, as preload decreases, the end-systolic points move to the left and downward. A line connecting these points ($D_n...D_1$) describes the pressure-volume relationship at end-systole. This end-systolic pressure-volume relationship (ESPVR) is in fact a graphic description of myocardial contractility. Figure 2-12A demonstrates that the slope of the ESPVR line represents contractility. All other factors being equal, a shift in the

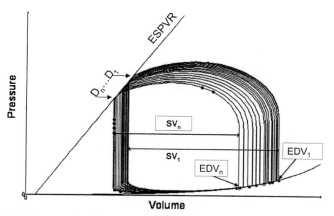

FIGURE 2-11 The effect of decreasing preload on the pressure-volume loop. As volume is removed, successive loops move toward the left from the 1st loop to the *n*th loop. The *n*th loop has less end-diastolic volume (EDV_n) and stroke volume (SV_n) than the 1st loop. Point *D* represents end-systole for each PV loop 1...*n*. The family of points $D_{1...n}$ fall on a line that represents the end-systolic pressure-volume relationship (ESPVR). Thus it can be seen that the diastolic compliance relationship and the ESPVR define the limits within which the ventricle responds to changes in preload. (Figure generated by the Heart Simulator, courtesy of Marc Dickstein, MD, and Daniel Burkhoff, MD, Columbia University.)

line upward to the left indicates increased contractility, where EF and SV are increased for a given end-diastolic pressure-volume relationship (EDPVR). A shift in the ESPVR down to the right is consistent with decreased myocardial contractility. SV and EF are decreased for a given EDPVR point. Thus, for a family of preload loops, contractility is defined by the ESPVR.[4]

In a sick child experiencing progressive reductions in contractility, all other factors would not remain equal. Various compensatory responses would take place including fluid retention, vasoconstriction, and tachycardia. Figure 2-12*B* demonstrates the effects of fluid retention leading to preload augmentation in a child who has experienced a progressive reduction in contractility. In this example, the fluid retention leads to a restoration of stroke volume and systolic pressures at the expense of higher end-diastolic volume and pressure.

Afterload

In the Starling muscle strip preparation, the concept of afterload is straightforward. It is the weight against which the fiber contracts. It is the mass that resists contraction. The magnitude of muscle shortening is directly related to the afterload, so that with increasing afterload, shortening is decreased and slowed. Afterload reduction increases fiber shortening. This concept is deceptively simple, and transferring this by analogy to the intact heart is potentially full of pitfalls and not at all straightforward. One reason for this is that it is not the load on the muscle strip that is important, but rather the stress, which is load per cross-sectional area. This is important in translation to the intact heart. Thus the concept of ventricular stress (a function of both load and geometry) is important in considering the in vivo determinants of afterload.[240,276] It should be remembered that the one-dimensional concept of systemic vascular resistance as afterload is only a gross approximation of afterload and has gained use only because it is a measurable parameter of cardiovascular function. The concept of afterload can be generalized as any factor that resists the ejection of blood from the heart. There are several determinants of afterload in the intact heart:

1. *Impedance* of the vasculature, which is related to the elastance of the great vessels and the resistance of the smaller vessels. In children the latter is generally of greater significance.

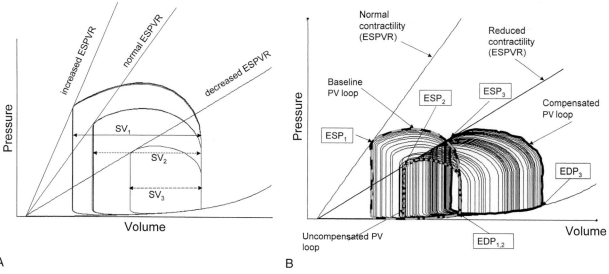

A   B

FIGURE 2-12 The effect of changing the end-systolic pressure-volume relationship (ESPVR). **A,** Pressure-volume (PV) loops are depicted with increased, normal, or decreased ESPVR (contractility) while all other variables (preload, afterload, heart rate) are held constant. The stroke volume (width of the PV loop) falls progressively (SV_1 to SV_3) with the reduction in ESPVR. Similarly, systolic pressure (height of the PV loop) decreases as ESPVR is reduced. **B,** In vivo, PV relationships showing progressive reduction in ESPVR (contractility) followed by preload augmentation secondary to fluid retention. The initial progression of PV loops from "baseline" (dashed PV loop) to "uncompensated" (dotted PV loop) shows the reduction in stroke volume and end-systolic pressure (ESP_1 to ESP_2). Fluid retention (preload augmentation) leads to a series of PV loops from "uncompensated" to "compensated," resulting in an increasing stroke volume and end-systolic pressure (ESP_2 to ESP_3). This compensation is achieved at the expense of higher end-diastolic pressure (EDP_3) and volume. (Figure generated by the Heart Simulator, courtesy of Marc Dickstein, MD, and Daniel Burkhoff, MD, Columbia University.)

2. The *ejection pressure* is also important and is in part determined by the vascular resistance. The end-systolic pressure is the major determinant of this factor.

3. *Ventricular outflow tract obstruction* can increase the load against which the heart must work. Thus valvular stenosis significantly affects ventricular afterload.

4. *Ventricular wall stress* is also a major determinant of afterload. Laplace's law simply states that the circumferential wall stress (T) is equal to the pressure (P) times the radius (r) divided by twice the wall thickness (t):

$$T = (P \times r) \, / \, 2t$$

In the heart, which is exposed to pressure from the outside (pericardial or intrathoracic pressure) and the inside (intraluminal pressure), the pressure that is important is the transmural pressure or

$$LV_{tm} = LV \text{ intraluminal} - LV \text{ extraluminal}$$
$$\text{(or pericardial)}$$

Although this is a simplification, several points are important to note. Wall stress increases with size, and thus volume loading increases wall stress. Therefore volume expansion increases afterload; that is, afterload is preload dependent. Additionally, hypertrophy by increasing the denominator of the Laplace equation, thickness, decreases wall stress. Finally, since transmural pressure is important, when intrathoracic pressure becomes more negative, say with inspiration, then transmural pressure and, therefore, afterload increase. This also partly explains why positive end-expiratory pressure (PEEP), which elevates intrathoracic pressure, may also act as afterload reduction for the heart (see Chapter 9). This effect accounts in part for the beneficial effect of PEEP in cardiogenic pulmonary edema.

5. *Inertia.* Preload not only acts to increase wall stress, but also provides an inertial mass against which the heart must work to eject blood; the greater the mass, the greater the inertia and therefore the greater the afterload. Again, afterload is preload dependent. All of these effects, as they increase afterload, decrease SV for a given contractility and preload. This apparent change in cardiac function with increasing afterload (i.e., decreased SV and EF for a given preload) can be understood by analyzing the effects of afterload on the pressure-volume relationship.

The effect of afterload on the pressure-volume loop is shown in Figure 2-13. As afterload is increased and the heart ejects to a higher pressure, the pressure-volume point for aortic valve opening moves up along the pressure axis. Systole occurs from this point. If preload remains constant, ejection occurs to a higher end-systolic point and SV is decreased. Preload augmentation will improve SV but at a higher end-diastolic point on the diastolic compliance curve. If the heart does not compensate for this increased afterload, or if decreased contractility results, the ESPVR will shift down to the right and the heart will be functioning in a lower inotropic state, that is, decreased SV and EF for a given end-diastolic pressure-volume point.

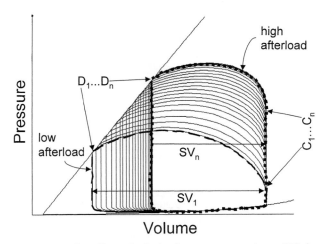

FIGURE 2-13 The effect of afterload on pressure volume (PV) loops assuming constant end-diastolic compliance and end-systolic pressure-volume relationship (ESPVR). A series of PV loops is shown beginning with low afterload (dashed line) and ending with high afterload (dotted line). Progressive increases in afterload lead to aortic valve opening at progressively higher pressures ($C_1...C_n$). Similarly, aortic valve closure occurs at progressively higher end-systolic pressures ($D_1...D_n$). The increase in afterload is associated with a reduction in stroke volume ($SV_1...SV_n$). (Figure generated by the Heart Simulator, courtesy of Marc Dickstein, MD, and Daniel Burkhoff, MD, Columbia University.)

Venous Return

Normally, the heart passively pumps all of the venous return it receives. It has tremendous preload reserve and can increase cardiac output threefold with increasing venous return. Under most conditions, it is venous return that determines cardiac output. Considering that venous return determines cardiac output, understanding what regulates venous return becomes the key to understanding what regulates cardiac output. Venous return is determined by the sum of the venous return from each organ. This in turn is, in the steady state, equal to the blood flow to each organ. What determines the individual blood flows? Each vascular bed determines its own blood flow, with few exceptions (the skin and most notably the pulmonary circulation). This is based on the fact that most vascular beds change their vascular resistance to regulate flow through the organ. If there is increasing metabolic demand by an organ, flow increases to meet this demand, venous return from the organ increases, and in turn venous return to the heart increases. Thus cardiac output is the sum of the flow through individual autoregulating vascular beds that are all determining their own flow in independent fashion. Thus cardiac output (CO) is determined by venous return (VR), which is:

$$CO = VR = \sum_{head}^{toe} (MBF, CBF, RBF, \text{muscle BF, skin BF,}$$
$$\text{splanchnic BF} \dots)$$

where MBF, CBF, and RBF represent myocardial, cerebral, and renal blood flow, respectively.

Only when this is overridden by neuroendocrine influences that override autoregulatory influences from each organ does CO begin to limit the blood flow to the body and individual systems. This is frequently the situation in the pediatric ICU.

Venous return to the heart can be graphically displayed, as shown in Figure 2-14. VR decreases with increasing right atrial

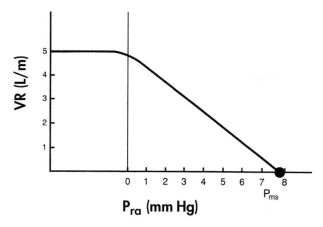

FIGURE 2-14 The normal venous return curve. Venous return (VR) is on the ordinate in L/min, and the abscissa shows right atrial pressure (P_{ra}) in mm Hg. Mean systemic pressure (P_{ms}) is between 7 and 8 mm Hg. The slope of this curve is proportional to the resistance to venous return. Maximum venous return occurs at a right atrial pressure (P_{ra}) around 0 mm Hg. Further decreases in atrial pressure below 0 do not augment venous return.

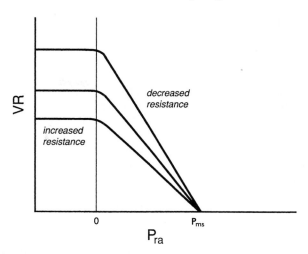

FIGURE 2-15 The effect of changing resistance on the venous return (VR) curve. Steeper slopes and higher plateaus of the VR curve can be achieved with decreased venous resistance. Thus decreasing resistance to venous return increases venous return and thus cardiac output (CO). P_{ms}, mean systemic pressure; P_{ra}, right atrial pressure.

pressure (P_{ra}). When P_{ra} is high enough, VR stops, as shown by the VR curve intercept on the abscissa. All flow is determined by a pressure gradient and resistance to flow (Ohm's law). The pressure gradient for VR is the difference between the downstream pressure, P_{ra}, and some upstream pressure. When these two pressures are the same, there can be no VR. Thus the abscissa intercept of the VR curve represents the upstream pressure for VR. This pressure has been variously called the dead pressure (the pressure measured at any point in the circulation when the heart stops), the mean circulatory filling pressure, and, perhaps most usefully, the mean systemic pressure (P_{ms}). It is the mean weighted pressure throughout the circulation when the pump (heart) is removed. It represents the capacitance and the relative filling of the entire circulation, both venous and arterial sides. This pressure can be increased by increasing intravascular volume or translocating fluid from the peripheral to the central circulation (vasoconstriction). It is an increase in the pressure gradient for VR, by increasing P_{ms}, which increases VR and therefore CO in response to a volume transfusion. This is preload augmentation. It is important to realize that if a volume transfusion increases P_{ms} and P_{ra} the same amount, VR will remain constant and CO will not increase. This occurs when the ventricle is on the steep part of its compliance curve, and a relatively small increase in volume leads to a large increase in ventricular EDP reflected by an increase in P_{ra}. If tricuspid incompetence is induced with volume and the P_{ra} increase is greater than P_{ms} increase, CO will actually decrease with volume loading, because VR is actually decreased. The VR curve also explains why, as intrathoracic pressure increases with positive pressure ventilation (PPV), cardiac output may fall. This is because P_{ra} increases and thus the pressure gradient for VR is decreased. VR falls and in turn CO falls.

Now consider what happens as P_{ra} decreases. VR increases and thus CO is augmented by a falling or decreased P_{ra}. The slope of the VR curve represents the resistance to VR: It varies as venous resistance changes. High-resistance states will decrease the height of the plateau, thus decreasing the maximal CO achievable (Fig. 2-15). The augmentation of CO

with falling P_{ra} is readily seen during spontaneous inspiration. As intrathoracic pressure falls, P_{ra} falls and VR is augmented. This transiently increases CO and is the converse of the situation described with PPV. When P_{ra} is elevated, this can be quite dramatic and explains the steep fall in jugular venous distension seen with inspiration in patients who have pericardial tamponade. It should be noted that the plateau of this curve occurs at around zero (or atmospheric) pressure. This is caused by inflow limitation around the thoracic inlet. The veins at the entrance to the thorax in the neck and abdomen are exposed to atmospheric pressure. As their intraluminal pressure falls below atmospheric, the transmural pressure becomes negative and the vessels collapse. Thus flow is limited until pressure builds up with continuing VR and the vein again opens to allow flow. This type of resistance that depends on surrounding pressure is called a Starling resistor. Flow limitation at the thoracic inlet explains why CO cannot be increased by decreasing P_{ra} below atmospheric pressure.

It is worth stating again that increased P_{ra} decreases VR and thus CO. This seems counterintuitive to the clinician who frequently, albeit illogically, considers it clinically beneficially to increase P_{ra}. Volume expansion will increase preload, but as mentioned it will increase VR and CO only if P_{ms} increases by more than P_{ra}. The conceptualization of P_{ra} as preload is what is mistaken. In fact understanding the VR curve indicates that anything that increases P_{ra} without increasing P_{ms} will decrease cardiac output. This is precisely what happens when the ventricular compliance (or elastance) characteristics are modified or inotropy is altered. If the heart becomes stiffer, or if contractility is impaired, the same ventricular EDV will be maintained at a higher P_{ra} and VR will decrease. As preload falls, CO will be impaired. Conversely, if afterload falls or contractility increases, the ventricle will function at lower EDP and atrial pressures, which permits augmentation of VR. Thus inotropes may additionally act by allowing increased EDV at lower filling pressures and thus augment VR. Understanding these aspects of the venous return curve is essential in managing critically ill children.

Veno-Cardiac Coupling

It is now necessary to consider coupling venous return and cardiac output. The cardiac function curve described previously, at essentially the same ESPVR relationship, describes the relationship between cardiac output and ventricular filling. It is obvious that over any given time period the VR and the CO must be equal. Thus the intercept of the VR curve and the CO curve in the steady state defines the circulation at any given time (Fig. 2-16). This point is called the equilibrium point (EP). This graphic relationship represents the simultaneous solution of the complex relationships that are described for cardiac function and vascular function. Figure 2-17 shows the effect of intravascular volume expansion, which increases P_{ms}. The VR curve shifts up to the right and a new equilibrium is established. The result is a greater CO and slightly higher P_{ra}, with an increased gradient for VR. Hemorrhage has the opposite effect. Figure 2-18 represents the effect of decreased contractility (or increased afterload). The cardiac function curve shifts down to the right along the same VR curve. At equilibrium P_{ra} is much greater and CO is decreased because the pressure gradient for VR is decreased. The chronic physiologic adaptation to this situation is to increase the P_{ms} by fluid retention, and this is the situation in heart failure.

Cardiac-Arterial Coupling

An analogous situation exists for the systemic arterial circulation, but the forces involved are different. Ohm's law,

$$\text{Resistance} = \text{Perfusion Pressure} / \text{Flow}$$

indicates that an increase in arterial resistance from vasoconstriction increases pressure. At the same time, a significant increase in resistance raises afterload to the heart and hence decreases cardiac output, unless compensatory mechanisms increase contractility and heart rate. It is important to realize that this system is much less sensitive than the venous coupling

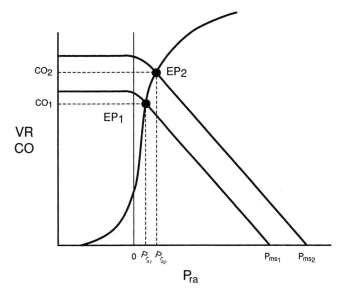

FIGURE 2-17   The effect of increase in mean systemic pressure (P_{ms}) on venous return (VR) and cardiac output (CO). The VR curve shifts to the right in a parallel fashion, and a new equilibrium point (EP_2) is established. Cardiac output is increased along the same cardiac function curve, and right atrial pressure marginally increases. P_{ra}, right atrial pressure.

in regulating cardiac output. On the venous side a pressure change of 1 or 2 mm Hg can alter cardiac output significantly. In fact, Guyton estimates a decrease of 14% in cardiac output for every 1 mm Hg decrease in P_{ms}-P_{ra}.[117] On the arterial side, pressure changes of 30 to 40 mm Hg may not alter function significantly, due to the great inotropic reserve of

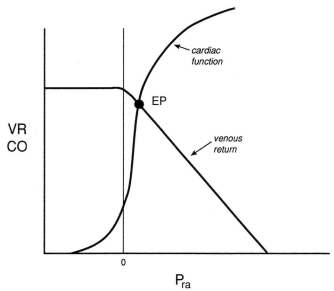

FIGURE 2-16   A graphical analysis of the cardiac function (Starling) curve with a venous return (VR) curve. At any given time, venous return must equal cardiac output (CO), and the simultaneous solution of the two equations is represented by the equilibrium point (EP). P_{ra}, right atrial pressure.

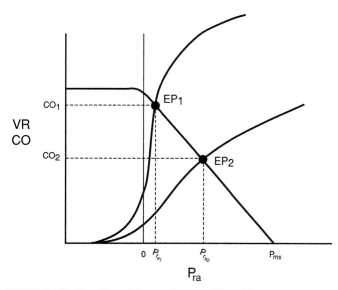

FIGURE 2-18   The effect of decreased contractility with a constant venous return (VR) curve. The cardiac function curve shifts downward to the right, establishing a new equilibrium point (EP_2) and at much higher right atrial pressure (P_{ra_2}) and a lower cardiac output (CO). Thus comparing Figures 2-17 and 2-18, it can be seen that right atrial pressure can increase under circumstances where the cardiac output either increases or decreases. Interpretation of right atrial pressure as preload is invalid without taking into account mean systemic pressure (P_{ms}) and the cardiac function relationship. P_{ra}, right atrial pressure.

the myocardium when healthy. Conversely, in the impaired myocardium, small increases in afterload may seriously affect cardiac output.

These concepts of venous and arterial coupling to cardiac function can be generalized to the left and right ventricle. Cardiac output and venous return are closely interconnected and must be taken together, whenever a therapeutic intervention is considered. Because the vasculature plays a major role in cardiovascular function and the regulation of cardiac output, a detailed discussion of regulation of vascular tone follows.

REGULATION OF SYSTEMIC VASCULAR TONE

Regulation of systemic vascular tone involves complex integration of the effects of neural, hormonal, and local control mechanisms on vascular myocyte function. Multiple mediator systems summate on the vascular myocyte to determine systemic vascular resistance, the distribution of the cardiac output, nutrient flow to the various vascular beds, and ultimately local tissue perfusion. In the normal state, local demands determine local flow. However, in critically ill children these normal homeostatic mechanisms become deranged and the local regulation of the circulation is overridden. In acutely stressful circumstances, these elements act in concert to defend the blood pressure and to supply critical organs (brain, myocardium) with adequate nutrient and oxygen delivery. Each vasoregulatory element has been studied in isolation, but the in vivo response must ultimately be finely tuned and coordinated in order to provide optimal growth, development, and response to stress. An understanding of how the vasculature and cardiac function are coupled depends on an understanding of the regulation of vascular tone.

Neural innervation of the systemic vasculature undergoes developmental maturation from prenatal life through adulthood. This development includes enhanced fine control of vascular responses by neocortical areas, increased modulation of afferent signals, and maturation of descending cortical inputs at the level of the spinal cord. With age and disease, these neural factors may be altered.

Autoregulation

Autoregulation is the ability of regional circulations to maintain a constant flow over a wide range of perfusion pressures (Fig. 2-19). As perfusion pressure falls, local vasodilation occurs, decreasing resistance and thus maintaining flow. Many regional vascular beds demonstrate autoregulation; however, this property varies with age and with disease states. Moreover, different vascular beds autoregulate by different mechanisms. Autoregulation is a local phenomenon, generally independent of neural or circulating humoral control.[145] The organs most frequently cited as demonstrating autoregulatory activity include the brain, myocardium, kidneys, and retina. These are "survival organs," essential for the stress response. Beyond autoregulation, there are other local influences that augment regional blood flow during increased metabolic activity or cardiac output.

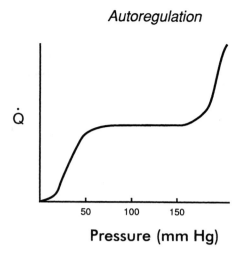

Autoregulation

FIGURE 2-19 The generalized autoregulatory curve of flow ($\dot{Q}$) versus pressure. Flow remains constant over a wide range of perfusion pressures (from 50 to 150 mm Hg in an adult vascular bed shown here). Loss of autoregulation would imply a linear relationship between pressure and flow. The autoregulatory curve is shifted toward the left in neonates, but the pressure limits are unknown.

The local mechanisms involved in autoregulation include myogenic, metabolic, and flow-dependent regulation. Myogenic mechanisms refer to the property of the arterial wall to sense alterations in intravascular pressure and mediate vasoconstriction when pressure is high, and vasorelaxation when pressure is reduced. The theorized "mechanoreceptor" of the vessel wall is unidentified; however, such a mechanism demands the presence of an afferent receptor capable of sensing pressure changes, wall tension, or stress. Proposed mechanosensing mechanisms include cytoskeleton associated protein kinases, integrin-cytoskeletal interactions, stretch-sensitive ion channels, and systems that generate reactive oxygen species in response to deformation.[6] The presence of this myogenic mechanism is advantageous in that organs continue to receive nutrients as required during lower pressure states and are protected from the harmful effects of hypertension.

Metabolic local control may contribute to autoregulation by multiple mechanisms to maintain oxygen delivery. As oxygen delivery falls with decreased regional perfusion, this elicits or allows increased concentrations of vasoactive metabolites to accumulate. Therefore, if oxygen delivery is decreased, increased levels of potassium, lactate, or adenosine may accrue and mediate vasodilation. As blood flow increases to normal, washout of these mediators occurs and vasodilation is maintained or reduced. Although these increases in metabolic products contribute to exercise-induced vasodilation, the evidence linking their contribution to autoregulation is less strong. Further, these factors would not appear to explain hypertension-induced vasoconstriction, unless the microenvironment can respond to alterations in these factors in the opposite direction.

Flow-dependent regulation refers to the coupling of changes in blood flow velocity to changes in vessel caliber. This mechanism may include secretion of vasoactive products from large vessels acting on arteriolar microvasculature or by "autocrine" action of microvessels responding to changes in shear stress. Regardless, this mechanism still requires presence of a mechanoreceptor or flow-sensor. The mechanisms of flow-dependent regulation are currently the focus of many research laboratories. It is possible that many vasoactive substances are involved, including endogenous endothelially released nitric oxide (NO) and endothelins, as well as physicochemical changes in ion channel and cell membrane structure that mediate changes in signal transduction mechanisms via regulation of intracellular ions and transmembrane electric potential.

The vascular sites of autoregulation include the precapillary arterioles and likely the larger arterioles (more than 100 μm) in many vascular beds. Evidence of the action of larger arterioles being dynamically involved in local regulation is found in the cerebral vasculature of the cat[122] and renal interlobar arterioles.[121] Furthermore local microvessel application of acetylcholine and bradykinin can induce ascending vasodilation in larger arteries proximal to the site of application. This suggests that micro- and macro-vessel communication may be involved in autoregulation.

Just as the mechanisms involved in autoregulation are debatable, the developmental aspects of appearance and threshold for autoregulation are unclear. Autoregulation is apparent in the newborn cerebrovascular and renovascular beds. Regulation of coronary blood flow and myocardial perfusion in the newborn is not well characterized. Cerebral blood flow is maintained at a lower level in newborns (40 mL/min/100 g) than in adults (60 mL/min/100 g),[211] and the distribution of blood flow is not identical. Although cerebral perfusion is considered critical, the actual threshold cerebral metabolic rate for oxygen in newborns without sustaining neurologic injury has been questioned.[8] It is clear that autoregulation to hypercapnia is impaired in newborn animals.[124] It is also likely that autoregulation is less effective in certain areas after brain injury secondary to hypoxia or trauma. The influences of cardiopulmonary bypass (CPB) and hypothermia on cerebral autoregulation are currently under intense study.

Renal autoregulation is quite different from cerebral autoregulation. First, it is unclear when renal autoregulation appears in infants. Conflicting evidence has been obtained: Piglets do not have autoregulatory capacity; but puppies do within a few weeks of birth.[228] Furthermore, although the kidney is the local sensor of blood flow, it is less sensitive to changes in blood gas composition than the brain in its effector responses. It is possible that the kidney need not have such fine control of autoregulation for delivery of oxygen, since its flow is luxurious and more in concert with its function as a filtering excretory organ. Nevertheless, ischemia or hypertension will result in injury to the kidney when regulatory mechanisms are insufficient.

Integrated neurohumoral and local mediators contribute to autoregulation in each vascular bed to different degrees. The global response to stress sometimes overwhelms the local autoregulatory mechanisms in certain regions. In severe hemorrhagic hypotension, cardiac output falls dramatically, and cerebral ischemia mediates an integrated neurohumoral response to rescue the brain and myocardium at expense to other organs. The powerful sympathetic vasoconstriction and neurally mediated release of epinephrine mediate an autotransfusion of remaining circulating volume into the central circulation. Cutaneous flow is significantly reduced, capacitance vessels constrict, and the celiomesenteric and renal beds also develop large increases in vascular resistance.

If circulating volume is not restored, multiple organ failure will result as each organ is unable to defend against the powerful "cardiocerebroprotective" reflexes.

Local Regulation of Vascular Tone

Local vessel tone and its autocrine and paracrine regulation are increasingly recognized as important in vascular control. Local myocyte tone is modified by oxygen, local gas tensions, flow, and locally released substances that may have both local (autocrine, paracrine) and distant (endocrine) effects on the circulation. The endothelium is an extremely responsive and highly active metabolic tissue that responds to perfusion pressure, phasic (or pulsatile) pressure, hypoxia, hypercapnia, and acidosis. It releases multiple mediators that have autocrine, paracrine, and endocrine effects, and as such plays a central role in the regulation and integration of the cardiovascular system. Our understanding of autoregulation is becoming increasingly clear as we further elucidate these local factors and mechanisms.

Vascular responses are classified as those responses that appear not to require intact perivascular or CNS regulation or result from circulating humoral influences. The unveiling of the metabolically active endothelium has explained many mechanisms involved in local vascular responses, but a great deal has yet to be learned. The sensors of local hypoxia, acidosis, energy depletion, and potassium accumulation are poorly understood. However, the response mechanisms are being elucidated and include actions of adenosine, regulation of prostaglandin synthesis, nitric oxide, and modulation of vascular tone by multiple different ion channels. The vascular endothelium secretes a large number of molecules that influence the tone of the systemic vasculature. These paracrine substances are responsible for many of the responses of the local microcirculation.

REGULATION OF VASCULAR TONE BY THE ENDOTHELIUM

ATP-Sensitive Potassium Channels

There are a number of different potassium channel subtypes involved in maintaining the electrophysiologic homeostasis of the cell. The ATP-sensitive potassium channel most likely functions to prevent depletion of ATP and protect the cell from irreparable impairment of energy metabolism.[205] Increasing the total outward potassium current shortens the action potential by hyperpolarization, and thereby reduces calcium influx through voltage-gated calcium channels. This diminishes intracellular calcium release and contraction, consequently conserving ATP.[319] These ATP-sensitive potassium channels are present in many cell types: pancreatic β-cells, skeletal muscle, vascular and other smooth muscle, neurons, endothelium, and renal epithelium, as well as myocardial cells.[56,319] Recently, the molecular structure of ATP-sensitive potassium channels has been identified and their clinical importance recognized.[41,56,78] The chief characteristic of ATP-sensitive potassium channels is their inhibition by intracellular ATP. These inhibitory effects result from ATP binding to the inwardly rectifying potassium channel subunit.

A number of endogenous and pharmacologic mediators activate ATP-sensitive potassium channels. The adenylate cyclase/cAMP/protein kinase A second messenger system, as well as the activation of protein kinase G by its signaling pathway (cGMP), seem to be responsible for phosphorylation of the ATP-sensitive potassium channel, thus activating the channel.[41,319] Agents that have shown the ability to activate the cAMP second messenger pathway include β-adrenergic agents, adenosine, vasoactive intestinal polypeptide, and calcitonin gene-related peptide. Nitric oxide may relax smooth muscle by a number of mechanisms, one of which is due to activation of these channels by the activation of protein kinase G. Prostacyclin also hyperpolarizes and relaxes vascular smooth muscle by activating ATP-sensitive potassium channels.[41] Nucleotide diphosphates, in the company of magnesium, activate ATP-sensitive potassium channels in various tissues, including vascular smooth muscle.[41,319] Pharmacologic agents that open the ATP-sensitive potassium channel by attaching to the sulphonylurea receptor subunit include pinacidil, diazoxide, and cromakalin.[319] Finally, septic shock, acidosis, ischemia, and hypoxia also seem to activate ATP-sensitive potassium channels, presumably by endotoxin or NO release, pH-dependent effects, adenosine release, and ATP depletion, respectively.[41] The clinical implications have only recently been appreciated.

The ATP-sensitive potassium channels play an important role in the regulation of arterial tone and other clinically important features of cardiovascular pathophysiology. They operate as mediators of the vascular response to a variety of pharmacologic and endogenous vasodilators, as well as compromised nutrient delivery and metabolic activity, that can directly increase blood flow to different tissues.[56] ATP-sensitive potassium channels have also been found in human pulmonary artery smooth muscle cells.[78] Not only does calcium influx stimulate smooth muscle contraction, but also smooth muscle cell growth.[78] ATP-sensitive potassium channels, through prevention of cell depolarization by potassium efflux, may inhibit cell growth as well as smooth muscle contraction.[78] Yuan and colleagues[320] found that a rise in cytosolic calcium, in addition to triggering cell contraction, rapidly increased nuclear calcium concentrations and promoted cell proliferation by shifting quiescent cells into the cell cycle and by driving the proliferating cells through mitosis. Thus increased calcium concentration may also contribute to the hypertrophy of small pulmonary arteries and muscularization of pulmonary arterioles, which are major features of primary pulmonary hypertension.[320] Angiotensin II, endothelin-1, phenylephrine, norepinephrine, and peptide growth factors have been reported to promote myocardial remodeling (myocardial hypertrophy and fibrosis) by increasing intracellular Ca^{++}. This increased intracellular Ca^{++} leads to activation of protein kinase C, which subsequently generates a chain of events that activates ribosomal proteins. These activated ribosomal proteins initiate protein synthesis and, consequently, cellular hypertrophic changes.[247] Sanada and colleagues[247] found that pharmacologic activators of ATP-sensitive potassium channels reduced myocardial hypertrophy in rats treated with an inhibitor of NO synthesis, N^w-nitro-L-arginine methyl ester, that resulted in activation of protein kinase C and the renin-angiotensin system. ATP-sensitive potassium channels appear to play a role in preventing myocardial hypertrophy, as well as causing vasodilation and protecting tissues from ischemic injury.

Another example of how ATP-sensitive potassium channels may be important is seen with the use of cardioplegia for CPB operations. Cardioplegia that contains a high potassium concentration gives rise to electromechanical arrest to protect the myocardium during CPB operations. Hyperkalemic solutions elevate intracellular calcium concentrations in isolated guinea pig ventricular myocytes.[168] This elevated intracellular calcium may lead to cellular dysfunction and contribute to myocardial damage in various pathophysiologic conditions associated with hyperkalemia, such as cardioplegic arrest. During cardioplegia, the myocardium is globally ischemic with a reduced production of ATP. A modest increase in intracellular calcium, in this situation, may represent an added load on the energy-dependent calcium-homeostatic mechanisms and may make cardiac cells more susceptible to reperfusion injury and diastolic dysfunction.[168] Lopez and colleagues[168] found that potassium channel opening drugs, such as aprikalim and nicorandil, prevent hyperkalemic solutions from increasing intracellular calcium by keeping the membrane potential below the gating level of voltage-gated calcium channels and inhibiting calcium entry. The opening of ATP-sensitive potassium channels with aprikalim has been associated with cardioprotection in isolated ischemic rabbit hearts.[225] Modulating ATP-sensitive potassium channels may provide a means of reducing ischemic damage to the myocardium and lessening the potentially deleterious increases in intracellular calcium associated with hyperkalemic cardioplegia.[168]

Although our understanding of the roles for ATP-sensitive potassium channels has greatly increased, studies evaluating the efficacy of ATP-sensitive potassium channel modulating agents in human patients are lacking.

Prostaglandins

Prostaglandins are synthesized throughout the circulation by the vascular endothelium and have moderate to profound local vascular regulatory influences. Prostaglandin synthesis is also found in vascular smooth muscle. Endothelium from large arteries, veins, and the microcirculation can synthesize prostaglandins. Hypoxic vasodilation is at least in part dependent on endothelial generation of prostaglandins.[55] Martin and colleagues[180] have shown that hypoxia increases prostacyclin release from vascular endothelium. The two major vasodilating prostaglandins are PGI_2 and PGE_2. PGE_1 (alprostadil) is a therapeutic agent to maintain or reestablish ductus arteriosus patency. Intense investigation over 30 years has revealed a growing number of prostaglandins, as well as organ-specific sites of synthesis and actions.

Intravenous (IV) $PGF_{2\alpha}$ infusion causes pulmonary and mesenteric vasoconstriction; however, no effect is seen on the kidney. PGE_2 or PGI_2 infusions cause vasodilation of the gastrointestinal tract and renal vascular beds. PGI_2 elicits pulmonary vasodilation. The use of synthetic prostacyclin analogues is now common practice in the management of pulmonary hypertension.[3,104,169,312] Various prostaglandins are involved in cerebral vascular responses to many stimuli,[14,54,259] including seizures and hypoxia, and possibly in autoregulation.

Prostaglandin E_1 infusions are used clinically to maintain ductus arteriosus patency and lower pulmonary vascular pressures. After CPB, PGE_1 infusions have been used to improve right ventricular performance by reduction of pulmonary pressures and right ventricular afterload. PGE_1 is given only by infusion since it is rapidly metabolized in the first pass through the lungs. Systemic vasodilation may also occur and hypotension may result. PGE_1 infusions may cause irritability, fever, apnea, and a number of other side effects.

Renal blood flow is sensitive to prostaglandin synthesis inhibitors, and acute renal failure has resulted from use and overdose of nonsteroidal antiinflammatory agents.[47,274] In premature infants where the persistently patent ductus arteriosus results in heart failure, indomethacin effectively closes the ductus. The major undesirable side effects of this treatment include renal insufficiency, thrombocytopenia, and bleeding.

Nitric Oxide

Nitric oxide is an important mediator of local vasodilation. Its actions include neurotransmission, relaxation of vascular smooth muscle contractile mechanisms, inhibition of platelet aggregation (and possibly prostaglandin synthesis), and complex chemical interactions with free radicals. Each of these actions may be involved in vascular regulation. Multiple isoforms of nitric oxide synthase (NOS) have been identified. Constitutive NOS is constantly present and probably involved in vascular regulation on a minute-to-minute basis in many microcirculatory beds. Age- and pathology-related changes in the expression, activation, or function of NOS may be related to hypertension, stroke, and various other cardiovascular diseases. Inducible NOS is another isoform that is expressed in macrophages and vascular smooth muscle cells when stimulated by infectious agents and by cytokines.[152] NO acts as a potent immune effector in the host defense.

The nitrovasodilators work via release of NO. Until 1980 the mechanism of action of these important agents was obscure. Still more is to be learned before the differences in action of sodium nitroprusside and nitroglycerin can be understood. Both agents mediate vasodilation but appear to have different hemodynamic profiles. Sodium nitroprusside elicits more profound arterial vasodilation and more significant blood pressure changes than nitroglycerin. Both agents act as coronary and cerebral vasodilators.

Inhaled NO is used in patients of all ages with pulmonary hypertension from a variety of causes. However, at this time, the FDA has only approved the use of NO for use in the neonate with persistent pulmonary hypertension. In this age group, it improves oxygenation and reduces the need for extracorporeal membrane oxygenation.[65,66,111,140] Inhaled NO also seems to improve oxygenation in children with acute hypoxemic respiratory failure.[87] The use of inhaled NO has also been advocated in patients with pulmonary hypertension after heart transplantation and other cardiac surgeries.[13,197] Nevertheless, enthusiasm for inhaled NO may be waning because of its questionable ability to improve survival.[66,172] Furthermore there is concern that inhaled NO may increase endothelin-1 levels and that this increase in endothelin-1 may be responsible for the rebound pulmonary hypertension that is occasionally seen when inhaled NO is discontinued.[222]

Endothelin

Endothelins are the most potent vasoconstrictor peptides. They are synthesized and released primarily by vascular endothelial cells. These peptides activate endothelin receptors on vascular smooth muscle cells. Since the discovery of endothelin in 1988, three isoforms (1, 2, and 3) and two receptor subtypes (A and B) have been identified.[318]

Endothelin is synthesized not only in the endothelium, but also in other tissues. Of the three isoforms, the most widely distributed, most studied, and most potent is endothelin-1. It is found in vascular and endocardial endothelial cells; mesangial, glomerular, and tubular epithelial cells in the kidney; and macrophages.[139,280] The endothelin-2 isoform has been detected primarily in renal tissue and appears particularly plentiful in renal adenocarcinoma, and also in the gastrointestinal tract. Finally, while endothelin-3 localizes primarily to the central nervous system, it is also found throughout the kidney.[139]

The precursors of all three endothelin isoforms have been traced to distinct genes. Preproendothelin-1 is encoded on human chromosome 6p23-24, preproendothelin-2 is encoded on human chromosome 1p34, and preproendothelin-3 is encoded on human chromosome 20q13.2-13.3.[139] The preproendothelins (203-amino-acids) are cleaved at two sites by a neutral endopeptidase to generate biologically inactive precursors, "big endothelins" (39-amino-acid prohormone). These are ultimately converted to mature peptides (21-amino-acid polypeptide) by endothelin-converting enzymes (metalloproteases).[139,318] Endothelin-converting enzyme-1, which is the earliest identified enzyme in this family, remains essential to endothelin processing. It is encoded on chromosome 1p36 and has at least four isoforms (1a, 1b, 1c, and 1d).[139] There is some thought that endothelin-converting enzyme-1 plays a role in fetal development. Mice with a deletion mutation of the endothelin-converting enzyme-1 gene have defects in specific neural crest–derived tissues, including brachial arch-derived craniofacial structures, aortic arch arteries, and the cardiac outflow tract.[139] Defects in synthesis of endothelin-1 may play a part in the category of human CATCH22 defects.[139]

The release and expression of endothelin appear to be modulated by a number of diverse stimuli. Factors that stimulate endothelin production include TGF_β, angiotensin II, interleukin-1, thrombin, adrenaline, prostaglandin $F_{2\alpha}$, low shear stress, fluid mechanical strain, pressure, and endothelin itself.[24,139] Endothelin synthesis is downregulated by vasodilators/anticoagulants such as NO, prostacyclin, heparin, atrial natriuretic peptide, and high shear stress.[139]

The cell response to endothelin is determined by binding to specific cell surface receptors, type A and B. Endothelin receptor type A has a higher affinity for endothelin-1 and endothelin-2, but less for endothelin-3. Endothelin receptor type B binds all three isopeptides with just about equal affinity. The endothelin receptor type A is found in vascular smooth muscle cells and encourages vasoconstriction and enhances cell proliferation.[139] The vasoconstriction is initiated through a multistep activation of phospholipase C, inositol triphosphate, and phosphokinase C. These peptides induce the opening of Ca^{++} channels and a rise in intracellular $[Ca^{++}]$, stimulating further Ca^{++}-induced Ca^{++} release.[139] The type B endothelin receptor is found on endothelial cells as well as vascular smooth muscle cells. It is the predominant receptor subtype in the renal tubule cells and is also present in aorta, brain, and lung tissues.[139] In contrast to the endothelin receptor type A, the type B endothelin receptors are thought to mediate vasodilation by encouraging release of prostaglandins (PGI_2) and NO from endothelium and potentiating NO-stimulated cGMP.[139] The biologic effects of endothelins are defined by the relative population of each receptor, which varies among tissues and cell types.[139] Endothelin plays a role in a number of diseases, including congestive heart failure (CHF). Endothelin-1 has been implicated in heart failure, myocardial infarction, atherosclerosis, hypertension, primary pulmonary hypertension, preeclampsia, cerebrovascular disease, acute and chronic renal failure, and cyclosporin-induced renal vasoconstriction.[139,214] Endothelin-1 induces expression of a number of proto-oncogenes that can promote endothelial smooth muscle cell proliferation, characteristically seen in atherosclerosis. In patients with CHF, high endothelin-1 levels are associated with elevated left ventricular end-diastolic volume, left atrial pressure, and pulmonary artery pressure.[24] Endothelin-1 has potent effects on the growth of hemodynamic-overload-induced cell hypertrophy, fibroblasts, and vascular smooth muscle cells and has inotropic properties as well. It mediates hypertrophy of ventricular myocytes from angiotensin II and norepinephrine stimulation.[280] Endothelin-1 plays an important part in the complex mechanisms responsible for the end-stage organ damage in chronic CHF.[308] Patients with myocardial infarction have very high endothelin-1 plasma levels, and these high concentrations are associated with an increased 1 year mortality.[214] In patients with pulmonary hypertension, plasma levels of endothelin-1 are elevated. In patients with cerebral hemorrhage, increased concentrations of endothelin-1 and endothelin-3 have been reported in cerebrospinal fluid.[24] These widespread effects suggest unique opportunities for therapeutic intervention.

Since the discovery of endothelin and its many effects, investigators have targeted the endothelin receptors A and B for therapeutic interventions. A number of peptide and nonpeptide molecules have been designed to block these receptors.[24] Medications, such as the mixed endothelin receptor type A and B antagonist, bosentan, have shown promising results in patients with CHF, systemic hypertension, and pulmonary hypertension. Bosentan significantly reduces mean arterial, pulmonary artery, right atrial, and pulmonary artery wedge pressures, and increases cardiac and stroke volume index in adults with CHF.[280] Further understanding of the endothelin system will increase our therapeutic options for control of the vasculature.

NEURAL REGULATION OF THE SYSTEMIC VASCULATURE

CNS control of the vasculature is highly complex and includes an extensive array of afferent receptors responding to perturbations in homeostasis. Multiple levels (spinal cord, brainstem, subcortical and neocortical areas) of control and modulation of afferent and efferent signals and a sophisticated network of effectors, including the heart, vascular smooth muscle, and endocrine glands, constitute this sophisticated system.

Cardiovascular Afferents

Afferent signals from the cardiovascular system involved in regulation of systemic blood flow and tone include carotid and aortic baroreceptors and chemoreceptors, pulmonary afferent receptors, cardiac afferent fibers, and perivascular nerves. When blood pressure falls, the firing rate of the arterial baroreceptors diminishes. This is interpreted by the CNS as a reduction in blood pressure; the CNS then augments sympathetic output to increase heart rate and vascular tone. In an integrated response at the level of the brainstem, the vagus nerve carrying cardiodecelerator output is diminished, which further allows the heart rate to rise. Conversely, with the appearance of systemic hypertension, the carotid baroreceptors increase their firing rate. This is perceived by the CNS as hypertension, prompting it to increase vagal tone, diminish sympathetic cardiac efferent response, and decrease sympathetic vasoconstrictor tone to the systemic vasculature. These responses are coordinated at the level of the brainstem and the nucleus tractus solitarius (NTS), which receives modulating input from neocortical and subcortical structures.

Baroreceptors

Baroreceptors are vascular sensors of blood pressure located in the carotid sinus and aortic arch, along with the walls of the left and right atria. Baroreceptor output increases with stretch (increased pressure). With hypotension, there is a diminished baroreceptor output. Baroreceptor firing sends an afferent signal to the cardioinhibitory centers of the brainstem, which produces vasodilation and decreased heart rate and decreased inotropic state of the heart. When hypotension develops, there is less baroreceptor output (afferent signal), and thus release of inhibition of the vasomotor center, which results in vasoconstriction and increased inotropic stimulation of the heart. Second, there is a decrease in the excitation of the cardioinhibitory center and therefore a reduction in vagal tone. This reduction in parasympathetic outflow and enhancement in generalized sympathetic activity leads to a positive inotropic and chronotropic effect, with generalized sympathetic vasoconstriction to defend the blood pressure.

It has recently become clear that the vascular endothelium modulates baroreceptor function in a paracrine fashion. The local production of prostacyclin by the endothelium in response to stretch increases baroreceptor sensitivity. Thus stretch-induced endothelial upregulation of neural activity via this mechanism can significantly enhance baroreceptor sensitivity and cardiovascular responses. Endothelial prostacyclin release has the effect of increasing baroreceptor activity and increasing cardioinhibitory center activity. In addition, there is evidence that the injured endothelium releases a baroreceptor inhibitory factor that blunts baroreceptor responses.

Endothelial injury, such as occurs in sepsis, after CPB, or in chronic hypertension and CHF, may seriously impair baroreceptor regulatory mechanisms. In this setting, irregular control of blood pressure and integration of circulatory function is at least in part due to endothelial dysfunction.

Venous vasoconstriction results in increased cardiac preload. Sympathetic outflow increases cardiac contractility and heart rate. This is accompanied by an increase in arterial vascular tone (cardiac afterload). Each of these components tends to return the blood pressure to normal. The aortic and carotid baroreceptors act both independently and in synergy. Maximal response to stress is achieved with the integration of all baroreceptor input. The vasoconstrictor response is not homogeneous throughout all vascular beds. Certain organs, including the brain, myocardium, and kidneys, autoregulate blood flow within a wide range of blood pressures. Vasoconstriction is most severe in the cutaneous, skeletal muscle, and splanchnic vascular beds, and thus flow to the autoregulated vascular beds is preserved during hemorrhage.

Arterial Chemoreceptors

Arterial chemoreceptors are found within the carotid body and respond to PaO_2, $PaCO_2$, and pH. As PaO_2 falls to 50 mm Hg, the nervous system responds with increasing ventilation. Neurally mediated release of adrenal epinephrine results in increased blood pressure.[204] Acidemia and hypercarbia also result in hypertension via neurally mediated vasoconstriction and release of catecholamines. Chemoreceptor afferents ascend to many sites within the brainstem, including the NTS. It is unclear whether the chemoreceptor and baroreceptor responses integrate to the same final brainstem nuclei, but it is likely that these responses are closely related and regulated. The chemoreceptors probably have little function during the nonstressed state and become activated when arterial blood chemistry is abnormal. It is still unclear how the chemoreceptor response to hypoxia associated with cyanotic CHD is altered, and whether the response is normal after surgical correction.

Cardiac afferent fibers also arise in the atria. These receptors are presumed to be important in monitoring venous pressure. Activation of atrial stretch mediates integrated neural responses including tachycardia and vasodilation to the kidneys, as well as release of natriuretic peptides. Natriuretic peptides, released from the atria, ventricles, and other sites, have been found to play an important role in the homeostasis of the cardiovascular system during CHF.[21,143,173,299] Vagal mechanoreceptor afferents originate within the ventricles. When stimulated, these may evoke profound bradycardia and systemic hypotension, known as the Bezold-Jarisch reflex. Cardiac sympathetic afferents are present and felt to be responsible for the perception of cardiac pain.

Cardiovascular Efferents

Central nervous system sympathetic control consists of highly organized multicircuit pathways, including the neocortex, hypothalamus, and brainstem nuclei. Afferent signals from carotid and aortic baroreceptors and chemoreceptors initiate responses within the hypothalamus and brainstem. These responses are directed to the NTS in the brainstem. From the NTS, sympathetic signals descend in the spinal cord and synapse in the intermediolateral column. These efferent signals are further modulated and processed and extend efferent signals to target organs, including the vasculature, via the sympathetic ganglia.

During CPB with deep hypothermia, cerebral autoregulation is impaired. Also, hypothermia and anesthetic agents alter CNS integration of protective cardiovascular reflexes. It is well known that organized brainstem reflexes are impaired

by hypothermia; hence the requirement of a minimum body temperature before neurologic examination for determination of brain death.

Autonomic control of this systemic vasculature is achieved via both the sympathetic and parasympathetic systems. Sympathetic output is derived from preganglionic neurons whose cell bodies lie primarily within the intermediolateral columns of the spinal cord. These preganglionic fibers are both myelinated and unmyelinated. Some of these fibers terminate at paravertebral sympathetic ganglia; others traverse greater distances to periaortic locations (celiac, superior mesenteric, and inferior mesenteric ganglia). Other preganglionic fibers extend to the adrenal medulla where chromaffin cells act as the postganglionic neurons.

Organization of sympathetic fibers is complex and demonstrates convergence (fibers from many levels converging at specific ganglia) and divergence (fibers from a single level splitting to innervate many ganglia). This architecture may allow for redundancy in case of injury and extremely fine control over regional processes (including vascular regulation). At the ganglia, preganglionic nerves release acetylcholine, which acts primarily upon postganglionic nicotinic cholinergic receptors. This activates postganglionic neurons, which in turn may release one of multiple neurotransmitters, most frequently norepinephrine. These other neurotransmitters include neuropeptides,[134] neuropeptide Y,[249,250] adenosine, and ATP,[52] among others (Table 2-1). Some ganglion cells innervate cerebral vasculature.[120] The vagus nerve innervates the heart and gastrointestinal smooth muscle but appears to have significantly less input in control of vascular tone. The balance of both limbs of the autonomic nervous system, as well as the fine control mechanisms found in the sympathetic nervous system, provide for balanced control of cardiovascular regulation.

Sympathetic stimulation results in generalized vasoconstriction via the action of norepinephrine on alpha-adrenergic receptors on blood vessels. Norepinephrine, epinephrine, and other vasoactive compounds are also secreted by the adrenal medulla in response to sympathetic stimulation. High-intensity sympathetic stimulation diminishes mesenteric smooth muscle peristalsis and decreases mesenteric blood flow secondary to activation of the renin-angiotensin system and the action of angiotensin II.

Table 2-1 Neurotransmitters Potentially Involved in Vascular Regulation

Norepinephrine
Acetylcholine (Ach)
Adenosine triphosphate (ATP)
Dopamine
Neuropeptide Y (NPY)
Substance P
Angiotensin II
Vasopressin
Bombesin
Galactin
Enkephalins
Serotonin
Calcitonin gene-related peptide (CGRP)
Vasoactive intestinal polypeptide (VIP)
Cholecystokinin
Oxytocin
Somatostatin

Parasympathetic efferent impulses are carried via the cranial and sacral nerves. These include the oculomotor, facial, glossopharyngeal, vagal, and sacral nerves. Cell bodies of parasympathetic nerves are located in brainstem nuclei and in the intermediolateral column of the spinal cord. These preganglionic nerves synapse at remote ganglia or within the wall or structure of target organs. Again, acetylcholine is the major neurotransmitter at parasympathetic ganglia.

Vasoregulation by the autonomic nervous system is accomplished via generalized changes in sympathetic tone and more controlled, region-specific responses. During hemorrhagic hypotension, generalized vasoconstriction is seen to preserve or return blood pressure to normal. However, autoregulation occurs to protect the brain and myocardium. The adrenal medulla and neurohypophysis receive increased flow. Skeletal muscle can also selectively receive increased perfusion during exercise.

Pharmacologic or anatomic disruption of the neural innervation of the cardiovascular system results in loss of the integrated responses referred to previously. Epidural and spinal anesthetic agents limit afferent as well as efferent neural signals from reaching their target end organs (including vasculature). Opioids have been demonstrated to alter afferent input at the spinal level[105] and may work within the brain and spinal cord by modulation of both afferent input and efferent responses.

Neurally mediated efferent actions include sympathetic and parasympathetic regulation of heart rate (chronotropy), conduction time (dromatropy), and contractility (inotropy). This highly complex system can be altered by central nervous system sedatives. Such sedatives and centrally acting antihypertensive agents act by reducing sympathetic output from brainstem nuclei and other cortical modulating centers. Many potent agents can reduce or ablate the response even to brain ischemia. It has recently been suggested that complete loss of integrated sympathetic control of the cardiovascular system may be used as a marker of brain death in children.[109] However, loss of brain function does not completely ablate all cardiovascular reflexes, some of which are mediated exclusively at the spinal level.[310]

Sympathetic neurovascular control functioning via ganglionic nicotinic cholinergic receptors can be blocked by nicotinic antagonists (i.e., trimethaphan or curare), resulting in failure to propagate the sympathetic signals and thereby induce vasodilation. Epidural local anesthetics also block the axonal conduction of preganglionic fibers. These agents can be used therapeutically to induce vasodilation and improve regional blood supply during ischemia from sepsis[286] or Kawasaki disease.[93]

Modulation of the usual neurovascular control mechanisms occurs with prolonged increases in neurotransmitter release (or pharmacologic supplementation). Receptors may internalize, change from high- to low-affinity states, or otherwise become downregulated. In septic shock, there appears to be disruption of normal signal transduction mechanisms, which interfere with the homeostatic response to hypotension. These observations partially explain why increasing doses of pharmacologic vasopressor support are required during prolonged therapy. Use of vasopressor agents to manage these responses is covered in Chapter 7.

Another limb of the neurovascular effector circuit includes sympathetic innervation of the adrenal medulla. Here the effector organ promptly responds to sympathetic stimulation by increased secretion of norepinephrine, epinephrine, and other vasoactive products. Stimulation of the adrenal releases potent constrictor agents to defend the blood pressure. Catecholamines and other vasoactive hormones constitute the humoral control mechanisms of the systemic vasculature, and adrenal secretion can be modulated by many agents.[146,287]

HUMORAL CONTROL OF THE SYSTEMIC VASCULATURE

Humoral control of systemic vasculature is affected by many circulating or paracrine substances that demonstrate vasoregulatory activity. Not all of these agents are truly endocrine hormones acting at distant sites. The multiple neurotransmitters and circulating vasoactive agents presented here (see Table 2-1) function via cell membrane receptors activating signal transduction mechanisms that elicit changes in vascular tone. The many neurovascular neurotransmitters reviewed here are included because they offer basic understanding of newly developing vasoactive agents in the laboratory. The release of representative vasoactive hormones from the brain, neurohypophysis, adrenal medulla and cortex, and endothelium is reviewed. Receptor systems and their ligands are presented together.

Vasoactive compounds released by neurons include the classically described adrenergic (norepinephrine) and cholinergic (acetylcholine) ligands of the sympathetic and parasympathetic nervous systems. This traditional description has now been enhanced by the elegant work of many investigators including:

1. Demonstration of co-secretion of neurotransmitters in certain perivascular beds, such as norepinephrine and ATP
2. Effects of neuromodulators: neurosecretory substances that enhance or diminish the release or activity of better-described neurotransmitters, without apparent intrinsic activity themselves
3. Documentation of apparent paradoxical activity of certain agents at low versus high concentrations
4. Paradoxical effect of agents when endothelium is present as opposed to absent

By investigation of multiple regional vascular beds in vivo and ex vivo, the principles of finely tuned vascular responses and control are being elucidated. The vasoactive endogenous compounds can be categorized by structure, including monoamines, peptides, prostaglandins, purines, kinins, and NO, among others. Within each group, there may exist vasodilators and vasoconstrictors; some compounds exhibit both activities, and some are active only in the presence of other agents. The major (but not exhaustive) categories of receptor-ligand systems are discussed in the following sections.

Adrenergic Receptors

Great advances in adrenergic receptor pharmacology have been made over the past decades and have provided a wealth of clinically useful agents. Adrenergic receptors of the systemic vasculature include alpha$_1$, alpha$_2$, beta$_1$, beta$_2$, beta$_3$, and dopamine$_{1-5}$ receptors. Each of the alpha-receptor groups has been further subtyped and is the focus of intense investigation to enable an understanding of regional vascular control. New understanding of receptor subtypes, location, and changes with disease and age offers promise of tailoring agents to specific needs and further advancing clinical care.

Alpha$_1$ adrenoreceptors mediate vasoconstriction. This receptor class activates G-proteins, which enhance phospholipase C activity, and increase IP$_3$ and cytoplasmic Ca^{++} concentrations, which mediate vascular smooth muscle contraction.[188] The receptor is tonically activated by perivascular nerve release of norepinephrine. Circulating epinephrine and dopamine also stimulate this response. In hemorrhagic or cardiogenic shock, it is common to observe a profoundly vasoconstricted systemic vasculature that is responding to intense sympathetic nerve release of norepinephrine and circulating epinephrine. Other alpha$_1$-active agents include methoxamine and phenylephrine. Alpha$_1$-mediated vasoconstriction can be so intense as to induce regional ischemia; hence the axiom that adequate circulating volume should be present before use of alpha-active agents. Although developmental differences in perivascular innervation are present from infancy to adulthood, the systemic vasculature of the child clearly responds to alpha agents in a manner similar to that in adults, as is evidenced by the clinical use of epinephrine, norepinephrine, and phenylephrine. Developmental maturation of receptor location has been studied in animals, but much more work remains to be done.[314]

Alpha$_2$ receptors are generally considered prejunctional in location, along with their presence in the CNS. Activation of alpha$_2$ receptors causes a decrease in intracellular cAMP and inhibits release of norepinephrine. This loss of norepinephrine release causes vasodilation. The mechanism of action of alpha$_2$ agents is via the G$_i$ protein, a regulatory protein that changes the interaction of the receptor complex interaction with adenylate cyclase, inhibiting formation of cAMP.[187] Clonidine is a currently available alpha$_2$ agonist in the United States. Multiple subtypes of alpha-adrenergic receptors have been found, and newer understanding of the alpha system may provide more specific therapeutic agents.

Beta-adrenergic receptors have been identified in at least three subtypes (beta$_1$, beta$_2$, and beta$_3$). Activation of beta$_1$ receptors causes an increase in intracellular cAMP, which in turn activates cAMP-dependent protein kinase. Through further phosphorylations, an increase in intracellular free Ca^{++} occurs, with resultant increased inotropy, and enhanced myocardial relaxation in diastole. Beta$_2$-receptor activation also results in increased cAMP and activation of cAMP-dependent kinases. In both vascular and bronchiolar smooth muscle, this initiates a decrease in intracellular calcium concentration and myorelaxation.

Atypical beta receptors have also been found and are thought to be involved in thermogenesis, lipolysis, and intrinsic sympathomimetic activity.[94] It is speculated that atypical beta-adrenergic receptors may be present on the human heart, but it is unclear what role these may play.[148] Further elucidation of location and subtypes of adrenergic receptors will possibly provide greater understanding and development of clinically useful agonists and antagonists.

Dopamine receptors also have been classified. There are now five (D$_{1-5}$) subsets of dopamine receptors recognized, all of which are G-protein linked.[9,294] D$_1$ receptors mediate vasorelaxation and have been implicated in the vasodilation of the renal vasculature during low-dose dopamine infusion.[88] Dopamine receptors are increasingly recognized as playing a role in hypertension and neurobiology.[88,294] Presynaptic and postsynaptic receptor locations may explain regional differences of vasodilation and vasoconstriction. D$_2$ receptors are found within the CNS and influence release of many hormones, including prolactin and beta-endorphin. Dopamine also has both alpha- and beta-adrenergic receptor effects. Although dopamine remains a staple of cardiovascular management, the putative renovascular effects are marginal and the value of "low-dose" dopamine highly questionable.[179]

Serotonin

Serotonin, also known as 5-hydroxytryptamine (5-HT), is a potent vasoactive monoamine. Serotonin is a putative neurotransmitter of perivascular neurons, with actions on differing regional vascular beds in various species. Serotonin vascular receptors have been identified. Serotonin may be active at a variety of receptors, including the 5-HT$_{1A-D}$, 5-HT$_2$, 5-HT$_3$, and adrenergic receptors (alpha, beta, and dopamine). The variety of receptors that may be activated by serotonin probably explains in part the various findings of vasoconstrictor and vasodilator influences seen from serotonin. Further, presynaptic serotonin receptors have been found on adrenergic nerve fibers in blood vessels. These may also be responsible for inhibition of release of norepinephrine and may explain the regional vascular differences seen in serotonin application.[224]

Investigations have revealed the presence of 5-HT$_{1D}$ receptors in human basilar artery and primate and dog cranial arteries. These receptors have likewise been found in human dura mater vessels. One recent pharmacologic advance in manipulation of regional systemic vasculature is the introduction of sumatriptan, a 5-HT$_{1D}$ agonist that induces vasoconstriction of cranial vasculature, ameliorating the symptoms of migraine. This is a notable clinical accomplishment in the application of a basic science discovery of regional distribution of receptors and the transfer of this knowledge to treatment of a common malady. Using this paradigm, investigations are continuing to define regional vascular receptors and develop specific agonists and antagonists to manipulate these vascular beds.

Acetylcholine

Acetylcholine (ACh) is the primary ganglionic neurotransmitter of both limbs of the autonomic nervous system and functions as a postganglionic neurotransmitter for the parasympathetic nervous system. Although it is primarily involved in exocrine gland secretion, neural release of ACh may evoke minor vasodilation as well.[34] Although the contribution of ACh as a neurotransmitter to neurovascular control is probably small, cholinergic vasodilator nerves have been demonstrated. These are restricted to specific vascular beds, including skeletal muscle, genitalia, and some intracranial arteries. A revelation in control of the vasculature has resulted from the apparent paradoxical constricting and dilating properties of ACh. This is discussed more fully in the section on NO.

ACh is not in clinical use due to its profound negative inotropic, chronotropic, and vasorelaxant properties. Endogenous circulating ACh levels are practically unmeasurable, and any ACh that does enter the circulation is metabolized immediately by circulating plasma cholinesterases unless large doses are used. Cholinergic antagonists do provide selective hemodynamic effects. Atropine (a muscarinic antagonist) increases heart rate, and nicotinic antagonists (e.g., trimethaphan, curare) have ganglionic blocking properties that reduce sympathetic outflow.

Purinergic Activity

Purinergic receptors are present in many vascular beds and are activated by adenosine and ATP. ATP acts as a cotransmitter with norepinephrine in certain tissues. As further subtyping of purinoceptors has been accomplished, it has become apparent that ATP can have both vasoconstrictor and vasodilator actions.[53] Adenosine is in widespread use for treatment of supraventricular tachycardia. It is a potent coronary vasodilator and in large doses reduces systemic vascular resistance.

Vasoactive Intestinal Peptide, Neuropeptide Y, and Vasoactive Peptides

Vasoactive intestinal peptide (VIP) is one of many potent peptides active in vascular regulation. Others include calcitonin gene-related peptide (CGRP), substance P, endothelin(s), oxytocin, arginine vasopressin, angiotensin, neuropeptide Y (NPY), and adrenocorticotropic hormone (ACTH). VIP is a vasodilating neurotransmitter found in the gastrointestinal tract and blood vessel walls.[246] It has now been studied in many species and vascular beds and may play a role in cerebral vasodilation and in co-secretion with ACh to promote exocrine gland blood flow and secretion.[171] Perivascular neuropeptides have been studied in developmental animal models and demonstrate significant variation from in utero to senescence.[74,189] These findings suggest potential opportunities to influence regional vascular flow selectively at different ages.

Neuropeptide Y is another peptide (36-amino acid) neurotransmitter demonstrating significant vasoconstriction in the cerebral and systemic vasculature.[100,283] It is released along with norepinephrine as a neurotransmitter of sympathetic nerves and is also released from the adrenal medulla tonically and during stress. Although no clinical application of these findings has been found, further investigations are in progress.

Angiotensin

The renin-angiotensin-aldosterone system is a significant regulator of systemic vascular tone. In response to diminished renal perfusion, the kidney secretes renin, an enzyme that catalyzes the transformation of angiotensinogen to angiotensin I. The latter undergoes further cleavage by angiotensin-converting enzyme (ACE) to yield the octapeptide angiotensin II. Angiotensin II demonstrates potent vasoconstrictor properties, stimulates norepinephrine release from sympathetic nerve terminals, reduces vagal tone, and elicits secretion of aldosterone from adrenocortical glomerulosa cells.[108,143] In turn, aldosterone promotes water and sodium retention and increases the excretion of potassium in the kidney.[143] Angiotensin II also stimulates secretion of arginine vasopressin from the neurohypophysis, further protecting and reexpanding the circulating blood volume by water retention.[108] Recently, a cardiac renin-angiotensin system that interacts with the autonomic nervous system has been shown to have profound direct and indirect actions on cardiac function, metabolism, and growth.[84]

Angiotensin II acts primarily as a potent vasoconstrictor of the systemic vasculature and efferent arterioles of the renal vasculature. Angiotensin II mediates constriction by stimulation of voltage-dependent Ca^{++} channels and the IP_3/DAG second messenger system to cause an influx of calcium into smooth muscle cells to induce contraction.[37] Inhibition of ATP-sensitive potassium channels by angiotensin II has also been reported to play a role in vasoconstriction.[41] Inhibitors of ACE (e.g., captopril, enalaprilat) are excellent antihypertensives and are used effectively in CHF to reduce systemic vascular resistance.

Arginine Vasopressin

Vasodilatory shock due to the vascular smooth muscle failing to constrict has been associated with many causes, such as sepsis, tissue hypoxia, and severe tissue ischemia. Several mechanisms have been proposed. In a review of vasodilatory shock by Landry and Oliver,[158] activation of ATP-sensitive potassium channels in the plasma membrane of vascular smooth muscle, induction of nitric oxide synthase, and deficiency of the hormone arginine vasopressin (AVP) have been implicated as causative factors for vasodilatory shock. Of these three mechanisms, arginine-vasopressin deficiency has generated the most recent clinical interest.

Arginine vasopressin (or antidiuretic hormone [ADH]) is a nine amino acid peptide that functions not just as a hormone of water reabsorption at the renal distal tubules, but also as a vasoconstrictor. There are three types of receptors that respond to AVP: V_{1a}, V_{1b}, and V_2 receptors. V_{1b} receptors are found only in pituitary vessels and stimulate antidiuretic hormone release. V_1 subtype AVP receptors are coupled to the IP_3/DAG second messenger system. Nonetheless, in the rat kidney V_1 receptors have been shown to release NO in response to stimulation with AVP.[130] The V_2 receptors are found mainly in the kidney and control fluid homeostasis by water and urea permeability and sodium transport. The V_2 receptor, found in the renal collecting duct, reduces free water loss by activating the cAMP second messenger system.[289] Finally, V_{1a} receptors are found in vascular smooth muscle throughout the body and on a number of other cells. The V_{1a} receptors are coupled to the IP_3/DAG second messenger system as well and increase cytoplasmic Ca^{++}, thus causing contraction of the actin and myosin filaments.[33,163] This results in increased SVR and arterial blood pressure. While AVP has been known for more than 70 years to cause vasoconstriction, recent knowledge of its clinical effect on vascular muscle constriction, namely activation of the V_{1a} receptors during refractory hypotension, has encouraged AVP's recent clinical use.

At low plasma concentrations of AVP (1 to 7 pg/mL [0.9 to 6.5 pmol/L]), regulation of renal collecting duct permeability occurs. With higher plasma concentrations (10 to 200 pg/mL

[9 to 187 pmol/L]), vasoconstriction occurs.[158] AVP deficiency has been identified as a cause of refractory septic shock. In a study by Landry and colleagues,[157] adults with septic shock had lower plasma levels of AVP (mean of 3.1 pg/mL) than adults with cardiogenic shock (mean of 22.7 pg/mL). Similar low plasma levels were found in children requiring vasopressors for septic shock by Choi and colleagues.[64] The mean plasma vasopressin level was 5.3 pg/mL (normal range = 1.0 to 13.3 pg/mL), indicating that there was a relative plasma vasopressin deficiency.[64] A mechanism proposed by Morales and colleagues[193] is that extended or marked periods of hypotension cause central nervous system depletion of AVP. This relative deficiency of AVP accompanied by persistent hypotension, hypoperfusion, and lactic acidosis results in NO production by the release of inflammatory mediators. Exposure to endotoxin or inflammatory cytokines (such as interleukin-1 or tumor necrosis factor) produces the expression of the inducible isoform (iNOS), which is calcium-independent, and generates large and sustained amounts of NO from many cell types, including endothelial cells.[191] The cellular acidosis that results may cause myocyte hyperpolarization via ATP-sensitive potassium channels that prevent voltage-gated Ca^{++} channels from opening. Thus calcium influx into the myocyte stops. Consequently, this causes resistance to catecholamines and a progressive worsening of vasodilatory hypotension, hypoperfusion, and lactic acidosis.[193]

Replacement of AVP in situations that are associated with its deficiency has shown promising results. A number of adult studies have shown beneficial effects on blood pressure and urine output with low-dose infusions of AVP (0.04 U/min) in vasodilatory septic shock refractory to catecholamine infusions.[175,290] It also appears that AVP has similar effects in adults following CPB and late hemorrhagic shock.[192,193] While there are no reported plasma AVP levels in adults following CPB, Rosenzweig and colleagues[238] identified 3 of 11 children with AVP deficiency and 1 child with a relative AVP deficiency following CPB. Furthermore, in dogs, Morales and colleagues showed AVP deficiency in the late phases of hemorrhagic shock.[192]

In children there have been fewer reports of AVP treatment. Rosenzweig and colleagues[238] studied children (age 3 days to 15 years) with underlying heart disease treated with AVP after surgery (dose ranging from 0.0003 to 0.002 U/kg/minute). The systolic, diastolic, and mean blood pressure increased and the inotrope score improved in 9 of 11 children. The two children that died had severely depressed cardiac function before the administration of AVP.[238] Similar results have been found in two other pediatric reports.[163,271]

The reported dosages of AVP infusions range from 0.0003 to 0.008 U/kg/minute in children. There is concern for the side effects of the vasoconstrictor activity of AVP. While there has been animal evidence and theoretical concern for myocardial ischemia (due to coronary vasoconstriction), pulmonary hypertension, and skin or intestinal ischemia, the studies using AVP infusions for refractory shock have not reported these effects.[175,193,290] The few studies in children have not reported adverse effects. The report by Rosenzweig and colleagues[238] suggests that elevating the blood pressure with AVP, through increased SVR, causes increased afterload that may not be optimal for the impaired left ventricle. While there have been no apparent clinical side effects from its use,

AVP should be used in appropriate situations and with care until larger, prospective studies have been completed to further assess its efficacy and safety, especially in children.

Natriuretic Peptides

Natriuretic peptides (NPs) function as both hormones and neurotransmitters. There are three types of NPs. The release of NPs appears to be in response to hemodynamic stress, and they have favorable effects on the myocardium. A-type natriuretic peptide (ANP) is secreted primarily from the atrial myocardium in response to atrial dilation but has been found to be secreted from the ventricular myocardium as well in response to diastolic dysfunction.[282] B-type natriuretic peptide (BNP) is produced and released almost completely by the ventricular myocardium in response to elevated end-diastolic pressure and volume. In a study of patients with cardiac amyloidosis and diastolic dysfunction, Takemura and colleagues[282] showed almost transmural myocardial expression of ANP and BNP, but with more prominence in the endocardial side than the epicardial side. These findings suggest that hemodynamic stress, particularly during the diastolic phase due to diastolic dysfunction, is essential for the overexpression of ventricular natriuretic peptides.[282] C-type natriuretic peptide (CNP) is produced and released by endothelial cells in response to shear stress. In a failing myocardium, NPs improve load conditions by their diuretic, natriuretic, and venous and arterial dilation properties.[21,185] This vasorelaxing action seems to be secondary to cGMP generation.

NPs are also particularly potent dilators of the pulmonary circulation constricted by hypoxia. There is also some evidence that these peptides inhibit the renin-angiotensin system, sympathetic nervous system, and endothelin pathway.[49,72,244] Brunner-La Rocca and colleagues[49] found that infusions of BNP in healthy adults and adults with CHF reduced pulmonary capillary pressure and mean arterial pressure without a concurrent increase in norepinephrine. They concluded that BNP demonstrated sympathoinhibitory effects. It was further hypothesized that these effects may be the result of baroreceptor reflex modulation, renin inhibition, angiotensin II antagonism, or cGMP activation.[49] NPs may also have direct and indirect antimitotic effects on the heart and blood vessels.[185] For example, Schirger and colleagues[248] found that BNP inhibited isolated human aortic vascular smooth muscle cell proliferation. ANP and CNP have also been found to possess antimitogenic actions in vascular smooth muscle cells through the natriuretic peptide A and B receptors, respectively, both of which are linked to particulate guanylate cyclase and the generation of cGMP. NPs may play an important role in the inhibition of atheroma formation and maintaining endothelial function in patients with atherosclerosis.[248] Furthermore ANP has been shown to possess antiinflammatory potential. ANP has been shown to inhibit the lipopolysaccharide (LPS)-induced nitric oxide synthase in macrophages in an autocrine fashion and reduce TNF_α secretion in macrophages. It also seems to attenuate the release of interleukin 1β.[149] Because of these physiologic effects, NPs are being increasingly used in the therapy and diagnosis of CHF, and as prognostic indicators for CHF.

Synthetic recombinant human BNP, such as nesiritide, improves function and alleviates the signs and symptoms of volume overload and cardiac decompensation. Colucci and colleagues[72] performed a randomized, double-blinded placebo-controlled study of nesiritide in adults with CHF. Nesiritide caused a significant dose-dependent decrease in pulmonary capillary wedge pressure, right atrial pressure, systemic vascular resistance, and systolic pressure; a moderate increase in cardiac index; and no substantial change in the heart rate.[72] Another means of increasing NPs in the circulation is by inhibiting neutral endopeptidase (NEP), which is responsible for the metabolism of NPs.[174] Preliminary reports have shown encouraging effects of NEP inhibitors on hemodynamics, symptoms, and exercise time in adults with CHF.[185]

BNP is used as both a diagnostic and prognostic tool. BNP, largely of ventricular origin, is released from the ventricles in proportion to intraventricular pressure or wall tension. This increase in wall tension causes various electrophysiologic abnormalities, thereby favoring arrhythmogenesis in the failing heart. Myocardial stretch, credited to volume overload, slows conduction, enhances refractoriness, and triggers after depolarizations and ventricular ectopic beats.[26] Elevated serum BNP levels are being used indirectly to identify increased myocardial wall tension and confirm the diagnosis of congestive heart failure in adults.[173] This also allows the identification of a patient group with higher risk of sudden death due to arrhythmias.[26] Evaluation of the diagnostic and prognostic efficacy of serum BNP levels in children is limited; however, there have been reports of elevated BNP in children with congestive heart failure.[207]

Glucocorticoid Receptors

It is well established that cardiac and vascular smooth muscle glucocorticoid receptors exist and are essential for optimal myocyte function. Glucocorticoids bind to receptors in the cytoplasm and this complex is transported to the nucleus, where it binds with high affinity to DNA. The interaction elicits transcription of many genes, and these gene products regulate the content and rate of transcription of messenger RNA.[295] The target genes activated included enzymes, regulatory proteins, and other cellular constituents.

Lack of stimulation of glucocorticoid receptors results in altered hemodynamic performance. Without the steroid-responsive gene products, myocardial and vascular smooth muscle contractile mechanisms are impaired. This results in lower than expected cardiac output, low systemic vascular resistance, and altered responses to standard vasoactive adrenergic agents. Occult hypocortisolism should be considered in the child unresponsive to standard vasopressor (alpha- and beta-adrenergic) therapy. This has become increasingly clear in the postoperative infant who may have relative hypocortisolemia and in critically ill neonates. It is not known whether other vasoconstrictor mechanisms are glucocorticoid dependent.

DISTRIBUTION OF CARDIAC OUTPUT

Many target tissues modify their response locally by multiple mechanisms to provide homeostasis. For example, the kidney will conserve water and sodium in response to increased vasopressin and decreased ANP. Low renal blood flow will cause release of renin, and the angiotensin II formed will act as a vasopressor and stimulate aldosterone secretion to further conserve sodium. Other examples include inadequate myocardial or cerebral flow. The myocardial response to inadequate myocardial blood flow elicits coronary vasodilation to protect the whole body from pump failure. Inadequate cerebral perfusion pressure elicits the powerful baroreceptor reflex and selective systemic vasoconstriction.

The distribution of cardiac output changes with development. The most dramatic alteration occurs with birth, where combined ventricular output changes to series output and each ventricle must perform the work previously accomplished as a combined output. Except in the case of anatomic abnormalities allowing shunting between the pulmonary and systemic circuits, the pulmonary blood flow and right ventricular output now equal the systemic blood flow and left ventricular output. Control of pulmonary blood flow is discussed in Chapter 3. Select control mechanisms of distribution of regional blood flow in the periphery are discussed subsequently.

Each organ has specific vascular receptors responsive to neural innervation and circulating hormones. The presence and degree of response to these signals differ in each regional vascular bed. Furthermore, although regional blood flow is usually dictated by local oxygen requirements, there are notable exceptions, including the carotid body, adrenal medulla, neurohypophysis, and kidneys. The carotid body, an afferent sensor, has a luxurious blood flow of nearly 2000 mL/min/100 g of tissue, certainly beyond its metabolic requirements. It is believed that this flow provides high-quality and instantaneous presentation of cardiovascular function for exquisitely sensitive neural reflexes to mediate any necessary changes.

In the fetus, salt and water homeostasis and excretion of nitrogen and organic acids are managed by the uteroplacental unit. In utero, renal vascular resistance is high; however, shortly after birth a dramatic decrease in renal vascular resistance allows increased renal flow, and the newborn kidney begins to assume these functions. Renal blood flow autoregulation appears early in life and provides for salt and water homeostasis by maintenance of a constant glomerular filtration rate (GFR). The newborn kidneys receive only 4% to 10% of cardiac output. This increases to approximately 20% of cardiac output in adulthood, the purpose of which is primarily to remove organic wastes and to achieve salt and water balance.[116] Again, oxygen delivery is not the critical metabolic component driving this significant renal blood flow.

The adrenal medulla also receives high blood flow, which is apparently not necessitated by oxygen requirements for metabolic or secretory function.[42] This is likely related to the need for urgent entry of catecholamines into the circulation during stress.

CARDIOVASCULAR DYSFUNCTION

Circulatory dysfunction occurs when the cardiovascular system is unable to deliver oxygen and nutrients to the tissues at a rate that fulfills their metabolic demands; that is, supply is inadequate for demand. When the cardiovascular system fails, many of the mechanisms that regulate the circulation (described in detail previously) are activated in a compensatory fashion. These compensatory mechanisms establish a new equilibrium point within the cardiovascular system and, if adequate, may restore supply to match demand to compensate for shock. Alternatively, the cardiovascular stress may be so acute or so severe that compensatory mechanisms are inadequate or have inadequate time to develop before supply falls below the critical level at which permanent tissue damage occurs. Cardiovascular failure can occur acutely or chronically. When there is an acute failure of supply to match demand, shock occurs. When chronic cardiovascular failure exists, supply cannot meet necessary increases in demand (limitation of exercise tolerance, growth failure) and compensatory mechanisms are functioning at or near their maximum merely to maintain subsistence delivery. This occurs in CHF.

In general, compensatory mechanisms protect critical metabolic areas, such as the brain and myocardium, at the expense of the peripheral circulation; however, it must be remembered that the compensatory mechanisms are not necessarily benign. As they progress to their fullest, these may oppose adequate cardiovascular function and lead to a worsening state by further impairing myocardial contractility or preventing adequate circulation to critical vascular beds. These compensatory mechanisms are critically balanced in newborns, in which there are greater basal oxygen demands, greater basal metabolic requirements, and a circulatory system that has difficulty responding to increased needs. We will first address chronic CHF, as this is frequently an underlying substrate for children who present to the ICU, especially those with CHD. The compensatory mechanisms that arise as a result of chronically compromised cardiovascular function are frequently the background for the acute cardiovascular dysfunction that is often seen in postoperative surgical patients. Early circulatory embarrassment may be characterized as low cardiac output syndrome, but as this continues shock becomes evident. The remainder of the discussion will focus on acute circulatory embarrassment and include areas of cardiovascular impairment not necessarily related to cardiovascular surgery but with which surgeons, intensivists, and cardiologists should be familiar in the critical care setting.

CONGESTIVE FAILURE

The pathophysiologic responses and compensatory mechanisms in chronic CHF have widespread systemic consequences. Causes of heart failure in children are listed in Table 2-2. These include congenital abnormalities that give rise to volume or pressure overload and primary myocardial diseases such as glycogen storage diseases, mucopolysaccharidoses, and endomyocardial fibroelastosis. Although ischemic heart disease leads the list in adults, this is an uncommon cause of CHF in children. Even so, anomalous coronary artery, Kawasaki disease, and periarteritis nodosa can cause ischemic heart disease in children, and ischemia plays a role in postoperative myocardial decompensation.

Factors that lead to cardiac failure can be separated into five general categories: (1) decreased muscle contractile function, (2) volume overload, (3) pressure overload, (4) diastolic dysfunction, and (5) changes in the systemic and pulmonary vasculature.[213,217] Changes in sarcomere function may be due to loss of sarcomeres, infarction and ischemia, or otherwise impaired sarcomere function, which is common in cardiac failure. Decreased contractility results from all the factors that contribute to cardiac failure. This decreased contractility is manifested by a decreased rate of development of contractile force,

Table 2-2　Causes of Heart Failure

Heart Rate Abnormalities
Supraventricular tachycardia (SVT)
Bradycardia
Ventricular arrhythmias

Congenital Heart Disease

Cardiomyopathies
Hypoxia
Metabolic disorders
　Hypoglycemia
　Hypocalcemia
　Acidosis
　Thyroid disorders
　Hypothermia
　Glycogen storage diseases
　Carnitine deficiency
　Mucopolysaccharidoses
　Endomyocardial fibroelastosis

Infectious Disorders
Sepsis
Myocarditis: viral or bacterial

Drug Intoxications

Neuromuscular Diseases
Duchenne's muscular dystrophy
Friedreich's ataxia

Vascular Diseases
Kawasaki disease
Polyarteritis nodosa
Embolism (cardiac or pulmonary)
Acute rheumatic fever

Trauma
Cardiogenic shock
Direct cardiac trauma

decreased shortening, and decreased velocity of shortening. Along with these, abnormalities in myosin ATP also cause decreased contractility.[252] Different myosin isoforms are also seen in chronically overloaded hearts. These alterations in the function of myosin ATP and the contraction-relaxation sequence ultimately impair myocardial contractile function.[166] They occur in the advanced stages of all types of cardiac failure. Furthermore there are clearly demonstrated abnormalities in the sarcolemma and sarcoplasmic reticulum in CHF.[213] These may contribute to the decreased velocity of shortening, the duration of the action potential, and changes in calcium transients. In addition mitochondrial abnormalities and abnormal calcium metabolism have also been reported.[213,215] All of these abnormalities cause abnormal calcium handling by the subcellular components and sarcoplasmic reticulum in the myocyte, which ultimately impairs contractile function. Abnormal calcium transients also impair diastolic function. Prolonged calcium transients, increased cytosolic calcium during diastole, and delayed decline in cytosolic calcium concentration can lead to both passive myocardial stiffness and delayed active relaxation.[323]

There are differences between volume overload and pressure overload.[57,213,217] Children who have left-to-right shunting, such as in ASD, VSD, or patent ductus arteriosus, may eventually develop heart failure characterized by increased ventricular volume and ventricular dilation.[113] This dilation leads to increased wall stress (via Laplace mechanisms), myocardial hypertrophy, increased oxygen consumption, abnormal oxygen delivery relationships, ischemia, and ultimately decreased contractility. As the compliance characteristics of the heart decline and diastolic pressures increase, diastolic dysfunction occurs with preload limitations. Pressure overload, characterized by valvular obstruction such as aortic stenosis, pulmonary stenosis, and pulmonary hypertension, has an even more deleterious effect on contractile function. In fact, in several experiments contractile function of isolated myocytes and papillary muscles is markedly impaired by pressure overload. There is a significant change in myosin isoforms and much slower myosin ATPase activity.[123,268] Downregulation of both the biochemical and functional bases of contraction occurs. The chronically pressure-overloaded heart responds with hypertrophy and increased wall thickness, which eventually results in decreased cardiac output and inadequate systemic oxygen delivery.

The importance of systolic function with decreased contractility has been widely recognized. Nevertheless, impaired diastolic function with impaired relaxation, elevated diastolic filling pressures, and impaired ventricular filling during diastole (with the consequences of these three) has become better recognized.[89] Diastolic heart failure presents with symptoms and signs of heart failure, but adequate ejection fraction is maintained and there is abnormal diastolic function.[322] Diastole consists of the stage during which the myocardium loses its ability to generate force or shorten and reverts to an unstressed length and force. Diastolic dysfunction takes place when these processes are prolonged, slowed, or incomplete.[322] Diastolic dysfunction has the effect of elevating the resting tension curve (see Fig. 2-5) and thus limiting diastolic function and stroke volume. Impaired diastolic function occurs in many settings, but particularly in the hypertrophied heart. It is due to changes in the connective tissue collagen matrix and the arrangement of muscle bundles within the heart. Changes in the myosin isotypes may lead to delayed relaxation and diastolic dysfunction on a nonanatomic basis, which, however, may still critically limit stroke volume. This is characteristic of both ischemic and hypertrophied muscle and plays a significant role in the myocardial dysfunction in postoperative cardiac patients. Patients with impaired diastolic function are more at risk for preload limitation during tachycardia. Clearly, restrictive cardiomyopathies and pericardial disease with pericardial restriction also impair diastolic function and limit ventricular filling. Diastolic dysfunction responds well to afterload reduction.[89,217]

A further major factor altering cardiovascular function in CHF is deranged peripheral vascular responses.[160] Systemic vasoconstriction occurs in all forms of advanced CHF. This results from compensatory mechanisms (discussion to follow) such as increased circulating catecholamines and angiotensin; however, it has recently become appreciated that endothelial impairment is also widespread in CHF.[90] This endothelial impairment was first recognized over 20 years ago when it was noticed that in severe CHF muscle blood flow did not increase in response to hand-grip exercise.[165,307] Thus, there appeared to be a primary failure of dilation in the muscle beds. It is usual for the muscle beds during exercise to increase blood flow by 15 to 20 times; however, in patients with CHF this may be limited to a factor of two or three.[160] Furthermore this does not correlate with resting left ventricular dysfunction and is not improved by inotropic agents that

improve cardiac function.[181] Linked with the realization of the role of endothelium in CHF is the demonstration that there is a derangement in vascular endothelial function. In multiple peripheral vascular beds, there is a widespread depression of vessels to respond to NO released by vasodilators such as acetylcholine and bradykinin.[153] Others have reported that although there is impaired response to NO release, there is perhaps an increased baseline release of NO.[147] This decreased tonic response may be a necessary factor in counteracting systemic vasoconstrictor action in heart failure and in maintaining some local flow. The impairment in endothelial function limits cardiovascular reserve. Furthermore, circulating endothelin is also increased in chronic failure, and the increase in circulating endothelin levels correlates with the severity of CHF,[178,273] thus serving as a marker of endothelial dysfunction in vascular disease. Additionally, diseases of deranged endothelium have increased endothelin levels. The effects of this increased circulating endothelin on the vasculature and multiple organ function are widespread.[273] The effects of deranged vascular tone (although initially compensatory in maintaining perfusion pressures) ultimately lead to increased afterload for an already impaired myocardium. In advanced stages, further decompensation with severe vasoconstriction and impaired myocardial function occurs. Despite this endothelial dysfunction, the vascular smooth muscle appears to be responsive to nitrovasodilators. Thus, therapies directed at restoring or replacing endothelial dysfunction may improve cardiovascular function in advanced states of heart failure and explain why afterload reduction is so beneficial.

Compensatory Mechanisms

There are both acute and chronic compensatory mechanisms for heart failure. Acutely, the heart rate increases because of increased sympathetic activity and circulating catecholamines. Stroke volume may be preserved by salt and water retention, which augments preload. Alterations in endothelial function and circulating catecholamines lead to vasoconstriction and increased afterload, which preserves perfusion pressure to organs at the expense of cardiac function.

There are also compensatory mechanisms aimed at preserving myocardial function. A long-term response to myocardial failure is myocardial hypertrophy.[213] As stated previously, the Laplace relationship indicates that myocardial oxygen tension, via myocardial wall tension, is related to ventricular diameter and thickness. As the heart dilates, wall stress increases and oxygen consumption increases, as well as the work required for contraction, unless there is a compensatory increase in muscle thickness.[113] Thus, teleologically, hypertrophy is a response to increased wall stress. This important compensatory mechanism occurs in either volume or pressure overload. Unfortunately, although this is beneficial at an early stage, hypertrophied heart muscle is not accompanied by increased capillary density and myocardial blood flow, and hence eventually outgrows its blood supply. It is therefore more at risk for ischemic injury. This impaired oxygen supply-delivery relationship leads to worsening of contractile function in the hypertrophied muscles, and ultimately this compensatory mechanism leads to a loss of contractility. This impairment in ventricular oxygen supply-demand relationships can be seen with increasing failure and hypertrophy. Oxygen extraction slowly increases.

This is limited because normal extraction is near 75% of maximal. With further hypertrophy it is not surprising that subendocardial ischemia, further impaired contractile function, and scarring can occur. This has been demonstrated in the developing heart.[177,213] It is important to notice that at very early stages (in utero and perinatal), pressure overload (valvular obstruction) may actually be accompanied by true myocardial hyperplasia and presumably by increased myocardial perfusion as well. If this is the case, the neonatal myocardium (at this developmental stage) may be less prone to damage caused by imbalances of oxygen and supply-demand ratios.[213]

Neurohumoral Alterations in Heart Failure

Neurohumoral alterations in heart failure have been well described and are primarily directed at preload augmentation and optimizing myocardial function.[99] It is interesting that in the failing heart, primary mechanisms for increasing or maintaining cardiac output are directed at maintaining mean circulatory filling pressure (P_{ms}). P_{ms} represents the filling of the entire vasculature and is determined by both vascular tone and intravascular volume. Thus, vasoconstrictor forces increase P_{ms}, at least transiently, and fluid retention increases P_{ms}. The neurohumoral forces that are acutely involved include the renin-angiotensin system, increased circulating catecholamines, alpha- and beta-adrenergic neural activity (directly on the vasculature), and changes in natriuretic factor (NF) and arginine vasopressin secretion. The complex neurohumoral response leads to both sodium and water retention, increasing myocardial preload by increasing mean circulatory filling pressure, leading potentially to cardiac dilation and enhanced contractility via the Frank-Starling mechanism. The natural compensatory mechanism for impaired contractility is preload augmentation. Preload augmentation is limited by the diastolic compliance characteristics of the heart (see Fig. 2-11). If EDPs increase as much as P_{ms}, the pressure gradient for venous return is not increased and preload remains the same but at a higher EDP. This is clearly deleterious. It should be noted, as mentioned previously regarding neonates with decreased compliance, that the mechanisms that increase myocardial preload may actually lead to CHF more rapidly in neonates than in adults. Thus, pulmonary edema and fluid retention may develop relatively earlier in neonates than in older patients.

The sympathetic nervous system, activated via baroreceptors found in the left ventricle, carotid sinus, aortic arch, and renal afferent arterioles, acts as an early compensatory mechanism that provides inotropic support and maintains cardiac output in CHF. Sustained sympathetic stimulation activates the renin-angiotensin system and the secretion of arginine vasopressin, endothelins, and other neurohormones to cause an increase in venous and arterial tone, an increased plasma norepinephrine concentration, and a progressive retention of salt and water.[143,251] Chronic elevation in the concentration of catecholamines leads to a decreased ability of the myocardium to respond to the catecholamines by a downregulation of beta-receptors and desensitization. Myocardial adrenergic activity is impaired by this decreased beta-receptor density, affinity, and responsiveness to adrenergic stimulation. Furthermore, excessive sympathetic activity is associated with cardiac myocyte apoptosis, hypertrophy,

and focal myocardial necrosis. In an attempt to improve the falling cardiac output in CHF, the compensatory mechanisms signal a progressive decline in the myocardial function.[143,251] Beta-adrenergic blocking medications have been used successfully in adults with CHF to prevent the effects of chronic adrenergic stimulation.[16,110] There have been far fewer studies in children, but the results have been encouraging. Laer and colleagues[154] evaluated 15 children with CHF that was the result of dilated cardiomyopathy (10 children) and congenital heart disease (5 children), and who were being treated with ACE inhibitors and digoxin at the beginning of the study. They found that oral carvedilol added to standard drug therapy in children with CHF was well tolerated and associated with better ventricular function and clinical symptom scores.[154]

Activation of the renin-angiotensin system causes increased concentrations of renin, angiotensin II, and aldosterone. Angiotensin II is a potent vasoconstrictor of the renal (efferent arterioles) and systemic circulation, where it stimulates the release of norepinephrine from sympathetic nerve terminals, inhibits vagal tone, and promotes the release of aldosterone. In addition, angiotensin II is thought to have mitogenic effects on the cardiac myocytes. The resultant cardiac remodeling may lead to a decrease in size of the capillary network relative to that of the myocardium, thus predisposing the patient to ischemic insults. Aldosterone in turn leads to the retention of sodium and water and the increased excretion of potassium.[143,251]

Neurohormones, such as arginine vasopressin, endothelins, natriuretic peptides, and endothelial hormones, are involved in the balance of myocardial function in CHF as well. Arginine vasopressin causes antidiuresis and vascular smooth muscle constriction, which augments preload and afterload. Endothelins, potent vasoconstrictors secreted from endothelium and other tissues, are increased in CHF and have been used in the prognostic evaluation of patients with CHF. Natriuretic peptides are released from the atrial and ventricular myocardium and vascular endothelium in response to volume expansion and pressure overload to act as physiologic antagonists to the effects of angiotensin II, aldosterone, arginine vasopressin, and endothelins. They cause constriction of glomerular efferent arterioles and dilation of afferent arterioles to increase the glomerular filtration rate and decrease sodium reabsorption in the collecting duct, thereby enhancing sodium and water excretion.[143,251,255]

Other endothelial hormones involved in CHF include NO, prostacyclin and prostaglandin E_1, bradykinin, and TNF-α. Constitutive NO synthetase (NOS) of endothelial cells is responsible for generation of NO, to decrease afterload and improve tissue perfusion. In CHF, NOS activity appears to be reduced.[143,251] Arachadonic acid derivatives, prostaglandin E_1 and prostacyclin, are also increased in CHF and are involved in maintaining glomerular filtration. Bradykinin, generated from the kallikrein-kinin system, promotes natriuresis and vasodilation, as well as stimulates the production of prostaglandins. Finally, TNF-α is elevated in cachectic patients with chronic CHF and has been implicated in the development of endothelial abnormalities, myocardial depression, and increases in NOS activity in vascular smooth muscle.[143,251]

The role of cardiac and systemic neurohumoral mechanisms in maintaining cardiac output in CHF is complex. Despite the detrimental effects of many of the neurohormones secreted in response to the failing myocardium, their absence would hasten the myocardial dysfunction seen in patients with CHF.

ACUTE CIRCULATORY DYSFUNCTION IN SHOCK

Shock is a clinical state of acutely inadequate or deranged circulatory function, with inadequate substrate (O_2, glucose) delivery to and energy production by the tissues. Ultimately, if uncorrected, the shock state progresses to irreversible cell damage, collapse of all homeostatic mechanisms, and death. The cardiovascular system is the focal point in shock, because cardiovascular malfunction eventually occurs in all shock states.

Inadequate energy production can result from inadequate substrate uptake, inadequate substrate delivery, and inadequate substrate utilization. Uptake impairment (environmental deprivation) such as in hypoxia, primary pulmonary disease, and intrapulmonary or intracardiac shunting will limit oxygen uptake and, if severe, will lead to cardiovascular collapse and shock. Inadequate substrate delivery will occur when inadequate substrate is taken into or distributed throughout the body. Inadequate delivery is due to poor cardiac performance or disturbed vascular tone. Absolute inadequate circulating blood volume is often the primary cause of shock (hypovolemic shock), especially in the postoperative state. Relatively inadequate volume may be present when the capacitance of the circulatory system is increased (distributive and septic shock). Although hypotension is frequently seen in shock, hypotension is not the sine qua non of shock in children. Many patients have failing cellular energy production or utilization while the blood pressure is maintained by homeostatic mechanisms. These defense mechanisms reach a limit and fail, and hypotension ensues. Shock is present before this hypotension occurs. Conversely, hypotension does not define shock. For example, controlled hypotension is used during many surgical procedures without accruing an energy deficit. Perfusion pressures lower than normal are routine during CPB, but shock is not present.

Although shock is ultimately a metabolic problem (cellular energy deficiency), regulation and pathology of the circulatory system are central to the pathophysiology. The traditional circulatory approach is the most useful in guiding monitoring and therapeutic manipulation. An understanding of oxygen delivery and cellular physiology is necessary; however, the current understanding of cellular bioenergetics does not afford any proven therapeutic modality at the cellular level at this time. Manipulation of the circulatory state remains the best approach to optimizing cellular recovery.

The complex array of regulatory systems designed to maintain adequate perfusion pressure and blood flow become perturbed in shock. Some of these homeostatic mechanisms are local (autoregulatory, autocrine, and paracrine), while others are mediated by an integrated response of the sympathetic nervous system. The endocrine system elaborates a number of hormones that regulate vascular tone and blood volume. Recently, the central role of the vascular endothelium in the regulation of vasomotor tone, both locally and distantly, has been recognized. This multisystem, integrated response to stress is critical for survival. It is activated by a wide variety of stimuli including hemorrhage, endotoxemia, and anaphylaxis. This highly adaptive group of responses is valuable as temporary defense under stress, but it may lead to deleterious effects on vital organs that, if not treated aggressively, will impair long-term survival.

With acute hemorrhage, systolic, diastolic, and pulse pressures all decrease. An initial sympathetically mediated increase in vascular tone compensates for decreased circulating volume. This increased tone results in weak peripheral pulses, with the available cardiac output shunted toward major vital organs instead of the extremities. Capillary filling is decreased, and pallor or an ashen appearance of the skin is obvious. Patients are tachypneic, tachycardiac, and agitated. The agitation arises from both inadequate cerebral blood flow (oxygen delivery) and increased systemic levels of catecholamines in response to hypotension. As further hemorrhage occurs and cardiac output falls, inadequate cerebral blood flow leads to altered mentation and ultimately unconsciousness. This is a desperate situation with only minutes available for resuscitation.

In the canine model of hemorrhagic shock, the use of controlled hemorrhage, to a constant pressure reservoir, with blood pressure maintained at 30% to 40% of control, has provided useful insights into the responses to hemorrhagic shock.[311] In this study, after the period of acute hemorrhage, blood volume loss into the reservoir continued to increase for 1 to 2 hours, indicating that vasoconstriction and compensatory mechanisms were operating. After this 2-hour period, blood began to return to the animal, indicating an increasing capacitance of the vascular space. After several hours of this significant hypotension, there was a period beyond which even additional massive transfusion did not result in survival of the animal. This marked the onset of irreversible shock. Thus hypovolemic hypotension per se becomes irreversible within hours.

In the first hours of acute hemorrhage, major compensatory responses include baroreceptor and chemoreceptor reflexes, cerebral ischemic responses, and activation of the endocrine system to release vasoactive substances. In early hemorrhagic shock the hematocrit is unchanged, since there has been no autotransfusion of extracellular fluid into the circulating volume. This will occur slowly. Hemodilution will also occur when non-blood-containing resuscitation fluids are administered. As a result of decreased renal perfusion, there is stimulation of the renin-angiotensin-aldosterone axis. Finally, with significant hypotension, Starling forces are altered, leading to reabsorption of fluid from the extravascular space into the circulating volume.

During hemorrhagic shock, there is a marked increase in adrenomedullary blood flow. This increase is thought to be important in facilitating release of catecholamines into the systemic circulation in response to shock. Eventually, with severe hemorrhage, intense renal vasoconstriction occurs and kidney perfusion becomes inadequate. As blood pressure falls below the lower limits of the autoregulatory potential, myocardial and cerebral blood flow become inadequate, and these critical organs also fail.

Humoral Responses in Shock

The endocrine system maintains an integrated balance during homeostasis. When hypotension occurs, humoral responses to this stress play an important role in host defenses. Circulating levels of epinephrine and norepinephrine are significantly increased (50-fold and 10-fold, respectively). Both agents increase myocardial contractility and increase vascular systemic tone in most organs. Corticotropin-releasing factor increases and causes ACTH release, resulting in increased systemic glucocorticoid levels. This provides increased glucocorticoids for the vascular and myocardial receptors, which are required for optimal contractile responses. Both glucocorticoids and catecholamines raise blood glucose, which is necessary because glucose supplies are utilized in stressed tissues, owing to lack of oxygen delivery and adaptation for energy production via anaerobic metabolism.

As hypotension ensues, there is less distension of the right and left atrial walls. This lack of distension inhibits the secretion of NP, a natriuretic and diuretic hormone. A decrease in synthesis, release, and action of NP results in further water and salt conservation. When renal perfusion pressure is diminished, there is an increased release of renin, which in turn stimulates conversion of angiotensinogen to angiotensin I. In turn, increased angiotensin I is converted to angiotensin II, an extremely potent vasoconstrictor. Angiotensin II also stimulates aldosterone secretion, which will act to increase absorption of sodium by the renal tubules.

When hypothalamic perfusion pressure falls or serum osmolality increases, a rise in circulating AVP occurs. AVP has many functions. As a circulating hormone, it is a potent vasoconstrictor and acts at the renal tubules to increase reabsorption of water. AVP also acts as a neurotransmitter and may be involved in integrating the hypothalamic-sympathetic response to stress.

Endothelial Injury

The endothelium regulates vascular function.[313] First, it elaborates vasodilators such as NO and prostacyclin, and vasoconstrictors such as the endothelins, which directly regulate vascular smooth muscle tone by both local (paracrine) and distant (endocrine) effects. The endothelial metabolism of circulating vasoactive substances such as angiotensin, catecholamines, and eicosanoids also contributes to the regulation of vascular tone. The second major way in which the endothelium modulates vascular function is by maintaining vascular integrity. Not only is the structural integrity of the endothelium important in regulating permeability, but the endothelium also plays a crucial role in solute and water transport into the interstitium. Thus, endothelial injury and dysfunction lead to increased transcapillary transudation and interstitial edema. The latter then impairs gas and nutrient flow to the parenchymal cells of the individual organs. Oxygen must diffuse through the interstitium from the red cell to the organ parenchymal cells; interstitial edema impairs this process. Endothelial injury with vascular leakage leads to further hypoxic injury. Finally, endothelial injury affects blood flow, which can lead to red cell clumping, hemostasis, sludging, platelet aggregation, neutrophil clumping, and obstruction of the microcirculation, with resultant ischemia. With severe endothelial destruction, the alveolocapillary basement membrane, which is the common basement membrane between the endothelium and the alveolar epithelium, becomes injured and fragmented. When this is particularly

severe, frank alveolar flooding and hemorrhagic pulmonary edema occur. Transudation of this fluid inactivates alveolar surfactant, and further deterioration of gas exchange results. Endothelial injury is ubiquitous in critical illness and not surprisingly the consequences are legion.[230]

It has been demonstrated that, in a fashion analogous to the vascular endothelium, the endocardium also alters myocardial function.[264] Brutsaert[50] first demonstrated that endocardial removal and damage have a negative inotropic effect on the myocardium. The realization that endocardial damage can negatively affect myocardial function may be important for the stunned myocardium in post-CPB cardiopulmonary performance.[128,155] Thus, widespread endothelial injury after CPB may also be responsible for myocardial dysfunction. Circulating myocardial depressant factors may be no more than factors that cause endothelial injury and thus also injure the endocardial endothelium, causing impaired myocardial function.[155] These studies have been extended by Mebazaa and colleagues,[186] who have demonstrated that the endocardium is capable of altering myocardial function by generation of endothelin, which is an inotrope. Additionally, the endocardial endothelium generates a negative inotropic substance that desensitizes the myocardial myocyte to calcium. The endocardium is also a rich source of eicosanoids and NO, which may have both direct paracrine effects on the myocardium and downstream endocrine effects on myocardial afterload. Thus, an understanding of endothelial injury is important not only for an understanding of the microcirculatory and vascular tone derangements that follow CPB, but also for an understanding of myocardial myocyte function and mechanics after CPB.[128] It can be seen that the factors that injure the endothelium have significant ramifications on integrated circulatory function.

After CPB, microcirculatory function is deranged throughout the body. The postsurgical systemic inflammatory response plays a significant role in mediating this injury.[155] This impaired microcirculatory function is to a great extent due to endothelial injury. This endotheliopathy occurs in every organ system and is the common pathologic condition of the post-CPB state. Endothelial injury impairs both vasoreactivity and vascular integrity at the microcirculatory level and underlies the pathology in all the individual organ systems such as the myocardium, lung, kidneys, and CNS. Thus, the common unifying concept of circulatory derangement and multiple organ system dysfunction in the post-CPB state requires an understanding of how endothelial injury occurs.[155,313]

The endothelium is injured in numerous ways during cardiac surgery and CPB.[155,297] Surgery itself initiates a systemic inflammatory response that targets the endothelium and gives rise to widespread endothelial dysfunction. CPB itself has long been known to activate complement. C3a and C5a complement activation stimulates circulating neutrophils, activating them to express endothelial adhesion molecules (LECAMS, ICAMS, and ELAMS) and thus interact with the endothelium. This binding and interaction of the neutrophil with the endothelium forms protected microenvironments in which free radicals, cathepsins, elastases, and pepsins released by the neutrophils can destroy the endothelium and alter endothelial function. In addition, CPB activates tumor necrosis factor (TNF) and interleukins 1 and 6 (and almost certainly other interleukins and cytokines). The activation of these mediators of the systemic inflammatory response by a combination of surgery and CPB accounts for the widespread organ system dysfunction seen after cardiac surgery.[155]

Clearly, circulating cytokines induce endothelial injury, alter microvascular function, and ultimately affect both vascular and myocardial function. The effects of this widespread endothelial injury are legion. For example, the loss of baseline production of NO causes increased pulmonary vascular and systemic vascular resistance, and decreased regulation in the microcirculation. This results in altered tissue perfusion, parenchymal injury, and multiple organ dysfunction. This is only one example of how common endothelial injury underlies pulmonary dysfunction, myocardial dysfunction, renal dysfunction, and almost certainly cerebral dysfunction in the post-CPB state. Apart from NO, multiple other vasoregulatory systems are disrupted. Ischemia and reperfusion and hypothermia-induced injury aggravate this endotheliopathy.

This construct suggests the need for endothelial protection.[313] Strategies to protect the endothelium from injury include steroids, which inhibit complement activation and some of the effects of the cytokines; specific interference with oxygen free radical generation; and inhibition of neutrophil degranulation. Removal of neutrophils from the circulation is beneficial in decreasing CPB-induced injury. Blocking neutrophil adherence and inhibition of adhesion molecules to the endothelium by the use of monoclonal antibodies such as CD11-CD18 also decreases CPB-induced injury. Therapies specifically directed toward preserving endothelial function may improve outcome in sepsis, systemic inflammatory shock syndrome, CPB, deep hypothermic arrest, and surgery, and may decrease postoperative complications and the duration of convalescence.

Is Shock an Endotheliopathy?

Increasing recognition of the critical involvement of the endothelium in cardiovascular regulation, along with increasing demonstration that the endothelium appears to be a target organ in critical illness, has led to the recognition that the pathophysiology of shock state is related to this endotheliopathy.[292,297,313] After CPB, hypoperfusion, sepsis, and severe hypothermia, multiple mediator systems, including tumor necrosis factor, interleukins, and other cytokines, are activated and cause endothelial dysfunction. This endothelial injury would be expected to alter coagulation profiles; affect regulation of vasomotor tone with loss of critical vasodilators, prostacyclin, and NO; and destroy the endothelial barrier function, leading to altered Starling mechanisms. Vascular endothelial dysfunction occurs in hypertension, heart failure, ischemia, and reperfusion, and in multiple organ systems including the heart, kidney, and brain. The widespread pathophysiologic effects of this endothelial dysfunction must be taken into account in every critically ill child.[313] The ramifications of this dysfunction are foremost for vascular tone. For example, after hypovolemic shock or CPB, endothelial impairment leads to the loss of vasodilator function from loss of NO and prostacyclin production. This causes elevated systemic vascular resistance, poor peripheral perfusion, and multiple organ dysfunction from impaired organ perfusion. This transiently stunned endothelium may recover within 12 to 24 hours, restoring the normal endothelial dilatory tone.

Physiologic therapy for this would include nitrovasodilators and phosphodiesterase inhibitors; thus, nitroglycerin, nitroprusside, and milrinone may be routinely indicated after cardiac surgery.

Another result of endothelial derangement may be hypersecretion of vasoactive substances. For example, in chronic CHF, endothelin appears to be elevated and involved in the circulatory disturbances that occur in heart failure.[178,273] Acute elevations of other endothelial vasoconstrictors and endothelially produced products almost certainly play an important role. Impaired endothelial metabolism of catecholamines and angiotensin would lead to further disturbances of circulatory homeostasis. There appears to be agreement that there is increased production of NO in septic shock. This is almost certainly not from the endothelium, but rather from phagocytes and vascular smooth muscle cells. Lipopolysaccharide causes an increase in inducible NOS and massive NO release. Although this clearly occurs in cytokine-activated shock, such as in septic shock, its role in hypovolemic and cardiogenic shock seems less important.

The coagulation cascade is finely balanced on the endothelium. The endothelium generates and activates a host of procoagulant and anticoagulant factors. Perturbation of the endothelium, not surprisingly, leads to perturbation of the coagulation cascade. It has become increasingly evident that disseminated intravascular coagulation is indeed evidence of widespread endothelial dysfunction. Thus, coagulopathies and thrombocytopenia are clinical findings of endothelial dysfunction and clearly have ramifications in postoperative surgical patients and in children suffering from shock.

Finally, endothelial dysfunction causes barrier breakdown. Endothelial tight junctions and endothelial cell barriers are potent factors in the Starling forces. The net transudation of fluid across the capillary endothelial membrane (Q) is governed by the Starling forces. Below is the Lawrence Papenheimer modification of the Starling equation, which describes the balance of transcapillary fluid flux regulated by hydrostatic pressures (P_{mv} [microvascular hydrostatic pressure] – P_{pmv} [the perivascular] or [interstitial microvascular pressure]) and the oncotic forces (π_{mv} [intravascular oncotic pressure] – π_{pmv} [perivascular oncotic pressure]). K_{fc} is the filtration coefficient, which is determined by the endothelial function, and σ is the reflectance coefficient, which is determined by collagen and connective tissue network characteristics.

$$Q = K_{fc} \left[(P_{mv} - P_{pmv}) - \sigma (\pi_{mv} - \pi_{pmv}) \right]$$

Endothelial dysfunction alters the filtration coefficient, leading to perturbed endothelial barrier function. Widespread interstitial edema and third spacing is a well-recognized result of endothelial dysfunction that frequently takes 24 to 36 hours to recover after routine CPB. In the presence of hemorrhagic shock, hypoxia, ischemia, or ongoing cytokine activation, this endothelial barrier dysfunction may be quite prolonged and lead to severe interstitial edema and pulmonary edema for many days.

These widespread consequences of this multifaceted endothelial dysfunction occur in virtually all states of circulatory shock. Although the exact clinical picture and the duration of endothelial impairment may vary among the various causes of shock, endothelial function is common to them all.

Endothelial protective measures such as prostacyclin infusion, monoclonal antibodies directed at CD18 or ICAM-1 to prevent neutrophil adherence and neutrophil-induced damage and the administration of L-arginine[279] may be useful adjunctive therapies and improve recovery after cardiac surgery and in systemic inflammatory response syndrome (SIRS).

Oxygen Utilization

Oxygen is the most limited substrate carried by the circulation.[258] It is clear that total absence of oxygen delivery results in neurologic and myocardial sequelae in a matter of minutes. Other tissues may be more resistant but eventually succumb to lack of oxygen for energy production. Approximately 90% of cellular oxygen supply is consumed by the mitochondria for oxidative metabolism of carbohydrates and other energy sources. Oxygen is also an obligatory cofactor for non-energy-producing enzymes in the production of oxygen free radicals and other labile compounds.

Early in the hypoxic or ischemic state, energy production is limited, but mitochondrial processes remain intact. More lengthy hypoxic-ischemic insults eventually destroy mitochondrial machinery. When the mitochondria are irreversibly damaged by lack of oxygen, the cell is beyond repair and survival. Further, any cells suffering from ischemic damage will develop edema due to loss of energy for Na^+-K^+ ion exchange pumps. This edema potentially impairs already limited oxygen delivery to adjacent cells. Therefore, even a discrete area of injury can be significantly enlarged with secondary injury.

Oxygen delivery ($\dot{D}O_2$) is the product of cardiac output (CO) and arterial oxygen content (CaO_2):

$$\dot{D}O_2 = CO \times CaO_2$$

Oxygen consumption ($\dot{V}O_2$) can be calculated from the Fick equation ($CmvO_2$ = mixed venous oxygen content):

$$\dot{V}O_2 = CO \times (CaO_2 - CmvO_2)$$

In shock, inadequate oxygen delivery occurs because of decreased cardiac output or maldistribution of blood flow. Hypermetabolic states (sepsis, hyperthermia) may also increase oxygen requirements and may result in a cellular oxygen deficiency even with normal or greater than normal blood flow and oxygen delivery. This dysfunctional oxygen metabolism is worsened by the fact that mitochondrial oxygen utilization is impaired in septic shock.[76]

The relationship of oxygen delivery and consumption has been investigated in many conditions, including postoperative surgical patients, patients with acute respiratory distress syndrome (ARDS), sepsis, and hemorrhage.[31,32,81,82,170,260,261,298] Physiologically, oxygen consumption is independent of oxygen delivery above a certain critical point and over a wide range (Fig. 2-20). Below this critical point, oxygen consumption becomes limited by delivery, that is, it is delivery dependent. In critically ill patients, including children, oxygen consumption appears to become delivery dependent over a wide range of oxygen delivery. The relationship becomes linear and there is no plateau phase, and thus no critical point. This appears to be true whether the critically ill child is suffering from shock, sepsis, or ARDS or is in the postoperative state. Many investigators have attempted to determine if this limited

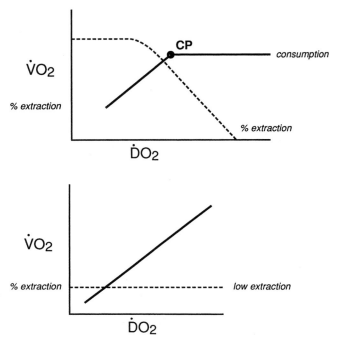

FIGURE 2-20   The top panel shows the normal relationship between oxygen consumption ($\dot{V}O_2$) and oxygen delivery ($\dot{D}O_2$). At a critical point (CP), consumption becomes delivery dependent. The oxygen extraction ratio is also shown as a percent versus delivery. The bottom panel represents the situation in critically ill patients. Consumption is delivery dependent, and extraction is low and constant.

oxygen delivery state is a unique pathologic feature of shock. Bihari and colleagues[31] reported that when oxygen delivery was increased by administration of prostacyclin, the prostacyclin-induced increase in oxygen uptake was greater in patients who subsequently died than in survivors. In survivors, the oxygen extraction ratio fell and mixed venous oxygen tension increased, as would be expected in a normal physiologic state. In patients who died, the extraction ratio actually rose and mixed venous oxygen tension remained the same. These data strikingly demonstrated that those patients in whom oxygen consumption becomes delivery dependent have a grave prognosis, and this severe physiologic derangement is associated with a poor outcome.

This pathologic supply dependency of oxygen consumption has suggested the need to maintain and enhance oxygen delivery in critically ill patients. Although it is a significant contributor, limited oxygen delivery is not the entire answer. Investigations attempting to augment oxygen delivery to improve oxygen utilization have had mixed results in improving patient morbidity and mortality.[81,82,119,272] The work of Shoemaker and colleagues[260,261] has probably most significantly demonstrated the efficacy of increasing oxygen delivery. Their studies have demonstrated that through the use of inotropic agents and augmentation of cardiac output with greater than normal oxygen delivery, which was associated with increased oxygen consumption, clinically significant decreased mortality and morbidity resulted. This has contributed to our realization that oxygen delivery and consumption must be critically evaluated in each critically ill child. Because pathologic occurrence of delivery-dependent oxygen consumption may be a factor in many illnesses, optimization of oxygen delivery is an important component of therapy. This can be checked by monitoring mixed venous oxygen tensions. Ideally, oxygen consumption should be measured and oxygen delivery increased until oxygen consumption reaches a plateau. This may be difficult in critically ill children and requires invasive monitoring. An indication of the underlying response to increased oxygen delivery can be obtained by monitoring mixed venous oxygen tension and acid-base balance. Interventions that increase mixed venous oxygen content are probably associated with the normal physiologic relationship or indicate that the patient has achieved adequate coupling of oxygen consumption and delivery.

CAUSES OF SHOCK

Shock is most frequently classified by the predominant pathophysiology present (Table 2-3). However, the predominant pathophysiology may change with time in the development of a persistent shock state. Further, shock may be considered in stages: compensated, uncompensated, and irreversible.

When the heart is the primary failing organ, cardiogenic shock results. Compensatory mechanisms maintain blood

Table 2-3   Classification of Shock

Cardiogenic
  Congenital heart disease
  Ischemic heart disease
    Anoxia
    Kawasaki disease
  Traumatic
  Infectious cardiomyopathies
  Drug toxicity
  Tamponade
Hypovolemic
  Dehydration
    Gastroenteritis
    Deprivation
    Heat stroke
  Burns
  Hemorrhage
Distributive
  Anaphylaxis
  Neurogenic
  Drug toxicity
  Septic
Neurogenic
Obstructive
  Left-sided
  Right-sided
  Tamponade
Septic Shock
Miscellaneous
  Heat stroke
  Pulmonary embolism
    Blood
    Air
    Fat
  Adrenal insufficiency
  Drug overdose
    Barbiturates
    Beta-antagonists

pressure (via vasoconstriction) at the cost of peripheral organ perfusion, to maintain blood flow to the brain and myocardium. When the child has experienced loss of circulating blood volume as the primary etiology, this is hypovolemic shock. The cardiovascular system will compensate to maintain blood pressure with increased cardiac performance but without adequate preload. Eventually, without adequate circulating volume, the heart and brain will be deprived of sufficient nutrient delivery. Neurogenic shock refers to loss of sympathetic nervous system regulation of the cardiovascular system. This may be due to catastrophic head injury or spinal injury or secondary to pharmacologic agents (e.g., local anesthetics) in the spinal fluid or epidural space. Some presentations of shock occur via mixed pathophysiology, including dysregulation of the heart and vascular control, as in septic shock and anaphylaxis. Each of these categories is discussed subsequently.

Eventually, compensatory mechanisms fail or inadequate perfusion of many organs results in accumulation of toxic products within the body, which further impairs cardiovascular function. Additionally, endothelial injury causes increased capillary permeability, which further reduces circulating volume and initiates a cycle of progressive cellular and organ dysfunction. After acute compensatory mechanisms are exhausted, the blood pressure will fall and inadequate perfusion and nutrient delivery will be exacerbated. This is uncompensated shock and it lasts only minutes to hours. If not treated aggressively, this progresses beyond an undefined meridian to become irreversible. No single biochemical or physiologic marker denotes the onset of irreversible shock. It is recognized by clinicians as that physiologic state that is unresponsive to all manipulations to support and promote homeostasis. Irreversible shock may last for minutes and result in cardiopulmonary collapse, but more frequently a state occurs in which the patient slowly loses previous improvements in physiologic signs. Biochemical evidence accumulates demonstrating onset of progressive multiorgan failure. This may occur over hours to days. Early recognition of and intervention for the compensated shock state may prevent further progression into the uncompensated and irreversible stages.

Hypovolemic Shock

The child with CHD may be the victim of trauma and hemorrhagic shock, as any other child. Hypovolemic shock can also result from vomiting and diarrhea, particularly in a child with underlying chronic disease, including CHD. Gastrointestinal bleeding can also result from hypoperfusion gastritis, ulcer formation, or ectopic tissue. Infants are at particularly significant risk. The ultimate result of the loss of circulating volume is inadequate organ perfusion. Even with a satisfactory or optimal cardiac performance, without preload, inadequate cardiac output will result. This may occur even with normal blood pressure, since the compensatory capabilities of the sympathetic nervous system are so significant. During this state, organ oxygen debt begins to accrue and the cells shift from aerobic (38 ATP/glucose) to much less energy-producing anaerobic metabolism (2 ATP/glucose). Eventually, a H^+ load will become sufficient to be excreted from cells and cause measurable systemic acidosis. Increased glucose utilization occurs, and infants and small children will exhaust their limited glucose/glycogen reserves. For these reasons, in children with impaired cardiac function, preload must be optimized. If the inadequate circulating volume is not restored, the progressive inadequate organ perfusion results in multiple organ failure. Urgent goals of therapy are to restore circulating volume and oxygen-carrying capacity. This will restore organ perfusion and oxygen delivery, and if therapeutic intervention occurs before degradation of cellular machinery, it will avoid the onset of organ failure.

Infants and children have a greater acute compensatory reserve than adults and can tolerate loss of as great as 30% of blood volume without hypotension. Adults become progressively more hypotensive starting at 15% loss. However, this acute compensation is short lived, and if hypotension occurs, the child is in life-threatening danger. Acute volume loss in the perioperative period may be occult and progressive if coagulopathy occurs. Since many anesthetic agents and hypothermia blunt the natural cardiovascular defenses, the child may succumb more quickly than anticipated. With the extensive monitoring and multiple tubes and drains that are used postoperatively after repair of CHD, extreme vigilance for blood loss is necessary.

Cardiogenic Shock

Cardiogenic shock is broadly defined as acute circulatory dysfunction caused by inadequate heart function. In pediatric critical care, cardiogenic shock is most frequently associated with cardiac surgery. The deleterious effects of CPB, ischemia, direct myocardial trauma, dysrhythmias, and tamponade lead to shock. Other children with unrepaired congenital defects may progress through advancing stages of heart failure in a subacute or chronic fashion to present in cardiogenic shock. Antineoplastic therapeutic agents (anthracyclines), radiation or idiopathic cardiomyopathies are occasionally seen. Underlying systemic conditions (mucopolysaccharidoses and glycogen storage diseases) eventually infiltrate the heart and result in heart failure. Hypermetabolic states also result in heart failure and shock (e.g., catecholamine-induced cardiomyopathy of pheochromocytoma and thyrotoxicosis). Rarely, a child will suffer acute myocardial infarction, or myocardial rupture or contusion secondary to trauma. Obstructive lesions to ventricular inflow and outflow (such as interrupted aortic arch or obstructive cardiomyopathy) can also be included here and are considered below.

As ventricular performance decreases for a given preload, stroke volume decreases. To compensate, heart rate increases. In infants, there is little capacity for improving maximal force (and thus stroke volume) during stress. Therefore, increased cardiac output relies on increased heart rate. When this compensatory activity fails, shock supervenes. If a stressed infant or child develops significant bradycardia without the capability of increasing stroke volume, cardiac output falls and shock ensues. Conversely, when tachydysrhythmias such as supraventricular tachycardia (SVT) or junctional ectopic tachycardia (JET) develop, there may be insufficient diastolic filling time to maintain sufficient stroke volume. Bradycardia and JET are poorly tolerated, and if not corrected, these dysrhythmias are progressively life threatening.

As cardiac failure progresses, multiple compensatory mechanisms occur (similar to hemorrhagic shock), but these become pathophysiologic and increase strain on the poorly functioning heart. The sympathetic nervous system acts as an integrated effector system that:

- Increases heart rate (± inotropy)
- Augments release of adrenomedullary catecholamines
- Increases adrenal aldosterone production and renal Na^+ reabsorption
- Increases vascular tone (afterload) (arterial > venous)
- Increases renin and angiotensin II release
- Increases vasopressin levels

These responses are activated within minutes and persist for hours to days until normal cardiac function is restored. If heart failure persists, this compensation may antagonize cardiac function by increased afterload (systemic vascular resistance), furthering its already weakened state. With augmented sympathetic nervous system activity, increased circulating catecholamines are present at sympathomyocyte junctions. As increased levels of these receptor ligands persist, beta-adrenergic receptor down regulation occurs.[38] This makes the heart less responsive to further stimulation and may explain how long-term increases in catecholamines eventually result in cardiomyopathy. Beta$_3$-adrenergic receptors have significant metabolic, anti-obesity, and insulinogenic effects but have also been found in the heart and circulation.[27,106] These receptors, which also respond to endogenous ligands, do not appear to internalize or down regulate to long-term exposure of catecholamines. They may also modulate a negative inotropic state and have been implicated in CHF.[106,107] As more knowledge of the actions of these receptors is gained, they may offer a new therapeutic approach.

Management of Cardiogenic Shock

Specific therapeutic goals in treatment of cardiogenic shock are to alleviate the etiology if possible, minimize cardiac oxygen demand, increase myocardial oxygen delivery, and blunt systemic responses to shock (such as compensatory sympathetic responses).

Treatment of cardiogenic shock includes use of pharmacologic agents to improve cardiac contractility (see Chapter 7). However, this therapy increases myocardial oxygen consumption and risks furthering myocardial ischemia and necrosis. Although dobutamine has been promoted as least injurious, the fact that it increases myocardial oxygen consumption while it may lower myocardial perfusion pressure at least suggests caution. Different practitioners favor different agents or combinations of agents. As newer agents have become available that work via non-beta-adrenergic mechanisms, it is possible to improve myocardial performance by alternate mechanisms when maximal beta-adrenergic stimulation has been achieved. Some of these agents (e.g., amrinone, milrinone) act via phosphodiesterase inhibition, which slows the breakdown of cyclic nucleotides and supports contractility.[72,159]

Use of nitrovasodilators is important to diminish the elevated systemic vascular tone and cardiac afterload. These agents (sodium nitroprusside and nitroglycerin) act by means of generation of NO or a related compound and mediate increases in cyclic GMP in vascular smooth muscle, resulting in relaxation.[190] This may reduce workload on the heart and thereby improve cardiac output. These agents are preferred postoperatively to the longer-acting ACE inhibitors, owing to their short half-lives.

Right ventricular failure may be responsive to decreasing PVR. This is accomplished with mild hyperventilation, hyperoxia, and alkalosis. Pharmacologic agents that decrease PVR include PGE_1, prostacyclin, and isoproterenol. Reports demonstrate the efficacy of inhaled NO,[233,235] and calcium channel antagonists (e.g., diltiazem) are currently in use in adult patients. Mechanical assistance is sometimes necessary to support infants and children in shock after CPB. This may include extracorporeal membrane oxygenation (ECMO), ventricular assist devices, or an intraaortic balloon pump and is discussed in Chapter 20.

Endocardial-Myocardial Failure

The critical interaction of endocardial-myocardial communication is being increasingly recognized. The endocardium is not merely a smooth-layered inner surface of the heart that acts as a conduit and to prevent platelet aggregation. It is now clear that the endocardium is a physiologically dynamic tissue that releases vasodilating prostanoids, NO, and vascular contracting factors, and modulates myocardial contractile tissue.[50,128,186,256]

With this rapidly advancing knowledge, it is clear that subendocardial ischemia risks loss of endothelial function. Further, with loss of pulsatile shear forces of circulating blood during CPB and hypothermic stresses, endothelial histologic changes are seen. As these histologic findings most probably herald functional changes, an understanding of these mechanisms of injury may advance the therapeutic options. Further, intracardiac suction systems disrupt circulating erythrocytes and leukocytes, and expose endocardial surfaces to the vacuum-induced shear forces and intracellular contents of disrupted cells.

Myocardial necrosis from global ischemia or oxygen debts during CPB or mismatched $\dot{D}O_2/\dot{V}O_2$ probably occurs more frequently than is diagnosed. In the post-CPB period, myocardial necrosis probably represents a very small percentage of tissue. However, as the myocardium is required to perform active work, this may worsen the state of other ischemic tissue until it also dies. When the cardiac performance is clinically inadequate, inotropic agents are often used to improve performance. This may aggravate already endangered myocardial tissue.

Right Ventricular Failure

Right ventricular failure is a more common problem in children than adults. Children far less frequently suffer from obstructive coronary artery disease (left ventricle affected), and many adults never advance to biventricular disease. In children, many obstructive lesions eventually result in right ventricular hypertrophy. Also, the right ventricle is used as the systemic ventricle for repair of hypoplastic left heart syndrome, and the longevity of the right ventricle used in this manner is unknown.[206] During CPB, the right ventricle is often the least hypothermic of the four chambers and may be at greater risk of ischemic damage. The approach to many complex repairs also includes right ventriculotomy. Pulmonary hypertension may coexist in the perioperative period, further challenging the right ventricle. For these reasons, the right ventricle is at particular risk for failure in infants and children; because of its strategic importance, when right ventricular performance is impaired, circulatory function is critically impaired.

As right ventricular failure occurs, septal motion into the left ventricle will decrease left ventricular outflow and increase left ventricular work. This is due to decreased EDV and lack of coordinated contribution of septal tissue to ejection. Cardiac output decreases further and venous return is impaired. Hepatic and splanchnic bed engorgement occurs. As cardiac output falls, compensatory sympathetic nervous system responses are invoked, as discussed previously.

Obstructive Shock

Obstructive shock is a paradigm invoked to relate all lesions capable of impairing forward cardiac output, thereby causing total body ischemia. These obstructions can be within the heart or extrinsic to the heart (within the pericardium, thorax, or great vessels).

Left-Sided Lesions

Obstruction of pulmonary venous return at the level of the pulmonary veins or the left atrium results in inadequate preload for the left ventricle. These obstructions include pulmonary venous hypoplasia, the membrane and embryonic remnants found in cor triatriatum, and valvular mitral stenosis. Any of these lesions results in inadequate left ventricular filling and inadequate cardiac output. Left ventricular outflow can be impaired by lesions of the ventricular septum (asymmetric septal hypertrophy), subaortic stenosis, or aortic valvular stenosis. Any of these lesions can provide significant resistance to left ventricular outflow, which necessitates increased left ventricular work to achieve adequate pressure to generate cardiac output. In asymmetric septal hypertrophy, the greater the contractility of the left ventricle, the greater is the resistance to outflow, because the muscular bundle increasingly obstructs the outflow tract. This dynamic obstruction requires restraint in use of inotropic agents until it is surgically corrected.

Aortic stenosis may present in infancy with critical stenosis resulting in severe left ventricular failure and shock, with dependency on the patency of the ductus arteriosus for systemic blood flow. Valvular stenosis is frequently associated with a bicuspid aortic valve and abnormal prenatal left ventricular development. Milder degrees of stenosis may be well tolerated and medically followed until surgical criteria are met. The significant increased wall tension imposed on the left ventricle contributes to inadequate subendocardial blood flow, and ischemia may develop insidiously, requiring close follow-up and eventually necessitating surgical repair of the lesion.

Supravalvular aortic stenosis, seen in Williams syndrome, can also present with significant obstruction to left ventricular outflow. Further, in the arch of the aorta, coarctation can present a significant obstructive lesion to cause shock. These patients, as well as patients with an interrupted aortic arch, are patent ductus dependent for blood flow to the descending aorta. As ductal flow decreases, these patients will present with shock. Discussion of these lesions is found in Chapters 26 and 27.

Dissection of the aorta can also cause an acute presentation of obstructive shock. These dissections may be acute as a result of trauma or may occur in patients with congenital syndromes of connective tissue disease such as Marfan syndrome.

Right-Sided Lesions

Impaired systemic venous return to the right side of the heart also diminishes preload to the left side. Tricuspid stenosis and pulmonic valvular stenosis prevent adequate pulmonary blood flow and result in cyanosis. In Ebstein's anomaly and tricuspid valve atresia, survival is compatible only with an alternative route of pulmonary blood flow. Left atrial, right atrial, right ventricular, and pulmonary vascular thrombosis or embolism can also result in obstructive shock. These lesions will prevent adequate left-sided return, and pulmonary embolism also induces right ventricular failure with bowing of the septum to the left, aggravating left ventricular outflow.

Tamponade

Cardiac tamponade is characterized by extrinsic resistance to ventricular diastolic relaxation. This impairs ventricular inflow and prevents adequate diastolic volume for ejection. Multiple lesions may be responsible for tamponade, including pericarditis, hemopericardium, pneumopericardium, severe pneumomediastinum, and tension pneumothorax. Fluid collections in the thorax (hydrothorax, hemothorax, chylothorax) can also embarrass cardiac function through a thoracic impedance mechanism. Each of these etiologies must be sought when a patient appears to be showing signs and symptoms of inadequate cardiac output.

Distributive Shock

Vascular tone is dynamic and highly integrated. The needs of each organ are regulated by various components: local mediators, neurovascular control, and humoral mechanisms. The delicate and highly integrated nature of vascular control allows for coordinated physiologic responses to various situations, including vigorous exercise and digestion, and responses to pathophysiologic states such as hypovolemia and hypoxia.

Distributive shock is a state of loss of this integrated control of the systemic vasculature. This may be due to loss of neurovascular control (neurogenic shock) or secondary to humoral mechanisms as in anaphylaxis with release of histamine, and loss of responsiveness of the vasculature to normal control mechanisms as a component of septic shock. Relatively inadequate circulating volume may be present when the systemic vasculature is excessively dilated. Hypotension results when the systemic vasculature does not respond to sympathetic innervation. Although circulating volume is normal and cardiac function may be adequate or supranormal, the systemic capacitance exceeds available volume and blood pressure falls. This may occur with administration of ganglionic blocking agents (trimethaphan) or sympatholytic agents (clonidine), anesthetics, or adrenergic blockers (e.g., prazosin, phentolamine, thorazine). Further, this situation is a major component of anaphylaxis, often mediated by histamine release. Other commonly used agents also release histamine, including morphine, neuromuscular blocking agents (curare), and many other drugs.[131,194,239]

Anaphylaxis is a state induced by the host response to a foreign antigen, with resultant production of immunoglobulin E (IgE). This reaction initiates a cascade of complex mechanisms invoking release of mediators from neutrophils, mast cells, eosinophils, and basophils. Complement is activated along with release of histamine, bradykinin, leukotrienes C_4 and D_4, eosinophilic chemotactic factor, and other vasoactive compounds. The ultimate clinical picture is one of severe vasodilation and hypotension. Cardiac performance may be directly impaired by some of these mediators (histamine and others), and preload is diminished secondary to venous pooling. The inability of homeostatic mechanisms to augment cardiac output and return the vascular tone to normal necessitates urgent resuscitation. Life-threatening bronchospasm or laryngospasm may be coexistent with the cardiovascular effects of this response. These patients require urgent volume resuscitation, vasopressor support (usually epinephrine), and airway management.

Almost any pharmacologic agent may act as a hapten that invokes an immune response and IgE production. This may result in anaphylaxis upon repeated exposure to the triggering agent or a related substance. The cross-reactivity of the many penicillin-related agents is well known, as well as the potential for reaction to the cephalosporin antibiotics. NPH insulin contains protamine, which has been suggested as a trigger for reactions to protamine after its administration at discontinuation of cardiopulmonary bypass.

Latex allergy and anaphylaxis have been increasingly recognized and reported in children and adults. Whether this is due to more frequent exposure of patients to latex from surgical procedures or environmental exposure, or due to changes in manufacturing processes and quality control, is debated. Anaphylaxis may occur upon exposure to latex in the operating room, catheterization laboratory, ICU, and any other facility where the child may come in contact with latex.

Children may also be exposed to other agents that produce a distributive shock state. These may include intoxications (accidental or self-inflicted) or iatrogenic exposures. Profound systemic vasodilation accompanies the use of large doses of major tranquilizers, barbiturates, and antihypertensives. Severe hypoglycemia, hypocalcemia, and hypermagnesemia may also result in vasodilation and hypotension, which require urgent recognition and therapy.

Neurogenic Shock

Neurogenic shock usually refers to loss of integrated sympathetic nervous system control over the cardiovascular system. Without sympathetic innervation, the parasympathetic innervation of the heart (vagus nerve) is left without antagonism. This results in bradycardia and diminished contractility. When the sympathetic innervation of the vascular system is lost, the capacitance increases dramatically (decreased systemic vascular resistance) and relative hypovolemia is present. This loss of sympathetic tone is the most dramatic representation of the complex integrity of vascular control. Neurogenic shock occurs from trauma to the cervical spinal cord, neural conduction blockade of the spinal and sympathetic outflow (spinal and epidural anesthesia), and catastrophic head injury. Although closed head trauma does not directly result in hypotension, premortal injury with loss of sympathetic centers in the hypothalamus and brainstem results in a pattern of neurogenic shock. In situations where myocardial function is unimpaired, administration of alpha-1 agonists like phenylephrine or norepinephrine recovers vascular tone, reduces the vascular capacitance, and improves the relative hypovolemia induced by the loss of vascular tone. Fluid administration improves the relative hypovolemia without affecting the vascular tone and is also effective in neurogenic shock.

Neurologic injury during cardiac surgery most likely involves the vagus and phrenic nerves and does not encompass loss of sympathetic outflow. These nerves can be injured by stretch, cold injury from ice solution, or transection. Also, despite intact neural activity, the heart and vasculature may respond poorly if hypothermia is present or if metabolic derangements persist (hyponatremia, hypocalcemia, hypomagnesemia, hypoglycemia, acidosis). After CPB, diffuse catastrophic neurologic injury may be heralded by hyperpyrexia, seizures, and excessive sympathetic activity, only to be followed by loss of central sympathetic tone. This portends a grim prognosis.

Another unique denervation situation is present after cardiac transplantation: The heart is denervated of both sympathetic and parasympathetic systems. The autonomous pacemakers of the donor heart will be the new natural heart rate, and contractility will also be unresponsive to nervous system activity. Nevertheless the heart will respond to endogenous circulating catecholamines and exogenous pharmacologic stimulants, of which isoproterenol is the most commonly used. Fortunately, it has been shown that reinnervation of the heart does occur over a period of years, with completion of reinnervation at 15 years after transplantation. This improves myocardial contractile function and response to exercise.[23] After cardiac transplantation, however, the nervous system control of vascular response should be unimpeded. There may be inappropriate bradycardia, which will respond to inotrope/chronotrope administration, and blood pressure and cardiac output should normalize.

Septic Shock

Septic shock is a clinical syndrome that results from the body's disproportionate inflammatory and procoagulation response to infection. It occurs during gram-negative and gram-positive bacteremia, fungemia, or viremia. Commonly responsible infectious agents are listed in Table 2-4. Shock may also be present when no microorganism is circulating but release of toxin has occurred, or when an inappropriate or excessive host immune response is activated. While there is a degree of ambiguity with regard to the definition of sepsis and its classification, cytokines, other inflammatory mediators, and coagulation factors have been found to play an important role in sepsis and may be used to better define the spectrum of sepsis in the future. The ongoing coagulopathy and consumption of coagulation factors present in sepsis and septic shock also play an important role in septic shock and are the target of many recent therapeutic investigations. Even when criteria of septic shock are not completely fulfilled, the hyperdynamic systemic inflammatory response syndrome may be present (Table 2-5) and heralds impending shock if not aggressively managed.[36]

Table 2-4 Pathogens Causing Septic Shock

Neonates
E. coli
Klebsiella species
Enterococcus species
Group B beta-hemolytic streptococci
Herpes simplex
Listeria monocytogenes
Staphylococcus aureus

Infants
Streptococcus pneumoniae
Neisseria meningitidis
Staphylococcus aureus
Haemophilus influenzae (non-typable)

Children
Enterobacteriaceae
Neisseria meningitidis
Staphylococcus aureus
Streptococcus pneumoniae

Immunocompromised Hosts
Candida species
Aspergillus species
Enterobacteriaceae
Pseudomonas species
Staphylococcus aureus
Staphylococcus epidermidis

The concept of the systemic inflammatory response syndrome (SIRS) has become a cornerstone of critical care medicine, both adult and pediatric.[5,48,86] Systemic release of inflammatory mediators occurs in critical illness apart from sepsis and infection, including in trauma, surgery, and shock from other states. Nevertheless the significant similarities in the pathways to tissue damage, endothelial dysfunction, cardiovascular dysregulation, and ongoing tissue damage with multiple organ dysfunction syndrome (MODS) have supported the concept of SIRS as a leading pathophysiologic unifier in critical care medicine. Although definitions are continually evolving, the general concept of fever, inflammation, and tissue damage gave rise to the concept of SIRS. Newer definitions seek to further define this syndrome (severe SIRS, SIRS without infection). This unifying concept has given rise to new theories in management of critically ill patients. The similarities between septic shock and SIRS should be remembered during the following discussion.

The septic state is characterized by early hyperdynamic cardiovascular function, which progresses to impaired or inadequate myocardial performance. Intravascular volume becomes inadequate for an increased systemic capacitance. The vascular smooth muscle is inappropriately unresponsive to vasoconstrictors, and maldistribution of cardiac output occurs, allowing organ and tissue ischemia to worsen. Beyond the physiologic characteristics of sepsis, there appears to be an oxygen utilization defect, whereupon cells do not extract or utilize oxygen appropriately even when delivered.[76]

Sepsis is a life-threatening condition in children and adults alike. Multiple alterations in cellular bioenergetics occur. Hemodynamic alterations in sepsis are well described and include tachycardia, arterial and venous dilation, relative or absolute hypovolemia, and abnormal cardiac function. Vascular dysfunction in sepsis presents as globally reduced

Table 2-5 Definitions of Infections and Inflammatory Syndromes

Infection	Microbial phenomenon characterized by an inflammatory response to the presence of microorganisms or the invasion of normally sterile host tissue by those organisms
Bacteremia	The presence of viable bacteria in the blood
Systemic inflammatory response syndrome	Systemic inflammatory response to a variety of severe clinical insults; the response is manifested by two or more of the following conditions: Temperature > 38° or < 36° C Heart rate > 90 beats/min Respiratory rate > 20 breaths/min or $PaCO_2$ < 32 mm Hg (< 4.3 kPa) WBC > 12,000 cells/mm³, < 4000 cells/mm³, or 10% immature (band) forms
Sepsis	Systemic response to infection, manifested by two or more of the following conditions as a result of infection: Temperature > 38° or < 36° C Heart rate > 90 beats/min Respiratory rate > 20 breaths/min or $PaCO_2$ < 32 mm Hg (< 4.3 kPa) WBC > 12,000 cells/mm³, < 4000 cells/mm³, or 10% immature (band) forms
Severe sepsis	Sepsis associated with organ dysfunction, hypoperfusion, or hypotension; hypoperfusion and perfusion abnormalities may include, but are not limited to, lactic acidosis, oliguria, or an acute alteration in mental status.
Septic shock	Sepsis with hypotension, despite adequate fluid resuscitation, along with the presence of perfusion abnormalities that may include, but are not limited to, lactic acidosis, oliguria, or an acute alteration in mental status; patients who are on inotropic or vasopressor agents may not be hypotensive at the time that perfusion abnormalities are measured.
Hypotension	A systolic blood pressure of < 90 mm Hg or a reduction of > 40 mm Hg from baseline in the absence of other causes for hypotension
Multiple organ dysfunction syndrome	Presence of altered organ function in an acutely ill patient such that homeostasis cannot be maintained without intervention

Hemodynamic values are based on adult data. Age-appropriate values should be used for children. WBC, white blood cell count.
From American College of Chest Physicians/Society of Critical Care Medicine Consensus Conference: Definitions for sepsis and organ failure and guidelines for the use of innovative therapies in sepsis. *Crit Care Med* 1992;20:864–874; with permission.

systemic vascular resistance. Although many vascular beds are dilated, there appear to be areas of microcirculatory vasoconstriction, resulting in a maldistribution of oxygen and nutrient delivery. The mechanisms involved are unclear. Damage to endothelium may occur primarily or may be secondary to the release of many compounds from neutrophils. Many inflammatory mediators have been implicated as causes of endothelial damage, including prostaglandins, leukotrienes, NO, tumor necrosis factor, and interleukins.[221]

The systemic vasculature appears to progress to a state of less vascular tone and greater capacitance. Permeability of microvasculature is also altered. Three mechanisms for this vasodilation during sepsis and the later phases of other shock states have been proposed. They include activation of the inducible form of NOS, activation of ATP-sensitive potassium channels, and vasopressin deficiency. Along with the induction of the macrophage isoform of NOS in sepsis, the constitutive isoform(s) of NOS also increases. NO activates myosin light-chain phosphatase by directly activating cGMP. It may also cause vasodilation by activating calcium-sensitive potassium channels in the plasma membrane of vascular smooth-muscle cells. These potassium channels are thought to be sensitive to the influx of cytosolic calcium, and once the calcium activates them, they hyperpolarize the plasma membrane and prevent further vasoconstriction. Although early work in septic, hypotensive animals using inhibitors of NOS has demonstrated improved arterial pressure, an improved outcome has not been a consistent finding.[201] This is also true in human studies.[68,223] Another proposed mechanism of vasodilation is activation of ATP-sensitive potassium channels. The opening of these channels allows an efflux of potassium, thus hyperpolarizing the plasma membrane and preventing the entry of calcium into the cell. These ATP-sensitive

potassium channels are activated by decreases in the cellular ATP concentration and by increases in the cellular concentrations of hydrogen ions and lactate. Thus, under circumstances of increased tissue metabolism or tissue hypoxia, these channels cause vasodilation. A final mechanism for vasodilation is vasopressin hormone deficiency. Vasopressin appears to act on the vasculature in a number of ways. It directly inactivates the ATP-sensitive potassium channels in vascular smooth muscle, potentiates the vasoconstrictor effects of norepinephrine, blunts the increase in cGMP induced by natriuretic peptides and NO, and decreases the synthesis of inducible NOS that is initiated by lipopolysaccharide. With the intense osmotic stimulation and, possibly, continuous baroreflex stimulation seen in septic shock and late stages of other shock states, neurohypophyseal stores of vasopressin may be exhausted.[158]

Although the sympathetic nervous system is responsive with greater activity, the vasculature appears to be less responsive to adrenergic stimulation.[18] An uncoupling of receptor-contractile element response appears to play a role.[263] However, appearance of endogenous inhibitors of contractile mechanisms (e.g., opioid peptides, NO) may contribute to this reduced responsiveness.[103] A loss of constitutive vasoconstrictive factors might also explain the vasodilated state. Regional vascular responses to sepsis have been investigated[203,243] as well as the response to inhibitors of prostaglandin synthesis and other mediators. Current investigations are focusing on the cellular and molecular mechanisms of the loss of receptor-mediated responses and inhibition of contractile elements.

The regional dysregulation impairs oxygen delivery to cells, and most therapy for sepsis is aimed at restoring or augmenting cardiorespiratory function and oxygen delivery.

Nonetheless, many patients progress to multiple organ failure and death. Because inflammatory and procoagulant host responses to infection are closely related, new therapies are being targeted at controlling the host-mediator response. Inflammatory cytokines, including TNF-α, IL-1β, and IL-6, are able to activate coagulation and inhibit fibrinolysis, whereas the procoagulant thrombin is capable of initiating multiple inflammatory pathways. The end result may be diffuse endovascular injury, multiorgan dysfunction, and death.[28] The host response to microbial invasion appears to be at least a significant contribution to mortality, but inhibitors of inflammatory mediator action (monoclonal antibodies to TNF, soluble receptors to TNF, and interleukin receptor antagonists) have failed to show benefit in clinical trials.[1,209,221] Nevertheless, inhibition of tumor necrosis factor remains an important target in preventing SIRS-induced injury.[7] A number of other studies have targeted the procoagulant response. The diffuse thrombus formation throughout the microcirculation compromises tissue perfusion to critical organs and causes multiorgan dysfunction. Recent studies utilizing high-dose antithrombin III and recombinant tissue factor pathway inhibitor to prevent diffuse coagulation in adults with severe sepsis have not shown improved outcomes.[2,306] Nevertheless, the PROWESS Study Group recently published modestly encouraging results for administration of human activated protein C (APC) in severe sepsis.[28] APC appears to intervene at multiple points during the systemic response to infection. It exerts an antithrombotic effect by inactivating factors Va and VIIIa, limiting the generation of thrombin. As a result of decreased thrombin levels, the inflammatory, procoagulant, and antifibrinolytic response induced by thrombin is reduced. APC also exercises an antiinflammatory effect by inhibiting the production of inflammatory cytokines (IL-1β, and IL-6) by monocytes and reducing the rolling of monocytes and neutrophils on injured endothelium by binding selectins.[28] APC indirectly enhances the fibrinolytic response by inhibiting plasminogen-activator inhibitor 1. The PROWESS Study Group showed an absolute reduction of mortality by 6.1% with administration of APC during the 28-day study period, when compared to a placebo group, and a significant reduction in serum IL-6 and D-dimer levels.[28] The adults that benefited the most from APC were the ones with the highest mortality risk. However, APC demonstrated a higher risk of serious bleeding than in the placebo group.[28] Because of its thrombolytic activity, contraindications to APC include active internal bleeding or trauma and intracranial pathology that create an unacceptable risk of life-threatening bleeding. In an open label, nonrandomized trial by Barton and colleagues, it was found that the pharmacokinetics, pharmacodynamic effects, and safety profile of APC in pediatric patients are similar to those previously published for adult patients. A large, phase 3, randomized, placebo-controlled study is ongoing, but the current literature does not support routine use of APC for children with septic shock at this time.[20]

Pathophysiology

The pathophysiology of septic shock has been described best for gram-negative bacteremia, but parallel events occur in progression of the shock state caused by gram-positive bacteria, fungus, rickettsia, and viral infections.[221] Each of the many organisms responsible form a nidus of infection, which may be in peripheral tissue or have direct access to the bloodstream via an intravascular catheter. As proliferation of the organism continues, there is continued release of increasing quantities of endotoxin or exotoxins into the bloodstream. These toxins elicit a host response comprising release of endogenous mediators from monocytes and activated macrophages, endothelial cells, and lymphocytes.[220] Along with the release of these mediators, there may be changes in gene expression within endothelial cells and myocytes, which are responsible for progressive organ dysfunction.[51,75,221,296] No organ is spared, since the endothelium is present in all. The most vital organs affected include the heart and lungs, CNS, kidneys, and gastrointestinal tract, along with the liver. Endothelial injury or metabolic responses are responsible for activation of the coagulation system, which will also become dysfunctional.[278]

The cardiovascular function in septic shock among adults and teenagers is often hyperdynamic initially, with apparently normal or elevated cardiac output and oxygen delivery, low systemic vascular resistance, and decreased arteriovenous oxygen difference. With systemic vasodilation, the patient appears warm, with bounding pulses and well perfused. However, infants and young children with septic shock are more likely to present with low cardiac output and increased systemic vascular resistance. The child may experience normal mentation or mild agitation, irritability, or restlessness. Fever is frequent but not universal. The autonomic nervous system is activated and there is increased heart rate and respiratory rate and decreased splanchnic perfusion. Urine output may appear satisfactory but will taper off as the glomerular filtration rate begins to decline with less renal blood flow.

Although the cardiovascular system appears hyperdynamic, and tachycardia is mediated via the sympathetic nervous system and adrenal catecholamines, ventricular function is abnormal. Left and right ventricles become dilated and the ejection fraction is diminished.[200,208,216,221] Increasing preload may augment stroke volume, but the contractile curve has shifted down and to the right. The etiology of the impaired myocardial function is probably multifactorial.

Extensive investigations in animal models and administration of small doses of endotoxin to humans have provided much information. Endotoxin or gram-positive bacteria injected into animals produce the same cardiovascular responses seen in septic shock.[199] Host molecules such as TNF and interleukins partially mediate the dysfunction initiated by endotoxin.[30,221] Global myocardial ischemia has also been implicated as the cause of myocardial depression in sepsis. Cunnion and associates[79] measured coronary blood flow during septic shock in humans and found that patients in septic shock appear to have adequate coronary blood flow. This argues against myocardial depression being due to ischemia. Circulating cardiodepressant factors have been found in the serum of patients in septic shock.[219,229] These are lipid soluble, low-molecular-weight compounds that demonstrate negative inotropic activity on beating cells in culture.[79] One or more of these host molecules may be responsible for the impaired cardiac performance noted.

Macrophages, endothelium, and endocardium are stimulated by TNF or endotoxin to produce NO. Along with its ability to vasodilate, NO is a direct negative inotrope in cell culture.[39,97] Augmented gene expression of NOS may be responsible for endocardial-mediated myocardial dysfunction.

Changes in vascular smooth muscle responsiveness to adrenergic agonists have been noted during sepsis. Circulating antagonists of the alpha-adrenergic receptor (mediating vasoconstriction) have not been found. However, dissociation of the adrenergic receptor from its signal transduction mechanism may be responsible for impaired response of the smooth muscle contractile mechanisms.[58,321] G-protein linked mechanisms and several others have been postulated as mediating receptor responsiveness in sepsis.[182,210,254]

Prostaglandin and leukotriene metabolism is also affected in sepsis. The imbalance created between the vasoconstrictor and vasodilator prostanoids may be responsible for pulmonary hypertension, as well as maldistribution of blood flow in the systemic circulation.[221] Local changes in endothelial function and production of prostanoid mediators may explain microvascular dysregulation with apparent adequate oxygen delivery in the macrocirculation, which is never available to cells due to microvascular plugging, or constriction.[221]

Cellular Metabolism

Beyond the cardiovascular and endothelial perturbations that occur in septic shock, much research has focused on the cellular metabolic effects that occur and explain the lack of oxygen utilization even when oxygen has been delivered in appropriate quantities.[135] The physiologic description of sepsis being a "delivery-dependent" oxygen consumption state has fostered the popular notion that sepsis induces cellular hypoxia by inadequate oxygen delivery.[316] However, many other metabolic abnormalities have also been noted, and, further, when a potential oxygen debt has been alleviated, there are continuing cellular metabolic derangements. Investigators have looked more closely at cellular physiology to determine if there are defects in energy-producing pathways, excessive energy utilization, or dysregulation of energy production.[76,135] When inadequate oxygen is available, cellular pathways move to anaerobic metabolism, with an increased generation of lactate. The formation of lactate does not necessarily correspond with increased H^+ production. The acidosis that often accompanies excessive lactate production is due to increased ATP utilization within the cells. When ATP is utilized, it is through a hydrolytic reaction that releases one H^+ ion for each ATP hydrolyzed.

Elevated lactate levels in children after cardiac surgery have been found to be associated with a high mortality in critically ill children.[125] Nevertheless there has been some disagreement over the usefulness of monitoring lactate levels after cardiac surgery.[126,195,262] One study, in support of its usefulness, showed that an elevated postoperative lactate level of more than 4.2 mmol/L had a positive predictive value of 100% and a negative predictive value of 97% for postoperative death.[262] Another study noted that a change in lactate level of more than 3 mmol/L during CPB had a sensitivity of 82% and a specificity of 80% for mortality, but the positive predictive value was low.[195] Finally, one study showed a positive predictive value of 32%.[126] While it seems that there is some conflict as to the validity of serum lactate levels as prognostic indicators in the postoperative period for children

after cardiac surgery, this measurement may be a stronger indicator of outcome when other tests, such as mixed venous saturation, and clinical signs and symptoms are taken into account.

Lactate levels are often, but not consistently, elevated in sepsis.[135] In addition increasing oxygen delivery does not always improve the hyperlactatemia.[300] It has also been reported that sepsis impairs cellular pyruvate dehydrogenase, an enzyme that regulates metabolism of glucose. More recent studies demonstrate that alterations occur within the glycolytic pathway and that increased glycolytic activity may occur even when the cells are not oxygen deprived.[293,317]

Hotchkiss and others[136,137,144,265] have used phosphorus 31 nuclear magnetic resonance (NMR) spectroscopy to examine cellular bioenergetics. In multiple elegant studies studying separate organ energetics, these investigators have been unable to demonstrate any depletion of high-energy phosphates early in the course of sepsis in laboratory animals. This appears to be true in both the brain and the heart during periods in which clinical symptoms of nervous system involvement or heart failure occur. These findings raise the possibility of direct sepsis-induced dysregulation of other cellular functions, rather than limitation of oxygen delivery.[76] As our understanding of gene expression during sepsis improves, and our ability to look at enzyme function at the cellular level is more precise, we may begin to elucidate the true biochemical irregularities induced by sepsis.

Most therapy employed for sepsis centers on cardiopulmonary support and oxygen delivery. Sepsis results from the complex interaction among endothelium, inflammatory cells, multiple mediators, coagulation factors, metabolic pathways, cellular organelles, cellular ion channels, and hormones. To reduce the morbidity and mortality of sepsis, future therapies must focus on multiple points and their interactions.

Miscellaneous Causes of Shock

Less frequent causes of shock include multiple endocrine etiologies, severe anemia, acute metabolic derangements, anaphylactic reactions, and drug overdoses. Endocrine pathology includes adrenal insufficiency, hypothyroidism, hyperthyroidism, and pheochromocytoma.

Adrenal insufficiency may present as shock in an insidious fashion. In adrenal insufficiency, lack of glucocorticoid production results in impaired myocardial performance and smooth muscle responsiveness to stimuli for constriction. Both cardiac myocytes and vascular smooth muscle cells have cytoplasmic glucocorticoid receptors.[295] Activation of these receptors by endogenous glucocorticoids appears essential for optimal contractile force generation. In adrenal insufficiency, not only will orthostatic hypotension occur secondary to volume depletion (as cortisol also has mineralocorticoid properties), but there is also inadequate cardiac output and vascular responsiveness to sympathetic stimulation. A child with adrenal insufficiency may appear to be suffering from distributive or cardiogenic shock. The most common cause for adrenal insufficiency is acute withdrawal from exogenous pharmacologic steroid therapy, with insufficient weaning for recovery of the hypothalamic-pituitary-adrenal axis. Adrenal hemorrhage may occur with overwhelming sepsis (Waterhouse-Friderichsen syndrome) or secondary to ischemia.[67]

Hypothyroidism has been characterized for decades as an occult etiology of heart failure, and in children it can also be elusive. The child who remains vasopressor dependent or requires assisted ventilation without obvious cause should be suspected of being hypothyroid. Hyperthyroidism and pheochromocytoma appear to induce a hyperdynamic state, which results in either fatigue or receptor downregulation, and shock. After a period of compensatory activity, the patient begins to demonstrate signs of cardiovascular failure. With hyperpyrexia, excessive fluid losses, and exhausted cardiovascular compensation, the child may become subacutely or acutely disoriented and hypovolemic, and suffer cardiopulmonary arrest.

Hypocalcemia, acute or secondary to hypoparathyroidism, may also impair cardiac and vascular smooth muscle contractility and needs to be considered early in the care of the child after correction of congenital heart defects. Hypocalcemia, when it occurs, is not primarily due to hypoparathyroidism, but more frequently from Ca^{++} chelation by citrate and ethylenediaminetetraacetic acid (EDTA) used as blood preservatives. Infants with congenital anomalies of the great vessels may have hypoparathyroidism and immunodeficiency (DiGeorge syndrome). These infants may require continuous calcium supplementation in the perioperative period to maintain cardiac function, vascular smooth muscle contractility, and respiratory muscle sufficiency and to prevent tetany and seizures.

Severe hemolytic anemia will place severe stress on the cardiopulmonary system to improve oxygen delivery. This may occur as a result of "jetting" around artificial valves, and occasionally the hemolysis may be severe. Patients with severe anemia (hemoglobin as low as 1.5 g/dL) have been reported to survive, but signs and symptoms of heart failure and shock were clearly present. Therapy is directed at improving oxygen carrying capacity by slow, cautious transfusion while avoiding the consequences of fluid overload.

Anaphylaxis is a catastrophic presentation of reaction by host immune response to a foreign material. Anaphylaxis will present with severe vasodilation and hypotension, and may or may not evoke cardiac failure; it may or may not occur upon the first presentation of an agent. Similarly, some drugs will result in moderately severe release of histamine, which will cause vascular dilation and possibly impaired myocardial performance. One such drug is vancomycin. When anaphylaxis is suspected, the initiating agent should be stopped and removed if possible, and intense cardiovascular support may be required for minutes to hours as the body begins to recover from this insult. Blood transfusion reactions may also cause hemodynamic instability.

Protamine used to reverse the anticoagulant effect of heparin may induce severe, life-threatening pulmonary hypertension with right ventricular failure, decreased venous return to the left ventricle, and shock. Urgent therapy involves stopping protamine administration, use of pulmonary vasodilator therapy, and improving cardiac output and systemic blood pressure; it may necessitate a return to CPB.

Many pharmacologic agents can result in cardiovascular collapse, including sedatives such as barbiturates (direct negative inotropic agents), chloral hydrate (ventricular dysrhythmias), beta-blockers, calcium channel blockers, alpha-adrenergic blockers, and many others. Barbiturates act as cardiac depressants along with other anesthetic agents. Any of these agents in sufficient dose may cause cardiogenic or mixed cardiogenic/distributive shock. It is vital to review the list of medications and concentrations of medications being received by the patient to make sure that accurately prescribed and appropriate doses are being used.

THERAPEUTIC STRATEGIES

Intensive care for children with critical heart disease includes sophisticated ventilatory support, monitoring, and therapeutic manipulation of the hemodynamic status. With a wealth of therapeutic modalities available, the clinician sets goals to achieve optimal cardiac function and systemic blood flow, and improved organ blood flow. This must be done while minimizing cardiac and other organ ischemia. Medical therapy may optimize the patient's condition preoperatively for the stress of surgical intervention and provide necessary support after surgery. Children with uncompensated heart failure can be returned to a state of compensation, allowing discharge from the ICU. Despite maximal pharmacotherapy, some children require complex circulatory assist technology, which may include ECMO, aortic balloon pump, or ventricular assist devices. These technologies are discussed in Chapter 21.

This chapter cannot address all the issues involved in the treatment of the various shock states. Detailed therapy for many of these conditions is the subject of multiple chapters throughout this book. Our purpose here is to briefly outline general principles underlying the treatment of all cardiovascular dysfunction and to address some specific therapeutic tools.

Respiratory Care

In all forms of resuscitation, it is essential to ensure that the airway and respiratory status are secure. Because further hypoxia, caused by airway involvement, sudden respiratory arrest, or respiratory failure, can catastrophically worsen the outcome from shock, early intervention is indicated. In addition, circulatory dysfunction involves the respiratory muscles and can lead to impaired respiratory muscle function.[15] In children, respiratory compensation occurs but can deteriorate rapidly in the face of acute circulatory dysfunction, leading to either apnea or inability to maintain adequate ventilation. The addition of respiratory failure to cardiovascular failure should be assiduously avoided. For these reasons, oxygen is required for all patients with circulatory impairment and should be immediately provided. Acute cardiovascular decompensation, such as may occur in the ICU, should be responded to by the initiation of 100% inspired oxygen, at least transiently until the child's hemodynamic status is stabilized. If there is the slightest question of impending respiratory failure or airway compromise, the airway should be secured by endotracheal intubation. Postoperatively, the addition of a thoracotomy and pulmonary trauma generally require intubation and ventilation. Nevertheless, it cannot be too strongly emphasized that, even if children are capable of breathing on their own and have a normal airway, intubation and ventilatory support should be continued until the hemodynamic status is certainly secured and hemodynamic stability can be relied on. If there is any potential for acute deterioration, such as cardiac dysrhythmias or hypotension, it is wise to provide mechanical ventilatory support until this has been adequately addressed. Mechanical ventilation alleviates the metabolic and energy demands of breathing (in some cases by as much as 20% to 30%) and removes the negative intrathoracic pressure and its effects on cardiac afterload. Cautious weaning of children from mechanical ventilation after cardiac surgery or in other shock states is necessary to ensure that they can tolerate the work of breathing and the effects of cardiorespiratory interactions. Once airway, breathing, and oxygenation are assured, specific cardiovascular therapy for shock should be rapidly initiated.

Treating the Underlying Condition

In any form of shock, the underlying and inciting condition must be addressed in addition to the general measures taken. For example, in septic shock the appropriate antibiotics must be administered in the appropriate doses. In obstructive shock, although hemodynamic support may be temporizing, surgery or catheter-based intervention is essential. Also, in patients with hypoplastic left heart syndrome, the low cardiac output cannot be adequately alleviated without some pulmonary-to-systemic shunt, such as medically opening the ductus arteriosus, or definitive surgery. Attempts to treat shock are merely temporizing and should not be unduly prolonged before surgical intervention.

Because brief periods of hypotension and hypoperfusion gravely alter the prognosis, great attention is focused on the blood pressure. In children with septic shock, early aggressive volume replacement improves survival, especially for those children receiving more than 40 mL/kg of fluid in the first hour of presentation to the emergency department.[58] This successful philosophy of early management of septic shock has been shown in a recent adult study on early goal-directed therapy in severe sepsis and septic shock by Rivers and colleagues. By tightly controlling CVP (8 to 12 mm Hg), MAP (≥ 60 and $90 \geq$ mm Hg), and central venous oxygen saturation ($\geq 70\%$) by aggressive fluid resuscitation, use of vasoactive and inotropic agents, and maintaining a hematocrit of 30% or greater, a statistically significant reduction of in-hospital mortality rate was found.[234] The central venous oxygen saturation reasonably approximates the mixed venous oxygen saturation found in the main pulmonary artery. By using the central venous oxygen saturation as an indicator of balance between systemic oxygen delivery and oxygen demand, this study emphasizes that the maintenance of blood pressure certainly is a first goal in the therapy of any type of shock; however, it is not the end point. Adequate blood pressure may exist with inadequate cardiac output and insufficient oxygen delivery. It should be remembered that blood pressure is the product of systemic resistance and the cardiac output, which is the product of stroke volume times heart rate. Bearing this in mind, it is important that an optimal heart rate and rhythm be assured. The issue of heart rate and cardiac output in the shock state or in states of acute circulatory dysfunction is discussed in Chapter 8.

Stroke Volume

Stroke volume is determined by preload, afterload, and contractility, as discussed. In treating a child with inadequate

circulatory function, all of these factors must be considered. Specific therapeutic modalities should be selected to address each issue. Additionally, many therapeutic interventions will affect multiple parameters and full understanding of their action is necessary. For example, inotrope therapy, which also increases heart rate, may not be acting by increasing contractility, but merely by increasing cardiac output through increased heart rate. Also, the use of an inotrope that improves myocardial function and compliance characteristics, thus lowering right atrial pressure, does not necessarily mean that preload has been decreased. Indeed, the lower right atrial pressure may allow increased stroke volume, for reasons discussed previously. Thus, when any therapeutic intervention is made, its effect on all of the parameters that determine blood pressure and cardiac output must be considered.

Preload

In the setting of inadequate preload, vascular damage, abnormal plasma oncotic pressure, and perturbed endothelial barrier function, the selection of fluid for intravascular volume is complex.[115,141,142,202,301,304,305] It is now commonplace to say that the battle between the choice of crystalloid and colloid has raged for many years in critical care.[80,167] Surely this is based on the fact that both intravascular volume expansion approaches have merit. Because clinical settings occur in which it is appropriate to give crystalloid or colloid, the clinician must be familiar with both sides of this argument.[83,96] The physician who deals with the postoperative cardiac patient must additionally be familiar with the many years of clinical trials comparing crystalloid and colloid solutions in the management of circulatory compromise.[141,301]

As the Starling equation states, the hydrostatic and oncotic pressures are important. It is the filtration coefficient (K_{fc}) that is related to vessel permeability to small molecules that is significantly altered in shock states. As seen in the Starling equation, the reflection coefficient (σ) represents the ability of the capillary membrane to prevent large molecules, such as plasma proteins, from crossing.[141] In shock states with significant endotheliopathy, the use of colloids when σ is altered is not helpful.

Shock caused by volume loss produced by burns, severe sepsis, or CPB occurs in part because of free transudation of colloids into the interstitial space.[141] This increases perimicrovascular oncotic pressures and tends to decrease the effectiveness of intravascular fluid expansion. In this clinical setting, it may not be quite so beneficial to give colloid-bearing fluids because they will leak and aggravate the problem. Interstitial fluid abnormalities and interstitial edema are part of the shock process and not determined by the type of fluid replacement. Furthermore, it is possible to have inadequate circulating blood volume in the face of edema, and edema itself does not indicate fluid overload.

There is experimental evidence of varying degrees of quality that supports both sides of the argument. The goal of fluid therapy is to maintain adequate preload without increasing edema. The advantages of the use of crystalloids are ready availability, lack of complications, low cost, and physiologic compatibility. The advantages of colloids are that (allegedly) they maintain intravascular volume longer and decrease the amount of edema (Table 2-6). From the outset, it should be realized

Table 2-6 Crystalloid Versus Colloid

CRYSTALLOID	
Pros	**Cons**
Inexpensive, readily available, no risk of anaphylaxis, physiologically compatible, replete interstitial space, readily diuresed	Limited intravascular volume expansion: < 30% for any clinically significant period of time; increased interstitial fluid, increased edema
COLLOID	
Pros	**Cons**
Prolonged intravascular retention, maintenance of colloid oncotic pressure, theoretically reduced interstitial fluid and edema	Expensive, anaphylaxis, coagulopathic, risk of infections, increased perimicrovascular oncotic pressure and hence leak from intravascular space

that in most shock states intravascular volume is not the only parameter disturbed by abnormalities in fluid and electrolyte balance. In hemorrhagic shock, the interstitial space also becomes depleted of both electrolytes and fluids, owing to autotransfusion. This necessitates resuscitation to maintain interstitial fluid volume as well. The derangements that occur in more chronic forms of circulatory insufficiency, such as chronic CHF when there may be a total body excess of fluid and electrolytes, are more complex. This problem is compounded by the fact that it is extremely difficult in the emergent situation to tell the difference between low output cardiac failure due to impaired contractility with high filling pressures and low output due to preload limitation, which in the injured heart may also be associated with high filling pressures.

Crystalloid Versus Colloid

In analysis of both crystalloid and colloid therapy in clinical trials, it was concluded that after trauma or in instances when the capillaries demonstrated increased permeability, resuscitation with crystalloids was most efficacious.[141] In other circumstances, including major elective surgery, there was a suggestion that mortality rates were lowered by the use of colloids. In a meta-analysis of select, adult, randomized trials of crystalloid versus colloid resuscitation by Choi and colleagues,[63] it was concluded that there was no overall difference in pulmonary edema, mortality, or length of stay between isotonic crystalloid and colloid resuscitation. Interestingly, they did find a statistically significant difference in mortality for trauma patients in favor of crystalloid resuscitation upon subgroup analysis.[63] Another important systematic review of randomized controlled trials by the Cochrane Injuries Group Albumin Reviewers found that there was a relative risk of death with albumin administration of 1.68 (95% CI of 1.26 to 2.23) compared to crystalloid solutions in critically ill patients with hypovolemia, burns, or hypoalbuminemia.[138] Nonetheless, it is difficult to interpret these meta-analyses because of the inclusion of heterogeneous groups of disease processes and resuscitation fluids.

There have been numerous studies supporting either crystalloid or colloid and the controversy still continues after 20 years of trials. The desired end point should determine the use of fluids. In the immediate postoperative period, if pure hypovolemia is the problem (not complicated by coagulopathy, bleeding diathesis, or demonstrable hypoproteinemia), then crystalloid is the fluid of choice. In children at risk for hypoglycemia, in infants younger than 6 months to 1 year of age, and in those who have had demonstrable hypoglycemia, dextrose-containing solutions should be used. When pure 5% or 10% dextrose is used, less than 10% of this fluid will remain in the intravascular space for an hour or so. Thus, the contribution to sustained intravascular volume expansion is minimal. Isotonic solutions such as saline or Ringer's lactate provide better intravascular filling, with 25% to 30% of crystalloid infusion remaining in the circulation for 1 to 2 hours. The use of hypertonic saline solutions has also been advocated, and small volumes of hypertonic solutions have produced improvement after hemorrhagic and septic shock.[141,212,301,303] The fear of sodium overload in the post-CPB period limits the use of these solutions, although some centers have reported the early use of hypertonic saline solutions in the immediate post-CPB period.[301] The risk of these lies in sodium overload, and their use in neonates with poor sodium handling is probably contraindicated.

Colloids may be indicated in profound hypoproteinemia or hypoalbuminemia, or when replacement therapy is indicated.[115] If bleeding diathesis is present or if there is difficulty in coagulation, fresh frozen plasma is the colloid of choice. The most expensive colloids are albumin and fresh frozen plasma.[115,141,304,305] Other colloids, including hydroxyethyl starches such as hetastarch, are less expensive and provide prolonged volume expansion with 50% to 75% remaining intravascular for longer than 1 hour. The dextrans have all but been abandoned for use in children due to fears of coagulopathy, impaired renal function, and risk of anaphylaxis.[202] It is our recommendation to replace intravascular volume via an approach similar to that taken for blood component therapy. When it is salt and water that is lacking, as in most cases, crystalloid solutions are adequate. If hypoproteinemia or coagulopathy persists, these should be appropriately restored, realizing that they are adding intravascular volume. If the hematocrit is unacceptably low, blood transfusion is the preferred fluid for intravascular volume expansion.

The use of blood products in volume augmentation should be guided by hematocrit, intravascular volume, and the type of fluid loss. Clearly, in acute hemorrhagic shock, replacement with whole fresh blood is ideal. Patients who are hemodiluted with low hematocrit and protein content after CPB should receive whole fresh blood or component therapy, including packed red cells and fresh frozen plasma as indicated. Administration of large volumes of packed red cells without concurrent administration of fresh frozen plasma may result in a dilutional coagulopathy.

The practitioner must be familiar with the agents available for intravascular volume expansion and their complications.[115,141,142,202,301,304,305] It must also be remembered that in hypoperfused patients with inadequate preload, it is not which fluid, but how much to give to restore the circulation, that is the primary focus of attention. This is optimally given when 5 to 10 mL/kg of intravascular volume expansion is administered and the critically ill child is closely observed for the physiologic response (i.e., improved peripheral perfusion and urinary output, decreased heart rate, increased blood pressure and perfusion pressure, improved level of consciousness, and optimized filling pressures). Boluses may be repeated every 5 to 10 minutes. Be aggressive.[58,118] Consideration should be given to colloids when volume expansion approaches total blood volume. A task force of the American College of Critical Care Medicine has developed a specific algorithm for fluid administration and other therapies in septic shock[59] (Fig. 2-21).

The trend in filling pressures may be more important than the absolute numbers, and these must be interpreted with regard to the patient's underlying cardiac status. It is even possible for intravascular volume expansion to lead to decreased cardiac filling pressures. For example, in the severely clamped-down, hypovolemic patient with a poorly perfused myocardium who is encountering a high afterload, the intravascular volume expansion may well decrease cardiac afterload as systemic vascular resistance is reduced and improve myocardial perfusion, leading to better myocardial dynamics and increased cardiac output at lower cardiac filling pressures. Despite the fall in filling pressures, preload (and diastolic volumes) will have been increased; however, because of improved compliance characteristics, the relationships of the myocardium will have changed and filling pressures may actually be lower.

In the setting of CHF, fluid therapy will initially, albeit transiently, increase cardiac output and oxygenation, but may ultimately be deleterious. To differentiate between shock

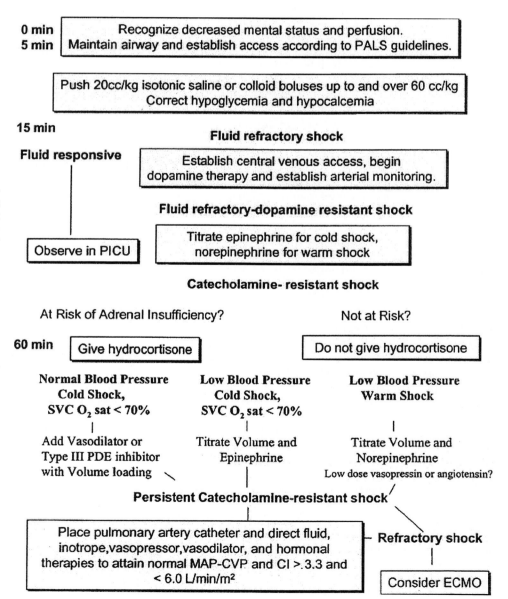

FIGURE 2-21 Recommendations for stepwise management of hemodynamic support in infants and children with septic shock. Goals include normal perfusion and perfusion pressure (mean arterial pressure–central venous pressure [MAP-CVP]). Proceed to next step if shock persists. CI, cardiac index; ECMO, extracorporeal membrane oxygenation; PALS, pediatric advanced life support; PDE, phosphodiesterase; PICU, pediatric intensive care unit; SVC O₂, superior vena cava oxygen. (From Carcillo JA, Fields AI: American College of Critical Care Medicine Task Force Committee Members: Clinical practice parameters for hemodynamic support of pediatric and neonatal patients in septic shock. Crit Care Med 30:1365–1378,2002; with permission.)

caused by CHF and other forms of shock, the cardiovascular system should be examined for evidence of heart failure, signs of hepatomegaly and neck vein distension. An empiric way to determine whether a patient will benefit from increased intravascular volume and perhaps higher right-sided pressures is to provide firm right upper quadrant abdominal pressure while observing the right atrial and blood pressure. This may transiently increase venous return and thus right atrial pressure. If this is not accompanied by a satisfactory increase in blood pressure or a fall in heart rate, or indeed appears to be deleterious to the patient, then the limit of fluid therapy has probably been attained.

Common errors in the therapy for hemodynamic insufficiency of any cause, and often in the ICU after cardiac surgery, are the use of dilute fluids, too little fluid, or an inadequate rate of fluid replacement. Quite high filling pressures (greater than 10 mm Hg) may be required in some children after cardiac surgery to assure adequate ventricular filling. When right-sided filling pressures in excess of 15 cm H_2O are required, this may indicate that myocardial function is critically impaired or that there is obstruction to right ventricular outflow. In the setting of high right atrial pressure, it may not be possible to achieve adequate venous return, and low cardiac output must be treated by other means.

Afterload

Blood pressure is generally preserved by maintaining high systemic vascular resistance, and this may be the situation in patients in cardiogenic shock, late septic shock, or hypovolemic shock, and in those who have undergone cardiac surgery. Although this works as an acute mechanism to maintain perfusion pressures, it is at the expense of noncritical peripheral vascular beds, and it increases myocardial oxygen consumption because of the high myocardial afterload. Although this is transiently beneficial, it may frequently be deleterious; thus, efforts to decrease afterload may be indicated and are virtually always required in the face of compromised cardiac function. After cardiac surgery in a patient with adequate blood pressure but poor peripheral perfusion, high systemic vascular resistance, and a clamped-down peripheral circulation, therapy includes preload augmentation, improved contractility, and afterload reduction. Of course, in patients with some forms of distributive shock, anaphylaxis, or septic shock, when systemic vascular resistance may be low and the blood pressure is low because of this, the direct approach of increasing vessel tone and systemic vascular resistance, while at the same time attempting to augment preload satisfactorily, is appropriate. Whenever possible, steps made to decrease afterload are indicated in patients with circulatory compromise and elevated systemic vascular resistance. For example, milrinone has proven beneficial in children with septic shock[19] and is widely used to support contractility and reduce both systemic and pulmonary artery pressures after cardiac surgery.[62,132]

Nitrovasodilators are useful in decreasing afterload (vascular impedance) and increasing venous vascular capacitance (decreasing preload). These effects decrease myocardial work, and by decreasing preload, these decrease left ventricular end-diastolic pressure, volume, and wall tension, which improves ventricular blood flow, oxygen balance, and myocardial performance.

Nitrovasodilators (nitroprusside, nitroglycerin, isosorbide dinitrate) function via generation of NO. This molecule activates guanylate cyclase–generating cGMP, which mediates smooth muscle relaxation (vascular and bronchial). Nitroprusside and nitroglycerin both dilate venous and arterial vasculature,[40,69] but different patterns are seen: nitroprusside with significant venous and arterial effects, and nitroglycerin with a greater change in venous capacitance than arterial. Our current understanding of the NO system does not explain the difference in patterns. It is possible that site-specific enzymes are required for the generation of NO from each of these agents. Both agents are used in dosages of 0.5 to 10 mcg/kg/minute.

Contractility

Increasing contractility in the setting of impaired circula-tory function is relatively straightforward. The use of potent inotropic agents such as dopamine and dobutamine, as well as the phosphodiesterase inhibitor milrinone and the more potent agent epinephrine, provide a reasonable armamentarium for increasing myocardial contractility. It should be noted that an increase in cardiac contractility is always accompanied by increased oxygen demanded by the myocardium. Thus, the potential risk of delayed healing and myocardial ischemia exists to limit their use. These agents are individually covered in Chapter 7. The selection of the appropriate inotrope depends on their side effects, the severity of shock, and what is particularly needed. See Figure 2-18 for illustration of the effect of an inotrope on contractility, cardiac output, and right atrial pressure. In low cardiac output, dopamine at 10 mcg/kg/minute is started. This causes some increase in systemic vascular resistance and probably has minimal effect on venous return; however, there is a shift in the cardiac function curve upward to the left. A new equilibrium (EP_2 to EP_1) is achieved with an increased cardiac output for a given venous return at a lower right atrial pressure (P_{ra1}). This demonstrates that in general, when inotropes are administered, a fall in right atrial pressure and heart rate reflects a salutary effect with increased cardiac output and almost certainly improved perfusion.

The adrenergic agent for inotropic support should be chosen with the response of the pulmonary and systemic vasculature in mind. For example, norepinephrine will not only provide some positive inotropic and chronotropic support ($beta_1$ action) but also strong alpha-adrenergic support, increasing vascular impedance and systemic blood pressure. There is sometimes a need to provide positive inotropy and vasoconstrictor support of the blood pressure while adequate preload is being restored.

In other situations, the systemic vasculature requires relaxation (or decreases in afterload) along with positive inotropic support. As the vascular impedance is reduced, there is a relief of myocardial work. Dopamine and dobutamine ($beta_1$, $beta_2$ action) accomplish these goals when used in the range of 1 to 10 mcg/kg/minute.

Isoproterenol ($beta_1$, $beta_2$) and epinephrine ($alpha_1$, $beta_1$, $beta_2$) augment cardiac activity while causing vasorelaxation (isoproterenol > epinephrine). Each agent increases myocardial oxygen consumption along with myocardial performance. In addition, careful titration is required so that peripheral vasodilation does not lower diastolic pressure sufficiently to impair coronary blood flow. As higher-dose epinephrine is used, its alpha-adrenergic receptor activity is seen and vasoconstriction appears. Not only the agent, but also its dosage must be considered in selecting the appropriate inotropic support.

Milrinone is a derivative of amrinone and has 10 to 75 times the inotropic potency of its progenitor.[19] As a bipyridine compound, milrinone inhibits phosphodiesterase III to cause increased intracellular cAMP in myocytes and vascular smooth muscle cells. The result is increased myocardial inotropy and vascular smooth muscle relaxation.[17,19,133] Myocardial oxygen consumption is not increased. Despite its frequent use and study in adults, milrinone does not have a long track record in children. Nevertheless, there have been a few studies to support its use in myocardial dysfunction due to sepsis and cardiac surgery.[17,19,62,132] In pediatric patients with septic shock, Barton and colleagues demonstrated increases in cardiac index, stroke volume index, left ventricular stroke work index, and right ventricular stroke work index, and decreases in systemic vascular resistance index and pulmonary vascular resistance index.[19] In other studies of infants and children after cardiac surgery, improved myocardial function and reduced systemic vascular resistance were also noted.[17,62] These results suggest that milrinone is beneficial for both systolic and diastolic dysfunction, as well as increased pulmonary and systemic vascular resistance. Recent work has shown that the beneficial effects of milrinone are dose related. In the largest double-blinded, placebo-controlled trial in chidren, Hoffman and colleagues[132] found that high-dose milrinone (75 mcg/kg bolus followed by an infusion of 0.75 mcg/kg/min), compared to placebo, significantly reduced the risk of low cardiac output syndrome in infants and children following cardiac surgery. The recommmended dosage of milrinone is a 50 mcg/kg bolus (over 5 to 15 minutes), followed by a continuous infusion of 0.5 mcg/kg/minute.[17,63] However, continuous infusions, without a bolus, of 0.25 to 1.0 mcg/kg/minute have been used in some centers.[227]Although milrinone has been reported to cause side effects such as thrombocytopenia, Hoffman and colleagues[132] demonstrated that milrinone use in infants and children following cardiac surgery was safe and found no increased risk of thrombocytopenia or arrhythmias.

Combined therapy may be useful to augment cardiac contractility and may include the combination of an adrenergic agent and a phosphodiesterase III inhibitor, because they act by different mechanisms to improve cardiac output. Ca^{++} may be a useful adjunct when hypocalcemia is present. Multiple-combination pharmacotherapy for the treatment of pulmonary hypertension includes agents such as PGE_1, phosphodiesterase inhibitors, NO, and nitrovasodilators (see Chapter 3).

Adjuncts to the Treatment of Shock

Bicarbonate Therapy

The routine use of sodium bicarbonate to treat metabolic acidosis is no longer widely accepted.[98,232] The deleterious effects of bicarbonate are (1) hyperosmolarity; (2) intraventricular hemorrhage in small infants (long recognized); (3) acute intracellular and cerebrospinal fluid acidosis due to the rapid movement of CO_2 through membranes without balancing bicarbonate; (4) sodium overload, if excessive; (5) and reduction of serum

ionized calcium, which may depress myocardial contractility. In the face of these risks, the lack of clear demonstration of efficacy further decreases the justification for its use.[98] These drawbacks are balanced against the supposed deleterious effects of the metabolic acidosis on the functioning of multiple enzymes, vascular resistance, and myocardial contractility. In contrast to these concerns is clinical experience.

Children with diabetic ketoacidosis, children treated for acute respiratory distress syndrome with permissive hypercapnia, or children who present with respiratory failure often have a markedly low pH without hemodynamic collapse. This suggests that the hemodynamic instability seen in patients with SIRS from sepsis or CPB is multifactorial and not solely due to a low pH. Furthermore, much of the literature demonstrates that bicarbonate therapy during cardiopulmonary resuscitation leads to increased respiratory acidosis and is potentially deleterious. Direct applicability of these data to a more chronic hypoperfusion status is less clear. Correction of metabolic acidosis increases systemic vascular resistance and decreases pulmonary vascular resistance. Sodium bicarbonate correction of metabolic acidosis also removes the need for respiratory compensation for metabolic acidosis and decreases work of breathing. It is well known that base deficits greater than −10 mEq/L are associated with a poor outcome and lactic acidosis is associated with a mortality of 60% to 90%, even in the face of maximal supportive therapy.[98] Nevertheless, sodium bicarbonate has not been demonstrated to improve the hemodynamic depression thought to be caused by metabolic acidemia.[98] The use of bicarbonate merely masks the problem and does not resolve it.

Bicarbonate supplementation, if used, should be given slowly in 1 to 2 mEq/kg boluses at no greater concentration than 0.5 to 1 mEq/mL due to the risk of a transient fall in mean arterial pressure and rise in intracranial pressure possibly related to its hypertonicity or an increase in CNS pCO_2.[98] The amount of bicarbonate required to half-correct metabolic acidosis is determined by the formula:

$0.3 \times$ Body weight (kg) $\times$ Base deficit
$$= \text{mEq of sodium bicarbonate.}$$

This serves as a rough guide. If metabolic acidosis persists or grows more severe, ongoing tissue ischemia is certainly present. Metabolic acidosis may be addressed by continuous bicarbonate infusion; however, if hyperosmolarity or hypernatremia occurs, dialysis (either peritoneal or hemofiltration) may be indicated to correct both the acidosis and the hypernatremia. Nonetheless, this should be carefully considered due to the fact that there is a lack of evidence to support sodium bicarbonate use even in the most critically ill patients.[98]

Calcium and Magnesium

Hypocalcemia and hypomagnesemia have a number of undesired effects. Symptoms of hypocalcemia include hypotension, tetany, seizures, muscle weakness, and cardiac rhythm disturbances. Hypomagnesemia causes tremor, muscle twitching, irritability, nystagmus, convulsions, cardiac arrhythmias, and electrocardiogram (ECG) abnormalities. The cardiac effects and convulsions are thought to be due to hypocalcemia associated with the hypomagnesemia.[150] These effects may complicate the care of children with congenital heart disease.

Hypocalcemia should be anticipated in the post-CPB period, after blood transfusions, after bicarbonate therapy, and with specific congenital disorders associated with congenital heart disease. The hypocalcemia that occurs after CPB may be due to the heparin and blood used in the circuit. Urban and colleagues noted that heparin caused a decrease in mean arterial pressure and systemic vascular resistance after an intravenous bolus and showed that it was related to an acute lowering of ionized calcium levels.[291] Blood used for transfusion, or during CPB, is usually anticoagulated and preserved with citrate. Citrate chelates calcium and can cause ionized hypocalcemia with a concomitant drop in blood pressure.[277] Bicarbonate reduces the amount of circulating ionized calcium by causing calcium to bind to albumin in a more alkalotic environment. The congenital disorders associated with hypocalcemia include DiGeorge syndrome and velocardiofacial syndrome. They are usually associated with a chromosome 22q11.2 microdeletion and have been placed in the category of the CATCH 22 phenotype. The features corresponding to this acronym include cardiac defects, abnormal facies, thymus hypoplasia, cleft palate, hypocalcemia. and the chromosome 22 microdeletion. Children with CATCH 22 will present with hypocalcemia from hypoparathyroidism due to hypoplasia or aplasia of the parathyroid glands. The congenital heart defects that are associated with CATCH 22 include conotruncal anomalies, such as tetralogy of Fallot and aortic arch abnormalities, aberrant subclavian arteries, and vascular rings.[281] These defects appear to be due to developmental defects of the first through fourth embryonal brachial arches and pharyngeal pouches.

Hypocalcemia has been associated with dysfunction of the cardiovascular system. Calcium plays a key role in the excitation and contraction of cardiac muscle fibers. There have been reports of impaired myocardial function and prolongation of the QT interval with hypocalcemia.[72,77] Stulz and colleagues[277] found reduced ventricular performance and decreased SVR in hypocalcemic dogs undergoing CPB. Desai and associates[85] reported similar results in acutely ill adults with hypocalcemia. There have also been reports of ventricular fibrillation, torsade de pointes, and prolongation of the QT interval in hypocalcemic patients.[151,269]

Calcium must be replaced under these circumstances. Nevertheless, rapid administration of calcium must be avoided because it can cause bradycardia. Treatment with either calcium chloride or calcium gluconate, administered via central access when possible, is indicated to correct systemic hypocalcemia.

Hypomagnesemia is often found in connection with hypocalcemia and also should be replaced. The mechanism leading to hypocalcemia in hypomagnesemia is controversial. Several factors have been proposed such as end organ unresponsiveness to parathyroid hormone (PTH); impaired synthesis and/or release of PTH; and impaired formation of 25-dihydroxyvitamin D_3.[257] Calcium infusions raise serum concentration of calcium and may increase contractility. This increased contractility is more pronounced when converting hypocalcemia to eucalcemia than in increasing normal concentration of Ca^{++} to hypercalcemia.[92] However, there is some thought that in patients after cardiac surgery calcium raises the blood pressure by increasing the vascular tone and subsequently the SVR. This increase in blood pressure may be at the cost of reduced cardiac output.[60,196]

Further evaluation of the clinical significance and outcome will clarify this issue.

Phosphorus

Hypophosphatemia is also a frequent occurrence postoperatively. Again this may be due to dilutional effects, deranged intracellular shifts, and increased cellular permeability. Urinary and gastrointestinal losses aggravate hypophosphatemia. Hypophosphatemia can be associated with impaired response to vasopressor medications, myocardial and respiratory muscle depression, and thus impaired oxygen delivery.[35] It should be considered in any patient with continuously compromised myocardial function or respiratory failure, despite what appears to be adequate therapy. Phosphorus administration has been reported to be beneficial in hypophosphatemic patients with septic shock.[35]

Steroids

Corticosteroids, like other steroid hormones, exert their influence by controlling the rate of protein synthesis by stimulating transcription of RNA. Corticosteroids influence carbohydrate metabolism, protein metabolism, lipid metabolism, electrolyte and water balance, the cardiovascular system, skeletal muscle, the CNS, and the formed elements of the blood; possess antiinflammatory properties; and affect various organs and tissues in a wide variety of ways. Because of the cardiovascular and antiinflammatory effects, corticosteroids have often been used during CPB and to treat shock.

The cardiovascular effects of corticosteroids are secondary to the regulation of renal sodium ion excretion, capillary permeability, vasomotor responses of small vessels, and cardiac output. Corticosteroid-induced hypertension may be the result of prolonged, excessive sodium retention and/or edema within the wall of the arterioles (reducing their lumina and increasing peripheral vascular resistance). Another possibility is that salt retention, or the mineralocorticoid effect of corticosteroids, sensitizes blood vessels to pressor agents, in particular angiotensin and circulating catecholamines.[61] The antiinflammatory effects of corticosteroids include inhibition of the early phase of the inflammatory process (fibrin deposition, capillary dilation, migration of leukocytes to the inflamed area, and phagocytic activity) and the late phase of the inflammatory process (edema, capillary proliferation, fibroblast proliferation, and collagen deposition). The most important factor in the antiinflammatory effect of glucocorticoids may be the ability to inhibit the recruitment of neutrophils and monocytes-macrophages.[61]

In clinical practice, steroids have been used as a therapeutic agent to counterbalance the effects of SIRS from CPB and shock. The initiation of CPB exposes blood to large areas of synthetic material that trigger complement activation (both classic and alternative pathways) and activate platelets, neutrophils, monocytes, and macrophages. Coagulation, fibrinolysis, and the kallikrein cascade are stimulated, thus increasing blood levels of various cytokines (tumor necrosis factor, interleukins, and so forth), impairing endothelial function, and increasing endothelial permeability. Nevertheless, steroids have no routine role in the therapy for shock states. If acute adrenal insufficiency (Waterhouse-Friderichsen syndrome) is suspected, stress doses of steroids can be administered, but pharmacologic doses are not indicated. A recent prospective, randomized, double-blinded, placebo-controlled study showed treatment for 7 days with low-dose hydrocortisone and fludrocortisone significantly reduced the incidence of death in adults with septic shock and relative adrenal insufficiency without increasing adverse events.[12] In patients subject to CPB and the subsequent associated SIRS, steroids such as methylprednisolone reliably and beneficially alter the balance of proinflammatory and anti-inflammatory mediators. Even so, there is still controversy over whether suppression of SIRS is clinically beneficial. In meta-analysis of steroid use during CPB by Chaney, nine prospective, randomized, double-blinded, placebo-controlled studies were analyzed. Specific hemodynamic benefits (increased cardiac index, decreased SVR) were associated with the use of the drug, but there was an increased need for postoperative pressors. From a pulmonary perspective, the use of methylprednisolone in this setting did not offer any benefit and may have been detrimental. The drug did not reliably prevent decreased postoperative pulmonary compliance or increased $P(A-a)O_2$ and may have delayed postoperative extubation for undetermined reasons. Finally, methylprednisolone was unable to beneficially affect perioperative fluid balance, but did increase perioperative glucose levels that may be associated with increased morbidity.[61] In a randomized, prospective, double-blinded study of 29 children, Bronicki and colleagues[46] found that 1 mg/kg of dexamethasone administered before CPB caused an eightfold decrease in serum interleukin-6 levels and a greater than three-fold decrease in tumor necrosis factor-alpha after CPB. Complement C3a and absolute neutrophil count were not affected by dexamethasone. The mean rectal temperature for the first 24 hours postoperatively was significantly lower in the group given dexamethasone than in controls, and dexamethasone-treated children required less fluid during the first 48 hours. Compared with controls, dexamethasone-treated children had significantly lower alveolar-arterial oxygen gradients during the first 24 hours and required less mechanical ventilation.[46] In conclusion, while steroids are commonly used in shock and CPB, their efficacy remains controversial.

Glycosides

Traditionally, glycosides have been given as an inotropic agent, but slow onset of action, arrhythmogenicity, unreliable serum levels, and negative chronotropic action limit their use in the acute setting of CHF. Digoxin is less frequently used, in view of the development of short-acting, potent cardiovascular agents. Its use has been relegated to the chronic outpatient management of impaired myocardial contractility.

Prostaglandins

Prostaglandin infusions are currently used to maintain patency of the ductus arteriosus for ductus-dependent lesions and to reduce pulmonary hypertension after CPB. PGE_1 (alprostadil) infusion often provides lifesaving systemic blood flow through the ductus arteriosus when congenital left-sided obstructive lesions are present (i.e., hypoplastic left heart syndrome, critical aortic stenosis, interrupted aortic arch, coarctation). Although this is only temporizing, these infants can be in a much more advantageous preoperative condition and with a higher

likelihood of surviving surgical repair without multiple organ failure secondary to preoperative, long-standing, critical ischemia. The dose of PGE_1 used is 0.05 to 0.4 mcg/kg/minute. The usual dose is 0.1 mcg/kg/minute, but it is reduced to the lowest effective dosage to minimize adverse effects. Fever, apnea, thrombocytopenia, hypotension, generalized edema, and other side effects have been reported. Also, the response to PGE infusion may diminish with time, and nonresponders have been documented. The use of prostaglandin infusion to treat pulmonary hypertension is covered in Chapter 3.

Angiotensin-Converting Enzyme Inhibitors

The renin-angiotensin-aldosterone system plays a major role in the neurohumoral response to myocardial systolic dysfunction. The primary derivative, angiotensin II, is responsible for the direct vasoconstriction, discharge of norepinephine, inhibition of vagal tone, and release of aldosterone that is seen in CHF. The consequence of aldosterone release is the retention of water and sodium.[143] Furthermore, angiotensin II is responsible for myocyte hypertrophy and stimulation of cardiac fibroblast activity.[44,108] Myocardial hypertrophy and fibrosis results and this subsequently impairs systolic function and increases diastolic stiffness.[44] Angiotensin-converting enzyme (ACE) inhibitors are a group of agents that interfere with normal ACE activity, preventing the transformation of angiotensin I to angiotensin II. This results in lower angiotensin II levels, with resultant vasodilation and decrease in synthesis and secretion of aldosterone.

Clinically, ACE inhibitors have been used to offset the effects of neurohumoral response to the failing myocardium and reduce the afterload in hearts with valvular regurgitation to improve cardiac output. Most children demonstrated improvements in left-to-right shunting, suggesting a possible benefit of this agent in children with heart failure secondary to large left-to-right shunts. Along with the antihypertensive action, the relaxation of the systemic vasculature improves myocardial performance by reducing myocardial afterload. ACE inhibitors have also been shown to affect cardiac remodeling by reversing myocardial hypertrophy and fibrosis.[43] This not only improves systolic function, but also improves diastolic function. ACE inhibitors have become indispensable in the management of CHF and valvular regurgitation.

THE POST–CARDIOPULMONARY BYPASS CIRCULATION

In restoring the circulation after cardiopulmonary bypass and surgical repair of congenital heart disease, general principles apply. The goals of hemodynamic monitoring and therapy include the following:

1. Attaining circulatory sufficiency for systemic oxygen delivery
2. Maintaining myocardial oxygen balance
3. Providing support during recovery from CPB and the stress of surgery, reestablishing water and salt balance and neurologic function, including thermostasis, and assessing any other organ failure
4. Initiating nutritional support

Cardioplegia and hypothermic CPB do not provide complete myocardial and other organ protection. Ischemic injury may still occur. Further myocardial injury results if a ventriculotomy is required for surgical repair. Atriotomy and a transvalvular approach to the ventricles cause less ventricular injury; however, atrial or valvular dysfunction may occur. With the multiple potential causes of cardiac dysfunction, it is essential to be prepared to provide inotropic support. An inverse relationship exists between mortality and postoperative cardiac output after repair of CHD.[218] After cardiac transplantation the heart may demonstrate sufficient contractility, but still require chronotropic support. Many agents are advocated for inotropic support, including adrenergics (epinephrine, dopamine, dobutamine, norepinephrine, isoproterenol), phosphodiesterase inhibitors (amrinone and milrinone, which raise intracellular cAMP), Ca^{++} infusion, and glycosides. Any agent that increases the myocardial intracellular cAMP or Ca^{++} concentration will augment inotropy.

Concomitant therapy, along with vasoactive agents to manipulate the vasculature, includes assisted ventilation; analysis of, and support of, heart rate and rhythm (pharmacologic or pacemaker); nutritional support; and analgesia for adequate pain management.

When children return from the operating room, they are frequently hypothermic, peripherally hypoperfused, tachycardiac, and acidotic. In addition the volume status is uncertain. Within the next few hours, it will be necessary to completely assess circulatory function and begin to correct the hemodynamic status. Many problems are caused by a hypercatecholaminergic status after cardiac surgery, which increases myocardial oxygen consumption and whole body oxygen demands. This is clearly deleterious. Adequate analgesia, sedation, and perhaps muscle relaxation are required in the early postoperative period to blunt the effects of the stress response.

Hypothermia must be corrected reasonably early. Hypothermic patients are also peripherally vasoconstricted and at a metabolic disadvantage. This additional stress to the recovering heart can precipitate or prolong low output states. Therefore, temperature homeostasis and rewarming are essential. This can be achieved by overhead radiant warmers and hot water circulating beds, and should not be overlooked in the postoperative state. As children rewarm, they vasodilate, not surprisingly. Their vascular capacitance will increase, and additional preload will be required. Afterload will also fall and blood pressure support, first with preload augmentation, will be required. Patients who become hypotensive with rewarming are markedly hypovolemic, and fluid resuscitation is essential. The high peripheral vascular tone and uncertain volume status; impaired contractility due to bypass ischemia, SIRS, and direct trauma; impaired endothelial function with an increased interstitial third space; impaired vascular control; and unknown fluid needs present a challenging scenario. The appropriate therapy for all patients is to maintain adequate oxygenation and oxygen delivery to prevent further injury and incur minimal cost to the myocardium, while awaiting recovery of the endothelium in the hypermetabolic postoperative state.

Assessing volume status in this circumstance may be difficult because the peripheral circulation is constricted, the myocardium is impaired, and filling pressures may appear to be adequate (or even high), despite inadequate preload.

Therapy should be directed at dilating and filling the circulation to maintain mean circulatory filling pressures, blunting the effects of high levels of circulating catecholamines and peripheral vasoconstriction, augmenting preload, and minimizing myocardial oxygen consumption. Afterload reduction, provided by both mechanical ventilation and IV vasodilators such as milrinone or nitroglycerin, is a logical and natural choice for any child after cardiac surgery. If hypotension with mild vasodilation ensues, this indicates that the patient is hypovolemic and requires preload supplementation. If this state is allowed to persist, further myocardial impairment can be expected with further elevated filling pressures, decreased preload, and impaired cardiac output; thus, there may be an ongoing vicious cycle from which the child cannot recover. Central hyperthermia is an extreme manifestation of this status. With decreased or absent peripheral perfusion, in a hypermetabolic state, core hyperthermia is due to failure to dissipate heat via the impaired countercurrent exchange mechanisms for cooling. Quite striking hyperthermia can occur postoperatively (greater than 40°C). This may be a manifestation of extremely poor cardiac output, and will certainly worsen the situation. Again, therapy is directed at preload augmentation, afterload reduction, and contractility therapy. Because of endothelial barrier dysfunction, third spacing can be expected, and edema routinely occurs in this setting. For this reason, mechanical respiratory support may be necessary until the endothelial defects resolve, the circulation becomes stable, and the third space begins to mobilize, sometime between 24 and 48 hours after surgery.

Cardiac Tamponade

Acute deterioration in hemodynamic status, despite what appears to be adequate volume, perfusion, and pressors, should lead to an aggressive search for cardiac tamponade. Plugging of mediastinal drains, hematoma formation, or even ventilatory abnormalities can tamponade the heart in the postoperative state even though the pericardium is no longer intact. This should be expected in the presence of a pulsus paradoxus, high venous pressures, and signs of an acute low-output state with decreased heart sounds. Echocardiography may be very helpful. Emergent reopening of the chest wound in the postoperative patient or pericardiocentesis in the medical patient is lifesaving.

CONCLUSION

New insights into the anatomy, physiology, and pharmacology of the developing cardiovascular system and its interaction with other organ systems have provided greater understanding of the action of currently available therapeutic agents and the development of more novel and specific agents. Much more needs to be learned to understand and intervene in the pathology of the cardiovascular system of the child. Congenital cardiovascular defects and their therapy demand a breadth of knowledge of the pathophysiology and available therapies, and an experienced clinician. Through the research of pharmacologists, physiologists, cell and molecular biologists, and clinicians, the development of new therapeutic agents and management strategies to modulate the cardiovasculature and its interactions with other organs will undoubtedly continue to advance.

References

1. Abraham E, Matthay MA, Dinarello CA, et al: Consensus conference definitions for sepsis, septic shock, acute lung injury, and acute respiratory distress syndrome: Time for a reevaluation. *Crit Care Med* 28:232–235, 2000.

2. Abraham E, Reinhart K, Svoboda P, et al: Assessment of the safety of recombinant tissue factor pathway inhibitor in patients with severe sepsis: A multicenter, randomized, placebo-controlled, single-blind, dose escalation study. *Crit Care Med* 29:2081–2089, 2001.

3. Adatia I: Recent advances in pulmonary vascular disease. *Curr Opin Pediatr* 14:292–297, 2002.

4. Ahmed SS, Regan TJ: Are pressure-volume relations at end-systole a reflection of left ventricular myocardial contractility? *Angiology* 34:137–148, 1983.

5. Alberti C, Brun-Buisson C, Goodman SV, et al: European Sepsis Group: Influence of systemic inflammatory response syndrome and sepsis on outcome of critically ill infected patients. *Am J Respir Crit Care Med* 168:77–84, 2003.

6. Ali MH, Schumacker PT: Endothelial responses to mechanical stress: Where is the mechanosensor? *Crit Care Med* 30:S198–206, 2002.

7. Altavilla D, Squadrito F, Serrano M, et al: Inhibition of tumour necrosis factor and reversal of endotoxin-induced shock by U-83836E, a "second generation" lazaroid in rats. *Br J Pharmacol* 124:1293–1299, 1998.

8. Altman DI, Perlman JM, Volpe JJ, Powers WJ: Cerebral oxygen metabolism in newborns. *Pediatrics* 92:99–104, 1993.

9. Amenta F, Ricci A, Rossodivita I, et al: The dopaminergic system in hypertension. *Clin Exp Hypertens* 23:15–24, 2001.

10. Anderson PAW: Immature myocardium, fetal, neonatal, and infant cardiac disease. In Moller J, Neal W (eds): *Fetal, Neonatal, and Infant Cardiac Surgery.* Norwalk, CT, Appleton & Lange, p 35, 1990.

11. Anderson PAW: The heart and development. *Semin Perinatol* 20:482–509, 1996.

12. Annane D, Sebille V, Charpentier C, et al: Effect of treatment with low doses of hydrocortisone and fludrocortisone on mortality in patients with septic shock. *JAMA* 288:862–871, 2002.

13. Ardehali A, Hughes K, Sadeghi A, et al: Inhaled nitric oxide for pulmonary hypertension after heart transplantation. *Transplantation* 72:638–641, 2001.

14. Armstead WM, Mirro R, Busija DW, Leffler CW: Opioids and the prostanoid system in the control of cerebral blood flow in hypotensive piglets. *J Cereb Blood Flow Metab* 11:380–387, 1991.

15. Aubier M, Trippenbach T, Roussos C: Respiratory muscle fatigue during cardiogenic shock. *J Appl Physiol* 51:499–508, 1981.

16. Azevedo ER, Kubo T, Mak S, et al: Nonselective versus selective beta-adrenergic receptor blockade in congestive heart failure: Differential effects on sympathetic activity. *Circulation* 104:2194–2199, 2001.

17. Bailey JM, Miller BE, Lu W, et al: The pharmacokinetics of milrinone in pediatric patients after cardiac surgery. *Anesthesiology* 90:1012–1018, 1999.

18. Baker CH, Sutton ET, Zhou Z, Reynolds DG: Reduced microvascular adrenergic receptor activity due to opioids in endotoxin shock. *Circ Shock* 32:101–112,1990.

19. Barton P, Garcia J, Kouatli A, et al: Hemodynamic effects of i.v. milrinone lactate in pediatric patients with septic shock: A prospective, double-blinded, randomized, placebo-controlled interventional study. *Chest* 109:1302–1312, 1996.

20. Barton P, Kalil AC, Nadel S, et al: Safety, pharmacokinetics, and pharmacodynamics of drotrecogin alfa (activated) in children with severe sepsis. *Pediatrics* 113:7–17, 2004.

21. Baughman KL: B–type natriuretic peptide: A window to the heart. *N Engl J Med* 347:158–159, 2002.

22. Baylen BG, Agata Y, Padbury JF, et al: Hemodynamic and neuroendocrine adaptations of the preterm lamb left ventricle to acutely increased afterload. *Pediatr Res* 26:336–342, 1989.

23. Bengel FM, Ueberfuhr P, Schiepel N, et al: Effect of sympathetic reinnervation on cardiac performance after heart transplantation. *N Engl J Med* 345:731–738, 2001.

24. Benigni A, Remuzzi G: Endothelin antagonists. *Lancet* 353:133–138, 1999.

25. Benson DW Jr, Hughes SF, Hu N, Clark EB: Effect of heart rate increase on dorsal aortic flow before and after volume loading in the stage 24 chick embryo. *Pediatr Res* 26:438–441, 1989.

26. Berger R, Huelsman M, Strecker K, et al: B-type natriuretic peptide predicts sudden death in patients with chronic heart failure. *Circulation* 105:2392–2397, 2002.

27. Berlan M, Galitzky J, Montastruc JL: Beta 3-adrenoceptors in the cardiovascular system. *Fundam Clin Pharmacol* 9:234–239, 1995.

28. Bernard GR, Vincent JL, Laterre PF, et al: Recombinant human protein C Worldwide Evaluation in Severe Sepsis (PROWESS) study group: Efficacy and safety of recombinant human activated protein C for severe sepsis. *N Engl J Med* 344:699–709, 2001.

29. Berridge MJ: Inositol trisphosphate and calcium signalling. *Nature* 361:315–325, 1993.

30. Beutler B, Milsark IW, Cerami AC: Passive immunization against cachectin/tumor necrosis factor protects mice from lethal effect of endotoxin. *Science* 229:869–871, 1985.

31. Bihari D, Smithies M, Gimson A, Tinker J: The effects of vasodilation with prostacyclin on oxygen delivery and uptake in critically ill patients. *N Engl J Med* 317:397–403, 1987.

32. Bland RD, Shoemaker WC, Abraham E, Cobo JC: Hemodynamic and oxygen transport patterns in surviving and nonsurviving postoperative patients. *Crit Care Med* 13:85–90, 1985.

33. Blatter LA, Wier WG: Agonist–induced [Ca2+]i waves and Ca(2+)-induced Ca2+ release in mammalian vascular smooth muscle cells. *Am J Physiol* 263:H576–586, 1992.

34. Bloom SR, Edwards AV: Vasoactive intestinal peptide in relation to atropine resistant vasodilation in the submaxillary gland of the cat. *J Physiol* 300:41–53, 1980.

35. Bollaert PE, Levy B, Nace L, et al: Hemodynamic and metabolic effects of rapid correction of hypophosphatemia in patients with septic shock. *Chest* 107:1698–1701, 1995.

36. Bone RC: Abnormal cellular metabolism in sepsis: A new interpretation. *JAMA* 267:1518–1519, 1992.

37. Bosnjak ZJ: Ion channels in vascular smooth muscle: Physiology and pharmacology. *Anesthesiology* 79:1392–1401, 1993.

38. Bouvier M, Hausdorff WP, De Blasi A, et al: Removal of phosphorylation sites from the beta 2-adrenergic receptor delays onset of agonist-promoted desensitization. *Nature* 333:370–373, 1988.

39. Brady AJ, Poole-Wilson PA, Harding SE, Warren JB: Nitric oxide production within cardiac myocytes reduces their contractility in endotoxemia. *Am J Physiol* 263:H1963–1966, 1992.

40. Braunwald E: Vasodilator therapy: A physiologic approach to the treatment of heart failure. *N Engl J Med* 297:331–333, 1977.

41. Brayden JE: Functional roles of KATP channels in vascular smooth muscle. *Clin Exp Pharmacol Physiol* 29:312–316, 2002.

42. Breslow MJ, Tobin JR, Mandrell TD, et al: Changes in adrenal oxygen consumption during catecholamine secretion in anesthetized dogs. *Am J Physiol* 259:H681–688, 1990.

43. Brilla CG, Funck RC, Rupp H: Lisinopril-mediated regression of myocardial fibrosis in patients with hypertensive heart disease. *Circulation* 102:1388–1393, 2000.

44. Brilla CG: Renin-angiotensin system mediated mechanisms: Cardioreparation and cardioprotection. *Heart* 84:i18–19, 2000.

45. Bristow MR, Ginsburg R, Umans V, et al: Beta 1- and beta 2-adrenergic-receptor subpopulations in nonfailing and failing human ventricular myocardium: Coupling of both receptor subtypes to muscle contraction and selective beta 1-receptor down-regulation in heart failure. *Circ Res* 59:297–309, 1986.

46. Bronicki RA, Backer CL, Baden HP, et al: Dexamethasone reduces the inflammatory response to cardiopulmonary bypass in children. *Ann Thorac Surg* 69:1490–1495, 2000.

47. Brooks PM, Day RO: Nonsteroidal antiinflammatory drugs: Differences and similarities. *N Engl J Med* 324:1716–1725, 1991.

48. Brun-Buisson C: The epidemiology of the systemic inflammatory response. *Intensive Care Med* 26:S64–74, 2000.

49. Brunner-La Rocca HP, Kaye DM, et al: Effects of intravenous brain natriuretic peptide on regional sympathetic activity in patients with chronic heart failure as compared with healthy control subjects. *J Am Coll Cardiol* 37:1221–1227, 2001.

50. Brutsaert DL, Meulemans AL, Sipido KR, Sys SU: Effects of damaging the endocardial surface on the mechanical performance of isolated cardiac muscle. *Circ Res* 62:358–366, 1988.

51. Bukh A, Martinez-Valdez H, Freedman SJ, et al: The expression of c-fos, c-jun, and c-myc genes is regulated by heat shock in human lymphoid cells. *J Immunol* 144:4835–4840, 1990.

52. Burnstock G, Kennedy C: A dual function for adenosine 5′-triphosphate in the regulation of vascular tone: Excitatory cotransmitter with noradrenaline from perivascular nerves and locally released inhibitory intravascular agent. *Circ Res* 58:319–330, 1986.

53. Burnstock G: Integration of factors controlling vascular tone: Overview. *Anesthesiology* 79:1368–1380, 1993.

54. Busija DW, Khreis I, Chen J: Prostanoids promote pial arteriolar dilation and mask constriction to oxytocin in piglets. *Am J Physiol* 264:H1023–1027, 1993.

55. Busse R, Forstermann U, Matsuda H, Pohl U: The role of prostaglandins in the endothelium-mediated vasodilatory response to hypoxia. *Pflugers Arch* 401:77–83, 1984.

56. Cao K, Tang G, Hu D, Wang R: Molecular basis of ATP-sensitive K+ channels in rat vascular smooth muscles. *Biochem Biophys Res Commun* 296:463–469, 2002.

57. Carabello BA, Zile MR, Tanaka R, Cooper G 4th: Left ventricular hypertrophy due to volume overload versus pressure overload. *Am J Physiol* 263:H1137–1144, 1992.

58. Carcillo JA, Davis AL, Zaritsky A: Role of early fluid resuscitation in pediatric septic shock. *JAMA* 266:1242–1245, 1991.

59. Carcillo JA, Fields AI: American College of Critical Care Medicine Task Force Committee Members: Clinical practice parameters for hemodynamic support of pediatric and neonatal patients in septic shock. *Crit Care Med* 30:1365–1378, 2002.

60. Castillo W, Quintos M, Wong P, et al: Calcium chloride infusion in infants following cardiac surgery does not improve hemodynamics. *Crit Care Med* 30:A156, 2002.

61. Chaney MA: Corticosteroids and cardiopulmonary bypass: A review of clinical investigations. *Chest* 121:921–931, 2002.

62. Chang AC, Atz AM, Wernovsky G, et al: Milrinone: Systemic and pulmonary hemodynamic effects in neonates after cardiac surgery. *Crit Care Med* 23:1907–1914, 1995.

63. Choi PT, Yip G, Quinonez LG, Cook DJ: Crystalloids versus colloids in fluid resuscitation: A systematic review. *Crit Care Med* 27:200–210, 1999.

64. Choi SJ, Jeffries HE, Newth CJ, et al: Vasopressin deficiency in pediatric septic shock. *Am J Respir Crit Care Med* 165:A157, 2002.

65. Christou H, Van Marter LJ, Wessel DL, et al: Inhaled nitric oxide reduces the need for extracorporeal membrane oxygenation in infants with persistent pulmonary hypertension of the newborn. *Crit Care Med* 28:3722–3727, 2000.

66. Clark RH, Kueser TJ, Walker MW, et al: Low-dose nitric oxide therapy for persistent pulmonary hypertension of the newborn. Clinical Inhaled Nitric Oxide Research Group. *N Engl J Med* 342:469–474, 2000.

67. Claussen MS, Landercasper J, Cogbill TH: Acute adrenal insufficiency presenting as shock after trauma and surgery: Three cases and review of the literature. *J Trauma* 32:94–100, 1992.

68. Cobb JP: Use of nitric oxide synthase inhibitors to treat septic shock: The light has changed from yellow to red. *Crit Care Med* 27:855–856, 1999.

69. Cohn JN, Franciosa JA: Vasodilator therapy of cardiac failure (first of two parts). *N Engl J Med* 297:27–31, 1977.

70. Colan SD, Parness IA, Spevak PJ, Sanders SP: Developmental modulation of myocardial mechanics: Age- and growth-related alterations in afterload and contractility. *J Am Coll Cardiol* 19:619–629, 1992.

71. Colucci WS, Elkayam U, Horton DP, et al: Nesiritide Study Group: Intravenous nesiritide, a natriuretic peptide, in the treatment of decompensated congestive heart failure. *N Engl J Med* 343:246–253, 2000.

72. Colucci WS, Wright RF, Braunwald E: New positive inotropic agents in the treatment of congestive heart failure: Mechanisms of action and recent clinical developments. 2. *N Engl J Med* 314:349–358, 1986.

73. Connor TB, Rosen BL, Blaustein MP, et al: Hypocalcemia precipitating congestive heart failure. *N Engl J Med* 307:869–872, 1982.

74. Cowen T, Haven AJ, Wen-Qin C, et al: Development and ageing of perivascular adrenergic nerves in the rabbit: A quantitative fluorescence histochemical study using image analysis. *J Auton Nerv Syst* 5:317–336, 1982.

75. Craig EA, Gross CA: Is hsp70 the cellular thermometer? *Trends Biochem Sci* 16:135–140, 1991.

76. Crouser ED, Julian MW, Blaho DV, Pfeiffer DR: Endotoxin-induced mitochondrial damage correlates with impaired respiratory activity. *Crit Care Med* 30:276–284, 2002.

77. Csanady M, Forster T, Julesz J: Reversible impairment of myocardial function in hypoparathyroidism causing hypocalcaemia. *Br Heart J* 63:58–60, 1990.

78. Cui Y, Tran S, Tinker A, Clapp LH: The molecular composition of K(ATP) channels in human pulmonary artery smooth muscle cells and their modulation by growth. *Am J Respir Cell Mol Biol* 26:135–143, 2002.

79. Cunnion RE, Schaer GL, Parker MM, et al: The coronary circulation in human septic shock. *Circulation* 73:637–644, 1986.

80. D'Ambra MN, Philbin DM: Con: Colloids should not be added to the pump prime. *J Cardiothorac Anesth* 4:406–408, 1990.

81. Danek SJ, Lynch JP, Weg JG, Dantzker DR: The dependence of oxygen uptake on oxygen delivery in the adult respiratory distress syndrome. *Am Rev Respir Dis* 122:387–395, 1980.

82. Dantzker DR, Foresman B, Gutierrez G: Oxygen supply and utilization relationships: A reevaluation. *Am Rev Respir Dis* 143:675–679, 1991.

83. De Bruin WJ, Greenwald BM, Notterman DA: Fluid resuscitation in pediatrics. *Crit Care Clin* 8:423–438, 1992.

84. De Mello WC, Danser AH: Angiotensin II and the heart: On the intracrine renin-angiotensin system. *Hypertension* 35:1183–1188, 2000.

85. Desai TK, Carlson RW, Thill-Baharozian M, Geheb MA: A direct relationship between ionized calcium and arterial pressure among patients in an intensive care unit. *Crit Care Med* 16:578–582, 1988.

86. Despond O, Proulx F, Carcillo JA, Lacroix J: Pediatric sepsis and multiple organ dysfunction syndrome. *Curr Opin Pediatr* 13:247–253, 2001.

87. Dobyns EL, Cornfield DN, Anas NG, et al: Multicenter randomized controlled trial of the effects of inhaled nitric oxide therapy on gas exchange in children with acute hypoxemic respiratory failure. *J Pediatr* 134:406–412, 1999.

88. Doggrell SA: The therapeutic potential of dopamine modulators on the cardiovascular and renal systems. *Expert Opin Investig Drugs* 11:631–644, 2002.

89. Dougherty AH, Naccarelli GV, Gray EL, et al: Congestive heart failure with normal systolic function. *Am J Cardiol* 54:778–782, 1984.

90. Drexler H, Hayoz D, Munzel T, et al: Endothelial function in chronic congestive heart failure. *Am J Cardiol* 69:1596–1601, 1992.

91. Driscoll DJ, Gillette PC, Ezrailson EG, Schwartz A: Inotropic response of the neonatal canine myocardium to dopamine. *Pediatr Res* 12:42–45, 1978.

92. Drop LJ, Scheidegger D: Plasma ionized calcium concentration: Important determinant of the hemodynamic response to calcium infusion. *J Thorac Cardiovasc Surg* 79:425–431, 1980.

93. Edwards WT, Burney RG: Use of repeated nerve blocks in management of an infant with Kawasaki's disease. *Anesth Analg* 67:1008–1010, 1988.

94. Feve B, Emorine LJ, Lasnier F, et al: The human beta 3–adrenergic receptor: Relationship with atypical receptors. *Am J Clin Nutr* 55:215S–218S, 1992.

95. Feldman AM: Modulation of adrenergic receptors and G-transduction proteins in failing human ventricular myocardium. *Circulation* 87:IV27–34, 1993.

96. Filston HC: Fluid and electrolyte management in the pediatric surgical patient. *Surg Clin North Am* 72:1189–1205, 1992.

97. Finkel MS, Oddis CV, Jacob TD, et al: Negative inotropic effects of cytokines on the heart mediated by nitric oxide. *Science* 257:387–389, 1992.

98. Forsythe SM, Schmidt GA: Sodium bicarbonate for the treatment of lactic acidosis. *Chest* 117:260–267, 2000.

99. Francis GS, Goldsmith SR, Levine TB, et al: The neurohumoral axis in congestive heart failure. *Ann Intern Med* 101:370–377, 1984.

100. Franco-Cereceda A, Liska J: Neuropeptide Y Y1 receptors in vascular pharmacology. *Eur J Pharmacol* 349:1–14, 1998.

101. Friedman WF: The intrinsic physiologic properties of the developing heart. *Prog Cardiovasc Dis* 15:87–111, 1972.

102. Friedman WF: The intrinsic properties of the developing heart. In Friedman WF, Lesch M, Sonnenblick EH (eds): *Neonatal Heart Disease*. Orlando, Fla., Grune & Stratton, pp 21–49, 1973.

103. Furman WL, Menke JA, Barson WJ, Miller RR: Continuous naloxone infusion in two neonates with septic shock. *J Pediatr* 105:649–651, 1984.

104. Galie N, Manes A, Branzi A: Emerging medical therapies for pulmonary arterial hypertension. *Prog Cardiovasc Dis* 45:213–224, 2002.

105. Gaumann DM, Yaksh TL, Tyce GM: Effects of intrathecal morphine, clonidine, and midazolam on the somato-sympathoadrenal reflex response in halothane-anesthetized cats. *Anesthesiology* 73:425–432, 1990.

106. Gauthier C, Langin D, Balligand JL: Beta 3-adrenoceptors in the cardiovascular system. *Trends Pharmacol Sci* 21:426–431, 2000.

107. Gauthier C, Leblais V, Moniotte S, et al: The negative inotropic action of catecholamines: Role of beta 3-adrenoceptors. *Can J Physiol Pharmacol* 78:681–690, 2000.

108. Givertz MM: Manipulation of the renin-angiotensin system. *Circulation* 104:E14–18, 2001.

109. Goldstein B, DeKing D, DeLong DJ, et al: Autonomic cardiovascular state after severe brain injury and brain death in children. *Crit Care Med* 21:228–233, 1993.

110. Goldstein S: Benefits of beta-blocker therapy for heart failure: Weighing the evidence. *Arch Intern Med* 162:641–648, 2002.

111. Golombek SG: The use of inhaled nitric oxide in newborn medicine. *Heart Dis* 2:342–347, 2000.

112. Gootman PM: Perinatal neural regulation of cardiovascular function. In Gootman N, Gootman P (eds): *Perinatal Cardiovascular Function*. New York, Marcel Dekker, pp 265–328, 1983.

113. Graham TP Jr: Ventricular performance in congenital heart disease. *Circulation* 84: 2259–2274, 1991.

114. Graham TP Jr, Jarmakani MM: Evaluation of ventricular function in infants and children. *Pediatr Clin North Am* 18:1109–1132, 1971.

115. Griffel MI, Kaufman BS: Pharmacology of colloids and crystalloids. *Crit Care Clin* 8:235–253, 1992.

116. Gruskin AB, Edelmann CM Jr, Yuan S: Maturational changes in renal blood flow in piglets. *Pediatr Res* 4:7–13, 1970.

117. Guyton AC: *Textbook of Medical Physiology*. Philadelphia, WB Saunders, 1981.

118. Han YY, Carcillo JA, Dragotta MA, et al: Early reversal of pediatric-neonatal septic shock by community physicians is associated with improved outcome. *Pediatrics* 112:793–799, 2003.

119. Hankeln KB, Gronemeyer R, Held A, Bohmert F: Use of continuous noninvasive measurement of oxygen consumption in patients with adult respiratory distress syndrome following shock of various etiologies. *Crit Care Med* 19:642–649, 1991.

120. Hara H, Hamill GS, Jacobowitz DM: Origin of cholinergic nerves to the rat major cerebral arteries: Coexistence with vasoactive intestinal polypeptide. *Brain Res Bull* 14:179–188, 1985.

121. Harder DR, Gilbert R, Lombard JH: Vascular muscle cell depolarization and activation in renal arteries on elevation of transmural pressure. *Am J Physiol* 253:F778–781, 1987.

122. Harder DR: Pressure-dependent membrane depolarization in cat middle cerebral artery. *Circ Res* 55:197–202, 1984.

123. Harigaya S, Schwartz A: Rate of calcium binding and uptake in normal animal and failing human cardiac muscle: Membrane vesicles (relaxing system) and mitochondria. *Circ Res* 25:781–794, 1969.

124. Harper AM: Autoregulation of cerebral blood flow: Influence of the arterial blood pressure on the blood flow through the cerebral cortex. *J Neurol Neurosurg Psychiatry* 29:398–403, 1966.

125. Hatherill M, McIntyre AG, Wattie M, Murdoch IA: Early hyperlactataemia in critically ill children. *Intensive Care Med* 26:314–318, 2000.

126. Hatherill M, Sajjanhar T, Tibby SM, et al: Serum lactate as a predictor of mortality after paediatric cardiac surgery. *Arch Dis Child* 77:235–238, 1997.

127. Heilbrunn SM, Shah P, Bristow MR, et al: Increased beta-receptor density and improved hemodynamic response to catecholamine stimulation during long-term metoprolol therapy in heart failure from dilated cardiomyopathy. *Circulation* 79:483–490, 1989.

128. Henderson AH, Lewis MJ, Shah AM, Smith JA: Endothelium, endocardium, and cardiac contraction. *Cardiovasc Res* 26:305–308, 1992.

129. Hill JR, Rahimtulla KA: Heat balance and the metabolic rate of newborn babies in relation to environmental temperature; and the effect of age and of weight on basal metabolic rate. *J Physiol* 180:239–265, 1965.

130. Hirata Y, Hayakawa H, Kakoki M, et al: Receptor subtype for vasopressin-induced release of nitric oxide from rat kidney. *Hypertension* 29:58–64, 1997.

131. Hirshman CA, Peters J, Cartwright-Lee I: Leukocyte histamine release to thiopental. *Anesthesiology* 56:64–67, 1982.

132. Hoffman TM, Wernovsky G, Atz AM, et al: Efficacy and safety of milrinone in preventing low cardiac output syndrome in infants and children after corrective surgery for congenital heart disease. *Circulation* 107:996-1002, 2003.

133. Hoffman TM, Wernovsky G, Atz AM, et al: Prophylactic intravenous use of milrinone after cardiac operation in pediatrics (PRIMACORP) study. Prophylactic intravenous use of milrinone after cardiac operation in pediatrics. *Am Heart J* 143:15–21, 2002.

134. Hollenberg SM, Cunnion RE, Parillo JE: The effect of tumor necrosis function on vascular smooth muscle: In vitro studies using rat aortic rings. *Chest* 100:1133–1137, 1991.

135. Hotchkiss RS, Karl IE: Reevaluation of the role of cellular hypoxia and bioenergetic failure in sepsis. *JAMA* 267:1503–1510, 1992.

136. Hotchkiss RS, Long RC, Hall JR, et al: An in vivo examination of rat brain during sepsis with 31P-NMR spectroscopy. *Am J Physiol* 257:C1055–1061, 1989.

137. Hotchkiss RS, Rust RS, Dence CS, et al: Evaluation of the role of cellular hypoxia in sepsis by the hypoxic marker [18F] fluoromisonidazole. *Am J Physiol* 261:R965–972, 1991.

138. Human albumin administration in critically ill patients: Systematic review of randomised controlled trials. Cochrane Injuries Group Albumin Reviewers. *BMJ* 317:235–240, 1998.

139. Hunley TE, Kon V: Update on endothelins: Biology and clinical implications. *Pediatr Nephrol* 16:752–762, 2001.

140. Hurford WE: Inhaled nitric oxide. *Respir Care Clin N Am* 8:261–279, 2002.

141. Huskisson L: Intravenous volume replacement: Which fluid and why? *Arch Dis Child* 67:649–653, 1992.

142. Imm A, Carlson RW: Fluid resuscitation in circulatory shock. *Crit Care Clin* 9:313–333, 1993.

143. Jackson G, Gibbs CR, Davies MK, Lip GY: ABC of heart failure: Pathophysiology. *BMJ* 320:167–170, 2000.

144. Jepson MM, Cox M, Bates PC, et al: Regional blood flow and skeletal muscle energy status in endotoxemic rats. *Am J Physiol* 252:E581–587, 1987.

145. Johnson PC: Autoregulation of blood flow. *Circ Res* 59:483–495, 1986.

146. Jordan DA, Miller ED Jr: Subarachnoid blockade alters homeostasis by modifying compensatory splanchnic responses to hemorrhagic hypotension. *Anesthesiology* 75:654–661, 1991.

147. Katz SD, Biasucci L, Sabba C, et al: Impaired endothelium-mediated vasodilation in the peripheral vasculature of patients with congestive heart failure. *J Am Coll Cardiol* 19:918–925, 1992.

148. Kaumann AJ: Is there a third heart beta-adrenoceptor? *Trends Pharmacol Sci* 10:316–320, 1989.

149. Kiemer AK, Vollmar AM: The atrial natriuretic peptide regulates the production of inflammatory mediators in macrophages. *Ann Rheum Dis* 60 (Suppl 3):68–70, 2001.

150. Kingston ME, Al-Siba'i MB, Skooge WC: Clinical manifestations of hypomagnesemia. *Crit Care Med* 14:950–954, 1986.

151. Klasaer AE, Scalzo AJ, Blume C, et al: Marked hypocalcemia and ventricular fibrillation in two pediatric patients exposed to a fluoride-containing wheel cleaner. *Ann Emerg Med* 28:713–718, 1996.

152. Koide M, Kawahara Y, Tsuda T, et al: Expression of nitric oxide synthase by cytokines in vascular smooth muscle cells. *Hypertension* 23:I45–48, 1994.

153. Kubo SH, Rector TS, Bank AJ, et al: Endothelium-dependent vasodilation is attenuated in patients with heart failure. *Circulation* 84:1589–1596, 1991.

154. Laer S, Mir TS, Behn F, et al: Carvedilol therapy in pediatric patients with congestive heart failure: A study investigating clinical and pharmacokinetic parameters. *Am Heart J* 143:916–922, 2002.

155. Laffey JG, Boylan JF, Cheng DC: The systemic inflammatory response to cardiac surgery: Implications for the anesthesiologist. *Anesthesiology* 97:215–252, 2002.

156. Lambert DG: Signal transduction: G proteins and second messengers. *Br J Anaesth* 71:86–95, 1993.

157. Landry DW, Levin HR, Gallant EM, et al: Vasopressin deficiency contributes to the vasodilation of septic shock. *Circulation* 95:1122–1125, 1997.

158. Landry DW, Oliver JA: The pathogenesis of vasodilatory shock. *N Engl J Med* 345:588–595, 2001.

159. Lawless S, Burckart G, Diven W, et al: Amrinone pharmacokinetics in neonates and infants. *J Clin Pharmacol* 28:283–284, 1988.

160. Le Jemtel TH, Katz SD, Sonnenblick EH: Peripheral circulatory response in cardiac failure. *Hosp Pract (Off Ed)* 26:75–82, 1991.

161. Lefkowitz RJ, Caron MG, Stiles GL: Mechanisms of membrane-receptor regulation: Biochemical, physiological, and clinical insights derived from studies of the adrenergic receptors. *N Engl J Med* 310:1570–1579, 1984.

162. Legato MJ: Cellular mechanisms of normal growth in the mammalian heart. II. A quantitative and qualitative comparison between the right and left ventricular myocytes in the dog from birth to 5 months of age. *Circ Res* 44:263–279, 1979.

163. Liedel JL, Meadow W, Nachman J, et al: Use of vasopressin in refractory hypotension in children with vasodilatory shock: Five cases and a review of the literature. *Pediatr Crit Care Med* 3:15–18, 2002.

164. Lister G, Walter TK, Versmold HT, et al: Oxygen delivery in lambs: Cardiovascular and hematologic development. *Am J Physiol* 237:H668–675, 1979.

165. Litchfield RL, Kerber RE, Benge JW, et al: Normal exercise capacity in patients with severe left ventricular dysfunction: Compensatory mechanisms. *Circulation* 66:129–134, 1982.

166. Lompre AM, Schwartz K, d'Albis A, et al: Myosin isoenzyme redistribution in chronic heart overload. *Nature* 282:105–107, 1979.

167. London MJ: Pro: Colloids should be added to the pump prime. *J Cardiothorac Anesth* 4:401–405, 1990.

168. Lopez JR, Jahangir R, Jahangir A, et al: Potassium channel openers prevent potassium-induced calcium loading of cardiac cells: Possible implications in cardioplegia. *J Thorac Cardiovasc Surg* 112:820–831, 1996.

169. Lowson SM, Doctor A, Walsh BK, Doorley PA: Inhaled prostacyclin for the treatment of pulmonary hypertension after cardiac surgery. *Crit Care Med* 30:2762–2764, 2002.

170. Lucking SE, Williams TM, Chaten FC, et al: Dependence of oxygen consumption on oxygen delivery in children with hyperdynamic septic shock and low oxygen extraction. *Crit Care Med* 18:1316–1319, 1990.

171. Lundberg JM: Evidence for coexistence of vasoactive intestinal polypeptide (VIP) and acetylcholine in neurons of cat exocrine glands. Morphological, biochemical and functional studies. *Acta Physiol Scand Suppl* 496:1–57, 1981.

172. Lundin S, Mang H, Smithies M, et al: Inhalation of nitric oxide in acute lung injury: Results of a European multicentre study. The European Study Group of Inhaled Nitric Oxide. *Intensive Care Med* 25:911–919, 1999.

173. Maisel AS, Krishnaswamy P, Nowak RM, et al: Breathing Not Properly Multinational Study Investigators: Rapid measurement of B-type natriuretic peptide in the emergency diagnosis of heart failure. *N Engl J Med* 347:161–167, 2002.

174. Maki T, Nasa Y, Yamaguchi F, et al: Long-term treatment with neutral endopeptidase inhibitor improves cardiac function and reduces natriuretic peptides in rats with chronic heart failure. *Cardiovasc Res* 51:608–617, 2001.

175. Malay MB, Ashton RC Jr, Landry DW, Townsend RN: Low-dose vasopressin in the treatment of vasodilatory septic shock. *J Trauma* 47:699–703, 1999.

176. Manasek FJ: Organization, interactions, and environment of heart cells during myocardial ontogeny. In Berne RM (ed): *Handbook of Physiology, Section 2: The Cardiovascular System, Vol. I, The Heart.* Bethesda, MD, American Physiology Society, 1983.

177. Manohar M, Bisgard GE, Bullard V, et al: Regional myocardial blood flow and myocardial function during acute right ventricular pressure overload in calves. *Circ Res* 44:531–539, 1979.

178. Margulies KB, Hildebrand FL Jr, Lerman A, et al: Increased endothelin in experimental heart failure. *Circulation* 82:2226–2230, 1990.

179. Marik PE: Low-dose dopamine: A systematic review. *Intensive Care Med* 28:877–883, 2002.

180. Martin LD, Barnes SD, Wetzel RC: Acute hypoxia alters eicosanoid production of perfused pulmonary artery endothelial cells in culture. *Prostaglandins* 43:371–382, 1992.

181. Maskin CS, Forman R, Sonnenblick EH, et al: Failure of dobutamine to increase exercise capacity despite hemodynamic improvement in severe chronic heart failure. *Am J Cardiol* 51:177–182, 1983.

182. Matsuda N, Hattori Y, Akaishi Y, et al: Impairment of cardiac beta-adrenoceptor cellular signaling by decreased expression of G (s alpha) in septic rabbits. *Anesthesiology* 93:1465–1473, 2000.

183. Mays PK, Bishop JE, Laurent GJ: Age-related changes in the proportion of types I and III collagen. *Mech Ageing Dev* 45:203–212, 1988.

184. McCormack J, Gelband H, Villafane J, et al: In vivo demonstration of maturational changes of the chronotropic response to alpha-adrenergic stimulation. *Pediatr Res* 24:50–54, 1988.

185. McMurray J, Pfeffer MA: New therapeutic options in congestive heart failure: Part I. *Circulation* 105:2099–2106, 2002.

186. Mebazaa A, Mayoux E, Maeda K, et al: Paracrine effects of endocardial endothelial cells on myocyte contraction mediated via endothelin. *Am J Physiol* 265:H1841–1846, 1993.

187. Michell RH: Post-receptor signalling pathways. *Lancet* 1:765–768, 1989.

188. Minneman KP: Alpha 1-adrenergic receptor subtypes, inositol phosphates, and sources of cell Ca^{2+}. *Pharmacol Rev* 40:87–119, 1988.

189. Mione MC, Dhital KK, Amenta F, Burnstock G: An increase in the expression of neuropeptidergic vasodilator, but not vasoconstrictor, cerebrovascular nerves in aging rats. *Brain Res* 460:103–113, 1988.

190. Moncada S, Palmer RM, Higgs EA: Nitric oxide: Physiology, pathophysiology, and pharmacology. *Pharmacol Rev* 43:109–142, 1991.

191. Moncada S: The 1991 Ulf von Euler Lecture: The L-arginine–nitric oxide pathway. *Acta Physiol Scand* 145:201–227, 1992.

192. Morales D, Madigan J, Cullinane S, et al: Reversal by vasopressin of intractable hypotension in the late phase of hemorrhagic shock. *Circulation* 100:226–229, 1999.

193. Morales DL, Gregg D, Helman DN, et al: Arginine vasopressin in the treatment of 50 patients with postcardiotomy vasodilatory shock. *Ann Thorac Surg* 69:102–106, 2000.

194. Moss J, Rosow CE, Savarese JJ, et al: Role of histamine in the hypotensive action of d-tubocurarine in humans. *Anesthesiology* 55:19–25, 1981.

195. Munoz R, Laussen PC, Palacio G, et al: Changes in whole blood lactate levels during cardiopulmonary bypass for surgery for congenital cardiac disease: An early indicator of morbidity and mortality. *J Thorac Cardiovasc Surg* 119:155–162, 2000.

196. Murdoch IA, Qureshi SA, Huggon IC: Perioperative haemodynamic effects of an intravenous infusion of calcium chloride in children following cardiac surgery. *Acta Paediatr* 83:658–661, 1994.

197. Murthy KS, Rao SG, Prakash KS, et al: Role of inhaled nitric oxide as a selective pulmonary vasodilator in pediatric cardiac surgical practice. *Indian J Pediatr* 66:357–361, 1999.

198. Nassar R, Reedy MC, Anderson PA: Developmental changes in the ultrastructure and sarcomere shortening of the isolated rabbit ventricular myocyte. *Circ Res* 61:465–483, 1987.

199. Natanson C, Danner RL, Elin RJ, et al: Role of endotoxemia in cardiovascular dysfunction and mortality: *Escherichia coli* and *Staphylococcus aureus* challenges in a canine model of human septic shock. *J Clin Invest* 83:243–251, 1989.

200. Natanson C, Fink MP, Ballantyne HK, et al: Gram-negative bacteremia produces both severe systolic and diastolic cardiac dysfunction in a canine model that simulates human septic shock. *J Clin Invest* 78:259–270, 1986.

201. Nava E, Palmer RM, Moncada S: Inhibition of nitric oxide synthesis in septic shock: How much is beneficial? *Lancet* 338:1555–1557, 1991.

202. Nearman HS, Herman ML: Toxic effects of colloids in the intensive care unit. *Crit Care Clin* 7:713–723, 1991.

203. Nishijima MK, Breslow MJ, Miller CF, Traystman RJ: Effect of naloxone and ibuprofen on organ blood flow during endotoxic shock in pig. *Am J Physiol* 255:H177–184, 1988.

204. Nishijima MK, Breslow MJ, Raff H, Traystman RJ: Regional adrenal blood flow during hypoxia in anesthetized, ventilated dogs. *Am J Physiol* 256:H94–100, 1989.

205. Noma A: ATP-regulated K^+ channels in cardiac muscle. *Nature* 305:147–148, 1983.

206. Norwood WI, Lang P, Hansen DD: Physiologic repair of aortic atresia–hypoplastic left heart syndrome. *N Engl J Med* 308:23–26, 1983.

207. Oana S, Terai M, Tanabe M, et al: Plasma brain natriuretic peptides and renal hypertension. *Pediatr Nephrol* 14:813–815, 2000.

208. Ognibene FP, Parker MM, Natanson C, et al: Depressed left ventricular performance: Response to volume infusion in patients with sepsis and septic shock. *Chest* 93:903–910, 1988.

209. Ohlsson K, Bjork P, Bergenfeldt M, et al: Interleukin-1 receptor antagonist reduces mortality from endotoxin shock. *Nature* 348:550–552, 1990.

210. Ohta A, Sitkovsky M: Role of G-protein-coupled adenosine receptors in downregulation of inflammation and protection from tissue damage. *Nature* 414:916–920, 2001.

211. Olesen J, Paulson OB, Lassen NA: Regional cerebral blood flow in man determined by the initial slope of the clearance of intra-arterially injected 133Xe. *Stroke* 2:519–540, 1971.

212. Oliveira RP, Velasco I, Soriano F, Friedman G: Clinical review: Hypertonic saline resuscitation in sepsis. *Crit Care* 6:418–423, 2002.

213. O'Loughlin MP, Fisher DJ: Mechanisms of congestive heart failure. In Garson A Jr, Bricker JT, McNamara DG (eds): *The Science and Practice of Pediatric Cardiology*. Philadelphia, Lea & Febiger, pp 244–249, 1990.

214. Omland T, Lie RT, Aakvaag A, et al: Plasma endothelin determination as a prognostic indicator of 1-year mortality after acute myocardial infarction. *Circulation* 89:1573–1579, 1994.

215. Panagia V, Michiel DF, Khatter JC, et al: Sarcolemmal alterations in cardiac hypertrophy due to pressure overload in pigs. In Abel FL, Newman WH (eds): *Functional Aspects of the Normal, Hypertrophied, and Failing Heart*. Boston, Martinus Nijhoff, 1984.

216. Parker MM, McCarthy KE, Ognibene FP, Parrillo JE: Right ventricular dysfunction and dilation, similar to left ventricular changes, characterize the cardiac depression of septic shock in humans. *Chest* 97:126–131, 1990.

217. Parmley WW: Pathophysiology of congestive heart failure. *Clin Cardiol* 15 Suppl 1:I5–12, 1992.

218. Parr GV, Blackstone EH, Kirklin JW: Cardiac performance and mortality early after intracardiac surgery in infants and young children. *Circulation* 51:867–874, 1975.

219. Parrillo JE, Burch C, Shelhamer JH, et al: A circulating myocardial depressant substance in humans with septic shock: Septic shock patients with a reduced ejection fraction have a circulating factor that depresses in vitro myocardial cell performance. *J Clin Invest* 76:1539–1553, 1985.

220. Parrillo JE, Parker MM, Natanson C, et al: Septic shock in humans: Advances in the understanding of pathogenesis, cardiovascular dysfunction, and therapy. *Ann Intern Med* 113:227–242, 1990.

221. Parrillo JE: Pathogenetic mechanisms of septic shock. *N Engl J Med* 328:1471–1477, 1993.

222. Pearl JM, Nelson DP, Raake JL, et al: Inhaled nitric oxide increases endothelin-1 levels: A potential cause of rebound pulmonary hypertension. *Crit Care Med* 30:89–93, 2002.

223. Petros A, Bennett D, Vallance P: Effect of nitric oxide synthase inhibitors on hypotension in patients with septic shock. *Lancet* 338:1557–1558, 1991.

224. Phillips CA, Mylecharane EJ, Shaw J: Mechanisms involved in the vasodilator action of 5-hydroxytryptamine in the dog femoral arterial circulation in vivo. *Eur J Pharmacol* 113:325–334, 1985.

225. Pignac J, Bourgouin J, Dumont L: Cold cardioplegia and the K⁺ channel modulator aprikalim (RP 52891): Improved cardioprotection in isolated ischemic rabbit hearts. *Can J Physiol Pharmacol* 72:126–132, 1994.

226. Rahko PS: Comparative efficacy of three indexes of left ventricular performance derived from pressure-volume loops in heart failure induced by tachypacing. *J Am Coll Cardiol* 23:209–218, 1994.

227. Ramamoorthy C, Anderson GD, Williams GD, Lynn AM: Pharmacokinetics and side effects of milrinone in infants and children after open heart surgery. *Anesth Analg* 86:283–289, 1998.

228. Reddy GD, Gootman N, Buckley NM, et al: Regional blood flow changes in neonatal pigs in response to hypercapnia, hemorrhage and sciatic nerve stimulation. *Biol Neonate* 25:249–262, 1974.

229. Reilly JM, Cunnion RE, Burch-Whitman C, et al: A circulating myocardial depressant substance is associated with cardiac dysfunction and peripheral hypoperfusion (lactic acidemia) in patients with septic shock. *Chest* 95:1072–1080, 1989.

230. Reinhart K, Bayer O, Brunkhorst F, Meisner M: Markers of endothelial damage in organ dysfunction and sepsis. *Crit Care Med* 30:S302–312, 2002.

231. Reithmann C, Gierschik P, Jakobs KH: Stimulation and inhibition of adenylyl cyclase. *Symp Soc Exp Biol* 44:207–224, 1990.

232. Rhee KH, Toro LO, McDonald GG, et al: Carbicarb, sodium bicarbonate, and sodium chloride in hypoxic lactic acidosis: Effect on arterial blood gases, lactate concentrations, hemodynamic variables, and myocardial intracellular pH. *Chest* 104:913–918, 1993.

233. Rich GF, Murphy GD Jr, Roos CM, Johns RA: Inhaled nitric oxide: Selective pulmonary vasodilation in cardiac surgical patients. *Anesthesiology* 78:1028–1035, 1993.

234. Rivers E, Nguyen B, Havstad S, et al: Early Goal-Directed Therapy Collaborative Group: Early goal-directed therapy in the treatment of severe sepsis and septic shock. *N Engl J Med* 345:1368–1377, 2001.

235. Roberts JD, Polaner DM, Lang P, Zapol WM: Inhaled nitric oxide in persistent pulmonary hypertension of the newborn. *Lancet* 340:818–819, 1992.

236. Rolph TP, Jones CT: Regulation of glycolytic flux in the heart of the fetal guinea pig. *J Dev Physiol* 5:31–49, 1983.

237. Romero TE, Friedman WF: Limited left ventricular response to volume overload in the neonatal period: A comparative study with the adult animal. *Pediatr Res* 13:910–915, 1979.

238. Rosenzweig EB, Starc TJ, Chen JM, et al: Intravenous arginine-vasopressin in children with vasodilatory shock after cardiac surgery. *Circulation* 100:II182–186, 1999.

239. Rosow CE, Moss J, Philbin DM, Savarese JJ: Histamine release during morphine and fentanyl anesthesia. *Anesthesiology* 56:93–96, 1982.

240. Ross J Jr: Afterload mismatch and preload reserve: A conceptual framework for the analysis of ventricular function. *Prog Cardiovasc Dis* 18:255–264, 1976.

241. Rubin K, Tingstrom A, Hansson GK, et al: Induction of B-type receptors for platelet-derived growth factor in vascular inflammation: Possible implications for development of vascular proliferative lesions. *Lancet* 1:1353–1356, 1988.

242. Rudolph AM: Myocardial growth before and after birth: Clinical implications. *Acta Paediatr* 89:129–133, 2000.

243. Ruokonen E, Takala J, Kari A, et al: Regional blood flow and oxygen transport in septic shock. *Crit Care Med* 21:1296–1303, 1993.

244. Ry SD, Andreassi MG, Clerico A, et al: Endothelin-1, endothelin-1 receptors and cardiac natriuretic peptides in failing human heart. *Life Sci* 68:2715–2730, 2001.

245. Sagawa K: The end-systolic pressure-volume relation of the ventricle: Definition, modifications and clinical use. *Circulation* 63:1223–1227, 1981.

246. Said SI, Mutt V: Polypeptide with broad biological activity: Isolation from small intestine. *Science* 169:1217–1218, 1970.

247. Sanada S, Node K, Asanuma H, et al: Opening of the adenosine triphosphate-sensitive potassium channel attenuates cardiac remodeling induced by long-term inhibition of nitric oxide synthesis: Role of 70-kDa S6 kinase and extracellular signal-regulated kinase. *J Am Coll Cardiol* 40:991–997, 2002.

248. Schirger JA, Grantham JA, Kullo IJ, et al: Vascular actions of brain natriuretic peptide: Modulation by atherosclerosis and neutral endopeptidase inhibition. *J Am Coll Cardiol* 35:796–801, 2000.

249. Schmidt RE, McAtee SJ, Plurad DA, et al: Differential susceptibility of prevertebral and paravertebral sympathetic ganglia to experimental injury. *Brain Res* 460:214–226, 1988.

250. Schmidt RE, Plurad DA, Roth KA: Effects of chronic experimental streptozotocin-induced diabetes on the noradrenergic and peptidergic innervation of the rat alimentary tract. *Brain Res* 458:353–360, 1988.

251. Schrier RW, Abraham WT: Hormones and hemodynamics in heart failure. *N Engl J Med* 341:577–585, 1999.

252. Schwartz K, Lecarpentier Y, Martin JL, et al: Myosin isoenzymic distribution correlates with speed of myocardial contraction. *J Mol Cell Cardiol* 13:1071–1075, 1981.

253. Scopes JW: Metabolic rate and temperature control in the human baby. *Br Med Bull* 22:88–91, 1966.

254. Seasholtz TM, Gurdal H, Wang HY, et al: Desensitization of norepinephrine receptor function is associated with G protein uncoupling in the rat aorta. *Am J Physiol* 273:H279–285, 1997.

255. Semigran MJ, Aroney CN, Herrmann HC, et al: Effects of atrial natriuretic peptide on myocardial contractile and diastolic function in patients with heart failure. *J Am Coll Cardiol* 20:98–106, 1992.

256. Shah AM, Mebazaa A, Wetzel RC, Lakatta EG: Novel cardiac myofilament desensitizing factor released by endocardial and vascular endothelial cells. *Circulation* 89:2492–2497, 1994.

257. Shalev H, Phillip M, Galil A, et al: Clinical presentation and outcome in primary familial hypomagnesaemia. *Arch Dis Child* 78:127–130, 1998.

258. Shepherd AP, Granger HJ, Smith EE, Guyton AC: Local control of tissue oxygen delivery and its contribution to the regulation of cardiac output. *Am J Physiol* 225:747–755, 1973.

259. Shibata M, Leffler CW, Busija DW: Pial arteriolar constriction following cortical spreading depression is mediated by prostanoids. *Brain Res* 572:190–197, 1992.

260. Shoemaker WC, Appel PL, Kram HB: Tissue oxygen debt as a determinant of lethal and nonlethal postoperative organ failure. *Crit Care Med* 16:1117–1120, 1988.

261. Shoemaker WC, Appel PL, Waxman K, et al: Clinical trial of survivors' cardiorespiratory patterns as therapeutic goals in critically ill postoperative patients. *Crit Care Med* 10:398–403, 1982.

262. Siegel LB, Dalton HJ, Hertzog JH, et al: Initial postoperative serum lactate levels predict survival in children after open heart surgery. *Intensive Care Med* 22:1418–1423, 1996.

263. Silverman HJ, Penaranda R, Orens JB, Lee NH: Impaired beta-adrenergic receptor stimulation of cyclic adenosine monophosphate in human septic shock: Association with myocardial hyporesponsiveness to catecholamines. *Crit Care Med* 21:31–39, 1993.

264. Smith JA, Shah AM, Fort S, Lewis MJ: The influence of endocardial endothelium on myocardial contraction. *Trends Pharmacol Sci* 13:113–116, 1992.

265. Song SK, Hotchkiss RS, Karl IE, Ackerman JJ: Concurrent quantification of tissue metabolism and blood flow via 2H/31P NMR in vivo. III. Alterations of muscle blood flow and metabolism during sepsis. *Magn Reson Med* 25:67–77, 1992.

266. Sonnenblick EH, Strobeck JE: Current concepts in cardiology: Derived indexes of ventricular and myocardial function. *N Engl J Med* 296:978–982, 1977.

267. Sonnenblick EH: Myocardial ultrastructure in the normal and failing heart. In Braunwald E (ed): *The Myocardium: Failure and Infarction.* New York, HP Publishing, 1974.

268. Sordahl LA, Wood WG, Schwartz A: Production of cardiac hypertrophy and failure in rabbits with Ameroid clips. *J Mol Cell Cardiol* 1:341–344, 1970.

269. Soroker D, Ezri T, Szmuk P, et al: Perioperative torsade de pointes ventricular tachycardia induced by hypocalcemia and hypokalemia. *Anesth Analg* 80:630–633, 1995.

270. Squire JM: *Molecular Mechanisms in Muscular Contraction: Topics in Molecular and Structural Biology.* Boca Raton, Fla., CRC Press, 1990.

271. Starc TJ, Rosenzweig EB, Landry DW, et al: Emergency use of vasopressin in children with vasodilatory shock due to sepsis or after bypass. *Crit Care Med* 28:A71, 2000.

272. Steffes CP, Bender JS, Levison MA: Blood transfusion and oxygen consumption in surgical sepsis. *Crit Care Med* 19:512–517, 1991.

273. Stevenson LW, Fonarow GC: Endothelin and the vascular choir in heart failure. *J Am Coll Cardiol* 20:854–857, 1992.

274. Stillman MT, Schlesinger PA: Nonsteroidal anti-inflammatory drug nephrotoxicity: Should we be concerned? *Arch Intern Med* 150:268–270, 1990.

275. Streeter DD Jr, Hanna WT: Engineering mechanics for successive states in canine left ventricular myocardium. II. Fiber angle and sarcomere length. *Circ Res* 33:656–664, 1973.

276. Strobeck JE, Sonnenblick EH: Myocardial contractile properties and ventricular performance. In Fozzard HA, Haber E, Jennings RB (eds): *The Heart and Cardiovascular System: Scientific Foundations.* New York, Raven Press, p 31, 1986.

277. Stulz PM, Scheidegger D, Drop LJ, et al: Ventricular pump performance during hypocalcemia: Clinical and experimental studies. *J Thorac Cardiovasc Surg* 78:185–194, 1979.

278. Suffredini AF, Harpel PC, Parrillo JE. Promotion and subsequent inhibition of plasminogen activation after administration of intravenous endotoxin to normal subjects. *N Engl J Med* 320:1165–1172, 1989.

279. Suschek CV, Schnorr O, Hemmrich K, et al: Critical role of L-arginine in endothelial cell survival during oxidative stress. *Circulation* 107:2607–2614, 2003.

280. Sutsch G, Kiowski W: Endothelin and endothelin receptor antagonism in heart failure. *J Cardiovasc Pharmacol* 35:S69–73, 2000.

281. Sykes KS, Bachrach LK, Siegel-Bartelt J, et al: Velocardiofacial syndrome presenting as hypocalcemia in early adolescence. *Arch Pediatr Adolesc Med* 151:745–747, 1997.

282. Takemura G, Takatsu Y, Doyama K, et al: Expression of atrial and brain natriuretic peptides and their genes in hearts of patients with cardiac amyloidosis. *J Am Coll Cardiol* 31:754–765, 1998.

283. Tatemoto K, Carlquist M, Mutt V: Neuropeptide Y—a novel brain peptide with structural similarities to peptide YY and pancreatic polypeptide. *Nature* 296:659–660, 1982.

284. Teitel DF, Sidi D, Chin T, et al: Developmental changes in myocardial contractile reserve in the lamb. *Pediatr Res* 19:948–955, 1985.

285. Thoma R: *Textbook of General Pathology.* London, Adam & Charles Black, 1895.

286. Tobias JD, Haun SE, Helfaer M, Nichols DG: Use of continuous caudal block to relieve lower-extremity ischemia caused by vasculitis in a child with meningococcemia. *J Pediatr* 115:1019–1021, 1989.

287. Tobin JR, Breslow MJ, Traystman RJ: Fentanyl and midazolam-mediated changes in adrenal blood flow and catecholamine secretion. *Anesthesiology* 79:A641, 1993.

288. Tomec RJ, Hoppel CL: Carnitine palmitoyltransferase in bovine fetal heart mitochondria. *Arch Biochem Biophys* 170:716–723, 1975.

289. Trinder D, Phillips PA, Stephenson JM, et al: Vasopressin V1 and V2 receptors in diabetes mellitus. *Am J Physiol* 266:E217–223, 1994.

290. Tsuneyoshi I, Yamada H, Kakihana Y, et al: Hemodynamic and metabolic effects of low-dose vasopressin infusions in vasodilatory septic shock. *Crit Care Med* 29:487–493, 2001.

291. Urban P, Scheidegger D, Buchmann B, Skarvan K: The hemodynamic effects of heparin and their relation to ionized calcium levels. *J Thorac Cardiovasc Surg* 91:303–306, 1986.

292. Vallet B: Bench-to-bedside review: Endothelial cell dysfunction in severe sepsis: A role in organ dysfunction? *Crit Care* 7:130–138, 2003.

293. Vary TC: Increased pyruvate dehydrogenase kinase activity in response to sepsis. *Am J Physiol* 260:E669–674, 1991.

294. Velasco M, Contreras F, Cabezas GA, et al: Dopaminergic receptors: A new antihypertensive mechanism. *J Hypertens* 3:S55–58, 2002.

295. Venkatesh VC, Ballard PL: Glucocorticoids and gene expression. *Am J Respir Cell Mol Biol* 4:301–303, 1991.

296. Verrier B, Muller D, Bravo R, Muller R: Wounding a fibroblast monolayer results in the rapid induction of the c-fos proto-oncogene. *EMBO J* 5:913–917, 1986.

297. Verrier ED: The vascular endothelium: Friend or foe? *Ann Thorac Surg* 55:818–819, 1993.

298. Villar J, Slutsky AS, Hew E, Aberman A: Oxygen transport and oxygen consumption in critically ill patients. *Chest* 98:687–692, 1990.

299. Villarreal D, Freeman RH, Reams GP: Natriuretic peptides and salt sensitivity: Endocrine cardiorenal integration in heart failure. *Congest Heart Fail* 8:29–36, 48, 2002.

300. Vincent JL, Dufaye P, Berre J, et al: Serial lactate determinations during circulatory shock. *Crit Care Med* 11:449–451, 1983.

301. Vincent JL: Fluids for resuscitation. *Br J Anaesth* 67:185–193, 1991.

302. Vincent RN, Click LA, Williams HM, et al: Esmolol as an adjunct in the treatment of systemic hypertension after operative repair of coarctation of the aorta. *Am J Cardiol* 65:941–943, 1990.

303. Wade CE: Hypertonic saline resuscitation in sepsis. *Crit Care* 6:397–398, 2002.

304. Wagner BK, D'Amelio LF: Pharmacologic and clinical considerations in selecting crystalloid, colloidal, and oxygen-carrying resuscitation fluids, Part 1. *Clin Pharm* 12:335–346, 1993.

305. Wagner BK, D'Amelio LF: Pharmacologic and clinical considerations in selecting crystalloid, colloidal, and oxygen-carrying resuscitation fluids, Part 2. *Clin Pharm* 12:415–428, 1993.

306. Warren BL, Eid A, Singer P, et al: KyberSept Trial Study Group: Caring for the critically ill patient: High-dose antithrombin III in severe sepsis: A randomized controlled trial. *JAMA* 286:1869–1878, 2001.

307. Weber KT, Kinasewitz GT, Janicki JS, Fishman AP: Oxygen utilization and ventilation during exercise in patients with chronic cardiac failure. *Circulation* 65:1213–1223, 1982.

308. Wei CM, Lerman A, Rodeheffer RJ, et al: Endothelin in human congestive heart failure. *Circulation* 89:1580–1586, 1994.

309. Weil SR, Russo PA, Heckman JL, et al: Pressure-volume relationship of the fetal lamb heart. *Ann Thorac Surg* 55:470–475, 1993.

310. Wetzel RC, Setzer N, Stiff JL, Rogers MC: Hemodynamic responses in brain dead organ donor patients. *Anesth Analg* 64:125–128, 1985.

311. Wetzel RC, Tobin JR: Shock. In Rogers MC (ed): *Textbook of Pediatric Intensive Care.* Baltimore, Williams & Wilkins, pp 563–613, 1992.

312. Wetzel RC: Aerosolized prostacyclin: In search of the ideal pulmonary vasodilator. *Anesthesiology* 82:1315–1317, 1995.

313. Wetzel RC: The intensivist's system. *Crit Care Med* 21:S341–344, 1993.

314. Whitsett JA, Noguchi A, Moore JJ: Developmental aspects of alpha- and beta-adrenergic receptors. *Semin Perinatol* 6:125–141, 1982.

315. Winegrad S: Regulation of cardiac contractile proteins: Correlations between physiology and biochemistry. *Circ Res* 55:565–574, 1984.

316. Wolf YG, Cotev S, Perel A, Manny J: Dependence of oxygen consumption on cardiac output in sepsis. *Crit Care Med* 15:198–203, 1987.

317. Wolfe RR, Jahoor F, Herndon DN, Miyoshi H: Isotopic evaluation of the metabolism of pyruvate and related substrates in normal adult volunteers and severely burned children: Effect of dichloroacetate and glucose infusion. *Surgery* 110:54–67, 1991.

318. Yanagisawa M, Kurihara H, Kimura S, et al: A novel potent vasoconstrictor peptide produced by vascular endothelial cells. *Nature* 332:411–415, 1988.

319. Yokoshiki H, Sunagawa M, Seki T, Sperelakis N: ATP-sensitive K+ channels in pancreatic, cardiac, and vascular smooth muscle cells. *Am J Physiol* 274:C25–37, 1998.

320. Yuan JX, Aldinger AM, Juhaszova M, et al: Dysfunctional voltage-gated K+ channels in pulmonary artery smooth muscle cells of patients with primary pulmonary hypertension. *Circulation* 98:1400–1406, 1998.

321. Zhou ZZ, Jones SB: The vascular response to adrenergic stimulation in pithed rats following endotoxin. *Circ Shock* 32:55–66, 1990.

322. Zile MR, Brutsaert DL: New concepts in diastolic dysfunction and diastolic heart failure: Part I: Diagnosis, prognosis, and measurements of diastolic function. *Circulation* 105:1387–1393, 2002.

323. Zile MR, Brutsaert DL: New concepts in diastolic dysfunction and diastolic heart failure: Part II: Causal mechanisms and treatment. *Circulation* 105:1503–1508, 2002.

Chapter 3

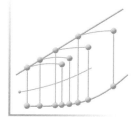

Regulation of Pulmonary Vascular Resistance and Blood Flow

LYNN D. MARTIN, MD, DANIEL NYHAN, MD, and
RANDALL C. WETZEL, MBBS, MBA

INTRODUCTION

The pulmonary circulation critically affects cardiopulmonary function in children with cardiovascular disease. Perioperatively, pulmonary vascular function profoundly influences morbidity and mortality in children undergoing repair of congenital heart defects. Normally, the pulmonary circulation conducts the entire cardiac output at a pressure less than 20% of systemic vascular pressure. Pulmonary vascular tone alters right ventricular function by changing right ventricular afterload and also affects left ventricular preload. Thus, the low resistance pressure-flow characteristics of the pulmonary circulation are essential not only for preserving efficient gas exchange and deterring the formation of pulmonary edema, but also for ensuring efficient cardiovascular performance. The pulmonary circulation's unique role is underscored by the fact that its response to a variety of physiologic and pharmacologic stimuli is often different from that of the systemic circulation. Because of its central position in the circulation, the pulmonary circulation plays an important role in determining the outcome of many diseases. Perhaps this is most clearly seen in persistent pulmonary hypertension of the newborn, when the pulmonary circulation fails to adapt to the extrauterine environment, and oxygenation, ventilation, cardiac output, and pulmonary function are critically impaired.

It is now abundantly clear that the pulmonary vascular endothelium is central to the integration of pulmonary vascular function. The endothelium, originally considered only a passive, semi-permeable barrier, is now recognized as an intensely metabolically active organ with profound local and systemic effects. To alter pulmonary vascular smooth muscle tone, all circulating substances, whether endogenous or exogenous, must interact with or cross the endothelium. The endothelial cell with its vast array of receptors, enzymes, and transport proteins, continuously in contact with circulating blood components, facilitates and modulates these interactions.

The strategic location of the pulmonary endothelium in series with the systemic circulation, linked with its ability to selectively alter levels of many circulating vasoactive substances, enables profound modulation of cardiovascular function by the pulmonary circulation. Due to its role in the regulation of pulmonary vascular smooth muscle tone and thus pulmonary blood flow, the endothelium will be the major focus of this chapter. Understanding the production and/or modulation of vasoactive substances by the endothelium and the alteration of endothelial function by multiple physiologic stimuli such as hypoxia and flow is central to managing children with heart disease. Particular emphasis will be placed on examining the endothelium's role in the effects of flow and pressure associated with congenital heart defects and on the morphology and function of the pulmonary circulation. Finally, a brief discussion of both conventional and experimental therapies for pulmonary hypertension, as it relates to children, will be provided.

DEVELOPMENT OF THE PULMONARY CIRCULATION

A principal feature of the normal growth and development of the lungs is continuous remodeling of the pulmonary vasculature throughout fetal, transitional, neonatal, and childhood periods. This section will review recent information regarding the normal structural maturation of the pulmonary circulation, which governs the functional behavior of the pulmonary circulation. These changes are particularly relevant to the transitional circulation. As before, the focus will be on the cell biology of the vessel wall and its relation to the structural and functional adaptations necessary for the transition from fetal to extrauterine life.

Structural Development

Morphologic development of the pulmonary vasculature affects the physiologic changes that occur in the perinatal period. Much of the understanding of the structure and regulation of the fetal pulmonary circulation comes from experiments done in fetal lambs or more recently in rats and mice. An important fact to consider is that the action, distribution, and ontogeny of the various mediators of transition may not be the same in humans as they are in animals; however, data derived from animals have historically correlated well with those obtained from humans.[71]

Embryology

The lungs are present by 28 days of gestation as paired diverticula of the foregut. Distinct buds for the lobes of the lung are present by the 35th day of gestation. The vascular supply to the lung buds consists of paired segmental arteries arising from the dorsal aorta cephalad to the celiac artery. These connections normally involute but may persist in association with pulmonary atresia to form anomalous arterial supplies to the lungs. The sixth pair of aortic arches gives branches to the vascular plexus of the developing lung at 32 days of gestation. The basic pattern of the pulmonary vasculature is established by the 50th day of gestation. The left sixth aortic arch gives rise to the main pulmonary artery, the proximal part of the hilar branches, and the ductus arteriosus. The right sixth aortic arch provides the proximal part of the right pulmonary artery.

Intrapulmonary arterial development mirrors that of the airways, the preacinar vessels follow the development of the airways, and the intraacinar vessels follow that of the alveoli.[124] The full adult complement of connecting airways and preacinar arteries is present by the 16th week of gestation.[125] Thereafter, the preacinar muscular arteries grow in size and length throughout gestation; however, there is little change in medial wall thickness. In contrast, the nonmuscular intraacinar vessels and alveoli develop mainly after birth. Morphologically recognizable alveoli are typically not evident until about eight weeks after birth. Thus, the relative lack of muscles in the intraacinar vessels may facilitate diffusion of gas through thin-walled airways, thereby increasing the surface area for gas exchange.

Vasculogenesis (de novo organization of blood vessels by in situ differentiation of endothelial precursors [angioblasts] from the mesoderm) is the first morphogenic process leading to development of the pulmonary vasculature. The angioblasts migrate, adhere, and form vascular channels that become arteries, veins, or lymphatics depending on the local factors within the mesenchyme.[192] Angioblasts differentiate into endothelium and either contribute to the expression of smooth muscle phenotype in the surrounding mesenchyme or recruit existing smooth muscle cells to the forming vessel. This process is then followed by angiogenesis (budding, sprouting, and branching of the existing vasculature to form new vessels). Local growth factors (fibroblast growth factors, transforming factor β, platelet-derived growth factor, and insulin-like growth factor) appear to play an important role in vascular development and cell differentiation in the developing lung.[192] Recent studies suggest that nitric oxide (NO) may act as a crucial signal in the angiogenic response to growth factors by terminating proliferation and promoting differentiation.[13]

Vascular Smooth Muscle Development

Early in lung development, the embryonic endothelial channels acquire a smooth muscle layer, thereby providing the means to generate vascular tone and regulate blood flow. During this time, the smooth muscles themselves undergo structural changes. Expression of actin and myosin, the two contractile proteins, is developmentally regulated. At least four heavy-chain myosin isoforms have been identified: two contractile and two synthetic in nature.[74] As development of the vascular bed progresses, a transition occurs from the synthetic isoform to the smooth muscle-specific contractile isoform. Increased expression of the synthetic isoforms in the fetus may contribute to the rapid hyperplasia of the neonatal vascular wall observed in response to stress.[192] Immediately after birth, mechanisms to slow smooth muscle cell replication and maintain it at a low level must be in place. A large list of growth inhibitors have been proposed as prospective candidates, including NO and natriuretic peptide.

Structure of Fetal Pulmonary Vessels

Fetal pulmonary arteries have cuboidal endothelial cells and a thicker muscular layer relative to the external diameter than do similar arteries in the adult. This increased muscularity is generally believed to be responsible for the increased vasoreactivity and elevated vascular resistance found in the fetal pulmonary vasculature. The medial smooth muscle layer is most prominent in the fifth- and sixth-generation arteries.[127] Toward the periphery of the lung, a region of incomplete muscularization replaces the completely encircling smooth muscle of the media.[237] Further distally in arteries larger than capillaries, an incomplete pericyte layer within the endothelial basement membrane replaces the muscle. In partially muscular small arteries, cells intermediate in position and structure between pericytes and mature smooth muscle cells are found. These are precursor smooth muscle cells that under certain conditions, such as hypoxia, rapidly differentiate into mature smooth muscle cells.[183] During the last trimester, the number of small blood vessels in the lung increases 40-fold, while the wet lung weight increases fourfold.[167] Thus, the number of blood vessels per unit of lung increases 10-fold, a process that prepares the lungs to accommodate the 10-fold increase in blood per unit of lung that occurs at birth.

Structural Adaptation to Extrauterine Life

Following birth the pulmonary vasculature undergoes continuous remodeling. Within the first 5 minutes of life, dilation and recruitment of small muscular arteries within the acinar region occur and are associated with a reduction in pulmonary artery pressure and resistance.[117] Endothelial cells become less cuboidal and more elongated with fewer surface projections and less overlap (Fig. 3-1).[116] The vascular smooth muscle becomes more fusiform and less globular with decreased density of endoplastic reticulum and increased density of myofilaments.[116] These structural adaptations result in functionally less compliant arteries.[109] Furthermore the increase in oxygen tension that occurs with ventilation relieves this pulmonary vasoconstrictor stimuli acting on many arteries. By the third day of life, the wall thickness of the small muscular preacinar arteries relative to their external diameter has fallen to adult values. Reduction in wall thickness of larger arteries is more gradual, declining to adult levels by 3 to 4 months of age. Changes in these arteries are the result of arterial dilation, although there may be regression of muscle mass after removal of the high-pressure state. Postnatal changes in the structure of the pulmonary vessels proceed only if pulmonary artery pressure falls to normal, low values. If pulmonary hypertension is sustained after birth, as in certain congenital heart defects, regression of fetal muscularization fails to occur.

Maturation of the pulmonary vascular bed continues postnatally. Intraacinar arterial and alveolar development are most rapid during the first 18 months of life and continue through childhood. Thereafter, alveoli increase in size until growth of the chest wall is complete. During infancy and childhood, the distribution of muscles in the intraacinar vessels gradually extends along the arterial tree into peripheral vessels. Muscles reach arterioles at the alveolar duct level by late childhood and arterioles of the alveolar wall level by adulthood.[125] The structure of the artery is partially determined by the diameter of the vessel, as muscle extends to the vessels of the same size in the fetus as in the adult, but to a more proximal level in the arterial pathway. Thus, a muscular terminal bronchiolar artery of a newborn is the same diameter as a muscular alveolar wall artery of the adult.

Functional Development

There are several important functional differences between the intrauterine and extrauterine pulmonary vasculature. In the fetus, the pulmonary vascular resistance diverts the majority of right ventricular output away from the lungs, through the patent ductus arteriosus and foramen ovale into the descending aorta and thus to the placenta for oxygenation. The elevated pulmonary vascular resistance of the fetus is attributed to the compression of the vessels by the nonaerated (fluid-filled) lungs and lack of rhythmic distention,[71] the presence of low resting alveolar and arteriolar oxygen tensions (hypoxic pulmonary vasoconstriction), and a different balance between vasoconstricting and vasodilating mediators than in the postnatal lung. Due to new vessel growth and increase in the size of the existing vessels during gestation, the resting pulmonary vasculature resistance decreases progressively; however, baseline resistance still remains greater than that of adults. Recent studies have demonstrated a reduced potential for vasoconstriction in fetal pulmonary vascular muscle compared to newborns or adults.[19] Therefore, the higher pulmonary vascular resistance in utero is not the result of greater pulmonary vascular smooth muscle mass or of increased muscle contractility.

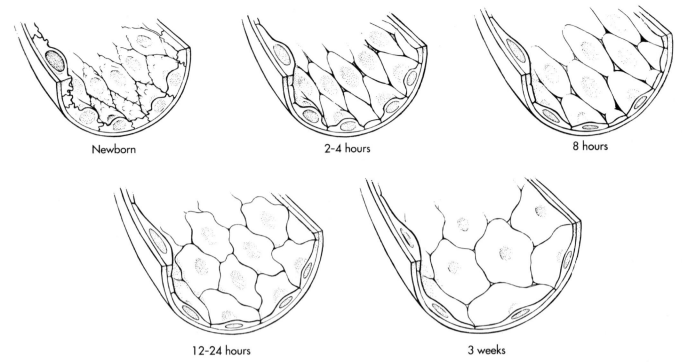

FIGURE 3-1 Developmental changes in the endothelium. This figure shows three-dimensional views of the endothelium at five developmental stages. Note the changes in longitudinal and transverse cross-sectional morphology of the cells—with cells in general becoming less plump, more spread out, with greater surface to volume ratios with increasing age. Metabolic activity and flow characteristics of the endothelial cells change with development. (Adapted from Allen KM, Haworth SG: Impaired adaptation of pulmonary circulation to extrauterine life in newborn pigs exposed to hypoxia: an ultrastructural study. *J Pathol* 150:205–212, 1986.)

Because the fetal pulmonary vasculature responds readily to vasodilators, the high-resistance, low-flow state is probably maintained in part by a predominance of active vasoconstriction.[59] The change in the balance of vasoconstricting and vasodilating mediators in the transition from the fetal to neonatal environment will be discussed further.

Mediators of High Pulmonary Vascular Tone

Eicosanoids Metabolites of arachidonic acid (known as eicosanoids) are C_{20} polyunsaturated fatty acids derived from lipid membranes to produce a variety of vasoactive and inflammatory mediators. Arachidonic acid is degraded by three enzymatic pathways: a) the cyclooxygenase pathway that produces prostenoids, b) the lipoxygenase pathway that produces leukotrienes, and c) an NADPH-dependent cytochrome P-450 epoxygenase pathway. The initiating step of eicosanoid metabolism is release of arachidonic acid from the acyl position of phospholipids in the cell membrane. This requires activation of phospholipase A_2 and is the rate-limiting step for prostaglandin biosynthesis (Fig. 3-2).

Arachidonic acid is readily oxygenated by the heme-dependent, microsomal glycoprotein enzyme, cyclooxygenase, to form the prostaglandin endoperoxides (PGG_2 and PGH_2) (Fig. 3-3). The cyclic prostaglandin endoperoxides are unstable intermediates that spontaneously hydrolyze to form several prostaglandins (PGD_2, PGE_2, and $PGF_{2\alpha}$). In vascular tissues, prostacyclin synthetase converts PGH_2 to prostacyclin (PGI_2). Prostacyclin is also unstable, with a half-life of about 3 minutes,

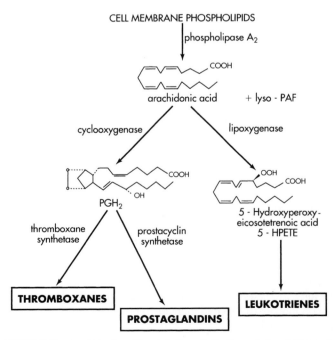

FIGURE 3-2 Arachidonic acid metabolism. Activation of phospholipase A leads to free arachidonate release from membrane triglycerides. This is metabolized by cyclooxygenase and lipoxygenase enzyme systems to members of the leukotrienes and prostaglandin families.

and spontaneously hydrolyzes to an inactive form (6 keto $PGF_{1\alpha}$). Endothelial cells are the most active producers of PGI_2.[292]

Prostacyclin production is regulated by both intracellular and extracellular factors (Fig. 3-4). Physiologic alterations in cell membranes increase prostacyclin production. Flow, with its associated shear stress, is the most significant physiological stimulus for prostacyclin production in vivo. Cultured mono-layers of endothelial cells produce bursts of prostacyclin in response to step increases in shear stress.[100] Importantly, cyclic changes in lung volume associated with breathing and mechanical ventilation also increase PGI_2 production.[296] Numerous circulating and local factors also stimulate endothelial prostacyclin production (Table 3-1). Prostacyclin affects physiologic function by activation of adenylate cyclase, thereby increasing intracellular cAMP. Increased cAMP inhibits platelet aggregation and decreases vascular smooth muscle tone.

Thromboxane A_2 (TXA_2) is the major vasoconstrictor cyclooxygenase product that also causes platelet aggregation. Its formation from endoperoxides is catalyzed by the enzyme thromboxane synthase (Fig. 3-5). Acetylcholine (normally a vasodilator) causes endothelium-dependent contractions in

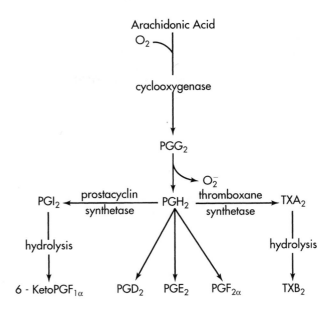

FIGURE 3-3 Arachidonic acid prostaglandin metabolism. PG, prostaglandin; TX, thromboxane.

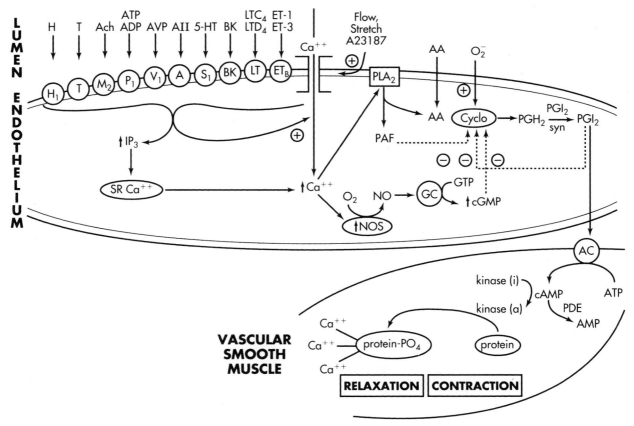

FIGURE 3-4 Regulation of endothelial prostacyclin synthesis and release. Multiple vasoactive agents circulating within the vascular lumen act at the endothelial cell membrane through either specific receptors or calcium ion channels to increase intracellular calcium. Ultimately, activation of phospholipase A_2 and cyclooxygenase initiates the eicosanoid cascade. Prostacyclin (PGI_2) then diffuses from the endothelial cell and acts on adenylate cyclase (AC) on the smooth muscle membrane to activate protein kinases that lead to phosphorylation and smooth muscle relaxation. H, histamine; T, thrombin; Ach, acetylcholine; AVP, arginine vasopressin; AII, angiotensin-II; 5-HT, 5-hydroxytryptamine (serotonin); BK, bradykinin; LT, leukotrienes; ET, endothelins; PLA_2, phospholipase A_2; PAF, platelet activating factor; *AA*, arachidonic acid; NO, nitric oxide; NOS, nitric oxide synthase; *GC*, guanylate cyclase; *IP₃*, inositol triphosphate; Cyclo, cyclooxygenase; SR, smooth endoplasmic reticulum; H_1, histamine type 1 receptor; S_1, serotonin type 1 receptor; T, thrombine receptor; BK, bradykinin receptor; M_2, muscarinic type 2 receptor; LT, leukotriene receptor; P_1, purinergic type 1 receptor; ET_B, endothelin type B receptor; V_1, vasopressin type 1 receptor; A, angiotensin receptor; AC, adenylate cyclase.

the aorta of adult spontaneously hypertensive but not normotensive rats of the same age.[173] This response can be prevented by inhibitors of phospholipase A_2 (PLA_2) and cyclooxygenase, but not inhibitors of PGI_2 and TXA_2 synthase. In contrast, TXA_2/endoperoxide (PGH_2) receptor antagonists prevent the endothelium-dependent contraction to acetylcholine in the aorta of the spontaneously hypertensive rat, indicating that PGH_2 is the mediator (see Fig. 3-5).[149] Activation of cyclooxygenase leads not only to the production of prostaglandins, but to the generation of superoxide ions. Superoxide ions and other free radicals are potential mediators of endothelium-dependent contraction. These free radicals may induce vasoconstriction via their inactivation and disruption of EDNO (endothelium derived nitric oxide) and PGI_2 (prostacyclin) production.[150] Thus, PGH_2-induced vasoconstriction may occur from either direct TXA_2/PGH_2 receptor stimulation or free radical production with subsequent inactivation of endothelial-derived vasodilators (EDNO, PGI_2).

Leukotrienes are lipid metabolites of arachidonic acid. Initially isolated in lung perfusates, they were presumed to have a role as mediators of anaphylaxis and identified as the slow-reacting substance of anaphylaxis (SRS-A). They were subsequently identified as leukotriene C_4 (LTC_4), leukotriene D_4 (LTD_4), and leukotriene E_4 (LTE_4).[249] The initial step in the biosynthesis of leukotrienes is the generation of arachidonic acid by PLA_2 (Fig. 3-6), followed by the incorporation of molecular oxygen into arachidonic acid by 5-lipoxygenase, resulting in the formation of 5-HPETE. This is subsequently converted into the unstable epoxide leukotriene A_4 (LTA_4) that is rapidly metabolized into either leukotriene B_4 (LTB_4) by a hydroxylase or into LTC_4 by conjugation with glutathione via glutathione transferase. The removal of γ-glutamyl residue

Table 3-1   Factors Affecting PGI_2 Biosynthesis

Factors Increasing Synthesis
Acetylcholine
Angiotensin I & II
Bradykinin
Calcium ionophore (A23187)
Interleukin-1 (IL-1)
Leukotrienes (LTC_4, LTD_4)
Mechanical stress (stretch, shear)
Nucleotides (ATP/UTP)
Platelet activating factor
Prostaglandins (PGG_2, PGH_2)
Serotonin
Thrombin
Thromboxane (TXB_2)
Trypsin

Factors Decreasing Synthesis
Fibroblast growth factor
Heparin
Interleukin-6 (IL-6)
Nitric oxide

Factors with Variable Response
Arachidonic acid
Endothelin
Histamine
Neuropeptide Y

of LTC_4 by transpeptidase leads to the formation of LTD_4, which can be converted into LTE_4 and leukotriene F_4 (LTF_4). LTC_4, LTD_4, LTE_4, and LTF_4 are collectively known as the sulfidopeptide leukotrienes because of the presence of the sulphur-containing amino acid cystine. The enzymatic steps resulting in the synthesis of LTD_4 and LTE_4 from LTC_4 represent conversion

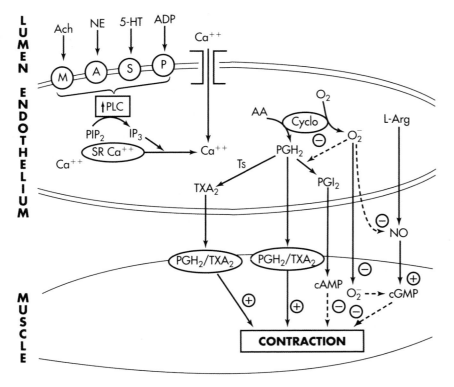

FIGURE 3-5 The regulation and interrelationships of thromboxane release. Acetylcholine (Ach), norepinephrine (NE), 5-hydroxytryptamine (5-HT), and adenosine diphosphate (ADP) act on their respective muscarinic (M), adrenergic (A), serotoninergic (S), and purinergic (P) cell membrane receptors to increase phospholipase C (PLC) activity, converting the phosphatidylinositol biphosphate (PIP_2) to inositol triphosphate (IP_3), which increases release of calcium from the smooth endoplasmic reticulum. This activates cyclooxygenase (Cyclo), leading to formation of PGH_2 from arachidonic acid (AA) and subsequently thromboxane (TXA_2) via thromboxane synthase (Ts). Both of these diffuse through the interstitial space to act on the vascular smooth muscle receptors and cause contraction. Of note is the superoxide (O_2^-) generation from cyclooxygenase also has an inhibitory effect on nitric oxide (NO) and thus blunts NO induced cyclic GMP dependent vasorelaxation and prostacyclin (PGI_2) and cyclic AMP–dependent vasorelaxation.

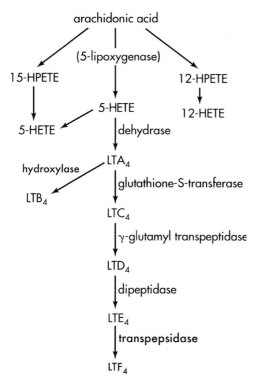

FIGURE 3-6 Leukotriene synthesis from arachidonic acid. HETE, Hydroxy-eicosatetraenoic acid; HPETE, hydroperoxyeicotetronic acid.

of one mediator into another and not simply an inactivation pathway. All three of these mediators are rapidly converted into inactive metabolites via nonspecific proteases.

Leukotrienes stimulate the production of PGI_2 from cultured endothelial cells via the stimulation of PLA_2 activity.[40] The increase in PGI_2 production is due to stimulation of the leukotriene receptor on the endothelial cell. Leukotriene receptor stimulation also results in the release of EDNO.[65]

The exact role of arachidonic acid and its metabolites in the fetal and neonatal pulmonary circulation remains controversial. Arachidonic acid constricts the pulmonary circulation of the fetus and the newborn.[278] Blocking prostaglandin or thromboxane synthesis does not decrease vascular resistance,[43] suggesting that these metabolites are not primarily responsible for the high resistance in the fetus. Others have shown that prostaglandins may have effects on the transition of the pulmonary circulation from intrauterine to extrauterine life.[98] Several lines of evidence suggest that leukotrienes are pulmonary vasoconstrictors in the fetus and neonate.[163] Leukotriene receptor antagonists increase fetal pulmonary blood flow and decrease pulmonary vascular resistance, suggesting a role in the physiologic control of fetal pulmonary circulation.[265] Other investigators have demonstrated increased leukotriene production in fetal versus neonatal animals.[134] Finally, LTD_4 increased pulmonary artery pressure and resistance when administered intravenously.[253] These studies suggest a physiologic role for leukotrienes in maintaining pulmonary vasoconstriction and thereby a low pulmonary blood flow in the normal fetus. However, questions about the nonselectivity of the leukotriene antagonists keep the physiologic role of the leukotrienes uncertain.[80]

Hypoxia The level of oxygen to which small pulmonary arteries are exposed is important in regulating pulmonary blood flow and resistance both in utero and postnatally.[71] The mechanisms responsible for the oxygen-dependent changes in pulmonary vascular tone are not fully understood but appear to be locally mediated and likely involve in part regulation of nitric oxide, endothelin, and prostacyclin.[180,258,259] Fetal oxygen levels are normally 17 to 20 mm Hg, at which the pulmonary circulation is maximally constricted.[246] Ventilation of the fetal lungs with nitrogen by itself, with no increase in oxygen tension, reduces pulmonary vascular resistance. A further fall occurs when oxygen is added to the gas mixture. The response of the pulmonary vasculature to alterations in oxygen tension varies with gestational age.[169,191] Thus oxygen, via alteration in the release of vasoactive substances, a direct effect on vascular smooth muscle, or the combination, decreases pulmonary vascular resistance and increases blood flow at birth.

Endothelin In 1985 Hickey and associates were the first to describe an endothelium derived constricting factor (EDCF) from bovine aortic endothelial cells that caused slowly developing and long-lasting vasoconstriction in isolated arterial rings.[121] This peptide, EDCF, was subsequently isolated, purified, and identified as a 21 amino acid peptide in an elegant series of experiments and called endothelin (ET).[306] This peptide is the most potent vasoconstrictor known. The biologically active 21 amino acid polypeptide is synthesized as a much larger (203 amino acid) protein precursor (preproendothelin—ppET) that requires biological processing. The 203 amino acid sequence of ppET-1 is processed in the cytoplasm (Fig. 3-7). An intermediate form designated proendothelin or big endothelin (big ET) has 92 amino acid residues. Big ET is converted to ET in the extracellular space by a recently recognized endothelin-converting enzyme (ECE).[154] ECE is located both in cytosol and membrane portions of endothelial cells.[289] The mechanism of release of endothelin from the endothelial cell remains unclear. Regardless of the precise mechanism, ET secretion appears to be polar (i.e., basement membrane secretion > luminal secretion).[286]

Southern blot analysis of human genomic DNA reveals three distinct genes that encode three distinct ET peptides termed endothelin-1 (ET-1), endothelin-2 (ET-2), and endothelin-3 (ET-3) (Fig. 3-8).[139] The isopeptides show different biological activities. The rank order for vasoconstricting activities is ET-1 = ET-2 > ET-3. Following intravenous injection of ET-1, there is a brief decrease in systemic blood pressure followed by a prolonged pressor response.[310] The initial dilator response is thought to be endothelium-dependent. ET-3 is the most potent dilator of these peptides (ET-3 > ET-1 = ET-2).[288] Measurable levels of ET-1 or ET-3 mRNA have been detected by northern blot analysis and in situ hybridization in many tissues from many species; however, ET-2 gene expression has been detected only in the mouse intestine.[248] Although ET-1 is stable in the blood, it is quickly eliminated from the circulation with a half-life of approximately seven minutes. Clearance occurs predominantly in the pulmonary and renal circulations.[261]

Endothelin binds to specific receptors. The discovery of the various ET isoforms and the diverse biological functions elicited by them suggested the existence of more than one ET receptor, which has subsequently been identified. One receptor

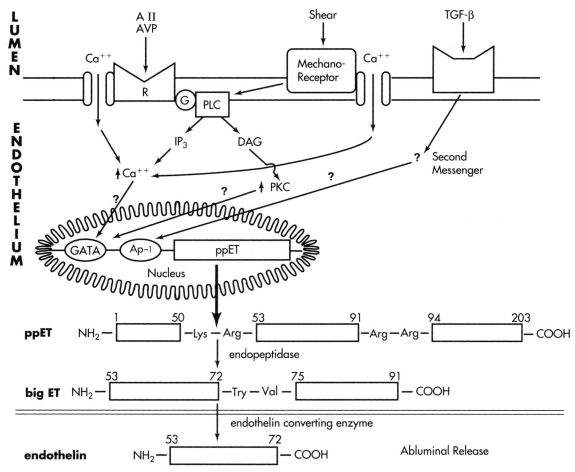

FIGURE 3-7 Regulation of endothelial endothelin production. Multiple intraluminal stimuli, including circulating vasoactive agents (angiotensin II [AII], argine vasopressin [AVP]), shear stress, and inflammatory cytokines, act through cell membrane receptors (R), which are frequently G-protein linked to inositol triphosphate (IP₃) and diacylglycerol (DAG). Intracellular activation of phosphokinase C (PKC) stimulates nuclear signaling via several recognized proto motor sequences (GATA, ATI) leading to synthesis of messenger RNA preproendothelin that is translated into preproendothelin (ppET). ppET is metabolized by an intracellular endopeptidase into big endothelin (big ET), as a post-translational change. Endothelin converting enzyme on the endothelial cell membrane cleaves big ET to endothelin for abluminal release. Endothelin is also released into the vascular lumen through a similar process at the luminal cell membrane. TGF-β, transforming growth factor β.

with a high specificity for ET-1 (ET_A receptor) represents the vascular smooth muscle receptor and mediates vasoconstriction.[11] The second receptor binds all isoforms of the peptide (ET_B receptor), is not expressed in vascular smooth muscle cells, and appears to represent the endothelial receptor linked to the production of PGI_2 and EDNO.[272] More recently, some investigators have suggested the presence of two distinct subtypes of the ET_B receptor.[211,260] These investigators have suggested that the ET_{B1} receptor mediates vasodilatation and the ET_{B2} receptor mediates vasoconstriction. The neonatal pulmonary circulation has predominately ET_A receptors, although ET_{B1} and probably ET_{B2} receptors are also present.

The precise mechanism of vasoconstriction and pressor responses induced by ET remains unclear. Vasoconstriction appears to be mediated through two distinct intracellular signal transduction systems (Fig. 3-9). These pathways include G-protein–regulated opening of calcium channels[310] and phospholipase C (PLC) activation.[274] In addition, PLA_2 activation by endothelin produces vasoconstrictor eicosanoids (PGH_2, TXA_2), which account for at least a portion of the sustained constrictor response.[238] Smooth muscle or endothelial ET elicits a prompt increase in intracellular free calcium concentration due to stimulated release by inositol

triphosphate (IP₃).[230,274] A later sustained phase in the ET-induced intracellular free calcium ion increase is ascribed to the influx of extracellular calcium that is abolished by calcium channel blockade.[274] Thus, the mechanism(s) of ET-induced vasoconstriction is multifactorial.

Since the initial discovery of the endothelins, many laboratories have studied their molecular biology, diverse biologic actions, and potential physiologic and pathologic significance. Endothelin-1 appears to play an important role in the physiology of the transitional pulmonary circulation via constriction of pulmonary arteries and veins.[287] Circulating levels of immunoreactive ET-1 are high in the fetus and decrease steadily in the postnatal period.[168] This finding may be due to endothelial-derived NO secretion. The low oxygen tension in the fetus will inhibit the production of NO.[161] This study also showed that NO can suppress ET-1 synthesis. Thus, lower levels of NO will result in higher amounts of circulating endothelin and increased vascular resistance. Other investigators have demonstrated that fetal ductal constriction and the resulting pulmonary hypertension are associated with increased ET-1 mRNA and decreased ET_B receptor expression without change in ET_A or ECE levels.[141] This model of pulmonary hypertension was used to show that

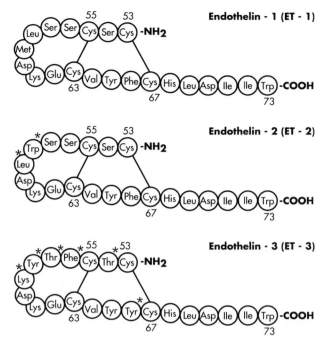

FIGURE 3-8 The amino acid sequences of the endothelin polypeptide family. The residues denoted by an asterisk indicate differences from the ET-1 sequence.

pulmonary hypertension can be attenuated by endothelin receptor blockade or ECE inhibition.[140,141] From these data, it is clear that endothelin plays a significant role in the regulation of pulmonary vascular tone in the fetus and newborn.

Mediators of the Transitional Circulation

At birth, the function of gas exchange must transfer from the placenta to the newborn's lungs. The onset of ventilation and the separation of the placenta result in rapid and dramatic circulatory adjustments to allow adequate pulmonary blood flow. These structural and functional adaptations produce an immediate decrease in pulmonary vascular resistance and an eightfold to 10-fold increase in pulmonary blood flow. As a consequence of the increased blood flow, pulmonary venous return is increased, which results in the reversal of the pressure difference between the right and left atria, functionally closing the foramen ovale. This is followed by removal of the placenta and an increase in the systemic vascular resistance. Finally, the ductus arteriosus and dluctus venosus functionally close over a period of several hours (anatomic closure occurs after several days), thereby separating the pulmonary and systemic circulations and establishing the normal postnatal circulatory pattern.

The stimuli with the most important role in decreasing pulmonary vascular resistance at birth are expansion and ventilation of the lungs with gas and the increase in

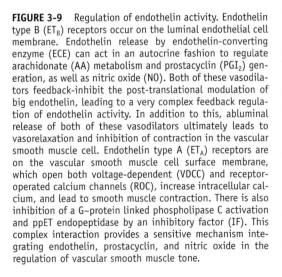

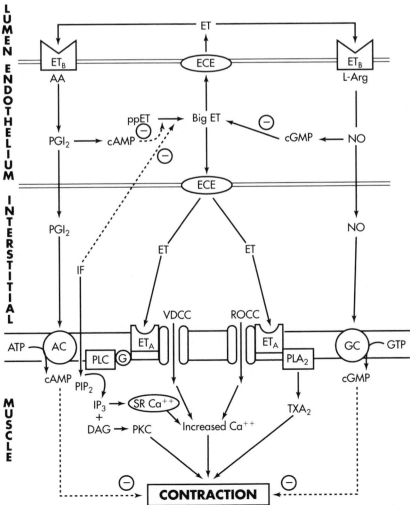

FIGURE 3-9 Regulation of endothelin activity. Endothelin type B (ET$_B$) receptors occur on the luminal endothelial cell membrane. Endothelin release by endothelin-converting enzyme (ECE) can act in an autocrine fashion to regulate arachidonate (AA) metabolism and prostacyclin (PGI$_2$) generation, as well as nitric oxide (NO). Both of these vasodilators feedback-inhibit the post-translational modulation of big endothelin, leading to a very complex feedback regulation of endothelin activity. In addition to this, abluminal release of both of these vasodilators ultimately leads to vasorelaxation and inhibition of contraction in the vascular smooth muscle cell. Endothelin type A (ET$_A$) receptors are on the vascular smooth muscle cell surface membrane, which open both voltage-dependent (VDCC) and receptor-operated calcium channels (ROC), increase intracellular calcium, and lead to smooth muscle contraction. There is also inhibition of a G–protein linked phospholipase C activation and ppET endopeptidase by an inhibitory factor (IF). This complex interaction provides a sensitive mechanism integrating endothelin, prostacyclin, and nitric oxide in the regulation of vascular smooth muscle tone.

oxygen tension. Each of these stimuli alone will decrease pulmonary vascular resistance (PVR) and increase pulmonary blood flow (PBF).[236,275] Ventilation of the fetal lung without changes in arterial oxygen or carbon dioxide tension will increase pulmonary blood flow to approximately 66%. Increases in perfusate oxygen tension will decrease PVR in isolated, perfused fetal lungs.[42] Hyperbaric oxygen breathing by the ewe will decrease PVR and increase PBF in fetal lambs to levels comparable to those after birth.[191] The largest effects on PVR and PBF are seen with ventilation using supplemental oxygen.[192]

Multiple mediators modulate PVR and blood flow during the transition from fetal to neonatal life. In addition to the structural changes of the pulmonary circulation noted earlier, the ability to release specific mediators and maturation of the specific receptor systems determine the changing responses to multiple stimuli. The pulmonary vascular endothelium plays a central role in the regulation of the perinatal pulmonary circulation through this paracrine function. Multiple homeostatic mechanisms determine the overall balance between endothelial-derived vasoconstricting and vasodilating factors. The principal endothelial vasodilating mediators are nitric oxide and prostaglandins.

Nitric Oxide Acetylcholine stimulates muscarinic receptors on endothelial cells to release one or more substances that result in relaxation of the underlying vascular smooth muscle.[78] This endothelial derived relaxing factor (EDRF) is a labile, extremely potent relaxing factor with a biologic half-life of between 6 and 50 seconds in oxygenated, aqueous medium.[105] The production and/or stability of EDRF is decreased in both high and low oxygen tensions.[50,78] In 1986, Furchgott and Ignarro simultaneously recognized the remarkable similarities between the biological properties of EDRF and nitric oxide (NO).[136] The chemical and pharmacological identification of EDRF from cultured aortic endothelial cells as NO by Palmer occurred the following year.[209] Subsequently, the chemical and pharmacological similarities between EDRF and EDNO released from intact arteries and veins were reported.[136]

NO is derived from the terminal guanidine nitrogen atom of L-arginine by the enzyme now called nitric oxide synthase (NOS) (Fig. 3-10).[187] NOS occurs in multiple cell lines in at least three different isoforms.[187] One isoform of NOS (type III or eNOS) has been isolated in both the cytosolic and membrane fractions of endothelial cells.[76] This enzyme is calcium and calmodulin dependent.[31,76] This enzyme can be isolated and cloned from bovine and human endothelium.[144,255] A second isoform (type II or iNOS) isolated in macrophages is cytokine inducible and appears to be calcium independent.[251] Studies utilizing mass spectrometry and $^{18}O_2$ (the radioactive isotope of oxygen) showed that the enzyme incorporates molecular oxygen into both NO and citrulline.[166] The third isoform of NOS (type I or nNOS) in cerebral neurons is calcium and calmodulin dependent.[29,76]

Many different physiologic, pharmacologic, and pathologic factors alter EDNO production and/or its effect on vascular smooth muscle tone (Tables 3-2 and 3-3). These include receptor and non–receptor-mediated stimuli, agents that (1) inhibit EDNO production, (2) inactivate EDNO that is released, and (3) suppresse its receptor (guanylate cyclase). Many of these stimulators and inhibitors were used in studies to understand the biochemistry and identity of EDNO.

Nitric oxide activates guanylate cyclase, which converts guanosine triphosphate (GTP) to cyclic guanosine monophosphate (cGMP) (see Fig. 3-10). Cyclic GMP causes vascular relaxation by decreasing the concentration of free calcium in vascular smooth muscle cytosol. This decrease in intracellular calcium occurs through multiple mechanisms including decreased calcium influx through receptor operated calcium channels, a reduction in the release of intracellular calcium, and a stimulation of active calcium efflux.[228,229] Endothelium-dependent cGMP accumulation in vascular smooth muscle occurs with all agents that release EDNO, across species, and in a variety of circulations.[137,187] Endothelium dependent relaxations are inhibited by methylene blue, an agent that inhibits guanylate cyclase activation.[177] The correlation between EDNO induced vasodilatation and cGMP accumulation in vascular smooth muscle has established cGMP accumulation as a useful bioassay for the detection of EDNO.

Chemical instability endows EDNO with one of the most important properties of a local mediator or autocoid; that is, rapid termination of action so that the biologic effect remains localized. The short biochemical half-life of several seconds makes it an ideal autocoid. Another mechanism of termination of NO's action and perhaps conservation of NO is the rapid binding to oxyhemoglobin. This serves to prevent luminally released EDNO from eliciting vasodilatation downstream. Furthermore, EDNO is rapidly oxidized to nitrite and nitrate in the presence of oxyhemoglobin. Finally, an additional mechanism of NO inactivation could be the concomitant generation and release of superoxide ions from vascular endothelial cells, smooth muscle cells, and phagocytic cells.

EDNO plays a critical role in developmental pulmonary vascular physiopathology. Stimulating endogenous NO production mimics transition by dialating the fetal pulmonary vasculature. Pulmonary vasodilatation by acetylcholine in fetal lambs can be blocked by arginine analogs and restored by excess L-arginine.[69,276] This suggests that acetylcholine is stimulating eNOS. Blockade of NOS activity in fetal lambs 10 days before birth results in pulmonary hypertension following delivery.[72] Although the exact mechanism is uncertain, oxygen is an important stimulus for EDNO production during transition. Both basal and stimulated NO release increase with increasing oxygen tension in intrapulmonary arteries isolated from near-term fetal lambs.[257] Arginine analogs block virtually the entire increase in fetal pulmonary blood flow caused by hyperbaric oxygenation without ventilation.[277]

All three isoforms of NOS are present and developmentally regulated in the fetal lung.[191,201,310] Rhythmic distention of the lungs without changing oxygen tension increased eNOS mRNA expression in lung tissue.[23] Oxygen ventilation caused a further increase in eNOS mRNA and increased eNOS protein expression. The ability of oxygen to modulate NOS expression appears late in gestation.[256] The maximized expression at birth may optimize the capacity for NO-mediated pulmonary vasodilatation. Further work using fetal lamb endothelial cell cultures demonstrated that exposure to 95% oxygen and shear stress increased eNOS mRNA and protein expression. These data suggest that both oxygen and shear stress induce eNOS expression and likely contribute to pulmonary vasodilation. The flow-stimulated increase in shear stress will augment basal EDNO release, facilitating pulmonary vasodilation as pulmonary blood flow increases

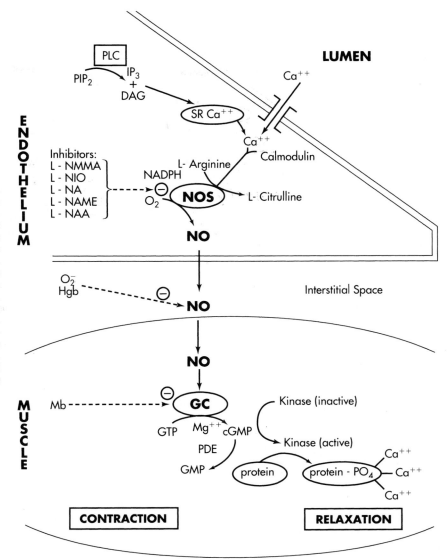

FIGURE 3-10 Synthesis of nitric oxide by endothelial cells. Multiple endothelial cell receptors lead to activation of calcium channels and increase intracellular calcium, which, with calmodulin, activates nitric oxide synthase to convert L-arginine to L-citrulline. The co-factors are oxygen and NADPH. Nitric oxide (NO) diffuses across the endothelial cell membrane into the smooth muscle cells, activating soluble guanylate cyclase (GC). GC converts GTP to cyclic GMP, which activates protein kinases, leading to phosphorylation and smooth muscle relaxation. Inhibitors are shown on the left side of the figure. Inside the endothelial cells, blocking nitric oxide synthase, are L-N-monomethyl arginine (L-NMMA), N-imino-ethyl–L-ornithine (L-NIO), L-nitroarginine (L-NA), L-nitroarginine methyl ester (L-NAME), and L-nitro amino argine (L-NAA). In the interstitial space, superoxide radical (O_2^-) and hemoglobin (Hgb) scavenge NO. In the muscle, methylene blue (MB) inhibits guanylate cyclase.

at birth. Finally, endogenous NO is known to upregulate eNOS gene expression in fetal pulmonary artery endothelial cells, providing a positive feedback loop in late gestation.[256]

In contrast to NOS expression noted earlier, in vivo and in vitro studies demonstrate a diminished ability to stimulate the fetal pulmonary vascular endothelium to increase NO production.[3] Fetal pulmonary artery rings have diminished EDNO activity when compared to that in postnatal animals.[1,3]

The endothelium-dependent vasodilatory potency increases between 115 and 140 days gestation, suggesting that maturational changes in endothelial cell function may contribute to circulatory changes associated with birth and differences in pulmonary vasoreactivity. In contrast, the fetus responds normally

Table 3-2   Factors Increasing EDNO Production

Thrombin	Calcium ionophore A23187
ATP, ADP	Shear stress
Serotonin	Arachidonic acid
Acetylcholine	Alkalosis
Norepinephrine	Trypsin
Vasopressin	Melittin
Bradykinin	LTC$_4$, LTD$_4$
Histamine	ET-1, ET-3
Substance P	Tumor necrosis factor
Vasoactive intestinal peptide	Platelet-derived growth factor

Table 3-3   Factors Decreasing EDNO Effect

Decrease Synthesis	Inactivate Nitric Oxide
Hypoxia	Hemoglobin
L-NMMA	Myoglobin
L-NAME	Hyperoxia
L-NIO	Oxygen free radicals
L-NAA	Nordihydroguaiaretic acid
Receptor Inhibitor	Eicosatetraynoic acid
Methylene blue	Oubain
	Hydroquinone
	Phenidone
	Dithiothreitol
	Pyrogallol
	BW 755 C
	Catecholamines

to endothelium-independent agonists such as sodium nitroprusside and inhaled NO.[3,155]

The age-related increase in endothelium-dependent relaxation may also be due to changes in the sensitivity of the underlying vascular smooth muscle.[310] For example, expression of soluble guanylate cyclase is higher in late-gestation and newborn rats than in adult rats.[24] This finding may explain in part the stronger response to inhaled nitric oxide commonly observed in newborn patients. Recent data suggest similar gestational regulation of the enzyme (cGMP-specific phosphodiesterase—PDE_5) expression and activity that is responsible for metabolism of NO's byproduct (cGMP). Expression of PDE_5 increases during gestation and the immediate newborn period in several species.[114,250] In addition, inhibitors of PDE_5 dilate the pulmonary vasculature of normal fetal lambs.[27,310]

Prostacyclin Eicosanoids, especially prostacyclin (PGI_2), have been proposed as mediators of the transition from intrauterine to neonatal environment. Prostacyclin production in the whole lung increases dramatically during late gestation and the early postnatal period.[4] Perhaps this is due to the onset of breathing, which stimulates pulmonary endothelial PGI_2 production and plays a major role in the decrease in pulmonary vascular resistance seen at birth.[70,234] Furthermore, the increase in pulmonary blood flow is blunted by inhibitors of prostaglandin synthesis during ventilation of fetal lungs.[279] This finding is more prominent in the preterm than the near-term fetus. This may be due in part to a decrease in the activity of adenylate cyclase, the effector mechanism producing dilation to PGI_2, as the fetus approaches term.[257] The increase in pulmonary blood flow at birth, through increased shear stress, further increases PGI_2 release, thus augmenting these vasodilatory responses. Another potential factor associated with the increase in PGI_2 during this period is the upregulation of constitutive cyclooxygenase.[28] Physiologic levels of estrogen enhance cyclooxygenase-1 mRNA and protein content in fetal lamb pulmonary artery endothelial cell cultures.[147] These factors all enhance the capacity for prostaglandin-mediated vasodilation in the newborn lung.

The effect of oxygen on prostaglandin production in the fetal and newborn lung is complex. Increased oxygen tension increases PGI_2 synthesis in isolated fetal pulmonary arteries.[257] Indomethacin, an inhibitor of prostaglandin synthesis, does not block the increase in fetal pulmonary blood flow or decrease in PVR in response to hyperbaric oxygen exposure.[190] In postnatal lambs, acute hypoxia directly stimulates cyclooxygenase gene expression and prostaglandin (PGI_2 and PGE_2) synthesis in endothelium and isolated lungs.[101,200,258] Hypoxic stimulation of prostacyclin synthesis may be greater in the immediate newborn period than later in life, thus providing a protective mechanism against excessive hypoxic vasoconstriction.[98] Maturational changes in the functional characteristics of other prostaglandins have also been described. For example, PGD_2 is a pulmonary vasodilator in utero but is a pulmonary vasoconstrictor in the newborn and adult with the degree of vasoconstriction increasing with maturation.[35,212] In summary, it appears that prostaglandins, especially PGI_2, are important in the mediation of pulmonary vasodilation in response to rhythmic distention of the lung,

but not to oxygen, and that this effect is enhanced in the preterm more so than the near-term fetus.

Platelet Activating Factor Platelet activating factor (PAF) is a biologically active phospholipid initially described as an albumin bound material produced by rabbit basophils that stimulated the release of histamine from platelets. PAF (acetyl glycerol ether phosphorylcholine) has received a great deal of attention as a potential mediator of cell communication and activation in a diverse group of pathophysiological processes.[117] Some of these physiologic effects include platelet activation and aggregation, neutrophil activation, neutrophil adherence, and alteration in vascular smooth muscle tone.

Platelet activating factor synthesis by endothelial cells is not constitutive but occurs rapidly following appropriate receptor stimulation. There are two hypothetical pathways for PAF production: the "remodeling" pathway and the "de novo" pathway (Fig. 3-11); however, the former is the predominant pathway in endothelial cells.[298] Phospholipase A_2 is the key enzyme in this pathway. The same agonists that cause arachidonate release stimulate PAF release from endothelial cells.[216] To date, the exact signal transduction mechanisms resulting in PAF release remain uncertain. Thus far, it is clear that changes in intracellular calcium play a key role in arachidonic metabolism and PAF production.[298] When endothelial cells are exposed to agonists or calcium ionophores in a calcium free buffer, arachidonic metabolism and PAF production are only a fraction of that seen when calcium is present.[216] The increase in intracellular Ca^{++} levels results in PLA_2 activation with subsequent release of PAF and arachidonic acid (Fig. 3-12).

The response of vascular smooth muscle to PAF is complex, related not only to species but also to circulation. This response is further complicated by the fact that PAF production is linked to arachidonate metabolites (PGI_2 and TXA_2) that modulate the effect of PAF on vascular smooth muscle tone. For example, TXA_2 production amplified the initial pulmonary vasoconstrictive response to PAF, but subsequent responses to PAF were not affected by thromboxane synthase inhibitors, suggesting that PAF has direct vascular effects.[280] In addition, PAF administration intravenously is associated with increased pulmonary vascular resistance that is either partially or completely blocked by cyclooxygenase inhibitors, suggesting that the predominant effect is secondary to the release of TXA_2.[178] Other investigators have noted a predominantly vasodilatory response to PAF in the pulmonary vasculature when administered in very low concentration.[179] These divergent responses could be related to differences in dose, species, or possibly selective receptor subtype stimulation.[119]

Recent studies suggest that PAF may play a physiologic role in the high basal systemic and pulmonary vascular tone in the fetus. Circulating levels of PAF drop significantly after delivery and oxygenation in lambs.[133] Because PAF is rapidly metabolized by PAF acetylhydrolase, studies demonstrating decreased levels of this enzyme in the neonatal period that approach adult values by 6 weeks of age suggest that the neonate may be at increased risk for pathophysiologic processes mediated by PAF.[33]

Other Potential Mediators Several other substances may play a significant role in regulation of pulmonary vascular tone and blood flow during transition. For example, oxygenation

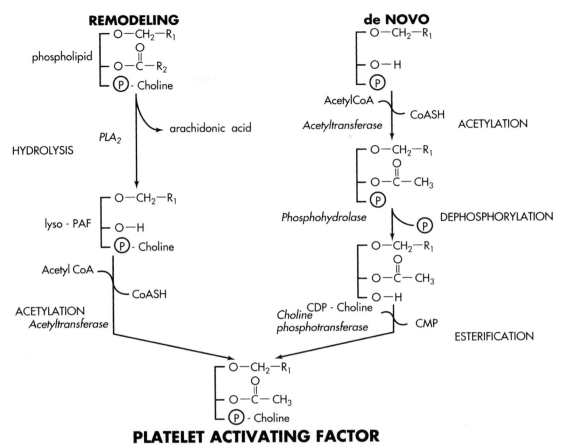

PLATELET ACTIVATING FACTOR

FIGURE 3-11 The two biosynthetic pathways of platelet activating factor (PAF). Both the de novo and remodeling pathways are shown. In the remodeling pathway, a cell membrane phospholipid precursor has an Sn2 position fatty acid hydrolyzed from it by phospholipase A_2 (PLA_2), yielding, in most cases, arachidonic acid and lyso-PAF. This is acetylated by acetyl CoA and acetyltransferase to platelet activating factor (PAF). In the de novo pathway, a glycerophosphate is first acetylated at the Sn2 position and then dephosphorylated and by esterification with choline phosphotransferase yields platelet activating factor. In endothelial cells the overwhelmingly dominant pathway is the remodeling pathway.

of fetal lambs stimulates bradykinin production that produces vasodilation in the intact fetus.[77] This vasodilatory response to bradykinin in the fetal pulmonary circulation appears to be due to the production of both PGI_2 and EDNO. Oxygenation also increases red blood cell adenosine triphosphate (ATP), which has been shown to act as a dilator in the fetal pulmonary vasculature and is a potential stimulus for EDNO production.[159,267] Increased synthesis and release of ATP appear to play a role in the pulmonary vasodilation following birth-related stimuli.[158] Plasma ATP levels increase in the

FIGURE 3-12 Agonist-receptor interaction and PAF. Receptor activation leads to both G-protein phospholipase D (GPLD) and phospholipase C (PLC) activation that, via diacylglycerol (DAG) and inositol triphosphate (IP_3), cause smooth endoplasmic reticular release of calcium. This activates phospholipase A_2, leading to hydrolysis of membrane bound phospholipid into arachidonic acid (AA) and platelet activating factor (PAF).

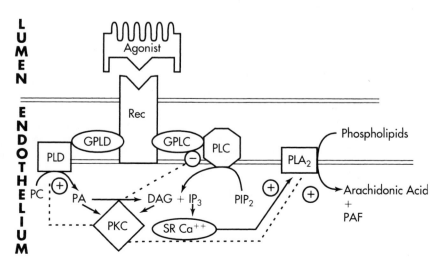

lung following ventilation with oxygen, but not with ventilation alone. Purine receptor antagonists block the vasodilation to oxygen in fetal lambs.[157] Atrial natriuretic peptide (ANP) causes pulmonary vasodilation in the fetus.[1,3] Circulating levels of ANP are elevated in the early postnatal period.[291] The increased pulmonary venous return, associated with the increase in blood flow at birth, causes atrial distention, thereby stimulating ANP release and augmenting cGMP-mediated vasodilation. Despite these limited data, the physiologic role of ANP in the transition of the pulmonary circulation is unclear. Finally, adrenomedullin, a pulmonary vasodilating peptide found in several peripheral tissues, has been found to be elevated shortly after birth with the levels corresponding to the degree of birth stress (defined as vaginal delivery or low arterial pH).[26] These findings suggest a physiologic role for adrenomedullin in the vascular adaptation of the newborn.

Ductus Arteriosus

In contrast to the pulmonary circulation, the ductus arteriosus actively constricts in response to the high oxygen postnatal environment. Involvement of the eicosanoids in this active postnatal vasoconstriction was initially suggested by experiments in which cyclooxygenase inhibitors (aspirin, indomethacin) initiated closure of the ductus arteriosus. Vasoconstriction of the ductus by cyclooxygenase inhibition, sensitivity of the fetal ductus to relaxant effects of PGE_2 both in vitro and in vivo,[202] and the demonstration that the ductus arteriosus possesses prostenoid synthetic enzymes[224] support the role for vasodilatory prostenoid, particularly PGE_2 in utero, in maintenance of ductal patency. This in utero modulation of the caliber of the ductus arteriosus also appears to involve the competition of enzyme activity for substrate (PGH_2) and the down regulation of pulmonary catabolic enzymes that would facilitate survival of circulating hormonal PGE_2.[217] Finally, endogenous PGE_2 inhibits the ability of the ductus to contract in response to increased oxygen tension, thus strengthening the hypothesis that circulating levels of PGE_2 may be important in the prenatal maintenance of ductal patency.

Increased oxygen tension with the first breath initiates functional closure of the ductus, a response that is independent of neural influences. Whether oxygen acts directly on ductal vascular smooth muscle cell or has its effect via a chemical mediator resulting in ductal closure is continually debated. Evidence suggests that an arachidonic metabolite catalyzed by cytochrome P-450 is involved in the active vasoconstriction of the ductus.[202] Inhibitors of the cytochrome P-450 pathway all relax the constricted ductus. Other vasoconstricting substances may also be involved in postnatal ductus closure. Endothelin induces long-lasting constriction of isolated ductus arteriosus from mature lambs at low oxygen tensions in relatively low doses.[44] The fact that plasma concentrations of endothelin are elevated at term further supports a potential role of endothelin in the closure of the ductus arteriosus at birth.

REGULATION OF PULMONARY BLOOD FLOW DISTRIBUTION

Regulation of pulmonary blood flow has ramifications with regard to oxygen delivery affecting both ventilation/perfusion matching and cardiovascular function. Regional changes in PVR alter the relative distribution of blood flow within the lung, altering ventilation-perfusion relationships and thus gas exchange. A localized increase in PVR in a hypoxic atelectatic lung results in blood flow diversion to better ventilated regions of the lung and improved gas exchange. A sound understanding of the relationship between pulmonary artery pressure, cardiac output, and pulmonary vascular resistance when vascular smooth muscle tone is constant is essential to recognizing the impact of active vasoconstriction. When cardiac output decreases and pulmonary artery pressure remains the same or increases, then active vasoconstriction must have occurred. Anytime cardiac output increases and the pressure gradient for pulmonary perfusion remains constant or decreases, the tone must have decreased. A variety of physiologic and pharmacologic stimuli may cause active vasomotion of the pulmonary circulation; however, many of these active events may be modified by compensatory, passive mechanisms. In this section mechanisms that alter the distribution of pulmonary blood flow will be discussed.

Passive Influences

In the past, the pulmonary circulation was generally regarded as a largely passive circuit in which blood flow regulation and distribution are predominantly determined by gravity-dependent hydrostatic gradients.[295] Using new high-resolution methods and experiments in both low and high gravity conditions, investigators showed that pulmonary perfusion is much more heterogeneous than that predicted by hydrostatic gradients.[84] These results emphasize the geometry of the pulmonary vascular tree as the primary determinant of pulmonary blood flow distribution. This new perspective has rekindled an interest in examining the factors determining regional pulmonary blood flow and indicates that the topographic distribution of pulmonary blood flow has not been completely resolved. The following discussion of the regulation of pulmonary blood flow distribution will first focus on the "classic" gravity-dependent hydrostatic pressure model. This will be followed by the "new" data from the high-resolution studies.

Gravity-Dependent Distribution

Gravitational forces have been thought of as the principal factor affecting the distribution of pulmonary blood flow. The right ventricle imparts kinetic energy to the blood in the pulmonary artery, which is dissipated by a vertical, gravity-dependent, hydrostatic gradient. At some height above the heart the absolute pressure in the pulmonary artery (P_{pa}) becomes less than atmospheric. At this point, alveolar pressure (P_A), which is equivalent to atmospheric pressure, exceeds P_{pa} and pulmonary venous pressure (P_{pv}), and the vessels in this region of the lung collapse (West zone 1). Further down the hydrostatic gradient, when P_{pa} exceeds P_A, blood flow begins (West zone 2). The pressure gradient for blood flow at this level in the lung is determined by alveolar pressure, that is, the mean P_{pa} minus P_A difference, rather than the more conventional P_{pa} minus P_{pv} difference. The relationship between blood flow and the alveolar pressure has been characterized as a waterfall effect. The blood flow is proportional to the difference between P_{pa} and P_A, regardless of the downstream pressure (P_{pv}). Therefore, the driving pressure (P_{pa} minus P_A) and blood flow increase linearly down this region of the lung. Eventually a region in the lung is reached in which P_{pv} exceeds P_A (West zone 3), and blood flow is determined by the pulmonary arteriovenous pressure difference (P_{pa} minus P_{pv}). Gravity causes both P_{pa} and P_{pv} to increase by a similar amount; therefore, the vessels remain permanently open and the perfusion pressure is constant. When pulmonary vascular pressures are extremely high, fluid transudate filters into the interstitial compartment. When this fluid formation exceeds lymphatic clearance, this interstitial fluid will eliminate the normal negative tension on extra-alveolar vessels. Eventually the pulmonary interstitial pressure (P_{isf}) becomes positive and exceeds P_{pv} (West zone 4).[295] In zone 4, blood flow is regulated by arterial to interstitial pressure difference, which is smaller than arterial to venous pressure difference. Hence, zone 4 conditions will have decreased blood flow compared to zone 3 conditions. All of the zones are depicted in Figure 3-13.

The relative distribution of these zones within the lung is not constant. Both pulmonary flow and ventilation are cyclic phenomena. Any given anatomic site in zone 2 may actually be in either zone 1 or zone 3 conditions depending upon whether the patient is in cardiac systole or diastole or in inspiration or expiration. Furthermore, many commonly encountered clinical phenomena alter these relationships (shock, emboli, increased intrathoracic pressure).

As P_{pa} and P_{pv} increase, three changes take place in the pulmonary circulation: 1) recruitment or opening of previously unperfused vessels, 2) distention of previously perfused vessels, and 3) transudation of fluid from excessively distended vessels. Recruitment occurs when P_{pa} and P_{pv} increase from low to moderate levels, while distention of these vessels occurs when P_{pa} and P_{pv} increase from moderate to high levels. These are two compensatory mechanisms within the pulmonary circulation to maintain low intravascular pressures at increased flows. Finally, when P_{pa} and P_{pv} increase from high to very high levels, transudation with the development of pulmonary interstitial edema or frank alveolar edema occurs. These factors are responsible in part for the curvilinear nature of the pressure-flow relationships of the pulmonary vasculature.

Gravity-Independent Distribution

The pulmonary vasculature can best be visualized as a two-compartment system: 1) a fixed structure that is the primary determinant of regional perfusion; and 2) a variable component

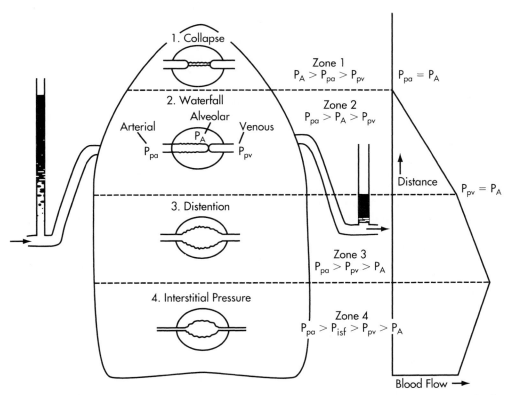

FIGURE 3-13 The four zones of the lung. Schematic diagram showing distribution of blood flow in the upright lung. In zone 1, alveolar pressure (P_A) exceeds pulmonary artery pressure (P_{pa}) and no flow occurs because the intra-alveolar vessels are collapsed by the compressing alveolar pressure. In zone 2, arterial pressure exceeds alveolar pressure, but alveolar pressure exceeds venous pressure (P_{pv}). Flow in zone 2 is determined by the arterial-alveolar pressure difference ($P_{pa} - P_A$) and has been likened to an upstream river waterfall over a dam. Since P_{pa} increases down zone 2 and P_A remains constant, the perfusion pressure increases and flow steadily increases down the zone. In zone 3, pulmonary venous pressure exceeds alveolar pressure, and flow is determined by the arterial-venous pressure difference ($P_{pa} - P_{pv}$), which is constant down this portion of the lung. However, the transmural pressure across the wall of the vessel increases down this zone, so that the caliber of the vessels increases (resistance decreases) and, therefore, flow increases. Finally, in zone 4, pulmonary interstitial pressure becomes positive and exceeds both pulmonary venous pressure and alveolar pressure. Consequently, flow in zone 4 is determined by the arterial-interstitial pressure difference ($P_{pa} - P_{isf}$). (Benumof JL: Respiratory physiology and respiratory function during anesthesia. In Miller RD (ed): *Anesthesia*, ed 3, New York: Churchill Livingstone, 1990, with permission.)

that acts on top of the fixed structure and is affected by local factors. The fixed structure is best characterized using a fractal geometry model, a mathematical science used to describe "natural objects." The variable component of the vasculature can be influenced by passive (such as recruitment and/or distention described previously) and active regional factors (see vasoregulation section). The relative contribution of the fixed and variable components of the pulmonary vasculature to pulmonary perfusion heterogeneity can be measured.

Perfusion Heterogeneity Reed and Wood[235] were the first to suggest the importance of the geometry of the pulmonary vascular tree as a meaningful determinant of blood flow distribution. They were able to find differences in blood flow at equal hydrostatic pressures and concluded that factors other than pulmonary arterial, venous, and alveolar pressures affect the distribution of blood flow. Numerous other investigators have also found gravity-independent discrepancy.[15,102,107,108] New techniques providing high-resolution measurements of pulmonary perfusion have confirmed a large degree of spatial heterogeneity of blood flow.[84] These observations have provided insight into the mechanisms matching heterogeneous perfusion to organ function and cellular needs. Until recently, the observed heterogeneity of pulmonary perfusion was interpreted within the context of the gravitational model as random noise. Fractal analysis demonstrated that this "error" can be recognized as a fundamental property of the biological system. Fractal analysis permits characterization of processes or structures that are not easily represented by the traditional analytic tools.

Fractals A fractal structure or process can be loosely defined as having a characteristic form that remains constant over a magnitude of scales. In simplistic terms, a structure is fractal if its small-scale form appears similar to its large-scale form. This is the quality of self-similarity or scale-independence. Although a fractal structure is similar across many scales of resolution, its apparent size or length is dependent on the ruler size to measure it.

Pulmonary blood flow distribution was first characterized by fractal methods in dogs.[90] The fractal nature of pulmonary blood flow has subsequently been documented in a number of laboratories and multiple species.[34,84,182] Pulmonary blood flow is spatially correlated with neighboring regions of lung (high-flow regions are adjacent to other high-flow regions and low-flow regions are next to other low-flow regions). This relationship between flows to pairs of lung pieces can be quantified using the correlation coefficient. The spatial correlation $[\rho(d)]$ is the correlation between blood flow to one piece at one position and a second position displaced from the first by a distance $[d]$. The correlation coefficient has a range of $-1.0 \leq \rho(d) \leq 1.0$ where $\rho(d) = 1.0$ indicates a perfect positive correlation between pairs, $\rho(d) = -1.0$ means a perfect negative correlation between pairs, and $\rho(d) = 0$ indicates a random association between pairs. A strong positive correlation is noted for neighboring pieces of lung blood flow.[84] To test the hypothesis that the fractal distribution and spatial correlation of pulmonary perfusion are due to the branching pattern of the pulmonary vasculature, investigators have modeled blood flow using a dichotomously branching tree.[89] This simplified model of pulmonary perfusion produces blood flow distributions and fractal dimensions similar to those seen in experimental animals. When expanded to three dimensions, the fractal model is able to explain the high local correlations in blood flow and the decreasing correlation as distance increases.[91] The self-similar (fractal) branching model of a pulmonary vascular system optimizes the cost-function relationships while closely approximating physiologic and morphometric data.[165] Fractal analysis provides a mechanism for capturing both the richness of the physiologic structure and its function in a single model.

Temporal Heterogeneity Pulmonary perfusion is obviously a dynamic system. Therefore, it stands to reason that perfusion to regions within the lung may change over time. Temporal changes in regional pulmonary perfusion at 20-minute intervals in anesthetized dogs were not random, with temporal flow patterns grouped together.[88] Groups were more tightly clustered in space than expected by chance alone. In addition, statistical clustering methods demonstrated that regulation of blood flow on a large scale (lobar arteries), and fractal analyses suggested regulation existed on a smaller scale (arterioles). Studies conducted in awake dogs daily for 5 days revealed that high-flow pieces were always high flow and low-flow pieces remained low flow every day.[87] This long-term stability supports the hypothesis that regional perfusion is determined primarily by a fixed structure such as the geometry of the pulmonary vasculature rather than a local passive process or vasoactive regulators.

Relative Contribution of Gravity Despite the fact that the gravity-dependent hydrostatic gradient models have dominated the direction and interpretation of pulmonary perfusion studies in the past, recent high-resolution methods,[86,126,182] as well as experiments in both microgravity[218] and macrogravity[127] environments continue to show that the pulmonary blood flow distribution is much more heterogeneous than can be explained by gravity alone. Although studies in many different species have confirmed these findings, some argue that these observations may not apply to humans. For instance, Hughes[132] proposes that gravity may not be as important a determinant of pulmonary blood flow distribution in quadrupeds when compared to the bipedal human. In an attempt to respond to this question, high-resolution methods were used on baboons. These primates have a pulmonary vascular tree that parallels the human system from its gross structure to the degree of muscularization at the arterial and venous level.[152] Gas exchange and hemodynamic responses to hypoxia[104] as well as postural changes[120] are identical to those of humans. Once again the high-resolution methods showed that pulmonary perfusion had a strong positive correlation regardless of posture (and therefore also gravity-dependent hydrostatic gradients).[85] Regions that were high flow in the upright position were also high flow in the head down position. Pulmonary perfusion heterogeneity was greatest in the upright posture and least in the prone position. With use of multiple-stepwise regression, it was estimated that 7%, 5%, and 25% of perfusion heterogeneity were due to gravity in the supine, prone, and upright posture, respectively. Therefore, it appears that gravity, although important, is not the predominant determinant of pulmonary perfusion distribution in upright primates.

Other Factors Other gravity-independent factors have also been identified that can influence pulmonary blood flow distribution and vascular tone. Primary among these are lung volume, cardiac output, and intrathoracic pressure. Each will be briefly reviewed.

Lung Volume. The volume of the normal lung at the end of a normal exhalation without a pressure differential between atmosphere and alveoli is defined as functional residual capacity (FRC). FRC depends on the balance of opposing static forces acting on the respiratory system. The intrinsic elastic properties of the lung favor a reduction in volume, while the natural tendency of the chest wall to recoil outward favors expansion. It is this balance between the elastic properties of the lung and chest wall that determines end-expiratory lung volume (EELV). In the physiologic resting condition, EELV and FRC are the same. Pulmonary vascular resistance is a function of lung volume.[299] As lung volume increases above FRC, total PVR increases due to compression of intraalveolar vessels. An increase in PVR below FRC has been demonstrated to occur secondary to hypoxic vasoconstriction of the large extraalveolar vessels.[20] These relationships are apparent when ventilation is occurring spontaneously or mechanically with positive pressure. It should be emphasized that total pulmonary vascular resistance is lowest when EELV equals FRC.

Cardiac Output. Vascular resistance is an expression of the relationship between driving pressure and flow (Poiseuille's law). In the pulmonary circulation, the driving pressure is the difference between mean pulmonary artery and downstream pressure, either P_A or P_{pv} (or P_{isf}), while the flow is defined as the right ventricular output. Passive changes in the diameter of the pulmonary vessels can be induced by increases in flow (right ventricular output) and/or by elevations of left atrial pressure. Therefore, pulmonary vascular resistance tends to fall as flow increases. Lower resistance at higher flows is further augmented by the fact that previously unperfused vessels are recruited as cardiac output and/or left atrial pressure increase.

Intrathoracic Pressure. Changes in lung volume directly affect PVR. Lung volume is determined by the difference between alveolar pressure and intrathoracic pressure (i.e., transpulmonary pressure—P_{tp}). Thus, major changes in intrathoracic pressure can significantly alter pulmonary vascular resistance. PVR determines right ventricular afterload, thus profoundly influencing right ventricular and ultimately left ventricular function. For example, consider a PEEP producing an alveolar pressure of 30 cm H_2O and a pleural pressure (P_{pl}) of 12 cm H_2O (i.e., P_{tp} of 18 cm H_2O). The same afterload on the right ventricle would be produced at the end of a spontaneous inspiration with a P_{pl} of −18 cm H_2O and an alveolar pressure in equilibrium with atmosphere (i.e., P_{tp} of −18 cm H_2O). Normal tidal volume inspiration from FRC produces insignificant increases in pulmonary vascular resistance and right ventricular afterload. In contrast, large tidal volumes or normal tidal volumes from an elevated EELV (asthma or PEEP) may significantly increase pulmonary vascular resistance and right ventricular afterload.

Pulmonary Vasoregulation

Definition

The term vasoregulation refers to the innumerable regulatory mechanisms that control the tone of vascular smooth muscle (VSM). Tone itself is ultimately determined by the activation of contractile mechanisms within the VSM cell. Vasoregulatory mechanisms can be categorized into those that reside locally and those that represent systemic neurohumoral influences. Teleologically, we would predict that local control mechanisms predominate in organs that are vital to the organism's survival, for example, the heart. Conversely, nonvital organs are likely to have vasoregulatory mechanisms that are predominately systemic, for example, the skin. Regulation of blood flow to the lungs does not fall neatly into either end of this spectrum. In contrast to systemic regional vascular beds, the pulmonary circulation must accommodate all of the cardiac output. Local regional control of blood flow within the lung is, however, as clearly important. This is best illustrated by the influence of hypoxia on the pulmonary circulation (hypoxic pulmonary vasoconstriction). Pulmonary vasoregulatory mechanisms are independent of mechanical influences on the pulmonary circulation. The latter include the effects of changes in lung volume, intrathoracic pressure, gravity, etc. These are considered in the preceding section.

The influence of pulmonary blood flow per se, and changes therein, on measurements of pulmonary vascular resistance represents a potential confounding variable in investigations of pulmonary vasoregulatory mechanisms. This pitfall and methods to address it are discussed in the next section, as are the spectrum of research approaches investigating pulmonary vasoregulatory mechanisms.

Investigative Models of the Pulmonary Circulation and Pulmonary Vasoregulation

The models used to investigate the pulmonary circulation and vasoregulatory mechanisms range from those that use in vivo whole organism conscious models to those that are cellular, subcellular/molecular biology, and genetic. Each approach has its own specific advantages and disadvantages. In general, models utilizing the whole organism are likely to furnish data that represent an integrated response. Nevertheless, such models are limited in their ability to provide detailed mechanistic information. In contrast, cellular and subcellular research approaches do provide detailed insights into mechanisms, but their significance may have to be tempered by the recognition that specific mechanisms and pathways may be modulated in an integrated system.

Changes in pulmonary blood flow can result in passive, nonvasoactive changes in calculated pulmonary vascular resistance if the relationship between pressure and flow in the pulmonary circulation is not rectilinear. There are considerable data on the pulmonary circulation to indicate that the relationship between pressure and flow is, in fact, not rectilinear.[170] The implications of this are clearly illustrated in Figure 3-14. In circumstances where the relationship between pressure and flow is not rectilinear, and there exists a positive pressure intercept at zero flow, changes in flow per se can result in changes in calculated pulmonary vascular resistance.

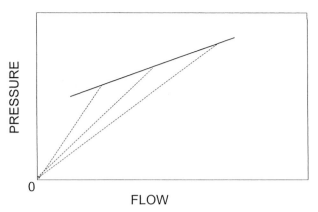

FIGURE 3-14 Influence of the nonrectilinear relationship between pressure and flow in the pulmonary circulation on one point calculations of pulmonary vascular resistance. The dotted lines represent a calculated PVR, which is assumed to pass through the origin. However, extrapolation of the solid line indicates a positive pressure of zero flow and represents the three pressure flow in vivo.

Pulmonary vascular resistance is calculated from the quotient of pressure and flow and is represented by the tangent of the angle connecting flow with zero. The limitations inherent in this approach can be overcome by either a) measuring pressures over a large range of flows, both before and following an intervention designed to investigate the role of a predetermined regulatory mechanism, or b) using a system where pulmonary flow is kept constant and vasoactive interventions will manifest themselves as changes in pressure.

Mediators, Modulators, Regulatory, and Counterregulatory Mechanisms

These terms, and what they imply in any particular setting, are potentially confusing. Indeed, use of the term "mediator" may be overly simplistic in that it implies a monotonic or linear interpretation of the role of a particular molecule/receptor (see subsequent discussion). Moreover, these terms should be interpreted in the context of whether the resultant effects occur acutely or chronically. Finally, these mechanisms may represent either adaptive or maladaptive responses of the organism to a stress stimulus and this may be situational. Both extracellular and intracellular signaling pathways are involved in these processes. A brief review of some key biologic principles underlying signaling is necessary to understand the complexities of vasoregulation.

Signaling, both extracellular and intracellular, allows cells to communicate with their environment. In this context, the environment could refer to the immediately adjacent milieu, remote segments of the organ, or the organism itself. Signaling pathways provide a means of communication and are intrinsic to homeostasis. A cartoon of a signaling pathway is depicted in Figure 3-15. This signaling pathway is represented as a linear sequence. This representation is far removed from what happens in biology. In biological systems there are multiple signaling pathways, some known, many yet unknown. These pathways branch and interconnect with one another. Moreover, these pathways loop both backward, providing

negative feedback mechanisms, and forward on themselves. Simply stated, biologic signaling pathways demonstrate communication within and between pathways (intra- and extrapathway "crosstalk," respectively), as denoted in Figure 3-15. These features of biologic signaling systems confer many advantages. Indeed, the term "advantage" is an understatement in that these features represent necessities in biologic systems. Otherwise, biologic systems would disintegrate. These features of signaling pathways result in at least three important biologic effects:

1. Negative feedback mechanisms provide a basis for preventing a response from getting out of control (runaway signaling).
2. Crosstalk offers the potential for amplifying and diverging a signal if and when this is necessary.
3. Feedback loops both within and between pathways provide the opportunity to fine-tune a response to a biologic stimulus.

The term "regulation" usually refers to the process whereby a single messenger initiates a response. The same messenger may concurrently initiate a more slowly developing but different response, the biologic result of which is the opposite to that of the acute response. This is referred to as counterregulation. Runaway signaling is prevented by counterregulation, which conceptually can occur at the following levels:

1. The receptor (the same messenger may bind to different receptor subtypes, each of which has different or perhaps even opposite effects; β-agonist stimulation of different β-adrenergic subtypes is a well-known example);
2. The receptor-coupling mechanisms in the cell membrane; for example, β-adrenergic receptors may be coupled to G-proteins that can be either inhibitory (G_i) or stimulatory (G_s)[266,304];
3. The signaling pathway (negative feedback either within or between pathways; for example, cyclic AMP inhibition of receptor/membrane coupling and cytosolic calcium inhibition of adenyl cyclase exemplify the former, while ATP modulation of L-type sarcolemmal calcium channels and calcium facilitation of voltage-dependent calcium channels [VDCCs][62] typify the latter); or
4. The contractile proteins (influence of pH on the binding of and response to calcium).[143,264]

Thus, considering the complexity of biological signaling pathways, it is perhaps overly simplistic to suggest that a single molecule and pathway mediate the response to a specific stimulus. The integrated response is likely to be modulated by any one of several interacting pathways. The response of the cell to a stimulus in the short term is likely to represent an adaptive response to the environment. The same stimulus, if prolonged, may result in genotypic or phenotypic changes that are maladaptive and ultimately fatal. This phenomenon is increasingly recognized in heart failure.[151] There may exist an analogous situation in the pulmonary circulation where activated signaling pathways may initially result in vasoactive changes, but the same stimulus, if protracted (chronic), may contribute to the trophic changes observed in pulmonary hypertension.

Pulmonary Vascular Heterogeneity

The lungs receive blood flow from both the pulmonary and the bronchial circulations. These communicate and under

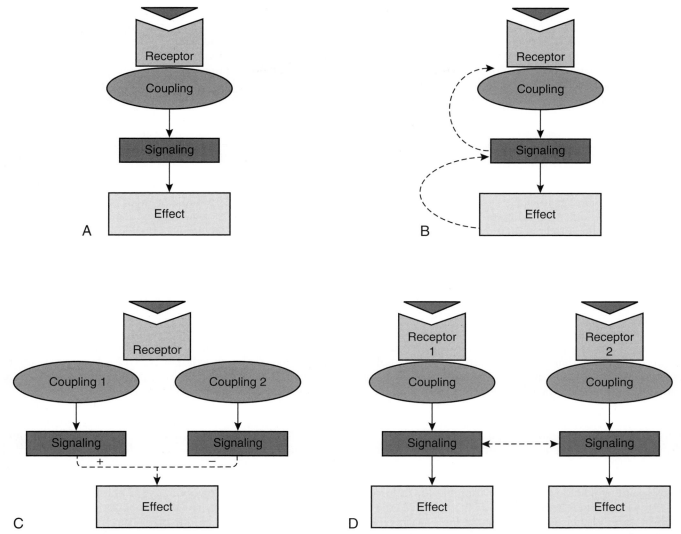

FIGURE 3-15 Cartoon of signaling illustrating a simple linear pathway **(A)**; feedback loops and intrapathway crosstalk **(B)**; activation of a common membrane receptor with coupling to two different signaling pathways and interpathway crosstalk **(C)**; and activation of two different membrane receptor types by the same agonist and the resultant signal pathway activation **(D)**.

physiological conditions, the bronchial circulation, account for less than 5% physiologic shunt. The pulmonary vasculature has several unique features that distinguish it from all systemic vascular beds. Its low pressures in physiologic states and its accommodation of all the cardiac output are obvious. Less evident is the anatomic and functional heterogeneity exhibited by the pulmonary vasculature. This has resulted in the use of terms such as alveolar/extraalveolar/corner vessels, zonal conditions, and recruitment and distention to describe features of pulmonary blood flow.

The terms "alveolar" and "extraalveolar" are almost self-explanatory. The former refers to the pulmonary microvessels involved in gas exchange, while the latter refers to larger, elastic, and muscular pulmonary arteries that branch and eventually give rise to alveolar gas exchanging vessels. The term "corner vessels" is a functional description used in models to characterize the pulmonary circulation and refers to pulmonary microvessels adjacent to, or at the corners of, neighboring alveoli.[82] They are not involved in gas exchange but may subserve a nutritional role for the lung parenchyma and provide pulmonary flow even in lung regions subject to zone 1 conditions. The term "zonal conditions" refers to pressures (pulmonary artery, alveolar, pulmonary venous) that determine blood flow in pulmonary alveolar vessels engaged in gas exchange. (The latter were discussed earlier; see gravity-dependent distribution section.) Recruitment implies the opening of pulmonary vessels not hitherto accommodating flow. Distension refers to the changes in vessel diameter and tone that accompany increases in pulmonary blood flow in vessels that are already perfused and thus alter vascular cross-sectional area and resistance.

The contribution of the pulmonary arterial tree, the microvasculature, and the pulmonary venous circulation to overall pulmonary vascular resistance is in contrast to that which exists in the systemic circulation. In the latter, the vast majority of resistance to flow resides within the systemic arterioles. In the pulmonary circulation, the arterioles are also important contributors to pulmonary vascular resistance and are subject to complex vasoactive control mechanisms, but the microvascular vessels and the pulmonary veins also contribute importantly to total pulmonary vascular resistance.

Vasoregulatory influences in the pulmonary vasculature have been shown to exhibit right/left differences. In vitro measurements of tension in pulmonary arterial rings from swine demonstrate important differences in endothelial-dependent relaxation in vessel rings procured from the right lung when compared to the left.[145] Impaired right-sided vasorelaxation was observed with both receptor-dependent (acetylcholine, bradykinin) and receptor-independent (A23187) endothelial-dependent vasodilators. In contrast, rings from both right and left lungs exhibited identical relaxation to the endothelial-independent vasodilator, sodium nitroprusside, indicating that the differential response resides in the endothelium. Inhibition of NO production failed to abolish the differential right/left response to acetylcholine. In contrast, cyclooxygenase pathway inhibition with indomethacin abolished this right/left differential response to endothelial-dependent vasodilators. This indicates that the impaired response in the right lung is likely due to a relative excess of vasoconstrictor products of the cyclooxygenase pathway.

Heterogeneity also exists within each lung's vasculature. With use of porcine pulmonary vessels ranging in size from 1.7 to 0.2 mm internal diameter (elastic conduit vessels → resistance vessels), Boels and coworkers demonstrated significant differences in endothelial-dependent relaxation to acetylcholine depending on vessel size.[25] In contrast, bradykinin was able to relax all vessel segments independent of size. Furthermore, these workers also demonstrated an age dependence of the response to acetylcholine. For example, acetylcholine caused contraction in porcine fetal pulmonary vessel rings. Thus, the evidence indicates that one's observations regarding pulmonary vasoregulation may be influenced by a) the lung vessels being studied (right vs. left), b) the size of the vessels, c) the specific agonist used in one's investigations, and d) the age of the species under investigation.

Vascular Smooth Muscle

Regulation of Contraction While vascular smooth muscle (VSM) has many features in common with skeletal and cardiac muscle, it has several unique features that distinguish it from either and confers on it the ability to perform its own unique functions. Smooth muscle cells are usually oblong in shape, measuring 2 to 5 microns in diameter and 20 to 500 microns in length. Importantly, smooth muscle can be divided into a) multi-unit smooth muscle, where fibers are independently innervated (this type of smooth muscle tends not to exhibit spontaneous contraction, does not have basal tone, and responds to phasic stimulation); and b) single-unit smooth muscle that acts like a syncytium with impulse propagation facilitated by gap junctions. A stimulus spreads beyond the initial effector smooth muscle cell and the smooth muscle behaves functionally as one. VSM falls into the latter category.

As in skeletal and cardiac muscle, contraction in VSM depends ultimately on crossbridge formation between actin and myosin. VSM differs from skeletal muscle in that the rate of tension development is slower, but the tension developed is maintained for a longer time. Molecular studies indicate that tension is maintained even when intracellular calcium concentration [Ca++]i and myosin light chain (MLC) phosphorylation are decreasing. The molecular mechanisms underlying this observation have not yet been determined. This mechanical phenomenon whereby tension is maintained with slowly cycling crossbridges is referred to as a "latch state" and requires low but ongoing calcium presence and MLC phosphorylation. Even though the mechanism is unclear, the phenomena are energy efficient in that tension is maintained with low actinomyosin ATPase activity and low ATP consumption. This contrasts with skeletal muscle where crossbridges are either in a low (relaxation) or a high (contraction) "affinity state." This requires high energy consumption and is referred to as a "rigor state." This is a complex process and is reviewed in detail elsewhere.[73,129,232] Crossbridging between actin and myosin is profoundly influenced by the extent to which MLCs are phosphorylated and the activity of actinomyosin ATPase (which provides the energy required for contraction). The extent to which MLC are phosphorylated is determined by the activity of kinases (promoting phosphorylation) and phosphatases (promoting dephosphorylation).

The key to understanding VSM contraction/relaxation is understanding the mechanisms that determine phosphorylation and dephosphorylation of MLC. It is necessary to understand how these protein kinases and phosphatases are themselves regulated. We will return to this later.

Phosphorylation of MLC is the pivotal step in the regulation of contraction of VSM (Fig. 3-16). The phosphorylated form of MLC interacts with actin to form crossbridges and generate contraction. MLC kinase phosphorylates and MLC phosphatase dephosphorylates MLC. MLC kinase activity is highly regulated by the calcium-calmodulin complex. In contrast, our understanding of how MLC phosphatase is regulated is far less complete. However, modulation of MLC phosphatase activity may be one of the mechanisms underlying agonist-induced calcium sensitization in VSM (the observation whereby the contractile response is altered in the setting of constant calcium concentration).

Regulation of Vascular Smooth Muscle Calcium Concentration

Mechanisms Increasing [Ca++]i Regulation of calcium in vascular smooth muscle has been reviewed by Orallo.[205] Calcium combines with calmodulin to form a calcium-calmodulin (Ca++-calmodulin) complex. This activates MLC kinase, converting it from an inactive to an active form. The activity of Ca++-calmodulin itself, and thus its ability to modulate MLC kinase and the subsequent steps leading to VSM contraction, are profoundly influenced by [Ca++]i. Cytosolic calcium concentration at rest is ~0.1 mm/L but may increase 100-fold during contraction. Cytosolic calcium concentration is the net result of calcium entry into and extrusion from the cytoplasm. The source, routes of entry and exit, and mechanisms controlling each of these are discussed separately.

Cytosolic calcium concentrations can increase either by entry from outside the cell across the sarcolemma or by release from the sarcoplasmic reticulum (SR). In general, extracellular calcium is a more important source of cytosolic

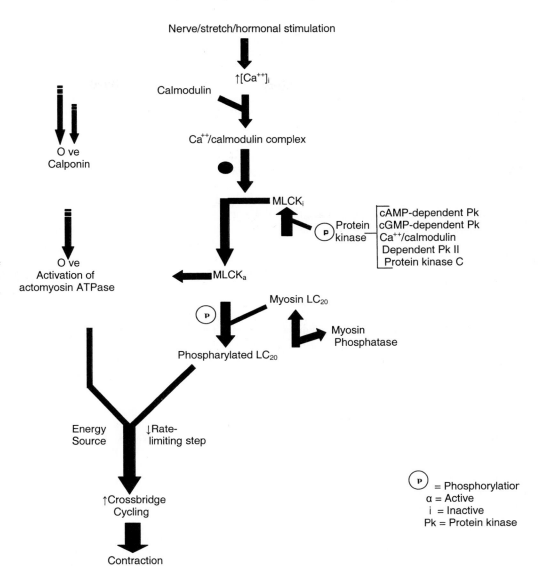

FIGURE 3-16 Central role of calcium and the calcium-calmodulin complex in modulating myosin light chain (MLC) activity and smooth muscle contraction.

calcium in VSM than is the SR. This contrasts with cardiac myocytes, where SR calcium is the main source of cytosolic calcium. Calcium is released from the SR by the entry of calcium into the cytoplasm adjacent to the foot process/ryanodine receptor(s). Multiple types of ryanodine receptors are expressed in VSM[197] component of the SR. This phenomenon is known as calcium-induced calcium release (CICR). As illustrated in Figure 3-17, influx of calcium across the sarcolemma can occur via:

Calcium channels (long or L-type) that are voltage-dependent, which are known as voltage-dependent calcium channels (VDCCs);
Nonspecific cation channels (NSCCs);
Receptor-operated channels (ROCs); and
Sodium calcium exchange.

Although there are six subtypes of VDCCs, in VSM, L-type calcium channels are the only ones that are considered important. In contrast to other excitable tissue, where sodium is important in generating action potentials, calcium is the major ion involved in action potential generation in VSM. The gating characteristics of VSM membrane calcium channels

result in relatively slow, but prolonged, entry of calcium. This explains the prolonged action potential with a plateau phase. Depolarization of VSM results in calcium influx via VDCCs and ultimately VSM contraction. Conversely, hyperpolarization impairs calcium entry, inhibits contraction, and thus causes vasorelaxation. The threshold potential for calcium entry via VDCCs is −40 mV. Calcium entry via L-type calcium channels may be important in maintaining basal tone. Various stimuli, including neurotransmitters and stretch, can increase (rendering the inside of the cell less negative relative to the outside) the resting membrane potential toward the threshold potential necessary to open VDCCs. The net result is calcium entry and VSM contraction.

The contribution of other sarcolemma channels (NSCCs, ROCs, sodium calcium exchange) to changes in $[Ca^{++}]_i$, their interaction with VDCCs, and their effects on Ca^{++} release from the SR are complex and depend on the stimulus and the VSM under study (systemic vs. pulmonary, arteriolar vs. venous, size of the vessel, etc.).

The contribution of non-VDCCs to increases in intracellular calcium is unmasked in the presence of L-type calcium channel blockers (for example, verapamil). Under these conditions, agonist (for example, norepinephrine) induced contractions are impaired but not abolished. This is in contrast to potassium-induced contractions that are completely abolished by L-type calcium channel blockers because the response to K+ is exclusively dependent on calcium entry via VDCCs. Similar differential responses to agonist vs. KCl stimulation are found if the external medium is rendered calcium free. These results indicate that, following agonist stimulation, intracellular calcium is increased by mechanisms that are VDCC-dependent and -independent. Further studies by various groups using selective blockers of L-type (VDCC) and non-L-type calcium channels, kinetic calcium measurements, permeabilized and nonpermeabilized preparations, indicate the following:

Calcium entry does occur via NSCCs during agonist stimulation;

NSCCs are coupled to L-type/VDCCs, and the latter are activated during agonist stimulation;

Calcium entry via non-L-type channels can cause calcium-induced calcium release from a ryanodine-sensitive pool in the SR;

Agonist-induced activation of sarcolemma receptor operated channels results in phospholipase-C activation via a G-protein mechanism;

Calcium influx across the sacrolemma is influenced by the calcium concentration/load in the VSM cell or, perhaps more accurately, in "restricted" spaces within the VSM (calcium capacitance);

Depletion of SR calcium activates plasma membrane store-operated calcium channels (SOCCs) facilitating calcium entry into the cell[81];

Intracellular calcium can increase calcium entry via VDCCs (facilitation) by a mechanism that is mediated by Ca++-calmodulin-dependent protein-kinase II phosphorylation.[62]

Phospholipase-C catalyzes the formation of 1,2 diacylglycerol and inositol 1,4,5 triphosphate (IP$_3$). IP$_3$ causes calcium release from the SR (see Fig. 3-17). Calcium in the SR is functionally compartmentalized and its release from the SR is signal specific, for example, the ryanodine-sensitive and the IP$_3$-sensitive pools. Finally, calcium (either entering from outside the cell or being released from the SR) is now recognized to be functionally compartmentalized in the cytoplasm itself. The calcium in the cytoplasm can be divided into that which is adjacent to the contractile proteins and causing contraction (contractile pool) and that which resides between the sarcolemma and the SR and does not cause contraction (noncontractile pool). Again, the change in calcium concentration in either compartment may be stimulus-specific. Thus, the mechanisms by which a specific agonist (e.g., α-adrenergic agonists, muscarinic agonists, prostenoids, angiotensin-II, endothelin-1, histamine) increases [Ca++]$_i$ and causes VSM contraction are complex and specific to the agonists under study.[148] Studies investigating the role of the sodium-calcium exchange mechanisms are inconsistent and tissue-specific. Thus, their physiologic importance is unclear. Indeed, this mechanism may contribute to calcium extrusion from the cell if serum calcium concentration is elevated.

Mechanisms Decreasing [Ca++]$_i$ Relaxation in vascular smooth muscle occurs when [Ca++]$_i$ is decreased by either extrusion across the sarcolemma or re-uptake of calcium by the SR and mitochondria. The primary mechanisms responsible for extrusion and re-uptake of calcium are illustrated in Figure 3-18. Extrusion of Ca++ across the sarcolemma occurs via the following mechanisms:

Calcium-magnesium ATPase pump that is modulated by the calcium-calmodulin complex (negative feedback mechanism);

Sodium-calcium exchange pump driven by the concentration gradient for sodium. The contribution of this mechanism may vary depending on the type of VSM.

Re-uptake of calcium by the SR is highly regulated. A calcium ATPase pump in the SR facilitates re-uptake of calcium. This is an energy-dependent process requiring ATP. Phospholamban inhibits calcium re-uptake by the SR. Phosphorylation of phospholamban inhibits the latter's inhibitory effects and, as a result, increases calcium re-uptake. Phosphorylation of phospholamban is promoted by cAMP-dependent kinases. Moreover, cAMP-dependent kinases (as well as cGMP kinases) have direct effects on the calcium ATPase pump via protein kinase C. The net result of

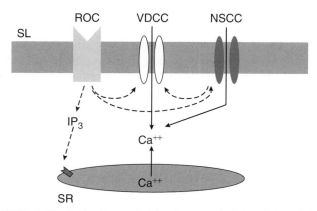

FIGURE 3-17 Mechanisms underlying increases in intracellular calcium concentration. NSCC, nonspecific calcium channels; ROC, recepter operated channels; SL, sarcolemma; SR, sarcoplasmic reticulum; VDCC, voltage-dependent calcium channels.

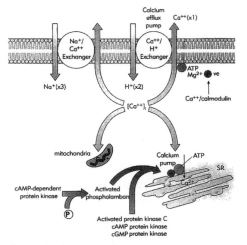

FIGURE 3-18 Mechanisms underlying decreases in intracellular calcium concentration. (From O'Beirne HA, Hopkins PM: Smooth muscle. In Hemmings HC Jr, Hopkins PM [eds]: *Foundations of Anesthesia: Basic and Clinical Services.* Phildelphia: Mosby, 2000; with permission.)

activation of these mechanisms is to promote calcium re-uptake by the SR. The mitochondria also take up calcium, but in the form of calcium phosphate. The contribution of this latter mechanism to rhythmic contraction and relaxation is unclear. It may play a role under conditions of cellular calcium overload (e.g., ischemia, anoxia).

Calcium Sensitivity This is a complex area and will be only briefly reviewed. For a more complete discussion, see reference 148.

Calcium sensitivity refers to the phenomenon of an altered contractile response at the same $[Ca^{++}]_i$. This altered response is not explained by changes between MLC phosphorylation and contraction but rather by changes in the relationship between calcium and MLC phosphorylation. In other words, the extent to which MLC is phosphorylated can be altered by other mechanisms, even when $[Ca^{++}]_i$ is constant. Several mechanisms have been proposed (Fig. 3-19). These include modulation of the following:

MLC kinase phosphorylation by calcium-calmodulin dependent myosin kinase 2 (Note: phosphorylation of MLC kinase inhibits this enzyme, thus inhibiting its ability to phosphorylate MLC. Phosphorylation of MLC kinase inhibits contraction; however, phosphorylation of MLC increases contraction);

MLC phosphatase activity;

Free calmodulin levels in the cell cytoplasm; and

Actin response distal to MLC.

The calcium-calmodulin complex activates MLC. The calcium-calmodulin complex also activates MLC kinase 2. MLC kinase 2 phosphorylates MLC kinase and inhibits its activity, an indirect effect opposite to the direct effect of the calcium-calmodulin complex per se. Thus, this is a classic negative feedback loop. Clearly, the indirect effect has to differ either quantitatively and/or temporally from the direct effect. Under baseline conditions, there is a balance between these counter-regulatory mechanisms. MLC kinase activity could be altered

even in the presence of constant $[Ca^{++}]_i$ if agonists modulate MLC kinase 2 and, thus, phosphorylation of MLC kinase.

Phosphorylation of MLC phosphatase also inactivates this enzyme, which increases MLC phosphorylation and increases contraction.

It had been hitherto assumed that calmodulin was not rate limiting and was readily diffusable within the cytoplasm. More recent studies indicate that less than 5% of calmodulin is readily diffusable and that calmodulin is compartmentalized in several intracellular pools with different affinities for agonist and ion (e.g., $[Ca^{++}]_i$)-induced mobilization. Thus, it is entirely possible that modulation of calmodulin could modulate the activity of MLC kinase, even if $[Ca^{++}]_i$ is constant.

Finally, sensitivity, as defined, could be altered distal to MLC kinase-MLC (i.e., actin). This mechanism of altering sensitivity would be independent of phosphorylation. Actin-binding proteins (e.g., calponin, caldesmon) could be responsible for this mechanism. Calponin may modulate the sensitivity of actin at any specific level of MLC activity. Caldesmon is a second regulatory protein, the precise role of which has not yet been well defined.[148]

Stimuli Promoting Vascular Smooth Muscle Relaxation The second messenger cyclic nucleotides (cAMP and cGMP) are important relaxant signals in VSM. By definition, the membrane potential modulates VDCCs and, thus, the balance of contraction-relaxation. Depolarization activates VDCCs causing calcium influx and contraction, while hyperpolarization inhibits VDCCs and promotes relaxation. The role of hyperpolarizing stimuli in the context of endothelium-derived hyperpolarizing factor (EDHF) and hypoxic pulmonary vasoconstriction is discussed subsequently. Intracellular cAMP is increased following G-coupled receptor stimulation (e.g., β-receptor agonist stimulation, vasodilator prostaglandins). cGMP is increased by NO, atrial natriuretic peptides, and nitro-vasodilators. The potential sites of action of protein kinase A are illustrated in Figure 3-20. Inhibition of MLC phosphorylation by cyclic nucleotide has been demonstrated, but it is unclear if this mechanism is important physiologically.[284] In contrast, it is clear that cyclic nucleotides uncouple the increase in MLC phosphorylation from the increase in $[Ca^{++}]_i$ and that this is a physiologically important mechanism underlying the effects of cyclic nucleotide mediated vasodilation. Cyclic nucleotide inhibition of contraction extends beyond the effect on Ca^{++}-calmodulin complex. Cyclic GMP-dependent protein kinase modulates MLC phosphatase[269] promoting dephosphorylation of MLC (see Fig. 3-19). Thus, NO/cGMP not only decreases $[Ca^{++}]_i$ but also decreases sensitivity. Finally, as illustrated in Figure 3-18, cyclic nucleotides promote calcium re-uptake by the SR and inhibit receptor-induced IP3-mediated calcium release from the SR.

Pulmonary Vascular Smooth Muscle Function

Extracellular Signaling and Modulation of Vascular Smooth Muscle Function VSM is subject to a vast array of regulatory influences. These can be categorized into autocrine, paracrine, and endocrine influences (Fig. 3-21), and those that result from autonomic nervous system neurotransmitter release. The endothelial cell acts as a paracrine organ, releasing from its abluminal surface vasoactive substances that

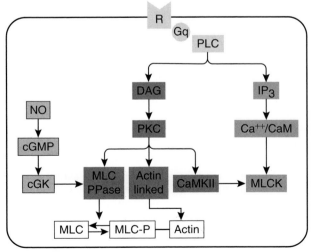

FIGURE 3-19 Mechanisms underlying changes in calcium sensitivity. Ca++/CaM, calcium calmodulin complex; CGK, cyclic GMP dependent protein kinase; cGMP, cyclic GMP; DAG, diacylglycerox; Gq, G-protein; IP3, inositol triphosphate; MLC, myosin light chain; MLCK, myosin light chain kinase 2; MLCPPase, MLC phosphatase; NO, nitric oxide; PKC, protein kinase C; PLC, phospholipase C; R, receptor

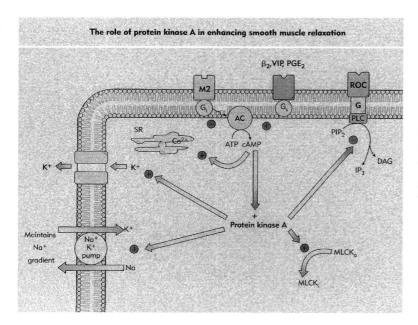

FIGURE 3-20 Influence of cyclic nucleotides and protein kinase A on mechanisms that regulate intracellular calcium and MLC kinase. (From O'Beirne HA, Hopkins PM: Smooth muscle. In Hemmings HC Jr, Hopkins PM [eds]: *Foundations of Anesthesia: Basic and Clinical Services*. Phildelphia: Mosby, 2000; with permission.)

modulate underlying VSM tone. These molecules are released by the endothelium following biophysical and/or biochemical stimulation of its adluminal surface (see Fig. 3-21). Moreover, the pulmonary vascular endothelium is increasingly recognized for its importance as a metabolic organ, transforming molecules from an inactive (or weakly active) form to an active form (e.g., angiotensin-I is catalyzed to angiotensin-II by converting enzyme). Finally, the vascular endothelium likely plays an important role in attenuating the effects of molecules that act directly on VSM.

Several important vasodilator and vasoconstrictor substances are produced by the endothelium (see Fig. 3-21). Their potential roles in the systemic vasculature, especially in the coronary vasculature, are well documented. NO, prostacyclin, and endothelial-derived hyperpolarizing factor (EDHF) can relax pulmonary VSM. Vasoconstrictor products of the cyclooxygenase pathway and the endothelin family can constrict pulmonary VSM. It has been clearly demonstrated that these substances have the capacity to modulate VSM. Nevertheless, their physiologic importance is more difficult to elucidate. This commentary applies even to NO, whose many physiologic and pathologic roles continue to be aggressively investigated.

The biochemical pathways underlying pulmonary vascular endothelial cell NO production are similar to those in the systemic vasculature. NO is produced by the enzymatic conversion of L-arginine to L-citrulline. Endothelial nitric oxide synthase (eNOS) is constitutively expressed and accounts for basal NO production. Importantly, endogenous NO production is most significant in small, precapillary pulmonary arteries and to a lesser degree in small veins and larger pulmonary arteries.[66,243] This contribution of basal NO production to maintenance of low pulmonary vascular resistance is probably modest.[60] In the pulmonary circulation, inhibition of NOS under nonstimulated conditions produces only modest increases in pulmonary vascular resistance. NO is likely more important in modulating the pulmonary vascular

response to acute and chronic pharmacological and pathological stimuli. It is now generally agreed that the endothelium does not mediate HPV and that hypoxic pulmonary vasoconstriction (HPV) can occur in pulmonary vessels whose endothelial cells are denuded either pharmacologically or mechanically. Acute hypoxia actually results in increased NO production when the endothelium is intact (perhaps via alterations in local shear stress). The increased NO production actually attenuates the direct VSM effects of hypoxia. Studies of the role of eNOS in models of chronic pulmonary hypertension (e.g., that which occurs following hypoxia or monocrotaline) and studies of human pulmonary hypertension indicate that NO production is increased rather than decreased. This would be consistent with the premise that endothelial cell dysfunction is not a primary component in these processes. Rather, increased NO production reflects a compensatory mechanism, especially in the important small precapillary resistance pulmonary vessels. This compensatory mechanism is incomplete in that pulmonary hypertension is still present, but it does indicate that pulmonary VSM cells have the capacity to respond to NO in these conditions (at least in their early or intermediate stages). Herein lies the basis for increasing vascular NO activity as a therapeutic paradigm.

The role of NO has been more completely elucidated in the systemic circulations, and it is unclear what role they may play in pulmonary vascular disease. For example, in the systemic circulation:

1. Although overall arginine concentrations indicate that NO production should not be substrate limited, the concentration of L-arginine within intracellular microdomains (caveolae) may indeed be rate limiting, especially in the presence of endogenous inhibitors of NO, for example, asymmetric dimethyl arginine [ADMA];
2. Under certain conditions eNOS production of NO can be decreased and that of the superoxide radical increased, attenuating or even reversing the vasorelaxant effect; and

Endothelium-derived vasoactive substances

Vasodilator substances

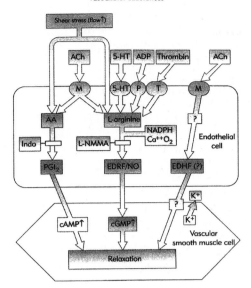

Vasocontracting factors (EDCFs)

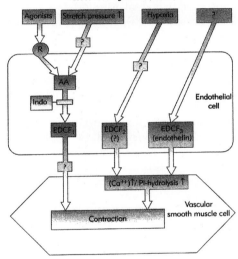

FIGURE 3-21 Extracellular mechanisms that modulate vascular muscle function. (From Nyhan D, Blanck TJJ: Cardiac physiology. In Hemming HC Jr, Hopkins PM [eds]: *Foundations of Anesthesia:* Basic Sciences for Clinical Practice. Philadelphia: Mosby, 2000; with permission.)

3. Radicals from any source (NOS, NADPH oxidase system) can rapidly scavenge NO, rendering it inactive.[105] In the systemic vasculature, at least, the NADPH oxidase system is no longer viewed as being confined to VSM cells in that a gp91-phox containing NADPH oxidase system similar to that in leukocytes has recently been described in endothelial cells.[99,208] Overall, the concept of oxidative stress in both normal and abnormal cardiovascular function, including pulmonary vascular function, has broad experimental support.[103,104]

It has been clearly demonstrated in both the systemic and pulmonary circulations that endothelial stimulation (e.g., with a calcium ionophore, acetylcholine, bradykinin, etc., which increase endothelial cell calcium-calmodulin) will cause vasorelaxation of underlying VSM, even following combined pharmacologic inhibition of NO/cGMP-dependent and prostacyclin/cAMP-dependent pathways. This vasorelaxation is associated with hyperpolarization of VSM (involving calcium sensitive potassium channels), and thus, the putative transmitter has been called EDHF. Although the responsible molecule has not been identified, epoxide products of the cytochrome P-450 system may play a role.[32] It is likely that there is more than one EDHF.[219] Also, myoendothelial gap junctions may be important in this mechanism of vasorelaxation.[75] The latter may account for the difficulty in identifying the biochemical substance using classic bioassay approaches. Although EDHFs may act in concert with NO, they may be the predominant endothelial dependent vasodilator mechanism in small vessels and microvessels. The contribution of EDHFs to the maintenance of low pulmonary vascular resistance has not been quantitated.

Hypoxic Pulmonary Vasoconstriction The fundamental mechanisms underlying contraction are similar across all VSM cells. Nevertheless, the extent to which a contraction is modulated will vary from one vascular bed to another and even regionally within a vascular bed. Moreover, the same stimulus may in fact evoke opposite responses in different VSM cells (contraction versus relaxation). This reflects differential sensing and signaling rather than fundamental differences in the mechanisms underlying contraction. This phenomenon is best illustrated by the differential responses of the pulmonary and systemic vessels to hypoxia. Hypoxia causes pulmonary vasoconstriction and pulmonary VSM contraction but causes systemic vasodilatation and systemic VSM relaxation. Hypoxic pulmonary vasoconstriction (HPV) is most pronounced in lobar pulmonary arteries ranging in size from 30 to 300 μm. HPV is not dependent on the autonomic nervous system or the endothelial cell. HPV is abolished by removal of calcium from the extracellular medium and by L-type calcium-channel blockers (e.g., verapamil). This indicates that VDCCs are critical in mediating HPV. Pulmonary VSM cells, like VSM cells elsewhere, contract following MLC phosphorylation and crossbridge formation with actin. The innumerable interactive mechanisms described previously ([Ca^{++}]$_i$, calcium-calmodulin, sensitivity, cyclic nucleotides, etc.) determine the net contractile response in pulmonary VSM. Hypoxia and acidosis are potent stimuli for this response. The precise mechanisms (cellular oxygen sensing and coupling to initial intracellular signaling) have not been completely elucidated (ATP and products of the cytochrome P-450 system have been proposed),[114] nor has an explanation for the opposite response in systemic vessels.

All VSM cells have at least one voltage-dependent potassium channel (K_v) that is activated by depolarization.[17,39,196] K_v channels can be modulated by pH[7] and hypoxia. Some insights into the possible mechanisms responsible for HPV can be gleaned from studies of intracellular acidosis and/or hypoxia in pulmonary and coronary VSM cells and in carotid body glomus cells. In type-1 glomus cells from the carotid body, hypoxia decreases potassium current in voltage-dependent potassium channels, promoting membrane depolarization and contraction. In patch-clamp studies of single pulmonary VSM cells, Berger and coworkers demonstrated that intracellular acidosis decreased potassium currents in voltage gated potassium channels (but not in ATP sensitive or calcium-activated potassium channels).[21] This results in a decrease in resting membrane potential (toward the threshold potential for VDCCs) with activation of VDCCs, calcium entry, and contraction. Intracellular acidosis had the opposite effects in VSM cells isolated from coronary arteries. In these latter cells, intracellular acidosis increased potassium currents in voltage-dependent potassium channels, increasing the resting membrane potential (hyperpolarization) and inhibiting contraction. Thus, voltage-dependent potassium channels are important in acidosis-induced coronary dilation. Recently, in contrast, Shimizu demonstrated that these voltage-dependent potassium channels (and, indeed, several other classes of potassium channels) do not contribute to hypoxia-induced coronary vasodilatation.[262] The role of voltage-dependent potassium channels in HPV was investigated directly by Post[214] and Yaun.[307] They demonstrated inhibition of K_v by hypoxia in pulmonary VSM cells. Hypoxic inhibition of K_v depolarizes the VSM and activates VDCCs (Fig. 3-22).

The influence of different K^+ channels (K_v, Kca^{++}, K_{ATP}, $K_{i/R}$) on membrane potential and, thus, on VDCCs and calcium influx into VSM is increasingly recognized. They provide a basis for the apparent disparate observations between different vascular beds (e.g., systemic vasodilatation mediated by activation of K_{ATP} channels vs. HPV affected by inhibition of K_v). Moreover, subtypes of K^+ channels (several families of K_v have been identified[196,240]) may provide an explanation for differential responses within the same vessel. One specific family of K_v may be particularly important in HPV. K_v 3.1 channels are thought to play an important physiologic role in excitable tissues.[79] For example, in the central nervous system they enable rapid neuronal discharge by inhibiting action potential duration and refractory period. Inhibition of K_v 3.1 by hypoxia would impair neuronal function and metabolism, thus serving as an adaptive mechanism. Osipenko and colleagues recently demonstrated that K_v 3.1b are expressed in pulmonary artery VSM.[207] Moreover, electrophysiologic and pharmacologic channel inhibition studies demonstrated that K^+ currents in K_v 3.1b channels (but not

other K_v channels, for example, K_v 1.1, 1.2, and 1.5) were inhibited by hypoxia. Importantly, these investigators confirmed their observations in membrane patches devoid of cytoplasm, indicating a membrane limited mechanism (either a direct effect of hypoxia on the channel or an effect on an immediately adjacent molecule/sensor that alters the channel). It is unlikely that there is only one oxygen-sensitive channel because there are non-K^+ channels that respond to hypoxia, and, as described, not all K^+ channels respond to hypoxia.[210] Multiple chemical substances have been claimed at various times to mediate HPV. These substances are more correctly viewed as probably being responsible for the variability in the HPV response across species, condition, age, gender, and so forth.

It is now widely recognized that all mammalian cells can sense oxygen concentration. The mechanisms responsible for oxygen sensing are an area of intense investigation. Nevertheless, these mechanisms remain undetermined,[210] and it is unknown if oxygen sensing mechanisms differ with acute vs. chronic exposure, in excitable vs. nonexcitable tissue, and within the vasculature across different vascular beds.[254] Recent approaches to this area have utilized genetic tools in simple organisms, for example, *Drosophila*. These studies have demonstrated a pivotal role for cGMP kinase and/or nitric oxide synthase (NOS) in oxygen homeostasis in this organism.[310] Following the isolation of a specific constitutively expressed mitochondrial isoform of NOS, which can inhibit mitochondrial respiration during hypoxia, it has been proposed (as a model) that hypoxia may simultaneously cause vasodilatation mediated by release of heme-bound cytoplasmic NO (increasing blood flow) and decrease oxygen consumption by inhibition of the mitochondrial cytochrome-oxidase system.[96] This is unproven, and its applicability to the pulmonary vasculature has not been explored. Considering the importance of oxygen homeostasis, it is likely, especially in complex organisms, that multiple signaling pathways with intra- and inter-pathway crosstalk modulatory influences will in the future be identified.[254] Their specific profile is likely to be tissue-specific.

Reactive Oxygen Species   A "radical" refers to an atom or molecule that contains an unpaired electron. Although much is unknown about how radicals exert their effects, the term "reactive" indicates a propensity to combine with important biological molecules. For example, the radical NO readily reacts with metal and thiol-containing proteins, which are part of ion channels (calcium-dependent potassium channels), receptors (NMDA), enzymes (guanylate cyclase), and transcription factors (nuclear factor, beta kappa).[53] Radicals that contain oxygen are referred to as "reactive oxygen species" (ROS). NO is an important example. Another important ROS is superoxide (O_2^-). Superoxide can be interconverted to other ROS (hydrogen peroxide and hydroxyl) and can also form secondary reactive species (peroxynitrite).[16] Almost all cell types in the vasculature have been shown to both produce and be regulated by ROS.[103,270]

Several cell types in the lung, including endothelial and VSM cells, produce superoxide. Any one or more of several enzymes, depending on the cell type, the stimulus, and the prevailing conditions can form superoxide. For example, under physiologic conditions, NOS will form the radical NO,

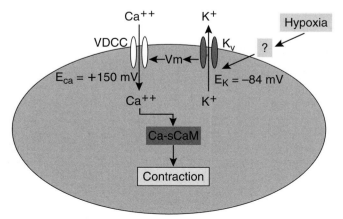

FIGURE 3-22   Mechanism underlying hypoxic pulmonary vasoconstriction (inhibition of K_v channels).

but under conditions of substrate limitation (i.e., L-arginine deficiency), NOS will generate superoxide.[310]

Superoxide is produced by lung tissue under basal conditions.[53] Increased production of superoxide and other reactive oxygen species and perturbations in the balance between ROS generation and scavenging (e.g., by superoxide dismutase) are likely critical in many lung conditions. Cellular superoxide dismutase is widely distributed in the lungs and is subject to complex regulation. Disturbances in ROS generation and/or superoxide dismutase may be important in mediating the lung injury associated with hypoxia, hyperoxia, ischemia reperfusion, and lung transplantation conditions.[53]

ROS in general, and superoxide specifically, can modulate both vessel contraction[131] and permeability. Superoxide increases contraction of pulmonary vessels/rings. It has been demonstrated that several mechanisms underlie this effect, including 1) destruction of NO released by the endothelial cell[171] or generated from NO donors[175]; 2) inhibition of endothelial cell calcium signaling and NOS activity[310]; 3) superoxide inhibition of protein kinase-C facilitated calcium re-uptake by the SR; and 4) superoxide inhibition of inositol 3-phosphate breakdown.[271] Finally, the role of ROS, scavengers of ROS, the regulation of each in the pulmonary vasculature under both physiologic and pathologic conditions, and the contribution to the pathogenesis of lung disease are only beginning to be understood.

PULMONARY VASCULAR DISEASE

Interactions between the endothelium and smooth muscle activity determine the functional features of the pulmonary circulation.[285] In disease, over time, these interactions result in hyperplasia, hypertrophy, smooth muscle differentiation and migration into the subendothelium, which cause altered pulmonary vascular structure, resistance, and reactivity. It is this interplay that determines both the resistance and reactivity of the pulmonary circulation. It is important to differentiate "resistance" from "reactivity." Although these concepts are frequently associated, that is, high resistance is often associated with high reactivity, this is not always the case. Reactivity is defined as a change in smooth muscle tone in response to a stimulus. It depends upon the intrinsic vascular smooth muscle response and its modulation by endothelial and nonendothelial responses. These same factors may or may not be the determinants of baseline pulmonary vascular resistance at any given time. For example, PVR decreases drastically at birth, while reactivity to many stimuli does not change. The effect of various modulators of pulmonary vascular smooth muscle tone on resistance and reactivity at any given developmental stage is quite complex. This complex interplay between structure and function has been studied in fetal, neonatal, and adult sheep.[2,98] Hypoxia in utero is associated with not only an increase in pulmonary vascular resistance but also a prolonged, blunted response to both vasoconstrictor and vasodilatory stimuli.[2]

Despite highly muscularized pulmonary arterioles, the onset of ventilation at birth leads to an abrupt decrease in baseline resistance and rapid changes in the biochemical milieu that produce a marked attenuation of hypoxic reactivity.

At two weeks of age, the baseline resistance has decreased further as muscularization involutes. Despite this fall in baseline resistance and decreased muscularization, pulmonary vasoresponsiveness to hypoxia at the small arteriolar level in the pulmonary circulation is more pronounced than at birth.[97] Thus, in the perinatal period, biochemical factors appear to blunt vasoreactivity and reduce resistance, whereas attenuated muscularization is not necessarily associated with a decreased reactivity at two weeks of age.[67,97,98] It is in this setting of rapid postnatal structural and functional changes in the pulmonary circulation that we will begin to examine diseases of the pulmonary vasculature. Pulmonary hypertension may be the result of abnormally increased muscularization, decreased vasodilatory activity, increased vasoconstrictor activity, or any combination of these.

Neonatal Pulmonary Vascular Disease

Failure or delay of the normal postnatal fall in pulmonary vascular resistance results in persistent pulmonary hypertension of the newborn, also called persistent fetal circulation. The elevated pulmonary vascular resistance causes right-to-left shunting across the patent foramen ovale and/or ductus arteriosus, resulting in hypoxemia and acidosis. Failure of the pulmonary vascular resistance to decrease at birth may be the result of pulmonary hypoplasia (underdevelopment) such as seen with congenital diaphragmatic hernia or oligohydramnios, an abnormal extension of muscle into peripheral arteries caused by an intrauterine stress (maldevelopment) or a perinatal insult (maladaptation) such as meconium aspiration and/or hypoxia, which leads to failure of the normal vasodilatory mediator systems.

Underdeveloped

Underdevelopment of the pulmonary arterial bed in utero occurs in disorders associated with lung hypoplasia, such as congenital diaphragmatic hernia, oligohydramnios, and thoracodystrophy. Alveolar capillary dysplasia is a syndrome of underdevelopment of the pulmonary capillary bed characterized by severe hypoxemia and pulmonary hypertension in the newborn that is unresponsive to therapeutic intervention.[8] This syndrome has been associated with congenital heart disease.[164] For this group of syndromes, peripheral arteries are reduced in proportion to the decrease in total alveolar number and the diminished lung volume. Both the diminished cross-sectional area of the pulmonary circulation and the resultant severe hypoxemia and hypercarbia cause increased resistance to pulmonary blood flow after birth. A pathologic study has suggested that there are morphologic, morphometric, and biochemical differences between pulmonary hypoplasias of differing etiologies.[195] This study nicely demonstrated that impairment in early gestation (before 16 weeks) results in both reduced bronchiolar branching and retarded acinar development, while processes at later stages influence only acinar development. Both intrathoracic compression by the herniated abdominal viscera and humoral growth factors are involved in the pathogenesis of pulmonary hypoplasia associated with congenital diaphragmatic hernia.[92]

Maldeveloped

Maldevelopment of the pulmonary circulation is associated with normal growth of the pulmonary vessels but excessive and precocious in utero muscularization of peripheral pulmonary arteries that increases resistance to blood flow. Accelerated in utero muscularization of pulmonary circulation is associated with fatal meconium aspiration and with congenital heart defects associated with elevated pulmonary venous pressure. Chronic alveolar hypoxia is the most frequently used experimental technique to study maldevelopment of the pulmonary vascular circulation. Chronic hypoxia or intrauterine constriction of the ductus arteriosus by cyclooxygenase inhibitors is also associated with increased muscularization of the pulmonary arteries.

The underlying mechanisms of these changes appear to be intrauterine hypoxia and stress causing sustained vasoconstriction and failure of the normal mechanisms regulating arterial muscularization. The anatomic changes include increased deposition of collagen and elastin in the adventitia and aberrant pulmonary vascular smooth muscle proliferation and maturation in the media. Again, the endothelium plays a central role in initiating and regulating these anatomic responses. Endothelial cells produce growth factors such as platelet-derived growth factor, endothelial cell derived growth factor, insulin-like growth factor 1, and fibroblast growth factor that regulate cellular proliferation.[64] These and other growth factors are released in response to decreased oxygen tension and induce pulmonary vascular smooth muscle cell proliferation. Both protein kinase-C (PKC) dependent and independent mechanisms appear to be involved in this proliferative response.[54] One potential mediator of this PKC dependent pathway is endothelin, which stimulates DNA synthesis and production of messenger RNA in vascular smooth muscle via PLC mediated production of IP_3 and diacylglycerol (DAG) that result in PKC stimulation.[273]

Besides cellular proliferation, chronic hypoxia also alters smooth muscle cell protein synthesis, receptor expression, and enzyme activities.[268] Down regulation of beta-adrenergic receptors and augmented G-protein–dependent adenylate cyclase activity have been associated with chronic hypoxia and may contribute to the structural changes observed in the pulmonary vasculature. Finally, soluble factors generated by vascular smooth muscle appear to be responsible for the increased production of collagen in the hypertensive arteries.[45]

Maladapted

Postnatal failure of the small preacinar muscular arteries to dilate represents maladaptation of the pulmonary vasculature. This may occur in infants with perinatal stress from a variety of causes such as hypoxia, hemorrhage, asphyxia, sepsis, or aspiration. Correction of the primary disturbance is the most successful method to reverse this pathologic state. The pathophysiologic basis for the failure of the pulmonary arteries to dilate remains poorly understood, but it may be related to abnormal vascular receptors or altered release and/or response to vasoactive mediators. For example, ET-1 levels have been shown to be elevated in persistent pulmonary hypertension of the newborn.[244] Conventional medical management of this syndrome consists of routine measures utilized in pulmonary hypertensive states including hyperventilation, sedation, and use of vasodilators such as nitric oxide. Others have suggested that mechanical hyperventilation may be detrimental.[310] In patients who fail to respond to conventional medical management, other therapeutic modalities such as high frequency oscillation, extracorporeal membrane oxygenation (ECMO), and inhaled NO have proven successful.[198]

Congenital Heart Disease

Many congenital cardiac lesions are associated with pulmonary vascular disease and pulmonary hypertension. These can be roughly divided into two broad categories: high flow lesions and obstructive lesions. Due to the more common nature of the high flow lesions, the majority of the discussion will be centered on high flow pulmonary hypertensive states and the nature of the vascular changes seen. New information about the cell biology of the vessel wall involved in the pathophysiologic mechanisms in these high-flow states will be briefly discussed.[61,221]

High Flow States

Determinants of Pulmonary Hypertension Congenital cardiac defects that have been associated with pulmonary hypertension include large ventricular atrial septal defect, atrioventricular septal defect and truncus arteriosus. In these lesions, there is initially left-to-right shunting. Later, with progressive elevation in pulmonary vascular resistance, a reversal of the shunt and cyanosis may occur. The pathologic basis for this clinical entity, known as Eisenmenger's syndrome, is the development of structural changes in the peripheral pulmonary arteries, which is described as "pulmonary vascular obstructive disease." Among the different congenital cardiac defects with left-to-right shunts and even among patients with the same abnormality, the incidence of this complication and its rate of progression vary considerably. Virtually all patients with uncorrected atrioventricular canal defects develop severe and irreversible pulmonary vascular disease if uncorrected; however, this complication is rarely seen with secundum atrial septal defects. The progressive nature of these diseases has led to earlier surgical repair. If surgical repair is carried out in the first year of life, the increase in pulmonary vascular resistance rarely persists. If it is delayed beyond two years, persistent elevation and progressive disease are likely. Finally, the combination of septal defects with high pulmonary blood flow and left-sided obstructive lesions such as coarctation or mitral valve disease increases the risk of severe elevations in pulmonary vascular resistance early in life.

Assessment of Pulmonary Hypertension Defining the patient with a specific congenital cardiac lesion who will develop pulmonary vascular disease is difficult. Clinical and radiologic manifestations are apparent only with advanced disease. Electrocardiography and radionuclide studies are relatively nonspecific. To date the most definitive method to assess the risk of rapidly progressive pulmonary vascular disease remains early cardiac catheterization. Criteria have been established to distinguish patients in whom, even after repair, persistent elevations in pulmonary resistance are likely. The measurement of PVR is influenced by a variety of factors, including inspired oxygen tension, sedation, lung disease, and others. Thus, in certain cases, in addition to the hemodynamic assessment, an evaluation of the structural state of the pulmonary circulation can provide useful information.

Wedge angiographic techniques have been developed to assess the structural state of the pulmonary vasculature. Quantitative pulmonary wedge angiographic studies predict a broad range of vascular abnormalities.[226] The abruptness of tapering correlates with the degree of abnormality in the peripheral arteries and is associated with persistent elevation in pulmonary vascular resistance after surgical repair.[227] When wedge angiogram and the hemodynamic assessment of the pulmonary vascular resistance appear discrepant or are difficult to interpret, analysis of lung biopsy tissue to predict potential for reversibility of the disease and risk of operation has also been utilized.[225]

Nature of Pulmonary Vascular Changes Heath and Edwards were the first to describe the progressive structural changes in the pulmonary circulation associated with high pulmonary blood flow and pressure. The Heath-Edwards changes began with qualitative descriptions of medial hypertrophy (grade I) and progression to cellular intimal proliferation (grade II). The latter is due to the migration of vascular smooth muscle cells from the media into the subendothelium, where they produce an extensive matrix of glycosaminoglycans, collagen, and elastin. Lumen occlusion from intimal hyperplasia is grade III. Grade IV represents the formation of dilation complexes and plexiform lesions resulting from medial thinning and atrophy and the development of small bypass channels around occluded vessels. Grades V and VI are terminal changes, grade V being angiomatoid formation and grade VI is fibrinoid necrosis. Grade III is thought to be partially reversible at best, in that some degree of elevated pulmonary vascular resistance will likely persist.

Realizing that features related to the growth and development of the pulmonary circulation would likely be perturbed in infants with congenital heart defects, Hislop and Reed studied postmortem lungs. They found that both the normal features of postnatal pulmonary vascular development and the abnormalities associated with chronic high flow states could be quantitatively assessed.[123] A more recent study confirmed the finding that pulmonary vascular disease, secondary to high blood flow, begins soon after birth with abnormal pulmonary vascular remodeling. If pulmonary artery pressure is allowed to remain elevated, pulmonary vascular obstructive disease develops.[109] The severity of altered growth and development of the pulmonary vasculature correlated with the hemodynamic state. Three progressively severe stages were seen.[221] Grade A is characterized by extension of muscle into distal, normally nonmuscular vessels. This change is associated with increased pulmonary blood flow and elevated pulse pressure but normal mean pulmonary artery pressure. The mechanism of extension of muscle involves differentiation of precursor to mature smooth muscle cells. Grade B is medial hypertrophy of the more proximal muscular arteries and is associated with an increased mean pulmonary artery pressure. This reflects an increase in both smooth muscle cell size and number. Grade B can be subdivided into mild and severe groups based on the degree of medial wall thickness

(mild = 1.5–2 times normal thickness, severe ≥ 2 times normal). Grade C represents reduced concentration of distal vessels and is associated with increased pulmonary vascular resistance. It represents failure of arterial multiplication to keep up with alveolar proliferation, although loss of distal vessels may also be occurring. The severity of these morphometric abnormalities is uniform throughout the lungs, although some subtle regional differences have been observed.[115] To what extent abnormal growth and structural remodeling of the pulmonary circulation are permanent and result in functional impairment was determined by correlating these features with postoperative hemodynamic behavior.[227] Patients with grade A or mild grade B changes had normal pulmonary artery pressures in the early postoperative period. The majority of patients with more severe medial hypertrophy (severe grade B or Heath-Edwards I) had elevated pulmonary artery pressures. Grade C may be found with Heath-Edwards grade I, is common with grade II, and is invariable with grade III. In general, features of grade III or greater correlate with severe elevations in pulmonary vascular resistance that is refractory to vasodilators. This severity of disease has generally been considered to be irreversible; however, the use of long-term vasodilator therapy in chronic pulmonary hypertension has been associated with arrested progression or even regression of structurally advanced pulmonary vascular disease.[14] Thus, the use of pathologic markers for clinical decision making may need reevaluation. The complexities of evaluating patients with pulmonary vascular disease secondary to congenital heart defects have recently been reviewed.[22]

Pulmonary Reactivity One of the most difficult challenges facing pediatric intensivists is to understand and control the reactive pulmonary circulation in the early postoperative period following repair of congenital heart defects. The "pulmonary hypertensive crisis" is thought to be a result of, in part, altered interactions of the vascular endothelium with platelets and leukocytes, which, following cardiopulmonary bypass and hypothermia, more easily aggregate, degranulate, and release potent vasoconstrictors such as thromboxane and leukotrienes. The effects of cardiopulmonary bypass are discussed in Chapter 20. Furthermore, the endothelium, with its basic antithrombogenic and vasodilatory properties, is injured during cardiopulmonary bypass. Evidence for endothelial injury has been suggested by alterations in the pulmonary clearance of norepinephrine, serotonin, and PGE_1 following cardiopulmonary bypass.[83,111] Cardiopulmonary bypass has also been associated with an increase in biologic activity of factor VIII and a decrease in antithrombin III values, suggesting a degree of pulmonary endothelial damage.[283] Cardiopulmonary bypass has also been associated with increases in microvascular endothelial permeability.[199] Recent information demonstrates a diminished endothelium-dependent pulmonary vasodilatory response to acetylcholine following cardiopulmonary bypass, providing further evidence for pulmonary endothelial dysfunction after bypass.[293] Studies from specimens obtained from heart-lung transplantation in four patients with Eisenmenger's syndrome demonstrated an impaired endothelium-dependent vasodilatory response to acetylcholine, indicating endothelial dysfunction.[56] In summary, the pulmonary hyperreactivity typically seen in postoperative cardiac patients appears to be due to a combination of endothelial dysfunction and platelet and neutrophil activation with mediator release, superimposed upon chronically altered endothelial and muscular structural and functional changes that promote hyperreactivity.

Mechanisms of Vascular Changes Endothelial cells are continuously subjected to hemodynamic forces associated with flow (pressure, shear stress). These profoundly influence endothelial structure and function. In fact, nearly every endothelial function is affected by flow. Fluid shear stress is associated with elongation along the axis of flow and redistribution of the cytoskeleton. Shear stress has been associated with cytoskeleton production, which appears necessary to maintain focal contact and adherence of the endothelium to the basement membrane.[290] Increased shear stress stimulates the release of platelet-derived endothelial growth factor[130] and tissue plasminogen activator resulting in increased fibrinolytic activity.[55] In an elegant series of experiments over the past decade, Rabinovich and coworkers[221] demonstrated that endothelial injury in response to high flow and/or pressure results in a loss of endothelial barrier function, thereby allowing a serum factor into the subendothelium that induces endogenous vascular elastase (EVE). This enzyme causes the release of several growth factors (e.g., basic fibroblast growth factor and transforming growth factor β) from precursor or mature smooth muscle cells that induce smooth muscle hypertrophy and proliferation along with increases in connective tissue protein (e.g., collagen and elastin) synthesis. Tenascin, a matrix glycoprotein that amplifies these responses, is also released. These mediators result in differentiation of precursor cells to mature smooth muscle in normally nonmuscular small peripheral arteries.

Scanning and transmission electron microscopy have been used to identify structural changes in pulmonary vascular endothelium associated with chronically altered flow states.[223] The hypertensive endothelium is coarse relative to the normotensive endothelium and interacts abnormally with marginating blood elements, such as platelets and leukocytes. Transmission electron microscopy reveals increased density of the microfilament bundles and rough endoplasmic reticulum. The former suggests altered cytoskeleton function that may serve to keep the endothelium well anchored to the subendothelium, while the latter indicates an increase in protein synthesis and metabolic activity, as described earlier.

Flow also significantly affects endothelial release of vasoactive substances. Flow increases the release of vasodilator substances PGI_2 and EDNO.[100,213,245] The release of these vasoactive substances appears to be flow (shear stress) and not pressure related.[204] Recent investigations suggest that chronically elevated blood flow further enhances EDNO release from endothelium.[186] The effect of flow on endothelin release is less clear. The net endothelial response to increases in flow and shear stress is vasodilatory.

Other endothelial functions are altered in the chronic high flow states. Endothelial cells from hypertensive pulmonary arteries stain densely for immunoperoxidase stain to Factor VIII.[222] However, the Factor VIII being synthesized lacks biological activity, due to a deficiency of high molecular weight components. It appears that the endothelium in patients with congenital heart defects and pulmonary hypertension may actually be less conducive to platelet adhesion and formation of platelet-fibrin microthrombi.

The endothelium's regulation of the pulmonary circulation and the vascular response to injury suggests that hemodynamic disturbances and pulmonary vascular changes associated with high pulmonary blood flow are an expression of endothelial cell dysfunction. Anatomic discontinuity of the endothelial layer, as well as metabolic dysfunction due to injury, allows the nonselective passage of plasma or cellular constituents into the arterial wall, exposing vascular smooth muscle to higher concentrations of vasoactive substances. Disturbed signal transduction by damaged endothelial cells alters smooth muscle cell responsiveness and vascular reactivity. Although actively antithrombogenic and immunologically neutral, the endothelium has the capacity to become procoagulant and involved in immune-related reactions. The endothelium is not merely a target, but actively participates in events associated with inflammation and vascular damage. Alteration in endothelial interactions with circulating cellular elements, such as platelets and leukocytes, results in the release of mediators that affect vascular tone, permeability, and proliferation.

In summary, the high flow congenital heart defects alter endothelial structure and function, thereby affecting their interaction with marginating blood elements. These abnormalities lead to degradation of the basement membrane and extracellular matrix, encouraging the differentiation of precursor cells to mature smooth muscle cells. Although there is an interrelationship between endothelial and smooth muscle changes, smooth muscle also responds directly to abnormal pressure, flow, and oxygen tension.[220] In the muscular arteries, increased elastase activity leads to breakdown of elastin and potentially other extracellular matrix proteins, which facilitates transfer of growth factors and mitogens leading to smooth muscle hyperplasia and collagen deposition. These alterations in endothelial function and vessel wall thickness increase intrinsic vascular resistance and vasoreactivity and ultimately lead to pulmonary hypertension.

Obstructive Vascular Disease

All forms of left heart obstruction can present with cyanosis secondary to right-to-left ductal shunting. Obstruction at any site from the pulmonary venous capillaries to the ascending aorta can cause cyanosis. Pulmonary venous stenosis, total anomalous pulmonary venous connection with obstruction, cor triatriatum, mitral stenosis or atresia, left ventricular hypoplasia, critical aortic stenosis or atresia, interrupted aortic arch, and coarctation of the aorta must be considered. Meticulous two-dimensional echocardiographic examination allows the diagnosis to be made in the majority of situations.

Pulmonary Disease

Diseases of the pulmonary parenchyma also lead to alterations in the pulmonary vasculature. Both acute and chronic alterations in lung function result in pulmonary vascular disease. Again, the pulmonary endothelium plays a central role. Endothelial injury in acute respiratory distress syndrome has been associated with marked alterations in the physiology and morphology of the pulmonary vasculature.[310] Endothelium-dependent pulmonary artery relaxations in vitro are impaired in arteries of patients with end-stage obstructive lung disease and appear to be associated with the development of pulmonary hypertension in this disorder.[57] Congenital abnormalities of the lung are also associated with pulmonary vascular disease and hypertension. By far the most common pediatric pulmonary anomaly associated with pulmonary vascular disease remains bronchopulmonary dysplasia.

Chronic Lung Disease

Chronic lung disease of infancy, better known as bronchopulmonary dysplasia (BPD), is associated with pulmonary vascular disease and pulmonary hypertension. In fact, pulmonary hypertension contributes significantly to the morbidity and mortality of BPD. Medial smooth muscle hyperplasia with extension of the muscle into more peripheral arteries and occasional obliteration of vessels by fibrosis is the common finding in patients with severe bronchopulmonary dysplasia.[5] The medial hypertrophy ultimately causes increased pulmonary vascular resistance and pulmonary hypertension. This diffuse and severe lung injury frequently leads to intrapulmonary shunting with associated worsening of hypoxemia, pulmonary hypertension, and ultimately myocardial failure. Therefore, treatment for this disorder is directed at the underlying lung disease and resolution of the hypoxemia. Prevention of hypoxemia, via the administration of supplemental oxygen, has been associated with improvements in hemodynamic status and long-term outcomes.[5] Unfortunately, not all children respond to supplemental oxygen, and a trial of pharmacological vasodilators may be indicated.[30]

Chronic Hypoxemia

Chronic hypoxemia, regardless of etiology, is associated with increased pulmonary vascular resistance and ultimately pulmonary hypertension. The most common clinical example of this is seen in patients with chronic upper airway obstruction and obstructive sleep apnea. This has been recognized particularly in patients with Down syndrome.[172] Relief of the airway obstruction may be associated with improvement in cardiovascular function over time.[263] Recurrent global hypoxemia leads to increased pulmonary vascular resistance and pressure that may result in right heart failure and cor pulmonale. Furthermore, the chronic fatigue state, in association with obesity, impairs daytime lung function and plays a major role in the development of pulmonary hypertension in obstructive sleep apnea patients. Therefore, chronic hypoxemia, from whatever etiology (lung disease, airway disease), can be ultimately associated with increased pulmonary vascular resistance and pulmonary hypertension.

THERAPY OF PULMONARY HYPERTENSION

The diverse etiologies of pulmonary hypertension and the myriad of mediator systems involved suggest that no single treatment will be uniformly effective for this condition. Unfortunately, few controlled comparisons of treatment regimens have been carried out. Once pulmonary hypertension has been diagnosed, therapeutic efforts should be simultaneously directed towards the specific treatment of the inciting cause suspected as well as towards the reduction of pulmonary vascular resistance.

Conventional Management

Conventional medical management of pulmonary hypertension can be divided into three broad categories: general supportive care and sedation, hyperventilation, and pharmacologic vasodilators.

General Supportive Care

General supportive care comprises measures that are routinely provided to any patient in a critical care unit. These include oxygen administration with positive pressure mechanical ventilation when needed to maintain normocarbia, correct acid/base abnormalities, and maintain normal temperature and blood pressure. In this group of patients, the avoidance and/or suppression of stressful stimuli by the administration of sedatives, analgesics, and/or anesthetics with neuromuscular paralysis is particularly important.[122] In fact, studies suggest that blunting of the intraoperative stress response by high-dose narcotic anesthesia reduces postoperative complications and mortality.[10] The maintenance of a normal blood pressure and cardiac output, via the administration of fluids and inotropic agents when indicated, also falls into the routine supportive care category.

Hyperventilation

Hyperventilation to produce respiratory alkalosis with mechanical positive pressure ventilation is a classic treatment for pulmonary hypertension. Respiratory alkalosis causes a relatively selective relaxation of the constricted pulmonary circulation in animals and humans.[174,193] The pulmonary circulation appears to sense hydrogen ion concentration and not arterial or alveolar carbon dioxide tension.[189] Thus, a therapeutic effect might best be achieved by a combination of metabolic and respiratory maneuvers designed to decrease hydrogen ion concentration.

The mechanism of the alkalosis-induced decrease in pulmonary vascular resistance is multifactorial. Reduced intracellular hydrogen ion concentration inhibits pulmonary vascular smooth muscle calcium permeability.[162] Vigorous cycling of the lungs to induce respiratory alkalosis promotes prostacyclin release.[110,296] Efforts to use high ventilator pressures and rapid rates in patients with nonhomogeneous lung disease are usually frustrated by massive pulmonary barotrauma. Furthermore, the high intrathoracic pressures associated with mechanical hyperventilation may lead to compromised cardiovascular function and exacerbate the hypoxemia, thereby limiting this treatment regimen. Thus, increasing hydrogen ion concentration with administration of sodium bicarbonate to create a metabolic alkalosis may be effective for treatment of pulmonary hypertension postoperatively.[36]

Vasodilator Therapy

Attempts to use vasodilator drugs or block endogenous vasoconstrictor release have resulted in the understanding that no single drug will likely be found to treat all the problems in every pulmonary hypertensive patient. Intravenous vasodilator therapy is limited by the fact that to date no selective pulmonary vasodilators are widely available for clinical intravenous use. Many drugs have been tried, but none have been consistently found safe and effective.

Alpha-Adrenergic Antagonists Alpha-adrenergic blocking agents inhibit alpha-adrenergic–mediated response known to cause vasoconstriction. Many drugs in this class have received special attention in the treatment of pulmonary hypertension. Tolazoline is the most widely used, particularly in neonatal patients. Results vary from dramatic, acute reductions in pulmonary vascular resistance and pressure to no significant response or, occasionally, detrimental decreases in systemic blood pressure. Tolazoline infusions have been reported to be beneficial in the treatment of pulmonary hypertension in infants and children following cardiac surgery.[252] The high incidence of untoward side effects, in particular systemic hypotension, limits the utility of this class of agents.

Nitrovasodilators Organic nitrates and related compounds, in particular sodium nitroprusside, are direct vascular smooth muscle relaxants, via an increase in intracellular cGMP. Nitroprusside vasodilates both arterial and venous vascular smooth muscle equally. Nitroglycerin appears to preferentially act as a venous vasodilator. Most studies in the pulmonary circulation have demonstrated a reduction in pulmonary vascular resistance and pressure with subsequent increases in pulmonary blood flow and cardiac output.[138] As with all the vasodilators, the principal adverse effect is systemic hypotension. Sodium nitroprusside administration in large doses over extended periods also is associated with cyanide toxicity. The loss of endogenous production following endothelial injury may lead to enhanced vascular reactivity (supersensitivity) to nitroprusside.[187,188]

Beta-Adrenergic Agonists Recognition that beta-adrenergic receptor activation is linked to increased intracellular cAMP and subsequent vascular smooth muscle relaxation prompted the use of these agents for the treatment of pulmonary hypertension. Isoproterenol, or any beta-adrenergic agonist, relaxes most varieties of smooth muscle, including bronchial and vascular smooth muscle. The majority of studies suggest that isoproterenol is an active pulmonary vasodilator.[47] Utility of this agent is limited by its nonselective beta-receptor specificity, stimulating both beta$_1$ and beta$_2$ receptors. The principal side effects are related to beta$_1$ stimulation and positive inotropic and chronotropic responses. Dobutamine also provides some mild benefit. Low diastolic pressures, which may impair myocardial perfusion while increasing myocardial and systemic oxygen demand, are a serious complication of these drugs.

Prostaglandins Two endogenous prostaglandins (PGE$_1$ and PGI$_2$) have similar structures and properties, the most significant of which is their potent vasodilatory effects. The first to be identified, PGE$_1$, has been utilized widely to maintain patency of the ductus arteriosus in ductal dependent cardiac lesions. This agent has been extensively studied as a pulmonary vasodilator in patients with pulmonary hypertension.[118] Prostacyclin (PGI$_2$) is more potent than PGE$_1$ and appears to be equally efficacious as a pulmonary vasodilator.[153,252] Prostacyclin analogues are useful for treating established

primary pulmonary hypertension. Furthermore, as with all the previous vasodilators discussed, this class of compounds lack pulmonary specificity and are limited by their systemic side effects when delivered intravenously. More recent studies have demonstrated a selective pulmonary vasodilation with aerosolized delivery.[113,184,203,297]

Calcium Channel Blockers The overwhelming physiologic and biochemical evidence of the substantial role of calcium in the regulation of smooth muscle contractions suggests that this class of compounds may be beneficial. Numerous studies have reported the pulmonary vasodilating properties of the calcium channel blocking drugs. Differences in the pharmacologic characteristics result in variability in hemodynamic, electrophysiologic, and vasodilation effects of these agents. These drugs may be beneficial in a subgroup of patients with long-standing primary or secondary pulmonary hypertension in which reductions in pulmonary artery pressure and resistance improved long-term survival.[239] Nifedipine has been the most widely studied in the treatment of pulmonary hypertension. Little has been published about calcium channel blockers in acute postoperative pulmonary hypertensive patients. Unfortunately, serious adverse side effects, such as sinus arrest, profound systemic hypotension, decreased myocardial contractility, and alterations in ventilation-perfusion relationships have been reported.

Nonconventional Management

The complex pathophysiology and potentially life-threatening nature of pulmonary hypertension continues to frustrate the clinician. In children who fail to respond to conventional medical management, clinicians will at times opt for experimental therapies in an attempt to improve patient outcomes. It must be emphasized that these therapies are experimental and should not become components of routine practice until further rigorous randomized clinical trials are performed. With these limitations in mind, we will review several options that may be available to clinicians in this select group of critically ill patients now or in the near future.

Mechanical Ventilation

Occasionally, nonconventional modes of mechanical ventilation may be utilized in an attempt to maintain or improve pulmonary gas exchange while maintaining or decreasing adverse effects on cardiovascular function. An example of this is high frequency ventilation (HFV) following cardiac surgery, used to maintain oxygenation and gas exchange at, in theory, lower peak and mean airway pressures, thus providing less limitation in cardiac preload. Not surprisingly, in situations in which HFV meets these goals, cardiovascular function is better.[181] Unfortunately, most studies demonstrating improvement in cardiac output with HFV have failed to use comparable levels of mean airway pressure during conventional ventilation and HFV. Studies in which mean airway pressures and/or intrathoracic pressures were matched between trials of HFV and conventional ventilation failed to demonstrate any salutary effect of HFV on cardiac output.

Another possible example is the use of airway pressure release ventilation (APRV). In APRV, airway pressures are intermittently decreased or "released" from a preset continuous positive airway pressure (CPAP) level to a lower pressure. Therefore, lung volumes transiently decrease allowing gas to exit the lungs passively, augmenting alveolar ventilation. Experimental models suggest better maintenance of cardiovascular function with APRV when compared to conventional ventilation.[231] This finding was subsequently confirmed in a case report in which a patient with severe ARDS showed marked improvement in cardiac output when switched from conventional mechanical ventilation to APRV.[63] Unfortunately, pediatric experience is limited to experimental models only.[176]

Experimental Vasodilators

The search continues for a selective intravenous pulmonary vasodilating agent. Promising candidates include magnesium sulfate, adenosine, adenosine triphosphate (ATP), and endothelin receptor antagonists. Magnesium sulfate activates adenylate cyclase as well as suppresses the release of catecholamines. This cation also directly reduces the responsiveness of smooth muscle to sympathomimetic amines and non-sympathomimetic vasopressors. These properties are responsible for the vascular dilation seen with its administration. Magnesium sulfate has been shown to have beneficial effects on oxygenation and gas exchange in newborns with severe persistent pulmonary hypertension of the newborn (PPHN).[6] Its use in children with pulmonary hypertension has not been reported. Adenosine and ATP have also been used in experimental models of pulmonary hypertension. Because of their rapid clearance in the pulmonary circulation, intravenous infusions of these agents have been reported to be relatively selective pulmonary vasodilators.[68,160] More recently, an open label, phase I study evaluating the safety and efficacy of an endothelial cell endothelin receptor (ET_A) antagonist in infants with postoperative pulmonary hypertension was published.[215] This agent decreased both systemic and pulmonary pressures (pulmonary > systemic) with an accompanying increase in right ventricular stroke index and cardiac output. The routine use of any of these agents awaits further clinical trials.

Recently, Sildenafil, a phosphodiesterase-5 inhibitor widely used for erectile dysfunction, has been reported to be efficacious in the treatment of pulmonary hypertension when given orally in adults. We have used this drug (0.5–1.0 mg/kg, every six hours) in our cardiac ICU to lower pulmonary vascular resistance and to facilitate weaning infants from iNO. Systemic effects seem minimal. The place of this orally active pulmonary vasodilator in children with heart disease is not yet clear. An aerosol prostacyclin preparation, Iloprost, has recently been licensed for the inhalational treatment of pulmonary hypertension. Its use in children is limited and it can be expected to be absorbed and to have some, although minimal, systemic effects. These drugs have been used in combination in adults with pulmonary hypertension and provide the potential for outpatient therapy without vascular access for pulmonary hypertension.

Inhaled Nitric Oxide

Of all the nonconventional modalities potentially available in the near future, inhaled nitric oxide (iNO) appears to have the most promise for routine therapy of acute life-threatening pulmonary hypertension. Because of its rapid inactivation by hemoglobin, iNO appears to be the first truly selective pulmonary vasodilator available for clinical use. iNO is delivered only to alveoli that are ventilated. It therefore improves rather than worsens ventilation-perfusion matching. Inhaled nitric oxide relaxes vascular smooth muscle in a manner identical to the endogenously released EDNO, i.e., activation of guanylate cyclase with production of cGMP. Multiple non-controlled studies have demonstrated beneficial effects in infants with PPHN. Based on these results, multicenter randomized trials in term and near-term newborns with hypoxemic respiratory failure have been completed.[198,241,294] Most studies demonstrate improved oxygenation and deceased pulmonary artery pressure without systemic effects; however, the clinical response may be heterogeneous.[282] To date, no study evaluating the use of iNO has demonstrated an improved survival rate in neonates. One study was able to demonstrate a positive correlation between early response to NO and patient outcome, perhaps related to the reversible nature of the condition.[95] Several studies have shown a significant decrease in the use of extracorporeal life support in the NO treated patients.[42,128,198] Based primarily on this finding, the US Food and Drug Administration has approved the use of inhaled nitric oxide for neonates and infants with hypoxemic respiratory failure and pulmonary hypertension.

Inhaled nitric oxide has also been studied in children and adults with severe hypoxemic respiratory failure. As in neonates, the response to NO in children is variable. Several studies demonstrated short-term improvements in oxygenation,[48,58,233] although one group was not able to document this improvement at 24 hours.[48] A phase II study in adults has also documented improved oxygenation; however, primary outcome variables (mortality, ventilator-free days) were improved only in patients receiving 5 ppm NO.[52] Because of this lack of benefit in the outcome variables in the studies to date, the use of NO has not been approved in children or adults with hypoxemic respiratory failure.

iNO has been used extensively in children with pulmonary hypertension following repair of congenital cardiac defects.[46,93,94,146,185,194,242] In a variety of cardiac defects, the majority of studies show a reduction in pulmonary arterial pressure. The reduction in pulmonary artery pressure is frequently proportional to the degree of elevation in pulmonary artery pressure. Others have used a trial of NO as a diagnostic test to differentiate pulmonary vasospasm from pulmonary vascular obstruction in postoperative patients.[18] The two small, randomized controlled trials published thus far have yielded conflicting results. One study demonstrated that 80 ppm NO selectively reduced mean pulmonary artery pressure in patients with postoperative mean pulmonary arterial pressures greater than 50% of mean systemic arterial pressures.[247] In contrast, Day and colleagues[49] failed to show any benefit with 20 ppm NO in postoperative patients. Further studies demonstrating clinical benefits will be needed before NO use will be approved for this patient population.

A recently recognized problem has been the rebound of pulmonary hypertension upon weaning and/or withdrawal of inhaled NO.[12] This obviously can have serious adverse hemodynamic consequences postoperatively.[38] The etiology of this rebound is unknown; however, some have speculated that exogenous NO may suppress endogenous production of EDNO.[93,94] Other possible explanations include modulation of endogenous pulmonary vasoconstrictors or other vasodilators as well as altered membrane receptor function on vascular smooth muscle cells. Recently, the rebound pulmonary hypertension has been attenuated with dipyridamole, a cyclic guanosine monophosphate-specific phosphodiesterase inhibitor, which blocks the hydrolysis of cGMP in vascular smooth muscle.[140–142] Thus, increased breakdown of NO-stimulated cGMP via increased phosphodiesterase activity may contribute to this clinical phenomenon.

Extracorporeal Support

Mechanical circulation support devices, including the intraaortic balloon pump, uni- and biventricular support devices, and extracorporeal circulation, have all taken a prominent role in postoperative cardiac surgery care (see Chapter 21). Due to size limitations, a small number of mechanical circulatory support devices are available for pediatric patients with cardiovascular failure. With the dissemination and widespread use of extracorporeal membrane oxygenation (ECMO) for neonates with reversible cardiorespiratory disease, this modality has recently received greater utilization in children following repair of congenital heart disease.[206] Due to the transient nature of the injury from cardiopulmonary bypass and surgical repair, it appears plausible that this modality may be of benefit in a select group of patients. Two retrospective series have been reported in which the use of ECMO resulted in a 40% to 60% survival in patients previously thought to have a 100% mortality rate.[51,156] Complications include bleeding, neurologic injury, and multiple organ system failure. Long-term follow-up of children requiring postoperative mechanical circulatory assist has been favorable, although neurologic impairment was more common in the smaller critically ill patients.[135] Due to the high resource demand and invasive nature of this procedure, ECMO must be used selectively. Unfortunately, identifying the appropriate population of children is quite difficult. Two recent studies have suggested serum lactate levels alone or in combination with central venous oxygen saturation may be useful in early identification of patients with a high risk of mortality.[37,281] No controlled prospective clinical studies have been attempted to demonstrate the clinical utility of this invasive, labor-intensive technology.

CONCLUSIONS

The pulmonary circulation provides both an enigma and a great challenge for the physician who cares for children with congenital heart disease. The pathologic changes within the pulmonary circulation often become the critical limitation of the cardiovascular system. The pulmonary circulation's far-reaching effects on cardiovascular performance range from hypoxia, right ventricular failure, and increased right-to-left intracardiac shunting to globally decreased cardiac output. The episodic nature of acute pulmonary hypertension, especially perioperatively, in the setting of cardiovascular compromise can prove rapidly fatal. For these reasons, pediatricians have been perennially interested in controlling, modifying, and decreasing pulmonary vascular resistance and preventing its acute elevation. In the past, the armamentarium with which this could be done was limited and nonspecific.

Our understanding of this critical situation has been greatly enhanced over the past few years. New insights into the endothelial regulation of the pulmonary circulation have not only explained changes that occur with development, cardiovascular disease, and chronic hypoxia, but also suggest exciting new therapeutic approaches that are specifically directed at the pulmonary circulation. Most recently, for failure of the pulmonary circulation, which had required total ECMO to provide some hope of recovery, we now have the promising advent of a specific therapy in the form of iNO. Nitric oxide not only decreases pulmonary vascular tone, but also, by virtue of being delivered to ventilated alveoli, lowers pulmonary vascular tone in the precise location required to enhance perfusion where it is most beneficial. Although there is still a great deal to be learned about nitric oxide toxicity, methods of delivery, and the clinical settings in which it will be beneficial, it represents the culmination of years of painstaking research, delineating the role of the endothelium in pulmonary vascular regulation.

References

1. Abman SH, Accurso FJ: Sustained fetal pulmonary vasodilation with prolonged atrial natriuretic factor and GMP infusions. *Am J Physiol* 260:H183–H192, 1991.
2. Abman SH, Accurso FJ, Wilkening RB, Meschia G: Persistent fetal pulmonary hypoperfusion after acute hypoxia. *Am J Physiol* 253:H941–H948, 1987.
3. Abman SH, Chatfield BA, Rodman DM, et al: Maturational changes in endothelium-derived relaxing factor activity of ovine pulmonary arteries in vitro. *Am J Physiol* 260:L280–L285, 1991.
4. Abman SH, Stenmark KR: Changes in lung eicosanoid content during normal and abnormal transition in perinatal lambs. *Am J Physiol* 262:L214–L222, 1992.
5. Abman SH, Wolfe RR, Accurso FJ, et al: Pulmonary vascular response to oxygen in infants with severe bronchopulmonary dysplasia. *Pediatrics* 75:80–84, 1985.
6. Abu-Osba YK, Galal O, Manasra K, Rejjal A: Treatment of severe persistent pulmonary hypertension of the newborn with magnesium sulphate. *Arch Dis Child* 67:31–35, 1992.
7. Ahn DS, Hume JR: pH regulation of voltage-dependent K+ channels in canine pulmonary arterial smooth muscle cells. *Pflugers Arch* 433:758–765, 1997.
8. Al-Hathlol K, Phillips S, Seshia MK, et al: Alveolar capillary dysplasia. Report of a case of prolonged life without extracorporeal membrane oxygenation (ECMO) and review of the literature. *Early Human Dev* 57:85–94, 2000.
9. Allen KM, Haworth SG: Impaired adaptation of pulmonary circulation to extrauterine life in newborn pigs exposed to hypoxia: an ultrastructural study. *J Pathol* 150:205–212, 1986.
10. Anand KJ, Hickey PR: Halothane-morphine compared with high-dose sufentanil for anesthesia and postoperative analgesia in neonatal cardiac surgery [see comments]. *N Engl J Med* 326:1–9, 1992.
11. Arai H, Hori S, Aramori I, et al: Cloning and expression of a cDNA encoding an endothelin receptor. *Nature* 348:730–732, 1990.
12. Atz AM, Adatia I, Wessel DL: Rebound pulmonary hypertension after inhalation of nitric oxide. *Ann Thorac Surg* 62:1759–1764, 1996.
13. Babaei S, Teichert-Kuliszewska K, Monge J-C, et al: Role of nitric oxide in the angiogenic response in vitro to basic fibroblast growth factor. *Circ Res* 82:1007–1015, 1998.
14. Barst RJ: Recent advances in the treatment of pediatric pulmonary artery hypertension. *Pediatr Clinics North Am* 46:331–345, 1999.
15. Beck KC, Rehder K: Differences in regional vascular conductance in isolated dog lungs. *J Appl Physiol* 61:530–538, 1986.
16. Beckman JS, Beckman TW, Chen J, et al: Apparent hydroxyl radical production by peroxynitrite: implications for endothelial injury from nitric oxide and superoxide. *Proc Natl Acad Sci USA* 87:1620–1624, 1990.
17. Beech DJ, Bolton TB: A voltage-dependent outward current with fast kinetics in single smooth muscle cells isolated from rabbit portal vein. *J Physiol Lond* 412:397–414, 1989.

18. Beghetti M, Morris K, Cox P, et al: Inhaled nitric oxide differentiates pulmonary vasospasm from vascular obstruction after surgery for congenital heart disease. *Intens Care Med* 25:1126–1130, 1999.

19. Belik J, Halayko A, Rao K, Stephens N: Pulmonary vascular smooth muscle: biochemical and mechanical developmental changes. *J Appl Physiol* 71:1129–1135, 1991.

20. Benumof JL: Mechanism of decreased blood flow to atelectatic lung. *J Appl Physiol* 46:1047–1048, 1979.

21. Berger MG, Vandier C, Bonnet P, et al: Intracellular acidosis differentially regulates K_v channels in coronary and pulmonary vascular muscle. *Am J Physiol* 275 (Heart Circ Physiol) 44:H1351–H1359, 1998.

22. Berger RMF: Possibilities and impossibilities in the evaluation of pulmonary vascular disease in congenital heart defects. *Eur Heart J* 21:17–27, 1999.

23. Black SM, Johengen MJ, Ma ZD, et al: Ventilation and oxygenation induce endothelial nitric oxide synthase gene expression in the lungs of fetal lambs. *J Clin Invest* 100:1448–1458, 1997.

24. Bloch KD, Filippov G, Sanchez LS, et al: Pulmonary soluble guanylate cyclase, a nitric oxide receptor, is increased during the perinatal period. *Am J Physiol* 272:L400–L406, 1997.

25. Boels PJ, Deutsch J, Gao B, Haworth SG: Maturation of the response to bradykinin in resistance and conduit pulmonary arteries. *Cardiovasc Res* 44:416–428, 1999.

26. Boldt T, Luukkainen P, Fyhrquist F, et al: Birth stress increases adrenomedullin in the newborn. *Acta Paediatr* 87:93–94, 1998.

27. Braner DA, Fineman JR, Chang R, Soifer SJ: M&B 22948, a cGMP phosphodiesterase inhibitor, is a pulmonary vasodilator in lambs. *Am J Physiol* 264:H252–H258, 1993.

28. Brannon TS, MacRitchie AN, Jaramillo MA, et al: Ontogeny of cyclooxygenase-1 and cyclooxygenase-2 gene expression in ovine lung. *Am J Physiol* 274:L66–L71, 1998.

29. Bredt DS, Snyder SH: Isolation of nitric oxide synthetase, a calmodulin-requiring enzyme. *Proc Natl Acad Sci USA* 87:682–685, 1990.

30. Brownlee JR, Beekman RH, Rosenthal A: Acute hemodynamic effects of nifedipine in infants with bronchopulmonary dysplasia and pulmonary hypertension. *Pediatr Res* 24:186–190, 1988.

31. Busse R, Mulsch A: Calcium-dependent nitric oxide synthesis in endothelial cytosol is mediated by calmodulin. *FEBS Lett* 265:133–136, 1990.

32. Campbell WB, Gebremedhin D, Pratt RF, et al: Identification of epoxyeicosatrienoic acids as endothelium-derived hyperpolarizing factors. *Circ Res* 78:415–423, 1996.

33. Caplan MS, Hsueh W, Sun XM, et al: Circulating plasma platelet activating factor in persistent pulmonary hypertension of the newborn. *Am Rev Resp Dis* 142:1258–1262, 1990.

34. Caruthers SD, Harris TR: Effects of pulmonary blood flow on the fractal heterogeneity in sheep lungs. *J Appl Physiol* 77:1474–1479, 1994.

35. Cassin S, Tod M, Philips J, et al: Effects of prostaglandin D2 on perinatal circulation. *Am J Physiol* 240:H755–H760, 1981.

36. Chang AC, Zucher HA, Hickey PR, Wessel DL: Pulmonary vascular resistance in infants after cardiac surgery: role of carbon dioxide and hydrogen ion. *Crit Care Med* 23:568–574, 1995.

37. Charpie JR, Dekeon MK, Goldberg CS, et al: Serial blood lactate measurements predict early outcome after neonatal repair or palliation for complex congenital heart disease. *J Thorac Cardiovasc Surg* 120:73–80, 2000.

38. Christenson J, Lavoie A, O'Connor M, et al: The incidence and pathogenesis of cardiopulmonary deterioration after abrupt withdrawal of inhaled nitric oxide. *Am J Respir Crit Care Med* 161:1443–1449, 2000.

39. Clapp LH, Gurney AM: Outward currents in rabbit pulmonary artery cells dissociated with a new technique. *Exp Physiol* 76:677–693, 1991.

40. Clark MA, Littlejohn D, Conway TM, et al: Leukotriene D4 treatment of bovine aortic endothelial cells and murine smooth muscle cells in culture results in an increase in phospholipase A2 activity. *J Biol Chem* 261:10713–10718, 1986.

41. Clark RH, Kueser TJ, Walker MW, et al: Low-dose nitric oxide therapy for persistent pulmonary hypertension of the newborn. Clinical Inhaled Nitric Oxide Research Group. *N Engl J Med* 342:469–474, 2000.

42. Clarke WR, Gause G, Marshall BE, Cassin S: The role of lung perfusate PO2 in the control of the pulmonary vascular resistance of exteriorized fetal lambs. *Respir Physiol* 79:19–31, 1990.

43. Clozel M, Clyman RI, Soifer SJ, Heymann MA: Thromboxane is not responsible for the high pulmonary vascular resistance in fetal lambs. *Pediatr Res* 19:1254–1257, 1985.

44. Coceani F, Armstrong C, Kelsey L: Endothelin is a potent constrictor of the lamb ductus arteriosus. *Can J Physiol Pharmacol* 67:902–904, 1989.

45. Crouch EC, Parks WC, Rosenbaum JL, et al: Regulation of collagen production by medial smooth muscle cells in hypoxic pulmonary hypertension. *Am Rev Respir Dis* 140:1045–1051, 1989.

46. Curran RD, Mavroudis C, Backer C, et al: Inhaled nitric oxide for children with congenital heart disease and pulmonary hypertension. *Ann Thorac Surg* 60:1765–1771, 1995.

47. Daoud FS, Reeves JT, Kelly DB: Isoproterenol as a potential pulmonary vasodilator in primary pulmonary hypertension. *Am J Cardiol* 42:817–822, 1978.

48. Day RW, Allen EM, Witte MK: A randomized, controlled study of the 1-hour and 24-hour effects of inhaled nitric oxide therapy in children with acute hypoxemic respiratory failure. *Chest* 112:1324–1331, 1997.

49. Day RW, Hawkins JA, McGough EC, et al: Randomized controlled study of inhaled nitric oxide after operation for congenital heart disease. *Ann Thorac Surg* 69:1907–1912, 2000.

50. De Mey JG, Vanhoutte PM: Anoxia and endothelium-dependent reactivity of the canine femoral artery. *J Physiol (Lond)* 335:65–74, 1983.

51. Delius RE, Bove EL, Meliones JN, et al: Use of extracorporeal life support in patients with congenital heart disease [comment] [see comments]. *Crit Care Med* 20:1216–1222, 1992.

52. Dellinger RP: Effects of inhaled nitric oxide in patients with acute respiratory distress syndrome: results of a randomized phase II trial. Inhaled Nitric Oxide in ARDS Study Group. *Crit Care Med* 26:15–23, 1998.

53. Demiryurek AT, Wadsworth RM: Superoxide in the pulmonary circulation. *Pharm Ther* 84:355–365, 1999.

54. Dempsey EC, McMurtry IF, O'Brien RF: Protein kinase C activation allows pulmonary artery smooth muscle cells to proliferate to hypoxia. *Am J Physiol* 260:L136–L145, 1991.

55. Diamond SL, Sharefkin JB, Dieffenbach C, et al: Tissue plasminogen activator messenger RNA levels increase in cultured human endothelial cells exposed to laminar shear stress. *J Cell Physiol* 143,144:364–371, 1990.

56. Dinh-Xuan AT, Higenbottam TW, Clelland CA, et al: Impairment of endothelium-dependent pulmonary-artery relaxation in chronic obstructive lung disease. *N Engl J Med* 324:1539–1547, 1991.

57. Dinh-Xuan AT, Higenbottam TW, Clelland CA, et al: Impairment of pulmonary endothelium-dependent relaxation in patients with Eisenmenger's syndrome. *Br J Pharmacol* 99:9–10, 1990.

58. Dobyns EL, Cornfield DN, Anas NG, et al: Multicenter randomized controlled trial of the effects of inhaled nitric oxide therapy on gas exchange in children with acute hypoxemic respiratory failure. *J Pediatr* 134:406–412, 1999.

59. Dukarm RC, Steinhorn RH, Morin FC III: The normal pulmonary vascular transition at birth. *Clin Perinatol* 23:711–726, 1996.

60. Dupuis J, Langleben D, Stewart DJ: Pulmonary hypertension. In Rubanyi GM (ed): *Patholophysiology and Clinical Applications of Nitric Oxide*, Part B. Amsterdam: Harwood Academic, 1999, pp. 267–282.

61. Durmowicz AG, Stenmark KR: Mechanisms of structural remodeling in chronic pulmonary hypertension. *Pediatr Rev* 20:e91–e102, 1999.

62. Dzhura I, Wu Y, Colbran RJ, et al: Calmodulin kinase determines calcium-dependent facilitation of L–type calcium channels. *Nat Cell Biol* 2:173–177, 2000.

63. Falkenhain SK, Reilley TE, Gregory JS: Improvement in cardiac output during airway pressure release ventilation. *Crit Care Med* 20:1358–1360, 1992.

64. Fanburg BL: Relationship of the pulmonary vascular endothelium to altered pulmonary vascular resistance. State of the art. *Chest* 93:101S–105S, 1988.

65. Fedyna JS, Snyder DW, Aharony D, et al: Pharmacologic characterization of the contractile activity of peptide leukotrienes in guinea-pig pulmonary artery. *Prostaglandins* 39:541–558, 1990.

66. Ferrario L, Amin HM, Sugimori K, et al: Site of action of endogenous nitric oxide on pulmonary vasculature in rats. *Pflugers Arch* 432:523–527, 1996.

67. Fike CD, Hansen TN: Hypoxic vasoconstriction increases with postnatal age in lungs from newborn rabbits. *Circ Res* 60:298–310, 1987.

68. Fineman JR, Crowley MR, Soifer SJ: Selective pulmonary vasodilation with ATP-MgCl$_2$ during pulmonary hypertension in lambs. *J Appl Physiol* 69:1836–1842, 1990.

69. Fineman JR, Heymann MA, Soifer SJ: N-Omega-nitro-L-arginine attenuates endothelium–dependent pulmonary vasodilation in lamb. *Am J Physiol* 260:H1299–H1306, 1991.

70. Fineman JR, Soifer SJ, Heymann MA: Regulation of pulmonary vascular tone in the perinatal period. *Annu Rev Physiol* 57:115–134, 1995.

71. Fineman JR, Soifer SJ, Heymann MA: The role of pulmonary vascular endothelium in perinatal pulmonary circulatory regulation. *Semin Perinatal* 15:58–62, 1991.

72. Fineman JR, Wong J, Morin FC III, et al: Chronic nitric oxide inhibition in utero produces persistent pulmonary hypertension in newborn lambs. *J Clin Invest* 93:2675–2683, 1994.

73. Fisher AJ, Smith CA, Thoden J, et al: Structural studies of myosin: nucleotide complexes: a revised model for the molecular basis of muscle contraction. *Biophys J* 68:19s–28s, 1995.

74. Fisher SA, Ikebe M: Developmental and tissue distribution of expression of nonmuscle and smooth muscle isoforms of myosin light chain kinase. *Biochem Biophys Res Commun* 217:696–703, 1995.

75. Fleming I: Myoendothelial gap junctions: the gap is there, but does EDHF go through it? *Circ Res* 86:249–250, 2000.

76. Forstermann U, Pollock JS, Schmidt HH, et al: Calmodulin-dependent endothelium-derived relaxing factor/nitric oxide synthase activity is present in the particulate and cytosolic fractions of bovine aortic endothelial cells. *Proc Natl Acad Sci USA* 88:1788–1792, 1991.

77. Frantz E, Soifer SJ, Clyman RI, Heymann MA: Bradykinin produces pulmonary vasodilation in fetal lambs: role of prostaglandin production. *J Appl Physiol* 67:1512–1517, 1989.

78. Furchgott RF, Zawadzki JV: The obligatory role of endothelial cells in the relaxation of arterial smooth muscle by acetylcholine. *Nature* 288:373–376, 1980.

79. Gan L, Kaczmarek LK: When, where, and how much? Expression of the KV 3.1 potassium channel in high-frequency firing neurons. *J Neurobiol* 37:69–79, 1998.

80. Gause G, Baker R, Cassin S: Specificity of FPL 57231 for leukotriene D4 receptors in fetal pulmonary circulation. *Am J Physiol* 254:H120–H125, 1988.

81. Gibson A, McFadzean I, Wallace P, Wayman CP: Capacitative Ca^{2+} entry and the regulation of smooth muscle tone. *TiPS* 19:266–269, 1998.

82. Gil J: The normal pulmonary microcirculation. In Fishman AP (ed): The Pulmonary Circulation: Normal and Abnormal. Philadelphia: University of Pennsylvania Press, 1990, pp. 3–16.

83. Gillis CN, Cronau LH, Greene NM, Hammond GL: Removal of 5-hydroxytryptamine and norepinephrine from the pulmonary vascular space of man: influence of cardiopulmonary bypass and pulmonary arterial pressure on these processes. *Surgery* 76:608–616, 1974.

84. Glenny RW: Blood flow distribution in the lung. *Chest* 114:8S–16S, 1998.

85. Glenny RW, Bernard S, Robertson HT, Hlastala MP: Gravity is an important but secondary determinant of regional pulmonary blood flow in upright primates. *J Appl Physiol* 86:623–632, 1999.

86. Glenny RW, Lamm WJ, Albert RK, Robertson HT: Gravity is a minor determinant of pulmonary blood flow distribution. *J Appl Physiol* 71:620–629, 1991.

87. Glenny RW, McKinney S, Robertson HT: The spatial pattern of pulmonary blood flow distribution is stable over days. *J Appl Physiol* 82:902–907, 1997.

88. Glenny RW, Polissar NL, McKinney S, Robertson HT: Temporal heterogeneity of regional pulmonary perfusion is spatially clustered. *J Appl Physiol* 79:986–1001, 1995.

89. Glenny RW, Robertson HT: Fractal modeling of pulmonary blood flow heterogeneity. *J Appl Physiol* 70:1024–1030, 1991.

90. Glenny RW, Robertson HT: Fractal properties of pulmonary blood flow: characterization of spatial heterogeneity. *J Appl Physiol* 69:532–545, 1990.

91. Glenny RW, Robertson HT: A computer simulation of pulmonary perfusion in three dimensions. *J Appl Physiol* 79:357–369, 1995.

92. Glick PL, Siebert JR, Benjamin DR: Pathophysiology of congenital diaphragmatic hernia. I. Renal enlargement suggests feedback modulation by pulmonary derived renotropins—a unifying hypothesis to explain pulmonary hypoplasia, polyhydramnios, and renal enlargement in the fetus/newborn with congenital diaphragmatic hernia. *J Pediatr Surg* 25:492–495, 1990.

93. Goldman AP, Delius RE, Deanfeld JE, et al: Nitric oxide might reduce the need for extracorporeal support in children with critical postoperative pulmonary hypertension. *Ann Thorac Surg* 62:750–755, 1996.

94. Goldman AP, Haworth SG, Macrae DJ: Does inhaled nitric oxide suppress endogenous nitric oxide production? *J Thorac Cardiovasc Surg* 112:541–542, 1996.

95. Goldman AP, Tasker RC, Hosiasson S, et al: Early response to inhaled nitric oxide and its relationship to outcome in children with severe hypoxemic respiratory failure. *Chest* 112:752–758, 1997.

96. Goligorsky MS: Making sense out of oxygen sensor. *Circ Res* 86:824–826, 2000.

97. Gordon JB, Hortop J, Hakim TS: Developmental effects of hypoxia and indomethacin on distribution of vascular resistances in lamb lungs. *Pediatr Res* 26:325–329, 1989.

98. Gordon JB, Tod ML, Wetzel RC, et al: Age-dependent effects of indomethacin on hypoxic vasoconstriction in neonatal lamb lungs. *Pediatr Res* 23:580–584, 1988.

99. Görlach A, Brandes RP, Nguyen K, et al: A gp91phox containing NADPH oxidase selectively expressed in endothelial cells is a major source of oxygen radical generation in the arterial wall. *Circ Res* 87:26–32, 2000.

100. Grabowski EF, Jaffe EA, Weksler BB: Prostacyclin production by cultured endothelial cell monolayers exposed to step increases in shear stress. *J Lab Clin Med* 105:36–43, 1985.

101. Green RS, Leffler CW: Hypoxia stimulates prostacyclin synthesis by neonatal lungs. *Pediatr Res* 18:832–835, 1984.

102. Greenleaf JF, Ritman EL, Sass DJ, Wood EH: Spatial distribution of pulmonary blood flow in dogs in left decubitus position. *Am J Physiol* 227:230–244, 1974.

103. Griendling KK, Sorescu D, Ushio-Fukai M: NAD(P)H oxidase: role in cardiovascular biology and disease. *Circ Res* 86:494–501, 2000.

104. Griendling KK, Ushio-Fukai M: NADH/NADPH oxidase and vascular function. *Trends Cardiovasc Med* 7:301–307, 1997.

105. Gryglewski RJ, Palmer RM, Moncada S: Superoxide anion is involved in the breakdown of endothelium-derived vascular relaxing factor. *Nature* 320:454–456, 1986.

106. Guenter CA, McCaffree DR, Davis LJ, Smith VS: Hemodynamic characteristics and blood gas exchange in the normal baboon. *J Appl Physiol* 25:507–510, 1968.

107. Hakim TS, Dean GW, Lisbona R: Effect of body posture on spatial distribution of pulmonary blood flow. *J Appl Physiol* 64:1160–1170, 1988.

108. Hakim TS, Lisbona R, Dean GW: Gravity-independent inequality in pulmonary blood flow in humans. *J Appl Physiol* 63:1114–1121, 1987.

109. Hall SM, Haworth SG: Onset and evolution of pulmonary vascular disease in young children: abnormal postnatal remodeling studied in lung biopsies. *J Pathol* 166:183–193, 1992.

110. Hammerman C, Aramburo MJ: Effects of hyperventilation on prostacyclin formation and on pulmonary vasodilation after group B beta-hemolytic streptococci-induced pulmonary hypertension. *Pediatr Res* 29:282–287, 1991.

111. Hammond GL, Cronau LH, Whittaker D, Gillis CN: Fate of prostaglandins E(1) and A(1) in the human pulmonary circulation. *Surgery* 81:716–722, 1977.

112. Hanson KA, Burns F, Rybalkin SD, et al: Developmental changes in lung cGMP phosphodiesterase-5 activity, protein, and message. *Am J Respir Crit Care Med* 158:279–288, 1998.

113. Haraldsson A, Kieler-Jensen N, Nathorst-Westfelt U, et al: Comparison of inhaled nitric oxide and inhaled aerosolized prostacyclin in the evaluation of heart transplant candidates with elevated pulmonary vascular resistance. *Chest* 114:780–786, 1998.

114. Harder DR, Narayanan J, Birks EK, et al: Identification of a putative microvascular oxygen sensor. *Circ Res* 76:54–61, 1996.

115. Haworth SG: Pulmonary vascular disease in different types of congenital heart disease. Implications for interpretation of lung biopsy findings in early childhood. *Br Heart J* 52:557–571, 1984.

116. Haworth SG, Hall SM, Chew M, Allen K: Thinning of fetal pulmonary arterial wall and postnatal remodeling: ultrastructural studies on the respiratory unit arteries of the pig. *Virchows Arch [A] Pathol Anat Histopathol* 411:161–171, 1987.

117. Haworth SG, Hislop AA: Adaptation of the pulmonary circulation to extra-uterine life in the pig and its relevance to the human infant. *Cardiovasc Res* 15:108–119, 1981.

118. Heerdt PM, Weiss CI: Prostaglandin E1 and intrapulmonary shunt in cardiac surgical patients with pulmonary hypertension [published erratum appears in *Ann Thorac Surg* 50(2):337, 1990]. *Ann Thorac Surg* 49:463–465, 1990.

119. Henson PM, Barnes PJ, Banks-Schlegel SP: NHLBI workshop summary. Platelet-activating factor: role in pulmonary injury and dysfunction and blood abnormalities. *Am Rev Respir Dis* 145:726–731, 1992.

120. Herman CM, Homer LD, Horwitz DL: Effects of sedation and posture on pulmonary gas exchange in the baboon. *J Appl Physiol* 30:498–501, 1971.

121. Hickey KA, Rubanyi G, Paul RJ, Highsmith RF: Characterization of a coronary vasoconstrictor produced by cultured endothelial cells. *Am J Physiol* 248:C550–C556, 1985.

122. Hickey PR, Hansen DD, Wessel DL, et al: Blunting of stress responses in the pulmonary circulation of infants by fentanyl. *Anesth Analg* 64:1137–1142, 1985.

123. Hislop A, Haworth SG, Shinebourne EA, Reid L: Quantitative structural analysis of pulmonary vessels in isolated ventricular septal defect in infancy. *Br Heart J* 37:1014–1021, 1975.

124. Hislop A, Reid L: Intra-pulmonary arterial development during fetal life—branching pattern and structure. *J Anat* 113:35–48, 1972.

125. Hislop A, Reid L: Pulmonary arterial development during childhood: branching pattern and structure. *Thorax* 28:129–135, 1973.

126. Hlastala MP, Bernard S, Erickson HH, et al: Pulmonary blood flow distribution in standing horses is not dominated by gravity. *J Appl Physiol* 81:1051–1061, 1996.

127. Hlastala MP, Chornuk MA, Self DA, et al: Pulmonary blood flow redistribution by increased gravitational force. *J Appl Physiol* 84:1278–1288, 1998.

128. Hoffman GA, Ross GA, Day SE, et al: Inhaled nitric oxide reduces the utilization of extracorporeal membrane oxygenation in persistent pulmonary hypertension of the newborn. *Crit Care Med* 25:352–359, 1997.

129. Horowitz A, Menice CB, Laporte R, et al: Mechanisms of smooth muscle contraction. *Physiol Rev* 76:967–1003, 1996.

130. Hsieh HJ, Li NQ, Frangos JA: Shear stress increases endothelial platelet-derived growth factor mRNA levels. *Am J Physiol* 260:H642–H646, 1991.

131. Hu N, Packer CS, Rhoades RA: Reactive oxygen-mediated contraction in pulmonary arterial smooth muscle: cellular mechanisms. *Can J Physiol Pharmacol* 69:383–388, 1991.

132. Hughes JM: Pulmonary blood flow distribution in exercising and in resting horses [editorial]. *J Appl Physiol* 81:1062–1070, 1996.

133. Ibe BO, Hibler S, Raj JU: Platelet-activating factor modulates pulmonary vasomotor tone in the perinatal lamb. *J Appl Physiol* 85:1079–1085, 1998.

134. Ibe BO, Raj JU: Endogenous arachidonic acid metabolism by calcium ionophore stimulated ferret lungs. Effect of age, hypoxia. *Lab Invest* 66:370–377, 1992.

135. Ibrahim AE, Duncan BW, Blume ED, Jonas RA: Long-term follow-up of pediatric cardiac patients requiring mechanical circulatory support. *Ann Thorac Surg* 69:186–192, 2000.

136. Ignarro LJ, Byrns RE, Buga GM, Wood KS: Endothelium-derived relaxing factor from pulmonary artery and vein possesses pharmacologic and chemical properties identical to those of nitric oxide radical. *Circ Res* 61:866–879, 1987.

137. Ignarro LJ: Biological actions and properties of endothelium-derived nitric oxide formed and released from artery and vein. *Circ Res* 65:1–21, 1989.

138. Ilbawi MN, Idriss FS, DeLeon SY, et al: Hemodynamic effects of intravenous nitroglycerin in pediatric patients after heart surgery. *Circulation* 72:II101–II107, 1985.

139. Inoue A, Yanagisawa M, Kimura S, et al: The human endothelin family: three structurally and pharmacologically distinct isopeptides predicted by three separate genes. *Proc Natl Acad Sci USA* 86:2863–2867, 1989.

140. Ivy DD, Kinsella JP, Abman SH: Endothelin blockade augments pulmonary vasodilation in the ovine fetus. *J Appl Physiol* 81:2481–2487, 1996.

141. Ivy DD, Kinsella JP, Ziegler JW, Abman SH: Dipyridamole attenuates rebound pulmonary hypertension after inhaled nitric oxide withdrawal in postoperative congenital heart disease. *J Thorac Cardiovasc Surg* 115:875–882, 1998.

142. Ivy DD, Le Cras TD, Horan MP, Abman SH: Increased lung preproET-1 and decreased ET-B receptor gene expression in fetal pulmonary hypertension. *Am J Physiol* 274:L535–L541, 1998.

143. Jacobus WE, Pores IH, Lucas SK, et al: Intracellular acidosis and contractility in the normal and ischemic heart as examined by 31P NMR. *J Mol Cell Cardiol* 14 (Suppl 3):13–20, 1982.

144. Janssens SP, Simouchi A, Quertermous T, et al: Cloning and expression of a cDNA encoding human endothelium-derived relating factor/nitric oxide synthase. *J Biol Chem* 267:22694, 1992.

145. Johnson LR, Dodam JR, Laughlin MH: Endothelium-dependent relaxation differs in porcine pulmonary arteries from the left and right caudal lobes. *J Appl Physiol* 88:827–834, 2000.

146. Journois D, Pouard P, Mauriat P, et al: Inhaled nitric oxide as a therapy for pulmonary hypertension after operations for congenital heart defects. *J Thorac Cardiovasc Surg* 107:1129–1135, 1994.

147. Jun SS, Chen Z, Pace MC, Shaul PW: Estrogen upregulates cyclooxygenase-1 gene expression in ovine fetal pulmonary artery endothelium. *J Clin Invest* 102:176–183, 1998.

148. Karaki H, Ozaki H, Hori M, et al: Calcium movements, distribution, and functions in smooth muscle. *Pharmacol Rev* 49:157–200, 1997.

149. Kato T, Iwama Y, Okumura K, et al: Prostaglandin H2 may be the endothelium-derived contracting factor released by acetylcholine in the aorta of the rat. *Hypertension* 15:475–481, 1990.

150. Katusic ZS, Vanhoutte PM: Superoxide anion is an endothelium-derived contracting factor. *Am J Physiol* 257:H33–H37, 1989.

151. Katz AM: Maladaptive hypertrophy and the cardiomyopathy of overload: familial cardiomyopathies. In Katz AM (ed): *Heart Failure: Pathophysiology, Molecular Biology, and Clinical Management.* Philadelphia: Lippincott, Williams & Wilkins, 2000, pp 277–310.

152. Kay MJ: Comparative morphologic features of the pulmonary vasculature in mammals. *Am Rev Respir Dis* 128:S52–S57, 1983.

153. Kermode J, Butt W, Shann F: Comparison between prostaglandin E1 and epoprostenol (prostacyclin) in infants after heart surgery. *Br Heart J* 66:175–178, 1991.

154. Kimura S, Kasuya Y, Sawamura T, et al: Conversion of big endothelin-1 to 21-residue endothelin-1 is essential for expression of full vasoconstrictor activity: structure-activity relationships of big endothelin-1. *J Cardiovasc Pharmacol* 13:S5–7, 1989.

155. Kinsella JP, Ivy DD, Abman SH: Ontogeny of NO activity and response to inhaled NO in the developing ovine pulmonary circulation. *Am J Physiol* 267:H1955–H1961, 1994.

156. Klein MD, Shaheen KW, Whittlesey GC, et al: Extracorporeal membrane oxygenation for the circulatory support of children after repair of congenital heart disease. *J Thorac Cardiovasc Surg* 100:498–505, 1990.

157. Konduri GG, Gervasio CT, Theodorou AA: Role of adenosine triphosphate and adenosine in oxygen-induced pulmonary vasodilation in fetal lambs. *Pediatr Res* 33:533–539, 1993.

158. Konduri GG, Mital S, Gervasio CT, et al: Purine nucleotides contribute to pulmonary vasodilation caused by birth-related stimuli in the ovine fetus. *Am J Physiol* 272:H2377–H2384, 1997.

159. Konduri GG, Theodorou AA, Mukhopadhyay A, Deshmukh DR: Adenosine triphosphate and adenosine increase the pulmonary blood flow to postnatal levels in fetal lambs. *Pediatr Res* 31:451–457, 1992.

160. Konduri GG, Woodard LL: Selective pulmonary vasodilation by low-dose infusion of adenosine triphosphate in newborn lambs. *J Pediatr* 119:94–102, 1991.

161. Kourembanas S, McQuillan LP, Leung GK, et al: Nitric oxide regulates the expression of vasoconstrictors and growth factors by vascular endothelium under both normoxia and hypoxia. *J Clin Invest* 92:99–104, 1993.

162. Krampetz IK, Rhoades RA: Intracellular pH: effect on pulmonary arterial smooth muscle. *Am J Physiol* 260:L516–L521, 1991.

163. Kulik TJ, Lock JE: Leukotrienes and the immature pulmonary circulation. *Am Rev Respir Dis* 136:220–222, 1987.

164. Lane JR, Siwik E, Preminger T, et al: Prospective diagnosis of alveolar capillary dysplasia in infants with congenital heart disease. *Am J Cardiol* 84:618–620, 1999.

165. Lefevre J: Teleonomical optimization of a fractal model of the pulmonary arterial bed. *Theor Biol* 102:225–248, 1983.

166. Leone AM, Palmer RM, Knowles RG, et al: Constitutive and inducible nitric oxide synthases incorporate molecular oxygen into both nitric oxide and citrulline. *J Biol Chem* 266:23790–23795, 1991.

167. Levin DL, Rudolph AM, Heymann MA, Phibbs RH: Morphological development of the pulmonary vascular bed in fetal lambs. *Circulation* 53:144–151, 1976.

168. Levy M, Tulloh RM, Komai H, et al: Maturation of the contractile response and its endothelial modulation in newborn intrapulmonary arteries. *Pediatr Res* 38:25–29, 1995.

169. Lewis AB, Heymann MA, Rudolph AM: Gestational changes in pulmonary vascular responses in fetal lambs in utero. *Circ Res* 39:536–541, 1976.

170. Linehan JH, Dawson CA: Pulmonary vascular resistance (P:Q relations). In Fishman AP (ed): *The Pulmonary Circulation: Normal and Abnormal.* Philadelphia: University of Pennsylvania Press, 1990, pp 41–56.

171. Liu Q, Wiener CM, Flavahan NA: Superoxide and endothelium-dependent constriction to flow in porcine small pulmonary arteries. *Br J Pharmacol* 124:331–336, 1998.

172. Loughlin GM, Wynne JW, Victorica BE: Sleep apnea as a possible cause of pulmonary hypertension in Down syndrome. *J Pediatr* 98:435–437, 1981.

173. Luscher TF, Vanhoutte PM: Endothelium-dependent contractions to acetylcholine in the aorta of the spontaneously hypertensive rat. *Hypertension* 8:344–348, 1986.

174. Malik AB, Kidd BS: Independent effects of changes in H+ and CO2 concentrations on hypoxic pulmonary vasoconstriction. *J Appl Physiol* 34:318–323, 1973.

175. Marczin N, Ryan US, Catravas JD: Methylene blue inhibits nitrovasodilator- and endothelium-derived relaxing factor-induced cyclic GMP accumulation in cultured pulmonary arterial smooth muscle cells via generation of superoxide anion. *J Pharmacol Exp Ther* 264:170–179, 1992.

176. Martin LD, Wetzel RC, Bilenki AL: Airway pressure release ventilation in a neonatal lamb model of acute lung injury. *Crit Care Med* 19:373–378, 1991.

177. Martin W, Villani GM, Jothianandan D, Furchgott RF: Selective blockade of endothelium-dependent and glyceryl trinitrate–induced relaxation by hemoglobin and by methylene blue in the rabbit aorta. *J Pharmacol Exp Ther* 232:708–716, 1985.

178. McCormack DG, Barnes PJ, Evans TW: Platelet-activating factor: evidence against a role in hypoxic pulmonary vasoconstriction. *Crit Care Med* 18:1398–1402, 1990.

179. McMurtry IF, Morris KG: Platelet-activating factor causes pulmonary vasodilation in the rat. *Am Rev Respir Dis* 134:757–762, 1986.

180. McQuillan LP, Leung GK, Marsden PA, et al: Hypoxia inhibits expression of eNOS via transcriptional and posttranscriptional mechanisms. *Am J Physiol* 267:H1921–H1927, 1994.

181. Meliones JN, Bowe EL, Dekeon MK, et al: High-frequency jet ventilation improves cardiac function after the Fontan procedure. *Circulation* 84:III364–III368, 1991.

182. Melsom MN, Flatebo T, Kramer-Johansen J, et al: Both gravity and non-gravity dependent factors determine regional blood flow within the goat lung. *Acta Physiol Scand* 153:343–353, 1995.

183. Meyrick B, Reid L: The effect of continued hypoxia on rat pulmonary arterial circulation. An ultrastructural study. *Lab Invest* 38:188–200, 1978.

184. Mikhail G, Gibbs J, Richardson M, et al: An evaluation of nebulized prostacyclin in patients with primary and secondary pulmonary hypertension. *Eur Heart J* 18:1499–1504, 1997.

185. Miller OI, Celermejer DS, Deanfield JE, Macrae DJ: Very low-dose inhaled nitric oxide: a selective pulmonary vasodilator after operations for congential heart disease. *J Thorac Cardiovasc Surg* 108:487–494, 1994.

186. Miller VM, Vanhoutte PM: Enhanced release of endothelium-derived factor(s) by chronic increases in blood flow. *Am J Physiol* 255:H446–H451, 1988.

187. Moncada S, Palmer RM, Higgs EA: Nitric oxide: physiology, pathophysiology, and pharmacology. *Pharmacol Rev* 43:109–142, 1991.

188. Moncada S, Rees DD, Schulz R, Palmer RM: Development and mechanism of a specific supersensitivity to nitrovasodilators after inhibition of vascular nitric oxide synthesis in vivo. *Proc Natl Acad Sci USA* 88:2166–2170, 1991.

189. Morin FC III: Hyperventilation, alkalosis, prostaglandins, and pulmonary circulation of the newborn. *J Appl Physiol* 61:2088–2094, 1986.

190. Morin FC III, Egan EA, Norfleet WT: Indomethacin does not diminish the pulmonary vascular response of the fetus to increased oxygen tension. *Pediatr Res* 24:696–700, 1988.

191. Morin FC III, Egan EA: Pulmonary hemodynamics in fetal lambs during development at normal and increased oxygen tension. *J Appl Physiol* 73:213–218, 1992.

192. Morin FC III, Stenmark KR: Persistent pulmonary hypertension of the newborn. *Am J Respir Crit Care Med* 151:2010–2032, 1995.

193. Morray JP, Lynn AM, Mansfield PB: Effect of pH and pCO2 on pulmonary and systemic hemodynamics after surgery in children with congenital heart disease and pulmonary hypertension. *J Pediatr* 113:474–479, 1988.

194. Morris GN, Lowson SM, Rich GF: Transient effects of inhaled nitric oxide for prolonged postoperative treatment of hypoxemia after surgical correction of total anomalous pulmonary venous return. *J Thorac Cardiovasc Anesth* 9:713–716, 1995.

195. Nakamura Y, Harada K, Yamamoto I, et al: Human pulmonary hypoplasia. Statistical, morphological, morphometric, and biochemical study. *Arch Pathol Lab Med* 116:635–642, 1992.

196. Nelson MT, Quayle JM: Physiological roles and properties of potassium channels in arterial smooth muscle. *Am J Physiol* 268:C799–C822, 1995.

197. Neylon CB, Richards SM, Larsen MA, et al: Multiple types of ryanodine receptor/Ca2+ release channels are expressed in vascular smooth muscle. *Biochem Biophys Res Comm* 215:814–821, 1995.

198. NINOS: Inhaled NO in full-term and nearly full-term infants with hypoxic respiratory failure. *N Engl J Med* 336:597–604, 1997.

199. Nolop KB, Braude S, Taylor KM, Royston D: Epithelial and endothelial flux after bypass in dogs: effect of positive end-expiratory pressure. *J Appl Physiol* 62:1244–1249, 1987.

200. North AJ, Brannon TS, Wells LB, et al: Hypoxia stimulates prostacyclin synthesis in newborn pulmonary endothelium by increasing cyclooxygenase-1 protein. *Circ Res* 75:33–40, 1994.

201. North AJ, Star RA, Brannon TS, et al: Nitric oxide synthase type I and type III gene expression are developmentally regulated in rat lung. *Am J Physiol* 266:L635–L641, 1994.

202. Olley PM, Coceani F: Lipid mediators in the control of the ductus arteriosus. *Am Rev Respir Dis* 136:218–219, 1987.

203. Olschewski H, Ghofrani HA, Walmrath D, et al: Inhaled prostacyclin and iloprost in severe pulmonary hypertension secondary to lung fibrosis. *Am J Respir Crit Care Med* 160:600–607, 1999.

204. Onohara T, Okadome K, Yamamura S, et al: Simulated blood flow and the effects on prostacyclin production in the dog femoral artery. *Circ Res* 68:1095–1099, 1991.

205. Orallo F: Regulation of cytosolic calcium levels in vascular smooth muscle. *Pharmacol Ther* 69:153–171, 1996.

206. O'Rourke PP: Use of extracorporeal life support in patients with congenital heart disease: state of the art? [editorial; comment]. *Crit Care Med* 20:1199–1200, 1992.

207. Osipenko ON, Tate RJ, Gurney AM: Potential role for Kv3.1b channels as oxygen sensors. *Circ Res* 86:534–540, 2000.

208. Pagano PJ: Vascular gp91phox—beyond the endothelium. *Circ Res* 87:1–3, 2000.

209. Palmer RM, Ferrige AG, Moncada S: Nitric oxide release accounts for the biological activity of endothelium-derived relaxing factor. *Nature* 327:524–526, 1987.

210. Perez-Garcia MT, Lopez-Lopez JR: Are K_v channels the essence of O2 sensing? *Circ Res* 86:490–491, 2000.

211. Perreault T, Baribeau J: Characterization of endothelin receptors in newborn piglet lung. *Am J Physiol* 268:L607–L614, 1995.

212. Perreault T, Coe JY, Olley PM, Coceani F: Pulmonary vascular effects of prostaglandin D2 in newborn pig. *Am J Physiol* 258:H1292–H1310, 1990.

213. Pohl U, Busse R: Pulsatile perfusion stimulates the release of endothelial autacoids. *J Appl Physiol* 1:215–235, 1986.

214. Post JM, Hume JR, Archer SL, et al: Direct role for potassium channel inhibition in hypoxic pulmonary vasoconstriction. *Am J Physiol* 31:C882–C890, 1992.

215. Prendergast B, Newby DE, Wilson LE, et al: Early therapeutic experience with the endothelin antagonist BQ-123 in pulmonary hypertension after congenital heart surgery. *Heart* 82:505–508, 1999.

216. Prescott SM, Zimmerman GA, McIntyre TM: Human endothelial cells in culture produce platelet-activating factor (1-alkyl-2-acetyl-sn-glycero-3-phosphocholine) when stimulated with thrombin. *Proc Natl Acad Sci USA* 81:3534–3538, 1984.

217. Printz MP, Skidgel RA, Friedman WF: Studies of pulmonary prostaglandin biosynthetic and catabolic enzymes as factors in ductus arteriosus patency and closure. Evidence for a shift in products with gestational age. *Pediatr Res* 18:19–24, 1984.

218. Prisk GK, Guy HJB, Elliot AR, West JB: Inhomogeneity of pulmonary perfusion during sustained microgravity on SLS-1. *J Appl Physiol* 76:1730–1738, 1994.

219. Quilley J, Fulton D, McGiff JC, et al: Hyperpolarizing factors. *Biochem Pharmacol* 54:1059–1070, 1997.

220. Rabinovitch M: Investigational approaches to pulmonary hypertension. *Toxicol Pathol* 19:458–469, 1991.

221. Rabinovitch M: Pulmonary hypertension: pathophysiology as a basis for clinical decision making. *J Heart Lung Transplant* 18:1041–1053, 1999.

222. Rabinovitch M, Andrew M, Thom H, et al: Abnormal endothelial factor VIII associated with pulmonary hypertension and congenital heart defects. *Circulation* 76:1043–1052, 1987.

223. Rabinovitch M, Bothwell T, Hayakawa BN, et al: Pulmonary artery endothelial abnormalities in patients with congenital heart defects and pulmonary hypertension. A correlation of light with scanning electron microscopy and transmission electron microscopy. *Lab Invest* 55:632–653, 1986.

224. Rabinovitch M, Boudreau N, Vella G, et al: Oxygen-related prostaglandin synthesis in ductus arteriosus and other vascular cells. *Pediatr Res* 26:330–335, 1989.

225. Rabinovitch M, Castaneda AR, Reid L: Lung biopsy with frozen section as a diagnostic aid in patients with congenital heart defects. *Am J Cardiol* 47:77–84, 1981.

226. Rabinovitch M, Keane JF, Fellows KE, et al: Quantitative analysis of the pulmonary wedge angiogram in congenital heart defects. Correlation with hemodynamic data and morphometric findings in lung biopsy tissue. *Circulation* 63:152–164, 1981.

227. Rabinovitch M, Keane JF, Norwood WI, et al: Vascular structure in lung tissue obtained at biopsy correlated with pulmonary hemodynamic findings after repair of congenital heart defects. *Circulation* 69:655–667, 1984.

228. Rapoport RM, Draznin MB, Murad F: Endothelium-dependent relaxation in rat aorta may be mediated through cyclic GMP-dependent protein phosphorylation. *Nature* 310:174–176, 1983.

229. Rapoport RM, Draznin MB, Murad F: Mechanisms of adenosine triphosphate-, thrombin-, and trypsin-induced relaxation of rat thoracic aorta. *Circ Res* 55:468–479, 1984.

230. Rapoport RM, Stauderman KA, Highsmith RF: Effects of EDCF and endothelin on phosphatidylinositol hydrolysis and contraction in rat aorta. *Am J Physiol* 258:C122–C131, 1990.

231. Rasanen J, Downs JB, Stock MC: Cardiovascular effects of conventional positive pressure ventilation and airway pressure release ventilation. *Chest* 93:911–915, 1988.

232. Rayment I, Holden HM, Whittaker M, et al: Structure of the actin-myosin complex and its implications for muscle contraction. *Science* 261:58–65, 1993.

233. Ream RS, Hauver JF, Lynch RE, et al: Low-dose inhaled nitric oxide improves the oxygenation and ventilation of infants and children with acute hypoxemic respiratory failure. *Crit Care Med* 27:989–996, 1999.

234. Redding GJ, McMurtry I, Reeves JT: Effects of meclofenamate on pulmonary vascular resistance correlate with postnatal age in young piglets. *Pediatr Res* 18:579–583, 1984.

235. Reed JH Jr, Wood EH: Effect of body position on vertical distribution of pulmonary blood flow. *J Appl Physiol* 28:310–311, 1970.

236. Reid DL, Thornburg KL: Pulmonary pressure-flow relationships in the fetal lamb during in utero ventilation. *J Appl Physiol* 69:1630–1636, 1990.

237. Reid L: Structure and function in pulmonary hypertension: new perceptions. *Chest* 89:279–288, 1986.

238. Reynolds EE, Mok LL: Role of thromboxane A2/prostaglandin H2 receptor in the vasoconstrictor response of rat aorta to endothelin. *J Pharmacol Exp Ther* 252:915–921, 1990.

239. Rich S, Kaufmann E, Levy PS: The effect of high doses of calcium-channel blockers on survival in primary pulmonary hypertension [see comments]. *N Engl J Med* 327:76–81, 1992.

240. Roberds SL, Tamkun MM: Cloning and tissue-specific expression of five voltage-gated potassium channel cDNAs expressed in rat heart. *Proc Natl Acad Sci USA* 88:1798–1802, 1991.

241. Roberts JD Jr, Fineman JR III, Morin FC, et al: Inhaled nitric oxide and persistent pulmonary hypertension of the newborn. The Inhaled Nitric Oxide Study Group. *N Engl J Med* 336:605–610, 1997.

242. Roberts JD Jr, Lang P, Bigatello LM, et al: Inhaled nitric oxide in congenital heart disease. *Circulation* 87:447–453, 1993.

243. Roos CM, Rich GF, Uncles DR, et al: Sites of vasodilation by inhaled nitric oxide vs sodium nitroprusside in endothelin-constricted isolated rat lungs. *J Appl Physiol* 77:51–57, 1994.

244. Rosenberg AA, Kennaugh J, Koppenhafer SL, et al: Elevated immunoreactive endothelin-1 levels in newborn infants with persistent pulmonary hypertension. *J Pediatr* 123:109–114, 1993.

245. Rubanyi GM, Vanhoutte PM: Flow-induced release of endothelium-derived relaxing factor. *Am J Physiol* 250:H1145–H1149, 1986.

246. Rudolph A: Fetal and neonatal pulmonary circulation. *Annu Rev Physiol* 41:383–395, 1979.

247. Russell IA, Zwass MS, Fineman JR, et al: The effects of inhaled nitric oxide on postoperative pulmonary hypertension in infants and children undergoing surgical repair of congenital heart disease. *Anes Analg* 87:46–51, 1999.

248. Saida K, Mitsui Y, Ishida N: A novel peptide, vasoactive intestinal contractor, of a new (endothelin) peptide family. Molecular cloning, expression, and biological activity. *J Biol Chem* 264:14613–14616, 1989.

249. Samuelsson B, Hammarstrom S, Murphy RC, Borgeat P: Leukotrienes and slow reacting substance of anaphylaxis (SRS-A). *Allergy* 35:375–381, 1980.

250. Sanchez LS, de la Monte SM, Filippov G, et al: Cyclic-GMP-binding, cyclic GMP specific phosphodiesterase (PDE5) gene expression is regulated during rat pulmonary development. *Pediatr Res* 43:163–168, 1998.

251. Schini VB, Vanhoutte PM: Inhibitors of calmodulin impair the constitutive but not the inducible nitric oxide synthase activity in the rat aorta. *J Pharmacol Exp Ther* 261:553–559, 1992.

252. Schranz D, Zepp F, Iversen S, et al: Effects of tolazoline and prostacyclin on pulmonary hypertension in infants after cardiac surgery. *Crit Care Med* 20:1243–1249, 1992.

253. Schreiber MD, Heymann MA, Soifer SJ: The differential effects of leukotriene C4 and D4 on the pulmonary and systemic circulations in newborn lambs. *Pediatr Res* 21:176–182, 1987.

254. Semenza GL: Perspective on oxygen sensing. *Cell* 98:281–284, 1999.

255. Sessa WC, Harrison JK, Barber CM, et al: Molecular cloning and expression of a cDNA encoding endothelial cell nitric oxide synthase. *J Biol Chem* 267:15274–15276, 1992.

256. Shaul P: Ontogeny of nitric oxide in the pulmonary vasculature. *Semin Perinatol* 21:381–392, 1997.

257. Shaul PW, Campbell WB, Farrar MA, Magness RR: Oxygen modulates prostacyclin synthesis in ovine fetal pulmonary arteries by an effect on cyclooxygenase. *J Clin Invest* 90:2147–2155, 1992.

258. Shaul PW, Farrar MA, Magness RR: Oxygen modulation of pulmonary arterial prostacyclin synthesis is developmentally regulated. *Am J Physiol* 262:H621–H628, 1993.

259. Shaul PW, Farrar MA, Zellers TM: Oxygen modulates endothelium-derived relaxing factor production in fetal pulmonary arteries. *Am J Physiol* 262:H355–H364, 1992.

260. Shetty S, Okada T, Webb R, et al: Functionally distinct endothelin B receptors in vascular endothelium and smooth muscle. *Biochem Biophys Res Comm* 191:459–464, 1993.

261. Shiba R, Yanagisawa M, Miyauchi T, et al: Elimination of intravenously injected endothelin-1 from the circulation of the rat. *J Cardiovasc Pharmacol* 13:S98–S101, 1989.

262. Shimizu S, Bowman PS, Thorne G, Paul RJ: Effects of hypoxia on isometric force, intracellular Ca^{2+}, pH, and energetics in porcine coronary artery. *Circ Res* 86:862–870, 2000.

263. Sie KC, Perkins JA, Clarke WR: Acute right heart failure due to adenotonsillar hypertrophy. *Int J Pediatr Otorhinol* 41:53–58, 1997.

264. Smith GL, Austin C, Crichton C, et al: A review of the actions and control of intracellular pH in vascular smooth muscle. *Cardiovas Res* 38:316–331, 1998.

265. Soifer SJ, Loitz RD, Roman C, Heymann MA: Leukotriene end organ antagonists increase pulmonary blood flow in fetal lambs. *Am J Physiol* 249:H570–H576, 1985.

266. Steinberg SF: The molecular basis for distinct B-adrenergic receptor subtype actions in cardiomyocytes. *Circ Res* 85:1101–1111, 1999.

267. Steinhorn RH, Morin FC III, Van Wylen DG, et al: Endothelium-dependent relaxations to adenosine in juvenile rabbit pulmonary arteries and veins. *Am J Physiol* 266:H2001–H2006, 1994.

268. Stenmark KR, Aldashev AA, Orton EC, et al: Cellular adaptation during chronic neonatal hypoxic pulmonary hypertension. *Am J Physiol* 261:97–104, 1991.

269. Surks HK, Mochizuki N, Kasi Y, et al: Regulation of myosin phosphatase by a specific interaction with cGMP-dependent protein kinase Ia. *Science* 286:1583–1587, 1999.

270. Suzuki YJ, Ford GD: Redox regulation of signal transduction in cardiac and smooth muscle. *J Mol Cell Cardiol* 31:345–353, 1999.

271. Suzuki YJ, Ford GD: Superoxide stimulates IP_3-induced Ca^{2+} release from vascular smooth muscle sarcoplasmic reticulum. *Am J Physiol* 262:H114–H116, 1992.

272. Takayanagi R, Kitazumi K, Takasaki C, et al: Presence of non-selective type of endothelin receptor on vascular endothelium and its linkage to vasodilation. *FEBS Lett* 282:103–106, 1991.

273. Takuwa N, Takuwa Y, Yanagisawa M, et al: A novel vasoactive peptide endothelin stimulates mitogenesis through inositol lipid turnover in Swiss 3T3 fibroblasts. *J Biol Chem* 264:7856–7861, 1989.

274. Takuwa Y, Kasuya Y, Takuwa N, et al: Endothelin receptor is coupled to phospholipase C via a pertussis toxin–insensitive guanine nucleotide–binding regulatory protein in vascular smooth muscle cells. *J Clin Invest* 85:653–658, 1990.

275. Teitel DF, Iwamoto HS, Rudolph AM: Changes in the pulmonary circulation during birth-related events. *Pediatr Res* 27:372–378, 1990.

276. Tiktinsky MH, Cummings JJ, Morin FC III: Acetylcholine increases pulmonary blood flow in intact fetuses via endothelium-dependent vasodilation. *Am J Physiol* 262:H406–H410, 1992.

277. Tiktinsky MH, Morin FC III: Increasing oxygen tension dilates fetal pulmonary circulation via endothelium-derived relaxing factor. *Am J Physiol* 265:H376–H380, 1993.

278. Tod ML, Cassin S: Perinatal pulmonary responses to arachidonic acid during normoxia and hypoxia. *J Appl Physiol* 57:977–983, 1984.

279. Tod ML, Yoshimura K, Rubin LJ: Indomethacin prevents ventilation-induced decreases in pulmonary vascular resistance of the middle region in fetal lambs. *Pediatr Res* 29:449–454, 1991.

280. Toyofuku T, Kobayashi T, Koyama S, Kusama S: Pulmonary vascular response to platelet-activating factor in conscious sheep. *Am J Physiol* 255:H434–H440, 1988.

281. Trittenwein G, Pansi H, Graf B, et al: Proposed entry criteria for postoperative cardiac extracorporeal membrane oxygenation after pediatric open heart surgery. *Artif Organs* 23:1010–1014, 1999.

282. Turbow R, Waffarn F, Yang L, et al: Variable oxygenation response to inhaled nitric oxide in severe persistent pulmonary hypertension of the newborn. *Acta Paediatr* 84:1305–1308, 1995.

283. Turner-Gomes SO, Andrew M, Coles J, et al: Abnormalities in von Willebrand factor and antithrombin III after cardiopulmonary bypass operations for congenital heart disease. *J Thorac Cardiovasc Surg* 103:87–97, 1992.

284. Van Riper DA, Weaver BA, Stull JT, Rembold CM: Myosin light chain kinase phosphorylation in swine carotid artery contraction and relaxation. *Am J Physiol* 168:H2466–H2475, 1995.

285. Veyssier-Belot C, Cacoub P: Role of endothelial and smooth muscle cells in the pathophysiology and treatment management of pulmonary hypertension. *Cardiovasc Res* 44:274–282, 1999.

286. Wagner OF, Christ G, Wojta J, et al: Polar secretion of endothelin-1 by cultured endothelial cells. *J Biol Chem* 267:16066–16068, 1992.

287. Wang Y, Coceani F: Isolated pulmonary resistance vessels from fetal lambs. Contractile behavior and responses to indomethacin and endothelin-1. *Circ Res* 71:320–330, 1992.

288. Warner TD, Mitchell JA, de Nucci G, Vane JR: Endothelin-1 and endothelin-3 release EDRF from isolated perfused arterial vessels of the rat and rabbit. *J Cardiovasc Pharmacol* 13:S85–S88, 1989.

289. Warner TD, Mitchell JA, D'Orleans-Juste P, et al: Characterization of endothelin-converting enzyme from endothelial cells and rat brain: detection of the formation of biologically active endothelin-1 by rapid bioassay. *Mol Pharmacol* 41:399–403, 1992.

290. Wechezak AR, Wight TN, Viggers RF, Sauvage LR: Endothelial adherence under shear stress is dependent upon microfilament reorganization. *J Cell Physiol* 139:136–146, 1989.

291. Weil J, Bidlingmaier F, Dohlemann C, et al: Comparison of plasma atrial natriuretic peptide levels in healthy children from birth to adolescence and in children with cardiac diseases. *Pediatr Res* 20:1328–1331, 1986.

292. Weksler BB, Marcus AJ, Jaffe EA: Synthesis of prostaglandin I2 (prostacyclin) by cultured human and bovine endothelial cells. *Proc Natl Acad Sci USA* 74:3922–3926, 1977.

293. Wessel DL, Adatia I, Giglia TM, et al: Use of inhaled nitric oxide and acetylcholine in the evaluation of pulmonary hypertension and endothelial function after cardiopulmonary bypass. *Circulation* 88:2128–2138, 1993.

294. Wessel DL, Adatia I, Van Marter LJ, et al: Improved oxygenation in a randomized trial of inhaled nitric oxide for persistent pulmonary hypertension of the newborn. *Pediatrics* 100:E7, 1997.

295. West JB, Dolbry CT, Naimark A: Distribution of blood flow in isolated lung: relations to vascular and alveolar pressures. *J Appl Physiol* 19:713–724, 1964.

296. Wetzel RC, Gordon JB, Gregory TJ, et al: High-frequency ventilation attenuation of hypoxic pulmonary vasoconstriction. The role of prostacyclin. *Am Rev Respir Dis* 132:99–103, 1985.

297. Wetzel RC: Aerosolized prostacyclin: In search of the ideal pulmonary vasodilator. *Anesthesiology* 82:1315–1317, 1995.

298. Whatley RE, Nelson P, Zimmerman GA, et al: The regulation of platelet-activating factor production in endothelial cells. The role of calcium and protein kinase C. *J Biol Chem* 264:6325–6333, 1989.

299. Whittenberger JL, McGregor M: Influence of state of inflation of the lung on pulmonary vascular resistance. *J Appl Physiol* 15:878–882, 1960.

300. Wiklund L, McGregor CGA, Miller VM: Effects of prolonged exposure to oxygen-derived free radicals in canine pulmonary arteries. *Am J Physiol* 270:H2184–H2190, 1996.

301. Wingrove JA, O'Farrell PH: Nitric oxide contributes to behavioral, cellular, and developmental responses to low oxygen in drosophila. *Cell* 98:105–114, 1999.

302. Wung JT, James LS, Kilchevsky E, James E: Management of infants with severe respiratory failure and persistence of the fetal circulation, without hyperventilation. *Pediatrics* 76:488–494, 1985.

303. Xia Y, Dawson VL, Dawson TM, et al: Nitric oxide synthase generates superoxide and nitric oxide in arginine-depleted cells leading to peroxynitrite-mediated cellular injury. *Proc Natl Acad Sci USA* 93:6770–6774, 1996.

304. Xiao R-P, Cheng H, Zhou Y-Y, et al: Recent advances in cardiac β(2)-adrenergic signal transduction. *Circ Res* 85:1091–1100, 1999.

305. Xue C, Reynolds PR, Johns RA: Developmental expression of NOS isoforms in fetal rat lung: implication for transitional circulation and pulmonary angiogenesis. *Am J Physiol* 270:L88–L100, 1996.

306. Yanagisawa M, Kurihara H, Kimura S, et al: A novel potent vasoconstrictor peptide produced by vascular endothelial cells [see comments]. *Nature* 332:411–415, 1988.

307. Yuan X-J, Goldman W, Tod ML, et al: Hypoxia reduces potassium current in cultured rat pulmonary but not mesenteric arterial myocytes. *Am J Physiol* 264:L116–L123, 1993.

308. Zapol WM, Jones R: Vascular components of ARDS. Clinical pulmonary hemodynamics and morphology. *Am Rev Respir Dis* 136:471–474, 1987.

309. Zellers TM, Vanhoutte PM: Endothelium-dependent relaxations of piglet pulmonary arteries augment with maturation. *Pediatr Res* 30:176–180, 1991.

310. Ziegler JW, Ivy DD, Fox JJ, et al: Dipyridamole potentiates pulmonary vasodilation induced by acetylcholine and nitric oxide in the ovine fetus. *Am J Respir Crit Care Med* 157:1104–1110, 1998.

Chapter 4

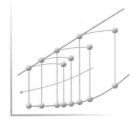

Renal Function and Heart Disease

BARBARA A. FIVUSH, MD, ALICIA M. NEU, MD,
RULAN PAREKH, MD, MS, LYNNE G. MAXWELL, MD,
LORRAINE C. RACUSEN, MD, JEANNETTE R.M. WHITE, MD, PhD,
and DAVID G. NICHOLS, MD, MBA

INTRODUCTION

Some form of renal dysfunction is a common accompaniment of heart disease. Indeed, congenital heart surgery is the most common cause of acute renal failure in infancy.[81] The risk of death increases sharply once renal failure occurs. Virtually all therapies for cardiac dysfunction involve some modulation of salt and water handling by the kidneys. For these reasons, this chapter focuses on interrelationships between cardiac output, renal perfusion, and handling of salt and water by the kidneys. In addition to these pathophysiologic considerations, we shall discuss the current use of diuretics, angiotensin-converting enzyme (ACE) inhibitors, and various renal replacement therapies. The hemodynamic and renal effects of surgery and cardiopulmonary bypass/deep hypothermic arrest are addressed in Chapter 20. The hemodynamic effects of inotropes and vasodilators used to treat congestive heart failure (CHF) are discussed in Chapter 7.

113

VASOMOTOR BALANCE IN THE KIDNEY

In the normal kidney, the delicate balance between vasodilator and vasoconstrictor effects favors vasodilation, allowing normal renal blood flow (RBF), glomerular filtration rate (GFR), and salt and water handling. The spectrum of renal dysfunction syndromes associated with heart disease, ranging from oliguria and fluid retention to prerenal azotemia to frank renal failure, reflects a disruption of the vasomotor balance with increased vasoconstrictor effects. Several signaling molecules govern the balance between renal vasodilation and vasoconstriction.

Renal Vasodilation

Atrial Natriuretic Peptide and Brain Natriuretic Peptide

The natriuretic peptides make up a family of polypeptide hormones that regulate blood volume. These peptides originate in the atria and the brain. The subsequent discussion focuses on atrial natriuretic peptide (ANP), because of the greater body of pediatric and developmental data on ANP than on brain natriuretic peptide (BNP).

ANP is a major renal vasodilator hormone. ANP levels are closely tied to the extent of circulating volume expansion, because ANP is produced by the endothelial cells of both atria in response to atrial distention, which occurs after expansion of the circulating blood volume. This peptide hormone produces natriuresis, diuresis, vasodilation, and hypotension via guanylate cyclase–linked membrane receptors.

The effects of ANP depend on the age of the patient and duration of volume expansion. The newborn appears to be relatively insensitive to the natriuretic and diuretic effects of ANP after volume expansion.[110] The decreased ANP response may arise from decreased ANP secretion (despite the volume stimulus) or reduced neonatal ANP receptor-binding capacity.[14,110] This decreased ANP response may play a role in the diminished ability of the newborn to tolerate volume overload.

In the presence of *acute* volume overload and atrial distention, there is increased ANP secretion, which is associated with subsequent natriuresis and diuresis, resulting in the restoration of normal salt and water balance. However, in established CHF, natriuresis and diuresis are diminished, despite increased ANP levels.[73] Paradoxically, avid sodium and water retention occurs in severe CHF despite elevated ANP levels. This results from decreased renal responsiveness to endogenous ANP.

Prostaglandin E_2 and I_2

Intrarenal vasodilatory prostaglandins such as prostaglandin E_2 (PGE_2) and I_2 are important in maintaining RBF in the face of systemic vasoconstriction. With low cardiac output, systemic blood pressure is maintained by release of vasoconstrictor substances including angiotensin II and vasopressin.[50,104] Intrarenal vasodilatory prostaglandins appear to counteract the effects of these vasoconstrictor compounds in experimental models of CHF.[6,93,107,131] The net effect of PGE_2 is to preserve RBF and salt excretion.[10] Patients with CHF have high levels of prostaglandins in the circulation,[21] and inhibitors of prostaglandin synthesis may precipitate acute renal failure in patients with marginal circulatory status.[40,83,126] This supports a role for vasodilatory prostaglandins in ameliorating the effects of systemic vasoconstrictors at the afferent arteriole, thereby maintaining glomerular blood flow.

Nitric Oxide, Bradykinin, Adrenomedullin

Nitric oxide (NO) has a basal vasodilatory effect in the kidney. Blockade of basal NO synthesis results in decreases in RBF and GFR.[4] The balance between NO and angiotensin II may be responsible for maintenance of the renal circulation.[109] NO appears to be an important component, or even the final common pathway, for other vasodilator pathways including those involving adrenomedullin and the angiotensin II receptor subtype 2–bradykinin system.

Bradykinin dilates the renovascular bed. Blockade of the renin-angiotensin system with angiotensin-converting enzymes (ACE) inhibitors decreases both systemic and glomerular capillary pressures, not only by lowering angiotensin II levels but also by increasing bradykinin levels.[127] Recent data suggest that the angiotensin II receptor is divided into two subtypes (AT1 and AT2). AT1 blockade with drugs, such as losartan or candesartan, appears to lead to increased circulating levels of angiotensin II (or its metabolites), which is free to bind to the AT2 receptor subtype. The subsequent AT2 activation initiates a vasodilator cascade involving bradykinin, NO, and cyclic guanosine 5-monophosphate.[111]

Adrenomedullin is the most recently described renal vasodilator.[59] Adrenomedullin causes an increase in RBF, which can be attenuated by inhibition of nitric oxide synthase, suggesting that the vasodilatory effect of adrenomedullin is mediated by NO.[80] Increased concentrations of this peptide appear to be associated with a variety of cardiovascular diseases including CHF, hemorrhagic shock, septic shock, and pulmonary hypertension. Moderate elevations of adrenomedullin concentration may be beneficial in promoting salt and water excretion in heart failure or pulmonary vasodilation in pulmonary hypertension.[84] In septic shock, significant elevations in adrenomedullin correlate with severity of hypotension.[88]

Renal Vasoconstriction

Renin-Angiotensin-Aldosterone System

The renin-angiotensin-aldosterone system (RAAS) performs an essential role in regulation of systemic blood pressure and renal vascular resistance in normal and diseased states. The juxtaglomerular apparatus in the kidney contains the modified smooth muscle cells that synthesize and release renin. Renin converts angiotensinogen to angiotensin I, which, in turn, is converted to angiotensin II by the action of ACE (Fig. 4-1). Angiotensin II stimulates the secretion of aldosterone from the adrenal cortex. Within this system, angiotensin II is the major vasoconstrictor. RAAS acts as an integrated feedback loop system to defend circulating blood volume and pressure. Any decrease in intraarterial blood volume decreases renal artery pressure and increases renal nerve discharge. Both events stimulate increased renin secretion from the juxtaglomerular apparatus. The resultant increase in angiotensin II constricts

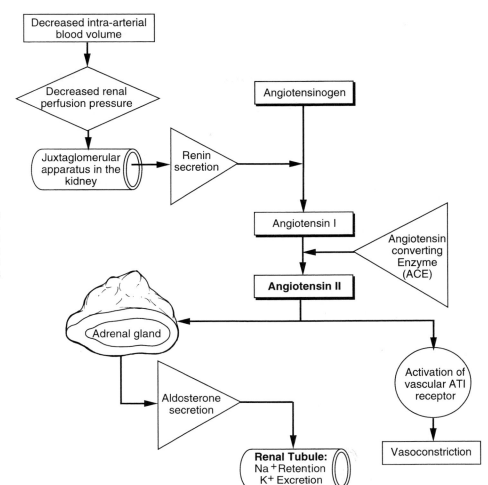

FIGURE 4-1 Integrated feedback loop of the renin-angiotensin-aldosterone system (RAAS). A reduction in blood volume or renal perfusion pressure leads to a cascade of events, which ultimately restore blood volume and perfusion pressure. Angiotensin II is central to this cascade.

systemic vessels primarily by activating the angiotensin II sub-receptor type 1 (AT1). The increased aldosterone levels promote sodium and water retention and potassium excretion by the kidney. The reduction in vascular capacity by vasoconstriction combines with salt and water retention to restore blood volume and renal perfusion pressure. The activity of RAAS depends on age. Newborns have a very active RAAS with increased renin gene expression, angiotensin II expression, and plasma renin activity.[121] The greater activity of RAAS in the newborn may explain the newborn's increased sensitivity to ACE inhibitors.

Endothelial Vasoconstrictors: Endothelin, Thromboxane A₂, Prostaglandin H₂

The vascular endothelium plays a critical role in the maintenance of GFR during hypoperfusion. Endothelial cells produce vasoactive substances that control the caliber and resistance of intrarenal vessels. It is likely that an altered balance of vasodilator and vasoconstrictor agents, caused at least in part by endothelial injury, underlies the alterations in renal perfusion and GFR that occur with hypoperfusion.

The injured endothelium is a source of several vasoconstrictors implicated in acute renal failure (ARF).[118,130]

These include the potent vasoconstrictor endothelin[49] and products of the cyclooxygenase pathway, including thromboxane A₂, prostaglandin H₂, and superoxide anions.[118,130] Plasma endothelin levels are elevated in patients with ARF, due to increased production as well as release, and they decline with recovery.[118,130] Infusion of anti-endothelin antibody in a branch of the renal artery in ischemic ARF in the rat produces increased single nephron GFR and renal plasma flow and decreased afferent and efferent arteriolar resistance when compared to controls with ischemia but without anti-endothelin antibody.[63] This provides evidence that local endothelial endothelin production in the kidney is an important pathogenic factor in ischemic renal injury. Endothelins 1 and 3, and endothelin receptors ETA and ETB, are found in the kidney; ETA is dominant in vessels, ETB in tubules. The ETA receptor is vasoconstrictive; ETB is vasodilatory via linkage to NO generation.[36] Inhibition of both ETA and ETB receptors ameliorates acute injury.[31] However, blockade of both may have deleterious effects on long-term kidney function, potentially via growth factor and cytokine effects.[32,106]

Thromboxane A₂, a cyclooxygenase metabolite of arachidonic acid, is synthesized by thromboxane synthetase in glomerular, tubular, and endothelial cells. This compound produces smooth muscle constriction and platelet aggregation, and stimulates cellular proliferation and extracellular matrix production. RBF decreases in experimental models with exaggerated renal thromboxane production.[16,62,95,107] In vitro, thromboxane-mimetic agents cause an increase in renal vascular resistance and mesangial cell contraction.[17,27] Hechtman and others[56,61,66] have documented increased thromboxane release following transient renal artery ligation. Pretreatment with thromboxane synthetase inhibitors prevented the increase in serum creatinine and acute tubular necrosis seen in this model. There is evidence that thromboxane may in part mediate renal injury due to oxygen free radicals in ischemia/reflow.[5,57]

Stress Hormone Response

Catecholamines and arginine vasopressin (antidiuretic hormone, ADH) decrease RBF and GFR. The infant with heart disease may encounter a variety of stimuli that increase the release of these stress hormones. Common stimuli include hypovolemia, hypoxia, hypercarbia, hypothermia, and pain.

RENAL RESPONSES DURING CARDIAC DYSFUNCTION

Pathophysiology of Salt and Water Retention

Cardiac dysfunction may generate a series of neural, vascular, and renal events that combine to produce the picture of CHF. As cardiac output decreases, reflex sympathetic activation results in redistribution of blood flow away from the kidney (to the heart and brain) and redistribution of blood flow within the kidney. Plasma norepinephrine levels are elevated significantly in patients with CHF. The resultant renal vasoconstriction decreases peritubular capillary and ultimately renal interstitial hydrostatic pressure. Systemic vasoconstriction increases systemic, peritubular capillary, and renal interstitial oncotic pressure. The net effect of reduced interstitial hydrostatic pressure and increased interstitial oncotic pressure is to augment salt and water reabsorption by the kidney (Fig. 4-2).

Cardiac dysfunction also leads to several hormonal stimuli that stimulate salt and water retention. Decreased RBF

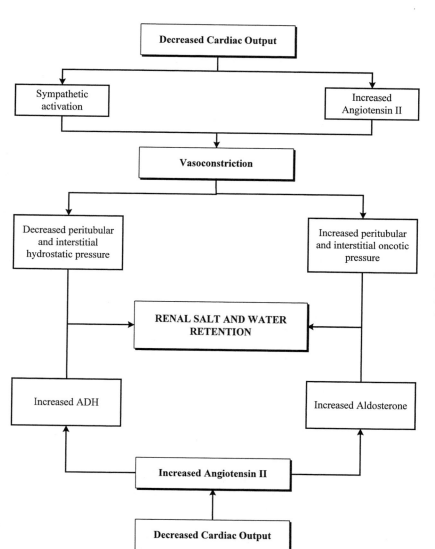

FIGURE 4-2   Pathophysiology of salt and water retention in the child with cardiac dysfunction. Note the combination of physical factors (hydrostatic and oncotic pressure changes) with hormonal stimuli (antidiuretic hormone and aldosterone).

activates the RAAS. Angiotensin II stimulates the release of arginine vasopressin (ADH) from the brain and aldosterone from the adrenal cortex. ADH increases water absorption from the distal tubule, while aldosterone promotes tubular sodium and water retention.

Under normal circumstances, ANP promotes salt and water excretion, which tends to counteract the effects of ADH and aldosterone. Children and adults with CHF have increased ANP levels but are resistant to the renal effects of ANP.[47] The extent of the increase in ANP correlates with severity of right or left ventricular dysfunction and may predict mortality.[77,122] In addition to disease state, surgical technique may affect atrial distention and ANP levels. Total cavopulmonary connection for the Fontan operation is associated with lower ANP levels than the atriopulmonary connection; and patients with a cavopulmonary connection appear to have better outcomes.[132]

Angiotensin and Aldosterone Effects on the Heart

Research in the past decade has shown that angiotensin and aldosterone not only exhibit vascular and renal effects, but also affect tissue repair and remodeling of the heart (Fig. 4-3). The extracellular fibrillar collagen network of the myocardium helps maintain tissue integrity as well as systolic and diastolic pump function. Elevations of circulating and myocardial angiotensin II and aldosterone first result in an adaptive response to myocardial injury by promoting wound healing. However, chronic elevation of angiotensin II and aldosterone produces myocardial fibrosis, in part because of the accumulation of extracellular matrix proteins,[13] analogous to fibrogenic effects in the kidney.[22,78]

Myocardial injury or possibly myocardial stretch from pressure or volume overload upregulates the RAAS in the heart. Renin, angiotensinogen, and angiotensinogen-converting enzyme are upregulated within the myocyte.[134] There is also increased uptake of renin and angiotensinogen from the circulation. The net effect of upregulation and increased uptake of RAAS components is to increase cardiac angiotensin II levels.[67,105] Angiotensin II binds to AT1 subreceptors to trigger myocyte hypertrophy and apoptosis.[67] In addition to the direct effect of angiotensin II on the myocyte through AT1 activation, programmed cell death also occurs because angiotensin II activates the p53 tumor suppressor gene, which encodes a protein that upregulates proapoptotic genes (Bax) and downregulates antiapoptotic genes (Bcl-2) in the myocyte. These molecular events may explain the myocyte apoptosis in the failing human heart.[84]

Aldosterone also affects the cardiac extracellular matrix in heart failure. The mineralocorticoid receptor is expressed in cardiac myocytes.[133] Following activation of the mineralocorticoid

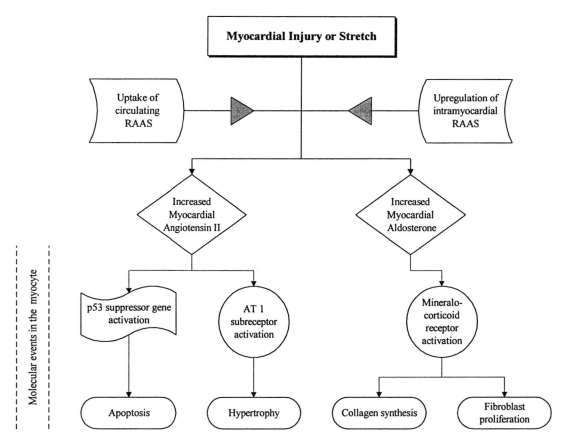

FIGURE 4-3   Molecular events following myocardial injury or stretch lead to elevated intramyocardial angiotensin II and aldosterone levels. In turn these hormones activate receptors or upregulate genes, which results in myocyte hypertrophy, fibrosis, and apoptosis.

receptor, aldosterone stimulates cardiac collagen synthesis and fibroblast proliferation.[11] Treatment with spironolactone, an aldosterone receptor antagonist, reduces the left ventricular volume and mass, suggesting that aldosterone contributes to ventricular dilation and hypertrophy in heart failure.[134]

Management

Management of salt and water retention is a vital component of the care of most children with critical heart disease. The complex and interrelated adaptations of the renal and neuroendocrine systems described previously often dictate a combination of therapies including diuretics, ACE inhibitors, AT1 receptor antagonists, and mineralocorticoid receptor antagonists.

Diuretics

Furosemide is the most commonly used diuretic in the child with critical heart disease. It is a "loop" diuretic, which primarily inhibits electrolyte reabsorption in the ascending limb of the loop of Henle, but also in the distal renal tubule. Furosemide may also produce renal vasodilation, which promotes diuresis. The diuresis begins within 1 hour of intravenous administration and results in urinary loss of all electrolytes. However, chloride and potassium losses deserve particular attention. Chloride and potassium losses frequently produce a hypokalemic, hypochloremic metabolic alkalosis.

The dosing strategy for furosemide depends on the clinical scenario and the patient's age. Fluid accumulation in the first 72 hours after open-heart surgery is generally treated with furosemide 1 mg/kg intravenously every 4 to 12 hours. Shorter dosing intervals should be used with caution in the newborn, in whom elimination of furosemide is delayed. Continuous furosemide infusion (0.1 mg/kg per hour) may achieve nearly equivalent total urine output over 24 hours as the intermittent regimen.[72] Although either intermittent or continuous furosemide is usually safe in this setting, the continuous regimen may permit diuresis with a lower total furosemide dose and greater hemodynamic stability even if the furosemide is started within 6 hours of surgery.[72]

Thiazide diuretics can be used to manage the child with chronic heart failure as an alternative to furosemide. Alternatives to furosemide deserve consideration, because furosemide activates the RAAS, which may contribute to myocardial remodeling and fibrosis.[97] Thiazides act by inhibiting sodium and chloride reabsorption in the distal convoluted tubule and a portion of the ascending limb of the loop of Henle. The diuresis peaks approximately 4 hours after administration and may last for 12 hours. Like furosemide, thiazides may produce hyponatremia and hypokalemia. However, in contrast to furosemide, thiazides may lead to hypercalcemia, hyperuricemia, or hyperglycemia. Typical dosages for chlorothiazide are 10 to 20 mg/kg per day orally divided once or twice daily.

Spironolactone, an aldosterone-receptor antagonist, has reemerged as an important component of congestive heart failure therapy. Spironolactone is a potassium-sparing diuretic. Its use declined during the 1980s and 1990s as ACE inhibitors combined with loop diuretics (with or without digoxin) became

standard therapy for CHF. Because aldosterone secretion is triggered by angiotensin II, it was presumed that ACE inhibition would prevent the secondary hyperaldosteronemia associated with heart failure. However, studies showed that ACE inhibitors accomplished only transient suppression of aldosterone secretion in many patients—a situation termed "aldosterone-escape."[116] The potential causes of aldosterone-escape include impaired hepatic metabolism of aldosterone in patients with heart failure, angiotensin-independent mechanisms for aldosterone release, and possibly genetic predisposition.[3,15,92]

A large randomized controlled trial has added powerful evidence to the theoretical arguments for aldosterone antagonism in patients with heart failure. The Randomized Aldactone Evaluation Study (RALES) showed that spironolactone added to standard therapy of an ACE inhibitor and a loop diuretic significantly reduced the risk of hospitalization or death for adults with heart failure compared to standard therapy alone.[98] To date there have been no similar large controlled trials in children, but the combination of laboratory and adult data suggests that spironolactone should be included in the therapy for children with heart failure.

The dose of spironolactone in children is 1 to 3 mg/kg per day orally taken as a single dose or divided in up to four doses. The major adverse reaction to spironolactone is hyperkalemia, and it is therefore contraindicated in patients with anuria, renal failure, or preexisting hyperkalemia.

Although still in clinical trials, ANP therapies may become an important approach to diuretic therapy for heart failure. Intravenous infusion of ANP causes a transient increase in urine output and cardiac output without activation of the RAAS.[82] Another approach to ANP therapy for heart failure involves inhibition of the enzyme neutral endopeptidase, which is responsible for the degradation of ANP. Oral candoxatril (after hydrolysis in the liver to candoxatrilat) is a specific neutral endopeptidase inhibitor that has a diuretic effect equivalent to furosemide 20 mg per day in adults with mild heart failure.[90] Further studies will be required to understand the role of endopeptidase inhibition in the treatment of heart failure, because not all endopeptidase inhibitors have produced a beneficial effect in heart failure.[91]

Angiotensin-Converting Enzyme Inhibitors

The prominent role of angiotensin II in the pathogenesis of heart failure makes inhibition of ACE a rational component of therapy. Heart failure from poor contractile function or left-to-right shunts and pulmonary overcirculation may indicate the need for ACE inhibition. Patients with moderate cardiac dysfunction after heart surgery may benefit from relief of systemic vasoconstriction by the use of an ACE inhibitor. A special situation is the child with single ventricle and bidirectional cavopulmonary anastomosis, in whom perioperative administration of an ACE inhibitor may decrease pleural effusions after surgery.[117]

Most experience with ACE inhibition in children has come from captopril (0.15 to 0.5 mg/kg twice to four times daily). Since captopril may cause hypotension, it is wise to begin with the lowest dose and increase daily as tolerated. This is especially true in the newborn. Because captopril is excreted by the kidney, the dose must be adjusted in patients with renal insufficiency. Enalapril is an alternative to captopril with the advantage of requiring only once or twice daily administration. Although there is no published pediatric experience yet, angiotensin subreceptor type 1 antagonists (e.g., losartan, valsartan, candesartan) may find a role in pediatric heart failure management by blocking the specific angiotensin II receptor rather than relying on ACE inhibition to prevent angiotensin II formation.

ACUTE RENAL FAILURE

Congenital heart disease surgery is the most common cause of ARF in the newborn.[81] Hypovolemia, hypotension, hypoxemia, hypercarbic acidosis, hypothermia, and other critical events in the perioperative period of the patient with congenital heart disease increase the risk of renal failure. Renal vasoconstriction and decreased renal perfusion represent the common denominator of the events leading to renal failure in the cardiac population. Depending on the duration and severity of the triggering event, the renal response will present either as prerenal azotemia, with little or no structural damage to the kidney, or as ARF, with tissue injury particularly involving the renal tubules. Postrenal failure secondary to obstruction of the genitourinary tract is uncommon in children with critical heart disease but should be excluded if the etiology of renal failure is unclear. Oliguria or anuria is the cardinal sign of renal failure.

Prerenal Azotemia

Severe dehydration or a moderate decrease in cardiac output, RBF, and GFR for other reasons increases renal vascular resistance before significant structural injury to the kidney ensues. Prerenal azotemia is the result and is characterized by avid salt and water reabsorption in the renal tubules. The patient becomes oliguric (<1 mL/kg/hr) and exhibits a characteristic urine and serum chemistry pattern (Table 4-1). The fractional excretion of sodium (urine/plasma Na^+ ÷ urine/plasma creatinine) decreases to less than 1%. Urine osmolality

Table 4-1 Typical Laboratory Data to Distinguish Prerenal Azotemia from Acute Renal Failure

Parameter	Prerenal Azotemia	Acute Renal Failure
Urine$_{Na}$ (mmol/L)	<20	>40
FE$_{Na}$ (%)	<1	>3
U/P osmolality ratio	>1.5	1–1.5
BUN/creatinine ratio	>20:1	10–15:1
Urine specific gravity	>1.020	~1.010
RI (Doppler ultrasound)	<0.71	>0.71

FE$_{Na}$, fractional excretion of sodium; U, urine; P, plasma; Na, sodium; BUN, blood urea nitrogen; Cr, creatinine; RI, resistive index based on renal blood flow velocity measured by Doppler ultrasound.[54]

$$FE_{Na} = \frac{U_{Na} \times P_{Cr}}{P_{Na} \times U_{Cr}} \times 100$$

$$RI = \frac{Peak\ systolic\ velocity - End\ diastolic\ velocity}{Mean\ velocity}$$

and specific gravity are elevated (>600 mOsm and >1.020, respectively). The serum urea nitrogen (SUN) increases disproportionately compared to serum creatinine, with a SUN/creatinine ratio of greater than 20:1.

This condition is rapidly reversible if fluid volume expansion and/or inotropic support normalize renal perfusion. The child with heart disease requires especially careful titration of fluid administration in this setting. In the postoperative period, additional fluid is given to optimize filling pressures in the hope of increasing urine output. Repeated small (5 mL/kg) aliquots are safer than a large bolus (20 mL/kg). Fluid administration is halted when the calculated fluid deficit has been replaced, the desired urine output has been achieved, or filling pressures have reached an upper limit (typically central venous pressure 10 to 15 mm Hg and left atrial pressure 10 to 12 mm Hg).

Dopamine is the drug most commonly considered in the management of prerenal azotemia, once hypovolemia has been repaired. Although infants and children very commonly receive an inotropic agent after cardiac surgery, dopamine should be specifically considered if urine output is poor. Of the commonly used inotropes, only dopamine (0.5 to 2.0 mcg/kg per minute) improves renal blood flow through direct renal vasodilation mediated by dopaminergic (DA1 and DA2) receptors.[25,38,49] The increase in RBF is associated with an increase in GFR and fractional excretion of sodium.[35] Higher doses (5 to 10 mcg/kg per minute) stimulate β1 receptors in the heart, leading to increased cardiac output (see Chapter 7 on Pharmacology). Dopamine increases natriuresis and diuresis even in the absence of improved RBF, an effect thought to be due to direct inhibition of tubular sodium reabsorption.[44] A combination of loop diuretics and dopamine may have a synergistic effect.[69,70]

The beneficial physiologic effects of low-dose dopamine have fed the hope that it would prevent or treat renal failure, which is associated with high mortality rates in the intensive care unit. No randomized controlled trial has addressed this question in postoperative pediatric cardiac patients. However, data from a large randomized controlled trial in adults as well as a meta-analysis of several smaller trials have shown convincingly that low-dose dopamine does *not* prevent or treat ARF in adults.[7,58] Thus, pending similar trials in children, it appears that dopamine should not be used with the expectation of preventing or treating acute renal failure. It remains a useful drug to increase cardiac output in low output states and to promote diuresis in patients with fluid overload.

Fenoldopam is the most recent addition to the family of drugs with specific dopamine DA1 receptor agonist properties. It also stimulates alpha$_2$-adrenergic receptors and leads to systemic vasodilation and specifically renal vasodilation. The treatment of malignant hypertension constitutes the approved indication for fenoldopam in adults. Animal data suggest that fenoldopam preserves RBF, GFR, and natriuresis in the face of severe hypovolemia.[41] This finding has led to interest in fenoldopam as a potential renoprotective drug during renal ischemia. To date, there is no large-scale, published experience with fenoldopam in children.

Mannitol is not used in the treatment of CHF or ARF but is frequently administered before or during cardiopulmonary bypass to protect renal function from the deleterious effects of the low and non-pulsatile flow. These factors and hypothermia combine to redistribute the reduced RBF from the outer cortex to the inner cortex, which reduces GFR.[124]

Mannitol acts as an osmotic diuretic. It begins exerting its effect in the proximal tubule. The increase in osmolarity of the tubular fluid leads to a passive increase in water excretion. Mannitol increases RBF either directly because of increased plasma volume (by drawing water intravascularly from the extracellular fluid), or by increasing prostaglandin production and vasodilating the renal cortical vasculature.[53] Increased blood volume alone is not the sole explanation for improved urine output, because experimental volume expansion with saline improves RBF without improving GFR, whereas mannitol improves both. The improvement in GFR and RBF with mannitol is associated with a decrease in both afferent and efferent arteriolar resistance, which may be mediated in part by prostaglandin release, because the effect is blunted by previous treatment with inhibitors of prostaglandin synthesis.[55] The prophylactic administration of mannitol attenuates the decrease in GFR and urine output in the settings of experimental[53] and clinical renal ischemia (aortic cross-clamp, cardiopulmonary bypass). Depending on the dose, addition of mannitol to the cardiopulmonary bypass priming solution may promote diuresis during the early postoperative period.[29] Careful maintenance of adequate intravascular volume and electrolyte balance during the early postoperative period is necessary when large doses of mannitol have been added to the cardiopulmonary bypass priming solution.

Clinical studies comparing prophylactic mannitol or furosemide with maintenance of adequate intravascular volume during cardiopulmonary bypass showed no reduction in the incidence of postoperative renal dysfunction using either therapy.[23,100] Most studies have been done in adults and are remarkable for the low incidence of postoperative renal dysfunction in both control and diuretic patients when compared to previous retrospective studies. With improved monitoring and intraoperative preservation of renal function, it has become clear that postoperative acute renal failure occurs predominantly in patients in whom cardiac output remains inadequate for prolonged periods.[43]

Acute Renal Failure from Renal Tubular Cell Injury

While the term acute tubular necrosis (ATN) is embedded firmly in medical jargon, it no longer accurately characterizes the pathogenesis of ARF from renal parenchymal injury, because sublethal tubular cell injury (rather than necrosis) may cause the clinical picture of ARF. The major triggers of renal parenchymal injury in the child with critical heart disease include shock, drug toxicity, and sepsis. The triggering event creates a scenario in which several subsequent insults such as renal ischemia, reduced glomerular permeability, "backleak" of glomerular filtrate into the interstitium, and/or tubular obstruction from cellular swelling or debris lead to actual acute renal failure.

Ultimately, prolonged renal hypoperfusion will result in tissue hypoxia, cellular adenosine triphosphate depletion, and failure of tubular cell function. If more marked reduction in GFR with filtration failure or other factors such as tubular

obstruction supervene, the patient may become anuric. A minority of patients may present with nonoliguric renal failure, defined as rapidly increasing serum creatinine in the face of normal urine output. This condition is difficult to diagnose without a high index of suspicion and close monitoring of serum creatinine.

Tubular cell injury is manifested initially by alterations in mitochondrial function and loss of regulation of intracellular electrolytes, as membrane integrity and function of intracellular ion pumps are compromised. Calcium, sodium, and chloride accumulate in the cell, while potassium and phosphate levels decrease.[74,113,115] Morphologically, the earliest alterations are ultrastructural, with swelling and disruption of mitochondrial cristae, and alterations in cell membranes, including blebbing and loss of microvilli from the apical surface and loss of organization in basolateral infoldings.[101] These early changes are sublethal and potentially reversible. Advanced changes, including condensation within and disruption of mitochondria, nuclear changes, and loss of plasma membrane integrity, are irreversible and reflect cell death. Alterations in cell cytoskeleton and attachment factors may also lead to exfoliation of sublethally injured cells.[102]

The diagnosis of ARF is suspected when a triggering event is followed by oliguria. The diagnosis is established by noting the typical changes in serum and urine chemistries, which include increasing serum creatinine and BUN, urine/plasma osmolality ratio of 1.0–1.5, urine sodium greater than 40 mmol/L, and fractional excretion of sodium greater than 3% (see Table 4-1). A variety of potentially life-threatening electrolyte abnormalities, such as hyperkalemia, hyperuricemia, hyperphosphatemia, and hypocalcemia, also offer clues to the presence of ARF. The immediate medical management of ARF requires preventing or treating these electrolyte abnormalities and limiting fluid intake to a volume equal to the urine output plus insensible losses (Table 4-2).

Table 4-2 Noninvasive Management of Fluid and Electrolyte Complications in Acute Renal Failure

Condition	Management
Hyperkalemia K$^+$ > 6.0 mEq/L (mmol/L)	Calcium chloride 10 mg/kg/dose IV* Bicarbonate 1 mEq/kg/dose IV† 25% dextrose 2 mL/kg IV (0.5 g/kg) plus regular insulin 0.1 unit/kg IV Kayexalate 1 g/kg PR or NG
Hypocalcemia Ionized Ca^{++} < 0.9 mmol/L	Calcium chloride 10 mg/kg/dose IV
Hyperuricemia Uric acid > 9.0 mg/dL (>0.5 mmol/L)	Allopurinol 10 mg/kg/day PO or NG ÷ TID‡ (25%–33% of maintenance rate + urine output replacement)
Fluid restriction	(25%–33% of maintenance rate + urine output replacement)

*Calcium chloride should be given via a central venous line to avois extravasation and tissue necrosis.
†Bicarbonate is not compatible with calcium chloride. Flush between injections.
‡Allopurinol dose must be adjusted in renal failure. The patient may require early dialysis, because hydration and alkalinization are important components of hyperuricemia therapy, which may not be tolerated by the cardiac patient.

INVASIVE MANAGEMENT OF ACUTE RENAL FAILURE

Indications

Often, medical management fails to control ARF and sodium, potassium, and water overload occur. The indications for initiating dialysis therapy in the postoperative cardiac patient are not always clear. The following guidelines may be helpful in determining which children will benefit from dialysis therapy:

1. Hypervolemia: volume overload with evidence of pulmonary edema or hypertension, particularly in the setting of impaired myocardial function after cardiopulmonary bypass. High filling pressures may serve as a guide to the need for dialysis.
2. Hyperkalemia: potassium greater than 6.5 mEq/L despite conservative measures or greater than 6.0 mEq/L in a hypercatabolic patient. All postoperative patients are hypercatabolic.
3. Metabolic acidosis: persistent metabolic acidosis with a serum HCO_3 less than 10 mEq/L and arterial pH less than 7.2, with no response to therapy.
4. Azotemia: elevated BUN level greater than 150 mg/dL or lower if rapidly increasing or associated with symptoms (change in mental status, bleeding, pericardial rub).
5. Neurologic complications: presence of neurologic symptoms and signs secondary to uremia or electrolyte imbalance.
6. Calcium and phosphorus imbalance: symptomatic hypocalcemia with tetany or seizures, in the presence of high serum phosphate.

In some circumstances, earlier dialysis may be warranted. For example, patients who have recently undergone cardiac surgery or have impaired myocardial function may not tolerate the degree of hypervolemia or hyperkalemia that a patient with normal cardiac function might tolerate.[76] Pulmonary edema may prevent appropriate respiratory compensation for metabolic acidosis and, therefore, force initiation of dialysis therapy for the fluid overloaded, acidotic patient. Conditions that result in a hypercatabolic state such as cardiac surgery, fever, or sepsis may necessitate earlier dialysis. Finally, early initiation of dialysis could be considered in the face of prolonged oliguria to allow adequate nutrition.

Once the decision has been made to dialyze, the specific form of therapy most beneficial to the individual needs to be determined. Options include peritoneal dialysis (PD), hemodialysis (HD), continuous arteriovenous hemofiltration (CAVH), and continuous venovenous hemofiltration (CVVH). The relative benefits and potential complications of each of these modalities are listed in Table 4-3.

Peritoneal Dialysis

Principles and Considerations of Peritoneal Dialysis

The functional PD system consists of three basic components: (1) the abdominal vasculature, (2) the semi-permeable peritoneal membrane, and (3) the peritoneal cavity. The peritoneal cavity is a potential space into which dialysis solution is

Table 4-3 Comparison of Peritoneal Dialysis, Hemodialysis, Continuous Arteriovenous Hemofiltration, and Continuous Venovenous Hemofiltration

Parameter	PD	HD	CAVH	CVVH
Indications				
Fluid removal	+	++	++	++
Urea and creatinine clearance	+	++	+	++
Potassium clearance	++	++	+	++
Complications				
Need for heparinization	–	+	+	+
Bleeding	–	+	+	+
Disequilibrium	–	+	–	–
Peritonitis	+	–	–	–
Pancreatitis	+	–	–	–
Protein loss	++	–	–	–
Hypotension	+	++	+	+
Decreased cardiac output	+	+	+	+
Respiratory compromise	+	possible	–	–
Vessel thrombosis		+	+	+
Hyperglycemia	possible	–	–	–
Lactic acidosis	possible	–	possible	–
Other infection		+	+	+
Inguinal hernia	+	–	–	–
Electrolyte imbalance	+	+	+	+

CAVH, continuous arteriovenous hemofiltration; CVVH, continuous venovenous hemofiltration; HD, hemodialysis; PD, peritoneal dialysis.
Modified from Maxwell LG, Colombani PM, Fivush, BA: Renal, endocrine, and metabolic failure. In Rogers, MC (ed): *Textbook of Pediatric Intensive Care*, 2nd ed, vol II. Baltimore: Williams and Wilkins, 1992, p 1152.

instilled. Diffusion of solute occurs bidirectionally across the peritoneal membrane as a consequence of many variables, including solute concentration gradient, blood supply to the peritoneal cavity, dialysate composition, and dialysate distribution.[30] The movement of solvent is determined predominantly by osmotic gradients. Most of the previous variables can be modified, maximizing the benefits of this system for the specific needs of the postoperative cardiac patient with ARF. In children, the higher ratio of the peritoneal surface area to body mass results in very efficient PD, sufficient to achieve desired solute and solvent clearance.[76]

There are very few contraindications to the initiation of acute PD.[1] These include infection of the abdominal wall, significant bowel distention, and communication between the chest and abdominal cavity. PD is quite useful in patients who have unstable hemodynamics or bleeding disorders (see Table 4-3).

Access for Peritoneal Dialysis

The relative ease with which PD catheters may be inserted is one of its benefits.[30,76] There are two different approaches to PD access.[1] The first involves the placement of an acute PD catheter. With no cuff to seal its entry point, this catheter can safely be maintained in children for only approximately 72 hours.[20] Additionally, there are no internal sutures to stabilize this somewhat rigid catheter. This type of acute PD catheter can be inserted at the bedside. The lack of a cuff, however, makes the risk of peritonitis great and necessitates frequent catheter changes. The technique for placement of an acute PD catheter is by Seldinger technique or a trocar to direct catheter insertion. The trocar method is not commonly used due to higher risk for intraabdominal complications.[103] The Cook PD catheters are available in sizes from 5F to 11.5F (Cook Critical Care, Bloomington, IN) and may be placed easily by Seldinger technique. Before placement, a Foley catheter should be inserted into the bladder, and an ultrasound performed to ensure complete bladder drainage. The acute PD catheter can then be safely placed through the linea alba of the rectus sheath 2 to 3 cm below the umbilicus in the midline, with the tip of the catheter directed toward the pelvic gutter.[12]

Another approach is placement of a permanent PD catheter that has a cuff and an internal absorbable suture.[1,28,30,76] These catheters can be used immediately postoperatively, and the cuff significantly decreases the risk of infection. Additionally, this type of catheter can remain in place indefinitely, a useful feature because postoperative cardiac patients may require dialysis over a long period. Unfortunately, the presence of the cuff necessitates operative placement and anesthesia. However, we have been able to place these catheters at the bedside with appropriate anesthesia support. The distal tip of the catheter should be placed in the pelvic gutter to allow for optimal flow. Some centers place PD catheters prophylactically during the cardiac surgery in high-risk patients.[114] There are a vast array of commercially available cuffed catheters for PD access. Because of the size of the abdominal cavity in children, we use single-cuff infant or pediatric catheters exclusively for children who weigh less than 30 kg. If the child weighs more than 30 kg, a double-cuff catheter can be used. This approach has a low complication rate from either placement or infection.

Equipment and Initiation of Peritoneal Dialysis

After placement, either type of PD catheter can be used immediately with any of a number of available dialysis systems. Most of these systems consist of Y-tubing with separate inflow and outflow segments. An infant PD set, the Gesco Dialy-Nate Set (Utah Medical Products, Midvale, UT) can be tolerated by even the smallest infant. The Gesco set requires changing every 48 hours. In our institution, a modification of the Baxter system is used for acute PD (Baxter Healthcare Corp., Deerfield, IL).[99] Alternatively a peritoneal dialysis cycler can be used.[88]

Commercial dialysis fluid is readily available for initiation of PD. The Baxter solution (Baxter HealthCare Corp., Deerfield, IL) for PD contains 132 mEq/L of sodium, 3.5 mEq/L of calcium, 0.5 mEq/L of magnesium, 96 mEq/L of chloride, and 40 mEq/L of lactate. There are three different dextrose concentrations available: D1.5%, D2.5%, and D4.25%. Increasing the dextrose concentration of the dialysis fluid increases the ultrafiltrate volume per pass. Low calcium dialysate is also commercially available, but rarely indicated in the acute setting. Commercially available dialysate solutions contain a relatively low concentration of sodium and also contain lactate. The presence of lactate may not be well tolerated in children with impaired liver function or lactic acidosis. In these circumstances, a bicarbonate-based solution can be used (Table 4-4).

Table 4-4 Electrolyte Composition of Dialysate Solutions

Electrolyte Concentration	Commercially Available Peritoneal Dialysis Solution (1.5% dextrose)	Calcium-Based Filtered Replacement Fluid or Dialysate*	Phosphorus-Based Filtered Replacement Fluid or Dialysate*
Na (mEq/L)	132	140†	140†
K (mEq/L)	0	0–5	0–5
Cl (mEq/L)	96–102	100	100
HCO₃ (mEq/L)	0	40	40
Lactate (mEq/L)	40	0	0
Ca (mEq/L)	3.5	3.0–4.0	0
PO₄ (mEq/L)	0	0	2‡
Mg (mEq/L)	0.5–1.5	0.5–1.5	0.5–1.5
Dextrose (g/L)	15	0–2.0	0–2.0

*Solutions made in the pharmacy with sterile water as the base.
†Sodium concentration is maintained at 140 with both NaCl and NaHCO₃.
‡K₃PO₄ 2 mEq/L provides 2 mEq/L of potassium and 4 mg/dL of phosphorus.
Reprinted with permission from Parekh RS, Bunchman TE: Dialysis support in the pediatric intensive care unit. *Adv Ren Replace Ther* 3(4):326, 1996.

Several important steps go into the treatment of pediatric cardiac patients receiving PD. Unless core cooling is the objective (e.g., junctional ectopic tachycardia), all PD fluid should be warmed to 38°C before instillation into the peritoneal cavity. This can be accomplished by using either a "K-pad" (Aquamatic k-20, American Hospital Supply Corp., Valencia, CA) or a radiant warmer over the dialysate bag or tubing. PD should be initiated with small volumes—approximately 20 mL/kg per pass over the first several days. This allows the catheter's tunnel to heal and avoids catheter leaks. Maintaining the child in the supine position during the initiation phase will minimize intraabdominal pressure and prevent leakage of dialysis fluid.[89] The pass volume is increased as tolerated to a range of 40 to 50 mL/kg per pass usually by the end of the first week of dialysis (Fig. 4-4). The final dialysate volume and the pass frequency, or the time the fluid remains in the abdomen (dwell time), will vary, depending on the specific needs of the patient. Table 4-5 provides general guidelines for optimizing ultrafiltration and solute clearance. In the volume-overloaded postoperative cardiac patient, it is often reasonable to use rapid cycling therapy with hourly cycles and a higher dextrose solution. Alternatively, in the patient with azotemia, longer intraperitoneal dwell times may be necessary for efficient clearance of urea to occur.

During the first 72 hours of PD therapy, heparin may be added to the dialysis fluid at a concentration of 250 U/L. Subsequent heparin usage is necessary only if there is persistent fibrin in the dialysis effluents. Prophylactic antibiotics may be administered intraperitoneally at the time the catheter is placed but are not generally indicated thereafter. White blood cell counts, differentials, and cultures of dialysis effluents are monitored daily as long as the child remains in the hospital; this allows early identification of peritonitis.

As mentioned previously, occasionally it may be necessary to modify the peritoneal dialysis fluid because of hyponatremia and/or the presence of liver dysfunction or lactic acidosis (see Table 4-4).[85] In addition, with continued rapid cycling, hypokalemia may occur. This is of particular concern

MANAGEMENT OF PERITONEAL DIALYSIS

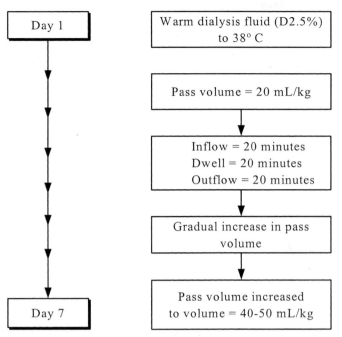

Day 1

Warm dialysis fluid (D2.5%) to 38° C

Pass volume = 20 mL/kg

Inflow = 20 minutes
Dwell = 20 minutes
Outflow = 20 minutes

Gradual increase in pass volume

Pass volume increased to volume = 40-50 mL/kg

Day 7

FIGURE 4-4 Algorithm for management of peritoneal dialysis.

in a postoperative cardiac patient, and potassium may be added to the dialysis fluid at a concentration of 3 to 4 mEq/L to maintain the serum potassium in normal range.

Complications of Peritoneal Dialysis

Even if the catheter has been placed appropriately, primary catheter dysfunction can occur. With an acute catheter, this is often a consequence of omentum wrapped around the catheter. In this situation, fluid can enter the abdominal cavity slowly on inflow, but there is usually poor outflow during the drain phase of the cycle. If this is the problem, it is likely that the catheter will need to be replaced. Partial omentectomies may be routinely performed when permanent catheters are placed to decrease this complication. Dysfunction can also occur as a consequence of fibrin in the catheter lumen. There have been reports of success in salvaging these catheters with the infusion of streptokinase.[8]

Table 4-5 Approaches to Optimizing Ultrafiltration and Solute Clearance During Peritoneal Dialysis

To Improve Ultrafiltration	To Improve Solute Clearance
Increase glucose concentration	Increase dialysate volume
Increase frequency of cycles	For potassium and urea: Increase frequency of cycles
Increase dialysate volume`	For phosphorus: Decrease frequency of cycles

Unfortunately, infection may occur during acute PD and can present as either peritonitis or exit site infection.[20,89,112] Screening for peritonitis should be performed by obtaining frequent white blood cell counts, differentials, and cultures of dialysis effluents. Peritoneal cell counts greater than 100 white blood cells per high power field or the presence of greater than 50% neutrophils on the differential is suggestive of bacterial peritonitis. Peritonitis, when detected early, is usually successfully treated with intraperitoneal antibiotics. Catheter loss occurs rarely as a consequence of infection. Additionally, exit site infections usually respond well to topical antibiotics and vigorous local care.

A special concern in the postoperative cardiac patient with impaired myocardial function on a ventilator is further cardiac or respiratory compromise as a consequence of large peritoneal dialysis volume (see Table 4-3).[18,112,129] It is critical to monitor blood pressure and arterial blood gases closely in this situation. It appears that PD volume is a critical factor for these complex patients. In our experience, infants with critical heart disease can tolerate pass volumes of up to 40 mL/kg, but it is prudent to begin with pass volumes of 10 mL/kg. An arterial line can be extremely useful and should be maintained in the majority of these patients.[76] The hemodynamics and pulmonary compliance usually improve as fluid removal is accomplished with peritoneal dialysis.[128]

Hydrothorax may constitute another potential complication in the cardiac patient undergoing PD. If a chest tube is in place, this complication may result in an excess of chest tube drainage and inadequate PD. To diagnose this suspected complication, simultaneous measurement of glucose in the chest tube drainage, PD effluent, and serum should be performed. If a hydrothorax is present, the glucose concentration in the chest drainage and dialysis effluent will be comparable and typically higher than that in serum. In patients without a chest tube, it may be necessary to perform a diagnostic and therapeutic thoracentesis. If a hydrothorax is confirmed, the peritoneal catheter should be placed to straight drain, which may relieve the hydrothorax and the associated potential for respiratory compromise.

Hemodialysis

HD involves two primary processes, diffusion and ultrafiltration, which occur across a manmade semi-permeable membrane between blood and dialysate compartments.[71] Subsequently, multiple factors significantly impact the diffusion of a substance from blood to dialysate, including solute concentration in blood and dialysate, surface area and permeability characteristics of the dialyzer, and the blood and dialysis flow rate. The primary determinant of ultrafiltration is the hydrostatic pressure generated across the membrane. At present, HD technology is fairly advanced and the hydrostatic pressure differential can be easily manipulated, with predictable fluid removal.[33]

The cardiovascular burden of HD—large solute and solvent shifts, rapid blood flow rate, and significant extracorporeal blood volume—may be poorly tolerated in children with cardiac disease.[60] Additionally, significant hypoxemia may occur during HD, making these patients poor candidates for this aggressive therapy (see Table 4-3).[60] Extreme caution must be used during the initiation phase of HD to avoid overzealous correction of metabolic and fluid derangements associated with ARF.

Hemodialysis Access

HD can be performed in most infants and children because of recent advances in HD access.[30,76] Access can be achieved with either two catheters or one double-lumen catheter in the venous circulation. In newborn infants, umbilical artery vessels may be used, or the catheters may be placed in separate access sites such as the femoral or subclavian veins. In general, if the child weighs less than 7 kg, it will be necessary to place two separate catheters for HD. If the child weighs more than 7 kg, it may be possible for a double-lumen catheter to be safely placed. The double-lumen catheter size should be at least 7F. The efficiency of HD increases with higher flow rates; therefore, the largest catheter possible for a given size child is indicated. In patients who weigh more than 12 kg, placing catheters as large as 9F to 10F is successful. There are many commercially available catheters with these dimensions and of varying lengths. Catheters from Shiley Inc. (Irvine, CA), Quinton Instruments Co. (Seattle, WA), and Medical Components Inc. (Harleysville, PA) give good results. For more specifics on appropriate catheter size and access location, see Table 4-6.

Equipment and Initiation of Hemodialysis

There are many available dialysis machines suitable for children. New machines, using bicarbonate buffer and variable dialysate sodium concentration, have resulted in dramatically improved HD results and should be exclusively used in the postoperative cardiac patient. Additionally, new volumetric technology has allowed very fine regulation of volume removal during this procedure and has improved dialysis even further in complex pediatric patients, particularly those with cardiac dysfunction.[33]

The particular circuit and dialyzer chosen for a given patient are predominantly determined by patient size. The volume of the extracorporeal circuit (blood tubing and dialyzer) should not exceed 10% of the child's calculated blood volume.[119] Neonatal lines (Fresenius USA Inc., Concord, CA) have an 18-mL blood volume, pediatric lines (Fresenius USA Inc., Concord, CA) have a 56-mL volume, and adult lines (C.D. Medical Inc., Miami Lakes, FL) are 120 to 150 mL in volume. The F3 dialyzer (Fresenius) is a hollow fiber dialyzer that has a surface area of 0.35 m² and a blood volume of only 30 mL and is made of polysulfone. This dialyzer is well tolerated by very small infants. The CA50 (Baxter HealthCare Corp., Deerfield, IL) is also a hollow fiber dialyzer, made of cellulose acetate, with a surface area of 0.5 m² and a blood volume of 38 mL. This particular dialyzer yields good clearance and ultrafiltration in small patients as well. A vast array of dialyzers are available for acute HD in patients who weigh more than 20 kg. Neonatal tubing is indicated for any child who weighs less than 13 kg, and pediatric tubing is well tolerated by patients between 13 and 30 kg. In children who weigh more than 30 kg, any standard adult blood tubing is acceptable. See Table 4-6 for specific HD protocols. If the patient weighs less than 5 kg, it is often necessary to prime the tubing and dialyzer with albumin, whole blood, or fresh frozen plasma (not packed cells), which is given to the patient as the dialysis is initiated. If a child weighs more than 5 kg, the small size of available extracorporeal circuits makes whole blood priming unnecessary.

The highly efficient nature of HD causes rapid solute and solvent shifts and, therefore, requires extreme caution during initiation.[75] If correction is too rapid, dialysis disequilibrium

Table 4-6   Equipment for Acute Hemodialysis

| Patient (kg) | DIALYZER | | TUBING | | Total Volume (mL) | Access and Catheters |
	Type	Volume (mL)	Type	Volume (mL)		
Neonate to 6 kg	F3	30	Neonatal	18	48	If no umbilical vessels, two separate sites—femoral artery or vein and superior vena cava (SVC)—with 4F, 5F, or 6F (2–4 in) lines or double-lumen (Cook/Med Comp) 7F (4 in).
7–12	CA 50 or	38	Neonatal	18	56	Double-lumen (Cook/Med Comp) 7F (4 in) or (Med Comp) 9F (4.75 in) in internal jugular, or femoral vessel.
	F4 (Fresenius)	44	Neonatal	18	62	
13–18	F4 (Fresenius)	44	Pediatric	56	100	Double-lumen (Med Comp) 9F (4.75 in) or double-lumen 8F (Arrow International) in internal jugular, or femoral vessel.
19–28	F6 (Fresenius)	83	Pediatric	56	139	Double-lumen (Med Comp) 9F (4–6 in) as above.
> 29	F6 (Fresenius) or	83	Adult	150	233	Double-lumen (Med Comp) 11F (4.75–6 in) or double-lumen 10F (Arrow International).
	SCE 90 (CD Medical)	85	Adult	150	235	

Modified from Maxwell LG, Colombani PM, Fivush BA: Renal, endocrine, and metabolic failure. In Rogers, MC (ed): *Textbook of Pediatric Intensive Care*, 2nd ed, vol II. Baltimore: Williams and Wilkins, 1992, p 1152.

syndrome occurs with resultant seizures. With this in mind, mannitol may be infused over the first hour or two of HD[75] to maintain serum osmolality. The use of mannitol can also be considered in patients with elevated sodium. Urea clearance should be kept below 30% to 40% during the first two to three dialysis procedures.[75] A specific dialysis prescription including blood flow rate and treatment time should be selected that is compatible with this goal. Children can tolerate blood flow rates in the range of 4 to 5 mL/kg per minute. However, during the initiation phase flow rates as low as 2 to 3 mL/kg per minute are recommended. By the third HD run, the blood flow rates can be increased to 5 mL/kg per minute. Net ultrafiltration rate should not exceed 0.2 mL/kg per minute to prevent hemodynamic compromise.

Heparin requirements are difficult to predict accurately for critically ill children who require HD. Many of these children have associated coagulopathies and are relatively anticoagulated. We rely upon frequent activated clotting times (ACT Hemochron Model no. 801, Edison, NJ) to guide systemic heparinization, and we attempt to maintain an activated clotting time (ACT) in the range of 120 to 150 seconds throughout the dialysis run. Often, acutely ill children receive no heparin through the entire procedure. However, if heparin is needed, a dose of 10 to 30 U/kg is given as a bolus, and then an hourly rate of 10 to 20 U/kg per hour is initiated with frequent measurement of ACT to prevent excessive anticoagulation.

Complications of Hemodialysis

It is imperative to carefully control the rate of HD. Rapid shifts in osmolarity result in disequilibrium and possibly cause increased intracranial pressure.[19,64] Because HD is pump-driven, air embolus, hemolysis, and blood loss may occur. Built-in safety features of the dialysis machine minimize these risks (see Table 4-3).

Continuous Arteriovenous Hemofiltration and Continuous Venovenous Hemofiltration

In the past, the use of continuous arteriovenous hemofiltration (CAVH) and continuous venovenous hemofiltration (CVVH) in critically ill infants and children was limited by difficulties in obtaining and maintaining vascular access and the poor availability of appropriately sized equipment. Recent advances in equipment and growing experience in this patient population have now made continuous hemofiltration a very practical option in the infant and young child with ARF. These therapies are particularly attractive in the patient with hemodynamic instability. In addition, these therapies can be helpful in the treatment of oliguric patients in need of better nutritional support, postoperative cardiac patients,[42] and septic patients. Because hemofiltration is a gentle form of continuous renal replacement therapy, it does not appear to adversely affect cardiac output or pulmonary function (see Table 4-3).[65,123] Finally, unlike HD, it does not appear to be associated with significant activation of the complement system,[39,54] making it an extremely useful therapy for the postoperative cardiac patient with volume overload and abnormal renal function.[68]

Access

Because CAVH is driven by the patient's mean arterial pressure, it requires both arterial and venous access. Ideal CAVH catheters should be short in length and large in diameter to provide as little resistance to flow as possible. In small infants who require CAVH, 4F catheters are acceptable for adequate flow and are safely placed in the femoral vessels. Larger children, however, should have at least a 5F catheter placed. The problems of arterial access and adequate mean arterial pressure have severely limited the utility of CAVH except as an adjunct to extracorporeal membrane oxygenation (ECMO). CVVH has become the preferred continuous technique. CVVH, a pump-driven therapy, requires only venous access. As described previously for HD, either a double-lumen venous catheter or two separate catheters can be used. Additionally, the largest possible sized catheters should be placed to assure optimal efficiency (see Table 4-6).

Equipment and Initiation

Because CVVH is a pump-driven therapy, specialized tubing is required for the circuit (Fig. 4-5). The Baxter bm11 Blood Monitor Pump (Baxter HealthCare Corp., Deerfield, IL) has commercially available pediatric tubing, which requires a priming volume of only 37 mL (Nextron, Fairfield, CT).

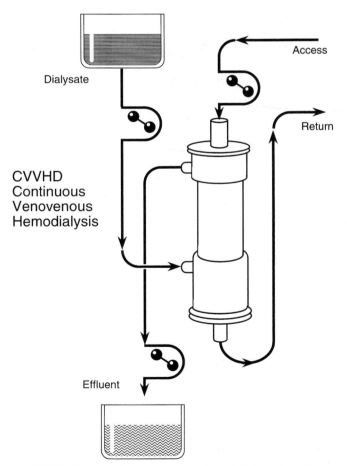

FIGURE 4-5 Continuous venovenous hemodialysis equipment.

Table 4-7 CAVH/CVVH Circuit Volumes and Hemofilter Properties

Patient Size (kg)	Hemofilter	Properties/Surface Area	Printing Volume	Line Volume
<10	Amicon Minifilter Plus	Polysulfone/0.07 m²	15 mL	CAVH—6 mL CVVH—37 mL
10–20	Renaflo II HF 400	Polysulfone/0.3 m²	28 mL	CAVH—14 mL CVVH—37 mL
>20	Renaflo II HF 700	Polysulfone/0.71 m²	53 mL	CAVH—20.3 mL CVVH—110 mL
	or Hospal Multiflow 60	Acrylonitrile and sodium methallyl sulfonate copolymer/0.6 m²	48 mL	CAVH—20.3 mL CVVH—90 ± 10 mL

CAVH, continuous arteriovenous hemofiltration; CVVH, continuous venovenous hemofiltration.

Another system is the Prisma (GAMBRO Healthcorp, Lakewood, CO). However, the only tubing currently available requires a priming volume of 90 ± 10 mL. The choice of hemofilter is based on the CVVH system used and the size and needs of the patient. With the Baxter system, we currently use the Renaflo II HF 400 (Minnetech, Minneapolis, MN) for patients weighing less than 20 kg, and the HF 700 for patients greater than 20 kg. With the Prisma circuit, the filter is an AN-69 membrane (Multiflow 60, Gambro Renal Care, Lakewood, CO). This biocompatible membrane is contraindicated for use in patients taking ACE inhibitors due to excess bradykinin production. The membrane activates prekallikrein and Hageman factor, which results in bradykinin formation. Excess bradykinin leads to vasodilation and subsequent hypotension. Table 4-7 details the required circuit volumes and hemofilter properties for both CAVH and CVVH.

Generally, continuous anticoagulation is necessary to maintain patency of CAVH/CVVH systems. ACT monitoring during therapy ensures adequate anticoagulation and determines the dose of heparin. A baseline ACT guides the initial heparin dose. In general, an ACT between 170 and 200 seconds is maintained.[30] Severely ill children who require CAVH or CVVH may maintain an ACT in this range without any heparinization. Other methods of anticoagulation include citrate, prostacyclin, low-molecular-weight heparin, and serine protease inhibitors.

Once CAVH/CVVH is begun, the goal is to remove excess fluid from the volume-overloaded patient. Hemodynamic compromise is avoided by carefully monitoring the rate at which the plasma ultrafiltrate is generated. With CAVH, an intravenous (IV) infusion pump may be attached to the ultrafiltrate drainage tubing to serve as a controller. The controller is then set so that the combined ultrafiltrate and urinary output exceeds the patient's intake by 5% to 10% of the patient's body weight per day. With CVVH, the Baxter system also requires an IV infusion pump to control the ultrafiltration rate. The relative inaccuracy of the infusion pump in this setting makes it imperative to monitor the dialysate effluent in a graduated cylinder to determine precise output. Conversely, the Prisma system monitors and controls the ultrafiltration rate internally, thus allowing for more controlled ultrafiltration.

One of the advantages of CVVH is the ability to reliably determine and adjust the blood flow rate through the hemofilter. The principles for determining blood flow rate for CVVH are similar to those already outlined for HD. However, because the risk for disequilibrium is lower than that with HD, higher blood flow rates may be used, and rates as high as 5 to 10 mL/kg/min are often well tolerated.

Complications of Continuous Arteriovenous Hemofiltration/Continuous Venovenous Hemofiltration

Hemofiltration is a very gentle form of continuous renal replacement therapy and as such has no absolute contraindications. Hypotension may occur as a consequence of hypovolemia from hemofiltration without appropriate volume replacement (see Table 4-3).[30] To avoid this, the cardiorespiratory status should be monitored frequently. It is important to measure hourly ultrafiltration volume, urinary volume, and hourly input to assure that significant swings in volume do not occur.[30]

Significant electrolyte losses must be anticipated with CAVH/CVVH. Frequent electrolyte monitoring is important to balance these losses. In most cases where hemofiltration has continued for longer than 48 hours, hypokalemia develops, and intravenous replacement is necessary. In general, all non–protein-bound substances freely traverse the semipermeable membrane of the hemofiltration cartridge, resulting in depletion of various substances.

Last, it is often necessary for systemic anticoagulation to be continuous to maintain hemofiltration. It is important to monitor for evidence of external bleeding, particularly at access sites. Inadequate anticoagulation may cause clotting of the hemofilter cartridge. If this occurs, there will be significant blood loss in the circuit, which must be replaced by transfusion.

Continuous Arteriovenous Hemodiafiltration/Continuous Venovenous Hemodiafiltration

Standard hemofiltration may not provide sufficient solute clearance in the patient with significant uremia or electrolyte abnormality. In this circumstance, two approaches to improve solute clearance may be used. The first is to provide filtration replacement fluid, either before or after the hemofilter (see Fig. 4-5). In this method, clearance occurs primarily by convection. The replacement fluid is typically standard peritoneal dialysis fluid, Lactated Ringer's, or a bicarbonate-based solution (see Table 4-4). Another approach is to add countercurrent dialysis. That is, dialysis fluid is introduced into the hemofiltration cartridge, where it surrounds the blood-filled capillary lumen (see Fig. 4-5). The exposure of the blood to dialysate as it traverses the cartridge enhances diffusion dramatically, increasing the clearance of electrolytes. Standard peritoneal dialysis solution or a bicarbonate-based solution can be used (see Table 4-4). The fluid can also be manipulated to regulate any metabolic imbalance that may arise. Because continuous arteriovenous hemodiafiltration (CAVH-D) and continuous venovenous hemodiafiltration (CVVH-D) are continuous therapies, hypokalemia should be anticipated, and often potassium (4 mEq/L) must be added to the dialysis solution.

This therapy has been extremely well tolerated and is very helpful for children requiring intensive dialysis. The gentle continuous nature of hemofiltration and the additional clearance obtained by dialysate makes this an exciting new therapy, one that will probably be used with increasing frequency in postoperative cardiac children.

Continuous Arteriovenous Hemodiafiltration on Extracorporeal Membrane Oxygenation

In patients who require either ultrafiltration or solute clearance while on ECMO, placing a hemofilter within the circuit is quite simple and very efficient, due to the large blood flow rates and consistent heparinization. Although the hemofilter may be placed in series with the oxygenator, if placed in parallel, there may be compromise of blood flow to the oxygenator, as the hemofilter presents a possible shunt through a lower resistance circuit. In addition, the excess blood flow through this smaller system may cause it to rupture. As ECMO flows are being weaned, an obligatory blood flow rate through the hemofiltration system must be added into whatever would be considered the minimum (or idling) ECMO pump rate. The minimum ECMO pump rate should not fall below the sum of the flow rate through the hemofilter (~150 mL/min) and the ECMO pump idle rate (~10%–20% of calculated cardiac output). Finally, the hemofiltration system is another source of air entry into the ECMO circuit. Because air embolism may be fatal, extreme care is required.

POTENTIAL OUTCOMES AND FUTURE DIRECTIONS

Immediate postoperative management of the infant or child requires a multidisciplinary approach with involvement of specialty services for optimal outcome. Additionally, the preoperative condition of the patient, the intraoperative course, and the underlying cardiac defect have a major impact on the ultimate postoperative course.

Unfortunately, despite meticulous management of the patient in the perioperative phase, acute renal failure will develop in some children after surgery. In one study, ARF developed in 2.5% of patients after cardiac surgery.[45] Survival of patients with renal failure is quite variable; in the cited study, the rate was only 35%.[45] The reason for this poor survival is that the ARF is often a marker of poor perioperative condition and hemodynamic instability. It is not the ARF itself that leads to morbidity and mortality, but the continued poor cardiac function in children that is ultimately fatal.[38]

Fortunately, the postoperative cardiac patients who are treated aggressively with dialysis and in whom cardiac function improves can be expected to have reasonable renal recovery. Chronic renal impairment is uncommon in children who recover from acute hemodynamic instability.

One avenue of investigation is the use of hormones and growth factors to speed recovery from acute renal injury. Epidermal growth factor stimulates morphologic and functional recovery following both ischemic and toxic insults in rats.[17,87] Hepatocyte growth factor and insulin-like growth factor-1 (IgG-1) accelerate repair and improve survival.[51,79] IgG-1 has demonstrated preservation of renal function postoperatively,[34] although it does not appear to reverse established renal failure.[46]

Additional new pharmacologic options may become available for preservation of renal function.[37,125] Calcium channel blockers have been used in clinical studies and may have effects on the vasculature as well as cytoprotective effects in the renal tubule. While some studies report that these agents prevent acute tubular necrosis,[26,86] these results are controversial.[2,9] Xanthine oxidase inhibitors and oxygen free radical scavengers, as well as ANP with dopamine, have been efficacious in experimental models of ischemic injury. A full understanding of the potential role of these therapies must await large randomized controlled trials.[9]

Finally, a renal tubular assist device has been developed to be placed in an extracorporeal continuous hemoperfusion circuit in series with a hemofilter.[48] It is hoped that this device may substitute for cellular and metabolic functions of the renal tubule to optimize renal replacement therapy. This sophisticated strategy might ultimately have particular efficacy in the pediatric population.

References

1. Alexander S: Dialysis in children. In Nolph K (ed): *Peritoneal Dialysis.* Boston: Kluwer Academic, 1990, pp 343–364.
2. Amar D, Fleisher M: Diltiazem treatment does not alter renal function after thoracic surgery. *Chest* 119:1476–1479, 2001.
3. Ayers CR, Davis JO, Lieberman F, et al: The effects of chronic hepatic venous congestion on the metabolism of d,l-aldosterone and d-aldosterone. *J Clin Invest* 41:884–895, 1962.
4. Ballevre L, Solhaug MJ, Guignard JP: Nitric oxide and the immature kidney. *Biol Neonate* 70(1):1–14, 1996.
5. Baud L, Nivez MP, Chansel D, Ardaillou R: Stimulation by oxygen radicals of prostaglandin production by rat renal glomeruli. *Kidney Int* 20:332–339, 1981.
6. Baylis C, Brenner BM: Modulation by prostaglandin synthesis inhibitors of the action of exogenous angiotensin II on glomerular ultrafiltration in the rat. *Circ Res* 43:889–898, 1978.
7. Bellomo R, Chapman M, Finfer S, et al: Low-dose dopamine in patients with early renal dysfunction: A placebo-controlled randomised trial. Australian and New Zealand Intensive Care Society (ANZICS) Clinical Trials Group. *Lancet* 356:2139–2143, 2000.
8. Bergstein J, Andreoli S, West K, Grofeld J: Streptokinase therapy for occluded Tenckhoff catheters in children on CAPD. *Perit Dial Int* 8:137–139, 1988.
9. Bock HA, Brunner FP, Torhorst J, Thiel G: Failure of verapamil to protect from ischaemic renal damage. *Nephron* 57:299–305, 1991.
10. Breyer MD, Breyer RM: Prostaglandin E receptors and the kidney. *Am J Physiol Renal Physiol* 279(1):F12–F23, 2000.
11. Brilla CG, Zhou G, Matsubara L, Weber KT: Collagen metabolism in cultured adult rat cardiac fibroblasts: response to angiotensin II and aldosterone. *J Mol Cell Cardiol* 26:809–820, 1994.
12. Bunchman TE: Acute peritoneal dialysis access in infant renal failure. *Perit Dial Int* 16:S509–S511, 1996.

13. Burlew BS, Weber KT: Connective tissue and the heart. Functional significance and regulatory mechanisms. *Cardiol Clin* 18(3):435–442, 2000.
14. Castro R, Leake RD, Ervin MG, et al: Ontogeny of atrial natriuretic factor receptors and cyclic GMP response in rabbit renal glomeruli. *Pediatr Res* 30:45–49, 1991.
15. Cicoira M, Zanolla L, Rossi A, et al: Failure of aldosterone suppression despite angiotensin-converting enzyme (ACE) inhibitor administration in chronic heart failure is associated with ACE DD genotype. *J Am Coll Cardiol* 37(7):1808–1812, 2001.
16. Coffman TM, Yarger WE, Klotman PE: Functional role of thromboxane production by acutely rejecting renal allografts in rats. *J Clin Invest* 75:1242–1248, 1985.
17. Coimbra TM, Cieslinski DA, Humes HD: Epidermal growth factor accelerates renal repair in mercuric chloride nephrotoxicity. *Am J Physiol* 259:F438–F443, 1990.
18. Conger JD, Robinette JB, Schrier RW: Smooth muscle calcium and endothelium-derived relaxing factor in the abnormal vascular responses of acute renal failure. *J Clin Invest* 82:532–537, 1988.
19. Davenport A, Will EJ, Davison AM: Early changes in intracranial pressure during haemofiltration treatment in patients with grade 4 hepatic encephalopathy and acute oliguric renal failure. *Nephrol Dial Transplant* 5:192–198, 1990.
20. Day RE, White RH: Peritoneal dialysis in children. Review of 8 years' experience. *Arch Dis Child* 52:56–61, 1977.
21. Dzau VJ, Packer M, Lilly LS, et al: Prostaglandins in severe congestive heart failure. Relation to activation of the renin-angiotensin system and hyponatremia. *N Engl J Med* 310:347–352, 1984.
22. Epstein M: Aldosterone as a mediator of progressive renal dysfunction: evolving perspectives. *Intern Med* 40:573–583, 2001.
23. Etheredge EE, Levitan H, Nakamura K, Glenn WL: Effect of mannitol on renal function during open-heart surgery. *Ann Surg* 161:53–62, 1965.
24. Favre L, Glasson P, Vallotton MB: Reversible acute renal failure from combined triamterene and indomethacin: a study in healthy subjects. *Ann Intern Med* 96:317–320, 1982.
25. Feltes TF, Hansen TN, Martin CG, et al: The effects of dopamine infusion on regional blood flow in newborn lambs. *Pediatr Res* 21:131–136, 1987.
26. Ferguson CJ, Hillis AN, Williams JD, et al: Calcium-channel blockers and other factors influencing delayed function in renal allografts. *Nephrol Dial Transplant* 5:816–820, 1990.
27. Fifer MA, Molina CR, Quiroz AC, et al: Hemodynamic and renal effects of atrial natriuretic peptide in congestive heart failure. *Am J Cardiol* 65:211–216, 1990.
28. Fine RN: Peritoneal dialysis update. *J Pediatr* 100:1–7, 1982.
29. Fisher AR, Jones P, Barlow P, et al: The influence of mannitol on renal function during and after open-heart surgery. *Perfusion* 13:181–186, 1998.
30. Fivush B, Porter C: Pediatric dialysis therapy. In Solez K, Racusen L (eds): *Acute Renal Failure.* New York: Marcel Dekker, Inc., 1991, pp 417–432.
31. Forbes JM, Leaker B, Hewitson TD, et al: Macrophage and myofibroblast involvement in acute renal failure is attenuated by endothelin receptor antagonists. *Kidney Int* 55:198–208, 1999.
32. Forbes JP, Hewitson TD, Becker GJ, Jones CL: Simultaneous blockade of endothelin A and B receptors in ischemic acute renal failure is detrimental to long-term function. *Kidney Int* 59:1333–1341, 2001.
33. Francisco LL: High efficiency dialysis. *Kidney* 21:7–11, 1988.
34. Franklin SC, Moulton M, Sicard GA, et al: Insuline-like growth factor I preserves renal function postoperatively. *Am J Physiol Renal Physiol* 272:F257–F259, 1997.
35. Furman WR, Summer WR, Kennedy TP, Sylvester JT: Comparison of the effects of dobutamine, dopamine, and isoproterenol on hypoxic pulmonary vasoconstriction in the pig. *Crit Care Med* 10:371–374, 1982.
36. Gariepy CE, Ohuchi T, Williams SC, et al: Salt-sensitive hypertension in endothelin-B receptor deficient rats. *J Clin Invest* 105:925–933, 2000.
37. Farwood S: New pharmacologic options for renal preservation. *Anesthesiol Clin North Am* 18:753–771, 2000.
38. Girardin E, Berner M, Rouge JC, et al: Effect of low dose dopamine on hemodynamic and renal function in children. *Pediatr Res* 26:200–203, 1989.
39. Hakim RM, Breillatt J, Lazarus JM, Port FK: Complement activation and hypersensitivity reactions to dialysis membranes. *N Engl J Med* 311:878–882, 1984.
40. Halliday HL, Hirata T, Brady JP: Indomethacin therapy for large patent ductus arteriosus in the very low birth weight infant: results and complications. *Pediatrics* 64:154–159, 1979.

41. Halpenny M, Markos F, Snow HM, et al: Effects of prophylactic fenoldopam infusion on renal blood flow and renal tubular function during acute hypovolemia in anesthetized dogs. *Crit Care Med* 29(4):855–860, 2001.
42. Heney D, Brocklebank JT, Wilson N: Continuous arteriovenous haemofiltration in the newlyborn with acute renal failure and congenital heart disease. *Nephrol Dial Transplant* 4:870–876, 1989.
43. Hilberman M, Derby GC, Spencer RJ, Stinson EB: Sequential pathophysiological changes characterizing the progression from renal dysfunction to acute renal failure following cardiac operation. *J Thorac Cardiovasc Surg* 79:838–844, 1980.
44. Hilberman M, Maseda J, Stinson EB, et al: The diuretic properties of dopamine in patients after open-heart operation. *Anesthesiology* 61:489–494, 1984.
45. Hilberman M, Myers BD, Carrie BJ, et al: Acute renal failure following cardiac surgery. *J Thorac Cardiovasc Surg* 77:880–888, 1979.
46. Hirschberg R, Kopple J, Lipsett P, et al: Multicenter trial of recombinant human insulin-like growth factor 1 in patients with acute renal failure. *Kidney Int* 55:2423–2432, 1999.
47. Holmstrom H, Hall C, Stokke TO, Thaulow E: Plasma levels of N-terminal proatrial natriuretic peptide in children are dependent on renal function and age. *Scand J Clin Lab Invest* 60(2):149–159, 2000.
48. Humes HD, Buffington DA, McKay SM, et al: Replacement of renal function with a tissue engineered kidney in uremic animals. *Nat Biotechnol* 17:451–455, 1999.
49. Hunley TE, Kon V: Endothelin in ischemic acute renal failure. *Curr Opin Neph Hypertens* 6(4):394–400, 1997.
50. Ichikawa I, Pfeffer JM, Pfeffer MA, et al: Role of angiotensin II in the altered renal function of congestive heart failure. *Circ Res* 55:669–675, 1984.
51. Igawa T, Matsumoto K, Kanda S, et al: Hepatocyte growth factor may function as a renotropic factor for regeneration in rats with acute renal injury. *Am J Physiol* 265: F61–F69, 1993.
52. Izumi M, Sugiura T, Nakamura H, et al: Differential diagnosis of prerenal azotemia from acute tubular necrosis and prediction of recovery by Doppler ultrasound. *Am J Kidney Dis* 35(4):713–719, 2000.
53. Johnston PA, Bernard DB, Perrin NS, Levinsky NG: Prostaglandins mediate the vasodilatory effect of mannitol in the hypoperfused rat kidney. *J Clin Invest* 68:127–133, 1981.
54. Kaplan AA, Toueg S, Kennedy TL: Complement kinetics during continuous arteriovenous hemofiltration: studies with a new polysulfone hemofilter. *Blood Purif* 6:27–36, 1988.
55. Kashgarian M, Siegel NJ, Ries AL, et al: Hemodynamic aspects in development and recovery phases of experimental postischemic acute renal failure. *Kidney Int Suppl* 6:S160–S168, 1976.
56. Kaufman RP Jr, Anner H, Kobzik L, et al: A high plasma prostaglandin to thromboxane ratio protects against renal ischemia. *Surg Gynecol Obstet* 165:404–409, 1987.
57. Kaufman RP Jr, Klausner JM, Anner H, et al: Inhibition of thromboxane (Tx) synthesis by free radical scavengers. *J Trauma* 28:458–464, 1988.
58. Kellum JA, Decker JM: Use of dopamine in acute renal failure: A meta-analysis. *Crit Care Med* 29:1526–1531, 2001.
59. Kitamura K, Kangawa K, Kawamoto M, et al: Adrenomedullin: a novel hypotensive peptide isolated from human pheochromocytoma. *Biochem Biophys Res Commun* 192:553–560, 1993.
60. Kjellstrand C, Pru C, Jahnke N, Danin T: Acute renal failure. In Drukker W, Parsons F, Maher J (eds): *Replacement of Renal Function by Dialysis.* Boston: Martinus Nijhoff, 1983, pp 514–535.
61. Klausner JM, Paterson IS, Kobzik L, et al: Vasodilating prostaglandins attenuate ischemic renal injury only if thromboxane is inhibited. *Ann Surg* 209:219–224, 1989.
62. Klotman PE, Smith SR, Volpp BD, et al: Thromboxane synthetase inhibition improves function of hydronephrotic rat kidneys. *Am J Physiol* 250:F282–F287, 1986.
63. Kon V, Yoshioka T, Fogo A, Ichikawa I: Glomerular actions of endothelin in vivo. *J Clin Invest* 83:1762–1767, 1989.
64. Krane NK: Intracranial pressure measurement in a patient undergoing hemodialysis and peritoneal dialysis. *Am J Kidney Dis* 13:336–339, 1989.
65. Lauer A, Alvis R, Avram M: Hemodynamic consequences of continuous arteriovenous hemofiltration. *Am J Kidney Dis* 12:110–115, 1988.
66. Lelcuk S, Alexander F, Kobzik L, et al: Prostacyclin and thromboxane A₂ moderate postischemic renal failure. *Surgery* 98:207–212, 1985.
67. Leri A, Claudio PP, Li Q, et al: Stretch-mediated release of angiotensin II induces myocyte apoptosis by activating p53 that enhances the local

renin-angiotensin system and decreases the Bcl2-to-Bax protein ratio in the cell. *J Clin Invest* 101:1326–1342, 1998.

68. Lieberman KV, Nardi L, Bosch JP: Treatment of acute renal failure in an infant using continuous arteriovenous hemofiltration. *J Pediatr* 106:646–649, 1985.

69. Lieberthal W, Levinsky NG: Treatment of acute tubular necrosis. *Semin Nephrol* 10:571–583, 1990.

70. Lindner A: Synergism of dopamine and furosemide in diuretic-resistant, oliguric acute renal failure. *Nephron* 33:121–126, 1983.

71. Lowrie E, Hamper C, Merrill J: Physical principles in hemodialysis. In Bailey G (ed): *Hemodialysis: Principles and Practice.* New York: Academic Press, 1972, pp 196–210.

72. Luciani GB, Nichani S, Chang AC, et al: Continuous versus intermittent furosemide infusion in critically ill infants after open-heart operations. *Ann Thorac Surg* 64(4):1133–1139, 1997.

73. Margulies KB, Heublein DM, Perrella MA, Burnett JC Jr: ANP-mediated renal cGMP generation in congestive heart failure. *Am J Physiol* 260:F562–F568, 1991.

74. Mason J, Beck F, Dorge A, et al: Intracellular electrolyte composition following renal ischemia. *Kidney Int* 20:61–70, 1981.

75. Mauer SM, Lynch RE: Hemodialysis techniques for infants and children. *Pediatr Clin North Am* 23:843–856, 1976.

76. Maxwell LG, Colombani PM, Fivush BA: Renal, endocrine, and metabolic failure. In Rogers MC (ed): *Textbook of Pediatric Intensive Care.* Baltimore: Williams and Wilkins, 1992, pp 1182–1234.

77. McDonagh TA, Cunningham AD, Morrison CE, et al: Left ventricular dysfunction, natriuretic peptides, and mortality in an urban population. *Heart* 86(1):21–26, 2001.

78. Mezzano SA, Ruiz-Ortega M, Egido J: Angiotensin II and renal fibrosis. *Hypertension* 38:635–638, 2001.

79. Miller SB, Martin DR, Kissane J, Hammerman MR: Insulin-like growth factor I accelerates recovery from acute ischemic renal injury in the rat. *Proc Natl Acad Sci* 89:11876–11880, 1992.

80. Miura K, Ebara T, Okumura M, et al: Attenuation of adrenomedullin-induced renal vasodilation by NG-nitro L-arginine but not glibenclamide. *Br J Pharmacol* 115:917–924, 1995.

81. Moghal NE, Brocklebank JT, Meadow SR: A review of acute renal failure in children: incidence, etiology and outcome. *Clin Nephrol* 49(2):91–95, 1998.

82. Munzel T, Drexler H, Holtz J, et al: Mechanisms involved in the response to prolonged infusion of atrial natriuretic factor in patients with chronic heart failure. *Circulation* 83:191–201, 1991.

83. Muther RS, Potter DM, Bennett WM: Aspirin-induced depression of glomerular filtration rate in normal humans: role of sodium balance. *Ann Intern Med* 94:317–321, 1981.

84. Nagaya N, Nishikimi T, Horio T, et al: Cardiovascular and renal effects of adrenomedullin in rats with heart failure. *Am J Physiol* 45:R213–R218, 1999.

85. Nash MA, Russo JC: Neonatal lactic acidosis and renal failure: the role of peritoneal dialysis. *J Pediatr* 91:101–105, 1977.

86. Neumayer HH, Junge W, Kufner A, Wenning A: Prevention of radio-contrast-media-induced nephrotoxicity by the calcium channel blocker nitrendipine: a prospective randomised clinical trial. *Nephrol Dial Transplant* 4:1030–1036, 1989.

87. Nigam S, Lieberthal W: Acute renal failure III. The role of growth factors in renal regeneration and repair. *Am J Physiol* 279:F3–F11, 2000.

88. Nishio K, Akai Y, Murao Y, et al: Increased plasma concentrations of adrenomedullin correlate with relaxation of vascular tone in patients with septic shock. *Crit Care Med* 25:953–957, 1997.

89. Nolph KD, Lindblad AS, Novak JW: Current concepts. Continuous ambulatory peritoneal dialysis. *N Engl J Med* 318:1595–1600, 1988.

90. Northridge DB, Newby DE, Rooney E, et al: Comparison of the short-term effects of candoxatril, an orally active neutral endopeptidase inhibitor, and frusemide in the treatment of patients with chronic heart failure. *Am Heart J* 138(6 Pt 1):1149–1157, 1999.

91. O'Connor CM, Gattis WA, Gheorghiade M, et al: A randomized trial of ecadotril versus placebo in patients with mild to moderate heart failure: the U.S. Ecadotril Pilot Safety Study. *Am Heart J* 138:1140, 1999.

92. Okubo S, Niimura F, Nishimura H, et al: Angiotensin-independent mechanism for aldosterone synthesis during chronic extracellular fluid volume depletion. *J Clin Invest* 99:855–860, 1997.

93. Oliver JA, Sciacca RR, Pinto J, Cannon PJ: Participation of the prostaglandins in the control of renal blood flow during acute reduction of cardiac output in the dog. *J Clin Invest* 67:229–237, 1981.

94. Olivetti G, Abbi R, Quaini F, et al: Apoptosis in the failing human heart. *N Engl J Med* 336:1131–1141, 1997.

95. Papanicolaou N, Hatziantoniou C, Bariety J: Selective inhibition of thromboxane synthesis partially protected while inhibition of angiotensin II formation did not protect rats against acute renal failure induced with glycerol. *Prostaglandins Leukotr Med* 21:29–35, 1986.

96. Parekh RS, BunchmanTE: Dialysis support in the pediatric intensive care unit. *Adv Ren Replace Ther* 3(4):326, 1996.

97. Patel A, Smith FG: Dose-dependent cardiovascular, renal, and endocrine effects of furosemide in conscious lambs. *Can J Physiol Pharmacol* 75(9):1101–1107, 1997.

98. Pitt B, Zannad F, Remme WJ, et al: The effect of spironolactone on morbidity and mortality in patients with severe heart failure. *N Engl J Med* 341:709–717, 1999.

99. Popovich RP, Moncrief JW, Nolph KD, et al: Continuous ambulatory peritoneal dialysis. *Ann Intern Med* 88:449–456, 1978.

100. Powers SR, Boba A, Hostnik W, Stein A: Prevention of postoperative acute renal failure with mannitol in 100 cases. *Surgery* 55:15–23, 1964.

101. Racusen LC: Structural correlates of renal electrolyte alterations in acute renal failure. *Miner Electrolyte Metab* 17:72–88, 1991.

102. Racusen LC: Alterations in tubular epithelial cell adhesion and mechanisms of acute renal failure. *Lab Invest* 67:158–165, 1992.

103. Reznick VM, Griswold WR, Peterson BM, et al: Peritoneal dialysis for acute renal failure in children. *Pediatr Nephrol* 5:715–717, 1991.

104. Riegger GA, Liebau G, Kochsiek K: Antidiuretic hormone in congestive heart failure. *Am J Med* 72:49–52, 1982.

105. Ruzicka M, Skarda V, Leenen FHH: Effects of ACE inhibitors on circulating versus cardiac angiotensin II in volume overload-induced cardiac hypertrophy in rats. *Circulation* 92:3568–3573, 1995.

106. Safirstein R: Endothelin: The yin and yang of ischemic acute renal failure. *Kidney Int* 59:1590–1591, 2001.

107. Schlondorff D, Ardaillou R: Prostaglandins and other arachidonic acid metabolites in the kidney. *Kidney Int* 29:108–119, 1986.

108. Schrier RW, Hensen J: Cellular mechanism of ischemic acute renal failure: role of Ca^{2+} and calcium entry blockers. *Klin Wochenschr* 66:800–807, 1988.

109. Sigmon DH, Carretero OA, Beierwaltes WH: Plasma renin activity and the renal response to nitric oxide synthesis inhibition. *J Am Soc Nephrol* 3:1288–1294, 1992.

110. Silberbach M, Stejskal E, Foker J, et al: Newborn cardiorenal dynamics: a state of atrial natriuretic peptide unresponsiveness. *Am J Physiol* 261:H2069–H2074, 1991.

111. Siragy HM, Carey RM: Angiotensin type 2 receptors: potential importance in the regulation of blood pressure. *Curr Opin Nephrol Hypertens* 10(1):99–103, 2001.

112. Smith WG, Patel KR, Briggs JD, Junor BJ: Continuous ambulatory peritoneal dialysis and pulmonary function. *Scott Med J* 28:355–356, 1983.

113. Snowdowne KW, Freudenrich CC, Borle AB: The effects of anoxia on cytosolic free calcium, calcium fluxes, and cellular ATP levels in cultured kidney cells. *J Biol Chem* 260:11619–11626, 1985.

114. Sorof JM, Stromberg D, Brewer ED, et al: Early initiation of peritoneal dialysis after surgical repair of congenital heart disease. *Pediatr Nephrol* 13:641–645, 1999.

115. Spencer AJ, LeFurgey A, Ingram P, Mandel LJ: Elemental microanalysis of organelles in proximal tubules. II. Effects of oxygen deprivation. *J Am Soc Nephrol* 1:1321–1333, 1991.

116. Struthers AD: Aldosterone escape during angiotensin-converting enzyme inhibitor therapy in chronic heart failure. *J Cardiac Failure* 2:47–54, 1996.

117. Thompson LD, McElhinney DB, Culbertson CB, et al: Perioperative administration of angiotensin converting enzyme inhibitors decreases the severity and duration of pleural effusions following bi-directional cavopulmonary anastomosis. *Cardiol Young* 11(2):195–200, 2001.

118. Tomita K, Ujiie K, Nakanishi T, et al: Plasma endothelin levels in patients with acute renal failure. *N Engl J Med* 321:1127, 1989.

119. Trachtman H, Hackney P, Tejani A: Pediatric hemodialysis: A decade's (1974–1984) perspective. *Kidney Int* 30:515–522, 1986.

120. Tsutamoto T, Wada A, Maeda K, et al: Effect of spironolactone on plasma brain natriuretic peptide and left ventricular remodeling in patients with congestive heart failure. *J Am Coll Cardiol* 37:1228–1233, 2001.

121. Tufro-McReddie A, Gomez RA: Ontogeny of the renin-angiotensin system. *Semin Nephrol* 13:519–530, 1993.

122. Tulevski LL, Groenink M, Van Der Wall EE, et al: Increased brain and atrial natriuretic peptides in patients with chronic right ventricular pressure overload: correlation between plasma neurohormones and right ventricular dysfunction. *Heart* 86(1):27–30, 2001.

123. Tuman KJ, Spiess BD, McCarthy RJ, et al: Effects of continuous arteriovenous hemofiltration on cardiopulmonary abnormalities during anesthesia for orthotopic liver transplantation. *Anesth Analg* 67:363–369, 1988.

124. Utley JR, Todd EP, Wachtel CC, et al: Effect of hypothermia, hemodilution, and pump oxygenation on organ water content and blood flow. *Surg Forum* 27:217–219, 1976.

125. Venkataraman R, Kellum JA: Novel approaches to the treatment of acute renal failure. *Expert Opin Invest Drugs* 9:2579–2592, 2000.

126. Walshe JJ, Venuto RC: Acute oliguric renal failure induced by indomethacin: possible mechanism. *Ann Intern Med* 91:47–49, 1979.

127. Weir MR, Henrich WL: Theoretical basis and clinical evidence for differential effects of angiotensin-converting enzyme inhibitors and angiotensin II receptor subtype 1 blockers. *Curr Opin Nephrol Hypertens* 4:403–411, 2000.

128. Werner HA, Wensley DF, Lirenman DS, LeBlanc JG: Peritoneal dialysis in children after cardiopulmonary bypass. *J Thorac Cardiovasc Surg* 113:64–68, 1997.

129. Winchester JF, Traveira Da Silva AM: Pulmonary function and peritoneal dialysis. *Int J Artif Organs* 4:267–269, 1981.

130. Yanagisawa M, Kurihara H, Kimura S, et al: A novel potent vasoconstrictor peptide produced by vascular endothelial cells. *Nature* 332:411–415, 1988.

131. Yared A, Kon V, Ichikawa I: Mechanism of preservation of glomerular perfusion and filtration during acute extracellular fluid volume depletion. Importance of intrarenal vasopressin-prostaglandin interaction for protecting kidneys from constrictor action of vasopressin. *J Clin Invest* 75:1477–1487, 1985.

132. Yoshimura N, Yamaguchi M, Oshima Y, et al: Suppression of the secretion of atrial and brain natriuretic peptide after total cavopulmonary connection. *J Thorac Cardiovasc Surg* 120(4):764–769, 2000.

133. Zennaro MC, Farman N, Bonbalet, JP, Lombes M: Tissue-specific expression of and messenger ribonucleic acid isoforms of the human mineralocorticoid receptor in normal and pathological states. *J Clin Endocrinol Metab* 82:1345–1352, 1997.

134. Zhang X, Dostal DE, Reiss K, et al: Identification and activation of autocrine renin-angiotensin system in adult ventricular myocytes. *Am J Physiol* 269:H1791–H1802, 1995.

Chapter 5

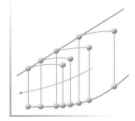

Splanchnic Function and Heart Disease

DAVID G. NICHOLS, MD, MBA, DYLAN STEWART, MD,
ANTONIO DE MAIO, PhD, and CHARLES N. PAIDAS, MD, MBA

INTRODUCTION

The splanchnic circulation is composed of the blood flow originating from the celiac, superior mesenteric, and inferior mesenteric arteries and is distributed to all abdominal viscera. The splanchnic circulation receives over 25% of the cardiac output and contains a similar percentage of the total blood volume under normal conditions. Thus, the splanchnic circulation can act as a site of regulation of distribution of cardiac output and also as a blood reservoir (Fig. 5-1). Multiple regulatory pathways are involved in the distribution of the splanchnic circulation. This chapter will be limited to the intestinal and hepatic circulations because of their functional importance, and particularly because they are sites of dysregulation during pathologic conditions and surgical stresses, such as cardiopulmonary bypass (CPB).

BASIC SCIENCE OF THE SPLANCHNIC CIRCULATION

Intestinal Circulation

Anatomy

The mesenteric arteries branch into multiple serosal arteries, which provide intestinal blood flow. These serosal arteries course from the mesenteric to the antimesenteric surface of the intestine, where they penetrate the muscular layer, giving rise to the submucosal and mucosal vasculature. The terminal arteriolar branches supply blood flow to the intestinal villus. This circulatory arrangement is of particular interest, because of the proximity of the arteriole and the venule in the villus, which creates a considerable countercurrent exchange of oxygen. Thus, an oxygen gradient is produced between the base and tip of the villus (Fig. 5-2). The potential for arteriovenous shunting and the complex plexus of capillaries contribute to making the distal portions of the villus prone to ischemia. This lability of flow at the villous tip is readily

131

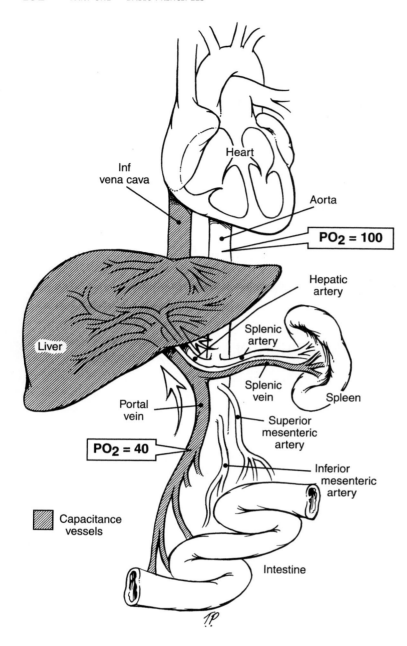

PO2 = 100

PO2 = 40

Capacitance vessels

Heart
Inf vena cava
Aorta
Hepatic artery
Splenic artery
Liver
Splenic vein
Spleen
Portal vein
Superior mesenteric artery
Inferior mesenteric artery
Intestine

FIGURE 5-1 Schematic representation of the splanchnic circulation. Total flow to the splanchnic viscera is controlled by resistance vessels in the mesenteric and hepatic arterial systems. The venous effluents from the splanchnic viscera converge to form the portal vein, which supplies approximately 75% of the total blood supply to the liver. This portal blood is not only high in substrate concentrations resulting from intestinal absorption but also tends to contain bacteria and endotoxin. Under normal circumstances, these are cleared by the resident macrophages of the liver, the Kupffer cells. The venular circulations of the intestines and the liver have a very large blood volume capacity and can thus have a very significant impact on circulating volume and venous return (see text). *PO2,* Partial pressure of oxygen.

evident in studies examining the progression of mucosal injury to a graded ischemic insult.[68]

Physiology

The balance of systemic constrictor and local dilatory mechanisms regulates intestinal blood flow. Systemic activation of sympathetic nerves results in vasoconstriction of the intestinal vasculature and decreased splanchnic blood flow. Catecholamines and other circulating factors, such as angiotensin II, also contribute to the constrictor response. Substances released from the intrinsic nonadrenergic noncholinergic (NANC) nerves largely mediate the dilatory mechanisms. These include neurotransmitters, adenosine, substance P, and nitric oxide. All of these factors, with the probable exception of substance P, may be released by nonneural tissue. The constrictor mechanisms act globally on the entire splanchnic circulation, whereas dilators work locally to affect alterations in the distribution of blood flow, particularly between the mucosal and muscular portions of the intestine (see Fig. 5-2). In addition, low concentrations of nitric oxide may also have other potent effects, such as antithrombosis and antiadhesion of leukocytes.[22]

Unlike the circulating catecholamines and angiotensin II, the constrictor effects of endothelin most likely act in a paracrine fashion. Endothelin-1 and endothelin-3 mediate both vasoconstriction and vasodilation in the intestinal blood vessels and cause contraction of intestinal smooth muscle.[7] Endothelin-A receptors mediate the contractile response, while the endothelin-B receptors mediate both contraction and relaxation, the latter via coupling to nitric oxide synthase.[52]

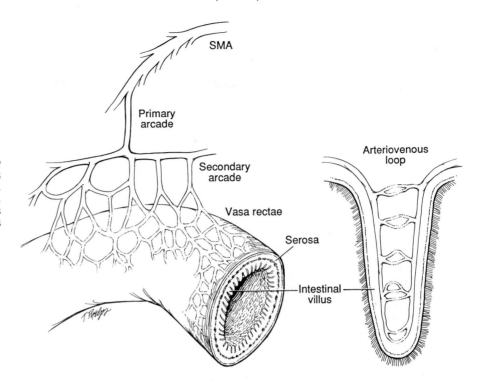

FIGURE 5-2 The superior mesenteric artery (SMA) divides into primary and secondary arcades followed by multiple divisions into vasa rectae. The vasa rectae penetrate the serosa, submucosa, and mucosa. Ultimately, the intestinal villus is supplied by an arteriovenous loop. The venous blood supply parallels the arterial system.

Hepatic Circulation

Anatomy

The terminal portions of the hepatic circulation are arranged in a series of repeating functional units called acini or lobules, depending on whether the portal triad or the central vein is used as the anatomic reference point. The basic unit is approximately 0.5 mm in diameter and consists of a portal venular inflow, a network of sinusoids, and a hepatic venular outflow. Blood flow through these subunits is fairly uniform during normal conditions.

The portal vein provides approximately 75% of the blood supply to the liver. This volume is equal to the total blood flow of the other splanchnic viscera, because it is formed from their venous effluent. Portal vein perfusion pressures are low (about 10 mm Hg), and portal blood is relatively oxygen-poor. The low perfusion pressure requires a low vascular resistance to accommodate the relatively high portal venous blood volume. In contrast, the hepatic artery, which supplies the remaining 25% of total hepatic blood flow, is oxygen-rich (mimics the partial pressure in systemic arterial blood) and perfuses the liver at systemic arterial pressure. Because the hepatic artery flow joins the portal venous system in the portal venules or directly in the hepatic sinusoid, arterial resistance must remain high to maintain a sufficient pressure drop to prevent retrograde flow through the portal vein.[38]

Physiology

Regulation of Hepatic Blood Flow Blood flow is unidirectional from the portal to the central vein within the sinusoidal beds of the hepatic lobule. Because the oxygen content is low, a significant oxygen gradient is established.[25] This situation results in relative centrilobular hypoxia, even under normal conditions. During conditions of low flow, this gradient becomes greater, and overt ischemia can develop in the centrilobular areas. The tendency toward ischemia may produce *centrilobular necrosis*, the hallmark of low flow injury in the liver.

The regulation of total portal blood flow lies primarily upstream in the resistance vessels of the intestine during normal conditions. Although intra- or post-hepatic diseases have relatively little influence on the total volume of portal blood flow, they can have great significance on the distribution of blood flow and portal pressure. In patients with chronic disease (i.e., cirrhosis), severe disruption of acinar blood flow results in portal hypertension. This leads to the development of extrahepatic shunts. Under these conditions, a substantial portion of portal blood can re-enter the circulation without first flowing through the liver. Total liver blood flow may not be affected before the development of extrahepatic shunts, which develop over days to weeks. However, heterogeneous distribution of blood flow can exist earlier as a result of intrahepatic shunts, which may impair liver function. In addition to shunting blood, contraction of intrahepatic vessels may cause substantial pooling of blood within the liver and mesenteric veins, resulting in a loss of circulating blood volume.

Systemic Venous Hypertension and Increased Outflow (Downstream) Pressure of the Liver The portal circulation, with low perfusion pressures, is sensitive to elevation of outflow (downstream) pressures. The site of increased pressure may occur anywhere along the pathway from the sinusoid to the hepatic vein to the right heart. Three cell types line the sinusoid: the endothelial cell, the Kupffer cell, and the hepatic stellate cell. All three cell types are capable of secreting vasoactive substances. Among the various vasoactive substances, endothelin-1 is a prominent vasoconstrictor of endothelial cells and hepatic stellate cells, leading to contraction of the hepatic sinusoid during shock.[62] In addition, sinusoidal contraction resulting in increased portal venous pressures has been associated with CPB. Cytokines, such as interleukin-1 and tumor necrosis factor; arachidonic acid metabolites including the thromboxanes, leukotrienes, and platelet activation factor; neutrophil products such as oxygen free radicals and peptidases; and endothelin-1 seem to mediate this process.[84] Sinusoidal perfusion failure is associated with impairment of the hepatic mitochondrial redox state, cholestasis, enzyme release from the liver, and hepatocyte necrosis.[63]

Systemic venous pressure elevation represents another cause of increased downstream pressure for the hepatic microcirculation. This increase in systemic venous pressure may arise from a variety of derangements such as clot in the great veins, right heart failure, tricuspid valve insufficiency, or pulmonary hypertension. A failing Fontan circulation in the patient with a univentricular heart represents a specific cause of systemic venous hypertension. Because the increase in downstream pressure originates in the heart or great vessels, there is a diffuse increase in systemic capillary pressure in addition to the increase in hepatic vein and sinusoidal pressure. Therefore the manifestations are more generalized with hepatomegaly, ascites, pleural effusions, and edema.

Liver dysfunction secondary to high right-sided venous pressure is associated with decreased hepatic blood flow and oxygen delivery. The increased hepatic venous pressure produces pressure atrophy of hepatocytes and perisinusoidal edema. These effects summate to create the classic pathological picture of centrilobular necrosis.

Hypotension and the Hepatic Artery Buffer Response

Even mild hypotension compromises splanchnic and therefore portal blood flow. However, total liver blood flow and hepatic oxygen delivery are preserved until hypotension becomes severe. Oxygen delivery is maintained as a result of a compensatory increase in hepatic artery flow. This compensation is termed the hepatic artery buffer response. Besides hypotension, any condition that results in a decrease in portal blood flow, such as CPB, will invoke a hepatic artery buffer response.[39] Although this arterial buffer response preserves total oxygen delivery, the response does not appear to be regulated by the metabolic needs of the hepatic parenchyma.[38,39] Rather, hepatic arterial resistance is sensitive to changes in the volume of the portal circulation. A vasodilator substance such as adenosine is likely released from hepatocytes at a constant rate. This substance is washed out of the interstitium, so that it does not accumulate, when portal flow is normal or elevated. When portal blood flow decreases, the vasodilator substance accumulates in the vicinity of the hepatic arterial resistance vessels, causing vasodilation and increased flow in the hepatic artery vascular bed. Other vasoactive agents such as nitric oxide and angiotensin II may also contribute to regulation of total liver blood flow in this setting.

EFFECTS OF CARDIOPULMONARY BYPASS ON THE SPLANCHNIC CIRCULATION

Overview

A number of factors may play a role in the regulation of hepatic and splanchnic blood flow and organ function during CPB for congenital heart surgery (Box 5-1). A decrease in splanchnic perfusion, as reflected by decreased gastric mucosal pH (pHi), is associated with early postoperative life-threatening complications.[4] Bypass technique, duration, and mediator release affect splanchnic perfusion.

Physiologic Factors

Bypass flow rate is the major determinant of portal and hepatic arterial blood flow during CPB. Failure to maintain normotension or high flow rates during CPB may jeopardize hepatic blood flow. Normothermic CPB causes a 50% decrease in hepatic blood flow during nonpulsatile bypass in dogs perfused at a lower than normal blood pressure.[15] Under these experimental conditions, hepatic blood flow decreases less than portal venous blood flow. Ostensibly, the hepatic artery buffer maintains hepatic flow during low CPB pump flow by increasing the contribution of hepatic arterial blood flow at a time when portal venous flow decreases.[45,83] This is true for any body temperature or perfusion technique. Conversely, portal venous flow improves more consistently by use of a higher flow rate, in keeping with previous studies showing the sensitivity of portal flow during conditions of decreased cardiac output.

The presence of a potent vasoconstrictor, especially in the setting of diminished cardiac output, during or after cardiac surgery may place the splanchnic circulation at risk for ischemia. Vasoactive mediators that may be released during cardiac surgery include angiotensin II,[35] vasopressin,[84] thromboxane A_2 and B_2,[13,87] and catecholamines, including epinephrine and norepinephrine[84] and the endothelins. All these substances may cause vasoconstriction, a potentially catastrophic event in the face of an already diminished oxygen delivery. Clinically, the presence of the hepatic buffer to maintain total hepatic flow when portal venous flow falls, and the maintenance of portal flow during high-flow CPB,

---

BOX 5-1 *Effects of Cardiopulmonary Bypass on Splanchnic Function*

↑ Extracellular fluid
↑ Exchangeable Na^+, ↓ K^+
↓ O_2 delivery
↑ O_2 consumption
↑ Hepatic venous lactate and pyruvate
Hyperglycemia (hypothermic CPB, 24° C–28° C)

Upward arrow, increases; downward arrow, decreases; Na^+, sodium ions; K^+, potassium ions; O_2, oxygen; CPB, cardiopulmonary bypass.

may account for the relatively low incidence of gastrointestinal complications after bypass.[15]

The effect of CPB pulsatility on hepatic blood flow depends on the CPB flow rate and temperature. Although some investigators show better preservation of hepatic blood flow by pulsatile bypass perfusion,[15,47] Mathie[47] did not observe any change in hepatic flow as long as the CPB flow rate was maintained at a high level. Pulsatile CPB decreases systemic vascular resistance and increases hepatic blood flow during hypothermia.[17,18,54,59] The beneficial effects of pulsatile flow may be apparent only when low-flow CPB is used. Angiotensin II levels increase during and after CPB in dogs[69] and adults, an increase that may be accentuated by nonpulsatile bypass and low perfusion rates.[78] The increase in angiotensin II levels during CPB may depend on the baseline preoperative angiotensin level, because angiotensin II levels actually decreased from very high preoperative levels following CPB in children.[5]

Changes in both PaO_2 and $PaCO_2$ have been shown to affect hepatic blood flow. Hypoxemia causes a mild constriction of the hepatic artery, an effect probably mediated by sympathetic stimulation.[46] Hyperoxia does not appear to alter hepatic blood flow.[32] Acidosis constricts hepatic artery flow but simultaneously dilates portal flow. Total hepatic blood flow will either increase or decrease depending on whether the constrictor or dilator effects predominate.[31,46] Hypocapnia decreases both hepatic artery and portal blood flow in dogs.[33] However, there are no data on the effect of hypocapnia on hepatic blood flow in infants undergoing congenital heart surgery.

A general decrease in core temperature unrelated to CPB has little effect on hepatic arterial blood flow but increases intestinal[29] and therefore portal[9,55] blood flow. When flow is kept constant during CPB, the same increase in portal and intestinal blood flow in response to a decrease in core temperature would be expected. Lowering the core temperature from 37°C to 28°C decreases oxygen consumption by 50%.[28] However, hypothermia impairs splanchnic oxygen extraction and may have deleterious effects on splanchnic function during hypothermic CPB.[8,72]

Rewarming after CPB may also affect oxygen delivery. Rewarming is characterized by a decrease in oxygen delivery and an increase in oxygen consumption.[37] This uncoupling of oxygen delivery and consumption may be responsible for the lactic acidosis that occurs after CPB. During rewarming, there is a generalized increase in sympathetic nervous system activity, resulting in increased levels of circulating norepinephrine.[77] Selective rewarming of either the spinal cord or the hypothalamus decreases splanchnic oxygen delivery in animal models. Spinal or hypothalamic warming results in increased splanchnic sympathetic nervous system output, and thus superior mesenteric artery vasoconstriction.[67] The effects of core rewarming on splanchnic blood flow, mucosal blood flow, and hepatic function have not been fully elucidated.

CPB affects hepatic lactate metabolism. Decreased peripheral oxygen delivery and increased oxygen consumption result in increased lactic acid levels both during and after cardiac bypass. In normal circumstances, hepatic lactate clearance is highly effective,[1] but this clearance capacity is saturated in the presence of very high systemic lactate levels when hepatic blood flow is less than 25% of normal.[53]

> **BOX 5-2** *Predisposing Factors That Define Patient at High Risk for Splanchnic Dyshomeostasis*
>
> Hypotension
> Prolonged shock
> Prolonged cardiopulmonary bypass
> Vasopressor support
> Postoperative low cardiac output
> High right-sided venous pressure
> Acidosis
> Prematurity

Hepatic venous lactate and pyruvate levels have been shown to increase during the first 30 minutes of CPB.[26] The combination of a rise in both lactate and pyruvate with a relatively constant lactate-pyruvate ratio suggests that there is not only an increase in anaerobic metabolism, but also a possible alteration in the activity of key enzymes such as pyruvate dehydrogenase.[26]

Although prospective data are not available, several retrospective studies reveal that most major gastrointestinal complications occur in CPB patients who experience episodes of hypotension or prolonged shock, particularly when pressor support is required (Box 5-2). Centrilobular hepatocellular necrosis, cholestasis, and intestinal ischemia are perhaps the most common complications, but other disorders such as gastritis, pancreatitis, and intestinal hemorrhage also occur with increased frequency in these critically ill patients.

CLINICAL CONDITIONS

Congenital Malformations

Certain congenital syndromes combine heart disease and intestinal atresia. The infant with Down syndrome (see also Chapter 46 on Syndromes and Congenital Heart Defects) may have an intracardiac defect combined with duodenal atresia. Bilious vomiting and less commonly abdominal distention suggest the possibility of bowel obstruction, which is confirmed with the classic double bubble sign on abdominal radiograph. The long-term survival rate for duodenal atresia is 86% with virtually all deaths occurring among patients who also had complex cardiac disease.[11]

Intestinal malformations occur in 40% of patients with the visceral heterotaxia syndromes (also called asplenia/polysplenia or Ivemark syndrome, see Chapter 46). While intestinal malrotation is the most common anomaly, gastric volvulus, preduodenal portal vein, esophageal hiatal hernia, and biliary atresia may also occur. The cardiac disease in this population is very complex. Those with asplenia syndrome (right atrial isomerism) demonstrate atrioventricular canal defect, double outlet right ventricle, transposition of the great arteries, anomalous pulmonary venous return, and pulmonary stenosis or atresia. Bilateral superior vena cavae are usually present. The subgroup with polysplenia syndrome (left atrial isomerism) usually have the combination of ventricular septal defect, atrial septal defect, and pulmonic stenosis. The inferior vena cava is usually interrupted. Instead, a dilated azygous venous system connects the infra-diaphragmatic veins with the superior vena cava. The normal visceral asymmetry is absent in this population (particularly in the asplenia group) so that the liver is midline and the stomach is on the side opposite to the cardiac apex. Thus, a chest and abdominal radiograph immediately suggest the diagnosis. Given the complexity of the heart disease and the immune deficiency associated with asplenia/polysplenia, the addition of intestinal obstruction leads to a very high (90%) mortality rate.[56]

The Alagille syndrome links congenital heart disease with liver disease. This is an autosomal dominant disorder with variable expressivity characterized not only by liver and heart abnormalities but also by a characteristic facies, butterfly vertebrae, corneal opacities, renal disease, and intracranial bleeding.[19] Mutations in the Jagged 1 (JAG1) gene form the genetic basis of this syndrome, although only 70% of Alagille patients will have a detectable JAG1 mutation. JAG1 encodes a ligand in the Notch signaling pathway, which is involved in cell fate determination.[49] Alagille patients typically exhibit right heart obstructive lesions ranging from peripheral pulmonic stenosis to tetralogy of Fallot. Cholestasis distinguishes the liver disease in this syndrome, which may progress to liver failure. Liver transplantation may be necessary because of intractable pruritus and failure to thrive. Elevated right heart pressure from peripheral pulmonic stenosis is not a contraindication for liver transplantation.[60]

Splanchnic Complications Associated with Specific Cardiac Operations

Etiology

The multiple etiologic factors that produce splanchnic complications with cardiac surgery or CPB are poorly understood (Box 5-3). The prevailing hypothesis is that ischemia/reperfusion injury plays a major role. This is supported by the clinical observation that most splanchnic complications occur in the setting of hypotension or overt shock. The involvement of other factors such as microemboli, toxins, infectious agents, and vasopressors is suggested by the fact that complications do not develop in all patients who experience hypotension or shock. These splanchnic complications can occur without a previous episode of hypotension. Likewise, there does not appear to be a specific splanchnic target organ, although the liver and the intestinal tract appear to be the

---

> **BOX 5-3** *Congenital Cardiac Anomalies Commonly Associated with Splanchnic Complications*
>
> Transposition of the great vessels
> Hypoplastic left heart syndrome
> Tricuspid atresia
> Tetralogy of Fallot
> Pulmonary atresia
> Ventricular septal defect (large left-to-right shunt)
> Coarctation of the aorta

---

most vulnerable. Table 5-1 presents some of the potential complications associated with certain operative procedures.

Postcoarctectomy Syndrome

The postcoarctectomy syndrome may develop after repair of coarctation of the aorta. It consists of abdominal pain and systemic hypertension sometimes accompanied by vomiting, ileus, and melena. The syndrome appears to be less common if the repair is carried out in infancy. The etiology appears to be a necrotizing arteritis, which develops after coarctectomy permits a sudden increase in mesenteric vascular pressures. The syndrome is reversible after bowel rest and control of hypertension.

Protein-Losing Enteropathy (PLE)

Protein-losing enteropathy consists of intestinal protein loss leading to hypoalbuminemia, diarrhea, edema, ascites, pleural effusions, lymphopenia, immunoglobulin deficiency, and hypercoagulability. It was originally described as a complication of baffle obstruction in the Mustard procedure,[37] but it is now seen most commonly after the Fontan operation.[12] It may also be a manifestation of right heart failure secondary to congenital or acquired valvular disease,[76] constrictive pericarditis,[64,85] or cardiomyopathy.[81]

The pathogenesis of PLE is unclear. It is believed that a chronically elevated systemic venous pressure is transmitted to the mesenteric veins, resulting in lymphangiectasia and protein loss into the gastrointestinal tract. This explanation appears to apply to many but not all patients with PLE, because PLE develops in some Fontan patients who have normal systemic venous pressures.[51] Conversely, except for the Fontan group, PLE usually does not develop in patients with elevated systemic venous pressures. Other factors that may combine with the Fontan operation to predispose to PLE include having the anatomic right ventricle as the systemic ventricle (e.g., hypoplastic left heart syndrome) and prolonged CPB time (>140 minutes).[66] Because prolonged CPB is known to release inflammatory cytokines and cause reperfusion injury, it is plausible that prolonged CPB combined with elevated systemic venous pressures may lead to a vascular or lymphatic injury of the intestinal tract.

Protein-losing enteropathy is uncommon within the first few months after the Fontan operation.[14] However, after several years of follow-up, 7% to 10% of Fontan patients have protein-losing enteropathy or hypoproteinemia.[16] Once the diagnosis has been established, the prognosis is guarded with a 5-year survival rate of 46% to 59%.[20,51]

The diagnostic evaluation for diarrhea in patients after the Fontan procedure may include endoscopy. On occasion, lymphangiectasias resulting from obstruction to lymphatic drainage may be visualized in the jejunum. Small bowel biopsy reveals dilated lacteals. In the face of a consistent history and physical findings, the diagnosis of PLE is supported by determination of fecal alpha$_1$ antitrypsin. This protein accounts for approximately 4% to 5% of total serum protein and is resistant to both intestinal and bacterial proteolysis. It is excreted intact in the stool and therefore can be quantitated as a marker of protein loss from the bowel.

Table 5-1 Splanchnic Complications Following Pediatric Cardiac Operations

Cardiac Pathology/Operation	Splanchnic Complication	Risk Factors (Perioperative)	Reference
Cardiopulmonary Bypass Group			
Hypoplastic left heart syndrome/Norwood	Mesenteric ischemia	Hypotension Cardiac arrest within 48 hr of mesenteric ischemia Vasopressors	27
Tricuspid atresia/Fontan TOF/repair AV canal/repair Pulmonary atresia/repair and valve	Acute hepatic failure	Elevated CVP Low cardiac output	34
Single ventricle/modified Fontan Tricuspid atresia/modified Fontan Mitral atresia/modified Fontan	Acute hepatic failure	Low cardiac output Low urinary output	48
VSD/repair TOF/repair ASD/repair	Perforated peptic ulcer UGI bleed	Hypotension Hypoxia	24
VSD/repair ASD/repair	UGI bleeding—gastric Stress ulceration	None reported	42
Transposition/Mustard Tricuspid atresia/Fontan	Protein-losing enteropathy	SVC obstruction SVC/IVC obstruction	37,70
Non-Cardiopulmonary Bypass Group			
Coarctation of aorta Subclavian flap	Peptic ulcers	Hemoconcentration	36
Coarctation Subclavian flap	Perforated peptic ulcer	None	40
Coarctation/end-to-end anastomosis	Renal failure	Associated cardiac anomalies	21
Nonoperated Group			
Hypoplastic left heart PDA + CHF	Mesenteric ischemia	Low birth weight Major associated anomalies	2,71

CVP, central venous pressure; AV, atrioventricular; TOF, tetralogy of Fallot; VSD, ventricular septal defect; UGI, upper gastrointestinal; ASD, atrial septal defect; SVC, superior vena cava; IVC, inferior vena cava; AVR, aortic valve replacement; PDA, patent ductus arteriosus; CHF, congestive heart failure.

Various medical and surgical treatment regimens have been used for PLE. Edema may be treated symptomatically with diuretics, 25% albumin infusion, and a diet high in protein and medium chain triglycerides. Angiotensin-converting enzyme (ACE) inhibitors may reduce systemic afterload and improve ventricular function. Intravenous or subcutaneous heparin (5000 to 7500 IU/m²/day) has improved PLE over the course of weeks in some cases.[3] Similarly, some patients respond to oral prednisone (2 mg/kg/day) with clinical and histologic improvement.[86] High-dose spironolactone (2 to 5 mg/kg/day) has also been found to be clinically efficacious for PLE.[70] Patients with PLE should undergo cardiac catheterization to evaluate overall hemodynamics and correct anatomic lesions such as pulmonary artery stenoses or aortopulmonary collateral vessels. If medical therapy has failed and no correctable anatomic lesions are found, the options include (1) fenestration to create a communication between the lateral tunnel or baffle and the atrium, (2) "Fontan-takedown" to restore the bidirectional Glenn anastomosis, and (3) heart transplantation.

Intestinal Ischemia and Necrotizing Enterocolitis

Gut ischemia, bacterial translocation, and bowel infarction represent a sequence of events in the premature infant that has been termed necrotizing enterocolitis (NEC). Similar findings may rarely arise in the full-term infant, particularly if there is underlying heart disease. Some authors have argued that intestinal ischemia in the full-term infant with heart disease should be considered a separate entity from conventional NEC in the premature.[27] However, most consider this as simply another manifestation of NEC, because the signs and symptoms are indistinguishable (Table 5-2).[44,50]

Regardless of the target population (premature versus cardiac), the end result is the same. Bowel ischemia progresses to infarction, bacterial translocation, sepsis, and multiple organ dysfunction syndrome if these conditions are undiagnosed or untreated. The clinical presentation typically includes abdominal distention, absent bowel activity, and lower gastrointestinal bleeding (see Table 5-2).

The diagnosis of NEC is difficult, and delay often results in death of the patient. Clinical findings usually begin with an increased abdominal girth. Occasionally, stools are grossly bloody. Fever, persistent tachycardia, and abdominal tenderness may be present. Flank edema, abdominal wall cellulitis, and limb edema are usually seen as late findings. Bowel sounds are absent or hypoactive. Suggestive laboratory data include metabolic acidosis, hyperkalemia, hyponatremia, leukocytosis with a left shift, thrombocytopenia, and hemoconcentration. Fluid resuscitation does not resolve these clinical and laboratory disorders. Flat plate and left lateral

Table 5-2   Modified Bell Staging Criteria for Necrotizing Enterocolitis

Stage	Classification	Systemic Signs	Intestinal Signs	Radiologic Signs
1a	Suspected NEC	Temperature instability, apnea, bradycardia, lethargy	Elevated residuals, emesis, mild abdominal distention, guaiac-positive stool	Normal or intestinal dilation, mild ileus
1b	Suspected NEC	Same as 1a	Bright-red blood from rectum	Same as 1a
2a	Proven NEC— mildly ill	Same as 1b	Same as 1b, plus absent bowel sounds, with or without abdominal tenderness	Intestinal dilation, ileus, pneumatosis intestinalis
2b	Proven NEC— moderately ill	Same as 2a, plus mild metabolic acidosis, mild thrombocytopenia	Same as 2a, plus definite abdominal tenderness, with or without abdominal cellulitus or right lower quadrant mass	Same as 2a, plus portal vein gas with or without ascites
3a	Advanced NEC— severely ill, bowel intact	Same as 2b, plus hypotension, bradycardia, severe apnea, combined respiratory and metabolic acidosis, disseminated intravascular coagulation, and neutropenia	Same as 2b, plus signs of generalized peritonitis, marked tenderness and abdominal distention	Same as 2b, plus definite ascites
3b	Advanced NEC—severely ill, bowel perforated	Same as 3a	Same as 3a	Same as 3a, plus pneumoperitoneum

From McElhinney DB, Hedrick HL, Bush DM, et al: Necrotizing enterocolitis in neonates with congenital heart disease: Risk factors and outcomes. *Pediatrics* 106:1080–1087, 2000, with permission.

decubitus radiographs may show distended intestinal loops, pneumatosis intestinalis, portal or biliary air, or pneumoperitoneum. Computed tomography scan of the abdomen supports these findings.[6] The presence of pneumoperitoneum is an absolute indication for laparotomy. Combinations of hyponatremia despite adequate fluid resuscitation, persistent left shift of the white blood cell count, thrombocytopenia, and metabolic acidosis are relative indications for laparotomy.[82] Doppler ultrasonography is helpful to identify flow in the aorta and superior mesenteric artery and vein roots.[57] However, because the pathologic condition is nonocclusive ischemia, flow to vessels beyond 3 to 4 cm from the root of the superior mesenteric artery is difficult to image by Doppler techniques. Gastric tonometry with mucosal pH measurement has been assessed in children as a method for diagnosing intestinal ischemia but has met with limited success.[57] Angiography[10] and selective infusion of either papaverine or glucagon have not been evaluated in a large prospective pediatric series.

The increased incidence of NEC (3% to 7%) in the cardiac population clearly points to heart disease as a risk factor.[43,50] It greatly exceeds the incidence of 0.3 per 1000 recorded in the largest surveillance study of greater than 500,000 live-birth infants.[61] Nevertheless, premature infants still have the highest incidence of NEC (10% to 17%).[80]

While cardiac disease in general is a risk factor for NEC, univentricular heart disease and especially the hypoplastic left heart syndrome stand out. In addition, prostaglandin E$_1$ (PGE$_1$) administration increases the risk of NEC independent of univentricular heart disease.[74] The risk of NEC with PGE$_1$ administration may be dose-dependent and requires doses greater than 0.05 mcg/kg/minute.[50] Other anatomic lesions have also been reported in association with NEC including truncus arteriosus, aortopulmonary window, transposition of the great arteries, and coarctation of the aorta.

The pathophysiology of NEC in the cardiac infant presumably entails intestinal hypoperfusion. Diastolic run-off and low diastolic pressures in truncus arteriosus and aortopulmonary window may contribute to intestinal hypoperfusion.

Perioperative shock in the infant with hypoplastic left heart syndrome or critical coarctation might lead to the same result. Finally, the therapeutic interventions with PGE$_1$, cardiac catheterization, or umbilical artery catheters might compromise gut perfusion.

In the absence of a clear indication for laparotomy, management is generally resuscitative and supportive. Enteral feeding is withheld and aggressive intravenous (IV) volume replacement instituted. A nasal or orogastric tube is mandatory for gastrointestinal decompression. Broad-spectrum antibiotic therapy is instituted. Operative intervention is reserved for specific complications, such as perforation or hemorrhage. The mortality rate is very high following laparotomy in infants who have undergone congenital heart surgery.[41]

The operative approach is generally via a supraumbilical transverse incision through both rectus muscles. All necrotic bowel is resected and a primary anastomosis performed if the infant is hemodynamically stable and the intestinal blood supply adequate. Otherwise, resection and diverting stomas are indicated. If lesions do not appear to be transmural or appear patchy throughout the midgut and no resection is necessary, a second-look laparotomy may be indicated within 24 to 48 hours. Intraoperative evaluation of mesenteric blood supply is feasible using Doppler imaging and fluorescein, but once again the technology has marginal sensitivity and specificity and has not been evaluated in infants by a prospective randomized format.

Hepatic Complications

Ischemic Hepatitis

Ischemic hepatitis or "shock liver" may occur as a result of decreased total hepatic blood flow secondary to low cardiac output, shock, or cardiac arrest.[23] Serum transaminase levels peak in less than 48 hours and are usually accompanied by two- to four-fold elevations in total serum bilirubin. A coagulopathy may result, usually resolving within 10 days. A liver biopsy is not necessary to confirm the diagnosis; however, histopathology typically reveals centrilobular hepatocellular necrosis. Extreme liver injury resulting from prolonged shock or sepsis may produce total infarction of an entire lobe or the entire liver without evidence of vascular occlusion. In contrast to ischemic hepatitis, patients with fulminant hepatic failure show a rapid decrease in serum transaminase levels, an increase in total bilirubin, and a worsening coagulopathy. Ischemic hepatitis and viral or drug-induced hepatitis can be differentiated from fulminant hepatic failure by noting the presence of underlying illness, such as congestive heart failure (CHF) or a low-flow state, as well as the rapid decrease (over 7 to 10 days) in serum transaminase levels.

Acute Hepatic Failure

Acute hepatic failure develops in less than 1% of children after cardiac surgery.[34] It typically occurs in the setting of multiple organ dysfunction following severe hypotension or shock. The histopathologic pattern consists of progressive centrilobular hepatocellular necrosis.[58,74] In contrast to the periportal hepatocytes, cells in the centrilobular region are particularly sensitive to hypoperfusion because of their position in the hepatic acinus.[25] Chronic passive venous congestion, typically secondary to high right-sided venous pressure, increases the risk of ischemic injury and centrilobular necrosis.

The child with acute hepatic failure exhibits jaundice, obtundation progressing to coma, and a coagulopathy. Biochemical studies reveal hypoglycemia, hyperbilirubinemia, markedly elevated serum transaminase levels, and an elevated serum ammonia level. Acute renal failure occurs commonly.

Treatment is supportive. The obtunded patient requires airway protection. Hypoglycemia is corrected. Salt and water intake is restricted. Therapies aimed at lowering the serum ammonia level include lactulose, laxatives, and dietary manipulation (protein restriction of 1 g/kg/day protein). If these measures fail, continuous venovenous hemofiltration may lower ammonia levels, but it has not been shown to alter outcome. Despite the coagulopathy in acute hepatic failure, fresh frozen plasma administration is hazardous, because the attendant protein load may increase serum ammonia levels.

The mortality rate in the setting of acute hepatic failure after congenital heart surgery exceeds 50%, because cardiorespiratory, renal, or neurologic dysfunction is almost always present as well.[73] Survivors regain nearly normal liver function with only mild liver enzyme and coagulation abnormalities.[30] However, most survivors have residual neurologic deficits.

Pancreatitis

Elevated serum amylase levels are relatively common after congenital heart surgery, occurring in up to 34% of patients.[79] However, proper interpretation of hyperamylasemia requires careful attention to amylase isoenzymes and to specific age references. Salivary amylase may raise total amylase concentrations but has no association with pancreatic injury. A greater than tenfold increase in pancreatic amylase after cardiac surgery implies frank pancreatitis, which carries a significant mortality rate of 21%.[79] Risk factors include age greater than 1 year, homograft implantation, and heart transplantation.

In addition to blood testing, the postoperative diagnosis of pancreatitis in children depends on clinical suspicion and radiologic studies. Swelling of the pancreas and surrounding tissue is seen on ultrasonography or computed tomography (CT) scan. Ultrasonography is less reliable than CT in detecting peripancreatic fluid. Fluid resuscitation, antacid therapy, and nasogastric decompression are mainstays of therapy in children. Parenteral nutrition and antibiotics are reserved for selected patients whose disease process does not respond to these other supportive measures.

References

1. Ahlborg G, Felig P, Hagenfeldt L, et al: Substrate turnover during prolonged exercise in man. Splanchnic and leg metabolism of glucose, free fatty acids, and amino acids. *J Clin Invest* 53:1080–1090, 1974.
2. Allen HA, Haney PJ: Left ventricular outflow obstruction and necrotizing enterocolitis. *Radiology* 150:401–402, 1984.
3. Bendayan I, Casaldaliga J, Castello F, Miro L: Heparin therapy and reversal of protein-losing enteropathy in a case with congenital heart disease. *Pediatr Cardiol* 21:267–268, 2000.
4. Bichel T, Kalangos A, Rouge JC: Can gastric intramucosal pH (pHi) predict outcome of paediatric cardiac surgery? *Paediatr Anaesth* 9:129–134, 1999.
5. Booker PD: Angiotensin II concentrations and gut mucosal perfusion in infants undergoing cardiopulmonary bypass. *J Cardiothorac Vasc Anesth* 13:446–450, 1999.
6. Brandt LJ, Boley SJ: AGA technical review on intestinal ischemia. American Gastrointestinal Association. *Gastroenterology* 118:954–968, 2000.
7. Burgener D, Laesser M, Treggiari-Venzi M, et al: Endothelin-1 blockade corrects mesenteric hypoperfusion in a porcine low cardiac output model. *Crit Care Med* 29:1615–1620, 2001.
8. Cain SM, Bradley WE: Critical O_2 transport values at lowered body temperatures in rats. *J Appl Physiol* 55:1713–1717, 1983.
9. Chapman BJ, Munday KA, Wilson RA: The effect of hypothermia on the circulation of the rat. *J Physiol (Lond)* 254:51P–52P, 1976.
10. Clark RA, Gallant TE: Acute mesenteric ischemia: Angiographic spectrum. *AJR* 142:555–562, 1984.
11. Dalla Vecchia LK, Grosfeld JL, West KW, et al: Intestinal atresia and stenosis: A 25-year experience with 277 cases. *Arch Surg* 133:490–496, 1998.
12. Davidson JD, Waldmann TA, Goodman DS, Gordon RS: Protein-losing gastroenteropathy in congestive heart failure. *Lancet* 1:899, 1961.
13. Davies GC, Sobel M, Salzman EW: Elevated plasma fibrinopeptide A and thromboxane B₂ levels during cardiopulmonary bypass. *Circulation* 61:808–814, 1980.
14. Davis CA, Driscoll DJ, Perrault J, et al: Enteric protein loss after the Fontan operation. *Mayo Clin Proc* 69:112–114, 1994.
15. Desai JB, Mathie RT, Taylor KM: Hepatic blood flow during cardiopulmonary bypass in the dog: A comparison between pulsatile and nonpulsatile perfusion. *Life Support Syst* 2(suppl 1):303–305, 1984.
16. Driscoll DJ, Offord KP, Feldt RH, et al: Five- to fifteen-year follow-up after Fontan operation. *Circulation* 85:469–496, 1992.
17. Dunn J, Kirsh MM, Harness J, et al: Hemodynamic, metabolic, and hematologic effects of pulsatile cardiopulmonary bypass. *J Thorac Cardiovasc Surg* 68:138–147, 1974.
18. Ellis EN, Brouhard BH, Conti VR: Renal function in children undergoing cardiac operations. *Ann Thorac Surg* 36:167–172, 1983.
19. Emerick KM, Rand EB, Goldmuntz E, et al: Features of Alagille syndrome in 92 patients: Frequency and relation to prognosis. *Hepatology* 29:822–829, 1999.
20. Feldt RH, Driscoll DJ, Offord KP, et al: Protein-losing enteropathy after the Fontan operation. *J Thorac Cardiovasc Surg* 112:672–680, 1996.
21. Fenchel G, Steil E, Seybold-Epting W, et al: Repair of symptomatic aortic coarctation in the first three months of life. Early and late results after resection and end-to-end anastomosis and subclavian flap angioplasty. *J Cardiovasc Surg (Torino)* 29:257–263, 1988.
22. Gaboury J, Niu X, Kubes P; Nitric oxide inhibits numerous features of mast cell–induced inflammation. *Circulation* 93:318–326, 1996.

23. Garland JS, Werlin SL, Rice TB: Ischemic hepatitis in children: Diagnosis and clinical course. *Crit Care Med* 16:1209–1212, 1988.

24. Gilbert JW, Morrow AG: Gastrointestinal bleeding after cardiovascular operations in children. *Surgery* 47:685–689, 1960.

25. Gumucio JJ: Hepatocyte heterogeneity: The coming of age from the description of a biological curiosity to a partial understanding of its physiological meaning and regulation. *Hepatology* 9:154–160, 1989.

26. Hampton WW, Townsend MC, Schirmer WJ, et al: Effective hepatic blood flow during cardiopulmonary bypass. *Arch Surg* 124:458–459, 1989.

27. Hebra A, Brown MF, Hirschl RB, et al: Mesenteric ischemia in hypoplastic left heart syndrome. *J Pediatr Surg* 28:606–611, 1993.

28. Hegnauer AH, D'Amato HE: Oxygen consumption and cardiac output in the hypothermic dog. *Am J Physiol* 178:138, 1954.

29. Hellon R: Thermoreceptors. In Fozzard HA, Solano RJ (eds): *Handbook of Physiology. Section 2: The Cardiovascular System.* Bethesda, Md: American Physiological Society, 1983, pp 659–673.

30. Heying R, Seghaye MC, Grabitz RG, et al: Mid-term follow-up after multiple system organ failure following cardiac surgery in children. *Acta Paediatr* 88:1238–1243, 1999.

31. Hughes RL, Mathie RT, Campbell D, Fitch W: Effect of hypercarbia on hepatic blood flow and oxygen consumption in the greyhound. *Br J Anaesth* 51:289–296, 1979.

32. Hughes RL, Mathie RT, Campbell D, Fitch W: Systemic hypoxia and hyperoxia, and liver blood flow and oxygen consumption in the greyhound. *Pflugers Arch* 381:151–157, 1979.

33. Hughes RL, Mathie RT, Fitch W, Campbell D: Liver blood flow and oxygen consumption during hypocapnia and IPPV in the greyhound. *J Appl Physiol* 47:290–295, 1979.

34. Jenkins JG, Lynn AM, Wood AE, et al: Acute hepatic failure following cardiac operation in children. *J Thorac Cardiovasc Surg* 84:865–871, 1982.

35. Kampp M, Lundgren O, Nilsson NJ: Extravascular shunting of oxygen in the small intestine of the cat. *Acta Physiol Scand* 72:396–403, 1968.

36. Konrad RM: Gastroduodenal haemorrhage and perforation following cardiovascular surgery in children. *Arch Dis Child* 38:158–160, 1963.

37. Krueger SK, Burney DW, Ferlic RM: Protein-losing enteropathy complicating the Mustard procedure. *Surgery* 81:305–306, 1977.

38. Lautt WW, Greenway CV: Conceptual review of the hepatic vascular bed. *Hepatology* 7:952–963, 1987.

39. Lautt WW: Relationship between hepatic blood flow and overall metabolism: The hepatic arterial buffer response. *Fed Proc* 42:1662–1666, 1983.

40. Lawhorne TW Jr, Davis JL, Smith GW: General surgical complications after cardiac surgery. *Am J Surg* 136:254–256, 1978.

41. Leitman IM, Paull DE, Barie PS, et al: Intra-abdominal complications of cardiopulmonary bypass operations. *Surg Gynecol Obstet* 165:251–254, 1987.

42. Lepley D, Weisel W, Gorman WC: Massive gastrointestinal bleeding as a complication of open heart surgery in children. *Dis Chest* 42:446–448, 1962.

43. Leung MP, Chau KT, Hui PW, et al: Necrotizing enterocolitis in neonates with symptomatic congenital heart disease. *J Pediatr* 113:1044–1046, 1988.

44. Martinez-Tallo E, Claure N, Bancalari E: Necrotizing enterocolitis in full-term or near-term infants: Risk factors. *Biol Neonate* 71:292–298, 1997.

45. Mathie R, Ohri S, Batten J, et al: Hepatic blood flow during cardiopulmonary bypass operations: The effect of temperature and pulsatility. *J Thorac Cardiovasc Surg* 114:292–293, 1997.

46. Mathie RT, Blumgart LH: Effect of denervation on the hepatic haemodynamic response to hypercapnia and hypoxia in the dog. *Pflugers Arch* 397:152–157, 1983.

47. Mathie RT: Hepatic blood flow during cardiopulmonary bypass. *Crit Care Med* 21:S72–S76, 1993.

48. Matsuda H, Covino E, Hirose H, et al: Acute liver dysfunction after modified Fontan operation for complex cardiac lesions. Analysis of the contributing factors and its relation to the early prognosis. *J Thorac Cardiovasc Surg* 96:219–226, 1988.

49. McCright B, Lozier J, Gridley T: A mouse model of Alagille syndrome: Notch2 as a genetic modifier of Jag1 haploinsufficiency. *Development* 129:1075–1082, 2002.

50. McElhinney DB, Hedrick HL, Bush DM, et al: Necrotizing enterocolitis in neonates with congenital heart disease: Risk factors and outcomes. *Pediatrics* 106:1080–1087, 2000.

51. Mertens L, Hagler DJ, Sauer U, et al: Protein-losing enteropathy after the Fontan operation: An international multicenter study. PLE study group. *J Thorac Cardiovasc Surg* 115:1063–1073, 1998.

52. Minchenko AG: Endothelin-1, endothelin receptors and ecNOS gene transcription in vital organs during traumatic shock in rats. *Endothelium* 6:303–314, 1999.

53. Mizock BA: The hepatosplanchnic area and hyperlactatemia: A tale of two lactates. *Crit Care Med* 29:447–449, 2001.

54. Mori A, Watanabe K, Onoe M, et al: Regional blood flow in the liver, pancreas and kidney during pulsatile and nonpulsatile perfusion under profound hypothermia. *Jpn Circ J* 52:219–227, 1988.

55. Nagano K, Gelman S, Bradley EL Jr, Parks D: Hypothermia, hepatic oxygen supply-demand, and ischemia-reperfusion injury in pigs. *Am J Physiol* 258:G910–G918, 1990.

56. Nakada K, Kawaguchi F, Wakisaka M, et al: Digestive tract disorders associated with asplenia/polysplenia syndrome. *J Pediatr Surg* 32:91–94, 1997.

57. Nicoloff A, Williamson K, Taylor L, Porter J: Duplex ultrasonography in evaluation of splanchnic artery stenosis. *Surg Clin North Am* 77:339–355, 1997.

58. Nunes G, Blaisdell FW, Margaretten W: Mechanism of hepatic dysfunction following shock and trauma. *Arch Surg* 100:546–556, 1970.

59. Ohri S, Bowles C, Mathie R, et al: Effect of cardiopulmonary bypass perfusion protocols on gut tissue oxygenation and blood flow. *Ann Thorac Surg* 64:163–170, 1997.

60. Ovaert C, Germeau C, Barrea C, et al: Elevated right ventricular pressures are not a contraindication to liver transplantation in Alagille syndrome. *Transplantation* 72:345–347, 2001.

61. Palmer SR, Biffin A, Gamsu HR: Outcome of neonatal necrotizing enterocolitis: Results of the BAPM/CDSC surveillance study, 1981–1984. *Arch Dis Child* 64:388–394, 1989.

62. Pannen BH, Schroll S, Loop T, et al: Hemorrhagic shock primes the hepatic portal circulation for the vasoconstrictive effects of endothelin-1. *Am J Physiol Heart Circ Physiol* 281:H1075–H1084, 2001.

63. Pannen BHJ, Koehler N, Hole B, et al: Protective role of endogenous carbon monoxide in hepatic microcirculatory dysfunction after hemorrhagic shock. *J Clin Invest* 102: 1220–1228, 1998.

64. Peterson VP, Hastrup J: Protein losing enteropathy in constrictive pericarditis. *Acta Med Scand* 173:401, 1963.

66. Powell AJ, Gauvreau K, Jenkins KJ, et al: Perioperative risk factors for development of protein-losing enteropathy following a Fontan procedure. *Am J Cardiol* 88:1206–1209, 2001.

67. Proppe DW: Alpha-adrenergic control of intestinal circulation in heat-stressed baboons. *J Appl Physiol* 48:759–764, 1980.

68. Revelly J, Ayuse T, Brienza N, et al: Endotoxic shock alters distribution of blood flow within the intestinal wall. *Crit Care Med* 24:1345–1351, 1996.

69. Richardson PDI, Wirthington PG: The effects of intraportal injection of noradrenaline, adrenaline, vasopressin, and angiotensin on the hepatic portal vascular bed of the dog: Marked tachyphylaxis to angiotensin. *Br J Pharmacol* 59:293–301, 1977.

70. Ringel RE, Peddy JB: Effect of high-dose spironolactone on protein-losing enteropathy in patients with Fontan palliation of complex congenital heart disease. *Am J Cardiol* 91:1031–1032, 2003.

71. Santulli TV, Schullinger JN, Heird WC, et al: Acute necrotizing enterocolitis in infancy: A review of 64 cases. *Pediatrics* 55:376–387, 1975.

72. Schumacker PT, Rowland J, Saltz S, et al: Effects of hyperthermia and hypothermia on oxygen extraction by tissues during hypovolemia. *J Appl Physiol* 63:1246–1252, 1987.

73. Seghaye MC, Engelhardt W, Grabitz RG, et al: Multiple system organ failure after open heart surgery in infants and children. *Thorac Cardiovasc Surg* 41:49–53, 1993.

74. Sherlock S: Hepatic transplantation. *South Med J* 80:357–361, 1987.

75. Singh GK, Fong LV, Salmon AP, Keeton BR: Study of low dosage prostaglandin usages and complications. *Eur Heart J* 15:377–381, 1994.

76. Strober W, Cohen LS, Waldmann TA, Braunwald E: Tricuspid regurgitation: A newly recognized cause of protein losing enteropathy, lymphocytopenia and immunologic deficiency. *Am J Med* 44:842, 1968.

77. Sun L, Adams D, Delphin E, et al: Sympathetic response during cardiopulmonary bypass: Mild versus moderate hypothermia. *Crit Care Med* 25:1990–1993, 1997.

78. Taylor KM, Bain WH, Russell M, et al: Peripheral vascular resistance and angiotensin II levels during pulsatile and nonpulsatile cardiopulmonary bypass. *Thorax* 34:594–598, 1979.

79. Tikanoja T, Rautiainen P, Leijala M, et al: Hyperamylasemia after cardiac surgery in infants and children. *Intensive Care Med* 22:959–963, 1996.

80. Uauy RD, Fanaroff AA, Korones SB, et al: Necrotizing enterocolitis in very low birth weight infants: Biodemographic and clinical correlates. National Institute of Child Health and Human Development Neonatal Research Network. *J Pediatr* 119:630–638, 1991.

81. Valberg LS, Corbett W, McCorriston JR, Parker JO: Excessive loss of plasma protein into the gastrointestinal tract associated with primary myocardial disease. *Am J Med* 39:668, 1965.

82. Veith FJ, Webber WB, Karl RC, Deysine M: Diagnostic peritoneal lavage in acute abdominal disease: Normal findings and evaluation in 100 patients. *Ann Surg* 166:290–295, 1967.

83. Waldhausen JA, Lombardo CR, McFarland JA: Studies of hepatic blood flow and oxygen consumption during total cardiopulmonary bypass. *Surgery* 46:1118–1127, 1959.

84. Wan S, LeClerc J, Vincent J: Inflammatory response to cardiopulmonary bypass: Mechanisms involved and possible therapeutic strategies. *Chest* 112:676–692, 1997.

85. Wilkinson P, Pinto B, Senior JR: Reversible protein losing enteropathy with intestinal lymphangiectasia secondary to chronic constrictive pericarditis. *N Engl J Med* 273:1178, 1965.

86. Zellers TM, Brown K: Protein-losing enteropathy after the modified Fontan operation: Oral prednisone treatment with biopsy and laboratory proved improvement. *Pediatr Cardiol* 17:115–117, 1996.

87. Zhang J, Bauer M, Clemens MG: Hepatic portal circulation in normal rat liver is not regulated by nitric oxide. *FASEB J* 8:A1063, 1994.

Chapter 6

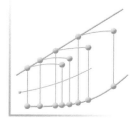

Cerebral Function and Heart Disease

ROBERT CHARLES TASKER, MD, MBBS

INTRODUCTION

Over the past 40 years, developments in the technology of intraoperative and postoperative supportive therapy have enabled major cardiothoracic operative advances. Although these changes have led to a progressive decrease in cardiac

143

morbidity and mortality, acute neurologic insult and the sequelae of operative repair, in a population of children now of increasingly younger age,[40] remain a major concern to all those involved in clinical care. The majority of children undergoing open-heart surgery are thankfully free of adverse consequences; however, a significant number suffer permanent neurologic sequelae and neurodevelopmental dysfunction. The focus of this chapter is a review of not only the recognition and management of specific neuropathologic problems related to cardiac surgery, but also the wider perspective of unique neurology in this patient population.

CENTRAL NERVOUS SYSTEM DISEASE AND NONOPERATED CONGENITAL HEART DISEASE

Irrespective of neurologic events related to the period of cardiac surgery, cerebral complications can be encountered in a proportion of children with congenital heart disease. These are potentially wide-ranging and include acute processes such as cerebral embolization and cerebrovascular accidents, as well as the more insidious effects on the process of neurodevelopment and the acquisition of "milestones."

Developmental Delay

Cognitive Function

The cognitive development of children with congenital heart disease is usually normal. Historically, at a time when corrective surgery was deferred to an older age, cognitive functions in children with cyanotic heart disease was, in comparison with acyanotic children, more often abnormal.[214] Over 40 years ago, it was appreciated that such neurodevelopmental delay appeared to be a result of undernutrition and chronic hypoxemia.[139] However, even from the more recent era of undertaking early or neonatal corrective surgery, some infants may already have hypotonia, failure to thrive, and delayed development.[169] Many mechanisms for such difficulties are possible and include associated malformations, the long-term consequence of anoxic events, prolonged seizures, and infarcts, as well as chronic hypoxia.[63,156] For example, in 1984, the role of hypoxia was suggested by an observation in young children with transposition of the great vessels. The age at which surgery was performed was inversely related to the cognitive level attained,[169] suggesting that postponement of definitive surgical repair may be associated with impairment of higher brain functions. In 1985, O'Dougherty and colleagues[178] reported that chronic hypoxia in cyanotic children was associated with impaired motor function, inability to sustain attention, and low academic achievement. These well-studied and now clinically "historical" observations on neurodevelopmental morbidity were reported in children with chronic insults such as hypoxia, pulmonary hypertension, and congestive cardiac failure. They are perhaps now becoming less significant in the present-day context of early (often prenatal) diagnosis and total repair even before the end of infancy. In this regard, the cognitive development of infants who have undergone open-heart surgery will be discussed in a later section (see Long-Term Neurologic Sequelae).

Underlying Neurogenetic Anomalies

Of equal importance to the effect of congenital heart disease on cognitive function, however, is the possibility of an associated neurogenetic anomaly, impaired developmental potential, or brain malformation in some very young patients. These possibilities are more frequent in children with congenital heart disease than in the general population. For example, in a prospective observational study of 56 neonates assessed before open-heart surgery, Limperopoulos and colleagues[137] found that neurobehavioral and neurologic abnormalities could be identified in greater than half of the cohort, and included hypotonia, hypertonia, jitteriness, motor asymmetries, and absent suck. Poor state regulation (62%) and feeding difficulties (34%) also were commonly observed. Three of the 56 patients had seizures, 38% had microcephaly, and 12% had macrocephaly. Preoperative abnormalities in head size (microcephaly), neurological examination, and motor control are strong predictors of long-term neurologic disability in infants with congenital heart disease who undergo later operative repair.[136] Preoperative magnetic resonance imaging (MRI) scans on newborns with complex congenital heart disease have shown a 4% incidence of brain hemorrhage, an 8% incidence of infarction, and a 17% incidence of periventricular leukomalacia.[145] Periventricular leukomalacia affects the differentiating oligodendrocyte and is characterized by focal necrosis in deep white matter around the lateral ventricles. It is associated with developmental delay, learning deficits, and attention deficit disorder.

Brain malformations may include both major and minor abnormalities, and, as noted previously,[137] microcephaly is common. On cerebral ultrasound scanning of the neonatal brain, preoperative abnormalities have been seen in some 10% to 60% of cases[126,155,241] and include, most commonly, findings such as ventriculomegaly, linear echodensities in the basal ganglia and thalamus, and cerebral atrophy. Brain anomalies are especially frequent with endocardial cushion defects because of their association with Down syndrome, but they are also sometimes found with coarctation of the aorta or aortic stenosis. Coarctation is associated with cerebral aneurysms and may also produce cerebral hemorrhage in their absence (see subsequent discussion).[74] The APOE ε2 polymorphism, which is present in 8% of the population, appears to be associated with an increased risk of developmental delay 1 year after congenital heart surgery.[78] All of these anomalies may be more obvious in those with an easily recognizable pattern of malformation (Table 6-1)[156,246] than in those with a subtle or isolated disorder of brain development. While the causes of brain injury are, in our clinical setting, often multifactorial, the likelihood of such preexisting single gene or contiguous gene defect should not be overlooked. For example, velocardiofacial, DiGeorge, and CATCH 22 syndromes are due to deletions of chromosome 22q11,[188] and it has been reported that deletions of 22q11 may be involved in 5% of all newborns with heart defects.[85] Also, dominantly inherited supravalvuvar aortic stenosis and sporadic Williams syndrome are both due to gene deletion at the elastin gene locus on chromosome 7.[70] In conditions such as those with the spectrum of velocardiofacial syndrome, the potential is present for learning difficulties, mental retardation, and psychiatric disorders[235] as well as brain anomalies[159] even in the absence of systemic or cardiopulmonary bypass–related

Table 6-1 Cardiac Disease and Central Nervous System Involvement in Various Patterns of Congenital Malformation

Pattern of Disease	Cardiac Defects	Central Nervous System Involvement
Chromosome Abnormality Syndromes		
Trisomy 21 (Down syndrome)	40% with anomalies	Mental deficiency
Hypotonia	Atrioventricular septal defect	
Flat facies	VSD	
Slanted palpebral fissures	PDA	
Small ears	ASD	
	Aberrant subclavian artery	
Trisomy 18	>50%	Mental deficiency
Clenched hands	VSD	Hypertonia (postneonatal period)
Short sternum	ASD	Diminished response to sound
Low arch dermal ridge patterning (fingertips)	PDA	
	10%–50%	Facial palsy
	Bicuspid aortic ± pulmonic valves	Paucity of myelination
	Nodularity of valve leaflets	Microgyria
	PS	Cerebellar hypoplasia
	Coarctation of aorta	Defect of corpus callosum
	<10%	Hydrocephalus
	Anomalous coronary artery	Meningomyelocele
	TGA	
	Tetralogy of Fallot	
	Coarctation of aorta	
	Aberrant subclavian artery	
Trisomy 13	>50%	Severe mental deficiency
Defects of eye, nose, lip, and forebrain	VSD (80%)	Holoprosencephaly type defect with varying
Polydactyly	PDA	degrees of incomplete forebrain, olfactory
Narrow hyperconvex fingernails	ASD	bulb, and optic nerve development
		Minor motor seizures
		Hypsarrhythmia
Trisomy 9 mosaic syndrome	>67%	Severe mental deficiency
Joint contractures	Various	
Low-set malformed ears		
5p– syndrome	>30%	Mental deficiency
Cat-like cry in infancy	Various	Microcephaly
Downward slant palpebral fissures		Hypotonia
9p– syndrome	30%–50%	Severe mental deficiency
Hypoplastic supraorbital ridge	VSD	Trigonocephaly
Upslanting palpebral fissures	PDA ± PS	
Craniosynostosis		
13q– syndrome	33%–67%	Mental deficiency
Thumb hypoplasia	Various	Microcephaly with tendency to trigonocephaly
Eye defects		and holoprosencephaly
High nasal bridge		
Cat-eye syndrome	>33%	Mild mental deficiency, some normal
Coloboma of iris	TAPVR	
Downslanting palpebral fissures	LSVC	
Anal atresia		
XO syndrome	>20%	Mean IQ 95 (low verbal)
Short female	Bicuspid aortic valve	Perceptive hearing loss—50%
Broad chest with wide-spaced nipples	Coarctation of aorta	
Congenital lymphedema or its residua	Valvular AS	
Very Small Stature, Not Skeletal Dysplasia		
De Lange syndrome	>30%	Seizures—20%
Synophrys	VSD	
Thin downturning upper lip		
Micromelia		
Rubinstein-Taybi syndrome	>33%	IQ range, 17–86
Broad thumbs and toes	VSD	Stiff unsteady gait
Slanted palpebral fissures	PDA	Electroencephalography abnormality
Hypoplastic maxilla		

LSVC, left superior vena cava; TAPVR, total anomalous pulmonary venous return.

(Continued)

Table 6-1 Cardiac Disease and Central Nervous System Involvement in Various Patterns of Congenital Malformation–*cont'd*

Pattern of Disease	Cardiac Defects	Central Nervous System Involvement
Moderate Small Stature		
Williams syndrome Typical facies Prominent lips	Supravalvular AS Peripheral pulmonary artery stenosis PS VSD ASD (renal artery stenosis, hypertension hypoplasia of aorta)	IQ range, 41–80 (perceptual and motor function more reduced than verbal and memory)
Noonan syndrome Webbing of neck Pectus excavatum Cryptorchidism	PS due to thickening or dysplasia Septal defect PDA Branch stenosis of pulmonary artery	25% mental retardation
Facial-Limb Defect as Major Feature		
Velocardiofacial syndrome	75% VSD 40%–50% Right aortic arch 15%–20% Tetralogy of Fallot 15%–20% Aberrant left subclavian artery	IQ range, 70–90
Environmental Etiologic Agent		
Fetal alcohol effects Prenatal onset growth deficiency Short palpebral fissures	VSD ASD	Mean IQ, 63 Microcephaly Fine motor dysfunction—weak grasp Poor eye-hand coordination ± tremulousness Irritability in infancy
Fetal trimethadione effects	Septal defects Tetralogy of Fallot	Mental deficiency Speech disorder
Fetal rubella Deafness Cataracts	PDA Peripheral PS Septal defects	Mental deficiency Microcephaly Deafness
Miscellaneous		
CHARGE association	Tetralogy of Fallot PDA DORV + AV canal VSD ASD Right-sided aortic arch	Most have shown some degree of mental deficiency ± CNS defect, and visual or auditory handicap
Meckel-Gruber syndrome Polydactyly Cystic dysplasia of kidneys Encephalocele	Occasional Septal defect PDA Coarctation of aorta PS	Microcephaly with sloping forehead Cerebral and cerebellar hypoplasia Posterior or dorsal encephalocele
Zellweger syndrome High forehead with flat facies Hypotonia	PDA Septal defect	Gross defects in early brain development Macrogyria and polymicrogyria Incomplete white matter myelination

VSD, Ventricular septal defect; PDA, patent ductus arteriosus; ASD, atrial septal defect; PS, pulmonary stenosis; TGA, transposition of the great arteries; AS, aortic stenosis; AV canal, atrioventricular canal; DORV, double outlet right ventricle.
Compiled from references 156 and 246.

factors. Furthermore, it is possible that these problems, dysmorphology of the heart and brain, may be linked, given the suggestion that individuals with velocardiofacial syndrome have a distinct pattern of regional brain dysmorphology affecting frontal lobes and left parietal lobe gray matter.[68]

Acute Neurologic Events

Episodic Cyanosis and Convulsions

Hypercyanotic spells ("Tet spells") constitute a major complication of cyanotic heart disease and may be seen in as many as 10% to 20% of such children. The episodes occur most frequently in children between 6 months and 3 years of age and are precipitated by exertion, feeding, or defecation.

They are marked by hyperpnea and a sudden increase in the previous level of cyanosis reflecting decreased pulmonary blood flow and increased right-to-left shunting. Consciousness may be decreased and a generalized convulsion may occur in severe cases.[238] Electroencephalography (EEG) early on and during these severe attacks shows large amplitude slow activity and not spike discharges, indicating that such seizures result from anoxia rather than underlying epilepsy.[48] In some cases, the cyanotic attack may be followed by the features of an acute cerebrovascular accident.

Cerebrovascular Events

Historically, in unrepaired cyanotic congenital heart disease, cerebrovascular events occurred during the first 20 months of life in 75% of patients. Tetralogy of Fallot and transposition of the great vessels accounted for 90% of all such cases.[44,191] Infarcts could occur spontaneously, especially in children younger than 2 years of age,[233] and often appeared following an attack of cyanosis and dyspnea. Children with low hemoglobin concentrations were at particular risk for arterial events, whereas a high hematocrit was more common in venous thrombosis.[238] Overall, venous thrombi were more common than arterial occlusions.[24] They were particularly correlated with dehydration and a high hematocrit, whereas arterial infarcts were often observed in patients with iron-deficiency anemia. Both, however, may be associated with increased blood viscosity.[44] Rarely, in tetralogy of Fallot, paradoxical embolization can occur from an inferior vena cava thrombus to the cerebral arteries.[80]

Arterial Infarction The clinical features of arterial infarction, in most cases, do not differ whether they result from thrombosis or embolism and are manifested by the sudden appearance of neurologic deficit in the territory of one major cerebral vessel.[104] In children with cyanotic congenital heart disease the majority of arterial infarcts are due to occlusions mainly located in the territory of the middle cerebral artery, but other large vessels may be involved. Hemiplegia of sudden onset is the usual clinical presentation but other focal deficits such as hemianopia or aphasia may be seen (Table 6-2). Weakness is maximal immediately after onset, and flaccidity is the rule.[77] Spasticity and pyramidal tract signs appear later. The degree of recovery is extremely variable with a substantial change being expected during the first 2 or 3 weeks of recovery. Subsequently, further slow progress may continue for several months. Seizures may also accompany the acute episode; in approximately 10% of children, they can follow the attack after a latent period of 6 months to 5 years. Approximately 20% of children, particularly those who incur a cerebrovascular accident during the early years of life, are left mentally retarded.[44]

Venous Thrombosis Venous thrombosis is difficult to distinguish from stroke of arterial origin. Historically, the children most susceptible to this problem were those with cyanotic disease, especially those younger than 1 year of age.[44,186] Typically, such children were polycythemic (but with red blood cell indices showing hypochromasia and microcytosis), and the onset of cerebral pathology was often precipitated by dehydration. Cerebral symptoms included headache, visual disturbance, seizures, and an alteration in the level of consciousness. The clinical features included papilledema and focal neurology such as hemiparesis, hemianopia, and aphasia. A fluctuating course is not unusual, and the clinical evolution depends on the extent and location of parenchymal damage, which is usually hemorrhagic in type. If the venous infarction is extensive, the intracranial pressure will be raised. Treatment is difficult but should include general supportive measures such as correcting dehydration and treating any systemic infection that might be present. Overhydration should be avoided, as severe cerebral edema is usually present. The latter is treated, if necessary, with supportive endotracheal intubation and conservative therapy. The potential role of local thrombolysis and mannitol therapy has not been fully evaluated in an "evidenced-based" manner, and so their use should be deferred and restricted to the involvement of appropriately appointed experts.

Bacterial Endocarditis and Cerebral Embolism Acute hemiplegia may also be the result of embolism due to bacterial endocarditis in patients with congenital intracardiac shunts (see Chapter 45). Most frequently, these emboli are to the lungs or the brain. Although most patients show hematuria because of embolization to the kidneys, cerebral embolization may rarely be the presenting clinical feature. Evidence for cerebral embolization can be a sudden disturbance of consciousness, hemiparesis, seizures, or aphasia. In this regard, cranial MRI findings in patients with infective endocarditis

Table 6-2 Main Features of Supratentorial Arterial Occlusion

Arterial Territory	Region of Ischemia	Clinical Findings
Internal carotid	Whole or part of territory of middle cerebral artery.	Hemiplegia
		Hemianopia
	Rarely territories of both middle and anterior cerebral arteries.	Unilateral sensory deficit
		Aphasia if dominant hemisphere
		Partial involvement with only incomplete hemiplegia is not rare
Middle cerebral	Convexity of hemisphere, except paramedial aspect and occipital lobe, insula, part of temporal lobe, internal capsule and basal ganglia, and orbital aspect of frontal lobe.	Hemiplegia with upper limb predominance
		Hemianopia
		Aphasia if dominant hemisphere
Anterior cerebral	Medial aspect of hemisphere, and paramedial aspect of their convexity.	Hemiplegia predominating on the lower limb
	Anterior part of the internal capsule and basal ganglia.	
Anterior choroidal	Optic tract, posterior limb of internal capsule, cerebral peduncle, and pallidum.	Hemiplegia
		Visual field defects
	Variable involvement of thalamus, caudate, and lateral geniculate body.	Dysarthria
		Ataxia sometimes
Thalamostriate	Caudate, putamen, and internal capsule.	Hemiplegia: motor, sensory, or mixed
		No hemianopia
		Language disturbances sometimes
Posterior cerebral	Lower part of temporal lobe, posterior part of thalamus, subthalamic nuclei, superior cerebellar peduncle, optic radiations, and occipital lobe.	Homonymous hemianopia
		Ataxia
		Hemiparesis
		Vertigo

indicate that multiple brain lesions are seen in most patients with, the most common finding being cortical branch infarction, usually involving the distal middle cerebral arterial tree.[16] Other pathologies include numerous small embolic lesions lodged in the supratentorial gray-white junction, multiple parenchymal macroabscesses, and cerebritis. The specific diagnosis and management of this condition rely on blood cultures, appropriate antibiotic treatment, and in some instances anticoagulation.

Mitral Valve Prolapse Mitral valve prolapse, a relatively common familial disorder, has also been suggested as a rare cause of recurrent transient ischemic attacks[113] and acutely abnormal neurology involving any vascular territory, including the retinal vessels. There is, however, a clinical paradox between the large number of persons with mitral valve prolapse in the general population who remain healthy and a subpopulation of patients with cerebral complications in association with mitral valve prolapse.[101] This is an important issue, not least because of the practical implications for prophylaxis. A recent case-control study has made some progress in answering this question.[82] Two hundred and thirteen patients younger than 45 years old with transient ischemic attack or documented ischemic stroke and 263 controls were studied. Mitral valve prolapse was present in 4 of 213 young patients with stroke (1.9%), as compared with 7 of the 263 controls (2.7%); prolapse was present in 2 of 71 patients (2.8%) with otherwise unexplained stroke. The crude odds ratio for mitral valve prolapse among patients who had strokes, as compared with those who did not have strokes, was 0.59 (95% confidence interval, 0.12 to 2.50; $p = 0.62$) after adjustment for age and gender. The authors therefore concluded that, when using currently accepted echocardiographic criteria for the diagnosis of mitral valve prolapse, they could not demonstrate an association between the presence of mitral valve prolapse and acute ischemic neurologic events in young people.

Cardiac Catheterization and Other Etiologies Thromboembolic complications may rarely be seen after cardiac catheterization, particularly in those investigated in the first few months of life. In such instances, there appears to be a predilection for the vertebrobasilar territories[50,66] suggesting local trauma to vessels as a source of the embolic material. However, in the case of balloon angioplasty in children, more generalized changes may occur: for example, a decrease in middle cerebral artery blood flow velocity by approximately 63% during the inflation cycle.[200]

Finally, acute cerebrovascular ischemia may result from the presence of carotid and cerebral arterial stenoses, as in a recent report on a child with Williams syndrome who suffered a cerebrovascular accident,[10] which reiterates the need for a complete neurovascular assessment of all such patients.

Brain Abscesses

Brain abscesses are rare before the age of 2 years, perhaps because they develop on previous small infarcts.[243] The incidence of this complication is still significant in developing countries where most children with cyanotic heart disease go uncorrected. The morbidity and mortality in this population is related to the degree of cyanosis.[73] The clinical presentation

Table 6-3 Symptoms and Neurologic Findings in Patients with Brain Abscess and Congenital Heart Disease

Symptoms	Neurologic Signs
Headache and/or vomiting	Lateralizing signs
Seizures	Papilledema
Fever	Hemiparesis
Listlessness	Increased deep tendon reflexes
Disorientation	Extensor plantar responses
Neck pain	Pupillary changes
	Stupor
	Neck stiffness
	Aphasia
	Homonymous hemianopia
	Localized percussion tenderness of skull

Compiled from references 196 and 243.

can be progressive, with initially minimal neurologic signs subsequently becoming readily apparent (Table 6-3).[196,243] Unfortunately, papilledema is of little value in the diagnosis of brain abscess in patients with cyanotic heart disease, because the retinal vessels in these patients are frequently engorged and tortuous with blurring of the disc margins even in the "normal" state.[190] Overall, persistent fever appears to be the most common mode of presentation.

Examination of the cerebrospinal fluid (CSF) reveals an increased protein concentration and a variable pleocytosis. Radioisotope brain scans, computed tomography (CT), and MRI are important tools that enable accurate diagnosis and localization of the infection. Cranial CT with contrast enhancement is an effective technique for differentiating infarction from abscess. An acute infarction often is not demonstrated, whereas an abscess has characteristic ring enhancement with surrounding cerebral edema. In patients with cyanotic heart disease, abscesses may be multiloculated and solitary in 42% and 48% of cases, respectively.[192] Multiple abscesses may be present in approximately 20% to 30% of cases,[39,117] and the frontal lobe, followed by the parietal lobe, are the most common sites of abscess localization.

Because it is often practically difficult to differentiate a brain abscess from an intracranial vascular accident, it has been suggested that systemic antibiotics be given to all patients with suspected stroke.[128] The initial treatment depends heavily on the proper selection of antimicrobial therapy with good intracranial penetration and covering a wide spectrum of organisms, as abscesses often have a mixed bacterial flora including some anaerobic organisms. Unfortunately, in more than one third of patients, pus from abscesses is sterile on culture.[39] However, when organisms are grown from abscesses in children with cyanotic heart disease, viridans, microaerophilic, or anaerobic streptococci predominate.[31]

If bacterial endocarditis is present, unusual organisms may also be present. Historically, initial antibiotic treatment comprised intravenous chloramphenicol, ampicillin, or methicillin and, at times, also an aminoglycoside. Now, the third-generation cephalosporins are widely used, though when possible, all such therapy should be guided by available antibiotic sensitivities. Antibiotics should be continued for 4 to 5 weeks, and the therapeutic response can be monitored by serial cranial imaging, which often continues to demonstrate ring enhancement for several weeks.

Brain abscess, especially in the early phase of cerebritis, may respond to antimicrobial therapy without surgical drainage.[31] Abscesses larger than 2 cm in diameter in deep-located or parietal-occipital regions should be aspirated immediately and repeatedly, mainly using CT-guided methods, to decrease intracranial pressure and avoid intraventricular rupture of brain abscess.[43,223] Irrespective of surgical puncture, however, continued medical treatment is certainly needed to achieve a complete cure, with disappearance of the capsule on cranial CT scan. In patients in whom the diagnosis of cerebral abscess has been in some doubt but antibiotics have been started, the antibiotics can be discontinued if the cranial CT scan fails to show any evidence of an abscess after 1 week.

Brain abscesses may produce severe cerebral edema, and management of this problem is of utmost importance. Also, seizures may complicate the acute disease process and should be treated vigorously. If the abscess causes significant mass effect, irrespective of size of abscess, surgery may be life-saving, although the mortality rate in this subgroup may be particularly high.[223] In such patients, evolution to intraventricular rupture of the brain abscess may herald a poorer prognosis, particularly because of the increased operative and anesthetic risk in these patients. Overall, the mortality rate for brain abscess is now around 10%,[6] with sequelae including epilepsy (30% to 40%), which is usually of the partial type; localized neurologic deficits; hydrocephalus; and mental retardation. The latter may, however, be more related to the underlying congenital cardiac pathology rather than the abscess itself.[5,105]

Intracranial Arterial Aneurysms

Individuals with a variety of congenital heart disorders may be at an increased risk of intracranial aneurysm development and cervicocephalic arterial dissection, particularly in adolescence. For example, in a large series of noninfectious intracranial aneurysms and cervicocephalic dissections seen in patients with congenital heart disease over a 23-year period, Schievink and colleages[205] found the following. Congenital heart disease was diagnosed in three (8%) of 36 children with intracranial aneurysms, in five (0.3%) of 1994 adults with intracranial aneurysms, in one (4%) of 25 children with cervicocephalic arterial dissections, and in five (2%) of 250 adults with cervicocephalic arterial dissections. The congenital heart disorders consisted of complex cardiac anomalies in three patients (truncus arteriosus, transposition of the great arteries, and tricuspid atresia in one patient each), pulmonic valve or arterial stenosis in two patients, aortic coarctation in four patients, and bicuspid aortic valve in five patients. Only one of these patients had an intracranial aneurysm and coarctation of the aorta, although this association has been well documented elsewhere.[74,146] The pathogenesis of this association may be attributable to an abnormality of the neural crest, because this region is of major importance in early cardiac development and in the derivation of the muscular arteries of the head and neck.

In patients with an arterial aneurysm, hemorrhagic stroke is the presenting clinical manifestation in the majority of cases, and this may be preceded by premonitory "pseudotumoral"

symptoms such as severe focal headache, meningeal signs, or transient neurological deficits.[151] Seizures may also be the first clinical manifestation of aneurysm.[79] All children suspected of intracranial hemorrhage should undergo cranial imaging for anatomic localization. Four-vessel angiography will provide complete information on the circle of Willis and collateral circulation. In this regard, noninvasive alternatives, such as MR angiography and CT angiography, should not be considered as "gold-standard" techniques, as they have reported sensitivies and specificities for detection of 76% to 98% and 85% to 100%, respectively.[242] (These techniques function even worse for the detection of aneurysms less than 5 mm diameter, which account for up to one third of unruptured aneurysms.) Once detected, surgical treatment is the usual therapy, although with the miniaturization of devices and catheters, as well as improvements in embolic materials, interventional endovascular therapy is growing as part of the multimodal approach to management.[232]

Cerebral-Cardiac Interaction

In addition to the effects of heart disease on the brain, the reciprocal effects of brain disease on the heart should be considered. For the purpose of discussion, these fall into two categories: those involving excess stimulation of the sympathetic nervous system, and the effects of gross intracerebral shunting.

Neurogenic Hemodynamic Problems

Intracranial pathology may cause abnormalities of pulse, blood pressure, and vascular resistance. For example, the hypertension and bradycardia of the Cushing's reflex in patients with increased intracranial pressure represent the classic example of this phenomenon, which is mediated by excessive sympathetic nervous system activity.[124] Sympathetic hyperactivity after intracranial hypertension may also result in pulmonary hypertension, intrapulmonary shunting, and neurogenic pulmonary edema.[157]

Cardiac electrical disturbances are also seen after a variety of neurologic problems, especially brain hemorrhage. In adults, the electrocardiographic (ECG) changes in association with intracerebral lesions have been known for over 50 years.[34,38] Approximately 98% of adults with subarachnoid hemorrhage will exhibit new-onset cardiac arrhythmias,[221] and 4% will display deadly torsade de pointes.[54] Approximately 77% of patients with intracerebral hemorrhage and 22% of patients with cerebral infarction will also exhibit new-onset arrhythmias.[132]

Clinical studies in stroke patients, compared with controls, demonstrate a significant increase in cardiac arrhythmias,[174] an elevation of serum cardiac enzymes, particularly CPK-MB,[175] and raised plasma catecholamines, particularly norepinephrine, not associated with increases of cortisol, which suggests a hypersympathetic state.[165,166]

The etiology of these neurogenic hemodynamic problems has been elucidated by both experimental and clinical studies. Laboratory studies indicate that involvement of the insula by experimental cerebral infarction appears to be crucial in mediating these cardiac complications.[91,217] Also, right as opposed to left hemisphere involvement represents risks for cardiac complications with increased plasma norepinephrine levels. Furthermore, there is a significantly increased QT interval when right is compared with left hemisphere infarction.[92] In humans, stimulation of the right insula increases sympathetic cardiovascular tone, whereas parasympathetic increases are more frequent during left insula stimulation. For example, in epileptic patients undergoing temporal lobectomy, pressor responses coupled with an increase in heart rate are more frequently encountered on right insular cortex stimulation.[181] Left insular stimulation engenders bradycardia and depressor responses. It is suggested that right middle cerebral artery infarction disinhibits insular function, resulting in increased sympathetic cardiovascular tone and the cardiac consequences of stroke.[182] In a study to compare the effects of right-sided and left-sided neck surgery,[183] postoperative QT prolongation occurred only after right-sided neck dissection. Moreover, 9% of these patients developed torsade de pointes or cardiac arrest.

The treatment of patients with neurogenic hemodynamic changes requires treatment of the underlying cause of increased intracranial pressure, if possible, in addition to general measures to lower intracranial pressure such as mechanical ventilation, diuretics, and sedation. Even though the Cushing's reflex and neurogenic pulmonary edema are mediated by systemic vasoconstriction, systemic vasodilators should be avoided because they lead to increased cerebral blood flow and worsening intracranial hypertension. The more delayed neurogenic hemodynamic changes, such as the development of cardiomyopathy, can be due to chronic changes in circulatory and tissue levels of catecholamines. Hence, the driving cerebral pathology should be sought and if possible rectified.

Intracranial Shunting: Aneurysm of the Great Vein of Galen

Aneurysms of the vein of Galen are rare and result from direct communication between one or several cerebral arteries and the vein. Anatomically, the most striking feature is dilatation of the vein of Galen, or sometimes the straight sinus—although this is secondary to the arteriovenous fistulae.[140]

The clinical signs are closely related to the age of the patient. The clinical syndromes produced by primary aneurysms fall into four main groups[8]: (1) neonates with severe cardiac failure and a cranial bruit; (2) neonates or infants initially with mild heart failure, then craniomegaly 1 to 6 months later, and a cranial bruit; (3) infants with craniomegaly and a cranial bruit; (4) older children presenting with headache, exercise syncope, and intracranial calcification around the pineal. On cranial CT, the vein of Galen aneurysm appears as a round midline high absorption mass just above and behind the third ventricle. This is connected to a prominent straight sinus and torcula.

There are many cerebral complications associated with vein of Galen aneurysms including spontaneous thrombosis, hemorrhage, and hydrocephalus.[152,173] In general, the earlier the malformation presents, the more dramatic its course. Sometimes, cerebrovascular steal may also occur.[90] The problems associated with vascular steal include visual deterioration, seizures, and significant brain parenchymal loss.

In regard to the cardiac complications of vein of Galen aneurysms, cardiac failure is the most common problem, and

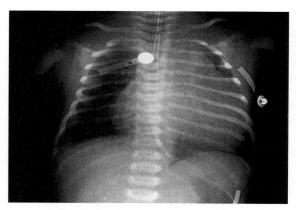

FIGURE 6-1　Chest radiograph of an infant with a vein of Galen aneurysm. There is marked cardiomegaly, which resolved once the cranial angiomatous malformation was embolized.

it is due to high flow through the malformation after the postnatal circulation has been established (Fig. 6-1). There is, however, the possibility that there may be a coexistent congenital heart defect. McElhinney and colleagues[148] reviewed 23 patients (12 neonates) with congenital heart disease and a vein of Galen aneurysm: six of these had sinus venosus atrial septal defect and nine had aortic coarctation. The importance of this association should not be underestimated, because there exists the potential for serious complications such as paradoxical embolization. Also, the overrepresentation of certain cardiac defects suggests that the association may be related to factors other than chance alone. Given this association, full echocardiographic evaluation with attention to the aortic arch is very important.

The morbidity and mortality rate of vein of Galen aneurysms is strongly dependent on age at presentation. In the neonate, a high morbidity and mortality rate is present, mostly related to the development of intractable congestive heart failure. Historically, the quality of survival in infants with this condition has also been very poor due to the development of progressive congestive heart failure, myocardial lesions, intractable seizures, hydrocephalus, and mental retardation.[56] Subependymal hemorrhage may occur after attempts at ventriculoperitoneal shunting for hydrocephalus, and the resultant brain damage may be widespread. In the older infant prognosis is guarded, and in a few cases, spontaneous thrombosis has been reported. In children with low-flow fistulas and an angiomatous network supplying the vein of Galen, the prognosis will depend on the severity and extent of their clinical problems, such as intracerebral steal.

In this context, the management of neonatal vein of Galen malformation requires multidisciplinary intervention with transcatheter embolization, ventricular shunting, and neurosurgical resection.[33,75] The development of a new generation of micropuncture systems for the femoral artery and of microcatheters for intracranial navigation has improved the anatomic and clinical results in infants.[143] It is, therefore, now possible to substantially decrease the severity of intracranial arteriovenous shunting in most cases by using a combination of transarterial and transvenous approaches.[28,95] The aim of such therapy is to obliterate or reduce central midline arteriovenous shunting which, hopefully, will eliminate the sump effect of the arteriovenous fistulas and relieve the brain from chronic venous hypertension due to arterialization of the dural sinuses. However, in many instances—particularly in very young infants—supportive treatment of heart failure and seizures may be needed before cerebrovascular therapy can be undertaken. If the patient also has a coexisting heart defect, then treatment is even more complicated. In these circumstances, it is more usual for the vein of Galen malformation to be the dominant lesion, so treatment of the central lesion should take precedence.

SEQUELAE OF CARDIAC SURGERY

In children, complications of cardiac surgery are one of the major sources of neurodevelopmental sequelae of congenital heart disease.[72] Despite this fact, the exact incidence of neurologic sequelae in children is generally unknown, although there are some indications from more recent prospective clinical studies.[20,22,144,155] For example, in one institution[155] over a period of 3 years (1989–1992), of 91 consecutive full-term infants who underwent 100 episodes of hypothermic cardiopulmonary bypass surgery, there was the following frequency of neurologic complications: reduced level of alertness at discharge from the hospital, 19%; seizures, 15% (70% of which were focal); severe hypotonia, 11% before surgery, and 7% at discharge from hospital; generalized pyramidal findings, 7%; asymmetry of tone, 5%; and chorea that did not persist, 11%. A retrospective analysis of 543 children who underwent cardiac surgery between 1994 and 1999 revealed symptoms of cerebral damage in 6.3% of the cohort.[237] The most significant predictors of symptomatic cerebral damage included complex malformations and postoperative metabolic acidosis (pH < 7.35).

Taking a practical clinical perspective, Ferry[72] categorized the presentation and time course of these complications into acute and chronic forms (Table 6-4). In children, the most prominent of the acute complications are focal and generalized

Table 6-4   The Clinical Presentation and Time Course of Acute and Chronic Neurologic Sequelae of Cardiac Surgery

Acute Postoperative Problems	Long-term Sequelae
Seizures	Seizure disorders
Altered level of consciousness	Mental retardation
Focal neurologic signs	Cerebral palsy
Hemiparesis	Motor deficits
Gaze palsy	Paraplegia
Altered muscle tone	Learning disorders
Movement disorders	Communication disorders
Athetoid posturing	Hearing loss
Choreiform	Language disorder
Behavior problems	Communicating hydrocephalus
Irritability	
Organic mental changes	
Spinal cord infarction	
Peripheral nervous system injury	
Horner's syndrome	
Brachial plexus neuropathy	
Vocal cord paralysis	

See reference 72.

seizures, intracranial hemorrhage, and spinal cord infarction. The chronic or late sequelae of cardiac surgery include mental retardation, cerebral palsy, gait disorders, seizures, and learning disorders.

Acute Neurologic Problems

The acute neurologic complications that can occur during or immediately after the operation include coma or lesser disturbances in the level of consciousness, seizures (generalized, focal, or multifocal), abnormalities in muscle tone, hemiparesis, organic mental syndromes, dyskinesias, gaze palsies, and personality changes.[32,155] In the immediate postoperative period these problems may be difficult to assess, because of the confounding effects of anesthesia and pharmacologic muscle relaxation.

Altered Level of Consciousness

When anoxic brain damage has been extensive, patients do not recover consciousness postoperatively. In general, persistent acute neurologic symptoms and signs reflect a period of impaired cerebral perfusion (local or generalized) or embolization during the time of bypass or postoperative period. Brain MRI may show abnormalities of periventricular leukomalacia, infarction, or hemorrhage early in the postoperative period after complex congenital heart surgery.[145] After several months most lesions, particularly those of periventricular leukomalacia, have resolved. When MRI findings of diffuse hypoxic ischemic injury persist after months, the accompanying neurological exam reveals mental retardation and cerebral palsy.[154]

Focal Infarction and Fontan Procedures An important subgroup of patients who may be at increased risk for postoperative focal infarction or strokes are those children who have had the Fontan procedure. A review of 645 patients who underwent the procedure over a 15-year period (1978 to 1993) identified 17 patients (2.6%; 95% confidence interval of 1.4% to 3.8%) who suffered a stroke.[61] The risk period for stroke in this population extended from the first postoperative day to 32 months after the Fontan procedure. In such patients, there may be a number of anatomic and physiologic factors that enhance the risk of thromboembolic complications and cardiogenic stroke.[160] Possible predisposing factors include demographic and surgical factors (e.g., patient age at operation, type of Fontan procedure performed, type of material used for the conduit, and use of valved or nonvalved conduits),[201] hemodynamic factors (e.g., arrhythmias, right-to-left shunts, polycythemia, and low cardiac output),[51] and abnormalities in the humoral coagulation systems.[45,46]

On a practical point these predominantly historical associations have raised the question of whether prophylactic anticoagulation with warfarin or antiplatelet agents should be used after Fontan procedures.[15,160,208] However, as yet, no consensus is to be found in the literature or in routine clinical practice as to the optimal type or duration of anticoagulation. Consequently, a wide variety of prophylactic anticoagulant regimens is currently in use.

Global Insult In the case of more general insult to the brain, global cerebral hypoperfusion may result from a variety of problems, such as incorrect cannulae placement, prolonged cardiopulmonary bypass, or inadequate perfusion pressure in the perioperative period.

Currently the most effective means of protecting the brain from cardiopulmonary bypass–induced or total circulatory arrest–induced injury is hypothermia.[193] However, in the context of cardiopulmonary bypass in children, what constitutes adequate cerebral perfusion pressure during hypothermia remains to be defined. The periods or events of particular concern, when the brain is at increased risk of neurologic insult, are the active cooling period; the period of low-flow cardiopulmonary bypass or total circulatory arrest; and the period during weaning and separation from cardiopulmonary bypass. Because these events are potentially central to perioperative neuropathologic changes, the basis for the neuroprotective strategies used in these patients will be reviewed more fully in a later section of this chapter.

Seizures

In early studies performed before the advent of cranial CT scanning, it was suggested that seizures were a frequent problem following surgery that involved profound hypothermia and circulatory arrest. For example, in 1984, Ehyai and colleagues[67] reported that 15 of 165 infants and young children (9%; 95% confidence interval of 4.7% to 13.5%) who underwent surgical correction of congenital heart defects using profound hypothermic and circulatory arrest experienced generalized or focal seizures postoperatively. In two thirds of these patients, there was no obvious etiology for the seizures, which occurred 24 to 48 hours following surgery, and there was no relation to the type of cardiac lesion or to the duration of the hypothermia and circulatory arrest. These seizures responded to anticonvulsant therapy, and the children did not have seizures or neurologic abnormalities on long-term follow-up. It is possible that some of these cases would have shown CT scan abnormalities and that some residual learning deficits might have been present if looked for.

In more recent series (1995–1997), the incidence of postoperative clinical seizures has been lower and fairly consistent, approximately 3% to 6%.[20,64,71] Despite this apparent improvement, however, the clinically relevant issue to consider is, what do such seizures represent? For example, in infants undergoing correction for transposition of the great arteries, postoperative combined EEG and video monitoring indicate that seizures appear to be representative of early, cardiopulmonary bypass–related brain injury.[102,197] In 171 infants undergoing either deep hypothermic circulatory arrest or low-flow cardiopulmonary bypass, the incidence of EEG seizures (20%) was more than three times that of clinical seizures (6%).[102] Most infants with EEG seizures had multiple seizures beginning between 13 and 36 hours postoperatively, and they lasted between 6 seconds and 980 minutes. The EEG seizures were localized most commonly to the frontal and central regions of the brain. The factors found to be associated with EEG seizures included use of deep hypothermic circulatory arrest, longer duration of circulatory arrest, and diagnosis of ventricular septal defect. On examining the relationship between these early EEG phenomena and neurodevelopmental outcome at ages 1 and 2½ years, there

were a number of significant findings.[197] At 1 year, children with early postoperative EEG seizures had a lower psychomotor development index, they were more likely to have an abnormal neurologic examination, and they were more likely to have MRI abnormalities. At 2½ years, children with EEG seizures had worse neurodevelopmental outcome with lower scores in several areas of function.

Clinically, when confronted with a patient with seizures in the postoperative period, all possible etiologies should be sought (e.g., infection, electrolyte disturbances, and cerebrovascular injury). So-called postpump seizures, usually seen in infants, are typified by certain characteristics that differentiate them from posthypoxic seizures.[63] As noted previously,[102] the onset is typically between 13 and 36 hours after surgery, which is later than seizures seen in the context of hypoxia-ischemia. Also, the typical clinical course is predictable. These seizures are confined to a relatively brief postoperative period; they have an abrupt onset and occur in series; and, although they have the potential for progression to status epilepticus, after several days the tendency for recurrence quickly diminishes.

All seizures should be treated with antiepileptic therapy. Some seizures, however, particularly if focal, may be difficult to control, despite the use of large doses of antiepileptic medication. Rarely, some patients may progress to West syndrome, with infantile spasms, hypsarrhythmia, and developmental delay.[59]

Spinal Cord Infarction

Ischemic spinal cord injury may occur not only following repair of coarctation of the aorta but also in open-heart surgery, following vascular collapse. For example, in 1985, among eight such patients, Puntis and Green[195] found that three had coarctation of the aorta repair, in which clamping of distal collateral vessels had previously been reported to lead to spinal cord injury. The other patients had variable risk factors, such as low-output failure postoperatively or emergency clamping of the aorta for hemostasis. Neurologic recovery was poor, with residual hemiparesis and bladder and bowel dysfunction in all but one survivor. In this series, the presumptive causative factors included local spinal cord hypoperfusion, microemboli, and postoperative hypotension leading to regional ischemia.

The incidence of this complication after coarctation repair is known, albeit now largely historical. In the 1980s, two institutions reported their historical experiences of spinal cord injury, which were remarkably similar: two of 138 patients (upper limit of 95% confidence interval is 3.4%) seen over a period of 22 years[219]; and none of 91 patients (upper limit of 95% confidence interval is 3.3%) seen over a period of 18 years.[18] However, in 1987, a United Kingdom and Ireland national inquiry[119] into the rate of paraplegia associated with operations of the aorta found that there were 16 such patients in a total of 5492 operations undertaken by 74 surgeons, an incidence of 0.3% (95% confidence interval of 0.2 to 0.4%). Fourteen of these instances followed primary operations, one occurring suddenly and permanently 1 month after operation. The remaining two followed second or third operations for coarctation, and in neither case was any form of bypass used.

In regard to the pathogenesis of ischemia-induced paraplegia, the potential for damage to the spinal cord arises on account of its variable, disrupted, and sometimes precarious blood supply. The blood supply of the spinal cord is derived from the anterior spinal artery, which provides a rich anastomotic network. This artery is supplied by branches of the vertebral arteries, radicular branches from each of the intercostal arteries, and other collateral vessels. In most individuals the anterior spinal artery is a continuous vessel, but in some people it is discontinuous. Because much of the blood supply to the anterior spinal artery arises from the cervical vessels and lower thoracic and upper lumbar vessels (the latter through the great radicular arteries, particularly of Adamkiewicz), possibly clamping of the aorta or of intercostal vessels for operative procedures may interfere appreciably with the blood supply to an isolated segment of the thoracic spinal cord, with consequent ischemic transection.

Intracranial Hemorrhage

Although a variety of intracranial hemorrhages and hematomas can occur following cardiac surgery, the incidence of this problem or the frequency of a particular lesion is not available from a large series of recently managed patients. Historical studies in limited numbers of children[107,108] have reported epidural and subdural hematoma to be the most common hemorrhagic lesion seen, but subarachnoid and intracerebral hemorrhages have also been noted. The pathogenesis is not fully understood but may be related to intraoperative anticoagulation, hypertonic perfusion, excessive diuresis, and venous or arterial hypertension during or after cardiopulmonary bypass. Generally, the neurologic course is similar to that of other patients with intracranial space-occupying lesion, and fundamental neurosurgical management principles for the treatment of this potentially reversible process should be observed.

Peripheral Nerve Lesions

A variety of peripheral nervous system lesions have been reported in adults following open-heart surgery.[133] These include brachial radiculoplexopathy; mononeuropathies of the saphenous, common peroneal, and ulnar nerves; singultus (secondary to phrenic nerve injury); unilateral vocal cord paralysis; Horner's syndrome; and facial neuropathy. The presumed causes include trauma associated with jugular venous cannulation, stretching of nerve roots due to positioning, trauma from cauterization, nerve compression at susceptible sites, or traction on nerves. Most of the deficits resolve in 6–8 weeks. Phrenic nerve paralysis is the most common clinically significant peripheral nerve lesion in infants who have undergone heart surgery. Additionally, transient Horner's syndrome and brachial plexus neuropathies have been seen in the pediatric age group, particularly after difficult jugular vein cannulation in the small infant.[72]

Long-Term Neurologic Sequelae

In contrast to the early period following cardiac surgery, the exact incidence of long-term or delayed neurologic sequelae of cardiac surgery, such as mental retardation, cerebral palsy, gait disorders, seizures, speech disorders, hearing loss, and learning disorders, is poorly characterized.

Delayed Choreoathetoid Syndrome

The onset of acute chorea is dramatic, profoundly disturbing, and fortunately rare with modern cardiac care. In the majority of children the clinical picture is rather stereotyped. It would appear that the reported cases are all in early childhood, and the onset is, in general, from 1 to 7 days after cardiac surgery with deep hypothermia, extracorporeal circulation, and circulatory arrest.*

Rarely, in older children, other movement problems may occur. For example, Singer and colleagues[215] reported the case of an adolescent boy in whom a variety of simple and complex motor and vocal tics (Tourette-like syndrome) developed, along with inattentiveness and obsessive-compulsive behaviors after cardiac surgery with cardiopulmonary bypass and profound hypothermia.

Clinical Features Bergouignan and colleagues[23] in 1961 were the first to describe the clinical findings and outcome of choreoathetoid syndrome in children after cardiac surgery with deep hypothermia, extracorporeal circulation, and cardiorespiratory arrest. In such patients, choreoathetoid movements mainly involving the limbs and orofacial musculature appear within the first postoperative week. Oral feeding is often impaired because of the abnormal movements of the tongue and oropharyngeal musculature. Muscle hypotonia, irritability, and abnormal conjugate eye movements or paralysis are common. These various clinical features have been incorporated into a clinical syndrome: the CHAP syndrome consists of Choreoathetosis and orofacial dyskinesias, Hypotonia, Affective changes, and Pseudobulbar signs.

On clinical inspection, the choreoathetosis can be seen to affect the face, bulbar muscles, and all four limbs, which may be followed by a Parkinson-like state.[25] Its severity progresses over 1 to 3 weeks. Tone seems to be poor in both trunk and limbs, with reflexes being either normal or suppressed. In relation to eye movements, there may be supranuclear ophthalmoplegia or downward gaze deviation.[198,245] Last, seizures during the acute phase have also been observed by a number of authors.[32,52,149] There appear to be no specific findings observed in the CT scans, CSF examination, or EEG that could be related to abnormal movements.

Natural History The onset of the abnormal movements occurs during the first 7 postoperative days and is either abrupt or follows a period in which the child exhibits a paucity of spontaneous movement. Although it is possible that in some of these cases the onset may have been suppressed by heavy sedation in the immediate postoperative period, in most patients there was a clear period of normality beforehand. The evolution of the movement disorder, after acute presentation, is that the abnormality can fade away in a few weeks or months or it can be permanent, although a decrease in intensity is often noticed.[23,41,52,109,149,198,245,247] Most recently, Gherpelli and colleagues[81] reported complete

---

*See references 23, 41, 47, 52, 81, 83, 86, 109, 127, 149, 198, 245, 247.

resolution of the abnormal movements in six of nine children, which is a better outcome than reported by previous authors[23,52,109,149,247] who found more than 50% of persistent, although sometimes less severe, choreoathetoid movements during follow-up. Age, however, may have a significant bearing on the type and natural history of the movement disorder. Wong and colleagues[247] noted two different forms of the choreoathetoid syndrome depending on age. A mild transient form of choreoathetosis developed in eight younger patients (median age 4.3 months), all of whom survived and had complete resolution of symptoms. A severe persistent form of the condition developed in 11 older patients (median age 16.8 months). The mortality rate was 46% in the severely affected group. The mildly affected patients all survived.

Long-term follow-up data are difficult to interpret in these patients because the series reported are small. Nevertheless, neurologic sequelae appear to include a high incidence of chronic neurodevelopmental deficits among patients with severe choreoathetosis in the immediate postoperative period.[20,23,41,57,58,62,109] These chronic deficits affect language, attention, memory, and motor function (persistent dyskinesia). It is unknown whether any specific treatment modifies the evolution of the condition. For example, symptomatic therapy with haloperidol, with or without benzodiazepines, has been useful in some patients, as it allows, apparently, earlier oral feeding because of improvement in oropharyngeal movements, and in some cases there is also improvement in the restlessness.[81] However, such treatment should be used with caution, for as short a time as possible, and only by experts familiar with this therapy, because of the potential chronic and irreversible adverse motor effects. Last, any optimism about treatment should be tempered by the experience reported by Medlock and colleagues,[149] who used haloperidol in five children with persistent choreoathetosis and observed a beneficial response in only one. Similarly, none of the five patients reported by Robinson and colleagues,[198] and none of the four patients reported by Wical and Tomasi,[245] responded conclusively to drug therapy, including haloperidol, valproic acid, and diphenhydramine.

Epidemiology The incidence of choreoathetoid syndrome after open-heart surgery is unknown but appears to be rare. In 1990, in North America, Ferry[72] reported that it was recognized in only 3 of 6 major pediatric cardiac surgery units that performed a mean of 450 operations per year. In 1990, DeLeon and colleagues[52] reported that eight of 758 children (1%; 95% confidence limits of 0.4 to 1.8%) undergoing an intracardiac operation under cardiopulmonary bypass and hypothermia developed choreoathetosis 3 to 7 days postoperatively. Similarly in 1993, Medlock and colleagues[149] reported that, during a period of 10 years, out of 668 children (aged 8 to 34 months) who underwent open-heart surgery with cardiopulmonary bypass, eight (1.2%; 95% confidence limits of 0.4 to 2%) developed postpump chorea within 2 weeks of surgery.

Pathophysiology The pathophysiology of choreoathetoid syndrome after open-heart surgery is uncertain. Deep hypothermia seems to be a possible factor because the reports began after the institution of this method of neuroprotection. Neuropathology studies of this condition are limited. In the 1960s, Bjork and Hultquist[25,26] described the histopathologic findings in the brains of four children who died within 102 days after cardiac surgery with deep hypothermia and cardiorespiratory arrest. They found a marked decrease in the number of ganglion cells of the globus pallidus, with similar but less pronounced changes in the putamen. Chaves and Scaltsas-Persson[41] described hypoxic neuronal degeneration and capillary proliferation in the basal ganglia in one patient. Kupsky and colleagues[127] reported the neuropathology in another two children. Examination of the brain showed neuronal loss, reactive astrocytosis, and degeneration of myelinated fibers (without frank necrosis) in the globus pallidus, primarily the outer segment, with sparing of other regions commonly susceptible to hypoxic-ischemic necrosis. Robinson and colleagues,[198] however, could not find any histologic abnormality in a child who died 5 months postoperatively who still had mild choreoathetoid movements at the time of death.

The precise neuroanatomic localization and pathogenesis of this condition are unknown, but presumably the basal ganglia and deep subcortical structures are involved, with the underlying etiology being poor regional perfusion. For example, most affected patients have cyanotic heart disease with systemic to pulmonary collateral vessels arising from the head and neck raising the possibility of a cerebrovascular steal phenomenon leading to regional brain ischemia.[247] Alternatively, hypocapnia-induced cerebral vasoconstriction during the rewarming period may be the significant factor in limiting basal ganglia perfusion. Curless and colleagues[47] described three patients who developed choreoathetosis after cardiopulmonary bypass with hypothermia: none had significant hypotension or hypoxemia, but all had hypocapnia and respiratory alkalosis during the rewarming period. This regional localization is supported by imaging of cerebral perfusion.[60] In 11 children who had a movement disorder after hypothermic cardiac surgery, perfusion defects were identified using single photon emission computed tomography (SPECT) with technetium-99m hexamethylpropylene amine oxime. Perfusion defects of the deep gray matter and cortex were seen in six and nine of the 11 patients, respectively. For both cortical and subcortical defects a strong right-sided predilection was present. Last, it is also possible that other biochemical variables may be involved in pathogenesis of this condition, including calcium and glucose homeostasis. But the delayed onset of neurologic deficits seems, most likely, to suggest an alteration of neurotransmitter status.

Neuropsychologic Sequelae

In infants and young children cardiac surgery may have consequences on development with the result that cognitive function is impaired. On long-term follow-up, the exact incidence of this problem is difficult to ascertain, mainly because of a general lack in neuropsychological studies with adequate preoperative and postoperative assessments. Furthermore, such studies are fraught with methodologic shortcomings. These include problems related to the sample (small number, patient heterogeneity, varying socioeconomic levels, preoperative intelligence quotient [IQ], and preexisting neurologic disorder), the surgery (timing, complexity, duration, type of bypass equipment, and potential for embolization), the postoperative period (variations of postoperative care and infection), and the follow-up assessment (lack of precise psychometric test batteries in younger children; poor choice of tests; reliance on summary IQ scores; failure to assess attention, memory, language processing, and academic achievement).

Historically, studies of neurodevelopmental outcome after pediatric cardiac surgery have shown a variety of cognitive, behavioral, and linguistic deficits.[27,55,220,244,248] The IQ in children after congenital heart surgery is typically reported as normal or low average with a broad range around the mean.[21,177]

In the modern era, the effect of neonatal open-heart surgery has been of particular concern. In this regard, prolonged circulatory arrest is thought to be one of the factors responsible for subsequent neurocognitive impairment,[27,59,94,170,177] and the risk of impairment has been reported to increase if deep hypothermic circulatory arrest exceeds 45 to 50 minutes.[94,244,248] In the largest prospective study examining the role of deep hypothermic circulatory arrest on cognitive function, 171 neonates were randomized to receive either a predominant deep hypothermic circulatory arrest strategy or a predominant low-flow cardiopulmonary bypass strategy during the arterial switch operation.[20,22,170] At 4 years of age, neither full-scale IQ scores nor overall neurologic status were related to duration of deep hypothermic circulatory arrest. Other abnormalities, however, such as oromotor apraxia, gross and fine motor coordination, and cranial nerve and brainstem abnormalities were related to prolonged deep hypothermic circulatory arrest.

A subgroup of particular note is the school-aged or adolescent survivors of staged palliation for hypoplastic left heart syndrome. Mahle and colleagues[144] conducted a cross-sectional questionnaire (115 of 138 eligible children) and neuropsychological (28 of 34 local children) study of school-aged survivors of staged palliation for hypoplastic left heart syndrome. On questioning, the majority of parents or guardians described their child's health as good (34%) or excellent (45%) and their academic performance as average (42%) or above average (42%). Of note, one third of the children were receiving some form of special education. On cognitive testing, mental retardation (IQ below 70) was found in 18% of the patients. However, whether these problems relate to preoperative abnormalities or to repeated surgery is difficult to assess, as multivariate analysis identified the presence of preoperative seizures as the only factor associated with lower full scale IQ scores.

Last, there is the issue of long-term psychological well-functioning in survivors of surgical correction for congenital heart disease, and three recent studies suggest that some patients with congenital heart disease are at risk of long-term behavioral or emotional maladjustment. Bellinger and colleagues[21] found that, in 171 patients with transposition of the great arteries 2½ years after neonatal surgery, the predominant use of circulatory arrest during the arterial switch operation was associated with more internalizing and externalizing problem behaviors. Alden and colleagues[7] assessed 31 children 11.5 years, on average, after surgery for transposition of the great arteries: 19% had clinically significant child psychiatric symptoms, which is slightly more than expected. Utens and colleagues[239] applied the Child Behavior Checklist to 125 children (aged 10 to 15 years) with operated congenital heart disease. Higher Child Behavior Checklist problem scores were associated with a greater number of heart operations and deep hypothermic circulatory arrest (below 22° C). "Internalizing" problems were associated with a greater number of heart operations, deep hypothermic circulatory arrest, younger gestational age at birth, low systemic oxygen saturation, and older age at surgical repair. "Externalizing" problems were associated with only a greater number of heart operations.

Other Late Sequelae

Other late neurologic sequelae are also seen as a complication of cardiac surgery. In the past, there has been a surprisingly high incidence of hearing loss in children with congenital heart disease,[11] which may or may not be related to surgery. As many as 25% of children aged 3 days to 12 years suffered hearing loss that was not associated with otitis media with effusion. More data,[180] however, also point to the possibility of developmental and maturational abnormalities, particularly in infants younger than 1 year of age with cyanotic congenital heart disease and chronic hypoxemia. Finally, vertebrobasilar ischemia after a Blalock-Taussig anastomosis can be the result of significant subclavian steal, but this is rare.[129]

PATHOGENESIS AND CEREBROPROTECTION

Clinical and laboratory research have implicated two major causes of cerebral injury after cardiac surgery, which are inadequate cerebral perfusion and embolization.

Inadequate Cerebral Perfusion

The cause of inadequate cerebral perfusion and the pathogenesis of related cerebral damage after cardiopulmonary bypass have been discussed by numerous authors.[193] Inadequate cerebral perfusion can result from a variety of factors that have to do with cooling and extracorporeal support during surgery. Unfortunately, these are difficult to assess, as there is, in general, lack of consistency in management (i.e., procedures, equipment, and practices) across institutions.

Perfusion Techniques

Autoregulation of total cerebral blood flow and its implications for global neurologic function are a critical issue. The blood gas strategy, either pH-stat (temperature corrected) or alpha-stat (temperature uncorrected), is a major determinant of cerebral perfusion during cardiopulmonary bypass. The basic principles governing these two strategies are discussed in Chapter 19 on Monitoring. The effects of pH-stat and alpha-stat blood gas management on cerebral perfusion and function are discussed in Chapter 20 on Cardiopulmonary Bypass. In regard to extracorporeal support, there are, currently, three main techniques used during open-heart surgery in infants and children.

Deep Hypothermic Circulatory Arrest Deep hypothermic circulatory arrest is undertaken when the patient has been cooled via surface and core cooling to a nasopharyngeal temperature of 15°C to 22°C. At this time, the patient is disconnected from the heart-lung machine and surgery performed in a bloodless field.

Deep hypothermic circulatory arrest can have significant effects on intracranial hemodynamics via effects on cerebral blood flow and intracranial pressure. These changes may occur both during the surgical procedure and for a significant period after surgery, with the consequence of changes or disruption in normal cerebral oxygenation and metabolism, and ensuing ischemia. For example, Greeley and colleagues[87] studied 67 infants and children undergoing cardiac surgery and cardiopulmonary bypass who received a standard anesthetic technique in which vasoactive or cerebroprotective agents were avoided. The cerebral blood flow was measured using the xenon-133 clearance technique. Patients were grouped based on different cardiopulmonary bypass techniques: repair during moderate-hypothermic bypass at 25°C to 32°C; repair during deep-hypothermic bypass at 18°C to 22°C; and repair with total circulatory arrest at 18°C. The effects of temperature, circulatory arrest, and rewarming on cerebral blood flow were studied. There was a significant correlation of cerebral blood flow with temperature during cardiopulmonary bypass: cerebral blood flow decreased significantly under hypothermic conditions in all groups compared with prebypass levels under normothermia. In all but the total circulatory arrest group, cerebral blood flow returned to baseline levels in the rewarming phase of cardiopulmonary bypass and exceeded baseline levels after bypass. Importantly, in the group undergoing total circulatory arrest, no significant increase in cerebral blood flow was observed during rewarming after total circulatory arrest (32 ± 12 minutes) or after weaning from cardiopulmonary bypass. Last, in this group, and in contrast to observations in the other groups, there was also an association between cerebral blood flow and mean arterial pressure, suggesting that the flow of blood may be pressure passive and no longer autoregulated.[231] Taken together, cerebral ischemia may thus ensue, either during or after the period of circulatory arrest.

Biochemical evidence of cerebral ischemia during deep hypothermic circulatory arrest has been shown in two clinical studies. Rossi and colleagues[202] studied 24 infants who underwent deep hypothermic circulatory arrest and seven children undergoing cardiovascular procedures without extracorporeal circulation or circulatory arrest. Jugular bulb venous catheter samples were used to assess regional biochemical changes in levels of brain-type creatine kinase (CK-BB, an index of cerebral ischemia, as release of this enzyme occurs during an ischemic insult to the brain). Infants undergoing circulatory arrest had a significant arteriovenous difference for CK-BB, with higher concentrations in the jugular venous effluent. The peak level occurred, on average, 127 minutes after reperfusion. van der Linden and colleagues[240] studied 17 patients undergoing congenital heart surgery during profound hypothermia. Following total circulatory arrest, lactate levels in jugular venous blood were higher than the arterial levels from the beginning of rewarming and until 3 hours after the end of cardiopulmonary bypass.

Low-Flow Cardiopulmonary Bypass In normal-flow cardiopulmonary bypass a heart-lung machine provides support at 100 to 150 mL/kg/minute (2.4 to 3.2 L/min/m²).

Varying degrees of hypothermia can then be used to provide cerebral and myocardial protection. Low-flow cardiopulmonary bypass with deep hypothermia is similar to the techniques of deep hypothermic circulatory arrest, where the patient is cooled to below 20°C. However, at this time, in contrast to circulatory arrest, the extracorporeal support cannulae are left in place, and the heart-lung machine continues to provide perfusion, albeit with flows at 25% to 50% (50 mL/kg/minute to as low as 25 mL/kg/minute) of the calculated normothermic flow rate.

In comparison with deep hypothermic circulatory arrest, low-flow cardiopulmonary bypass may, theoretically, maintain some cerebral blood flow. However, at the extreme of the low-flow state, the effects of the two techniques on cerebral blood flow are indistinguishable.[36,203,231] Also, the effect of temperature on cerebral blood flow and cerebral metabolism is not of the same magnitude: in the former the temperature relationship is linear, and in the latter it is exponential. The net result is that cerebral blood flow becomes, relatively, more luxuriant at deep hypothermic temperatures, and flow-metabolism coupling is lost. At normothermia the mean ratio of cerebral blood flow to cerebral metabolic rate is 20:1, and at deep hypothermia the ratio increases to 75:1 (Fig. 6-2),[88] which is of major importance when low-flow cardiopulmonary bypass is used. Therefore if adequate cerebral oxygen delivery were supplied, low-flow cardiopulmonary bypass could theoretically provide an indefinite period of effective cerebral perfusion. As shown in Table 6-5,[88,121] using data from infants and children, Kern and coworkers[121] have predicted that at hypothermic temperatures typically used during deep hypothermic cardiopulmonary bypass, flow rates as low as 8 mL/kg/minute should meet cerebral demands.

Clinical experience suggests that circulatory arrest during deep hypothermia is safe for approximately 50 to 60 minutes. A more precise method of predicting safe limits for total circulatory arrest based on brain metabolism has been

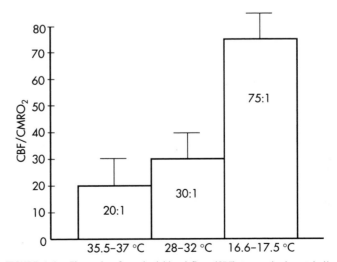

FIGURE 6-2 The ratio of cerebral blood flow (CBF) to cerebral metabolic rate for oxygen (CMRO₂) increases with decreasing temperature using alpha-stat blood gas management. At normothermia the CBF:CMRO₂ ratio is 20:1, at moderate hypothermia 30:1, and at deep hypothermia 75:1. CBF becomes increasingly luxuriant at lower temperatures, allowing for the safe implementation of low-flow cardiopulmonary bypass. (From Kern FH, Greeley WJ, Ungerleider RM: The effects of bypass on the developing brain. *Perfusion* 8:49, 1993; with permission.)

Table 6-5 Calculation of Minimal Pump Flow Rates during Hypothermic Bypass

MPFRt = 100 mL/kg/min x $(0.0194e^{0.1171(t)})/(0.0194e^{0.1171(37°C)})$

Temperature (°C)	$CMRO_2$ (mL/100 g/min)	Predicted MPFR (mL/kg/min)
37	1.48	100
32	0.823	56
30	0.654	44
28	0.513	34
25	0.362	24
20	0.201	14
18	0.159	11
15	0.112	8

The equation in the top panel is the suggested equation defining minimal pump flow rate for any temperature (t) (MPFRt). The lower panel solves the equations for mean cerebral metabolism for oxygen ($CMRO_2$) and the minimal predicted pump flow rate (MPFR) for the hypothermic temperature (t) during cardiopulmonary bypass in children.
See reference 121.

described by Greeley and colleagues.[88] For the brain, the metabolic reduction induced by hypothermia is described by the temperature coefficient, or Q10—the ratio of brain metabolism measured at two temperatures separated by 10°C. The data in children suggest that hypothermia decreases the cerebral metabolic rate for oxygen by a mean of 3.6 for every 10°C reduction in temperature. If one assumes that at normal temperature the brain can tolerate an ischemic period of 3 to 5 minutes, then at a brain temperature of 15°C (using Q10 data), brain metabolism is sufficiently reduced to allow for a "safe" circulatory arrest period of 53 to 90 minutes. However, central to these calculations is the assumption that cerebral cooling is uniform and complete, which may not always be achieved (see subsequent discussion).

As already alluded to, there may be a "no-flow" phenomenon during extreme low-flow cardiopulmonary bypass. In this regard, studies in infants have demonstrated that with profound hypothermic circulatory arrest, and extreme low-flow states, intracranial pressure can increase to 18 mm Hg.[35,222] Furthermore, Taylor and colleagues,[231] in a study of 25 neonates and infants, found that, during profound hypothermia, in nine patients there was no cerebral blood flow detectable when the cerebral perfusion pressure (i.e., the numerical difference between the mean arterial and mean intracranial pressures) fell to a critical level of 9 ± 2 mm Hg. No relationship was found between pump flow rates and the critical cerebral perfusion pressure at which cerebral blood flow was lost. It is also of note that in two patients cerebral blood flow was lost at pump flow rates of 28% and 33% of normal. It seems advisable, therefore, to maintain mean arterial pressure above 20 mm Hg and avoid pump flow rates below 25% of normal flow rates, thereby ensuring cerebral perfusion pressures above 12 mm Hg during low-flow cardiopulmonary bypass.

Finally, to give the preceding discussion a clinical context, the results of a recent randomized clinical trial suggest that low-flow bypass may be more advantageous in regard to early developmental outcome.[21] In this study, Bellinger and colleagues[21] compared the Bayley Scales of Infant Development at 1 year of age in 171 infants with transposition of the great arteries who underwent the arterial switch operation using either predominantly total circulatory arrest or predominantly low-flow cardiopulmonary bypass. The children randomized to the circulatory arrest group scored lower than those assigned to the low-flow bypass group. Responses to parental questionnaires completed when the children were 2½ years old indicated that the children in the circulatory arrest group, especially those with a ventricular septal defect, also exhibited poorer expressive language and were considered to display more internalizing and externalizing problem behaviors.

Pulsatile Cardiopulmonary Bypass Continuous pulsatile flow during cardiopulmonary bypass is provided with the assistance of a synchronous pump. Potentially, cerebral blood flow could be improved by this technique. However, studies in adults have not proven its usefulness in improving neurologic outcomes. For example, Murkin and colleagues[163,164] compared the neuropsychological outcome of 316 adults undergoing extracorporeal circulation with or without pulsatile flow. Even though the use of pulsatile perfusion was associated with decreased incidences of myocardial infarction, death, and major complications, the incidence of stroke (2.5%) did not differ between the groups. Furthermore, pulsatility had no effect on the incidence of cognitive or other neurologic dysfunction.

Induced-Hypothermia Strategy

In regard to cerebroprotection during cardiac surgery, the most important factor before and after the period of circulatory arrest or low-flow is hypothermia. Unfortunately, there is a paucity of clinical information on cooling during cardiopulmonary bypass in children.

The Adequacy of Brain Cooling If cooling is going to be depended upon as the main strategy for cerebroprotection during cardiac surgery, then the adequacy and thoroughness of brain cooling during bypass is the first aspect of management that it is necessary to consider. The variability in the effectiveness of brain cooling appears to depend on biologic, mechanical, and technical factors.

The adequacy of cerebral perfusion during the cooling phase may be an important factor. Greeley and colleagues[88] found significantly higher cerebral oxygen extractions and cerebral metabolic rates in approximately 10% of patients undergoing congenital heart surgery despite their having been cooled to nasopharyngeal and rectal temperatures of 18°C. Three of these patients went on to have significant neurologic dysfunction despite a relatively short period of circulatory arrest. A likely explanation suggested by the authors was that inadequate cerebral perfusion resulted in inefficient brain cooling and the existence of temperature gradients throughout the brain.

Mechanical factors may contribute to inadequate cerebral perfusion. Kern and colleagues[120] found low jugular venous oxygen saturation despite cooling to 15°C to 17°C to be more likely in those with modified aortic cannula placement, such as patients undergoing the arterial switch procedure for transposition of the great arteries. In this instance, the aortic cannula is placed as far from the aortic root as possible, to facilitate coronary transfer, that is, in a position where the tip of the aortic cannula may promote preferential flow down the aorta or induce "steal" flow away from the cerebral circulation. However, an alternative view about the presence of non-homogeneous brain cooling occurring as a result of standard techniques has been put forward by Kurth and colleagues.[130] These authors used near-infrared spectroscopy (NIRS) to study kinetic changes in cerebrovascular hemoglobin oxygen saturation ($HbO_2\%$) in 17 neonates undergoing cardiac surgery as they were cooled to 15° C, underwent total circulatory arrest, and were rewarmed. They found that $HbO_2\%$ in brain vasculature increased during the initial 8 minutes of cardiopulmonary bypass as nasopharyngeal temperature decreased and then remained constant until circulatory arrest. After the onset of circulatory arrest, cerebrovascular $HbO_2\%$ decreased curvilinearly for 40 minutes, suggesting that cerebral rewarming during circulatory arrest rather than reperfusion was observed. And, because there was no rise in nasopharyngeal temperatures over this period, they concluded that non-homogeneous brain cooling was unlikely.

A minimum duration of cooling (>20 minutes) may be necessary to ensure uniform brain cooling to achieve adequate neuroprotection. Bellinger and colleagues[19] found that in infants with transposition of the great arteries undergoing deep hypothermic circulatory arrest, for core cooling periods of less than 20 minutes' duration (11 to 18 minutes), shorter cooling periods were associated with lower developmental scores on follow-up. Also, it was noted that, within this range of cooling period, an increase of 5 minutes of core cooling was associated with a 26-point improvement in score. Similarly, Wong and colleagues[247] found that, in comparison with 17 diagnosis- and age-matched historical controls, 19 patients who developed choreoathetosis after cardiac surgery had shorter duration (22 ± 7 versus 40 ± 29 minutes, $p = 0.053$) of cooling before the onset of deep hypothermic circulatory arrest.

Cerebral Vulnerability after Hypothermic Circulatory Arrest
Following circulatory arrest, there is evidence in infants that a brief period of cold reperfusion may be beneficial,[13,116,199] and in rabbits a slower rate of rewarming may be of value.[69] Together, these studies suggest that the process of rewarming the brain after deep hypothermic circulatory arrest may also be a critical period in terms of potential for injury.

More recently, the time course of this period of vulnerability has been studied using a variety of techniques to characterize the physiology and cerebral effects.[49,62,64,179,189,242] O'Hare and colleagues[179] used the Doppler assessment of cerebral blood flow velocity to determine how long cerebral hypoperfusion persisted after profound hypothermic circulatory arrest. Ten infants undergoing congenital heart disease surgery were divided into two groups based on the pump modality that was used: mild hypothermic cardiopulmonary bypass or deep hypothermic bypass with circulatory arrest. The study demonstrated that, in comparison with controls, a sustained reduction in the middle cerebral artery blood flow velocity pattern followed deep hypothermic circulatory arrest. This postoperative abnormality persisted for the time course of the study (i.e., 4 hours), despite the adequacy of cerebral perfusion pressures, and supports the concept of a prolonged unreactive cerebrovascular bed. These physiologic changes, occurring after deep hypothermic circulatory arrest, have

also been further characterized biochemically by Pesonen and colleagues.[189] In 10 children cerebral venous oxygen desaturation occurred between 2 and 6 hours after surgery in association with arteriovenous, transcerebral differences in hypoxanthine and lactoferrin, suggesting delayed impairment of cerebral oxygenation and the coexistence of abnormal energy state and neurophil activation. du Plessis and colleagues[62] used NIRS to study the relationship between cerebral intravascular (hemoglobin) and mitochondrial (cytochrome aa3) oxygenation in 63 infants (aged 1 day to 9 months) undergoing deep hypothermic repair of congenital heart defects. With rewarming and reperfusion following circulatory arrest, there was dissociation in the recovery of intravascular oxygenation and oxidized cytochrome aa3. The recovery of oxidized cytochrome aa3 was delayed, and even after 60 minutes of reperfusion only 46% of the infants had recovered to baseline levels. These effects were more pronounced in infants older than 2 weeks of age and suggest a prolonged impairment of intrinsic mitochondrial function, or of delivery of intravascular oxygen to the mitochondrion, or some combination of these two effects. Last, using postoperative EEG monitoring as an endpoint in a single-center randomized controlled trial of acid-base management in infants undergoing deep hypothermic cardiopulmonary bypass, du Plessis and colleagues[64] challenged the notion that the alpha-stat strategy was superior to the pH-stat strategy for organ protection. Relevant to the current discussion is that these authors found the alpha-stat strategy to be associated with longer recovery times to first EEG activity (mean ± SD, 38 ± 33 versus 29 ± 14 minutes; hazard ratio = 1.54, 95% confidence interval of 1.03 to 2.30, $p = 0.03$), which is of similar time course to the abnormalities described previously.

The management options for the cerebral vulnerability phase are limited. Every effort should be made to preserve adequate cardiac output and cerebral oxygen delivery. Modified ultrafiltration after cardiopulmonary bypass may be beneficial for a host of reasons, one of which is improved cerebral recovery.[216]

Microembolization and Massive Air Embolism

Microembolization during cardiopulmonary bypass has been well documented in adults and historically was regarded by many as a major cause of postoperative cerebral dysfunction and damage.[3,4,30,141,162] Various types of microemboli are formed during cardiopulmonary bypass (Table 6-6), and they can be detected in the arterial inflow line. Many solid microemboli made up of platelet and leukocyte aggregates are resistant to deaggregation and can be formed despite apparently

Table 6-6 Types of Microemboli Formed during Cardiopulmonary Bypass

Host-derived	Foreign Material
Platelets	Particulate matter
Leukocytes	Insoluble calcium products
Muscle fragments	Antifoam particles
Lipid droplets	Air
Protein	Oxygen

adequate heparinization.[207] Gaseous emboli may be generated by the pump oxygenator and these can be detected by various means, including echo ultrasound and transesophageal echocardiography. Microemboli of oxygen can arise during oxygenation of the blood,[171] or air emboli can result from incomplete defoaming of the blood in the bubble oxygenators.[218] Microemboli may also arise from residual air left in the heart during the surgical procedure. Massive air embolism, although rare during heart surgery, can lead to devastating neurologic complications, with a significant instantaneous mortality.[158] If cerebral air embolism is recognized intraoperatively, it can be treated by reinstituting cardiopulmonary bypass or employing hyperbaric oxygen therapy.

Cerebral Hypoperfusion and Neuroprotection

Many agents have been suggested as potential therapies to limit or prevent the development of brain damage after an ischemic insult. Behind all such notions, however, one should remember that the pathophysiology varies greatly among the different types of cerebral damage (global versus regional; anoxic versus hypoxic) seen in the cardiac surgery patient (see previous discussion). Because an increasingly younger population of patients are undergoing surgery, the particular emphasis of this section will be the phenomena of cerebral hypoperfusion and potential mechanisms for protection against hypoxic-ischemic injury in the developing brain.

Phases of Neuronal Injury

From the neonatal period onward, significant alterations occur in the brain. As well as increases in size and myelination, there are changes in the brain's complexity. There are changes in the total number of neurons, synapses, established neural connections, and the distribution and number of excitatory amino acid receptors, for example, the N-methyl-D-aspartate (NMDA) ionophore. Cerebrovascular control mechanisms are well developed by the time of normal birth, and the healthy infant can regulate cerebral hemodynamics in the face of alterations of blood pressure and blood gas tension, although these mechanisms are easily disrupted by hypoxic-ischemic injury.

The metabolic cascades induced during and following ischemia have been described in detail by many authors. The initiating event, a decrease in local cerebral blood flow below a critical threshold, results in progressive pathophysiologic changes that culminate in neurodegeneration. These acute ischemia-induced processes can be divided into three important phases based on major movements in cellular ions (Fig. 6-3).[142] First is a phase of metabolic depression, occurring within minutes of an insult, with rapid decrease in electrical activity and suppression of neurotransmission (phase 1). At a cellular ionic level, there is a slow increase in extracellular potassium concentration ($[K^+]_e$) from approximately 3 mmol/L up to 8 to 10 mmol/L. At least two types of K^+ channel appear to be responsible for this change in K^+ conductance, one activated by an increase in intracellular calcium concentration ($[Ca^{++}]_i$) and the other activated by a decrease in adenosine triphosphate (ATP), the ATP-sensitive K^+ channel (K_{ATP}). The second phase is characterized by almost complete energy failure and anoxic depolarization (phase 2). It starts abruptly when an $[K^+]_e$ of 8 to 10 mmol/L triggers, within seconds, a rapid transition to an $[K^+]_e$ of 50 to 70 mmol/L. Once this depolarization has occurred there follows a loss of sodium (Na^+) and calcium (Ca^{++}) ion gradients and a release of various neurotransmitters into the extracellular space, including glutamate, aspartate, and dopamine. The sudden increase in membrane permeability, which has resulted in this transition, may be attributable to the opening of voltage-gated K^+, Na^+, and Ca^{++} channels.

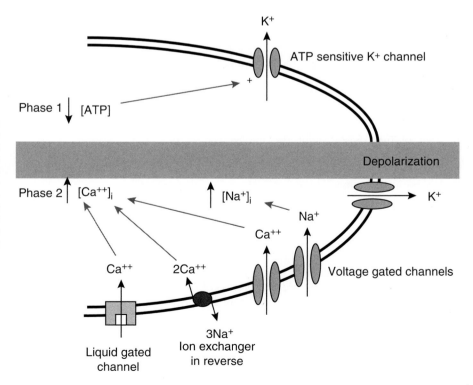

FIGURE 6-3 Schematic illustration of cellular ionic changes occurring during the ischemia-induced periods of metabolic depression with bioenergetic stress (phase 1) and complete energy failure with anoxic depolarization (phase 2). Where [ATP] is the concentration of adenosine triphosphate; $[Ca^{++}]_i$ and $[Na^+]_i$ are the intracellular concentrations of calcium and sodium, respectively; and [K^+] is potassium. (From Tasker RC: Pharmacological advance in the treatment of acute brain injury. *Arch Dis Child* 81:90–95, 1999; with permission.)

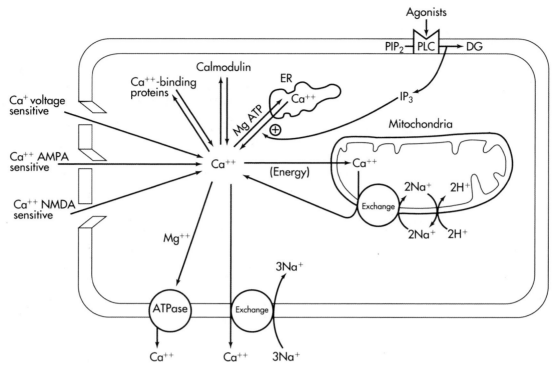

FIGURE 6-4 Calcium homeostasis in a neuron. Calcium influx is regulated by voltage-sensitive and ligand (glutamate)–sensitive channels named after their most potent synthetic agonists (NMDA and AMPA). PIP_2—phosphatidyl inositol diphosphate; PLC—phospholipase C; DG—diacylglcerol; IP_3—inositol triphosphate. Energy-dependent regulation of intracellular calcium $[Ca^{++}]_i$ is via an ATP-dependent pump; translocation for Na^+ ions, and uptake into endoplasmic reticulum (ER) and mitochondria. Energy-dependent calcium homeostasis occurs via buffering of calcium ions by calmodulin and other intracellular proteins (calbindin, parvalbumin).[98]

Calcium ions, however, may also enter neurons through ligand-gated ion channels, such as the NMDA ionophore (Fig. 6-4).[98] This latter route of entry does not depend on a net increase in endogenous levels of the receptor ligands, glutamate and aspartate, because either cellular energy failure or depolarization can also open the channel in the absence of neurotransmitter. (Another mechanism whereby Ca^{++} may move into the cell is as a result of a functional reversal of the Na^+-Ca^{++} ion exchanger, which instead of moving Ca^{++} out of the cell is driven to work in reverse by a high $[Na^+]_i$, thus further increasing $[Ca^{++}]_i$.) The third, and final, phase marks a period of neurodegeneration (phase 3), which may be played out over many hours or even days.[123] In this regard, a number of hypotheses about the mechanism of neuronal injury have been proposed, and include excitatory amino acid neurotoxicity;[204] disturbed function in mitochondria[2] or endoplasmic reticulum,[187] or both;[213] and, Ca^{++}-mediated toxicity.[125,212] At an ionic level, initially, the cell membrane is fully depolarized with high $[Ca^{++}]_i$: these two derangements are able to trigger a number of degradative processes either on their own or in combination with any of the above mechanisms (Fig. 6-5).[210,211] As to which of these mechanisms predominates in a particular insult, there are a variety of factors that may be important in determining the specific process of neurodegeneration (e.g., the intensity and time course of the insult, whether or not a period of recovery or reperfusion occurs, and whether or not irreversible cell swelling—an important process leading to necrosis starting during phase 1—has also resulted).[172]

Considering the relationship between excitatory amino acid system activation and energy failure, the brain of immature animals is known to be generally more resistant to anoxia and ischemia than that of adults. This is attributed to low cerebral energy consumption in immature brains and to a more delayed energy failure.[65,228,236] It has been suggested that

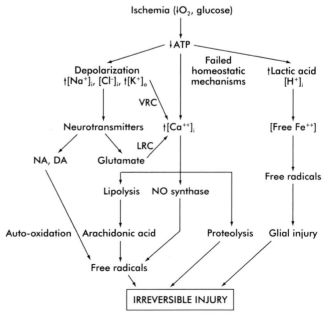

FIGURE 6-5 Potential mechanisms of ischemic brain damage. ATP, Adenosine triphosphate; VRC, voltage-regulated calcium channels; LRC, ligand-regulated calcium channels; NA, noradrenaline (norepinephrine); DA, dopamine; NO, nitric oxide.[210]

when the severity of a hypoxia-ischemia insult is comparable in the immature and adult brain, the former is less likely to develop energy failure severe enough to activate its excitatory amino acid system. However, once the excitatory amino acid system is activated in the immature brain, because of intrinsically exaggerated postsynaptic excitatory activities, it could have more devastating effects than in the adult brain.[99]

Rescue and Protective Treatments

The recognition of complex hemodynamic, electrophysiologic, and biochemical cascades involved in the process of brain injury has provided a framework for the development of pharmacologic and metabolic interventions before, during, and after cerebral ischemia, each designed to prevent or ameliorate neuronal death or injury.

Glucose Supplementation In laboratory studies, the potential role of glucose supplementation rescue treatment has been considered. Pretreating immature animals with glucose prolongs survival during hypoxia by maintaining brain ATP and phosphocreatine levels.[106] In marked contrast, however, in juvenile and adult animals, elevated levels of blood glucose during ischemia aggravate the severity of the brain damage,[194] which may lead to cerebral infarction when associated with an accumulation of lactic acid above a critical point (16 to 20 mmol/kg). Concerning the more clinically useful 'rescue-therapy,' one neonatal animal model using posthypoxic glucose supplementation reduced hypoxic-ischemic brain damage,[100] although the mechanism of protection was not fully understood and the "window of opportunity" was not generally characterized. From a practical standpoint, the perioperative team should seek to control the serum glucose tightly in a normal range.

Inhibitors of Cerebral Metabolism Hypothermia, which generally depresses metabolism, is currently by far the most effective and commonly used means of inhibiting cerebral metabolism during cardiopulmonary bypass. Hypothermia appears to depress general cerebral metabolism, whereas drugs, such as barbiturates, depress only that part related to active electrical function.[153] It is hypothermia's protective effect at the cellular level that seems to enable the brain to tolerate prolonged periods of circulatory arrest.

Hypothermia enhances the brain's tolerance of ischemia by slowing ATP depletion and lactic acid formation.[93,209,230,249] However, it also induces an acid shift in intracellular pH, which may be important in regard to neuroprotection.[230] Lowering body temperature $2°$ C to $5°$ C (mild to moderate hypothermia) may protect the brain by attenuating the peri-ischemic release of excitatory amino acid neurotransmitters.[37] In this regard, it is of interest that, in immature animals, lowering body temperature $5°$ C provides as much partial protection against hypoxia-ischemia induced brain damage as pretreatment with the NMDA receptor antagonist, dizocilpine maleate (MK-801).[110] Recent in vivo evidence also indicates that, in addition to a 30%–40% decrease in cerebral metabolism, a temperature of $31°$ C is associated with an increased fraction of glucose metabolism shunted through the pentose phosphate pathway.[118] Stimulation of the pentose phosphate pathway (or hexose monophosphate shunt) in neutrophils generates sufficient protons for lowering intracellular pH.[89] Such a mechanism may, therefore, account for the ameliorating effect of hypothermia: that is, production of nicotinamide adenine dinucleotide phosphate (NADPH) which has tissue-protective effects by maintaining membrane potential, and ion transport, and by removing membrane-toxic oxygen radicals.[17]

The mechanism by which drug agents acting on brain metabolism protect the brain is believed to be partly due to their ability to reduce the cerebral metabolic rate for oxygen ($CMRO_2$). Isoflurane decreases $CMRO_2$, primarily by suppressing cortical electrical activity. Barbiturates, known to reduce $CMRO_2$ in a dose-dependent manner (but only down to the point of isoelectric EEG), have also been shown to protect the brain during incomplete ischemia.[150] Midazolam, a short-acting water-soluble benzodiazepine, in sufficient dosage also profoundly depresses $CMRO_2$.[176] Accordingly, it may be an alternative to barbiturates for cerebral protection. Isoflurane, a volatile anesthetic, has also been used to protect the brain during incomplete ischemia.[167,168] Isoflurane produces an isoelectric EEG in humans at hemodynamically tolerable concentrations (2.4%).

Channel Blockers and Other Neuroprotective Drugs The theory of pharmacologic neuroprotection posits the existence of agents that will minimize the effects of ischemia on the brain. The focus of much animal laboratory work in neuroprotection has been on focal ischemia—stroke—models in mature animals, in which treatment is given during or after an artery supplying the brain has been occluded, or during both periods. And, to a lesser extent, studies have also been conducted in immature animals. In all such studies, the aim of the neuroprotective maneuver is to influence the ischemia-induced cascade so as to maximize the proportion of (previously) ischemic brain that will survive and recover. To date, many pharmacological approaches, or combination of approaches, have been applied to animal models with beneficial effects, which seemed to promise efficacy in patients. Unfortunately, experience through the 1990s demonstrated that the process of converting a promising drug effect in the laboratory to a clinically useful test product was fraught with difficulty. Translation to clinical practice was not forthcoming. In stroke therapy, only thrombolysis with recombinant tissue plasminogen activator[234] and antiplatelet therapy with aspirin[42,111,161] proved to be effective for acute stroke. Other agents (NMDA receptor antagonists and other channel blockers), although in advanced stages of clinical development, were, in a number of instances, withdrawn during clinical trial with, in some cases, results still to be published.

The challenge for the future, therefore, is to bridge the gap between preclinical research and clinical utility. There is also the continued need for new therapeutic ideas, which may require defining endogenous homeostatic neuroprotective defense mechanisms, or even the development of better models that mimic the clinical entities seen in our practice.[229]

NEUROLOGIC MONITORING AND MANAGEMENT

As already discussed, the process of cardiopulmonary bypass with or without circulatory arrest puts the brain at significant risk for neurologic injury. Concern over the potential development of cerebral injury has prompted the use of various intraoperative and postoperative monitoring techniques, with the supposition that early identification may result in early remedy and the avoidance of brain damage. There is, however, no clinical evidence that once a cerebral insult has occurred, monitoring of whatever form alters the eventual outcome. Sadly, many of these techniques merely make us more sophisticated observers of events usually having an unrelenting course. There is perhaps some merit, though, in that we may be able to evaluate prognosis and, in time, the effects of new therapies. Furthermore, monitoring helps to make us aware of when injury occurs and may, therefore, focus future investigations on specific times of injury prevention.

Markers of Cerebral Injury

For years there has been a quest for markers of cerebral injury, which in our population of patients could be used before, during, and after surgery. The current markers may be separated into three categories: neuroimaging, brain metabolism and blood flow, and biochemical. As with previous sections, the developing brain will be a particular emphasis.

Neuroimaging

The advantages of MRI over CT scan for brain imaging include the lack of ionizing radiation; greater sensitivity to blood flow, edema, hemorrhage, and myelination; lack of beam-hardening artifacts; and easier differentiation between gray and white matter. Magnetic resonance imaging of the brain is being used in some centers.[72] For example, McConnell and colleagues[147] assessed MRIs in 12 acyanotic patients and 6 cyanotic patients. Fifteen of these patients survived cardiac surgery, having undergone moderate hypothermic cardiopulmonary bypass using a nonpulsatile membrane oxygenator, and completed both the preoperative and postoperative images. Ten of the preoperative images were interpreted as normal. One third (five of 15) of the patients showed ventriculomegaly and dilatation of the subarachnoid spaces on preoperative imaging. Fourteen of

the 15 patients showed measurable increase in ventricular volumes and subarachnoid spaces when the preoperative and postoperative images were compared. Four patients in the study developed postoperative subdural hematomas. One patient had a preoperative white matter infarct and another developed a postoperative infarct. Interestingly, the age at which these infants were assessed meant that such structural abnormalities detected by MRI were "subclinical," that is, no neurologic symptom or deficit was found on examination, probably because the child's neurodevelopment was not sufficiently matured to express the deficit. The measurable ventricular enlargement and dilatation of the subarachnoid spaces suggest that brain parenchymal volumes actually diminished, because there were no concomitant changes in cranial dimensions. Whatever the reason for these changes, this study showed an alarming incidence of brain pathology. The fact that most of the findings were "subclinical" highlights the crudeness of our more conventional neurologic evaluation.

Brain Metabolism and Blood Flow

An early marker of cerebral injury after an insult may be changes in the brain energy state or brain metabolism. These can be assessed by magnetic resonance spectroscopy or by the use of various metabolic tracers, as in the case of positron emission tomography (PET). Magnetic resonance spectroscopy can be used clinically to measure the concentration of ATP, phosphocreatine, and inorganic phosphate, as well as the intracellular pH in the brain. These metabolites reflect the level of tissue and cellular energy. Any significant alteration in cerebral blood flow or metabolism that produces an energy change can therefore be assessed noninvasively. Distinctive spectra are observed over brain regions with infarction and changes in oxygenation (Fig. 6-6).[53] Positron emission tomography has also been used as a clinical and research tool for measuring cerebral oxygen and glucose extraction.[57,60] However, the potential diagnostic and prognostic value of this tool in the cardiac surgical population has not yet been fully realized.

Alterations in global cerebral blood flow and regional distribution, impairment of autoregulation, and changes in

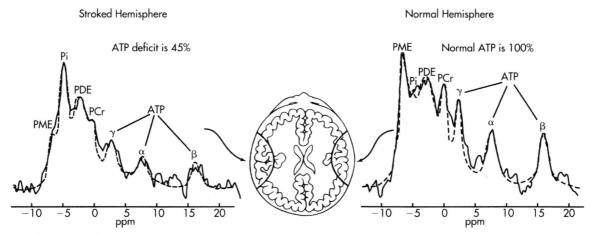

FIGURE 6-6   An illustration of NMR signals from two hemispheres of the neonatal brain, in which hypoxia and ischemia selectively affected the left hemisphere. The significant feature of the spectrum is that hydrolysis of ATP has occurred in one hemisphere. Two types of traces are presented—the original data and the computer fitting of the same data. The cranial CT scan showed an infarct in the left hemisphere. (From Delivoria-Papadopoulos M, Chance B: 31-PNMR in the newborn. In Guthrie RD [ed]: *Neonatal Intensive Care*. New York, Churchill Livingstone, 1986; with permission.)

blood flow pulsatility may all be markers of brain injury, available in the first 24 to 48 hours after an insult. Three techniques that are currently being used are ^{133}Xe clearance, assessment of Doppler flow velocities, and PET. And, as discussed in previous sections of this chapter, there has been a major clinical research effort to apply these assessments of cerebral blood flow measurement to neonates and young infants at risk for brain injury following cardiac surgery.

Biochemical Markers

Among the readily available clinical biochemical markers, metabolic acidosis secondary to lactate accumulation in the first 24 hours after surgery appears to be the most useful predictor of subsequent neurologic injury. In particular, a pH <7.35 and a lactate >40 mg/dL significantly increase the odds of a newborn sustaining a diagnosis of brain damage after cardiac surgery.[237]

There has also been growing interest in the clinical measurement of two proteins that may serve as markers of brain-related complications after cardiac surgery. The assumption is that these proteins are released from neuronal and astroglial cells, respectively, and not from any other cell type—such as fat, for example. It is hoped that they might be specific for brain injury, but there are some data to suggest an extracerebral source during cardiopulmonary bypass.[9]

Neuron-Specific Enolase Neuron specific enolase is an enzyme involved in glycolysis, which is localized in neurons and axonal processes. Potentially, it escapes into the blood and CSF at the time of neural injury. For example, in 200 adults undergoing cardiac surgery, Isgro and colleagues[112] determined, with a prospective study design, serum levels of neuron specific enolase before the operation, right after the operation, and 48 hours later. Fifty patients undergoing general surgical treatment were used as controls. Preoperatively, serum levels of the enzyme were low in all patients. The early postoperative measurements indicated a significant increase in levels in the cardiac rather than the general surgical patients. In 17 out of the 200 cardiac patients a neurological complication occurred and elevated levels were found in 16 of these 17 patients, with the highest concentrations being measured in 7 patients exhibiting the most severe neurological complications (i.e., transient ischemic attacks and stroke). The authors therefore suggested that, in addition to its value in detecting cerebral injury, neuron specific enolase might also be of prognostic value.

In children undergoing cardiac surgery with cardiopulmonary bypass, however, the predictive value of neuron specific enolase has been questioned. Schmitt and colleagues[206] measured serum neuron specific enolase before and up to 102 hours after cardiac surgery with cardiopulmonary bypass in 27 children. In 11 children CSF neuron specific enolase was also measured at 48 and 66 hours after surgery. In common with the adult study[112] described earlier, elevated serum neuron specific enolase seemed to indicate brain injury associated with cardiopulmonary bypass surgery. However, low concentration of the enzyme in the postoperative CSF samples questioned the neuronal origin of the elevated serum levels. (It should be noted that the enzyme is also found in erythrocytes.) Additionally, normal postoperative CSF enzyme levels were found in two children with surgery-related neurologic sequelae.

S-100 Protein Experimentally, the release of neuron-specific astroglial S-100 protein to the CSF is a marker of cerebral damage. Recently, a number of clinical studies have been undertaken in children undergoing cardiac surgery.[1,12,114,138] In an observational study of 97 children, Lindberg and colleagues[138] found that serum concentrations of S-100 protein before cardiac operation were highest in neonates. Children with Down syndrome, regardless of age, had basal levels comparable to those in neonates. Immediately after extracorporeal circulation there was an increase in serum S-100 protein concentration, and multivariate regression analysis showed that the difference in concentration was significant with respect to age, perfusion time, and the use of circulatory arrest. The authors rightly concluded that if such a biochemical parameter were to be of value in the early identification of postperfusion cerebral injuries then there was need for age-matched reference values as well as the necessity for taking into consideration perfusion time. Ashraf and colleagues[12] found that, in comparison with 12 infants undergoing cardiopulmonary bypass, the serum S-100 protein levels in 12 neonates undergoing total circulatory arrest were significantly higher 24 hours after surgery. However, in light of the cited study by Lindberg and colleagues,[138] this result should be interpreted with caution, as the total circulatory arrest group were younger and experienced a longer perfusion time than the cardiopulmonary bypass group.

Given the limitation of these studies, Abdul-Khaliq and colleagues[1] sought to identify appropriate clinical controls. In their institution routine biochemical monitoring of S-100 protein was undertaken. The authors therefore compared the release pattern of serum S-100 protein in infants and children with and without neurologic abnormalities after corrective cardiac operations. Data from infants undergoing corrective surgery for coarctation of the aorta without cardiopulmonary bypass (64 infants) served for control values. The utility of measuring serum S-100 protein levels appeared to be supported by the observation that higher serum concentrations—more than 2 standard deviations—than the peak S-100 values in controls were found in four infants with neurologic and cardiac complications. Most recently, however, Jensen and colleagues[114] have reported their serial serum findings in 17 cardiac surgical and 31 noncardiac surgical patients. In both groups of patients, a significant increase in S-100 concentrations was observed during surgery, although the increase in the cardiopulmonary bypass group was higher. None of these patients developed signs of neurological sequelae, and so the clinical significance of this change has to be reconsidered. For the time being, at least, it could be argued that open-heart surgery with cardiopulmonary bypass initiates a "normal" and insignificant transient release (albeit marked) of S-100 protein into the circulation.

Monitors of Intra- and Postoperative Changes in Cerebral Function

Based on a number of studies certain periods of cardiopulmonary bypass have been identified during which the brain is at increased risk of neurological injury. These periods include the active cooling period, the period of low-flow bypass or total circulatory arrest, and the period during weaning and separation from bypass. Rightly, investigation of cerebral function during the intraoperative and postoperative period requires the reliable measurement of cerebral blood flow, cerebral metabolism, and cerebral electrical activity. In the latter, depression of activity is a function of the duration of continuous circulatory arrest, and an impaired metabolic recovery from such changes may be an excellent marker of cerebral injury after circulatory arrest. In the context of the previous section, a variety of methodologies have been used in cardiac surgery patients.[122] The topic of this section will be restricted to the noninvasive techniques that have the potential for clinical cerebral electrophysiologic and hemodynamic monitoring.

Electroencephalography

Standard EEG The technique of EEG assessment of children undergoing cardiac surgery has been available for over 40 years.[184] Conventional EEG provides information about cortical brain activity, at the time of recording. Multiple factors may affect the level of such activity, and in the context of pediatric cardiac surgery, the signals reflect the summed effects of brain temperature, cerebral perfusion, metabolic state, anesthesia, and drug action on the normal background activity expected for age or stage of brain development.[14,96,97,103] Unfortunately, while the technique itself is quite sensitive, the changes observed are generally not that specific, particularly when one considers that deep hypothermia alone will lead to the disappearance of EEG activity. Despite these failings, in the resuscitated and warmed deeply comatose child, perhaps the most useful application of EEG is in prognostication. In this regard, Pampiglione and Harden[185] reported in 1968 four distinct EEG patterns of prognostic value in children that were seen in the first 24 hours after resuscitation from cardiac arrest (Fig. 6-7).

Signal-Processed EEG Other EEG techniques, involving signal processing of cortical activity, have also been employed in intraoperative and postoperative care.[224,226] There are, however, major limitations with such approaches, which necessitate the continued use of intermittent conventional EEG assessment. Most experience has been with the use of the cerebral function monitor (CFM) or cerebral function

analyzing monitor (CFAM) and the compressed spectral array (CSA).

The CFM/CFAM displays changes in EEG amplitude (Fig. 6-8). In brief, after detection by one or two isolation preamplifiers on extension cables, the EEG signal is divided between several circuits. These include an asymmetric band-pass filter (band width 1-27 Hz) with an output that is used for amplitude and frequency analysis, two circuits of conventional EEG filters, two circuits for signal overload detection, and a single circuit that may be used for the detection of muscle activity at the recording electrodes. The output is displayed as an on-line paper trace showing distribution of weighted amplitude (logarithmic scale—upper portion of output trace), percentage activity in frequency bands (beta 8 to 13 Hz, alpha >14 Hz, theta 4 to 7 Hz, delta <3 Hz—lower portion of output trace), as well as the percentage activity below a preset amplitude (suppression) of a single EEG channel (or two channels alternately) (Fig. 6-8). The automated frequency analysis can be performed on signals as small as 1 μV peak to peak amplitude. Amplitude distribution is computed for signals in the range 0.63 to 220 μV peak to peak, with a second range of 1.9 to 660 μV. In addition, electrode impedance (0 to 20 kOhms) is constantly displayed on a channel that will also indicate electrical interference.

The CSA depicts condensed EEG amplitudes at different frequencies during periodic sampling intervals. The spectral analysis is performed with the fast Fourier transform, and the power (amplitude²) of the various frequencies that constitute the signal is displayed.

With the earlier mentioned forms of monitoring (CFM/CFAM or CSA), a fall in amplitude and slowing of frequency (Fig. 6-8) and the appearance of paroxysmal activity can be identified. However, in the case of paroxysmal activity, not all of the "electrical seizures" will be documented by the CFAM channels being monitored if the patient has a variable focus or multifocal discharges (Figs. 6-8 and 6-9).[29,225] This may be a particular problem in young patients with seizures and status epilepticus complicating cerebral hypoperfusion state.[227] Certain EEG phenomena may also be followed during extracorporeal cooling and rewarming in both adults and children.[84,134] However, what is done with this information remains a contentious point. Apart from optimizing general systemic care, and appropriately treating seizures, there are as

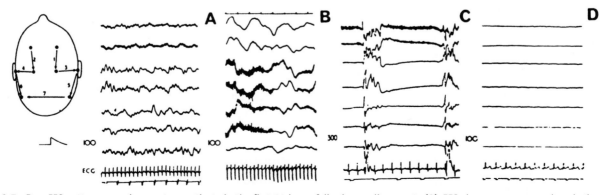

FIGURE 6-7 Four EEG patterns seen in comatose patients in the first 24 hours following cardiac arrest. **(A)** EEG shows some excess slow rhythms; **(B)** diffuse d-wave activity without faster frequencies; **(C)** intermittent activity in which prolonged periods of marked EEG attenuation are interrupted by briefer bursts of irregular activity; **(D)** isoelectric EEG. Patterns C and D are prognostically very poor with the usual outcome of death. (From Pampiglione G, Harden A: Resuscitation after cardiopulmonary arrest: Prognostic evaluation of early electroencephalographic findings. *Lancet* 1:1216–1265, 1968; with permission.)

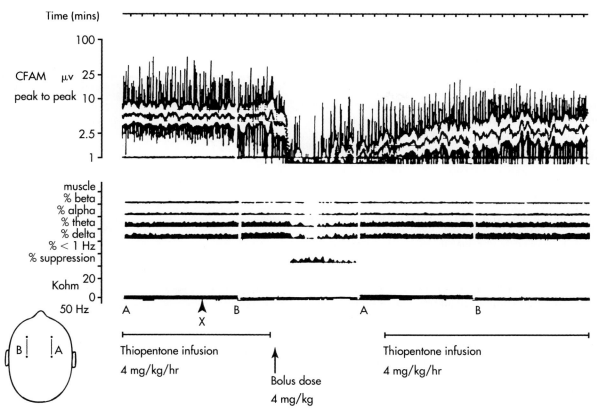

FIGURE 6-8 CFAM trace (10-minute epochs recorded alternately from each hemisphere, A and B) over a 40-minute period in a 5-year-old girl with seizures. A transient fall in amplitude and slowing of frequency are seen following an intravenous bolus dose of thiopentone. "X" indicates the last of five focal seizures clinically observed involving the left arm and angle of mouth. No paroxysmal changes are seen in the critical area being monitored. (From Tasker RC, Byrd SG, Harden A, Matthew DJ: The cerebral function analysing monitor in paediatric medical intensive care: Applications and limitations. *Intensive Care Med* 16:60–68, 1990; with permission.)

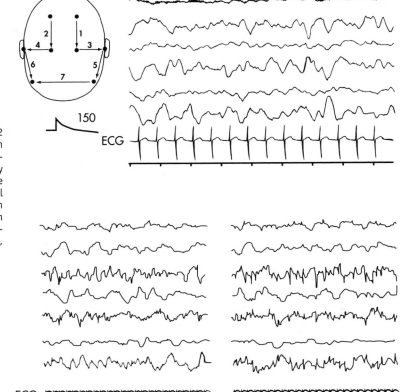

FIGURE 6-9 Contrasting EEG features in two infants aged 12 and 14 months with focal seizures following cardiac surgery. In the upper trace, irregular slow activities are seen over right temporal regions, where an infarct was subsequently demonstrated by cranial CT scan. In the lower trace, persistent discharges over the right temporal regions are not, presumably indicating local disturbance—the cranial CT scan was normal (note the change in paper speed compared with the upper traces—1.5 cm/s). (From Boyd SG, Harden A: Clinical neurophysiology of the central nervous system. In Brett EM [ed]: *Paediatric Neurology*. New York, Churchill Livingstone, 1991, pp 717–795; with permission.)

yet no specific pharmacotherapies that could reverse the effects of a damaging insult. Concerning prognosis, the signal-processed EEG findings can be used to indicate the need for more complete electrophysiological investigation (e.g., formal EEG and evoked potentials), which can then be interpreted in the framework of recognizable patterns and constellations of reversibility and irreversibility.

Multimodality Evoked Potentials Evoked potentials are sensitive prognostic tools in young infants at risk for developmental disability. Limperopoulos and colleagues[135] undertook somatosensory and brain stem auditory evoked potentials before and after cardiac surgery in 58 consecutively managed infants and newborns. The results showed that perioperative somatosensory evoked potential abnormalities were more common in newborns (11 of 27; 95% confidence interval of 22 to 61%) than in infants (4 of 31; 95% confidence interval of 4 to 30%) with congenital heart defects. Brain stem conduction times were within normal limits in all subjects. Importantly, all newborns with abnormal somatosensory evoked potentials had abnormal neurologic examinations both perioperatively and again 1 year after open-heart surgery. Also, in all of the newborns with abnormal somatosensory evoked potentials, standard developmental assessments at 1-year indicated deficits in one or more domains. Taken together, these findings indicate the potential importance of such monitoring.

Near-Infrared Spectroscopy

Since the initial description of NIRS[115] in 1977 there have been a variety of studies applying this technique to the noninvasive monitoring of intracerebral dynamics during and after cardiopulmonary bypass.[14,49,62,130,131]

Near-infrared spectroscopy depends on the relative transparency of biological tissue to light in the near-infrared spectrum. Three compounds that absorb light at these wavelengths are present in variable concentrations in the brain: oxyhemoglobin (HbO_2), deoxyhemoglobin (Hb), and cytochrome-c oxidase ($CytO_2$). Transillumination of the intact head offers the possibility of continuous noninvasive monitoring, by using suitable algorithms to convert changes in the attenuation of transmitted light into changes in [HbO_2], [Hb], and [$CytO_2$]. As already discussed in previous sections of this chapter, this technology has been used mainly as a tool in clinical research. The place of NIRS in the wider practice of perioperative cardiac care has yet to be defined. However, there are some indications that including NIRS in a battery of neurophysiologic monitoring for pediatric cardiac surgery may decrease the incidence of postoperative neurologic sequelae and reduce the length of stay.[14]

Postoperative Care

Seizures, focal neurological signs, and an unexpected depressed level of consciousness may all be features of significant neurological insult. As discussed in previous sections of the chapter, these features of an acute neurological process may be masked by concomitant sedation and paralysis. Obviously the priority in all patients having cardiac surgery must be good cardiopulmonary care, with meticulous attention to hemodynamic status. Diastolic hypotension may be a

Table 6-7 Management of Patient Who Fails to Lighten or Awaken Following Cardiac Surgery

Clinical Process	Examination—Investigation
1. Review	
All drugs administered	Chart review
Metabolic status	Temperature
	Blood glucose, calcium, sodium
	Blood pressure
2. Assess full neurology	Clinical trends
Failure to move or respond	Peripheral nerve stimulation
Comatose	Peripheral neurophysiology
Focal motor signs	EEG
Seizures	Evoked potentials
	CT scan or MRI
	CT scan
	EEG
	CT scan
3. If deeply comatose and flaccid with no spontaneous movement	Drug level screening
Institutional protocol for "brain death" assessment	Clinical evaluation
	± adjunctive tests:
	EEG
	Blood flow study

EEG, electroencephalography; CT, computed tomography; MRI, magnetic resonance imaging.

particular risk factor for periventricular leukomalacia, the most common brain MRI abnormality after neonatal cardiac surgery.[76] A concerted effort should be made to attend to a regular neurological examination. In those patients in whom this is not possible because of the necessary drugs administered, attention should be given to the possibility of unappreciated (and uncontrolled) seizures or continuing cerebral insult from poor cerebral perfusion—factors that of themselves will contribute to any primary neurological injury.

Anticonvulsant therapy for seizures or treatment of any metabolic derangement causing seizures should be administered promptly. Because the anticonvulsant medications may aggravate hemodynamic compromise in the immediate postoperative period, they should be administered slowly, in incremental doses, and under continuous hemodynamic surveillance. Airway and ventilatory support with continued intubation may be necessary due to the seizures themselves or obtundation from anticonvulsant medications. Poor cerebral perfusion and the development of cytotoxic cerebral edema with raised intracranial pressure will require the support for that problem. Tables 6-7 and 6-8 outline some of the management protocols that may be followed in these instances.

CONCLUSIONS

Infants and children with heart disease have a unique spectrum of neurologic disease. Newer technologies and a wider appreciation of cerebral physiology mean that we now understand more about the prevention of problems, particularly brain injury after open-heart surgery. The challenge for the future, however, is to bridge the gap between new therapeutic ideas and clinical utility.

Table 6-8 Anticonvulsant Therapy

Therapy	Anticonvulsant	Patient	Intravenous Dose	Blood Level
First-line	Diazepam	Neonatal	0.2–0.4 mg/kg	
		Infant/child	0.2–0.4 mg/kg	
		Adult	10 mg	
	or			
	Lorazepam	Infant/child	0.1–0.2 mg/kg	
		Adult	4–8 mg	
	or			
	Phenytoin	Neonatal	20 mg/kg	10–20 mcg/mL
		Infant/child	20 mg/kg	
		Adult	15–20 mg/kg (up to 1000 mg)	
Second-line	Phenytoin (if not already given)	As above		10–20 mcg/mL
	Phenobarbital	Neonatal	20 mg/kg	10–40 mcg/mL
		Infant/child	20 mg/kg	
	Thiopental		2–8 mg/kg load (increments of 2 mg/kg) 1–10 mg/kg/hr maintenance (under EEG control)	

References

1. Abdul-Khaliq H, Alexi-Meskhishvili V, Lange PE: Serum S-100 protein levels after pediatric cardiac surgery: A possible new marker for postperfusion cerebral injury. *J Thorac Cardiovasc Surg* 117:843–844, 1999.
2. Abe K, Aoki M, Kawagoe J, et al: Ischemic delayed neuronal death: A mitochondrial hypothesis. *Stroke* 26:1478–1489, 1995.
3. Aberg T, Kihlgren M: Cerebral protection during open-heart surgery. *Thorax* 32:525–533, 1977.
4. Aberg T, Ronquist G, Tyden H, et al: Adverse effects on the brain in cardiac operations as assessed by biochemical, psychometric, and radiologic methods. *J Thorac Cardiovasc Surg* 87:99–105, 1984.
5. Aebi C, Kaufmann F, Schaad UB: Brain abscess in childhood: Long-term experiences. *Eur J Pediatr* 150:282–286, 1991.
6. Aicardi J: Infectious diseases. In: *Diseases of the Nervous System. Clinics in Developmental Medicine*, 2nd ed. London: Mac Keith Press, 1998, p 392.
7. Alden B, Gilljam T, Gillberg C: Long-term psychological outcome of children after surgery for transposition of the great arteries. *Acta Paediatr* 87:405–410, 1998.
8. Amacher AL, Shillito J: The syndromes and surgical treatment of aneurysms of the great vein of Galen. *J Neurosurg* 39:89–97, 1973.
9. Anderson RE, Hansson LO, Nilsson O, et al: Increase in serum S100A1-B and S100BB during cardiac surgery arises from extracerebral sources. *Ann Thorac Surg* 71:1512–1517, 2001.
10. Ardinger RH Jr, Goertz KK, Mattioli LF: Cerebrovascular stenoses with cerebral infarction in a child with Williams syndrome. *Am J Med Genet* 51:200–202, 1994.
11. Arnold SA, Brown OE, Finitzo T: Hearing loss in children with congenital heart disease: A preliminary report. *Int J Pediatr Otorhinolaryngol* 11:287–293, 1986.
12. Ashraf S, Bhattacharya K, Tian Y, Watterson K: Cytokine and S100B levels in paediatric patients undergoing corrective cardiac surgery with or without total circulatory arrest. *Eur J Cardiothorac Surg* 16:32–37, 1999.
13. Astudillo R, van der Linden J, Ekroth R, et al: Absent diastolic cerebral blood flow velocity after circulatory arrest but not after low flow in infants. *Ann Thorac Surg* 56:515–519, 1993.
14. Austin EH 3rd, Edmonds HL Jr, Auden SM, et al: Benefit of neurophysiologic monitoring for pediatric cardiac surgery. *J Thorac Cardiovasc Surg* 114:707–715, 717, 1997.
15. Balling G, Vogt M, Kaemmerer H, et al: Intracardiac thrombus formation after the Fontan operation. *J Thorac Cardiovasc Surg* 119:745–752, 2000.
16. Bakshi R, Wright PD, Kinkel PR, et al: Cranial magnetic resonance imaging findings in bacterial endocarditis: The neuroimaging spectrum of septic brain embolization demonstrated in twelve patients. *J Neuroimaging* 9:78–84, 1999.
17. Baquer NZ, Hothersall JS, McLean P: Function and regulation of the pentose phosphate pathway in brain. *Curr Top Cell Regul* 29:265–289, 1988.
18. Behl PR, Sante P, Blesovsky A: Isolated coarctation of the aorta: Surgical treatment and late results. Eighteen years' experience. *J Cardiovasc Surg (Torino)* 29:509–517, 1988.
19. Bellinger DC, Wernovsky G, Rappaport LA, et al: Cognitive development of children following early repair of transposition of the great arteries using deep hypothermic circulatory arrest. *Pediatrics* 87:701–707, 1991.
20. Bellinger DC, Jonas RA, Rappaport LA, et al: Developmental and neurological status of children after heart surgery with hypothermic circulatory arrest or low-flow cardiopulmonary bypass. *N Engl J Med* 332:549–555, 1995.
21. Bellinger DC, Rappaport LA, Wypij D, et al: Patterns of developmental dysfunction after surgery during infancy to correct transposition of the great arteries. *J Dev Behav Pediatr* 18:75–83, 1997.
22. Bellinger DC, Wypij D, Kuban KC, et al: Developmental and neurological status of children at 4 years of age after heart surgery with hypothermic circulatory arrest or low-flow cardiopulmonary bypass. *Circulation* 100:526–532, 1999.
23. Bergouignan M, Fontan F, Trarieux M: Syndromes, choréiformes, de l'enfants au decours, de l'interventiones, cardiochirurgicales, sous hypothermie profonde. *Rev Neurol (Paris)* 105:48, 1961.
24. Berthrong M, Sabiston DC, Jr: Cerebral lesions in congenital heart disease. *Bull Hopkins Hosp* 89:384, 1951.
25. Bjork VO, Hultquist G: Brain damage in children after deep hypothermia for open-heart surgery. *Thorax* 15:284–291, 1960.
26. Bjork VO, Hultquist G: Contraindications to profound hypothermia in open-heart surgery. *J Thorac Cardiovasc Surg* 44:1–13, 1962.
27. Blackwood MJ, Haka-Ikse K, Steward DJ: Developmental outcome in children undergoing surgery with profound hypothermia. *Anesthesiology* 65:437–440, 1986.
28. Borthne A, Carteret M, Baraton J, et al: Vein of Galen vascular malformations in infants: Clinical, radiological and therapeutic aspect. *Eur Radiol* 7:1252–1258, 1997.
29. Boyd SG, Harden A: Clinical neurophysiology of the central nervous system. In Brett EM (ed): *Paediatric Neurology*. New York: Churchill Livingstone, 1991, p 717.
30. Branthwaite MA: Prevention of neurological damage during open-heart surgery. *Thorax* 30:258–261, 1975.
31. Brook I: Brain abscess in children: Microbiology and management. *J Child Neurol* 10:283–288, 1995.
32. Brunberg JA, Reilly EL, Doty DB: Central nervous system consequences in infants of cardiac surgery using deep hypothermia and circulatory arrest. *Circulation* 50:II60–II68, 1974.
33. Brunnelle F: Arteriovenous malformation of the vein of Galen in children. *Pediatr Radiol* 27:501–513, 1997.
34. Burch GE, Meyers R, Abildskov JA: A new electrocardiographic pattern observed in cerebrovascular accidents. *Circulation* 9:719–723, 1954.

35. Burrows FA, Hillier SC, McLeod ME, et al: Anterior fontanel pressure and visual evoked potentials in neonates and infants undergoing profound hypothermic circulatory arrest. *Anesthesiology* 73:632–636, 1990.

36. Burrows FA, Bissonnette B: Cerebral blood flow velocity patterns during cardiac surgery utilizing profound hypothermia with low-flow cardiopulmonary bypass or circulatory arrest in neonates and infants. *Can J Anaesth* 40:298–307, 1993.

37. Busto R, Globus M-YT, Dietrich WD, et al: Effect of mild hypothermia on ischemia–induced release of neurotransmitter and free fatty acids in rat brain. *Stroke* 20:904–910, 1989.

38. Byer E, Ashman R, Toth LA: Electrocardiograms with large upright T-waves and long Q-T intervals. *Am Heart J* 33:796–799, 1947.

39. Chakraborty RN, Bidwai PS, Kak VK, et al: Brain abscess in cyanotic congenital heart disease. *Indian Heart J* 41:190–193, 1989.

40. Chang R-KR, Chen AY, Klitzner TS: Factors associated with age at operation for children with congenital heart disease. *Pediatrics* 105:1073–1081, 2000.

41. Chaves E, Scaltsas-Persson I: Severe choreoathetosis (CA) following congenital heart disease (CHD) surgery. *Neurology* 38:284, 1988.

42. Chinese Acute Stroke Trial (CAST) Collaborative Group: Randomized placebo-controlled trial of early aspirin use in 20000 patients with acute ischaemic stroke. *Lancet* 349:1641–1649, 1997.

43. Ciurea AV, Stoica F, Vasilescu G, Nuteanu L: Neurosurgical management of brain abscesses in children. *Child's Nerv Syst* 15:309–317, 1999.

44. Cottrill CM, Kaplan S: Cerebral vascular accidents in cyanotic congenital heart disease. *Am J Dis Child* 125:484–487, 1973.

45. Cromme-Dijkhuis AH, Henkens CMA, Bijleveld CMA, et al: Coagulation factor abnormalities as possible thrombotic risk factors after Fontan operations. *Lancet* 336:1087–1090, 1990.

46. Cromme-Dijkhuis AH, Hess J, Hahlen K, et al: Specific sequelae after Fontan operation at mid- and long-term follow-up. Arrhythmia, liver dysfunction, and coagulation disorders. *J Thorac Cardiovasc Surg* 106:1126–1132, 1993.

47. Curless RG, Katz DA, Perryman RA, et al: Choreoathetosis after surgery for congenital heart disease. *J Pediatr* 124:737–739, 1994.

48. Daniels SR, Bates SR, Kaplan S: EEG monitoring during paroxysmal hyperpnea of tetralogy of Fallot: An epileptic or hypoxic phenomenon? *J Child Neurol* 2:98–100, 1987.

49. Daubeney PE, Smith DC, Pilkington SN, et al: Cerebral oxygenation during paediatric cardiac surgery: Identification of vulnerable periods using near infrared spectroscopy. *Eur J Cardiothorac Surg* 13:370–377, 1998.

50. Dawson DM, Fischer EG: Neurologic complications of cardiac catheterization. *Neurology* 27:496–497, 1977.

51. Day RW, Boyer RS, Tait VF, Ruttenberg HD: Factors associated with stroke following the Fontan procedure. *Pediatr Cardiol* 16:270–275, 1995.

52. DeLeon S, Ilbawi M, Arcilla R, et al: Choreoathetosis after deep hypothermia without circulatory arrest. *Ann Thorac Surg* 50:714–719, 1990.

53. Delivoria-Papadopoulos M, Chance B: 31-P NMR spectroscopy in the newborn. In Guthrie RD (ed): *Neonatal Intensive Care*. New York: Churchill Livingstone, 1986.

54. Di Pasquale G, Pinelli G, Andreoli A, et al: Torsade de pointes and ventricular flutter-fibrillation following spontaneous cerebral subarachnoid hemorrhage. *Int J Cardiol* 18:163–172, 1988.

55. Dickinson DF, Sambrooks JE: Intellectual performance in children after circulatory arrest with profound hypothermia in infancy. *Arch Dis Child* 54:1–6, 1979.

56. Diebler C, Dulac O, Renier D, et al: Aneurysms of the vein of Galen in infants aged 2 to 15 months. Diagnosis and natural evolution. *Neuroradiology* 21:185–197, 1981.

57. Doyle LW, Nahmias C, Firnau G, et al: Regional cerebral glucose metabolism of newborn infants measured by positron emission tomography. *Dev Med Child Neurol* 25:143–151, 1983.

58. du Plessis AJ, Bellinger DC, Gauvreau K, et al: Neurologic outcome of choreoathetoid encephalopathy after cardiac surgery. *Pediatr Neurol* 27:9–17, 2002.

59. du Plessis AJ, Kramer U, Jonas RA: West syndrome following deep hypothermic infant cardiac surgery. *Pediatr Neurol* 11:246–251, 1994.

60. du Plessis AJ, Treves ST, Hickey PR, et al: Regional cerebral perfusion abnormalities after cardiac operations. Single photon emission computed tomography (SPECT) findings in children with postoperative movement disorders. *J Thorac Cardiovasc Surg* 107:1036–1043, 1994.

61. du Plessis AJ, Chang AC, Wessel DL, et al: Cerebrovascular accidents following the Fontan operation. *Pediatr Neurol* 12:230–236, 1995.

62. du Plessis AJ, Newburger J, Jonas RA, et al: Cerebral oxygen supply and utilization during infant cardiac surgery. *Ann Neurol* 37:488–497, 1995.

63. du Plessis AJ: Neurologic complications of cardiac disease in the newborn. *Clin Perinatol* 24:807–826, 1997.

64. du Plessis AJ, Jonas RA, Wypij D, et al: Perioperative effects of alpha-stat versus pH-stat strategies for deep hypothermic cardiopulmonary bypass in infants. *J Thorac Cardiovasc Surg* 114:991–1000, 1997.

65. Duffy TE, Kohle SJ, Vannucci RC: Carbohydrate and energy metabolism in perinatal rat brain: Relation to survival in anoxia. *J Neurochem* 24:271–276, 1975.

66. Easley RB, Lastra C, Tobias JD: Posterior cerebral circulation infarct following cardiac catheterization and balloon angioplasty in an adolescent. *Clin Pediatr (Phila)* 36:535–538, 1997.

67. Ehyai A, Fenichel GM, Bender HW Jr: Incidence and prognosis of seizures in infants after cardiac surgery with profound hypothermia and circulatory arrest. *JAMA* 252:3165–3167, 1984.

68. Eliez S, Schmitt JE, White CD, Reiss AL: Children and adolescents with velocardiofacial syndrome: A volumetric MRI study. *Am J Psychiatry* 157:409–415, 2000.

69. Enomoto S, Hindman BJ, Dexter F, et al: Rapid rewarming causes an increase in the cerebral metabolic rate for oxygen that is temporarily unmatched by cerebral blood flow. A study during cardiopulmonary bypass in rabbits. *Anesthesiology* 84:1392–1400, 1996.

70. Ewart AK, Morris CA, Atkinson D, et al: Hemizygosity at the elastin locus in a developmental disorder, Williams syndrome. *Nat Genet* 5: 11–16, 1993.

71. Fallon P, Aparicio JM, Elliott MJ, Kirkham FJ: Incidence of neurological complications of surgery for congenital heart disease. *Arch Dis Child* 72:418–422, 1995.

72. Ferry PC: Neurologic sequelae of open-heart surgery in children. An "irritating question." *Am J Dis Child* 144:369–373, 1990.

73. Fischbein CA, Rosenthal A, Fischer EG, et al: Risk factors of brain abscess in patients with congenital heart disease. *Am J Cardiol* 34:97–102, 1974.

74. Freedom RM: Cerebral vascular disorders of cardiovascular origin in infants and children. In Edwards MBS, Hoffman HJ (eds): *Cerebral Vascular Disease in Children and Adolescents*. Baltimore: Williams and Wilkins, 1989, p 423.

75. Friedman DM, Madrid M, Berenstein A, et al: Neonatal vein of Galen malformations: Experience in developing a multidisciplinary approach using an embolization treatment protocol. *Clin Pediatr (Phila)* 30:621–629, 1991.

76. Galli KK, Zimmerman RA, Jarvik GP, et al: Periventricular leukomalacia is common after neonatal cardiac surgery. *J Thorac Cardiovasc Surg* 127: 692–704, 2004.

77. Garcia JH, Pantoni L: Strokes in childhood. *Semin Pediatr Neurol* 2: 180–191, 1995.

78. Gaynor JW, Gerdes M, Zackai EH, et al: Apolipoprotein E genotype and neurodevelopmental sequelae of infant cardiac surgery. *J Thorac Cardiovasc Surg* 126:1736–1745, 2003.

79. Gerosa M, Licata C, Fiore DL, Iraci G: Intracranial aneurysms of childhood. *Child's Brain* 6:295–302, 1980.

80. Geva T, Frand M, Benjamin P, Hegesh J: Cerebral embolization from an inferior vena cava thrombus in tetralogy of Fallot. *Pediatr Cardiol* 11:44–46, 1990.

81. Gherpelli JL, Azeka E, Riso A, et al: Choreoathetosis after cardiac surgery with hypothermia and extracorporeal circulation. *Pediatr Neurol* 19:113–118, 1998.

82. Gilon D, Buonanno FS, Joffe MM, et al: Lack of evidence of an association between mitral-valve prolapse and stroke in young patients. *N Engl J Med* 341:8–13, 1999.

83. Gingold M, Bodensteiner J, Hogg J, Chung E: Hypoxia-induced CHAP syndrome. *J Child Neurol* 10:70–72, 1995.

84. Glaria AP, Murray A: Monitoring brain function during cardiothoracic surgery in children and adults at two levels of hypothermia. *Electroencephalogr Clin Neurophysiol* 76:268–270, 1990.

85. Glover TW: CATCHing a break on 22. *Nat Genet* 10:257–258, 1995.

86. Greeley WJ, Ungerleider RM, Smith LR, Reves JG: The effects of deep hypothermic cardiopulmonary bypass and total circulatory arrest on cerebral blood flow in infants and children. *J Thorac Cardiovasc Surg* 97:737–745, 1989.

87. Greeley WJ, Ungerleider RM, Kern FH, et al: Effects of cardiopulmonary bypass on cerebral blood flow in neonates, infants, and children. *Circulation* 80:1209–1215, 1989.

88. Greeley WJ, Kern FH, Ungerleider RM, et al: The effect of hypothermic cardiopulmonary bypass and total circulatory arrest on cerebral metabolism in neonates, infants, and children. *J Thorac Cardiovasc Surg* 101:783–794, 1991.

89. Grinstein S, Furuya W: Cytoplasmic pH regulation in phorbol ester–activated human neutrophils. *Am J Physiol* 251:C55–C65, 1988.

90. Grossman RI, Bruce DA, Zimmerman RA, et al: Vascular steal associated with vein of Galen aneurysm. *Neuroradiology* 26:381–386, 1984.

91. Hachinski VC, Smith KE, Silver MD, et al: Acute myocardial and plasma catecholamine changes in experimental stroke. *Stroke* 17:387–390, 1986.

92. Hachinski VC, Oppenheimer SM, Wilson JX, et al: Asymmetry of sympathetic consequences of experimental stroke. *Arch Neurol* 49:697–702, 1992.

93. Hagerdal M, Harp J, Siesjö BK: The effect of induced hypothermia upon oxygen consumption in the rat brain. *J Neurochem* 24:311–316, 1975.

94. Haka-Ikse K, Blackwood MJA, Steward DJ: Psychomotor development of infants and children after profound hypothermia during surgery for congenital heart disease. *Dev Med Child Neurol* 20:62–70, 1978.

95. Halbach VV, Dowd CF, Higashida RT, et al: Endovascular treatment of mural-type vein of Galen malformations. *J Neurosurg* 89:74–80, 1998.

96. Harden A, Ashton BM: EEG studies during acidaemia and alkalaemia in children undergoing cardiac surgery. *Electroencephalogr Clin Neurophysiol* 22:128–135, 1967.

97. Harden A, Glaser GH, Pampiglione G: Electroencephalographic and plasma electrolyte changes after cardiac surgery in children. *Br Med J* 4:210–213, 1968.

98. Harris RJ, Symon L, Branston NM, Bayhan M: Changes in extracellular calcium activity in cerebral ischaemia. *J Cereb Blood Flow Metab* 1:203–209, 1981.

99. Hattori H, Wasterlain CG: Excitatory amino acids in the developing brain: Ontogeny, plasticity, and excitotoxicity. *Pediatr Neurol* 6:219–228, 1990.

100. Hattori H, Wasterlain CG: Posthypoxic glucose supplement reduces hypoxic-ischemic brain damage in the neonatal rat. *Ann Neurol* 28:122–128, 1990.

101. Heck AF: Neurologic aspects of mitral valve prolapse. *Angiology* 40:743–751, 1989.

102. Helmers SL, Wypij D, Constantinou JE, et al: Perioperative electroencephalographic seizures in infants undergoing repair of complex congenital cardiac defects. *Electroencephalogr Clin Neurophysiol* 102:27–36, 1997.

103. Hicks RG, Poole JL: Electroencephalographic changes with hypothermia and cardiopulmonary bypass in children. *J Thorac Cardiovasc Surg* 81:781–786, 1981.

104. Hilal SK, Solomon GE, Gold AP, Carter S: Primary cerebral arterial occlusive disease in children. I. Acute acquired hemiplegia. *Radiology* 99:71–86, 1971.

105. Hirsch JF, Roux FX, Sainte-Rose C, et al: Brain abscess in childhood. A study of 34 cases treated by puncture and antibiotics. *Child's Brain* 10:251–265, 1983.

106. Holowach-Thurston J, Hauhart RE, Jones EM: Anoxia in mice: Reduced glucose in brain with normal or elevated glucose in plasma and increased survival after glucose treatment. *Pediatr Res* 8:238–243, 1974.

107. Humphreys RP, Hoffman HJ, Mustard WT, Trusler GA: Cerebral hemorrhage following heart surgery. *J Neurosurg* 43:671–675, 1975.

108. Hungxi S, Xiaoquin H, Kongsoon L: Intracranial hemorrhage and hematoma following open-heart surgery. In Becker R, Katz J, Polonius MJ (eds): *Psychopathological and Neurological Dysfunctions Following Open-Heart Surgery.* New York: Springer-Verlag, 1982, p 293.

109. Huntley DT, al-Mateen M, Menkes JH: Unusual dyskinesia complicating cardiopulmonary bypass surgery. *Dev Med Child Neurol* 35:631–636, 1993.

110. Ikonomidou C, Mosinger JL, Olney JW: Hypothermia enhances protective effect of MK-801 against hypoxic/ischemic brain damage in infant rats. *Brain Res* 487:184–187, 1989.

111. International Stroke Trial Collaborative Group: The International Stroke Trial (IST): A randomized trial of aspirin, subcutaneous heparin, both, or neither among 19435 patients with acute ischaemic stroke. *Lancet* 349:1569–1581, 1997.

112. Isgro F, Schmidt C, Pohl P, Saggau W: A predictive parameter in patients with brain related complications after cardiac surgery? *Eur J Cardiothorac Surg* 11:640–644, 1997.

113. Jackson AC, Boughner DR, Barnett HJ: Mitral valve prolapse and cerebral ischemic events in young patients. *Neurology* 34:784–787, 1984.

114. Jensen E, Sandstrom K, Andreasson S, et al: Increased levels of S-100 protein after cardiac surgery with cardiopulmonary bypass and general surgery in children. *Paediatr Anaesth* 10:297–302, 2000.

115. Jobsis FF: Noninvasive, infrared monitoring of cerebral and myocardial oxygen sufficiency and circulatory parameters. *Science* 198:1264–1267, 1977.

116. Jonassen AE, Quaegebeur JM, Young WL: Cerebral blood flow velocity in pediatric patients is reduced after cardiopulmonary bypass with profound hypothermia. *Thorac Cardiovasc Surg* 110:934–943, 1995.

117. Kagawa M, Takeshita M, Yato S, Kitamura K: Brain abscess in congenital cyanotic heart disease. *J Neurosurg* 58:913–917, 1983.

118. Kaibara T, Sutherland GR, Colbourne F, Tyson RL: Hypothermia: Depression of tricarboxylic acid cycle flux and evidence for pentose phosphate shunt upregulation. *J Neurosurg* 90:339–347, 1999.

119. Keen G: Spinal cord damage and operations for coarctation of the aorta: Aetiology, practice, and prospects. *Thorax* 42:11–18, 1987.

120. Kern FH, Jonas RA, Mayer JE Jr, et al: Temperature monitoring during CPB in infants: Does it predict efficient brain cooling? *Ann Thorac Surg* 54:749–754, 1992.

121. Kern FH, Greeley WJ, Ungerleider RM: The effects of bypass on the developing brain. *Perfusion* 8:49–54, 1993.

122. Kern FH, Greeley WJ, Ungerleider RM: The assessment of cerebral function during pediatric cardiopulmonary bypass. *Perfusion* 8:63–70, 1993.

123. Kirino T: Delayed neuronal death in the gerbil hippocampus following ischemia. *Brain Res* 239:57–69, 1982.

124. Kocsis B, Fedina L, Pasztor E: Effect of preexisting brain ischemia on sympathetic nerve response to intracranial hypertension. *J Appl Physiol* 70:2181–2187, 1991.

125. Kristiàn T, Siesjö BK: Calcium in ischemic cell death. *Stroke* 29:705–718, 1998.

126. Krull F, Latta K, Hoyer PF, et al: Cerebral ultrasonography before and after cardiac surgery in infants. *Pediatr Cardiol* 15:159–162, 1994.

127. Kupsky WJ, Drozd MA, Barlow CF: Selective injury of the globus pallidus in children with post-cardiac surgery choreic syndrome. *Dev Med Child Neurol* 37:135–144, 1995.

128. Kurlan R, Griggs RC: Cyanotic congenital heart disease with suspected stroke. Should all patients receive antibiotics? *Arch Neurol* 40:209–212, 1983.

129. Kurlan R, Krall RL, Deweese JA: Vertebrobasilar ischemia after total repair of tetralogy of Fallot: Significance of subclavian steal created by Blalock-Taussig anastomosis. Vertebrobasilar ischemia after correction of tetralogy of Fallot. *Stroke* 15:359–362, 1984.

130. Kurth CD, Steven JM, Nicolson SC, et al: Kinetics of cerebral deoxygenation during deep hypothermic circulatory arrest in neonates. *Anesthesiology* 77:656–661, 1992.

131. Kurth CD, Steven JM, Nicolson SC: Cerebral oxygenation during pediatric cardiac surgery using deep hypothermic circulatory arrest. *Anesthesiology* 82:74–82, 1995.

132. Lavy S, Yaar I, Melamed E, Stern S: The effect of acute stroke on cardiac functions as observed in an intensive stroke care unit. *Stroke* 5:775–780, 1974.

133. Lederman RJ, Breuer AC, Hanson MR, et al: Peripheral nervous system complications of coronary artery bypass graft surgery. *Ann Neurol* 12:297–301, 1982.

134. Levy WJ: Quantitative analysis of EEG changes during hypothermia. *Anesthesiology* 60:291–297, 1984.

135. Limperopoulos C, Majnemer A, Rosenblatt B, et al: Multimodality evoked potential findings in infants with congenital heart defects. *J Child Neurol* 14:702–707, 1999.

136. Limperopoulos C, Majnemer A, Shevell MI, et al: Predictors of developmental disabilities after open heart surgery in young children with congenital heart defects. *J Pediatr* 141:51–58, 2002.

137. Limperopoulos C, Majnemer A, Shevell MI, et al: Neurologic status of newborns with congenital heart defects before open heart surgery. *Pediatrics* 103:402–408, 1999.

138. Lindberg L, Olsson AK, Anderson K, Jogi P: Serum S-100 protein levels after pediatric cardiac operations: A possible new marker for postperfusion cerebral injury. *J Thorac Cardiovasc Surg* 116:281–285, 1988.

139. Linde LM, Rasof B, Dunn OJ: Mental development in congenital heart disease. *J Pediatr* 71:198–203, 1967.

140. Litvak J, Yahr MD, Ransohoff J: Aneurysms of the great vein of Galen and midline cerebral arteriovenous anomalies. *J Neurosurg* 17:945, 1960.

141. Loop FD, Szabo J, Rowlinson RD, Urbanek K: Events related to microembolism during extracorporeal perfusion in man: Effectiveness of in-line filtration recorded by ultrasound. *Ann Thorac Surg* 21:412–420, 1976.

142. Lutz PL, Nilsson GE: *Neuroscience Intelligence Unit: The Brain without Oxygen*, 2nd ed. Springer-Verlag: Heidelberg, 1997.

143. Lylyk P, Vinuela F, Dion JE, et al: Therapeutic alternatives for vein of Galen vascular malformations. *J Neurosurg* 78:438–445, 1993.

144. Mahle WT, Clancy RR, Moss EM, et al: Neurodevelopmental outcome and lifestyle assessment in school-aged and adolescent children with hypoplastic left heart syndrome. *Pediatrics* 105:1082–1089, 2000.

145. Mahle WT, Tavani F, Zimmerman RA, et al: An MRI study of neurological injury before and after congenital heart surgery. *Circulation* 106:I109–I114, 2002.

146. Matson DD: Intracranial arterial aneurysms in childhood. *J Neurosurg* 23:578–583, 1965.

147. McConnell JR, Fleming WH, Chu WK, et al: Magnetic resonance imaging of the brain in infants and children before and after cardiac surgery. A prospective study. *Am J Dis Child* 144:374–378, 1990.

148. McElhinney DB, Halbach VV, Silverman NH, et al: Congenital cardiac anomalies with vein of Galen malformations in infants. *Arch Dis Child* 78:548–551, 1998.

149. Medlock MD, Cruse RS, Winek SJ, et al: A 10-year experience with postpump chorea. *Ann Neurol* 34:820–826, 1993.

150. Meyer FB, Sundt TM Jr, Yanagihara T, Anderson RE: Focal cerebral ischemia: Pathophysiologic mechanisms and rationale for future avenues of treatment. *Mayo Clin Proc* 62:35–55, 1987.

151. Meyer FB, Sundt TM Jr, Fode NC, et al: Cerebral aneurysms in childhood and adolescence. *J Neurosurg* 70:420–425, 1989.

152. Meyers PM, Halbach VV, Phatouros CP, et al: Hemorrhagic complications in vein of Galen malformations. *Ann Neurol* 47:748–755, 2000.

153. Michenfelder JD: The interdependency of cerebral functional and metabolic effects following massive doses of thiopental in the dog. *Anesthesiology* 41:231–236, 1974.

154. Miller G, Mamourian AC, Tesman JR, et al: Long-term MRI changes in brain after pediatric open heart surgery. *J Child Neurol* 9:390–397, 1994.

155. Miller G, Eggli KD, Contant C, et al: Postoperative neurologic complications after open heart surgery on young infants. *Arch Pediatr Adolesc Med* 149:764–768, 1995.

156. Miller G, Vogel H: Structural evidence of injury or malformation in the brains of children with congenital heart disease. *Semin Pediatr Neurol* 6:20–26, 1999.

157. Milley JR, Nugent SK, Rogers MC: Neurogenic pulmonary edema in childhood. *J Pediatr* 94:706–709, 1979.

158. Mills NL, Ochsner JL: Massive air embolism during cardiopulmonary bypass. Causes, prevention, and management. *J Thorac Cardiovasc Surg* 80:708–717, 1980.

159. Milnick RJ, Bello JA, Shprintzen RJ: Brain anomalies in velo-cardio-facial syndrome. *Am J Med Genet* 54:100–106, 1994.

160. Monagle P, Cochrane A, McCrindle B, et al: Thromboembolic complications after Fontan procedures—the role of prophylactic anticoagulation. *J Thorac Cardiovasc Surg* 115:493–498, 1998.

161. Multicentre Acute Stroke Trial—Italy (MAST-I) Group: Randomized controlled trial of streptokinase, aspirin, and combination of both in treatment of acute ischaemic stroke. *Lancet* 346:1509–1514, 1995.

162. Muraoka R, Yokota M, Aoshima M, et al: Subclinical changes in brain morphology following cardiac operations as reflected by computed tomographic scans of the brain. *J Thorac Cardiovasc Surg* 81:364–369, 1981.

163. Murkin JM, Martzke JS, Buchan AM, et al: A randomized study of the influence of perfusion technique and pH management strategy in 316 patients undergoing coronary artery bypass surgery. I. Mortality and cardiovascular morbidity. *J Thorac Cardiovasc Surg* 110:340–348, 1995.

164. Murkin JM, Martzke JS, Buchan AM, et al: A randomized study of the influence of perfusion technique and pH management strategy in 316 patients undergoing coronary artery bypass surgery. II. Neurologic and cognitive outcomes. *J Thorac Cardiovasc Surg* 110:349–362, 1995.

165. Myers M, Norris JW, Hachinski VC: Plasma norepinephrine in stroke. *Stroke* 12:200–204, 1981.

166. Myers MG, Norris JW, Hachinski VC, et al: Cardiac sequelae of acute stroke. *Stroke* 13:838–842, 1982.

167. Newberg LA, Michenfelder JD: Cerebral protection by isoflurane during hypoxemia or ischemia. *Anesthesiology* 59:29–35, 1983.

168. Newberg LA, Milde JH, Michenfelder JD: The cerebral metabolic effects of isoflurane at and above concentrations that suppress cortical electrical activity. *Anesthesiology* 59:23–28, 1983.

169. Newburger JW, Silbert AR, Buckley LP, Fyler DC: Cognitive function and age at repair of transposition of the great arteries in children. *N Engl J Med* 310:1495–1499, 1984.

170. Newburger JW, Jonas RA, Wernovsky G, et al: A comparison of the perioperative neurologic effects of hypothermic circulatory arrest versus low-flow cardiopulmonary bypass in infant heart surgery. *N Engl J Med* 329:1057–1064, 1993.

171. Nicks R: Arterial air embolism. *Thorax* 22:320–326, 1967.

172. Nicotera P, Leist M, Manzo L: Neuronal cell death: A demise with different shapes. *Trends Pharmacol Sci* 20:46–51, 1999.

173. Nikas DC, Proctor MR, Scott RM: Spontaneous thrombosis of vein of Galen aneurysmal malformation. *Pediatr Neurosurg* 31:33–39, 1999.

174. Norris JW, Froggatt GM, Hachinski VC: Cardiac arrhythmias in acute stroke. *Stroke* 4:392–396, 1978.

175. Norris JW, Hachinski VC, Myers MG, et al: Serum cardiac enzymes in stroke. *Stroke* 10:548–553, 1979.

176. Nugent M, Artru AA, Michenfelder JD: Cerebral metabolic, vascular and protective effects of midazolam maleate: Comparison to diazepam. *Anesthesiology* 56:172–176, 1982.

177. Oates RK, Simpson JM, Turnbull JA, Cartmill TB: The relationship between intelligence and duration of circulatory arrest with deep hypothermia. *J Thorac Cardiovasc Surg* 110:786–792, 1995.

178. O'Dougherty M, Wright FS, Loewenson RB, Torres F: Cerebral dysfunction after chronic hypoxia in children. *Neurology* 35:42–46, 1985.

179. O'Hare B, Bissonnette B, Bohn D, et al: Persistent low cerebral blood flow velocity following profound hypothermic circulatory arrest in infants. *Can J Anaesth* 42:964–971, 1995.

180. Okutan V, Demirkaya S, Lenk MK, et al: Auditory brainstem responses in children with congenital heart disease. *Pediatr Int* 41:620–623, 1999.

181. Oppenheimer SM, Gelb AW, Girvin JP, Hachinski VC: Cardiovascular effects of human insular stimulation. *Neurology* 42:1727–1732, 1992.

182. Oppenheimer S: The anatomy and physiology of cortical mechanisms of cardiac control. *Stroke* 24:3–5, 1993.

183. Otteni J, Pettecher T, Bronner C, et al: Prolongation of the QT interval and sudden cardiac arrest following right radical neck dissection. *Anesthesiology* 59:358–361, 1983.

184. Pampiglione G: Electroencephalographic and metabolic changes after surgical operations. *Lancet* II:263, 1965.

185. Pampiglione G, Harden A: Resuscitation after cardiocirculatory arrest. Prognostic evaluation of early electroencephalographic findings. *Lancet* 1:1261–1265, 1968.

186. Parsons CG, Astley R, Burrows FG, Singh SP: Transposition of great arteries. A study of 65 infants followed for 1 to 4 years after balloon septostomy. *Br Heart J* 33:725–731, 1971.

187. Paschen W, Doutheil J: Disturbances of the functioning of endoplasmic reticulum: A key mechanism underlying neuronal cell injury? *J Cereb Blood Flow Metab* 19:1–18, 1999.

188. Payne RM, Johnson MC, Grant JW, Strauss AW: Toward a molecular understanding of congenital heart disease. *Circulation* 91:494–504, 1995.

189. Pesonen EJ, Peltola KI, Korpela RE, et al: Delayed impairment of cerebral oxygenation after deep hypothermic circulatory arrest in children. *Ann Thorac Surg* 67:1765–1770, 1999.

190. Peterson RA, Rosenthal A: Retinopathy and papilledema in cyanotic congenital heart disease. *Pediatrics* 49:243–249, 1972.

191. Phornphutkul C, Rosenthal A, Nadas AS, Berenberg W: Cerebrovascular accidents in infants and children with cyanotic congenital heart disease. *Am J Cardiol* 32:329–334, 1973.

192. Prusty GK: Brain abscess in cyanotic heart disease. *Indian J Pediatr* 60:43–51, 1993.

193. Pua HL, Bissonnette B: Cerebral physiology in paediatric cardiopulmonary bypass. *Can J Anaesth* 45:960–978, 1998.

194. Pulsinelli WA, Waldman S, Rawlinson D, Plum F: Moderate hyperglycemia augments ischemic brain damage: A neuropathologic study in the rat. *Neurology* 32:1239–1246, 1982.

195. Puntis JW, Green SH: Ischaemic spinal cord injury after cardiac surgery. *Arch Dis Child* 60:517–520, 1985.

196. Raimondi AJ, Matsumoto S, Miller RA: Brain abscess in children with congenital heart disease. I. *J Neurosurg* 23:588–595, 1965.

197. Rappaport LA, Wypij D, Bellinger DC, et al: Relation of seizures after cardiac surgery in early infancy to neurodevelopmental outcome. Boston Circulatory Arrest Study Group. *Circulation* 97:773–779, 1998.

198. Robinson RO, Samuels M, Pohl KR: Choreic syndrome after cardiac surgery. *Arch Dis Child* 63:1466–1469, 1988.

199. Rodriguez RA, Austin EH 3rd, Audenaert SM: Postbypass effects of delayed rewarming on cerebral blood flow velocities in infants after total circulatory arrest. *J Thorac Cardiovasc Surg* 110:1686–1690 (discussion 1690–1691), 1995.

200. Rodriguez RA, Hosking MC, Duncan WJ, et al: Cerebral blood flow velocities monitored by transcranial Doppler during cardiac catheterizations in children. *Cathet Cardiovasc Diagn* 43:282–290, 1998.

201. Rosenthal D, Friedman A, Kleinman S, et al: Thromboembolic complications after Fontan operations. *Circulation* 92:II287–293, 1995.

202. Rossi R, Ekroth R, Lincoln C, et al: Detection of cerebral injury after total circulatory arrest and profound hypothermia by estimation of specific creatine kinase isoenzyme levels using monoclonal antibody techniques. *Am J Cardiol* 58:1236–1241, 1986.

203. Rossi R, van der Linden J, Ekroth R, et al: No flow or low flow? A study of the ischemic marker creatine kinase BB after deep hypothermic procedures. *J Thorac Cardiovasc Surg* 98:193–199, 1989.

204. Rothman S: Synaptic release of excitatory amino acid neurotransmitter mediates anoxic neuronal death. *J Neurosci* 4:1884–1891, 1984.

205. Schievink WI, Mokri B, Offpgras DG, et al: Intracranial aneurysms and cervicocephalic arterial dissections associated with congenital heart disease. *Neurosurgery* 39:685–689, 1996.

206. Schmitt B, Bauersfeld U, Schmid ER, et al: Serum and CSF levels of neuron-specific enolase (NSE) in cardiac surgery with cardiopulmonary bypass: A marker of brain injury? *Brain Dev* 20:536–539, 1998.

207. Shaw PJ: Neurological complications of cardiovascular surgery: II. Procedures involving the heart and thoracic aorta. *Int Anesthesiol Clin* 24:159–200, 1986.

208. Shirai LK, Rosenthal DN, Reitz BA, et al: Arrhythmias and thromboembolic complications after the extracardiac Fontan operation. *J Thorac Cardiovasc Surg* 115:499–505, 1998.

209. Siesjö BK: *Brain Energy Metabolism.* Chichester: John Wiley & Sons, 1978.

210. Siesjo BK: Cerebral circulation and metabolism. *J Neurosurg* 60:883–908, 1984.

211. Siesjo BK, Bengtsson F: Calcium fluxes, calcium antagonists, and calcium-related pathology in brain ischemia, hypoglycemia, and spreading depression: A unifying hypothesis. *J Cereb Blood Flow Metab* 9:127–140, 1989.

212. Siesjö BK: Pathophysiology and treatment of focal cerebral ischemia. Part I: Pathophysiology. *J Neurosurg* 77:169–184, 1992.

213. Siesjö BK, Hu B, Kristiàn T: Is the cell death pathway triggered by the mitochondrion or the endoplasmic reticulum? *J Cereb Blood Flow Metab* 19:19–26, 1999.

214. Silbert A, Wolff PH, Mayer B, et al: Cyanotic heart disease and psychological development. *Pediatrics* 43:192–200, 1969.

215. Singer HS, Dela Cruz PS, Abrams MT, et al: A Tourette-like syndrome following cardiopulmonary bypass and hypothermia: MRI volumetric measurements. *Mov Disord* 12:588–592, 1997.

216. Skaryak LA, Kirshbom PM, DiBernardo LR, et al: Modified ultrafiltration improves cerebral metabolic recovery after circulatory arrest. *J Thorac Cardiovasc Surg* 109:744–752, 1995.

217. Smith KE, Hachinski VC, Gibson CJ, Ciriello J: Changes in plasma catecholamine levels after insula damage in experimental stroke. *Brain Res* 375:182–185, 1986.

218. Solis RT, Noon GP, Beall AC Jr, DeBakey ME: Particulate microembolism during cardiac operation. *Ann Thorac Surg* 17:332–344, 1974.

219. Sorland SJ, Rostad H, Forfang K, Abyholm G: Coarctation of the aorta. A follow-up study after surgical treatment in infancy and childhood. *Acta Paediatr Scand* 69:113–118, 1980.

220. Stevenson JG, Stone EF, Dillard DH, Morgan BC: Intellectual development of children subjected to prolonged circulatory arrest during hypothermic open heart surgery in infancy. *Circulation* 50:5–suppl II:9, 1974.

221. Stober T, Anstatt TH, Sen S, et al: Cardiac arrhythmias in subarachnoid hemorrhage. *Acta Neurochir* 93:37–44, 1988.

222. Stow PJ, Burrows FA, McLeod ME, Coles JG: The effects of cardiopulmonary bypass and profound hypothermic circulatory arrest on anterior fontanel pressure in infants. *Can J Anaesth* 34:450–454, 1987.

223. Takeshita M, Kagawa M, Yato S, et al: Current treatment of brain abscess in patients with congenital cyanotic heart disease. *Neurosurgery* 41:1270–1278 (discussion 1278–1279), 1997.

224. Talwar D, Torres F: Continuous electrophysiologic monitoring of cerebral function in the pediatric intensive care unit. *Pediatr Neurol* 4:137–147, 1988.

225. Tasker RC, Boyd SG, Harden A, Matthew DJ: EEG monitoring of prolonged thiopentone administration for intractable seizures and status epilepticus in infants and young children. *Neuropediatrics* 20:147–153, 1989.

226. Tasker RC, Boyd SG, Harden A, Matthew DJ: The cerebral function analysing monitor in paediatric medical intensive care: Applications and limitations. *Intens Care Med* 16:60–68, 1990.

227. Tasker RC, Boyd SG, Harden A, et al: The clinical significance of seizures in critically ill young infants requiring intensive care. *Neuropediatrics* 22:129–138, 1991.

228. Tasker RC, Sahota S, Williams SR: Bioenergetic recovery following ischemia in brain slices studied by 31P-NMR spectroscopy: Differential age effect of depolarization mediated by endogenous nitric oxide. *J Cereb Blood Flow Metab* 16:125–133, 1996.

229. Tasker RC: Pharmacological advance in the treatment of acute brain injury. *Arch Dis Child* 81:90–95, 1999.

230. Tasker RC, Sahota S, Williams SR: Hypercarbia or mild hypothermia, only when not combined, improve postischemic bioenergetic recovery in neonatal rat brain slices. *J Cereb Blood Flow Metab* 20:612–619, 2000.

231. Taylor RH, Burrows FA, Bissonnette B: Cerebral pressure-flow velocity relationship during hypothermic cardiopulmonary bypass in neonates and infants. *Anesth Analg* 74:636–642, 1992.

232. terBrugge KG: Neurointerventional procedures in the pediatric age group. *Childs Nerv Syst* 15:751–754, 1999.

233. Terplan KL: Brain changes in newborns, infants and children with congenital heart disease in association with cardiac surgery. Additional observations. *J Neurol* 212:225–236, 1976.

234. The National Institute of Neurological Disorders and Stroke rt-PA Stroke Study Group: Tissue plasminogen activator for acute ischemic stroke. *N Engl J Med* 333:1581–1587, 1995.

235. Thomas JA, Graham JM: Chromosome 22q11 deletion syndrome: An update and review for the primary pediatrician. *Clin Pediatr* 5:253–286, 1997.

236. Thurston JH, McDougal DB Jr: Effect of ischemia on metabolism of the brain of the newborn mouse. *Am J Physiol* 216:348–352, 1969.

237. Trittenwein G, Nardi A, Pansi H, et al: Early postoperative prediction of cerebral damage after pediatric cardiac surgery. *Ann Thorac Surg* 76:576–580, 2003.

238. Tyler HR, Clark DB: Cerebro-vascular accidents in patients with congenital heart disease. *Arch Neurol Psychiatry* 77:483, 1957.

239. Utens EM, Verhulst FC, Duivenvoorden HJ, et al: Prediction of behavioural and emotional problems in children and adolescents with operated congenital heart disease. *Eur Heart J* 19:801–807, 1998.

240. van der Linden J, Astudillo R, Ekroth R, et al: Cerebral lactate release after circulatory arrest but not after low flow in pediatric heart operations. *Ann Thorac Surg* 56:1485–1489, 1993.

241. van Houten JP, Rothman A, Bejar R: High incidence of cranial ultrasound abnormalities in full-term infants with congenital heart disease. *Am J Perinatol* 13:47–53, 1996.

242. Wardlaw JM, White PM: The detection and management of unruptured intracranial aneurysms. *Brain* 123:205–221, 2000.

243. Weil ML: Infections of the nervous system. In Menkes JH (ed): *Textbook of Child Neurology.* Philadelphia: Lea & Febiger, 1990.

244. Wells FC, Coghill S, Caplan HL, Lincoln C: Duration of circulatory arrest does influence the psychological development of children after cardiac operation in early life. *J Thorac Cardiovasc Surg* 86:823–831, 1983.

245. Wical BS, Tomasi LG: A distinctive neurologic syndrome after induced profound hypothermia. *Pediatr Neurol* 6:202–205, 1990.

246. Wiedemann H-R, Kunze J, Grosse F-R: *Clinical Syndromes,* 3rd ed. Baltimore: Mosby-Wolfe, 1997.

247. Wong PC, Barlow CF, Hickey PR, et al: Factors associated with choreoathetosis after cardiopulmonary bypass in children with congenital heart disease. *Circulation* 86:II 118–126, 1992.

248. Wright JS, Hicks RG, Newman DC: Deep hypothermic arrest: Observations on later development in children. *J Thorac Cardiovasc Surg* 77:466–468, 1979.

249. Yager JY, Asselin J: Effect of mild hypothermia on cerebral energy metabolism during the evolution of hypoxic-ischemic brain damage in the immature rat. *Stroke* 27:919–926, 1996.

Chapter 7

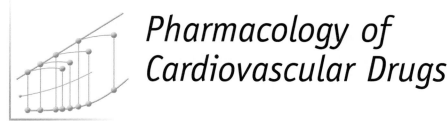

Pharmacology of Cardiovascular Drugs

SARAH TABBUTT, MD, PhD, MARK A. HELFAER, MD, and DAVID G. NICHOLS, MD, MBA

INTRODUCTION

The triad of preload, afterload, and inotropic state of the heart determines cardiac output, which is defined as the product of stroke volume and heart rate. The parasympathetic and sympathetic nervous systems balance inotropy (contractility), chronotropy (heart rate), and lusitropy (myocardial relaxation). An understanding of the anatomy, physiology, and molecular biology of the sympathetic and parasympathetic nervous systems forms the basis of pharmacologic manipulation of the cardiovascular system. This chapter presents basic principles and clinical applications of continuous intravenous and inhaled therapies that affect the inotropy, chronotropy, and afterload of the cardiovascular system. Antiarrhythmic drugs are presented in Chapter 8, "Pediatric Arrhythmias."

AUTONOMIC CONTROL OF THE CARDIOVASCULAR SYSTEM

Sympathetic (Adrenergic) Control

Sympathetic Neuroanatomy

Autonomic control of the cardiovascular system is determined by the sympathetic and parasympathetic inputs. The cell bodies of the preganglionic sympathetic neurons are located in the anterolateral gray matter of the spinal cord from T1 to L3.

The preganglionic cell bodies receive inputs from the vasomotor center in the brainstem that travel through the bulbospinal tract in the intermediolateral column of the spinal cord. Preganglionic axons synapse with postganglionic neurons at sympathetic ganglia, which are collected into two paravertebral chains, three abdominal prevertebral ganglia (celiac, superior mesenteric, and inferior mesenteric ganglia), and left and right cervical ganglia (inferior, middle, and superior cervical ganglia). The inferior cervical ganglion is often fused with the first thoracic ganglion to form the stellate ganglion. The postganglionic fibers to the myocardium arise from the cervical ganglia and the first four thoracic paravertebral ganglia, whereas postganglionic fibers to blood vessels may arise from cervical, paravertebral, or prevertebral ganglia, depending on the location of the blood vessel.

The neurotransmitter at sympathetic ganglia is acetylcholine, whereas norepinephrine is the neurotransmitter released from the sympathetic postganglionic nerve terminal (Fig. 7-1). The metabolic pathway leading to the formation of norepinephrine begins with the active transport of tyrosine into the axoplasm where it is converted to L-DOPA and dopamine (Fig. 7-2). Dopamine is taken up into synaptic vesicles and converted to norepinephrine. Once an action potential leads to the influx of Ca^{++} into the nerve terminal, norepinephrine is released into the synaptic cleft by exocytosis.

Sympathetic innervation to the adrenal gland differs from other sympathetic nerves both anatomically and metabolically. Preganglionic fibers to the celiac ganglion are collected into the greater splanchnic nerve, which travels to the adrenal gland. Sympathetic stimulation releases acetylcholine at the axon terminal of the greater splanchnic nerve, which in turn leads to the release of epinephrine and norepinephrine from adrenomedullary cells. Epinephrine release is possible because the adrenal medulla contains the enzyme phenylethanolamine N-methyltransferase, which converts norepinephrine to epinephrine. Hence, sympathetic stimulation results in local release of norepinephrine to areas with sympathetic innervation, in addition to the release of circulating epinephrine (20%) and norepinephrine (80%) from the adrenal medulla, which produces widespread effects to areas not directly innervated by sympathetic fibers.

Adrenoreceptors

Endogenous neurohormones (e.g., epinephrine and norepinephrine) and exogenous adrenergic drugs exert their cardiovascular effects by combining with adrenergic receptors in the heart and vasculature. Although genes for at least nine distinct adrenoreceptor subclasses have been identified and cloned,[56,64,82,123,124,138,184,211] the clinical pharmacology of adrenergic drugs is still largely based on the four classic receptor subtypes: alpha$_1$, alpha$_2$, beta$_1$, and beta$_2$. Norepinephrine and epinephrine are agonists for alpha and beta receptors in the vasculature and the myocardium. Myocardial adrenergic receptors are primarily (80% to 85%) of the beta subclass.[37,73] Stimulation of the myocardial beta receptor leads to increased sinus node firing rate, more rapid atrioventricular conduction, and increased myocardial contractility. Alpha$_1$ receptors constitute a minority of the total adrenergic receptors in ventricular myocardium. Stimulation of alpha$_1$ receptors also has a positive inotropic effect. The central cellular mechanism

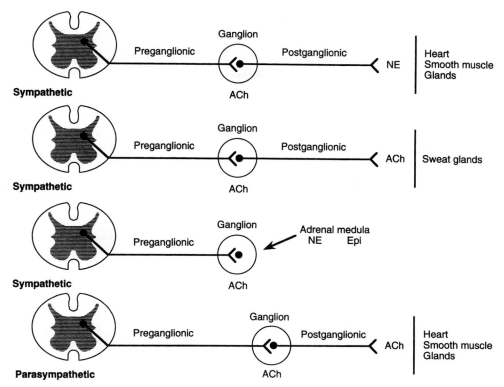

FIGURE 7-1 Neurotransmitters for the sympathetic and parasympathetic nervous system. ACh, acetylcholine; NE, norepinephrine; Epi, epinephrine. (Modified from Merrin RG: Autonomic nervous system pharmacology. In Miller RD [ed]: *Anesthesia.* New York: Churchill Livingstone, 1990; with permission.)

underlying increased myocardial contractility is an increase in intracellular Ca^{++} concentration (or perhaps availability) in response to stimulation of adrenergic receptors in the sarcolemma. This process is initiated and amplified by a membrane-bound transduction system consisting of adrenergic receptors, guanine nucleotide-binding proteins (G proteins), and the effector enzyme adenyl cyclase.[127]

Vascular smooth muscle contains mainly $beta_2$ and $alpha_1$ receptors with $beta_2$ agonism leading to vasodilation and $alpha_1$ agonism to vasoconstriction. Norepinephrine has only a small effect on $beta_2$ receptors but is a potent $alpha_1$ agonist leading to intense vasoconstriction. Conversely, low concentrations of epinephrine are sufficient to stimulate $beta_2$ receptors, whereas higher epinephrine concentrations are required for $alpha_1$ receptor stimulation.

Recognition of a negative feedback mechanism within the sympathetic nervous system led to the identification of an $alpha_2$ receptor subclass. $Alpha_2$ receptors are found primarily in pre- and postganglionic sympathetic nerve terminals to peripheral vasculature and within the central nervous system (CNS).[200] While stimulation of postganglionic $alpha_2$ receptors leads to vasoconstriction, the overall effect of an $alpha_2$ agonist such as clonidine is sympathetic inhibition because norepinephrine secretion is inhibited from the preganglionic nerve terminal and/or sympathetic outflow is decreased from the CNS.

Myocardial Beta$_1$ and Beta$_2$ Receptors Myocardial adrenergic receptors in the non-ailing heart are 65% $beta_1$ and 20% $beta_2$.[38] Norepinephrine, the dominant endogenous cardiac neurotransmitter, has 30 to 50 times greater affinity for the $beta_1$ compared with the $beta_2$ receptor. Thus, in the non-failing heart, $beta_1$ is the predominant regulator of contractility and heart rate.[85] Activation of myocardial $beta_1$ and $beta_2$ receptors results in increased inotropy and chronotropy.[159] The different adrenoreceptor subclasses use different G proteins and second messengers. In the case of the beta receptor, the major events in this process consist of a first messenger (e.g., epinephrine) binding to a $beta_1$ or $beta_2$ receptor, which produces a conformational change in the receptor, so that it can activate the stimulatory G protein (Gsα) (Fig. 7-3). The G protein functions as a transducer of the signal by activating the effector enzyme adenyl cyclase. Activation of adenyl cyclase amplifies the signal through the production of the second messenger, cyclic adenosine monophosphate (cAMP). Finally, cAMP activates protein kinase A, leading to phosphorylation of a variety of cAMP-dependent proteins, which ultimately effect excitation-contraction coupling. Because cAMP is broken down by phosphodiesterase, inhibition of phosphodiesterase raises cAMP levels and increases myocardial contractility (see section on phosphodiesterase inhibitors).

Among the proteins activated by protein kinase A is the L-type, voltage-sensitive calcium channel in the sarcolemmal membrane. Activation of this calcium channel allows entry of a small amount of extracellular calcium into the cell, which binds to the ryanodine receptor (RyR2) on the sarcoplasmic reticulum. Binding of calcium to the ryanodine receptor triggers the release of micromolar amounts of calcium from sarcoplasmic reticulum into the cytoplasm. This process is known as calcium-induced calcium release (CICR), which initiates contraction by binding to the troponin complex, a series of regulatory proteins on the actin molecule. The conformational changes within the troponin complex reverse the inhibition of actin and myosin, thereby allowing contraction

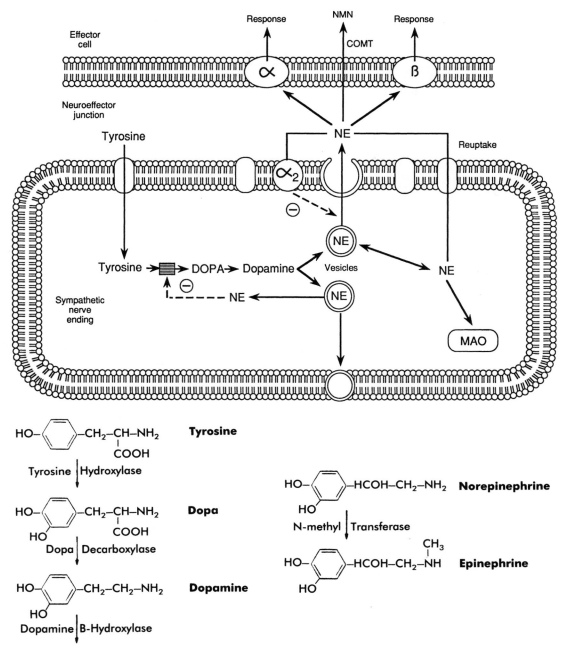

FIGURE 7-2 Catecholamine metabolism at the sympathetic nerve ending. The sympathetic nerve ending is separated from an effector cell by the neuro-effector junction. The effector cell may be cardiac or vascular smooth muscle. Tyrosine is taken up actively into the sympathetic nerve ending and hydroxy-lated in a rate-limiting step to DOPA. DOPA is converted to dopamine. Dopamine is taken up into vesicles where it is converted to norepinephrine (NE). NE may be stored in vesicles or released into the neuroeffector junction by exocytosis. From the neuroeffector junction, NE may (1) stimulate alpha or beta recep-tors, (2) enter the effector cell where it is degraded by catechol-o-methyltransferase (COMT) to normetanephrine (NMN), or (3) stimulate alpha receptors in the sympathetic nerve ending membrane leading to inhibition of NE exocytosis. Alternatively, NE undergoes reuptake into the sympathetic nerve ending, where it is either stored or broken down by monoamine oxidase (MAO) within mitochondria.

to take place. Relaxation of the myocardial fiber becomes possible, when re-uptake of cytosolic calcium into sarco-plasmic reticulum occurs via energy-dependent sarcoplasmic reticulum/endoplasmic reticulum calcium ATPase (SERCA) pumps. Any drug that improves myocardial fiber contractil-ity must either increase the concentration of intracellular calcium or increase the sensitivity of the myocardial fiber to calcium.

Vascular Beta$_2$ Receptors Beta$_2$ adrenergic receptors in the vascular smooth muscle mediate dilation and relaxation. Activation of the beta$_2$ vascular receptor similarly results in increased intracellular cAMP. However, here cAMP inhibits myosin light chain kinase resulting in vascular smooth muscle relaxation (Fig. 7-4).[169] Due to stoichiometric differences between myocardial and peripheral vascular beta$_2$ receptors, beta$_1$ selective antagonists such as pindolol have peripheral

FIGURE 7-3 Major components of signal transduction within the cardiomyocyte. First messenger (epinephrine, E) binds to the beta$_1$ adrenoreceptor (βAR). The resultant conformational change in the stimulatory G protein (Gsα) activates the effector enzyme adenyl cyclase, which increases production of the second messenger, cyclic AMP (cAMP). cAMP activates protein kinase A (PKA), which phosphorylates the L-type calcium channel to allow calcium entry into the cytoplasm. Calcium binding to the ryanodine receptor (RYR2) on the sarcoplasmic reticulum (SR) results in calcium efflux from SR to raise cytoplasmic calcium levels to micromolar levels. Calcium efflux from SR could also be accomplished by norepinephrine (NE) binding to the alpha adrenergic receptor (α$_1$ receptor) leading to a conformational change in the Gαq protein, which activates phospholipase C (PLC). PLC breaks down membrane-bound phospholipids to produce inositol triphosphate (IP$_3$) and diacylglycerol (DAG). IP$_3$ binds to the IP3R2 calcium release channel on SR (or endoplasmic reticulum) resulting in calcium efflux. The final step to effect muscle fiber contraction requires binding of calcium to troponin I to disinhibit the contractile apparatus.

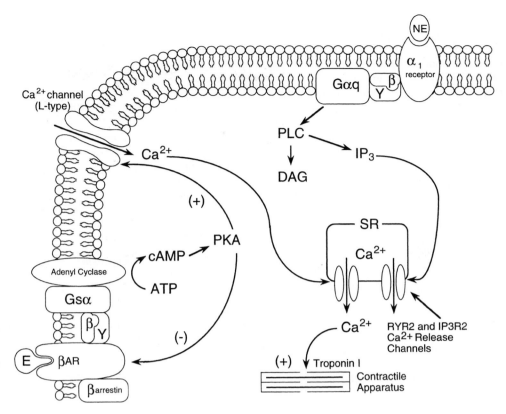

vascular beta$_2$ agonist activity without myocardial beta$_2$ agonist activity[114] theoretically improving its therapeutic benefits in heart failure.[38]

Myocardial and Vascular Alpha Receptors Alpha$_1$ receptors constitute 13% to 15% of the adrenergic receptors in ventricular myocardium.[38] Alpha$_1$ agonists activate a different pathway. Once an alpha$_1$ agonist binds to the alpha$_1$ receptor, a different G protein (G$_{αq}$) is activated and, in turn, activates phospholipase C (see Fig. 7-3). The activated phospholipase C hydrolyzes membrane-bound phospholipids to inositol

triphosphate (IP$_3$) and diacylglycerol (DAG). IP$_3$ stimulates the release of Ca^{++} from sarcoplasmic reticulum. DAG activates protein kinase C and subsequent phosphorylation of intracellular proteins, which regulate cell responsiveness.

Adrenoreceptors in Heart Failure Circulating levels of norepinephrine are raised in heart failure.[55,231] There is a selective downregulation in the number of myocardial beta$_1$ receptors without a change in the number of beta$_2$ or alpha$_1$ receptors, resulting in an increased percentage of the latter two receptors (47% beta$_1$, 25% beta$_2$, and 28% alpha$_1$).[37,40,73,129]

FIGURE 7-4 Cellular mechanisms of actions of vasodilators. Kinase, myosin light chain kinase.[169]

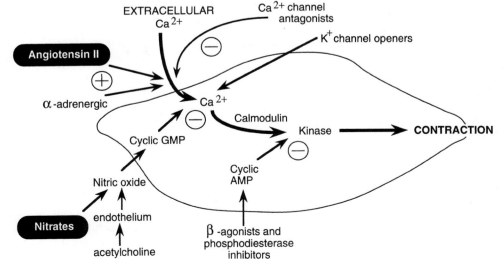

Either increased receptor destruction or decreased receptor synthesis (or both) may cause downregulation.[210] In addition, uncoupling of the beta$_2$ receptor from the G protein–adenylate cyclase complex prevents effective signal transduction.[38] A another proposed mechanism of beta-receptor desensitization involves sequestration or internalization of the receptor away from the cell surface. In contrast to downregulation, sequestration permits recycling the receptor back to the cell surface once chronic beta agonist exposure has ceased.[103]

Cardiopulmonary bypass (CPB) with aortic cross-clamping is a potent stimulus for release of myocardial norepinephrine.[185] This could explain myocardial beta-adrenergic desensitization observed in children following CPB with aortic cross-clamping, which is postulated to result from beta-receptor uncoupling.[206]

As a result of beta$_1$ downregulation and beta$_2$ uncoupling, inotropic drugs fail to yield previously attainable levels of hemodynamic support in conditions of heart failure, or following CPB with aortic cross-clamp.[103,160,206]

Adrenoreceptors and Exogenous Agonists Similar to chronic exposure to elevated endogenous norepinephrine in heart failure, chronic administration of exogenous agonists induces downregulation of beta receptors.[160] Animal studies indicate that after 7 days of isoproterenol (beta$_1$ and beta$_2$ agonist), beta$_2$ receptors are decreased 60%–80% while beta$_1$ receptors remain unchanged.[154,254]

Parasympathetic Control

The parasympathetic innervation to the heart is provided by the vagus nerve. The long preganglionic fibers synapse in ganglia within the heart from which very short postganglionic fibers travel to the sinus node, atrioventricular (AV) node, and cardiomyocytes. Acetylcholine is the neurotransmitter released by both preganglionic and postganglionic parasympathetic nerve terminals (see Fig. 7-1). Myocardial muscarinic receptors are predominantly of the M2 subtype.[39] Vagal (cholinergic) stimulation depresses cardiac rate and contractile function by limiting the accumulation of intracellular Ca^{++}.

Negative inotropic effects are mediated by activation of inhibitory receptors in the sarcolemma. The two best-studied inhibitory receptor systems in the human heart include the muscarinic (M2) receptor and the adenosine A$_1$ receptor.

Muscarinic receptor density is 2- to 2.5-fold greater in the atria than in the ventricles in contrast to the uniform distribution of beta receptors.[39] Muscarinic receptors are bound to an inhibitory G protein (G$_i$). Activation of this receptor leads to inhibition of adenylate cyclase activity and the subsequent decrease in intracellular cAMP levels.[39] Muscarinic agonists may also stimulate opening of K$^+$ channels in atrial pacemaker cells, leading to K$^+$ influx and hyperpolarization of the cell membrane.[191] The latter mechanism may also be linked to G proteins and account for the bradycardic effect of muscarinic drugs.[177]

Similarly, the transmembrane adenosine A$_1$ receptor is coupled to inhibitory G protein. Activation of the adenosine A$_1$ receptor in the myocardium decreases cardiac oxygen demand by opening sarcolemmal K$^+$ channels resulting in decreased heart rate and decreased contractility. In addition, activation of adenosine A$_1$ receptors antagonizes beta-adrenergic stimulation by inhibiting the formation of cAMP by adenylate cyclase. Thus, the adenosine A$_1$ receptor mediates the negative chronotropic, inotropic, and anti–beta adrenergic effects of adenosine.[218]

Transplanted Heart

Cardiac transplantation results in near complete sympathetic and parasympathetic denervation, leaving inotropy and chronotropy dependent on circulating endogenous norepinephrine and exogenous inotropes. The denervated heart has an increased responsiveness to isoproterenol[250] and dobutamine,[35] which may reflect upregulation of beta-adrenergic receptors.[139]

INOTROPIC DRUGS

Dopamine

Mechanism

Dopamine is a sympathomimetic amine capable of directly stimulating beta$_1$ and alpha$_1$ receptors. It also functions indirectly as an intermediary in the enzymatic pathway leading to the production of norepinephrine and epinephrine. Twenty-five percent of infused dopamine is used to produce endogenous norepinephrine.[95] In addition, dopamine receptors are found in the coronary, renal, mesenteric, and cerebral arteries. Dopamenergic-1 (DA$_1$) receptors are postsynaptic and result in vasodilation. Dopamenergic-2 (DA$_2$) receptors are presynaptic and result in vasodilation due to inhibition of release of norepinephrine. At low concentrations (1–3 mcg/kg/min), dopamine interacts with the dopaminergic receptors located in the renal, mesenteric, and coronary vascular beds causing vasodilation. At moderate infusion rates (5–8 mcg/kg/min), dopamine acts directly on the beta$_1$ receptor resulting in beta$_1$ agonism as well as indirectly releasing norepinephrine from the nerve terminals. At higher infusion rates (>20 mcg/kg/min), dopamine interacts with alpha$_1$ receptors in the vasculature (Table 7-1).[86]

Metabolism

Thirty percent of plasma dopamine is protein bound.[11] Dopamine is degraded by two enzyme systems: COMT (catechol-o-methyltransferase) and MAO (monoamine oxidase).

Pharmacokinetics

The pharmacokinetics of dopamine in children are not clearly characterized because of the individual variability. In a heterogeneous group of pediatric intensive care unit patients, the t$_{1/2}$ α, (distribution half-life) was 1.8 ± 1.1 minutes, and the t$_{1/2}$ β, (elimination half-life) was 26 ± 14 minutes.[71] These kinetics were unaffected by liver or renal disease[71]; however, others[166,251] have reported reduced dopamine clearance rates in the presence of hepatic or renal disease. The variable clearance rates for dopamine underscore the great interindividual variability, such that estimation of plasma dopamine levels based on the infusion rate is difficult in a given child.

Concomitant administration of dobutamine may affect dopamine clearance. In the presence of dobutamine, dopamine

Table 7-1   Dopamine Pharmacology

	DOSE (mcg/kg/min)		
	2–5	5–10	>15
Receptor	DA$_1$, DA$_2$	beta$_1$	alpha$_1$
Major Effects	Renal, coronary, mesenteric vasodilation	↑ CI	↑ SVR, ↑ PVR
Indications	Low urine output (e.g., after CPB)	Low cardiac output	Low BP with low SVR (e.g., septic shock) Preterm infant
Major Complications		Arrhythmia Extravasation and tissue necrosis	

Upward arrow, increases; CI, cardiac index; SVR, systemic vascular resistance; PVR, pulmonary vascular resistance; CPB, cardiopulmonary bypass; BP, blood pressure; DA$_1$, dopaminergic-1; DA$_2$, dopaminergic-2.

clearance increases linearly as the dopamine infusion rate is raised.[71] Conversely, dopamine clearance was not affected by infusion rate in patients who received dopamine alone.

Age may affect dopamine clearance. Children younger than 2 years of age clear dopamine twice as fast as those older than 2 years.[166] This may explain the fact that infants require a higher dopamine infusion rate to achieve an effect equivalent to that found in older children and adults.

Pharmacodynamics

Although there is wide variability between patients, the hemodynamic effects of dopamine are dose dependent, with renal vasodilation evident at low infusion rates, increased inotropy at moderate infusion rates, and increased vascular resistance at higher infusion rates (see Table 7-1). Infusion of dopamine at 5 mcg/kg/min causes a 17% rise in the cardiac index and a 70% rise in renal plasma flow (Fig. 7-5).[87] Because the rise in the glomerular filtration rate is not as great as the increase in renal plasma flow, the filtration fraction falls. The overall impact is that the "functional renal reserve" is restored. This is, in a sense, "luxury perfusion," because, on balance, the renal oxygen supply and demand ratio is raised, making renal ischemia less likely. Therefore, urinary sodium excretion increases.[88]

Clinical correlation of the impact of low-dose dopamine on urine output and creatinine clearance in pediatrics is less clear. Although case studies support the use of low-dose dopamine to augment urine output,[140] the literature remains equivocal.[180] The cardiac (but not the renal) effects of dopamine are diminished with propranolol, which may reflect dopamine activation of renal DA receptors and myocardial beta$_1$ receptors (Fig. 7-6).[87] Despite high circulating levels of atrial natriuretic factor levels, renal circulation is vasoconstricted after cardiac surgery in children and urinary sodium excretion is reduced.[88] Thus, following cardiac bypass, dopamine can improve renal perfusion.

Augmentation of cardiac index with dopamine is dose dependent with individual variablility. There is little, if any, cardiovascular improvement with lower doses of dopamine (2.5 mcg/kg/min), but cardiac index increases once dopamine infusion rates exceed 5 mcg/kg/min (see Fig. 7-5).[87] The effects of dopamine on heart rate appear to be dose dependent, so that tachycardia contributes significantly to the rise in cardiac index at infusion rates greater than 7.5 mcg/kg/min,[132,223,247] but not at 5 mcg/kg/min[87,132,223] In adults with cardiac dysfunction, dopamine lowers systemic

vascular resistance in doses up to 10 mcg/kg/min.[132,223] At greater than or equal to 10 mcg/kg/min, the systemic vascular resistance increases.[132] Dopamine increases the myocardial oxygen consumption, but it also increases oxygen delivery, leaving the coronary sinus and mixed venous oxygen saturation unchanged.[15]

Management of the hypotensive premature infant represents a special circumstance in which dopamine infusions have been used. Systemic hypotension is associated with cerebral injury in very low birth weight infants.[148] Although there is no significant difference between dopamine and dobutamine in the incidence of periventricular leukomalacia, grade III to IV intraventricular hemorrhage, or mortality,

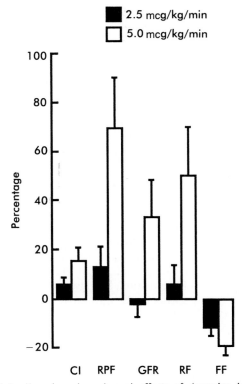

FIGURE 7-5 Hemodynamic and renal effects of dopamine infusion at 2.5 and 5 mcg/kg/min. CI, cardiac index; RPF, renal plasma flow; RF, renal fraction of cardiac output; FF, filtration fraction; GFR, glomerular filtration rate. (From Girardin E, Berner M, Rouge JC, et al: Effect of low dose dopamine on hemodynamic and renal function in children. *Pediatr Res* 26:200–3, 1989; with permission.)

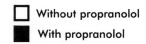

□ Without propranolol

■ With propranolol

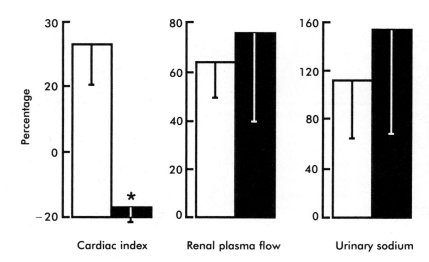

FIGURE 7-6 Effects of propranolol pretreatment on hemodynamic and renal response to dopamine infusion at 5 mcg/kg/min. Propranolol diminishes the increase in cardiac output but has no effect on renal plasma flow or urinary sodium. (From Girardin E, Berner M, Rouge JC, et al: Effect of low dose dopamine on hemodynamic and renal function in children. *Pediatr Res* 26:200–203, 1989; with permission.)

dopamine is more successful than dobutamine in short-term blood pressure elevation.[121,149,196,227] Premature infants seem to require higher doses than children and adults for an equivalent inotropic effect[67,68]; however, they demonstrate alpha effects at lower doses.[213,253]

Indications

Common scenarios for administration of dopamine include (1) low cardiac output following cardiac surgery, (2) septic shock with low cardiac output and low systemic vascular resistance, and (3) premature infants with hypotension. (See also Chapter 4 on renal function.)

Side Effects and Complications

The major complications of dopamine therapy in children are extravasation and arrhythmia. Infiltration of a peripheral intravenous line and extravasation of the infusion may result in tissue necrosis and gangrene. Several case reports document effective therapy for tissue ischemia from dopamine extravasation with application of topical 2% nitroglycerin ointment.[248] Local vasodilation should be observed within 15 to 30 minutes of application. Mild hypotension may result from this therapy. Others have infiltrated the alpha blocker phentolamine (Regitine) into the affected area with complete resolution of tissue ischemia.[221] Dopamine is preferentially administered into a central vein to reduce the risk of this complication.

Supraventricular tachydysrhythmias have been reported after dopamine infusion in infants and children.[99] Risk factors include a preexisting supraventricular rhythm disturbance and high-dose dopamine (10 to 20 mcg/kg/min).[99] Increased frequency of premature ventricular beats occurs at dopamine greater than 5 mcg/kg/min.[132]

Dobutamine

Mechanism

Dobutamine is a synthetic catecholamine, that improves the inotropic state of the heart with little effect upon chronotropy (Fig. 7-7). Dobutamine acts primarily on beta$_1$ receptors, with some beta$_2$ and alpha effect. Unlike dopamine, dobutamine does not release norepinephrine. Dobutamine used clinically contains two enantiomeric forms. The (−) isomer is a potent alpha agonist, causing an increase in vascular resistance. However, the (+) isomer is a potent beta agonist as well as an alpha antagonist, which blocks the effects of the (−) isomer.[199]

FIGURE 7-7 Chemical structure of dobutamine.

Metabolism

Dobutamine is metabolized by glucuronidation via COMT.

Pharmacokinetics

The pharmacokinetics of dobutamine in children remains controversial. Most studies indicate that plasma dobutamine concentration rate is linearly related to infusion rate in the individual patient, consistent with a first-order pharmacokinetic model.[27,103] Others have shown nonlinear or bi-exponential pharmacokinetics.[11,209] Schwartz and colleagues[209] studied a heterogeneous group of patients in the pediatric intensive care unit who were receiving dobutamine (1 to 25 mcg/kg/min). They report a two compartment model with a $t_{1/2}$ α of 1.65 ± 0.2 minutes and a $t_{1/2}$ β of 25.8 ± 11.5 minutes. Half-lives did not correlate with age, weight, gender, disease state, or duration of dobutamine infusion. The half-lives were shorter when dopamine was co-administered.[209] The different pharmacokinetic models that have emerged for dobutamine may be explained in part by the greater than five-fold inter-subject variability in dobutamine clearance.[27] This variability is not a function of different underlying disease states, since it is also seen in healthy children receiving dobutamine infusion.[27]

There seems to be a shift in the dose-response curve in younger (less than 1 year old) children. Thus, younger children need a higher dose than adults to achieve the same pharmacologic effect.[174]

Pharmacodynamics

The myocardial effects of dobutamine are not completely explained by its beta$_1$ adrenergic receptor stimulation. Interestingly, there is an increase in cardiac index from an increase in stroke volume index without a significant increase in heart rate.[66,132,133,174] At low infusion doses (less than 5 mcg/kg/min), children experience a decrease in pulmonary capillary wedge pressure and an increase of cardiac output and blood pressure without an increase in heart rate (Table 7-2).[26,66,100] At higher doses (greater than 5 mcg/kg/min), there is an associated increase in heart rate (Fig. 7-8).[66,100] Systemic vascular resistance is either unchanged[66] or decreased[132,174] after dobutamine. There is no effect on pulmonary vascular resistance.[66,174]

Following cardiopulmonary bypass in children, dobutamine has a more pronounced chronotropic effect with a significant increase in heart rate and no increase in stroke volume associated with the increase in cardiac index at doses greater than 4 mcg/kg/min.[34]

Indications

Dobutamine is particularly useful for patients with depressed left ventricular function and elevated left ventricular filling pressure who are not hypotensive (e.g., dilated cardiomyopathy), and patients with hemodynamically significant aortic or mitral regurgitation requiring afterload reduction and inotropy.

Table 7-2   Dobutamine Pharmacology

	DOSE (mcg/kg/min)		
	0.5–2.5	5	7.5–10
Receptor	beta	beta	beta
Major Effects	↑ CI	↑ SVI	↑ SVI
	↓ PCWP	↑ CI	↑ CI
	↑ BP	↓ PCWP	↑ BP
		→ HR	↑ → HR
		→ PVR	→ PVR
		↓ → SVR	↓ → SVR
Indications	Severe mitral regurgitation		
	LV diastolic dysfunction (dilated cardiomyopathy)		
Major Complications	Arrhythmias		

Upward arrow, increases; downward arrow, decreases; rightward arrow, no change; CI, cardiac index; SVR, systemic vascular resistance; PVR, pulmonary vascular resistance; BP, blood pressure; HR, heart rate; SVI, stroke volume index; PCWP, pulmonary capillary wedge pressure.

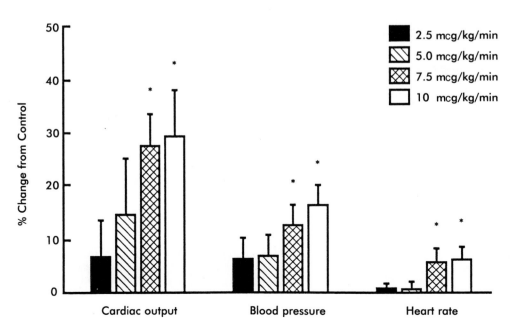

FIGURE 7-8 Effects of dobutamine infusion on cardiac output, blood pressure, and heart rate at different infusion rates in children. Note the increase in cardiac output and blood pressure with dopamine infusion at greater than 5 mcg/kg/min. (From Habib DM, Padbury JF, Anas NG, et al: Dobutamine pharmacokinetics and pharmacodynamics in pediatric intensive care patients. *Crit Care Med* 20:601-8, 1992; with permission.)

Side Effects and Complications

Dobutamine causes less arrhythmia than epinephrine or isoproterenol.

Phosphodiesterase Inhibitors

Mechanism

Amrinone and milrinone are bipyridine derivatives (Fig. 7-9) that inhibit cyclic nucleotide phosphodiesterase (III)[107] resulting in increased cAMP in myocardial and vascular muscle. This action is independent of beta blockade, histamine-2 receptor blockade, muscarinic blockade, ganglionic blockade, or reserpine administration.[4] Phosphodiesterase III is cAMP-specific and has a low K_m for this substrate.[114] The resultant increase in cAMP produces an increase in intracellular ionic calcium concentration,[104] and therefore improved myocardial contractility by increasing calcium transit and myofilament binding.[70] In the systemic vasculature, increased cAMP results in relaxation, decreasing afterload.

Phosphodiesterase III inhibitors may have antiinflammatory effects in septic shock. In vitro, cardiac myocytes exposed to tumor necrosis factor–alpha (TNF-alpha) have a reduced contractile response to epinephrine compared with controls, whereas myocytes exposed to TNF-alpha have an augmented contractile response to phosphodiesterase III inhibitor compared with controls.[168] Production of TNF-alpha and IL-1-beta in rabbits exposed to endotoxin is significantly attenuated by phosphodiesterase (III) inhibition (amrinone or vesnarinone). In addition, the diastolic dysfunction seen with endotoxin alone was significantly improved in animals receiving phosphodiesterase (III) inhibition.[220] Thus, in vitro studies support the use of phosphodiesterase (III) inhibitors, not only for their inotropic and arterial vasodilatory effects, but also for a potentially direct antiinflammatory role.

Metabolism

Amrinone is primarily excreted unchanged in the urine, but some is metabolized by glucuronidation and acetylation.[236] Milrinone elimination is primarily renal. Amrinone is light sensitive and should not be mixed in glucose.

Pharmacokinetics

The dose equivalent of amrinone is 15 to 20 times that of milrinone. For infants and children, the loading dose of amrinone is 1 to 3 mg/kg followed by an infusion at 5 to 15 mcg/kg/min,[130] while the loading dose for milrinone is 50 mcg/kg with an infusion at 0.5 to 1 mcg/kg/min. Amrinone elimination

in adults is 3 to 4 hours, in children 5 to 6 hours, and in newborns 12 to 44 hours.

Milrinone pharmacokinetics in pediatrics has been studied primarily following cardiac surgery. Unlike amrinone, milrinone does not bind to the bypass circuitry.[182] Milrinone kinetics seem to fit best to a three component model[10] with a steady state volume of distribution of 900 mL/kg in infants and 700 mL/kg in children.[10,182] The elimination clearances for milrinone following cardiopulmonary bypass are 2.6 to 3.8 mL/kg/min for infants and 5.6 to 5.9 mL/kg/min for children.[10,182] These clearance rates in infants and children are two- to threefold greater than milrinone clearance in adults and explain the higher infusion rates (0.5 to 1 mcg/kg/min) needed to maintain therapeutic levels in the pediatric population.[182]

Pharmacodynamics

In adults with significant chronic congestive failure, amrinone improves cardiac index, reduces left ventricular filling pressures, and improves the speed of contraction. These beneficial consequences are seen without significant side effects such as tachycardia.[134] After open-heart surgery in adults, cardiac index increases and heart rate increases, while pulmonary capillary wedge pressure, right atrial pressure, and systemic and pulmonary vascular resistance all decrease with amrinone[89] or milrinone[74,75,118] administration. These findings were most pronounced in those individuals with heart failure.[75] Following cardiac surgery in neonates both amrinone and milrinone have been shown to increase cardiac index and heart rate, and to decrease both pulmonary and systemic vascular resistance (Figs. 7-10 and 7-11).[50,244]

The vasodilatory effects of amrinone may depend on the level of pulmonary vascular resistance (PVR) before treatment. Administration of amrinone to children with left-to-right intracardiac shunts resulted in a more dramatic decrease in PVR in those patients with baseline elevation of their pulmonary artery pressures and PVR compared with those with normal pulmonary artery pressures and PVR.[190] Similarly, in

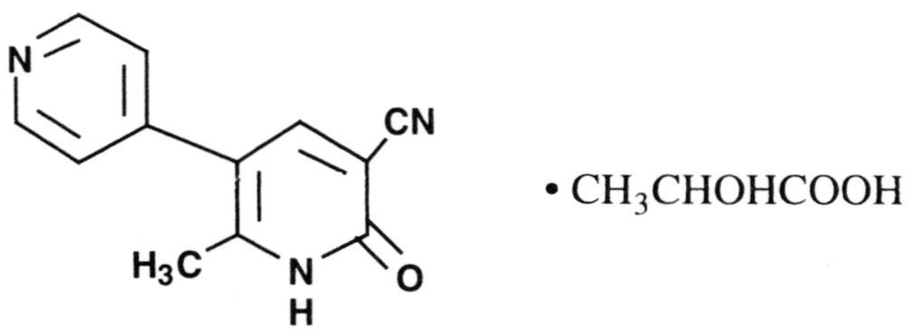

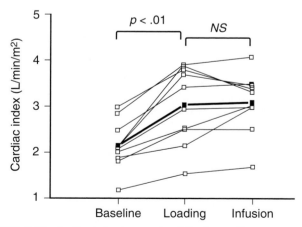

FIGURE 7-10 Cardiac index in neonates following cardiac surgery, with milrinone loading (50 mcg/kg) and infusion (0.5 mcg/kg/min). NS, nonsignificant; solid squares, mean values; open squares, individual values. (From Chang AC, Atz AM, Wernovsky GW, Burke RP: Milrinone: Systemic and pulmonary hemodynamic effects in neonates after cardiac surgery. *Crit Care Med* 23:1907-14, 1995; with permission.)

• CH₃CHOHCOOH

FIGURE 7-9   Chemical structure of milrinone.

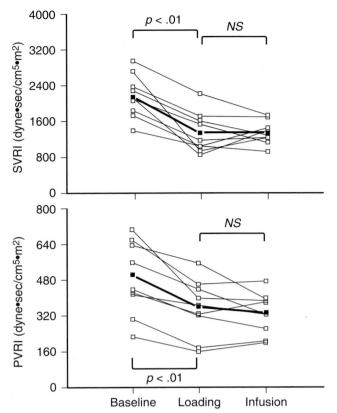

FIGURE 7-11 Systemic (top) and pulmonary (bottom) vascular resistance indexes in neonates following cardiac surgery, with milrinone loading (50 mcg/kg) and infusion (0.5 mcg/kg/min). NS, nonsignificant; solid squares, mean values; open squares, individual values. (From Chang AC, Atz AM, Wernovsky GW, Burke RP: Milrinone: Systemic and pulmonary hemodynamic effects in neonates after cardiac surgery. *Crit Care Med* 23:1907–14, 1995; with permission.)

adults following cardiac surgery, patients with increased PVR had a greater reduction in PVR with milrinone than those with normal PVR.[75]

Barton and colleagues[16] administered milrinone to children with nonhyperdynamic septic shock and demonstrated that milrinone significantly increased cardiac index, increased stroke volume index, and increased oxygen delivery while decreasing systemic and pulmonary vascular resistance and not affecting heart rate.

Indications

Amrinone and milrinone are excellent following cardiac surgery to augment inotropy and decrease systemic vascular resistance during periods of low cardiac output (Table 7-3). Hoffman and colleagues[106] demonstrated in a double-blinded, placebo-controlled multicenter trial in infants and children following corrective heart surgery (n = 227) that milrinone (0.75 mcg/kg/min) significantly decreased the incidence of low cardiac output syndrome compared with placebo (Fig. 7-12). They are also excellent agents for dilated cardiomyopathy due to myocarditis, graft rejection, or sepsis- associated cardiac dysfunction. Milrinone can improve cardiac index and oxygen delivery in children with nonhyperdynamic septic shock.[16] Preliminary data suggest that some phosphodiesterase inhibitors, including amrinone, reduce systemic inflammatory response by reducing tumor necrosis factor and interleukin-1.[229]

Side Effects and Complications

Hypotension is the most frequent cardiovascular side effect due to the vasodilatory properties noted above. It may be prevented by administering the loading dose slowly (over 10 to 20 minutes) and/or by concomitant volume expansion. Alternatively, a lower loading dose may be given. Milrinone and amrinone should be avoided in patients with severe left or right heart outflow tract obstruction because of the risk that fixed outflow tract obstruction in the presence of vasodilation may compromise coronary perfusion.

Amrinone can rarely cause thrombocytopenia, arrhythmia, and hepatotoxicity. Thrombocytopenia is mediated by nonimmune peripheral platelet destruction, the specific mechanism of which is unclear. There is no correlation between thrombocytopenia and amrinone dose, plasma concentration, or duration of administration.[193] The amrinone metabolite, N-acetylamrinone, has been implicated in the development of thrombocytopenia, because the plasma concentration of N-acetylamrinone is higher in thrombocytopenic patients.[193] Thrombocytopenia has been reported with milrinone in patients following cardiac surgery, but there was no nonsurgical control group.[182] Other studies found no effect of milrinone on platelet count or function.[117] Thrombocytopenia does not represent an absolute contraindication to the use of amrinone; rather, clinical judgment should be applied.

Table 7-3 Phosphodiesterase Inhibitor Pharmacology

Parameter	Amrinone		Milrinone
Loading dose	1–3 mg/kg		20–50 mcg/kg
Infusion	5–20 mcg/kg/min		0.2–1 mcg/kg/min
Major Effects		Increase cardiac index	
		Increase heart rate (following caridac surgery)	
		Decrease pulmonary vascular resistance	
		Decrease systemic vascular resistance	
Indications		Postoperative cardiac surgery	
		Dilated cardiomyopathy	
		Nonhyperdynamic septic shock	
Major Complications	Hypotension with loading dose		Hypotension with loading dose
	Thrombocytopenia		Possible thrombocytopenia
	Rare arrhythmia		Rare arrhythmia

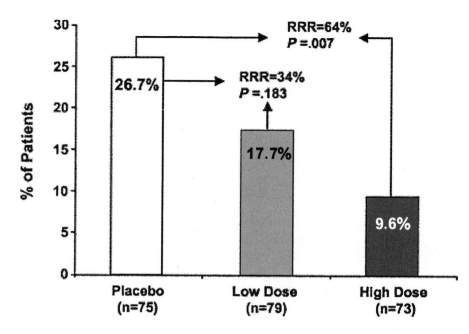

FIGURE 7-12 Primary end point: development of low cardiac output syndrome (LCOS)/death in the first 36 hours (pre-protocol population, n = 227). Therapy for LCOS was defined as an increase in pharmacological support (100% over baseline), addition of a new inotropic agent, initiation of extracorporeal life support, or mechanical pacing. High-dose milrinone was 0.75 mcg/kg/min. Low-dose milrinone was 0.25 mcg/kg/min. (From Hoffman TM, Wernovsky G, Atz AM: Efficacy and safety of milrinone in preventing low cardiac output syndrome in infants and children after corrective surgery for congenital heart disease. *Circulation* 107:996–1002, 2003, with permission.)

Epinephrine

Mechanism

Epinephrine is a mixed beta$_1$ and beta$_2$ agonist at low doses and an alpha agonist at higher doses. Thus, it functions as combined inotrope and chronotrope, and at higher doses, as a vasoconstrictor.

Metabolism

The enzyme systems COMT and MAO (see Fig. 7-2) degrade epinephrine.

Pharmacokinetics

Limited data exist on the pharmacokinetics of epinephrine in children. Epinephrine infusion rates designed to increase myocardial contractility (0.03 to 0.2 mcg/kg/min) yield plasma epinephrine levels of 670 to 9430 pg/mL.[77] Plasma epinephrine concentrations vary linearly with epinephrine infusion rate, suggesting first-order kinetics. Clearances rates for epinephrine range from 15.6 to 79.2 mL/kg/min and are similar to those for dopamine and dobutamine.[77] The half-life of epinephrine is approximately 2 minutes.

Pharmacodynamics: Continuous Infusion

Epinephrine is used frequently in the management of children with septic shock or low cardiac output syndrome after cardiac surgery when other inotropic agents have failed. Despite this clinical application of the drug, no large clinical series on continuous epinephrine infusion for children in shock have been published.

Epinephrine infusion (3 to 30 mcg/min) improves oxygen delivery by increasing cardiac index without increasing systemic vascular resistance in adults with septic shock unresponsive to fluid resuscitation.[131,157] After open-heart surgery, adult patients demonstrate a marked increase in cardiac output at infusion rates of 0.02 to 0.08 mcg/kg/min.[203]

Epinephrine infusion in instrumented newborn piglets increased cardiac index and mixed venous oxygen content in a linear fashion. As infusion rates increase, alpha$_1$ agonist effects predominate and systemic vascular resistance is increased.[12] At the highest infusion rates, systemic vascular resistance is greatly increased and cardiac index begins to fall.[12,48] Newborns may be more susceptible than adults to myocardial injury including sarcolemmal rupture and mitochondrial Ca^{++} granule deposition after prolonged high-dose epinephrine infusion.[48]

The pulmonary vascular bed contains alpha and beta$_2$ receptors, so that pulmonary vasoconstriction (alpha stimulation) or vasodilation (beta$_2$ stimulation) can be expected depending on a variety of circumstances.[108] The effects of epinephrine infusion on pulmonary blood flow and pulmonary vascular resistance depend, in part, on the epinephrine infusion rate,[12] duration of exposure to epinephrine,[59] the presence of hypoxia,[137,179] and the preexisting pulmonary vascular tone.[146] At low and medium doses (<0.8 mcg/kg/min), epinephrine decreases PVR and increases pulmonary blood flow. Ventilation-perfusion mismatch may result.[28] Higher doses appear to raise PVR if the pre-infusion PVR was normal. Conversely, if the pre-infusion PVR was elevated by either hypoxia or sepsis, even high dose epinephrine administration (1 to 3.5 mcg/kg/min) may yield predominantly beta$_2$ adrenergic stimulation and pulmonary vasodilation.[137,146,179] For example, administration of an epinephrine bolus following cardiopulmonary bypass in newborn lambs with single-ventricle physiology created in utero results is a dramatic increase in the ratio of pulmonary to systemic blood flow (Q_p/Q_s).[183]

The effects of epinephrine infusion on regional blood flow have been evaluated primarily in animal studies. In adult sheep, renal vascular resistance increases in a dose-dependent manner with epinephrine infusion.[30] Similarly, newborn piglets demonstrate decreased superior mesenteric artery, hepatic, and renal blood flow with epinephrine (less than 3 mcg/kg/min).[33,53] Further data in sheep suggest that the reduction in renal blood flow with epinephrine is not dependent on age.[161] Following cardiac surgery in adults, epinephrine administration (0.04 mcg/kg/min) reduces the ratio of renal blood flow to cardiac index, whereas this ratio is not changed with dobutamine (2 to 8 mcg/kg/min) and is improved with dopamine (4 mcg/kg/min).[203]

Pharmacodynamics: Cardiac Arrest

Epinephrine is still considered the drug of choice in cardiopulmonary resuscitation (CPR) and is given as a bolus in doses that stimulate alpha-adrenergic receptors (see Chapter 13 on Cardiopulmonary Resuscitation). In a witnessed pediatric cardiac arrest, the standard initial dose of epinephrine is 10 mcg/kg. Although the administration of high-dose epinephrine (100 mcg/kg) has been controversial in the past,[43,90,91,223,224] a recent randomized controlled trial indicates that high-dose epinephrine may actually worsen outcomes after cardiac arrest in children.[175] The proximity to the heart of access for medication delivery and the indication for epinephrine will impact the dose. If 10mcg/kg is ineffective, higher doses may be considered. Bolus administration of epinephrine to a compromised myocardium is likely to result in ventricular fibrillation.

In an infant animal model of cardiopulmonary resuscitation, continuous infusion of epinephrine (4 mcg/kg/min) resulted in improved myocardial and cerebral blood flow.[205] This finding has been replicated in an adult CPR model.[150]

Epinephrine can be administered down the endotracheal tube resulting in good serum levels (Fig. 7-13).[51] The suggested endotracheal dose is 100 mcg/kg, ten times the recommended intravenous dose.[5]

Indications

Patients with depressed ventricular function, low cardiac output, and systemic hypotension can benefit from epinephrine infusion, particularly when dopamine alone is insufficient. It should be avoided in patients at high risk for ventricular arrhythmia.

Side Effects and Complications

The most serious side effect of epinephrine is ventricular arrhythmia. Myocarditis, hypokalemia, and hypercapnia, particularly in the presence of inhaled anesthetics such as halothane, predispose patients to ventricular arrhythmia during epinephrine administration. Hypokalemia and hyperglycemia represent the most common metabolic side effects during epinephrine administration. Serum K^+ decreases as a result of K^+ uptake into muscle after beta$_2$ receptor stimulation. Hyperglycemia results from suppressed insulin release as well as increased glycogenolysis and gluconeogenesis. Epinephrine should be administered only through central venous access due to risk of severe skin necrosis with extravasation.

Norepinephrine

Mechanism

Norepinephrine is an endogenous catecholamine that is the neurotransmitter at sympathetic postganglionic fibers

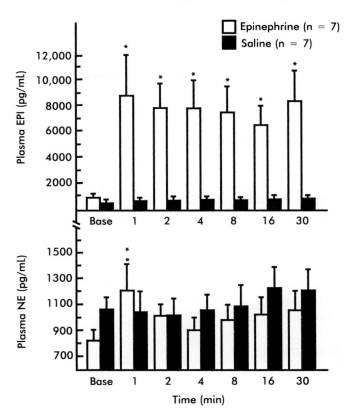

FIGURE 7-13 Plasma epinephrine (EPI) and norepinephrine (NE) levels before and after administration of epinephrine via endotracheal tube. (From Chernow B, Holbrook P, D'Angona DS, et al: Epinephrine absorption after intratracheal administration. *Anesth Analg* 63:829–32, 1984; with permission.)

(see Fig. 7-1). It has potent beta$_1$ and alpha stimulating effects. In contrast to epinephrine, norepinephrine has only minor effects on beta$_2$ receptors.

Metabolism

The enzyme systems COMT and MAO degrade norepinephrine.

Pharmacokinetics

Similar to epinephrine, norepinephrine has a short half-life. After secretion of norepinephrine by the nerve endings, most of it is reabsorbed (where MAO can degrade it); the remainder diffuses into the bloodstream where it remains active for at most minutes. Local tissue degradation occurs via COMT.

Pharmacodynamics

The clinical effects of norepinephrine administration are mainly increased cardiac index and increased vascular (systemic and pulmonary) resistance. Several adult studies have suggested that norepinephrine is useful in increasing systemic blood flow in patients with hyperdynamic septic shock.[143,201]

Indications

Norepinephrine is useful in vasodilatory shock that is not responsive to dopamine or epinephrine. It can augment coronary blood flow by increasing systemic diastolic pressure, at the expense of increasing afterload. It should be used via central venous access only.

Side Effects and Complications

Extravasation can result in tissue necrosis.

Isoproterenol

Mechanism

Isoproterenol is a synthetic catecholamine in which an iso-propyl substituent has been added to the amino terminus of norepinephrine (Fig. 7-14). Isoproterenol is a nonspecific beta agonist with no alpha-adrenergic activity and therefore increases inotropy, chronotropy, and systemic and pulmonary vasodilation.

Metabolism

The major degradative pathway for isoproterenol is via COMT.

Pharmacokinetics

Postoperative cardiac patients require significantly lower infusion rates than reactive airway disease patients to achieve clinical effect.[186] The steady-state plasma concentration normalized to infusion rate is higher (2.1 ± 0.3 vs. 1.7 ± 0.4 ng/mL), and the clearance rate is lower (33.2 ± 4.9 vs. 48.4 ± 7.3 mg/kg/min) in the cardiac patient group.[186]

Pharmacodynamics

In vitro, isoproterenol has greater positive inotropic effects in newborns than in adults.[165] Systolic blood pressure is increased. Diastolic and mean blood pressures are decreased because of systemic vasodilation.[165] Experiments in lambs, with and without aortopulmonary shunts, demonstrated that while isoproterenol increased myocardial and systemic oxygen consumption, it also increased oxygen delivery so that systemic mixed venous saturation increased and coronary sinus saturation was maintained (Figs. 7-15 and 7-16).[15] This effect was more significant with isoproterenol (0.1 mcg/kg/min) than with dopamine (10 mcg/kg/min).[15]

The effective dosage range is 0.05 to 1 mcg/kg/min.

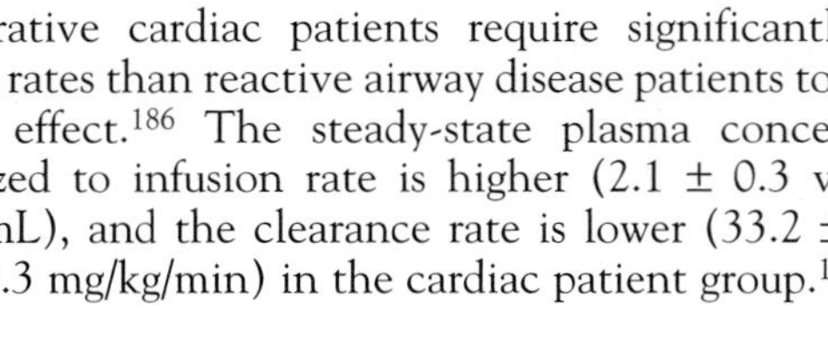

Isoproterenol

FIGURE 7-14 Chemical structure of isoproterenol.

Indications

Isoproterenol may increase ventricular escape rate in cases of complete heart block. It is used to maintain heart rate and decrease afterload immediately following heart transplantation. Isoproterenol can be used for beta-blockade overdose for postoperative cardiac patients managed with preoperative beta blockade. Isoproterenol may be administered through peripheral intravenous access.

Side Effects and Complications

Arrhythmia, both atrial and ventricular, can occur with iso-proterenol. Isoproterenol should be avoided in patients with hypertrophic cardiomyopathy, fixed outflow tract obstruction, or compromised coronary blood flow, as it can increase myocardial oxygen consumption and decrease coronary perfusion pressure. When it is used to stabilize complete heart block or effects of beta blockade, hypotension can occur if the isoproterenol fails to effectively increase the heart rate. Due to potential risk of myocardial ischemia,[141,151] isoproterenol has been replaced by the more beta$_2$ specific terbutaline in treatment of the child with status asthmaticus.

Calcium

In the past, calcium was routinely administered in situations where improved cardiac function was needed. In vitro testing of isolated myocardial preparations reveals that baseline myocardial contractility in newborns is significantly less than that in adults. In newborn lambs with single ventricle physiology, Reddy[183] and colleagues demonstrated that administration of calcium (10 mg/kg of calcium chloride) significantly increased systolic blood pressure and decreased Q_p:Q_s prebypass (Table 7-4). The maximal inotropic effect of calcium in the newborn was significantly greater than in adults, perhaps because of a lower intracellular calcium concentration.[165] The best indicator of hypocalcemia is ionized rather than total serum calcium. Calcium is of particular importance in newborns with congenital heart disease, particularly those with conotruncal abnormalities, who are at increased risk of 22q11 deletion and associated hypoparathyroidism.

The role of calcium administration in the absence of documented hypocalcemia remains problematic. Studies in adults have suggested that calcium is ineffective in the face of refractory asystole,[225] yet of potential benefit in a subset of patients with refractory electromechanical dissociation.[226] Current CPR guidelines discourage use of calcium for treatment of asystole and recommend its use in cases of hyperkalemia, hypermagnesemia, and calcium channel blocker overdose.[5]

Significant hypocalcemia is very common in critically ill children and may be due to relative or absolute hypoparathyroidism. Hypocalcemia is associated with poor outcome in critically ill children.[47] On the other hand, modestly low calcium levels are not related to impaired cardiac function. Furthermore, slow infusions of calcium in this setting do not improve cardiac performance.[42] Calcium seems to play a more critical role following cardiac surgery. In adults following cardiopulmonary bypass, calcium increases blood pressure without improving cardiac index.[195] However, in infants and

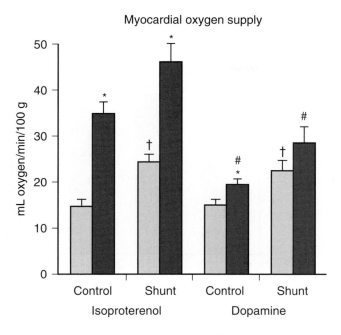

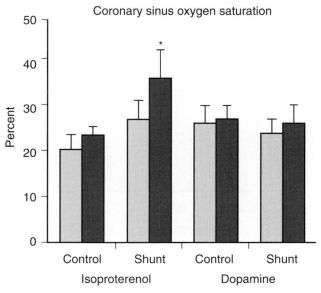

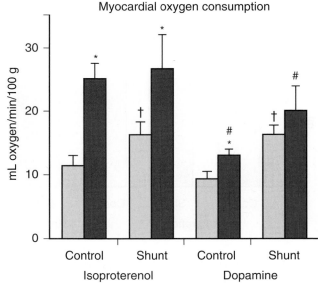

FIGURE 7-15 Myocardial oxygen supply, myocardial oxygen consumption, and coronary sinus oxygen saturation in control lambs (control) and lambs with aortopulmonary shunt (shunt) during the baseline period (shaded bars) and during the infusion period (solid bars). *$P < .05$ compared with baseline values. †$P < .05$ compared with control lambs at baseline. #$P < .05$ compared with changes in the isoproterenol group. The conversion factor from milliters O_2 to micromol O_2 is 0.02241. Data are presented as mean value ± SEM. (From Bartelds B, Gratama JW, Meuzelaar KJ, et al: Comparative effects of isoproterenol and dopamine on myocardial oxygen consumption, blood flow distribution and total body oxygen consumption in conscious lambs with and without an aortopulmonary left to right shunt. *J Am Coll Cardiol* 31:473–81, 1998; with permission.)

children, maintaining ionized calcium levels is important for maintaining blood pressure and cardiac output, perhaps due to relatively diminished intracellular calcium stores, or perhaps due to the relative increased volume of transfused citrated blood products.

Thyroid Hormone

Thyroid hormone directly affects inotropy and peripheral vascular resistance. Thyroxine (T4) is synthesized by the thyroid gland and converted by deiodinase enzymes to the active compound triiodothyronine (T3). T3 increases synthesis of the fast alpha-myosin heavy chain, increases sarcoplasmic reticulum Ca++ adenosine triphosphatase, and increases intracellular cAMP, resulting in increased inotropy and decreased peripheral vascular resistance.[94]

Thyroid hormone abnormalities are well documented in children following cardiac surgery[18,32,41,94] and in adults following cardiac bypass,[22] post–myocardial infarction, and with severe congestive heart failure.[102] Specifically, T3 is decreased. T4 and thyrotropin (TSH) are normal or decreased, while reverse T3 is increased. In adults with congestive heart failure, a low T3:reverse T3 index was associated with lower cardiac index, elevated filling pressures, and poorer outcome.[102] The label *euthyroid sick syndrome* describes this constellation of abnormal thyroid function tests in a clinically euthyroid patient who is suffering from critical illness. The mechanism for the euthyroid sick syndrome appears to involve decreased peripheral conversion of T4 to T3, decreased clearance of reverse T3 generated from T4, and decreased binding of thyroid hormones to thyroid binding globulin.

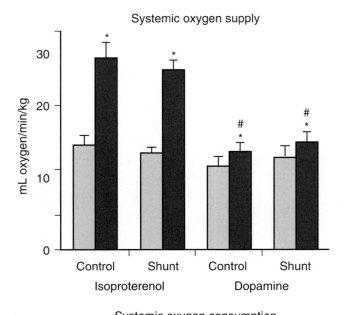

Systemic oxygen supply

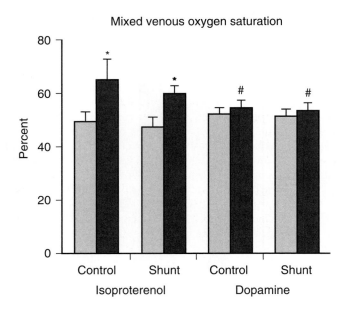

Mixed venous oxygen saturation

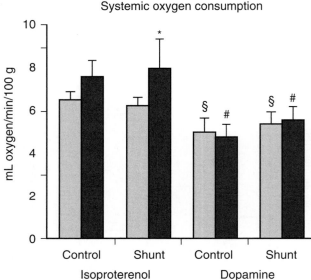

Systemic oxygen consumption

FIGURE 7-16 Systemic oxygen supply, total body oxygen consumption, and mixed venous oxygen saturation in control lambs (control) and lambs with aortopulmonary shunt (shunt) during the baseline period (shaded bars) and during the infusion period (solid bars). *$P < .05$ compared with baseline values. §$P < .05$ compared with control lambs at baseline. #$P < .05$ compared with changes in the isoproterenol group. Data are presented as mean value ± SEM. (From Bartelds B, Gratama JW, Meuzelaar KJ, et al: Comparative effects of isoproterenol and dopamine on myocardial oxygen consumption, blood flow distribution and total body oxygen consumption in conscious lambs with and without an aortopulmonary left to right shunt. *J Am Coll Cardiol* 31:473–81, 1998; with permission.)

Table 7-4 Prebypass and Postbypass Hemodynamic Measurements Before and After Administration of Calcium

	PAP (mm Hg)	SAP (mm Hg)	Qp (mL/min/kg body weight)	Qs (mL/min/kg body weight)	Qp:Qs	PVR (mm Hg/min/kg)	SVR (mm Hg/min/kg)
Before bypass							
Pre-calcium	31.7 ± 5.4	55.5 ± 11.6	249 ± 30	130 ± 39	2.09 ± 0.80	0.101 ± 0.031	0.41 ± 0.15
Post-calcium	32.0 ± 5.4	59.0 ± 12.5	268 ± 26†	150 ± 41**	1.90 ± 0.58††	0.100 ± 0.025	0.38 ± 0.14††
After bypass							
Pre-calcium	28.6 ± 4.4	51.7 ± 8.8	238 ± 55	149 ± 49	1.71 ± 0.55	0.101 ± 0.027	0.34 ± 0.14
Post-calcium	28.9 ± 4.0	58.0 ± 7.8††	268 ± 62†	174 ± 50**	1.60 ± 0.44	0.090 ± 0.025**	0.32 ± 0.11

*Neonatal lambs with single ventricle physiology created in utero (Damus-Kaye-Stansel, main pulmonary artery ligation, and placement of 5-mm aortopulmonary shunt) had direct measurement of systemic and pulmonary blood flow both before and after cardiopulmonary bypass 48 to 72 hours postnatally. Administration of calcium (calcium choride 10 mg/kg) increased systemic arterial pressure both pre- and postbypass and decreased Qp:Qs pre-bypass.
†$P < 0.001$
**$P < 0.0001$, relative to preadministration values.
††$P < 0.05$
Data presented are mean values ± SD.
PAP, pulmonary artery pressure; PVR, pulmonary vascular resistance; Qp, indexed pulmonary blood flow; Qp:Qs, pulmonary:systemic blood flow ratio; Qs, indexed systemic blood flow; SAP, systemic arterial pressure; SVR, systemic vascular resistance.
From Reddy VM, Liddicoat JR, McElhinney DB, et al: Hemodynamic effects of epinephrine, bicarbonate and calcium in the early postnatal period in a lamb model of single-ventricle physiology created in utero. *J Am Coll Cardiol* 28:1877–1883, 1996; with permission.

Controversy exists over the efficacy of thyroid hormone therapy in the setting of compromised cardiac function. Administration of T3 (0.8 mcg/kg bolus followed by 0.113 mcg/kg/hr infusion) to adults for 6 hours immediately following coronary artery bypass surgery significantly increased cardiac index and decreased systemic vascular resistance, compared with the placebo control, but did not affect inotropic requirements or perioperative mortality or morbidity.[122] In contrast, using a similar dose of T3 in a similar population of adults immediately following coronary artery bypass graft surgery, Bennett-Guerrero and colleagues[22] found no significant change in cardiac index or systemic vascular resistance. Administration of T3 (0.7 mcg/kg followed by 0.17 mcg/kg/hr) for 6 hours to adults with severe congestive heart failure (ischemic or idiopathic cardiomyopathy) resulted in increased cardiac output and decreased systemic vascular resistance without a change in filling pressures or systemic or pulmonary artery pressures (Fig. 7-17).[101] Currently T3 seems more beneficial in the setting of congestive heart failure or dilated cardiomyopathy. Bettendorf and colleagues[31] found that T3 administration to infants increased cardiac index during the first 24 hours after cardiac surgery compared to the placebo group. This effect was most pronounced if the infants had undergone prolonged cardiopulmonary bypass (> 1.8 hours). By 72 hours, the T3 and placebo groups had similar cardiac indices and T3 levels. Further investigations of thyroid hormone analogs may prove useful.

Digoxin

Mechanism

Digoxin is a cardiac glycoside, which increases the force and velocity of myocardial systolic contraction. Cardiac glycosides achieve this effect by inhibition of the Na^+-K^+ ATPase in the cardiomyocyte, which results in increased intracellular Na^+ concentration. As intracellular Na^+ increases, intracellular Ca^{++} also increases through a Na^+-Ca^{++} exchange mechanism. Contractile force and velocity depend on the concentration of and sensitivity to Ca^{++} in the contractile apparatus. Digoxin's ability to drive the Na^+-Ca^{++} exchanger may be limited in the immature heart.[176]

Metabolism

Digoxin undergoes metabolism in the liver and limited enterohepatic circulation. In addition, bacteria in the large intestine may metabolize the drug. Unmetabolized digoxin and metabolites are then excreted in urine and feces. Impaired renal function prolongs the elimination half-life of digoxin.

Pharmacokinetics

Absorption of oral digoxin from the gastrointestinal tract is essentially complete, but plasma concentrations of the drug may vary considerably from one individual to another.

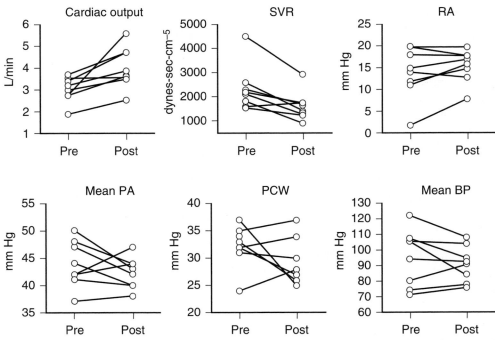

FIGURE 7-17 Hemodynamic parameters at baseline (pre) and 2 hours after (post) initial triiodothyronine bolus (0.7 mcg/kg) followed by infusion (0.2 mcg/kg/hr) in adults with congestive heart failure. There is a significant increase in cardiac output at 2 hours (3 ± 0.6 to 4 ± 1 L/min, *P* = .03), with a reduction in systemic vascular resistance (2291 ± 1022 to 1664 ± 629 dynes × s × cm⁻⁵, *P* = .02) without change in other parameters. BP, arterial blood pressure; PA, pulmonary artery pressure; PCW, pulmonary capillary wedge pressure; RA, right atrial pressure; SVR, systemic vascular resistance. (From Hamilton MA, Stevenson LW, Fonarow GC, et al: Safety and hemodynamic effects of intravenous triiodothyronine in advanced congestive heart failure. *Am J Cardiol* 81:443-7, 1998; with permission.)

The onset of action after an oral dose occurs within 30 to 120 minutes and peaks at about 6 to 8 hours. The effects of intravenous digoxin begin after 5 to 30 minutes. The elimination half-life in patients with normal renal function ranges between 26 and 45 hours.

Pharmacodynamics

Digoxin has mild to moderate inotropic effects and is the only oral inotropic agent currently in widespread use. Hemodynamic effects include increase contractility, cardiac output, and renal perfusion.[119] Some of these beneficial effects may arise from neurohumoral modulation including decreased plasma renin activity, attenuated sympathetic drive, and improved baroreceptor sensitivity. While there are some data to suggest that the hemodynamic and neurohumoral effects of digoxin translate to clinical benefits in adults,[187] there are no such randomized controlled studies in children.

Indications

Digoxin may be used to treat children with congestive heart failure or supraventricular tachyarrhythmias. The antiarrhythmic applications of this drug are discussed in Chapter 8. Patients with systolic ventricular dysfunction may benefit from the addition of digoxin (Table 7-5) to an overall anticongestive regimen including diuretic and angiotensinconverting enzyme inhibitor agents. Appropriate candidates have mild to moderate ventricular dysfunction with stable blood pressure and perfusion. Some examples include infants and children with large left-to-right shunts or dilated cardiomyopathy. Digoxin should be used with caution in hypertrophic cardiomyopathy due to the known association with accessory pathways. There is relative contraindication for the use of digoxin in the presence of atrioventricular block, sinus bradycardia, ventricular tachycardia, Wolff-Parkinson-White syndrome, hypokalemia, hypercalcemia, hypomagnesemia, or renal insufficiency.

Side Effects and Complications

Dysrhythmias constitute the most serious manifestation of digitalis toxicity and include atrioventricular block as well as

Table 7-5   Oral Digoxin* Total Digitalizing (loading) Dose and Maintenance Doses in Children with Normal Renal Function

Age	TDD(mcg/kg)[†]	MD (mcg/kg/day) ÷ q 12 h
Premature	20–30	5–7.5
Term	25–35	6–10
1 m–2 y	35–60	10–15
2–5 y	30–40	7.5–10
5–10 y	20–35	5–10
> 10 y	10–15	2.5–5[††]

MD, Maintenance dose; TDD, total digitalizing (loading) dose.
*IV doses are 80% of the oral doses.
[†]Give half the TDD, then divide the remainder into two doses and administer q 8 hours. Obtain an electrocardiograph before each digitalizing dose.
[††]Teenagers may receive maintenance digoxin as a once-daily dose.

Table 7-6   Treatment Algorithm for Digitalis Intoxication

- Discontinue digitalis preparations
- Correct hypokalemia if necessary (KCl 0.5 mEq/kg IV over 1 hour)
- Give Fab fragments of purified digitalis antibodies (Digibind) for acute, life-threatening intoxication
  - If serum digoxin level is unknown: Digibind 10 vials (380 mg) IV over 1 hour
  - If cardiac arrest: Digibind 10 vials IV bolus
- Give esmolol (see Table 7-7) or lidocaine (1 mg/kg IV) for ventricular tachycardia, if Digibind fails
- Use cardiac pacing for life-threatening heart block, if Digibind fails

ventricular and supraventricular tachyarrhythmias. Although adults may exhibit nausea and vomiting as the first sign of digitalis toxicity, children usually present with dysrhythmia as the first sign of toxicity. The most common precipitating factors are hypokalemia or various drug interactions. Amiodarone, calcium channel blockers, and quinidine decrease digoxin clearance and may raise serum digoxin concentrations to toxic levels. Diuretics, amphotericin, and corticosteroids may precipitate hypokalemia and digitalis toxicity. The therapeutic and toxic digoxin levels are highly variable, especially in infants. However, in general, a serum digoxin concentration of 1 to 2 ng/mL represents the therapeutic range. Table 7-6 illustrates the treatment algorithm for digitalis intoxication.

BETA BLOCKADE

Esmolol

Mechanism

Esmolol {(±)-Methyl   p-[2-hydroxy-3-(isopropylamino) propoxy] hydrocinnamate hydrochloride} is a relatively specific beta$_1$ antagonist.

Metabolism

Esmolol undergoes rapid hydrolysis by red cell esterases.

Pharmacokinetics

Initial pharmacokinetic data in children indicate a faster elimination (t$_{1/2}$ 2.7 to 4.5 min) than reported in adults.[58,245,246]

Pharmacodynamics

Esmolol is a relatively selective beta$_1$ antagonist (Table 7-7). Dosing should be determined by therapeutic response. Esmolol is usually administered as a loading dose (100 to 500 mcg/kg) followed by an infusion (100 to 1000 mcg/kg/min).[58,245] The anti-arrhythmic properties of esmolol are described elsewhere (see Chapter 8).

Table 7-7   Esmolol Pharmacology

Loading Dose	100–500 µg/kg
Infusion	50–1000 µg/kg/min
Mechanism	Beta$_1$ blockade
Major Effects	Decreased heart rate
	Decreased blood pressure
Indications	Supraventricular tachycardia
	Postcoarctectomy hypertension
	Dynamic subvalvar outflow tract obstruction
Major Complications	Bradycardia
	Hypotension
	Bronchospasm
	Hypoglycemia

Indications

A common indication for esmolol in pediatric heart disease is control of postoperative hypertension after coarctation repair. Persistent hypertension, or paradoxical hypertension, occurs in 63% to 100% of patients during the postoperative period following surgical coarctation repair.[105,192,212] Studies in children demonstrate a significant increase in systolic blood pressure during the first 24 hours after surgery, followed by a significant rise in diastolic blood pressure over the subsequent 1 to 3 days. Theories on the etiology of postoperative hypertension include activation of the sympathetic nervous system and/or the renin-angiotensin system. Norepinephrine levels are elevated following coarctation repair compared with other surgeries of similar magnitude.[84,212] Similarly, renin levels are significantly elevated in the first 4 postoperative days following coarctation repair, compared with other surgical controls.[84] The use of beta blockade in children during the perioperative period for coarctation repair results in a significant decrease in systolic and diastolic blood pressure, and in plasma renin activity.[84] Esmolol, specifically, has been shown to control hypertension in children following coarctation repair.[222,235,246]

Beta blockade has been demonstrated to improve survival in pediatric patients with symptomatic hypertrophic cardiomyopathy.[171] Although the long-term mechanism of beta blockade in hypertrophic cardiomyopathy most likely differs from the short-term mechanism, esmolol can be used to test the child's hemodynamic stability on beta-blockade before transitioning to an oral beta blocker with a longer half-life. Theoretically, esmolol can increase ventricular filling time and augment cardiac output. Similarly, it can improve antegrade blood flow in infants following balloon dilation of critical or severe pulmonary stenosis, with significant right-to-left atrial shunting. Esmolol can help treat hypercyanotic spells in tetralogy of Fallot.[167] Esmolol can be used for pheochromocytoma after effective alpha blockade has been established to prevent unopposed alpha-adrenergic stimulation and severe hypertension.

Side Effects and Complications

Extravasation can cause tissue necrosis. The current maximum recommended peripheral infusion concentration is 20 mg/mL. Esmolol can induce bronchospasm or hypoglycemia. Administration to infants who are also receiving a calcium channel blocker can precipitate severe hypotension and cardiac arrest.

Carvedilol

Carvedilol is a nonselective beta-receptor and alpha$_1$-receptor antagonist. In addition, carvedilol is a strong antioxidant.[76] Carvedilol is effectively absorbed after oral administration. It is 98% protein bound with a t$_{1/2}$ of 7 to 10 hours in adults. Adult dosing for carvedilol is 3.125 to 6.25 mg twice daily. If tolerated, it can be increased to a recommended maximum of 50 mg twice daily. Pediatric dosing is recommended at 0.08 mg/kg to 0.75 mg/kg twice daily.[44]

Carvedilol has been shown to be effective therapy for chronic heart failure. Upregulation of the sympathetic nervous system is associated with congestive heart failure, and this increased adrenergic activity (increased cardiac workload, increased oxygen consumption, etc.) may be associated with the progression of heart failure. Carvedilol attenuates the beta-adrenergic activity, and, in addition, as an alpha$_1$ blocker, it reduces ventricular afterload by lowering blood pressure and may play a role in cardiac remodeling and reducing hypertrophy.

A large (n = 1094) double-blind, placebo-controlled trial comparing placebo to carvedilol in adults with chronic heart failure concurrently treated with digoxin, diuretic, and angiotensin-converting enzyme inhibitor showed a significant reduction in mortality (7.8% vs. 3.2%) and in cardiovascular related hospitalizations (27% reduction).[172]

A pilot study of the use of carvedilol (average final maintenance dose of 0.46 mg/kg twice daily) in addition to digoxin diuretic, and angiotensin-converting enzyme inhibitor for pediatric heart failure due to cardiomyopathy (n = 37) or congenital heart disease (n = 9) found a significant improvement in ventricular shortening fraction (16.2% to 19%, p = 0.005) and New York Heart Association class.[44] Azeka and associates[9] also found in a small (n = 22) randomized, prospective, double-blind, placebo-controlled trial in pediatric patients with heart failure that carvedilol improved left ventricular ejection fraction (17.8% to 34.6%, p = 0.001). Results of the Pediatric Randomized Carvedilol Trial in Heart Failure are not yet available.[214]

Side effects including dizziness (19%), hypotension (14%), and headache (14%) occur in about 54% of pediatric patients with heart failure at the doses noted above.[44]

VASODILATION

Basic Principles

The work that the heart must perform is proportional to the pressure (ΔP) against which it must pump multiplied by the volume (V) that it pumps.

$$\text{Work} = \Delta P \times V$$

Decreasing the pressure against which the heart pumps decreases the work of the heart. The pressure against which the heart pumps is best understood as afterload, and it is proportional to systemic or pulmonary pressures. A more elaborate model accounts for the fact that the systemic ventricle must raise the potential energy of the blood from the level at which it exists in the thorax to one that exists in the descending aorta. Therefore, the change in pressure will be proportional to the mean arterial pressure in the descending aorta, subtracted from the intrathoracic pressure (ΔP) (see Chapter 9, "Pericardial Effusion and Tamponade"). Thus, positive pressure ventilation (which increases intrathoracic pressure) decreases the work that the heart must perform to bring blood to the descending aorta. Pharmacological reduction of afterload can be attained by administration of an arterial vasodilator.

Nitroprusside

Nitroprusside was discovered in 1850 and introduced into clinical use in 1974.[98,173]

Mechanism

In vitro data suggest that nitroprusside causes release of nitric oxide, which then reacts with a variety of thiols to produce unstable S-nitrosothiols, which are potent activators of guanylate cyclase. This, in turn, causes a rise in intracellular cyclic guanosine monophosphate (cGMP), which activates cGMP-dependent protein kinases and ultimately leads to smooth muscle relaxation and vasodilation.[109] An alternative theory based upon experimentation of cerebral vessels under cranial windows has been advanced. This hypothesis suggests that nitrovasodilators activate sensory fibers to release calcitonin gene related peptide, which in turn relaxes (cerebral) vascular smooth muscle by activating guanylate cyclase and raising intracellular cGMP.[239]

Metabolism

Nitroprusside metabolism occurs in a series of steps (Fig. 7-18). One of the five cyanide (CN^-) ions in the nitroprusside molecule is inactivated by the formation of methemoglobin. The remaining four CN^- ions usually combine with thiosulfate to form thiocyanate (SCN^-). This reaction is mediated by the hepatic and renal mitochondrial enzyme rhodanase. A cofactor in this reaction is vitamin B_{12}.[232]

Pharmacokinetics

Nitroprusside has a rapid onset and elimination ($t_{1/2}$ less than 5 minutes). Thiocyanate is excreted in the urine ($t_{1/2}$ 4 to 7 days). Nitroprusside is light sensitive and can be administered through peripheral intravenous access.

Pharmacodynamics

Nitroprusside is a mixed vasodilator that results in afterload reduction (arterial vasodilation) and preload reduction (venous vasodilation). It has no direct cardiac effects (Table 7-8). The dose (0.5 to 8 mcg/kg/min) should be titrated to effect. Nitroprusside (0.2 to 6 mcg/kg/min) has been shown to be safe and effective in neonates.[20,21]

Indications

Ventricular dysfunction has been evaluated as a potential indication for nitroprusside administration, but the results

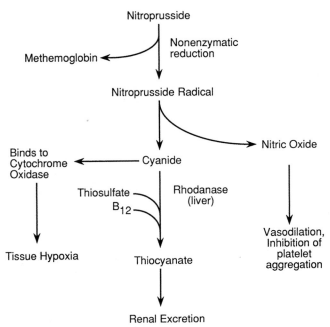

FIGURE 7-18   Metabolic pathway for the degradation of nitroprusside.

depend greatly on the etiology of heart failure. Patients with a primary myocardial dysfunction such as dilated cardiomyopathy may improve while receiving nitroprusside.[63] Presumably, afterload reduction improves diastolic function of the left ventricle such that left-sided filling pressures are lowered. Similarly, children with mitral regurgitation benefit from nitroprusside administration[17] with reduced SVR and enhanced forward cardiac output.[162]

   Low cardiac output syndrome after open-heart surgery is an indication for nitroprusside. In this setting, nitroprusside is combined with an inotrope and may require volume expansion to maintain preload. Nitroprusside, supplemented by blood transfusion to maintain filling pressure, significantly

Table 7-8   Nitroprusside Pharmacology

Dose (mcg/kg/min)	0.5–8
Mechanism	Direct smooth muscle relaxation
Major Effects	Venous and arteriolar vasodilation
	Decreases SVR, PVR
	Decreases preload
Indications	Hypertensive emergencies
	Deliberate hypotension technique during major surgery
	Blood pressure control after coarctation repair
	Afterload reduction after cardiac surgery
Major Complications	Severe hypotension
	Tachycardia
	Compromised cardiac output in preload-dependent physiology
	Hypertension after weaning nitroprusside
	Ventilation:perfusion mismatch
	Increase Q_p:Q_s in infants with large left-to-right shunt
	Cyanide and thiocyanate intoxication

SVR, systemic vascular resistance; PVR, pulmonary vascular resistance.

increases cardiac index in children with low output syndrome following cardiac surgery.[6,24] The addition of epinephrine (0.15 to 0.45 mcg/kg/min) to nitroprusside (2 to 11 mcg/kg/min) further augments the cardiac index without increasing systemic vascular resistance.[24]

Hypertensive emergencies can be effectively managed with nitroprusside. The major advantage of nitroprusside in this setting is the gradual and controlled manner in which blood pressure can be decreased. Nitroprusside infusion avoids neurologic complications associated with bolus administration of vasodilators such as diazoxide and hydralazine. Progressive increases in cardiac index in children with hypertensive crisis receiving nitroprusside may simulate nitroprusside tachyphylaxis in that higher nitroprusside doses are required to achieve equivalent blood pressure control.[194] Nitroprusside has been demonstrated to be a safe and useful therapy for hypertensive crisis[78,96] in the pediatric population. In addition, nitroprusside can be used alone or in conjunction with esmolol for systemic hypertension following coarctation repair.

Controlled hypotension during surgery associated with massive blood loss represents another indication for nitroprusside infusion. Examples of such operations include spinal fusion[21] and intracranial procedures. The technique of deliberate hypotension seeks to lower mean arterial pressure but maintain constant end-organ blood flow. Beta blockade in addition to nitroprusside may be required to prevent significant tachycardia and achieve effective deliberate hypotension.

Side Effects and Complications

The major side effects of nitroprusside are predictable from its hemodynamic and metabolic properties. Profound systemic hypotension can occur with a sudden bolus. Several precautions are necessary. Invasive arterial pressure monitoring allows immediate detection of sudden hypotension. Patients should have large-bore intravenous access established so that intravascular volume can be expanded rapidly. If necessary, children can be placed in the Trendelenburg position, which shifts blood volume to the central circulation and restores adequate blood pressure. Discontinuation of nitroprusside may produce rebound hypertension, which may be aggravated by increased SVR, hypervolemia, or tachycardia.

Nitroprusside can worsen ventilation:perfusion mismatch resulting in hypoxemia, particularly in patients with pulmonary edema or lung disease.

Cyanide and, to a lesser extent, thiocyanate toxicities are the most feared metabolic complications. If thiosulfate or rhodanase levels are inadequate in the face of high nitroprusside infusion rates, free CN^- may accumulate and lead to tissue hypoxia by binding to cytochrome oxidase and inhibiting oxidative phosphorylation. Patients with cyanide toxicity exhibit a metabolic acidosis in spite of adequate oxygen delivery and increased mixed venous saturation due to decreased oxygen consumption. Thiocyanate is normally excreted in the urine, but when this compound accumulates, psychosis and convulsions ensue. Although thiocyanate toxicity is unusual in children with normal hepatic and renal function,[125] prolonged high-dose administration of nitroprusside increases the risk of toxicity. Initial treatment for cyanide toxicity

Table 7-9 Sodium Nitrite and Sodium Thiosulfate Doses for Treatment of Cyanide Poisoning from Nitroprusside Toxicity

Hemoglobin (g/dL)	Initial dose of 3% Sodium Nitrite* (mL/kg IV)	Initial dose of 25% Sodium Thiosulfate† (mL/kg IV)
8	0.22	1.10
10	0.27	1.35
12	0.33	1.65
14	0.39	1.95

*Maximum initial dose is 10 mL
†Maximum initial dose is 50 mL

consists of breaking amyl nitrite pearls onto gauze and having the patient inhale the vapors. In adults, this temporizing measure is followed by 300 mg (10 mL of a 3% solution) of sodium nitrite at a rate of 2.5 to 3 mL/min and 12.5 mg of sodium thiosulfate as 50 mL of a 25% solution.[29] Pediatric dosages depend on the child's hemoglobin concentration (Table 7-9). In adults, 12.5-mg hydroxocobalamin administered over 30 minutes prevented accumulation of cyanide and acidosis.[57] Co-administration of thiosulfate with nitroprusside may decrease the risk of cyanide toxicity in adults and children.

Nitroglycerin

The mechanism of action of nitroglycerin is thought to be the same as described for nitroprusside. In contrast to nitroprusside, the major effect of nitroglycerin is dilation of the venous capacitance vessels with lesser effects on arterioles. Hence, right and left atrial pressures are reduced. Pulmonary and systemic arterial pressures may also fall, and reflex tachycardia may occur. Nitroglycerin is not as effective as nitroprusside in lowering blood pressure in healthy children undergoing major surgery.[249] In adult patients with myocardial ischemia, nitroglycerin has been shown to improve ischemia based upon electrocardiographic findings presumably because of improvement in the ratio of myocardial oxygen supply and demand.[54] Likewise, in adults after coronary artery bypass surgery, nitroglycerin can be as effective as nitroprusside in treating postoperative hypertension. However, nitroglycerin has a more favorable effect upon pulmonary gas exchange, increasing the alveolar-arterial O_2 gradient ($AaDO_2$) only modestly, whereas nitroprusside administration was associated with a significant rise in $AaDO_2$.

Low cardiac output syndrome after cardiac surgery has been treated with nitroglycerin.[23] Children were investigated who had undergone cardiac surgery and had low cardiac indexes (less than 2.5 L/min/m²) with left atrial pressures of 10 to 14 mm Hg. Administration of nitroglycerin (initial dose of 0.1 mcg/kg/min, doubled every 5 minutes until the left atrial pressure fell 30%) resulted in a significant improvement of cardiac index. In those 10 children with adequate intravascular volume who did not require inotropic support, there was an improvement of cardiac function without a significant change in either heart rate or mean arterial blood pressure (Fig. 7-19). These investigators could not determine whether these salutary effects of nitroglycerin were due to

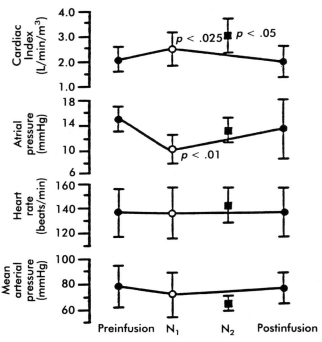

FIGURE 7-19 Hemodynamic effects of nitroglycerin infusion in children after cardiac surgery. There is a significant increase in cardiac index and a fall in atrial pressures during nitroglycerin infusion (N_1). A further increase in cardiac index is noted in four patients during nitroglycerin infusion and preloading (N_2). (From Benson LN, Bohn D, Edmonds JF, et al: Nitroglycerin therapy in children with low cardiac index after heart surgery. *Cardiovasc Med* 4:207–15, 1979; with permission.)

improvements in myocardial oxygen supply (via coronary vasodilation and improved myocardial regional blood flow) or blood transfusion (made possible by the vasodilation) or decreased myocardial oxygen demand (by reduction of afterload).[23] Recent work indicates that endothelin-1, which is elevated following cardiac surgery in infants and children, results in coronary vasoconstriction that is reversed by nitroglycerin.[144]

Nitroglycerin has been used as a pulmonary vasodilator in children with variable success depending on the etiology and duration of pulmonary hypertension. Successful pulmonary vasodilation has been achieved after the arterial switch procedure for transposition of the great arteries[60] and after closure of intracardiac left-to-right shunts.[110] Although the nitroglycerin dosage has ranged from 2 to 10 mcg/kg/min, significant lowering of pulmonary pressure has required infusion rates 5 mcg/kg/min or more. Conversely, nitroglycerin was not effective in lowering pulmonary artery pressure and resistance in a neonatal sepsis model.[198] Taken together, these data suggest that nitroglycerin at higher doses may be useful for some cases of reactive pulmonary hypertension; however, fixed pulmonary vascular disease, sepsis, and chronic lung disease do not respond. Nitric oxide inhalation has replaced nitroglycerin infusion where isolated pulmonary vasodilation is the sole desired effect.

Patients with persistent or regressed aneurysms following Kawasaki syndrome demonstrate decreased coronary vasodilation to nitroglycerin both at the site of the regressed aneurysm[153,228] and at angiographically normal coronary segments.[228] The diminished reactivity to nitroglycerin suggests fixed stenosis or ongoing vasculitis with endothelial dysfunction

in some patients who appear to have recovered from the acute phase of Kawasaki syndrome.

Nesiritide

Nesiritide is the human recombinant form of B natriuretic peptide (BNP). BNP is a hormone that is released from ventricular myocytes subjected to increased volume stretch. The circulating BNP then binds to natriuretic peptide receptors (NPRs), which are linked to guanylate cyclase and lead to increased intracellular concentrations of cyclic guanosine monophosphate (cGMP). BNP leads to a variety of physiologic effects primarily in vascular smooth muscle (vasodilation) and in the kidney (natriuresis and diuresis). In addition, BNP decreases the synthesis of a variety of hormones associated with congestive heart failure (CHF) including norepinephrine, endothelin-1, as well as angiotensin and aldosterone. BNP does not have inotropic or chronotropic effects. Nesiritide, like endogenous BNP, is metabolized by neutral endopeptidase into inactive fragments.

To date there are no pediatric trials of nesiritide. Adult studies have used a loading dose of 2 mcg/kg IV bolus followed by an infusion at 0.005 to 0.01 mcg/kg/min. When higher infusion rates are desired, a 1 mcg/kg bolus is usually followed by an infusion rate increase of 0.005 mcg/kg/min. Based on the "Vasodilation in Acute CHF" (VMAC) study, new boluses followed by infusion rate increases should not take place more frequently than every 3 hours.[181] The maximum infusion rate is 0.03 mcg/kg/min.

Nesiritide is indicated for the treatment of acute decompensated congestive heart failure in patients who are dyspneic at rest. It produces venous (at lower doses) and arterial (at higher doses) vasodilation. Stroke volume and cardiac index increase without any effect on heart rate, inotropic state, or myocardial oxygen consumption. Other beneficial effects in the CHF patients include mild diuresis and natriuresis, as well as decreased aldosterone and endothelin-1 secretion. Nesiritide may be more effective and associated with fewer side effects in the treatment of acute congestive heart than either nitroglycerin or dobutamine in normotensive adults.[219] Hypotension is the major acute side effect of nesiritide. Recent meta-analyses have raised the concern of increased risk of renal dysfunction or death at 30 days after treatment with nesiritide, although there are no conclusive data from large controlled trials. The drug should not be administered in hypotensive patients or in patients with fixed stroke volume (e.g., cardiac tamponade, obstructive cardiomyopathy).

Enalaprilat

Enalaprilat is an intravenous form of angiotensin-converting enzyme (ACE) inhibitor. ACE converts angiotensin I to angiotensin II, which is a potent systemic vasoconstrictor. Hence, administration of ACE inhibitor lowers SVR and increases venous capacitance. Blood pressure does not change significantly if cardiac output can increase to compensate for the fall in SVR.

In adults with congestive heart failure secondary to ischemic heart disease, enalaprilat administered either as a bolus or continuous infusion improves hemodynamics and oxygen delivery, although it had no impact on cardiac index.[178]

With the exception of treatment of acute hypertensive crisis, there are no data on the use of enalaprilat in children. Extrapolation of the indications for enalaprilat can be made from the oral ACE inhibitors. Captopril has been used successfully in three patient populations: congestive heart failure in dilated cardiomyopathy, congestive heart failure in large left-to-right shunts, and systemic hypertension. A hypereninemic state and, consequently, increased angiotensin levels characterize all of these conditions. Congestive heart failure symptoms and signs diminish in the majority of patients with dilated cardiomyopathy during the first month of therapy with captopril.[17] These children experience a decrease in SVR that is balanced by an increase in cardiac index so that systemic blood pressure is usually unchanged.[19]

In contrast, patients with CHF due to *restrictive* cardiomyopathy usually do not respond favorably to captopril.[19] Cardiac output does not increase to compensate for the fall in SVR, and these children experience systemic hypotension.

Infants with large left-to-right shunts (e.g., VSD) and CHF may have a favorable response to captopril.[204,215,217] The hemodynamic response depends on the baseline SVR, so that infants with increased SVR (greater than 20 U/m^2) as well as increased pulmonary-to-systemic flow ratio (Q_p:Q_s) and pulmonary artery pressure are most likely to achieve a reduction in Q_p:Q_s after captopril.[217]

Captopril has been used for children with renal hypertension. The antihypertensive effects are seen after repeated doses over the course of several days. In these patients, the mean initial dose was 1.3 mg/kg/day and the mean sustaining dose was 2.2 mg/kg/day.[36]

There are few significant complications from ACE inhibitors. Hypotension is the major hemodynamic complication. It is more common at high doses and in young infants. Blood pressure should be monitored closely at the start of captopril therapy, and dosages are increased gradually. Renal insufficiency occurs rarely.[217] The mechanism is thought to be a reduction in efferent arteriolar tone, which is needed to maintain adequate glomerular filtration.[86]

Prostacyclin

Prostacyclin (prostaglandin I_2, epoprostenol) is an antithrombotic agent and a potent systemic and pulmonary artery vasodilator.[45,46,116,234] Prostacyclin has resulted in pulmonary vasodilation in infants who were resistant to the pulmonary vasodilatory effects of tolazoline.[207] Prostacyclin has a sufficiently short (3 to 5 minute) half-life such that the effects can be titrated enabling testing of efficacy during right heart catheterization for pulmonary artery hypertension (PAH).[13] Children with primary PAH who respond to prostacyclin demonstrate a decrease in pulmonary vascular resistance (PVR) and an increase in cardiac index.[14,233] Prostacyclin is a nonspecific arterial vasodilator and therefore can significantly decrease systemic vascular resistance[233] resulting in profound systemic hypotension.

Among adults with primary pulmonary hypertension, outpatient prostacyclin therapy lowers pulmonary vascular resistance and improves symptoms over a mean follow-up period of 17 months.[145] Tolerance to prostacyclin, as manifested by return of symptoms, could be corrected by increasing the dose. Similarly, long-term (mean 21 months)

prostacyclin therapy in children with primary PAH resulted in a 59% decrease in PVR and a 42% increase in cardiac index.[14] The dosages for prostacyclin infusion have ranged between 2 and 20 ng/kg/min with most studies suggesting an effective dosage at 5 ng/kg/min.[116,197] Side effects of long-term prostacyclin therapy include diarrhea, flushing, headache, nausea, vomiting, and line-related sepsis.[14]

Taken together, these data indicate that although prostacyclin has prominent vasodilatory properties on the pulmonary circulation, it falls short of the objective of selective pulmonary vasodilation, and systemic hypotension may result. However, in responsive patients, prostacyclin is an effective therapy for PAH, delaying and perhaps avoiding lung transplantation.

Prostaglandin E$_1$

Mechanism

Prostaglandins are members of the eicosanoid family and are derived from essential fatty acids with arachidonic acid being the precursor. Prostaglandin E$_1$ (PGE$_1$) is a potent vasodilator and specifically maintains patency of the ductus arteriosus in the fetus and newborn. The exact mechanism of PGE$_1$ vasodilation specific to the ductus arteriosus is not well delineated. However, in other tissues, PGE$_1$ appears to result in dose-related increases in nitric oxide and nitric oxide synthase.[72] PGE$_1$ also acts as an inhibitor of platelet aggregation.[113]

Metabolism

PGE$_1$ is nearly completely metabolized on first pass through the pulmonary circulation to 13,14-dihydro-15-keto-PGE$_1$.

Pharmacodynamics

The usual starting dose is 0.05 mcg/kg/min, which can be doubled every 15 to 30 minutes up to 0.2 mcg/kg/min until a clinical response is achieved. Maximal response occurs 15 minutes to 4 hours after start of the infusion.[81] Once the duct is open, patency can usually be maintained with doses of 0.01 to 0.025 mcg/kg/min. Newborns up to a month of age may still respond to PGE$_1$ infusion as long as ductal closure is not complete.[81,136,237]

Indications

The major indication for PGE$_1$ is maintaining patency of the ductus arteriosus in infants with congenital heart disease (CHD). Ductal-dependent CHD includes lesions with inadequate pulmonary blood flow, inadequate systemic blood flow, and inadequate mixing (Table 7-10). The introduction of PGE$_1$ into clinical practice in 1976 allowed stabilization and recovery of newborns with nearly all ductal-dependent cardiac lesions prior to repair or palliation of complex congenital heart lesions.[81]

Newborns with right-sided obstructive lesions may have ductal-dependent pulmonary blood flow and present with cyanosis and paucity of pulmonary blood flow by chest radiograph. Cyanosis will improve dramatically with initiation of PGE$_1$.[65]

Infants with left-sided obstructive lesions may have ductal-dependent systemic blood flow and present with systemic

Table 7-10   Ductal-Dependent Lesions Requiring Stabilization with Prostaglandin E₁ Infusion

Parameter	Ductal-Dependent Pulmonary Blood Flow	Ductal-Dependent Systemic Blood Flow	Inadequate Mixing
Presenting Symptoms	Cyanosis	Shock	Cyanosis
Lesions	Severe tetralogy of Fallot	Hypoplastic left heart syndrome	Transposition of the great arteries
	Pulmonary atresia with intact ventricular septum	Critical aortic stenosis	Taussig-Bing double-outlet right ventricle
	Critical pulmonary stenosis	Interrupted aortic arch	
	Severe Ebstein's anomaly	Critical coarctation	
	Single ventricle with severe pulmonary stenosis or atresia	Single ventricle with severe aortic stenosis or atresia	

hypoperfusion and shock. PGE₁ administration usually results in resolution of acidosis and increased pulses.[65]

Newborns with transposition of the great arteries (TGA), with or without a VSD, will have ductal-dependent mixing if the intracardiac shunting is inadequate. A subset of these patients with nearly intact atrial septum will present with early shock; however, a majority of infants with TGA present with isolated cyanosis. Initiation of PGE₁ will help stabilize these patients until a balloon atrial septostomy can be performed.

Thus, PGE₁ is an appropriate initial therapy for any newborn presenting with cyanosis who is not responsive to oxygen (absence of pulmonary pathology by chest radiograph), or who has evidence of systemic hypoperfusion and weak or absent pulses without an obvious alternative etiology of shock (e.g., sepsis, metabolic disease). A few cardiac lesions cannot be stabilized by PGE₁ therapy alone, and infants with these lesions will rapidly progress to shock. These include the following: (1) Total anomalous pulmonary venous return with obstruction requires surgical repair or stabilization on veno-arterial extracorporeal membrane oxygenator. Administration of PGE₁ to these patients can worsen symptoms.[163] (2) Hypoplastic left heart syndrome with intact atrial septum requires opening of the atrial septum in the catheterization laboratory or operating room. (3) TGA with inadequate intracardiac shunting requires emergent balloon atrial septostomy.

Side Effects and Complications

Side effects of PGE₁ include primarily hypotension, temperature elevation, edema, and hypoventilation.[135] These complications were more common with intra-aortic versus intravenous administration. Respiratory depression, including apnea, occurred in 12% of children and was most common in infants with a birth weight less than 2 kg.[135] Thus, premature infants, those requiring high-dose PGE₁, or those with inadequate observation time on PGE₁ may benefit from a secure airway for transportation. PGE₁ also causes pulmonary vasodilation at a dose as low as 0.05 to 0.1 mcg/kg/min with an increase in pulmonary blood flow in patients with pulmonary hypertension.[238]

Nitric Oxide

Mechanism

Nitric oxide (NO) is a free radical, originally described as endothelium-derived relaxing factor, that has widespread effects including relaxation of vascular smooth muscle. NO is endogenously produced by conversion of L-arginine to L-citrulline by nitric oxide synthase (NOS). Various isoforms of NOS have been identified in a variety of cell types.[115,155] Of particular interest from a cardiovascular standpoint is the production of NO in vascular endothelial cells. NO functions by activating guanylate cyclase and increasing cGMP resulting in relaxation of constricted vascular smooth muscle.

Pharmacokinetics

NO has a half-life of seconds. Binding to hemoglobin inactivates NO with an affinity 1500 times greater than the binding of carbon monoxide by hemoglobin.[152] The nitrosylhemoglobin compound is converted to methemoglobin, which is ultimately reduced to ferrous hemoglobin by the enzyme methemoglobin reductase. Because of the rapid inactivation by hemoglobin, inhaled nitric oxide never reaches the systemic circulation and does not produce systemic vasodilation.

Pharmacodynamics

The rapid pharmacokinetics of this agent allow an inhaled form of this drug to be used as a specific pulmonary vasodilator. Animal studies have shown that NO dilates the pulmonary vasculature in the face of pulmonary vasoconstriction induced by a thromboxane endoperoxide analogue or by hypoxia.[83] The selective reduction of PVR using inhaled NO compared with intravenous nitroprusside in vasoconstricted lambs is nicely demonstrated in Figure 7-20.[80] Inhalation of nitric oxide or a NO-releasing compound (especially S-nitroso-N-acetylpenicillamine) produces bronchodilation in a dose-dependent manner. This result was obtained in guinea pigs with bronchospasm induced by methacholine infusion.[69] The implications of these findings are that the combination of inhaled nitric oxide–induced vasodilation and bronchodilation may improve ventilation-perfusion.

Indications

There are several current clinical indications for inhaled NO therapy. The most extensive clinical trials of NO are for treatment of *persistent pulmonary hypertension of the newborn* (PPHN). As a result of extensive clinical trials of NO in neonates with PPHN, inhaled NO has recently received Food and Drug

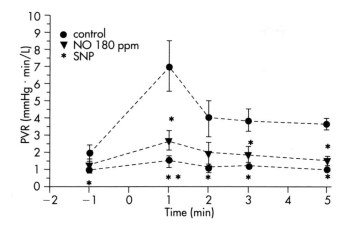

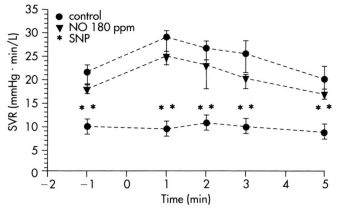

FIGURE 7-20 Effects of inhaled nitric oxide (NO) and sodium nitroprusside (SNP) on pulmonary vascular resistance (PVR) and systemic vascular resistance (SVR). Vasoconstriction was produced by bolus injection of protamine 5 minutes after heparin injection in lambs. Nitric oxide selectively prevents the increase in PVR but not SVR. Nitroprusside has a non-selective effect. (From Fratacci MD, Frostell CG, Chen TY, et al: Inhaled nitric oxide. A selective pulmonary vasodilator of heparin-protamine vasoconstriction in sheep. *Anesthesiology* 75:990–9, 1991; with permission.)

Administration (FDA) approval. PPHN is a syndrome characterized by pulmonary hypertension with right-to-left shunt at the patent ductus arteriosus and/or the patent foramen ovale. It occurs in association with meconium aspiration, hypoplastic lungs, hyaline membrane disease, or in utero hypoxia, or it can be idiopathic. Under normal circumstances, pulmonary endothelial cells release increasing amounts of nitric oxide as gestation progresses.[1] Newborns with PPHN may have diminished nitric oxide synthesis.[49] Several randomized prospective trials in infants with PPHN demonstrate improved oxygenation with NO but have differing outcome (death, ECMO) results depending on inclusion criteria and ventilation strategies. Wessel and colleagues[243] compared inhaled NO with conventional ventilation to a control group with the option of high frequency oscillatory ventilation (HFOV) and found that although there was no difference in mortality or the need for ECMO, systemic oxygenation was improved in the group receiving NO. In a multicenter trial, Roberts and colleagues[188] demonstrated that in conventionally ventilated patients, inhaled NO (80 ppm) increased systemic oxygenation,

decreased requirement for ECMO, but did not affect mortality compared with controls. Davidson and colleagues[61] found that in conventionally ventilated patients, NO (5 to 80 ppm) improved oxygenation but did not significantly alter the incidence of ECMO or death compared with controls. The Neonatal Inhaled Nitric Oxide Study Group compared NO (20 ppm) to control (100% FiO$_2$), with 55% of each group requiring HFOV, and found NO improved oxygenation ($P <$ 0.001), decreased the oxygenation index ($P < 0.001$), decreased need for ECMO ($P = 0.014$), but did not affect mortality ($P = 0.6$) compared with controls.[230] Although most of these studies excluded patients with lung hypoplasia (diaphragmatic hernia) or sepsis, they seem more resistant to nitric oxide than other causes of PPHN.[120] Collectively, these trials suggest that the term infant with hypoxic respiratory failure (not caused by diaphragmatic hernia) should receive NO (20 ppm) inhalation therapy.

The use of NO in patients with *congenital heart disease* has been demonstrated. Patients with pulmonary hypertensive congenital heart disease demonstrated a significant decrease in PVR without a change in SVR both before and after cardiopulmonary bypass.[242] Roberts and colleagues measured changes in PVR in infants with increased pulmonary blood flow due to intracardiac shunting under conditions of high FiO$_2$, NO, and NO plus high FiO$_2$ compared with low FiO$_2$ controls. High FiO$_2$, NO (80 ppm), and the combination all increased pulmonary blood flow and significantly decreased PVR compared with controls. A large subset of these patients had trisomy 21.[189] Due to its rapid onset and short half-life, NO is an excellent agent for evaluation of pulmonary vascular reactivity to determine candidacy for surgical repair. Similarly, in patients with severe congestive heart failure, NO testing in the catheterization laboratory can be helpful in determining pulmonary reactivity and eligibility for heart transplantation (reactive pulmonary hypertension) versus combined thoracic organ transplantation (nonreactive pulmonary hypertension). In the absence of intracardiac shunting, patients with pulmonary hypertension and left ventricular failure have been shown to demonstrate a significant decrease in pulmonary artery pressures and PVR, and increased left atrial pressures (or pulmonary capillary wedge pressures) without change in cardiac index.[2] Administration of NO to patients with left ventricular failure must be done with caution, as the ventricle may not tolerate potential increased preload.

NO can be helpful in controlling *postoperative pulmonary hypertension*. Postoperative pulmonary hypertension may reflect filtration of inflammatory mediators activated by cardiopulmonary bypass (with or without hypothermic circulatory arrest), hypoxic pulmonary vasoconstriction, or pulmonary endothelial cell dysfunction from increased preoperative pulmonary blood flow or following CPB. Wessel and colleagues[240] demonstrated that pulmonary vasodilation produced by acetylcholine is lost in the post-bypass period, whereas inhaled nitric oxide remains an effective pulmonary vasodilator. This difference may reflect inability of the pulmonary endothelial cell to produce adequate NO in response to acetylcholine following CPB. Other investigators have demonstrated effectiveness of NO at lowering pulmonary artery pressure and improving hemodynamics following congenital heart surgery in infants and children.[111,202]

Although both hyperventilation (pH 7.5 ± 0.03, pCO_2 32.3 ± 5.4 mm Hg) and inhaled NO (40 ppm) improve postoperative pulmonary hypertension in children,[158] inhaled NO therapy has the theoretical advantage of avoiding the higher ventilatory support and possible decreased cerebral blood flow that may be associated with the hyperventilation strategy. The clinical implications are significant. Patients with postoperative right ventricular dysfunction may benefit from the right ventricular afterload reduction provided by NO.[208] Patients with reactive preoperative pulmonary hypertension (i.e., those with atrioventricular septal defects, total anomalous pulmonary venous return) who are at risk for early postoperative pulmonary hypertensive crises may be stabilized with NO.[93,111]

Side Effects and Complications

Delivery systems have now been developed to deliver inhaled NO at concentrations of 1 to 80 ppm via conventional ventilator, high-frequency oscillators, intraoperative anesthesia machine, face mask, or nasal cannula.[241] An appropriate scavenging system is necessary to avoid environmental production of the highly toxic nitrogen dioxide (NO_2) [$2NO + O_2 = 2NO_2$].[79] Chemiluminescence monitoring can be used to detect NO_2.[126] Standards from the Occupational Safety and Health Administration limit NO_2 exposure to less than 5 ppm.[164] Current clinically used NO doses have not led to detection of nitrogen dioxide in the airway; however, the extent of nitrogen dioxide formation in the lung is unknown.

Methemoglobin (reference range 0% to 5%) is a metabolic byproduct of nitric oxide inhalation. Inhalation of nitric oxide 80 ppm for 23 hours in lambs raises methemoglobin to a maximum level of 3%.[252] Patients receiving 40 to 80 ppm NO for a median of 40 hours had methemoglobin levels of 2.5 ± 0.4% with 18% of patients with levels greater than 4.6%.[241] Other studies have shown no elevation in methemoglobin with prolonged administration of 20 to 80 ppm NO.[2,111]

VASOCONSTRICTORS

Phenylephrine

Phenylephrine is an $alpha_1$ agonist with very little beta effect. Its major action is systemic and pulmonary arterial vasoconstriction, increasing SVR and systemic arterial pressure (systolic, diastolic, and mean). Reflex bradycardia can occur. The increase in pulmonary artery pressure is less pronounced than the increase in aortic pressure.

Phenylephrine has been used in a variety of settings. Bolus (10 mcg/kg) and/or continuous (2 to 5 mcg/kg/min) intravenous phenylephrine have been used to reverse and treat the hypercyanotic spells of tetralogy of Fallot. By increasing the systemic vascular resistance in excess of the pulmonary vascular resistance, this $alpha_1$ agonist lessens right-to-left ventricular shunting and improves arterial oxygenation.[170,216]

Septic shock with low SVR has been considered an indication for phenylephrine in adults. In a small series of patients, oxygen delivery, oxygen consumption, stroke volume index, and urine output all increased after phenylephrine infusion.[97] Phenylephrine is rarely used in pediatric septic shock.

Arginine-Vasopressin

Arginine-vasopressin (or antidiuretic hormone) is a neuropeptide secreted by the posterior pituitary gland in response to increases in serum osmolality or decreases in plasma volume. At low concentrations, vasopressin causes free water retention by the kidney. At higher concentrations, vasoconstriction occurs.[142]

Adults with vasodilatory septic shock have been shown to have low vasopressin plasma levels.[128] Vasopressin (0.04 U/min) improves arterial blood pressure by increasing systemic vascular resistance without affecting cardiac index in adults with vasodilatory septic shock.[142] Similarly, adults with vasodilatory shock following cardiac surgery have inappropriately low serum vasopressin concentrations and demonstrate increased mean arterial pressure with vasopressin (0.09 ± 0.05 U/min).[7,156] Vasopressin has also been shown to improve systemic blood pressure without affecting cardiac index in post-cardiac surgery patients with milrinone-induced vasodilation and hypotension.[92]

In children, plasma levels of vasopressin following congenital cardiac surgery appear to be elevated compared with preoperative levels.[3,8] However, infants and children with acceptable cardiac function but vasodilatory shock following cardiac surgery that is refractory to inotropes and vasopressors demonstrate a significant increase in systemic blood pressure with vasopressin infusion (0.0003 to 0.002 U/kg/min).[192]

Thus, vasopressin should be considered in the patient with adequate cardiac function but severe vasodilatory shock that is not responsive to dopamine or epinephrine.

CONCLUSION

The interplay between clinical trial and molecular biology has been particularly fruitful in the understanding and design of cardiovascular drugs. Elucidation of adrenal receptor desensitization, cloning of receptor genes, and the effects of nitric oxide are some of the examples of important biologic developments that now affect clinical care. In the future, cardiovascular therapy will become more specific and safer as further insights into basic mechanisms are developed.

References

1. Abman SH, Chatfield BA, Hall SL, McMurtry IF: Role of endothelium-derived relaxing factor during transition of pulmonary circulation at birth. Am J Physiol 259:H1921–H1927, 1990.
2. Adatia I, Perry S, Landzberg M, et al: Inhaled nitric oxide and hemodynamic evaluation of patients with pulmonary hypertension before transplantation. J Am Coll Cardiol 25:1656–1664, 1995.
3. Agnoletti G, Scotti C, Panzali AF, et al: Plasma levels of atrial natriuretic factor (ANF) and urinary excretion of ANF, arginine vasopressin and catecholamines in children with congenital heart disease: Effect of cardiac surgery. Eur J Cardiothorac Surg 7:533–539, 1993.
4. Alousi AA, Farah AE, Lesher GY, Opalka CJ Jr: Cardiotonic activity of amrinone—Win 40680 [5-amino-3,4′-bipyridine-6-(1H)-one]. Circ Res 45:666–677, 1979.

5. Anonymous. Guidelines 2000 for cardiopulmonary resuscitation and emergency cardiovascular care. Part 10: Pediatric advanced life support. The American Heart Association in collaboration with the International Liaison Committee on Resuscitation. *Circulation* 102:I291–I342, 2000.

6. Appelbaum A, Blackstone EH, Kouchoukos NT, Kirklin JW: Afterload reduction and cardiac output in infants early after intracardiac surgery. *Am J Cardiol* 39:445–451, 1977.

7. Argenziano M, Chen JM, Choudhri AF, et al: Management of vasodilatory shock after cardiac surgery: Identification of predisposing factors and use of a novel pressor agent. *J Thorac Cardiovasc Surg* 116:973–980, 1998.

8. Ationu A, Singer DR, Smith A, et al: Studies of cardiopulmonary bypass in children: Implications for the regulation of brain natriuretic peptide. *Cardiovasc Res* 27:1538–1541, 1993.

9. Azeka E, Franchini Ramires JA, et al: Delisting of infants and children from the heart transplantation waiting list after carvedilol treatment. *J Am Coll Cardiol* 40:2034–2038, 2002.

10. Bailey JM, Miller BE, Lu W, et al: The pharmacokinetics of milrinone in pediatric patients after cardiac surgery. *Anesthesiology* 90:1012–1018, 1999.

11. Banner W Jr, Vernon DD, Minton SD, Dean JM: Nonlinear dobutamine pharmacokinetics in a pediatric population. *Crit Care Med* 19:871–873, 1991.

12. Barrington K, Chan W: The circulatory effects of epinephrine infusion in the anesthetized piglet. *Pediatr Res* 33:190–194, 1993.

13. Barst RJ: Recent advances in the treatment of pediatric pulmonary artery hypertension. *Pediatr Clin North Am* 46:331–345, 1999.

14. Barst RJ: Vasodilator therapy for primary pulmonary hypertension in children. *Circulation* 99:1197–1208, 1999.

15. Bartelds B, Gratama JW, Meuzelaar KJ, et al: Comparative effects of isoproterenol and dopamine on myocardial oxygen consumption, blood flow distribution and total body oxygen consumption in conscious lambs with and without an aortopulmonary left to right shunt. *J Am Coll Cardiol* 31:473–481, 1998.

16. Barton P, Garcia J, Kouatli A, et al: Hemodynamic effects of IV milrinone lactate in pediatric patients with septic shock. *Chest* 109:1302–1312, 1996.

17. Beekman RH, Rocchini AP, Dick M 2nd, et al: Vasodilator therapy in children: Acute and chronic effects in children with left ventricular dysfunction or mitral regurgitation. *Pediatrics* 73:43–51, 1984.

18. Belgorosky A, Weller G, Chaler E, et al: Evaluation of serum total thyroxine and triiodothyronine and their serum fractions in nonthyroidal illness secondary to congenital heart disease. Studies before and after surgery. *J Endocrinol Invest* 16:499–503, 1993.

19. Bengur AR, Beekman RH, Rocchini AP, et al: Acute hemodynamic effects of captopril in children with a congestive or restrictive cardiomyopathy. *Circulation* 83:523–527, 1991.

20. Benitz WE, Malachowski N, Cohen RS, et al: Use of sodium nitroprusside in neonates: Efficacy and safety. *J Pediatr* 106:102–110, 1985.

21. Bennett NR, Abbott TR: The use of sodium nitroprusside in children. *Anaesthesia* 32:456–463, 1977.

22. Bennett-Guerrero E, Jimenez JL, White WD, et al: Cardiovascular effects of intravenous triiodothyronine in patients undergoing coronary artery bypass graft surgery. *JAMA* 275:687–692, 1996.

23. Benson LN, Bohn D, Edmonds JF, et al: Nitroglycerin therapy in children with low cardiac index after heart surgery. *Cardiovasc Med* 4:207–215, 1979.

24. Benzing G 3rd, Helmsworth JA, Schreiber JT, Kaplan S: Nitroprusside and epinephrine for treatment of low output in children after open-heart surgery. *Ann Thorac Surg* 27:523–528, 1979.

25. Benzing G 3rd, Helmsworth JA, Schrieber JT, et al: Nitroprusside after open-heart surgery. *Circulation* 54:467–471, 1976.

26. Berg RA, Donnerstein RL, Padbury JF: Dobutamine infusions in stable, critically ill children: Pharmacokinetics and hemodynamic actions. *Crit Care Med* 21:678–686, 1993.

27. Berg RA, Padbury JF, Donnerstein RL, et al: Dobutamine pharmacokinetics and pharmacodynamics in normal children and adolescents. *J Pharmacol Exp Ther* 265:1232–1238, 1993.

28. Berk JL, Hagen JF, Koo R: Effect of alpha and beta adrenergic blockade on epinephrine induced pulmonary insufficiency. *Ann Surg* 183:369–376, 1976.

29. Berlin CM Jr: The treatment of cyanide poisoning in children. *Pediatrics* 46:793–796, 1970.

30. Bersten AD, Rutten AJ, Summersides G, Ilsley AH: Epinephrine infusion in sheep: Systemic and renal hemodynamic effects. *Critical Care Med* 22:994–1001, 1994.

31. Bettendorf M, Schmidt KG, Grulich-Henn J, et al: Tri-iodothyronine treatment in children after cardiac surgery: A double-blind, randomized, placebo-controlled study. *Lancet* 356:529–534, 2000.

32. Bettendorf M, Schmidt KG, Tiefenbacher U, et al: Transient secondary hypothyroidism in children after cardiac surgery. *Pediatric Research* 41:375–379, 1997.

33. Bigam DL, Barrington KJ, Jirsch DW, Cheung PY: Effects of a continuous epinephrine infusion on regional blood flow in awake newborn piglets. *Biology of the Neonate* 73:198–206, 1998.

34. Bohn DJ, Poirier CS, Edmonds JF, Barker GA: Hemodynamic effects of dobutamine after cardiopulmonary bypass. *Crit Care Med* 8:367–371, 1980.

35. Borow KM, Neumann A, Arensman FW, Yacoub MH: Cardiac and peripheral vascular responses to adrenoceptor stimulation and blockade after cardiac transplantation. *J Amer Coll Cardiol* 14:1229–1238, 1989.

36. Bouissou F, Meguira B, Rostin M, et al: Long term therapy by captopril in children with renal hypertension. *Clin Exp Hypertens* 8A:841–845, 1986.

37. Bristow MR, Minobe W, Rasmussen R, et al: Alpha-1 adrenergic receptors in the nonfailing and failing human heart. *J Pharmacol Exp Ther* 247:1039–1045, 1988.

38. Bristow MR: Pathophysiologic and pharmacologic rationales for clinical management of chronic heart failure with beta-blocking agents. *Am J Cardiol* 71:12–22C, 1993.

39. Brodde OE, Broede A, Daul A, et al: Receptor systems in the nonfailing human heart. *Basic Res Cardiol* 87:1–14, 1992.

40. Brodde OE, Zerkowski HR, Doetsch N, et al: Myocardial beta-adrenoreceptor changes in heart failure: Concomitant reduction in beta$_1$- and beta$_2$-adrenoreceptor function related to the degree of heart failure in patients with mitral valve disease. *J Am Coll Cardiol* 14:323–331, 1989.

41. Brogan TV, Bratton SL, Lynn AM: Thyroid function in infants following cardiac surgery: Comparative effects of iodinated and noniodinated topical antiseptics. *Critical Care Med* 25:1583–1587, 1997.

42. Broner CW, Stidham GL, Westenkirchner DF, Watson DC: A prospective, randomized, double-blind comparison of calcium chloride and calcium gluconate therapies for hypocalcemia in critically ill children. *J Pediatr* 117:986–989, 1990.

43. Brown CG, Martin DR, Pepe PE, et al: A comparison of standard-dose and high-dose epinephrine in cardiac arrest outside the hospital. The Multicenter High-Dose Epinephrine Study Group. *N Engl J Med* 327:1051–1055, 1992.

44. Bruns LA, Chrisant MK, Lamour JM, et al: Carvedilol as therapy in pediatric heart failure: An initial multicenter experience. *J Pediatr* 138:505–511, 2001.

45. Bush A, Busst C, Booth K, et al: Does prostacyclin enhance the selective pulmonary vasodilator effect of oxygen in children with congenital heart disease? *Circulation* 74:135–144, 1986.

46. Bush A, Busst C, Knight WB, Shinebourne EA: Modification of pulmonary hypertension secondary to congenital heart disease by prostacyclin therapy. *Am Rev Respir Dis* 136:767–769, 1987.

47. Cardenas-Rivero N, Chernow B, Stoiko MA, et al: Hypocalcemia in critically ill children. *J Pediatr* 114:946–951, 1989.

48. Caspi J, Coles JG, Benson LN, et al: Age-related response to epinephrine-induced myocardial stress. A functional and ultrastructural study. *Circulation* 84: III394–III399, 1991.

49. Castillo L, de Rojas T, Chapman T, et al: Nitric oxide synthesis is decreased in persistent pulmonary hypertension of the newborn. *Pediatr Res* 33:20A, 1993.

50. Chang AC, Atz AM, Wernovsky G, et al: Milrinone: Systemic and pulmonary hemodynamic effects in neonates after cardiac surgery. *Crit Care Med* 23:1907–1914, 1995.

51. Chernow B, Holbrook P, D'Angona DS Jr, et al: Epinephrine absorption after intratracheal administration. *Anesth Analg* 63:829–832, 1984.

52. Chernow B, Rainey TG, Lake CR: Endogenous and exogenous catecholamines in critical care medicine. *Crit Care Med* 10:409–416, 1982.

53. Cheung PY, Barrington KJ, Pearson RJ, et al: Systemic, pulmonary and mesenteric perfusion and oxygenation effects of dopamine and epinephrine. *Am J Resp & Critical Care Med* 155:32–37, 1997.

54. Chiariello M, Gold HK, Leinbach RC, et al: Comparison between the effects of nitroprusside and nitroglycerin on ischemic injury during acute myocardial infarction. *Circulation* 54:766–773, 1976.

55. Chidsey CA, Braunwald E, Morrow AG: Catecholamine excretion and cardiac stores of norepinephrine in congestive heart failure. *Am J Med* 39:442–451, 1965.

56. Cotecchia S, Schwinn DA, Randall RR, et al: Molecular cloning and expression of the cDNA for the hamster α_1- adrenergic receptor. *Proc Natl Acad Sci USA* 85:7159–7163, 1988.

57. Cottrell JE, Casthely P, Brodie JD, et al: Prevention of nitroprusside-induced cyanide toxicity with hydroxocobalamin. *N Engl J Med* 298:809–811, 1978.

58. Cuneo BF, Zales VR, Blahunka PC, Benson DW Jr: Pharmacodynamics and pharmacokinetics of esmolol, a short-acting beta-blocking agent, in children. *Pediatr Cardiol* 15:296–301, 1994.

59. Cutaia M, Porcelli RJ: Pulmonary vascular reactivity after repetitive exposure to selected biogenic amines. *J Appl Physiol* 55:1868–1876, 1983.

60. Damen J, Hitchcock JF: Reactive pulmonary hypertension after a switch operation. Successful treatment with glyceryl trinitrate. *Br Heart J* 53:223–225, 1985.

61. Davidson D, Barefield ES, Kattwinkel J, et al: Inhaled nitric oxide for the early treatment of persistent pulmonary hypertension of the term newborn: A randomized, double-masked, placebo-controlled, dose-response, multicenter study. *Pediatrics* 101:325–334, 1998.

62. Deal JE, Barratt TM, Dillon MJ: Management of hypertensive emergencies. *Arch Dis Child* 67:1089–1092, 1992.

63. Dillon TR, Janos GG, Meyer RA, et al: Vasodilator therapy for congestive heart failure. *J Pediatr* 96:623–629, 1980.

64. Dixon RA, Kobilka BK, Strader DJ, et al: Cloning of the gene and cDNA for mammalian beta-adrenergic receptor and homology with rhodopsin. *Nature* 321:75–79, 1986.

65. Donahoo JS, Roland JM, Kan J, et al: Prostaglandin E1 as an adjunct to emergency cardiac operation in neonates. *J Thorac Cardiovasc Surg* 81:227–231, 1981.

66. Driscoll DJ, Gillette PC, Duff DF, et al: Hemodynamic effects of dobutamine in children. *Am J Cardiol* 43:581–585, 1979.

67. Driscoll DJ, Gillette PC, Ezrailson EG, Schwartz A: Inotropic response of the neonatal canine myocardium to dopamine. *Pediat Res* 12:42–45, 1978.

68. Driscoll DJ, Gillette PC, Lewis RM, et al: Comparative hemodynamic effects of isoproterenol, dopamine, and dobutamine in the newborn dog. *Pediat Res* 13:1006–1009, 1979.

69. Dupuy PM, Shore SA, Drazen JM, et al: Bronchodilator action of inhaled nitric oxide in guinea pigs. *J Clin Invest* 90:421–428, 1992.

70. Earl CQ, Linden J: Biochemical mechanisms for the inotropic effect of the cardiotonic drug milrinone. *J Cardiovasc Pharmacol* 8:864–872, 1986.

71. Eldadah MK, Schwartz PH, Harrison R, Newth CJ: Pharmacokinetics of dopamine in infants and children. *Crit Care Med* 19:1008–1011, 1991.

72. Escrig A, Marin R, Mas M: Repeated PGE1 treatment enhances nitric oxide and erection responses to nerve stimulation in the rat penis by upregulating constitutive NOS isoforms. *J Urology* 162:2205–2210, 1999.

73. Feldman AM: Modulation of adrenergic receptors and G-transduction proteins in failing human ventricular myocardium. *Circulation* 87:IV27–34, 1993.

74. Fenek RO: Intravenous milrinone following cardiac surgery: I. Effects of bolus infusion followed by variable dose maintenance infusion. The European Milrinone Multicentre Trial Group. *J Cardiothor Vasc Anesth* 6:554–562, 1992.

75. Fenek RO: Intravenous milrinone following cardiac surgery: II. Influence of baseline hemodynamics and patient factors on therapeutic response. The European Milrinone Multicentre Trial Group. *J Cardiothor Vasc Anesth* 6:563–567, 1992.

76. Feuerstein G, Yue TL, Ma X, Ruffolo RR: Novel mechanisms in the treatment of heart failure: Inhibition of oxygen radicals and apoptosis by carvedilol. *Prog Cardiovasc Dis* 41:17–24, 1998.

77. Fisher DG, Schwartz PH, Davis AL: Pharmacokinetics of exogenous epinephrine in critically ill children. *Crit Care Med* 21:111–117, 1993.

78. Fleischmann LE: Management of hypertensive crisis in children. *Pediatric Annals* 6:410–414, 1977.

79. Francoe M, Troncy E, Blaise G: Inhaled nitric oxide: Technical aspects of administration and monitoring. *Crit Care Med* 26:782–796, 1998.

80. Fratacci MD, Frostell CG, Chen TY, et al: Inhaled nitric oxide. A selective pulmonary vasodilator of heparin-protamine vasoconstriction in sheep. *Anesthesiology* 75:990–999, 1991.

81. Freed MD, Heymann MA, Lewis AB, et al: Prostaglandin E1 infants with ductus arteriosus-dependent congenital heart disease. *Circulation* 64:899–905, 1981.

82. Frielle T, Collins S, Daniel KW, et al: Cloning of the cDNA for the human beta 1-adrenergic receptor. *Proc Natl Acad Sci USA* 84:7920–7924, 1987.

83. Frostell C, Fratacci MD, Wain JC, et al: Inhaled nitric oxide. A selective pulmonary vasodilator reversing hypoxic pulmonary vasoconstriction. *Circulation* 83:2038–2047, 1991.

84. Gidding SS, Rocchini AP, Beekman R, et al: Therapeutic effect of propranolol on paradoxical hypertension after repair of coarctation of the aorta. *N Engl J Med* 312:1224–1228, 1985.

85. Gilbert EM, Olsen SL, Renlund DG, Bristow MR: Beta-adrenergic receptor regulation and left ventricular function in idiopathic dilated cardiomyopathy. *Am J Cardiol* 71:23C–29C, 1993.

86. Gilman AG, Rall TW, Nies AS, et al (eds): *The Pharmacological Basis of Therapeutics*. New York: Pergamon Press, 1990.

87. Girardin E, Berner M, Rouge JC, et al: Effect of low dose dopamine on hemodynamic and renal function in children. *Pediatr Res* 26:200–203, 1989.

88. Girardin EP, Berner ME, Favre HR, et al: Atrial natriuretic factor after heart operations in children. Relation to hemodynamic and renal parameters. *J Thorac Cardiovasc Surg* 102:526–531, 1991.

89. Goenen M, Pedemonte O, Baele P, Col J: Amrinone in the management of low cardiac output after open heart surgery. *Am J Cardiol* 56:33B–38B, 1985.

90. Goetting MG, Paradis NA: High dose epinephrine in refractory pediatric cardiac arrest. *Crit Care Med* 17:1258–1262, 1989.

91. Goetting MG, Paradis NA: High-dose epinephrine improves outcome from pediatric cardiac arrest. *Ann Emerg Med* 20:22–26, 1991.

92. Gold J, Cullinane S, Chen J, et al: Vasopressin in the treatment of milrinone-induced hypotension in severe heart failure. *Am J Cardiol* 85:506–508, 2000.

93. Goldman AP, Delius RE, Deanfield JE, et al: Nitric oxide might reduce the need for extracorporeal support in children with critical postoperative pulmonary hypertension. *Ann Thorac Surg* 62:750–755, 1996.

94. Gomberg-Maitland M, Frishman WH: Thyroid hormone and cardiovascular disease. *Am Heart J* 135:187–196, 1998.

95. Goodall M, Alton H: Metabolism of 3-hydroxytyramine (dopamine) in human subjects. *Biochem Pharmacol* 17:905–914, 1968.

96. Gordillo-Paniagua G, Velasquez-Jones L, Martini R, Valdez-Bolanos E: Sodium nitroprusside treatment of severe arterial hypertension in children. *J Pediatr* 87:799–802, 1975.

97. Gregory JS, Bonfiglio MF, Dasta JF, et al: Experience with phenylephrine as a component of the pharmacologic support of septic shock. *Crit Care Med* 19:1395–1400, 1991.

98. Guiha NH, Cohn JN, Mikulic E, et al: Treatment of refractory heart failure with infusion of nitroprusside. *N Engl J Med* 291:587–591, 1974.

99. Guller B, Fields AI, Coleman MG, Holbrook PR: Changes in cardiac rhythm in children treated with dopamine. *Crit Care Med* 6:151–154, 1978.

100. Habib DM, Padbury JF, Anas NG, et al: Dobutamine pharmacokinetics and pharmacodynamics in pediatric intensive care patients. *Crit Care Med* 20:601–608, 1992.

101. Hamilton MA, Stevenson LW, Fonarow GC, et al: Safety and hemodynamic effects of intravenous triiodothyronine in advanced congestive heart failure. *Am J Cardiol* 81:443–447, 1998.

102. Hamilton MA, Stevenson LW, Luu M, Walden JA: Altered thyroid hormone metabolism in advanced heart failure. *J Am Coll Cardiol* 16:91–95, 1990.

103. Harding SE, Brown LA, Wynne DG, et al: Mechanisms of beta-adrenoreceptor desensitization in the failing human heart. *Cardiovasc Resear* 28:1451–1460, 1994.

104. Hayes JS, Bowling N, Boder GB, Kauffman R: Molecular basis for the cardiovascular activities of amrinone and AR-L57. *J Pharmacol Exp Ther* 230:124–132, 1984.

105. Ho ECK, Moss AJ: The syndrome of mesenteric arteritis following surgical repair of aortic coarctation. *Pediatrics* 49:40–45, 1972.

106. Hoffman TM, Wernovsky G, Atz AM: Efficacy and safety of milrinone in preventing low cardiac output syndrome in infants and children after corrective surgery for congenital heart disease. *Circulation* 107:996–1002, 2003.

107. Honerjager P, Schafer-Korting M, Reiter M: Involvement of cyclic AMP in the direct inotropic action of amrinone, biochemical and functional evidence. *Naunyn Schmiedebergs Arch Pharmacol* 318:112–120, 1981.

108. Hyman AL, Lippton HL, Kadowitz PJ: Autonomic regulation of the pulmonary circulation. *J Cardiovasc Pharmacol* 7:S80–95, 1985.

109. Ignarro LJ, Lippton H, Edwards JC, et al: Mechanism of vascular smooth muscle relaxation by organic nitrates, nitrites, nitroprusside and nitric oxide: Evidence for the involvement of S-nitrosothiols as active intermediates. *J Pharmacol Exp Ther* 218:739–749, 1981.

110. Ilbawi MN, Idriss FS, DeLeon SY, et al: Hemodynamic effects of intravenous nitroglycerin in pediatric patients after heart surgery. *Circulation* 72:II101–107, 1985.

111. Journois D, Pouard P, Mauriat P, et al: Inhaled nitric oxide as a therapy for pulmonary hypertension after operations for congenital heart defects. *J Thorac Cardiovasc Surg* 107:1129–1135, 1994.

112. Kariya T, Wille LJ, Dage RC: Biochemical studies on the mechanism of cardiotonic activity of MDL 17,043. *J Cardiovasc Pharmacol* 4:509–514, 1982.

113. Katzenschlager R, Weiss K, Rogatti W, et al: Interaction between prostaglandin E1 and nitric oxide (NO). *Thromb Res* 62:299–304, 1991.

114. Kaumann AJ, Lobnig BM: Mode of action of (-)-pinodolol on feline and human myocardium. *Br J Pharmacol* 89:207–218, 1986.

115. Kelly RA, Balligand JL, Smith TW: Nitric oxide and cardiac function. *Circ Res* 79:363–380, 1996.

116. Kermode J, Butt W, Shann F: Comparison between prostaglandin E1 and epoprostenol (prostacyclin) in infants after heart surgery. *Br Heart J* 66:175–178, 1991.

117. Kikura M, Lee MK, Safon RA, et al: The effects of milrinone on platelets in patients undergoing cardiac surgery. *Anesth Analges* 81:44–48, 1995.

118. Kikura M, Levy JH, Michelsen LG, et al: The effects of milrinone on hemodynamics and left ventricular function after emergence from cardiopulmonary bypass. *Anesth Analges* 85:16–22, 1997.

119. Kimball TR, Daniels SR, Meyer RA, et al: Effect of digoxin on contractility and symptoms in infants with a large ventricular septal defect. *Am J Cardiol* 68:1377–1382, 1991.

120. Kinsella JP, Abman SH: Inhalational nitric oxide therapy for persistent pulmonary hypertension of the newborn. *Pediatrics* 91:997–998, 1993.

121. Klarr JM, Faix RG, Pryce CJ, Bhatt-Mehta V: Randomized, blind trial of dopamine versus dobutamine for treatment of hypotension in preterm infants with respiratory distress syndrome. *J Pediatr* 125:117–122, 1994.

122. Klemperer JD, Klein I, Gomez M, et al: Thyroid hormone treatment after coronary-artery bypass surgery. *N Engl J Med* 333:1522–1527, 1995.

123. Kobilka BK, Dixon RA, Frielle T, et al: cDNA for the human beta 2-adrenergic receptor: A protein with multiple membrane-spanning domains and encoded by a gene whose chromosomal location is shared with that of the receptor for platelet-derived growth factor. *Proc Natl Acad Sci USA* 84:46–50, 1987.

124. Kobilka BK, Kobilka TS, Daniel K, et al: Chimeric alpha 2-, beta 2-adrenergic receptors: Delineation of domains involved in effector coupling and ligand binding specificity. *Science* 240:1310–1316, 1988.

125. Kunathai S, Sholler GF, Celermajer JM, et al: Nitroprusside in children after cardiopulmonary bypass: A study of thiocyanate toxicity. *Pediatr Cardiol* 10:121–124, 1989.

126. Laguenie G, Berg A, Saint-Maurice JP, Dinh-Xuan AT: Measurement of nitrogen dioxide formation from nitric oxide by chemiluminescence in ventilated children. *Lancet* 341:969, 1993.

127. Lambert DG: Signal transduction: G proteins and second messengers. *Br J Anaesth* 71:86–95, 1993.

128. Landry DW, Levin HR, Gallant EM, et al: Vasopressin deficiency contributes to the vasodilation of septic shock. *Circulation* 95:1122–1125, 1997.

129. Landzberg JS, Parker JD, Gauthier DF, Colucci WS: Effects of myocardial alpha 1-adrenergic receptor stimulation and blockade on contractility in humans. *Circulation* 84:1608–1614, 1991.

130. Lawless S, Burckart G, Diven W, et al: Amrinone in neonates and infants after cardiac surgery. *Crit Care Med* 17:751–754, 1989.

131. Le Tulzo Y, Seguin P, Gacouin A, et al: Effects of epinephrine on right ventricular function in patients with severe septic shock and right ventricular failure: A preliminary descriptive study. *Intensive Care Med* 23: 664–670, 1997.

132. Leier CV, Heban PT, Huss P, et al: Comparative systemic and regional hemodynamic effects of dopamine and dobutamine in patients with cardiomyopathic heart failure. *Circulation* 58:466–475, 1978.

133. Leier CV, Webel J, Bush CA: The cardiovascular effects of the continuous infusion of dobutamine in patients with severe cardiac failure. *Circulation* 56:468–472, 1977.

134. LeJemtel TH, Keung E, Sonnenblick EH, et al: Amrinone: A new non-glycosidic, non-adrenergic cardiotonic agent effective in the treatment of intractable myocardial failure in man. *Circulation* 59:1098–1104, 1979.

135. Lewis AB, Freed MD, Heymann MA, et al: Side effects of therapy with prostaglandin E1 in infants with critical congenital heart disease. *Circulation* 64:893–898, 1981.

136. Lewis AB, Takahashi M, Lurie PR: Administration of prostaglandin E1 in neonates with critical congenital cardiac defects. *J Pediatr* 93:481–485, 1978.

137. Lock JE, Olley PM, Coceani F: Enhanced beta-adrenergic-receptor responsiveness in hypoxic neonatal pulmonary circulation. *Am J Physiol* 240:H697–H703, 1981.

138. Lomasney JW, Lorenz W, Allen LF, et al: Expansion of the alpha 2-adrenergic receptor family: Cloning and characterization of a human alpha 2-adrenergic receptor subtype, the gene for which is located on chromosome 2. *Proc Natl Acad Sci USA* 87:5094–5098, 1990.

139. Lurie KG, Bristow MR, Reitz BA: Increased beta-adrenergic receptor density in an experimental model of cardiac transplantation. *J Thorac Cardiovasc Surg* 86:195–201, 1983.

140. Lynch SK, Lemley KV, Polak, MJ: The effect of dopamine on glomerular filtration rate in normotensive, oliguric premature neonates. *Pediatr Nephrol* 18:649–652, 2003.

141. Maguire JF, Geha RS, Umetsu DT: Myocardial specific creatine phosphokinase isoenzyme elevation in children with asthma treated with intravenous isoproterenol. *J Allergy Clin Immunol* 78:631–636, 1986.

142. Malay MB, Ashton RC Jr, Landry DW, Townsend RN: Low-dose vasopressin in the treatment of vasodilatory septic shock. *J Trauma* 47:699–704, 1999.

143. Martin C, Papazian L, Perrin G, et al: Norepinephrine or dopamine for the treatment of hyperdynamic septic shock? *Chest* 103:1826–1831, 1993.

144. McGowan FX Jr, Davis PJ, Siewers RD, del Nido PJ: Coronary vasoconstriction mediated by enothelin-1 in neonates. Reversal by nitroglycerin. *J Thorac Cardiovasc Surg* 109:88–97, 1995.

145. McLaughlin VV, Genthner DE, Panella MM, Rich S: Reduction in pulmonary vascular resistance with long-term epoprostenol (prostacyclin) therapy in primary pulmonary hypertension. *N Engl J Med* 338:273–277, 1998.

146. Meadow WL, Rudinsky BF, Strates E: Selective elevation of systemic blood pressure by epinephrine during sepsis-induced pulmonary hypertension in piglets. *Pediatr Res* 20:872–875, 1986.

147. Merrin RG: Autonomic nervous system pharmacology. In Miller RD (ed): *Anesthesia*. New York: Churchill Livingstone, 1990.

148. Miall-Allen VM, De Vries LS, Whitelaw AGL: Mean arterial blood pressure and neonatal cerebral lesions. *Arch Dis Child* 62:1068–1069, 1987.

149. Miall-Allen VM, Whitelaw AG: Response to dopamine and dobutamine in the preterm infant less than 30 weeks gestation. *Crit Care Med* 17:1166–1169, 1989.

150. Michael JR, Guerci AD, Koehler RC, et al: Mechanisms by which epinephrine augments cerebral and myocardial perfusion during cardiopulmonary resuscitation in dogs. *Circulation* 69:822–835, 1984.

151. Mikhail MS, Hunsinger SY, Goodwin SR, Loughlin GM: Myocardial ischemia complicating therapy of status asthmaticus. *Clin Pediatr* 26:419–421, 1987.

152. Million D, Zillner P, Baumann R: Oxygen pressure-dependent control of carbonic anhydrase synthesis in chick embryonic erythrocytes. *Am J Physiol* 261:R1188–1196, 1991.

153. Mitani Y, Okuda YR, Shimpo H, et al: Impaired endothelial function in epicardial coronary arteries after Kawasaki disease. *Circulation* 96:454–461, 1997.

154. Molenaar P, Smolich JJ, Russell FD, et al: Differential regulation of beta-1 and beta-2 adrenoceptors in guinea pig atrioventricular conducting system after chronic (-)-isoproterenol infusion. *J Pharmacol Exp Ther* 255:393–400, 1990.

155. Moncada S, Palmer RM, Higgs EA: Nitric oxide: Physiology, pathophysiology, and pharmacology. *Pharm Rev* 43:109–142, 1991.

156. Morales DL, Gregg D, Helman DN, et al: Arginine vasopressin in the treatment of 50 patients with postcardiotomy vasodilatory shock. *Ann Thor Surg* 69:102–106, 2000.

157. Moran JL, O'Fathartaigh MS, Peisach AR, et al: Epinephrine as an inotropic agent in septic shock: A dose-profile analysis. *Crit Care Med* 21:70–77, 1993.

158. Morris K, Beghetti M, Petros A, et al: Comparison of hyperventilation and inhaled nitric oxide for pulmonary hypertension after repair of congenital heart disease. *Crit Care Med* 28:2974–2978, 2000.

159. Motomura S, Reinhard-Zerkowski H, Daul A, Brodde OE: On the physiologic role of beta-2 adrenoreceptors in the human heart: In vitro and in vivo studies. *Am Heart J* 119:608–619, 1990.

160. Muntz KH, Zhao M, Miller JC: Downregulation of myocardial beta-adrenergic receptors. Receptor subtype selectivity. *Circ Res* 74:369–375, 1994.

161. Nakamura KT, Matherne GP, Jose PA, et al: Effects of epinephrine on the renal vascular bed of fetal, newborn, and adult sheep. *Pediatr Res* 23:181–186, 1988.

162. Nakano H, Ueda K, Saito A: Acute hemodynamic effects of nitroprusside in children with isolated mitral regurgitation. *Am J Cardiol* 56:351–355, 1985.

163. Neirotti RA, Alvarez CE, Campos MD, et al: Total anomalous pulmonary venous connection. *Scand J Thorac Cardiovasc Surg* 25:97–100, 1991.

164. NIOSH recommendation for occupational safety and health standards 1998. *MMWR* 37:1–29, 1988.

165. Nishioka K, Nakanishi T, George BL, Jarmakani JM: The effect of calcium on the inotropy of catecholamine and paired electrical stimulation in the newborn and adult myocardium. *J Mol Cell Cardiol* 13:511–520, 1981.

166. Notterman DA, Greenwald BM, Moran F, et al: Dopamine clearance in critically ill infants and children: Effect of age and organ system dysfunction. *Clin Pharmacol Ther* 48:138–147, 1990.

167. Nussbaum J, Zane EA, Thys DM: Esmolol for the treatment of hypercyanotic spells in infants with tetralogy of Fallot. *J Cardiothorac Anesth* 3:200–202, 1989.

168. Odeh M: Tumor necrosis factor-alpha as a myocardial depressant substance. *Int J Cardiol* 42:231–238, 1993.

169. Opie LH, Kaplan N, Poole-Wilson PA: Angiotension-converting enzyme inhibitors and conventional vasodilators. In Opie LH (ed): *Drugs for the Heart*, 4th ed. Philadelphia: WB Saunders, 1995.

170. Oshita S, Uchimoto R, Oka H, et al: Correlation between arterial blood pressure and oxygenation in tetralogy of Fallot. *J Cardiothorac Anesth* 3:597–600, 1989.

171. Ostman-Smith I, Wettrell G, Riesenfeld T: A cohort study of childhood hypertrophic cardiomyopathy. *J Am Coll Cardiol* 34:1813–1822, 1999.

172. Packer M, Bristow MR, Cohn JN, et al: The effect of carvedilol on morbidity and mortality in patients with chronic heart failure. U.S. Carvedilol Heart Failure Study Group. *N Engl J Med* 334:1349–1355, 1996.

173. Palmer RF, Lasseter KC: Sodium nitroprusside. *N Engl J Med* 292:294–296, 1975.

174. Perkin RM, Levin DL, Webb R, et al: Dobutamine: A hemodynamic evaluation in children with shock. *J Pediatr* 100:977–983, 1982.

175. Perondi MB, Reis AG, Paiva EF, et al: A comparison of high-dose and standard-dose epinephrine in children with cardiac arrest. *N Engl J Med* 350:1722-1730, 2004.

176. Phoon CK, Wu ST, Parmley WW: Digoxin's minimal inotropic effect is not limited by sodium-calcium exchange in the intact immature rabbit heart. *J Cardiovasc Pharmacol Ther* 2:97–105, 1997.

177. Pfaffinger PJ, Martin JM, Hunter DD, et al: GTP-binding proteins couple cardiac muscarinic receptors to a K channel. *Nature* 317:536–538, 1985.

178. Podbregar M, Voga G, Horvat M, et al: Bolus versus continuous low dose of enalaprilat in congestive heart failure with acute refractory decompensation. *Cardiology* 91:41–49, 1999.

179. Porcelli RJ, Cutaia MV: Pulmonary vascular reactivity to biogenic amines during acute hypoxia. *Am J Physiol* 255:H329–H334, 1988.

180. Prins I, Plotz FB, Uiterwaal CS, van Vught HJ: Low-dose dopamine in neonatal and pediatric intensive care: A systemic review. *Intensive Care Med* 27:206–210, 2001.

181. Publication Committee for the VMAC Investigators (Vasodilation in the Management of Acute CHF): Intravenous niseritide vs. nitroglycerin in the treatment of the decompensated congestive heart failure: A randomized controlled trial. *JAMA* 287:1531–1540, 2002.

182. Ramamoorthy C, Anderson GD, Williams GD, Lynn AM: Pharmacokinetics and side effects of milrinone in infants and children after open heart surgery. *Anesth Analg* 86:283–289, 1998.

183. Reddy VM, Liddicoat JR, McElhinney DB, et al: Hemodynamic effects of epinephrine, bicarbonate and calcium in the early postnatal period in a lamb model of single-ventricle physiology created in utero. *J Am Coll Cardiol* 28:1877–1883, 1996.

184. Regan JW, Kobilka TS, Yang-Feng TL, et al: Cloning and expression of a human kidney cDNA for an alpha 2-adrenergic receptor subtype. *Proc Natl Acad Sci USA* 85:6301–6305, 1988.

185. Reves JG, Karp RB, Buttner EE, et al: Neuronal and adrenomedullary catecholamine release in response to cardiopulmonary bypass in man. *Circulation* 66:49–55, 1982.

186. Reyes G, Schwartz PH, Newth CJ, Eldadah MK: The pharmacokinetics of isoproterenol in critically ill pediatric patients. *J Clin Pharmacol* 33:29–34, 1993.

187. Rich MW, McSherry F, Williford WO, Yusuf S: Digitalis Investigation Group. Effect of age on mortality, hospitalizations and response to digoxin in patients with heart failure: The DIG study. *J Am Coll Cardiol* 38:806–813, 2001.

188. Roberts JD Jr, Fineman JR, Morin FC III, et al: Inhaled nitric oxide and persistent pulmonary hypertension of the newborn. The Inhaled Nitric Oxide Study Group. *N Engl J Med* 336:605–610, 1997.

189. Roberts JD, Lang P, Bigatello LM: Inhaled nitric oxide in congenital heart disease. *Circulation* 87:447–453, 1993.

190. Robinson BW, Gelband H, Mas MS: Selective pulmonary and systemic vasodilator effects of amrinone in children: New therapeutic implications. *J Am Coll Cardiol* 21:1461–1465, 1993.

191. Robishaw JD, Foster KA: Role of G proteins in the regulation of the cardiovascular system. *Annu Rev Physiol* 51:229–244, 1989.

192. Rosenzweig SB, Starc TJ, Chen JM: Intravenous arginine-vasopressin in children with vasodilatory shock after cardiac surgery. *Circulation* 100:182–186, 1999.

193. Ross MP, Allen-Webb EM, Pappas JB, McGough EC: Amrinone-associated thrombocytopenia: Pharmacokinetic analysis. *Clin Pharmacol Ther* 53:661–667, 1993.

194. Rouby JJ, Gory G, Bourrelli B, et al: Resistance to sodium nitroprusside in hypertensive patients. *Crit Care Med* 10:301–304, 1982.

195. Royster RL, Butterworth JF 4th, Prielipp RC, et al: A randomized, blinded, placebo-controlled evaluation of calcium chloride and epinephrine for inotropic support after emergence from cardiopulmonary bypass. *Anesth Analg* 74:3–13, 1992.

196. Roze JC, Tohier C, Maingueneau C, et al: Response to dobutamine and dopamine in the hypotensive very preterm infant. *Arch Dis Child* 69:59–63, 1993.

197. Rubin LJ: Primary pulmonary hypertension. *N Engl J Med* 336:111–117, 1997.

198. Rudinsky BF, Komar KJ, Strates E, Meadow WL: Neither nitroglycerin nor nitroprusside selectively reduces sepsis-induced pulmonary hypertension in piglets. *Crit Care Med* 15:1127–1130, 1987.

199. Ruffolo RR Jr, Spradlin TA, Pollock GD, et al: Alpha and beta adrenergic effects of the stereoisomers of dobutamine. *J Pharmacol Exp Ther* 219:447–455, 1981.

200. Ruffolo RR Jr: Distribution and function of peripheral alpha-adrenoceptors in the cardiovascular system. *Pharmacol Biochem Behav* 22:827–833, 1985.

201. Ruokonen E, Takala J, Kari A, et al: Regional blood flow and oxygen transport in septic shock. *Crit Care Med* 21:1296–1303, 1993.

202. Russell IA, Zwass MS, Fineman JR, et al: The effects of inhaled nitric oxide on postoperative pulmonary hypertension in infants and children undergoing surgical repair of congenital heart disease. *Anesth Analg* 87:46–51, 1998.

203. Sato Y, Matsuzawa H, Eguchi S: Comparative study of effects of adrenaline, dobutamine and dopamine on systemic hemodynamics and renal blood flow in patients following open heart surgery. *Jpn Circ J* 46:1059–1072, 1982.

204. Scammell AM, Arnold R, Wilkinson JL: Captopril in treatment of infant heart failure: A preliminary report. *Int J Cardiol* 16:295–301, 1987.

205. Schleien CL, Dean JM, Koehler RC, et al: Effect of epinephrine on cerebral and myocardial perfusion in an infant animal preparation of cardiopulmonary resuscitation. *Circulation* 73:809–817, 1986.

206. Schranz D, Droege A, Broede A, et al: Uncoupling of human cardiac beta-adrenoceptors during cardiopulmonary bypass with cardioplegic cardiac arrest. *Circulation* 87:422–426, 1993.

207. Schranz D, Zepp F, Iversen S, et al: Effects of tolazoline and prostacyclin on pulmonary hypertension in infants after cardiac surgery. *Crit Care Med* 20:1243–1249, 1992.

208. Schulze-Neick I, Bultmann M, Werner H, et al: Right ventricular function in patients treated with inhaled nitric oxide after cardiac surgery for congenital heart disease in newborns and children. *Am J Cardiol* 80:360–363, 1997.

209. Schwartz PH, Eldadah MK, Newth CJ: The pharmacokinetics of dobutamine in pediatric intensive care unit patients. *Drug Metab Dispos Biol Fate Chem* 19:614–619, 1991.

210. Schwinn DA, Lomasney JW, Lorenz W, et al: Molecular cloning and expression of the cDNA for a novel alpha 1-adrenergic receptor subtype. *J Biol Chem* 265:8183–8189, 1990.

211. Schwinn DA: Adrenoceptors as models for G protein-coupled receptors: Structure, function and regulation. *Br J Anaesth* 71:77–85, 1993.

212. Sealey WC: Paradoxical hypertension after repair of coarctation of the aorta: A review of its causes. *Ann Thorac Surg* 50:323–329, 1990.

213. Seri I: Cardiovascular, renal, and endocrine actions of dopamine in neonates and children. *J Pediatr* 126:333–344, 1995.

214. Shaddy RE, Curtin EL, Sower B, et al: The Pediatric Randomized Carvedilol Trial in Children with Heart Failure: Rationale and design. *Am Heart J* 144:383–389, 2002.

215. Shaddy RE, Teitel DF, Brett C: Short-term hemodynamic effects of captopril in infants with congestive heart failure. *Am J Dis Child* 142:100–105, 1988.

216. Shaddy RE, Viney J, Judd VE, McGough EC: Continuous intravenous phenylephrine infusion for treatment of hypoxemic spells in tetralogy of Fallot. *J Pediatr* 114:468–470, 1989.

217. Shaw NJ, Wilson N, Dickinson DF: Captopril in heart failure secondary to a left to right shunt. *Arch Dis Child* 63:360–363, 1988.

218. Shryock JC, Belardinelli L: Adenosine and adenosine receptors in the cardiovascular system: Biochemistry, physiology and pharmacology. *Am J Cardiol* 79:2–10, 1997.

219. Silver MA, Horton DP, Ghali JK, Elkayam U: Effect of nesiritide versus dobutamine on short-term outcomes in the treatment of patients with acutely decompensated heart failure. *J Am Coll Cardiol* 39:798–803, 2002.

220. Silverman HJ, Penaranda R, Orens JB, Lee NH: Impaired beta-adrenergic receptor stimulation of cyclic adenosine monophosphate in human septic shock: Association with myocardial hyporesponsiveness to catecholamines. *Crit Care Med* 21:31–39, 1993.

221. Siwy BK, Sadove AM: Acute management of dopamine infiltration injury with Regitine. *Plast Reconstr Surg* 80:610–612, 1987.

222. Smerling A, Gersony WM: Esmolol for severe hypertension following repair of aortic coarctation. *Crit Care Med* 18:1288–1290, 1990.

223. Steen PA, Tinker JH, Pluth JR, et al: Efficacy of dopamine, dobutamine and epinephrine during emergence from cardiopulmonary bypass in man. *Circulation* 57:378–384, 1977.

224. Stiell IG, Hebert PC, Weitzman BN, et al: High-dose epinephrine in adult cardiac arrest. *N Engl J Med* 327:1045–1050, 1992.

225. Stueven HA, Thompson B, Aprahamian C, et al: Lack of effectiveness of calcium chloride in refractory asystole. *Ann Emerg Med* 14:630–632, 1985.

226. Stueven HA, Thompson B, Aprahamian C, et al: The effectiveness of calcium chloride in refractory electromechanical dissociation. *Ann Emerg Med* 14:626–629, 1985.

227. Subhedar NV, Shaw NJ: Dopamine versus dobutamine for hypotensive preterm infants. *Cochrane Libr* 1:1–19, 2000.

228. Suzuki A, Yamagishi M, Kimura K, et al: Functional behavior and morphology of the coronary artery wall in pateints with Kawasaki disease assessed by intravascular ultrasound. *J Am Coll Cardiol* 27:291–296, 1996.

229. Takeuchi K, del Nido PJ, Ibrahim AE, et al: Vesnarinone and amrinone reduce the systemic inflammatory response syndrome. *J Thorac Cardiovasc Surg* 117:375–382, 1999.

230. The Neonatal Inhaled Nitric Oxide Study Group: Inhaled nitric oxide in full-term and nearly full-term infants with hypoxic respiratory failure. *N Engl J Med* 336:597–604, 1997.

231. Thomas JA, Marks BH: Plasma norepinephrine in congestive heart failure. *Am J Cardiol* 41:233–243, 1978.

232. Tinker JH, Michenfelder JD: Sodium nitroprusside: Pharmacology, toxicology and therapeutics. *Anesthesiology* 45:340–354, 1976.

233. Turanlahti MI, Laitinen PO, Sarna SJ, Pesonen E: Nitric oxide, oxygen, and prostacyclin in children with pulmonary hypertension. *Heart* 79:169–174, 1998.

234. Vane JR, Botting RM: Pharmacodynamic profile of prostacyclin. *Am J Cardiol* 75:3A–10A, 1995.

235. Vincent RN, Click LA, Williams HM, et al: Esmolol as an adjunct in the treatment of systemic hypertension after operative repair of coarctation of the aorta. *Am J Cardiol* 65:941–943, 1990.

236. Ward A, Brogden RN, Heel RC, et al: Amrinone. A preliminary review of its pharmacological properties and therapeutic use. *Drugs* 26:468–502, 1983.

237. Ward KE, Pryor RW, Matson JR, et al: Delayed detection of coarctation in infancy: Implications for timing of newborn follow-up. *Pediatrics* 86:972–976, 1990.

238. Weesner KM: Hemodynamic effects of prostaglandin E1 in patients with congenital heart disease and pulmonary hypertension. *Cathet Cardiovasc Diagn* 24:10–15, 1991.

239. Wei EP, Moskowitz MA, Boccalini P, Kontos HA: Calcitonin gene-related peptide mediates nitroglycerin and sodium nitroprusside–induced vasodilation in feline cerebral arterioles. *Circ Res* 70:1313–1319, 1992.

240. Wessel DL, Adatia I, Giglia TM, et al: Use of inhaled nitric oxide and acetylcholine in the evaluation of pulmonary hypertension and endothelial function after cardiopulmonary bypass. *Circulation* 88:2128–2138, 1993.

241. Wessel DL, Adatia I, Thompson JE, Hickey PR: Delivery and monitoring of inhaled nitric oxide in patients with pulmonary hypertension. *Crit Care Med* 22:930–938, 1994.

242. Wessel DL: Inhaled nitric oxide for the treatment of pulmonary hypertension before and after cardiopulmonary bypass. *Crit Care Med* 21:S344–345, 1993.

243. Wessel DL, Adatia I, Van Marter LJ, et al: Improved oxygenation in a randomized trial of inhaled nitric oxide for persistent pulmonary hypertension of the newborn. *Pediatrics* 100:E7, 1997.

244. Wessel DL, Triedman JK, Wernovsky G, et al: Pulmonary and systemic hemodynamics of amrinone in neonates following cardiopulmonary bypass. *Circulation* 80:II488, 1989.

245. Wiest DB, Garner SS, Uber WE, Sade RM: Esmolol for management of pediatric hypertension after cardiac operations. *J Thorac Cardiovasc Surg* 115:890–897, 1998.

246. Wiest DB, Trippel DL, Gillette PC, Garner SS: Pharmacokinetics of esmolol in children. *Clin Pharmacol Ther* 49:618–623, 1991.

247. Williams DB, Kiernan PD, Schaff HV, et al: The hemodynamic response to dopamine and nitroprusside following right atrium–pulmonary artery bypass (Fontan procedure). *Ann Thorac Surg* 34:51–57, 1982.

248. Wong AF, McCulloch LM, Sola A: Treatment of peripheral tissue ischemia with topical nitroglycerin ointment in neonates. *J Pediatr* 121:980–983, 1992.

249. Yaster M, Simmons RS, Tolo VT, et al: A comparison of nitroglycerin and nitroprusside for inducing hypotension in children: A double-blind study. *Anesthesiology* 65:175–179, 1986.

250. Yusuf S, Theodoropoulos S, Mathias CJ, et al: Increased sensitivity of the denervated transplanted human heart to isoprenaline both before and after beta-adrenergic blockade. *Circulation* 75:696–704, 1987.

251. Zaritsky A, Lotze A, Stull R, Goldstein DS: Steady-state dopamine clearance in critically ill infants and children. *Crit Care Med* 16:217–220, 1988.

252. Zayek M, Wild L, Roberts JD, Morin FC 3rd: Effect of nitric oxide on the survival rate and incidence of lung injury in newborn lambs with persistent pulmonary hypertension. *J Pediatr* 123:947–952, 1993.

253. Zhang J, Penny DJ, Kim NS, et al: Mechanisms of blood pressure increase induced by dopamine in hypotensive preterm neonates. *Arch Dis Child Fetal Neonatal Ed* 81:F99–F104, 1999.

254. Zhao M, Muntz KH: Differential downregulation of beta-2 adrenergic receptors in tissue compartments of rat heart is not altered by sympathetic denervation. *Circ Res* 73:393–400, 1993.

PART TWO

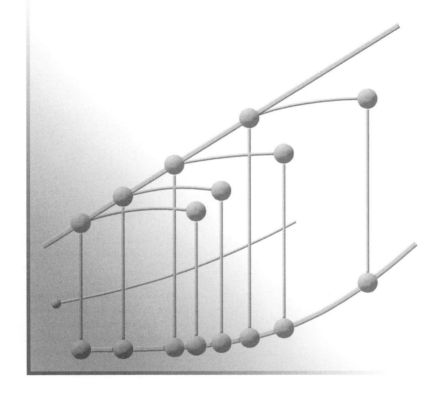

Special Problems

Chapter 8

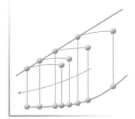

Pediatric Arrhythmias

RONALD J. KANTER, MD, MICHAEL P. CARBONI, MD,
and MICHAEL J. SILKA, MD

INTRODUCTION

Advances in treatment options combined with an improved understanding of the causes and mechanisms of cardiac arrhythmias now provide the means for improved care of young patients with disorders of the cardiac rhythm. The aims of this chapter are (1) to describe the physiology of the normal cardiac rhythm; (2) to describe the pathophysiology underlying abnormal heart rhythms; (3) to discuss the etiology and mechanisms of a variety of specific pediatric arrhythmias; (4) to examine the various pathologic states that generate the arrhythmogenic substrate for arrhythmias in children; and (5) to outline the pharmacologic, catheter-based, and device therapies now available to treat these disorders in children.

THE NORMAL CARDIAC RHYTHM AND ELECTROCARDIOGRAM

The normal cardiac rhythm is initiated by cells within the sinoatrial (SA) node, a crescent-shaped collection of cells situated in the lateral terminal groove of the right atrium at its junction with the superior vena cava. Sinus nodal cells depolarize spontaneously and trigger a wave of depolarization that spreads throughout both atria. Atrial electrical activation is manifest on the surface electrocardiographic (ECG) recording as the P wave. The morphology of the P wave is influenced by the site of origin of the activating stimulus, the size of the atria, and the rate of conduction of the electrical impulses throughout the atria. Although specialized conducting tracts or fibers from the SA node to the atrioventricular (AV) node have been reported and named (e.g., Bachmann, Wenckebach, Thorel internodal tracts), the histologic evidence for such tracts continues to be debated.[48]

The AV node is located in the medial right atrium within the muscular atrioventricular septum. Conduction through the AV node is slow, thus providing a significant delay between activation of the atria and the ventricles. This delay allows time for atrial contraction to contribute to the diastolic filling of the ventricles, thus providing AV synchrony. The atria and ventricles are otherwise electrically insulated from one another by fibro-fatty tissue planes, except at the site where the AV bundle (of His) penetrates the membranous septum. Within the ventricular septum, the His bundle divides into left and right bundle branches. The right bundle branch runs in the deep subendocardium of the interventricular septum until it emerges in the moderator band. The left bundle branch fans out broadly shortly after emerging on the left ventricular endocardial surface. The concept of discrete anterior and posterior fascicles is no longer considered accurate.

These large conduction fibers remain insulated from surrounding myocardium by sheaths of fibrous tissue until they have further divided into the Purkinje network of smaller fibers that conducts the wave of depolarization throughout the ventricular myocardium. Depolarization of the ventricles produces the QRS complex on the surface ECG. QRS morphology is influenced by the origin of the ventricular activation, the presence of conduction block or delay in the bundle branches, and the rate of electrical conduction within the ventricles. Repolarization of the ventricular myocardium is reflected by the ST segment and T wave. In summary, the PR, QRS, and QT intervals on the surface ECG provide measures of the rates of cardiac conduction and repolarization. The normal ranges of these intervals change with age as shown in Table 8-1.[15]

During normal sinus rhythm, the cells within the sinus node tissue spontaneously depolarize (a slowly rising membrane potential during phase 4) until they reach activation threshold (phase 0), at which time an action potential is generated, which initiates a cardiac beat (Fig. 8-1). Certain other cardiac tissues also spontaneously depolarize, albeit at a rate slower than that of the sinus node. Therefore, if the sinus node fails or slows markedly, other sites along the conduction path spontaneously depolarize and can initiate cardiac depolarization until the sinus rate resumes. The resultant rhythm is considered an "escape" beat or rhythm. The most common escape rhythm is an AV nodal (or junctional) escape rhythm. This may be a normal phenomenon, especially during sleep or in persons with high vagal tone. If the rate of depolarization of the conduction tissue below the sinus node becomes faster than the sinus rate, this may give rise to an accelerated escape rhythm. Escape rhythms that arise in the ventricles (idioventricular) are typically quite slow and erratic.

MECHANISMS OF ARRHYTHMIAS

The mechanisms most often responsible for cardiac arrhythmias are (1) failure of impulse formation, (2) conduction block, (3) reentrant excitation, (4) enhanced automaticity, and

Table 8-1 Normal Electrocardiographic Intervals in Children (defined as the 2nd through 98th percentile values)

Age	PR (msec, in lead II)	QRS (msec, in lead V₅)*	QT (msec, in lead V₅)
0–1 d	79–161	21–76	210–370
1–3 d	81–139	22–67	223–346
3–7 d	74–135	21–68	220–327
7–30 d	72–138	22–79	220–301
1–3 mo	72–130	23–75	222–317
3–6 mo	73–146	22–79	221–305
6–12 mo	73–157	25–76	218–324
1–3 yr	82–148	27–76	248–335
3–5 yr	84–161	31–72	264–354
5–8 yr	90–163	32–79	278–374
8–12 yr	87–171	32–85	281–390
12–16 yr	92–175	34–88	292–390

*The QRS duration was measured only in lead V₅ because the onset of the QRS is most sharply defined there. This measurement in a single lead underestimates the full QRS duration because in some cases the beginning or end of the QRS in lead V₅ may not deviate from the baseline and will not be detected.

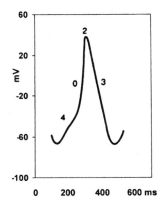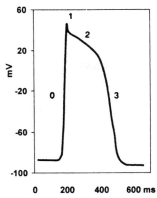

FIGURE 8-1 Cardiac action potentials from a sinus node cell (*left*) and a ventricular myocyte (*right*). The phases of the action potential are numbered. During phase 0, there is rapid depolarization, mediated by inward calcium flux in sinus node cells and the opening of sodium channels in myocytes. The early rapid repolarization (phase 1) seen in ventricular cells is the result of sodium channel inactivation and a transient outward potassium current. The plateau (phase 2) results from the balance of currents that depolarize the cell membrane, such as the inward calcium current, and currents that repolarize the membrane, principally outward potassium currents. The membrane repolarizes (phase 3) as potassium currents increase and drive the potential more negative. Unique to cells with automaticity such as the sinus node is a steady diastolic depolarization during phase 4. Once this depolarization reaches a threshold level, inward calcium currents are activated and phase 0 is initiated.

(5) triggered activity.[50] Reentry and block are abnormalities of impulse conduction; failure of impulse formation, enhanced automaticity, and triggered arrhythmias are abnormalities of impulse generation. One or more of these mechanisms underlie the specific cardiac arrhythmias.

Failure of impulse formation occurs when normal pacemaking tissue (i.e., the sinoatrial node) does not reach activation threshold at a rate commensurate with physiologic requirements. This may occur during moments of extreme vagotonia, such as when a newborn receives nasopharyngeal stimulation, or may occur as part of "sick sinus syndrome" chronically following atrial surgery.

Conduction block refers to the failure of an electrical impulse to travel its normal pathway to completely depolarize the atria and ventricles. Conduction block may be physiologic, as in atrial flutter or fibrillation where only a fraction of the atrial impulses conduct through the AV node or in the setting of augmented vagal tone that transiently produces AV block. A premature impulse may also fail to conduct at some level because adjacent tissue remains refractory to depolarization from the previous impulse. Conduction block may result from pathology such as ischemia, postoperative edema, infarction, or fibrosis and interrupt conduction at the level of sinoatrial or AV node, His bundle, or bundle branches. It may also be congenital as in congenital complete AV block.

Reentrant excitation is the most common cause of tachyarrhythmias. This is a mechanism for the self-propagation of a wavefront that repetitively travels the same conduction circuit. The conditions necessary to initiate and sustain reentrant arrhythmias include unidirectional block in one limb of the path (e.g., long refractory period at the site of block), sufficiently slow conduction around the other limb of the circuit such that the site of unidirectional block is recovered from refractoriness when the impulse returns, and capacity for retrograde conduction through the area of original

block (Fig. 8-2). The path may encircle inexcitable tissue such as surgical injury or scar from previous myocardial infarction or tissue fibrosis, or it may include normally excitable tissues with discrepant conduction properties such as occurs in AV nodal reentry or accessory pathway mediated tachycardias. In most cases, reentrant arrhythmias are readily inducible and terminable by programmed electrical stimulation with premature extra stimuli or rapid pacing.

Automaticity is a normal property of several different types of cardiac cells and consists of a gradual depolarization of resting membrane potential during diastole (phase 4) (see Fig. 8-1). Once activation threshold is attained, the rate of depolarization increases steeply (phase 0) and a full action potential ensues. Cells capable of automaticity include those in the sinus node, specialized regions of the atria, the atrioventricular node, and

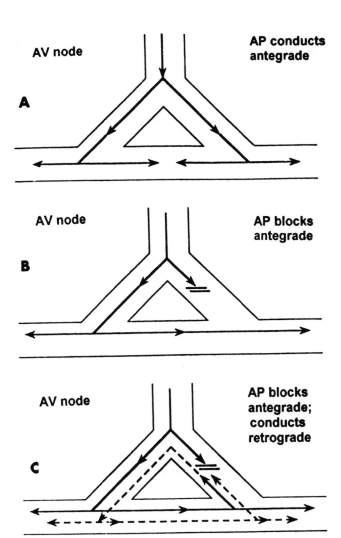

FIGURE 8-2 Mechanism of reentry arrhythmias. **(A)** Reentry requires two conduction pathways that may be anatomically or physiologically distinct, such as an AV node and an accessory pathway (AP). **(B)** Conduction block may occur in one pathway, such as an accessory pathway, with slow conduction over the other pathway, the AV node. **(C)** If this slowly conducted impulse travels retrograde over the previously blocked pathway, it will reenter the circuit and then initiate a regular tachycardia by repetitively circling the path. As an example of accessory pathway mediated tachycardia, the circuit would be antegrade unidirectional block in the accessory pathway with slow antegrade conduction over the AV node to the ventricle and return to the atrium due to retrograde conduction over the accessory pathway.

the His-Purkinje system. The cells with the most rapid diastolic depolarization, usually in the SA node, determine the heart rate. Abnormal automaticity may develop in cells that are not normally automatic, such as atrial and ventricular myocytes. Conditions that increase the likelihood of enhanced abnormal automaticity include ischemia, electrolyte imbalances, catecholamine excess, and certain drug toxicities. An abnormal automatic rhythm often exhibits a gradual increase in rate, or "warm-up," before becoming a regular tachycardia and a gradual deceleration before termination.[18]

Automatic rhythms can usually be transiently interrupted ("overdrive suppressed") by overdrive pacing or programmed extrastimuli, but they cannot be reliably initiated or terminated by these methods.

Triggered activity develops in the setting of low amplitude secondary depolarizations (afterdepolarizations) of the membrane potential during (phase 3) or after (phase 4) normal repolarization. If an afterdepolarization reaches the activation threshold potential, another action potential is triggered that is coupled closely to the first. If this second action potential is accompanied by another afterdepolarization, the process can be repetitive and give rise to a sustained arrhythmia. Early afterdepolarizations (EADs) are present during repolarization (phase 3) and arise as a result of enhanced calcium or sodium entry through sarcolemmal ion channels.[56,70] Conditions associated with EADs are often present in postoperative patients and include acidosis, hypoxia, hypokalemia, and a variety of antiarrhythmic agents. The development of sustained EAD-triggered ventricular arrhythmias is bradycardia dependent, with an increased frequency of EADs observed at slow rates or following pauses in the cardiac rhythm. Delayed afterdepolarizations (DADs) develop after the membrane potential has fully repolarized (phase 4) and are caused by intracellular calcium overload and a subsequent oscillatory uptake and release of calcium from the sarcoplasmic reticulum.[56] The prototypic arrhythmia associated with DADs is digitalis intoxication. Delayed afterdepolarization–triggered ventricular arrhythmias may also be associated with catecholamine excess and can be initiated by rapid pacing.

PEDIATRIC CLINICAL ARRHYTHMIAS

Using the mechanistic approach described previously, most cardiac arrhythmias in children are listed in Table 8-2. This categorization allows for a more rational approach to the selection of pharmacologic or interventional therapies. The following section will provide a general overview of specific rhythm abnormalities in children.

Bradyarrhythmias

Sinus Bradycardia

A lower limit of the normal heart rate has not been rigorously established for children. Estimates have been made from surveys in normal children using Holter monitoring and standard surface ECGs. The surface ECG estimates have tended to be higher than the Holter estimates in infants and young children, possibly due to anxiety associated with the placement of the ECG leads just before ECG recording. A guideline for the diagnosis of sinus bradycardia is shown in Table 8-3.

Table 8-2   Arrhythmia Types According to Mechanism

Bradycardias	Failure of impulse formation
	Sinus bradycardia
	Sinus node arrest
	Conduction block
	Sinus node exit block
	AV node block
	Bundle branch block
Tachycardias	Reentry
	Atrial flutter (macroreentry)
	Atrial fibrillation
	Sinus node reentry tachycardia
	AV node reentry tachycardia
	AV reciprocating tachycardia (including permanent form of junctional reciprocating tachycardia)
	Most ventricular tachycardia (including torsade de pointes?)
	Enhanced automaticity
	Some atrial ectopic tachycardias
	Junctional ectopic tachycardia
	Accelerated junctional rhythm
	Accelerated idioventricular rhythm
	Some ventricular tachycardias
	Triggered activity
	Some atrial ectopic tachycardias
	Digitalis toxicity
	Initiating beat of torsade de pointes?
	Some ventricular tachycardias
	Other mechanisms causing premature beats
	Supernormal conduction
	Parasystole

AV, atrioventricular.

Note that this guideline does not apply to children with fever or cardiac dysfunction or in the postoperative state, situations in which the "normal" heart rate is expected to be considerably higher. Thus, these relatively "normal" heart rates may be too slow and result in hypoperfusion or hypotension. In addition to a slow heart rate, the diagnosis of *sinus* bradycardia implies that the rhythm is regular and that the P wave originates in the sinus node. A "sinus" P wave is upright in leads I, II, and aVF, as the wave of depolarization spreads from high to low and from right to left in the atria. Furthermore, the P wave morphology should match that seen in a previous ECG, if available, when sinus rhythm was clearly present. Sinus bradycardia may occur in the intensive care unit (ICU) setting during airway suctioning, elevated intracranial pressure, hypoxia, hypoglycemia, hypercalcemia, and acidosis. Drugs in therapeutic or toxic doses (e.g., digoxin, beta-blockers, amiodarone) may also cause sinus bradycardia. Surgical injury or trauma to the sinus node may also result in persistent sinus bradycardia.

Table 8-3   Sinus Bradycardia in Children

Age	Rate (bpm)
Infants and children to 2 yr of age	<90
Children age 2–6 yr	<80
Children age 6–11 yr	<70
Children older than 11 yr	<60

bpm, beats per minute.

Sinus Arrest

Sinus arrest results from failure of impulse generation in the sinus node. It is manifested as a pause in the rhythm for a duration that is not a multiple of the sinus cycle length. If sinus arrest is prolonged, another automatic focus in the atria, AV node, or ventricles may become active and generate an escape rhythm that continues until sinus node function recovers. Pauses greater than 3 seconds warrant careful assessment and in some cases are an indication for permanent pacemaker implantation.[45]

Sinus Node Exit Block

High-grade sinus node exit block is diagnosed when the sinus node is discharging regularly but not all the impulses produce atrial depolarization. In second-degree type I (Wenckebach) SA block, the P-P intervals shorten on successive beats until exit block occurs and the P wave is absent (i.e., a "dropped" P wave). This occurs because the percent slowing of sinoatrial conduction tends to decrease during successive beats (i.e., the electrographically invisible "sinus discharge"-to-P wave interval increases proportionately less from beat to beat). The pause in the series of P waves is less than twice the duration of the P-P interval just before the pause. Frequently, second-degree type I SA block demonstrates a recurring pattern of groups of beats separated by pauses ("grouped beating"). In second-degree type II SA block, a pause in apparent sinus activity is present with a duration that is twice the sinus cycle length; the preceding P-P intervals do not vary. With second-degree SA exit block, a single P wave is usually absent, whereas with sinus arrest, the pauses are irregular and last up to several seconds. Higher grades of SA block are difficult to distinguish from sinus arrest unless the pause duration is an exact multiple of the sinus cycle length. Both exit block and sinus arrest are frequently seen following atrial surgeries such as the Mustard or hemi-Fontan procedures but may occasionally be seen in normal persons as a result of enhanced vagal tone.[13]

Atrioventricular Block

Atrioventricular block may be congenital, related to changes in autonomic tone, or develop in association with a number of disease states, as listed in Table 8-4. First-degree AV block is present when the PR interval is longer than the age-specific norm (see Table 8-1). As an isolated finding, first-degree AV block is benign and warrants no specific treatment or follow-up. When part of an evolving disease state or if there is associated bundle branch block, attention should be paid to the possible development of more advanced AV block.

Second-degree AV block is present when an atrial depolarization intermittently is not conducted to the ventricles resulting in the appearance of a "dropped beat." Mobitz type I second-degree AV block (Wenckebach AV conduction) exhibits a gradual prolongation of the PR interval before the nonconducted P wave (Fig. 8-3A). The pause that develops between QRS complexes is equal to or less than twice the interval between QRS complexes before block occurred. This type of AV block usually occurs within the AV node. If this rhythm occurs during sleep, it is usually benign and is due to enhanced parasympathetic tone. However, if it occurs during wakeful activities it may cause symptoms. In young children,

Table 8-4 Causes of Atrioventricular Block

Increased parasympathetic (vagal) tone	Airway suctioning Intubation Pain Bowel distention Vasovagal syncope
Metabolic disorders	Hypokalemia Hyperkalemia Hypomagnesemia Hypocalcemia Hypercalcemia Hypoglycemia
Associated with congenital heart disease	Heterotaxies, especially "polysplenia" Congenitally corrected transposition of the great arteries Persistent left SVC with absent right SVC
Postcardiac surgery	VSD, especially in congenitally corrected transposition AV canal Others, much more rarely
Congenital complete atrioventricular block	
Hypothermia	
Infectious diseases	Rubella Mumps Lyme disease Rocky Mountain spotted fever Chagas disease (Trypanosomiasis) Rheumatic fever Diphtheria Enteroviral myocarditis Perivalvular abscess
Myopathies	Myotonic dystrophy Duchenne's muscular dystrophy Polymyositis Kearns-Sayre syndrome
Medications	β-blockers Calcium channel blockers Digoxin Amiodarone Sotalol

AV, atrioventricular; SVC, superior vena cava; VSD, ventricular septal defect.

Wenckebach AV conduction has been reported to progress to more advanced degrees of AV block.[117]

Mobitz type II second-degree AV block is characterized by a constant PR interval over the several beats prior to a nonconducted P wave. Typically the block develops below the AV node in the His bundle (Fig. 8-3B). This rhythm most often develops in children with structural heart disease or following cardiac surgery but occasionally may present in structurally normal hearts with advanced conduction system disease. QRS prolongation or even frank bundle branch block may coexist. Unlike Mobitz I block, Mobitz II frequently progresses to complete heart block, and therefore it is critical to distinguish between these two conditions. Differentiating type I from type II Mobitz block when there is 2:1 AV block is not possible since changes in the PR interval cannot be assessed. In patients with a widened QRS, syncope, or structural heart disease, type II block should be highly suspected. Patients who have recurrent or persistent Mobitz II AV block and a low ventricular escape rate for longer than 7 days postoperatively require permanent pacemaker implantation.[45]

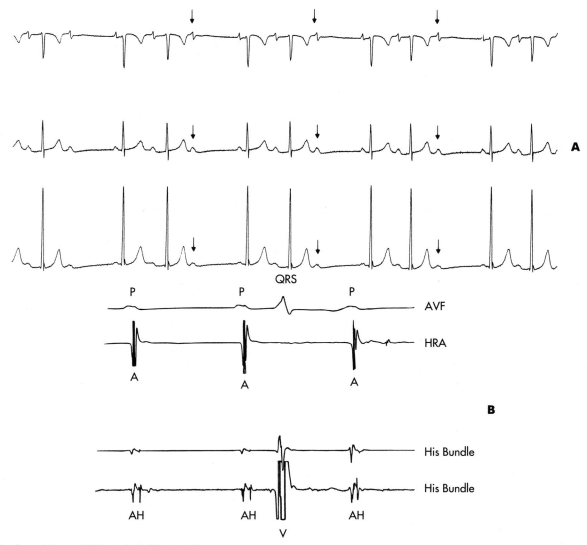

FIGURE 8-3 Second-degree AV block. **A,** Mobitz I AV block is manifested by a gradual prolongation of the P-R interval until an atrial beat is not conducted (arrow) to the ventricles. **B,** Infranodal second-degree AV block demonstrated by intracardiac electrogram recordings (paper speed 100 mm/sec). The top tracing is surface lead aVF. The middle tracing is an intracardiac electrogram from a catheter placed in the high right atrium (HRA) that shows regular atrial activity. The bottom two tracings are recorded from a catheter placed across the tricuspid valve in the region of the His bundle. This catheter shows atrial activation (A), the His bundle potential (H) but no ventricular activation (V) for the first and third beats. The second beat demonstrates normal AV conduction although the H-V interval is prolonged.

Third-degree or complete heart block (CHB) may be congenital or acquired and indicates that no atrial impulses are conducted to the ventricles (Fig. 8-4). The ventricular rate is maintained solely by escape pacemakers below the site of block in the AV node, His bundle, or fascicles. Congenital heart block is present in approximately 1 of every 20,000 live births.[77] One fourth to one half of cases are associated with structural heart disease, especially L-transposition of the great arteries and abnormalities of atrial and ventricular septum formation. In most patients without structural heart disease, there is an association with maternal anti-Ro (SS-A) or anti-La (SS-B) autoantibodies.[83,90] Presumably, these immunoglobin cross the placenta and mediate a cytotoxic immunological response within the AV node or His bundle. The precise mechanism has not been conclusively demonstrated. Acquired CHB most commonly develops as a complication of the surgical correction of congenital heart disease, especially in patients who require surgery near the AV node, such as ventricular septal defect (VSD) repair, AV canal repair, or tetralogy of Fallot. Postoperative CHB that persists for longer than 7 to 10 days following surgery generally will be persistent and is an absolute indication for permanent pacemaker implantation.[45,123]

The management of CHB is guided by the age of the patient, the degree of symptoms and whether it is acquired or congenital. The acute treatment of symptomatic CHB involves the use of chronotropic agents such as isoproterenol or atropine. *If medical therapy is not effective or insufficient, some form of temporary pacing should be initiated until permanent pacemaker implantation can be performed.* Patients with congenital CHB and a structurally normal heart may be completely asymptomatic, especially if their escape pacemaker has a relatively normal rate and increases with exercise.

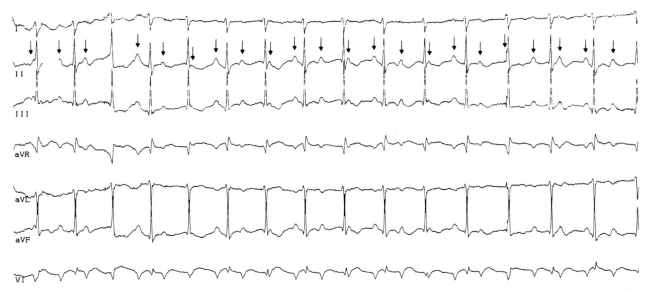

FIGURE 8-4 Complete heart block with atrioventricular dissociation. The atrial rate is 150/minute, indicated by arrows, which mark the P waves. The ventricular rate (88/minute) is completely regular and unrelated to the atrial rhythm.

However, if the escape rate is low and/or does not respond to increased sympathetic tone, patients may develop fatigue, exercise intolerance, syncope, or congestive heart failure. Newborns and infants with CHB and a ventricular rate less than 55 beats per minute should undergo pacemaker implantation regardless of symptoms because of an increased risk of sudden death.[77] In an older asymptomatic child with congenital CHB, pacemaker implantation should be considered if the average daytime heart rate is less than 40 beats per minute, if significant ventricular ectopy exists at rest or during exercise testing or if left ventricular dysfunction is present. Natural history studies have recently suggested that all patients with CHB should be considered for permanent pacing during the second or third decade of life, regardless of the absence of symptoms.[78] In contrast to congenital CHB, escape rhythms are erratic and unreliable when CHB is acquired. For this reason, the cardiac rhythm must be supported by permanent pacemaker implantation even if the patient is asymptomatic. In the acute postoperative setting, temporary pacing is used until the AV conduction returns or a permanent pacing system is implanted.

Tachyarrhythmias

Supraventricular Tachycardias

Sinus Tachycardia Sinus tachycardia is a regular non-reentrant tachycardia with sinus P waves. As with sinus bradycardia, the definition of sinus tachycardia has not been clearly established in children. Table 8-5 presents age-specific ranges of "normal" heart rates. In infants and children, sinus tachycardia generally does not exceed 230 beats per minute. Sinus tachycardia may indicate fever, hypovolemia, hypoxia, pain, hypercarbia, or myocardial failure. An unusual pathologic form of sinus tachycardia known as *inappropriate sinus tachycardia* may occur in teenage females. Also, sinus tachycardia may be present in a group of disorders collectively known as *postural orthostatic tachycardia syndrome*.

Sinus Node Reentrant Tachycardia Sinus node reentrant tachycardia resembles sinus tachycardia in that it is regular and has sinus morphology P waves. However, it is distinguished from sinus tachycardia by an abrupt initiation and termination compared with the gradual acceleration and deceleration of the heart rate in sinus tachycardia. Sinus node reentrant tachycardia, as its name implies, is mediated by a reentry circuit located within the region of the sinus node. An atrial reentrant tachyarrhythmia arising in the upper right atrium would have a similar P wave morphology. This is an uncommon arrhythmia in children, most commonly occurring after atrial surgery.

Atrial Flutter Atrial flutter is a rapid, regular atrial tachycardia with atrial rates ranging from 200 to 500 beats per minute in children. It is a macroreentry tachyarrhythmia frequently related to surgical incision or lines of conduction block following surgery for congenital heart disease. Less than 10% of

Table 8-5 Age-Specific Range of Normal Heart Rates in Children (defined as the 2nd through 98th percentile values)

Age	Heart Rate (bpm)
0–1 d	94–155
1–3 d	92–158
3–7 d	90–166
7–30 d	107–182
1–3 mo	120–179
3–6 mo	106–186
6–12 mo	108–168
1–3 yr	90–152
3–5 yr	73–137
5–8 yr	64–133
8–12 yr	63–130
12–16 yr	61–120

bpm, beats per minute.
From Davignon A, Rautaharju P, Boisselle E, et al: Normal ECG standards for infants and children. *Pediatr Cardiol* 1:123–152, 1979.

children with atrial flutter have a structurally normal heart.[34] Most have repaired or unoperated congenital heart disease or a cardiomyopathy.[54] In contrast to adults, in whom there are well-defined "p" waves, atrial flutter in children often has indistinct "f" waves or an isoelectric appearing baseline between QRS complexes (Fig. 8-5). Thus, it is important to consider a diagnosis of atrial flutter in the presence of an unexplained tachycardia without distinct P waves, particularly when occurring in a patient with congenital heart disease.

Different types of atrial flutter have been characterized based on f wave morphology and anatomic substrate.[107] Type I atrial flutter has a negative sawtooth pattern and type II a positive sawtooth pattern in lead II. Electrophysiologic mapping studies have demonstrated that the slow zone of conduction of the reentry circuit in both types of atrial flutter in adults passes between the tricuspid valve annulus and the ostium of the inferior vena cava.[27] The current nomenclature identifies these atrial flutters as *typical*, either counterclockwise atrial flutter (type I) or clockwise (type II). A similar circuit may rarely exist in children, as well. However, in the setting of structural or surgical heart disease involving the atria, critical isthmuses of slow conduction are often related to surgical incisions and adjacent areas of myocardium.[55] These types of atrial flutter are now called *intraatrial reentry tachycardia* or *incisional atrial tachycardia*. Catheter ablation has been of modest efficacy in the treatment of this arrhythmia.

Atrial Fibrillation Atrial fibrillation is a rapid, irregularly irregular rhythm with atrial rates ranging from 350 to 600 beats per minute. This rhythm appears to be mediated by multiple microreentry circuits scattered throughout the atria.[107] It may be paroxysmal or persistent. The ventricular response is irregular and is significantly slower than the atrial rate, due to slowed conduction through the AV node. In children, atrial fibrillation is much less common than atrial flutter. However, atrial fibrillation is an increasingly common problem in teenagers and adults with congenital heart disease, both for unoperated and postoperative patients. In the absence of congenital heart disease in older children and teenagers, atrial fibrillation may occur as a result of sudden hypervagotonia, in association with Wolff-Parkinson-White syndrome, or, rarely, as an isolated, familial disorder.

Atrial Ectopic Tachycardias Atrial ectopic tachycardias are recognized as regular narrow–QRS complex tachycardias with a P wave morphology that is different from the sinus P wave. As in sinus tachycardia, the P wave is usually temporally nearer to the succeeding (not the preceding) QRS, making this a *long R-P tachycardia*. The majority of cases are due to abnormal automaticity at a site within the atria different from the sinus node (ectopic).[10,44] Diagnosis of this arrhythmia is important, because chronic atrial tachycardia at rates greater than 125 beats per minute may lead to left ventricular dysfunction, so-called tachycardia-induced cardiomyopathy. Although some atrial tachycardias may resolve spontaneously, the majority of patients require therapy, especially if a cardiomyopathy has resulted.[76] Complete pharmacologic suppression with beta-blockers, digoxin, or type IA antiarrhythmic agents is frequently ineffective, prompting the use of type IC or III agents.[67] Cardioversion and atrial overdrive

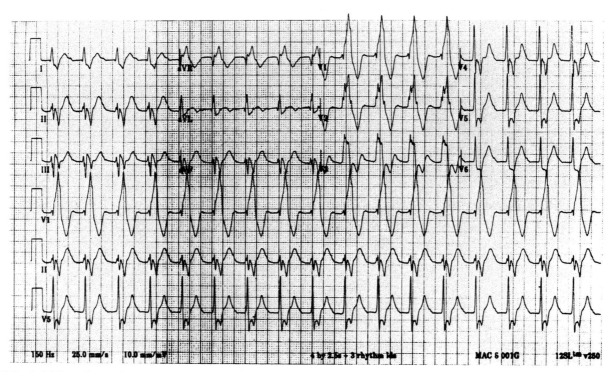

FIGURE 8-5 Atrial flutter in a patient with congenital heart disease. The presence of an unexplained tachycardia with no visible P waves is a common presentation of atrial flutter in these patients. The atrial rate is 204/minute with 2:1 AV block.

pacing will not terminate these tachycardias if the mechanism is enhanced automaticity or triggered. Radiofrequency catheter ablation has been demonstrated to be a safe and effective alternative.[121] Surgical ablation remains an option for children with refractory arrhythmias or multiple ectopic foci.[36]

Junctional Ectopic Tachycardia Junctional ectopic tachycardia (JET) is an uncommon tachycardia that results from abnormal automaticity within the AV node or His bundle regions[85,118] and therefore will not respond to cardioversion. The rate of JET is usually between 110 and 250 beats per minute, although rates as high as 370 have been reported. JET occurs in a rare congenital form in children younger than 6 months of age or more commonly following surgery for congenital heart disease (e.g., VSD, AVSD, Fontan operation, and tetralogy of Fallot). This rhythm is usually incessant and characterized by a narrow QRS complex, often with AV dissociation (Fig. 8-6). The onset (warm-up) and termination are gradual. The associated symptoms are dependent on the rate and duration of the tachycardia. JET is a serious postoperative rhythm disturbance and at times is associated with impaired hemodynamic performance and poor outcome following cardiac surgery. Because postoperative JET is often unresponsive to medical therapy, initial treatment should include reduction of adrenergic drugs, normalization of blood electrolyte concentrations, and atrial pacing at rates slightly faster than the JET rate (if possible) to restore AV synchrony and optimize cardiac output.[5] Medical therapy is often only successful in modest

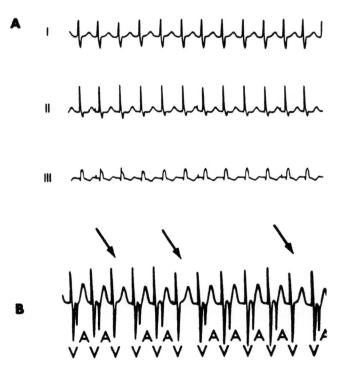

FIGURE 8-6 Junctional ectopic tachycardia (JET). **A,** ECG leads I, II, and III obtained 2 days following closure of an atrial and ventricular septal defect. The ventricular rate is 180/minute, with no apparent P waves. This ECG in the postoperative patient suggests JET. **B,** Combined surface ECG and atrial electrogram recording during tachycardia. The V-A relationship is irregular, with intermittent V-A block (arrows). This confirms the origin of the tachycardia as below the common AV node and that the atrium is not an essential component to sustain the tachycardia.

slowing of the rate but initial therapy with digoxin with or without a beta-blocker has been attempted. Failing this, procainamide, propafenone, flecainide, and amiodarone have all been shown to be variously effective to reduce the rate of tachycardia or restore sinus rhythm, although prohibitive hypotension may result from any of these drugs. Amiodarone appears to be most efficacious.[27] Different congenital heart surgery centers also use surface cooling (33° C to 35° C) and paralysis to slow the junctional rate and allow atrial overdrive pacing. The role of this intervention in the treatment algorithm for postoperative JET varies among centers. Surgical or radiofrequency catheter ablation of the bundle of His (and pacemaker implantation) is rarely necessary for refractory or severely symptomatic patients. Postoperative JET tends to be a transient rhythm that seldom persists longer than 48 to 72 hours. Hence, support of hemodynamics and cardiac rhythm during this interval is the primary strategy.

AV Nodal Reentrant Tachycardia AV nodal reentrant tachycardia (AVNRT) is the most common form of supraventricular tachycardia in adults and is not uncommon in children over 5 to 10 years of age. It usually occurs in the absence of other cardiac abnormalities. It is mediated by functionally discrepant zones of conduction within the region of the AV node. One of these pathways, the "fast" pathway, conducts impulses rapidly and has a relatively long refractory period. The other, or "slow," pathway has slower conduction velocity but a shorter refractory period. AVNRT is usually initiated by a premature atrial beat that blocks in the fast pathway but conducts over the slow pathway. If conduction down the slow pathway is sufficiently delayed, the fast pathway recovers and is able to conduct the impulse in the retrograde direction. At the atrial end of the fast pathway, the impulse can return down the slow pathway, and thus a cycle between these pathways is established that sustains the arrhythmia. The retrograde P wave usually occurs simultaneously with ventricular depolarization and may not be seen on the surface ECG. Hence, this is one of the "short R-P tachycardias." The most sensitive lead for detecting these P waves is V_1 where a slight deformation of the terminal portion of the QRS complex resembling a small R' wave is frequently visible. If atrial wires have been placed surgically or an esophageal lead is used, the recording of an atrial electrogram simultaneous with the surface QRS will help to diagnose this rhythm.

Atypical AVNRT develops in a small percentage of patients and is mediated by antegrade conduction along the "fast pathway" and retrograde conduction via the "slow pathway."[102] Since retrograde conduction (from ventricles to atria) in atypical AVNRT is slow, the R-P interval is long and P waves are readily apparent. They are negative in the inferior leads (II, III, aVF).

When presenting in the emergency department or intensive care unit, this tachycardia will respond to vagal maneuvers (such as an ice cloth over the upper half of the face), intravenous phenylephrine, or intravenous adenosine. With respect to chronic management, patients should be taught safe vagal maneuvers that can terminate the tachycardia at home. Chronic medical therapy is directed at slowing conduction in the AV node, and therefore digoxin, beta-blockers, and calcium-channel agents are often effective. In many centers, radiofrequency catheter modification of the slow pathway is considered first-line therapy. This approach eliminates a critical element of the reentry circuit and is curative.[51]

AV Reciprocating Tachycardia AV reciprocating tachycardia (AVRT) is the most common form of pathologic tachycardia in infants and young children. It is a reentry tachycardia that employs both the AV node and an accessory pathway connecting the atria and ventricles. If the accessory pathway is capable of conducting impulses in the antegrade direction during sinus rhythm, the surface ECG may show a delta wave (also described as ventricular preexcitation). Patients having episodes of AVRT and a delta wave while in sinus rhythm are said to have the Wolff-Parkinson-White syndrome (Fig. 8-7A). If a delta wave is not apparent on the surface ECG, the pathway is considered to be "concealed."

The most common form of AVRT is called "orthodromic" (Fig. 8-7B). Its circuit involves antegrade conduction over the AV node, followed by retrograde conduction over the accessory pathway. Orthodromic AVRT is paroxysmal in onset and is initiated by a premature atrial or ventricular beat or by sudden junctional rhythm. Since the ventricles are depolarized by normal conduction down the AV node, the QRS complexes are usually narrow, and a delta wave will not be present. The exception would be rate-dependent bundle branch block, in which the QRS is wide complex and must be differentiated from ventricular tachycardia. As in patients having typical variety of AVNRT, the surface ECG will manifest a short R-P interval (R-P interval < P-R interval). The morphology of the retrograde P wave during orthodromic AVRT is influenced by the location of the accessory pathway: Septal accessory pathways produce P waves that are similar to those seen in AVNRT; right-sided pathways produce P waves that are upright in leads I and aVL; left-sided pathways produce P waves that are inverted in leads I and aVL.

Antidromic AVRT occurs in less than 10% of patients with accessory pathways. It occurs when the atrial impulse is conducted to the ventricles via the accessory pathway and retrograde to the atria via the AV node. Since the ventricular activation is via the accessory pathway rather than the normal AV conduction system, the QRS during tachycardia is wide complex (see Fig. 8-7C) and appears maximally preexcited. In patients having Wolff-Parkinson-White (WPW) syndrome, there may be a similar ECG appearance during tachycardias that originate in the atria such as atrial flutter or fibrillation. The latter should always be suspected when there is an irregular, wide-complex tachycardia. Unlike antidromic AVRT, atrial tachycardias with a "bystander" preexcitation pattern will not respond to AV nodal blocking agents and may require cardioversion to prevent an unacceptably rapid ventricular response.

For acute termination of orthodromic AVRT, vagal maneuvers are the first line of therapy. Agents that act at the AV node (e.g., intravenous beta-blockers, digoxin, verapamil, adenosine) may be used in the setting of orthodromic AVRT with continuous ECG monitoring. In infants less than 1 year of age, verapamil and beta-blockers should not be used due to their negative inotropic effects.[26] Chronic therapy is aimed at impairing conduction in the AV node and/or accessory pathway and suppressing premature atrial and ventricular beats, which initiate tachycardia. Atrioventricular blocking agents are usually the first agent due to their more favorable risk-benefit profile. However, both digoxin and verapamil may shorten refractoriness in accessory pathways and therefore have the potential to increase the ventricular rate in response to atrial fibrillation or atrial flutter. They should not be prescribed in patients who have a delta wave while in sinus rhythm. The role of radiofrequency catheter ablation in these patients continues to change. It is generally agreed that this should be considered primary therapy in older children and teenagers who (1) were resuscitated from ventricular fibrillation; (2) are refractory to medical therapy; (3) cannot tolerate medical therapy due to side-effects or coexisting medical problems such as asthma; or (4) have an accessory pathway that has dangerous conduction properties, as determined during an electrophysiology study. Contemporary practice now includes catheter ablation in symptomatic patients as first-line therapy, especially if the patient is interested in athletic pursuits, military enrollment, or high-risk avocations.

Permanent Junctional Reciprocating Tachycardia Permanent junctional reciprocating tachycardia (PJRT) is a narrow-complex often incessant tachycardia with rates from 120 to 250 beats per minute, characterized by sudden onset and termination, negative P waves in leads II, III, and aVF, and a long R-P interval (Fig. 8-8).[21] It must be discriminated from atypical AVNRT and from some forms of atrial ectopic tachycardia. This arrhythmia is an unusual variant form of orthodromic AVRT. It is the most common form of incessant tachycardia in children but is uncommon in neonates and adults. When chronic, it may result in left ventricular dilatation and failure. The underlying mechanism is reentry with retrograde conduction over a slowly conducting accessory pathway most commonly located in proximity to the ostium of the coronary sinus. Digoxin, beta-blockers, and type IA antiarrhythmics are generally ineffective in terminating PJRT. Type IC agents and type III agents often provide partial but frequently incomplete suppression of tachycardia. Radiofrequency catheter ablation offers the potential for a definitive cure with a low risk of inadvertent high-grade AV block.[109]

Ventricular Tachyarrhythmias

Premature Ventricular Contractions Nonsustained arrhythmias of ventricular origin include single premature ventricular contractions (PVCs), two consecutive PVCs (couplets), and bigeminy (a PVC alternating with each sinus beat). A PVC is an ectopic beat that activates the ventricles before the wave of depolarization initiated by the normal sinus node reaches the ventricle. These beats are usually wider than the normal QRS complex (> 0.08 seconds in infants or > 0.09 msec in children older than 3 years) or at least different in morphology from the normal QRS complex. A widened QRS complex may also be seen with an aberrantly conducted supraventricular beat or when a supraventricular beat is conducted over an accessory pathway. A fusion beat results when the depolarization wavefront conducted to the ventricle from the sinus node collides with a wavefront emanating from an ectopic ventricular focus.

Up to 2% of normal children have PVCs on a routine ECG.[53] However, the same triggers that provoke PVCs may potentially cause sustained ventricular arrhythmias (Table 8-6), and thus careful evaluation is required to identify whether any of these

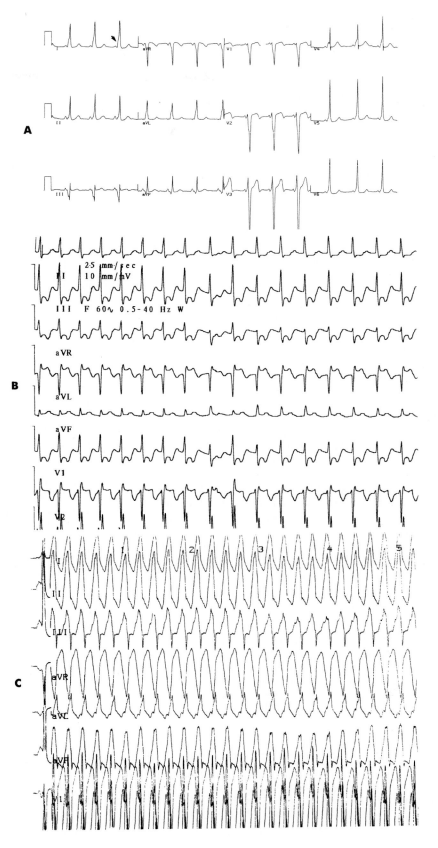

FIGURE 8-7 ECGs from a patient with the Wolff-Parkinson-White syndrome. During sinus rhythm **(A)**, there is antegrade conduction over both the AV node and the accessory pathway, resulting in ventricular preexcitation (arrow indicates delta wave). During orthodromic reciprocating tachycardia **(B)**, there is antegrade AV node conduction resulting in a normal QRS complex with retrograde conduction from the ventricle to atria completing the reentry circuit. Panel **(C)** demonstrates maximal preexcitation during antidromic reciprocating tachycardia with antegrade conduction via the accessory pathway and retrograde conduction over the AV node.

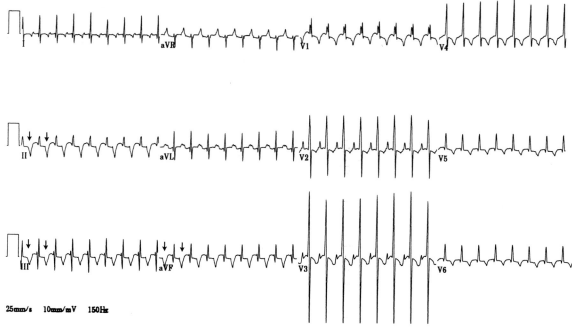

FIGURE 8-8   Permanent form of junctional reciprocating tachycardia with characteristic deeply inverted P waves in the inferior leads (II, III, aVF).

associated conditions are present. A Holter monitor quantifies the frequency and character of PVCs. In a child, PVCs occurring at a rate of more than 1 per minute are considered "frequent,"[32] although there is not a clear correlation between frequent PVCs and more serious ventricular arrhythmias. PVCs that have a constant morphology are considered uniform, and those with multiple morphologies are multiform. In children with a normal QT interval duration and a structurally normal heart by echocardiogram, uniform PVCs are usually benign and further testing is not indicated. Symptomatic ventricular ectopy in children may be further evaluated by exercise treadmill testing. The normal exercise response is a reduction in PVC frequency. If PVC frequency increases or if ventricular tachycardia develops, further evaluation is

indicated, as described later. In patients with structural heart disease, presyncope, or syncope, complex ventricular ectopy may serve as a marker for malignant ventricular arrhythmias; invasive evaluation may then be recommended.[100]

Ventricular Tachycardia   Ventricular tachycardia (VT) is a potentially life-threatening arrhythmia originating below the bundle of His. It is broadly defined as three or more consecutive beats arising from the ventricles at a rate exceeding 10% above the prevailing sinus rate. The QRS complex is usually widened except in infants and small children, in whom the QRS morphology may be narrow but distinct from the morphology seen during sinus rhythm. If the morphology of the QRS complex is uniform, the VT is considered monomorphic. If the QRS complexes vary, the VT is polymorphic. If polymorphic VT develops in the setting of a prolonged QT interval (see following text), the rhythm is termed "torsade de pointes." If VT lasts longer than 30 seconds, it is considered to be sustained; otherwise it is nonsustained.

Sustained VT in children most often develops in association with metabolic/electrolyte derangements, drug/toxin exposure, or myocardial abnormalities (see Table 8-6). VT may be the first manifestation of a cardiomyopathy in a young patient without clinical evidence of heart disease.[16] In children under the age of 3 years, sustained ventricular arrhythmias are rare, but when present, VT is often incessant (i.e., in VT for greater than 10% of the day) and associated with myocardial tumors.[39] In children and young adults with symptomatic VT, 85% have myocardial abnormalities.[69,80]

There are two types of VT that occur in otherwise normal hearts, usually during exercise.[127] The most common form has QRS complexes that usually have a left bundle branch morphology and an inferior axis in the frontal plane suggesting that the tachycardia arises in the right ventricular outflow tract. The underlying mechanism in most cases is triggered activity or enhanced automaticity (related to increased

Table 8-6   Causes of Ventricular Ectopy and Ventricular Tachycardia

Metabolic/Electrolyte Derangements	Hypoxia/ischemia
	Hypercarbia
	Hypothermia
	Acidosis
	Hypokalemia, hyperkalemia
Drug/Toxin Exposure	Any Class I or III antiarrhythmic agent
	Sympathomimetic agents (e.g., cocaine)
	Digitalis toxicity
	Drugs that prolong the QT interval (see Table 8-7)
Myocardial Abnormalities	Myocardial infarction
	Congenital heart disease
	Cardiomyopathy: dilated, hypertrophic, or restrictive
	Certain inborn errors of metabolism
	Certain neuromuscular disorders
	Myocarditis
	Myocardial tumors
Idiopathic	

sympathetic tone), and therefore the initial treatment for these children includes calcium channel blockers or beta-blockers.[49] The other form has a right bundle branch block QRS morphology and left axis deviation. Also known as fascicular VT, it uses a reentry mechanism and is one of the only forms of VT that may respond to verapamil, as well as to beta-blockers.

The diagnostic evaluation of VT begins with the appreciation that not all wide-complex tachycardias are VT. Supraventricular tachycardias conducting aberrantly to the ventricles or over an accessory pathway also have a wide QRS complex.[7] The diagnosis of VT is proven by the finding of AV dissociation, fusion beats, or capture beats. Careful differentiation of these possibilities is necessary before providing therapy. The cardiac anatomy and overall function should be evaluated by echocardiography. Cardiac catheterization and electrophysiology study is indicated for most children with sustained wide-complex tachycardia to further characterize abnormalities seen on the echocardiogram; to search for subtle anatomic or functional abnormalities, including the early stages of a cardiomyopathy; to accurately determine the mechanism of the wide-complex tachycardia; to evaluate the potential efficacy of antiarrhythmic drugs; and in some instances to perform radiofrequency catheter ablation of the tachycardia substrate. If the diagnosis remains uncertain, other tests may be considered: endomyocardial biopsy to detect myocarditis or certain types of cardiomyopathy; or MRI scan or right ventricular angiogram to detect RV dysplasia.

Therapeutic management of VT is determined by the etiology, hemodynamic stability, and age of the patient. Hemodynamically unstable arrhythmias should be treated by immediate electrical cardioversion. Reversible causes of VT, such as hypoxia or hyperkalemia, must be treated promptly. Pharmacologic therapy with class I or III antiarrhythmic agents alone or in combination can be employed for acute termination of VT and for chronic arrhythmia suppression.[32] Catheter ablation and surgical approaches are of limited efficacy, although tachycardia originating in the right ventricular outflow tract can be cured by radiofrequency catheter ablation in greater than 90% of cases.[79]

Torsade de Pointes Torsade de pointes is a form of polymorphic VT that develops in the setting of prolonged QT interval.[52] A partial list of the causes of QT prolongation, including both acquired and congenital forms, appears as Table 8-7. In some patients, QT prolongation is seen only intermittently or in relation to emotional or exertional stress. Torsade de pointes is characterized by the following features: (1) In a single ECG lead, the polarity of the QRS complexes repetitively twists around an isoelectric baseline; (2) the tachycardia frequently terminates spontaneously; and (3) infrequently the tachycardia sustains and/or degenerates into ventricular fibrillation.

Torsade de pointes may occur in the setting of sinus pauses especially in the presence of hypokalemia, or by sudden increases in sympathetic tone. The "pause-dependent" arrhythmias are often associated with a short cycle–long cycle–short cycle sequence of beats, as shown in Figure 8-9. The QRS complex following the long cycle (i.e., the pause) usually has a markedly prolonged QT interval and/or bizarre T wave morphology. In patients with "adrenergic-dependent" torsade de pointes, the catecholamine surge may be produced by exertion, fright, or startling noises, or it may exist as part of the stress response to cardiac surgery.

Table 8-7 Causes of QT Interval Prolongation

Congenital	Romano-Ward syndrome (autosomal dominant)
	Jervell and Lange-Nielsen syndrome (autosomal recessive)
Medications/Toxins	Anesthetic agents: enflurane, isoflurane, halothane
	Antiarrhythmic agents: Class IA (esp., quinidine) and Class III (esp., sotalol)
	Antibiotics/antifungals: erythromycin, trimethoprim-sulfamethoxazole, pentamidine, ketoconazole
	Psychiatric: phenothiazines, tricyclics, tetracyclics
	Antihistamines: terfenadine, astemizole
	Organophosphate insecticides
Metabolic Abnormalities	Hypokalemia
	Hypomagnesemia
	Hypocalcemia
	Hypothyroidism
	Hypothermia
	Liquid protein diets
Severe Bradycardia	Marked sinus bradycardia or sinus arrest
	High-grade atrioventricular block
Myocardial Diseases	Ischemia/infarction
	Myocarditis
	Cardiomyopathy
	HIV disease
Central Nervous System Disorders	Subarachnoid hemorrhage
	Intracranial trauma
	CNS tumor
	CNS infection
	Cerebrovascular occlusion

CNS, central nervous system; HIV, human immunodeficiency virus.

Prolonged torsade de pointes is always poorly tolerated hemodynamically and, if it does not spontaneously convert to sinus rhythm, will ultimately degenerate into ventricular fibrillation. Therefore, prompt direct current cardioversion should be performed. For frequently repeating episodes, initial treatment includes the correction of electrolyte abnormalities and elimination of medications that may have contributed to the QT prolongation (see Table 8-7). In the pause-dependent form, intravenous isoproterenol or cardiac pacing increases the heart rate and thereby shortens the QT interval, suppressing recurrent episodes of torsade. Intravenous magnesium has also proved effective in both terminating and suppressing torsade de pointes.[109] For the adrenergic form, chronic beta-blockade therapy represents initial management.

Ventricular Fibrillation Ventricular fibrillation (VF) is an extremely rapid and irregular ventricular arrhythmia with low amplitude QRS complexes. It may arise de novo (primary VF) or, more commonly, result from degeneration of hemodynamically unstable supraventricular or ventricular tachycardias. The majority of children who develop VF have experienced a severe metabolic or toxic event; have a structurally abnormal or severely injured heart; have WPW syndrome; or have prolonged QT syndrome or another of the newly discovered channelopathies, such as Brugada syndrome.[103] Initial treatment includes electrical defibrillation followed by rapid administration of lidocaine, amiodarone, or, less commonly now, procainamide (unless long QT interval) to suppress

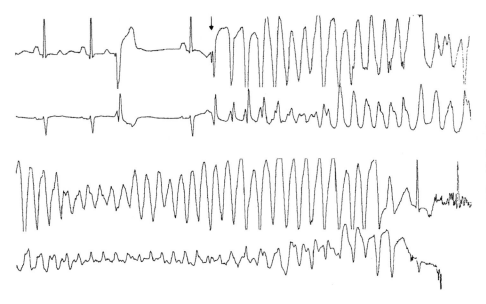

FIGURE 8-9 Torsade de pointes in a patient with the long QT syndrome. Two simultaneous ECG leads from a Holter monitor are shown (the strip is continuous). Following a long-short sequence that begins after a PVC (third beat), the T wave morphology changes markedly (arrow), and another PVC results in the initiation of polymorphic VT.

additional episodes of VF. Potential causes should then be identified and treated.

Other Arrhythmias

Sinus Arrhythmia

Sinus arrhythmia is an irregular rhythm originating in the sinus node characterized by variable PP intervals. All P waves are identical or nearly identical. In most children there is normal variability in PP intervals associated with the respiratory cycle (the rate increases with inspiration and decreases with expiration). Criteria for the normal range of sinus arrhythmia vary; in children, a variation in PP interval of 100% or more suggests sinus node dysfunction. Generally, sinus arrhythmia is at most mildly symptomatic (e.g., palpitations) and warrants no specific treatment. From a practical standpoint, sinus arrhythmia must be differentiated from pathologic sinus pauses that may be responsible for more significant symptoms, such as syncope.

Wandering Atrial Pacemaker

Wandering atrial pacemaker is an arrhythmia produced by the simultaneous and competing activity of three or more atrial pacemakers, one of which is usually the sinus node. It is an irregular rhythm characterized by variable P-wave morphology and PR intervals. As in sinus arrhythmia, the symptoms are mild and treatment is not indicated unless long pauses are present.

Accelerated Idioventricular Rhythm

In contrast to the slow ventricular rhythm seen in association with complete heart block and the rapid rate of VT, accelerated idioventricular rhythm (AIVR) is a rhythm originating within the ventricles that has a rate 10% or less faster than the prevailing sinus rate. It is generally well tolerated in children. AIVR may be seen in normal children or in the setting of myocardial ischemia in adults. Specific therapy is

usually not needed unless the patient is hemodynamically unstable. AIVR usually terminates when the excitable focus in the ventricle becomes less active or the sinus rate accelerates.

Atrioventricular Dissociation

Atrioventricular dissociation is a nonspecific term that merely indicates that the atrial and ventricular rates are different. Complete AV block exists when the atrial rate is faster than the ventricular, the rates are constant, and there is no relationship between atrial and ventricular events. More commonly, isorhythmic dissociation is present when two independent pacemakers (usually the sinus and AV nodes) beat at approximately the same rate and thereby compete for control of the cardiac rhythm. The dominant rhythm changes as one slightly slows or speeds its rate. This rhythm is commonly seen during inhalational anesthesia. It may also be seen in children with high resting vagal tone and no other abnormalities, or in patients with true sick sinus syndrome. Another example of AV dissociation is sinus rhythm with accelerated junctional rhythm and retrograde conduction block; this may be pathologic.

CLINICAL ENTITIES FREQUENTLY ASSOCIATED WITH ARRHYTHMIAS

This section deals with a variety of entities in which cardiac arrhythmias may play a prominent role in children and teenagers and which may come to the attention of the intensivist.

Neurocardiogenic Syncope

Neurocardiogenic syncope is not an arrhythmia but a symptom complex caused by a neurally mediated reflex response to upright posture, emotional stress, or fear.[6,106] It is discussed in this context because it is an important and underrecognized cause of syncope, is sometimes associated with profound bradycardia, and may result in ICU admission for evaluation. The triggers for this and related reflexes resulting in syncope include (1) venous pooling in the lower extremities that reduces venous return; (2) increased sympathetic tone in a variety of conditions (e.g., fear, sight of blood, emotion); (3) carotid sinus stimulation (carotid sinus hypersensitivity seen only in the elderly); (4) airway stimulation, which is particularly important during suctioning in the postoperative infant; (5) swallowing (deglutition syncope); (6) urination (postmicturition syncope); and (7) gastrointestinal upset (e.g., syncope in the setting of gastroenteritis).

In children and teenagers having neurocardiogenic syncope, postural changes or sympathetic surges cause vigorous cardiac contraction. This results in stimulation of ventricular mechanoreceptors and an increase in nonmyelinated C-fiber activity (Bezold-Jarisch reflex).[1] Afferent signals converge in the brainstem, and the efferent responses are abrupt withdrawal of peripheral sympathetic tone and an increase in parasympathetic tone mediated by the vagus nerve. This results primarily in hypotension due to profound peripheral vasodilation (the vasodepressor response), with or without bradycardia (the cardioinhibitory response). Some patients have only the vasodepressor component and develop syncope without a change in heart rate.

The diagnosis is often suggested by careful history taking that reveals a clear triggering event. Routine laboratory tests, including the 12-lead ECG, after neurocardiogenic syncope are usually normal. However, a 12-lead ECG should always be performed to help rule out less common but more serious causes of syncope, such as hypertrophic cardiomyopathy, WPW syndrome, and long QT syndrome. Head-up tilt table testing has emerged as the most useful diagnostic technique, although the predictive accuracy of this test is variable and greatly influenced by use of adjunctive drugs.[94,95] If a patient's premonitory symptoms and syncope are reproduced, if structural heart disease is absent, and if other etiologies have been ruled out, the diagnosis of neurocardiogenic syncope is made. In the presence of structural heart disease, bradyarrhythmias and tachyarrhythmias must be excluded before the diagnosis of neurocardiogenic syncope can be established.

Treatment is directed toward interrupting the reflex arc that mediates syncope. Options include the following:

Encouraging increased dietary sodium and water intake, which may be effective in less severe cases.

Oral salt tablets or fludrocortisone acetate (Florinef) to promote fluid retention and thereby blunt the reduction in venous return by upright posture.

Beta-blockers to inhibit vigorous left ventricular contraction.

Centrally acting agents, such as fluoxetine hydrochloride (Prozac), a serotonin reuptake antagonist, which may blunt the efferent response.

Vasoconstrictor agents, such as midodrine. This drug must be used with caution and never in the evening, due to risk of recumbent hypertension.

Disopyramide (Norpace) for both its negative inotropic effect and its vagolytic effect. This drug is not well tolerated in children due to undesirable vagolytic side effects.

Sudden Cardiac Death

Sudden cardiac death occurs in 1 to 14 pediatric patients per 100,000 patient years.[22,43] These events can be subdivided into three groups: (1) sudden infant deaths, (2) sudden deaths in patients with apparently normal hearts, and (3) sudden deaths in children known to have structurally abnormal hearts.

The cause of sudden infant death syndrome (SIDS) remains unclear and is probably multifactorial. Cardiac arrhythmias, central nervous system abnormalities, inborn errors of metabolism, central control of breathing, and pulmonary abnormalities have all been proposed. Large, prospective, population studies have provided conflicting results regarding a correlation between cardiac arrhythmias or QT interval prolongation and subsequent SIDS.[99,105] Objective parameters for risk assessment are not available.

Most sudden deaths in apparently normal children are heart related.[22] Autopsy studies have revealed the occult presence of hypertrophic cardiomyopathy, coronary artery anomalies, myocarditis, aortic rupture (usually in association with Marfan's syndrome), coronary aneurysms consistent with Kawasaki's disease, and aortic stenosis.[17,22] Other potential cardiac causes that would be undetectable on routine autopsy evaluation include primary ventricular tachycardia or fibrillation, ventricular fibrillation related to WPW syndrome, and torsade de pointes ventricular tachycardia related to the long QT syndromes. These will be further discussed later in the chapter. A history of syncope associated with exercise should raise the suspicion of a serious cardiac disorder.

Patients with certain known congenital or acquired heart diseases are at higher risk for sudden cardiac death than healthy children and teens.[30] Of 981 children with structural heart disease studied in a retrospective evaluation at the Texas Children's Hospital, 10% died suddenly.[31] Young patients at highest risk were those having pulmonary hypertension with unoperated congenital heart disease, postoperative tetralogy of Fallot, and cardiomyopathy. More than 75% of the patients who died had severely limited exercise capacity (New York Heart Association Class III or IV), cardiomegaly on chest radiography, or poor hemodynamics on cardiac catheterization. Sudden death occurred during sports activities in 22% and during sleep in 28%. In 62% of patients in whom the cause of death was known, a sudden tachycardia or bradycardia was responsible.

Myocarditis

Inflammation of the heart, or myocarditis, may be produced by infectious agents, radiation, chemicals (e.g., lead), pharmacologic agents (e.g., anthracyclines), cocaine, and metabolic disorders (e.g., uremia). The most common etiology is viral infection, especially coxsackievirus A and B, echovirus, influenza A_2, varicella, poliomyelitis, hepatitis B, and human immunodeficiency virus (HIV). The pathophysiology appears to involve virus-mediated triggering of an immune response targeted at myocytes in the weeks after the initial infection.

The clinical expression of myocarditis ranges from no symptoms to fulminant heart failure. In many patients, transient ECG abnormalities (sinus tachycardia, diminished voltages, and ST-segment and T-wave changes) accompany systemic viral infection, but other cardiac symptoms are absent. With more significant myocardial involvement, patients may report dyspnea, fatigue, palpitations, and chest discomfort. In some patients the first manifestation of myocarditis is a fatal ventricular arrhythmia; 5% to 10% of children dying suddenly have active myocarditis on postmortem examination.[112] Up to 10% of children with VT may have occult myocarditis.[92] It is generally felt that patients suspected as having myocarditis as the cause for left ventricular dysfunction should not be treated with digoxin due to its potentiating effect on ventricular tachycardia. Myocarditis that extends to the conduction system may produce AV block that is usually transient but may require temporary pacing. The diagnosis is established by an endomyocardial biopsy that demonstrates an interstitial inflammatory infiltrate and myocyte necrosis. Potentially effective treatment for viral myocarditis includes immunosuppressive therapy to modify the immune response. Circulatory support by extracorporeal membrane oxygenation may even be necessary during this acute phase when VT is present.

Wolff-Parkinson-White Syndrome

Accessory AV pathways are embryonic remnants of direct atrial and ventricular continuity present early in cardiogenesis.[24] During subsequent development, formation of the annulus fibrosus interrupts AV muscular continuity except in the region of the His bundle. AV connections that persist after formation of the annulus fibrosus potentially provide a substrate for tachycardias. Rarely, accessory pathways are inherited as an autosomal dominant trait.[116]

As previously noted, when anterograde conduction down an accessory pathway results in "preexcitation" of the ventricles, we say the patient has WPW. This is manifested on the ECG by a slurring of the upstroke of the QRS complex (the delta wave) and a shortening of the PR interval. On the 12-lead ECG, ventricular preexcitation may be confused with right or left bundle branch block, right or left ventricular hypertrophy, and anterior or posterior myocardial infarction. Algorithms have been developed to estimate the location of the accessory pathway from the morphology of the delta wave on a standard 12-lead ECG.

In addition to AV reciprocating tachycardia described previously, a minority of young persons having WPW are at peculiar risk of developing atrial fibrillation, especially during or following exercise. Unlike the normal AV node, the accessory pathway may permit a very rapid ventricular rate response, even predisposing to degeneration to ventricular fibrillation and sudden death. Digoxin may actually increase this risk due to its unpredictable effects on accessory pathway conduction characteristics (see earlier text). Any young person presenting with an irregular, wide-complex tachycardia should be assumed to have WPW and atrial fibrillation and should be managed accordingly. Furthermore, any patient having a history of syncope and an ECG demonstrating WPW pattern deserves urgent cardiology consultation.

Long QT Syndrome

The long QT syndrome (LQTS) is a heritable disorder of cardiac potassium or sodium channel protein structure and function. This entity is one of a group of "channelopathies" that clinically presents as recurrent syncope, seizures, or sudden death.[35,52] Cardiac arrhythmias are typically provoked by physical or emotional stress, although one type, "LQT3," causes sudden death during sleep.

Historically, two clinical variants of congenital long QT syndrome had been identified: an autosomal dominant form with normal hearing (Romano-Ward syndrome) and an autosomal recessive form with congenital deafness (Jervell and Lange-Nielsen syndrome). However, recent advances in molecular genetics have led to an explosion in our understanding of this group of disorders, with eight forms of LQTS thus far identified and the genetic loci (on chromosomes 11, 7, 3, 4, 21) and gene products known for seven of them.[119] Among the better understood of the LQTs' (types 1–3), relatively specific electrocardiographic patterns (of the T waves) and clinical triggers for torsades de pointes are being uncovered. It is hoped that genetic identification of susceptible patients will soon permit early treatment. Even "acquired long QT syndrome" may be due to minor channel defects that predispose to ventricular arrhythmias when exposed to certain medications or to metabolic derangements (see Table 8-7).

The pathogenesis of torsade de pointes in most patients having LQTS is probably related to exaggerated dispersion of ventricular refractoriness and catecholamine-induced early afterdepolarizations, which then initiates a malignant, rapid, reentrant ventricular tachycardia. The faulty ion channels predispose to this dispersion of refractoriness.

The LQTS should be suspected in any child with exertional or emotional syncope, especially if it associated with a seizure and not associated with a prodrome. Discriminating LQTS from pallid breath-holding spells in toddlers can be especially challenging. Most patients with congenital long QT syndrome become symptomatic by the age of 15 years.[96] The surface ECG is often diagnostic in demonstrating a markedly prolonged QT interval, especially if the T waves are broad and flat (LQTS1), double humped (LQTS2), or normal but delayed in onset (LQTS3). The QT interval should be measured from the onset of the QRS complex to the point of maximal change in the slope as the T wave merges with the baseline. An average of three consecutive sinus beats should be determined. The U wave, if present, should not be included in the measurement unless it merges with the T wave and is greater than one half the amplitude of the T wave. Since the QT interval normally varies with heart rate, a "corrected" QT interval (QT_c) is more diagnostic. The standard correction is achieved using Bazett's formula, defined as the QT interval divided by the square root of the preceding RR interval. Not unexpectedly, there is overlap of the distribution of QT_c intervals among carriers and noncarriers of the long QT gene.[68] The region of overlap is approximately 0.41 to 0.47 seconds; a QT_c interval greater than 0.47 seconds has a high specificity for the long QT syndrome.[120] Because of the difficulty in defining the long QT syndrome on the sole basis of the QT interval, additional diagnostic criteria have been proposed (Table 8-8).[98]

A 1993 retrospective multicenter international study described the clinical features of the long QT syndrome in 287 patients younger than 21 years of age (mean age at presentation is 6.8 years).[35] The longest QT interval was found in lead II in 82% of patients. A small subset (6%) of this group had a QT_c of less than 0.44 second and were identified because of symptoms and a positive family history. Forty-five percent presented with cardiac arrest, syncope, or a seizure, and 56% had symptoms related to exercise and/or emotion. A positive family history for a long QT interval was present in 60% and for cardiac arrest, syncope, or seizures in 39%. During electrophysiologic testing, 12% had inducible polymorphic VT, 7% had inducible nonsustained VT, 5% developed torsade de pointes during catecholamine infusion, and 2% had spontaneous torsade. Over 75% of patients were treated with beta-blockers, and of these 60% experienced effective suppression of ventricular arrhythmias. For patients with continued symptoms

Table 8-8 1993 Long QT Syndrome (LQTS) Criteria

Criteria	Points
ECG Findings*	
QT$_c$†	
> 0.47 sec	3
0.46–0.47 sec	2
0.45 sec (males)	1
Torsade de pointes	2
T wave alternans	1
Notched T waves (three leads)	1
Low heart rate for age‡	0.5
Clinical History	
Syncope	2
With stress	1
Without stress	0.5
Congenital deafness	
Family History§	
Definite LQTS‖	1
Unexplained sudden death in immediate	
family member younger than 30 yr	0.5

If sum of points is 0–1, the probability of having LQTS is low; if score is 2–3, the probability is intermediate; and if the score is 4 or greater, the probability is high.

* In the absence of secondary causes for ECG features.
† Calculated by Bazett's formula.
‡ Resting heart rate below the second percentile for age.
§ Cannot include the same family member in both of the following.
‖ Defined as an LQTS score of 4 or greater.
ECG, electrocardiograph; QTc, corrected QT interval.
From Schwartz PJ, Moss AJ, Vincent GM, Crampton RS: Diagnostic criteria for the long QT syndrome. An update. *Circulation* 88: 782–784, 1993.

on beta-blockers, nonpharmacologic therapies were used, including pacemaker implantation to prevent excessive brady-cardia (15%), left cardiac sympathetic denervation (high thoracic left sympathectomy) to alter autonomic input to the heart (2%), and defibrillator implantation to treat recurrent arrhythmias (1%). Within the first year of follow-up, cardiac arrest, syncope, or seizure developed in 10%. Over the first 5 years of follow-up, 8% died suddenly and two thirds of these patients were asymptomatic in the year before their death. Multivariate analysis revealed that a presenting QT$_c$ greater than 0.6 second and medication noncompliance were correlated with subsequent sudden death. The sudden death rate in those with a QT$_c$ greater than 0.6 second and medication noncompliance was 83% to 91% over a mean follow-up of 5 years.

Congenital Heart Disease

Children with congenital heart disease (CHD) are predisposed to atrial and ventricular arrhythmias both before and after surgical repair.[64,113,114] In general, atrial surgery increases the likelihood of sinus node dysfunction and atrial arrhythmias, and ventricular surgery is associated with ventricular tachyarrhythmias. Rhythm disturbances have a tendency to increase in frequency with the passage of time after cardiac surgery and in the presence of new or progressive hemodynamic deterioration. Late sudden death after cardiac surgery appears to be related to surgical scar in the ventricle and the complexity of the congenital lesion.[33] Sudden death occurs in less than 0.1% of patients after pulmonary valvotomy,[126] up to 4% after VSD repair,[126] 3% to 15% after atrial redirection operation for d-transposition of the great arteries (Mustard or Senning operations),[4,42,47,115] up to 5% after aortic valve

surgery,[126] 1.5% to 6% after tetralogy of Fallot repair,[12,57,79,81,87] and 18% after repair of truncus arteriosus with a single pulmonary artery.[29] Identifying criteria for risk stratifying these high-risk patients and for selecting which patients to treat with antiarrhythmic drugs or implantable defibrillators are not currently underway. Noninvasive ambulatory rhythm monitoring, signal averaged ECGs, exercise testing, and invasive electrophysiologic studies have all been used in an effort to determine such risk.[2] Children with corrected CHD who present with cardiac arrest, syncope, or presyncope should be referred to an electrophysiologist skilled in the treatment of patients with congenital heart disease.

Of interest to the intensivist are arrhythmias encountered in the immediate postoperative period following congenital heart surgery (see junctional ectopic tachycardia in the previous section). Sinus or junctional bradycardia is not uncommon after any right heart surgery in which there is a period of elevated right atrial pressure or other right atrial distortion. Accordingly, we often encounter this following AVSD surgery and during ECMO management even in the absence of congenital heart disease. Bradycardia may present in the absence of abnormal hemodynamics when damage to the sinus node or its blood supply occurs. This should be considered in patients having just undergone repair of complex anomalous pulmonary venous return, the hemi-Fontan operation, or the Fontan operation. Ventricular arrhythmias, on the other hand, are uncommon immediately postoperatively and may represent ongoing metabolic disturbance or occult oxygen myocardial supply/demand imbalance. New atrial or ventricular ectopy, especially several days remote from surgery, may warn of new hemodynamic problems, such as a patch or valve leaflet dehiscence or bacterial endocarditis.

Ebstein's anomaly is worthy of special comment. It is associated with WPW syndrome and right-sided accessory pathways in 10% of patients.[82] Most children requiring right heart surgery for this condition now undergo catheter ablation prior to surgery to reduce the postoperative arrhythmia risk. Nevertheless, other atrial and ventricular arrhythmias are common perioperatively in these complex patients.

Sudden asystole within hours or days of congenital heart surgery almost always invokes an urgent evaluation of the infant's or child's airway, consideration of cardiac tamponade or perforation, or other vagal stimuli. However, cases of the Bezold-Jarisch reflex due solely to myocardial overstretch and responsive only to atropine have been reported.[28] Hence, in the absence of other etiologies, atropine may be considered in such patients. Proof of efficacy should be followed by continuous infusion until the patient's hemodynamics have improved.

Hypertrophic Cardiomyopathy

Hypertrophic cardiomyopathy is a primary disorder of the contractile proteins of the myofibril. Grossly, it is characterized by marked thickening of the ventricular myocardium and some combination of hyperdynamic systolic function, left ventricular outflow tract obstruction, and diastolic dysfunction with pulmonary venous congestion. Over 50% of cases of hypertrophic cardiomyopathy are inherited (usually, autosomal dominant pattern with variable penetrance). Young patients present with a range of symptoms, including fatigue, exercise intolerance, chest pain, shortness of breath, syncope, and sudden death. Sudden death appears to be most common in children and young adults aged 10 to 35 years, and not infrequently occurs before the disease is recognized.[72] Approximately 40% of the deaths happen during or just after vigorous physical activities; in the remaining cases, patients were sedentary or engaged in light activities. Hypertrophic cardiomyopathy appears to be the most common cause of sudden death in young athletes.[74] Risk factors for sudden death include a family history of sudden death, a history of syncope, VT on Holter monitoring, and—in children—excessive ventricular hypertrophy.[73]

The cause of syncope or cardiac arrest in children and young adults appears to be myocardial ischemia and secondary ventricular arrhythmias.[19] Exercise thallium studies in 15 young patients ages 6 to 23 years with hypertrophic cardiomyopathy and a history of syncope or sudden death revealed inducible myocardial ischemia in all 15. Therapy with verapamil alone or in combination with a beta-blocker over a 23 ± 6–month follow-up period prevented symptomatic recurrences in 11 of the 15.[19]

Dilated Cardiomyopathy

Dilated cardiomyopathy is a heterogeneous group of conditions having in common diminished left ventricular systolic function. As many as 50% of affected individuals are now thought to have a heritable disorder of a myocyte protein, with dystrophin abnormality as the original protein identified. Of the remainder, many are thought to have a burned-out viral myocarditis. Patients present with fatigue, orthopnea, dyspnea on exertion, syncope, and sudden death. Both atrial (especially atrial fibrillation) and ventricular arrhythmias are commonly seen in children with dilated cardiomyopathy. Outpatient management with amiodarone is the safest antiarrhythmic drug in this patient group, because it does not have appreciable myocardial depressant properties. Those having the most severe left ventricular dysfunction appear to be at greatest risk for sudden death. A left ventricular ejection fraction less than 20% carries a 5-year survival rate of 50%[84] and justifies consideration of ICD implantation as a bridge to cardiac transplantation.

Intensive care unit management of these patients requires an aggressive approach to any ventricular ectopy. Normalization of hypoglycemia, hypoxia, and plasma electrolyte concentrations, including magnesium, is paramount. Judicious use of lidocaine is appropriate with the first signs of ectopy. Progression of ectopy to runs of ventricular tachycardia may require addition of intravenous amiodarone and consideration of cardiovascular support with an ECMO circuit as an emergency bridge to transplant. Although often necessary, all manner of pressor support is problematic due to proarrhythmic tendency.

Arrhythmogenic Right Ventricular Dysplasia

Arrhythmogenic right ventricular dysplasia (ARVD) is clinically characterized by ventricular arrhythmias and focally or globally dilated right ventricle. Pathologically, right ventricular myocardium is replaced by fibrofatty material, and there may be thinning of the right ventricular free wall, usually in a heterogeneous pattern.[23,71] The disease may be familial, and the pathogenesis has been shown to involve apoptosis in some cases.

Patients usually present between the second and fourth decades with cardiomegaly, monomorphic ventricular tachycardia, syncope, or sudden death. Arrhythmias are often provoked by exercise. The natural history of ARVD is progressive fatty

infiltration, deterioration in right ventricular function, and increased frequency of VT. The resting ECG may show right atrial abnormalities, incomplete right bundle branch block (RBBB), and T-wave inversions in the precordial leads. Electrophysiologic testing demonstrates inducible VT originating in the right ventricle (and therefore exhibiting a left bundle branch block [LBBB] morphology) in most patients. Echocardiography or radionuclide angiography may reveal right ventricular dysfunction and dilatation, and contrast angiography may show diffuse or segmental wall motion abnormalities in the right ventricle. Endomyocardial biopsy is usually normal, since the interventricular septum is less frequently involved, but occasionally may detect fatty tissue infiltration. The diagnosis may also be suspected from gated magnetic resonance imaging, because fat density is readily depicted and wall thinning is easily demonstrated.[91]

Treatment options include pharmacotherapy, surgical exclusion of involved portions of the right ventricle, implantable defibrillator,[9,68] or cardiac transplantation. Radiofrequency catheter ablation may only temporize, given the progressive nature of the disease process. The most effective pharmacologic agents appear to be beta-blockers and Class III antiarrhythmic drugs. Even in patients in whom defibrillators are implanted, drug therapy may be necessary to reduce the frequency of arrhythmic episodes. In refractory patients with malignant ventricular arrhythmias, cardiac transplantation should be considered.

ARVD may be a more frequent cause of sudden death in young athletes than had been appreciated and should be considered in all children and teenagers with ventricular tachycardia having a LBBB morphology, especially if concomitant right ventricular dilatation or dysfunction is present.[23]

DIAGNOSTIC METHODS FOR PEDIATRIC ARRHYTHMIAS

This section provides the clinician with an overview of the tools available for diagnosis of arrhythmias in the young. The first two sections are especially germane to the intensivist, as they represent the primary techniques used in the intensive care unit. A brief discussion of ambulatory event monitoring, exercise testing, tilt table testing, and formal electrophysiologic testing are included for completion's sake.

Electrocardiography

The standard 12-lead surface ECG serves several important roles. First, it may provide evidence for acute and serious cardiac pathology, including peaked T waves and broad QRS of hyperkalemia, ST-segment depression of myocardial ischemia, prolonged QT_c of hypocalcemia or hypokalemia, reduced voltages of large pericardial effusion or myocarditis, or new peaked P waves and RVH of a pulmonary embolus. Second, it may provide evidence for the presence of structural heart disease, especially in the newborn. Third, the ECG may add to the weight of evidence in the case of diagnostic dilemmas: the short PR interval and massive precordial QRS forces of Pompe's disease; or the mosque shape of the ST and T waves of hypothyroidism, as examples.

Most pertinent to this discussion, however, the ECG is the tool of choice to diagnose an ongoing arrhythmia, and the mechanism of the arrhythmia may be determined by careful examination. Close examination for the presence of ventricular preexcitation (i.e., a delta wave) or a prolonged QT_c interval may provide an immediate clue to the diagnosis. Each beat should be analyzed, with particular attention to each P wave and QRS complex and to the P and QRS relationship. The main limitation to the 12-lead ECG is that it provides only a brief look at the cardiac rhythm (10 seconds), unless a rhythm strip is also obtained.

The bedside ECG monitor provides the added benefit of continuous monitoring. To maximize the likelihood of determining the mechanism of an arrhythmia that develops or determining whether the arrhythmia is supraventricular or ventricular, at least two and preferably three ECG leads should be monitored. P waves are usually most evident in the inferior leads (II, III, aVF) and lead V_1. If the P wave is small or indistinct, one of the leads should be either of the following:

1. A Lewis lead, with the right arm electrode placed in the left second intercostal space and the left arm electrode placed in the left fourth intercostal space (both at the left sternal border). This configuration will maximize the P-wave amplitude; or
2. A modified V_1 lead, with the right arm lead near the left shoulder, the left arm lead in the usual V_1 position in the right second intercostal space, and the ground electrode near the right shoulder. This configuration also optimizes P-wave detection and frees the left precordium for application of patches or paddles for cardioversion.

Newer telemetry systems have sophisticated arrhythmia recognition algorithms, permitting recall of brief events and even full disclosure of all earlier patient rhythms. Paper strips of any arrhythmia should be promptly labeled, edited, and placed into the patient's chart so that this important documentation is not lost.

Direct Atrial and Ventricular Electrograms

Unlike outpatient or typical inpatient ward facilities, the intensive care unit is uniquely equipped to facilitate acquisition of direct cardiac electrical signals—from transesophageal or intracardiac electrode catheters or from epicardial wires, surgically placed at the conclusion of heart surgery. The ability to record electrograms from conductors attached to or adjacent to the heart provides a great deal of interpretive information in children having pathologic tachycardias and even bradycardias; information that may be impossible to obtain from the surface ECG.

Bipolar recordings from the electrodes in transvenous or transesophageal catheters, or from each pair of epicardial wires, may be attached to standard ECG recording devices or to intensive care unit monitors as follows: Attach one electrode connecting wire (or use alligator clamps if necessary) to the monitor's cable corresponding to "right arm" and the other electrode to the monitor's cable corresponding to "left arm." Be certain that the monitor's leg cables are appropriately attached to the patient (Fig. 8-10A). Lead I will represent a bipolar electrogram from the chamber in continuity with the bipolar catheter (or epicardial pair of wires). In the case of the transesophageal catheter, there will be sharp atrial and ventric-ular signals. In all other cases, if the chamber being viewed is atrial, there may be minimal ventricular signal,

making a simultaneous surface lead desirable; the surface QRS can serve as a ventricular reference. If the lead I, II, III montage is available, leads II and III will represent electrical fusion between the atrial electrogram and QRS, which will serve the same purpose. There are other methods of obtaining discrete cardiac electrograms using temporary pacing systems (Fig. 8-10B). Examples of bipolar and unipolar atrial electrograms with simultaneous ventricular references appear as Figure 8-11. These methods are invaluable for discriminating postoperative JET from sinus tachycardia or SVT, sinus bradycardia from nonconducted atrial bigeminy, and atrial flutter with 2:1 AV conduction from sinus tachycardia, to name a few. Simultaneous use of pharmacologic agents, such as adenosine, makes this technique even more powerful.

Ambulatory Rhythm Recording

The Holter monitor is a tool that generates a complete log of a patient's cardiac rhythm for 24-hour intervals and allows a more quantitative analysis of the type and frequency of arrhythmias. It also guarantees that a hard copy of any arrhythmias will be available for review, and it is therefore especially useful in patients with unknown arrhythmias or conditions that may be arrhythmic in origin and that occur very frequently. Because most arrhythmias in children are not daily events, newer, cordless, ambulatory monitors may be conveniently carried by older children and teenagers. They are applied to the patient's chest during symptoms, and when activated they will record the rhythm. Loop recorders are equally small devices but are constantly attached. When activated, they have the advantage of recording the rhythm during a period of time prior to activation, thus permitting documentation of brief events or events causing brief loss of consciousness.

Exercise Testing

Exercise testing on a treadmill or bicycle is an important component of the evaluation of patients with known or suspected cardiac arrhythmias, especially those with symptoms associated with excitement, fear, or physical exertion. Both bradyarrhythmias and tachyarrhythmias may be triggered by the exercise challenge. Further information regarding exercise capacity and exercise-induced ischemia is gained. Obviously, this is impractical immediately postoperatively and in children younger than 6 years of age.

Tilt Table Testing

Head-up tilt testing may be performed in children with recurrent syncope not thought to be related to primary heart disease. The patient is securely strapped to a table and raised one or more times to a head-up position 60 to 80 degrees from the horizontal. Testing is performed with simultaneous ECG monitoring, invasive or noninvasive blood pressure measurement, and intravenous (IV) access. The patient is first tilted upright for 20 to 60 minutes. If this trial fails to reproduce symptoms, additional trials may be performed during infusions of isoproterenol. A positive test reproduces the patient's premonitory symptoms and results in hypotension and syncope. Unfortunately, the predictive accuracy of this test is only fair.

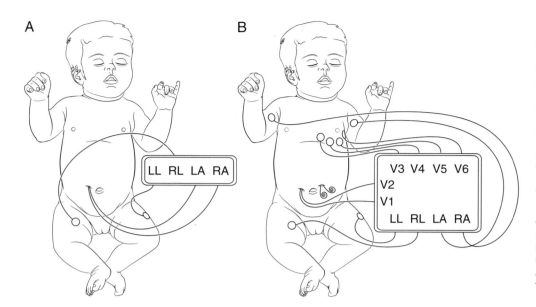

FIGURE 8-10 **A,** A method for recording a bipolar atrial electrogram involves connecting the atrial electrodes (or wires) to the right arm and left arm leads and leaving the leg leads connected to the right and left legs. The atrial electrogram is very prominent in lead I and observable, but less prominent, in the other limb leads. **B,** An alternate method for recording a unipolar atrial electrogram from temporary epicardial wires. This setup requires normal attachment of limb leads to establish a central Wilson terminus (plus V3). One atrial wire is connected to V1, the other to V2, and a V1-V2-V3 montage is recorded. Two unipolar atrial electrograms with large amplitude (far-field) ventricular electrograms will appear as V1 and V2. Compare this method with that described in the text.

Electrophysiology Study

The electrophysiology study is the most provocative means of tachyarrhythmia induction and permits thorough analysis of arrhythmias.[86] It plays an important role in the management of many cardiac arrhythmias. Typically, the study involves the placement of multiple multipolar catheters into the right heart from the femoral, internal jugular, and subclavian veins.[40] Catheters are used to pace the heart and to record electrograms from multiple sites in the heart in order to evaluate the conduction system and determine the mechanism of any induced arrhythmias. Standard pacing techniques used to evaluate the specialized conduction system and to induce pathologic tachycardias include the following:

1. Sinus node function can be evaluated by measurement of the sinus node recovery time (SNRT). The atrium is paced at a rate faster than the sinus rate for 30 seconds or more and then abruptly terminated. The time from the last paced atrial beat to the first spontaneous sinus beat defines the SNRT. This test does not have good

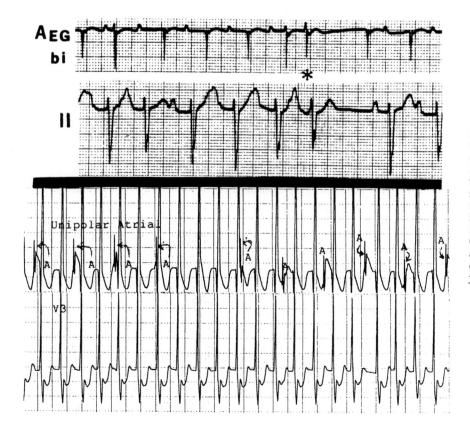

FIGURE 8-11 A comparison of techniques used to obtain epicardial atrial electrograms. On *top,* as described in the text and illustrated in Fig. 8-10A, bipolar atrial electrograms (AEGs) are much larger than the ventricular and must be compared with a surface lead (II) to identify the QRS. This technique readily identifies a nonconducted premature atrial beat (*). On the *bottom,* the technique shown in Figure 8-10B illustrates the easy identification of the QRS and atrial electrograms (A) in one lead, but the atrial signal may be dwarfed by the large ventricular one. This V1-V3 montage demonstrates postoperative junctional ectopic tachycardia.

predictive accuracy, and a normal SNRT does not rule out significant sinus node disease.

2. AV node function can be evaluated with atrial and ventricular pacing protocols. The anterograde conduction time through the AV node can be estimated by the AH interval recorded from a catheter lying along the tricuspid valve in the region of the His bundle. This interval is measured from the local atrial electrogram (A) to the onset of His bundle potential (H) (see Fig. 8-3B). With progressively faster atrial pacing, the normal AV node develops Mobitz I second-degree AVB that may not appear until the pacing rate exceeds 200 beats per minute.

3. The HV interval reflects His-Purkinje system conduction and is measured from the onset of the His bundle potential (H) to the earliest QRS deflection in any surface ECG lead. The normal HV interval in children is 30 to 50 milliseconds. A subnormal HV interval suggests the presence of an accessory pathway that is prematurely activating the ventricle, and a prolonged HV interval suggests infranodal conduction system disease.

4. Atrial or ventricular arrhythmias can be induced by pacing the atrium or ventricle via intravascular catheters placed in these chambers or through an esophageal lead. After pacing at a fixed rate for eight to ten beats, one or more premature extrastimuli are introduced. This method, called *programmed stimulation*, is an effective means of inducing reentry tachycardias. Triggered arrhythmias can sometimes be induced by rapid bursts of pacing at a critical rate, and automatic arrhythmias may be seen during catecholamine infusion.

5. Arrhythmia mapping can be accomplished with one of the catheters by systematically recording electrograms at multiple sites in one of the cardiac chambers or along the AV rings. This allows localization of a reentry circuit, a focus of an automatic tachycardia, or an accessory pathway. Once one of these critical sites is found, catheter ablation can be performed.

Indications for electrophysiologic study are constantly evolving. Our current indications include: (1) for specific purpose of radiofrequency catheter ablation for a previously documented tachycardia; (2) to characterize and possibly ablate a documented wide complex tachycardia; (3) following syncope in a patient who had undergone congenital heart surgery; (4) following resuscitated sudden death of unknown etiology; (5) for proof of efficacy of antiarrhythmic drugs in a patient with ventricular tachycardia; (6) to complete evaluation of palpitations, when noninvasive means have been repeatedly unsuccessful (esophageal study); and (7) occasionally, to evaluate level of second-degree AV block.

MANAGEMENT OF PEDIATRIC ARRHYTHMIAS

To this point, we have presented the mechanisms of arrhythmias, a catalog of arrhythmia types seen in young patients, disease entities often associated with arrhythmias in children, and methods available for their diagnosis. Now, discussion will predominately focus on the acute, intensive care management of pediatric arrhythmias with special attention to postoperative

arrhythmias in patients who have recently undergone surgery for congenital heart defects.

In the critical care setting, treatment must frequently occur before the specific cardiac diagnosis is made. This emergency therapy for cardiac arrhythmias in children, especially in the postoperative setting, will be most effective if cardiac arrhythmias are anticipated. Any evidence of bradycardias, tachycardias, or extrasystoles before the onset of a more serious arrhythmia may guide the selection of therapy. For life-threatening, acute tachyarrhythmias evidenced by an acute change in level of consciousness, impairment of peripheral perfusion, or hypotension, electrical cardioversion may take precedence over pharmacotherapy. Prophylactic pharmacotherapy (directed at the specific arrhythmia) may then be instituted, until the clinical situation warrants discontinuation. Coexisting medications must also be considered when treating cardiac arrhythmias, especially adrenergic agents, digoxin, and drugs known to affect blood electrolyte concentrations. Thus, when treating cardiac arrhythmias in the ICU, one must consider (1) preexisting rhythm disturbances, (2) the clinical setting, (3) the hemodynamic status, and (4) interaction with other drugs. When considering treatment for all arrhythmias, adequate oxygenation, correction of electrolyte disturbances, and adequacy of sedation are important factors.

This section will be an encyclopedic approach to treatment options.

Pharmacologic Treatment of Tachyarrhythmias and the Vaughan-Williams Classification

This widely used antiarrhythmic drug classification is based upon common actions of different agents (Table 8-9). These medications predominately affect ion currents responsible for various phases of the cardiac action potential (see Fig. 8-1). Some have their effect on the sympathetic and parasympathetic balance contributing to the persistence of cardiac arrhythmias. Several medications are effective through multiple mechanisms. The same mechanisms responsible for the antiarrhythmic effects may also be responsible for the side effects seen with antiarrhythmic medications.

Class I drugs inhibit inward depolarizing sodium channels, resulting in a slowed upstroke of the cardiac action potential and secondary alteration of action potential duration and refractoriness of excitable tissues. Class II agents block beta-adrenergic receptors altering the sympathetic influence on electrophysiologic properties of cardiac cells. Class III medications predominately block potassium channels resulting in prolonged phase 3 repolarization of the cardiac action potential. Class IV antiarrhythmics block calcium channels, which are the depolarizing channels in the sinoatrial and AV nodes.

Class IA Antiarrhythmic Drugs (Quinidine, Procainamide, and Disopyramide)

Of the Class IA agents, procainamide is the drug most often used in the intensive care setting in the United States, due to its availability in parenteral form. The primary action of procainamide is to block the inward sodium channel, with lesser repolarizing potassium channel blockade and vagolytic effects. It can be expected to prolong the cardiac action potential and refractory period of atrial, ventricular, and His-Purkinje cells. Conduction velocity is slowed and automaticity is decreased.

TABLE 8-9   Classification of Antiarrhythmic Agents

Class	Subclass	Drug	Pharmacologic Effect
I		Moricizine	Depression of rate of increase of action potential
	IA	Quinidine Procainamide Disopyramide	Increased AP duration, and increased atrial and ventricular ERP; increased JT interval; vagolytic action
	IB	Lidocaine, Mexiletine, Tocainide	Decreased AP duration but increased ventricular ERP; unchanged QRS complex; unchanged JT interval
	IC	Propafenone Flecainide (Encainide)	Depressed rate of increase of action potential, causing widening of QRS complex; unchanged AP duration, but increased atrial and ventricular ERP; unchanged JT interval
II		Beta-blockers	Inhibition of beta-adrenergic receptors
III		Amiodarone Sotalol Bretylium	Increased AP duration Increased JT interval
IV		Verapamil, Diltiazem	Blockade of Ca^{++} channels

ERP, end resting potential.

The major effect of these agents on the ECG is prolongation of the corrected QT interval (QT$_c$). The PR interval will prolong in the presence of preexisting His-Purkinje system disease. Likewise, procainamide slows the heart rate in the presence of sinus node dysfunction. Class IA drugs are most useful in treating all reentrant supraventricular tachycardias and some ventricular tachycardias. In the management of postoperative JET, procainamide in combination with hypothermia may be efficacious.[122]

The major noncardiac side effects limiting use of procainamide in the acute setting are nausea, vomiting, and central nervous system symptoms. These agents all have negative inotropic properties, especially disopyramide; and due to slight alpha-adrenergic blocking effects, they may also cause hypotension. Due to its vagolytic property, procainamide used in the setting of atrial fibrillation or rapid atrial tachycardia will accelerate AV nodal conduction resulting in a rapid ventricular response. In those instances, a beta-blocker or calcium channel blocking drug is also necessary. Prolongation of the QT$_c$ may predispose patients with an unstable ventricular myocardium to develop torsade de pointes. Thus, these Class I agents, although effective, have been superceded by other agents in most circumstances.

Class IB Antiarrhythmic Drugs (Phenytoin, Mexiletine, Lidocaine)

Lidocaine is a Class IB agent that is available in intravenous form in the United States and has classically been a part of Advanced Cardiac Life Support treatment algorithms for ventricular tachycardia and fibrillation. Its primary effects are to slow ventricular conduction and to raise the threshold for ventricular fibrillation.[41] It has little effect on atrial and nodal tissue. Lidocaine particularly depresses conductivity in injured or hypoxic myocardium, accounting for its efficacy immediately following myocardial infarction. It has mild negative inotropic effects. Heart block and decreased myocardial function are potential complications of lidocaine therapy in the postoperative period, although it is generally a well-tolerated drug. Central nervous system toxicity in the form of seizures, disorientation, drowsiness, agitation, and paresthesias can be expected at supratherapeutic blood levels, especially at levels in excess of 10 to 15 µg/mL.

Mexiletine and phenytoin are orally active agents effective at suppressing PVCs and ventricular arrhythmias, especially in patients having undergone ventriculotomy for repair of congenital heart defects and having abnormal hemodynamics (e.g., tetralogy of Fallot).[58,61] These agents may also be effective in the therapy of ventricular arrhythmias in certain patients with the long QT syndrome. Phenytoin is particularly useful for treating digoxin overdose by suppressing afterdepolarizations and digoxin-related ventricular arrhythmias. These oral agents do not depress ventricular function; however, intravenous phenytoin must be given very slowly due to tendency to cause hypotension.

Class IC Antiarrhythmic Drugs (Flecainide, Propafenone)

Flecainide and propafenone are Class IC agents,[11,59,61] which decrease the phase 0 slope and slow conduction velocities throughout the myocardium. They have the longest time constant for dissociation from sodium channels of any currently used drugs and therefore may exert their effects at rather slow heart rates. They are available only in oral form in the United States. They are efficacious in treating sustained and resistant ventricular tachyarrhythmias and refractory reentrant supraventricular tachycardias. Propafenone also has calcium channel and beta-blocking activity.[60] It has also been reported to be useful in treating junctional ectopic tachycardias.[61,107] These drugs can increase the PR interval and QRS duration. They have been associated with malignant proarrhythmia, so caution is required when using them, especially in children with impaired left ventricular function or previous cardiac surgery. Proarrhythmia may take the form of worsening of the index VT or SVT[25] or induction of an incessant, difficult to terminate, ventricular tachycardia. Proarrhythmia is usually related to higher doses, and careful monitoring of the rhythm and QRS duration is warranted.

Class II Antiarrhythmic Drugs (Beta-Blockers)

Class II agents are direct antagonists of beta-adrenergic receptors.[63] They decrease the slope of phase 4 of pacemaking tissues, thus reducing automaticity and lowering heart rates.[59,61] These agents typically prolong the PR interval slightly, shorten the QT$_c$ interval, and have little effect on QRS duration.

Beta-blockers increase the refractory period of the AV node and are used as chronic therapy to prevent those SVTs that use the AV node as a part of the tachycardia circuit. They are also used chronically to limit the ventricular rate response to atrial flutter and atrial fibrillation,[63] and intravenous preparations are used for immediate reduction in ventricular rate. They may also be useful in suppressing ventricular extrasystoles and those ventricular tachycardias seen in persons having no other heart disease. They have been shown to shorten the QT_c in certain patients with the long QT syndrome and are protective against development of potentially fatal torsade de pointes in most.

Propranolol is the prototypic drug in this class, having both β1 and β2 receptor–blocking effects. Esmolol, an intravenous agent that is ultra–short-acting, has a plasma half-life of 8 minutes, and is an excellent alternative when initiating beta-blockade therapy in postoperative or cardiomyopathic patients. It can be delivered in small IV boluses or as a rapidly accelerating IV infusion. When using these drugs in the acute care setting, side effects include depression of ventricular function, vasodilation and hypotension, and bradycardia. Intravenous use of these drugs may be especially hazardous in infants, and alternative agents should be considered. Extreme caution should also be used in patients with sinoatrial node dysfunction or advanced AV nodal disease. In patients with asthma, beta-blockers may precipitate small airway bronchospasm, and β1-specific blocking agents such as metoprolol are preferred.

Class III Antiarrhythmic Drugs (Amiodarone, Sotalol, Bretylium)

The Class III antiarrhythmic agents act principally by potassium channel blockade. Thus, they prolong repolarization and refractoriness of most cardiac tissues. Bretylium elevates the ventricular fibrillation threshold and is successful in suppressing recurrent ventricular arrhythmias in patients with myocardial injury or hypoxia.[3,8,62] Although bretylium is a peripheral vasodilator, it does not interfere with myocardial contractility. Amiodarone and sotalol have additional beta-adrenergic blocking effects,[11,88,104] and amiodarone has lesser sodium and calcium channel blocking effects. The ECG effects of these drugs are to increase the PR and QT intervals without affecting the QRS duration.

Bretylium has been used only as an intravenous preparation for hemodynamically unstable ventricular tachycardias and fibrillation and has been largely replaced by intravenous amiodarone. Oral sotalol and amiodarone are useful agents for chronic prevention of otherwise medically resistant ventricular tachycardia and almost any supraventricular tachycardia. They have unique efficacy in treating automatic tachycardias, such as atrial ectopic tachycardia.

Amiodarone is available as an intravenous preparation and is finding wider use in the intensive care setting. Studies have shown amiodarone to be quite effective against ventricular and supraventricular arrhythmias in the normal heart as well as postoperative arrhythmias in repaired congenital heart disease, especially hemodynamically significant JET. An intravenous load is administered over at least 30 to 45 minutes and may be repeated to achieve the desired effect. An infusion is needed to maintain the effect. Although there are no direct negative inotropic effects of amiodarone, alpha-adrenergic blocking properties and resultant hypotension may occur. Intravenous volume expansion or calcium chloride is used to treat secondary hypotension. Significant prolongation of the QT_c may occur, resulting in the development of torsade de pointes, and patients should be evaluated with serial ECGs. Additionally, amiodarone decreases conductivity of nodal tissues and may produce significant sinus bradycardia, sinus arrest, or variable AV block, especially if preexisting disease exists in those tissues. Temporary or permanent pacing may be needed. Long-term systemic side effects of amiodarone include phototoxicity, corneal deposits, altered thyroid function, and depressed liver function. Pulmonary interstitial fibrosis rarely occurs with prolonged chronic use, but shock lung may rarely occur in the acute setting. Treatment for these side effects consists of discontinuing the antiarrhythmic medication and supportive therapies. Unfortunately, amiodarone is very lipophilic and has an extremely long elimination half-life, making treatment of chronic side effects a problem.

Sotalol has combined beta-adrenergic and potassium channel blockade, making it a useful agent in the therapy of supraventricular and ventricular arrhythmias. Sotalol is an oral drug with similar electrophysiologic effects as amiodarone without the systemic toxicities. Sotalol causes QT interval prolongation, in a dose-related manner, increasing the risk of *torsade de pointes* to a greater extent than amiodarone. In addition, sinus bradycardia, sinus arrest, or AV block may occur, necessitating the placement of temporary or permanent pacing devices. The beta-blocking effects are responsible for other side effects such as decreased ventricular function, fatigue, dizziness, and syncope.

Class IV Antiarrhythmic Drugs (Calcium Channel Blockers)

The Class IV drugs are calcium channel inhibitors.[61] Verapamil is the most frequently used drug of this class in children, although it has more negative inotropic properties than other subclasses of calcium channel blockers, such as nifedipine and diltiazem.[125] These agents slow conduction in calcium channel-rich tissues such as the sinoatrial and AV nodes. Electrocardiographic effects may include sinus slowing and prolongation of the PR interval.

Before the availability of adenosine, intravenous verapamil was widely used to terminate AVNRT and AVRT. However, due to reports of hypotension, bradycardia, and cardiac arrest in infants, the use of intravenous verapamil fell out of favor and is best avoided in infants younger than 1 year of age.[26] Although all calcium channel blockers cause some degree of negative inotropy and peripheral vasodilation, diltiazem appears to be safer than verapamil and still provides excellent negative dromotropy. Both agents are excellent choices to slow the ventricular response in the presence of atrial fibrillation or flutter. The exception is in patients with WPW syndrome and atrial flutter or fibrillation; the ventricular response may actually be enhanced via the accessory pathway, due to *relative* block in the AV node, and therefore it is not indicated in this setting. Unless there is certainty that the tachycardia is supraventricular, calcium channel blockers should also not be used for wide-complex, regular tachycardias. Great care should be taken when using these agents in combination with beta-blockers due to their combined negative inotropic, chronotropic, and dromotropic effects.

Complications of calcium antagonists in the ICU setting are peripheral vasodilation, decreased myocardial contractility, sinus bradycardia, and atrioventricular block, any of which may lead to hypotension and shock.

Other Antiarrhythmic Drugs

Adenosine Adenosine is an endogenous nucleoside that in high dose produces sinus bradycardia and transient conduction block in the AV node.[89,113] This effect is mediated through specific membrane A_1 adenosine receptors coupled to adenylate cyclase and specific sarcolemmal potassium channels.[61] The transient effects are due to its rapid uptake and deamination by red blood cells, which result in a very short half-life (less than 10 seconds). The action of adenosine is antagonized by methylxanthines, including theophylline, and therefore patients receiving these medications may be relatively resistant to adenosine. The effects of adenosine are dose-dependent and time-dependent. Atrioventricular block usually develops within 10 to 30 seconds after an intravenous bolus injection. In general, accessory pathway conduction is not influenced by adenosine.

Clinically, intravenous adenosine will abruptly terminate approximately 90% of cases of reentrant tachycardias that involve the sinoatrial or AV nodes,[93] namely, sinus node reentry, AVRT, and AVNRT. Adenosine may also be useful for determining the mechanism of unknown arrhythmias.[89] Transient AV block by adenosine may reveal atrial flutter or other atrial tachycardias by blocking the ventricular response,[20] without affecting the primary arrhythmia mechanism. The failure of adenosine to terminate a wide-complex tachycardia suggests that the arrhythmia is VT or a preexcited atrial tachycardia rather than an aberrantly conducted SVT. Some forms of right ventricular outflow tract VT in the otherwise normal heart are also terminated by adenosine.

Adenosine is initially administered as a 50 to 100 mcg/kg rapid bolus into a large peripheral vein. Failing the initial dose, increasing doses up to 300 mcg/kg may be administered every 1 to 2 minutes as needed. Following tachycardia conversion, the initial escape rhythm may include PVCs, marked sinus bradycardia, AV block, and, rarely, atrial fibrillation. This drug should not be administered unless an external defibrillator is available. Systemic side effects are common but usually mild and short-lived; they include dyspnea, flushing, chest discomfort, bronchospasm, coughing, headache, and hypotension. In children with impaired contractility and uncertain volume status, cautious monitoring of blood pressure is necessary. Adenosine should be used with caution in patients with asthma. Since adenosine usually does not have significant or prolonged negative inotropic effects, it is preferable to verapamil in patients with impaired left ventricular function, concomitant beta-adrenergic blockade, or wide-complex tachycardia.

Digoxin The use of digitalis glycosides is time-honored,[61] and children are frequently receiving digoxin upon arrival to the intensive care unit. Its primary action is inhibition of membrane-bound Na^+-K^+ ATPase, with resultant intracellular calcium loading. Its primary cardiac electrophysiologic effect is AV conduction delay, related to its effect on calcium traffic, and by enhancing vagal influences. The glycosidic portion of the digoxin molecule enhances carotid sinus baroreceptor reactivity, which leads to increased vagal tone and decreased sympathetic tone. In addition, it appears to have a central parasympathetic influence. In ventricular muscle, digoxin shortens the action potential and decreases the VF threshold, thus explaining the tendency for digoxin to induce ventricular tachyarrhythmias. Digoxin slows the normal sinus rate, increases the PR interval, and causes visible alteration (coving) of the ST segments. QRS interval duration is unaffected, even at toxic doses. The QT interval may be shortened as a result of hastened ventricular repolarization.

Similar to calcium channel blockers, the major applications of digoxin are for treatment and prevention of reentrant supraventricular tachyarrhythmias that involve the sinoatrial or AV node and ventricular rate control in the presence of atrial flutter or fibrillation. Unlike verapamil, however, its AV node blocking effects are countered by physiologic periods of vagolysis or enhanced adrenergic states, as may occur during exercise. Systemic loading, even when administered parenterally, requires at least 12 to 16 hours; thus, its use in the ICU setting may be limited. Digoxin may precipitate ventricular ectopy and arrhythmias, especially in patients with an unstable electrolyte status. Digoxin also may shorten accessory pathway refractoriness in a patient with WPW syndrome, potentially increasing the ventricular rate response to atrial fibrillation. Therefore, electrophysiologists advise against the use of digoxin in patients with WPW.

Systemic signs of toxicity include visual disturbances, disorientation, anxiety, drowsiness, abdominal pain, hyperkalemia, nausea, and vomiting. Cardiac signs of toxicity are exclusively proarrhythmias: advanced sinoatrial and AV block in younger patients and, additionally, a variety of ventricular or atrial tachyarrhythmias in adults; however, any of these proarrhythmias may occur at any age. An SVT with AV conduction blockade is the classic sign of digoxin toxicity, and failure to recognize this and administration of additional doses of digoxin may be catastrophic. The biologic response to digoxin is variable, and therapeutic levels vary widely in children. Neonates may have artificially elevated levels due to maternal digoxin-like substances. Furthermore, the pharmacokinetics of digoxin are altered by multiple agents, including phenytoin, lidocaine, quinidine, and amiodarone,[61] and the dose of digoxin should be decreased in patients concomitantly receiving verapamil. The coincident use of digoxin with either verapamil or a beta-blocker may result in prohibitive bradycardia, although their coincident use is not absolutely contraindicated. These factors tend to limit the use of digoxin, which is no longer the drug of choice in patients having an SVT without a precise diagnosis.

Recognizing digoxin toxicity is important because the emergent use of digoxin-specific Fab fragments (Digibind) may be life-saving. Factors that predispose to digoxin toxicity include high serum level (suspect dosing error, intentional poisoning, renal disease, hypothyroidism, coexisting drugs), coexistent myocardial ischemia, myocarditis, hypoxemia, hypokalemia, hypercalcemia, alkalosis, and coincident use of adrenergic drugs. Indications for the use of Digibind include hyperkalemia, the new occurrence or worsening of a bradycardia, or the occurrence of a tachyarrhythmia in a patient in whom digoxin ingestion is known or strongly suspected. Serum concentrations may be misleading and should not be considered steady state unless the ingestion occurred at least 6 hours previously. Especially if there is a delay in Digibind administration, arrhythmias should be aggressively treated. Atrioventricular block should be treated with atropine or a temporary pacing catheter, and ventricular tachycardia with intravenous phenytoin or lidocaine. Hyperkalemia should be treated by standard means, excluding intravenous calcium. The dose of Digibind is calculated based on total body load of digoxin. If the amount of digoxin received is known, then 1 vial (40 mg) per 0.5 mg digoxin is given intravenously over 15 to 30 minutes. If a steady-state serum concentration is known, then calculate the total body load (TBL): TBL = serum concentration (ng/mL) × 5.6 × weight (kg)/1000, then administer 1 vial (40 mg) per 0.5 mg TBL. If digoxin toxicity is highly suspected and dose or level of digoxin is unknown, then 10 vials (400 mg) should be administered. A bolus injection may be given should cardiac arrest be imminent. Cardioversion may be necessary should the patient be unstable, although there is additional risk of this, because digoxin lowers the ventricular fibrillation threshold. Prophylactic administration of lidocaine is advisable in those cases.

Magnesium Anecdotal reports of the use of intravenous magnesium to treat torsade de pointes and ventricular arrhythmias associated with prolonged QT syndrome have indicated that this drug may have a role in the treatment of ventricular arrhythmias. Side effects of magnesium include hypotension and hypotonia, which may lead to respiratory complications. This drug should be considered for patients with ventricular arrhythmias and prolonged QT syndrome.

Treatment of Tachyarrhythmias Using Vagal Maneuvers

An abrupt increase in parasympathetic tone generated by a variety of vagal maneuvers can result in transient AV block that will terminate any reentry arrhythmia involving the SA or AV node. These include SA node reentry, AV node reentry, and AV reciprocating tachycardias. The maneuvers in Table 8-10 are most effective when used soon after the onset of symptoms, before sympathetic tone rises to a high level.[124] These simple maneuvers can be taught to most parents so that they can be applied even at home. Failing these maneuvers, pharmacological enhancement of vagal tone can be provided in the intensive care unit or emergency department using intravenous phenylephrine or edrophonium. Caveats to their use should be heeded, but phenylephrine, in particular, may be a good substitute for adenosine, if adenosine is contraindicated or not effective.

Table 8-10 Physical Maneuvers for Terminating AV Node–Dependent Supraventricular Tachycardias

Enhancement of vagal tone to the AV node	Exposure of upper half of face to ice water or ice in washcloth
	Finger in throat (gag maneuver)
	Right carotid sinus massage
Sudden volume/pressure changes to the right heart	Valsalva maneuver (has vagal component)
	Bearing down
	Squatting
	Gentle pressure to abdomen in an infant until he or she resists
	Turning patient upside down

AV, atrioventricular.

Treatment of Bradyarrhythmias

A wide array of pharmacologic and device treatment options exist for bradycardia encountered in the intensive care setting. It must be remembered that in infants and all patients with diminished systolic function, chronotropic support is particularly important, due to relatively reduced capacity for inotropic recruitment during periods of hemodynamic stress. It also must be remembered that bradycardia is age and situation dependent. A heart rate of 50 beats per minute may be tolerated in a young child but not in an infant. A heart rate of 90 beats per minute is not usually hemodynamically acceptable in an infant following cardiac surgery. Patients with decreased cardiac output (e.g., poor perfusion, hypotension, decreased urine output, mental status changes), or congestive heart failure, may require augmentation of heart rate to hasten recovery time and improve outcomes.

Pharmacologic Agents for Treatment of Bradycardia

Pharmacologic augmentation of heart rate is accomplished though the use of either vagolytic or β-adrenergic agents. Atropine is a vagolytic agent that substantially increases sinoatrial rate and improves AV conduction in most patients. However, impaired AV conduction due to surgical trauma or edema of the AV node may not be as responsive to atropine. Also, atropine is not expected to be effective treatment for impaired AV conduction caused by pathology below the level of the AV node (i.e., the bundle of His and bundle branches). It should be noted that immediately following cardiac transplant, bradycardia may not be responsive to atropine, because the heart has been at least temporarily denervated. Atropine has also been successfully used in the occasional infant with a severe Bezold-Jarisch reflex (myocardial overstretch) causing hypervagotonia/asystole following cardiac surgery.

Of the adrenergic agents, isoproterenol is the most widely used for pure heart rate augmentation, although epinephrine and norepinephrine also cause varying degrees of beta-receptor stimulation. Isoproterenol is a nonselective, pure beta-adrenergic agonist. As such, it increases both the chronotropic and the inotropic state of the heart. It also lowers systemic vascular resistance and, in certain settings of pulmonary arteriolar hypertension, may reduce pulmonary vascular resistance. Its major drawbacks include increase of myocardial and total body oxygen consumption, hyperglycemia, and increase of metabolic requirements by the injured myocardium. Therefore, its use must be weighed against the real potential for myocardial damage. Depending upon the etiology, isoproterenol may rapidly prove lifesaving by improving AV conduction. All catecholamines carry arrhythmogenic potential, and caution must be exercised in using these agents.

Temporary Electrical Pacing for Treatment of Bradycardia

Various methods of temporary cardiac pacing should be available in the intensive care setting for treatment of hemodynamically significant bradycardia in which drugs are either ineffective or not desirable. The method of artificial pacing should be selected based upon the mechanism of bradycardia, the extent of hemodynamic fragility, the anticipated duration of temporary pacing, and the patient's level of alertness and need for sedation. The methods of artificial pacing currently available include temporary transvenous, epicardial, transesophageal, and external transthoracic pacing. All of these methods can be used until appropriate rhythm is restored spontaneously or until a permanent pacing device can be implanted. In general, transthoracic and transesophageal pacing are the most noxious and require heavy sedation; transvenous requires central venous access and, therefore, carries risk of bacteremia and vascular or cardiac damage; and epicardial, of course, requires surgical exposure. Irrespective of the method of temporary pacing, it should be remembered that the ability for an electrical current to depolarize myocardium depends upon reasonably normal electrolyte (especially potassium) and acid-base status.

Other than the transthoracic (transcutaneous) pacing systems, all temporary pacing conductors consist of insulated wires that are connected to an external temporary pacing device. Although unipolar pacing is possible, it is painful and often difficult to accomplish. Therefore, most temporary pacing conductors are bipolar, consisting of at least two insulated wires within a catheter, with one serving as the cathode and the other, the anode. The typical pacing device can pace a single chamber (atrial or ventricular) or both chambers ("dual chamber"). Older devices allow one to set the pacing rate, the interval between paced atrial and paced or sensed ventricular events ("A-V delay"), the pacing output of each chamber (up to 20 milliamperes), and the device's capacity to sense intrinsic ventricular activity (ventricular "sensitivity"). These terms will be further discussed later in this chapter. Newer devices function similarly to permanent pacemakers with the ability to choose from a broader variety of pacing modes and refractory periods.

The pacing output is selected based upon the pacing threshold of the chamber paced. This is defined as the minimum output (usually programmable as current, in milliamperes) resulting in a propagated response (P or QRS on the monitor). Thresholds are determined by slowly decreasing the output until capture is lost. Determining whether a propagated response has occurred is aided by the presence of an arterial waveform, because, sometimes, the polarization energy from the pacing spike obscures the ability to identify a surface QRS. Typically, the output is maintained at two times the threshold, if possible. Thresholds should be measured at least daily. If, over time, the threshold increases toward the maximum output of the device, one should reverse the polarity of the pacing leads. This is accomplished by switching the cathodal and anodal wires from the conducting catheter to the opposite poles of the pacing device. Often, this will decrease the threshold slightly. Sensitivity refers to the size of the intrinsic cardiac signals (electrograms) that the device will recognize. If an intrinsic event is recognized by the pacing device sooner than the programmed low rate, and the pacing device is programmed to a demand mode, the pacing device will inhibit its output and restart the low-rate clock. Think of sensitivity as a wall that can be raised and lowered with the device on one side looking over at the intrinsic electrograms (atrial or ventricular). A higher sensitivity actually refers to a lower wall and the ability to recognize smaller intrinsic signals. The level of the wall is determined by the sensitivity setting on the device, measured in millivolts. The lower millivolt settings reflect a greater sensitivity. A setting should be selected that allows the device to see intrinsic impulses but not noncardiac electrical or motion artifacts (noise). The "asynchronous"

setting prevents all sensing by the device and paces at the chosen rate without inhibition by intrinsic beats. In pacemaker-dependent patients, batteries in the temporary pacing device should be replaced regularly (every day or two). This can be safely accomplished by swapping a fully charged device for the old device instead of changing batteries in the currently used device.

At the end of most open-heart operations, two pairs of pacing wires (one pair for an atrium and one for a ventricle) are sutured to the epicardial surface and tunneled through the skin in the subxyphoid region. They may then be used for temporary bipolar pacing, using the previously described programmable temporary pacing device. Typically, these temporary pacing wires may be used for about 2 weeks before the pacing thresholds increase to prohibitive levels. This mode of pacing is not painful to the patient.

Temporary transvenous pacing catheters are passed to the endocardial surface of the right ventricle through a venous sheath in the femoral, axillary, internal jugular, or subclavian vein. Connector cables are then attached to the external pacing device. Balloon-tipped, flow-directed, bipolar pacing catheters are available that allow easier placement of the catheter from the left subclavian or either internal jugular vein into the right ventricle. Fluoroscopy is not generally necessary when using these catheters, although echocardiography may provide guidance. Confirmation of lead placement can be performed by first observing adequate ventricular pacing and then performing chest radiograph. Permanent pacing leads can also be used for temporary pacing. The lead is placed as just described and attached to a permanent pacemaker that has been secured externally. Fluoroscopy is necessary for placement of these leads. Preformed, J-shaped temporary pacing catheters are also available for atrial pacing, but placing these also requires fluoroscopy. Other than in immediately postoperative patients (who already have temporary epicardial pacing wires), the need for *temporary* synchronous, atrioventricular pacing (i.e., requiring atrial and ventricular leads)—versus ventricular pacing alone—in the pediatric patient is limited. Such situations would more often benefit from temporary placement of a permanent atrial lead, using fluoroscopy.

Another method of cardiac pacing involves the use of a transesophageal pacing catheter passed through the nares and positioned posterior to the left atrium. Positioning can be confirmed by successful atrial pacing at a rate faster than the prevailing sinus rate—and then by chest radiograph. This method of pacing may be used for atrial overdrive pacing to terminate reentrant supraventricular tachycardias, for initiation and/or diagnostic evaluation of tachycardias, or for short-term chronotropic support in patients having intact AV conduction. Ventricular pacing is possible in smaller patients but is not practical given other alternatives. The energy necessary to afford atrial capture may require the use of portable electrophysiologic stimulators capable of increasing the duration over which each pulse is delivered (the pulse width)—usually to 10 msec—in addition to currents of at least 20 milliamperes (mA). Sensing of intrinsic atrial electrograms may be possible but is not usually necessary except in the case of diagnostic assessment of a rhythm. Pacing outputs should be set to 2 to 5 mA greater than the pacing threshold. If electrograms can be recorded, catheter positioning is best when the atrial electrograms are larger than the ventricular electrograms, but this may not always be obtained. The major risks of this technique relate to inadvertent passage of the catheter into the lower airway or mucosal bleeding. Transesophageal pacing may be painful—depending on the energy required to pace the heart. It should not be performed for any significant time.

Transthoracic pacing was developed by Paul Zoll, and the device bearing his name has become synonymous with the technique. The Zoll stimulator, and similar devices manufactured by other companies, generates a relatively large current at low voltage through the chest from large-surface skin patches placed on the surface of the chest and back or from the apex to the right shoulder. Several sizes of patches are now available for patients of nearly any size. Although the current density is low, as might be expected, this method of pacing also stimulates chest wall muscles to contract and is quite painful, requiring the patient to be sedated. This form of pacing is invaluable for patients with any kind of bradycardia who need immediate pacing. Even in the well-sedated infant, this method of pacing will result in skin damage if continued for more than a few hours. These devices are also capable of transcutaneous cardioversion or defibrillation through the patches, should the need arise.

INTENSIVE CARE UNIT APPROACH TO THE DIAGNOSIS AND TREATMENT OF ARRHYTHMIAS

This final section incorporates the definitions, concepts, and therapy options described previously to provide a systematic, arrhythmia-based approach to acute diagnosis and treatment. A compilation of antiarrhythmic drugs and dosing appears as Table 8-11. In addition, definitive treatment options are discussed, including catheter ablation, surgical ablation, and device implantation, because many patients are cared for pre- and postprocedure in the ICU.

Summary of Treatment of Bradyarrhythmias

Acute Stabilization

1. If the patient is hemodynamically unstable, is in heart failure, or develops ventricular arrhythmias as an escape rhythm, immediate measures should be taken to increase the heart rate, including one or more of the following:
   a. Atropine, 0.02 mg/kg IV bolus
   b. Isoproterenol
   c. Temporary pacing
      i. Ventricular pacing adequate in most situations.
      ii. Atrial pacing may be used if AV conduction is intact (reliable only with atrial epicardial wires, transvenous J-shaped temporary catheter, or a permanent pacemaker lead).
      iii. AV sequential pacing is beneficial when LV function is impaired (using epicardial wires or transvenous pacing catheters).
   d. Discontinue all sedatives and other medications that may contribute to bradycardia
   e. "Digibind" if AVB is caused by digitalis overdose

2. If the patient is hemodynamically stable:
   a. Discontinue sedatives and other medications that may contribute to bradycardia.
   b. Temporary pacing measures should be available if deterioration in clinical status.
   c. "Digibind" if hyperkalemia, second-degree AV block, tachyarrhythmias, and strong suspicion of digoxin overdose
3. Permanent pacemaker implantation if bradycardia is persistent and satisfies published recommendations (Table 8-12).

Permanent Pacemakers

Most children requiring permanent cardiac pacing have undergone operative treatment of CHD[65] or have congenital complete atrioventricular block (CAVB). Indications for permanent pacemaker implantation have been formulated[45] and modified for the pediatric age group (see Table 8-12). Children who require permanent pacing and who have been admitted to an intensive care unit prior to implantation usually fall into one of two categories: (1) CAVB just developed during congenital heart surgery; or (2) they had symptoms of low cardiac output (especially syncope or seizures) and were demonstrated to have a bradycardic syndrome.

Those healthcare providers who care for children with permanent pacemakers are well served to familiarize themselves with the terminology used to describe standard pacemaker programming. As developed by the Intersociety Commission for Heart Disease and the North American Society of Pacing and Electrophysiology (ICHD/NASPE), the five-letter pacemaker code is used internationally. The first letter specifies which cardiac chambers are paced: A(trium), V(entricle), or D(ual). The second letter denotes which chamber is sensed: again A, V, D, or O if no sensing is performed. The third position describes the pacemaker response to a sensed electrical event: I(nhibited), T(riggered), D(ual response), or O for no response. For example, in VVI mode, the pacemaker paces and senses only in the ventricle and is *inhibited* by intrinsic ventricular activity if that activity is sensed sooner than the next paced event would occur based upon the programmed lower rate. In DDD mode, a dual-chamber pacemaker senses and paces in both chambers. *Triggering* of a ventricular paced event will occur after an atrial event if there is no intrinsic ventricular event sensed during the postatrial programmed AV delay. Sensing of intrinsic atrial and/or ventricular events before the next expected paced event according to the programmed lower rate or AV delay, respectively, will *inhibit* the pacemaker output to the atrium or ventricle, respectively.

The only letter used in the fourth position from the ICHD/NASPE code that is of common interest in pediatrics is "R," which denotes rate responsiveness.[108] Most contemporary devices are capable of increasing the rate based upon certain sensor-dependent physical or true physiologic changes. The most common sensor is a piezoelectric crystal in the pulse generator that produces an output proportional to the patient's physical activity. All modern pacemakers have bidirectional telemetry that allows reprogramming of multiple parameters (i.e., pacing mode, voltage output, sensitivity) and retrieval of pacemaker or patient data.

Even without full familiarity with permanent pacing systems, the intensivist should be acquainted with certain issues

Table 8-11   Drug Therapy for Arrhythmias Commonly Used in the Intensive Care Unit

Drug	Dose	Route	Drug Level	Side Effects
Therapies for Supraventricular Tachycardia				
Adenosine	50–300 mcg/kg	Rapid IV bolus, every 1 min to effect		Hypotension, bradycardia, sinus arrest, atrial fibrillation, headache, chest pain, bronchospasm
Digoxin	Total digitalizing dose (TDD) (mcg/kg/24 hr) 　　　　　　PO　　IV/IM Premature　20　　15 Full term　30　　20 < 2 yr old　40–50　30–40 2–10 yr old　30–40　20–30 > 10 yr old　10–15　　8–12 Give ½ TDD initially, then ¼ TDD q 8–18 hrs × 2 doses Maintenance dose (mcg/kg/day) Premature　5　　　3–4 Full term　8–10　　6–8 < 2 yr old　10–12　6–8 2–10 yr old　8–10　6–8 > 10 yr old　2.5–5　2–3 If < 10 yrs old, BID dosing; otherwise, QD		1–3 ng/mL	Sinus bradycardia, AV node block, and less commonly, atrial and ventricular tachyarrhythmias, diarrhea, nausea, vomiting, somnolence
Edrophonium	0.04 mg/kg	IV × 3 to effect		Profound bradycardia Abdominal pain
Phenylephrine	0.5–5 mcg/kg, titrate to blood pressure	IV bolus to effect		Hypertension
Verapamil	0.05–0.15 mg/kg, over 3 minutes	Slow IV bolus; may repeat after 15 min	100–300 ng/mL	Hypotension; may treat with $CaCl_2$ 10% (see text)
Therapies for Ventricular Tachycardia				
Lidocaine	*IV Bolus:* 1 mg/kg, repeat in 10 min if necessary *Infusion:* 20–50 mcg/kg/minute	IV bolus, infusion	1–7 mcg/mL	Hypotension Seizure CNS depression
Bretylium	5 mg/kg bolus; repeat as necessary up to 10 mg/kg	IV bolus		Hypotension
Magnesium sulfate	15–30 mg/kg	IV bolus		Hypotension Lethargy
Phenytoin	*IV Load:* 1–2 mg/kg/5 min up to 15 mg/kg; not faster than 1 mg/kg/min *Maintenance:* 5–10 mg/kg/12 hr	IV bolus, PO	15–20 mcg/mL	AV block Hypotension
Therapies for Supraventricular Tachycardia and for Ventricular Tachycardia				
Esmolol	500 mcg/kg IV bolus, then 100–1000 mcg/kg/min Increase every 2 min to effect	IV infusion	0.15–0.2 mcg/mL	Hypotension Bronchospasm Worsening of CHF Hypoglycemia
Propranolol	0.01–0.1 mg/kg slow bolus	IV bolus	20–150 ng/mL	Hypotension, asystole, bronchospasm, worsening CHF, hypoglycemia
Amiodarone	*IV Load:* 5 mg/kg over 25–45 min, may repeat × 2 *IV Maintenance:* 0.42 mg/kg/hr *PO Load:* 10 mg/kg/day divided q 8–12 hrs × 7–10 days *PO Maintenance:* 5 mg/kg/day (max. 200–400 mg/day)	IV, PO		Acute (IV): Hypotension, torsade de pointes VT, nausea, sinus bradycardia or AV block if intrinsic conduction disease, note significant drug–drug interactions
Procainamide	*IV Load:* 5–15 mg/kg (not to exceed 1 mg/kg/min) *Infusion:* 20–80 mcg/kg/min	IV, PO	4–8 mcg/mL NAPA: 10–30 mcg/mL	Hypotension, torsade de pointes VT, nausea, sinus bradycardia or AV block if intrinsic conduction disease
Propafenone	200–600 mg/m²/day divided q 6–8 hr	PO (IV not available in U.S.)	Follow QRS duration (should not increase by > 25%)	Proarrhythmia, nausea, paresthesias, tremor, hypotension
Flecainide	3–6 mg/kg/day divided q 8–12 hr	PO (IV not available in U.S.)	0.2–1.0 mcg/mL	Proarrhythmia, vision changes, lightheadedness, nausea
Sotalol	2–6 mg/kg/day divided q 8–12 hr	PO		See propranolol, torsade de pointes VT
Therapies for Bradyarrhythmias				
Atropine	0.01 mg/kg (not < 0.1 mg)	IV, IM		Tachycardia, dry mouth, CNS effects, flushing
Isoproterenol	0.1–2.0 mcg/kg/min, titrated	IV infusion		Tachycardia, hypotension, nausea, PVCs

Table 8-12   Recommendations for Pacemaker Implantation in the Pediatric Age Range*

Class I: Concensus for Implantation

1. Advanced second- or third-degree AV block associated with symptomatic bradycardia, congestive heart failure, or low cardiac output.
2. Sinus node dysfunction with correlation of symptoms during age-inappropriate bradycardia. The definition of bradycardia varies with the patient's age and expected heart rate.
3. Postoperative advanced second- or third-degree AV block that is not expected to resolve or persists at least 7 days after cardiac surgery.
4. Congenital third-degree AV block with a wide QRS escape rhythm or ventricular dysfunction.
5. Congenital third-degree AV block in the infant with a ventricular rate <50 to 55 bpm or with congenital heart disease and a ventricular rate <70 bpm.
6. Sustained pause-dependent VT, with or without prolonged QT, in which the efficacy of pacing is thoroughly documented.

Class IIa: Conflicting Evidence, with Weight of Evidence in Favor of Implantation

1. Bradycardia-tachycardia syndrome with the need for long-term antiarrhythmic drug treatment other than digitalis.
2. Congenital third-degree AV block beyond the first year of life with an average heart rate <50 bpm or abrupt pauses in ventricular rate that are two or three times the basic cycle length.
3. Long QT syndrome with 2:1 AV or third-degree AV block.
4. Asymptomatic sinus bradycardia in the child with complex congenital heart disease with resting heart rate <35 bpm or pauses in ventricular rate >3 seconds.

Class IIb: Conflicting Evidence, with Inadequate or Incomplete Evidence Supporting Implantation

1. Transient postoperative third-degree AV block that reverts to sinus rhythm with residual bifascicular block.
2. Congenital third-degree AV block in the asymptomatic neonate, child, or adolescent with an acceptable rate, narrow QRS complex, and normal ventricular function.
3. Asymptomatic sinus bradycardia in the adolescent with congenital heart disease with resting heart rate <35 bpm or pauses in ventricular rate >3 seconds.

Class III: General Agreement That Implantation is Not Indicated

1. Transient postoperative AV block with return of normal AV conduction within 7 days.
2. Asymptomatic postoperative bifascicular block with or without first-degree AV block.
3. Asymptomatic type I second-degree AV block.
4. Asymptomatic sinus bradycardia in the adolescent with longest RR interval <3 seconds and minimum heart rate >40 bpm.

bpm, beats per minute.
*Modified from the Joint American Heart Association and American College of Cardiology position statement from 1998: Gregoratos G, Cheitlin MD, Conill A, et al: ACC/AHA guidelines for implantation of cardiac pacemakers and antiarrhythmia devices. A report of the America College of Cardiology/American Heart Association Task Force Report on Practice Guidelines. *J Am Coll Cardiol* 31:1175–1209, 1998.

pertinent to these patients. These include recognition of gross lead fracture, disconnection, or dislodgment by radiograph; basic knowledge of rhythm strip interpretation of pacemaker failure to capture, failure to output, failure to sense, and artifact; and wound management of the newly implanted or chronically infected pacemaker pocket. If a high frequency current is being used near the pacemaker (such as from an electrocautery system), a doughnut magnet should be taped over the pacemaker to prevent pacemaker inhibition, especially if the patient is pacemaker-dependent. A magnetic field closes an electronic device known as a reed switch, which interrupts the pacemaker's sensing ability, thus assuring output.

Summary of Treatment of Tachyarrhythmias

The following outlines combine diagnostic and therapeutic considerations, much as one encounters in the clinical setting. Although, in general, supraventricular tachycardias are hemodynamically well tolerated and ventricular tachycardias less well tolerated, every patient should be carefully evaluated with respect to end-organ perfusion: blood pressure, sensorium, urine output, and skin perfusion. Indeed, the child with idiopathic ventricular tachycardia and a normal heart may simply feel palpitations, whereas the teenager with tetralogy of Fallot and atrial flutter with 1:1 AV conduction may be in shock. Any patient suspected of having a reentrant tachycardia and who presents with altered level of consciousness and other evidence for shock should undergo emergent cardioversion.

If the patient's clinical status permits, a thoughtful diagnostic approach will usually yield a better opportunity to provide accurate, focused therapy. This approach should include a full 12-lead ECG at standard 25 mm/sec and perhaps one at 50 mm/sec to help identify subtle electrical signals. Use of esophageal, epicardial, or intracavitary electrograms may prove valuable to identify the atrial events and relate them to the QRS. A disciplined accounting of the regularity of rate, the atrial/ventricular relationship, the P wave morphology(ies), the QRS morphology(ies), historical information, and response to adenosine will usually yield the diagnosis.

Generally, narrow complex tachycardias are supraventricular in origin, and wide complex are ventricular in origin. Certainly, there are exceptions to this. For instance, SVT with bundle branch aberrancy will have a wide QRS, as will SVT using an accessory pathway in the anterograde direction, either as a component of antidromic reciprocating tachycardia or as an "innocent bystander" in some other SVT. Conversely, infants can have ventricular tachycardia in which the QRS appears to be narrow but is actually prolonged when compared to age-appropriate normal values; and ventricular tachycardia emanating from the ventricular septum may be associated with a relatively narrow QRS in patients of any age. Because of this potential overlap, when therapy for one type of tachycardia fails, the patient should be considered as having the other type.

The most difficult to manage tachycardias are incessant tachycardias that are unresponsive to drugs or to direct current cardioversion; radiofrequency ablation of the tachycardia substrate is the procedure of last resort. Two caveats apply here: (1) some patients have a reentrant SVT that does terminate with standard AV nodal blocking agents for one or a few beats, and, because of the prevailing electrophysiologic conditions, the patient goes right back into SVT. This may appear to be an incessant *automatic* tachycardia, but careful scrutiny of the termination will reveal the actual mechanism. That patient requires pharmacologic agents that influence other components of the reentrant circuit; (2) patients having primary atrial tachycardias and who are given an AV nodal blocking agent will appear to experience transient termination of the tachycardia. In fact, careful observation will reveal continuation of the abnormally fast P wave rate during the period of apparent termination. That patient also requires a different approach.

A final point worthy of emphasis is that the Class III agent amiodarone is gaining support in the acute management of tachyarrhythmias. In the 2000 Guidelines for Cardiopulmonary Resuscitation,[46] amiodarone has been added as an alternative therapy should the more traditional pharmacologic therapies or cardioversion fail. Amiodarone has been shown to be effective in treating most forms of tachycardia,[85,118] especially with incessant varieties or in the postoperative setting. Amiodarone should be considered when time and hemodynamic status prohibit the trial of multiple interventions. It is important to be aware that the termination of tachycardia with amiodarone may leave the patient with severe bradycardia or AV block requiring back-up pacing.

Diagnosis and Management of Narrow Complex Tachyarrhythmias

1. Regular 1:1 relationship between P & QRS and long R-P (QRS-P > P-QRS)
   a. Sinus tachycardia (briefly slows with adenosine)
      i. Consider presence of excessive beta-adrenergic therapy, low cardiac output, pain, anemia or fever, and treat underlying problem
   b. Sinus node reentry tachycardia (abrupt onset and termination; P wave axis and morphology identical to that observed in normal sinus rhythm)
      i. Vagal maneuvers
      ii. Adenosine, phenylephrine, edrophonium, esmolol, verapamil (if > 1 year old)
   c. Atrial tachycardia (paroxysmal or incessant; P-wave morphology distinct from sinus)
      i. Adenosine will terminate some tachycardias using reentry or triggered automaticity as the mechanism
      ii. Establish incessant nature of tachycardia by attempting atrial overdrive pacing to terminate tachycardia; start at 75% of tachycardia cycle length (CL=60,000/rate in beats per minute) and pace for 3 to 5 seconds; increase rate, as necessary
      iii. If incessant, evaluate ventricular function
      iv. If function normal, consider esmolol; if diminished ventricular function, start with digoxin
      v. Add class IC or III agent to that used from iv. Intravenous amiodarone is most efficacious, but propafenone or flecainide may be useful in stable patients capable of oral drug administration
      vi. Radiofrequency catheter ablation
2. Regular relationship between P and QRS and short R-P (QRS-P < P-QRS)
   a. AV reciprocating tachycardia (AVRT) (the P-wave morphology depends on the location of the accessory

pathway) and AV node reentry tachycardia (AVNRT):
   i. Vagal maneuvers
   ii. Adenosine, phenylephrine, edrophonium, or intravenous verapamil (if > 1 year old)
   iii. Atrial overdrive pacing for termination, especially if temporary epicardial wires in place
   iv. If patient is unstable and SVT immediately recurrent:
      (a) Intravenous esmolol or procainamide
      (b) Intravenous amiodarone
      (c) Radiofrequency catheter ablation
   v. If patient is stable and SVT immediately or frequently recurrent:
      (a) same as iv(a), or oral propranolol (verapamil or digoxin also acceptable if no delta wave with sinus beats)
      (b) Oral propafenone, flecainide, sotalol, or amiodarone
3. Nonsustained but incessant tachycardia: long R-P
   a. If 1:1 P & QRS relationship, may be atrial ectopic tachycardia or permanent form of junctional reciprocating tachycardia (PJRT = type of AVRT): See 1. c. iii., iv., v., vi.
   b. If P wave rate > QRS rate, must be atrial tachycardia: favors Class III agents
   c. If P wave rate = QRS rate, and P waves negative in II, III, aVF, likely PJRT: favors Class IC agents
4. Regular R-R interval with V-A dissociation, and QRS rate > P wave: JET
   a. Normalize blood electrolytes, and limit exogenous catecholamines
   b. Digoxin and atrial overdrive pace to permit AV synchrony, if possible
   c. If rate slowing is unsuccessful, add one of the following agents:
      i. Procainamide
      ii. Propafenone (only enteral formulation available in U.S.)
      iii. Amiodarone (may be the most effective)[85]
   d. Surface cooling to a rectal temperature of 33°C to 35°C. (plus paralysis to prevent shivering) may supercede "c" above or may be a useful adjunct to pharmacologic therapy. Its exact place in the treatment algorithm for JET is not completely established. In postoperative JET, the ultimate goal of therapy is to reduce the junctional rate to permit atrial pacing and allow AV synchronous activation. This generally means rate reduction to <180 beats per minute in infants and <150 beats per minute in older children.
   e. If the above fail and hemodynamic instability is present, consider His bundle catheter ablation and permanent pacemaker implantation
5. Irregularly irregular QRS rate with indistinct or "sawtooth" P waves: atrial fibrillation or flutter
   a. Obtain atrial electrograms to discriminate these rhythms
   b. Atrial fibrillation (always irregularly irregular atrial electrograms)
      i. If duration of tachycardia unknown or > 36 hours, transesophageal echo to assess for intra-atrial

thrombus (may be necessary in Fontan patients with atrial flutter, as well)
  ii. Ventricular rate control with intravenous esmolol, verapamil, or diltiazem
  iii. Synchronized direct current cardioversion
 c. Atrial flutter (regular atrial rate)
  i. Consider atrial overdrive pacing to terminate tachycardia
  ii. Pharmacologic cardioversion possible with Class IA, IC, or III agents (procainamide most commonly used); Class IA agents must always be accompanied by calcium- or β-adrenergic blocking agent
  iii. Synchronized direct current cardioversion

Diagnosis and Management of Wide Complex Tachyarrhythmias

The differential diagnosis of wide complex tachyarrhythmias includes VT, aberrantly conducted SVT, and SVT conducted antegrade over an accessory pathway. Useful methods for detecting SVT include vagal maneuvers or adenosine to transiently block conduction in the AV node. This will expose atrial flutter or atrial tachycardia and will terminate a reentry arrhythmia that uses the AV node as part of its reentry circuit. Specific therapy as outlined previously should be initiated. If the mechanism of the tachycardia remains unclear, it should be considered to be VT until proved otherwise.

1. If the patient is hemodynamically unstable or in heart failure, immediate measures should be taken to terminate the tachycardia, including one or more of the following:
 a. Prompt electrical cardioversion (2 J/kg) and repeat, if necessary
 b. Lidocaine, 1 mg/kg IV bolus, and, if necessary, repeat every 5 minutes for two additional doses; followed by an infusion of 20 to 50 mcg/kg/min
 c. Procainamide, 10 to 15 mg/kg infused over 30 to 60 minutes. If hypotension or the QRS widens, the infusion should be slowed
 d. Amiodarone, 5 mg/kg over 20 to 45 minutes, and may be repeated in tandem two additional times. Hypotension may be treated with intravenous calcium chloride, volume, or by slowing drug infusion. (This drug now supersedes procainamide in many algorithms.)
 e. Electrolyte abnormalities, acid-base balance, hypoxemia, and hypoglycemia should be corrected concomitantly
 f. Medications that may be aggravating ectopy should be stopped if possible
 g. Specific therapies for drug-induced ventricular tachycardia (e.g., "Digibind" and phenytoin for digoxin overdose; sodium bicarbonate [NaHCO₃] for tricyclic antidepressant overdose)
 h. Extracorporeal membrane oxygenation has been successfully used to support the circulation in instances of drug resistant, incessant ventricular tachycardia due to acute myocarditis
2. If the patient has a prolonged QT interval during sinus rhythm and develops incessant torsade de pointes, emergent electrical cardioversion (generally

asynchronous) is mandatory, followed by one or more of the following:
 a. Lidocaine, 1 mg/kg IV bolus, repeated every 5 minutes for two additional doses and then followed by an infusion of 20 to 50 mcg/kg/min
 b. Magnesium sulfate, 15 to 30 mg/kg IV bolus, followed by an infusion of 15 mg/kg/min
 c. If patient is bradycardic, pre- or postcardioversion, temporary pacing or judicious use of isoproterenol may be useful
 d. Correction of hypokalemia
3. If the patient is hemodynamically stable, metabolic factors and medications that may be aggravating ectopy should be corrected or stopped if possible. An attempt should be made to determine the mechanism of the arrhythmia so that directed therapy may be administered. If the diagnosis is ventricular tachycardia, a variety of agents may be efficacious and can be tested serially. Based upon a combination of the side-effect profiles and published efficacies, an example of a logical sequence of drug trials might include beta-blocker, mexiletine (or IV lidocaine), sotalol, procainamide, propafenone, and amiodarone. Individualized therapy is crucial; for example, ventricular tachycardias following right heart surgery are generally not responsive to Class IA agents but may be responsive to Class IB drugs. Patients with poor ventricular function may be especially prone to the proarrhythmic effects of Class IC agents.

Cardioversion and Defibrillation

For unstable patients with hypotension or altered mental status due to atrial or ventricular tachyarrhythmias, prompt cardioversion or defibrillation is indicated. Electrical energy is applied between two paddles or adhesive electrode patches placed on the chest or on the chest and back. The success of this procedure depends on its ability to fully depolarize the heart, thereby terminating most reentry tachyarrhythmias and allowing sinus rhythm to be restored. Automatic tachyarrhythmias persist despite cardioversion and may actually accelerate due to the release of endogenous catecholamines.

Cardioversion refers to a shock, usually in the range of 0.25 to 4 J/kg, that is delivered synchronously with the QRS complex of the surface ECG. Energy delivery synchronous with the QRS complex reduces the risk of conversion of the tachycardia to ventricular fibrillation. The lower energy range is generally used for atrial arrhythmias, and the upper energy range for ventricular arrhythmias. Defibrillation is a high-energy shock, usually 2 to 4 J/kg, delivered asynchronously for the treatment of ventricular fibrillation.

Permanent Implantable Defibrillators

For patients with a history of sudden cardiac death and those at high risk for lethal ventricular arrhythmias, and especially for those who have failed or are intolerant of antiarrhythmic agents, the implantable cardioverter-defibrillator (ICD) is recommended therapy. The basic components of these systems are (1) a lead system for sensing the ventricular rate; (2) a lead system for delivering energy to the heart; and (3) the generator housing the battery, capacitors, and electronic circuitry. The rate-sensing lead is either a bipolar endocardial lead placed in the right ventricular apex or an epicardial pair of sensing leads attached to a ventricle. The shocking leads include one or more coils, mesh patches, or metal arrays that may be epicardial (patches), intravascular (coils), or subcutaneous (arrays). Most contemporary systems involve a rate-sensing lead and shocking coil(s) that are incorporated into a single transvenous device, and the current is delivered between the coil(s) and the ICD outer can. This approach has the added benefit of not requiring a thoracotomy to place defibrillation patches. These systems can be implanted in children down to about 25 kg, although the ICD itself may have to be implanted in the abdominal wall and the lead tunneled down to it in the smaller patients.

ICDs deliver energy as a biphasic shock (i.e., with the conductors alternating over milliseconds as cathode, then anode), and most can be programmed to deliver up to 35 J. The current implantable devices (considered fourth generation) are multifunctional and can deliver not only high-energy shocks for defibrillation, but also low-energy shocks for synchronized cardioversion, or overdrive pacing for termination of sustained VT. Newer systems are capable of dual-chamber bradycardia pacing and can discriminate SVTs from VTs using a variety of recognition algorithms. These devices are fully programmable by means of telemetry and are capable of storing data that recall the device status, detected tachyarrhythmias, and delivered therapy.

Postoperative management of these patients is not complicated, but different systems will respond to magnet application in different ways. Consultation with an electrophysiologist should always accompany management of these patients. Also, their treatment modes should be inactivated just prior to exposure to high-frequency electromagnetic fields, such as electrocautery. Finally, like patients with pacemakers, patients with these devices may not undergo magnetic resonance imaging.

A 1993 retrospective international multicenter study summarized the use of ICDs in 125 patients younger than 20 years of age at the time of implantation.[101] The youngest child was 2 years old and weighed 9.7 kg. Patients presented with cardiac arrest (76%), recurrent ventricular arrhythmias (10%), or syncope (10%). Associated cardiovascular diseases included cardiomyopathy (58%) and CHD (18%). A subset of patients with no apparent structural heart disease had primary arrhythmias, including ventricular fibrillation (15%) and the long QT syndrome (11%). Complications included a single intraoperative death (0.8%), wound infection (3%), pericardial effusion (2%), pneumothorax (0.8%), and device erosion (2%). Over a mean follow-up period of 31 ± 23 months, 68% of patients experienced at least one ICD shock. Five patients underwent cardiac transplantation with the ICD serving as a bridge to transplant. Actuarial survival rates at 1, 2, and 5 years after implant were 95%, 93%, and 85%, respectively. Impaired left ventricular function was the principal risk factor for mortality in these patients after ICD implantation. This study demonstrates that children with life-threatening arrhythmias have frequent recurrences of these rhythms, and that ICDs provide effective therapy with low operative morbidity.

Catheter Ablation

Catheter ablation refers to the delivery of energy by a catheter directly into myocardium to damage a specific site within the heart and thereby eliminate or modify the electrophysiologic milieu. Radiofrequency energy in the 550-kHz range is most commonly used. Using a standard 4-mm tip catheter, hemispherical lesions approximately 4 mm in diameter can be created. This targeted energy can be used therapeutically for both automatic and reentry arrhythmias. The indications for this procedure vary according to the clinical circumstance and specific arrhythmia. Radiofrequency ablation has been safely employed in children of all ages,[111] and in children is used most often to ablate accessory pathways,[6,111] AV node reentry tachycardia, and atrial ectopic tachycardia; however, the spectrum of application of this modality is rapidly expanding and newer energy sources, including cryoablation, are currently being used as well.

Surgical Therapy for Arrhythmias

Surgical intervention for the treatment of cardiac arrhythmias is generally reserved for the rare patient who has failed pharmacologic and catheter ablation therapies.[39] Accessory AV pathways can be divided by an incision placed in the atrium just above the annulus of the mitral or tricuspid valve and extended at least 1 cm or more to each side of the presumed pathway location.[14] AVNRT can be eliminated by perinodal cryosurgery or perinodal surgical dissection.[14] Ectopic atrial tachycardias can be cured by excision or cryoablation of the arrhythmogenic focus after careful intraoperative mapping. VT arising from a single site in the right ventricle in an otherwise normal heart may be treated by surgical excision or cryoablation.

Two surgical techniques may be useful where other options are ineffective. For patients with the long QT syndrome and recurrent episodes of torsade de pointes despite medical therapy, left cervical sympathectomy with removal of all three left thoracic sympathetic ganglia increases survival rates and improves the quality of life.[97] Among patients having undergone the older style Fontan operations, medically resistant and complex atrial reentrant tachycardias and/or atrial fibrillation may be a daunting clinical problem. There is new experience with a surgical technique in which specific, anatomically based linear incisions or cryolesions in the right—and sometimes left—atrium eliminate the substrates for these arrhythmias.[75] This maze operation is being performed in combination with anatomic conversion to a more contemporary style of caval redirection to the pulmonary arteries (either lateral tunnel or extracardiac conduit).

References

1. Abboud FM: Ventricular syncope: Is the heart a sensory organ? *N Engl J Med* 320:390–392, 1989.
2. Alexander ME, Walsh EP, Saul JP, et al: Value of programmed ventricular stimulation in patients with congenital heart disease. *J Cardiovasc Electrophysiol* 10:1033–1044, 1999.
3. Anderson JL, Patterson E, Conlon M, et al: Kinetics of antifibrillatory effects of bretylium: Correlation with myocardial drug concentrations. *Am J Cardiol* 46:583–592, 1980.
4. Ashraf MH, Cotroneo J, DiMarco D, et al: Fate of long-term survivors of Mustard procedure (inflow repair) for simple and complex transposition of the great arteries. *Ann Thorac Surg* 42:385–389, 1986.
5. Bash SE, Shah JJ, Albers WH, Geiss DM: Hypothermia for the treatment of postsurgical greatly accelerated junctional ectopic tachycardia. *J Am Coll Cardiol* 10:1095–1099, 1987.
6. Benditt DG, Remole S, Milstein S, Bailin S: Syncope: Causes, clinical evaluation, and current therapy. *Annu Rev Med* 43:283–300, 1992.

7. Benson DW Jr, Smith WM, Dunnigan A, et al: Mechanisms of regular, wide QRS tachycardia in infants and children. *Am J Cardiol* 49:1178–1188.

8. Bernstein JG, Koch-Weser J: Effectiveness of bretylium tosylate against refractory ventricular arrhythmias. *Circulation* 45:1024–1034, 1972.

9. Blomstrom-Lundqvist C, Sabel KG, Olsson SB: A long term follow up of 15 patients with arrhythmogenic right ventricular dysplasia. *Br Heart J* 58:477–488, 1987.

10. Case CL, Gillette PC: Automatic atrial and junctional tachycardias in the pediatric patient: Strategies for diagnosis and management. *PACE* 16:1323–1335, 1993.

11. Case CL, Trippel DL, Gillette PC: New antiarrhythmic agents in pediatrics. *Pediatr Clin North Am* 36:1293–1320, 1989.

12. Chandar JS, Wolff GS, Garson A, et al: Ventricular arrhythmias in postoperative tetralogy of Fallot. *Am J Cardiol* 65:655–661, 1990.

13. Cohen ML, Wernovsky G, Vetter VL: Sinus node function after a systemically staged Fontan procedure. *Circulation* 98:II 352–358, 1998.

14. Cox JL: Surgery for cardiac arrhythmias. In Braunwald E (ed): *Heart Disease: A Textbook of Cardiovascular Medicine*, 4th ed. Philadelphia: WB Saunders, 1992, pp 295–322.

15. Davignon A, Rautaharju P, Boisselle E, et al: Normal ECG standards for infants and children. *Pediatr Cardiol* 1:123–152, 1979.

16. Deal BJ, Miller SM, Scagliotti D, et al: Ventricular tachycardia in a young population without overt heart disease. *Circulation* 73:1111–1118, 1986.

17. Denfield SW, Garson A Jr: Sudden death in children and young adults. *Pediatr Clin North Am* 37:215–231, 1990.

18. Dhala AA, Case CL, Gillette PC: Evolving strategies for managing atrial ectopic tachycardia in children. *Am Heart J* 74:283–286, 1994.

19. Dilsizian V, Bonow RO, Epstein SE, et al: Myocardial ischemia detected by thallium scintigraphy is frequently related to cardiac arrest and syncope in young patients with hypertrophic cardiomyopathy. *J Am Coll Cardiol* 22:796–804, 1993.

20. diMarco JP, Sellers TD, Lerman BB, et al: Diagnostic and therapeutic use of adenosine in patients with supraventricular tachyarrhythmias. *J Am Coll Cardiol* 6:417–425, 1985.

21. Dorostkar P, Silka MJ, Morady F, Dick M: Clinical course of persistent junctional reciprocating tachycardia. *J Am Coll Cardiol* 33:366–376, 1999.

22. Driscoll DJ, Edwards WD: Sudden unexpected death in children and adolescents. *J Am Coll Cardiol* 5:118B–121B, 1985.

23. Dungan WT, Garson A Jr, Gillette PC: Arrhythmogenic right ventricular dysplasia: A cause of ventricular tachycardia in children with apparently normal hearts. *Am Heart J* 102:745–750, 1981.

24. Dunnigan A: Development aspects and natural history of preexcitation syndromes. In Benditt DG, Benson DW (eds): *Cardiac Preexcitation Syndromes*. New York: Martinus Nijhoff, 1986, pp 21–29.

25. Echt DS, Liebson PR, Mitchell LB, et al: Mortality and morbidity in patients receiving encainide, flecainide, or placebo. The Cardiac Arrhythmia Suppression Trial. *N Engl J Med* 324:781–788, 1991.

26. Epstein ML, Kiel EA, Victorica BE: Cardiac decompensation following verapamil therapy in infants with supraventricular tachycardia. *Pediatrics* 75:737–740, 1985.

27. Feld GK, Fleck RP, Chen PS, et al: Radiofrequency catheter ablation for the treatment of human type 1 atrial flutter. Identification of a critical zone in the reentrant circuit by endocardial mapping techniques. *Circulation* 86:1233–1240, 1992.

28. Fullerton DA, St. Cyr JA, Clarke DR, et al: Bezold-Jarisch reflex in postoperative pediatric cardiac surgical patients. *Ann Thorac Surg* 52:534–536, 1991.

29. Fyfe DA, Driscoll DJ, DiDonato RM, et al: Truncus arteriosus with single pulmonary artery: Influence of pulmonary vascular obstructive disease on early and late operative results. *J Am Coll Cardiol* 5:1168–1172, 1985.

30. Garson A: Arrhythmias and sudden death. In Gillette PC, Garson A (eds): *Pediatric Arrhythmias: Electrophysiology and Pacing*. Philadelphia: WB Saunders, 1990, pp 630–636.

31. Garson A: Ventricular arrhythmias. In Gillette PC, Garson A (eds): *Pediatric Arrhythmias: Electrophysiology and Pacing*. Philadelphia: WB Saunders, 1990, pp 427–500.

32. Garson A Jr: Ventricular arrhythmias. In Gillette PC, Garson A (eds): *Pediatric Arrhythmias: Electrophysiology and Pacing*. Philadelphia: WB Saunders, 1990, pp 427–500.

33. Garson A Jr: Ventricular dysrhythmias after congenital heart surgery: A canine model. *Pediatr Res* 18:1112–1120, 1984.

34. Garson A Jr, Bink-Boelkens M, Hesslein PS, et al: Atrial flutter in the young: A collaborative study of 380 cases. *J Am Coll Cardiol* 6:871–878, 1985.

35. Garson A Jr, Dick M II, Fournier A, et al: The long QT syndrome in children. An international study of 287 patients. *Circulation* 87:1866–1872, 1993.

36. Garson A Jr, Moak JP, Friedman RA, et al: Surgical treatment of arrhythmias in children. *Cardiol Clin* 7:319–329, 1989.

37. Garson A Jr, Moak JP, Smith RT Jr, et al: Usefulness of intravenous propafenone for control of postoperative junctional ectopic tachycardia. *Am J Cardiol* 59:1422–1424, 1987.

38. Garson A Jr, Nihill MR, McNamara DG, et al: Status of the adult and adolescent after repair of tetralogy of Fallot. *Circulation* 59:1232–1240, 1979.

39. Garson A Jr, Smith RT Jr, Moak JP, et al: Incessant ventricular tachycardia in infants: Myocardial hamartomas and surgical cure. *J Am Coll Cardiol* 10:619–626, 1987.

40. Garson A Jr, Smith RT Jr, Moak JP: Invasive electrophysiologic studies in children. *Cardiol Clin* 4:551–563, 1986.

41. Gerstenblith G, Spear JF, Moore EN: Quantitative study of the effect of lidocaine on the threshold for ventricular fibrillation in the dog. *Am J Cardiol* 30:242–247, 1972.

42. Gewillig M, Cullen S, Mertens B, et al: Risk factors for arrhythmia and death after Mustard operation for simple transposition of the great arteries. *Circulation* 84:III-187–III-192, 1991.

43. Gillette PC, Garson A Jr: Sudden cardiac death in the pediatric population. *Circulation* 85:I64–I69, 1992.

44. Gillette PC, Garson A Jr: Electrophysiologic and pharmacologic characteristics of automatic ectopic atrial tachycardia. *Circulation* 56:571–575, 1977.

45. Gregoratos G, Cheitlin MD, Conill A, et al: ACC/AHA Guidelines for implantation of cardiac pacemakers and antiarrhythmia devices. A report of the American College of Cardiology/American Heart Association Task Force Report on Practice Guidelines. *J Am Coll Cardiol* 31:1175–1209, 1998.

46. Guidelines 2000 for Cardiopulmonary Resuscitation and Emergency Cardiovascular Care. Part 6: Advanced cardiovascular life support: 7D: The tachycardia algorithms. The American Heart Association in collaboration with the International Liaison Committee on Resuscitation. *Circulation* 102(8 Suppl):I158–I165, 2000.

47. Hayes CJ, Gersony WM: Arrhythmias after the Mustard operation for transposition of the great arteries: A long-term study. *J Am Coll Cardiol* 7:133–137, 1986.

48. Ho SY, Anderson RH. Embryology and anatomy of the normal and abnormal conduction system. In Gillette PC, Garson A (eds): *Pediatric Arrhythmias: Electrophysiology and Pacing*. Philadelphia: WB Saunders, 1990.

49. Hoch DH, Rosenfeld LE: Tachycardias of right ventricular origin. *Cardiol Clin* 10:151–164, 1992.

50. Hoffman BF, Rosen MR: Cellular mechanisms for cardiac arrhythmias. *Circ Res* 49:1–15, 1981.

51. Jackman WM, Beckman KJ, McClelland JH, et al: Treatment of supraventricular tachycardia due to atrioventricular nodal reentry, by radiofrequency catheter ablation of slow-pathway conduction. *N Engl J Med* 327:313–318, 1992.

52. Jackman WM, Friday KJ, Anderson JL, et al: The long QT syndromes: A critical review, new clinical observations and a unifying hypothesis. *Prog Cardiovasc Dis* 31:115–172, 1988.

53. Jacobsen JR, Garson A Jr, Gillette PC, McNamara DG: Premature ventricular contractions in normal children. *J Pediatr* 92:36–38, 1978.

54. Kalman JM, VanHare GF, Olgin JE, et al: Ablation of "incisional" reentrant atrial tachycardia complicating surgery for congenital heart disease. *Circulation* 93:502–512, 1996.

55. Kanter RJ, Papagiannis J, Carboni MP, et al: Radiofrequency catheter ablation of supraventricular tachycardia substrates after Mustard and Senning operations for d-transposition of the great arteries. *J Am Coll Cardiol* 35:428–441, 2000.

56. Kaseda S, Gilmour RF Jr, Zipes DP: Depressant effect of magnesium on early afterdepolarizations and triggered activity induced by cesium, quinidine, and 4-aminopyridine in canine cardiac Purkinje fibers. *Am Heart J* 118:458–466, 1989.

57. Katz NM, Blackstone EH, Kirklin JW, et al: Late survival and symptoms after repair of tetralogy of Fallot. *Circulation* 65:403–410, 1982.

58. Kavey RE, Blackman MS, Sondheimer HM: Phenytoin therapy for ventricular arrhythmias occurring late after surgery for congenital heart disease. *Am Heart J* 104:794–798, 1982.

59. Kelliher GJ, Kowey P, Engel T, et al: Clinical pharmacology of antiarrhythmic agents. *Cardiovasc Clin* 16:287, 1985.

60. Klitzner TS: Arrhythmias in the general pediatric population: An overview. *Pediatr Ann* 20:347–349, 1991.

61. Klitzner TS, Friedman WF: Cardiac arrhythmias: The role of pharmacologic intervention. *Cardiol Clin* 7:299–318, 1989.

62. Kniffen FJ, Lomas TE, Counsell RE, et al: The antiarrhythmic and antifibrillatory actions of bretylium and its *o*-iodobenzyl trimethylammonium analog, UM-360. *J Pharmacol Exp Ther* 192:120–128, 1975.

63. Kornbluth A, Frishman WH, Ackerman M: Beta-adrenergic blockade in children. *Cardiol Clin* 5:629–649, 1987.

64. Krongrad E: Postoperative arrhythmias in patients with congenital heart disease. *Chest* 85:107–113, 1984.

65. Kugler JD, Danford DA: Pacemakers in children: An update. *Am Heart J* 117:665–679, 1989.

66. Kugler JD, Danford DA, Deal BJ, et al: Radiofrequency catheter ablation for tachyarrhythmias in children and adolescents. (In conjunction with the Pediatric Electrophysiology Society). *N Eng J Med* 330:1481–1487, 1994.

67. Kunze KP, Kuck KH, Schluter M, Bleifeld W: Effect of encainide and flecainide on chronic ectopic atrial tachycardia. *J Am Coll Cardiol* 7:1121–1126, 1986.

68. Lemery R, Brugada P, Janssen J, et al: Nonischemic sustained ventricular tachycardia: Clinical outcome in 12 patients with arrhythmogenic right ventricular dysplasia. *J Am Coll Cardiol* 14:96–105, 1989.

69. Liberthson R, Brian A, McGovern M, et al: Electrophysiologic observations and survival analysis in children and young adults with symptomatic ventricular tachycardia or fibrillation. *Circulation Suppl* 72:197, 1985.

70. Marban E, Robinson SW, Wier WG: Mechanisms of arrhythmogenic delayed and early afterdepolarizations in ferret ventricular muscle. *J Clin Invest* 78:1185–1192, 1986.

71. Marcus FI, Fontaine GH, Guiraudon G, et al: Right ventricular dysplasia: A report of 24 adult cases. *Circulation* 65:384–398, 1982.

72. Maron BJ, Fananapazir L: Sudden cardiac death in hypertrophic cardiomyopathy. *Circulation* 85:I57–I63, 1992.

73. Maron BJ, Olivotto I, Spirito P, et al: Epidemiology of hypertrophic cardiomyopathy–related death: Revisited in a large non-referral-based patient population. *Circulation* 102:858–864, 2000.

74. Maron BJ, Roberts WC, McAllister HA, et al: Sudden death in young athletes. *Circulation* 62:218–229, 1980.

75. Mavroudis C, Backer CL, Deal BJ, Johnsrude CL: Fontan conversion to cavopulmonary connection and arrhythmia circuit cryoablation. *J Thorac Cardiovasc Surg* 115:547–556, 1998.

76. Mehta AV, Sanchez GR, Sacks EJ, et al: Ectopic automatic atrial tachycardia in children: Clinical characteristics, management and follow-up. *J Am Coll Cardiol* 11:379–385, 1988.

77. Michaelsson M, Engel MA: Congenital complete heart block: An international study of the natural history. *Pediatr Cardiol* 4:87–101, 1972.

78. Michaelsson M, Jonzon A, Riesenfeld T: Isolated congenital complete atrioventricular block in adult life: A prospective study. *Circulation* 92:442–449, 1995.

79. Morady F, Kadish AH, DiCarlo L, et al: Long-term results of catheter ablation of idiopathic right ventricular tachycardia. *Circulation* 82:2093–2099, 1990.

80. Morady F, Scheinman MM, Hess DS, et al: Clinical characteristics and results of electrophysiologic testing in young adults with ventricular tachycardia or ventricular fibrillation. *Am Heart J* 106:1306–1314, 1983.

81. Murphy JG, Gersh BJ, Mair DD, et al: Long-term outcome in patients undergoing surgical repair of tetralogy of Fallot. *N Engl J Med* 329:594–599, 1993.

82. Oh JK, Holmes DR Jr, Hayes DL, et al: Cardiac arrhythmias in patients with surgical repair of Ebstein's anomaly. *J Am Coll Cardiol* 6:1351–1357, 1985.

83. Olah KS, Gee H: Antibody mediated complete congenital heart block in the fetus. *PACE* 16:1872–1879, 1993.

84. Packer M, O'Connor CM, Ghali JK, et al, for the Prospective Randomized Amlodipine Survival Evaluation Study Group (PRAISE): Effect of amlodipine on morbidity and mortality in severe chronic congestive heart failure. *N Engl J Med* 335:1107–1114, 1996.

85. Perry JC, Knilans TK, Marlow D, et al: Intravenous amiodarone for life-threatening tachyarrhythmias in children and young adults. *J Am Coll Cardiol* 22:95–98, 1993.

86. Pickoff AS, Wolff GS, Tamer D, et al: Arrhythmias and conduction system disturbances in infants and children—recent advances and contributions of intracardiac electrophysiology. *Cardiovasc Clin* 11:203–219, 1980.

87. Quattlebaum TG, Varghese PJ, Neill CA, et al: Sudden death among postoperative patients with tetralogy of Fallot. A follow-up study of 243 patients for an average of twelve years. *Circulation* 54:289–293, 1975.

88. Rakita L, Sobol SM: Amiodarone in the treatment of refractory ventricular arrhythmias. Importance and safety of initial high-dose therapy. *JAMA* 250:1293–1295, 1983.

89. Ralston MA, Knilans TK, Hannon DW, Daniels SR: Use of adenosine for diagnosis and treatment of tachyarrhythmias in pediatric patients. *J Pediatr* 124:139–143, 1994.

90. Reed BR, Lee LA, Harmon C, et al.: Autoantibodies to SS-A/Ro in infants with congenital heart block. *J Pediatr* 103:889–891, 1983.

91. Ricci C, Longo R, Pagnan L, et al: Magnetic resonance imaging in right ventricular dysplasia. *Am J Cardiol* 70:1589–1595, 1992.

92. Rocchini AP, Chun PO, Dick M: Ventricular tachycardia in children. *Am J Cardiol* 47:1091–1097, 1981.

93. Ros SP, Fisher EA, Bell TJ: Adenosine in the emergency management of supraventricular tachycardia. *Pediatr Emerg Care* 7:222–223, 1991.

94. Ross BA, Hughes S, Anderson E, Gillette PC: Abnormal responses to orthostatic testing in children and adolescents with recurrent unexplained syncope. *Am Heart J* 122:748–754, 1991.

95. Samoil D, Grubb BP, Kip K, Kosinski DJ: Head-upright tilt table testing in children with unexplained syncope. *Pediatrics* 92:426–430, 1993.

96. Schwartz PJ, Locati EH, Moss AJ, et al: Left cardiac sympathetic denervation in the therapy of congenital long QT syndrome. A worldwide report. *Circulation* 84:503–511, 1991.

97. Schwartz PJ: Long QT syndrome. In Horowitz LN (ed): *Current Management of Arrhythmias*. Philadelphia: BC Decker, 1991, pp 194–198.

98. Schwartz PJ, Moss AJ, Vincent GM, Crampton RS: Diagnostic criteria for the long QT syndrome. An update. *Circulation* 88:782–784, 1993.

99. Schwartz PJ, Stramba-Badiale M, Segantini A, et al: Prolongation of the QT interval and the sudden infant death syndrome. *N Engl J Med* 338:1709–1714, 1998.

100. Seliem MA, Benson DW Jr, Strasburger JF, Duffy CE: Complex ventricular ectopic activity in patients less than 20 years of age with or without syncope, and the role of ventricular extrastimulus testing. *Am J Cardiol* 68:745, 1991.

101. Silka MJ, Kron J, Dunnigan A, Dick M II: Sudden cardiac death and the use of implantable cardioverter-defibrillators in pediatric patients. The Pediatric Electrophysiology Society. *Circulation* 87:800–807, 1993.

102. Silka MJ, Kron J, Halperin BD, McAnulty JH: Mechanisms of AV node reentrant tachycardia in young patients with and without dual AV node physiology. *Pacing Clin Electrophysiol* 17:2129–2133, 1994.

103. Silka MJ, McAnulty JH: Survival following ventricular fibrillation. In Quan L, Franklin WH (eds): *Ventricular Fibrillation: A Pediatric Problem*. Armonk, NY: Futura Publishing, 2000.

104. Singh BN: Amiodarone: Historical development and pharmacologic profile. *Am Heart J* 106:788–797, 1983.

105. Southall DP, Richards JM, Rhoden KJ, et al: Prolonged apnea and cardiac arrhythmias in infants discharged from neonatal intensive care units: Failure to predict an increased risk for sudden infant death syndrome. *Pediatrics* 70:844–851, 1982.

106. Sra JS, Jazayeri MR, Dhala A, et al: Neurocardiogenic syncope. Diagnosis, mechanisms, and treatment. *Cardiol Clin* 11:183–191, 1993.

107. Stanton MS, Miles WM, Zipes DP: Atrial fibrillation and flutter. In Zipes DP, Jalife J (eds): *Cardiac Electrophysiology*. Philadelphia: WB Saunders, 1990.

108. Sulke AN, Pipilis A, Henderson RA, et al: Comparison of the normal sinus node with seven types of rate responsive pacemaker during everyday activity. *Br Heart J* 64:25–31, 1990.

109. Ticho BS, Saul JP, Hulse JE, et al: Variable location of accessory pathways associated with the permanent form of junctional reciprocating tachycardia and confirmation with radiofrequency ablation. *Am J Cardiol* 70:1559–1564, 1992.

110. Tzivoni D, Banai S, Schuger C, et al: Treatment of torsade de pointes with magnesium sulfate. *Circulation* 77:392–397, 1988.

111. Van Hare GF, Lesh MD, Scheinman M, Langberg JJ: Percutaneous radiofrequency catheter ablation for supraventricular arrhythmias in children. *J Am Coll Cardiol* 17:1613–1620, 1991.

112. Vetter VL: Ventricular arrhythmias in patients with congenital heart disease. *Cardiovasc Clin* 22:255–273, 1992.

113. Vetter VL: Management of arrhythmias in children—unusual features. *Cardiovasc Clin* 16:329–358, 1985.

114. Vetter VL: Sudden death in children and adolescents. In Morganroth J, Horowitz LN (eds): *Sudden Cardiac Death*. New York: Grune & Stratton, 1985, pp 33–46.

115. Vetter VL, Tanner CS, Horowitz LN: Inducible atrial flutter after the Mustard repair of complete transposition of the great arteries. *Am J Cardiol* 61:428–435, 1988.

116. Vidaillet HJ Jr, Pressley JC, Henke E, et al: Familial occurrence of accessory atrioventricular pathways (preexcitation syndrome). *N Engl J Med* 317:65–69, 1987.

117. Villian E, Bonner D, Trigo C, et al: Outcome of, and risk factors for, second degree atrioventricular block in children. *Cardiol Young* 6:315–319, 1996.

118. Villain E, Vetter VL, Garcia JM, et al: Evolving concepts in the management of congenital junctional ectopic tachycardia. A multicenter study. *Circulation* 81:1544–1549, 1990.

119. Vincent GM, Timothy K, Fox J, et al: The inherited long QT syndrome: From ion channel to bedside. *Cardiol Rev* 7:44–55, 1999.

120. Vincent GM, Timothy KW, Leppert M, Keating M: The spectrum of symptoms and QT intervals in carriers of the gene for the long QT syndrome. *N Engl J Med* 327:846–852, 1992.

121. Walsh EP, Saul JP, Hulse JE, et al: Transcatheter ablation of ectopic atrial tachycardia in young patients using radiofrequency current. *Circulation* 86:1138–1146, 1992.

122. Walsh EP, Saul JP, Sholler GF, et al: Evaluation of a staged treatment protocol for rapid automatic junctional tachycardia after operation for congenital heart disease. *J Am Coll Cardiol* 29:1046–1053, 1997.

123. Weindling SN, Saul JP, Gamble WJ, et al: Duration of complete atrioventricular block after congenital heart disease surgery. *Am J Cardiol* 82:525–527, 1998.

124. Wellens HJJ, Brugada P, Penn OC, et al: Pre-excitation syndromes. In Zipes DP, Jalife J (eds): *Cardiac Electrophysiology*. Philadelphia: WB Saunders, 1990, pp 691–702.

125. Wit AL, Cranefield PF: Effect of verapamil on the sinoatrial and atrioventricular nodes of the rabbit and the mechanism by which it arrests reentrant atrioventricular nodal tachycardia. *Circ Res* 35:413–425, 1974.

126. Wolfe RR, Driscoll DJ, Gersony WM, et al: Arrhythmias in patients with valvar aortic stenosis, valvar pulmonary stenosis, and ventricular septal defect. Results of 24-hour ECG monitoring, *Circulation* 87:I89–I101, 1993.

127. Yabek SM: Ventricular arrhythmias in children with an apparently normal heart. *J Pediatr* 119:1–11, 1991.

Chapter 9

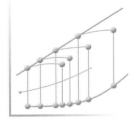

Pericardial Effusion and Tamponade

F. BENNETT PEARCE, MD, MASAO TAKATA, MD, PhD,
and JAMES L. ROBOTHAM, MD

INTRODUCTION

The physiology and pathophysiology of the pericardium have fascinated physiologists and clinicians for years. The functional significance of the pericardium has occasionally been overlooked, because patients with congenital absence of the pericardium may be asymptomatic,[126] or pericardiectomy in animals[177] or humans[52] may not produce clinical problems. Experiments, however, suggest that the pericardium may influence cardiac performance even under normal conditions. It is well known that the pericardium can affect hemodynamics in the disease state. Characteristic hemodynamic signs have been found in pericardial disease (e.g., pulsus paradoxus or Kussmaul's sign), suggesting that unique hemodynamic events take place in the presence of pericardial pathology.

This chapter covers pericardial effusion and tamponade in infants and children. Numerous etiologies of effusion and tamponade are known, and the common ones are covered. The pathologic processes of the pericardium are in themselves of concern, but the common hemodynamic consequences of these diseases are critically important for diagnosis and treatment of these patients. Thus special emphasis is put on understanding physiologic and pathophysiologic aspects of pericardial diseases. Finally, newer approaches to the normal pericardial space and the use of the pericardial space as a therapeutic delivery site are discussed.

ANATOMY AND PHYSIOLOGY OF THE PERICARDIUM

Anatomic Considerations

The pericardium consists of two layers. The inner visceral pericardium, also called epicardium, constitutes the external surface of the heart, whereas the outer parietal pericardium is a thin and semitransparent membrane enclosing the heart. The parietal layer is what is commonly referred to as the "pericardium." The space between the two layers is called the pericardial or intrapericardial space. Under normal physiologic conditions, only a small amount of fluid is present in the pericardial space, approximately 15 to 50 mL in humans.[6]

Thus the pericardium (i.e., parietal pericardium) is virtually in direct contact with the heart surface. The pericardium covers the heart and extends for a short distance onto the great vessels and the vena cavae. The pulmonary veins are extrapericardial.

The pericardium also is in intimate contact with other structures in the thorax. It is tethered by its reflection around the great vessels and fibrous connection with the vertebral column, sternum, and diaphragm. The outer surface of the pericardium is in direct contact with the pleura. The lungs constitute a space that envelops the heart and pericardium termed the *cardiac fossa*. The close relationship of the pericardium with the heart and lungs produces complex heart/pericardium/lung interactions, particularly during respiration. The elastic properties of the pericardium have been investigated in vitro in detail.[90,140,204] Figure 9-1 schematically illustrates a typical pressure/volume relationship of the whole pericardium. The pericardial tissue is initially very extensible, but it becomes much less compliant once it is stretched beyond a certain length, resulting in considerable elastic recoil force. This relationship is the result of the histology of the pericardium, which contains elastin fibers and collagen fibers. The collagen fibers are wavy at nonstretched lengths. As the pericardium is stretched, the less compliant collagen fibers straighten and gradually take up the load.[95,112] Thus the pericardium will exert increasing external constraining forces over the heart as the intrapericardial volume increases. The ligamentous attachments of the pericardium also play some role, as the pressure/volume curve of the in situ pericardium is less steep than that for the in vitro pericardium.[67]

Composition of Normal Pericardial Fluid

Pericardial fluid is classically defined as an ultrafiltrate of plasma and contains protein concentrations of 25% to 33% of plasma, with albumin being present to a greater extent than larger molecules.[76] Macromolecules appear to move through large pores or via transcytosis.[22] More is being learned about the composition of pericardial fluid in health and disease.

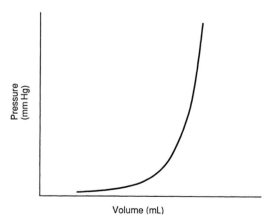

FIGURE 9-1 A schematic illustration showing a typical pressure-volume relationship of the whole pericardium obtained in animal experiments. A tube is inserted into the pericardial space of a dead animal with all the great vessels of the heart ligated. The total intrapericardial volume is varied by infusion of saline into the pericardial space, and the resultant changes in intrapericardial pressure are measured.

Pericardial fluid may contain cytokines, prostaglandins, atrial natriuretic peptide (in congestive heart failure), endothelin, and growth factors that may locally influence myocytes and vascular tissue.[7,91] The potential role of pericardial mesothelial cells as paracrine modulators of cardiac myocytes, and local, pulmonary, and systemic vascular endothelial and vascular smooth muscle cells has recently been explored.[121] The ability of the normal pericardium to act as a "reservoir" of pericardial mesothelial and cardiac endothelial humoral agents via lymphatic pathways for both local and remote actions has stimulated interest in using the pericardial space as a delivery site for therapeutic interventions.[12,58,121,125]

Pericardial Pressure

To assess the degree of constraining effect by the pericardium, measurement of pericardial pressure, the pressure over the heart below the parietal pericardium, is essential. However, the optimal technique for measurement is still controversial,[161] because under normal conditions, the pericardial pressure is not a simple "liquid" pressure but should rather be considered a "surface" pressure.[65,90,166,181]

The concept of liquid versus surface pressure is derived from analysis of pleural pressure in traditional pulmonary mechanics.[4,134] A liquid pressure is generalized hydrostatic pressure acting in the liquid. It can be measured with a fluid-filled cannula or transducer-tipped catheter and hence is familiar to clinicians. A surface pressure is a force per unit area acting over a surface or between two surfaces. It is equal to the sum of any liquid pressure and a "contact stress" (i.e., a regional pressure due to deformation forces produced by the apposition of two surfaces). Because the pericardium is in contact with the heart surface, the constraining forces are transmitted mainly in a form of contact stress. The pericardial surface pressure under physiologic conditions is thus higher than the pericardial liquid pressure. As pericardial fluid accumulates, the pericardium will lose its contact with the heart surface, and the pericardial pressure becomes equal to pericardial liquid pressure. A fluid-filled catheter inserted into the pericardial space would therefore underestimate the true pericardial pressure under normal, nontamponade conditions. In contrast, a flat flexible balloon inserted between the heart and pericardium is more sensitive to such contact forces.[4,134] Although the flat-balloon technique is not totally free from errors because of the distortion of the curved interface between the pericardium and the heart by the inserted balloon itself,[181,193] it is at present accepted by most investigators as a better method than a fluid-filled cannula of estimating pericardial surface pressure.[65,89,90,98,153,166,167,183,194] A fluid-filled catheter does provide a good estimation of pericardial pressure when an abnormally large pericardial fluid collection completely surrounds all four chambers of the heart.

Studies with flat balloons have identified some important characteristics of pericardial pressure. Pericardial pressure shows a phasic change within a cardiac cycle,[89,90,161,181,183] with its maximum near end diastole, its minimum near end systole, and a waveform similar to externally measured ventricular dimensions.[181] Moreover, significant regional differences were observed in pericardial pressure over various sites of the heart, particularly between the left (LV) and right ventricles (RV).[89,153,166,181] It can be demonstrated that the pericardial pressure is influenced by underlying ventricular volume, although the effect of the opposite ventricular volume may sometimes dominate.[166,181] Thus under normal physiologic conditions, pericardial pressure appears to have a regional nature, being influenced by local events occurring mainly in the immediately subjacent chamber.

Functions of the Pericardium

Various functions have been attributed to the pericardium.[6,169] These include (1) maintenance of the heart in a fixed position in the chest; (2) protection of the heart from infection, inflammation, or contiguous spread of malignancy from surrounding structures; (3) minimizing friction associated with cardiac motion; and (4) influencing cardiac dynamics by exerting external constraining forces over the heart. With an elevated heart volume, little question occurs that the pericardium limits cardiac filling and hence the preload of the heart. This concept is supported by experimental studies that evaluate changes in the pressure/volume relationship of the cardiac chambers before and after pericardiectomy[15,113,175] or studies using the flat-balloon technique.[65,89,90,153,166,167,181,183,194] When the heart volume is markedly elevated, the pericardium can prevent overdistention, myocardial hemorrhage, or worsening valvular insufficiency.[14,107] Acute cardiac overdistention will increase systolic ventricular wall tension and oxygen demand, because a thinner wall must develop a higher tension for a given chamber pressure, according to the LaPlace relationship. However, if cardiac dilation occurs chronically or a pericardial effusion develops over a long period, the pericardium will hypertrophy and enlarge, with the mechanical constraining effects of the pericardium remaining relatively unchanged.[66,113]

Some controversy exists over the extent of pericardial constraint over the heart under normal physiologic conditions and volumes. Studies using liquid-filled balloons reported that pericardial pressure is approximately equal to the right atrial (RA) or RV diastolic pressure.[166,194] The studies also found that the RV is working with a very low transmural pressure and that most of the right-sided cardiac filling is limited by the elastic recoil of the pericardium rather than the intrinsic stiffness of the RA and RV. These findings implied that the Frank-Starling relationship is not operative in the right heart. This is in contradistinction to the conventional wisdom that the sarcomere fiber length and degree of shortening are directly proportional. Other studies, using more flexible air-filled balloons,[65,89,153,181,165] found that the pericardial contribution to RV diastolic pressure would be one third to two thirds of the measured intracavitary pressure, implying that the right heart transmural pressure does vary more than the narrow ranges of pressure suggested by the liquid-balloon studies. The precise point at which the pericardium begins to limit the RV volume remains to be established. These studies have shown, however, that the pericardium exerts some constraining influence on RV filling, even at normal volume and pressure. Thus the pericardium should not be ignored in any patient who shows evidence of compromised cardiac performance.

Pericardial Versus Lung Constraint

Under physiologic closed-chest conditions, the lungs have direct contact with the pericardial surface, producing a focal

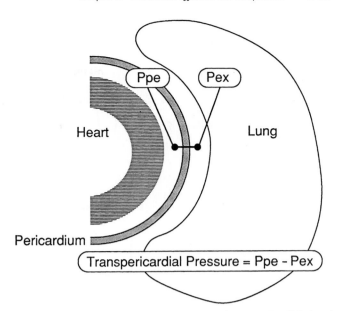

FIGURE 9-2 Relationships of the pericardial (Ppe), extrapericardial pleural (Pex), and transpericardial pressures. The pericardial pressure represents the total external constraint of the heart produced by the pericardium and the lung. It is the sum of the transpericardial pressure, i.e., pericardial constraint, and the extrapericardial pleural pressure, i.e., lung constraint.

pleural surface over the heart.[61,65,98,116,118,183,201] The total external constraint of the heart may be seen to have two components, a load produced by the elastic recoil of the pericardium (i.e., pericardial constraint) and a load produced by the focal pleural surface pressure around the heart (i.e., lung constraint). As illustrated in Figure 9-2, pericardial pressure actually includes the influence of the extrapericardial pressure (i.e., the lung constraint), thus representing the total external constraint of the heart. The difference between pericardial and extrapericardial pressures (i.e., transpericardial pressure [intrapericardial–extrapericardial]) reflects only the component contributed by the pericardial constraint. With positive-pressure ventilation (PPV), particularly with positive end-expiratory pressure (PEEP) or auto-PEEP leading to global or local lung overdistention, the influence of the lung constraint on cardiac performance would become apparent. This is most easily appreciated under conditions in which the rib cage is surgically opened, allowing atmospheric pressure to surround all thoracic structures. Even under these conditions, with the generalized intrathoracic pressure being almost zero, lung inflation can result in compression of the heart. The quantitative effect of pericardial versus lung constraint during PEEP has been evaluated by several studies.[65,98,183] Figure 9-3 illustrates the typical changes in simultaneously measured pericardial and extrapericardial pressures during PEEP.[183] With a PEEP of 0 cm H_2O, most of the pericardial pressure was contributed by the transpericardial pressure, reflecting an absence of lung constraint. In contrast, with increases in PEEP, the relative contribution of the extrapericardial pressure to the total pericardial pressure increased, and the relative contribution of the transpericardial pressure decreased, reflecting the predominance of lung constraint on ventricular filling.

With spontaneous respiration, pleural pressure is negative throughout the chest cavity. Thus cardiac filling is facilitated

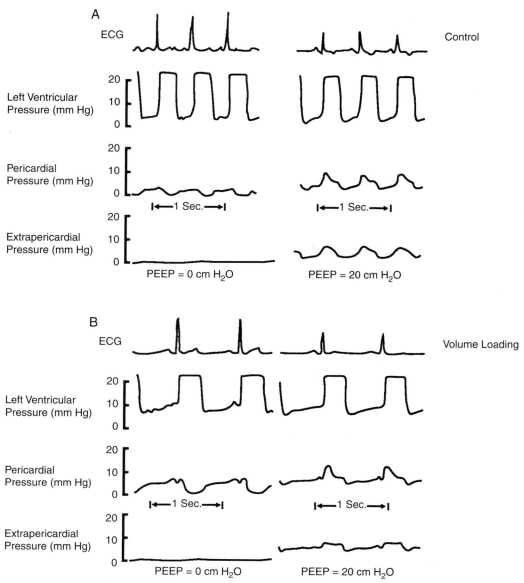

FIGURE 9-3 Changes in pericardial and extrapericardial pleural pressures over the left ventricle (LV) during positive end-expiratory pressure (PEEP) obtained in dog experiments. Two flat latex balloons were placed into the pericardial space over the LV to measure pericardial pressure and over the pericardium beneath the lung to measure extrapericardial pressure. With the chest closed, pressures were simultaneously recorded during application of PEEP under baseline volume conditions **(A)** and volume loaded conditions **(B).** With a PEEP of 0 cm H_2O, pericardial pressure was positive with a phasic change within a cardiac cycle, while extrapericardial pressure was approximately 0 mm Hg with minimal cardiac oscillations. With a PEEP of 20 cm H_2O, pericardial pressure increased. Under baseline volume conditions, extrapericardial pressure became positive and approached pericardial pressure with regard to its phasic values and waveform. Thus, the component of transpericardial pressure was markedly reduced. Under volume loaded conditions, extrapericardial pressure became positive and phasic but remained lower than pericardial pressure, with a substantial component of transpericardial pressure still present. *ECG,* electrocardiogram. (From Takata M, Robotham JL: Ventricular external constraint by the lung and pericardium during positive end-expiratory pressure. *Am Rev Respir Dis* 143:872–875, 1991; with permission.)

by the negative pleural pressure lowering RA pressure, which can increase venous return. However, despite the negative "generalized" intrathoracic pressure, if lung volume markedly increases (e.g., in bronchopulmonary dysplasia or respiratory syncytial virus [RSV] pneumonitis), focal compression of the heart can result, limiting cardiac filling. A radiographic "teardrop" heart can be seen in status asthmaticus despite markedly negative generalized pleural pressure, as measured with an esophageal balloon.[176] In this case, the lungs may impose a positive local surface pressure on the heart, which is not measured by the esophageal balloon, which "sees" neither the intrapericardial pressure nor the pressure applied by the lungs over the surface of the heart. The same principle may account for some component of the exercise limitation in patients with chronic obstructive lung disease in whom air trapping markedly increases at elevated respiratory rates. It appears that the lungs can act as a second pericardium as the lung volume increases during either positive- or negative-pressure ventilation.[183] Thus the heart can be constrained by the pericardium, lungs, or combination of the two. The external constraint by the lungs may explain why humans or animals are able to survive without the pericardium.

Pleural effusions may produce important cardiac constraint.[5] This has been shown in dogs and in humans, where echocardiographic signs of RA, RV, and LV diastolic collapse have been seen.[99,197,198] The ability of a pleural effusion to compromise cardiac filling should be borne in mind when evaluating patients with pericardial and pleural effusions in which the hemodynamic compromise seems out of proportion to the degree of pericardial fluid accumulation. Interestingly, in the canine model, the same degree of intrapericardial pressure elevation was better tolerated when caused by a pleural rather than a pericardial effusion.

Influence of the Pericardium on Ventricular Loading during Respiration

Respiration produces changes in ventricular loading conditions, which can result in profound effects on cardiac performance. The pericardium plays an important role in modulating such important cardiorespiratory interactions.[181] Negative intrathoracic pressure enhances systemic venous return.[179,182,184] RV volume increases with the increase in systemic venous return,[132,148] whereas LV volume decreases because of a mechanism known as diastolic ventricular interdependence.[25,29,34,135,136,152,202] As RV volume increases, if the expansion of the RV free wall is limited by its intrinsic stiffness or a relatively stiff pericardium, the increased volume displaces the ventricular septum leftward, producing a decrease in LV compliance and an impairment of LV filling. The decrease in LV preload due to ventricular interdependence is considered to be a major mechanism of pulsus paradoxus[110] (i.e., an inspiratory decrease in LV stroke volume). Although ventricular interdependence exists to a small degree without the pericardium present, the presence of the pericardium markedly enhances the degree of ventricular interdependence and pulsus paradoxus.[25,135]

A negative intrathoracic pressure also directly increases the LV afterload to the degree to which the LV pressure decreases relative to the extrathoracic compartments into which arterial blood is pumped (Fig. 9-4).[83,135,137] The decrease in pressure around the LV increases the transmural LV pressure, resulting in a decreased LV stroke volume. This increase in LV afterload is an alternative mechanism for the pathogenesis of pulsus paradoxus, which would act in concert with ventricular interdependence to decrease LV stroke volume (i.e., increased LV afterload combined with decreased LV preload). The importance of an increased afterload increases under conditions in which the LV is sensitive to small changes in afterload (e.g., heart failure or conditions with large negative pleural pressures, as in status asthmaticus or upper airway obstruction in croup, epiglottitis, or obstructive sleep apnea). Until recently, however, the role of the pericardium in modulating the effects of respiration on LV afterload had not been well defined.

Changes in pericardial and extrapericardial pressure have been studied experimentally by using flat balloons during negative intrathoracic pressure produced by phrenic nerve stimulation to stimulate a spontaneous inspiration.[181] The pericardial pressure over the LV did not decrease as much as the extrapericardial pleural or esophageal pressure, with an increase in transpericardial (intrapericardial − extrapericardial) pressure at both end systole and end diastole (Fig. 9-5). An enhanced systemic venous return during the inspiratory effort produces an increase in total ventricular volume, resulting in increased elastic recoil of the pericardium as it is distended and hence increased transpericardial pressure. Therefore with the presence of the pericardium, the true surrounding pressure over the LV is less negative than the imposed negative intrathoracic pressure. This implies that the degree of LV afterload produced by inspiration during spontaneous respiration is effectively attenuated by the pericardium.

This finding leads to an appreciation of a more generalized role of the pericardium. It has long been recognized that the pericardium modulates large increases in cardiac volume (e.g., preload). It can now be seen that the elastic recoil of the pericardium limits acute increases in preload *and* afterload. Thus a possible role of the pericardium is to limit acute changes in ventricular loading not only during respiration but also during any pharmacologic, neural, humoral, or mechanical perturbation. For example, during exercise, there are large swings in intrathoracic and abdominal pressure, increased sympathetic tone affecting both systemic and pulmonary vascular beds, and increased venous pumping from muscular activity, all of which result in acute changes in total venous return and biventricular afterloads. In such situations, the pericardium may prevent the overdistention of the heart and assist ventricular ejection by attenuating increases in LV afterload. The pericardium may play an important role in maintaining hemodynamic stability under a variety of physiologic and pathophysiologic conditions. In conditions associated with ventricular dysfunction in which the ratio of oxygen supply to demand is abnormal, limiting of increases in preload and afterload is generally considered therapeutic. The pericardium may perform this function.

PATHOPHYSIOLOGY OF PERICARDIAL EFFUSION AND TAMPONADE

Hemodynamic Profiles

Excessive accumulation of pericardial fluid due to any pathologic process leads to characteristic abnormalities (i.e., cardiac tamponade). The classic hemodynamic profile of severe cardiac tamponade includes elevation and equilibration of RV and LV diastolic pressures with the surrounding pericardial pressure, reduced cardiac output, hypotension, and pulsus paradoxus.[145] Progression of hemodynamic changes in tamponade proceeds in predictable fashion and has been divided into stages based on a large number of clinical observations.[147] In phase I tamponade, accumulation of pericardial fluid produces an increase in pericardial pressure, which in turn in increases the RV and LV diastolic pressures. Cardiac output is not usually compromised. The inspiratory decrease in systolic arterial pressure is present or increased but does not reach the diagnostic criterion of pulsus paradoxus (a decrease >10 mm Hg).[62,146] In phase II, the elevated pericardial pressure becomes equal to RV diastolic pressure but remains lower than LV diastolic pressure. The transmural RV diastolic pressure approaches 0 mm Hg and accounts for a significant decrease in cardiac output. The inspiratory decrease of arterial pressure is exaggerated, and pulsus paradoxus is observed in most but not all patients. In phase III tamponade, the

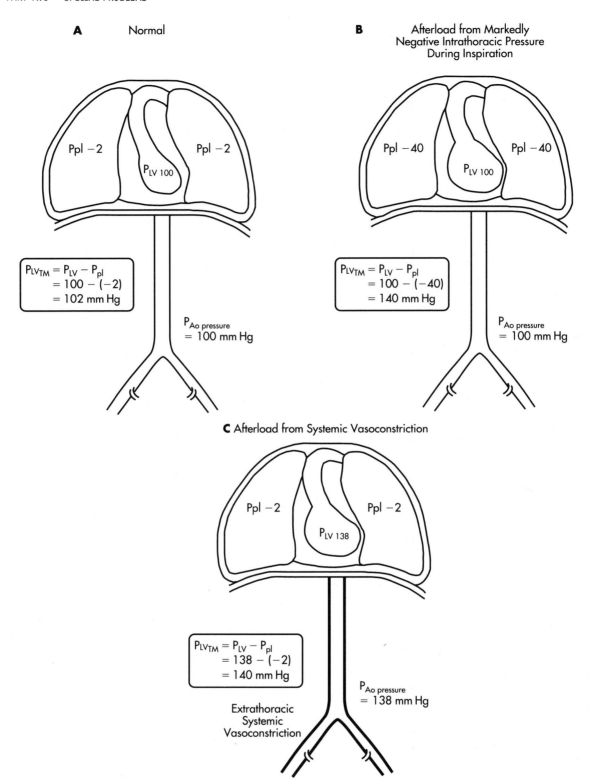

FIGURE 9-4 Afterload to the left ventricle (LV) is proportional to the transmural LV pressure (LV$_{TM}$) = LV cavitary pressure relative to atmosphere (P$_{LV}$) − intrathoracic or pleural pressure (P$_{pl}$). **A,** Normal. **B,** Increased P$_{LV_{TM}}$ (afterload) from negative intrathoracic pressures due to airway obstruction on inspiration. Note systolic P$_{LV}$ and extrathoracic aortic pressures remain normal. **C,** Increased P$_{LV_{TM}}$ (afterload) from systemic vasoconstriction leading to raised extrathoracic aortic and P$_{LV}$ pressures. Note pleural pressure remains normal.

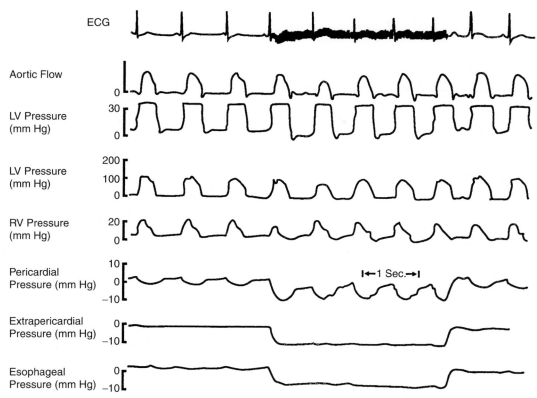

FIGURE 9-5 Changes in pericardial pressure, extrapericardial pleural pressure, and esophageal pressure during negative intrathoracic pressure in dog experiments. An electromagnetic flow probe was placed around the ascending aorta to measure flow, and micromanometer-tipped catheters were placed into the left ventricle (LV) and right ventricle (RV) for pressure measurement. The chest was closed airtight, and phrenic nerve stimulation as represented by the noise in electrocardiogram (ECG) was performed to produce negative intrathoracic pressure. The animal's airway was occluded to prevent changes in lung volume. Esophageal and extrapericardial pleural pressures show a quasi-square wave decrease with an amplitude of approximately −10 mm Hg. During the period of negative intrathoracic pressure, pericardial pressure does not fall as much as extrapericardial pleural and esophageal pressures, particularly at end-diastole, with an increased transpericardial pressure (pericardial − extrapericardial pleural pressure). Aortic flow shows a small decrease at the first beat and a large decrease at the second beat during negative intrathoracic pressure, i.e., pulsus paradoxus. (From Takata M, Mitzner W, Robotham JL: Influence of the pericardium on ventricular loading during respiration, *J Appl Physiol* 68:1640–1650, 1990; with permission.)

pericardial and RV diastolic pressures equilibrate with the LV diastolic pressure, and these pressure further increase together. Both the transmural RV and LV diastolic pressures become almost nil, consistent with minimal end-diastolic volumes. Cardiac output is severely compromised, and pulsus paradoxus is observed in almost all cases.

Compensatory mechanisms in response to reduced arterial pressure further contribute to the typical picture of tamponade. Baroreflex-induced systemic arteriolar vasoconstriction increases systemic vascular resistance to compensate for the hypotension. Vasoconstriction in the peripheral venous beds will increase the mean systemic pressure, compensating in part for the decreased gradient for venous return and hence reduced ventricular preload. Reflex tachycardia and increased contractility also help maintain cardiac output.[69]

Alteration in venous and atrial pressure waveforms in tamponade have been recognized since the original description of the syndrome in 1873.[110] The systolic x descent in the atrial/venous pressure curve is accentuated, whereas the diastolic y descent is attenuated.[142,145,163] Studies have demonstrated that, in addition to the changes in venous pressures, the associated waveforms of venous flows in venae cavae and pulmonary veins are altered by tamponade pathophysiology.

Venous flows into the atria are normally biphasic during the cardiac cycle (i.e., one peak during ventricular systole and the other during ventricular diastole). With experimentally produced tamponade, this biphasic flow pattern is replaced by a predominant systolic flow with an absent diastolic component,[18] as shown in Figure 9-6. These findings are consistent with several other studies in animals and humans that measured flow velocities in the superior vena cava (SVC) or hepatic vein by using Doppler echocardiography.[10,23,31,32,41,192]

Changes in Pericardial Constraint with Tamponade

An understanding of the quantitative and qualitative changes in the pericardial constraint can explain why these characteristic hemodynamic changes can take place in cardiac tamponade. The abnormal increase in the volume of the fluid in the pericardial space produces two conditions. First, the pericardial pressure markedly increases, owing to enhanced recoil forces of the pericardium produced by the increased intrapericardial volume. With progression of tamponade, the pericardial pressure approaches intraluminal atrial or ventricular diastolic pressures, resulting in the transmural RV and LV diastolic

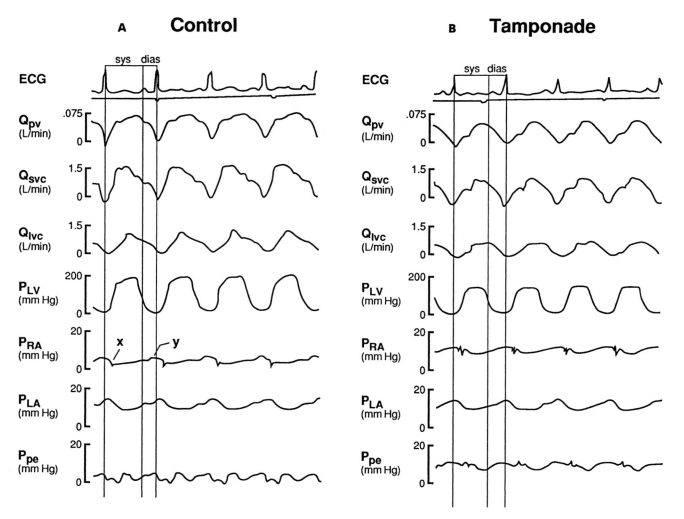

FIGURE 9-6   Changes in venous flow waveforms with an experimentally produced cardiac tamponade in dogs. The animal was instrumented with ultrasound flow probes to measure venous flows in superior vena cava (Q_{SVC}) and inferior vena cava (Q_{IVC}) and a branch of pulmonary vein (Q_{PV}), two micromanometer-tipped catheters into the left ventricle and right atrium (left ventricular pressure [P_{LV}] and right atrial pressure [P_{RA}], and a fluid-filled catheter in the pericardial space (P_{PE}). The vertical lines define systole (sys) and diastole (dias). In the control state **(A)**, the systolic x descent and diastolic y descent can be seen in P_{RA}. Both the systolic and diastolic components are present in Q_{PV}, Q_{SVC}, and Q_{IVC}. After the production of tamponade **(B)**, P_{PE} increased and cyclically decreases only during ventricular ejection. P_{RA} follows the changes in P_{PE}, i.e., the y descent disappears. The diastolic fraction of flow is markedly diminished for Q_{SVC} and Q_{IVC}, venous return to the right atrium being almost completely during ventricular systole. Q_{PV} also became predominantly systolic, but not to the same degree as observed in the venae cavae. P_{pe}, Pericardial pressure; P_{LA}, left atrial pressure. (From Beloucif S, Takata M, Shimada M, Robotham JL: Influence of pericardial constraint on atrioventricular interactions, *Am J Physiol* 263:H125–H134, 1992; with permission.)

pressures approaching zero. In the severe tamponade condition, the intraluminal atrial or ventricular diastolic pressures (i.e., the downstream pressures for venous return) are effectively determined by the pericardial pressure. Second, the normal physiologic regional inhomogeneities in pericardial pressure are abolished and replaced by a uniform liquid pressure because of a liquid column in the pericardial space. Effectively, changes in pericardial pressure on one area are transmitted to other areas instantaneously. These two unique conditions (i.e., the "elevated" and "uniform" pericardial pressures) appear to be necessary to produce the specific pathophysiologic hemodynamic events observed in tamponade.[18]

As the degree of tamponade increases, the "elevated" pericardial pressure limits venous return and cardiac filling as RA pressure increases. First, the RV preload and then the LV

preload are reduced, producing a profound decrease in cardiac output and hypotension. The "uniform" pericardial pressure constrains the four cardiac chambers all together, thereby enhancing chamber-to-chamber interactions. The enhancement of a "horizontal" chamber-to-chamber interaction (i.e., diastolic ventricular interdependence) would result in marked exaggeration of the normal inspiratory decrease in LV stroke volume and arterial pressure. Thus pulsus paradoxus occurs in nearly all cases of severe tamponade. Exceptions to this occur when abnormal communications exist between cardiac chambers (atrial septal defect [ASD];patent foramen ovale [PFO]), when there is alteration of normal ventricular pressure/volume relations (hypertrophic cardiomyopathy, severe aortic stenosis, aortic insufficiency),[62,146,192] or when there is decreased intravascular volume[9] (low-pressure tamponade). Pulsus paradoxus is not specific for tamponade and can be seen in chronic obstructive airway disease, pulmonary embolism, hypovolemia, RV infarction, restrictive cardiomyopathy, tense ascites, or extreme obesity.[42,43,84,117,159,192]

In addition to such horizontal interactions between cardiac chambers, a "vertical" chamber-to-chamber interaction between an atrium and an ipsilateral ventricle has been defined and termed *atrioventricular interaction*.[18]

The degree of such vertical atrioventricular interaction can be characterized by how the atrial and ventricular volume changes within a cardiac cycle are "coupled" to each other. With complete coupling during a cardiac cycle, filling and emptying of the atrium are 180 degrees out of phase with those of the ipsilateral ventricle (i.e., the atrium would fill only during ventricular ejection). An increased *and* uniform pericardial pressure would enhance such an atrioventricular interaction, leading to the specific changes in atrial pressure and venous flow waveforms classically recognized in tamponade.[18]

With tamponade, systolic ventricular ejection reduces the total intrapericardial volume (Fig. 9-7). The reduced total intrapericardial volume results in a decrease in the "uniform" liquid pericardial pressure all over the heart (i.e., not only over the ventricles but also over the atria). Because pericardial pressure effectively determines intraluminal atrial pressures,

the latter decrease along with the decrease in pericardial pressure (hence the prominent systolic x descent), resulting in antegrade systolic venous flow. If sufficient venous return can occur during systole to replace the ejected stroke volume, the decreased pericardial and atrial pressures increase to their previous levels by end systole, stopping further venous inflow. During diastole, atrial emptying and ventricular filling (i.e., intrapericardial volume transfer through atrioventricular valves) will not produce any change in the total intrapericardial volume. Therefore both pericardial and atrial pressures remain unchanged. If atrial pressure does not decrease, there is no y descent found and hence no gradient for diastolic venous inflow. Thus the nature of pericardial constraint in tamponade (i.e., quantitatively "elevated" and qualitatively "uniform" pericardial pressure) tightly couples changes in atrial and ventricular volumes within a cardiac cycle, and atrial filling is essentially concurrent with systolic ventricular emptying, with a large x descent during this time and an absent or diminished y descent.[18]

Tamponade Versus Constriction

A broad spectrum of pericardial diseases can be classified into two distinct entities, cardiac tamponade and constrictive pericarditis.[163] Constrictive pericarditis does occur but is rare in the pediatric age group.[122] However, analyses of similarities and differences between these two clinical syndromes may substantially facilitate our understanding of how the pericardium affects cardiac performance under pathologic conditions.

The hallmark of constrictive pericarditis is a densely thickened, noncompliant, fibrous, and adherent pericardium that restricts filling of cardiac chambers. Little question occurs that the pericardial constraint is markedly elevated in constrictive pathology, due to changes in the elastic property of the pericardium itself. The pericardial pressure in constriction should be elevated, if it can be appropriately measured in the adhesive pericardial space. Thus the hemodynamic changes in constrictive pericarditis have many similarities to those of cardiac tamponade (i.e., reduced cardiac output, hypotension, and elevated atrial and RV/LV diastolic pressures). This is not surprising, because the key pathophysiologic problem is common between the two forms of pericardial disease (i.e., an abnormally elevated pericardial constraint and pericardial pressure).

Despite these similarities, it has been documented and indeed has challenged physiologists and cardiologists for decades that considerable differences are present in hemodynamic profiles between cardiac tamponade and constrictive pericarditis.

For example, pulsus paradoxus is observed more often in tamponade than in constriction.[162] Kussmaul's sign[110] (i.e., a paradoxical inspiratory increase in RA pressure) is occasionally associated with constriction but rarely with tamponade.[142,144] In addition to this difference in respiratory-induced hemodynamic signs, differences exist in steady-state venous pressure and flow waveforms between tamponade and constriction. With tamponade, as described earlier, the systolic x descent in atrial pressure is accentuated, and the venous flows become predominantly systolic. With constriction, atrial pressure shows a prominent y descent with a relatively small x descent, and ventricular diastolic pressure often exhibits a "dip and plateau"

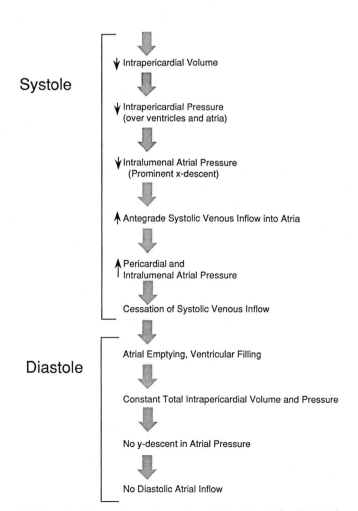

Systole

↓ Intrapericardial Volume

↓ Intrapericardial Pressure (over ventricles and atria)

↓ Intraluminal Atrial Pressure (Prominent x-descent)

↑ Antegrade Systolic Venous Inflow into Atria

↑ Pericardial and Intraluminal Atrial Pressure

Cessation of Systolic Venous Inflow

Diastole

Atrial Emptying, Ventricular Filling

Constant Total Intrapericardial Volume and Pressure

No y-descent in Atrial Pressure

No Diastolic Atrial Inflow

FIGURE 9-7 Atrioventricular interaction during tamponade. Changes in atrial pressure, volume, and flow during tamponade.

pattern (i.e., a steep transient decrease at early diastole followed by a relatively unchanged portion during late diastole).[143,163] Doppler studies in humans have demonstrated an enhanced diastolic venous flow with a relatively small systolic component.[23,32,82,114] These observations imply that the manner in which the pericardium constrains the heart may be quite different between tamponade and constriction, despite similarly increased pericardial pressure, thereby affecting the status of horizontal (i.e., ventricular interdependence) as well as vertical (i.e., atrioventricular interaction) cardiac chamber interactions.

Coupled Versus Uncoupled Pericardial Constraint

A coherent physiologic rationale to explain the hemodynamic differences between cardiac tamponade and constrictive pericarditis had been lacking until the recent proposal of "coupled versus uncoupled pericardial restraint."[180] In this theory, the nature of the pericardial constraint is classified as one of two types: (1) a *coupled* constraint exerted by uniform pericardial liquid pressure over all four cardiac chambers; and (2) an *uncoupled* constraint produced by independent and different local pericardial surface pressures over each cardiac chamber. The essence of this concept is that a coupled constraint restricts the volumes of all cardiac chambers together, whereas an uncoupled constraint independently restricts the volume of each cardiac chamber. As described earlier, under normal conditions, the pericardial pressure is essentially a regional surface pressure. With cardiac tamponade, the regional differences in pericardial pressure are abolished and replaced by a "uniform" liquid pressure. On the contrary, with constrictive pericarditis, most of the pericardium would still maintain its macroscopic contact with the heart surface, and the pericardial pressure should be of "regional" nature (i.e., related to the underlying chamber volume) unless a large amount of effusion is present in addition to constrictive pathology. It is thus reasonable to apply the coupled-versus-uncoupled constraint concept to the interpretation of hemodynamic events with cardiac tamponade and constrictive pericarditis.

Based on this framework, the effects of coupled versus uncoupled pericardial constraint on cardiac chamber interactions were studied extensively by mathematical model analyses.[180] Figure 9-8 illustrates an example of such analyses (i.e., analysis of atrioventricular interaction using an open-loop model of right heart circulation). The RA and RV were modeled by time-varying elastances (E_{ra} and E_{rv}) connected with systemic venous and pulmonary arterial impedances, and a "coupled" constraint was modeled by adding a single pericardial elastance (E_{pe}) over both the RA and RV, whereas an "uncoupled" constraint was modeled by adding two different pericardial elastances (E_{pera} and E_{perv}) on the RA and RV individually. Differential equations defining the model behavior were numerically solved on a computer, and the effects of increases in pericardial elastances were simulated (Fig. 9-9). With increases in coupled constraint (E_{pe}), the venous flow became a predominantly systolic flow, and the RA pressure showed a prominent x descent. With increases

COUPLED PERICARDIAL CONSTRAINT

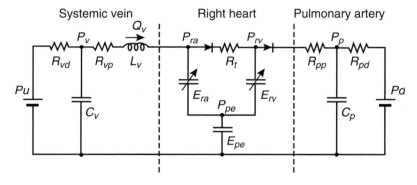

UNCOUPLED PERICARDIAL CONSTRAINT

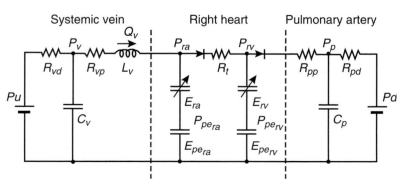

FIGURE 9-8 An electrical analog of the mathematical model of atrioventricular interaction with pericardial constraint. The model is a lumped, linear parameter, open-loop model of right heart circulation. The RA and RV were defined as time-varying elastances (E_{ra} and E_{rv}). The systemic venous system was modeled by an upstream pressure source (P_u) and a four-element venous impedance network including a capacitance (C_v), an inertance (L_v), and two resistances (R_{vd} and R_{vp}). The pulmonary arterial system consists of a three-element impedance network including a capacitance (C_p) and two resistances (R_{pp} and R_{pd}), and a downstream pressure source (P_d). Two one-way valves represented by diodes were interposed between E_{ra} and E_{rv} (tricuspid valve) and between E_{rv} and the pulmonary arteries (pulmonic valve). A resistance placed between E_{ra} and E_{rv} represents trans-tricuspid valve resistance (R_t). The driving force for flow in the model is provided by a pressure gradient between P_u and P_d, and periodic increases in E_{ra} and E_{rv} with the two competent valves. A coupled pericardial constraint was modeled by adding a "single" external elastance (E_{pe}) over both the right atrial and ventricular elastances (E_{ra} and E_{rv}), while an uncoupled pericardial constraint was modeled by adding two "separate" external elastances ($E_{pe_{ra}}$ and $E_{pe_{rv}}$) on E_{ra} and E_{rv}, respectively. P_p, pressure at the pulmonary arterial capacitance; P_{pe}, pericardial pressure over both RA and RV for coupled constraint; $P_{pe_{ra}}$, pericardial pressure over RA for uncoupled constraint; $P_{pe_{rv}}$, pericardial pressure over RV for uncoupled constraint; P_{ra}, RA pressure; P_{rv}, RV pressure; P_v, pressure at the systemic venous capacitance; Q_v, combined vena caval flow. (From Takata M, Harasawa Y, Beloucif S, Robotham JL: Coupled vs. uncoupled pericardial constraint: Effects on cardiac chamber interactions. *J Appl Physiol* 83:1799–1813, 1997; with permission).

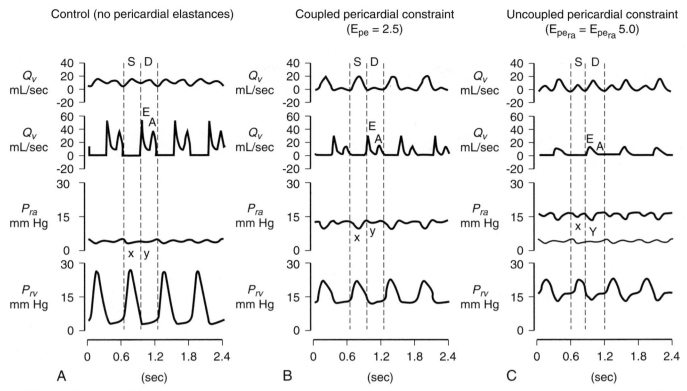

FIGURE 9-9   Simulation traces in the mathematical model of atrioventricular interaction, showing changes in combined vena caval flow (Q_v), tricuspid flow (Q_t), RA pressure (P_{ra}), and RV pressure (P_{rv}) with increases in pericardial constraint. **Panel A:** control condition with no pericardial constraint; **panel B:** increased coupled constraint; **panel C:** increased uncoupled constraint. A, atrial contraction component in tricuspid flow; D, ventricular diastole; S, ventricular systole; E, rapid filling wave in tricuspid flow; x, x descent in RA pressure; y, y descent in RA pressure. See text for further explanation. (From Takata M, Harasawa Y, Beloucif S, Robotham JL: Coupled vs. uncoupled pericardial constraint: Effects on cardiac chamber interactions. *J Appl Physiol* 83:1799–1813, 1997; with permission.)

in uncoupled constraint (E_{pera} and E_{perv}), the venous flow became a predominantly diastolic flow, with a markedly attenuated A wave in tricuspid flow. The RA pressure showed a prominent y descent, with a "dip and plateau" pattern in RV pressure. The model therefore well approximated the characteristic venous flow and pressure changes observed in pericardial diseases; increased coupled constraint accounted for the patterns in cardiac tamponade, and increased uncoupled constraint accounted for those in constrictive pericarditis.

Why do such characteristic flow and pressure patterns take place with the increased "uncoupled" constraint (i.e., constrictive pericarditis)? An intuitive explanation could be made when appreciating that with constriction, the pericardial pressure is "elevated" but still retains its "regional" nature, restricting volumes of each cardiac chamber independently. This is in contrast to the situation with tamponade, in which the pericardial pressure is "elevated" and becomes "uniform." Thus atrioventricular interaction in constriction should be much less than that in tamponade, with changes in atrial and ventricular volumes within a cardiac cycle not being coupled. During systole, ventricular ejection decreases the pericardial pressure over the ventricle but not over the atrium. The RA pressure shows little change during systole (diminished x descent), resulting in a small systolic venous flow. During diastole, the atrial emptying into the ventricle produces a decrease in pericardial pressure over the atrium. The resultant decrease in RA pressure (y descent) will enhance venous return, producing a diastolic antegrade venous flow. Ventricular filling

will occur mainly during early diastole when the tricuspid valve opens and the compliance of the ventricle is added to that of the atrium for the upstream venous beds, but it is rapidly attenuated because of the stiff RV and the RV pericardium, resulting in a dip-and-plateau pattern in ventricular pressures.

With the increased uncoupled constraint, the regional pericardium acts as if it were an additional free wall placed on either the RV or LV surface. Ventricular interdependence in constriction should be somewhat augmented, but not at all to the level observed with tamponade, which can produce an almost complete intrapericardial volume coupling between the two ventricles. Therefore pulsus paradoxus will not be very frequently observed with constrictive pericarditis. Similarly, a large inspiratory increase in venous return from the abdomen to the right heart, which is the key mechanism for pathogenesis of Kussmaul's sign,[110] would not be buffered by the left-sided compliances with constriction, resulting in a more manifest Kussmaul's sign. These explanations are supported by mathematical analyses of the volume elastance model of the effects of pericardium on ventricular interdependence.[180]

The coupled vs. uncoupled constraint concept thus offers a useful unifying theory to understand the pericardial constraint of the heart in normal and disease states and may provide insights from which better diagnostic and therapeutic strategies in pericardial disease can be developed. The analyses based on this concept,[18,180] together with previous experimental and clinical studies,[10,23,31,32,82,114] suggest that echocardiographic observations of atrioventricular volumes and flow patterns within a cardiac cycle may be useful in early diagnosis of tamponade or constrictive pathophysiology. Marked coupling between atrial and ventricular volume changes (i.e., reciprocal changes during a cardiac cycle) with dominant venous flow during ventricular systole suggests tamponade, whereas minimal changes in atrial volume and predominant flow during ventricular diastole suggests a constrictive process.

ETIOLOGY OF PERICARDIAL EFFUSION AND TAMPONADE

Pericardial effusion and tamponade are encountered in a variety of clinical settings. Pericardial effusion may consist of transudate (e.g., postpericardiotomy syndrome), exudate (e.g., purulent pericarditis), blood (e.g., chest trauma), air (e.g., pneumopericardium), chyle (idiopathic or postoperative chylopericardium), or even intravenous crystalloid solution (e.g., perforation of the RA or intrapericardial cava by a central venous catheter). Both inflammatory (pericarditis) and noninflammatory processes are responsible for abnormal fluid accumulation, as summarized in Table 9-1. Purulent pericarditis has become much less common in the era of antibiotics and routine vaccination against previously common bacterial pathogens. At present, pericardial effusion in children is most often associated with viral infection, systemic illness, or cardiac surgery. Zahn and colleagues.[207] reported in 1992 that

Table 9-1   Etiology of Pericardial Effusion and Tamponade

Infectious Pericarditis
Viral
Coxsackievirus B, echovirus, adenovirus, Epstein-Barr virus, mumps, varicella, poliomyelitis, hepatitis B, influenza (including post-vaccination), cytomegalovirus, measles, respiratory syncytial virus, human immunodeficiency virus
Bacterial/Tuberculous
Staphylococcus aureus, Haemophilus influenzae, Neisseria meningitidis, Streptococcus pneumoniae (including resistant forms), β-hemolytic streptococci, *Mycoplasma pneumoniae, Mycobacterium tuberculosis*
Fungal
Candida
Aspergillus
Pericarditis with Systemic Disease
Systemic Inflammatory Disease
Rheumatic fever, juvenile rheumatoid arthritis, systemic lupus erythematosus, ulcerative colitis, Kawasaki disease
Neoplasms
Leukemia, lymphoma, metastatic tumor, radiation pericarditis
Renal
End-stage renal disease, dialysis
Traumatic and Postoperative
Blunt chest trauma, central line malposition, catheterization/biopsy, rupture of coronary aneurysm (Kawasaki), early postoperative hemorrhage, postpericardiotomy syndrome, elevated venous pressure (post hemi- or completion Fontan), post cardiac transplantation
Miscellaneous and Drug-Related
Elevated central venous pressure
Superior vena cava syndrome, primary pulmonary hypertension and right ventricular failure, decompensated congestive heart failure
Drug-Related
Procainamide, hydralazine, penicillins, cromolyn, dantrolene, anthracyclines

among 41 children with nonpurulent pericardial effusions, the major etiologies were malignancy (20%), postpericardiotomy syndrome (17%), aseptic pericarditis (12%), and postoperative Fontan procedure (12%). A more recent report[189] of 94 drainage procedures in 73 children noted etiologies such as postoperative cardiac surgery (74%), infectious causes (6%), secondary to complications from interventional cardiac procedures (5.3%), malignancy (5.3%), lymphangiomatosis (2%), and two cases with idiopathic and one case each of trauma, collagen vascular disease, autoimmune polyglandular failure, and hypothyroidism. The two series represent etiologies of effusions that required drainage and may not represent the occurrence rates for effusions in general, many of which (especially idiopathic or viral and postpericardiotomy syndrome) do not require drainage.

Infectious Pericarditis

Viral

Acute pericarditis has usually been assumed to be viral in etiology, but in many cases, an etiologic virus is not detected.[39] For this reason, it also is known as aseptic or idiopathic pericarditis. An upper respiratory infection usually precedes the onset of symptoms by 10 days to 2 weeks.[39] Viral etiologies have been variously reported but also are difficult to confirm.[63] The technique of polymerase chain reaction (PCR) may identify the specific viral etiology.[151]

Other reported viral etiologies include coxsackievirus (generally considered to be the most common type), adenovirus, RSV, varicella, hepatitis B, and postinfluenza vaccine.[2,63,85,155,178] Pericardial disease has been reported with the broad spectrum of cardiac abnormalities associated with human immunodeficiency virus (HIV) infection and may occur from the virus itself or from opportunistic agents associated with HIV.[13,55,115,123]

Bacterial

Purulent pericarditis can be life-threatening, and patients with this illness are generally toxic appearing. The illness usually results from direct or hematogenous spread to the pericardium.[60] It rarely occurs in the absence of infection elsewhere. It appears to be a disease of children, especially infants and young children.[27,51,74] It also occurs as a result of direct penetrating injury or as a complication of operations on the heart, lungs, or esophagus. Its presence may not be suspected until late in the course of the disease, and a high incidence of tamponade is associated with bacterial pericarditis.[51] Effective treatment requires knowledge of the responsible microorganisms to make an appropriate choice of antibiotics.

The shift in the etiologic spectrum of purulent pericarditis related to antibiotic therapy has been documented.[100] In adults, the most common etiology is *Staphylococcus aureus* or gram-negative bacteria.[100] In children, *S. aureus* is currently the major pathogen.[60,63,131,196] In a review of purulent pericarditis in 162 children, 44% were due to *S. aureus*, 22% due to *Haemophilus influenzae*, 9% due to *Neisseria meningitidis*, and 6% to *Streptococcus pneumoniae*.[60] *S. aureus* pericarditis is often associated with osteomyelitis, pneumonia, or skin infections.[60,196] It continues to be a dangerous pathogen with a higher mortality than other pathogens.[27,60]

H. influenzae pericarditis is generally associated with respiratory infection and sometimes with meningitis. The average age of patients with *H. influenzae* pericarditis is approximately 5 years, similar to those with *H. influenzae* pneumonia and epiglottitis.[53] *H. influenzae* pericardial effusions have a tendency to form a thick, organized fibropurulent "peel," which adheres to the epicardial and pericardial membranes and may require surgical rather than percutaneous needle drainage.[21] Widespread and routine use of the vaccine against *H. influenzae* has markedly reduced the incidence of all forms of serious *H. influenzae* infection, including pericarditis.

N. meningitidis is responsible for a small number of cases. These are normally associated with meningococcemia and appear within a few days of hospitalization.[49] A purulent but sterile late-onset effusion may occur.[51]

Tuberculous

Tuberculous pericarditis, although rare in children in developed countries, remains an important cause of pericarditis in developing countries and in immunocompromised patients.[93,96] In addition, resistant strains emerging in association with HIV may make this a more frequent clinical entity even in developed countries.[28] It is a dominant cause of constrictive pericarditis worldwide.[122] It is rarely a primary infection and usually results from local extension from nearby structures or hematogenous spread.

Pericarditis with Systemic Disease

Pericarditis may be a manifestation of inflammatory carditis associated with systemic processes. Examples of this include acute rheumatic fever, juvenile rheumatoid arthritis, systemic lupus erythematosus, and Kawasaki disease.[37,46,129,205] Neoplastic disease is a major cause of pericarditis and pericardial effusion in both children and adults.[45,81,189,207] Pericardial diseases occur as a result of hematologic malignancies more commonly than as a result of metastatic processes in children. Neoplastic pericardial disease is frequently encountered in the hospital population, particularly in end-stage disease.[189,207] Pericardial effusion is common in patients with end-stage renal disease and may occur in patients on dialysis as well.[106,150]

Traumatic and Postoperative Pericardial Effusion

Chest trauma is a leading cause of cardiac tamponade in children.[16,71] Its presentation can be delayed in onset.[26] Many of these patients will have shock as a component of their presentation.[186] Recognition requires an index of suspicion along with an understanding of the signs of tamponade. Widening mediastinum on chest radiograph or electrocardiographic signs of cardiac contusion or both (sometimes without external evidence of thoracic trauma) along with elevated troponin[88] should raise the index of suspicion for tamponade, especially if the patient shows signs of hemodynamic instability after an initial period of stability. In acute trauma settings, combined rupture of the heart and pericardium can be more difficult to recognize because the signs of tamponade may not be seen.[120] Hemopericardium or effusion containing hyperalimentation solution can occur when a central venous catheter erodes through an intrapericardial caval vessel or cardiac chamber.[73,75,78] Myocardial injury during endomyocardial biopsy[138] (more frequently in the dilated cardiomyopathy/myocarditis patient than in the post-transplant patient) or during catheterization may occur.[200] The increase in the number of interventional procedures being done in the catheterization laboratory has resulted in an increase in the number of rescue pericardiocentesis procedures.[190] Hemopericardium may follow rupture of a coronary aneurysm in Kawasaki disease.[103]

After cardiac surgery, effusions related to postoperative oozing or bleeding may accumulate, particularly in the first 5 postoperative days.[8,47] These effusions are usually hemodynamically unimportant and usually resolve spontaneously.[47] These effusions, however, may become significant and may require urgent intervention. This is particularly true if anticoagulants are used in the postoperative period. The index of suspicion should therefore be higher in postoperative mechanical prosthetic valve recipients.[188]

The postoperative collection may be circumferential and in an intact pericardium may produce classic tamponade involving pathologic coupling, as discussed earlier. Localized, particularly posterior fluid accumulations may occur and may obstruct venous flow into the atria.[19,101,188] Either form of pericardial effusion may produce a clinical picture of profound shock, which may be difficult to distinguish from low cardiac output secondary to ventricular failure. Echocardiography is essential to make a bedside distinction.[188] Although "classic" tamponade with uniform fluid collection around the heart is readily diagnosed with transthoracic echocardiography, localized posterior collections of blood or thrombus may be more readily identified with transesophageal echocardiography.[20,94,188] Hence the diagnosis of localized pericardial clot must be kept in mind in patients who have signs of tamponade but have a negative transthoracic echocardiographic evaluation. Surgical exploration with evacuation of localized thrombus may be required. In addition to the success of echo-guided percutaneous needle drainage in circumferential effusions, a high degree of success in draining localized effusions with echo-guided needle/catheter-drainage techniques has been documented.[190] The composition of the localized fluid accumulation may affect the success of any attempted percutaneous drainage procedure.

"Posterior" or "local" tamponade is better understood as uncoupled restraint within the physiologic framework as presented earlier. These patients have been shown to have a prominent y descent in the right atrial pressure tracing, which is seen in constrictive pericarditis but is not typical of classic tamponade.[19]

Later-occurring pericardial effusions may be inflammatory (postpericardiotomy) or due to increased venous pressure, especially in patients after SVC–pulmonary artery connection (hemi-Fontan or bidirectional Glenn) or Fontan-type operations. Postpericardiotomy syndrome is the most common type of inflammatory pericarditis in the postoperative patient and may occur in adults and in children. It usually appears in children who have convalesced uneventfully until they begin to have low-grade fever, loss of appetite, or general discomfort. Nonspecific symptoms may occur in younger infants. It usually appears between 7 days and 2 months after the operation.[72] It is usually a self-limited process but recurrences may occur.[139] Etiologies are thought to be an immunologic response to a viral illness[54] or productions of autoantibodies against myocardial antigens after cardiac injury associated with open-heart surgery.[130] It may occur, however, in immunosuppressed patients after cardiac transplantation,[33,38] and some controversy exists over the role that antiheart antibodies play in the process.[203] Although the process usually responds to anti-inflammatory therapy and rarely requires drainage, patients with postpericardiotomy are represented in the largest reports of pericardiocentesis.[189,207]

Pericardial effusion may occur after Fontan or less commonly after cavopulmonary anastomosis. The effusions are usually transudative but may be chylous. Increased venous pressure is thought to be a principal factor in the pathogenesis. Prolonged drainage may indicate hemodynamic problems within the repair and should prompt consideration.[207]

Postoperative effusions may occur in patients after heart transplantation.[195] These may be due to the smaller donor heart within the chronically stretched recipient pericardium. Persistence of pericardial effusions after transplant has been correlated with both higher incidence and more severe histology of rejection.[40]

Miscellaneous and Drug-Related Pericardial Effusion

Various etiologies may act through the mechanism of increased central venous pressure. These may be SVC syndrome from central venous catheters,[108] presence of venous cannulae for extracorporeal membrane oxygenation,[109] pulmonary hypertension with RV failure,[87] and decompensated congestive heart failure.[97]

Drug-induced pericarditis may be a result of an immunologic mechanism with an inflammatory cause of the effusion. Systemic inflammatory or lupus-like symptoms may occur. Common etiologic agents include procainamide, hydralazine, penicillins, cromolyn, dantrolene, and anthracycline.[170] Withholding the responsible drug almost always results in clinical resolution, especially if the process is recent in onset.

CLINICAL MANIFESTATIONS

Symptoms and Physical Findings

Clinical findings of pericardial effusion depend on many factors (e.g., the cause, underlying systemic illness, rate and degree of accumulation of pericardial fluid, and age of the patient). The following description applies mainly to clinical findings of acute viral pericarditis with development of large/massive pericardial effusion.

The leading symptom of acute pericarditis is precordial pain, if the child is able to complain or give a history. The pain varies in severity but is normally relieved by leaning forward and is exacerbated by the supine position, inspiration, swallowing, and body motion. Radiation to the trapezius ridge is highly characteristic of pericardial pain. Low-grade fever usually develops (it is often >38°C in purulent pericarditis). Tachypnea and dyspnea may be observed when an early stage of tamponade is reached. In acute pericarditis, these symptoms are usually preceded by a viral prodrome or evidence of upper respiratory infection.

Except for the friction rub, physical findings are usually nonspecific until the accumulated pericardial fluid produces hemodynamic impairment.[160] The pericardial friction rub is a scratchy or creaky sound, likened to the sound of creaking leather or walking on snow. It also can be reproduced by rubbing hair between the fingers in close proximity to the ear. The rub may be triphasic during the cardiac cycle (i.e., one phase occurring during atrial systole, the next during ventricular systole, and the last during ventricular diastole).[173] It is most commonly heard over the lower left sternal border and may be augmented by the sitting position or inspiration, presumably because these maneuvers bring the heart closer to the chest wall.

Presumably the rub is the result of contact between fibrous adhesions within the pericardial space or contact between the inflamed parietal and visceral pericardium. In the case of a large effusion, the rub may still be audible[160] and possibly result from residual contact directly behind the heart or between the external parietal pericardium and surrounding structures.[172] The rub is considered highly characteristic of pericarditis.[172] It may vary in intensity during the process, and its absence does not rule out pericardial disease.[35,160]

Hemodynamic abnormalities encountered in pericarditis depend on the degree or phase of tamponade, as described earlier.[147] Pericardial effusion may be seen by echocardiography without hemodynamic impairment or with early impairment[160] before classic features of tamponade are seen.[192] With progression, cardiac sounds become muffled. Elevation of ventricular diastolic and venous pressures produces jugular venous distention and later hepatomegaly. Central venous pressure monitoring waveforms will demonstrate prominent ventricular systolic x descent and reduced ventricular diastolic y descent (see Fig. 9-6). Decreased LV stroke volume results in reflex tachycardia, vasoconstriction with poorly perfused extremities, progressively narrowing pulse pressure, decreased urinary output, and eventually hypotension. Beck's description of the "acute cardiac triad" in 1935 truncates these to three findings: (1) "a falling arterial pressure," (2) "a rising venous pressure," and (3) "a small, quiet heart."[17] Beck's triad is considered one of the characteristic findings in tamponade.

Pulsus paradoxus is considered another characteristic finding. The word *paradoxus* may be misleading, because pulsus paradoxus represents an exaggeration of the normal inspiratory decrease in blood pressure, as noted previously. Kussmaul originally used the term because he observed a decrease in the pulse volume despite the ("paradoxical") continued presence of a precordial impulse.[110]

For detection, the patient should be instructed to breathe normally because the augmented negative intrathoracic pressure during a deep inspiration may cause a falsely positive pulsus paradoxus. Upper or lower airway pathology may produce this problem. In general, an inspiratory decrease of arterial pressure of more than 20 mm Hg is highly suggestive of pericardial effusion with tamponade. The detection of pulsus paradoxus by sphygmomanometric technique is often difficult in children, and the precise diagnosis may require measurement of arterial pressure with an indwelling catheter. Alternatively, observation of pulse oximetry waveform with spontaneous respiration may be suggestive.[185] Palpation of the peripheral pulse that decreases perceptibly with inspiration should consideration of pulsus paradoxus and the attendant differential diagnosis, including tamponade.

Laboratory Findings

Chest roentgenography is nonspecific and may appear nearly normal, particularly with a rapidly accumulating effusion that is small in volume but nevertheless compressive. More commonly, a nonspecific enlargement of the cardiac silhouette is seen with loss of the contours of the component structures of the normal cardiac shadow. This produces the globular or water-bottle appearance. A rapidly increasing or unexplained enlargement in cardiac silhouette, or both, remains a common clue to pericardial disease. Clear pulmonary vascular markings (lack of pulmonary venous congestion) would support the diagnosis of pericardial effusion rather than congestive heart failure. The reason the pulmonary vasculature is not radiographically distended despite elevated venous pressure remains to be clearly elucidated, but the observation does suggest central compartment hypovolemia. When pericardial effusion is suspected, serial chest radiographs of identical technique may be helpful in defining a pattern of steadily increasing cardiac size, particularly in postoperative cardiac patients.

Electrocardiographic (ECG) recordings are often abnormal, and a classic pattern involving four stages of ST-segment elevation and T-wave inversion has been described.[174] These ECG changes are presumed to result from action of the pericardial fluid on the myocardium directly or from compression of the epicardial vessels by the effusion rather than due to any contribution from the electrically inert pericardium.[129,174] The electrophysiologic effects of components (particularly prostaglandins) of pericardial fluid have been investigated,[124,125] and in the future, their exact clinical role may be elucidated. Further, the clinical utility of the ST-T changes in the pediatric, particularly teenage, population may be confounded by the normal variant of early repolarization.[77] Regular alternation of QRS amplitude (i.e., electrical alternans) may occur in the presence of a large pericardial effusion and is the result of swinging or rotation of the heart within the fluid-filled pericardial space.[168] Low QRS voltage may be seen in the presence of a large pericardial effusion. Dysrhythmias were not common in a large series of acute pericarditis.[171] Atrial fibrillation is present in approximately one third of cases of constrictive pericarditis.[122]

Echocardiography has been used since its earliest clinical applications to assess pericardial disease.[59] It has assumed greater importance over time and, along with Doppler imaging, is the most important diagnostic test in the assessment of pericardial disease and its hemodynamic consequences. Because pericardial effusion may produce significant cardiac compression in the absence of classic findings such as Beck's triad, echocardiography is important in the diagnosis and management of pericardial effusion.[79]

Whereas most children can be imaged effectively with transthoracic echocardiography (Fig. 9-10), transesophageal echocardiography may be necessary to image loculated posterior effusions or clots, particularly in the early postoperative period.[19,101] Quantification of the amount of pericardial fluid present is subjective, but localized noncircumferential

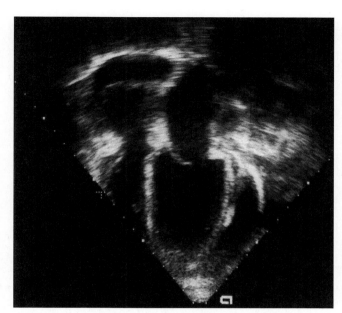

FIGURE 9-10 Two-dimensional echocardiogram of a moderate-sized, noncircumferential pericardial effusion in a postoperative cardiac transplant patient. Note the partial right atrial collapse.

(usually posterior) effusions are described as small, whereas circumferential effusions with anterior and posterior components are usually described as moderate to large, depending on the degree of epicardial/pericardial separation.[23] It is important to be mindful that small effusions (with rapid accumulation in a relatively stiff pericardium) can produce significant cardiac compression. Experience with echocardiography has produced methods to assess more accurately the degree of cardiac compression than a semiquantitative estimate of the amount of fluid present.[192]

Morphologic features that suggest tamponade include diastolic compression of the RA and RV.[11,105,154] RA collapse in late diastole likely represents vertical atrioventricular coupling as the atrium empties into the ventricle without simultaneous atrial filling (see earlier). These two echocardiographic signs are considered to reflect the almost negative transmural RA and RV diastolic pressures in tamponade. They are useful but have some limitations in sensitivity and specificity.

Additional morphologic features of tamponade include abnormal mitral valve motion,[158] inferior vena caval plethora without inspiratory collapse,[86] and swinging heart.[104] Because many children with congenital heart disease have elevated RV pressure and RV hypertrophy, it is important to keep in mind that RV collapse may not be present under these circumstances.[68,164]

Addition of Doppler analysis to the morphologic signs noted earlier has helped to refine further clinical diagnostic accuracy and confirm some of the previously noted laboratory observations of the hemodynamic patterns in tamponade.[10,23,31,32,41] These include inspiratory decreases in left ventricular filling producing delay in mitral valve opening, increased isovolumic relaxation time, and decreased mitral velocity. Reciprocal changes are noted on the right side. In expiration, the left-sided filling is increased with the increased extrapericardial pulmonary venous pressure compared with LA pressure. Opposite changes occur on the right side. In addition to these, predominant systolic antegrade venous flow with absent or retrograde diastolic flow are characteristic of tamponade physiology. All of these signs confirm the previously noted "coupling" between atria and ventricles in tamponade (i.e., atrial and ventricular filling and emptying being virtually of equal magnitude and 180 degrees out of phase).[18]

Other previously reported imaging modalities for the detection of the spectrum of pericardial disease include angiography, fluoroscopy, radionuclide angiography, computed tomography, and magnetic resonance imaging. Magnetic resonance imaging is quite helpful in assessing the pericardial thickness and is useful when constrictive pericarditis is in the differential.[119] Because constrictive pericarditis is rare in children and because transthoracic imaging produces diagnostic images in children, the other imaging modalities are not used often in pediatrics.

Hematologic and biochemical findings depend on the cause of the pericardial effusion. Leukocytosis with immature polymorphonuclear leukocyte predominance is normally present in purulent pericarditis, whereas lymphocytosis is often seen in viral pericarditis or postpericardiotomy syndrome. Erythrocyte sedimentation rate and acute-phase reactants are usually elevated. Cardiac enzyme levels may increase slightly owing to some inflammatory involvement of the myocardium. Cultures of blood, urine, spinal fluid, throat, nasopharynx, or stool should be evaluated for both bacterial and viral pathogens. Consideration should be given to testing for HIV. A purified protein derivative (PPD) test should be placed if tuberculous pericarditis is in the differential. Because pericarditis may be the initial manifestation of a systemic disease, a thorough workup, particularly for collagen vascular disease, should be considered.

Pericardial fluid samples obtained by pericardiocentesis should be sent for cell count, cytology, biochemistry (glucose, protein, lactate dehydrogenase), and latex agglutination studies, in addition to Gram and acid-fast stains, with appropriate cultures. Pericardial fluid PCR may be useful in selected cases, although the utility may depend on the organism being sought.[36,141] Cytologic examination should always be performed to exclude malignancy.

In purulent pericarditis, the pericardial fluid usually shows marked leukocytosis and may be frank pus. The protein level is usually elevated, and the glucose is usually low. In contrast, the fluid in idiopathic pericarditis may be straw colored or slightly bloody and usually has a predominance of mononuclear cells.

Pericardial biopsy (including percutaneous approaches) has been reported in adult series, but its role in children is uncertain.[80,209]

TREATMENT

Therapy for Pericardial Effusion

In addition to drainage of the pericardial fluid, supportive therapy is important. It is important in patients being prepared for drainage procedures, as well as in those with mild hemodynamic impairment who may ultimately be stabilized without a drainage procedure. These would include patients with postpericardiotomy syndrome and minimal hemodynamic impairment, who may respond quickly to anti-inflammatory therapy. Because a compressive effusion affects mainly preload, intravenous fluids may help stabilize the patient. Diuretics may worsen the patient's condition by further reducing preload. Cardiac output is maintained by reflex tachycardia and augmentation of contractility. Inotropic agents may be of some benefit. In more advanced stages of tamponade, blood pressure is maintained with peripheral vasoconstriction of both the venous and arterial beds. Accordingly, vasodilators should be avoided. With life-threatening tamponade, cardiorespiratory collapse may require endotracheal intubation and mechanical ventilation. Application of PPV, PEEP, or continuous positive airway pressure (CPAP) must be performed with great care, because the combination of increased intrathoracic pressure and increased lung volumes may further reduce systemic venous return and increase total external constraint of the heart.[183]

Technique of Pericardiocentesis

The technique of percutaneous pericardiocentesis has evolved from a "blind" emergency procedure that could not provide prolonged drainage into a safe procedure with the option of reliable long-term drainage.[191] An additional benefit of an indwelling pericardial catheter is that it will provide some information about how rapidly and how much fluid is being produced as it is aspirated over time (Fig. 9-11).[111] Echocardiography has helped to refine the procedure and is now an essential part of the technique (occasional emergencies may require that drainage be performed without simultaneous imaging). In a Mayo Clinic series, the improvements in pericardiocentesis resulted in reduced numbers of surgical procedures required to treat pericardial effusions.[188]

Pericardiocentesis is usually performed in the intensive care unit (ICU) or catheterization laboratory setting, but outpatient procedures have been reported.[50] It is usually performed with sedation and local anesthesia. Ideally the anesthesia or ICU staff is present to maintain adequate levels of sedation and to monitor the airway, avoiding if possible the need for PPV (see earlier).

Echocardiography is used to plan the procedure, determine the site of skin puncture, define the optimal needle course, anticipate the depth, and with echo-contrast injection, confirm intrapericardial location of the needle. A careful echocardiogram with particular attention to the transducer angulation (the ultimate needle angulation) is performed before the skin is prepped. The best site of puncture has been described as the point at which the largest fluid accumulation is closest to the body surface. In a retrospective pediatric series of 94 procedures in 73 patients at the Mayo Clinic, the optimal site of puncture was determined to be para-apical (68.1%), subxyphoid (17%), left axillary (5.3%), left parasternal (3.2%), right parasternal (2.1%), posterolateral (1.1%), or unspecified by procedure note (3.2%).[189] Other experienced centers find that the subxyphoid approach is still the most frequent.[111]

The needle should be of adequate length to reach the effusion (6 cm should be adequate), and many centers now use a Teflon-sheathed needle.[189] Commercially available kits contain needles, guide wires, dilators, and catheters[133]; examples are shown in Figure 9-12. Alternatively, the supplies can be assembled from items available in most hospitals (Table 9-2).[191]

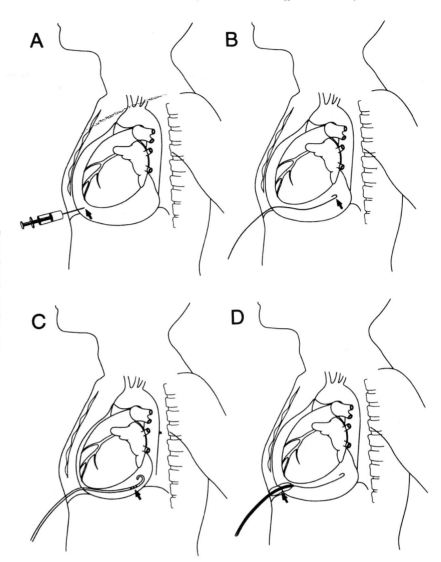

FIGURE 9-11 Schematic of pericardiocentesis technique. **A,** Introduction of needle (arrow). **B,** Passage of guide wire (arrow). **C,** Pigtail catheter in pericardial space (arrow). **D,** Balloon inflation to create pericardial-pleural space window (arrow). (From Lang P: Other catheterization laboratory techniques and interventions: Atrial septal defect creation, transseptal puncture, pericardial drainage, foreign body retrieval, exercise and drug testing. In Lock JE, Keane JF, Perry SF (eds): *Diagnostic and Interventional Catheterization in Congenital Heart Disease*. 2nd ed. Boston, Kluwer Academic Publishers, pp 256–258, 2000; with permission.)

The skin and deeper structures are infiltrated with 1% to 2% lidocaine after sterile prep. The needle is inserted at the site and with a predetermined trajectory with continuous gentle aspiration. The usual angle for the subxyphoid approach is 15 degrees above the skin.[168] If fluid is obtained, the Teflon sheath is advanced about 2 cm off of the needle, and the needle removed. The fluid may be bloody (56%) or nonbloody (44%).[189]

In the event of bloody fluid, confirmation of intrapericardial rather than intracardiac needle position is important. Bloody pericardial fluid is nonclotting; additionally, bloody pericardial fluid usually sinks to the bottom of a gauze sponge, whereas blood forms clots on the surface of the gauze.[111] Alternatively, a small amount (2 to 5 mL) of agitated saline contrast can be injected with echocardiographic monitoring from a separate site.[128,191] Dense opacification of the pericardial space confirms an intrapericardial position.

If a single drainage is planned, then the effusion is drained by repeated aspiration through the Teflon sheath or needle until echocardiography confirms adequate drainage. If prolonged drainage is required, a minimum of fluid is drained on penetration of the pericardium, leaving the largest possible epicardial/pericardial separation to facilitate safe passage of the guide wire and catheter. Once the guide wire is successfully passed, the Teflon catheter is removed, and a small stab incision is made in the skin. A dilator or sheath-dilator is then passed. The sheath is advocated by some[191] to facilitate passage of a pigtail catheter through the tissues without damage to the tip and to prevent the accidental removal of the wire from the pericardial space by the catheter during a difficult passage. (Others use a pigtail alone.[111,168]) The sheath is removed when the catheter tip is safely in the pericardial space. If necessary, another saline injection is performed to confirm the position of the catheter. The fluid is then drained as completely as possible by syringe suction. The catheter may then be flushed with saline to prevent catheter plugging, and intermittent drainage (frequency dependent on reaccumulation rate and hemodynamics; usual minimum, every 2 hours) is followed by sterile saline catheter flush to maintain catheter patency. This is preferred over continuous drainage for maintenance of catheter patency.

Balloon pericardiotomy has been used in adults and there is some experience in children.[187,208] Surgical drainage can be accomplished via a subxyphoid approach or laparoscopy.[102,149]

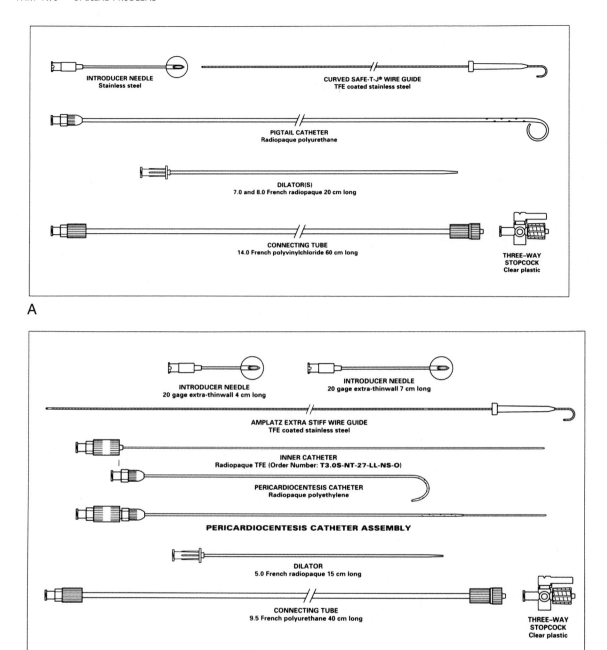

FIGURE 9-12 Commercially available **(A)** Lock and **(B)** Park pericardiocentesis sets. (Courtesy of Cook Incorporated, Bloomington, IN; with permission.)

Therapy for Specific Underlying Etiologies

Treatment of viral or idiopathic pericarditis involves bed rest and usually antiinflammatory doses of aspirin (50 to 75 mg/kg/day) or nonsteroidal antiinflammatory agents (NSAIDs). Refractory cases may require treatment with prednisone (2 mg/kg/day, maximum dose, 60 mg/day). Therapy with prednisone should be closely supervised and tapered as quickly as possible because of systemic side effects. Pericardial fluid drainage is needed in a minority of cases. Treatment of pericardial effusion due to postpericardiotomy syndrome is similar. Analgesics are sometimes used for accompanying chest pain. Idiopathic pericarditis usually subsides spontaneously or responds quickly to anti-inflammatory treatment, and persistence beyond 2 weeks should prompt a search for other causes.[160] Treatment for postpericardiotomy syndrome is usually given for 4 to 6 weeks. Late recurrence may occur in idiopathic/viral pericarditis and in postpericardiotomy syndrome.[139] Recurrent cases may respond to aspirin/NSAIDs or to prednisone. Colchicine has shown effectiveness at preventing recurrences in some studies including limited

Table 9-2 Equipment for Pericardiocentesis

Echocardiography machine and appropriate transducer(s)
Pericardiocentesis tray
  Povodone-iodine solution (skin antiseptic)
  Sterile transparent plastic drape (or sterile towels/eye sheet)
  25- and 20-gauge needle for local anesthetic administration
  1%–2% lidocaine
  Multiple 16–18 gauge, 5–8 cm length (polyTef-sheathed) needles
  Syringes (10–20 mL and one 60 mL)
  Specimen collection tubes—sterile
  Plastic tubing and three-way stopcock
  Scalpel (no. 11 blade)
  4 × 4 gauze pads
Other supplies
  Sheath introducer set
    Fine-gauge polyTef-coated floppy tipped guide wire
    Dilator and introducer sheath
  A standard pigtail angiocatheter (appropriate to sheath size) with
    multiple side-holes
  Fluid receptacle (1 L vacuum bottle)
  Manometer
  Dressings and antiseptic ointment
  Sterile isotonic saline
  Sterile gloves, mask, and gown

Adapted from Tsang TS, Freeman WK, Sinak LJ, Seward JB: Echocardiographically guided pericardiocentesis: Evolution and state-of-the-art technique. *Mayo Clin Proc* 73:647–652, 1998.

experience in children.[3,30,206] In another study of recurrent pericarditis in children, colchicine was not effective.[139]

Purulent pericarditis requires aggressive combined therapies with antibiotics, hemodynamic support, and pericardial drainage. Late detection may contribute to mortality.[60] Needle aspiration of the pericardium may provide temporary hemodynamic relief and a specimen for diagnosis, but adequate pericardial drainage may not be technically possible with needle techniques because of the fibropurulent nature of the effusion.[21] The approaches reported are subxyphoid, left anterior thoracotomy, and median sternotomy, and complete or partial pericardiectomy may be required to relieve cardiac compression.[1,56,64,102,127,157] Successful catheter drainage has been reported.[24,92]

In purulent pericarditis, initial antibiotic therapy should cover a broad spectrum including Staphylococci, *H. influenzae*, *S. pneumoniae*, and *N. meningitidis*. The emergence and local prevalence of highly resistant strains of *S. pneumoniae* and *S. aureus* may influence initial therapy. Duration of antibiotic therapy is usually 4 to 6 weeks. After successful treatment for purulent pericarditis, the possibility of constrictive pericarditis should be kept in mind.[51,60]

Tuberculous pericarditis should be treated with combination antituberculous therapy. Prednisone may be used in the early stages of tuberculous pericarditis to decrease inflammation and adhesions of the pericardium. Antituberculous therapy alone may not be effective. Percardiectomy may be required.[28]

In pericarditis associated with systemic illness, pericardiocentesis and cytologic studies, as well as systematic evaluation of other organ systems, are critical for accurate diagnosis. Without appropriate general management for the underlying illness, the treatment of pericardial pathology itself (i.e., with anti-inflammatory drugs and drainage of pericardial effusion) may not be effective.

THE FUTURE: PERICARDIAL THERAPEUTICS

In the past, access to the pericardium has been reserved for situations with excessive pericardial fluid. Thus the normal pericardial space has not been routinely used for the delivery of agents or for the study of pericardial or myocardial/pericardial physiology. New approaches to the normal pericardial space may provide access to study the hemodynamic physiology and the biochemical physiology of the pericardium and pericardial fluid.[121,156,199] The transatrial approach allows the study of the intact pericardium. Heretofore, study of pericardial pathology has been accomplished only through an instrumented (therefore not completely intact) pericardium.

Pericardial fluid has characteristics of a plasma ultrafiltrate, but it also varies significantly because of its conditioning by local vascular tissues and myocytes. The composition of pericardial fluid may be affected by disease stages such as congestive heart failure, as well as ischemia or pulmonary hypertension.[7,44,57,91,121] Samples in a human pericardial fluid bank may help in the understanding of pericardial fluid composition in health and disease.[48]

It was pointed out recently that as a site for therapeutics and drug delivery, the pericardium has several advantages over conventional intravascular therapy, including (1) access to perivascular tissue, (2) delivery into a low-turnover reservoir with minimal loss of agent into circulation, and (3) perfusion of atrial and ventricular epicardial tissue.[199] The ability to bypass the endothelium may have advantages in some circumstances. Pericardial gene delivery has been shown to be effective in experimental animals.[70] Experimental experience with intrapericardial administration of nitric oxide precursors and antiarrhythmic agents has been reported.[12,58]

References

1. Adebo OA, Adebonojo SA: Purulent pericarditis in children. *J Thorac Cardiovasc Surg* 88:312–313, 1984.
2. Adler R, Takahashi M, Wright HT Jr: Acute pericarditis associated with hepatitis B infection. *Pediatrics* 61:716–719, 1978.
3. Adler Y, Finkelstein Y, Guindo J, et al: Colchicine treatment for recurrent pericarditis: A decade of experience. *Circulation* 97:2183–2185, 1998.
4. Agostoni E: Mechanics of the pleural space. *Physiol Rev* 52:57–128, 1972.
5. Alam HB, Levitt A, Molyneaux R, et al: Can pleural effusions cause cardiac tamponade? *Chest* 116:1820–1822, 1999.
6. Altman C: Pericarditis and pericardial disease. In Garson A, Bricker J, Fisher D, et al (eds): *The Science and Practice of Pediatric Cardiology.* 2nd ed. Baltimore, Williams and Wilkins, 1998, pp 1795–1815.
7. Amano J, Suzuki A, Sunamori M, et al: Atrial natriuretic peptide in the pericardial fluid of patients with heart disease. *Clin Sci (Lond)* 85:165–168, 1993.
8. Angelini GD, Penny WJ, el-Ghamary F, et al: The incidence and significance of early pericardial effusion after open heart surgery. *Eur J Cardiothorac Surg* 1:165–168, 1987.
9. Antman EM, Cargill V, Grossman W: Low-pressure cardiac tamponade. *Ann Intern Med* 91:403–406, 1979.
10. Appleton CP, Hatle LK, Popp RL: Cardiac tamponade and pericardial effusion: Respiratory variation in transvalvular flow velocities studied by Doppler echocardiography. *J Am Coll Cardiol* 11:1020–1030, 1988.
11. Armstrong WF, Schilt BF, Helper DJ, et al: Diastolic collapse of the right ventricle with cardiac tamponade: An echocardiographic study. *Circulation* 65:1491–1496, 1982.
12. Ayers GM, Rho TH, Ben-David J, et al: Amiodarone instilled into the canine pericardial sac migrates transmurally to produce electrophysiologic effects and suppress atrial fibrillation. *J Cardiovasc Electrophysiol* 7:713–721, 1996.

13. Barbaro G: Cardiovascular manifestations of HIV infection. *Circulation* 106:1420–1425, 2002.

14. Bartle SH, Hermann HJ: Acute mitral regurgitation in man. Hemodynamic evidence and observations indicating an early role for the pericardium. *Circulation* 36:839–851, 1967.

15. Bartle SH, Hermann HJ, Cavo JW, et al: Effect of the pericardium on left ventricular volume and function in acute hypervolaemia. *Cardiovasc Res* 2:284–289, 1968.

16. Beaver BL, Laschinger JC: Pediatric thoracic trauma. *Semin Thorac Cardiovasc Surg* 4:255–262, 1992.

17. Beck CS: Two cardiac compression triads. *J Am Med Assoc* 104:714–716, 1935.

18. Beloucif S, Takata M, Shimada M, Robotham JL: Influence of pericardial constraint on atrioventricular interactions. *Am J Physiol* 263:H125–H134, 1992.

19. Beppu S, Tanaka N, Nakatani S, et al: Pericardial clot after open heart surgery: Its specific localization and haemodynamics. *Eur Heart J* 14:230–234, 1993.

20. Berge KH, Lanier WL, Reeder GS: Occult cardiac tamponade detected by transesophageal echocardiography. *Mayo Clin Proc* 67:667–670, 1992.

21. Blickman JG, Dunlop RW, Fulton DR: Diagnostic implications of the echocardiographically demonstrated pericardial peel. *Am Heart J* 119:965–998, 1990.

22. Bodega F, Zocchi L, Agostoni E: Macromolecule transfer through mesothelium and connective tissue. *J Appl Physiol* 89:2165–2173, 2000.

23. Borganelli M, Byrd BF III: Doppler echocardiography in pericardial disease. *Cardiol Clin* 8:333–348, 1990.

24. Bouwels L, Jansen E, Janssen J, et al: Successful long-term catheter drainage in an immunocompromised patient with purulent pericarditis. *Am J Med* 83:581–583, 1987.

25. Bove AA, Santamore WP: Ventricular interdependence. *Prog Cardiovasc Dis* 23:365–388, 1981.

26. Bowers P, Harris P, Truesdell S, Stewart S: Delayed hemopericardium and cardiac tamponade after unrecognized chest trauma. *Pediatr Emerg Care* 10:222–224, 1994.

27. Boyle JD, Pearce ML, Guze LB: Purulent pericarditis: Review of the literature and report of 11 cases. *Medicine* 40:119–144, 1961.

28. Bozbuga N, Erentug V, Eren E, et al: Pericardiectomy for chronic constrictive tuberculous pericarditis: Risks and predictors of survival. *Tex Heart Inst J* 30:180–185, 2003.

29. Brinker JA, Weiss JL, Lappe DL, et al: Leftward septal displacement during right ventricular loading in man. *Circulation* 61:626–633, 1980.

30. Brucato A, Cimaz R, Balla E: Prevention of recurrences of corticosteroid-dependent idiopathic pericarditis by colchicine in an adolescent patient. *Pediatr Cardiol* 21:395–396, 2000.

31. Burstow DJ, Oh JK, Bailey KR, et al: Cardiac tamponade: Characteristic Doppler observations. *Mayo Clin Proc* 64:312–324, 1989.

32. Byrd BF III, Linden RW: Superior vena cava Doppler flow velocity patterns in pericardial disease. *Am J Cardiol* 65:1464–1470, 1990.

33. Cabalka AK, Rosenblatt HM, Towbin JA, et al: Postpericardiotomy syndrome in pediatric heart transplant recipients: Immunologic characteristics. *Tex Heart Inst J* 22:170–176, 1995.

34. Cassidy SS, Wead WB, Seibert GB, Ramanathan M: Changes in left ventricular geometry during spontaneous breathing. *J Appl Physiol* 63:803–811, 1987.

35. Cayler GG, Haybi H, Riley HDJ, Simon JL: Pericarditis with effusion in infants and children. *J Pediatr* 63:262–272, 1963.

36. Cegielski JP, Devlin BH, Morris AJ, et al: Comparison of PCR, culture, and histopathology for diagnosis of tuberculous pericarditis. *J Clin Microbiol* 35:3254–3257, 1997.

37. Chang RW: Cardiac manifestations of SLE. *Clin Rheum Dis* 8:197–206, 1982.

38. Charitos CE, Kontoyannis DA, Nanas JN: Postpericardiotomy syndrome during intensive immunosuppression after cardiac transplantation. *Acta Cardiol* 55:95–97, 2000.

39. Christian HA: Nearly ten decades of interest in idiopathic pericarditis. *Am Heart J* 42:645–651, 1951.

40. Ciliberto GR, Anjos MC, Gronda E, et al: Significance of pericardial effusion after heart transplantation. *Am J Cardiol* 76:297–300, 1995.

41. Cohen ML: Experimental cardiac tamponade: Correlation of pressure, flow velocity, and echocardiographic changes. *J Appl Physiol* 69:924–931, 1990.

42. Cohen SI, Kupersmith J, Aroesty J, Rowe JW: Pulsus paradoxus and Kussmaul's sign in acute pulmonary embolism. *Am J Cardiol* 32:271–275, 1973.

43. Cohn JN, Pinkerson AL, Tristani FE: Mechanism of pulsus paradoxus in clinical shock. *J Clin Invest* 46:1744–1755, 1967.

44. Cortina A, Ambrose JA, Prieto-Granada J, et al: Left ventricular function after myocardial infarction: Clinical and angiographic correlations. *J Am Coll Cardiol* 5:619–624, 1985.

45. da Costa CM, de Camargo B, Gutierrez y Lamelas R, et al: Cardiac tamponade complicating hyperleukocytosis in a child with leukemia. *Med Pediatr Oncol* 33:120–123, 1999.

46. Dajani AS, Taubert KA, Gerber MA, et al: Diagnosis and therapy of Kawasaki disease in children. *Circulation* 87:1776–1780, 1993.

47. D'Cruz IA, Overton DH, Pai GM: Pericardial complications of cardiac surgery: Emphasis on the diagnostic role of echocardiography. *J Card Surg* 7:257–268, 1992.

48. Dickson TJ, Gurudutt V, Nguyen AQ, et al: Establishment of a clinically correlated human pericardial fluid bank: Evaluation of intrapericardial diagnostic potential. *Clin Cardiol* 22:I40–I42, 1999.

49. Dixon LM, Sanford HS: Meningococcal pericarditis in the antibiotic era. *Mil Med* 136:433–438, 1971.

50. Drummond JB, Seward JB, Tsang TS, et al: Outpatient two-dimensional echocardiography-guided pericardiocentesis. *J Am Soc Echocardiogr* 11:433–435, 1998.

51. Dupuis C, Gronnier P, Kachaner J, et al: Bacterial pericarditis in infancy and childhood. *Am J Cardiol* 74:807–809, 1994.

52. Ebert PA, Najafi H: The pericardium. In Sabiston DCJ, Spencer FC (eds): *Surgery of the Chest*. 5th ed. Philadelphia, WB Saunders, 1990, pp 1230–1249.

53. Echeverria P, Smith EW, Ingram D, et al: Hemophilus influenzae b pericarditis in children. *Pediatrics* 56:808–818, 1975.

54. Engle MA, Zabriskie JB, Senterfit LB, et al: Viral illness and the postpericardiotomy syndrome: A prospective study in children. *Circulation* 62:1151–1158, 1980.

55. Estok L, Wallach F: Cardiac tamponade in a patient with AIDS: A review of pericardial disease in patients with HIV infection. *Mt Sinai J Med* 65:33–39, 1998.

56. Farrow CD Jr, Brom AG, Nauta J: The surgical treatment of pericarditis: A follow-up study. *Dis Chest* 48:478–483, 1965.

57. Fazekas L, Horkay F, Kekesi V, et al: Enhanced accumulation of pericardial fluid adenosine and inosine in patients with coronary artery disease. *Life Sci* 65:1005–1012, 1999.

58. Fei L, Baron AD, Henry DP, Zipes DP: Intrapericardial delivery of L-arginine reduces the increased severity of ventricular arrhythmias during sympathetic stimulation in dogs with acute coronary occlusion: Nitric oxide modulates sympathetic effects on ventricular electrophysiological properties. *Circulation* 96:4044–4049, 1997.

59. Feigenbaum H, Zaky A, Waldhausen JA: Use of ultrasound in the diagnosis of pericardial effusion. *Ann Intern Med* 65:443–452, 1966.

60. Feldman WE: Bacterial etiology and mortality of purulent pericarditis in pediatric patients: Review of 162 cases. *Am J Dis Child* 133:641–644, 1979.

61. Fewell JE, Abendschein DR, Carlson CJ, et al: Mechanism of decreased right and left ventricular end-diastolic volumes during continuous positive-pressure ventilation in dogs. *Circ Res* 47:467–472, 1980.

62. Fowler NO: Pulsus paradoxus. *Heart Dis Stroke* 3:68–69, 1994.

63. Fowler NO, Manitsas GT: Infectious pericarditis. *Prog Cardiovasc Dis* 16:323–336, 1973.

64. Fredriksen RT, Cohen LS, Mullins CB: Pericardial windows or pericardiocentesis for pericardial effusions. *Am Heart J* 82:158–162, 1971.

65. Freeman GL, LeWinter MM: Determinants of intrapericardial pressure in dogs. *J Appl Physiol* 60:758–764, 1986.

66. Freeman GL, LeWinter MM: Pericardial adaptations during chronic cardiac dilation in dogs. *Circ Res* 54:294–300, 1984.

67. Freeman GL, Little WC: Comparison of in situ and in vitro studies of pericardial pressure-volume relation in dogs. *Am J Physiol* 251:H421–427, 1986.

68. Frey MJ, Berko B, Palevsky H, et al: Recognition of cardiac tamponade in the presence of severe pulmonary hypertension. *Ann Intern Med* 111:615–617, 1989.

69. Friedman HS, Lajam F, Zaman Q, et al: Effect of autonomic blockade on the hemodynamic findings in acute cardiac tamponade. *Am J Physiol* 232:H5–11, 1977.

70. Fromes Y, Salmon A, Wang X, et al: Gene delivery to the myocardium by intrapericardial injection. *Gene Ther* 683–688, 1999.

71. Fulton DR, Grodin M: Pediatric cardiac emergencies. *Emerg Med Clin North Am* 1:45–61, 1983.

72. Fyler DC: Pericardial disease. In Fyler DC (ed): *Nadas' Pediatric Cardiology*. Philadelphia, Hanley and Belfus, pp 363–368, 1992.

73. Garg M, Chang CC, Merritt RJ: An unusual case presentation: Pericardial tamponade complicating central venous catheter. *J Perinatol* 9:456–457, 1989.

74. Gersony WM, McCracken GH, Jr: Purulent pericarditis in infancy. *Pediatrics* 40:224–232, 1967.

75. Giacoia GP: Cardiac tamponade and hydrothorax as complications of central venous parenteral nutrition in infants. *JPEN J Parenter Enteral Nutr* 15:110–113, 1991.

76. Gibson AT, Segal MB: A study of the composition of pericardial fluid, with special reference to the probable mechanism of fluid formation. *J Physiol* 277:367–377, 1978.

77. Ginzton LE, Laks MM: The differential diagnosis of acute pericarditis from the normal variant: New electrocardiographic criteria. *Circulation* 65:1004–1009, 1982.

78. Green C, Yohannan MD: Umbilical arterial and venous catheters: Placement, use, and complications. *Neonatal Netw* 17:23–28, 1998.

79. Guberman BA, Fowler NO, Engel PJ, et al: Cardiac tamponade in medical patients. *Circulation* 64:633–640, 1981.

80. Gupta K, Mathur VS: Diagnosis of pericardial disease using percutaneous biopsy: Case report and literature review. *Tex Heart Inst J* 30:130–133, 2003.

81. Hancock EW: Neoplastic pericardial disease. *Cardiol Clin* 8:673–682, 1990.

82. Hatle LK, Appleton CP, Popp RL: Differentiation of constrictive pericarditis and restrictive cardiomyopathy by Doppler echocardiography. *Circulation* 79:357–370, 1989.

83. Hausknecht MJ, Brin KP, Weisfeldt ML, et al: Effects of left ventricular loading by negative intrathoracic pressure in dogs. *Circ Res* 62:620–631, 1988.

84. Hetzel PS, Wood EH, Burchell HB: Pressure pulses in the right side of the heart in a case of amyloid disease and in a case of idiopathic heart failure simulating pericarditis. *Mayo Clin Proc* 28:107–112, 1952.

85. Hildebrandt HM, Maassab HF, Willis PW: Influenza virus pericarditis. *Am J Dis Child* 104:579–582, 1962.

86. Himelman RB, Kircher B, Rockey DC, Schiller NB: Inferior vena cava plethora with blunted respiratory response: A sensitive echocardiographic sign of cardiac tamponade. *J Am Coll Cardiol* 12:1470–1477, 1988.

87. Hinderliter AL, Willis PW IV, Long W, et al: Frequency and prognostic significance of pericardial effusion in primary pulmonary hypertension. PPH Study Group. Primary pulmonary hypertension. *Am J Cardiol* 84:481–484, A10, 1999.

88. Hirsch R, Landt Y, Porter S, et al: Cardiac troponin I in pediatrics: Normal values and potential use in the assessment of cardiac injury. *J Pediatr* 130:872–877, 1997.

89. Hoit BD, Lew WY, LeWinter M: Regional variation in pericardial contact pressure in the canine ventricle. *Am J Physiol* 255:H1370–1377, 1988.

90. Holt JP, Rhode EA, Kines H: Pericardial and ventricular pressure. *Circ Res* 8:1171–1181, 1966.

91. Horkay F, Szokodi I, Selmeci L, et al: Presence of immunoreactive endothelin-1 and atrial natriuretic peptide in human pericardial fluid. *Life Sci* 62:267–274, 1998.

92. Houghton JL, Becherer PR: Haemophilus influenzae pericarditis successfully treated by catheter drainage. *South Med J* 80:766–768, 1987.

93. Hugo-Hamman CT, Scher H, De Moor MM: Tuberculous pericarditis in children: A review of 44 cases. *Pediatr Infect Dis J* 13:13–18, 1994.

94. Hutchison SJ, Smalling RG, Albornoz M, et al: Comparison of transthoracic and transesophageal echocardiography in clinically overt or suspected pericardial heart disease. *Am J Cardiol* 74:962–965, 1994.

95. Ishihara T, Ferrans VJ, Jones M, et al: Histologic and ultrastructural features of normal human parietal pericardium. *Am J Cardiol* 46:744–753, 1980.

96. Jaiyesimi F, Abioye AA, Antia AU: Infective pericarditis in Nigerian children. *Arch Dis Child* 54:384–390, 1979.

97. Kataoka H: Pericardial and pleural effusions in decompensated chronic heart failure. *Am Heart J* 139:918–923, 2000.

98. Kingma I, Smiseth OA, Frais MA, et al: Left ventricular external constraint: Relationship between pericardial, pleural and esophageal pressures during positive end-expiratory pressure and volume loading in dogs. *Ann Biomed Eng* 15:331–346, 1987.

99. Kisanuki A, Shono H, Kiyonaga K, et al: Two-dimensional echocardiographic demonstration of left ventricular diastolic collapse due to compression by pleural effusion. *Am Heart J* 122:1173–1175, 1991.

100. Klacsmann PG, Bulkley BH, Hutchins GM: The changed spectrum of purulent pericarditis: An 86 year autopsy experience in 200 patients. *Am J Med* 63:666–673, 1977.

101. Kochar GS, Jacobs LE, Kotler MN: Right atrial compression in postoperative cardiac patients: Detection by transesophageal echocardiography. *J Am Coll Cardiol* 16:511–516, 1990.

102. Kouchoukos NT, Blackstone EH, Doty DB, et al: Pericardial disease. In *Kirklin/Barratt-Boyes Cardiac Surgery*. 3rd ed. Philadelphia: Churchill Livingstone; 2003.

103. Koutlas TC, Wernovsky G, Bridges ND, et al: Orthotopic heart transplantation for Kawasaki disease after rupture of a giant coronary artery aneurysm. *J Thorac Cardiovasc Surg* 113:217–218, 1997.

104. Kronzon I, Cohen ML, Winer HE: Contribution of echocardiography to the understanding of the pathophysiology of cardiac tamponade. *J Am Coll Cardiol* 1:1180–1182, 1983.

105. Kronzon I, Cohen ML, Winer HE. Diastolic atrial compression: A sensitive echocardiographic sign of cardiac tamponade. *J Am Coll Cardiol* 2:770–775, 1983.

106. Kumar S, Lesch M: Pericarditis in renal disease. *Prog Cardiovasc Dis* 22:357–369, 1980.

107. Kuno Y: The significance of the pericardium. *J Physiol* 50:1–36, 1915.

108. Kurekci E, Kaye R, Koehler M: Chylothorax and chylopericardium: A complication of a central venous catheter. *J Pediatr* 132:1064–1066, 1998.

109. Kurian MS, Reynolds ER, Humes RA, Klein MD: Cardiac tamponade caused by serous pericardial effusion in patients on extracorporeal membrane oxygenation. *J Pediatr Surg* 34:1311–1314, 1999.

110. Kussmaul A: Ueber schwielige Mediastino-Pericarditis und den paradoxen Puls. *Klin Wochenschr* 10:443, 1873.

111. Lang P: Other catheterization laboratory techniques and interventions: atrial septal defect creation, transseptal puncture, pericardial drainage, foreign body retrieval, exersise and drug testing. In Lock JE, Keane JF, Perry SF (eds): *Diagnostic and Interventional Catheterization in Congenital Heart Disease*. 2nd ed. Boston, Kluwer Academic Publishers, pp 256–258, 2000.

112. Lanir Y: A structural theory for the homogeneous biaxial stress-strain relationships in flat collagenous tissues. *J Biomech* 12:423–436, 1979.

113. LeWinter MM, Pavelec R: Influence of the pericardium on left ventricular end-diastolic pressure-segment relations during early and later stages of experimental chronic volume overload in dogs. *Circ Res* 50:501–509, 1982.

114. Linden R, Byrd BF III: Superior vena cava Doppler: A non-invasive method for the diagnosis of pericardial disease. *Int J Cardiol* 16:145–153, 1987.

115. Lipshultz SE, Chanock S, Sanders SP, et al: Cardiovascular manifestations of human immunodeficiency virus infection in infants and children. *Am J Cardiol* 63:1489–1497, 1989.

116. Lloyd TC Jr: Respiratory system compliance as seen from the cardiac fossa. *J Appl Physiol* 53:57–62, 1982.

117. Lorell B, Leinbach RC, Pohost GM, et al: Right ventricular infarction. Clinical diagnosis and differentiation from cardiac tamponade and pericardial constriction. *Am J Cardiol* 43:465–471, 1979.

118. Marini JJ, Culver BH, Butler J: Mechanical effect of lung distention with positive pressure on cardiac function. *Am Rev Respir Dis* 124:382–386, 1981.

119. Masui T, Finck S, Higgins CB: Constrictive pericarditis and restrictive cardiomyopathy: Evaluation with MR imaging. *Radiology* 182:369–373, 1992.

120. May AK, Patterson MA, Rue LW III et al: Combined blunt cardiac and pericardial rupture: Review of the literature and report of a new diagnostic algorithm. *Am Surg* 65:568–574, 1999.

121. Mebazaa A, Wetzel RC, Dodd-o JM, et al: Potential paracrine role of the pericardium in the regulation of cardiac function. *Cardiovasc Res* 40:332–342, 1998.

122. Mehta A, Mehta M, Jain AC: Constrictive pericarditis. *Clin Cardiol* 22:334–344, 1999.

123. Milei J, Grana D, Fernandez Alonso G, Matturri L: Cardiac involvement in acquired immunodeficiency syndrome—a review to push action. The Committee for the Study of Cardiac Involvement in AIDS. *Clin Cardiol* 21:465–472, 1998.

124. Miyazaki T, Pride HP, Zipes DP: Prostaglandins in the pericardial fluid modulate neural regulation of cardiac electrophysiological properties. *Circ Res* 66:163–175, 1990.

125. Miyazaki T, Zipes DP: Pericardial prostaglandin biosynthesis prevents the increased incidence of reperfusion-induced ventricular fibrillation produced by efferent sympathetic stimulation in dogs. *Circulation* 82:1008–1019, 1990.

126. Moore R: Congenital deficiency of the pericardium. *Arch Surg* 11:765, 1925.

127. Morgan RJ, Stephenson LW, Woolf PK, et al: Surgical treatment of purulent pericarditis in children. *J Thorac Cardiovasc Surg* 85:527–531, 1983.

128. Muhler EG, Engelhardt W, von Bernuth G: Pericardial effusions in infants and children: Injection of echo contrast medium enhances the safety of echocardiographically-guided pericardiocentesis. *Cardiol Young* 8:506–508, 1998.

129. Nadas AS, Levy JM: Pericarditis in children. *Am J Cardiol* 7:109–117, 1961.

130. Nomura Y, Yoshinaga M, Haraguchi T, et al: Relationship between the degree of injury at operation and the change in antimyosin antibody titer in the postpericardiotomy syndrome. *Pediatr Cardiol* 15:116–120, 1994.

131. Okoroma EO, Perry LW, Scott LP III: Acute bacterial percarditis in children: Report of 25 cases. *Am Heart J* 90:709–713, 1975.

132. Olsen CO, Tyson GS, Maier GW, et al: Diminished stroke volume during inspiration: A reverse thoracic pump. *Circulation* 72:668–679, 1985.

133. Park SC, Pahl E, Ettedgui JA, et al: Experience with a newly developed pericardiocentesis set. *Am J Cardiol* 66:1529–1531, 1990.

134. Permutt S, Caldini P: Tissue pressures and fluid dynamics of the lungs. *Fed Proc* 35:1876–1880, 1976.

135. Peters J, Fraser C, Stuart RS, et al: Negative intrathoracic pressure decreases independently left ventricular filling and emptying. *Am J Physiol* 257:H120–131, 1989.

136. Peters J, Kindred MK, Robotham JL: Transient analysis of cardiopulmonary interactions. I. Diastolic events. *J Appl Physiol* 64:1506–1517, 1988.

137. Peters J, Kindred MK, Robotham JL: Transient analysis of cardiopulmonary interactions. II. Systolic events. *J Appl Physiol* 64:1518–1526, 1988.

138. Pophal SG, Sigfusson G, Booth KL, et al: Complications of endomyocardial biopsy in children. *J Am Coll Cardiol* 34:2105–2110, 1999.

139. Raatikka M, Pelkonen PM, Karjalainen J, Jokinen EV: Recurrent pericarditis in children and adolescents: Report of 15 cases. *J Am Coll Cardiol* 42:759–764, 2003.

140. Rabkin S, Berghause DG, Bauer HF: Mechanical properties of the isolated canine pericardium. *J Appl Physiol* 36:69–73, 1974.

141. Rana BS, Jones RA, Simpson IA: Recurrent pericardial effusion: The value of polymerase chain reaction in the diagnosis of tuberculosis. *Heart* 82:246–247, 1999.

142. Reddy PS: Hemodynamics of cardiac tamponade in man. In Reddy PS, Leon DF, Shaver JA (eds): *Pericardial Disease*. New York, Raven Press, pp 161–185, 1982.

143. Reddy PS: Hemodynamics of constrictive pericarditis. In Reddy PS, Leon DF, Shaver JA (eds): *Pericardial Disease*. New York, Raven Press, pp 275–297, 1982.

144. Reddy PS: The pathophysiology of pulsus paradoxus in cardiac tamponade. In Reddy PS, Leon DF, Shaver JA (eds): *Pericardial Disease*. New York, Raven Press, pp 215–230, 1982.

145. Reddy PS, Curtiss EI, O'Toole JD, Shaver JA: Cardiac tamponade: Hemodynamic observations in man. *Circulation* 58:265–272, 1978.

146. Reddy PS, Curtiss EI: Cardiac tamponade. *Cardiol Clin* 8:627–637, 1990.

147. Reddy PS, Curtiss EI, Uretsky BF: Spectrum of hemodynamic changes in cardiac tamponade. *Am J Cardiol* 66:1487–1491, 1990.

148. Robotham JL: Haemodynamic consequences of mechanical ventilation. *Acta Anesthesiol Scand* 36:7–52, 1987.

149. Rodriguez MI, Ash K, Foley RW, Liston W: Pericardio peritoneal window: Laparoscopic approach. *Surg Endosc* 13:409–411, 1999.

150. Rostand SG, Rutsky EA: Pericarditis in end-stage renal disease. *Cardiol Clin* 8:701–707, 1990.

151. Satoh T, Kojima M, Ohshima K: Demonstration of the Epstein-Barr genome by the polymerase chain reaction and in situ hybridisation in a patient with viral pericarditis. *Br Heart J* 69:563–564, 1993.

152. Scharf SM, Brown R, Saunders N, Green LH: Effects of normal and loaded spontaneous inspiration on cardiovascular function. *J Appl Physiol* 47:582–590, 1979.

153. Scharf SM, Brown R, Warner KG, Khuri S: Intrathoracic pressures and left ventricular configuration with respiratory maneuvers. *J Appl Physiol* 66:481–491, 1989.

154. Schiller NB, Botvinick EH: Right ventricular compression as a sign of cardiac tamponade: An analysis of echocardiographic ventricular dimensions and their clinical implications. *Circulation* 56:774–779, 1977.

155. Seddon DJ: Pericarditis with pericardial effusion complicating chickenpox. *Postgrad Med J* 62:1133–1134, 1986.

156. Seferovic PM, Ristic AD, Maksimovic R, et al: Initial clinical experience with PerDUCER device: Promising new tool in the diagnosis and treatment of pericardial disease. *Clin Cardiol* 22:I30–35, 1999.

157. Sethi GK, Nelson RM, Jenson CB: Surgical management of acute septic pericarditis. *Chest* 63:732–735, 1973.

158. Settle HP, Adolph RJ, Fowler NO, et al: Echocardiographic study of cardiac tamponade. *Circulation* 56:951–959, 1977.

159. Settle HP Jr, Engel PJ, Fowler NO, et al: Echocardiographic study of the paradoxical arterial pulse in chronic obstructive lung disease. *Circulation* 62:1297–1307, 1980.

160. Shabetai R: Acute pericarditis. *Cardiol Clin* 8:639–644, 1990.

161. Shabetai R: Pericardial and cardiac pressure. *Circulation* 77:1–5, 1988.

162. Shabetai R: The pathophysiology of pulsus paradoxus in cardiac tamponade. In Reddy PS, Leon DF, Shaver JA (eds): *Pericardial Disease*. New York, Raven Press, pp 215–230, 1982.

163. Shabetai R, Fowler NO, Guntheroth WG: The hemodynamics of cardiac tamponade and constrictive pericarditis. *Am J Cardiol* 26:480–489, 1970.

164. Silverman N: Postoperative evaluation. In Silverman N (ed): *Pediatric Echocardiography*. Baltimore, Williams and Wilkins, 1993.

165. Slinker BK, Ditchey RV, Bell SP, LeWinter MM: Right heart pressure does not equal pericardial pressure in the potassium chloride–arrested canine heart in situ. *Circulation* 76:357–362, 1987.

166. Smiseth OA, Frais MA, Kingma I, et al: Assessment of pericardial constraint in dogs. *Circulation* 71:158–164, 1985.

167. Smiseth OA, Scott-Douglas NW, Thompson CR, et al: Nonuniformity of pericardial surface pressure in dogs. *Circulation* 75:1229–1236, 1987.

168. Spodick DH: Acute cardiac tamponade. *N Engl J Med* 349:684–690, 2003.

169. Spodick DH: Macrophysiology, microphysiology, and anatomy of the pericardium: A synopsis. *Am Heart J* 124:1046–1051, 1992.

170. Spodick DH: Pericarditis in systemic diseases. *Cardiol Clin* 8:709–716, 1990.

171. Spodick DH: Frequency of arrhythmias in acute pericarditis determined by Holter monitoring. *Am J Cardiol* 53:842–845, 1984.

172. Spodick DH: Pericardial rub: A prospective, multiple observer investigation of pericardial friction in 100 patients. *Am J Cardiol* 35:357–362, 1975.

173. Spodick DH: Acoustic phenomena in pericardial disease. *Am Heart J* 81:114–124, 1971.

174. Spodick DH: In *Acute Pericarditis*. New York, Grune and Stratton, p 17, 1957.

175. Spotnitz HM, Kaiser GA: The effect of the pericardium on pressure-volume relations in the canine left ventricle. *J Surg Res* 11:375–380, 1971.

176. Stalcup SA, Mellins RB: Mechanical forces producing pulmonary edema in acute asthma. *N Engl J Med* 297:592–596, 1977.

177. Stray-Gundersen J, Musch TI, Haidet GC, et al: The effect of pericardiectomy on maximal oxygen consumption and maximal cardiac output in untrained dogs. *Circ Res* 58:523–530, 1986.

178. Streifler JJ, Dux S, Garty M, Rosenfeld JB: Recurrent pericarditis: a rare complication of influenza vaccination. *Br Med J (Clin Res Ed)* 283:526–527, 1981.

179. Takata M, Beloucif S, Shimada M, Robotham JL: Superior and inferior vena caval flows during respiration: pathogenesis of Kussmaul's sign. *Am J Physiol* 262:H763–70, 1992.

180. Takata M, Harasawa Y, Beloucif S, Robotham JL: Coupled vs. uncoupled pericardial constraint: Effects on cardiac chamber interactions. *J Appl Physiol* 83:1799–1813, 1997.

181. Takata M, Mitzner W, Robotham JL: Influence of the pericardium on ventricular loading during respiration. *J Appl Physiol* 68:1640–1650, 1990.

182. Takata M, Robotham JL: Effects of inspiratory diaphragmatic descent on inferior vena caval venous return. *J Appl Physiol* 72:597–607, 1992.

183. Takata M, Robotham JL: Ventricular external constraint by the lung and pericardium during positive end-expiratory pressure. *Am Rev Respir Dis* 143:872–875, 1991.

184. Takata M, Wise RA, Robotham JL: Effects of abdominal pressure on venous return: Abdominal vascular zone conditions. *J Appl Physiol* 69:1961–1972, 1990.

185. Tamburro RF, Ring JC, Womback K: Detection of pulsus paradoxus associated with large pericardial effusions in pediatric patients by analysis of the pulse-oximetry waveform. *Pediatrics* 109:673–677, 2002.

186. Tanaka H, Fujita T, Endoh Y, Kobayashi K: Pericardial tamponade type injury: A 17-year study in an urban trauma center in Japan. *Surg Today* 29:1017–1023, 1999.

187. Thanopoulos BD, Georgakopoulos D, Tsaousis GS, et al: Percutaneous balloon pericardiotomy for the treatment of large, nonmalignant pericardial effusions in children: Immediate and medium-term results. *Cathet Cardiovasc Diagn* 40:97–100, 1997.

188. Tsang TS, Barnes ME, Hayes SN, et al: Clinical and echocardiographic characteristics of significant pericardial effusions following cardiothoracic surgery and outcomes of echo-guided pericardiocentesis for management: Mayo Clinic experience, 1979–1998. *Chest* 116:322–331, 1999.

189. Tsang TS, El-Najdawi EK, Seward JB, et al: Percutaneous echocardiographically guided pericardiocentesis in pediatric patients: Evaluation of safety and efficacy. *J Am Soc Echocardiogr* 11:1072–1077, 1998.

190. Tsang TS, Freeman WK, Barnes ME, et al: Rescue echocardiographically guided pericardiocentesis for cardiac perforation complicating catheter-based procedures. The Mayo Clinic experience. *J Am Coll Cardiol* 32:1345–1350, 1998.

191. Tsang TS, Freeman WK, Sinak LJ, Seward JB: Echocardiographically guided pericardiocentesis: Evolution and state-of-the-art technique. *Mayo Clin Proc* 73:647–652, 1998.

192. Tsang TS, Oh JK, Seward JB: Diagnosis and management of cardiac tamponade in the era of echocardiography. *Clin Cardiol* 22:446–452, 1999.

193. Tsitlik JE, Halperin HR, Guerci AD, et al: Augmentation of pressure in a vessel indenting the surface of the lung. *Ann Biomed Eng* 15:259–284, 1987.

194. Tyberg JV, Taichman GC, Smith ER, et al: The relationship between pericardial pressure and right atrial pressure: An intraoperative study. *Circulation* 73:428–432, 1986.

195. Vandenberg BF, Mohanty PK, Craddock KJ, et al: Clinical significance of pericardial effusion after heart transplantation. *J Heart Transplant* 7:128–134, 1988.

196. Van Reken D, Strauss A, Hernandez A, Feigin RD: Infectious pericarditis in children. *J Pediatr* 85:165–169, 1974.

197. Vaska K, Wann LS, Sagar K, Klopfenstein HS: Pleural effusion as a cause of right ventricular diastolic collapse. *Circulation* 86:609–617, 1992.

198. Venkatesh G, Tomlinson CW, O'Sullivan T, McKelvie RS: Right ventricular diastolic collapse without hemodynamic compromise in a patient with large, bilateral pleural effusions. *J Am Soc Echocardiogr* 8:551–553, 1995.

199. Verrier RL, Waxman S, Lovett EG, Moreno R: Transatrial access to the normal pericardial space: A novel approach for diagnostic sampling, pericardiocentesis, and therapeutic interventions. *Circulation* 98:2331–2333, 1998.

200. Vitiello R, McCrindle BW, Nykanen D, et al: Complications associated with pediatric cardiac catheterization. *J Am Coll Cardiol* 32:1433–1440, 1998.

201. Wallis TW, Robotham JL, Compean R, Kindred MK: Mechanical heart-lung interaction with positive end-expiratory pressure. *J Appl Physiol* 54:1039–1047, 1983.

202. Wead WB, Norton JF: Effects of intrapleural pressure changes on canine left ventricular function. *J Appl Physiol* 50:1027–1035, 1981.

203. Webber SA, Wilson NJ, Fung MY, et al: Autoantibody production after cardiopulmonary bypass with special reference to postpericardiotomy syndrome. *J Pediatr* 121:744–747, 1992.

204. Wiegner AW, Bing OH, Borg TK, Caulfield JB: Mechanical and structural correlates of canine pericardium. *Circ Res* 49:807–814, 1981.

205. Yancey CL, Doughty RA, Cohlan BA, Athreya BH: Pericarditis and cardiac tamponade in juvenile rheumatoid arthritis. *Pediatrics* 68:369–373, 1981.

206. Yazigi A, Abou-Charaf LC: Colchicine for recurrent pericarditis in children. *Acta Paediatr* 87:603–604, 1998.

207. Zahn EM, Houde C, Benson L, Freedom RM: Percutaneous pericardial catheter drainage in childhood. *Am J Cardiol* 70:678–680, 1992.

208. Ziskind AA, Pearce AC, Lemmon CC, et al: Percutaneous balloon pericardiotomy for the treatment of cardiac tamponade and large pericardial effusions: Description of technique and report of the first 50 cases. *J Am Coll Cardiol* 21:1–5, 1993.

209. Ziskind AA, Rodriguez S, Lemmon C, Burstein S: Percutaneous pericardial biopsy as an adjunctive technique for the diagnosis of pericardial disease. *Am J Cardiol* 74:288–291, 1994.

Chapter 10

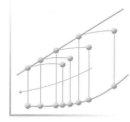

Anesthesia for Pediatric Cardiac Surgery

WILLIAM J. GREELEY, MD, MBA

INTRODUCTION

Pediatric cardiac anesthesia continues to evolve as an exciting and technically demanding subspecialty in which anesthetic management is based on sound physiologic principles. Congenital cardiovascular surgery and anesthesia are often performed under unusual physiologic conditions. Rarely in clinical medicine are patients exposed to such biologic extremes as during congenital heart surgery. Commonly, patients are cooled to 18° C, acutely hemodiluted by more than 50% of their extracellular fluid volume, and undergo periods of total circulatory arrest up to 1 hour. The ability to manage patients under these physiologic extremes is a vital function of the pediatric cardiovascular anesthesiologist.

Clearly, the perioperative management of these complex patients requires a group of physicians (surgeon, anesthesiologist, cardiologist, critical care specialist) and nurses working as a team. This team orientation is essential to achieve an optimal outcome. While the quality of the surgical repair, the effects of cardiopulmonary bypass, and postoperative care are the major determinants of outcome, meticulous anesthetic management is imperative. Ideally, despite the complexity of the patients and the marked physiologic changes attributed to cardiopulmonary bypass (CPB) and the surgical procedures, anesthetic care should never contribute substantially to morbidity or mortality.[58] The challenge is to understand the principles underlying the management of patients with congenital heart disease and apply them to clinical anesthesia.

PREOPERATIVE MANAGEMENT

Preoperative Evaluation

Caring for children with congenital heart disease presents the anesthesiologist with a wide spectrum of anatomic and physiologic abnormalities. Patients range from young, healthy, asymptomatic children having a small atrial septal defect (ASD) closed to the newborn infant with hypoplastic left heart syndrome requiring aggressive perioperative hemodynamic and ventilatory support. Intertwined with the medical diversity of these patients are the psychological factors affecting both the patient and the parents. Preparation of the patient and the family is time-consuming, but omitting or

267

compromising this aspect of patient care is a major deterrent to a successful outcome and patient/parental satisfaction. This approach mandates that cardiac surgeons, cardiologists, anesthesiologists, intensivists, and nurses work as a team in preparing the patient and the family for surgery and postoperative recovery. This team-oriented approach not only prepares the patient and family but also serves as a safeguard to prevent errors and omissions in the exacting perioperative care necessitated by the complexity of cardiac surgery for congenital heart disease. The preoperative visit offers the family the opportunity to meet the surgeon and anesthesiologist and to begin preparing the patient and family for surgery.

The preoperative evaluation should always start with a careful history and physical examination.[138] The history should concentrate on the cardiopulmonary system. Parents should be questioned about the general health and activity of their child. Fundamentally, a child's general health and activity will reflect cardiorespiratory reserve. Deficiencies may point toward cardiovascular or other systems that may influence anesthetic or surgical risk. It is important to determine whether the child has normal or impaired exercise tolerance. Is he or she gaining weight appropriately or exhibiting signs of failure to thrive on the basis of cardiac cachexia? Does the child exhibit signs of congestive heart failure (diaphoresis, tachypnea, poor feeding, recurrent respiratory infections)? Is there progressive cyanosis or new onset of cyanotic spells? Any intercurrent illness such as a recent upper respiratory tract infection or pneumonia must be ascertained. Lower respiratory tract infections may require a delay in proposed surgery, based on the negative impact that airway reactivity and elevations in pulmonary vascular resistance (PVR) may have on surgical outcome. Recurrent pneumonia is frequently associated with pulmonary overcirculation and altered lung compliance in patients with increased pulmonary blood flow. It is equally important to ascertain current medications, previous anesthetic problems, or family history of anesthetic difficulties. In the modern era of echocardiography and cardiac catheterization, physical examination rarely contributes additional anatomic information about the underlying cardiac lesion.

Careful review of the cardiac catheterization data and an understanding of its potential impact on the operative and anesthetic plan are essential. Cardiac catheterization is another modality to assess anatomy and physiologic function in congenital heart disease. Although many anatomic questions can now be reliably answered noninvasively, children with complex anatomic questions or those for whom physiologic data are required, catheterization remains a vital tool. Important catheterization data for the anesthesiologist include:

1. Child's response to sedative medications
2. Pressure and oxygen saturation in all chambers and great vessels
3. Location and magnitude of intra- and extra-cardiac shunt ($Q_p:Q_s$)
4. Pulmonary vascular resistance, systemic vascular resistance
5. Chamber sizes and function
6. Pulmonary vascular resistance
7. Distortion of systemic or pulmonary arteries related to prior surgery
8. Coronary artery anatomy

9. Anatomy, location and function of previously created shunts
10. Acquired or congenital anatomic variants that might have an impact on planned vascular access.

Careful review of the cardiac catheterization data and an understanding of its potential impact on the operative and anesthetic plan are essential. Not all the medical problems can be evaluated and corrected preoperatively; the surgeon, cardiologist, and anesthesiologist must discuss the potential management problems and any need for further evaluation or intervention before arrival in the operating room. Appropriate communication and cooperation between the two physicians will optimize patient care and facilitate perioperative clinical management. Typically, institutions have a regularly scheduled combined cardiology/cardiac surgery meeting to discuss candidates for surgery during which all of the essential information presented above is displayed and discussed. Such a meeting provides an invaluable opportunity for learning about specific surgical candidates as well as a continuing educational forum that promotes an interdisciplinary exchange directed at contemporary concepts in congenital heart disease and its treatment, both medical and surgical.[123]

Premedication

For infants between 6 and 9 months of age, pentobarbital (2 to 4 mg/kg) may be administered orally. A calm, cooperative, sedated child is the usual result. Children older than 9 months of age receive a benzodiazepine or a barbiturate as an oral premedication. Our current preference is midazolam 0.3 to 0.7 mg/kg orally 10 to 20 minutes before induction. The higher dose is used in the smallest patients. Alternatively, pentobarbital 4 mg/kg is administered 1 hour before induction. For infants younger than 6 months of age, no premedication is used.

INTRAOPERATIVE MANAGEMENT

Physiologic Monitoring

The monitoring used for any specific patient should depend on the child's condition and the magnitude of the planned surgical procedure. The perioperative monitoring techniques available are listed in Table 10-1. Noninvasive monitoring is placed before induction of anesthesia. In the crying child, patient, the anesthesiologist may elect to defer application of monitoring devices until immediately after the induction of anesthesia. Standard monitoring includes an electrocardiographic (ECG) system, pulse oximetry, capnography, precordial stethoscope, and an appropriate-sized blood pressure cuff (either oscillometric or Doppler). Additional monitoring includes an indwelling arterial catheter, temperature probes, and an esophageal stethoscope. Foley catheters are generally employed when surgical intervention entails cardiopulmonary bypass, might produce renal ischemia, or when the anesthetic management includes a regional technique associated with urinary retention. Some centers routinely employ central venous pressure monitoring for major cardiovascular surgery.[90] Alternatively, we typically use directly placed transthoracic atrial lines to obtain that information for separation from

Table 10-1 Monitoring of Organ Systems

Cardiopulmonary System
Esophageal stethoscope
Electrocardiogram
Standard seven-lead system, ST-T wave analysis, esophageal
  electrocardiographic lead
Pulse oximetry
Automated oscillometric blood pressure
Capnograph
Ventilator parameters
Indwelling arterial catheter
Central venous pressure catheter
Pulmonary artery catheter
Transthoracic pressure catheter
  Left or right atrium, pulmonary artery
Echocardiography with Doppler color flow imaging
  Epicardial or transesophageal
Central Nervous System
Peripheral nerve stimulator
Processed electroencephalography
Specialized
  Cerebral blood flow—xenon clearance methodology
  Cerebral metabolism—near-infrared spectroscopy, oxygen consumption
  Transcranial Doppler
  Jugular venous bulb oxygen saturation
  BIS monitor
Temperature
Nasopharyngeal, rectal, esophageal, tympanic
Renal Function
Foley catheter

cardiopulmonary bypass and the postoperative period. In that setting, the benefits of the information or access provided by percutaneous central venous pressure catheters in the pre-bypass period must be weighed against the risks they pose.

Continuous monitoring of arterial pressure is only possible through an indwelling intra-arterial catheter. In young children, cannulation of the radial artery with a 22-gauge catheter is preferred. In older children and adolescents, a 20-gauge catheter may be substituted. Careful inspection, palpation, and four-extremity noninvasive blood pressure determinations will ensure that previous or currently planned operative procedures, such as a previous radial artery cutdown, subclavian flap for coarctation repair, or a Blalock-Taussig shunt, do not interfere with the selected site of arterial pressure monitoring. Other sites available for cannulation include the ulnar, femoral, axillary, or umbilical (in neonates) arteries. Cannulation of the posterior tibial or dorsalis pedis arteries is not usually sufficient for complex operative procedures. Peripheral arterial catheters, principally of the distal lower extremities, function poorly after cardiopulmonary bypass and do not reflect central aortic pressure when distal extremity temperature remains low.[123]

Myocardial and cerebral preservation is principally maintained through hypothermia; therefore, the accurate and continuous monitoring of body temperature is crucial. Rectal and nasopharyngeal temperature are monitored, as they reflect core and brain temperature, respectively. Monitoring of esophageal temperature is a good reflection of cardiac and thoracic temperature. Tympanic probes, although a useful reflection of cerebral temperature, can cause tympanic membrane rupture.

Pulse oximetry and capnography provide instantaneous feedback concerning adequacy of ventilation and oxygenation. They are useful guides in ventilatory and hemodynamic adjustments to optimize $Q_p:Q_s$ before and after surgically created shunts and pulmonary artery bands. Peripheral vasoconstriction in patients undergoing deep hypothermia and circulatory arrest renders digital oxygen saturation probes less reliable. The use of a tongue sensor has been advocated in the newborn to provide a more central measure of oxygen saturation, with less temperature-related variability.[109]

The use of transthoracic right or left atrial catheters or transvenous superior van caval catheters is based on the individual disease process, physiologic state and surgical intervention. For example, in children undergoing a Fontan procedure for tricuspid atresia or univentricular heart, these measurements are especially useful. Following Fontan operation, pulmonary blood flow must occur without benefit of monitoring ventricular pumping. Subtle changes in preload, PVR, and pulmonary venous pressure influence pulmonary blood flow and thus systemic cardiac output. Data derived from systemic venous and left atrial pressure help distinguish the relative importance of intravascular volume (central venous pressure [CVP]), PVR (CVP–left atrial pressure [LAP] gradient), or ventricular compliance (LAP), each of which requires a different therapeutic approach.

Intraoperative Echocardiography

In recent years, newer techniques for monitoring patients during pediatric cardiovascular surgery have been introduced. The most promising of these techniques is echocardiography with Doppler color flow imaging. Several reports have described the usefulness of intraoperative echo-Doppler during congenital heart surgery.[18,49,92,93] Two-dimensional echocardiography combined with pulsed-wave Doppler ultrasound and color flow mapping is able to provide detailed morphologic as well as physiologic information in the majority of operative cases. Using echo-Doppler in the operating room, anatomic and physiologic data can be obtained before CPB, thus refining the operative plans. Prebypass echo-Doppler precisely defines anesthetic and surgical management.[94,133] Because of the unrestricted epicardial and transesophageal echocardiography (TEE) approaches in anesthetized patients, new findings are frequently discovered and management plans changed accordingly (Fig. 10-1). Postbypass echo-Doppler evaluation is able to immediately assess the quality of the surgical repair as well as assess cardiac function by examining ventricular wall motion and systolic thickening.[94,133] This technique can show residual structural defects after bypass, which can be immediately repaired in the same operative setting and prevents leaving the operating room with significant residual structural defects that will require reoperation at a later time (Fig. 10-2). By identifying patients with new right ventricular (RV) and left ventricular (LV) contraction abnormalities after bypass, as determined by a change in wall motion or systolic thickening, echo-Doppler provides guidance for immediate pharmacologic interventions. Importantly, postbypass ventricular dysfunction and residual structural defects identified by echo-Doppler are associated with an increased incidence of reoperation and higher morbidity and mortality rate.[132] Thus this monitoring tool is helpful in

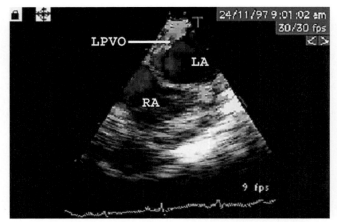

FIGURE 10-1 Intraoperative transesophageal echocardiogram (TEE) pre-cardiopulmonary bypass demonstrating left pulmonary vein obstruction (LPVO). Diagnosis of LPVO was not previously recognized in this patient with simple transposition of the great arteries, which required repair of the pulmonary veins while on cardiopulmonary bypass. LA, left atrium; RA, right atrium.

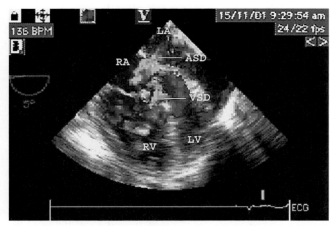

FIGURE 10-2 Postcardiopulmonary bypass transesophageal echocardio-gram (TEE) in a patient with showing a residual atrial (ASD) and ventricular septal defects (VSD). Residual defects were due to suture dehisence and required re-repair after going back on CPB.

assessing surgical outcome and identifying operative risk factors. Whether early identification of these abnormalities, which directs appropriate medical and surgical interventions, will improve outcome remains to be determined.

INDUCTION AND MAINTENANCE OF ANESTHESIA

The principles of intraoperative management of cardiothoracic surgical procedures are based on an understanding of the pathophysiology of each disease process and a working knowledge of the effects of the various anesthetic and other pharmacologic interventions on a particular patient's condition. Selecting an induction technique is dependent on the degree of cardiac dysfunction, the cardiac defect, and the degree of sedation provided by the premedication. In children with good cardiac reserve, induction techniques can be quite varied as long as induction is careful and well monitored. The titration of induction agents is more important than the specific anesthetic technique in patients with reasonable cardiac reserve. A wide spectrum of anesthetic induction techniques with a variety of agents has been used safely and successfully, such as sevoflurane and nitrous oxide; intravenous or intramuscular ketamine; or intravenous propofol, fentanyl, midazolam, or thiopental.[83,110,114] For neonates undergoing open-heart surgery, opioid-relaxant inductions are most prevalent while older children with sufficient cardiac reserve typically receive inhalation inductions with sevoflurane. The application of EMLA cream (emulsion of lidocaine 2.5% and prilocaine 2.5%) at the site of intravenous cannula insertion facilitates cannulation and minimizes patient pain and stress. Ketamine has been the most popular agent for anesthetic induction in patients with cyanotic conditions because it increases systemic vascular resistance and cardiac output thereby diminishing the magnitude of right-to-left shunting. Administration of ketamine can be given intravenously or

intramuscularly. An intramuscular injection may result in pain, agitation, and subsequent arterial desaturation.

Inhalation inductions are generally well tolerated by most children. An inhalation induction with sevoflurane can easily and safely be performed even in cyanotic patients such as tetralogy of Fallot. In these patients, who are at risk of right-to-left shunting and systemic desaturation, oxygenation is well maintained with a patent airway and normal ventilation.[42] Skilled airway management and efficiency of ventilation are an equally essential component of selection during anesthetic induction. While it is essential to understand the complexities of shunts and vascular resistance changes, airway and ventilation effects on the cardiovascular system are of primary importance during the induction of anesthesia.

After anesthetic induction, intravenous access is established or augmented as appropriate. A nondepolarizing muscle relaxant is usually administered and an intravenous opioid and/or inhalation agent chosen for maintenance anesthesia. The child is preoxygenated with 100% FiO$_2$ and a lubricated nasal endotracheal tube is carefully positioned. A nasal tube is usually selected because most patients require a period of postoperative mechanical ventilation and the nasal route provides greater stability and patient comfort compared to the oral route. Some degree of alveolar preoxygenation is recommended even in the infant whose systemic perfusion might be jeopardized by lowering PVR with resulting increase in pulmonary blood flow. This maneuver delays desaturation during intubation. If the child arrives in the operating room with an endotracheal tube in place, it is our practice to change it. Inspissated secretions in a tube with a small internal diameter can cause significant obstruction to gas flow. During periods of bypass when humidified ventilation is discontinued, significant endotracheal tube obstruction can occur. This can be minimized by placing a new endotracheal tube at the beginning of the procedure.

Due to the diverse array of congenital heart defects and surgical procedures, an individualized anesthetic management plan is essential. The maintenance of anesthesia in these patients depends on the age and condition of the patient, the nature of the surgical procedure, the duration of cardiopulmonary bypass, and the need for postoperative ventilation. An assessment of the hemodynamic objectives designed to lessen the pathophysiologic loading conditions should be developed for each patient taking advantage of the known qualitative effects of specific anesthetic agents and ventilatory strategies. These individualized plans must also integrate with the overall perioperative goals to configure the optimal anesthetic. In children with complex defects requiring preoperative inotropic and mechanical ventilatory support, a carefully controlled hemodynamic induction and maintenance anesthetic with a potent opioid is generally chosen. In patients with a simple ASD or ventricular septal defect (VSD), a potent inhalation agent is preferred as the principal anesthetic agent. This allows for early postoperative extubation and a less prolonged period of intensive care monitoring. More important than the specific anesthetic techniques and drugs is the skilled execution of the anesthetic plan taking into account patient response to drugs, the changes associated with surgical manipulation, and early recognition of intraoperative complications.

The reported changes in blood pressure and heart rate for the inhalation agents in normal children are observed in pediatric cardiac surgical patients as well. Although both halothane and isoflurane decrease blood pressure in neonates, infants, and children, the vasodilatory properties of isoflurane may improve overall myocardial contractility, compared to the effects of halothane.[96] Despite improved cardiac reserve with isoflurane, the incidence of laryngospasm, coughing, and desaturation during induction of anesthesia limits its use as an induction agent in children with congenital heart defects.[35] The use of potent inhalation agents as primary anesthetics should be reserved for the child with adequate cardiovascular reserve who is a candidate for early postoperative extubation. In these patients, the myocardial depression and hypotension associated with the use of inhalation agents is well tolerated. Examples include closure of an ASD or VSD, excision of a discrete subaortic membrane, pulmonic or aortic stenosis, ligation of a patent ductus arteriosus (PDA), and repair of coarctation of the aorta.

Sevoflurane offers a more tolerable aroma without the magnitude of myocardial depression that accompanies halothane.[116] Hemodynamically, sevoflurane tends to produce some tachycardia, particularly in older children, and preserve systemic arterial pressure.[71] Reductions in heart rate and systemic arterial pressure are more modest in infants anesthetized with sevoflurane when compared to halothane controls, while the former exhibit echocardiographic evidence of normal contractility and cardiac index.[63,139] Controversies continue to surround the potential toxic byproducts of sevoflurane anesthesia both related to patient metabolism as well as the production of Compound A in the anesthesia breathing circuit. While the importance of Compound A in adult practice remains uncertain, evidence suggests production of this toxin is significantly diminished in children.[36]

Children with complex congenital heart disease and limited cardiac reserve demand an anesthetic technique that provides hemodynamic stability. Inhalation agents are less well tolerated as a primary anesthetic in patients who have limited cardiac reserve, especially after cardiopulmonary bypass. Fentanyl and sufentanil are excellent induction and maintenance anesthetics for this group of patients. Low to moderate doses of these opioids can be supplemented with inhalation anesthetics. Adding low concentrations of inhalation agents to smaller doses of opioids shortens or eliminates the need for postoperative mechanical ventilation while maintaining the advantage of intraoperative hemodynamic stability. Postoperative mechanical ventilation will be required when a high-dose opioid technique is used. The hemodynamic effect of fentanyl at a dose of 25 mcg/kg with pancuronium given to infants in the postoperative period after operative repair of a congenital heart defect shows no change in left atrial pressure, pulmonary artery pressure, pulmonary vascular resistance, and cardiac index and a small decrease in systemic vascular resistance and mean arterial pressure.[59] Higher doses of fentanyl at 50 to 75 mcg/kg with pancuronium result in a slightly greater fall in arterial pressure and heart rate in infants undergoing repair for complex congenital heart defects.[57] Despite the wide safety margin exhibited by these opioids, a selected population of infants and children with marginally compensated hemodynamic function sustained by endogenous catecholamines may manifest more extreme cardiovascular changes with these doses. Fentanyl has also been shown to block stimulus-induced pulmonary vasoconstriction and contributes to the stability of the pulmonary circulation in neonates after congenital diaphragmatic hernia repair.[60] Thus the use of fentanyl may be extrapolated to the operating room where stabilizing pulmonary vascular responsiveness in newborns and young infants with reactive pulmonary vascular beds is crucial to weaning from cardiopulmonary bypass and stabilizing shunt flow.

CARDIOPULMONARY BYPASS

Differences Between Adult and Pediatric Cardiopulmonary Bypass

The physiologic effects of CPB on neonates, infants, and children are significantly different than in adults. (Table 10-2) During CPB, pediatric patients are exposed to different biologic extremes not seen in adults, including deep hypothermia (18°C to 20°C), hemodilution (3- to 15-fold greater dilution of circulating blood volume), low perfusion pressures (20 to 30 mm Hg), wide variation in pump flow rates (ranging from highs of 200 mL/kg/min to total circulatory arrest), and differing blood pH management techniques (α-stat or pH stat, or both sequentially). These parameters significantly differ from normal physiology and affect preservation of normal organ function during and after CPB. In addition to these prominent changes, subtle variations in glucose supplementation, cannula placement, presence of aortopulmonary collaterals, and patient age may also be important factors affecting organ function during cardiopulmonary bypass. Adult patients are infrequently exposed to these biologic extremes. In adult cardiac patients, temperature is rarely lowered below 25°C, hemodilution is more moderate, perfusion pressure is generally maintained at 50 to 80 mm Hg, flow rates are maintained at 50 to 65 mL/kg/minute and pH management strategy is less influential because of moderate

Table 10-2   Differences Between Cardiopulmonary Bypass in Adult and Pediatric Patients

Parameter	Adult patient	Pediatric patient
Hypothermic temperature	Rarely below 25°C–32°C	Commonly 18°C–20°C
Use of total circulatory arrest	Rare	Common
Pump prime: dilutional effects on blood volume	25%–33%	100%–200% (additional additives in pediatric primes)
Perfusion pressures	50–80 mm Hg	20–50 mm Hg
Influence of pH-STAT management strategy	Minimal at moderate hypothermia	Marked at deep hypothermia
Measured PaCO$_2$ differences	30–45 mm Hg	20–80 mm Hg
Glucose regulation	Hypoglycemia rare; requires significant hepatic injury	Hypoglycemia common; reduced hepatic glycogen stores
Hyperglycemia	Frequent; generally easily controlled with insulin	Less common; rebound hypoglycemia may occur

hypothermic temperatures and rare use of circulatory arrest. Variables such as glucose supplementation rarely pose a problem in adult patients due to large hepatic glycogen stores. Venous and arterial cannulae are larger and less deforming of the atria and aorta, and their placement more predictable. Although superficially similar, the conduct of CPB in children is considerably different from that in adults. One would therefore expect marked physiologic differences and sequelae in the response to CPB in the child (Table 10-3).

Prime Volume

The priming solutions used in pediatric cardiopulmonary bypass take on great importance because of the disproportionately large prime-volume to blood-volume ratio in children. In adults, the priming volume is equivalent to 25% to 33% of the patient's blood volume, whereas in neonates and infants, the priming volume may exceed the patient's blood volume by 200%. Even contemporary low-volume bypass circuits rarely reduce this figure much below 150% in the smallest neonates.

Therefore, care must be taken to achieve a physiologically balanced prime and limit the volume as much as possible. Most pediatric priming solutions, however, have quite variable levels of electrolytes, calcium, glucose, and lactate. Electrolytes, glucose, and lactate levels may be quite high if the prime includes large amounts of banked blood, or quite low if a minimal amount of banked blood is added. Calcium levels are generally very low in pediatric prime solutions; this may contribute to the rapid slowing of the heart with the initiation of bypass. The main constituents of the priming solution include crystalloid, banked blood (to maintain a temperature-appropriate hematocrit), and colloid. Other supplements that may be added to the prime are mannitol, a buffer (sodium bicarbonate or THAM), and steroids. Many institutions add colloid or fresh frozen plasma to the pump prime in neonates and small infants or use whole blood in the priming solution. Low concentrations of plasma proteins have been shown experimentally to impair lymphatic flow and alter pulmonary function by increasing capillary leak.[11,117] Although adding albumin to pump prime has not been

Table 10-3   Sequelae of Pediatric Cardiopulmonary Bypass

End-Organ Injury	Etiology/Signs
Renal injury	Organ immaturity, preexisting renal disease Post-cardiopulmonary bypass low CO, use of DHCA Renal dysfunction: characterized by reduced GFR and ATN
Pulmonary injury	Endothelial injury, increased capillary leak, complement activation, leukocyte degranulation Pulmonary dysfunction: characterized by reduced compliance, reduced FRC, and increased A-a gradient
Cerebral injury after DHCA	Loss of autoregulation, suppressed metabolism and cerebral blood flow, cellular acidosis, and cerebral vasoparesis CNS dysfunction: characterized by seizures, reduced developmental quotients, choreoathetosis, learning disabilities, behavioral abnormalities

DHCA, deep hypothermic circulatory arrest; CO, cardiac output; GFR, glomerular filtration rate; ATN, acute tubular necrosis; CNS, central nervous system; FRC, functional residual capacity; A-a, alveolar-arterial oxygen gradients.

shown to alter outcome in adults during CPB, one study has suggested that maintaining normal colloid osmotic pressure may improve survival in infants undergoing CPB.[51,89] The addition of fresh-frozen plasma or whole blood is an attempt to restore the level of procoagulants that are severely diluted with CPB in infants. For neonates and infants, blood must be added to the priming solution. Most institutions use packed red blood cells in their prime solution, however, some use whole blood. The use of whole blood supplements both red blood cells and the coagulation factors with a single donor exposure. In fact, low-volume bypass circuits may enable perfusionists and anesthesiologists to share a single unit of whole blood thereby limiting the donor exposure to one throughout the entire perioperative course. The addition of any blood products will cause a much higher glucose load in the prime. Hyperglycemia may increase the risk of neurologic injury if brain ischemia occurs. Mannitol is added to promote an osmotic diuresis and to scavenge oxygen free radicals from the circulation. Steroids are added to stabilize membranes to produce the theoretical advantage of reducing ion shifts during periods of ischemia. Steroids, however, may raise glucose levels and this may be detrimental if there is a period of cerebral ischemia. Steroids remain one of the more controversial additives in priming solutions.

Temperature

Hypothermic CPB is used to preserve organ function during cardiac surgery. Three distinct methods of CPB are used: moderate hypothermia (25°C–32°C), deep hypothermia (18°C–20°C), or deep hypothermic circulatory arrest (DHCA). The choice of method of bypass to use is based on the required surgical conditions, patient size, the type of operation, and the potential physiologic impact on the patient.

Moderate hypothermic CPB is the principal method of bypass employed for older children and adolescents. In these patients, venous cannulae are less obtrusive, and the heart can easily accommodate superior and inferior vena cava cannulation. Bicaval cannulation reduces right atrial blood return, and improves the surgeon's ability to visualize intracardiac anatomy. Moderate hypothermia may also be chosen for less demanding cardiac repairs in infants, such as an ASD or an uncomplicated VSD. Most surgeons are willing to cannulate the inferior and superior vena cavae in neonates and infants. However, in these patients this approach is technically more difficult and likely to induce brief periods of hemodynamic instability. Additionally, the pliability of the cava and the rigidity of the cannulas may result in caval obstruction, impaired venous drainage, and elevated venous pressure in the mesenteric and cerebral circulation.

Deep hypothermic cardiopulmonary bypass is generally reserved for neonates and infants requiring complex cardiac repair. However, certain older children with complex cardiac disease, or severe aortic arch disease benefit from deep hypothermic temperatures. For the most part, deep hypothermia is selected to allow the surgeon to operate under conditions of low-flow CPB or total circulatory arrest. Low pump flows (50 mL/kg/min) improve the operating conditions for the surgeon by providing a near bloodless field. DHCA allows the surgeon to remove the atrial and/or aortic cannula. Using this technique, surgical repair is more precise because of the bloodless and cannula-free operative field. Arresting the circulation, even at deep hypothermic temperatures, introduces the concern of how well deep hypothermia preserves organ function, with the brain being at greatest risk.[74]

Hemodilution

Although hemoconcentrated blood has an improved oxygen-carrying capacity, its viscosity reduces efficient flow through the microcirculation. With hypothermic temperatures, blood viscosity increases significantly and flow decreases. Hypothermia, coupled with the nonpulsatile flow of CPB, impairs blood flow through the microcirculation. Blood sludging, small vessel occlusion, and multiple areas of tissue hypoperfusion may result. Therefore, hemodilution is an important consideration during hypothermic CPB. The appropriate level of hemodilution for a given hypothermic temperature however, is not well defined. Because red blood cells serve as the major reservoir of oxygen during circulatory arrest, hematocrit values between 25% and 30% are generally preferred for deep hypothermia when this technique is used.

Currently, no evidence exists for defining the optimal hematocrit after weaning from CPB. Decisions concerning post-CPB hematocrits are made based on the patients post-repair function and anatomy. Patients with residual hypoxemia or those with moderate to severe myocardial dysfunction benefit from the improved oxygen carrying capacity of hematocrit levels of 40% or higher. Patients with a physiologic correction and excellent myocardial function may tolerate hematocrit levels of 20% to 25%.[84] In children with mild to moderate myocardial dysfunction, accepting hematocrit levels between these extremes seems prudent. Therefore, in patients with physiologic correction, moderately good ventricular function, and hemodynamic stability, the risks associated with blood and blood product transfusion should be strongly considered during the immediate postbypass period.

Initiation of Cardiopulmonary Bypass

Arterial and venous cannulation of the heart before initiating CPB may result in significant problems in the peribypass period. A malpositioned venous cannula has the potential for vena caval obstruction. The problems of venous obstruction are magnified during CPB in the neonate because arterial pressures are normally low (20 to 40 mm Hg), and large relatively stiff cannulas easily distort these very pliable venous vessels.[11,51,119] A cannula in the inferior vena cava may obstruct venous return from the splanchnic bed, resulting in ascites from increased hydrostatic pressure and/or directly reduced perfusion pressure across the mesenteric, renal, and hepatic vascular beds. Significant renal, hepatic, and gastrointestinal dysfunction may ensue and should be anticipated in the young infant with unexplained ascites. Similar cannulation problems may result in superior vena cava obstruction. This condition may be more ominous during bypass. Under these circumstances, three problems may ensue: (1) cerebral edema, (2) a reduction in regional or global cerebral blood flow, and (3) reduced proportion of pump flow reaching the cerebral circulation causing inefficient brain cooling. In the operating room, it is advisable either to monitor superior vena cava pressures via an internal jugular catheter or by looking at the patient's head for signs of puffiness or venous distension after initiating bypass. Discussions with the perfusionist regarding adequacy of venous return and/or large cooling gradients between the upper and lower body should alert the anesthesiologist and the surgeon to potential venous cannula problems. Patients with anomalies of the large systemic veins (persistent left superior vena cava or azygous continuation of an interrupted inferior vena cava) are at particular risk for problems with venous cannulation and drainage.

Problems with aortic cannula placement also occur. The aortic cannula may slip beyond the takeoff of the innominate artery and, therefore, selectively flow to the right side of the cerebral circulation. Also, the position of the tip of the cannula may promote preferential flow down the aorta or induce a Venturi effect to steal flow from the cerebral circulation. This problem has been confirmed during cerebral blood flow monitoring by the appearance of large discrepancies in flow between the right and left hemisphere after initiating CPB. Other clues to cannula misplacement include better cooling in the lower body than the upper body. The presence of large aortic to pulmonary collaterals, such as a large PDA, may also divert blood to the pulmonary circulation from the systemic circulation thereby reducing cerebral blood flow and the efficiency of brain cooling during CPB.[122] The surgeon should gain control of the ductus either prior to or immediately after instituting CPB to eliminate this problem and, if possible, large aortopulmonary collateral vessels should be embolized in the cardiac catheterization laboratory before the operative procedure. Neonates with significant aortic arch abnormalities (e.g., aortic atresia, interrupted aortic arch) may require radical modifications of cannulation techniques, such as placing the arterial cannula in the main pulmonary artery and temporarily occluding the branch pulmonary arteries to perfuse the body via the PDA, or even dual arterial cannulation of both the ascending aorta and main pulmonary artery. Such adaptations require careful vigilence to assure effective, thorough cooling of vital organs.

Once the aortic and venous cannulae are positioned and connected to the arterial and venous limb of the extracorporeal circuit, bypass is initiated. The arterial pump is slowly started and once forward flow is assured, venous blood is drained into the oxygenator. Pump flow rate is gradually increased until full circulatory support is achieved. If venous return is diminished, arterial line pressure high, or mean arterial pressure excessive, pump flow rates must be reduced. High line pressure and inadequate venous return are usually due to malposition or kinking of the arterial and venous cannulae, respectively. The rate at which venous blood is drained from the patient is determined by the height difference between the patient and the oxygenator inlet and the diameter of the venous cannula and line tubing. Venous drainage can be enhanced by increasing the height difference between the oxygenator and the patient or by using a larger venous cannula. Venous drainage can be reduced by either decreasing the height difference between the oxygenator and the patient or by partially clamping the venous line.

Once CPB begins, careful observation should be focused to assure appropriate circuit connections, myocardial perfusion and optimal cardiac decompression. Ineffective venous drainage can rapidly result in ventricular distension. This is especially true in infants and neonates where ventricular compliance is low and the heart is relatively intolerant of excessive preload augmentation. If ventricular distension occurs, pump flow must be reduced and the venous cannula repositioned. Alternatively, the heart may be decompressed by placing a cardiotomy suction or small vent in the appropriate chamber.

Deep Hypothermic Circulatory Arrest

Neonates and small infants weighing less than 8 to 10 kg who require extensive repair of complex congenital heart defects may have their repair using DHCA. This technique facilitates precise surgical repair under optimal conditions, free of blood or cannulas in the operative field, providing maximal organ protection, and often resulting in shortened total CPB time. The scientific rationale for the use of deep hypothermic temperatures rests primarily upon a temperature-mediated reduction of metabolism. Whole body and cerebral oxygen consumption during induced hypothermia decreases the metabolic rate for oxygen by a factor of 2 to 2.5 for every $10°$ C reduction in temperature.[91] These results are consistent with in vitro models, which relate temperature reduction to a decrease in the rate constant of chemical reactions. The reduction in oxygen supply during deep hypothermic low-flow CPB (DHCPB) is associated with preferential increases in vital organ perfusion (e.g., to the brain) and by increased extraction of oxygen.[32] Therefore, to some extent DHCPB exerts a protective effect by reducing the metabolic rate for oxygen, promoting preferential organ perfusion and increasing tissue oxygen extraction.

Extensive clinical experience using DHCA has shown the duration of safe circulatory arrest period may last 35 to 40 minutes.[74] Beyond this duration, the incidence of permanent and transient neurologic sequelae may increase. Both the duration of the arrest period and variations in perfusion technique during cooling and rewarming influence the development of these problems. The effects of deep hypothermia on tissue metabolism and oxygen consumption and extraction clearly do not explain the entire protective effect of safe DHCA, though. Cortical PO_2 and PCO_2 levels indicate basal cerebral metabolic activity during DHCA (i.e., anaerobic metabolism). During brain ischemia, excitatory amino acids (EAA) such as glutamate and aspartate are released and are putative mediators of ischemic damage.[5,33,61,105] Hypothermia has been shown to significantly decrease the release of EAA, suggesting another mechanism besides metabolism reduction for its protective effect.[10] In addition, membrane changes that transform a normal semiliquid to a semisolid form during hypothermia may act to prevent calcium influx during reperfusion and thereby account for additional protection noted in some experimental models.[126]

Although all organ systems are at risk for the development of ischemia and reperfusion injury, as manifested by lactate and pyruvate production during DHCA, the brain appears to be the most sensitive and the least tolerant of these effects. Brain stem and cortical evoked potentials as well as processed EEG are altered after DHCA.[9,55,81,107] The abnormalities in the evoked potentials appear to be related to the duration of DHCA and are attributed to altered metabolism.

During reperfusion after the arrest period cerebral blood flow (CBF) and metabolism remain depressed in neonates and small infants (Figs. 10-3 and 10-4).[48] Importantly, during the use of these extremes of temperature, it appears that autoregulation is lost and cerebral perfusion becomes highly dependent on the conduct of extracorporeal perfusion and presumably postbypass hemodynamic performance.

Current controversy exists regarding the immediate-term and long-term neuropsychologic effects of DHCA. Early reports regarding the long-term consequences of DHCA on brain development and intelligence were conflicting.[47] Transient neurologic dysfunction and other reversible cerebral injuries have been reported. These transient, subtle neuropsychologic disturbances have led investigators to examine more systematically the long-term outcome after DHCA.

More recently a number of more sophisticated studies examining the outcome after DHCA have been performed. In a randomized clinical trial comparing the incidence of brain injury following DHCA or low-flow CPB, DHCA was demonstrated to have longer EEG recovery times and a higher incidence of clinical seizures in the early postoperative period.[99] The DHCA group also had a higher incidence of neurologic abnormalities and poor motor function at one year of age, and poor expressive language and motor development at 2½ years, particularly in those who exhibited early postoperative seizures.[106] Reports from the same clinical trial have shown that the DHCA cohort has continued to have worse motor coordination and planning and speech abnormalities at 4 years of age.[3,4,137] Of interest, both the DHCA and low CPB groups have lower cognitive and motor performance compared to a general population. This latter finding suggests factors outside DHCA and low flow bypass but within the perioperative period, are associated with poor neuropsychologic development.

A recent clinical study has suggested pH-stat blood gas management strategy during CPB to be associated with an improved neuropsychologic outcome in children.[4] This study was a retrospective developmental study with a core of patients who have undergone surgery for transposition of the great artery. The authors found a strong positive correlation between arterial PCO₂ during cooling before circulatory rest

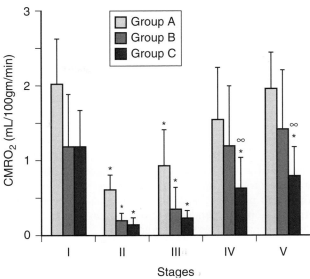

FIGURE 10-3 Bar chart of the changes in cerebral metabolism (CMRO₂) before, during, and after cardiopulmonary bypass in neonates and infants. Group A underwent repair using moderate hypothermic bypass at 28°C–32°C; group B, using deep hypothermic bypass with continuous flow at 18°C–22° C; group C, using deep hypothermic circulatory arrest at 18°C. Stage I, prebypass; Stages II and III, during hypothermic bypass; Stage IV, rewarmed on bypass; Stage V, after bypass. Note the reduction in cerebral metabolism in all groups during hypothermic CPB and the impaired cerebral metabolism after DHCA (group C). (Mean data 5 standard deviation; *P < 0.001, Stages II, III, IV, V versus I; 1 = P < 0.01; group C versus A, B.) (From Greeley WJ, Kern FH, Ungerleider RM, et al: The effect of hypothermic cardiopulmonary bypass and total circulatory arrest on cerebral metabolism in neonates, infants, and children. *J Thorac Cardiovasc Surg* 101:783–794, 1991.)

and developmental score. This suggested that children undergoing alpha-stat blood gas management strategy had a worse developmental outcome than where a pH-stat strategy was employed. In a randomized clinical trial of neonates undergoing cardiac surgery using deep hypothermic circulatory arrest, pH-stat management was noted to have faster EEG recovery times and fewer postoperative seizures compared to an alpha-stat bypass group.[29,67] Therefore, the beneficial effect of pH-stat management clinically remains preliminary.

DHCA Group

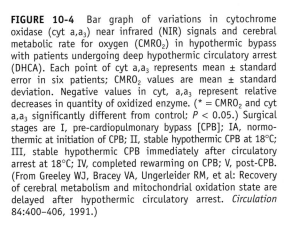

FIGURE 10-4 Bar graph of variations in cytochrome oxidase (cyt a,a₃) near infrared (NIR) signals and cerebral metabolic rate for oxygen (CMRO₂) in hypothermic bypass with patients undergoing deep hypothermic circulatory arrest (DHCA). Each point of cyt a,a₃ represents mean ± standard error in six patients; CMRO₂ values are mean ± standard deviation. Negative values in cyt, a,a₃ represent relative decreases in quantity of oxidized enzyme. (* = CMRO₂ and cyt a,a₃ significantly different from control; P < 0.05.) Surgical stages are I, pre-cardiopulmonary bypass [CPB]; IA, normothermic at initiation of CPB; II, stable hypothermic CPB at 18°C; III, stable hypothermic CPB immediately after circulatory arrest at 18°C; IV, completed rewarming on CPB; V, post-CPB. (From Greeley WJ, Bracey VA, Ungerleider RM, et al: Recovery of cerebral metabolism and mitochondrial oxidation state are delayed after hypothermic circulatory arrest. *Circulation* 84:400–406, 1991.)

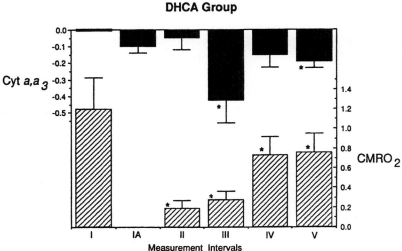

Certain experimental studies have also suggested the superiority of pH-stat strategy (Fig. 10-5). In one study, pH-stat animals had greater cerebral blood flow during cooling and better recovery of cerebral ATP and intracellular pH after arrest and reperfusion.[70] Brain water content was also less in the pH-stat group. These studies suggested that pH-stat CPB might have protective mechanisms due to an increased rate of brain cooling. In more recent experimental studies comparing pH-stat and alpha-stat cardiopulmonary bypass on cerebral oxygenation blood flow, cerebral protective effect of pH-stat management was demonstrated and indicated that the kinetics of cerebral deoxygenation might contribute to the mechanism of protection.[79,80,101] Clearly more work needs to be done in this area before pH-stat is definitively recommended.[46] (See Chapter 20 on cardiopulmonary bypass.) However, preliminary experimental and clinical studies suggest a superiority of this technique in certain patient groups, especially those with aortopulmonary collateral circulation.

Because of the potential for neurologic dysfunction after DHCA, some institutions use low-flow deep hypothermic CPB as an alternative technique.[14] Because low-flow bypass can produce ischemia if flow is too low and because it lengthens the CPB time, compared to DHCA, serious concerns over this technique have also arisen.[112,127] A experimental study demonstrated worse brain injury with low-flow bypass than with DHCA.[117]

Other factors such as surface cooling, anesthetic agents, and cerebral protective agents may influence and modify the effects of DHCPB and DHCA.[50,86] The potential use of certain pharmacologic agents such as anesthetic drugs, barbiturates, lidocaine, or calcium channel blockers is unknown. There are no clinical studies in children systematically examining the influence of these pharmacologic agents on cerebrovascular physiology or neurologic outcome. Therefore, the use of these agents remains entirely speculative and

unfounded. Clearly, further study of the long-term effects of DHCA on neuropsychologic outcome in children is necessary. Fundamental questions regarding DHCPB with low-flow versus DHCA also need to be further addressed. Equally important, the manner in which the patient is cooled and rewarmed may affect outcome,[44,72] and merits further investigation, even before the testing of pharmacologic drugs.

Discontinuation of Cardiopulmonary Bypass

When weaning from CPB, blood volume is assessed by direct visualization of the heart and monitoring right atrial or left atrial filling pressures. When filling pressures are adequate, the patient fully warmed, acid/base status normalized, heart rate adequate and sinus rhythm achieved, the venous drainage is stopped and the patient can be weaned from bypass. The arterial cannula is left in place so that a slow infusion of residual pump blood can be used to optimize filling pressures.[129] Myocardial function is assessed by direct cardiac visualization, and either a transthoracic left or right atrial catheter, a percutaneous internal jugular catheter, or by the use of intraoperative echocardiography. Pulse oximetry can also be used to assess the adequacy of cardiac output.[102] Low systemic arterial saturation or the inability of the oximeter probe to register a pulse may be a sign of very low output and high systemic resistance.[120]

After the repair of complex congenital heart defects, the anesthesiologist and surgeon may have difficulty separating patients from cardiopulmonary bypass. Under these circumstances, the differential diagnosis includes (1) an inadequate surgical result with a residual defect requiring repair, (2) pulmonary artery hypertension, and (3) right or left ventricular dysfunction. Two general approaches are customarily used, either independently or in conjunction with one another. An intraoperative cardiac catheterization can be performed to assess isolated pressure measurements from the various great vessels and chambers of the heart (i.e., catheter pullback measurements or direct needle puncture to evaluate residual pressure gradients across repaired valves, sites of stenosis and conduits, and oxygen saturation data to examine for residual shunts).[40] Alternatively, transesophageal echocardiography (TEE) may be used to provide an intraoperative image of structural or functional abnormalities to assist in the evaluation of the postoperative cardiac repair.[94,131] If structural abnormalities are found, the patient can be placed back on CPB and residual defects can be repaired before leaving the operating room (Fig. 10-6). Leaving the operating room with a significant residual structural defect adversely affects survival and increases patient morbidity.[94,131] For the anesthesiologist, TEE can rapidly identify right and left ventricular dysfunction and suggest the presence of pulmonary artery hypertension. In addition, TEE can identify regional wall motion abnormalities due to ischemia or intramyocardial air that will direct specific therapy and provide a means of assessing the results of these interventions.[45]

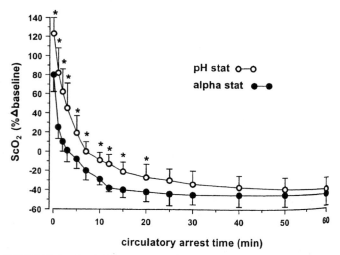

FIGURE 10-5 Cortical oxygen saturation (ScO_2) during deep hypothermic circulatory arrest in the pH-stat and the alpha-stat groups. The ScO_2 half-life during arrest was significantly greater in the pH-stat than in the α-stat group. (From Kurth CD, O'Rourke MM, O'Hara IB: Comparison of pH-stat and alpha-stat cardiopulmonary bypass on cerebral oxygenation and blood flow in relation to hypothermic circulatory arrest in piglets. *Anesthesiology* 89:110–118, 1998.)

MODIFIED ULTRAFILTRATION

One important factor affecting the morbidity and mortality after cardiac surgery in children is the effect of cardiopulmonary bypass. During the initiation of cardiopulmonary

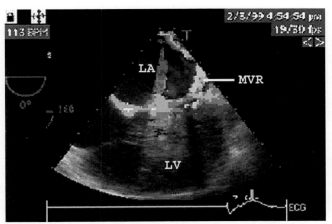

FIGURE 10-6 A postcardiopulmonary bypass transesophageal echocardiogram in a patient after mitral valve placement. Note the regurgitant jet representing a significant perivalvular leak requiring re-repair on CPB. LA, left atrium; LV, left ventricle; MVR, mitral valve regurgitation.

bypass considerable hemodilution occurs. This hemodilution is the result of the priming volume required for the CPB circuit. Under many circumstances this hemodilutional effect is intentional, decreasing blood viscosity and thereby preventing sludging when the patient is cooled to temperatures below 20° C. After CPB, hemodilution is associated with tissue edema and organ dysfunction. Because blood elements are exposed to the nonendothelialized circuitry of CPB, there is also a significant inflammatory response as result of CPB. Both these effects of hemodilution and inflammation are exaggerated in neonates, infants and young children due to their disproportionate exposure to the circuit relative to their body size. This inflammatory response leads to an increase in capillary permeability, leading to an overall increase in total body edema postoperatively.[98]

Efforts to reduce the hemodilution and inflammatory effects CPB included reducing priming volume, perioperative anti-inflammatory and diuretic therapies, and the use of postoperative peritoneal dialysis. The technique of modified ultrafiltration (MUF) was first used clinically as an alternative method to reduce the adverse effects of CPB in children.[97]

The technique of MUF is performed after cardiopulmonary bypass is complete and allows filtration of both the patient and remaining contents of the CPB circuit including the venous reservoir.[20,30,130] Using the MUF technique, an ultrafilter is interposed in the CPB circuit between the aortic arterial line and the venous cannula which is located in the right atrium. After weaning from CPB, the blood is removed from the patient via the aortic cannula and fed through the ultrafilter along with blood from the venous reservoir and oxygen. The outlet of the ultrafilter is fed to the right atrium of the patient. Blood flow through the ultrafilter approximates 200 mL/minute that is maintained by a roller pump. Suction is applied to the filter port of the ultrafilter resulting in an ultrafiltration rate of 100 to 150 mL/minute. A constant left atrial or right atrial pressure is maintained achieving continued hemodynamic stability in the patient. Ultrafiltration is carried out with end points either being time (15 to 20 minutes) or achieving a hematocrit value of approximately 40%.[130]

Ultrafiltration appears to offer two major advantages. First, total body water is reduced as a direct result of removing the ultrafiltrate.[97] This effect counteracts the hemodilution effects associated with the institution of CPB. In addition, the hematocrit is increased after CPB, enhancing oxygen delivery to the tissues. Secondly, MUF has been shown to remove some of the deleterious vasoactive substances associated with inflammatory response to CPB.[68,136] This effect is mediated by reducing circulating cytokines, which are associated with capillary leak syndrome. Examination of the ultrafiltrate shows that it contains low molecular weight, inflammatory mediators including C3A, C5A, interleukin-6A, interleukin-8A, tumor necrosis factor, myocardial depressant factor, and various other cytokines. Several studies have shown that compared to control patients, patients that have MUF after CPB have substantially less increase in total body water, less complement and interleukin release, require less blood transfusions and show a faster recovery of systolic blood pressure.[34,97,130]

In a clinical study examining the effect of MUF on left ventricular systolic function in children, MUF was associated with an increase in intrinsic left ventricular systolic function and a decrease in end-diastolic pressure, thereby improving left ventricular compliance.[22] In an experimental study MUF has also been demonstrated to improve cerebral blood flow, cerebral metabolic activity and cerebral oxygen delivery after DHCA (Fig. 10-7).[121] This latter effect acutely improves cerebral metabolism after DHCA, and may reduce and reverse the known deleterious effects of DHCA on brain function after CPB. In another clinical study further defining the benefits of MUF, MUF was demonstrated to reduce postoperative blood use, chest tube drainage, pleural effusions, and hospital stay in patients after cavopulmonary operations.[78]

An alternative to MUF is conventional ultrafiltration during rewarming period of CPB. In an experimental model examining MUF versus conventional ultrafiltration, modified ultrafiltration was alone effective in reducing weight gain and myocardial edema, and was associated with improving left ventricular function.[19] Possible complications of modified ultrafiltration include air embolus, patient cooling during ultrafiltration, and bleeding.[125] These theoretical and technical potential complications appear not to be of substantial concern. It is the view of most groups that the benefits of MUF far exceed the risk.[20]

In summary, MUF is a safe adjunct reversing the deleterious effects of hemodilution and the inflammatory response associated with cardiopulmonary bypass in children. Perioperative blood loss and blood use is significantly reduced when MUF is used. MUF also improves left ventricular function, systolic blood pressure, and increases oxygen delivery. Pulmonary compliance and brain function after CPB are also improved. Therefore, the use of MUF is becoming more routine in pediatric patients after CPB.

ANTICOAGULATION, HEMOSTASIS, AND BLOOD CONSERVATION

Modern pediatric cardiac anesthesia must include the principles and practice of effective anticoagulation, hemostasis, and

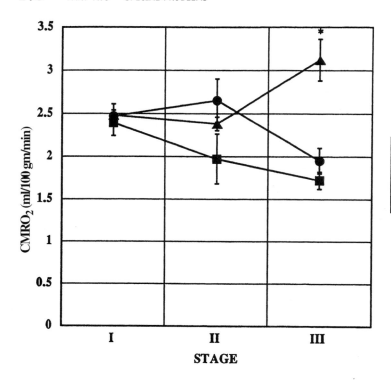

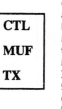

FIGURE 10-7 Cerebral metabolic rate for oxygen measurements ($CMRO_2$) before and after deep hypothermic circulatory arrest. Note the significant increase in $CMRO_2$ in the MUF animals compared with the control and transfusion groups at stage 3. CTL, control; MUF, modified ultrafiltration; TX, tranfusion. I, before cardiopulmonary bypass (CPB); II, 5 minutes after CPB; III, 25 minutes after CPB. (From Skaryak LA, Kirshbom PM, DiBernardo LR, et al: Modified ultrafiltration improves cerebral metabolic recovery after circulatory arrest. *J Thorac Cardiovasc Surg* 109:744–751, 1995.)

blood conservation. Bleeding after cardiopulmonary bypass remains a significant problem in pediatric cardiac surgery.[88] Continuing blood loss post-CPB requiring blood component replacement is associated with hemodynamic compromise as well as morbidity from multiple donor exposures. In pediatric patients, restoration of hemostasis has proved difficult; diagnosis of the problem and treatment are marginally effective.

Neonates, infants, and children undergoing cardiac surgery with CPB have a higher rate of postoperative bleeding than that seen in older patients.[88] This is due to several factors. First, there is disproportionate exposure to the nonendothelialized extracorporeal circuit, which produces an inflammatory-like response.[76] This inflammatory response to cardiopulmonary bypass is inversely related to patient age; the younger the patient the more pronounced the response.[43,76] As complement and platelet activation are linked to the activation of other protein systems in the blood (i.e., fibrinolytic), it is probable that this hemostatic activation, which results in impaired hemostasis and increased bleeding tendency, plays a major role during pediatric cardiac surgery. Second, the type of operations performed in neonates and infants usually involves more extensive reconstruction and suture lines, creating more opportunities for surgical bleeding than in adult cardiac patients. Operations are also frequently performed using deep hypothermia or circulatory arrest, which may further impair hemostasis.[26] Third, the immature coagulation system in neonates may also contribute to impaired hemostasis.[1] While procoagulant and factor levels may be reduced in young patients with congenital heart disease due to immature or impaired hepatosynthesis,[16] functional bleeding tendencies are usually not present before surgery. Finally, patients with cyanotic heart disease demonstrate an increased bleeding tendency before and after cardiopulmonary bypass.[56]

CPB is a significant thrombogenic stimulus requiring anticoagulation with heparin prior to CPB initiation. Heparin is usually administered empirically based on patient weight and its effect followed by activated clotting time (ACT) monitoring. Because heparin effect is primarily due to coupling with antithrombin III (AT III) and because there are age-related differences and quantitative differences in procoagulants and inhibitors, variability of heparin dosing and its effect have been a concern. High heparin sensitivity is observed in the first week of life and then decreases progressively until about 3 years of age when values approach those observed in adults.[130] These findings are consistent with evidence in infants of variable quantities of both procoagulants and inhibitors, especially prothrombin and AT III.[73] Heparin administration to the patient must also include a consideration of the quantity and composition of the priming volume for CPB, especially if fresh frozen plasma is added. We recommend a heparin dose of 200 U/kg plus an additional dose of 1 to 3 U/mL of prime, and maintaining the activated clotting time (ACT) above 400 seconds.

Heparin is neutralized with protamine dosed according to the quantity of heparin administered or based on body weight. Protamine excess may actually contribute to postoperative bleeding.[64] It appears that the protamine dose requirement is high for neonates and decreases with age. The relatively increased protamine requirement for young as compared to older children and adults is indicative of higher circulating heparin levels after CPB.[66] Delayed hepatic clearance of heparin due to organ immaturity and the predominant use of hypothermic circulatory arrest in the young will decrease metabolism and excretion of heparin. We typically administer 4 mg/kg protamine in neonates, while 2 mg/kg usually restores the ACT to baseline values in adolescents and adults.

Interpatient variability mandates some form of individual assessment to guide drug dose, to prevent excess protamine.[64]

Neonates and young infants with congenital heart disease will have low circulating levels of procoagulants and inhibitors. The thrombogenic and dilutional effects of CPB further contribute to hemostatic abnormalities after CPB. Formed blood elements such as leukocytes and platelets may be activated and procoagulants diluted by CPB. Furthermore, deep hypothermic circulatory arrest causes increased clotting and fibrinolytic activity. The lower the temperature, the higher the degree of hemostatic activation. Therefore, the causes of bleeding post-CPB are multifactorial. Injudicious use of blood products to correct individual coagulation abnormalities separately can further exacerbate dilution of existing procoagulants as well as carry the risks of multiple donor exposure. Because the transfusion of blood products is associated with numerous complications, transfusion is to be assiduously avoided, unless specifically indicated by impairment in tissue oxygenation or documented coagulopathies with clinically significant bleeding. All efforts at blood conservation during cardiac surgery should be routinely used by all members of the operative team, intraoperatively as well as postoperatively.

Bleeding after CPB is not an unusual occurrence. The surgeon should first attempt to identify any obvious source of surgical bleeding at the sites of repair. Next, adequate protamine reversal of heparin is assessed by measuring an ACT. In general, standard coagulation tests show a prolongation of the partial thromboplastin time (PTT), prothrombin time, hypofibrinogenemia, and dilution of other procoagulants as well as a prolonged bleeding time in many pediatric patients, with and without bleeding (Fig. 10-8). The most common reason for persistent bleeding is platelet dysfunction.[52,140] Under such circumstances, administration of platelets is warranted in the presence of bleeding. Routine administration of blood products to correct laboratory coagulation abnormalities in the absence of bleeding is never clinically

indicated. After platelets have been given and if bleeding is still present, reassessment and repeat platelet infusion or the administration of cryoprecipitate or fresh-frozen plasma may be beneficial. Under most circumstances, meticulous surgical technique, appropriate administration of protamine, adequate patient temperature, and platelet infusion will correct excessive bleeding. In neonates, excessive bleeding as well as the escalating dilutional effects of selective component therapy on the remaining procoagulants in small patients make the treatment of bleeding a difficult one. The use of fresh whole blood may be warranted under these circumstances. The administration of fresh whole blood (less than 48 hours old) after CPB can meet all the hematologic requirements with minimum donor exposure. The efficacy of whole blood in restoring hemostasis and reducing blood loss after CPB has been demonstrated in patients younger than 2 years of age undergoing complex surgical repairs.[88]

Many attempts have been made to reduce bleeding after cardiopulmonary bypass by pharmacologic interventions. Desmopressin acetate1[108,115] and the antifibrinolytics—aminocaproic acid (EACA) or tranexamic acid 180—have been tried with variable success in significantly reducing postoperative blood loss after cardiac surgery. However, the most impressive results have been demonstrated with the use of aprotinin.[113] A proteinase inhibitor, aprotinin has antifibrinolytic properties in low concentrations and acts as kallikrein inhibitor at higher levels. CPB causes increased kallikrein by contact activation, promoting thrombus and fibrin generation, which promotes fibrinolysis. The inhibition of kallikrein results in an inhibition of the contact phase of coagulation and the inhibition of fibrinolysis reduces bleeding. Reduced thrombin generation leads to a diminished platelet stimulation. Better-preserved platelet function has been described for patients with aprotinin.[110] Not surprisingly, then, aprotinin significantly reduces the intraoperative and postoperative blood loss in cardiac surgery.[24-28] Aprotinin use during pediatric

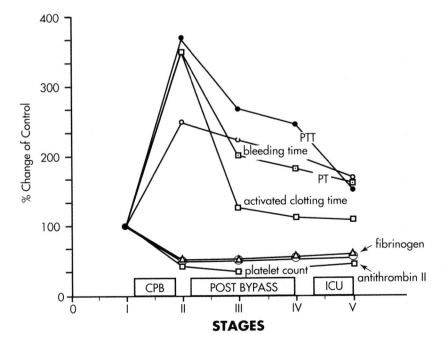

FIGURE 10-8 Plot of blood coagulation profile changes before, during, and after cardiopulmonary bypass (CPB) in 25 children. Clotting times and coagulant factors are shown as percent change from control. Stage I, baseline, before CPB; Stage II, post-CPB, before protamine reversal of heparin; Stage III, after protamine; Stage IV, just before leaving the operating room; stage V, after 3 hours in the intensive care unit (ICU). PTT, partial thromboplastin time; PT, prothrombin time.

cardiac surgery attenuates fibrinolytic activation in a dose-dependent fashion, reducing the formation of fibrin-split products.[21,26] Higher doses of aprotinin reduce thrombin/AT III complex and F1/F2 fibrin fragments, supporting the hypothesis of suppression of clotting activation with higher aprotinin doses and plasma concentrations. While several studies have demonstrated efficacy in reducing hemorrhage and donor exposures after congenital heart surgery, this benefit may not be evident with simple primary cardiac repairs (e.g., VSD, ASD, tetralogy of Fallot).[13,103] To date, the use of aprotinin for congenital heart surgery has been generally confined to certain patients requiring reoperation, for example, Ross procedure, as well as in cardiac/lung transplantation procedures.

The techniques of blood conservation must be continued during the postoperative period. Isolated coagulation abnormalities are often present in the uncomplicated postoperative cardiac patient. Usually these coagulation abnormalities self-correct during the first postoperative day and are not associated with excessive bleeding. Therefore, routine correction of these abnormalities with infusion of blood products is not warranted. Administration of blood products should not occur in the absence of clinical evidence of bleeding and the identification of a specific defect requiring targeted component therapy. Routine use of blood products for volume replacement is also to be avoided; lactated Ringer's or saline solution can be satisfactorily administered at a reduced cost without the hazards associated with transfusion.

POSTOPERATIVE PAIN MANAGEMENT

Regional anesthesia has been used for postoperative pain control in infants and children, after a thoracotomy, a sternotomy, and simple procedures requiring CPB.[104] This method avoids opioid-induced respiratory depression from intravenous doses of these drugs. The administration of opioids in the epidural space is a very effective approach to pain management. This technique is used in children for postoperative pain control when given in the epidural space via the caudal route as a "single shot" or via a small caudal catheter. Morphine or Dilaudid provide effective analgesia with a duration of 6 to 12 hours, with no significant respiratory depression. Caudal morphine 0.07 to 0.1 mg/kg diluted in 5 to 10 mL of sterile saline has been used with good success in our practice. The use of regional anesthesia for postoperative pain appears to be best suited for the child extubated in the early postoperative period. Relative contraindications of this technique include hemodynamic instability and patients with abnormal clotting profiles with continued active bleeding. Using this regional technique, better arterial oxygenation, a more rapid ventilator wean, and decreased postoperative respiratory complications may be expected. However, urinary retention occurs frequently in patients without a bladder catheter. Generally, no treatment of the latter is required. Children requiring a bilateral thoracosternotomy incision (i.e., clamshell for lung transplantation) merit consideration for a thoracic epidural analgesia. This technique significantly reduces the respiratory depression and pulmnary mechanics abnormalities that accompany the quantity of systemic opioids that would be necessary to provide adequate analgesia for these excruciatingly painful incisions. If the procedure

requires systemic heparinization, we will typically defer placement of these catheters until the heparin effect is neutralized. For patients undergoing heart/lung transplantation, a thoracic epidural can be placed early in the postoperative period (8 to 16 hours after surgery) to facilitate early extubation and excellent pain control. Recently, an epidural hematoma was reported in a patient with an epidural catheter after cardiac surgery using CPB.[111]

SPECIFIC ANESTHETIC CONSIDERATIONS

Anesthesia for Simple Open-Heart Procedures

Simple open-heart procedures include those defects that involve relatively straightforward surgical repair, uncomplicated hemodynamics, minimal to moderate postoperative intensive care, and mechanical ventilation. Examples include repairs of ASD, VSD, and some cases of tetralogy of Fallot in otherwise healthy children with good cardiopulmonary reserve. Patients with congestive heart failure and minimal reserve will require a different level of care, despite the relatively "simple" nature of the surgical procedure.

Specific anesthetic considerations for these patients, in addition to the general guidelines previously discussed, are predicated on the use of CPB, occasional use of DHCA, and the specific perioperative issues associated with these defects (Table 10-4). The anesthetic management can be divided into three phases: precorrection, immediate postcorrection, and postoperative. During the precorrection phase, the plans for premedication, induction and maintenance of anesthesia, and selection of monitors are based on the patient's physiology and plans for postoperative care. Premedication without opioid is selected for patients who will be extubated at the end of the procedure; opioid is added for those who will remain on mechanical ventilation. Inhalation induction is typically tolerated well, but special considerations should be made for patients with right-to-left shunting. The rise in arterial anesthetic concentration is slowed in patients with right-to-left shunting, since arterial (anesthetic-saturated) blood is diluted with blood that has not passed through the lungs; this effect is more pronounced with insoluble agents.[77,128] Patients with particularly high right ventricular outflow tract obstruction benefit from particular vigilance to adequate airway and ventilation, to prevent pulmonary hypertension, impaired pulmonary blood flow, and diminished left-sided filling. Aside from necessary preparation for airway management, agents to maintain SVR (phenylephrine) and reduce PVR (oxygen, halothane, opioid) should be readily available throughout the precorrection period, particularly during induction.

The level of monitoring also reflects the nature of the procedure: adequate intravenous access for fluid or blood transfusion anticipates the potential for bleeding; invasive pressure monitoring is established in preparation for CPB. Transthoracic atrial lines are placed before discontinuing CPB if the need for central pressure monitoring, or for delivery of intropic/hemodynamic infusions is anticipated. Simple PFO/secundum ASD closures do not typically require central catheters. Anesthetic maintenance comprises opioid, 10 to

Table 10-4 Intraoperative Hemodynamic Goals

Condition	HR	Contractility	Preload	Pulmonary Vascular Resistance	Systemic Vascular Resistance
Shunts					
L → R (all types)	normal	normal	↑	↑	↓
Ventricular Septal Defect R → L	normal	normal	normal	↓	↑
Obstructive					
Aortic stenosis	↓*	normal-↑	↑	normal	↑*
Aortic coarctation	normal	normal	↑	normal	↓
Mitral stenosis	↓	normal-↑	↑	normal-↓	normal
Pulmonary stenosis	↓	↑	↑	↓	normal
Dynamic subaortic obstruction	↓*	↓*	↑	normal	normal-↑
Dynamic subpulmonic obstruction	↓	↓*	↑	↓	normal
Regurgitant					
Aortic insufficiency	normal-↑	normal-↑	↑	normal	normal-↓
Mitral regurgitation	normal	normal-↑	↑	normal-↓	↓
Pulmonary insufficiency	normal-↑	normal	↑	↓	normal
Tricuspid regurgitation	normal	normal	↑	↓	normal

Many congenital heart defects include several of the above lesions; for dynamic outflow obstruction, an asterisk (*) marks the most important consideration.
Adapted from Steven JM, Nicolson SC: Congenital heart disease. In Greeley WJ (ed): *Atlas of Anesthesia, Vol VII: Pediatric Anesthesia.* New York, Harcourt Pub Ltd, 1999.

50 mcg/kg fentanyl, supplemented with inhalation anesthetic, depending on the anticipated time of extubation.

Atrial septal defects and ventricular septal defects require the use of CPB for access to the surgical site. Right atriotomy allows visualization of most ASDs, and, using a trans-tricuspid approach, some VSDs (membranous). Depending on the size of the defect, suture (for PFO), pericardial patch, or prosthetic material may be used for closure. This technique may be associated with atrial arrhythmias and conduction delay after repair. Some VSDs may not be visible through the tricuspid valve, such as malalignment, supracristal, and muscular; right or left ventriculotomy may be required for their closure. Consequences of ventricular incision include AV node dysfunction with various degrees of heart block, and ventricular myocardial dysfunction.

The numerous varieties of RV outflow obstruction in tetralogy of Fallot necessitate an individualized approach to each patient. Generally, right ventriculotomy enables repair of the VSD and excision of excess muscle proximal to the pulmonic valve; extension of the incision permits the placement of a patch across the annulus of the pulmonary valve to enlarge the RVOT. Insufficiency or regurgitation of the pulmonic valve may result. More complex cases of tetralogy of Fallot may require more extensive surgical intervention, and are considered separately in the following section.

With these relatively straightforward repairs, separation from CPB is achieved with minimal to no inotropic support. The potential for conduction disturbances, particularly after ventriculotomy, supports the placement of temporary epicardial pacing wires. Other immediate postcorrection issues include residual shunt and bleeding. Significant residual shunts, as assessed by intraoperative TEE, potentially necessitate return to CPB for reevaluation or re-repair. Bleeding can be monitored after sternal approximation with the use of a mediastinal drain placed to wall suction.

Factors to be evaluated for determining the level of postoperative care required include the need for mechanical ventilation, need for inotropic support, and the presence of other complications. Tables 10-5 and 10-6 list common postoperative issues by surgical site and procedure, respectively. Following simple ASD repair, many patients can be extubated immediately. Patients who have undergone VSD repair and simple tetralogy of Fallot repair typically remain on mechanical ventilation for 2 to 12 hours, depending on the type of repair. Dopamine at 3 mcg/kg/minute or less is used to assist recovery from mild ventricular dysfunction.

Anesthesia for Complex Open-Heart Procedures

Except for the correction of left-to-right shunts and uncomplicated tetralogy of Fallot repair, most open-heart procedures for congenital heart defects are considered complex for a number of reasons. The defects themselves involve more than one cardiac structure; the hemodynamics that ensue necessitate more complex medical and surgical approaches (Table 10-7). Despite the development of newer diagnostic techniques allowing for early detection of congenital heart disease, many patients present only when significant cardiovascular compromise has occurred. While the same framework of considerations as used for the simple procedures can be applied here, patients undergoing complex repairs tend to require higher levels of perioperative monitoring, and hemodynamic and ventilatory support.

In spite of these complexities, children who have only moderate symptoms undergo premedication and inhalation induction as for simple procedures, with intravenous placement after induction. Patients with cardiovascular compromise undergo intravenous induction without premedication, to allow for greater hemodynamic control. Nasotracheal intubation is

Table 10-5   Postoperative Complications by Procedure

Procedure	Extubation Time Frame	Postoperative Issues, Potential Problems
Percutaneous device closure (ASD, PDA)	Early	Residual shunt flow
Thoracoscopy	Early	Mild pain; atelectasis; pneumothorax, chylothorax, hemothorax; pleural effusion; inadvertent ligation of thoracic duct; injury to vagus/recurrent laryngeal nerve; sequelae of lateral decubitus position
Thoracotomy	Early-intermediate	Significant pain (impaired pulmonary mechanics if unresolved), atelectasis; other issues same as thoracoscopy; lung contusion from direct retraction
Median sternotomy	Early-late	Pericardial, pleural effusion; brachial plexus injury; phrenic nerve paresis (impaired diaphragmatic function); pain
Ventriculotomy	Intermediate-late	Ventricular arrhythmias, conduction delay, ventricular dysfunction
Atriotomy	Early-late	Atrial arrhythmias, conduction delay, sinoatrial and atrioventricular node dysfunction
Cardiopulmonary bypass	Early-late	Activation of inflammatory cascade; platelet dysfunction; bleeding; transfusion requirement; short- and long-term neurologic sequelae
Deep hypothermic circulatory arrest	Intermediate-late	Same as for cardiopulmonary bypass; higher incidence of short- and long-term neurologic sequelae

ASD, atrial septal defect; PDA, patent ductus arteriosus.

selected over the oral route to provide more postoperative comfort for the patient, and to minimize the likelihood of dislodgement. Invasive arterial monitoring is necessary for continuous blood pressure and frequent monitoring of arterial blood gases, hematocrit, and electrolytes, both in the operating room and in the intensive care unit. While the procedures share many of the same potential postoperative complications, such as bleeding, ventricular dysfunction, and arrhythmias, each type of case raises its own set of anesthetic issues. The encyclopedic list of complex defects precludes individual discussion; however, the unique physiologic and surgical features of the following lesions present considerations that can be extrapolated for similar defects. These unique defects are complex tetralogy of Fallot with abnormal pulmonary vasculature, univentricular heart, truncus arteriosus, and transposition of the great arteries. General precorrection hemodynamic goals for some defects are presented in Table 10-5; most complex lesions comprise a combination of the problems listed.

Of the diagnostic criteria for tetralogy of Fallot (malalignment VSD, overriding aorta, RV hypertrophy, and RV outflow obstruction), the RV outflow obstruction is the most variable in both degree and location. The spectrum ranges from dynamic subpulmonic obstruction with normal anatomy

distally to small pulmonary valve to absent pulmonary valve and arteries. In the latter cases, with diminutive or absent pulmonary arteries, pulmonary blood flow occurs either through a patent ductus arteriosus, or by aortopulmonary collateral circulation. These phenomena can be demonstrated with echocardiography, but are frequently evaluated with angiography before surgery. In addition, the 5% to 6% incidence of abnormal coronary anatomy, with the anterior descending artery originating from the right coronary artery and traversing the RV outflow tract, necessitates careful preoperative evaluation before RV outflow tract incision is planned.[31]

This physiology often results in protection of the pulmonary vasculature from overcirculation and the subsequent development of pulmonary vascular occlusive disease. Cyanosis and compensatory polycythemia are frequent findings in these patients. Depending on the size and inflow source of the pulmonary circulation, surgical options range from augmentation of small pulmonary arteries to reimplantation of aortopulmonary collaterals onto an RV-PA conduit. While these plans theoretically provide pulmonary blood flow, the small caliber of the vessels can result in high pulmonary vascular resistance. The decision to close the VSD may also impact postcorrection myocardial function. Right ventricular failure may result from elimination of systolic popoff, if VSD

Table 10-6   Postoperative Complications by Surgical Site

Specific Procedure	Postoperative Complication
Percutaneous device closure (ASD, PDA)	Residual shunt, delayed detection of cardiac perforation
Coarctation repair	Neurologic dysfunction from thoracic aortic cross-clamp
Arterial switch, anomalous coronary repair	Coronary insufficiency/myocardial ischemia
Atrial switch (Mustard, Senning)	Loss of sinus rhythm, venous baffle obstruction
Stage I for HLHS	Inadequate shunt (pulmonary) blood flow, aortic arch obstruction/coarctation
Stage II, III for HLHS	Arrhythmias, baffle or venous pathway obstruction, ventricular dysfunction
AV canal repair	AV valve dysfunction (stenosis/regurgitation) conduction disturbance
Truncus arteriosus repair	Semilunar valve dysfunction
Tetralogy of Fallot repair	Heart block, RV dysfunction, pulmonic regurgitation, residual RVOT obstruction
Resection subaortic membrane	Recurrence of subaortic obstruction

ASD, atrial septal defect; PDA, patent ductus arteriosus; HLHS, hypoplastic left heart syndrome; AV, atrioventricular; RV, right ventricular; RVOT, right ventricular outflow tract.

Table 10-7 Simple versus Complex Congenital Open-Heart Procedures: Anesthetic Considerations

Consideration	Simple Open Procedure	Complex Open Procedure
Preoperative evaluation	Growth history/symptoms, medications, CBC, ECG, echocardiogram	Growth history/symptoms, medications/inotropes, ventilatory support, CBC count, electrolytes ECG, echocardiogram, cardiac catheterization data, MRI
Premedication (>6 mo old)	Pentobarbital 4 mg/kg PO (+/− meperidine 3 mg/kg PO) **or** diazepam 0.05–0.1 mg/kg PO	Pentobarbital 4 mg/kg PO + meperidine 3 mg/kg PO **or** diazepam 0.05–0.1 mg/kg PO
Induction	Inhalation (if no IV)	Inhalation or intravenous
Maintenance	Fentanyl 10–50 mcg/kg* + pancuronium 0.1–0.4 mg/kg* + inhalation agent if ineeded	Fentanyl 50–75 mcg/kg* + pancuronium 0.4 mg/kg*
Antibiotics	Cefazolin 25 mg/kg IV **or** vancomycin 10 mg/kg IV (if PCN allergy)	Cefazolin 25 mg/kg IV **or** vancomycin 10 mg/kg IV (if PCN allergy)
Special monitors	Arterial line Two temperature sensors (central, peripheral) Urinary catheter +/− atrial lines +/− TEE	Arterial line Two temperature sensors (central, peripheral) Urinary catheter Atrial lines +/− TEE
Special techniques	CPB, occasional DHCA	CPB, frequent DHCA
Fluids	Pre-CPB: limited crystalloid Post-CPB: crystalloid, FWB or PRBCs†	Pre-CPB: limited crystalloid Post-CPB: FWB or PRBCs†
Inotropic/hemodynamic support	Dopamine 3 mcg/kg/min (not always needed)	Almost always: Dopamine 3 mcg/kg/min Occasional additions: epinephrine 0.05–0.2 mcg/kg/min milrinone (bolus +/− infusion) inhaled nitric oxide nitroprusside 0.5–5 mcg/kg/min
Postoperative mechanical ventilation	0–12 hr	6–24+ hr

*Total dose.
†Choice of FWB or PRBCs determined by hematocrit and amount of bleeding.
CBC, complete blood cell; ECG, electrocardiogram; MRI, magnetic resonance imaging; PCN, penicillin; TEE, transesophageal echocardiogram; CPB, cardiopulmonary bypass; DHCA, deep hypothermic circulatory arrest; FWB, fresh whole blood; PRBCs, packed red blood cells.

is closed, inducing a pressure load on the RV, which must now pump against potentially high pulmonary vascular resistance. Mechanisms to minimize PVR through a reconstructed pulmonary circulation include mild hypocapnia, high inspired oxygen concentration, adequate anesthesia/analgesia, and pharmacologic therapy. Agents useful for this purpose include inhaled nitric oxide, opioids, milrinone, dobutamine, and isoproterenol.

Mixing lesions present a distinct set of challenges to the anesthesiologist. Precorrection management is similar for these defects, the differences in surgical goals for each is reflected in the postcorrection care. The parallel, rather than series, nature of the systemic and pulmonary circulations necessitates medical therapy to balance flow through each. Examples include univentricular heart and truncus arteriosus. Surgery for univentricular heart is typically staged over time, to allow development of the pulmonary vasculature and maintain ventricular function. Following Stage I palliation, the parallel arrangement of systemic and pulmonary circulations is maintained. Repair of truncus arteriosus, by contrast, achieves repair in one operative encounter, and results in separation of the circulations into the normal serial arrangement. Particularly in the neonatal period, when a majority of these patients present, the reactivity of the pulmonary vasculature provides a useful way, in the precorrection period, to achieve balanced circulation (i.e., $Q_p:Q_s$ of 1). Because of this arrangement, pulmonary overcirculation implies systemic hypoperfusion; this may eventually result in diminished perfusion of end organs and acidosis. As previously noted, hypercapnia and low inspired oxygen concentration promote increases in PVR; these factors can be regulated by

altering inspired gas mixtures, with the addition of CO_2 or N_2. In the operating room, CO_2 is added to achieve an SpO_2 near 85%. Metabolic acidosis is treated by attempting to improve systemic flow, and, on occasion, intravenous sodium bicarbonate.

The infant with univentricular heart undergoing initial palliation (the first stage in the series of operations leading to Fontan physiology) to provide pulmonary blood flow requires special considerations. The use of an arterial-to-pulmonary artery shunt impacts the site of arterial cannulation. For a planned right modified Blalock-Taussig shunt, the right upper extremity is avoided. The diminutive size of the ascending aorta in hypoplastic left heart syndrome often preclude its cannulation and use for initiating bypass; an alternative strategy employs pulmonary artery cannulation, with subsequent snaring of the branch pulmonary arteries to allow systemic flow through the ductus arteriosus. Surgical repair reconfigures the pulmonary trunk into the neo-ascending aorta, such that this site can be recannulated after DHCA for reinitiating CPB. Depending on the size of the native aorta, homograft or prosthetic material is used for augmentation. An arterial-to-pulmonary artery shunt, either from the right subclavian or right carotid artery, will supply the pulmonary circulation. Occasionally, a centrally located shunt between the ascending aorta and the pulmonary artery may be used.

Separation from bypass is achieved once inotropic support is started, ventilation is initiated, and shunt flow is established. Issues that complicate postcorrection management in the operating room and the ICU include hypoxemia and metabolic acidosis. Hypoxemia following a Stage I palliation results from several factors including inadequate ventilation, impaired shunt flow, and high pulmonary vascular resistance. The placement of a fresh endotracheal tube with a large internal diameter, the process of suctioning the lungs before resuming ventilation after DHCA, and the use of a neonatal ventilator minimize the opportunity for inadequate ventilation. Impaired shunt flow can result from thrombus or kinking of the shunt, excessive length, or inadequate diameter. Manipulation of pulmonary vascular resistance, using ventilation, inspired oxygen concentrations, and pulmonary vasodilators may provide some improvement in oxygen saturation. Compression of vascular structures following chest closure occasionally diminishes pulmonary blood flow, and may require leaving the sternum open for 24 to 48 hours. While some metabolic acidosis is anticipated following separation from CPB, its persistence suggests impaired systemic perfusion, either from aortic arch obstruction, ventricular dysfunction, or severe AV valve regurgitation. Echocardiography assists in diagnosing these problems. Inotropic support and afterload reduction may improve systemic flow. Expectant management of mild arch obstruction may allow balloon dilatation in the cardiac catheterization laboratory at a later date; severe arch obstruction necessitates surgical revision.

Anesthesia for Closed-Heart Procedures

Early corrective repair in infancy has significantly reduced the number of noncorrective, palliative closed-heart operations. Corrective closed-heart procedures include PDA ligation and repair of coarctation of the aorta. Noncorrective closed-heart operations include pulmonary artery banding, and extracardiac shunts such as the Blalock-Taussig shunt. All these procedures are performed without CPB. Therefore, venous access and intra-arterial monitoring are important in evaluating and supporting these patients. A pulse oximeter remains an invaluable monitor during intraoperative management.

PDA ligation is typically performed through a left thoracotomy, although video-assisted thoracoscopic techniques are increasingly prevalent.[8,82] Physiologic management is that of a left-to-right shunt producing volume overload. Patients with a large PDA and low PVR generally present with excessive pulmonary blood flow and congestive heart failure. Neonates and premature infants also run the risk of having substantial diastolic runoff to the pulmonary artery, potentially impairing coronary perfusion. Thus, patients range from an asymptomatic healthy young child to the sick ventilator-dependent premature infant on inotropic support. The former patient allows for a variety of anesthetic techniques culminating in extubation in the operating room. The latter patient requires a carefully controlled anesthetic and fluid management plan. Generally a trial of medical management with indomethacin and fluid restriction is attempted in the premature infant prior to surgical correction. In the premature infant, transport to the operating room can be especially difficult and potentially hazardous, requiring great vigilance to avoid extubation, excessive patient cooling, or venous access disruption. For these reasons, many centers are now performing ligation in the neonatal intensive care unit. Intraoperatively, retractors may interfere with cardiac filling and ventilatory management so that hypotension, hypoxemia, and hypercarbia occur. Complications include inadvertent ligation of the left pulmonary artery or descending aorta, recurrent laryngeal nerve damage,

and excessive bleeding due to inadvertent PDA disruption. After ductal ligation in premature infants, worsening pulmonary compliance can precipitate a need for increased ventilatory support. Manifestations of an acute increase in LV afterload should be anticipated especially if LV dysfunction has developed preoperatively. More recently, PDA ligation has been performed in infants and children using thoracoscopic surgical techniques. This approach has the advantages of limited incisions at thoracoscopic sites, promoting less postoperative pain and discharge from the hospital the same day of surgery.

Coarctation of the aorta is a narrowing of the descending aorta near the insertion of the ductus arteriosus. Obstruction to aortic flow is the result and this may range from severe obstruction with compromised distal systemic perfusion to mild upper extremity hypertension as the only manifestation. Associated anomalies of both the mitral and aortic valves can occur. In the neonate with severe coarctation, systemic perfusion is dependent on right-to-left shunting across the PDA. In these circumstances, LV dysfunction is very common and PGE_1 is necessary to preserve sufficient systemic perfusion. Generally, a peripheral intravenous line and an indwelling arterial catheter, preferably in the right arm, are recommended for intraoperative and postoperative management. In patients with LV dysfunction, a central venous catheter may be desirable for pressure monitoring and inotropic support. The surgical approach is through a left thoracotomy, whereby the aorta is cross-clamped and the coarctation repaired with an on-lay prosthetic patch, a subclavian artery flap, or resection of the coarctation with an end-to-end anastomosis. During cross-clamp, we usually allow significant proximal hypertension (20% to 25% increase over baseline), based upon evidence that vasodilator therapy may jeopardize distal perfusion and promote spinal cord ischemia.[39] Intravascular volume loading with 10 to 20 mL/kg of crystalloid is given just before removal of the clamp. The anesthetic concentration is decreased, and additional blood volume support is given until the blood pressure increases. Postrepair rebound hypertension due to heightened baroreceptor reactivity is common and often requires medical therapy. After cross-clamp, aortic wall stress due to systemic hypertension is most effectively lowered by institution of beta-blockade with esmolol or α/β-blockade with labetolol.[23] Propranolol is useful in older patients but can cause severe bradycardia in infants and young children. Although it actually increases calculated aortic wall stress in the absence of beta blockade by accelerating dP/dT, the addition of sodium nitroprusside may become necessary to control refractory hypertension. Captopril or an alternative antihypertensive regimen is begun in the convalescent stage of recovery in those patients with persistent hypertension.

The management of infants undergoing placement of extracardiac shunts without cardiopulmonary bypass centers around similar goals as other shunt lesions: balancing pulmonary and systemic blood flow by altering $PaCO_2$, PaO_2, and ventilatory dynamics. Central shunts are usually performed through a median sternotomy, while Blalock-Taussig shunts may be performed through a thoracotomy or sternotomy. In patients in whom pulmonary blood flow is critically low, partial cross-clamping of the pulmonary artery required for the distal anastomosis causes further reduction of pulmonary blood flow and desaturation, necessitating meticulous monitoring of pulse oximetry. Careful application of the cross-clamp to avoid pulmonary artery distortion will help to maintain pulmonary blood flow. Under circumstances, in which severe desaturation and bradycardia occur with cross-clamping, CPB will be required for repair. Intraoperative complications include bleeding and severe systemic oxygen desaturation during chest closure, usually indicating a change in the relationship of the intrathoracic contents that results in distortion of the pulmonary arteries or kink in the shunt. Pulmonary edema may develop in the early postoperative period in response to the acute volume overload that accompanies the creation of a large surgical shunt. Measures directed at increasing PVR, such as lowering inspired O_2 to room air, allowing the $PaCO_2$ to rise, and adding PEEP are helpful maneuvers to decrease pulmonary blood flow until the pulmonary circulation can adjust. Decongestive therapy such as diuretics and digoxin may alleviate the manifestations of congestive heart failure. Under such circumstances, early extubation is inadvisable.

Pulmonary artery banding is used to restrict pulmonary blood flow in infants who are deemed uncorrectable either for anatomical or physiologic reasons. These patients are generally in congestive heart failure with reduced systemic perfusion and excessive pulmonary blood flow. The surgeon places a restrictive band around the main pulmonary artery to reduce pulmonary blood flow. Band placement is very imprecise and requires careful assistance from the anesthesia team to accomplish successfully. Many approaches have been suggested. We place the patient on 21 percent inspired oxygen concentration and maintain the $PaCO_2$ at 40 mm Hg, to simulate the postoperative state. Depending upon the malformation, a pulmonary artery band is tightened to achieve hemodynamic (e.g., distal pulmonary artery pressure 50% to 25% systemic pressure) and/or physiologic (e.g., $Q_p{:}Q_s$ approaching 1) goals. Should the attainment of these objectives produce unacceptable hypoxemia, the band is loosened.

Blalock-Hanlon atrial septectomy is now an uncommon procedure for enlarging an intra-atrial connection. This procedure is done by occluding caval flow and creating an intra-atrial communication through the atrial septum. In patients with hypoplastic left heart syndrome with an intact atrial septum, this procedure is life saving and must be performed within hours of birth. Balloon atrial septostomies (Rashkind procedure) and blade septectomies performed in the cardiac catheterization laboratory have replaced surgical intervention, except when left atrial size is very small or the atrial septum is thickened. Improved safety of CPB has led to the virtual elimination of such intracardiac procedures using inflow occlusion. Surgical septectomies, because they are currently confined to the most difficult subset, are rarely performed without benefit of CPB.

Anesthesia for Heart and Lung Transplantation

While perioperative management for thoracic organ transplantation is considered elsewhere in this text (see Chapter 16), the application of these procedures to children requires some specific modification. Differences include the characteristics of the candidates, preparation of these children, anesthetic management, surgical considerations, postbypass management, and outcome.

Even though some of the earliest heart transplants were performed for congenital heart malformations, this indication became rare by the early 1980s. In 1984, more than 60% of the few pediatric heart transplants were performed in patients with cardiomyopathy, usually adolescents. In the next decade, a dramatic rise in the number of infants and young children with congenital heart malformations treated with heart transplantation resulted in a marked shift in the demographics (Fig. 10-9).[65] By 1995, more than 70% of the children receiving heart transplants were younger than 5 years of age; half of those younger than 1 year. The overwhelming majority of these infants undergo transplant for congenital heart malformations for which reconstructive options either have failed or are not believed to exist.[65] The implications of this shift reach into every element of perioperative management.

Children considered for heart transplantation are more likely to have pulmonary hypertension than adults. Most adult transplant programs will not offer heart transplant therapy to patients with PVR over 6 Wood units × m^2.[75] The exclusion threshold in infants and children remains controversial. Some programs accept patients with PVR as high as 12 Wood units × m^2, particularly if the pulmonary vasculature responds to vasodilators such as oxygen, NO, calcium channel blockers, or prostacyclin.[38] Neonates are generally assumed to have elevated PVR, but outcome data from some programs suggest that the importance of this factor on postoperative outcome is substantially less in the first year of life, perhaps because the infant donor hearts, having recently undergone transitional circulation, are better prepared to cope with the right ventricular pressure load that elevated PVR imposes.[37]

The anesthetic plan for pediatric heart transplantation must accommodate a wide spectrum of pathophysiologies.

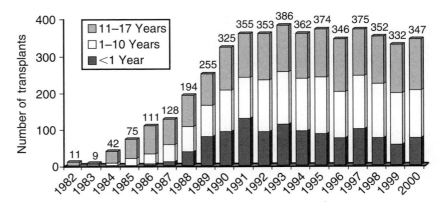

FIGURE 10-9 Demographic data for pediatric heart transplantation by age. Stacked bar graph illustrates the total number and age distribution for heart transplantation younger than 18 years. Note the rapid increase in transplants performed during the late 1980s with particular growth in the population of children aged 5 years and under. Having peaked in the mid-1990s, the total number of transplants (both adult and pediatric) has declined slightly, but the relative age proportions within the pediatric population remain relatively constant. (From Hosenpud JD, Bennett LE, Keck BM, et al: The Registry of the International Society for Heart and Lung Transplantation: Eighteenth Official Report–2001. *J Heart Lung Transplant* 20:805–815, 2001.)

Recipients with congenital heart malformations benefit from the same analysis of loading conditions and optimizing hemodynamics discussed previously. Although a few of these patients undergo heart transplant because the natural history of reconstructive heart surgery poses greater risk despite reasonable ventricular function, most candidates exhibit some manifestations of impaired ventricular performance. As such, they require careful titration of anesthetic agents with minimal myocardial depressant characteristics to avoid cardiovascular collapse. In this fragile population, even modest doses of opioids can be associated with marked deterioration in systemic hemodynamics, presumably by reducing endogenous catecholamine release. As with most congenital heart patients, skilled management of the airway and ventilation represent crucial elements in a satisfactory induction, particularly in the face of elevated PVR. No matter how elegant the anesthetic plan in conception and implementation, a certain proportion of these children will decompensate upon induction, necessitating resuscitative therapy.

While orthotopic heart transplantation poses some technical challenges in neonates and young infants, the replacement of an anatomically normal heart is less complex than several reconstructive heart procedures commonly performed at this age. However, the need to adapt this procedure to incorporate repair of major concurrent cardiovascular malformations requires the consummate skill and creativity that remains the province of the few exemplary congenital heart surgeons.[2,15] Having withstood extended ischemic periods, heart grafts are extraordinarily intolerant of superimposed residual hemodynamic loads that might accompany imperfect vascular reconstruction. The extensive vascular repair and, particularly in older children with longstanding hypoxemia, the propensity to coagulopathy together elevate hemorrhage to a major cause of morbidity and even mortality in pediatric heart transplantation. Nevertheless, once successfully implanted, these grafts will respond to physiologic factors that stimulate growth and adaptation in the developing infant and child.[141]

Management considerations during separation from CPB and the early postoperative period are primarily focused on three pathophysiologic conditions; myocardial preservation, denervation, and PVR. Even expeditious transplants usually force the heart to endure ischemic periods that exceed those encountered for reconstructive surgery. Although some centers believe the infant heart is more tolerant of extended ischemia,[37] these hearts will demonstrate a period of reperfusion injury and virtually all require pharmacologic and, in some cases, mechanical support. In addition, endogenous adaptive responses and exogenous pharmacologic agents that act via myocardial sympathetic activation are ineffective in the denervated graft. Since the majority of children presenting for heart transplantation exhibit some element of elevated PVR, even with isolated end-stage cardiomyopathy, the right ventricle of a newly implanted heart is particularly vulnerable to failure.

As such, ventilatory and pharmacologic interventions are usually configured to exert a favorable impact on PVR and provide inotropic and chronotropic support. Once the lungs are fully expanded, we ventilate to $PaCO_2$ values in the low 30s using a FiO_2 of 1. Virtually all recipients receive low-dose dopamine (3 to 5 mcg/kg/min) and isoproterenol (0.02 to 0.05 mcg/kg/min) to promote inotropy, chronotropy, and lower PVR. In the event that these do not provide sufficient inotropy in the face of more significant postischemic dysfunction, additional agents are added (e.g., milrinone, epinephrine). Most transplant centers have a specific regimen for immunosuppression to be initiated in the perioperative period. As with adults, pediatric transplant programs typically use triple drug immunosuppression with a calcinuerin inhibitor (e.g., cyclosporin, tacrolimus), antimetabolite (e.g., azathioprine), and steriod. Following an interval without rejection, some pediatric programs will taper and discontinue one or even two of these agents, particularly in neonates in whom they believe some element of tolerance develops.[6,12]

National statistics indicate that the outcome from pediatric heart transplant is slightly less favorable than comparable adult results.[65] The principle risk factors are age under 1 year and congenital heart defects. Because these factors are highly related (i.e., the vast majority of infants younger than 1 year of age undergo transplantation for congenital heart disease), it is difficult to determine the independent effect of age. Concurrent repair of structural cardiovascular anomalies substantially increases perioperative risk of hemorrhage, residual hemodynamic loading conditions, and right heart failure from elevated PVR. Taken together, infants younger than 1 year of age have an operative mortality (<30 days) of 24%, more that twice that of older children.[65] Beyond the early postoperative period, mortality rates are quite comparable for all age groups. Nevertheless, the sequelae of rejection and the consequences of the requisite immunosuppression result in significant ongoing morbidity and mortality. Since even the best transplant recipients have only achieved 28% 14-year survival, these procedures can only be considered palliative for children.[65]

Lung and heart-lung transplantation have achieved respectable operative survival in children.[7,17] They remain the only viable surgical therapy for infants and children with severe pulmonary vascular disease, and selected progressive pulmonary diseases. These remain uncommon procedures in pediatrics. Lung transplantation carries the additional morbidity of obliterative bronchiolitis, a debilitating small airway disease that results in gradual deterioration in flow-related pulmonary functions over time. Despite operative mortality that is currently less than 20%, the 3-year survival is only 50% to 60%.[17,65]

Anesthesia for Interventional or Diagnostic Cardiac Procedures

Advances in interventional and diagnostic cardiac catheterization techniques are significantly changing the operative and nonoperative approach to the patient with a congenital heart defect.[100,118] Nonoperative interventional techniques are being used instead of procedures requiring surgery and CPB for safe closure of secundum ASDs, VSDs, and PDAs. Stenotic aortic and pulmonic valves, recurrent aortic coarctations, and branch pulmonary artery stenoses can be dilatated in the catheterization lab, avoiding surgical intervention as well.[53,62,85,95] These techniques shorten hospital stay and are particularly beneficial to patients with recurrent coarctation and muscular or apical VSDs, who are at a higher risk during operative intervention. Many patients with complex cardiac defects are poor operative risks. Innovative interventional procedures improve vascular anatomy, reduce pressure loads on ventricle, and decrease the operative risk for these patients. For example, in tetralogy of Fallot with hypoplastic pulmonary arteries, balloon angioplasty and vascular stenting procedures create favorable pulmonary artery anatomy and reduce pulmonary artery pressure and right ventricular end-diastolic pressure. High-risk patients undergoing diagnostic evaluation of pulmonary artery hypertension in anticipation of heart-lung transplantation also require anesthetic management. Despite the attendant high risks of the procedure in these patients with suprasystemic RV pressure, these patients are best managed with general anesthesia and controlled ventilation.

Anesthetic management of interventional or diagnostic procedures in the catheterization lab must include the same level of preparation that would apply in caring for these patients in the operating room. The patients have the same complex cardiac physiology and, in some cases, greater physiologic complexity and less cardiovascular reserve because they are deemed high operative risks. Interventional catheterization procedures can impose acute pressure load on the heart during balloon inflation. Large catheters placed across mitral or tricuspid valves create acute valvular regurgitation or, in the case of a small valve orifice, transient valvular stenosis. When catheters are placed across shunts, severe reductions in pulmonary blood flow and marked cyanosis may occur.[62,87] The anesthetic plan must consider the specific cardiology objectives of the procedure and the impact of anesthetic management in facilitating or hindering the interventional procedure. In general, there are three distinct periods involved in an interventional catheterization: the data acquisition period, the interventional period, and the postprocedural evaluation period.

During the data acquisition period the cardiologist performs a hemodynamic catheterization to evaluate the need for and extent of the planned intervention. Catheterization data are obtained under normal physiologic conditions; that is, room air, physiologic $PaCO_2$, and spontaneous ventilation are preferred. Increased FiO_2 or changes in $PaCO_2$ may obscure physiologic data. During the procedural period, the patient is usually intubated and mechanically ventilated. A secured airway allows the anesthesiologist to concentrate on hemodynamic issues. Positive-pressure ventilation also reduces the risk of air embolism. During spontaneous ventilation a large reduction in intrathoracic pressure may entrain air into vascular sheaths and result in moderate to large pulmonary or systemic air emboli. Precise device placement is also facilitated with muscle relaxants that eliminate patient movements and controlled ventilation thereby reducing the respiratory shifting of cardiac structures. Substantial blood loss and changes in ventricular function occur commonly during the intervention. Blood volume replacement and inotropic support may be necessary during or immediately after the interventional procedure. In the postprocedural period, the success and the physiologic impact of the intervention are evaluated. Blood pressure, mixed venous oxygen saturation, ventricular end diastolic pressure, and cardiac output, when available, are used to assess the impact of the intervention. Persistent severe hemodynamic derangement indicates the need for intensive care unit monitoring and/or respiratory or cardiovascular support.

Because of the hemodynamic variability of many of these patients, as well as changing anesthetic requirements, continuous intravenous infusion with ketamine/midazolam or, more recently, propofol/alfentanil, are appropriate. Potent inhaled anesthetics are generally not used as the primary anesthetic and are reserved for adjunctive anesthesia. The success of these interventions will undoubtedly result in widespread availability and use over the next few years.

References

1. Andrew M, Paes B, Milner R, et al: Development of the human coagulation system in the full-term infant. *Blood* 70:165–172, 1987.
2. Bailey LL: Heart transplantation techniques in complex congenital heart disease. *J Heart Lung Transplant* 12:S168–175, 1993.
3. Bellinger DC, Jonas RA, Rappaport LA, et al: Developmental and neurologic status of children after heart surgery with hypothermic circulatory arrest or low-flow cardiopulmonary bypass. *N Engl J Med* 332:549–555, 1995.
4. Bellinger DC, Rappaport LA, Wypij D, et al: Patterns of developmental dysfunction after surgery in infancy to correct transposition of the great arteries. *J Dev Behav Ped* 18:75–83, 1997.
5. Benveniste H, Drejer J, Schousboe A, Diemer NH: Elevation of the extracellular concentrations of glutamate and aspartate in rat hippocampus during transient cerebral ischemia monitored by intracerebral microdialysis. *J Neurochem* 43:1369–1374, 1984.
6. Boucek MM, Kanakriyeh MS, Mathis CM, et al: Cardiac transplantation in infancy: donors and recipients. Loma Linda University Pediatric Heart Transplant Group. *J Pediatr* 116:171–176, 1990.
7. Bridges ND, Malory GB Jr, Huddleston CB, et al: Lung transplantation in children and young adults with cardiovascular disease. *Ann Thorac Surg* 59:813–820, 1995.
8. Burke RP, Wernovsky G, van der Velde M, et al: Video-assisted thoracoscopic surgery for congenital heart disease. *J Thorac Cardiovasc Surg* 109:499–508, 1995.
9. Burrows FA, Hillier SC, McLeod ME, et al: Anterior fontanel pressure and visual evoked potentials in neonates and infants undergoing profound hypothermic circulatory arrest. *Anesthesiology* 73:632–636, 1990.
10. Busto R, Globus MY, Dietrich WD, et al: Effect of mild hypothermia on ischemia-induced release of neurotransmitters and free fatty acids in rat brain. *Stroke* 20:904–910, 1989.
11. Byrick RJ, Kay JC, Noble WH: Extravascular lung water accumulation in patients following coronary artery surgery. *Can Anaesth Soc J* 24:332–345, 1977.
12. Canter CE, Moorhead S, Saffitz JE, et al: Steroid withdrawal in the pediatric heart transplant recipient initially treated with triple immunosuppression. *J Heart Lung Transplant* 13:74–79, 1994.
13. Carrel TP, Schwanda M, Vogt PR, Turina MI: Aprotinin in pediatric cardiac operations: a benefit in complex malformations and with high-dose regimen only. *Ann Thorac Surg* 66:153–158, 1998.
14. Castaneda AR, Mayer JE Jr, Jonas RA, et al: The neonate with critical congenital heart disease: repair—a surgical challenge. *J Thorac Cardiovasc Surg* 98:869–875, 1989.
15. Chartrand C, Guerin R, Kangah M, Stanley P: Pediatric heart transplantation: surgical considerations for congenital heart diseases. *J Heart Transplant* 9:608–616, 1990.
16. Colon-Otero G, Gilchrist GS, Holcomb GR, et al: Preoperative evaluation of hemostasis in patients with heart disease. *Mayo Clin Proc* 62:379–385, 1987.
17. Conte JV, Robbins RC, Reichenspurner H, et al: Pediatric heart-lung transplantation: intermediate-term results. *J Heart Lung Transplant* 15:692–699, 1996.
18. Cyran SE, Myers JL, Gleason MM, et al: Application of intraoperative transesophageal echocardiography in infants and small children. *J Cardiovasc Surg (Torino)* 32:318–321, 1991.
19. Daggett CW, Lodge AJ, Scarborough JE, et al: Modified ultrafiltration versus conventional ultrafiltration: a randomized prospective study in neonatal piglets. *J Thorac Cardiovasc Surg* 115:336–341, 1998.
20. Darling E, Nanry K, Shearer I, et al: Techniques of paediatric modified ultrafiltration: 1996 survey results. *Perfusion* 13:93–103, 1998.

21. Davies MJ, Allen A, Kort H, et al: Prospective, randomized, double-blind study of high-dose aprotinin in pediatric cardiac operations. *Ann Thorac Surg* 63:497–503, 1997.

22. Davies MJ, Nguyen K, Gaynor JW, Elliott MJ: Modified ultrafiltration improves left ventricular systolic function in infants after cardiopulmonary bypass. *J Thorac Cardiovasc Surg* 115:361–369, 1998.

23. DeSanctis RW, Doroghazi RM, Austen WG, Buckley JJ: Aortic dissection. *N Engl J Med* 317:1060–1067, 1987.

24. Dietrich W, Barankay A, Hahnel C, Richter JA: High-dose aprotinin in cardiac surgery: three years' experience in 1,784 patients. *J Cardiothorac Vasc Anesth* 6:324–327, 1992.

25. Dietrich W, Henze R, Barankay A, et al: High-dose aprotinin application reduces homologous blood requirement in cardiac surgery. *J Cardiothorac Anesth* 3:S79, 1989.

26. Dietrich W, Mossinger H, Spannagl M, et al: Hemostatic activation during cardiopulmonary bypass with different aprotinin dosages in pediatric patients having cardiac operations. *J Thorac Cardiovasc Surg* 105:712–720, 1993.

27. Dietrich W, Spannagl M, Jochum M, et al: Influence of high-dose aprotinin treatment on blood loss and coagulation patterns in patients undergoing myocardial revascularization. *Anesthesiology* 73:1119–1126, 1990.

28. Dietrich W, Spannagl M, Schramm W, et al: The influence of preoperative anticoagulation on heparin response during cardiopulmonary bypass. *J Thorac Cardiovasc Surg* 102:505–514, 1991.

29. du Plessis AJ: Neurologic complications of cardiac disease in the newborn. *Clin Perinatol* 24:807–826, 1997.

30. Elliott JJ: Ultrafiltration and modified ultrafiltration in pediatric open-heart operations. *Ann Thorac Surg* 56:1518–1522, 1993.

31. Fellows KE, Freed MD, Keane JF, et al: Results of routine preoperative coronary angiography in tetralogy of Fallot. *Circulation* 51:561–566, 1975.

32. Fox LS, Blackstone EH, Kirklin JW, et al: Relationship of brain blood flow and oxygen consumption to perfusion flow rate during profoundly hypothermic cardiopulmonary bypass. *J Thorac Cardiovasc Surg* 87:658–664, 1984.

33. Fox LS, Blackstone EH, Kirklin JW, et al: Relationship of whole body oxygen consumption to perfusion flow rate during hypothermic cardiopulmonary bypass. *J Thorac Cardiovasc Surg* 83:239–248, 1982.

34. Friesen RH, Campbell DN, Clarke DR, Tornabene MA: Modified ultrafiltration attenuates dilutional coagulopathy in pediatric open-heart operation: *Ann Thorac Surg* 65:1787–1789, 1997.

35. Friesen RH, Lichtor JL: Cardiovascular effects of inhalational induction with isoflurane in infants. *Anesth Analg* 62:411–414, 1983.

36. Frink EJ Jr, Green WB Jr, Brown EA, et al: Compound A concentrations during sevoflurane anesthesia in children. *Anesthesiology* 84:566–571, 1996.

37. Fukushima N, Gundry SR, Razzouk AJ, Bailey LL: Risk factors for graft failure associated with pulmonary hypertension after pediatric heart transplantation. *J Thorac Cardiovasc Surg* 107:985–989, 1994.

38. Gajarski RJ, Towbin JA, Bricker JT, et al: Intermediate follow-up of pediatric heart transplant recipients with elevated pulmonary vascular resistance index. *J Am Coll Cardiol* 23:1682–1687, 1994.

39. Gelman S, Reves JG, Fowler K, et al: Regional blood flow during cross-clamping of the thoracic aorta and infusion of sodium nitroprusside. *J Thorac Cardiovasc Surg* 85:287–291, 1983.

40. Gold JP, Jonas RA, Lang P, Castaneda A: Transthoracic intracardiac monitoring lines in pediatric surgical patients: A ten year experience. *Ann Thorac Surg* 42:185, 1986.

41. Greeley WJ, Bracey VA, Ungerleider RM, et al: Recovery of cerebral metabolism and mitochondrial oxidation state are delayed after hypothermic circulatory arrest. *Circulation* 84:400–406, 1991.

42. Greeley WJ, Bushman GA, Davis DP, Reves JG: Comparative effects of halothane and ketamine on systemic arterial oxygen saturation in children with cyanotic heart disease. *Anesthesiology* 65:666–668, 1986.

43. Greeley WJ, Bushman GA, Kong DL, et al: Effects of cardiopulmonary bypass on eicosanoid metabolism during pediatric cardiovascular surgery. *J Thorac Cardiovasc Surg* 95:842–849, 1988.

44. Greeley WJ, Kern FH, Ungerleider RM, et al: The effect of hypothermic cardiopulmonary bypass and total circulatory arrest on cerebral metabolism in neonates, infants, and children. *J Thorac Cardiovasc Surg* 101:783–794, 1991.

45. Greeley WJ, Kern FH, Ungerleider RM, Kisslo JA: Intramyocardial air causes right ventricular dysfunction after repair of a congenital heart defect. *Anesthesiology* 73:1042, 1990.

46. Greeley WJ, Ungerleider RM: Assessing the effect of cardiopulmonary bypass on the brain. *Ann Thorac Surg* 52:417–419, 1991.

47. Greeley WJ, Ungerleider RM: Assessing the effect of cardiopulmonary bypass on the brain. *Ann Thorac Surg* 52:417–419, 1991.

48. Greeley WJ, Ungerleider RM, Smith LR, Reves JG: The effects of deep hypothermic cardiopulmonary bypass and total circulatory arrest on cerebral blood flow in infants and children. *J Thorac Cardiovasc Surg* 97:737–745, 1989.

49. Hagler DJ, Tajik AJ, Seward JB, et al: Intraoperative two-dimensional Doppler echocardiography. A preliminary study for congenital heart disease. *J Thorac Cardiovasc Surg* 95:516–522, 1988.

50. Hammer GB: Pediatric thoracic anesthesia. *Anesth Analg* 92:1449–1464, 2001.

51. Haneda K, Thomas R, Breazeale DG, Dillard DH: The significance of colloid osmotic pressure during induced hypothermia. *J Cardiovasc Surg* (Torino) 28:614–620, 1987.

52. Harker LA: Bleeding after cardiopulmonary bypass. *N Engl J Med* 314:1446–1448, 1986.

53. Hellenbrand WE, Fahey JT, McGowan FX, et al: Transesophageal echocardiographic guidance for transcatheter closure of atrial septal defects. *Am J Cardiol* 66:207–213, 1990.

54. Henling CE, Carmichael MJ, Keats AS, Cooley DA: Cardiac operation for congenital heart disease in children of Jehovah's Witnesses. *J Thorac Cardiovasc Surg* 89:914–920, 1985.

55. Henriksen L, Barry DI, Rygg IH, Skovsted P: Cerebral blood flow during early cardiopulmonary bypass in man. Effect of procaine in cardioplegic solutions. *Thorac Cardiovasc Surg* 34:116–123, 1986.

56. Henriksson P, Varendh G, Lundstrom NR: Haemostatic defects in cyanotic congenital heart disease. *Br Heart J* 41:23–27, 1979.

57. Hickey PR, Hansen DD: Fentanyl- and sufentanil-oxygen-pancuronium anesthesia for cardiac surgery in infants. *Anesth Analg* 63:117–124, 1984.

58. Hickey PR, Hansen DD, Norwood WI, Castaneda AR: Anesthetic complications in surgery for congenital heart disease. *Anesth Analg* 63:657–664, 1984.

59. Hickey PR, Hansen DD, Wessel DL, et al: Pulmonary and systemic hemodynamic responses to fentanyl in infants. *Anesth Analg* 64:483–486, 1985.

60. Hickey PR, Hansen DD, Wessel DL, et al: Blunting of stress responses in the pulmonary circulation of infants by fentanyl. *Anesth Analg* 64:1137–1142, 1985.

61. Hickey PR, Wessel DL: Anesthesia for treatment of congenital heart disease. In Kaplan JA (ed): Cardiac Anesthesia. 2nd Ed. Grune & Stratton, Orlando, FL, 1987, p 635.

62. Hickey PR, Wessel DL, Streitz SL, et al: Transcatheter closure of atrial septal defects: Hemodynamic complications and anesthetic management. *Anesth Analg* 74:44–50, 1992.

63. Holzman RS, van der Velde ME, Kaus SJ, et al: Sevoflurane depresses myocardial contractility less than halothane during induction of anesthesia in children. *Anesthesiology* 85:1260–1267, 1996.

64. Horkay F, Martin P, Rajah SM, Walker DR: Response to heparinization in adults and children undergoing cardiac operations. *Ann Thorac Surg* 53:822–826, 1992.

65. Hosenpud JD, Bennett LE, Keck BM, et al: The Registry of the International Society for Heart and Lung Transplantation: Eighteenth Official Report–2001. *J Heart Lung Transplant* 20:805–815, 2001.

66. Jobes DR, Shaffer GW, Aitken GL: Increased accuracy and precision of heparin and protamine dosing reduces blood loss and transfusion in patients undergoing primary cardiac operations. *J Thorac Cardiovasc Surg* 110:36–45, 1995.

67. Jonas RA, Bellinger DC, Rappaport LA, et al: Relation of pH strategy and developmental outcome after hypothermic circulatory arrest. *J Thorac Cardiovasc Surg* 106:362–368, 1993.

68. Journois D, Pouard P, Greeley WJ, et al: Hemofiltration during cardiopulmonary bypass in pediatric cardiac surgery. *Anesthesiology* 81:1181–1189, 1994.

69. Kawashima Y, Yamamoto Z, Manabe H: Safe limits of hemodilution in cardiopulmonary bypass. *Surgery* 76:391–397, 1974.

70. Kawata H, Fackler JC, Aoki M, et al: Recovery of cerebral blood flow and energy state after hypothermic circulatory arrest versus low flow bypass in piglets. *J Thorac Cardiovasc Surg* 102:671–685, 1993.

71. Kern C, Erb T, Frei FJ: Haemodynamic responses to sevoflurane compared with halothane during inhalational induction in children. *Paediatr Anaesth* 7:439–444, 1997.

72. Kern FH, Jonas RA, Mayer JE Jr, et al: Temperature monitoring during infant CPB: Does it predict efficient brain cooling? *Ann Thorac Surg* 54:749–754, 1992.

73. Kern FH, Morana NJ, Sears J, Hickey PR: Coagulation defects in neonates during CPB. *Ann Thorac Surg* 54:541–546, 1992.

74. Kirklin JW, Barratt-Boyes BG (eds): Cardiac Surgery. 2nd Ed. Churchill Livingstone, New York, 1993.

75. Kirklin JK, Naftel DC, McGiffin DC, et al: Analysis of morbid events and risk factors for death after cardiac transplantation. *J Am Coll Cardiol* 11:917–924, 1988.

76. Kirklin JK, Westaby S, Blackstone EH, et al: Complement and the damaging effects of cardiopulmonary bypass. *J Thorac Cardiovasc Surg* 86:845–857, 1983.

77. Kirshbom RM, Skaryak LA, DiBernardo LR, et al: Effect of aortopulmonary collaterals on cerebral cooling and metabolic recovery during cardiopulmonary bypass and circulatory arrest. *Circulation*, 92:II490–494, 1995.

78. Koutlas TC, Gaynor JW, Nicolson SC, et al: Modified ultrafiltration reduces postoperative morbidity after cavopulmonary connection. *Ann Thorac Surg* 64:37–42, 1997.

79. Kurth CD, O'Rourke MM, O'Hara IB: Comparison of pH-stat and alpha-stat cardiopulmonary bypass on cerebral oxygenation and blood flow in relation to hypothermic circulatory arrest in piglets. *Anesthesiology* 89:110–118, 1998.

80. Kurth CD, O'Rourke MM, O'Hara IB, Uher B: Brain cooling efficiency with pH-stat and alpha-stat cardiopulmonary bypass in newborn pigs. *Circulation* 96:II358–363, 1997.

81. Kurth CD, Priestley M, Watzman HM, et al: Desflurane confers neurologic protection for deep hypothermic circulatory arrest in newborn pigs. *Anesthesiology* 95:959–964, 2001.

82. Laborde F, Folliguet T, Batisse A, et al: Video-assisted thoracoscopic surgical interruption: The technique of choice for patent ductus arteriosus. Routine experience in 230 pediatric cases. *J Thorac Cardiovasc Surg* 110:1681–1684, 1995.

83. Laishley RS, Burrows FA, Lerman J, Roy WL: Effects of anesthetic induction on oxygen saturation in cyanotic congenital heart disease. *Anesthesiology* 65:673–677, 1986.

84. Leone BJ, Spahn DR, Smith LR, et al: Acute isovolemic hemodilution and blood transfusion. Effects on regional function and metabolism in myocardium with compromised coronary blood flow. *J Thorac Cardiovasc Surg* 105:694–704, 1993.

85. Lock JE, Rome JJ, Davis R, et al: Transcatheter closure of atrial septal defects. Experimental studies. *Circulation* 79:1091–1099, 1989.

86. Mackensen GB, Sato Y, Nellgard B, et al: Cardiopulmonary bypass induces neurologic and neurocognitive dysfunction in the rat. *Anesthesiology* 95:1485–1491, 2001.

87. Malviya S, Burrows FA, Johnston AE, Benson LN: Anaesthetic experience with paediatric interventional cardiology. *Can J Anaesth* 36:320–324, 1989.

88. Manno CS, Hedberg KW, Kim HC, et al: Comparison of the hemostatic effects of fresh whole blood, stored whole blood, and components after open-heart surgery in children. *Blood* 77:930–936, 1991.

89. Marelli D, Paul A, Samson R, et al: Does the addition of albumin to the prime solution in cardiopulmonary bypass affect clinical outcome? *J Thorac Cardiovasc Surg* 98:751–756 1989.

90. Maxwell LG, Yaster M: Perioperative management issues in pediatric patients. *Anesthesiol Clin North America* 18:601–632, 2000.

91. Michenfelder JD, Theye RA: Hypothermia: effect of canine brain and whole-body metabolism. *Anesthesiology* 29:1107–1112, 1968.

92. Miller-Hance WC, Silverman NH: Transesophageal echocardiography (TEE) in congenital heart disease with focus on the adult. *Cardiol Clin* 18:861–892, 2000.

93. Muhiudeen IA, Roberson DA, Silverman NH, et al: Intraoperative echocardiography in infants and children with congenital cardiac shunt lesions: transesophageal versus epicardial echocardiography. *J Am Coll Cardiol* 16:1687–1695, 1990.

94. Muhiudeen IA, Roberson DA, Silverman NH, et al: Intraoperative echocardiography for evaluation of congenital heart defects in infants and children. *Anesthesiology* 76:165–172, 1992.

95. Mullins CE: Pediatric and congenital therapeutic cardiac catheterization. *Circulation* 79:1153–1159, 1989.

96. Murray D, Vandewalker G, Matherne GP, Mahoney LT: Pulsed Doppler and two-dimensional echocardiography: Comparison of halothane and isoflurane on cardiac function in infants and small children. *Anesthesiology* 67:211–217, 1987.

97. Naik SK, Knight A, Elliott MJ: A prospective randomized study of a modified technique of ultrafiltration during pediatric open-heart surgery. *Circulation* 84:III422–431, 1991.

98. Neuhof C, Walter D, Dapper F, et al: Bradykinin and histamine generation with generalized enhancement of microvascular permeability in neonates, infants, and children undergoing cardiopulmonary bypass surgery. *Pediatr Crit Care Med* 4:299–304, 2003.

99. Newburger JW, Jonas RA, Wernovsky G, et al: A comparison of the perioperative neurologic effects of hypothermic circulatory arrest versus low-flow cardiopulmonary bypass in infant heart surgery. *N Engl J Med* 329:1057–1064, 1993.

100. Odegard RC, DiNardo Ja, Tsai-Goodman B, et al: Anaesthesia considerations for cardiac MRI in infants and small children. *Pediatr Anaesth* 14:471–476, 2004.

101. O'Rourke MM, Nork KM, Kurth CD: Altered brain oxygen extraction with hypoxia and hypotension following deep hypothermic circulatory arrest. *Acta Neurochirurg* 70:78–79, 1997.

102. Oshita S, Uchimoto R, Oka H, et al: Correlation between arterial blood pressure and oxygenation in tetralogy of Fallot. *J Cardiovasc Anesth* 3:597–600, 1989.

103. Penkoske PA, Entwistle LM, Marchak BE, et al: Aprotinin in children undergoing repair of congenital heart defects. *Ann Thorac Surg* 60: S529–532, 1995.

104. Peterson KL, DeCampli WM, Pike NA, et al: A report of two hundred twenty cases of regional anesthesia in pediatric cardiac surgery. *Anesth Analg* 90:1014–1019, 2000.

105. Pulsinelli WA, Levy DE, Sigsbee B, et al: Increased damage after ischemic stroke in patients with hyperglycemia with or without established diabetes mellitus. *Am J Med* 74:540–544, 1983.

106. Rappaport LA, Wypij D, Bellinger DC, et al: Relation of seizures after cardiac surgery in early infancy to neurodevelopmental outcome. Boston circulatory Arrest Study Group. *Circulation* 97:773–779, 1998.

107. Rebeyka IM, Coles JG, Wilson GJ, et al: The effect of low-flow cardiopulmonary bypass on cerebral function: An experimental and clinical study. *Ann Thorac Surg* 43:391–396, 1987.

108. Reynolds LM, Nicolson SC, Jobes DR, et al: Desmopressin does not decrease bleeding after cardiac operation in young children. *J Thorac Cardiovasc Surg* 106:954–958, 1993.

109. Reynolds LM, Nicolson SC, Steven JM, et al: Influence of sensor site location on pulse oximetry kinetics in children. *Anesth Analg* 76:751–754, 1993.

110. Rivenes SM, Lewin MB, Stayer SA, et al: Cardiovascular effects of sevoflurane, isoflurane, halothane, and fentanyl-midazolam in children with congenital heart disease: An echocardiographic study of myocardial contractility and hemodynamics. *Anesthesiology* 94:223–229, 2001.

111. Rosen DA, Hawkinberry DW 2nd, Rosen KR: An epidural hematoma in an adolescent patient after cardiac surgery. *Anesth Analg* 98:966–969, 2004.

112. Rossi R, van der Linden J, Ekroth R, et al: No flow or low flow? A study of the ischemic marker creatine kinase BB after deep hypothermic procedures. *J Thorac Cardiovasc Surg* 98:193–199, 1989.

113. Royston D, Taylor KM, Bidstrup BP, Sapsford RN: Effect of aprotinin on need for blood transfusion after repeat open-heart surgery. *Lancet* 2:1289–1291, 1987.

114. Russell IA, Miller Hance WC, Gregory G, et al: The safety and efficacy of sevoflurane anesthesia in infants and children with congenital heart disease. *Anesth Analg* 92:1152–1158, 2001.

115. Salzman EW, Weinstein MJ, Weintraub RM, et al: Treatment with desmopressin acetate to reduce blood loss after cardiac surgery. *N Engl J Med* 314:1402–1406, 1986.

116. Sarner JB, Levine M, Davis PJ, et al: Clinical characteristics of sevoflurane in children. A comparison with halothane. *Anesthesiology* 82:38–46, 1995.

117. Scheller MS, Branson PJ, Cornacchia LG, Alksne JF: A comparison of the effects on neuronal Golgi morphology, assessed with electron microscopy, of cardiopulmonary bypass, low-flow bypass, and circulatory arrest during profound hypothermia. *J Thorac Cardiovasc Surg* 104: 1396–1404, 1992.

118. Schindler E, Muller M, Kwapisz M, et al: Ventricular cardiac-assist devices in infants and children: Anesthetic considerations. *J Cardiothorac Vasc Anesth* 17:617–621, 2003.

119. Schupbach P, Pappova E, Schilt W, et al: Perfusate oncotic pressure during cardiopulmonary bypass: optimum level as determined by metabolic acidosis, tissue edema, and renal function. *Vox Sang* 35:332–344, 1978.

120. Severinghaus JW, Spellman MJ Jr: Pulse oximeter failure thresholds in hypotension and vasoconstriction. *Anesthesiology* 73:532–537, 1990.

121. Skaryak LA, Kirshbom PM, DiBernardo LR, et al: Modified ultrafiltration improves cerebral metabolic recovery after circulatory arrest. *J Thorac Cardiovasc Surg* 109:744–751, 1995.

122. Spach MS, Serwer GA, Anderson PA, et al: Pulsatile aortopulmonary pressure-flow dynamics of patent ductus arteriosus in patients with various hemodynamic states. *Circulation* 61:110–122, 1980.

123. Stayer SA, Andropoulos DB, Russell A: Anesthetic management of the adult patient with congenital heart disease. *Anesthesiol Clin North Am* 21:653–673, 2003.

124. Stern DH, Gerson JI, Allen FB, Parker FB: Can we trust the direct radial artery pressure immediately following cardiopulmonary bypass? *Anesthesiology* 62:557–561, 1985.

125. Steven JM, Nicolson SC: Congenital Heart Disease. In Greeley WJ (ed): Atlas of Anesthesia, Vol. VII: Pediatric Anesthesia. Harcourt Pub Ltd, 1999.

126. Sutton LN, Clark BJ, Norwood CR, et al: Global cerebral ischemia in piglets under conditions of mild and deep hypothermia. *Stroke* 22:1567–1573, 1991.

127. Swain JA, McDonald TJ Jr, Griffith PK, et al: Low flow hypothermic cardiopulmonary bypass protects the brain. *J Thorac Cardiovasc Surg* 102:76–83, 1991.

128. Tanner GE, Angers DG, Barash PG, et al: Effect of left-to-right, mixed left-to-right, and right-to-left shunts on inhalational anesthetic induction in children: A computer model. *Anesth Analg* 64:101–107, 1985.

129. Thornburg KL, Morton MJ: Filling and arterial pressure as determinants of RV stroke volume in the sheep fetus. *Am J Physiol* 244:H656–H663, 1983.

130. Ungerleider RM: Effects of cardiopulmonary bypass and use of modified ultrafiltration. *Ann Thorac Surg.* 65:S35–S98, 1998.

131. Ungerleider RM: Decision making in pediatric cardiac surgery using intraoperative echo. *Int J Card Imaging* 4:33–35, 1989.

132. Ungerleider RM, Greeley WJ, Kanter RJ, Kisslo JA: The learning curve for intraoperative echocardiography during congenital heart surgery. *Ann Thorac Surg* 54:691–696, 1992.

133. Ungerleider RM, Kisslo JA, Greeley WJ, et al: Intraoperative prebypass and postbypass epicardial color flow imaging in the repair of atrioventricular septal defects. *J Thorac Cardiovasc Surg* 98:90–99, 1989.

134. Verghese ST, McGill WA, Patel RI, et al: Ultrasound-guided internal jugular venous cannulation in infants: a prospective comparison with the traditional palpation method. *Anesthesiology* 91:71–77, 1999.

135. Vieira A, Berry L, Ofoso F, Andrew M: Heparin sensitivity and resistance in the neonate: an explanation. *Thromb Res* 63:85–98, 1991.

136. Wang MJ, Chiu IS, Hsu CM, et al: Efficacy of ultrafiltration in removing inflammatory mediators during pediatric cardiac operations. *Ann Thorac Surg* 61:651–656, 1996.

137. Wernovsky G, Wypij D, Jonas RA, et al: Postoperative course and hemodynamic profile after the arterial switch operation in neonates and infants: A comparison of low-flow cardiopulmonary bypass versus circulatory arrest. *Circulation* 92:2226–2235, 1995.

138. Wessel, D: Managing low cardiac output syndrome after congenital heart surgery. *Crit Care Med* 29:S220–S230, 2001.

139. Woodey E, Pladys P, Copin C: Comparative hemodynamic depression of sevoflurane versus halothane in infants: an echocardiographic study. *Anesthesiology* 87:795–800, 1997.

140. Woodman RC, Harker LA: Bleeding complications associated with cardiopulmonary bypass. *Blood* 76:1680–1697, 1990.

141. Zales VR, Wright KL, Pahl E, et al: Normal left ventricular muscle mass and mass/volume ratio after pediatric cardiac transplantation. *Circulation* 90:II61–65, 1994.

Chapter 11

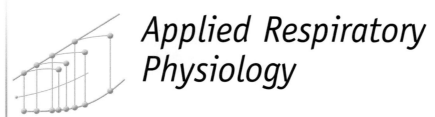

Applied Respiratory Physiology

LYNN D. MARTIN, MD, JON N. MELIONES, MD, MS, and
RANDALL C. WETZEL, MBBS, MBA

INTRODUCTION

It is not uncommon for clinicians who care for children with heart disease to underestimate the effect alterations in respiratory physiology have on cardiovascular performance. As a result of their intimate relationship within the thorax, the cardiovascular and respiratory systems cannot be thought of independently and should be considered to function as a single unit, the cardiorespiratory system. Cardiorespiratory interactions occur because the pulmonary and systemic circulations are in series and because the lungs and chest wall physically surround the heart and great vessels exposing them to intrathoracic pressure. Cardiorespiratory interactions cause significant changes in both cardiac and pulmonary function, including alterations of pulmonary blood flow and respiratory mechanics. For a variety of reasons, the effects of cardiorespiratory interactions are exaggerated in infants and children with heart disease. Therefore, providing effective respiratory support for children with critical heart disease requires an understanding of not only the physiology of the respiratory system under normal and pathologic conditions, but also the cardiorespiratory consequences of these processes. Providing respiratory support for infants and children with heart disease also requires a knowledge of the changes in respiratory physiology that occur in response to growth and how the presence of congenital cardiac disease alters respiratory mechanics.

This chapter will discuss the basic principles of respiratory physiology and pathophysiology and provide the foundation for determining respiratory support for infants and children with heart disease. The initial sections will focus on the respiratory physiology that is critical to pulmonary gas exchange and include: (1) the distribution of pulmonary blood flow, (2) the distribution of ventilation as a function of respiratory compliance, resistance, and time, (3) resting lung volume or functional residual capacity (FRC), and (4) the matching of ventilation and perfusion. In the final sections, respiratory pathophysiology and the alterations in respiratory physiology secondary to congenital cardiac disease will be discussed.

DISTRIBUTION OF PULMONARY BLOOD FLOW

The pulmonary vasculature can be modeled as having two components: (1) a fixed component that is the primary determinant of regional perfusion and (2) a variable component that acts on top of the fixed structure and is affected by local factors. The fixed structures can best be characterized using fractal geometry, a new mathematical science used to describe "natural objects."[26] The variable component of the vasculature can be influenced by passive and active regional factors such as recruitment and/or distention due to changing hydrostatic or driving pressures. Active factors such as vasomotion in response to shear stress or hypoxic vasoconstriction will influence regional perfusion. The relative contribution of both the fixed and variable components of the pulmonary circulation to pulmonary perfusion heterogeneity can be quantified. An in-depth discussion of these multiple influences regulating regional and global pulmonary perfusion can be found in Chapter 3.

Passive Pulmonary Blood Flow

Passive alterations in pulmonary vascular resistance and blood flow are the primary determinants of the distribution of pulmonary blood flow. In the majority of critically ill patients, the primary emphasis in critical care is placed on altering active pulmonary blood flow without a clear appreciation of the importance of passive pulmonary blood flow. Active pulmonary blood flow, however, cannot be fully appreciated without a sound understanding of the passive relationship that occurs between pulmonary artery pressure, alveolar pressure, and cardiac output.

For the past three decades, the pulmonary circulation has been generally regarded as a largely passive circuit in which blood flow distribution is predominantly determined by hydrostatic gradients. However, recent studies using high-resolution methods and experiments in microgravity and macrogravity environments have revealed an unexpected degree of perfusion heterogeneity. A classic description of pulmonary perfusion distribution based on gravity-dependent hydrostatic gradients will be followed by a brief discussion of the more recent work demonstrating greater degrees of heterogeneity of blood flow.

Gravity-Dependent Determinants of Blood Flow

For many years, it has been held that the primary determinant of the distribution of pulmonary blood flow is gravity. The right ventricle imparts kinetic energy to blood during systole and ejects a stroke volume into the pulmonary artery. The kinetic energy is dissipated in the lungs as blood in the pulmonary artery climbs a vertical column in the gravity-dependent lung. The pulmonary artery pressure, therefore, decreases by 1 cm H_2O per centimeter vertical distance up the lung (Fig. 11-1). The distribution of pulmonary blood flow to different lung segments is dependent upon the differences between three pressures in the lung: (1) intraalveolar pulmonary artery pressure (P_{pa}) or pulmonary capillary pressure, (2) alveolar pressure (P_A), and (3) venous pressure (P_{pv}). At some height above the heart, the absolute pressure in the pulmonary artery (P_{pa}) becomes less than zero (atmospheric).[75] At that point, P_A exceeds P_{pa} and P_{pv}. In this region, the pulmonary vessels are collapsed, due to the higher P_A, and blood flow ceases (West zone 1, $P_A > P_{pa} > P_{pv}$). Lung that undergoes ventilation but no perfusion does not contribute to gas exchange and is referred to as physiologic "dead space." Normally, very few of the lung units function as zone 1. Any factor that alters the P_{pa}/P_A relationship supporting the collapse of pulmonary vessels (i.e., $P_A > P_{pa}$ or $P_{pa}/P_A < 1$) will result in an increase in zone 1 lung. These conditions include an increase in P_A (application of positive pressure to the airways), or a reduction of P_{pa} (decreased cardiac output, shock, pulmonary emboli).

In regions of the lung where P_{pa} exceeds P_A and $P_A > P_{pv}$, perfusion occurs (West zone 2, $P_{pa} > P_A > P_{pv}$). Pulmonary arterial flow to this region is determined by the mean pulmonary artery versus alveolar pressure difference ($P_{pa} - P_A$).[62] Blood flow is independent of the venous (P_{pv}) or left atrial pressure. Since mean P_{pa} increases down the lung while mean P_A remains constant, the mean driving pressure ($P_{pa} - P_A$) increases and blood flow in the lower portions of the lung increases. In inferior segments of the lung, P_{pv} exceeds P_A and blood flow is governed by the pulmonary arteriovenous pressure difference ($P_{pa} - P_{pv}$) (West zone 3, $P_{pa} > P_{pv} > P_A$). The effects of gravity are equal on pulmonary artery and pulmonary venous pressure and both P_{pa} and P_{pv} increase at the same rate; thus the capillaries are permanently open and the perfusion pressure ($P_{pa} - P_{pv}$) is constant. However, since the increase in pleural pressure (P_{pl}) is less than the increase in P_{pa} and P_{pv}, the transmural distending pressure ($P_{pa} - P_{pl}$ and $P_{pv} - P_{pl}$) increases down zone 3. Therefore, the resistance is decreased, and for a given driving pressure, flow increases. Thus, flow increases at lower lung levels in zone 3. It must be realized that ventilation and pulmonary blood flow are constantly changing forces and any given portion of the lung may actually move in and out of zone 2 conditions and become either zone 1 or zone 3, depending upon whether the patient is in cardiac systole or diastole, inspiration or expiration, or spontaneous or positive pressure ventilation.

When pulmonary vascular pressures are extremely high, fluid transudate forms in the interstitial space. When fluid flow into the interstitial space exceeds the lymphatic clearance rate, fluid accumulates. This eliminates the normally present negative tension on the extraalveolar vessels. Pulmonary interstitial pressure (P_{isf}) eventually becomes positive and exceeds P_{pv} (West zone 4, $P_{pa} > P_{isf} > P_{pv} > P_A$).[62] In zone 4, pulmonary blood flow is regulated by the arteriointerstitial pressure difference ($P_{pa} - P_{isf}$). The arteriointerstitial pressure difference in zone 4 is less than the zone 3 difference ($P_{pa} - P_{pv}$); therefore, zone 4 blood flow is less than zone 3 blood flow.

Alterations of P_{pa} and P_{pv} not only cause changes in regional blood flow but also affect the microcirculation. Three gradual changes take place in the pulmonary circulation when P_{pa} and P_{pv} increase: (1) recruitment or opening of previously nonperfused vessels, (2) distention or widening of previously perfused vessels (increased cross-sectional area, less resistance), and (3) transudation of fluid at the capillary level.[52] Recruitment occurs when P_{pa} and P_{pv} are increased from low to moderate levels, distension occurs when P_{pa} and P_{pv} are increased from

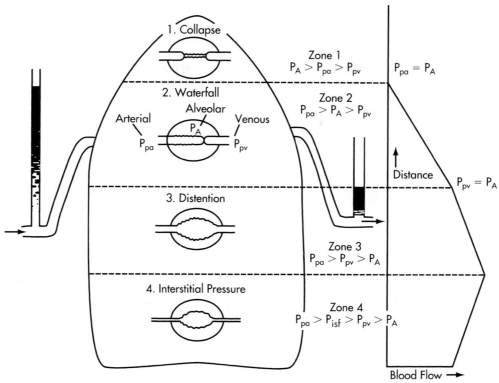

FIGURE 11-1   The four zones of the lung. Schematic diagram showing distribution of blood flow in the upright lung. In zone 1, alveolar pressure (P_A) exceeds pulmonary artery pressure (P_{pa}) and no flow occurs because the intraalveolar vessels are collapsed by the compressing alveolar pressure. In zone 2, arterial pressure exceeds alveolar pressure, but alveolar pressure exceeds venous pressure (P_{pv}). Flow in zone 2 is determined by the arterial-alveolar pressure difference ($P_{pa} - P_A$) and has been likened to an upstream river waterfall over a dam. Since P_{pa} increases down zone 2 and P_A remains constant, the perfusion pressure increases and flow steadily increases down the zone. In zone 3, pulmonary venous pressure exceeds alveolar pressure, and flow is determined by the arterial-venous pressure difference ($P_{pa} - P_{pv}$), which is constant down this portion of the lung. However, the transmural pressure across the wall of the vessel increases down this zone, so that the caliber of the vessels increases (resistance decreases), and therefore, flow increases. Finally, in zone 4, pulmonary interstitial pressure becomes positive and exceeds both pulmonary venous pressure and alveolar pressure. Consequently, flow in zone 4 is determined by the arterial-interstitial pressure difference ($P_{pa} - P_{isf}$). (From Benumof JL: Respiratory physiology and respiratory function during anesthesia. In Miller RD (ed): *Anesthesia*. New York: Churchill Livingstone, 1990; and West JB, Dollery CT, Heard BE: Increased pulmonary vascular resistance in the dependent zone of the isolated dog lung caused by perivascular edema. *Circ Res* 17:191, 1965.)

moderate to high levels, and finally, transudation occurs when P_{pa} and P_{pv} are increased from high to very high levels.

Gravity-Independent Determinants of Blood Flow

The first study to demonstrate that the geometry of the vascular bed is an important determinant of pulmonary blood flow distribution was made by Reed and Wood.[66] New techniques providing high-resolution measurements of pulmonary perfusion have confirmed a large degree of spatial heterogeneity, likely based on the architecture of the vasculature. Neighboring regions of lung have similar magnitudes of flow (i.e., high-flow regions are adjacent to other high-flow regions, while low-flow regions are adjacent to other low-flow regions).[25] This relationship can be quantified using correlation coefficients between flows to pairs of lung regions. The spatial correlation [$\rho(d)$] is the correlation between blood flow to one region at one position and blood flow to a second region displaced by distance d. The correlation can range from 1 (perfect positive correlation) to −1 (perfect negative correlation) with 0 indicating random association between pairs. When the spatial correlation of perfusion is determined for regional pulmonary perfusion, a positive correlation is found for neighboring regions. This spatial correlation is best modeled using fractal methods.[31] When extended to three dimensions, this fractal model is able to explain the high local correlations in blood flow and the decreasing correlation as distance increases.[32] Pulmonary perfusion has also been shown to have temporal variability.[29]

Recent studies utilizing these high-resolution methods[28,30,42] as well as experiments performed in both microgravity[65] and macrogravity[37] settings have demonstrated that pulmonary perfusion is far more heterogeneous than can be explained by gravity alone. Although multiple studies in different species have confirmed gravity-independent perfusion heterogeneity, these observations have not been made in man. Some investigators suggest that gravity is not an important determinant of pulmonary blood flow distribution in quadrupeds (a characteristic common to all species in these studies) because their posture produces smaller lung volumes.[41] Quadrupeds also have a more muscularized vascular system with a smaller proportion of their vascular resistance in the microvascular segments. In an attempt to overcome these potential problems, high-resolution methods were recently used in baboons (a species with pulmonary structures and physiology remarkably similar to man).[27] With the use of multiple-stepwise regression, gravity-dependent perfusion heterogeneity was estimated at 7%, 5%, and 25% in the supine, prone, and upright positions, respectively. Therefore, these recent high-resolution experiments continue to suggest that gravity is an important, but not predominant, determinant of pulmonary perfusion heterogeneity.

Pulmonary vascular resistance and blood flow are dependent on a variety of physiologic conditions including lung volume. The lung volume at the end of an expiration in normal lungs, when the pressure differential between the atmosphere and alveoli is zero, defines the functional residual capacity (FRC). Total pulmonary vascular resistance is increased when lung volume is either increased above or decreased below FRC (Fig. 11-2).[12,69,78] The increase in total pulmonary vascular resistance at lung volumes above FRC is due to a large increase in vascular resistance contributed by the small intraalveolar vessels, which are extended and compressed by the expanded alveolus and surrounding lung.[4] The increase in total pulmonary vascular resistance at lung volumes below FRC is due to hypoxic pulmonary vasoconstriction that occurs in collapsed alveoli and the tortuous course of the large extraalveolar vessels at low lung volumes.[3]

Functional residual capacity can be understood as the lung volume at which pulmonary vascular resistance is minimized. It is worth noting that lung compliance and resistance are also optimized at FRC, with compliance being the highest at FRC

and resistance being the lowest. Thus, in normal lungs, end-expiratory lung volume (EELV) is the same as FRC (EELV in normal lungs), and the work of ventilation and perfusion is minimized.

The relationship between lung volume and FRC is obviously variable. Tidal ventilation occurs from EELV (FRC in normal lungs), and thus pulmonary vascular resistance (PVR), airway resistance, and lung compliance cycle dynamically with ventilation. In disease states, EELV can be increased above FRC (obstructive disease) or decreased below FRC (restrictive disease). This pathologic EELV (EELV not equal to FRC) will alter PVR, compliance, and resistance.

Active Pulmonary Blood Flow

Total PVR expresses the relationship between flow and driving pressure (Ohm's law). In the pulmonary circulation the vessels are not rigid tubes, but expand as flow increases. Therefore, pulmonary vascular resistance is flow dependent and decreases as flow increases.[22] In addition, previously nonperfused vessels are recruited (opened) as cardiac output increases. Because of these physiologic principles, pulmonary vascular resistance is not precisely measured in the pulmonary circulation and the relationship between flow and pressure must be carefully assessed. Two situations, however, can occur in which pulmonary vascular resistance changes can be accurately measured. One condition is active pulmonary vasoconstriction that occurs when cardiac output is decreased and P_{pa} remains constant or is increased. Another is active pulmonary vasodilation, which can occur when cardiac output increases and P_{pa} remains constant or decreases.

A variety of physiologic or pharmacologic stimuli may cause alterations of the pulmonary circulation. One of the most frequently encountered is alveolar hypoxia. Alveolar hypoxia of a whole lung, lobe, or lobule of lung causes localized pulmonary vasoconstriction (see Chapter 3), referred to as a hypoxic pulmonary vasoconstriction (HPV). HPV is present in all mammalian species.[71] The mechanisms by which alveolar hypoxia cause pulmonary vasoconstriction remain unclear, although two theories have been proposed.[21,73] First, alveolar hypoxia may change the balance between vasoconstrictor substance(s) and vasodilator substance(s) elaborated from multiple potential sources (endothelium, smooth muscle, etc.), with the net result of vasoconstriction. Recent evidence suggests that HPV may in part be a result of a reduction of endothelium-derived nitric oxide. Second, hypoxia may stimulate the metabolic activity of pulmonary vascular smooth muscle, partially depolarizing the cell membrane, influencing excitation coupling, and causing ion fluxes that cause vasoconstriction. Thus, HPV appears to be due to hypoxia-induced modulation of vasoactive substances and/or a direct action on the pulmonary vascular smooth muscle. HPV may involve the entire lung or be limited to localized regions of the lung, depending on whether there is global or regional alveolar hypoxia.[49] Regional alveolar hypoxia causes locally increased vascular resistance and shunts blood toward normoxic lung with lower vascular resistance, thereby improving ventilation/perfusion matching. Global alveolar hypoxia results in an elevated mean P_{pa} and an increased workload for the right ventricle. Regional HPV is, therefore, a protective mechanism designed to optimize ventilation/perfusion matching,

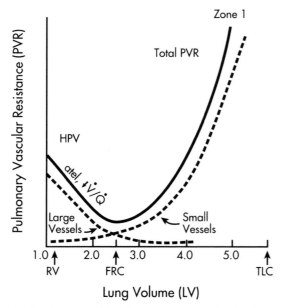

FIGURE 11-2   An asymmetrical U-shaped curve relates total pulmonary vascular resistance (PVR) to lung volume. The trough of the curve occurs when lung volume equals functional residual capacity (FRC). Total pulmonary resistance is the sum of resistance in small vessels (increased by increasing lung volume) and the resistance in large vessels (increased by decreasing lung volume). The endpoint for increasing lung volume (toward total lung capacity [TLC]) is the creation of zone 1 conditions, and the endpoint for decreasing lung volume (toward residual volume [RV]) is the creation of low $\dot{V}_A/\dot{Q}$ and atelectatic (atel) areas that have hypoxic pulmonary vasoconstriction (HPV). (From Benumof JL: Respiratory physiology and respiratory function during anesthesia. In Miller RD (ed): *Anesthesia*. New York: Churchill Livingstone, 1990.)

while global HPV is a maladaptive response and can lead to right ventricular dysfunction and failure.

DISTRIBUTION OF VENTILATION

Gravity-Dependent Determinants of Ventilation

The lung is a viscoelastic structure that is located inside and is supported by the chest wall. Gravity causes the lung to assume a globular shape with a relatively more negative pressure at the top and a more positive pressure at the base of the lung. The magnitude of the pleural pressure (P_{pl}) gradient depends on the density of the lung. Pleural pressure normally increases 7.5 cm H_2O from the top to the bottom of the adult lung.[39]

In normal lungs, P_A is equal throughout the lung and the P_{pl} gradient results in regional differences in transpulmonary pressure ($P_A - P_{pl}$). Where P_{pl} is most positive (i.e., least negative), the transmural pressure differences result in the alveoli being compressed and smaller than the apical alveoli.[53] Thus, small basal alveoli are on the mid-portion and the large apical alveoli are on the upper portion of a normal pressure-volume curve of the lung (Fig. 11-3). Dependent alveoli are relatively more compliant (have a greater volume change for a given change in pressure, i.e., steep slope), while nondependent alveoli are relatively less compliant (flat slope). Therefore, the majority of the tidal volume during normal ventilation is preferentially distributed to dependent alveoli, since these alveoli expand more per unit pressure change than do nondependent alveoli.

Gravity-Independent Determinants of Ventilation

Compliance

The relationship between the change in volume (ΔV) and change in distending pressure (ΔP) defines compliance. The elastic properties of the respiratory system and its components, the lungs and chest wall, are graphically defined by their respective volume-pressure relationships (Fig. 11-4). The total respiratory system compliance is determined by the compliance of the lungs and chest wall.[57] Lung compliance is determined by ΔV and the *transpulmonary* pressure gradient ($P_A - P_{pl}$, the ΔP for the lung). Chest wall compliance depends on ΔV and the *transmural* pressure gradient ($P_{pl} - P_{ambient}$, the ΔP for the chest wall). To determine the total respiratory compliance, ΔV and the *transthoracic* pressure gradient ($P_A - P_{ambient}$, the ΔP for the lung and chest wall together) must be known.

During certain modes of positive or negative pressure lung inflation, the transthoracic pressure gradient first increases to a peak value and then decreases to a lower plateau value. The peak transthoracic pressure is the pressure required to overcome both elastic and airway resistance (see following). The transthoracic pressure decreases to a plateau value because gas redistributes over time to alveoli with longer time constants. As the gas redistributes into an increased number

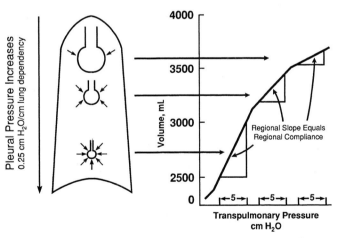

FIGURE 11-3 Pleural pressure increases 0.25 cm H_2O per centimeter down the lung. The increase in pleural pressure causes a fourfold decrease in alveolar volume. The caliber of the air passages also decreases as lung volume decreases. When regional alveolar volume is translated over to a regional transpulmonary pressure–alveolar volume curve, small alveoli are on a steep (*large slope*) portion of the curve, and large alveoli are on a flat (*small slope*) portion of the curve. Because the regional slope equals regional compliance, the dependent small alveoli normally receive the largest share of the tidal volume. Over the normal tidal volume range (lung volume increases by 500 mL from 2500 mL (normal functional residual capacity) to 3000 mL, the pressure-volume relationship is linear. Lung volume values in this diagram relate to the upright position. (From Benumof JL: Respiratory physiology and respiratory function during anesthesia. In Miller RD (ed): *Anesthesia*. New York: Churchill Livingstone, 1990.)

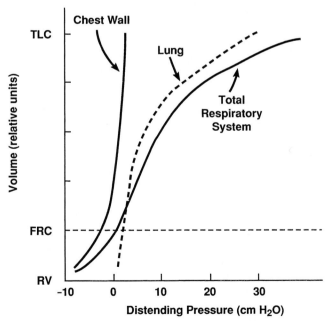

FIGURE 11-4 Pressure-volume relationships (i.e., compliance curves) of the chest wall, lung, and total respiratory system in the normal infant. At FRC, the distending pressures of the lung and chest wall are equal and opposite, resulting in the exertion of zero net distending pressure on the total respiratory system. At lung volumes in excess of FRC, the chest wall of the infant displays very high compliance characteristics relative to the adult counterpart. In addition, total respiratory system pressure-volume relationships display sigmoid characteristics, with compliance decreasing at either extreme of lung volume. RV, residual volume; FRC, functional residual capacity; TLC, total lung capacity. (Modified from Kendig EL, Chernick V: *Disorders of the Respiratory Tract in Children*. Philadelphia: WB Saunders, 1977, p 17.)

of alveoli, less pressure is generated by the same volume of gas, and the pressure decreases. Therefore, two measures of compliance can be made, dynamic and static. During positive pressure ventilation, *dynamic compliance* can be estimated by calculating the volume change (tidal volume) divided by the *peak* inspiratory pressure minus the end-expiratory pressure (PEEP). *Static compliance* can be approximated by measuring the change in volume divided by the *plateau* inspiratory pressure minus the end-expiratory pressure. Plateau pressure falls below peak inspiratory pressure because of gas redistribution; therefore, static compliance is greater than dynamic compliance. Static compliance is a better evaluation of the entire respiratory system, since the measurement reflects more of the gas exchanging alveoli.

The compliance relationship of the chest wall and lung units is sigmoidal. At the extremes of lung volumes, compliance decreases and a larger increase in peak inspiratory pressure is required to obtain similar changes in volume. Underinflation (atelectasis, hypoventilation, EELV < FRC) and over-expansion (asthma, excessive positive end expiratory pressure, EELV > FRC) should thus be avoided, since they require greater peak pressures to change lung volume.

The pressure-volume relationship of the alveolus is influenced by other factors, including alveolar geometry. The amount by which the pressure inside an alveolus (P, in dyn/cm^2) is above ambient pressure depends on the surface tension (*T*, in dyn/cm) and the radius of curvature of the alveolus (*R*, in cm) as expressed in the Laplace equation:

$$P = 2T/R$$

Using this relationship, the pressure inside small alveoli would be higher than inside large alveoli. Since small alveoli would have greater pressure than large ones, small alveoli would empty into larger ones, until theoretically, one gigantic alveolus would be left (Fig. 11-5A). This phenomenon does not occur in the lung because of the alterations in alveolar surface tension. The surface tension of the fluid lining the alveoli is variable and decreases as the surface area of the alveoli is reduced.[9] When alveolar size decreases, the surface tension of the lining fluid falls to a greater extent than the corresponding reduction of radius, so that the transmural pressure gradient (=2T/R) actually diminishes, not increases. Therefore, small alveoli do not discharge their contents into large alveoli (Fig. 11-5B) and the elastic recoil of the small alveoli is less than that of the large alveoli. Surfactant produced by type II alveolar pneumocytes is responsible for these unique surface tension characteristics and allows more uniform ventilation throughout the entire lung.

Alterations in chest wall and lung compliance are important conditions that require continuous evaluation in critically ill children. Although both an increase and a decrease in compliance can result in a change in lung volume, a reduction in compliance requires prompt identification and intervention. A decrease in intrinsic compliance of the lungs and/or chest wall will result in decreased total compliance and a reduction of lung volume for a given alveolar pressure and a decrease in FRC. In many clinical instances, this may necessitate the application of additional distending pressure (P_A) in the form of positive pressure ventilation and/or continuous positive airway pressures (CPAP/PEEP) to reestablish normal lung volumes.

Resistance

For gas flow to occur, a pressure gradient must be generated to overcome the nonelastic airway resistance of the lungs. Mathematically, resistance (*R*) is defined by the pressure gradient (ΔP) required to generate a given flow of gas ($\dot{V}$). Physically, resistance results from the friction during movement of gas molecules within the airways (airway resistance)

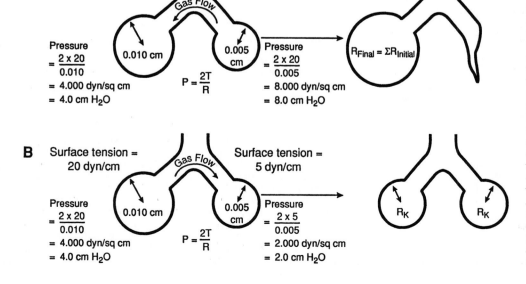

A   Surface tension (*T*) in both alveoli = 20 dyn/cm

Pressure
$= \dfrac{2 \times 20}{0.010}$
= 4.000 dyn/sq cm
= 4.0 cm H_2O

0.010 cm   0.005 cm

$P = \dfrac{2T}{R}$

Pressure
$= \dfrac{2 \times 20}{0.005}$
= 8.000 dyn/sq cm
= 8.0 cm H_2O

$R_{Final} = \Sigma R_{Initial}$

B   Surface tension = 20 dyn/cm

Surface tension = 5 dyn/cm

Pressure
$= \dfrac{2 \times 20}{0.010}$
= 4.000 dyn/sq cm
= 4.0 cm H_2O

0.010 cm   0.005 cm

$P = \dfrac{2T}{R}$

Pressure
$= \dfrac{2 \times 5}{0.005}$
= 2.000 dyn/sq cm
= 2.0 cm H_2O

R_K R_K

FIGURE 11-5 Relationship between surface tension (*T*), alveolar radius (*R*), and alveolar transmural pressure (*P*). A, Pressure relationship in two alveoli of different size but with the same surface tension in their lining fluids. The direction of gas flow will be from the higher pressure small alveolus to the lower pressure large alveolus. The net result is one large alveolus ($R_{Final} = \Sigma R_{Initial}$). B, Pressure relationship of two alveoli of different size when allowance is made for the expected changes in surface tension (less tension in smaller alveolus). The direction of gas flow is from the larger alveolus to the smaller alveolus until the two alveoli are of equal size and are volume stable (R_K). ΣR, sum of all individual radii; K, constant. (From Benumof JL: Respiratory physiology and respiratory function during anesthesia. In Miller RD (ed): *Anesthesia*. New York: Churchill Livingstone, 1990.)

as well as friction from motion of the lung and chest wall (tissue viscous resistance). These components make up the total nonelastic resistance of the respiratory system. Normally, airway resistance accounts for approximately 75% of total nonelastic resistance.[15] However, in conditions where respiratory pathophysiology alters tissue viscous resistance, airway resistance may be altered.

The pressure gradient (ΔP) along the airway is dependent upon the caliber of the airway and the rate and pattern of airflow. During laminar flow, the pressure drop down the airway is proportional to the flow. When flow exceeds a critical velocity, it becomes turbulent and the pressure drop down the tube becomes proportional to the square of the flow.[70] As flow becomes more turbulent, pressure increases more than flow, and resistance increases. Increased airway resistance requires a larger pressure gradient between the airway opening and the alveoli to maintain flow. During positive pressure ventilation, this requires the generation of higher inspiratory pressures to achieve similar ventilation, whereas during spontaneous breathing, a more negative intrapleural and alveolar pressure must be achieved to maintain similar ventilation. In both cases, the work required to produce adequate gas flow is increased.

Resistance of the airways is approximated by the diameter of the airway, the velocity of airflow, and the properties of inhaled gases. Resistance is determined by Poiseuille's law, which governs the laminar flow of gas in nonbranching tubes:

$$P = \dot{V}(8L\acute{\eta}/\pi r^4)$$

where P = pressure, $\dot{V}$ = flow, L = length, r = radius of the tube, and $\acute{\eta}$ is the viscosity of the gas.[10,24] Airway resistance is inversely proportional to the radius of the conducting airways raised to the fourth power during laminar flow and to the fifth power during turbulent flow.

Total airway resistance is determined by a number of factors including the cross-sectional area of the airway. The upper airway contributes nearly 50% of total airway resistance in infants and adults, and conditions that compromise the lumen of the upper airway can lead to an increase in total airway resistance.[38] In adults, this can be overcome by endotracheal intubation with a large endotracheal tube. In smaller patients who require high minute ventilation, airway resistance may actually increase after endotracheal intubation.[45] In the adult and adolescents, the peripheral airways have a large total cross-sectional area, and only 20% of total airway resistance is determined by airways < 2 mm.[63] Therefore, in adults, small airway disease may be considerable with little change in total airway resistance. In infants and children, however, small airways account for approximately 50% of total airway resistance, and diseases that alter small airways can lead to dramatic alterations in resistance and significant obstruction to gas flow (e.g., bronchiolitis).[16]

Airway resistance is also dependent on alterations in lung volume. When lung volume is increased above FRC, airway resistance increases by only a small amount.[1,15] In contrast, when lung volume is decreased below FRC, airway resistance increases dramatically. Airway resistance is also dependent on conducting airway patency. Intrathoracic conducting airways have a tendency to narrow on exhalation and open on inspiration. The result is an increase in airway resistance during exhalation. In conditions where total cross-sectional area is reduced and airway resistance increased, small airways collapse, and flow limitations occur during expiration. In these conditions, expiratory time must be lengthened to avoid gas trapping, alveolar over-distention, and dead space ventilation. In a pediatric swine model of acute respiratory distress syndrome, increasing tidal volumes, increasing PEEP levels, and the development of pulmonary overdistention all demonstrated detrimental effects on the cardiovascular system by increasing pulmonary vascular resistance and characteristic impedance while significantly decreasing cardiac output.[14]

Time Constants

The interaction between compliance and resistance largely determines the distribution of ventilation within the lungs. This relationship is defined as the product of the resistance (R) and compliance (C), which is the time constant (τ), measured in seconds:

$$\tau = R\left(\frac{cm\,H_2O}{L/sec}\right) \times C\left(\frac{L}{cm\,H_2O}\right)$$

The time constant defines the time required for each compartment to achieve a change in volume following the application or withdrawal of a constant distending pressure. It also describes the time required for the pressure within alveoli to equilibrate. As an example, a constant distending pressure applied to the airway overcomes airway resistance and expands the lung (elastic forces). The component of the distending pressure overcoming resistance to airflow is maximal initially and declines exponentially as airflow decreases. The component overcoming elastic forces increases proportional to the change in lung volume. Thus, the pressure required to overcome compliance is initially minimal, then increases exponentially with increasing lung volume. Lung volume approaches equilibrium according to an exponential function with the time course of change in these exponential curves being described by their time constant. Mathematically, 63% of lung inflation (or deflation) occurs in one time constant (Fig. 11-6).

Most causes of respiratory failure have widespread abnormalities in pulmonary resistance and compliance, resulting in striking inhomogeneity in regional time constants. Consequently, with normal tidal breathing, certain compartments fill and empty rapidly (short time constants) while others fill and empty slowly (long time constants). This inhomogeneity of time constants results in marked irregularities in the distribution of ventilation with abnormal gas exchange.[61,68] Under these conditions, successful positive pressure ventilation may require manipulation of inspiratory and expiratory time to allow more uniform distribution ("homogeneity") of ventilation among lung compartments. This strategy, described in Chapter 12, frequently improves ventilation/perfusion matching.

Work of Breathing

Work of breathing is defined as the energy necessary to perform tidal ventilation over a set unit of time. The work of breathing

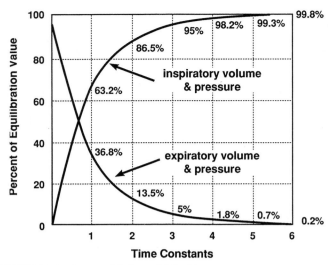

FIGURE 11-6 Exponential rise and fall of lung pressure and lung volume during inspiration and expiration expressed in terms of time constants. (From Chatburn RL: Principles and practice of neonatal and pediatric mechanical ventilation. *Respir Care* 36:569, 1991.)

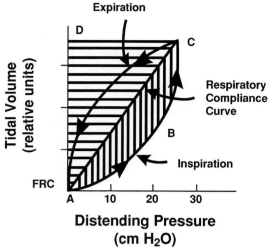

FIGURE 11-7 Inspiratory/expiratory pressure-volume loop recorded during respiratory cycle. The normal respiratory cycle entails the expenditure of work during inspiration to overcome resistive and elastic impedance to allow inflation of the lungs. Total work of breathing (pressure × volume) is defined by the sum of resistive work (area defined by ABC) plus elastic work (area defined by ACD). Total work of breathing (area defined by ABCD) is increased either by an increase in resistive properties of the respiratory system or by a decrease in respiratory compliance (*slope of line* between A and C). (From Goldsmith JP, Karotkin EH: *Assisted Ventilation of the Neonate*. Philadelphia: WB Saunders, 1981, p 29.)

is determined by the pressure-volume characteristics (compliance and resistance) of the respiratory system (Fig. 11-7). During breathing, work must be done to overcome the tendency of the lungs to collapse and chest wall to spring out (Fig. 11-7, area ADC), and the frictional resistance to gas flow that occurs in the airways (Fig. 11-7, area ABC). Work of breathing (Fig. 11-7, area ABCD) is increased by conditions that increase resistance or decrease compliance, or when respiratory frequency increases.

If minute volume is constant, the "compliance" work is increased when tidal ventilation is large and respiratory rate slow. The "resistance" work is increased when the respiratory rate is rapid and tidal ventilation decreased. When the

two components are summated and the total work plotted against the respiratory frequency, an optimal respiratory frequency that minimizes the total work of breathing can be obtained (Fig. 11-8). In children with restrictive lung disease (EELV < FRC, low compliance) and short time constants, the optimal respiratory frequency is increased, while children with obstructive lung diseases (EELV > FRC, high resistance) with long time constants have a lower optimal respiratory frequency.

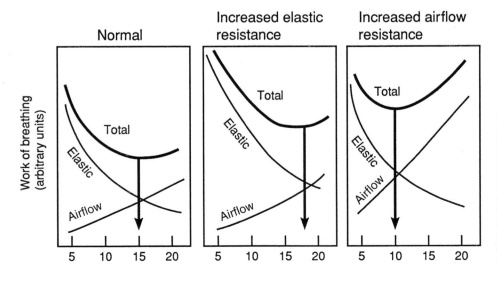

FIGURE 11-8 Diagrams show the work done against elastic and airflow resistance separately and summated to indicate the total work of breathing at different respiratory frequencies in adults. The total work of breathing has a minimum value at about 15 breaths/min under normal circumstances. For the same minute volume, minimum work is performed at higher frequencies with stiff (less compliant) lungs and at lower frequencies when the airflow resistance is increased. (From Nunn JF: *Applied Respiratory Physiology*. Boston: Butterworth, 1987, p 109.)

Lung Volumes and Airway Closure

Functional residual capacity is defined as the volume of gas remaining in the normal lungs at the end of an expiration, when $P_A = P_{ambient}$. FRC depends on the balance of the lungs' intrinsic elastic properties that favor reduction in volume and the natural tendency of the chest wall to recoil outward. Changes in the elastic properties of either of these components of the respiratory system alter FRC.

Total lung capacity (TLC) is the entire gas volume of the maximally spontaneously inflated pulmonary parenchyma and airways in the thorax. It provides the reference point for all other lung volumes and capacities (Fig. 11-9). Vital capacity defines the volume obtained by maximal expiration from TLC and is the maximum volume possible during spontaneous ventilation. As such, it provides a measure of ventilatory reserve.

A critical relationship occurs between the volume of gas remaining in the normal lungs at the end of expiration (FRC) and the volume of gas in the lung at which point conducting airways collapse, which is called the closing capacity (CC). Using the inert gas washout technique during maximal inspiratory and expiratory maneuvers, the point at which conducting airways in dependent lung regions begin to collapse can be identified and is referred to as CC.[11] If EELV falls below CC, or CC is elevated above EELV, these areas of lung collapse and do not participate in gas exchange. Diseases or conditions that either decrease EELV below CC or increase CC above EELV will result in maldistribution of ventilation and adversely affect ventilation perfusion matching.[64] In older children and adults, FRC is well above closing capacity. In contrast, during spontaneous ventilation in young infants, closing capacity exceeds FRC and regions of the lung are collapsed, resulting in ventilation/perfusion mismatch.[48] This observation explains, in part, the relative frequency with which young children with respiratory disease progress to acute respiratory failure.[56] Respiratory interventions play a crucial role in reestablishing the relationship between EELV and CC. In situations characterized by EELV < FRC (pulmonary edema, acute or infantile respiratory distress syndrome, and pneumonitis), CPAP or PEEP can be used to increase EELV toward (normal) FRC. In conditions with increased CC (bronchiolitis, asthma), bronchodilators and control of pulmonary secretions assist in reversing obstruction and decreasing EELV toward FRC.

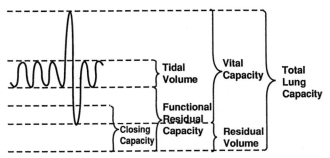

FIGURE 11-9 Functional components of lung volume. (From Scarpelli EM: *Pulmonary Physiology of the Fetus, Newborn, and Child*. Philadelphia: Lea & Febiger, 1975, p 27.)

Ventilation/Perfusion Matching

Matching of lung ventilation (V) and perfusion (Q) at the alveolar level is necessary for optimal gas exchange to occur. The ratio of ventilation to perfusion (V/Q) expresses the amount of ventilation relative to perfusion in any given lung region. Both pulmonary blood flow and ventilation increase with distance down the normal upright lung in a gravity-dependent manner (as discussed previously). Since blood flow increases more rapidly and from a much lower value than ventilation, V/Q decreases exponentially.

Ventilation/perfusion mismatch alters both arterial oxygen (PaO_2) and carbon dioxide ($PaCO_2$) tensions. Blood flow from underventilated alveoli (V/Q <1) tends to have increased $PaCO_2$ and decreased PaO_2. Blood flow from overventilated (V/Q >1) alveoli have lower $PaCO_2$ but cannot increase the PaO_2 due to the flat upper portion of the oxyhemoglobin dissociation curve. Thus, in conditions with ventilation/perfusion inequalities, carbon dioxide can be eliminated from the overventilated alveoli to compensate for the underventilated alveoli, but large alveolar to arterial oxygen gradients can occur. In fact, ventilation/perfusion (V/Q) mismatching is the major cause of hypoxemia associated with respiratory diseases. $PaCO_2$ may be normal or even low in response to compensatory hyperventilation for the hypoxemia.[58,76]

Ventilation-perfusion inequality can be altered by a variety of respiratory interventions that include increasing inspired oxygen or application of positive pressure to the airway. Increasing the concentration of inspired oxygen overcomes the alveolar arterial gradient in poorly ventilated alveoli (i.e., low V/Q lung compartments) resulting in improved oxygen content of the blood.

PHYSIOLOGY OF GAS AND FLUID EXCHANGE

Gas Properties

The primary function of the respiratory system is to transfer oxygen and carbon dioxide across the alveolar-capillary membrane. This process occurs in the terminal gas exchange unit (alveoli). The transfer of oxygen and carbon dioxide represents the summation of multiple interactions at the level of the alveoli and represents the fundamental process of gas exchange between inspired gases and pulmonary capillary blood. For a more thorough evaluation of these complex interactions, several excellent reviews are available.[10,18] The purpose of this section is not to be comprehensive, but rather to provide enough background to convey the basic principles of gas exchange.

The behavior of gases and the principles of gas exchange can be expressed by certain laws. The pressure exerted by a gas and its components is observed by Dalton's law. Dalton's gas law states that the pressure exerted by a group of gases is the sum of the partial pressure of these gases. This property defines the pressure exerted by the individual components of a gas mixture. At standard temperature (37° C) and at sea level (atmospheric pressure P_B = 760 mm Hg), air consists of

20.93% oxygen. Therefore, the partial pressure exerted by oxygen in air is:

$$P_{air}O_2 = (\% \ O_2 \ in \ air) \times atmospheric \ pressure \ (P_B)$$

$$P_{air}O_2 = 0.2093 \times 760 = 159 \ mm \ Hg$$

The partial pressure of oxygen, however, is altered before gas exchange at the alveolar level. When a gas is inhaled, it is warmed and saturated with water vapor. The partial pressure exerted by water vapor must be accounted for and varies with the temperature of the humidified gas, it is independent of pressure. At 37° C, the partial pressure of water vapor is 47 mm Hg. Therefore, by the time an inhaled gas has reached the level of the alveoli, the partial pressure of the gas has been reduced to 149 mm Hg ($0.2093 \times 760 - 47 \ mm \ Hg$).

At the alveolar level the percentage of carbon dioxide in the alveolus is normally about 5.6% and the partial pressure of alveolar carbon dioxide would be:

$$P_ACO_2 = (\% \ CO_2 \ in \ alveolus) \times (P_B - P_{water \ vapor})$$

$$P_ACO_2 = 0.056 \times (760 - 47 \ mm \ Hg) = 40 \ mm \ Hg$$

Under normal conditions, inspired gas is diluted by gas that remains in the alveoli after expiration. This gas contains water vapor and carbon dioxide. Therefore, the partial pressure of oxygen in the alveoli decreases. The sum of the partial pressures must equal the same total pressure, and any increase in partial pressure of a gas must be accomplished with a similar decrease in another gas. Under normal conditions, the respiratory quotient is 0.8 and the partial pressure of carbon dioxide is 40 mm Hg. Therefore, the partial pressure of oxygen at the alveolus is reduced.

$$P_AO_2 = PIO_2 - P_ACO_2/R,$$

where PIO_2 is the partial pressure of inspired oxygen and R is the respiratory quotient, or

$$P_AO_2 = 0.2093 \times (P_b - 47 \ mm \ Hg) - 40 \ mm \ Hg/0.8$$
$$= 99 \ mm \ Hg$$

This is known as the alveolar gas equation.

Alveolar Ventilation

When inspiration occurs, gas is drawn into the thorax and a portion of this gas is distributed to the alveoli. It is this portion of the inspired gas that determines alveolar ventilation. The remaining gas does not contribute to gas exchange and is referred to as dead space ventilation. Dead space ventilation can be defined by its location. Gas that does not contribute to gas exchange and is located in the conducting airways is referred to as "anatomic" dead space. This gas is incapable of gas exchange because of the anatomy of the conducting airways. Anatomic dead space in millimeters approximates the weight of the individual in pounds. The inspired gas that enters the alveolus and does not contribute to gas exchange is referred to as "alveolar" dead space. This distinction is essential, since anatomic dead space represents a portion of the gas exchange system that cannot exchange gas and does not change in an individual with a normal airway, whereas alveolar dead space is a portion of the respiratory system that receives gas but is not involved with gas exchange. This varies with lung perfusion. The total amount of the respiratory system

that does not participate in gas exchange is referred to as "physiologic" dead space.

$$V_D \ physiologic = V_D \ anatomic + V_D \ alveolar$$

The tidal volume is distributed between physiologic dead space and those alveoli that provide gas exchange referred to as alveolar ventilation (V alveolar).

$$Tidal \ volume = V_D \ anatomic + V_D \ alveolar + V \ alveolar$$

Under normal conditions, anatomic dead space is equal to physiologic dead space. An increase in alveolar dead space occurs in a variety of pathophysiologic conditions such as acute respiratory distress syndrome. In certain conditions, alveolar dead space may be recruited to exchange gas and, therefore, represents a potential area for supplemental gas exchange.

Assessments of alveolar ventilation provide insight into conditions of normal and abnormal cardiorespiratory physiology. The P_aO_2 is affected primarily by the presence of right-to-left intracardiac or intrapulmonary shunt and is not a good indicator of alveolar ventilation. The P_aCO_2 is less affected by shunting and is a more accurate assessment of alveolar ventilation than is the P_aO_2. The partial pressure of carbon dioxide in pulmonary capillary blood is 46 mm Hg, which differs only slightly from the partial pressure of arterial carbon dioxide ($P_aCO_2 = 40 \ mm \ Hg$). Therefore, a 50% reduction of pulmonary blood flow will result in only a 3 mm Hg increase in the partial pressure of carbon dioxide in arterial blood (P_aCO_2 from 40 mm Hg to 43 mm Hg). However, a 50% reduction in alveolar ventilation will result in a doubling of the partial pressure of carbon dioxide in arterial blood ($P_aCO_2 = 80 \ mm \ Hg$). An accurate estimation of alveolar ventilation through measurements of P_aCO_2 aids in the assessment of the adequacy of respiratory function in patients with hypoxia from right-to-left intracardiac shunting, while measurements of PaO_2 may not.

Alveolar-Capillary Membrane

The alveolar-capillary membrane is the gas exchanging surface that separates alveolar gas and capillary blood.[20] The alveolar side of the alveolar-capillary membrane is bounded by the epithelial cells. Underneath the epithelium is the epithelial basement membrane. The blood side of the alveolar-capillary membrane is the capillary endothelial cells and the endothelial basement membrane. At the alveolar-capillary membrane the basement membrane of the alveolar epithelial cells and the capillary endothelial cells are fused and, in health, watertight. The alveolar-capillary membrane is contiguous with the interstitial space that contains lymphatic channels and connective tissue. There are important differences between the epithelial and endothelial junctions that govern fluid flow. The junctions between the alveolar epithelial cells are tight whereas the endothelial cell junctions are loose and permit fluid transfer into the interstitium. The tight epithelial junctions help prevent the accumulation of intraalveolar fluid, that is, alveolar pulmonary edema.

Diffusion

Diffusion is defined as the energy-independent (passive) transfer of gas across the alveolar-capillary membrane. The Fick principle of diffusion governs the movements of gases across the alveolar-capillary membrane. Gases move from an area of high partial pressure to an area of lower partial pressure. The amount of gas diffusing across a semi-permeable membrane is dependent upon the partial pressure difference of the gas in the two locations (P_1–P_2), the surface area available for diffusion (A) and the diffusion coefficient (K), and is inversely related to the distance of diffusion (d):

Amount of gas diffusing (Q/min) = [(P_1 – P_2) × A × K]/d

Therefore, the propensity of a gas to diffuse across the alveolar-capillary membrane is dependent upon the partial pressure differences of the gas in the two locations and the diffusion coefficient of the gas (K).[60,62] The diffusion coefficient is directly dependent upon the solubility of the gas and inversely proportional to the square root of the molecular weight of the gas. With these formulas, it can be demonstrated that carbon dioxide has a much higher solubility than oxygen in water (24:1 at 30° C). Although the partial pressure difference of carbon dioxide between the alveolus and pulmonary capillary is small, carbon dioxide diffuses 20 times faster across the alveolar-capillary membrane than does oxygen because of its high solubility.

Oxygen Diffusion/Transport As blood enters the pulmonary capillaries, it begins the transfer of gases across the alveolar-capillary membrane. Red blood cells in the pulmonary capillaries are exposed to alveolar gas for approximately 0.75 seconds.[76] The pulmonary capillary transit time depends on the cardiac output and intrapulmonary blood volume. The transport of oxygen across the alveolar-capillary membrane begins immediately upon entry into the alveolar-capillary complex. When capillary blood first enters the alveolar-capillary gas exchange unit, there is a large gradient between the partial pressure of oxygen in the alveolus ($P_AO_2 = 100$ mm Hg) and in the capillary ($P_{capillary}O_2 = 40$ mm Hg). This results in an initial rapid diffusion of oxygen into the capillary. As oxygen diffuses into the capillary, the partial pressure of oxygen in capillary blood increases and the gradient for diffusion decreases resulting in a reduction in the diffusion rate over time. Although there is a reduction in oxygen transfer, the transfer of oxygen is not usually limited by diffusion, since oxygen transfer is rapid and the oxygen tension of pulmonary capillary blood approximates the oxygen tension of alveolar gas in the first 0.25 seconds.[77] Under normal conditions, little oxygen transfer occurs after the initial 0.25 seconds. This results in a 0.50-second "buffer," which provides extra time for diffusion to occur. Therefore, in most pathologic conditions, hypoxia does not occur from impaired diffusion.

In the absence of right-to-left intracardiac shunting, hypoxia most commonly results from ventilation-perfusion mismatch. This occurs when an alveolus receives inadequate ventilation compared to pulmonary blood flow (ventilation/perfusion < 1.0). When individual alveoli receive inadequate quantities of oxygen, P_AO_2 falls. The affected alveolus has less oxygen available for gas exchange, and a reduction in oxygen transfer occurs with resultant hypoxemia. To limit the development of arterial hypoxemia, the respiratory system has intrinsic mechanisms to enhance ventilation/perfusion matching. In conditions where alveolar ventilation is inadequate for perfusion, the low alveolar oxygen concentration results

in local vasoconstriction and a redistribution of flow to regions with a higher ventilation/perfusion ratio (hypoxic pulmonary vasoconstriction). In addition, lung regions with a low ventilation/perfusion ratio have high alveolar carbon dioxide concentration that dilates the lower airways and increases ventilation to these areas. In regions where the ventilation/perfusion ratio is high, the alveolar carbon dioxide level will be low and promote local airway constriction and a redistribution of airflow to lung units where ventilation/perfusion ratios approximate unity.

When the transfer of oxygen to the capillaries is complete, oxygen is carried in two forms: (1) oxygen dissolved in plasma, and (2) oxygen bound to hemoglobin. The amount of oxygen that is carried by the blood is referred to as the total oxygen content (CaO_2). Only a small portion of oxygen is dissolved in plasma. The majority of oxygen is carried bound to hemoglobin due to its high affinity for oxygen. One gram of hemoglobin can carry 1.39 mL of oxygen. For these reasons, the oxygen content (CaO_2) is critically dependent upon the arterial saturation (SaO_2) and hemoglobin (Hgb) concentration and relatively insensitive to the partial pressure of oxygen.

$$CaO_2 \, (mL \cdot dL^{-1}) = [1.39 \, (mL \cdot g^{-1}) \times Hgb \, (g \cdot dL^{-1}) \times SaO_2] + [0.003 (mL \cdot mm \, Hg^{-1} \cdot dL^{-1}) \times PaO_2 \, (mm \, Hg)]$$

The amount of oxygen that can be bound to hemoglobin is related to the partial pressure of oxygen in the blood and the affinity of hemoglobin for oxygen, known as the oxygen-hemoglobin dissociation curve. Factors that influence the affinity of hemoglobin for oxygen include pH, PCO_2, temperature, and the amount of 2,3-diphosphoglycerate (DPG) present. Alterations in the oxygen-hemoglobin dissociation curve occur at individual organ levels. At the tissue level, a decrease in pH, increase in PCO_2, increase in temperature, or increase in DPG results in a shift of the oxygen-hemoglobin dissociation curve to the right. This shift in the oxygen-hemoglobin dissociation curve allows an unloading of oxygen to tissues. At the alveolar level, the reverse occurs, and a shift to the left of the oxygen-hemoglobin dissociation curve occurs with increased hemoglobin affinity for oxygen and increased oxygen uptake by capillary blood.

Maintaining appropriate arterial oxygen content is an important concern in treating infants and children with congenital heart disease. Patients with intracardiac right-to-left shunting will not significantly increase their arterial saturation and oxygen content with the administration of inspired oxygen. In these conditions, a significant increase in oxygen carrying capacity can be obtained by raising the hemoglobin concentration. For a given arterial saturation, an increase in hemoglobin results in an increase in oxygen carrying capacity and oxygen delivery. Augmentation of oxygen carrying capacity by raising the hemoglobin levels is particularly advantageous in infants with anemia.

Carbon Dioxide Diffusion/Transport The diffusion of carbon dioxide is similar to the process that occurs with oxygen transfer. Carbon dioxide diffusion across the alveolar-capillary membrane is more rapid than oxygen diffusion due to the greater solubility of carbon dioxide. Carbon dioxide transport is dependent upon a variety of interactions in the red blood cell and plasma. The amount of carbon dioxide carried by the blood is dependent on its partial pressure and the presence of oxyhemoglobin. In the presence of oxyhemoglobin there will be a lower carbon dioxide content for a given partial pressure of oxygen. This results in the improved carbon dioxide removal as capillary blood becomes oxygenated. As blood is transported to peripheral tissues, carbon dioxide is taken up from the peripheral tissues and transported to the alveolus for gas exchange.

Fluid Transport

Starling's forces govern the flow of fluid in and out of the capillaries and interstitium.[6,7] The alveolar epithelium is relatively resistant to fluid movement whereas the endothelial membrane is more permeable. The force tending to push fluid out of the capillaries and into the interstitium is the hydrostatic pressure in the capillaries (P_{cap}). This is opposed by the hydrostatic pressure in the interstitium (P_{int}). The differences between these forces, $P_{cap} - P_{int}$, is the net effect of the hydrostatic forces. Under normal conditions, P_{cap} is greater than P_{int} and the net force promotes fluid movement out of the capillaries into the interstitium. The force tending to promote fluid entry into the capillaries and out of the interstitium is the colloid osmotic pressure difference between the capillaries and interstitium ($\pi_{cap} - \pi_{int}$). The balance of these forces is dependent on a number of factors, including the reflection coefficient (K), which delineates the ability of the capillary membrane to prevent the passage of proteins across the capillary membrane. The sum total of these forces defines the flow of fluid into the interstitium and is equal to the filtration rate (Q):

$$Q = K[(P_{cap} - P_{int}) - (\pi_{cap} - \pi_{int})]$$

Under normal conditions, the effect of Starling's forces is to promote a small amount of net flux of fluid into the interstitium that is promptly removed by lymphatics. In conditions of left atrial hypertension and/or left ventricular dysfunction (myocardial ischemia/infarction, cardiomyopathy, mitral stenosis) hydrostatic pressure in the pulmonary capillaries may increase dramatically ($P_{cap} \gg P_{int}$) and excessive fluid flows into the interstitium. The integrity of the alveolar-capillary membrane is essential to regulate the flow of fluid in the interstitium. Disruption of the alveolar-capillary membrane results in an increased permeability to large molecular weight proteins and massive fluid accumulation in the lung.

DEVELOPMENTAL CONSIDERATIONS

Effective respiratory support in children requires a fundamental understanding of the developmental changes in the static and dynamic components of respiratory mechanics.[1,15,55] Respiratory rate, inspiratory time, inspiratory flow, tidal volume, and mechanical properties of the respiratory system for a given age are the principal determinants of respiratory support in children. These developmental features of respiratory physiology limit the applicability of ventilatory equipment and approaches designed primarily for adults.

Respiratory Rate

Respiratory rate decreases from 30 to 60 breaths per minute (bpm) in neonates to the adult value of 12 to 16 bpm by mid-adolescence. Higher respiratory rates in neonates and young children are reflected in shorter inspiratory times. Normal inspiratory time in infants is between 0.4 and 0.5 seconds. In adults, the inspiratory time is approximately 1.25 seconds.[54]

Tidal Volume

Tidal volume relative to body weight changes little during development, that is, 6–8 mL/kg.[19,55] On an absolute basis, however, the range of tidal volume encountered in children changes by orders of magnitude with advancing age (e.g., 18 mL per breath in the newborn vs. 500 mL per breath in the adult).

Inspiratory Flow

Although the average inspiratory flow encountered in the smallest child is approximately 1.9 L/min,[54] peak inspiratory flows during periods of respiratory distress can approach 20 L/min.[1] This is in contrast to older children and adults, who can generate instantaneous peak flows between 300 and 600 L/min, despite a normal average inspiratory flow of 24 L/min.

Total Respiratory Compliance

Total respiratory compliance is the change in respiratory system volume per unit change in distending pressure. The absolute value of total respiratory compliance increases by a factor of 20 from the neonatal period through adolescence.[55] When total respiratory compliance is expressed on a relative basis as a function of lung volume or body weight (i.e., specific respiratory compliance), pediatric and adult values are remarkably similar (approximately 0.06 mL per centimeter H_2O per milliliter lung volume).

Total Respiratory Conductance

Total respiratory conductance, which is the reciprocal of total resistance, is flow per unit pressure change across the respiratory system. Total respiratory conductance increases from infancy to adulthood by a factor of 15.[19] Just as for total compliance, airway conductance normalized for unit lung volume or body weight is similar for infants and adults (0.24 to 0.28 mL/sec · cm H_2O/mL FRC).

Respiratory compliance and conductance define the mechanical forces required to inflate the lungs during positive pressure ventilation. Although the absolute values of compliance and conductance are much lower in the infant, when these are indexed to relative size, inspiratory flow, and tidal volume, they are similar to values found in adults. Therefore, comparable inspiratory pressures are required in infants and adults to assure adequate volume during positive pressure ventilation. Nevertheless, the low absolute compliance and high absolute resistance of the developing respiratory system require special attention in designing systems to deliver physiologic tidal volumes to children. Pediatric ventilators must deliver low inspiratory volumes under pressures comparable to those used in adults; consequently, estimates of tidal volume delivered during positive pressure ventilation in children are subject to gross error due to the relatively large volume of the ventilator systems.[54] The distribution of volume delivered by a positive pressure ventilator between the ventilator circuit (i.e., compressible volume) and the patient is determined by the relative compliance of the circuit and the patient.[35] In the presence of a compliant circuit, the delivered tidal volume may be significantly less than the set tidal volume. These large circuit compliance characteristics also give rise to decreased sensitivity of ventilator valve systems to spontaneous inspiratory efforts and delays in the delivery of assisted or synchronized positive pressure breaths.[50] These factors must be accounted for when providing mechanical ventilatory support for children.

ALTERATIONS IN RESPIRATORY PHYSIOLOGY SECONDARY TO CONGENITAL HEART DISEASE

Abnormalities in cardiovascular structure and function can lead to alterations in respiratory mechanics. The alterations in respiratory mechanics that develop in patients with congenital heart disease are a direct result of changes in pulmonary blood volume and pulmonary artery pressure. Both of these are dependent on the amount of pulmonary blood flow. Therefore, the changes that occur in respiratory mechanics can be classified depending upon the presence of increased or decreased pulmonary blood flow.

Increased Pulmonary Blood Flow

Congenital cardiovascular anomalies associated with increased pulmonary blood flow are due to a left-to-right intracardiac shunt. The respiratory derangements that occur in patients with increased pulmonary blood flow include (1) excessive pulmonary blood volume and (2) excessive pulmonary vascular pressures (Table 11-1).

In patients with excessive pulmonary blood volume, there is an increase in red blood cell mass in the pulmonary circulation.

The increased red blood cell mass results in perfusion to alveoli in excess of ventilation and hence ventilation/perfusion mismatch. When alveolar ventilation is inadequate for pulmonary blood flow, $P_{cap}O_2$ falls. If the ventilation/perfusion mismatch is significant, hypoxia will ensue. In many patients, the left-to-right intrapulmonary shunt is a result of excessive pulmonary blood volume, since lung volumes and EELV are not altered.[44,46,72] The alteration in respiratory mechanics may mimic what occurs in patients with atelectasis. The increased pulmonary blood volume can also cause alterations in respiratory mechanics by increasing lung weight. This results in a reduction of compliance and necessitates an increase in airway pressure to generate a given lung volume during positive pressure ventilation.

Excessive pulmonary blood flow can also modify respiratory mechanics by altering pulmonary vascular pressures.[46] Increased pulmonary blood flow results in an increase in pulmonary artery, capillary, and venous pressures, factors that favor the development of extravascular lung water. Extravascular fluid accumulation and alveolar atelectasis cause a loss of lung volume, a reduction of lung compliance, a decrease in tidal volume, and a compensatory increase in respiratory frequency.[40,44] Many of the manifestations of excessive extravascular lung water resolve with surgical correction of the underlying anomaly.[34] The decrease in lung compliance that occurs in patients with increased pulmonary blood flow has been correlated with the estimated blood volume on chest radiography, the ratio of pulmonary artery to aortic diameter determined by echocardiogram, and pulmonary artery pressures.[2,17,34,40]

Both large and small airway obstructions can occur in patients with increased pulmonary blood flow. Small airway obstruction results from intrinsic narrowing of the airways due to fluid collecting in the airway lumen or extrinsic compression from interstitial edema, or dilation of the pulmonary vasculature.[2] Large airway obstruction occurs when a dilated or high pressure vascular structure causes external compression of the airway lumen. Increased pulmonary blood flow combined with pulmonary artery hypertension causes dilation of the pulmonary arteries and left atrium and predisposes to large airway compression. Large airway obstruction results in a restriction to gas flow, primarily during exhalation. If airway obstruction becomes significant, increased work of breathing, increased respiratory frequency, and abnormalities

Table 11-1   Effects of Congenital Heart Disease on Respiratory Function

Blood Flow	Abnormality	Pathophysiology	Respiratory Abnormality
↑ Pulmonary Blood Flow	↑ Pulmonary blood volume	↓ V/Q R→L shunt	Hypoxia
		↑ Lung weight	↓ Compliance
	↑ P_{cap}	↑ Lung fluid accumulation	↓ Compliance
		Interstitial/alveolar edema	↓ Lung volumes ↑ Airway resistance
	↑ P_{pa}	Large airway obstruction	↑ Airway resistance
	↑ P_{la}	Small airway obstruction	↑ Airway resistance
↓ Pulmonary Blood Flow	↓ Pulmonary blood volume	↑ Dead space ventilation	Hypoxia
	Airway hypoplasia	↓ Lung weight	↑ Compliance
		Small airway obstruction	↑ Airway resistance

P_{cap}, Hydrostatic capillary pressure; P_{la}, left atrial pressure; P_{pa}, pulmonary artery pressure; R→L shunt, intrapulmonary right-to-left shunt; V/Q, ventilation/perfusion.

of gas exchange develop. When the obstruction is severe, inspiration may also be compromised. If dynamic hyperinflation occurs, chest radiographs will demonstrate increased lung volumes, and respiratory mechanics will delineate abnormalities of expiratory flow and increased airway resistance. In patients with large airway disease, application of PEEP may reduce the obstruction and "stent" the airway, pending medical or surgical intervention. Reduction of pulmonary artery volume and pressure reverses these abnormalities, provided tracheomalacia is not present.

Attempts have been made to correlate the alterations in respiratory mechanics with other signs of excessive pulmonary blood flow. Therapy should be directed at reversing the cause of the obstruction, since surgical interventions on the airways are frequently unsuccessful. Large airway obstruction can also occur when vascular structures proximal to an area of stenosis become dilated, compress the airways, and present in a similar manner.

Decreased Pulmonary Blood Flow

The effects of a right-to-left shunt and decreased pulmonary blood flow on respiratory mechanics are nearly opposite to those that occur in patients with increased pulmonary blood flow and are due to the reduction of pulmonary blood volume and arterial pressure. The decreased pulmonary blood volume results in a decrease in lung weight, an increase in lung compliance, and alterations in ventilation/perfusion matching.[2] When decreased pulmonary blood flow is present, ventilation occurs without perfusion and physiologic dead space increases.[47] The extent of the ventilation/perfusion mismatch is directly correlated with the severity of hypoxia.[23] The increase in dead space ventilation results in a decrease in ventilatory efficiency, which initiates compensatory mechanisms that include an increase in minute ventilation and a reduction in arterial carbon dioxide.[23,47]

Patients with decreased pulmonary blood flow may also develop hypoplasia of the airways.[78] If the airway hypoplasia is significant, a reduction of the airway lumen and an increase in airway resistance can occur.

Children with uncorrected or palliated cyanotic cardiac defects have chronic hypoxia, which results in a reduced ventilatory response to acute hypoxia. The magnitude of this blunting correlates with the severity of the chronic hypoxemia. These findings explain, in part, the recent observation that cardiac patients with chronic cyanosis have frequent and severe decreases in oxygen saturation during sleep.[36] Other studies demonstrated that these alterations are reversible with correction of the chronic hypoxemia.[8]

In summary, alterations in pulmonary mechanics are expected in nearly every child with congenital heart disease. These changes in mechanics can range from subclinical changes to overt respiratory system failure. Clinicians treating patients with congenital heart disease must take into account these changes in respiratory mechanics when applying mechanical ventilatory support for this patient population.

References

1. Auld PAM: Pulmonary physiology of the newborn infant. In Scarpelli EM (ed): *Pulmonary Physiology of the Fetus, Newborn, and Child.* Philadelphia: Lea & Febiger, 1975, p 140.

2. Bancalari E, Jesse MJ, Gelband H, Garcia O: Lung mechanics in congenital heart disease with increased and decreased pulmonary blood flow. *J Pediatr* 90:192–195, 1977.

3. Benumof JL: Mechanism of decreased blood flow to atelectatic lung. *J Appl Physiol* 46:1047–1048, 1979.

4. Benumof JL, Rogers SN, Moyce PR, et al: Hypoxic pulmonary vasoconstriction and regional and whole-lung PEEP in the dog. *Anesthesiology* 51:503–507, 1979.

5. Benumof JL: Respiratory physiology and respiratory function during anesthesia. In Miller RD (ed): *Anesthesia.* New York: Churchill Livingstone, 1990, pp 505–550.

6. Berne RM, Levy MN: Coronary circulation and cardiac metabolism. In Berne RM, Levy MN (eds): *Cardiovascular Physiology.* St. Louis: Mosby, 1981, pp 211–222.

7. Berner M, Rouge JC, Friedli B: The hemodynamic effect of phentolamine and dobutamine after open-heart operations in children: influence of the underlying heart defect. *Ann Thorac Surg* 35:643–650, 1983.

8. Blesa MI, Lahiri S, Rashkind WJ, Fishman AP: Normalization of the blunted ventilatory response to acute hypoxia in congenital cyanotic heart disease. *N Engl J Med* 296:237–241, 1977.

9. Brown ES, Johnson RP, Clements JA: Pulmonary surface tension. *J Appl Physiol* 14:717, 1959.

10. Bryan AC, Wohl MD: Respiratory mechanics in children. In Fishman AP (ed): *Handbook of Physiology.* Baltimore: Williams & Wilkins, 1986.

11. Burger EJ Jr, Macklem P: Airway closure: demonstration by breathing 100 percent O_2 at low lung volumes and by N_2 washout. *J Appl Physiol* 25:139–148, 1968.

12. Burton AC, Patel DJ: Effect on pulmonary vascular resistance of inflation of the rabbit lungs. *J Appl Physiol* 12:239, 1958.

13. Chatburn RL: Principles and practice of neonatal and pediatric mechanical ventilation. *Respir Care* 36:569, 1991.

14. Cheifetz IM, Craig DM, Quick G, et al: Increasing tidal volumes and pulmonary overdistention adversely affect pulmonary vascular mechanics and cardiac output in a pediatric swine model. *Crit Care Med* 26:710–716, 1998.

15. Chernick V, Avery ME: The functional basis of respiratory pathology. In Kendig EL Jr, Chernick V (eds): *Disorders of the Respiratory Tract in Children.* Philadelphia: WB Saunders, 1977, pp 3–61.

16. Connors AF Jr, McCaffree DR, Gray BA: Effect of inspiratory flow rate on gas exchange during mechanical ventilation. *Am Rev Respir Dis* 124:537–543, 1981.

17. Davies CJ, Cooper SG, Fletcher ME, et al: Total respiratory compliance in infants and young children with congenital heart disease. *Pediatr Pulmonol* 8:155–161, 1990.

18. England SJ: Current techniques for assessing pulmonary function in the newborn and infant: advantages and limitations. *Pediatr Pulmonol* 4:48–53, 1988.

19. Fisher BJ, Carlo WA, Doershuk CF: Pulmonary function from infancy through adolescence. In Scarpelli EM (ed): *Pulmonary Physiology: Fetus, Newborn, Child, and Adolescent.* Philadelphia: Lea & Febiger, 1990, p 421.

20. Fishman AP: Pulmonary edema. The water-exchanging function of the lung. *Circulation* 46:390–408, 1972.

21. Fishman AP: Hypoxia on the pulmonary circulation. How and where it acts. *Circ Res* 38:221–231, 1976.

22. Fishman AP: Dynamics of the pulmonary circulation. In Hamilton F (ed): *Handbook of Physiology. Section 2. Circulation.* Baltimore: Williams & Wilkins, 1963, p 1667.

23. Fletcher R: Relationship between alveolar deadspace and arterial oxygenation in children with congenital cardiac disease. *Br J Anaesth* 62:168–176, 1989.

24. Fredberg JJ, Glass GM, Boynton BR, Frantz ID: Factors influencing mechanical performance of neonatal high-frequency ventilators. *J Appl Physiol* 62:2485–2490, 1987.

25. Glenny RW: Spatial correlation of regional pulmonary perfusion. *J Appl Physiol* 72:2378–2386, 1992.

26. Glenny RW: Blood flow distribution in the lung. *Chest* 114:8S–16S, 1998.

27. Glenny RW, Bernard S, Robertson HT, Hlastala MP: Gravity is an important but secondary determinant of regional pulmonary blood flow in upright primates. *J Appl Physiol* 86:623–632, 1999.

28. Glenny RW, Lamm WJ, Albert RK, Robertson HT: Gravity is a minor determinant of pulmonary blood flow distribution. *J Appl Physiol* 71:620–629, 1991.

29. Glenny RW, Polissar NL, McKinney S, Robertson HT: Temporal heterogeneity of regional pulmonary perfusion is spatially clustered. *J Appl Physiol* 79:986–1001, 1995.

30. Glenny RW, Polissar L, Robertson HT: Relative contribution of gravity to pulmonary perfusion heterogeneity. *J Appl Physiol* 71:2449–2452, 1991.

31. Glenny RW, Robertson HT: Fractal modeling of pulmonary blood flow heterogeneity. *J Appl Physiol* 70:1024–1030, 1991.

32. Glenny RW, Robertson HT: A computer simulation of pulmonary perfusion in three dimensions. *J Appl Physiol* 79:357–369, 1995.

33. Goldsmith JP, Karotkin EH: *Assisted Ventilation of the Neonate.* Philadelphia: WB Saunders, 1981, p 29.

34. Griffin AJ, Ferrara JD, Lax JO, Cassels DE: Pulmonary compliance. An index of cardiovascular status in infancy. *Am J Dis Child* 123:89–95, 1972.

35. Hakanson DO: Positive pressure ventilation: Volume-cycled ventilators. In Goldsmith JP, Karotkin EH (eds): *Assisted Ventilation of the Neonate.* Philadelphia: WB Saunders, 1981, p 128.

36. Hiatt PW, Mahony L, Tepper RS: Oxygen desaturation during sleep in infants and young children with congenital heart disease. *J Pediatr* 121:226–232, 1992.

37. Hlastala MP, Chornuk MA, Self DA, et al: Pulmonary blood flow redistribution by increased gravitational force. *J Appl Physiol* 84:1278–1288, 1998.

38. Hogg JC: Age as a factor in respiratory disease. In Kendig EL Jr, Chernick V (eds): *Disorders of the Respiratory Tract in Children.* Philadelphia: WB Saunders, 1977, pp 177–187.

39. Hoppin FG Jr, Green ID, Mead J: Distribution of pleural surface pressure in dogs. *J Appl Physiol* 27:863–873, 1969.

40. Howlett G: Lung mechanics in normal infants and infants with congenital heart disease. *Arch Dis Child* 47:707–715, 1972.

41. Hughes JMB: Invited editorial on pulmonary blood flow distribution in exercising and resting horses. *J Appl Physiol* 81:1049–1050, 1996.

42. Kallas HJ, Domino KB, Glenny RW, et al: Pulmonary blood flow redistribution with low levels of positive end-expiratory pressure. *Anesthesiology* 88:1291–1299, 1998.

43. Kendig EL, Chernick V: *Disorders of the Respiratory Tract in Children.* Philadelphia: WB Saunders, 1977, p 17.

44. Lees MH, Way RC, Ross BB: Ventilation and respiratory gas transfer of infants with increased pulmonary blood flow. *Pediatrics* 40:259–271, 1967.

45. Lesouef PN, England SJ, Bryan AC: Total resistance of the respiratory system in preterm infants with and without an endotracheal tube. *J Pediatr* 104:108–111, 1984.

46. Levin AR, Ho E, Auld PA: Alveolar-arterial oxygen gradients in infants and children with left-to-right shunts. *J Pediatr* 83:979–987, 1973.

47. Lindahl SG, Olsson AK: Congenital heart malformations and ventilatory efficiency in children. Effects of lung perfusion during halothane anaesthesia and spontaneous breathing. *Br J Anaesth* 59:410–418, 1987.

48. Mansell A, Bryan C, Levison H: Airway closure in children. *J Appl Physiol* 33:711–714, 1972.

49. Marshall BE, Marshall C: Continuity of response to hypoxic pulmonary vasoconstriction. *J Appl Physiol* 49:189–196, 1980.

50. Martin LD, Rafferty JF, Wetzel RC, Gioia FR: Inspiratory work and response times of a modified pediatric volume ventilator during synchronized intermittent mandatory ventilation and pressure support ventilation. *Anesthesiology* 71:977–981, 1989.

51. Martin LD, Rafferty JF, Walker LK, Gioia FR: Principles of respiratory support and mechanical ventilation. In Rogers MC (ed): *Textbook of Pediatric Intensive Care.* Baltimore: Williams and Wilkins, 1992, pp 135–203.

52. Maseri A, Caldini P, Harward P, et al: Determinants of pulmonary vascular volume: recruitment versus distensibility. *Circ Res* 31:218–228, 1972.

53. Milic-Emili J, Henderson JA, Dolovich MB, et al: Regional distribution of inspired gas in the lung. *J Appl Physiol* 21:749–759, 1966.

54. Mushin WW, Rendell-Baker L, Thompson PW, Mapleson WW: Clinical aspects of controlled respiration. In *Automatic Ventilation of the Lungs.* Oxford: Blackwell Scientific, 1980, p 33–61.

55. Nelson NM: Neonatal pulmonary function. *Pediatr Clin North Am* 13:769–799, 1966.

56. Newth CJ: Recognition and management of respiratory failure. *Pediatr Clin North Am* 26:617–643, 1979.

57. Nunn JF: Elastic resistance to ventilation. In *Applied Respiratory Physiology.* Boston: Butterworth, 1977.

58. Nunn JF: Distribution of the pulmonary blood flow. In *Applied Respiratory Physiology.* Boston: Butterworth, 1977, p 274.

59. Nunn JF: *Applied Respiratory Physiology.* Boston: Butterworth, 1987, p 109.

60. O'Brodovich HM, Mellins RB, Mansell AL: Effects of growth on the diffusion constant for carbon monoxide. *Am Rev Respir Dis* 125: 670–673, 1982.

61. Pepe PE, Marini JJ: Occult positive end-expiratory pressure in mechanically ventilated patients with airflow obstruction: the auto-PEEP effect. *Am Rev Respir Dis* 126:166–170, 1982.

62. Permutt S, Bromberger-Barnea B, Bane HN: Alveolar pressure, pulmonary venous pressure and the vascular waterfall. *Med Thorac* 19:239, 1962.

63. Polgar G, Kong GP: The nasal resistance of newborn infants. *J Pediatr* 104:108, 1984.

64. Pontoppidan H, Geffin B, Lowenstein E: Acute respiratory failure in the adult. 1. *N Engl J Med* 287:690–698, 1972.

65. Prisk GK, Guy HJB, Elliot AR, West JB: Inhomogeneity of pulmonary perfusion during sustained microgravity on SLS-1. *J Appl Physiol* 76:1730–1738, 1994.

66. Reed JH, Wood EH: Effect of body position on vertical distribution of pulmonary blood flow. *J Appl Physiol* 28:303–311, 1970.

67. Scarpelli EM: *Pulmonary Physiology of the Fetus, Newborn, and Child.* Philadelphia: Lea & Febiger, 1975, p 27.

68. Simbruner G, Gregory GA: Performance of neonatal ventilators: the effects of changes in resistance and compliance. *Crit Care Med* 9:509–514, 1981.

69. Simmons DH, Linds CM, Miller JH, et al.: Relation of lung volume and pulmonary vascular resistance. *Circ Res* 9:465, 1961.

70. Sykes MK: The mechanics of ventilation. In Scurr C, Feldman S (eds): *Scientific Foundations of Anaesthesia.* Philadelphia: FA Davis, 1970, p 174.

71. Sylvester JT, Rock P: Acute hypoxic responses. In Bergofsky EH (ed): *Abnormal Pulmonary Circulation.* New York: Churchill Livingstone, 1986, pp 127–165.

72. Thorsteinsson A, Jonmarker C, Larsson A, et al: Functional residual capacity in anesthetized children: normal values and values in children with cardiac anomalies. *Anesthesiology* 73:876–881, 1990.

73. Weir EK: Does normoxic pulmonary vasodilation rather than hypoxic vasoconstriction account for the pulmonary pressor response to hypoxia? *Lancet* 1:476–477, 1978.

74. West JB, Dollery CT, Heard BE: Increased pulmonary vascular resistance in the dependent zone of the isolated dog lung caused by perivascular edema. *Circ Res* 17:191, 1965.

75. West JB, Dollery CT, Naimark A: Distribution of blood flow in isolated lung: Relation to vascular and alveolar pressures. *J Appl Physiol* 19:713, 1964.

76. West JB: Ventilation-perfusion ratio inequality and overall gas exchange. In *Ventilation/Blood Flow and Gas Exchange.* London: Blackwell Scientific, 1977, p 53–82.

77. West JB: *Ventilation/Blood Flow and Gas Exchange.* London: Blackwell Scientific Publications, 1977.

78. Wittenberger JL, McGregor M, Berglund E, et al: Influence of state of inflation of the lung on pulmonary vascular resistance. *J Appl Physiol* 15:878, 1960.

Chapter 12

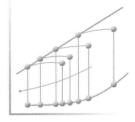

Respiratory Support for the Child with Critical Heart Disease

IRA M. CHEIFETZ, MD, LYNN D. MARTIN, MD,
JON N. MELIONES, MD, MS, and RANDALL C. WETZEL, MBBS, MBA

RESPIRATORY SUPPORT

Classification of Positive-Pressure Ventilators

A mechanical ventilator is a life-support system designed to replace or support lung function. A ventilator is designed to alter, transmit, and directly apply energy in a predetermined way to perform the work of the thorax and lungs. Nomenclature to classify the essential features of positive-pressure ventilators has been described by many authors and continues to be an area of confusion for practitioners not intimately involved in the design and development of ventilators.[24,110,118] A sound classification system provides a common knowledge-base of terms and concepts to facilitate the understanding, interpretation, and assessment of ventilator operating systems and performance characteristics. The classification system must be clinically relevant and accurately reflect the pattern of respiratory support a patient receives. Technological advances in the design, monitoring, and application of positive-pressure ventilation (PPV) mandate that classification systems be continually revised and updated to remain current. This section will present a classification system as it supports the clinical practice of ventilatory care.

Power Input/Transmission

Ventilator power input is either electrical or pneumatic (compressed gas). The transmission of input power is a function of the drive and control mechanisms of the ventilator. Ventilator classification focuses on the control variables, output parameters, and alarm systems as applied to their clinical utility. More specifically, clinicians focus on how each tidal volume is delivered to describe the type of respiratory support a patient receives.

Control Schemes and Control Variables

Ventilator control variables address the physical qualities adjusted, measured, and/or used to manipulate the various phases of the ventilatory cycle. The four general types of control variables are inspiratory flow pattern, limit, trigger, and cycle. Classifying ventilators with this system may seem cumbersome and challenging to practitioners who have used earlier systems; however, this system addresses new technological advances in ventilator operation, is based on the physiology of the ventilatory strategies, and provides a platform for new technology without confounding terminology.

Typically, the control variables remain constant despite changes in ventilatory load. Therefore, the ventilator sacrifices all other preset variables to keep the control variables constant despite changes in the patient's compliance and resistance.[15] Thus, the other variables are dependent variables. They depend on the controlled variable as well as changes in the patient's pulmonary compliance and resistance. Each manufacturer develops and refines its control scheme for the manipulation of these variables. Nevertheless, commonalities arise between ventilators which allow clinicians to describe the resultant respiratory patterns with common terminology.

Inspiratory Flow The inspiratory flow pattern sets the characteristics of gas flow during a positive-pressure breath and affects the distribution of that breath within the patient's respiratory system. Clinicians must consider several factors when selecting an inspiratory flow pattern for a given patient. Airway pressures are dependent upon the mechanical properties of the lungs and the movement of gas into the lungs. The airway pressures generated during inspiration increase as flow enters the respiratory system and encounters the resistance of the airways. The gas volume must also overcome the elastic recoil of the lung. Therefore, peak pressure = (flow)(R_{aw}) + (V_T)(elastance), where R_{aw} is the airway resistance and V_T is the tidal volume. The shape of the inspiratory flow pattern as it delivers the positive pressure breath determines the shape of the pressure curve and the peak pressure generated.[78] This can be predicted given knowledge of the characteristics of the various flow patterns and the pneumatic characteristics of the patient's lungs, as described following. As derived from the equation, the selection of an appropriate inspiratory flow pattern based upon the patient's pulmonary pathophysiology will improve the effectiveness of ventilation, reduce peak inspiratory pressure, optimize mean airway pressure, and promote patient-ventilator synchrony.[79]

Figure 12-1 illustrates typical inspiratory flow patterns available with positive-pressure ventilators.[102] Four inspiratory flow patterns exist. A sine wave pattern is generated by a variable flow with a rapid increase during the early phase of inspiration, a peak at mid-inspiration, then a decrease in flow until end-inspiration. A square wave pattern is produced by a constant flow of gas throughout inspiration. Ascending, accelerated flow patterns produce a ramp pattern with low flow at beginning inspiration and a linear increase in flow throughout inspiration with peak flow delivered at end-inspiration. Descending decelerated flow is a waveform characterized by peak flow at the beginning of inspiration and then a decrease in flow until end-inspiration. This decrease in flow can be either linear or curvilinear depending on the specific programming of the ventilator. The functional performance of the various types of inspiratory flow patterns remains constant across manufacturers but may be produced by dramatically different control schema. The flow pattern characteristics of a specific mechanical ventilator significantly influence the airway pressures generated. Clinicians should monitor inspiration/expiration (I:E) ratios when selecting flow patterns during volume limited ventilation and adjust the peak flow to maintain an appropriate inspiratory time.

Gas flow always takes the path of least resistance. Alterations in inspiratory flow pattern affect the distribution of gas flow based on the underlying pathophysiology and anatomical considerations of the respiratory system.

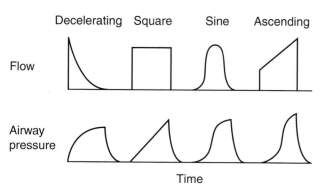

FIGURE 12-1 Tracings typical of the various inspiratory waveforms available with mechanical ventilators. Pressure control ventilation uses a descending waveform that results in lower peak and higher mean airway pressures. Volume control utilizes a square waveform. (Modified from Pontoppidan H, Geffin B, Lowenstein E: Acute respiratory failure in the adult. 3. *N Engl J Med* 287:799–806, 1972.)

Ascending (accelerating) flow patterns deliver the highest flow at end-inspiration when the effects of resistance and elastance are increased. Ascending flow patterns produce higher peak pressures compared to other flow patterns. A decelerating flow pattern has several advantages over an ascending pattern. Decelerating flow patterns deliver the highest flow at the beginning of inspiration when volume and elastance are low. Inspiratory flow then decreases during inspiration as delivered volume increases. Therefore, peak airway pressure is lower but mean airway pressure is higher with this flow pattern. In general, as the maximum flow moves from the beginning to the end of the inspiratory cycle, peak pressure increases and mean airway pressure decreases.

Flow patterns should be matched to the patient's clinical condition. In clinical situations where the patient has high airway resistance (asthma, tracheal stenosis, airway obstruction), peak airway pressures may be reduced by avoiding a flow pattern with high peak flow rates. In these patients, a square wave, constant flow pattern may generate a lower peak pressure than a descending flow pattern as a result of the decrease in peak flow. The actual effects in individual patients may vary widely. In contrast, respiratory pathology characterized by a low compliance may benefit from a descending flow pattern where the peak pressure is reduced but the mean airway pressure is increased. Variable flow ventilation (i.e., pressure control ventilation) utilizes a decelerating flow pattern, which can significantly decrease the peak inspiratory pressure and increase the mean airway pressure to recruit collapsed alveoli.[71,73,75]

Trigger The inspiratory phase of a breath can be initiated by (1) patient effort, as determined by a change in either pressure or flow in the ventilator circuit, or (2) time. Therefore, mechanical breaths may be pressure-, time-, or flow-triggered.[35,109] Flow triggering increases the sensitivity of the ventilator to the patient's spontaneous demands and decreases the response time of tidal volume delivery. The ventilator "sensitivity" determines the degree of inspiratory effort a patient must exert to trigger the ventilator to deliver a tidal volume. Ideally, this should be adjusted to -0.5 to -1.5 cm H_2O or 0.1 to 3.0 L/min of flow to minimize the patient's imposed work of breathing (WOBi). Some older neonatal ventilators trigger inspiration by an external sensor taped to the abdomen of the infant to sense respiratory movement and initiate inspiration ("impedance" trigger).

Cycle The cycle variable determines when inspiration ends. This variable is used as a feedback signal to terminate gas flow and to allow the patient to passively exhale. Time is the most common cycle variable for mechanical breaths (time cycled). Certain spontaneous breaths (pressure supported breaths, for example) can be flow cycled. In a flow cycled breath, the expiratory valve opens when inspiratory flow decreases to a preset percentage of peak inspiratory flow. This algorithm is generally preset, not adjustable, and varies among ventilators.

Limit During inspiration, pressure, volume, and flow increase above the end-expiratory values. Limit variables allow the clinician to control the upper limits of pressure and/or volume of the mechanical breath a patient receives; hence, the description "pressure limited" and "volume limited."

Ventilatory Modes

Using this terminology, a system can be developed that describes the ventilatory modes and specific breathing patterns used during PPV. Ventilatory modes may include mechanical breaths, spontaneous breaths, or a combination of both.

Mechanical Breaths

Assist control mode delivers a patient-triggered ventilator tidal volume with each spontaneous effort. In an assist control mode, the ventilatory rate is determined by the patient and, therefore, may be in excess of the preset control rate. When there is no spontaneous respiratory effort, the minimum ventilatory rate is that which is set by the clinician. Assist control modes should be contrasted with support modes of ventilation. In both modes, a predetermined level of support is adjusted by the clinician. In assisted modes the inspiratory time is determined by the clinician. In contrast, in supported modes, the inspiratory time is determined by the patient. Assist control breaths may be limited by either volume or pressure. A patient may receive volume control ventilation, where a predetermined minimum breath rate is delivered and breaths are volume limited, or pressure control ventilation, where a preset minimum breath rate is delivered along with a preset pressure limit.

Pressure regulated volume control (PRVC) combines the attributes of pressure control ventilation with a volume guarantee. In this mode, the ventilator guarantees a preset minute ventilation. In PRVC, the ventilator monitors the airway resistance and compliance of the lungs and adjusts the inspiratory pressure level via a predetermined algorithm to deliver a preset volume limit. PRVC provides the benefit of a stable minute ventilation while providing the opportunity to use a decelerating inspiratory flow pattern. This approach, in essence, utilizes the benefits of both volume control and pressure control ventilation. It has been shown to decrease peak inspiratory pressures in congenital heart diseasse (CHD) patients and reduce inspired oxygen concentration needs.[66]

Spontaneous Breaths

Spontaneous breathing may be supported with continuous positive airway pressure (CPAP), a mode in which the ventilator maintains a constant airway pressure throughout inspiration and expiration. A preset expiratory pressure limit prevents the patient from exhaling down to atmospheric pressure at end-expiration. Continuous or demand flow during inspiration maintains airway pressure above atmospheric pressure. Raising the expiratory pressure above atmospheric pressure increases end-expiratory lung volume (EELV) proportionate to the pressure applied and total respiratory compliance. The CPAP mode can be used alone or in conjunction with mechanical breaths. Of note, when used in combination with mechanical breaths, the term positive end-expiratory pressure (PEEP) is used instead of CPAP.

Pressure support ventilation (PSV) is a spontaneous breathing mode that can be used alone or in combination with other modes (synchronized intermittent mandatory ventilation [SIMV], CPAP). A preset level of inspiratory pressure is delivered above the baseline end-expiratory pressure with each spontaneous respiratory effort. PSV is initiated when pressure or flow decreases to the preset threshold level during inspiration. When this trigger is sensed by the ventilator, flow accelerates into the breathing circuit and increases proximal airway pressure to the preset pressure level. The pressure support breath is usually terminated when flow decreases to 25% of peak flow.[76] The tidal volume delivered in this mode will vary with changes in lung compliance, airway resistance, pressure support, and inspiratory time.

Volume support (VS) combines the benefits of pressure support ventilation with a volume guarantee during spontaneous breathing. The ventilator monitors airway resistance and pulmonary compliance and adjusts the pressure support level using a predetermined algorithm to deliver a preset minute ventilation. In this mode, the pressure used to deliver the tidal volume is automatically adjusted (a dependent variable).

Combined Breaths

Intermittent mandatory ventilation (IMV) and synchronized intermittent mandatory ventilaton (SIMV) modes combine mechanical breaths with spontaneous breaths. SIMV differs from IMV by synchronizing the initiation of the mechanical breaths with the patient's spontaneous effort. The use of non-synchronized IMV has dramatically decreased because the lack of patient-ventilator synchrony results in patient discomfort and increased work of breathing. Improvements in technology have enabled most ventilators to be synchronized to the patient's respiratory effort.

Flow for spontaneous breathing may be provided by a continuous flow of gas through the breathing circuit, a demand valve, or a combination of both. If PEEP is applied with continuous and demand flow, the spontaneous breaths become CPAP breaths. Pressure support is often administered in conjunction with SIMV.

Neonatal and Pediatric Ventilators

In this classification system, the mechanical breaths produced by most neonatal ventilators would be considered constant flow, time triggered, time cycled, and pressure limited breaths. Advances in neonatal ventilator design now provide the option of most modes that are available on pediatric and adult ventilators.[9] Improvements in calibration and the measurement of smaller volumes facilitate volume limited mechanical SIMV breaths with CPAP or pressure support for the spontaneous breaths.[1,70] Mechanical breaths can be pressure- or flow-triggered, time cycled, and volume or pressure limited. Spontaneous breaths are constant flow, CPAP or variable flow, pressure supported breaths.[124] The primary difference between neonatal and pediatric/adult ventilators is the range of flows and volumes the ventilator can deliver. Neonatal ventilators are able to deliver lower flows and volumes at faster rates, and deliver breaths with a shorter response time to patient-triggered effort. Pediatric ventilators are essentially the same ventilators used in adults, only at lower ranges of flow and volume.

As technology advances, the ventilator manufacturers are designing ventilators that are capable of ventilating patients ranging from small neonates to large adults. Table 12-1 contains the common classifications of mechanical ventilator breaths by mode of ventilation.

Output Waveform Analysis

Before waveform graphics became integral components of ventilator systems, ventilator monitoring was restricted to reading the ventilator's controls, digital monitors, and mechanical gauges as well as physical assessment. Detailed analysis of the patient/ventilator interface was, therefore, impossible. Technological advances now permit continuous monitoring of respiratory mechanics including displays of gas flow, volume delivery, and airway pressure. Output waveforms are a useful tool for understanding the characteristics of ventilator operation and provide a graphic display of the various modes of ventilation.[123] Waveform analysis can be used to optimize mechanical ventilatory support and analyze ventilator incidents and alarm conditions. Using this technology, it is possible to tailor the form of ventilatory support, improve patient-ventilator synchrony, reduce patient work of breathing, and calculate a variety of physiologic parameters related to respiratory mechanics.

The most useful waveforms are flow, pressure, and volume graphed over time. Convention dictates that positive values correspond to inspiration and negative values to expiration; horizontal axes represent time in seconds and vertical axes represent the measured variable in its common unit of measurement. Optimal measurements are obtained when the pressure and flow monitoring device is positioned between the endotracheal tube and the ventilator circuit.[20,123] Measurements may also be obtained from the inspiratory or expiratory limbs of the ventilatory circuit. Integration of intrapleural pressure from an esophageal balloon further enhances graphic data and enables assessment of the patient's work of breathing.

Table 12-1 Classification of Modes of Positive-Pressure Ventilation Used for Cardiac Patients

MODE	Mechanical Breath Variables			Spontaneous Breath Variables		
	Trigger	Cycle	Limit	Trigger	Cycle	Limit
Control ventilation	Time Flow Pressure	Time	Volume Pressure	—	—	—
Synchronized intermittent mandatory ventilation (SIMV)	Time Flow Pressure	Time	Volume Pressure	Flow Pressure	Flow	Pressure
Supported ventilation (PSV or VS)	—	—	—	Flow Pressure	Flow	Pressure Volume

PSV, pressure support ventilation; VS, volume support

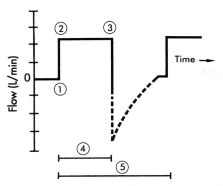

FIGURE 12-2 Inspiratory flow graphic of a square wave mechanical breath. 1 represents the initiation of flow from the ventilator; 2, peak inspiratory flow; 3, end inspiration; 4, inspiratory time; and 5, total cycle time. Positive deflections indicate flow from the ventilator to the patient. (Modified from MacIntyre NR, Ho L: Weaning mechanical ventilatory support. *Anesth Report* 3:211–215, 1990.)

During spontaneous breathing, patient effort, work of breathing, and the level of intrinsic PEEP are best evaluated using esophageal pressure measurements.[82]

In addition to plotting flow, pressure, and volume versus time, each of these parameters can be plotted against each other. Pressure-volume and flow-volume loops can be particularly helpful in assessing alterations in resistance or compliance, work of breathing, overdistention of the lung, and intrinsic PEEP (PEEP$_i$).

Flow Graphics

Flow sensors should be capable of measuring a wide range of flows (−300 to +150 L/min) and be resistant to motion artifact, moisture, and respiratory secretions.[78] The flow graphic has two distinct parts: inspiratory flow and expiratory flow. The inspiratory flow graphic displays the magnitude, duration, and flow pattern of the positive-pressure breath or spontaneous breath. Figure 12-2 is a theoretical inspiratory flow pattern of a continuous flow mechanical breath. In actual application, flow delivery mechanisms have response times that alter the shape of the flow graphic. These response times result in a positive slope at the start of inspiration and a negative slope at end-inspiration (Fig. 12-3). Graphical flow analysis can also be affected by back pressure in the patient-ventilator circuit. Third-generation ventilators with low internal compliance and increased driving pressures are less

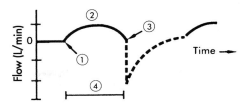

FIGURE 12-4 Inspiratory flow graphic of a spontaneous breath. 1 represents the start of inspiration; 2, peak inspiratory flow; 3, end inspiration; and 4, inspiratory time. Inspiratory flow from the patient to the ventilator by convention is represented as a positive deflection. (Modified from MacIntyre NR, Ho L: Weaning mechanical ventilatory support. *Anesth Report* 3:211–215, 1990.)

responsive to changes in back pressure, but significant alterations in lung compliance and airway resistance may affect the shape of the flow graphic.

The flow graphic of a spontaneous breath is demonstrated in Figure 12-4. The characteristic of the flow graphic is determined by the characteristics of the patient's inspiratory demand and the ventilatory support provided to the spontaneous breath (i.e., continuous flow CPAP, demand flow CPAP, and/or pressure support).

The expiratory flow of gas is passive for both mechanical and spontaneous breaths. (Although in some modes, e.g., PSV, the patient are able to forcibly exhale and thus assist exhalation.) The magnitude, duration, and pattern of the expiratory graphic are determined by the resistance of both the patient's respiratory system and the ventilator circuit. Important features of the ventilator circuit that affect the flow graphic include the size and length of the endotracheal tube, internal diameter and length of the ventilator circuit, resistance of the expiratory valve, and distensibility of the circuit itself. Figure 12-5 represents a typical expiratory flow graphic for a positive-pressure breath. The expiratory flow, by convention, is shown below the zero baseline. Since the characteristics of the patient circuit that affect the expiratory flow pattern are generally fixed, dramatic changes in the expiratory flow curve may be attributable to changes in the patient's compliance, resistance, or activity. For example, an increase in airway resistance due to obstructive disease or secretions may

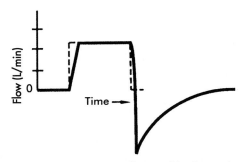

FIGURE 12-3 Constant inspiratory flow graphic of a mechanical breath, modified by ventilator response time. Note the phase shift and alteration in shape of the flow curve during inspiration. (Modified from MacIntyre NR, Ho L: Weaning mechanical ventilatory support. *Anesth Report* 3:211–215, 1990.)

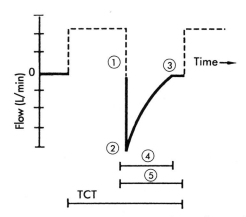

FIGURE 12-5 Representation of a normal expiratory flow graphic. 1 represents the start of expiration; 2, peak expiratory flow; 3, end expiratory flow; 4, duration of expiratory flow; and 5, expiratory time. Expiratory flow from the patient to the ventilator by convention is represented as a negative deflection. TCT, total cycle times. (Modified from MacIntyre NR, Ho L: Weaning mechanical ventilatory support. *Anesth Report* 3:211–215, 1990.)

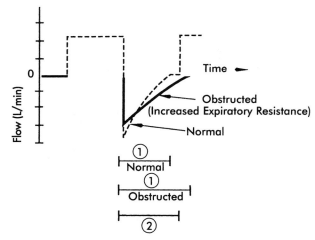

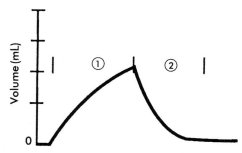

FIGURE 12-8 Volume graphic of a volume-control mechanical breath. 1 represents time for inspiration, while 2 represents expiratory time. The volume that is delivered to the patient during inspiration is the delivered inspiratory volume. The volume that returns during expiration is the expiratory volume. (Modified from MacIntyre NR, Ho L: Weaning mechanical ventilatory support. *Anesth Report* 3:211–215, 1990.)

FIGURE 12-6 Abnormal expiratory flow graphic in a patient with airway obstruction. The expiratory flow exceeds the available expiratory time, and exhalation is not complete. If expiratory time is short (as occurs in the expiratory waveform marked *obstructed*), premature termination of exhalation will occur with resultant gas trapping and increased dead space/tidal volume ratio. "Normal" time (1) equals normal patient expiratory time. "obstructed" time (1) is prolonged patient expiratory time secondary to obstruction. Time (2) represents mechanical time for expiration. (Modified from MacIntyre NR, Ho L: Weaning mechanical ventilatory support. *Anesth Report* 3:211–215, 1990.)

result in decreased peak expiratory flow, increased duration of flow, or failure of flow to return to baseline (Fig. 12-6).

Pressure Graphics

Although resistance of the endotracheal tube is a component of the pressure graphic, pressures measured are generally considered to reflect airway pressure (P_{aw}). In a typical pressure triggered breath from a demand-flow valve, there is a slight pressure drop at the beginning of inspiration, and the magnitude of the drop is proportionate to the patient's peak inspiratory flow rate, sensitivity of the demand valve, and response of the flow delivery system. (This pressure drop usually is not seen in a flow triggered breath.) During a mechanically supported breath, the peak inspiratory pressure is determined by the patient and circuit compliance, resistance, delivered tidal volume, and inspiratory flow (Fig. 12-7). Baseline pressure reflects the expiratory pressure in the circuit (i.e., PEEP or CPAP). The pressure-time graphic is useful for evaluating the stability of PEEP in the presence of an air leak.

Volume Graphics

Volume is generally measured by integrating the flow signal with inspiratory time (Fig. 12-8). The upsweep of the graphic represents the volume delivered to the patient and/or circuit. The downsweep of the graphic represents the total expiratory volume. Typically, inspiratory and expiratory volumes should be equal. Nevertheless, it is not uncommon in infants and children with uncuffed endotracheal tubes for the expiratory volume to be less than the inspiratory volume. An actual percentage leak can be calculated and may aid in the decision to change the endotracheal tube size.

Patient-Ventilator Synchrony

The timing sequence of various respiratory events can be determined by displaying volume, flow, and pressure over time (Figs. 12-9 and 12-10). Comparisons of all three graphics simultaneously facilitate analysis of ventilator-patient interactions. Ventilator dys-synchrony becomes evident when the timing and magnitude of flow, pressure, and volume are disproportionate or delayed.

Ventilator Parameters and Alarm Systems

Parameters In critically ill children, ventilator parameters should be measured and recorded by trained personnel approximately every 6 hours. Spontaneous tidal volume and respiratory rate are a reflection of circuit characteristics, respiratory system compliance and resistance, and respiratory muscle function. Assessment of mechanical tidal volume and preset rate assures delivery of the prescribed alveolar ventilation and facilitates detection of endotracheal or ventilator circuit leaks. Inspiratory time is selected by the clinician to facilitate patient comfort and synchronous breathing during PPV. The patient's age and respiratory pattern are major considerations in the selection of inspiratory time. Recommended inspiratory times by age group are as follows:

Newborns: 0.3 to 0.5 seconds
Toddlers: 0.5 to 0.75 seconds
Children: 0.75 to 1.0 seconds
Adults: 0.75 to 1.5 seconds

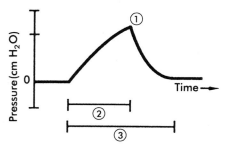

FIGURE 12-7 Pressure graphic of a valved-control mechanical breath. 1 represents the peak inspiratory pressure; 2 is the inspiratory time; and 3, duration of positive pressure. (Modified from MacIntyre NR, Ho L: Weaning mechanical ventilatory support. *Anesth Report* 3:211–215, 1990.)

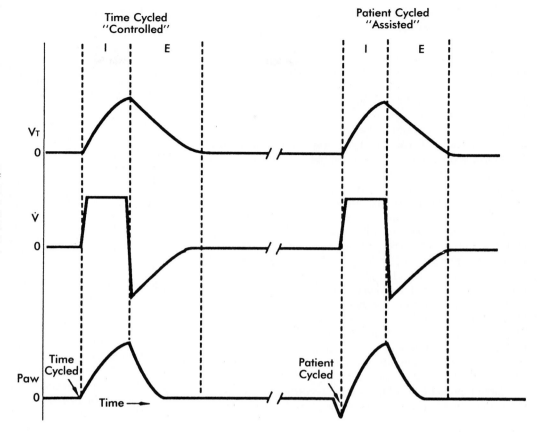

FIGURE 12-9 Graphical orientation of volume, flow, and pressure of mechanical volume control and volume assist breaths. E, expiratory; I, inspiration; Paw, airway pressure; $\dot{V}$, flow, V_T, tidal volume. (Modified from MacIntyre NR, Ho L: Weaning mechanical ventilatory support. *Anesth Report* 3:211–215, 1990.)

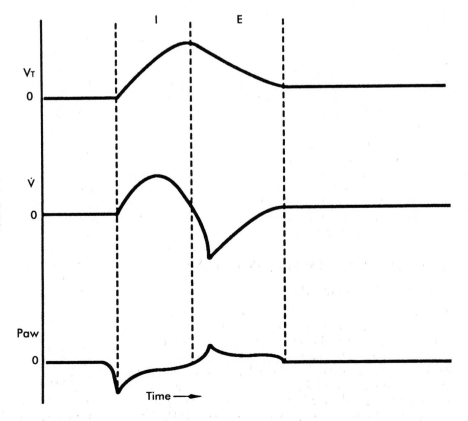

FIGURE 12-10 Graphical orientation of volume, flow, and pressure of a spontaneous breath. E, expiratory; I, inspiration; Paw, airway pressure; $\dot{V}$, flow; V_T, tidal volume. (Modified from MacIntyre NR, Ho L: Weaning mechanical ventilatory support. *Anesth Report* 3:211–215, 1990.)

Total cycle time is the time allotted for one complete inspiratory (I) and expiratory (E) cycle. I:E ratio is an expression of the set inspiratory time and the remaining expiratory cycle time. Recommended I:E ratios vary greatly with ventilator rate. Ratios of 1:2 or 1:3 are most desirable, but should be no lower than 1:1 in assisted ventilation to allow adequate time for exhalation. Peak flow should be titrated to the spontaneous demands of the patient.

Peak inspiratory pressures during volume-limited ventilation are a reflection of volume, flow, inspiratory time, airway resistance, and respiratory system compliance. Peak inspiratory pressures vary with alterations in the patient's respiratory physiology. The presence of airway secretions, bronchospasm, tubing kinks, pneumothorax, agitation, and decreased lung compliance all may increase peak inspiratory pressures. Decreased peak pressures reflect an air leak around the endotracheal tube, a leak in the ventilator circuit, or an improvement in the child's lung mechanics. Peak pressure is not an indicator of changes in patient condition with time-cycled, pressure-limited ventilation.

Mean airway pressure closely reflects alveolar pressure and is an important indicator of the degree of PPV required to achieve adequate oxygenation. Mean airway pressure is principally a function of inspiratory time and PEEP; however, tidal volume, peak inspiratory pressure, inspiratory flow pattern, and ventilator rate also play a role.

Plateau pressure is obtained by recording the pressure following an inspiratory hold maneuver. Plateau pressure reflects the compliance of the lung without gas flow and eliminates the airway resistance component. A pleateau pressure must be obtained with a constant inspiratory flow pattern and cannot be measured in the presence of an air leak.

Positive end-expiratory pressure is produced by closure of the ventilator expiratory valve. The volume of gas remaining in the lung is proportionate to the end-expiratory pressure and the patient's compliance. Increasing the volume of gas increases EELV.

Alarms Ventilator alarm systems have improved dramatically with microprocessor technology.[72] Input power alarms notify clinicians of changes in electrical or pneumatic supplies. Control circuit alarms notify the clinician of incompatible parameters or that the ventilator self-test has failed. Output alarms indicate unacceptable levels of ventilator output, including peak airway pressure, end-expiratory pressure, volume, flow, minute ventilation, respiratory rate, and inspired gas concentration. FiO_2 should be analyzed continuously with high and low alarm limits set to prevent inadvertent hypoxemia or hyperoxemia.

Nonconventional Modes of Ventilation

High-Frequency Ventilation

High-frequency ventilation (HFV) refers to a variety of technologies that use "low" tidal volumes and high ventilatory frequencies to minimize the effects of increased peak pressure. If HFV is to be effective, adequate alveolar ventilation must be provided despite delivered tidal volumes that may be less than dead space volume. HFV consists of a variety of ventilatory strategies including high-frequency oscillatory ventilation (HFOV) and high-frequency jet ventilation (HFJV).

High-Frequency Oscillatory Ventilation

HFOV utilizes an electrically powered piston diaphragm oscillator to alternate positive and negative pressures in the airway. With use of this diaphragm, tidal volumes between 1 and 3 mL/kg are generated with cycles ranging from 240 to 900 beats per minute (4 to 15 Hz). During HFOV, inspiration and expiration are both active and occur above and below the mean airway pressure baseline. HFOV has been used successfully in neonates with respiratory distress syndrome and children with acute respiratory distress syndrome (ARDS).[2,3,27,117] HFOV has also been used successfully in air leak syndrome in both neonates and children. Recently, HFOV has been approved for use in adults.

The exact mechanisms of gas exchange during HFOV remain controversial. The potential mechanisms include convective gas transport, coaxial flow, Taylor dispersion, molecular diffusion, and the Pendelluft effect.[17,22,42,56,61,93,114,126] Conventional bulk flow is responsible for gas delivery to the larger airways and potentially to the alveoli close to these larger airways. Coaxial flow is the bidirectional flow of gas in the airways at the same time. A net flow of gas can occur in one direction through the center of the airway and in the other direction in the area closer to the airway wall. Taylor dispersion describes gas flow along the front of a high-velocity gas flow. Gas transport occurs as a result of gas dispersion beyond the bulk flow front. Molecular diffusion is known to occur at the alveolar level during conventional ventilation, and enhanced diffusion may play a role during high-frequency ventilation. The Pendelluft effect is the phenomenon of intraunit gas mixing due to the impedance difference among lung units.

Any strategy that results in increased mean airway pressure may result in rapid transmission of the increased intrathoracic pressure to the cardiovascular structures, and subsequently to cardiovascular compromise. HFOV should be used with caution in patients with congenital heart disease associated with passive pulmonary blood flow and/or right ventricular dysfunction, since these patients may be sensitive to the resulting higher mean airway pressures. Because HFOV is not often used in patients following cardiac surgery, a further discussion of HFOV is beyond the scope of this chapter.

High-Frequency Jet Ventilation

Most HFJV systems use a high-pressure, air-oxygen gas source that generates gas flow. A rapid solenoid valve allows for flow interruption, which regulates the frequency of ventilation.[18] A reducing valve is present that allows adjustments of inspiratory driving pressure from 10 to 50 psi. The current US Food and Drug Administration–approved HFJV system (Bunnell Life Pulse Ventilator, Bunnell, Inc., Salt Lake City, UT) requires a second ventilator in tandem.

During HFJV, peak inspiratory pressures can be controlled from 8 to 50 cm H_2O, inspiratory time from 20 to 40 msec, and respiratory rate from 150 to 600 insufflations/min. The PEEP and sigh breaths are regulated by the tandem ventilator. Previously, a specific endotracheal tube was necessary for HFJV, which required reintubation. This is no longer required, as specific jet adapters are now used.

Effect on Gas Exchange Although the mechanism of gas exchange during HFJV has not been well defined, convection streaming and enhanced molecular diffusion are known to occur.[18] Simply defined, convection streaming is the flow of gas in a bulk flow manner to the level of the alveoli. Gas is injected into the airway at high speed during HFJV. The gas molecules located in the center of the inspired gas travel faster than those at the edges (asymmetric velocity profiles). Exhalation is passive and promoted by an extremely short inhalation time (20 to 40 msec) and long exhalation times. The exhaled gas travels at a slower velocity than the inspired gas. When exhaled gas encounters the rapidly moving inspired gas, it is extruded along the tracheal walls. The net result is continuous exhalation of gas around the inspired gas. Molecular diffusion is the rapid kinetic motion of molecules and occurs in the terminal bronchioles and alveoli. A variety of other theories have been proposed to explain the ability of HFJV to provide adequate ventilation at tidal volumes below dead space.[18]

Carbon Dioxide Elimination During PPV, manipulations in minute ventilation, ventilatory rate, and tidal volume allow alterations in CO_2 elimination. During HFJV, CO_2 elimination is governed by the relationship $(V_T)^a \times f^b$, where V_T = tidal volume, f = frequency.[41] In this relationship, a ranges from 1.5 to 2.5 and b from 0.5 to 1.0. Because $a > b$, alveolar ventilation during HFJV has a greater dependency on alterations in tidal volume than frequency.

The primary method of eliminating CO_2 during HFJV is by increasing the delivered tidal volume. Increasing the delivered tidal volume can be accomplished by increasing the inspiratory pressures during HFJV. This increases alveolar ventilation and may improve ventilation/perfusion matching. If atelectasis develops, increasing the PEEP (i.e., mean airway pressure) may help recruit lung volume. PEEP is adjusted during HFJV on the tandem ventilator. The tandem ventilator is usually set to administer 0 to 10 sigh breaths per minute. The sigh breath should be set at a peak pressure less than that set on the HFJV (HFJV breaths are not interrupted), and should not exceed 30 cm H_2O. In patients, sigh breaths are designed to prevent atelectasis and allow for appropriate recruitment of lung volume. Alternatively, EELV may be maintained without any sigh breaths if the PEEP (i.e., mean airway pressure) is titrated upward. When the $PaCO_2$ becomes elevated, increasing the HFJV peak pressure (i.e., tidal volume) may be necessary to increase alveolar ventilation.

During HFJV, tidal volume is dependent on the respiratory frequency, which also affects CO_2 elimination. When the respiratory frequency is increased, a reduction of tidal volume may occur, resulting in decreased tidal alveolar ventilation.[41] Therefore, under certain conditions, increasing the respiratory frequency may result in a reduction in alveolar ventilation. For these reasons, manipulations of tidal volume remain the most important determinate of alveolar ventilation during HFJV.

In premature infants, HFJV is initiated at frequencies of 360 to 480 insufflations/min. This can be accomplished since the premature lung has a short time constant and b approximates 1.0. In premature infants, increasing the respiratory frequency results in improved alveolar ventilation. In older patients and those with compliant lungs, the lung has a longer time constant and b approaches 0.5. In comparison to premature patients, increasing the respiratory frequency in older patients and patients with normal compliance results in a reduction of the delivered tidal volume and an overall reduction of alveolar ventilation. For these reasons, HFJV is

usually begun at a frequency of 240 to 300 insufflations/min in children with respiratory or cardiovascular dysfunction.

Lung Volumes During HFJV, lung volumes do not vary dramatically because peak pressures are low, inspiratory time is short, and mean airway pressure is constant. Mean lung volume is determined by the mean airway pressure. Therefore, lung volumes remain relatively static around the mean lung volume. During HFJV, oxygenation is primarily dependent upon mean airway pressures, and increasing mean airway pressures will increase lung volume and improve ventilation-perfusion ($\dot{V}/\dot{Q}$) matching. Mean airway pressure is most affected by increasing the PEEP on the tandem ventilator. Peak inspiratory pressure of the jet ventilator and the tidal volume and rate of the sigh breaths play a lesser role.

Effect on Cardiovascular Parameters The primary physiologic effect of HFJV is improved ventilation at equivalent mean airway pressures developed during conventional mechanical ventilation. Therefore, during HFJV the mean airway pressures can be reduced while maintaining alveolar ventilation and CO_2 clearance, thus limiting the potential adverse effects of positive intrathoracic pressure on cardiovascular performance.[18,85,91]

High-Frequency Jet Ventilation Setup The Bunnell Life Pulse Ventilator is set up in tandem with a positive pressure ventilator. For most infants and children with CHD, the HFJV is set at a rate of 240 to 300 and an inspiratory time of 20 msec. Peak inspiratory pressures and FiO_2 are set to similar values to those used during PPV. The positive-pressure ventilator is set in the SIMV mode at a rate of 0 to 10 breaths per minute and a delivered tidal volume of 6 to 8 cc/kg. The PEEP is set to similar values used during PPV. Adjustments are made according to the principles outlined in the previous sections.

Negative Pressure Ventilation

Negative pressure ventilation (NPV) can be used in patients after surgery for CHD and in pediatric patients with respiratory dysfunction.[64,111,112] Currently, NPV is usually performed using a chest cuirass that covers the patient's chest and abdomen. Negative pressure is generated within this cuirass. Such cuirass devices avoid the limitations of body tank devices (iron lung type devices), which are rarely used today. The advantage of NPV is that intubation is avoided, sedation requirements may be decreased, and systemic venous return may be improved. However, the disadvantage of NPV is that left ventricular afterload may be increased. The regulation of respiratory parameters during NPV, including inspiration/ expiration ratios, can be difficult. NPV is not routinely used in patients with CHD; however, it may be an effective technique in patients with passive pulmonary blood flow such as following Glenn shunt and Fontan procedures.[111,112]

CARDIORESPIRATORY INTERACTIONS

Providing adequate oxygenation can be accomplished only by understanding how the cardiorespiratory system functions as a unit and how alterations in the respiratory system lead to changes in cardiovascular function.

In patients with CHD, alterations in intrathoracic pressures are transmitted to cardiac structures and can dramatically alter cardiovascular performance. Alterations in cardiovascular performance may be more dramatic in neonates and children than in adults for a number of reasons. First, ventricular dysfunction can be particularly severe in infants and children after cardiac surgery. In infants, the myocardium is immature, intrinsically noncompliant, and surgical interventions frequently require transmyocardial incisions and intracardiac repair. Also, congenital cardiac surgery may require the placement of prosthetic material into the heart, which can disrupt normal myocardial architecture and function, resulting in myocardial injury, myocardial edema, and abnormal ventricular function. These factors cause the neonatal myocardium to be more sensitive to alterations in preload and afterload after cardiac surgery.

A second factor is myocardial wall tension. The myocardium of neonates and young children generates a low pressure. Therefore, small changes in intrathoracic pressure can lead to relatively large changes in transmural pressure ($P_{transmural} = P_{intracardiac} - P_{pleural}$). In contrast, the adult myocardium generates a higher intraventricular pressure resulting in only minimal changes in the transmural pressure for a given change in intrathoracic pressure. Transmural pressure affects cardiovascular performance since they contribute to myocardial wall tension.[95,105,106] Because changes in intrathoracic pressure result in a more dramatic change in myocardial wall tension, PPV has a more dramatic effect on ventricular function in infants and children compared to adults.

Finally, the pulmonary and systemic circulations of neonates and children are highly reactive to alterations in intrathoracic pressures. Minor changes in intrathoracic pressure and lung volume can alter the afterload imparted on the right and left ventricle resulting in altered ventricular wall stress and performance.

In the following sections, the effects of a variety of respiratory interventions on cardiac function will be enumerated. These sections are not designed to be all-inclusive, but rather to present cardiorespiratory interactions that are clinically relevant to physicians caring for infants and children with CHD. Interested readers are encouraged to review the references provided for a more in-depth review of this topic.[95-97,104]

Effect of Oxygen Administration

A primary goal of the cardiorespiratory system is to deliver oxygen to the tissues. One method to improve oxygen delivery is to increase the oxygen content of the blood by increasing the concentration of inspired oxygen. Oxygen administration results in an increase in both alveolar and arterial oxygen content. Alterations in alveolar and arterial oxygen content independently result in a reduction of pulmonary vascular resistance (PVR). Neonates are more sensitive to alterations in P_AO_2 and PaO_2 than adults. In conditions of increased afterload, a reduction of PVR will decrease right ventricular afterload and lead to an improvement of right ventricular function. These beneficial cardiorespiratory interactions may be used in the perioperative period to assist patients with right ventricular (RV) dysfunction.

A reduction of PVR is not always beneficial. The addition of inspired oxygen can lead to a reduction of PVR and may

increase pulmonary blood flow in the presence of a systemic-to-pulmonary shunt. In conditions of decreased pulmonary flow, this may improve oxygen delivery by increasing oxygen content. In situations of increased pulmonary flow (residual ventricular septal defect (VSD), large patent ductus arteriosus (PDA), hypoplastic left heart syndrome), the increase in pulmonary blood flow occurs at the expense of systemic flow, and a reduction in systemic oxygen delivery may occur. When oxygen delivery falls below a critical level, profound acidosis and death may occur.

Effect of Ventilatory Manipulations on Heart Rate

The institution of PPV has been shown to cause minor changes in heart rate. An increase in lung volume results in a reflex bradycardia that is modest at the usual tidal volumes employed in clinical practice. Excessive tidal volume ventilation will, however, result in a reflex bradycardia that may become clinically significant.

Effect of Ventilatory Manipulations on Right Ventricular Function

Important differences exist between the physiologic response of the right and left ventricles to alterations in intrathoracic pressures and lung volumes.[104] The right ventricle is extremely sensitive to alterations in intrathoracic pressure for a variety of reasons. Systemic venous return to the right atrium (RA) is passive and occurs as a result of a pressure gradient. When the RA pressure is 0 mm Hg or negative, the pressure gradient for venous return is greatest (Fig. 12-11). As RA pressure increases, there is a decreased pressure gradient for venous return, and RV preload falls. During spontaneous breathing, RA pressure is low, impedance to blood flow to

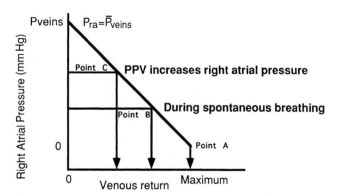

FIGURE 12-11 Venous return to the right heart occurs passively and is dependent on a pressure gradient from the systemic veins to the right atrium. When right atrial pressure (P_{ra}) is zero, there is no impedance to flow back to the right heart and venous return is maximum (Point A). As right atrial pressure is increased, and mean systemic pressure (P_{veins}) is held constant, there is a progressive reduction in venous return. When right atrial pressure exceeds mean systemic venous pressure, venous return ceases. During spontaneous breathing, right atrial pressure is low and systemic venous return is high (Point B). During positive pressure ventilation intrathoracic pressure and right atrial pressure increase resulting in a reduction of venous return (Point C). PPV, positive pressure ventilation; P_{ra}, right atrial pressure; P_{veins}, venous pressure; $\bar{P}_{veins}$, mean venous pressure. (Modified from Pontoppidan H, Geffin B, Lowenstein E: Acute respiratory failure in the adult. 1. *N Engl J Med* 287:690–698, 1972.)

the right heart is low, and venous return is high. Positive-pressure ventilation alters RV preload by increasing intrathoracic pressure. During PPV, the increase in intrathoracic pressure is transmitted to the right heart, resulting in an increase in RA pressure. The increase in RA pressure causes a decreased pressure gradient for venous return, and RV preload decreases. Therefore, PPV reduces RV output by decreasing RV preload.

One determinant of ventricular contractility is myocardial oxygen delivery. In the nonhypertensive right ventricle, coronary flow occurs primarily in systole and is dependent on the systolic pressure difference between the aorta and RV.[48] Because PPV results in increased RV pressure, the pressure difference between the aorta and RV is decreased, and RV coronary flow falls during inspiration. As a result, RV contractility, cardiac output, and oxygen delivery may decrease, especially when the RV end-diastolic pressure is also elevated. Myocardial blood flow is determined by the myocardial perfusion pressure, which depends on intrathoracic, aortic, and RV pressures. An increase in intrathoracic or RV systolic pressure, or a reduction in aortic pressure, will cause a reduction in RV myocardial blood flow. In the majority of clinical conditions, the pressure difference is such that aortic pressure far exceeds RV and intrathoracic pressure, and RV myocardial blood flow is relatively unaffected by PPV. In certain pathophysiologic conditions, including low aortic pressure (i.e., postoperatively), RV dysfunction, and increased intrathoracic pressures, these interactions can become clinically important. When these conditions are present, the adequacy of RV blood flow should be addressed and interventions taken to optimize RV perfusion. These interventions consist of minimizing peak and mean intrathoracic pressures, as well as increasing aortic pressure.

The RV has been shown to be exquisitely sensitive to changes in intrathoracic pressures that alter PVR. Neonates and infants are more sensitive to these changes than adult patients. Modifications of RV afterload through respiratory intervention, as described in a later section, are an important therapeutic option essential in infants and children with RV dysfunction.

Right ventricular afterload is influenced by a variety of intrathoracic processes. One modulator of RV afterload is lung volume (Fig. 12-12). Functional residual capacity (FRC) is the lung volume from which normal tidal ventilation occurs. In restrictive lung disease, diseases such as ARDS, pneumonia, and musculoskeletal abnormalities, EELV is less than the FRC (the normal EELV). At lung volumes above or below FRC, PVR is increased. When EELV is below FRC, vascular resistance is increased by hypoxic pulmonary vasoconstriction and the tortuous course of large- to medium-sized blood vessels that supply the lung; thus PVR is inceased.[11,12] As lung volume increases, the large vessels become linear, their capacitance increases, hypoxia subsides, and vascular resistance decreases. As lung volumes continue to increase above FRC, hyperexpansion of the alveoli and compression of the pulmonary capillaries occur, and vascular resistance increases.[26] The total PVR is the sum of these forces. PVR is elevated at low or high lung volumes and is the lowest when EELV equals functional residual capacity. Positive-pressure ventilation can promote a reduction of RV afterload in patients with low lung volumes by expansion of collapsed lung units and reducing vascular resistance. Alternatively, PPV can result in increased RV afterload

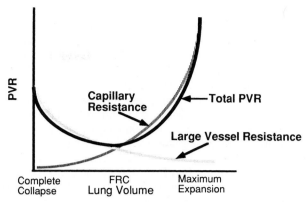

FIGURE 12-12 Pulmonary vascular resistance is dependent on lung volume and the sum of the resistance contributed by the large to medium sized pulmonary vessels and pulmonary capillaries. At lung volumes less than functional residual capacity, pulmonary vascular resistance is high due to hypoxic pulmonary vasoconstriction and the increased resistance contributed by the tortuous large and medium sized vessels. As lung volume increases, pulmonary vascular resistance falls. High lung volumes are associated with an increase in pulmonary vascular resistance due to increased resistance contributed by compression of the pulmonary capillaries. FRC, functional residual capacity, PVR, pulmonary vascular resistance. (Modified from West JB, Dolbry CT, Naimark A: Distribution of blood flow in isolated lung: Relation to vascular and alveolar pressures. *J Appl Physiol* 19:713, 1964.)

due to excessive alveolar expansion and compression of the capillaries.[26] In the normal lung, EELV is maintained at FRC to minimize pulmonary vascular and airway resistance as well as optimize lung compliance. Thus, at FRC the work of matching ventilation and perfusion is minimized. As EELV diverges from FRC the work of V̇/Q̇ matching increases. A primary goal of mechanical ventilation is to maintain EELV at or near FRC.

Effect of Ventilatory Manipulations on Left Ventricular Function

The changes that occur in left ventricular (LV) preload in response to PPV are well understood. Three physiologic principles have been proposed to explain why LV preload is decreased during PPV. First, the LV can eject only the quantity of blood that it receives from the RV.[98] Because right ventricular cardiac output is decreased during PPV, the LV receives a decreased quantity of blood, and LV preload falls. Second, RV afterload and RV systolic pressure increase during PPV.[95] The increase in right ventricular pressure results in conformational changes in the intraventricular septum and a decrease in LV compliance and LV preload. Finally, direct compression of the LV from increased intrathoracic pressure may further reduce preload. Under various circumstances, one or all of the mechanisms may reduce LV preload during PPV. LV intrinsic contractility is not generally altered by ventilatory interventions. When contractility is reduced during ventilatory manipulations, it is secondary to high airway pressures. Increased airway pressures reduce preload and alter afterload resulting in a reduction in cardiac output, myocardial oxygen delivery, and contractility.

LV afterload is altered by ventilator manipulations. One determinant of LV afterload is LV transmural pressure (LVTM).[96] LVTM can be approximated by the difference between the

LV systolic pressure and intrathoracic pressure ($LVTM = P_{LV} - P_{intrathoracic}$).[96,97] LVTM can be reduced by either decreasing aortic pressure and, therefore, LV pressure, or increasing intrathoracic pressure. During PPV, the increase in intrathoracic pressure is rapidly transmitted to the intrathoracic arterial system. LV wall tension remains the same, however, as both the LV pressure generated and the intrathoracic pressure generated are equal. For example, if LV transmural pressure = P_{LV} (100 mm Hg) – $P_{intrathoracic}$ (10 mm Hg) = 90 mm Hg, an increase in intrathoracic pressure by 30 mm Hg causes no net change in LV wall tension, as P_{LV} (130 mm Hg) – $P_{intrathoracic}$ (40 mm Hg) = 90 mm Hg. The extrathoracic arterial system also develops an increase in arterial pressure due to propagation of the increased arterial pressure. When the increase in intrathoracic pressure results in a significant increase in arterial pressure, aortic pressure will be autoregulated due to baroreceptor stimulation.[96,97] This results in a reflex decrease in aortic pressure, and a compensatory reduction of LV pressure occurs. When aortic pressure returns to baseline due to this reflex action, the LV systolic pressure falls and the transmural pressure gradient falls. Using the previous example, if $LVTM = P_{LV}$ (100 mm Hg) – $P_{intrathoracic}$ (10 mm Hg) = 90 mm Hg, with an increase in intrathoracic pressure by 30 mm Hg and a return of aortic pressure to 100 mm Hg, LV wall tension = P_{LV} (100 mm Hg) – $P_{intrathoracic}$ (40 mm Hg) = 60 mm Hg. Therefore, the end result of a persistent increase in intrathoracic pressure is a decrease in LVTM (decreased afterload), as a consequence of aortic pressure autoregulation. Thus, increased intrathoracic pressure decreases LV afterload.

Under usual clinical conditions, intrathoracic pressure is low compared to LV pressure, and inspiration occurs over only one to two cardiac cycles. This results in only minor phasic changes in LV afterload, and, hence, autoregulation may not occur. If intrathoracic pressure is high and the increased intrathoracic pressure occurs over multiple cardiac cycles, LV afterload can be reduced. Clinicians should be aware of these interactions, especially in neonates with LV dysfunction and concomitant respiratory dysfunction. Clinical signs that suggest that a patient may be experiencing these important cardiorespiratory interactions include wide fluctuations in arterial tracing during inspiration. If this is observed and improvements in LV performance are the goal, the clinician should consider respiratory strategies that optimize intrathoracic pressure to augment LV performance.

RESPIRATORY SUPPORT FOR CHILDREN WITH HEART DISEASE: A SYSTEMATIC APPROACH

The application of respiratory support for children with CHD requires balancing the effects of each respiratory intervention on the cardiovascular and respiratory systems. Because of the cardiorespiratory interactions that occur and the diversity of the conditions treated, a single, standardized approach is not appropriate. Respiratory strategies, therefore, should be designed to address the specific pathophysiologic condition of each patient. This section defines respiratory management strategies using the principles outlined previously. First, the initial respiratory support settings will be presented, then a systematic approach will be outlined for pathophysiologic respiratory and cardiovascular conditions.

Goals of Respiratory Support

When the goals of the respiratory system are not met by spontaneous breathing, artificial respiratory support is required.[54] Despite a wide variety of respiratory support, all types of support have two common goals: (1) optimize oxygen delivery by improving the oxygen content of blood (systemic arterial saturation) while decreasing the oxygen needs of the respiratory muscles (i.e., decrease the work of breathing); and (2) improve carbon dioxide elimination. Respiratory support should meet these goals while minimizing the deleterious effects of these interventions on other organ systems.

The initial ventilatory strategy for all patients should be one that is simple, meets the needs of the patient, provides the greatest benefit with the lowest risk for complications, and represents an approach that is familiar to the multidisciplinary intensive care team. The criteria for initiating PPV vary according to the intended goals and the needs of each child.

Perioperative Management

Respiratory support should be initiated when arterial hypoxemia ($SaO_2 < 90\%$ to 92% in the absence of right-to-left intracardiac shunt) and/or alveolar hypoventilation with resultant hypercapnia ($PaCO_2 > 60$ torr in neonates, $PaCO_2 > 55$ torr in children) exists despite pharmacologic therapy and oxygen administration. An additional indication exists when oxygen delivery is inadequate to meet tissue/organ oxygen demand. PPV has been shown to be useful in these conditions by reducing the work of breathing, which subsequently decreases respiratory muscle oxygen consumption and improves the oxygen supply/demand relationship. The beneficial effects of PPV are especially dramatic in patients who have abnormal pulmonary mechanics and in whom an average reduction of oxygen consumption of 25% is achieved.[19,40] PPV reduced lactic acid production in animals with circulatory shock, resulting in the redirection of circulation from respiratory muscles to vital organs.[8,129] The oxygen needs of the respiratory system are high in the newborn period, especially with acute respiratory failure. The withdrawal of either positive or negative pressure ventilatory support in neonatal animals with respiratory failure is associated with a marked alteration in cardiac output attributable to increased work of breathing.[113] For these reasons, it is not unusual for neonates with heart disease to require temporary ventilatory support until medical management can be optimized and the patient can adjust to the physiologic changes in the cardiorespiratory system that occur after birth.

Respiratory support in the postoperative period is an extension of the support initiated in the operating room (Fig. 12-13). Communication between the cardiovascular anesthesiologist, cardiac surgeon, and intensive care team is essential. Upon arrival in the intensive care unit (ICU), communication is directed at determining the surgical procedure, the integrity of the repair, the pathophysiology observed after surgery, and the potential for cardiovascular or respiratory dysfunction.

INITIAL VENTILATOR SETTINGS

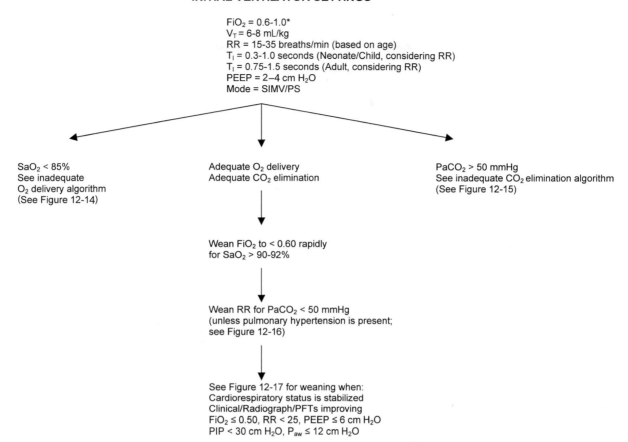

FiO_2 = 0.6-1.0*
V_T = 6-8 mL/kg
RR = 15-35 breaths/min (based on age)
T_I = 0.3-1.0 seconds (Neonate/Child, considering RR)
T_I = 0.75-1.5 seconds (Adult, considering RR)
PEEP = 2–4 cm H_2O
Mode = SIMV/PS

SaO_2 < 85%
See inadequate
O_2 delivery algorithm
(See Figure 12-14)

Adequate O_2 delivery
Adequate CO_2 elimination

$PaCO_2$ > 50 mmHg
See inadequate CO_2 elimination algorithm
(See Figure 12-15)

Wean FiO_2 to < 0.60 rapidly
for SaO_2 > 90-92%

Wean RR for $PaCO_2$ < 50 mmHg
(unless pulmonary hypertension is present;
see Figure 12-16)

See Figure 12-17 for weaning when:
Cardiorespiratory status is stabilized
Clinical/Radiograph/PFTs improving
FiO_2 ≤ 0.50, RR < 25, PEEP ≤ 6 cm H_2O
PIP < 30 cm H_2O, P_{aw} ≤ 12 cm H_2O

*For infants with single ventricle physiology, increased pulmonary
blood flow, and decreased systemic blood flow, a lower FiO_2 may be
indicated. (See text for more details.)

FIGURE 12-13   Decision-making algorithm designed for the initiation of positive-pressure ventilation in patients with two ventricles after uncomplicated cardiac surgery. Initial ventilatory settings are described, and reduction of ventilatory settings is dependent upon resolution of cardiorespiratory dysfunction. I_T, inspiratory time; Paw, mean airway pressure; PEEP, positive end-expiratory pressure; PFTs, pulmonary function tests; PIP, peak inspiratory pressure; RR, respiratory rate (frequency); V_T, tidal volume.

Next, a complete physical examination should be performed with particular attention to the adequacy of the cardiorespiratory system, including clinical assessments of cardiac output and respiratory function.

Patients who are extubated in the operating room or shortly after admission to the ICU should be monitored for the development of hypoxemia, hypercapnia, and/or increased work of breathing. After a period of time, if hypoxemia (SaO_2 < 90% to 92%) or hypercapnia ($PaCO_2$ > 60 torr) is progressive and refractory to conservative therapy (supplemental nasal/mask oxygen, chest physiotherapy), reintubation and the initiation of PPV may be required.

The development of a metabolic acidosis in the postoperative period that is refractory to medical therapy may require reintubation to optimize the oxygen supply/demand relationship. Nevertheless, one should be cautious when using metabolic acidosis as an indicator to institute PPV. Metabolic acidosis is treated by creating a compensatory respiratory alkalosis using PPV, since prescribing a respiratory alkalosis does not address the underlying pathophysiologic disturbance(s).

If the oxygen content is high and respiratory muscle oxygen consumption low, therapy should be directed at augmenting oxygen delivery by improving cardiac output, thereby directly treating the underlying cause of the metabolic acidosis. Mechanical ventilation can decrease oxygen consumption, increase oxygen content, and increase cardiac output, thus favorably altering the supply–demand relationship.

Inspired Oxygen Concentration

Postoperative patients transferred to the ICU on PPV are initially ventilated with an oxygen concentration of 0.60 to 1.0 (unless there is a small alveolar-arterial gradient). One important exception is a patient with single ventricle physiology with signs of increased pulmonary blood flow and decreased systemic blood flow, in which case a "lower" fraction of inspired oxygen is indicated. In these patients oxygen should be supplemented to maintain SaO_2 between 75% and 85%.

During transport, fluid shifts and changes in lung volume with resultant alveolar hypoventilation may occur. The initiation of high inspired oxygen concentrations provides a buffer against the development of hypoxia in patients at risk for ventilation/perfusion mismatch. Once patient transfer has been completed and stable hemodynamics achieved, weaning of the inspired oxygen should begin. Inspired oxygen is reduced when the SaO_2 is >92%, in the absence of a right-to-left intracardiac shunt. Certain conditions (e.g., pulmonary hypertension) may require prolonged administration of high concentrations of inspired oxygen. In the majority of patients, however, a rapid reduction of inspired oxygen to nontoxic levels (FiO_2 <0.50) while maintaining SaO_2 >92% can be accomplished over the initial 12 to 24 hours. The benefits of oxygen administration should be continually balanced against the risks. Arterial hypoxemia should not be tolerated, and a hypoxic patient should receive the appropriate oxygen necessary to reverse hypoxemia. If the patient does not tolerate a reduction of the inspired oxygen concentration to a nontoxic level (FiO_2 <0.50), an aggressive investigation into the etiology of the hypoxemia should be performed. Weaning of inspired oxygen below 0.50 will be discussed in the section on weaning from PPV.

Tidal Volume

In postoperative CHD patients, the delivered tidal volume (V_T) is one of the most important ventilatory parameters set during the initiation of PPV. The optimal V_T is determined by the patient's clinical condition and is adjusted during mechanical breaths by examination of the patient's chest excursions and/or by the use of a pneumotachometer placed at the endotracheal tube.[20] Too frequently, clinicians order a predetermined V_T without examining how effective this V_T moves gas in and out of the lungs. It is worth reiterating that the V_T set on the ventilator may be significantly higher than the V_T the patients actually receives (referred to as the delivered or effective V_T).[20,123] This is a result of the distensibility of the ventilator circuit, air leak, and circuit dead space.[13,20,38,49,83] This problem is magnified in neonates in whom a small change in V_T leads to a large percentage change in effective V_T.[20] For these reasons, the delivered V_T should be set on the ventilator using a pneumotachometer placed at the endotracheal tube (spontaneous breath V_T = 4 to 6 mL/kg, mechanical breath delivered V_T = 6 to 8 mL/kg). The V_T can then be titrated to provide adequate chest excursion and appropriate gas entry as determined by physical exam. The corroboration of adequate gas exchange is then obtained by blood gas analysis. The extremes of tidal volumes should be avoided unless specific pathophysiologic conditions warrant these strategies (see subsequent discussion).

Ventilator Frequency

The ventilator frequency in neonates and young children is initiated at 15 to 35 breaths per minute (bpm). When necessary, hyperventilation can usually be accomplished by increasing V_T but may rarely require increased ventilatory frequencies of greater than 35 bpm. The treatment for alveolar hypoventilation is outlined in the text that follows. Increases in ventilatory frequency above 35 bpm may be associated with inadvertent inverse ratio ventilation and subsequently increased EELV and pulmonary overdistention. These higher ventilatory rates should be used cautiously due to the potential detrimental effects of increased lung volume and intrinsic PEEP on gas exchange and cardiorespiratory performance.

Inspiratory Time

The inspiratory time is set between 0.3 and 1.0 seconds in infants and children, and between 0.75 and 1.5 seconds in adults. A reduction of the inspiratory time below 0.3 seconds does not allow adequate time for the distribution of gas to alveolar units. Prolongation of the inspiratory time in infants may result in an excessively high inspiratory/expiratory ratio. An excessive prolongation of inspiratory time can result in significant elevations in mean airway pressure, decreased venous return, and decreased cardiac output.[29]

Prolongation of the inspiratory time with an increased or reversed inspiratory/expiratory ratio has been advocated as a means of increasing mean airway pressure and recruiting low ventilation/perfusion compartments in diseases involving decreased compliance and lung volumes.[103] Oxygenation improves with elevation of mean airway pressure, regardless of the phasic pattern of airway pressure.[14] The application of PEEP elevates mean airway pressure with less risk of barotrauma and circulatory depression and is the preferred approach in patients with combined cardiovascular and respiratory disease.[92] The precise relationship between inspiratory and expiratory times during PPV must be tailored to address the patient's underlying pathophysiology. As a general guideline, deviation from normal physiologic respiratory patterns with regard to rate and inspiratory time should be avoided.

Positive End-Expiratory Pressure

The application of PEEP is an essential step in providing respiratory support for postoperative patients.[31,99–101] PEEP opens atelectatic regions of the lung, increases end-expiratory lung volume, improves ventilation/perfusion matching, and reduces right-to-left intrapulmonary shunting. The net effect of PEEP is improved oxygenation.[50,119,125] In postoperative patients, PEEP is initiated at 3 to 6 cm H_2O to recruit lung volume and prevent alveolar atelectasis. Increased PEEP should be used in specific conditions, which include (1) severe reductions in lung compliance (ARDS), or (2) excessive pulmonary blood flow in patients with shunt physiology. A reduction of PEEP to less than 3 cm H_2O may result in loss of lung volume with a reduction of compliance, increased PVR, and hypoxemia. High levels of PEEP (>10 cm H_2O) may result in overexpansion of normal lung units, reduced compliance, increased PVR, increased dead space ventilation, and ventilation/perfusion mismatch due to shunting of blood away from normal yet overexpanded alveoli to abnormal alveoli.[28,37,59,68,120,134] High PEEP should, therefore, be avoided unless specifically required for acute lung injury and must be appropriately monitored. In general, in the absence of intrinsic lung disease, children following cardiac surgery do not require PEEP greater than 6 cm H_2O.

Ventilator Mode

A volume-limited SIMV mode (with pressure support) is the preferred initial mode for most postoperative patients.

SIMV provides a stable minute ventilation synchronized with the patient and will reduce the chance of wide swings in ventilation (assuming the patient's spontaneous respiratory rate is relatively constant). A preset V_T will be delivered and peak inspiratory pressures will fluctuate as compliance changes. In the majority of postoperative patients, cardiovascular dysfunction is the dominant pathophysiologic disturbance, and respiratory dysfunction, while present, is usually self-limited. Therefore, volume-limited SIMV usually results in minimal swings in peak airway pressure and stable arterial blood gases, which supports the resolution of cardiovascular dysfunction during postoperative convalescence. As cardiovascular function improves, the respiratory sequelae will resolve. After improvements in cardiorespiratory function, the patient may be converted to full pressure-support ventilation to facilitate weaning. Infrequently, respiratory dysfunction may be severe and high peak airway pressures develop during the use volume-limited SIMV. In these conditions, alternative strategies such as variable flow ventilation (pressure control ventilation or pressure control/pressure support ventilation, or pressure regulated volume control)

should be considered to potentially minimize barotrauma and cardiovascular side effects while maximizing oxygen delivery.

Physiologic Conditions Requiring Alterations in Support

Inadequate Oxygen Delivery

When oxygen delivery is inadequate to meet tissue needs, metabolic acidosis develops. In the postoperative period, inadequate oxygen delivery is usually related to decreased cardiac output from myocardial dysfunction.

If inadequate oxygen delivery results from an intracardiac right-to-left shunt, respiratory interventions play a minor role and are directed at decreasing PVR and/or improving RV function. If the primary cause of the decreased oxygen delivery is a decreased arterial oxygen content, respiratory support is the primary intervention (Fig. 12-14). Alterations in oxygenation are, most commonly, a result of hypoventilation or ventilation/perfusion mismatch.

The transfer of oxygen from inhaled gas to the pulmonary capillaries is dependent upon inspired gas reaching the alveoli,

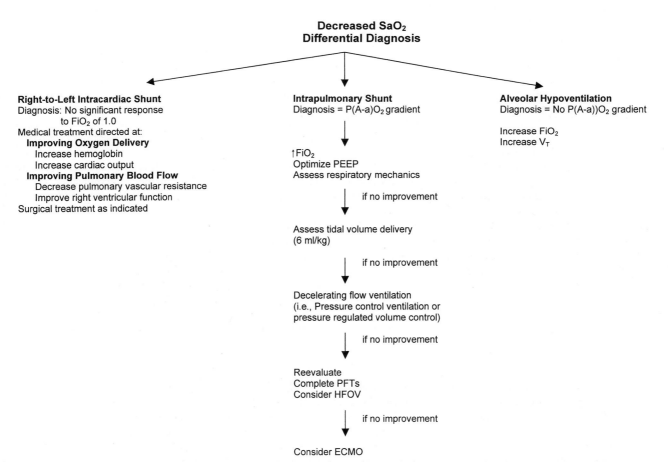

FIGURE 12-14 Decision-making algorithm for postoperative patients who develop decreased oxygen delivery during positive-pressure ventilation. Identification of the cause for the decreased oxygen delivery is the initial step in managing this pathophysiology. Causes of decreased SaO_2 include right-to-left intracardiac shunt or ventilation/perfusion mismatch. ECMO, extracorporeal membrane oxygenation; HFOV, high-frequency oscillatory ventilation; It, inspiratory time; PFTs, pulmonary functions' tests; PVR, pulmonary vascular resistance; RV, right ventricle.

pulmonary blood flow perfusing ventilated alveolar units, the presence of an adequate alveolar-to-capillary oxygen gradient, and the diffusion of oxygen across the alveolar-capillary membrane. Alterations in oxygen transfer occur when the P_{AO_2} in perfused alveolar units falls. This can occur as a result of alveolar hypoventilation (a reduction of P_{AO_2} in normally functioning alveolar units), low ventilation/perfusion ratio (P_{AO_2} falls because of an inability of inspired gas to reach perfused injured alveoli), or high ventilation/perfusion ratio (an inability of pulmonary blood to reach ventilated alveoli).

In the postoperative period, the cause for arterial hypoxemia is often ventilation/perfusion mismatch. Patients with ventilation/perfusion mismatch have restrictive lung disease secondary to alveolar atelectasis and a reduction in lung volumes. This condition can be inferred by demonstrating decreased chest excursion and crackles during inspiration. If the patient is spontaneously breathing, patient-ventilator dyssynchrony and tachypnea may be noted on clinical examination. Chest radiography demonstrates a reduction in lung volumes with evidence of atelectasis. Bedside respiratory mechanics can help to confirm a reduction in lung volumes by demonstrating a decrease in pulmonary compliance and a prolonged recruitment phase in the inspiratory limb of the pressure-volume curve. The diagnosis of a significant intrapulmonary shunt and hypoxemia from ventilation/perfusion mismatch is made by determining the alveolar-to-arterial oxygen gradient. When the patient breathes 100% oxygen for 15 to 30 minutes, the presence of a PaO_2 <400 mm Hg in the absence of intracardiac shunting indicates a clinically significant intrapulmonary shunt.

The systematic approach outlined for conditions with low ventilation/perfusion ratios is directed at decreasing intrapulmonary shunt by increasing lung volumes. Initially, this is accomplished by increasing PEEP to restore collapsed alveolar units and improve compliance. PEEP is increased until there is improvement in arterial hypoxemia or toxicity occurs.[94,120] Excessive PEEP may reduce cardiac output in some children. The reduction of cardiac output due to increasing PEEP is more dramatic in conditions of hypovolemia and/or myocardial dysfunction and can lead to a significant reduction in oxygen delivery.[28,59,120] A worsening of oxygenation has been reported with excessive PEEP, presumably because blood flow is shunted to poorly ventilated alveolar units from overdistended regions of the lung due to a local increase in PVR.[134] These potentially adverse cardiorespiratory effects of PEEP require clinicians to be cautious in applying PEEP levels greater than 10 cm H_2O in children with cardiovascular dysfunction.

During changes in PEEP, strict attention to respiratory parameters including V_T and compliance is warranted. If V_T falls below the level that provides adequate chest excursion, an increase in V_T may be required. If the patient demonstrates hypoxemia despite alterations in PEEP, the V_T should be increased to provide adequate V_T by exam and respiratory mechanics. If the peak airway pressure exceeds 30 to 32 cm H_2O, pressure control ventilation (i.e., decelerating inspiratory flow) should be considered. The use of a decelerating flow pattern will usually result in a lower peak airway pressure, a higher mean airway pressure, and improved oxygenation when compared to volume control ventilation (square wave, constant inspiratory flow). Pressure control ventilation provides a consistent peak pressure but varying V_T depending upon lung compliance. Rapid changes in compliance in either direction can result in wide swings in oxygenation and ventilation, which may be detrimental. For this reason, arterial blood gas measurements and respiratory parameters should be closely monitored during pressure control ventilation, and frequent reevaluation of the clinical condition is warranted. Once respiratory failure has improved and peak airway pressures are less than 30 to 32 cm H_2O, conversion to volume-limited ventilation may be performed to reduce the chance of fluctuations in ventilation. Another approach is to use a mode of ventilation that guarantees minute ventilation/tidal volume while providing a decelerating flow pattern. An example of this is pressure regulated volume control.

If arterial hypoxemia persists, reevaluation of the patient is required. The need for inspired oxygen (FiO_2) >0.60, PEEP > 6–10 cm H_2O, peak airway pressures >32 cm (H_2O_2), and mean airway pressures >15 cm H_2O, in the absence of intracardiac right-to-left shunt, indicates the presence of respiratory failure and may be associated with a poor prognosis in postoperative CHD patients. Physical examination, noninvasive testing, and invasive testing should be directed at reevaluating the possibility of a residual or previously undiagnosed right-to-left intracardiac shunt, inadequate pulmonary blood flow, or left heart abnormalities. If severe respiratory failure continues to be the etiology of the hypoxia, increasing the PEEP, increasing the inspiratory time, or changing to high-frequency ventilation should be considered. One must determine the effects of these maneuvers on cardiac output. This can be done noninvasively by echocardiography. Invasive evaluation includes the measurements of lactic acid and mixed venous saturation.[23,25] Both have been shown to be good indicators of global oxygen delivery.

Attempts have been made to physiologically define "optimal PEEP" in terms of total oxygen delivery. However, defining the optimal PEEP level strictly in terms of oxygen delivery has been criticized because decreased oxygen delivery secondary to a fall in cardiac output with high levels of PEEP can often be reversed by intravascular volume expansion and/or inotropes. Thus, a further enhancement of oxygen delivery may be achieved by higher levels of PEEP if cardiac output is otherwise maintained.[51,90,120,128] The level of PEEP associated with maximal oxygen delivery coincides best with the achievement of ideal lung volume and maximum total respiratory compliance.[120]

The application of "high" levels of PEEP (>10 to 12 cm H_2O), prolongation of the inspiratory time, and high-frequency ventilation, therefore, require continuous evaluation of the cardiorespiratory effects of these manipulations. If refractory hypoxia persists, one should consider high-frequency oscillatory ventilation or extracorporeal life support.

Increased Oxygen Consumption

Patient-ventilator dyssynchrony defines a condition where spontaneous inspiratory efforts by the patient are out of phase with positive pressure breaths delivered by the ventilator, resulting in the patient "fighting" the ventilator. During patient-ventilator dyssynchrony, WOB_i is increased, oxygen consumption of the respiratory muscles may be high, and a reduction in effective V_T may result. In addition, barotrauma may occur and cardiac afterload may be adversely affected. The clinical diagnosis is made by observing the patient breathing spontaneously with the ventilator or by monitoring airway graphics. If dys-synchrony continues, oxygenation and ventilation may deteriorate. When patient-ventilator dys-synchrony is significant, primary hypoxemia due to ventilation/perfusion mismatch, mucous plugging, pneumothorax, and reactive airways disease must be eliminated as the etiology. When these causes are eliminated, altering the ventilator mode, changing the inspiratory flow pattern, improving the ventilator trigger sensitivity, or increasing overall ventilator support may improve patient-ventilator synchrony. When manipulation in the ventilator parameters does not improve patient-ventilator synchrony, increased sedation should be attempted. When sedation is instituted/increased, spontaneous ventilation may reduce or cease, and thus, ventilatory support must be increased to ensure appropriate gas exchange. Persistence of dys-synchrony after these maneuvers may necessitate a trial of neuromuscular blockade. This is rarely required and should be reserved for patients with uncontrollable dys-synchrony and elevated airway pressures.

Following cardiac surgery the impaired myocardium can be "protected" by judicious management of mechanical ventilation. Obviously, if respiratory function is completely furnished by the ventilator, there will be no respiratory muscle effort. Subsequently, work of breathing, and the cardiac work associated with this, will be reduced. Using the ventilator to maintain the EELV near FRC will minimize the work of $\dot{V}/\dot{Q}$ matching. Preventing patient-ventilator dys-synchrony will prevent increased RV afterload and decreased preload while minimizing barotrauma. Finally, alleviation of LV afterload by eliminating negative intrathoracic pressure may also be beneficial.

Inadequate Carbon Dioxide Elimination

Another goal of the respiratory system is the removal of carbon dioxide generated from the tissue metabolic processes. When carbon dioxide elimination is inadequate, hypercapnia develops. Although hypoxemia is the most frequently observed abnormality in the immediate postoperative period, hypercapnia frequently occurs in the weaning phase. Hypercapnia can have profound effects on a variety of organ systems including alterations in pulmonary vascular resistance, myocardial performance, and catecholamine release. Inadequate carbon dioxide elimination is a result of inadequate minute ventilation or increased alveolar dead space.

Hypercapnia occurs if total minute ventilation is decreased or if dead space ventilation (V_D) is increased. The latter is more common in children with heart disease. Because dead space is ventilated but not perfused, lung, alterations in cardiac output and pulmonary perfusion can change dead space. In low cardiac output states, lung perfusion is low and hypercapnia in the face of normal total minute ventilation indicates increased V_D. If pulmonary perfusion can be increased in this setting, $PaCO_2$ should decrease (all other factors being the same). Because the lung is perfused primarily during expiration, an adequate expiratory time is critical. Therefore, increasing positive pressure ventilation may actually increase V_D and worsen hypercapnia if expiratory time is shortened. Collapsed alveoli require a higher transpulmonary pressure to increase their diameter in comparison to open alveolar units. Therefore, a given volume of inspired gas is distributed primarily to open alveoli, and overdistension may occur.

Overdistension compresses capillaries, decreases perfusion, and results in increased dead space ventilation (V_D). The volume of inspired gas that results in overdistention does not contribute to gas exchange and results in increased dead space ventilation and increased volutrauma. As a result of these abnormalities, alveolar minute ventilation (volume of gas involved in gas exchange per unit time) falls. Large to medium airway obstruction results from airway plugging with secretions or kinking of the endotracheal tube and represents a physical barrier preventing inspired gas from reaching the alveoli.

In all patients with hypercapnia, before the initiation of respiratory interventions, a comprehensive examination of the respiratory system is required. Patients with inadequate ventilation or obstruction of medium to large airways have a decreased gas entry to alveoli. The clinical manifestations will be dominated by decreased alveolar ventilation (V_A). Tachypnea and tachycardia will be present in the majority of patients with significant hypercapnia. Because patients with inadequate alveolar ventilation and hypercapnia increase work of breathing, they may also demonstrate patient-ventilator dyssynchrony. These patients attempt to compensate for an inadequate V_A by increasing the spontaneous rate and may fight the ventilator. The presence of hypercapnia can lead to systemic arterial hypertension and ventricular ectopy secondary to endogenous catecholamine release. Systemic hypertension, in this clinical scenario, should not be misinterpreted as patient agitation, and administration of sedatives should be avoided until arterial blood gas analysis, clinical assessment, and radiographic assessment are performed. If sedatives are administered to hypercapnic patients, a further reduction in alveolar ventilation may develop and a worsening of hypercapnia can be precipitated.

The examination of the respiratory system in patients with airway obstruction may demonstrate decreased chest excursion and expiratory wheezing. When inefficient ventilation is present, symmetric decreased breath sounds will be present. This is in contrast to patients with mechanical obstruction who may demonstrate asymmetric breath sounds. Chest radiographs in patients with inadequate effective alveolar minute ventilation demonstrate decreased lung volumes throughout all lung fields and diffuse atelectasis. If mechanical obstruction of the large to medium airways is the etiology, larger areas of hypoaeration will be present adjacent to areas of normal aeration. In extreme cases of large airway obstruction, total lobes of the lung can become collapsed.

The pathophysiology of small airway obstruction caused by bronchospasm differs from the previous causes for airway obstruction. When small airway obstruction from bronchospasm occurs, there is an inability of alveolar gas to be expelled from the lungs. This results in increased lung volumes, development of intrinsic PEEP, and an increase in dead space ventilation. On physical examination, these patients have evidence for increased lung volume and in extreme cases may have a barrel chest. A markedly prolonged expiratory phase, expiratory wheezing, and occasionally inspiratory wheezing will be present on auscultation. Chest radiography demonstrates hyperlucent areas of the lung and increased lung volumes. Respiratory mechanics are diagnostic and will show an increase in expiratory resistance and EELV greater than FRC.

The management of mechanical obstruction of the medium to large airways includes chest physiotherapy and suctioning. If this does not result in prompt resolution of

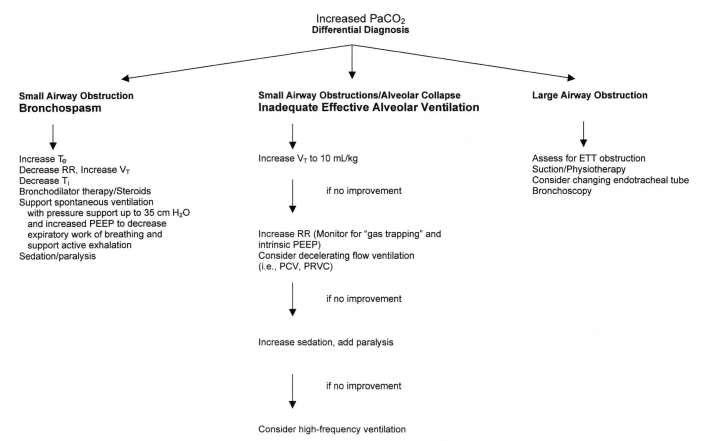

FIGURE 12-15   Decision-making algorithm designed for postoperative patients who develop increased $PaCO_2$. Elevated $PaCO_2$ is a result of inadequate alveolar ventilation. This can be categorized into pathology, which results in small or large airway obstruction or alveolar collapse. Strategies are then dependent upon the underlying pathophysiology. All approaches require an increase in effective alveolar ventilation. T_e, expiratory time; T_i, inspiratory time.

these symptoms, endotracheal tube change or bronchoscopy may be necessary. In the majority of postoperative patients, hypercapnia results from inadequate effective alveolar ventilation secondary to collapsed alveoli and small airways. When this occurs, an appropriate increase in V_T and/or PEEP may be required. Airway pressures should be monitored to ensure that they are not in the toxic range. If the measured V_T is appropriate, an increase in the respiratory frequency should be attempted. Continued hypercapnia may require an increase in sedation or neuromuscular blockade if patient-ventilator dys-synchrony is present.[38,45,47,119] In the presence of continued hypercapnia the V_T should be increased until hypercapnia resolves or until a peak airway pressure of 32 cm H_2O is reached. If hypercapnia continues, one should consider conversion to an alternative mode of ventilation to provide improved effective minute ventilation at a lower peak airway pressure (Fig. 12-15).

Patients with small airway disease require therapy directed at reversing bronchospasm, promoting the ability of retained alveolar gas to be exchanged with inspired gas, and increasing alveolar ventilation. The initial approach should be to increase the expiratory time by reducing the respiratory rate,

while maintaining the inspiratory time in the appropriate physiologic range. When the respiratory rate is reduced, the V_T may be increased to provide an adequate alveolar ventilation. If this does not allow adequate emptying of the alveoli, a reduction of inspiratory time can be attempted. Bronchodilator therapy should be considered early in the management of patients with CHD and small airway obstruction. In these patients, alveolar hyperexpansion and hypercapnia can result in dramatic alterations in cardiovascular function, and aggressive respiratory interventions are required to prevent the development of severe cardiorespiratory failure. Respiratory mechanics are recommended in all patients with significant gas trapping since a variety of management approaches may be necessary.

Therapy for Specific Pathophysiologic Conditions

Left Ventricular Dysfunction

In postoperative patients with LV dysfunction, cardiorespiratory interactions should be evaluated and directed at optimizing

LV function.[32,57,85,88] Because PPV decreases both venous return and LV afterload (which have contrasting effects on cardiac output), careful attention to hemodynamic function is required when ventilating children with LV dysfunction. Maintaining EELV near FRC while minimizing airway pressure will optimize LV function.

The positive end-expiratory pressure and tidal volume (6 to 8 mL/kg) should be titrated to prevent atelectasis. Thoracic pump augmentation of LV filling with the phasic increase in intrathoracic pressure may result in improved LV filling and output.[67,96,97] Thoracic augmentation of LV preload has been demonstrated in infants after surgery for CHD.[86] One potential side effect of thoracic augmentation is increased airway pressures with the risk of volutrauma/barotrauma. Therefore, when thoracic augmentation is used, particular attention should be given to the intrathoracic pressures required to augment LV filling. If high intrathoracic and airway pressures are required, high tidal volume ventilation should be suspended. To accomplish the lowest intrathoracic and mean airway pressures possible, low ventilatory rates are utilized along with short inspiratory time. In most cases, the cardiorespiratory risks of thoracic pump augmentation significantly outweigh the potential benefits.

In neonates and young children, postoperative tachycardia frequently occurs and an increase in intrathoracic pressure may be distributed over multiple cardiac cycles. When this occurs, thoracic augmentation is demonstrated during the initial beat after inspiration. In later beats following PPV there is a reduction in LV filling, and thoracic augmentation does not occur. To optimize thoracic augmentation, therefore, the increase in thoracic pressure should be distributed over two heartbeats; otherwise, side effects will develop and an actual reduction of LV filling can occur.

If patients with LV dysfunction develop pulmonary edema and decreased systemic oxygen saturation, oxygen content may fall and oxygen delivery will be further compromised. In these instances, the hemoglobin should be maintained at a high level and an increased level of inspired oxygen initiated. PEEP should be increased to improve oxygenation while being carefully titrated to ensure enhanced oxygen delivery.

Right Ventricular Dysfunction

Patients with RV dysfunction will benefit from manipulations of cardiorespiratory interactions to optimize RV preload and minimize RV afterload. In patients with RV dysfunction, PPV is initiated with a tidal volume of 6 to 8 mL/kg, a rate of 15 to 20 bpm, FiO_2 = 1.0, and a long expiratory time. RV afterload can be reduced by hyperoxygenation and alkalization if pulmonary hypertension is present. Since the majority of pulmonary blood flow occurs during expiration, inspiratory times should be short compared to expiratory times and low frequency ventilation used. PEEP should be set to maintain EELV and reduce PVR. It is important to maintain EELV near FRC because an EELV less than FRC will result in increased PVR. Patients with RV dysfunction are particularly sensitive to changes in intrathoracic pressure since cardiac output is preload-dependent. These may benefit from ventilation strategies that reduce intrathoracic pressure and increase preload such as reducing the mean airway pressure. This can be accomplished by minimizing end-expiratory

pressure, decreasing inspiratory time, and utilizing the mode of ventilation with the lowest intrathoracic pressure. The RV response to ventilatory manipulations is more dramatic in patients with concomitant hypovolemia because RV preload is already reduced. Therefore, strict attention to intravascular volume status is required in patients with RV dysfunction and elevated intrathoracic pressures. HFJV may be considered in patients with RV dysfunction who require mean airway pressures greater than 15 cm H_2O. HFJV may allow a reduction of mean airway pressure, improved RV preload, and increased RV cardiac output.[85]

Pulmonary Artery Hypertension

Therapy for pulmonary artery hypertension is directed at lowering pulmonary artery pressures and improving RV function by optimizing preload and contractility (Fig. 12-16).[21,36,80] Patients with elevated PVR are sensitive to changes in RV preload. Because of the increased afterload, the RV will require increased RV preload to maximize RV stroke volume. Therefore, these patients require an assessment of right-sided filling pressures and higher than usual filling pressures (RA pressure 10 to 12 mm Hg). As afterload increases, the end-systolic volume of the RV increases. An increase in RV diastolic and systolic volume can result in conformational changes of the intraventricular septum, which can cause a reduction of LV preload and, thus, stroke volume.[98] Patients with pulmonary hypertension frequently require inotropic agents to increase RV output. However, the use of inotropic agents in patients with pulmonary artery hypertension has had limited success. This may be related to the relative insensitivity of the RV to inotropes. Agents such as dopamine, epinephrine, and dobutamine have limited utility in treating patients with pulmonary hypertensive crisis, and these patients are more successfully treated by decreasing the RV afterload. Maintaining RV coronary perfusion pressure through inotropic support may be helpful because RV perfusion occurs primarily during systole.[130]

Therapy directed at reducing pulmonary hypertension consists of increasing pH, decreasing $PaCO_2$, increasing PaO_2 and P_AO_2, and optimizing intrathoracic pressures.[21,30,36,80] Increasing pH has been shown to significantly reduce PVR in a variety of studies. Drummond and colleagues demonstrated that by reducing $PaCO_2$ to 20 torr and increasing pH to 7.6, a consistent reduction of PVR is obtained in infants with pulmonary hypertension. In addition, maintaining serum bicarbonate levels to achieve a pH between 7.5 and 7.6 while maintaining a $PaCO_2$ of 40 torr resulted in a similar reduction in PVR.[67] However, the potentially adverse effects of these physiologic changes on the cerebral vasculature must be considered. Both an increase in pH and a reduction in $PaCO_2$ could independently result in a reduction in RV afterload. Other studies have shown that an increase in both alveolar oxygen (P_AO_2) and arterial oxygen (PaO_2) by increasing inspired oxygen concentration reduces PVR.[21,80] Increasing inspired oxygen in patients with intracardiac shunts may result in little change in PaO_2; however, a reduction in PVR may occur. This effect is related to an increase in P_AO_2 and demonstrates that an increase in both alveolar and arterial oxygen content can alter PVR. In animal studies, increasing inspired oxygen concentration has been shown to be a more

PULMONARY ARTERY HYPERTENSION

Diagnosis: Decreased oxygen delivery as a result of pulmonary hypertension and decreased right ventricular output

Treatment: Decrease right ventricular afterload

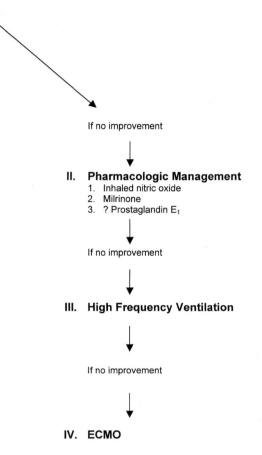

I. Ventilatory Strategy

1. Increase alveolar and arterial oxygen
   a. FiO_2
   b. Positive pressure ventilation
2. Assess respiratory mechanics for pulmonary over- or underinflation

If no improvement

II. Pharmacologic Management
1. Inhaled nitric oxide
2. Milrinone
3. ? Prostaglandin E_1

If no improvement

III. High Frequency Ventilation

If no improvement

IV. ECMO

FIGURE 12-16 Decision-making algorithm for postoperative patients with pulmonary artery hypertension. Manipulations of pH, FiO_2, and ventilatory mechanics are the most crucial.

potent pulmonary vasodilator in neonates compared to adults.[80] The use of inspired oxygen to reduce PVR has been useful in the ICU and is a frequent mode of interrogating pulmonary vascular responsiveness in the cardiac catheterization laboratory.[80] Another successful approach is the use of inhaled nitric oxide, described in detail in Chapter 7 on Pharmacology of Cardiovascular Drugs. While hyperventilation is effective at lowering pulmonary artery pressure and pulmonary vascular resistance in children with pulmonary hypertension after repair of congenital heart disease, it decreases cardiac output and increases systemic vascular resistance and should not be advocated.[87]

PPV is often required in patients with pulmonary artery hypertension. The effects of different types of ventilation on PVR are not well established. A reduction in mean airway pressure has been shown to reduce PVR.[85] Patients with pulmonary artery hypertension may benefit from hyperventilation, but because of the detrimental effects of elevated mean airway pressure on PVR and RV filling, mean airway pressure should be limited.[10] PEEP must be used judiciously in

these patients. High PEEP (>10 cm H_2O) or high mean airway pressure may result in alveolar overdistention and compression of the pulmonary capillaries with a resultant increase in PVR.[1] Therefore, the overall approach to these patients should be directed at providing the necessary amount of PEEP to maintain the lungs at functional residual capacity (see Fig. 12-12).

Several differences in lung physiology in infants lead to EELV less than FRC, increased closing capacity, and increased airway collapse during normal tidal breathing.[43,44,46,52] This process results in a ventilation/perfusion mismatch with segments of lung demonstrating perfusion without ventilation.[53] As these nonventilated lung segments become hypoxic, a secondary hypoxic response can develop, and PVR increases. Respiratory mechanics can be used to optimize tidal volume delivery and PEEP in these patients.

HFJV has been used in patients with pulmonary hypertension and RV dysfunction because of the detrimental effects of PPV on RV dynamics and the need for hyperventilation. HFJV should be ideally suited for patients with RV dysfunction and/or pulmonary artery hypertension because it may reduce mean airway pressure and PVR while maintaining a similar or lower $PaCO_2$.

Weaning from Positive-Pressure Ventilation

When PPV is required for a longer time than expected for the surgical procedure performed, a thorough investigation for the presence of residual cardiac disease or intercurrent illness is necessary. Weaning from PPV requires the patient to gradually assume the entire work of breathing. Understanding respiratory muscle performance in infants and children is necessary to manage withdrawal (weaning) from PPV.[89]

Successful weaning from PPV depends upon a variety of factors, including adequate cardiovascular function, the presence of satisfactory ventilatory reserve, and favorable pulmonary mechanics. During the weaning phase, the patient will have a gradual increase in respiratory muscle work, and if the cardiorespiratory system is unable to meet its goals, inadequate gas exchange with resultant hypoxemia and hypercapnia and inadequate oxygen delivery will occur (Fig. 12-17).

Oxygenation

Hypoxia during weaning from PPV usually results from ventilation/perfusion mismatch (intrapulmonary shunt). As PEEP and peak airway pressures are reduced, atelectasis may develop with resultant loss of lung volume and increased intrapulmonary shunt. Impaired gas exchange from right-to-left intrapulmonary shunting can be identified by the presence of an elevated alveolar-arterial oxygen tension gradient, $P_{(A-a)}O_2$. When hypoxemia is encountered, increasing the inspired oxygen concentration may be necessary. If the hypoxemia persists despite increased inspired oxygen, weaning must be terminated until the etiology of the hypoxemia is identified and corrected. If loss of lung volume is the etiology for the ventilation/perfusion mismatch, an increase in PEEP may be necessary and weaning suspended until improvements in pulmonary compliance are seen.

Oxygen Delivery

Abnormalities of respiratory mechanics lead to increased work of breathing. When the patient is sedated and receiving high levels of cardiorespiratory support, respiratory muscle oxygen consumption may be minimal. In contrast, in critically ill patients, 50% of total oxygen consumption may be used by the respiratory muscles in response to the increased workload.[40] Therefore, significant resolution of cardiorespiratory dysfunction must occur before weaning from PPV is performed. If marginal oxygen delivery and abnormal respiratory

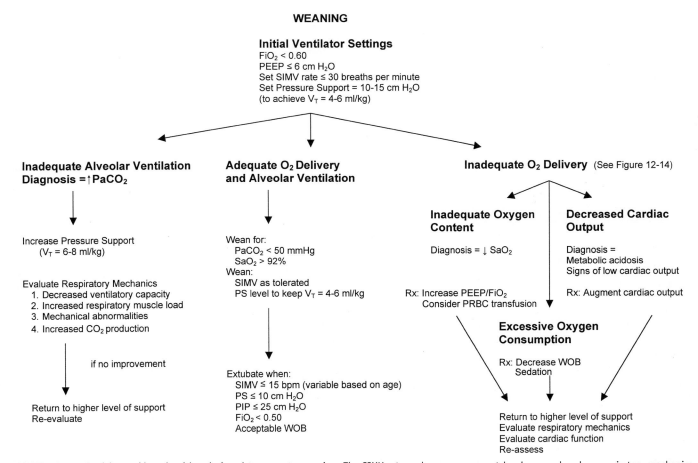

FIGURE 12-17 Decision-making algorithm designed to promote weaning. The SIMV rate and pressure support levels are reduced as respiratory mechanics improve. Weaning is terminated when inadequate oxygen delivery or inadequate alveolar ventilation (increased $PaCO_2$) occurs. When this occurs, the strategy is directed at treating reversible causes and supporting the cardiorespiratory system until resolution of cardiorespiratory dysfunction has occurred. PIP, peak inspiratory pressure; PS, pressure support; SIMV, synchronized intermittent mandatory ventilation; WOB, work of breathing.

mechanics are present, weaning may result in an imbalance between oxygen supply and demand, anaerobic metabolism, and metabolic acidosis.[129] The development of a metabolic acidosis during the weaning phase requires reinstitution of previous ventilatory support and an aggressive evaluation for the underlying pathophysiologic disturbance.

Carbon Dioxide Elimination

In infants and children, the most common cause of failure to wean from PPV is inadequate alveolar ventilation due to respiratory muscle pump failure. The etiology of respiratory muscle pump failure can be categorized into two causes: decreased ventilatory capacity and increased respiratory muscle load (Table 12-2). Respiratory muscle failure can be caused by a variety of events, including shock, hypoxemia, and hypercapnia. These conditions diminish the contraction of the diaphragm and may cause a decrease in V_T via impairment of excitation-contraction coupling by intracellular acidosis.[6,131,132] When the respiratory muscles cannot provide adequate alveolar ventilation, respiratory acidosis results from an inadequate effective tidal volume. The patient will attempt to compensate for the reduced V_T by increasing the respiratory frequency. The presence of hypercapnia despite a significant increase in respiratory frequency necessitates termination of weaning. Patients who require diuretic support may develop a metabolic alkalosis and a mild-to-moderate compensatory respiratory acidosis. These patients will have an increased $PaCO_2$ and normal (or possibly increased) pH, and weaning should continue provided the increased pH does not significantly reduce the respiratory drive.

Failure to wean from PPV can also occur from a variety of conditions that reduce ventilatory performance. Airway obstruction with lung hyperinflation from diseases such as bronchomalacia, bronchopulmonary dysplasia, airway compression by vascular structures, or chronic lung disease may occur.[133]

Table 12-2 Etiologies of Respiratory Pump Failure[84]

Decreased Ventilatory Capacity
Neurologic
Decreased respiratory center output
Cervical spinal cord surgery
Phrenic nerve dysfunction
Respiratory muscle
Hyperinflation
Malnutrition
Metabolic derangements
Decreased oxygen supply
Disuse atrophy
Fatigue
Abdominal wall defects
Increased Respiratory Muscle Load
Increased ventilatory requirements
Increased CO_2 production
Increased dead space ventilation
Inappropriately elevated ventilatory drive
Increased work of breathing
Decreased efficiency of breathing
Increased chest wall compliance
Respiratory pattern

Hyperinflation of the lungs leads to a flattened diaphragm and shortened fiber length, which results in a decreased transdiaphragmatic pressure generation. Additionally, tidal breathing occurs at the upper, less compliant portion of the pressure-volume curve of the lung.[122] Malnutrition[4,81] and metabolic derangements such as hypomagnesemia, hypophosphatemia, hypocalcemia, and may hypokalemia impair respiratory muscle performance and present as an inability to wean from ventilatory support.[5,7,33]

Disuse atrophy of the respiratory musculature occurs in premature infants after 12 days of PPV and may complicate weaning attempts.[65] Infants lack fatigue-resistant type I fibers and may be more susceptible to fatigue.[62] Phrenic nerve dysfunction or, less commonly, neurologic causes such as inadequate respiratory center output can cause failure to wean from PPV. Residual respiratory depressant drugs, such as opioids and benzodiazepines, may complicate weaning attempts. These patients hypoventilate but do not demonstrate increased work of breathing. Finally, the highly compliant chest wall and the rapid, shallow respiratory pattern of the neonate significantly decrease ventilatory efficiency, increase work of breathing, and may result in weaning failure.

Increased Ventilatory Requirements

Rarely, failure to wean from PPV can also occur when there are increased ventilatory requirements without adequate compensation. Increased ventilatory requirements may be a result of increased tissue CO_2 production necessitating increased alveolar ventilation to preserve normocapnia. Excessive carbohydrate calories during enteral and parenteral nutrition can cause hypercapnia due to excessive CO_2 production. In addition, CO_2 production increases with fevers (10% increase for each degree centigrade) and excessive muscle activity (seizures, shivering, rigor). Conditions that increase the ratio of physiologic dead space to tidal volume (V_D/V_T) such as reduced cardiac output, airway obstruction, or excessive positive airway pressure require an increase in minute ventilation to maintain effective ventilation and normocapnia. Increased dead space is common postoperatively, and virtually all children require minute ventilation greater than normal following surgery. Increased ventilatory requirements can also occur from other pathophysiologic conditions. Excessive respiratory drive from psychological stress, neurologic lesions, or pulmonary irritant receptor stimulation may lead to inappropriate hyperventilation and increased respiratory muscle load.

Techniques for Weaning

Following uncomplicated closed-heart or simple bypass procedures such as atrial septal closure or correction of aortic or pulmonary obstruction, extubation can occur shortly after surgery when the patient is awake and fully recovered from anesthesia.[108] This may occur in the pediatric ICU or the operating room. Other children may require more prolonged ventilation. Risk factors predicting the potential need for prolonged PPV include younger age (<10 months), longer cardiopulmonary bypass and aortic cross-clamp times, preoperative mechanical ventilatory requirement, greater than one surgical procedure, presence of pulmonary artery hypertension, and premature extubation requiring reintubation.[60] Preexisting pulmonary disease and severe systemic disease complicated by malnutrition may also prolong the need for ventilatory support. With good nursing care and the selection of an appropriate endotracheal tube, prolonged oral or nasal endotracheal intubation is a relatively safe alternative to tracheostomy in infants and children. Tracheostomy is usually performed after approximately 4 weeks of intubation for PPV or when a congenital or acquired airway lesion is documented.

Several techniques can be used to wean patients from PPV including t-tube weaning, synchronous intermittent mandatory ventilation, and supported modes of ventilation (i.e., pressure support ventilation or volume support ventilation). During the weaning phase, the patient assumes the work of breathing, which includes both patient demands and the demands imposed by the artificial respiratory support. The mechanically imposed work of breathing is a function of the endotracheal tube size, circuit size, inspiratory gas flow rate, and ventilator type. The work of breathing imposed by these factors can be quite substantial especially in the neonate who requires a small endotracheal tube. Any method of weaning ventilatory support must take these considerations into account. There are no well-controlled clinical trials that demonstrate a clear superiority for any one technique.[101a]

Despite this lack of definitive data, SIMV has emerged as the most common approach to weaning PPV in infants and children. The gradual reduction in SIMV rate allows the patient to slowly adjust to the increasing workloads with the withdrawal tailored to the capabilities of the patient. The appearance of respiratory distress, hypoxemia, or carbon dioxide retention of any point should temporarily halt further weaning efforts.

Pressure Support Ventilation   Pressure support ventilation was developed to improve weaning by assisting the patient's ventilation. PSV requires patient effort and the ability of the ventilator to appropriately sense the patient's effort. When a child initiates a breath, the ventilator senses the effort (pressure or flow trigger) and delivers a rapid increase in inspiratory gas flow until a preset pressure is achieved. Expiration begins when the exhalation valve opens as a predetermined parameter is reached, such as a decrease in inspiratory flow to 25% of peak flow. Termination of the breath is not related to volume, pressure, or time. The patient, therefore, retains control of the cycle length as well as the inspiratory flow, inspiratory time, and frequency. The patient's effort, the preset positive-pressure limit, and respiratory system impedance/compliance determine the delivered V_T. During PSV, the degree of machine support depends upon the level of preset pressure.[16] PSV decreases work of breathing imposed by mechanical factors and abolishes diaphragmatic muscle fatigue in selected patients who failed more "traditional" weaning attempts.[16] These findings may be related to the improved pressure-volume load characteristics that occur during PSV and the enhanced endurance conditioning of the diaphragm.[69,74] PSV has been used successfully in a variety of clinical conditions. In addition, PSV has been used to compensate for imposed mechanical work of breathing due to endotracheal tube impedance and inspiratory demand valves.[39]

The advantages of PSV over other forms of ventilation may be helpful in patients who are difficult to wean from PPV.

Two methods of weaning during PSV have been advocated.[58,77] In one method,[77] patients are initially ventilated at PS_{max} (pressure support level required to produce a full mechanical tidal volume breath). As clinical status dictates, the pressure support (PS) level is gradually decreased while respiratory rate and delivered tidal volume are closely monitored. In the second approach,[58] spontaneous intermittent PPV (SIMV) plus PS is used. The pressure support level is set to achieve a delivered tidal volume of 4 to 6 mL/kg (i.e., a "spontaneous" breath). As the cardiorespiratory system improves and sedation is decreased, the patient increases the number of spontaneous breaths, and the SIMV rate is reduced. As the SIMV rate is decreased, the pressure support level is decreased to maintain a delivered tidal volume of 4 to 6 mL/kg as pulmonary compliance improves. Patients who fail weaning will demonstrate tachypnea, tachycardia, ineffective gas exchange, and increased work of breathing.

Criteria for Extubation

Predicting successful extubation in infants and children presents unique challenges to the pediatric intensive care physician. Currently, there are no widely accepted criteria for predicting successful extubation in children. Methods used to predict extubation in adults such as respiratory frequency to tidal volume ratio,[121,136] CROP index (compliance, rate, oxygenation, and pressure),[136] t-piece trials, and negative inspiratory effort measurements[107] are either unreliable or not easily performed in children. Recently, a pediatric clinical study by Khan and colleagues characterized multiple predictors of extubation failure.[63] Unfortunately, these authors were unable to identify a single parameter or formula for predicting extubation in children and concluded that a combination of factors should influence any extubation decision.

Several studies have attempted to define criteria for extubation in children.[34,55,116,127] Hubble[55] demonstrated that the V_D/V_T ratio may be a useful, objective determinate of the readiness for extubation in infants and children. Shoults[115] was unable to find a correlation between maximum negative inspiratory airway pressure and successful removal of PPV in a group of neonates. In a group of older infants receiving postoperative PPV, the combination of a crying vital capacity >15 mL/kg and a maximum negative inspiratory airway pressure >45 cm H_2O accurately predicted successful discontinuation of ventilatory support. Failure to meet these criteria was associated with a failure to tolerate withdrawal of PPV and extubation.[115] In a separate study, Dicarlo[34] demonstrated a reduced mean lung compliance during the acute phase of ventilation. However, the primary determinants of the inability to extubate were an elevated airway resistance during the weaning phase and postoperative weight gain. In neonates weight gain may be an important determinate of the ability to extubate. Cardiopulmonary bypass in these patients results in increased interstitial fluid accumulation and weight gain, which may exceed 25% in the first 24 hours after bypass. Liberation from PPV is accomplished when postoperative weight has returned to 10% to 20% of preoperative values. This can be accomplished by vigorous diuresis in the postoperative period after the patient's hemodynamic status has been stabilized. Weaning should be considered when there has been adequate resolution of cardiovascular dysfunction, and respiratory mechanics have improved such that the work of breathing is not excessive.

Extubation of the trachea should be considered in the presence of normal arterial oxygenation and carbon dioxide elimination ($PaCO_2 < 45$ torr) on minimal ventilatory support (SIMV 5 to 10 breaths per minute, CPAP/PEEP 5 cm H_2O, PS 5 to 10 cm H_2O, and inspired oxygen < 0.40 to 0.50). Taken together with the previously mentioned indices of respiratory reserve, these criteria indicate the ability to tolerate independent ventilation with acceptable requirements for supplemental oxygen.

CONCLUSIONS

Respiratory support for infants and children with CHD requires a thorough understanding of cardiorespiratory performance. With use of the principles of cardiac function, respiratory physiology, and cardiorespiratory interactions, a management strategy can be developed that is matched to the pathophysiology of the patient. This strategy will vary depending upon the pathophysiology of the patient. The principles outlined in this chapter will allow clinicians the opportunity to maximize patient care and improve outcome variables.

References

1. Amitay M, Etches PC, Finer NN, Maidens JM: Synchronous mechanical ventilation of the neonate with respiratory disease. Crit Care Med 21:118–124, 1993.
2. Arnold JH, Hanson JH, Toro-Figuero LO, et al: Prospective, randomized comparison of high-frequency oscillatory ventilation and conventional mechanical ventilation in pediatric respiratory failure. Crit Care Med 22:1530–1539, 1994.
3. Arnold JH, Anas NG, Luckett P, et al: High frequency oscillatory ventilation in pediatric respiratory failure: A multicenter experience. Crit Care Med 28:3913–3919, 2000.
4. Arora NS, Rochester DF: Respiratory muscle strength and maximal voluntary ventilation in undernourished patients. Am Rev Respir Dis 126:5–8, 1982.
5. Aubier M, Murciano D, Lecocguic Y, et al: Effect of hypophosphatemia on diaphragmatic contractility in patients with acute respiratory failure. N Engl J Med 313:420–424, 1985.
6. Aubier M, Trippenbach T, Roussos C: Respiratory muscle fatigue during cardiogenic shock. J Appl Physiol 51:499–508, 1981.
7. Aubier M, Viires N, Piquet J, et al: Effects of hypocalcemia on diaphragmatic strength generation. J Appl Physiol 58:2054–2061, 1985.
8. Aubier M, Viires N, Syllie G, et al: Respiratory muscle contribution to lactic acidosis in low cardiac output. Am Rev Respir Dis 126:648–652, 1982.
9. Bandy KP, Hicks JJ, Donn SM: Volume-controlled ventilation for severe neonatal respiratory failure. Neo Intens Care 6:70–73, 1992.
10. Bash SE, Shah JJ, Albers WH, Geiss DM: Hypothermia for the treatment of postsurgical greatly accelerated junctional ectopic tachycardia. J Am Coll Cardiol 10:1095–1099, 1987.
11. Benumof JL: Mechanism of decreased blood flow to atelectatic lung. J Appl Physiol 46:1047–1048, 1979.
12. Benumof JL, Rogers SN, Moyce PR, et al: Hypoxic pulmonary vasoconstriction and regional and whole-lung PEEP in the dog. Anesthesiology 51:503–507, 1979.
13. Binda RE Jr, Cook DR, Fischer CG: Advantages of infant ventilators over adapted adult ventilators in pediatrics. Anesth Analg 55:769–772, 1976.
14. Boros SJ, Matalon SV, Ewald R, et al: The effect of independent variations in inspiratory-expiratory ratio and end expiratory pressure during mechanical ventilation in hyaline membrane disease: The significance of mean airway pressure. J Pediatr 91:794–798, 1977.
15. Branson RD, Chatburn RL: Technical description and classification of modes of ventilator operation. Respir Care 37:1026–1044, 1992.
16. Brochard L, Harf A, Lorino H, Lemaire F: Inspiratory pressure support prevents diaphragmatic fatigue during weaning from mechanical ventilation. Am Rev Respir Dis 139:513–521, 1989.
17. Brusasco V, Knopp TJ, Rehder K: Gas transport during high-frequency ventilation. J Appl Physiol 55:472–478, 1983.
18. Bunnell JB: High-frequency jet ventilation. Neo Intens Care 3:28–32, 1990.
19. Bursztein S, Taitelman U, De Myttenaere S, et al: Reduced oxygen consumption in catabolic states with mechanical ventilation. Crit Care Med 6:162–164, 1978.
20. Cannon ML, Cornell J, Tripp-Hamel DS, et al: Tidal volume measurements in infants should be obtained with a pneumotachometer located at the endotracheal tube. Am J Resp Crit Care Med 162:2109–2112, 2000.
21. Chang AC, Zucker HA, Hickey PR, Wessel DL: Pulmonary vascular resistance in infants after cardiac surgery: Role of carbon dioxide and hydrogen ion. Crit Care Med 23:568–574, 1995.
22. Chang HK: Mechanisms of gas transport during ventilation by high frequency oscillation. J Appl Physiol 56:553–563, 1984.
23. Charpie JR, Dekeon MK, Goldberg CS, et al: Serial blood lactate measurements predict early outcome after neonatal repair or palliation for complex congenital heart disease. J Thorac Cardiovasc Surg 120:73–80, 2000.
24. Chatburn RL: Classification of mechanical ventilators. Respir Care 37:1009–1025, 1992.
25. Cheifetz IM, Kern FH, Schulman SR, et al: Serum lactates correlate with mortality after operations for complex congenital heart disease. Ann Thorac Surg 64:735–738, 1997.
26. Cheifetz IM, Craig DM, Quick G: Increasing tidal volumes and pulmonary overdistention adversely affect pulmonary vascular mechanics and cardiac output in a pediatric swine model. Crit Care Med 26:710–716, 1998.
27. Clark RH, Gerstmann DR, Null DM, deLemos RA: Prospective randomized comparison of high-frequency oscillatory and conventional ventilation in respiratory distress syndrome. Pediatrics 89:5–12, 1992.
28. Colgan FJ, Nichols FA, Deweese JA: Positive end-expiratory pressure, oxygen transport, and the low-output state. Anesth Analg 53:538–543, 1974.
29. Cournand A, Motley HL, Werko L, Richards DW Jr: Physiological studies of the effects of intermittent positive pressure breathing on cardiac output in man. Am J Physiol 152:162, 1948.
30. Custer JR, Hales CA: Influence of alveolar oxygen on pulmonary vasoconstriction in newborn lambs versus sheep. Am Rev Respir Dis 132:326–331, 1985.
31. Dantzker DR, Brook CJ, Dehart P, et al: Ventilation-perfusion distributions in the adult respiratory distress syndrome. Am Rev Respir Dis 120:1039–1052, 1979.
32. Deal CW, Warden JC, Monk I: Effect of hypothermia on lung compliance. Thorax 25:105–109, 1970.
33. Dhingra S, Solven F, Wilson A, McCarthy DS: Hypomagnesemia and respiratory muscle power. Am Rev Respir Dis 129:497–498, 1984.
34. DiCarlo JV, Raphaely RC, Steven JM, Norwood WI, Costarino AT: Pulmonary mechanics in infants after cardiac surgery. Crit Care Med 20:22–27, 1992.
35. Donn SM, Nicks JJ, Becker MA: Flow-synchronized ventilation of preterm infants with respiratory distress syndrome. J Perinatology 14:90–94, 1994.
36. Drummond WH, Gregory GA, Heymann MA, Phibbs RA: The independent effects of hyperventilation, tolazoline, and dopamine on infants with persistent pulmonary hypertension. J Pediatr 98:603–611, 1981.
37. Dueck R, Wagner PD, West JB: Effects of positive end-expiratory pressure on gas exchange in dogs with normal and edematous lungs. Anesthesiology 47:359–366, 1977.
38. Epstein RA: The sensitivities and response times of ventilatory assistors. Anesthesiology 34:321–326, 1971.
39. Fiastro JF, Habib MP, Quan SF: Pressure support compensation for inspiratory work due to endotracheal tubes and demand continuous positive airway pressure. Chest 93:499–505, 1988.
40. Field S, Kelly SM, Macklem PT: The oxygen cost of breathing in patients with cardiorespiratory disease. Am Rev Respir Dis 126:9–13, 1982.

41. Fredberg JJ, Glass GM, Boynton BR, Frantz ID: Factors influencing mechanical performance of neonatal high-frequency ventilators. *J Appl Physiol* 62:2485–2490, 1987.

42. Fredberg JJ: Augmented diffusion in the airways can support pulmonary gas exchange. *J Appl Physiol* 49:232–238, 1980.

43. Garson A Jr, Gillette PC: Junctional ectopic tachycardia in children: Electrocardiography, electrophysiology and pharmacologic response. *Am J Cardiol* 44:298–302, 1979.

44. Gewillig MH, Lundstrom UR, Deanfield JE, et al: Impact of Fontan operation on left ventricular size and contractility in tricuspid atresia. *Circulation* 81:118–127, 1990.

45. Gibney RT, Wilson RS, Pontoppidan H: Comparison of work of breathing on high gas flow and demand valve continuous positive airway pressure systems. *Chest* 82:692–695, 1982.

46. Gillette PC, Kugler JD, Garson A Jr: Mechanisms of cardiac arrhythmias after the Mustard operation for transposition of the great arteries. *Am J Cardiol* 45:1225–1230, 1980.

47. Greenough A, Morley C, Davis J: Interaction of spontaneous respiration with artificial ventilation in preterm babies. *J Pediatr* 103:769–773, 1983.

48. Guyton AC: *Textbook of Medical Physiology.* Philadelphia: WB Saunders, 1981.

49. Haddad C, Richards CC: Mechanical ventilation of infant: Significance and elimination of ventilator compression volume. *Anesthesiology* 29:365–370, 1968.

50. Hammon JW Jr, Wolfe WG, Moran JF, et al: The effect of positive end-expiratory pressure on regional ventilation and perfusion in the normal and injured primate lung. *J Thorac Cardiovasc Surg* 72:680–689, 1976.

51. Hemmer M, Suter PM: Treatment of cardiac and renal effects of PEEP with dopamine in patients with acute respiratory failure. *Anesthesiology* 50:399–403, 1979.

52. Hickey PR, Hansen DD: Fentanyl- and sufentanil-oxygen-pancuronium anesthesia for cardiac surgery in infants. *Anesth Analg* 63:117–124, 1984.

53. Hickey PR, Hansen DD, Wessel DL, et al: Blunting of stress responses in the pulmonary circulation of infants by fentanyl. *Anesth Analg* 64:1137–1142, 1985.

54. Hickling KG: Ventilatory management of ARDS: Can it affect the outcome? *Intensive Care Med* 16:219–226, 1990.

55. Hubble CL, Gentile MA, Tripp DS, et al: Dead space to total ventilation ratio predicts successful extubation in infants and children. *Crit Care Med* 28:2034–2040, 2000.

56. Isabey D, Hart A, Change HK: Alveolar ventilation during high-frequency oscillation: Core dead space concept. *Respir Environ Exerc Physiol* 56:700–707, 1984.

57. Jenkins J, Lynn A, Edmonds J, Barker G: Effects of mechanical ventilation on cardiopulmonary function in children after open-heart surgery. *Crit Care Med* 13:77–80, 1985.

58. Kacmarek RM: Inspiratory pressure support: Does it make a clinical difference? *Intensive Care Med* 15:337, 1989.

59. Kanarek DJ, Shannon DC: Adverse effect of positive end-expiratory pressure on pulmonary perfusion and arterial oxygenation. *Am Rev Respir Dis* 112:457–459, 1975.

60. Kanter RK, Bove EL, Tobin JR, Zimmerman JJ: Prolonged mechanical ventilation of infants after open heart surgery. *Crit Care Med* 14:211–214, 1986.

61. Katz A, Gentile MA, Craig DM, et al: Heliox improves gas exchange during high-frequency oscillatory ventilation in a pediatric model of acute lung injury. *Am J Resp Crit Care Med* 164:260–264, 2001.

62. Keens TG, Bryan AC, Levison H, Ianuzzo CD: Developmental pattern of muscle fiber types in human ventilatory muscles. *J Appl Physiol* 44:909–913, 1978.

63. Khan N, Brown A, Venkataraman ST: Predictors of extubation success and failure in mechanically ventilated infants and children. *Crit Care Med* 24:1568–1579, 1996.

64. Klonin H, Bowman B, Peters M, et al: Negative pressure ventilation via chest cuirass to decrease ventilator-associated complications in infants with acute respiratory failure: A case series. *Respir Care* 45:486–490, 2000.

65. Knisely AS, Leal SM, Singer DB: Abnormalities of diaphragmatic muscle in neonates with ventilated lungs. *J Pediatr* 113:1074–1077, 1988.

66. Kocis KC, Dekeon MK, Rosen HK, et al: Pressure-regulated volume control vs volume control ventilation in infants after surgery for congenital heart disease. *Pediatr Cardiol* 22:233–237, 2001.

67. Koehler RC, Chandra N, Guerci AD, et al: Augmentation of cerebral perfusion by simultaneous chest compression and lung inflation with abdominal binding after cardiac arrest in dogs. *Circulation* 67:266–275, 1983.

68. Kumar A, Falke KJ, Geffin B, et al: Continuous positive-pressure ventilation in acute respiratory failure. *N Engl J Med* 283:1430–1436, 1970.

69. Leith DE, Bradley M: Ventilatory muscle strength and endurance training. *J Appl Physiol* 41:508–516, 1976.

70. MacDonald KD, Wagner WR: Infant synchronous ventilation. *J Respir Care Pract* :21–26, 1992.

71. MacIntyre N, Nishimura M, Usada Y, et al: The Nagoya conference on system design and patient-ventilator interactions during pressure support ventilation. *Chest* 97:1463–1466, 1990.

72. MacIntyre NR, Day S: Essentials for ventilator-alarm systems. *Respir Care* 37:1108–1112, 1992.

73. MacIntyre NR, Ho LI: Effects of initial flow rate and breath termination criteria on pressure support ventilation. *Chest* 99:134–138, 1991.

74. MacIntyre NR, Leatherman NE: Mechanical loads on the ventilatory muscles. A theoretical analysis. *Am Rev Respir Dis* 139:968–973, 1989.

75. MacIntyre NR, Leatherman NE: Ventilatory muscle loads and the frequency–tidal volume pattern during inspiratory pressure-assisted (pressure-supported) ventilation. *Am Rev Respir Dis* 141:327–331, 1990.

76. MacIntyre NR, Ho L: Weaning mechanical ventilatory support. *Anesth Report* 3:211–215, 1990.

77. MacIntyre NR: Weaning from mechanical ventilatory support: Volume-assisting intermittent breaths versus pressure-assisting every breath. *Respir Care* 33:121, 1988.

78. MacIntyre NR: *Graphical Analysis of Flow, Pressure, and Volume during Mechanical Ventilation.* Yorba Linda, CA: Bear Medical Systems, Inc., 1991.

79. MacIntyre NR: Patient-ventilator interactions: Dys-synchrony and imposed work loads. In: *Problems in Respiratory Care.* Philadelphia: Lippincott, 1991.

80. Malik AB, Kidd BS: Independent effects of changes in H^+ and CO_2 concentrations on hypoxic pulmonary vasoconstriction. *J Appl Physiol* 34:318–323, 1973.

81. Mansell AL, Andersen JC, Muttart CR, et al: Short-term pulmonary effects of total parenteral nutrition in children with cystic fibrosis. *J Pediatr* 104:700–705, 1984.

82. Marini JJ: Monitoring derived variables. *Resp Care* 37:1097–1107, 1992.

83. Martin LD, Rafferty JF, Wetzel RC, Gioia FR: Inspiratory work and response times of a modified pediatric volume ventilator during synchronized intermittent mandatory ventilation and pressure support ventilation. *Anesthesiology* 71:977–981, 1989.

84. Martin LD, Rafferty JF, Walker LK, Gioia FR: Principles of respiratory support and mechanical ventilation. In Rogers MC (ed): *Textbook of Pediatric Intensive Care.* Baltimore: Williams and Wilkins, 1992, pp 135–203.

85. Meliones JN, Bove EL, Dekeon MK, et al: High-frequency jet ventilation improves cardiac function after the Fontan procedure. *Circulation* 84:III364–368, 1991.

86. Meliones JN, Snider AR, Serwer GA, et al: Pulsed Doppler assessment of left ventricular diastolic filling in children with left ventricular outflow obstruction before and after balloon angioplasty. *Am J Cardiol* 63:231–236, 1989.

87. Morris K, Beghetti M, Petros A, et al: Comparison of hyperventilation and inhaled nitric oxide for pulmonary hypertension after repair of congenital heart disease. *Crit Care Med* 28:2974–2978, 2000.

88. Nelson NM: Neonatal pulmonary function. *Pediatr Clin North Am* 13:769–799, 1966.

89. Nichols DG: Respiratory muscle performance in infants and children. *J Pediatr* 118:493–502, 1991.

90. Qvist J, Pontoppidan H, Wilson RS, et al: Hemodynamic responses to mechanical ventilation with PEEP: The effect of hypervolemia. *Anesthesiology* 42:45–55, 1975.

91. Perez Fontan JJ, Heldt GP, Gregory GA: Mean airway pressure and mean alveolar pressure during high-frequency jet ventilation in rabbits. *J Appl Physiol* 61:456–463, 1986.

92. Perkin RM, Levin DL: Adverse effects of positive-pressure ventilation in children. In Gregory GA (ed): *Respiratory Failure in the Child.* New York: Churchill Livingstone, 1981, p 163.

93. Permutt S, Mitzner W, Weinmann G: Model of gas transport during high-frequency ventilation. *J Appl Physiol* 58:1956–1970, 1985.

94. Pick MJ, Hatch DJ, Kerr AA: The effect of positive end expiratory pressure on lung mechanics and arterial oxygenation after open heart surgery in young children. *Br J Anaesth* 48:983–987, 1976.

95. Pinsky MR: Determinants of pulmonary arterial flow variation during respiration. *J Appl Physiol* 56:1237–1245, 1984.

96. Pinsky MR, Summer WR: Cardiac augmentation by phasic high intrathoracic pressure support in man. *Chest* 84:370–375, 1983.

97. Pinsky MR, Summer WR, Wise RA, et al: Augmentation of cardiac function by elevation of intrathoracic pressure. *J Appl Physiol* 54:950–955, 1983.

98. Pinsky MR, Perlini S, Solda PL, et al: Dynamic right and left ventricular interactions in the rabbit: Simultaneous measurement of ventricular pressure-volume loops. *J Crit Care* 11:65–76, 1996.

99. Pontoppidan H, Geffin B, Lowenstein E: Acute respiratory failure in the adult. 3. *N Engl J Med* 287:799–806, 1972.

100. Pontoppidan H, Geffin B, Lowenstein E: Acute respiratory failure in the adult. 2. *N Engl J Med* 287:743–752, 1972.

101. Pontoppidan H, Geffin B, Lowenstein E: Acute respiratory failure in the adult. 1. *N Engl J Med* 287:690–698, 1972.

101a. Randolph AG, Wypij D, Venkataraman ST, et al: Effect of mechanical ventilator weaning protocols on respiratory outcomes in infants and children: A randomized control trial. *JAMA* 288:2561–2568, 2002.

102. Rau JL: Inspiratory flow patterns: The shape of ventilation. *Resp Care* 38:132–140, 1993.

103. Reynolds EO, Taghizadeh A: Improved prognosis of infants mechanically ventilated for hyaline membrane disease. *Arch Dis Child* 49:505–515, 1974.

104. Robotham JL, Lixfeld W, Holland L, et al: The effects of positive end-expiratory pressure on right and left ventricular performance. *Am Rev Respir Dis* 121:677–683, 1980.

105. Sagawa K: The end-systolic pressure-volume relation of the ventricle: Definition, modifications and clinical use. *Circulation* 63:1223–1227, 1981.

106. Sagawa K, Suga H, Shoukas AA, Bakalar KM: End-systolic pressure/volume ratio: A new index of ventricular contractility. *Am J Cardiol* 40:748–753, 1977.

107. Sahn SA, Lakshminarayan S: Bedside criteria for discontinuation of mechanical ventilation. *Chest* 63:1002–1005, 1973.

108. Schuller JL, Bovill JG, Nijveld A, et al: Early extubation of the trachea after open heart surgery for congenital heart disease. A review of 3 years' experience. *Br J Anaesth* 56:1101–1108, 1984.

109. Servant GM, Nicks JJ, Donn SM, et al: Feasibility of applying flow-synchronized ventilation to very low birth weight infants. *Resp Care* 37:249–253, 1992.

110. Shapiro BA: A historical perspective on ventilator management. *New Horizons* 2:8–18, 1994.

111. Shekerdemian LS, Bush A, Shore DF, et al: Cardiopulmonary interactions after Fontan operations: Augmentation of cardiac output using negative pressure ventilation. *Circulation* 96:3934–3942, 1997.

112. Shekerdemian LS, Shore DF, Lincoln C, et al: Negative pressure ventilation improves cardiac output after right heart surgery. *Circulation* 94:49–55, 1996.

113. Shepard FM, Arango LA, Simmons JG, Berry FA: Hemodynamic effects of mechanical ventilation in normal and distressed newborn lambs. A comparison of negative pressure and positive pressure respirators. *Biol Neonate* 19:83–100, 1971.

114. Sherer PW, Haselton FR: Convective exchange in oscillatory flow through bronchial-tree models. *J Appl Physiol* 53:1023–1033, 1982.

115. Shimada Y, Yoshiya I, Tanaka K, et al: Crying vital capacity and maximal inspiratory pressure as clinical indicators of readiness for weaning of infants less than a year of age. *Anesthesiology* 51:456–459, 1979.

116. Shoults D, Clarke TA, Benumof JL, Mannino FL: Maximum inspiratory force in predicting successful neonate tracheal extubation. *Crit Care Med* 7:485–486, 1979.

117. Simma B, Fritz M, Fink C, Hammerer I: Conventional ventilation versus high-frequency oscillation: Hemodynamic effects in newborn babies. *Crit Care Med* 28:227–231, 2000.

118. Smallwood RW: Ventilators—reported classifications and their usefulness. *Anaesth Intensive Care* 14:251–257, 1986.

119. Stark AR, Bascom R, Frantz ID: Muscle relaxation in mechanically ventilated infants. *J Pediatr* 94:439–443, 1979.

120. Suter PM, Fairley B, Isenberg MD: Optimum end-expiratory airway pressure in patients with acute pulmonary failure. *N Engl J Med* 292:284–289, 1975.

121. Tahvanainen J, Salmenpera M, Nikki P: Extubation criteria after weaning from intermittent mandatory ventilation and continuous positive airway pressure. *Crit Care Med* 11:702–707, 1983.

122. Tobin MJ: Respiratory muscles in disease. *Clin Chest Med* 9:263–286, 1988.

123. Tobin MJ: Monitoring of pressure, flow, and volume during mechanical ventilation. *Respir Care* 37:1081–1096, 1992.

124. Tokioka H, Kinjo M, Hirakawa M: The effectiveness of pressure support ventilation for mechanical ventilatory support in children. *Anesthesiology* 78:880–884, 1993.

125. Tyler DC: Positive end-expiratory pressure: A review. *Crit Care Med* 11:300–308, 1983.

126. Vengas JG, Hales CA, Strieder DJ: A general dimensionless equation of gas transport by high-frequency ventilation. *J Appl Physiol* 60:1025–1030, 1986.

127. Venkataraman ST, Khan N, Brown A: Validation of predictors of extubation success and failure in mechanically ventilated infants and children. *Crit Care Med* 28:2991–2996, 2000.

128. Venus B, Jacobs HK, Lim L: Treatment of the adult respiratory distress syndrome with continuous positive airway pressure. *Chest* 76:257–261, 1979.

129. Viires N, Sillye G, Aubier M, et al: Regional blood flow distribution in dog during induced hypotension and low cardiac output. Spontaneous breathing versus artificial ventilation. *J Clin Invest* 72:935–947, 1983.

130. Vlahakes GJ, Turley K, Hoffman JI: The pathophysiology of failure in acute right ventricular hypertension: Hemodynamic and biochemical correlations. *Circulation* 63:87–95, 1981.

131. Watchko JF, LaFramboise WA, Standaert TA, Woodrum DE: Diaphragmatic function during hypoxemia: Neonatal and developmental aspects. *J Appl Physiol* 60:1599–1604, 1986.

132. Watchko JF, Standaert TA, Woodrum DE: Diaphragmatic function during hypercapnia: Neonatal and developmental aspects. *J Appl Physiol* 62:768–775, 1987.

133. Weiner P, Suo J, Fernandez E, Cherniack RM: The effect of hyperinflation on respiratory muscle strength and efficiency in healthy subjects and patients with asthma. *Am Rev Respir Dis* 141:1501–1505, 1990.

134. Weisman IM, Rinaldo JE, Rogers RM, Sanders MH: Intermittent mandatory ventilation. *Am Rev Respir Dis* 127:641–647, 1983.

135. West JB, Dolbry CT, Naimark A: Distribution of blood flow in isolated lung: Relation to vascular and alveolar pressures. *J Appl Physiol* 19:713, 1964.

136. Yang KL, Tobin MJ: A prospective study of indexes predicting the outcome of trials of weaning from mechanical ventilation. *N Engl J Med* 324:1445–1450, 1991.

Chapter 13

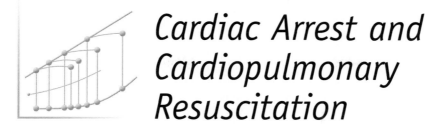

Cardiac Arrest and Cardiopulmonary Resuscitation

DONALD H. SHAFFNER, JR., MD, CHARLES L. SCHLEIEN, MD,
SCOTT M. ELEFF, MD, ELIZABETH A. HUNT, MD, MPH, and
DAVID G. NICHOLS, MD, MBA

333

EPIDEMIOLOGY OF CARDIOPULMONARY RESUSCITATION IN CHILDREN WITH HEART DISEASE

Location and Outcomes

Both the etiology and outcome of pediatric cardiac arrest vary depending on the location of the arrest. Among children who arrest outside the hospital, noncardiac causes predominate and the outcome remains very poor (<10% survival).[274] Conversely, cardiovascular disease is the most common cause of in-hospital arrest in children.[296,310,327] The rates of survival to discharge are higher after in-hospital arrests ranging from 13.7% in a large unselected pediatric intensive care unit (ICU) population to 44% in postoperative cardiac patients.[231,296] These limited data imply that caregivers of children with cardiovascular disease in the ICU need to be well trained in cardiopulmonary resuscitation (CPR) and may influence outcome favorably.

Risk Factors

Out-of-hospital arrests of cardiac origin comprise a very heterogeneous group of etiologies. The cardiac diseases associated with sudden cardiac death can be either previously recognized or unrecognized diseases (Table 13-1).[21] Children with repaired congenital heart disease constitute the largest group among the patients with previously recognized heart disease. For example, patients with tetralogy of Fallot and residual right ventricular outflow tract obstruction or pulmonary insufficiency and right ventricular volume overload may be at risk for ventricular dysrhythmias. Residual anatomic lesions may also play a role in the 4% of hypoplastic left heart syndrome patients who experience sudden cardiac death after the stage I Norwood operation.[194] Dysrhythmias may be another risk factor for post-discharge sudden cardiac death among hypoplastic left heart patients.[194] These examples underscore the importance of careful follow-up after congenital heart surgery, so that risk factors can be identified and corrected.

The group with previously unrecognized heart disease (see Table 13-1) is more challenging, because cardiac arrest may be the presenting sign of the abnormality. But even for these children, a careful assessment by the pediatrician or emergency department physician may prevent cardiac arrest. The children with previously unrecognized heart disease may have underlying structural (but silent) heart disease such as hypertrophic cardiomyopathy, coronary anomalies, or arrhythmogenic right ventricular dysplasia. Other patients have no structural heart disease, but rather have conduction system abnormalities such as long QT syndrome, Wolff-Parkinson-White syndrome, primary ventricular fibrillation, or unrecognized commotio cordis. Commotio cordis is an under-appreciated syndrome in which low energy impact to the chest wall such as from a baseball probably leads to ventricular fibrillation because of impact during the vulnerable period just before the peak of the T wave.[183]

Many of the entities in the group with previously unrecognized heart disease have an underlying genetic predisposition. Thus the physician may prevent cardiac arrest by carefully exploring the circumstance of any premature cardiac death among the child's first-degree relatives. A history of exertional chest pain or syncope should trigger a thorough family

Table 13-1   Underlying Cardiac Diagnoses in Children Presenting with Sudden Cardiac Death

PATIENTS AT RISK FOR OUT-OF-HOSPITAL CARDIAC ARREST FROM CARDIOVASCULAR DISEASE *(SUDDEN CARDIAC DEATH)*			
WITH PREVIOUSLY RECOGNIZED HEART DISEASE		**WITH PREVIOUSLY UNRECOGNIZED HEART DISEASE**	
Congenital	**Acquired**	**Structural Heart Disease**	**No Structural Heart Disease**
• Tetralogy of Fallot • Hypoplastic left heart syndrome • Transposition of the great arteries • Aortic stenosis • Single ventricle palliative procedures—Fontan, Glenn, hemi-Fontan • Marfan syndrome • Eisenmenger syndrome • Congenital (or postoperative) heart block	• Kawasaki syndrome • Dilated cardiomyopathy • Myocarditis	• Hypertrophic cardiomyopathy • Congenital coronary artery abnormalities • Arrhythmogenic right ventricular dysplasia • Myocarditis	• Long QT syndrome • Wolff-Parkinson-White syndrome • Primary ventricular tachycardia and ventricular fibrillation • Commotio cordis • Primary pulmonary hypertension

Modified from Berger S, Dhala A, Friedberg DZ: Sudden cardiac death in infants, children, and adolescents. *Pediatr Clin North Am* 46:221–234, 1990.

history, physical examination, electrocardiograph (ECG), and echocardiogram with the aim of uncovering the high-risk child before cardiac arrest occurs.

In-hospital arrests of cardiac origin occur most commonly in the postoperative patient after congenital heart surgery. Preoperative, intraoperative, and postoperative risk factors are associated with postoperative arrest in this population. The arrest victim is more likely to have required preoperative mechanical ventilation or prostaglandin administration. Intraoperatively, the arrest population has a longer mean aortic cross-clamp time (76 min vs. 51 min) and longer mean cardiopulmonary bypass time (124 min vs. 85 min).[311] A cardiopulmonary bypass time greater than 150 minutes is associated with a greater than 13-fold increased risk of a major adverse event such as cardiac arrest, emergency chest opening, multiple organ failure, or death (odds ratio [OR] 13.7, 95% confidence interval [CI]: 3.3–57.2).[97] Persistent hyperlactemia (> 4 mmol/L) during the first 8 hours after admission to the ICU predicts a major adverse event after congenital heart surgery.[97]

PHYSIOLOGY OF CARDIOPULMONARY RESUSCITATION

Recognition of the Need for Cardiopulmonary Resuscitation

The decision to initiate CPR in the ICU requires the recognition that a patient's vital signs are inadequate. An understanding of the cerebral and cardiac perfusion requirements in children is necessary to determine the adequacy of the vital parameters. Exact data are lacking to address these requirements for the wide range of patients' ages in the pediatric ICU. Specific pediatric experience and training are necessary to make decisions about these perfusion requirements because of the lack of definitive data. A lower rate of CPR in children receiving anesthetics by anesthesiologists trained in pediatric anesthesiology suggests that the knowledge of the appropriate hemodynamic variables in children may reduce the need for resuscitation.[154]

When insufficient oxygen delivery to the brain or heart occurs or the circulation is inadequate to deliver resuscitative drugs to the heart, then CPR should be started immediately. The presence of inadequate respiration or circulation should be evident in the patient undergoing invasive monitoring in the ICU. The gold standard for absent circulation in the absence of electronic monitoring had relied on carotid artery palpation in children and brachial artery palpation or chest auscultation in infants.[51,171] In recent years several studies have found the pulse check method to lack sensitivity and specificity as a diagnostic tool, particularly in the pre-hospital setting.[99,178] Furthermore a significant percentage of rescuers spend more than the recommended 5–10 seconds in search of a pulse. Therefore the most recent American Heart Association guidelines have dropped the requirement for a pulse check by lay rescuers in favor of determining the *signs of circulation* including breathing and movement.[4] Physicians should continue to check for pulselessness, but only as one item in a constellation of findings including apnea, flaccidity, cyanosis, and poor perfusion to determine the indication for CPR.

Reestablishment of Ventilation

The finding that exhaled air from the rescuer provides adequate oxygenation for the victim is the basis for bystander CPR when supplemental oxygen is not available.[103] Investigators exhaling *directly* into either the endotracheal tube or face mask of a paralyzed patient maintained arterial oxygen saturations greater than 90%.[103] One hundred percent oxygen administration by way of endotracheal intubation maximizes oxygen delivery to the vital organs during CPR. The need to optimize oxygen delivery outweighs the risk of oxygen toxicity in the setting of resuscitation. One hundred percent oxygen should be used whenever available.

Initially, researchers believed that closed-chest compressions alone provided adequate ventilation during CPR.[165] Unfortunately, soft tissue obstruction may prevent adequate ventilation in humans and necessitates intubation and positive pressure ventilation.[264] Endotracheal intubation is the standard means to assure ventilation by those who maintain training to do so. First responders should assist ventilation when appropriate through bag-mask ventilation, until someone trained in intubation is available. The American Heart Association requires bag-mask ventilation be mastered by all health care providers taking basic life support (BLS) and advanced life support (ALS) courses.[7] When endotracheal intubation is performed, the endotracheal tube (ETT) placement should be verified by the presence of end-tidal CO_2 (ETCO$_2$). This is especially important during CPR when the rate of inadvertent esophageal placement is higher than that in non-arrest situations.[28,29]

The demonstration of ETCO$_2$ after intubation reliably assures correct placement of the ETT in children.[28] Detection of ETCO$_2$ by a sensor in the breathing circuit indicates tracheal intubation. The lack of ETCO$_2$ implies esophageal intubation. Awaiting six respiratory cycles to assess for positive or negative ETCO$_2$ is recommended.[7] An esophageal intubation may initially show positive ETCO$_2$ due to CO_2 introduced into the esophagus with bag-mask ventilation prior to the intubation.[7] Decreased levels of pulmonary blood flow produced by CPR during cardiac arrest may give a false negative test for ETCO$_2$ in 15% of the measurements in correctly positioned intubations.[29] Measurable ETCO$_2$ after six breaths is proof of endotracheal intubation but the absence of ETCO$_2$ should be checked by visual inspection of the ETT placement because ETCO$_2$ may be very low until pulmonary circulation is restored, especially in infants. An ETT also provides access to the circulation for drug administration. Table 13-2 demonstrates the vascular access algorithm.

Five patterns of ventilation during chest compression have been investigated to determine the optimal pattern of ventilation during CPR.[341] The patterns investigated were no ventilation (oxygen only), continuous positive airway pressure, ventilation independent of compression, ventilation interposed between compressions, and ventilation synchronized with compression. All five patterns allow adequate oxygenation but vary in their effect on ventilation and hemodynamic pressures. Positive-pressure ventilation has hemodynamic impact due to the changes in intrathoracic pressure. Simultaneous compression and ventilation during CPR (SCV-CPR) gave the greatest improvement in blood

Table 13-2   Algorithm for Vascular Access during Cardiopulmonary Resuscitation

1. Three attempts at venous access*
2. Intraosseous line if unsuccessful at venous access
3. ETT route if no IV or IO access†
4. Cutdown saphenous or central line if no IV or IO line

*Use 5–10 mL of normal saline to flush drugs given through a peripheral line to ensure central delivery.
†Only give Lidocaine, Atropine, Naloxone, and Epinephrine by ETT.
ETT epinephrine administration requires 10 times IV dose.
Dilute ETT drugs to 5 mL in saline to help distribution to the distal bronchial tree.
ETT, endotracheal tube; IV, intravenous; IO, intraosseous.

flow and survival in dogs but no clear benefit of SCV-CPR has been shown in humans (see SCV-CPR section below). In unintubated patients, ventilation should be interposed between compressions to facilitate delivery, but it is unnecessary to synchronize ventilations with compressions in intubated patients (except in the newly born).[4]

Reestablishment of Circulation

Mechanisms of Blood Flow during Cardiopulmonary Resuscitation

Kouwenhoven and colleagues[165] proposed that external chest compression squeezed the heart between the sternum and the vertebral column forcing blood to be ejected. This assumption, of direct cardiac compression during external CPR, became known as the *cardiac pump mechanism* of blood flow during CPR. The cardiac pump mechanism proposes that the atrioventricular valves close during ventricular compression and that ventricular volume decreases, causing the ejection of blood. During chest relaxation, ventricular pressures fall below atrial pressures, allowing the atrioventricular valves to open and the ventricles to fill. This sequence of events resembles the normal cardiac cycle and occurs during direct cardiac compression in open-chest CPR.

Several observations of the hemodynamics during external CPR are inconsistent with the cardiac pump mechanism (Table 13-3). First, similar elevations in the arterial and venous intrathoracic pressures during closed-chest CPR suggest a generalized increase in intrathoracic pressure.[333] Second, reconstructing the integrity of the thorax in patients with flail sternum improves the blood pressure during CPR (a flail sternum should allow direct cardiac compression during closed-chest CPR).[260] Third, patients with ventricular fibrillation produce adequate blood flow to maintain consciousness by repetitive coughing or deep breathing.[74,138,219] These observations suggest a generalized increase in intrathoracic pressure may contribute to the production of blood flow during CPR. In fact, the demonstration that an increase in intrathoracic pressure without direct cardiac compression (i.e., a cough) can produce blood flow epitomizes the thoracic pump mechanism of blood flow during CPR. The existence of different mechanisms has lead to extensive research addressing the involvement of the cardiac and thoracic pump in blood flow during CPR.

Thoracic Pump Mechanism   Chest compressions during CPR generate almost equal pressures in the left ventricle, aorta, right atrium, pulmonary artery, airway, and the esophagus.[54,65,220,229,245,260,312] If all intrathoracic pressures are equal then suprathoracic arterial pressures must be higher than the suprathoracic venous pressures for cerebral perfusion to occur. Venous valves, either functional or anatomic, prevent the direct transmission of the elevation in intrathoracic pressure to the suprathoracic veins. These jugular venous valves are present in animals,[52,54,75,111,128,130,221,260] and humans,[55,120,121,221,229,312] undergoing CPR. This unequal transmission of the intrathoracic pressure to the suprathoracic vasculature establishes the gradient necessary for cerebral blood flow during closed-chest CPR.

During normal cardiac function, the lowest pressure in the circuit occurs on the atrial side of the atrioventricular valves. This low "downstream" pressure allows venous return to the pump. The extrathoracic shift of this low-pressure area to the cephalic side of the jugular venous valves during the thoracic pump mechanism implies the heart is merely a conduit during closed-chest CPR. Angiographic studies show blood passing from the vena cavae through the right heart to the pulmonary artery and from the pulmonary veins through the left heart to the aorta during a single chest compression.[65,220] Unlike normal cardiac activity and open-chest CPR, echocardiographic studies during closed-chest CPR in both dogs[65,220] and humans[63,255,339] have shown that the atrioventricular

Table 13-3   Comparison of Mechanisms of Blood Flow during Closed-Chest Compressions

Proposed Mechanism	Cardiac Pump	Thoracic Pump
Findings during compression	Sternum and spine compress heart	General increase in intrathoracic pressure
Atrioventricular valves	Closed	Open
Aortic diameter	Increases	Decreases
Blood movement	Left ventricle to aorta	Pulmonary veins to aorta
Ventricular volume	Decreases	Little change
Compression rate	Dependent	Little effect
Duty cycle	Little effect	Dependent
Compression force	Increases role	Decreases role
Clinical situations	Small chest	Large chest
	High compliance	Low compliance

valves are open during blood ejection. Also, unlike native cardiac activity and open-chest CPR, aortic diameter decreases instead of increases during blood ejection.[220,339] These findings during closed-chest CPR support the thoracic pump mechanism and are consistent with the heart as a passive conduit for blood flow.

Cardiac Pump Mechanism Although there is strong evidence for the thoracic pump mechanism during external chest compressions, there are specific situations when the cardiac pump mechanism predominates during closed-chest CPR. First, applying more force during chest compressions increases the likelihood of direct cardiac compression. Increasing the force of chest compressions in animals undergoing CPR, increases the closure of the atrioventricular valves implying more direct cardiac compression.[108,133] Second, a smaller chest size seems to allow more direct cardiac compression. Adult dogs with small chests have better hemodynamics during closed-chest CPR than dogs with large chests.[15] Third, the very compliant infant chest should permit more direct cardiac compression. During closed-chest CPR in an infant swine model, excellent blood flows are produced compared to most adult models.[275] Unlike the adult model, the addition of simultaneous ventilation with compression does not augment the flow produced during piglet CPR.[22] This failure of SCV-CPR to augment already high flows also occurs in small dogs.[15] The lack of contribution of SCV-CPR in the infant or small adult animal models implies that excellent compression (probably direct cardiac) occurs, and that additional intrathoracic pressure is of no benefit.

Some transesophageal echocardiography studies demonstrate closing of the atrioventricular valves during the compression phase of conventional CPR in adults.[142,167] These echocardiogram findings support the occurrence of cardiac compression during CPR in contrast to other studies showing the heart as a conduit. The above information suggests that either mechanism of blood flow may occur during CPR. There is no evidence to suggest that the cardiac and thoracic pump are mutually exclusive and varying CPR technique may alter the contribution of each (see CPR Methods subsequently).

The Distribution of Blood Flow during Cardiopulmonary Resuscitation

During CPR, total blood flow is decreased but redistribution optimizes perfusion of the heart and brain. This redistribution toward the vital organs should enhance outcome. The maintenance of myocardial blood flow during CPR promotes the return of spontaneous circulation. The maintenance of cerebral blood flow during CPR determines the quality of outcome. The distribution of blood flow to the brain during CPR depends on the development of three gradients: intrathoracic-suprathoracic, intracranial-extracranial, and caudal-rostral.

The first gradient, intrathoracic-suprathoracic, provides oxygenated blood from the chest to upper extremities and head. The presence of venous valves prevents transmission of intrathoracic pressure to the venous circulation. Either venous collapse, secondary to the elevated intrathoracic pressure, or closure of anatomic valves in the jugular system prevents transmission to the venous system.[111,221,260] When CPR is effective, arterial collapse does not occur and elevated intrathoracic

pressure is transmitted to suprathoracic arteries, thus providing suprathoracic blood flow.

The second gradient, intracranial-extracranial, directs flow away from the extracranial suprathoracic vessels and toward the intracranial vessels. Vasoconstrictors have little effect on intracranial vessels but do constrict extracranial vessels, effectively shunting blood to increase intracranial blood flow. Use of the vasoconstrictor epinephrine increases intracranial flow while decreasing cephalic skin, muscle, and tongue blood flows.[275]

The third gradient, caudal-rostral, occurs within the intracranial vessels. CPR alone seems to increase the distribution of flow to caudal areas of the brain. Ischemia preceding CPR significantly increases the distribution of flow to caudal areas.[211,286,287] This caudal redistribution also occurs in other models of global ischemia[146] and may provide relative sparing of the brain stem.

Myocardial blood flow does not have the advantage of the large extrathoracic pressure gradient that augments cerebral flow. The thoracic pump generates equal increases in all intrathoracic structures. This lack of a gradient results in poor myocardial blood flow during external chest compressions. Many studies show a much lower percentage of blood flow during closed-chest CPR for the myocardium compared to the cerebrum.[93,211,275]

The type of CPR influences the myocardial blood flow. Methods which are more likely to cause direct cardiac compression, such as high impulse CPR, result in unusually high myocardial blood flows.[93,196] Myocardial blood flow may be present only during relaxation[196] and correlates with "diastolic" pressure.[63] Conversely, myocardial blood flow may occur during compression and relate to "systolic" pressures.[211,275] Regional flow within the heart also changes during CPR. A shift in the ratio of subendocardial-subepicardial blood flow occurs. This ratio shifts from the normal 1.5:1 to 0.8:1 during CPR.[275] This ratio reverts to normal with epinephrine administration.

Blood flow, to organs other than the heart or brain, falls dramatically during CPR. The lack of valves in the infrathoracic veins leads to retrograde transmission of venous pressure and decreases the gradient for blood flow below the diaphragm in animals.[43] The reports of regional blood flows during CPR for several extrathoracic organs reveal small intestine 5% to 22%, pancreas 1% to 25%, liver 1% to 20%, kidney 1% to 12%, adrenal 12%, extremity muscle 1% to 5%, and spleen 0% to 3%, of pre-arrest flows.[160,211,288,328] The addition of abdominal compressions during CPR does not further compromise the infrathoracic organ blood flow.[160,328] The addition of epinephrine during closed-chest CPR almost completely eliminates flow to these already poorly perfused subdiaphragmatic organs (except the adrenal gland).[248]

Little data are available regarding pulmonary blood flow during CPR. Pulmonary blood flow occurs primarily at times of low intrathoracic pressure during closed-chest CPR.[65] High extrathoracic (primarily suprathoracic) venous pressure builds up during compression and results in pulmonary filling during relaxation as intrathoracic pressure falls.

Rate and Duty Cycle

The 1986 American Heart Association Guidelines for CPR and Emergency Cardiac Care recommended increasing the rate of chest compressions from 60 to 100 per minute.[3] This change represented a compromise between advocates of the thoracic pump mechanism and the cardiac pump mechanism.[109] The mechanics of these two theories of blood flow differ but a faster compression rate could augment both. It is necessary to understand the concepts of *compression rate*, *duty cycle*, and *compression force* to understand the mechanics of CPR.

Compression rate is the number of cycles per minute. *Duty cycle* is the ratio of the duration of the compression phase to the entire compression-relaxation cycle expressed as a percent. For example, at a rate of 30 compressions per minute (total cycle 2 seconds), a 1.2-second compression time produces a 60% duty cycle. The role of duty cycle differs between the two mechanisms of blood flow (see Table 13-3). *Compression force* is the pressure and the acceleration applied to the chest.

If direct cardiac compression generates blood flow (cardiac pump), then the force of the compression determines the stroke volume. Prolonging the compression (increasing the duty cycle) beyond the time necessary for full ventricular ejection fails to produce any additional increase in stroke volume in this model. In contrast, increasing the rate of compressions increases cardiac output, since a fixed ventricular blood volume ejects with each cardiac compression. Therefore, blood flow is rate sensitive but duty cycle insensitive in the cardiac pump mechanism.

If the thoracic pump produces blood flow, the reservoir of blood to be ejected is the large capacitance of the thoracic vasculature. With the thoracic pump mechanism, increasing both the force of compression and the duty cycle enhance flow. The longer duty cycles allow more time to empty the large intrathoracic vascular volume affected by the thoracic pump. Changes in compression rate do not affect flow over a wide range of rates.[136] Therefore, blood flow is duty cycle–sensitive but rate-insensitive in the thoracic pump mechanism.

Mathematical models of the cardiovascular system confirm that both the applied force and the compression duration determine blood flow with the thoracic pump mechanism.[26,135] Nevertheless, experimental animal data support both the thoracic pump and cardiac pump mechanisms as generating blood flow during closed-chest CPR. Discrepancies among the results of various studies may be attributed to differences in CPR models and compression techniques. These differences may involve issues of chest compliance and geometry, maturity of different animal species, or chest compression techniques. For example, either mechanism may be involved in an infant with a very compliant chest wall. Differences in techniques include the magnitude of sternal displacement, the compression force, the compression rate, and the duty cycle.

Several studies in dogs show a benefit of a fast compression rate (120 per minute) over slower rates during conventional CPR.[109,196,270] Studies in piglets,[83] puppies,[112] and humans[55,227,317] find no difference in the effectiveness of conventional CPR at various rates. A piglet CPR study found that duty cycle was the major determinant of cerebral perfusion pressure.[83] The duty cycle at which venous return becomes limited varies with age. Increasing duty cycle was more effective in two-week-old than eight-week-old piglets.[83]

The discrepancy between the importance of rate and duty cycle in various models by different investigators generates confusion. Increasing the rate of compressions during conventional CPR to 100 per minute satisfies both those who prefer the faster rates and those who support a longer duty cycle. This is true because it is physically easier for a rescuer to produce a 50% duty cycle at a rate of 100 than at 60 compressions per minute (holding compression is physically difficult at slow rates). This is the reason behind the change to an increased compression rate in the 1986 American Heart Association guidelines and its continued recommendation in 1992 and 2000.[4,5]

Chest Geometry

Chest geometry plays an important role in the ability of extrathoracic compressions to generate intrathoracic pressures. Shape, compliance, and deformability are chest characteristics with a significant impact during CPR. The age of the patient affects each of these characteristics. The change in these characteristics with age may explain some differences in CPR between the pediatric and adult animal models.

Chest Shape During anterior-to-posterior delivered compressions, the change in cross-sectional area (and intrathoracic pressure) of the chest relates to its shape.[84] The thoracic index refers to the ratio of the anteroposterior diameter to the lateral diameter. A keel-shaped chest, as in an adult dog, has a greater anteroposterior diameter and thus a thoracic index greater than one. A flat chest, as in a thin human, has a greater lateral diameter and thus a thoracic index of less than one. A circular chest would have a thoracic index of one. A circle with the same perimeter has a larger cross-sectional area than either of these elliptical chests. As the anteroposterior compression flattens a circle, it decreases the cross-sectional area and compresses the contents (increasing intrathoracic pressure). In contrast, as a keel-shaped chest approaches a circular shape, the cross-sectional area increases during the application of an anteroposterior compression (decreasing intrathoracic pressure). The cross-sectional area of the keel-shaped chest does not decrease until the compression continues past the circular shape to flatten the chest. This implies a threshold distance past which the compression must proceed before compressing intrathoracic contents (Fig. 13-1).[84] Thus the rounded, flatter chests of small dogs and pigs (and human infants) may require less displacement than the keel-shaped chests of adult dogs to generate thoracic ejection of blood. The rounded chest of small dogs improves the efficacy of external thoracic compression when compared to the keel-shaped adult dog.[15]

Chest Compliance As we age, the cartilage in our chests calcifies and the compliance changes. The stiffer, or less compliant, older chest may require greater compression force to generate the same anteroposterior displacement. Three-month-old swine require much greater pressure for anteroposterior displacement than their 1-month old counterparts.[84] The compliance of the chest not only affects the amount of displacement but also, what becomes compressed. Direct cardiac compression is more likely to occur in the more compliant chests of younger animals. Cerebral blood flow production in a piglet model of external CPR was much greater than expected when compared to the usual adult animal experience.[275] The more compliant infant chest may allow more direct cardiac compression, accounting for the high flows that resemble those produced by open-chest cardiac massage.

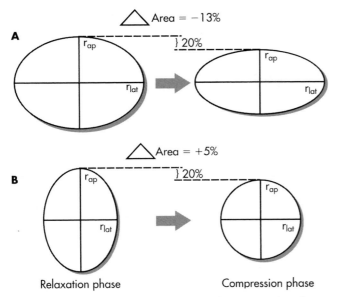

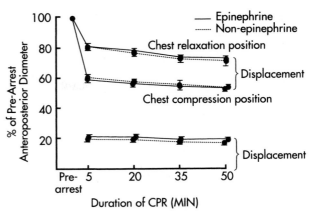

FIGURE 13-1 Changes in area of ellipses with constant circumference. Each ellipse is labeled with anteroposterior radius (r_{ap}) and lateral radius (r_{lat}), and a 20% anteroposterior compression is applied. Indicated change in areas equals relaxed area minus compressed area. **A,** Initial anteroposterior/lateral ratio, 0.7; and compression leads to positive ejection because relaxed area minus compressed area is negative. **B,** Initial anteroposterior/lateral ratio, 1.4; and compression toward a circular shape results in an increase in area. (From Dean JM, Koehler RC, Schleien CL, et al: Age-related changes in chest geometry during cardiopulmonary resuscitation. *J Appl Physiol* 62:2212–2219, 1987.)

FIGURE 13-2 Piston position during chest compression and relaxation phases of the cycle, and net piston displacement expressed as a percentage of pre-arrest anteroposterior chest diameter (12.0 ± 0.3 cm). Note that displacement was essentially unchanged over the 50-minute duration but that marked deformation occurred during the relaxation phase by 5 minutes and continued to further deform over the 50-minute period in both the epinephrine (*solid line*) and no epinephrine (*dashed line*) groups. (From Schleien CL, Dean JM, Koehler RC, et al: Effect of epinephrine on cerebral and myocardial perfusion in an infant animal preparation of cardiopulmonary resuscitation. *Circulation* 73:809–817, 1986. By permission of the American Heart Association, Inc.)

Chest Deformation Chest deformation occurs as CPR becomes prolonged. The chest flattens as compressions continue, producing larger decreases in cross-sectional area at the same displacement. While progressive deformation may lead to more direct cardiac compression, too much deformation may decrease the recoil of the chest wall and produce less effective compressions. A pediatric model of prolonged conventional CPR shows a progressive ineffectiveness of chest compressions over time (Fig. 13-2).[82,275] The permanent deformation of the chest in this model approaches 30% of the original anteroposterior diameter. Attempting to limit the deformation by increasing intrathoracic pressure from within during compression with SCV-CPR was ineffective.[22] Neither the amount of deformation nor the time to deterioration of flows was different. In an attempt to limit the production of deformation, investigators used a third mode of infant animal CPR with a thoracic vest to deliver compressions. The vest distributes compression force diffusely and greatly decreases permanent deformation (3% vs. 30%).[285] Unfortunately, the deterioration of blood flows with time still occurs and appears unrelated to the amount of deformation in this model. Thus, deterioration of effectiveness of CPR with time appears to be related to more than just chest deformation.

The relevance of chest geometry characteristics found in animal studies in relation to humans is unclear. Body weight, surface area, chest circumference, and chest diameter did not correlate with the aortic pressure produced during CPR in a study of nine adults already declared dead.[312] There has not been a direct comparison of adult and pediatric human CPR.

The increased compliance and deformability of the infant chest makes it likely that pediatric CPR would be more effective than in adults (as seen in animal models).

Maintenance of Circulation

Efficacy of Blood Flow during Cardiopulmonary Resuscitation

Blood flows produced by conventional closed-chest CPR without pharmacologic support are disappointingly low. The range of cerebral blood flow in dogs is 3% to 14% of pre-arrest levels.[30,147,162,188] Cerebral perfusion pressures are also low, 4% to 24% of pre-arrest levels in animals[30,160,188] and only 21 mm Hg in humans.[121] Myocardial blood flows in this basic CPR mode are also disappointingly low at 1% to 15% of pre-arrest levels in dogs.[54,136,162,188,328] Myocardial blood flow is directly related to myocardial perfusion pressure. Plotting myocardial blood flow in milliliters per minute per gram versus myocardial perfusion pressure in mm Hg gives a slope of 0.01 to 0.015.[248,328]

Besides pharmacologic support, several other factors affect cerebral and myocardial blood flow during CPR. These factors include age, intracranial pressure, duration of CPR, and duration of pre-resuscitation ischemia (Table 13-4). Age affects cerebral blood flow during closed-chest CPR. Two-week-old piglets have substantially higher cerebral blood flow (50% of pre-arrest) and slightly higher myocardial flow (17% of pre-arrest) than in adult models.[275] Two studies on older pigs showed comparable or lower cerebral blood flow but much lower myocardial flow (1% to 8% of pre-arrest).[43,288] No human data exist with blood flows at different ages during CPR.

Intracranial pressure can represent the downstream pressure for cerebral blood flow and, if elevated, decrease cerebral perfusion. Intracranial pressure increases in response to increasing intrathoracic pressure with closed-chest CPR.[257]

Table 13-4 Factors Relating to the Effectiveness of Cardiopulmonary Resuscitation

Factor	Relationship
Aortic diastolic pressure	↑ aortic diastolic pressure: ↑ MBF
End-tidal CO_2	↑ $ETCO_2$: ↑ MBF
Age	↑ age: ↓ CBF
ICP	↑ ICP: ↓ CBF
Duration of CPR	↑ duration CPR: ↓ CBF
Duration of ischemia	↑ duration ischemia: ↓ CBF

ICP, intracranial pressure; MBF, myocardial blood flow; $ETCO_2$, end-tidal carbon dioxide; CBF, cerebral blood flow; ↑, increase; ↓, decrease.

This relationship is linear and the value for the ratio of the change in intrathoracic pressure is 0.33.[130] These data imply that one third of the increase in intrathoracic pressure is transmitted to the intracranial pressure. There is no relation between the transmission of the intrathoracic pressure to the intracranial contents and the carotid or jugular pressures. The transmission can be partially blocked by occluding the cerebrospinal fluid or vertebral vein flow.[130] The rise in intracranial pressure with chest compressions is even greater when baseline intracranial pressure is elevated (two thirds of the intrathoracic pressure may be transmitted to the intracranial pressure). The efficacy of CPR deteriorates markedly in the face of elevated intracranial pressure.

Increased duration of CPR has a negative effect on cerebral blood flow and seems most detrimental in infant animal preparations.[275,288] The length of the ischemic period before CPR also has a negative effect on cerebral blood flow.[174,287] As the ischemic duration is increased the subsequent forebrain blood flow during CPR is reduced more than brainstem blood flow.[286,287] Hypothermia prevented the reduction of cortical reflow after short ischemic periods in a canine model.[286] It seems obvious that a short ischemic period and quick resuscitation would improve eventual outcome, but the cause of these effects on cerebral blood flow is unclear.

There appear to be thresholds for minimum vital organ blood flow during CPR. The inability to maintain blood flow during CPR above these thresholds results in organ malfunctions. In the heart, myocardial blood flow of 20 mL/minute/100 g of heart, or greater, is necessary for successful defibrillation in dogs.[130,265] In the brain, cerebral blood flow of greater than 15 to 20 mL/minute/100 g of brain is necessary to maintain normal electrical activity during CPR.[211]

Monitoring the Effectiveness of Cardiopulmonary Resuscitation

Monitoring the effectiveness of CPR is difficult. An adequate myocardial perfusion pressure is necessary to allow the heart to be restarted during CPR. The above data suggest that a myocardial blood flow of 20 mL/minute/100 g is necessary for return of spontaneous circulation. This flow would correlate with a myocardial perfusion pressure (MPP) of 20 mm Hg (aortic relaxation pressure – right atrial relaxation pressure). Data from CPR in humans show that a MPP of 15 mm Hg was necessary for, but did not guarantee, return of spontaneous circulation. Often right atrial relaxation pressure is low and the aortic "diastolic" pressure represents the myocardial perfusion pressure. Without an arterial line, detection of this

"diastolic" pressure is difficult during CPR. If an arterial line is present in a patient receiving CPR, the clinician can observe the effect of interventions on the "diastolic" blood pressure as a guide to maximizing performance and perhaps efficacy.

The measurement of venous oxygen saturation is described as a method to monitor the effectiveness of CPR. In humans, venous oxygen saturations correlated with the return of spontaneous circulation.[256,297] This observation may be of use in victims with central venous access during CPR.

Another method to monitor myocardial perfusion during CPR is to follow the production of end-tidal CO_2 ($ETCO_2$). $ETCO_2$ is particularly useful as a patient is more likely to have an ETT than either a central venous line or an arterial line. The amount of CO_2 exhaled depends on the amount of pulmonary blood flow. Generally as pulmonary blood flow increases, $ETCO_2$ levels rise. Therefore, as blood flow to the heart and lungs improves during CPR, $ETCO_2$ should rise. It is usual practice for a patient receiving CPR with an ETT in place to be hand-ventilated as opposed to receiving ventilation through the ventilator. It can be helpful to have a quantitative $ETCO_2$ monitor attached to the ETT while ventilating in order to guide effective CPR. During CPR a mean $ETCO_2$ less than 10 mm Hg is predictive of a poor outcome.[46,176,332] Alternatively an $ETCO_2$ greater than 15 mm Hg during CPR is predictive of resuscitation.[18,27] Thus, $ETCO_2$ monitoring is useful in determining the effectiveness of CPR and an $ETCO_2$ less than 10 to 15 mm Hg indicates the need to modify CPR to improve blood flow. $ETCO_2$ also serves as an indicator of undetected cardiac output during pulseless electrical activity,[18] the return of spontaneous circulation during CPR,[113] and the presence of spontaneous circulation during cardiopulmonary bypass.[116]

There are pitfalls in the monitoring of $ETCO_2$ during CPR. The administration of bicarbonate increases CO_2 production and may elevate $ETCO_2$ without a corresponding increase in pulmonary blood flow. The administration of epinephrine may decrease $ETCO_2$ despite an increase in the myocardial perfusion causing a misinterpretation that CPR has become less effective[200] (the cause of this brief fall in $ETCO_2$ with epinephrine is unclear). The contamination of disposable $ETCO_2$ detectors by resuscitation medications (epinephrine, atropine, or lidocaine) or gastric acid may decrease their accuracy in the assessment of CPR effectiveness or the detection of esophageal intubation.[214]

Conventional Cardiopulmonary Resuscitation Methods

Conventional CPR includes closed-chest-compressions delivered manually with ventilations interposed after every fifth compression. Table 13-5 shows basic life-support procedures. This system of CPR can be delivered in any setting without additional equipment and with a minimum of training. No large randomized study exists to demonstrate the superiority of any alternate mode of CPR over conventional CPR.

Rescuer fatigue is a major problem with manual CPR in the "field." Individual variation between rescuers performing manual CPR can be a problem in the field and in the lab. Mechanical devices are available to deliver chest compressions to overcome fatigue and to standardize compression delivery, but are not recommended for children.[4]

Table 13-5 Basic Life-Support Procedures[5]

Parameter	Newborn (<12 h)	Infant (<1 yr)	Child (1–8 yr)	Adult
Breathing	30 breaths/min	20 breaths/min	20 breaths/min	12 breaths/min
Pulse check	umbilical cord	brachial/femoral	carotid	carotid
Compress area	below nipples	lower $\frac{1}{3}$ sternum	lower $\frac{1}{3}$ sternum	lower $\frac{1}{2}$ sternum
Compress with	two fingers/encircle	two fingers/encircle	one hand	two hands
Depth	$\frac{1}{3}$ AP diameter	$\frac{1}{3}$–$\frac{1}{2}$ AP diameter	$\frac{1}{3}$–$\frac{1}{2}$ AP diameter	$\frac{1}{3}$–$\frac{1}{2}$ AP diameter
Rate	90/min	100/min minimum	100/min	100/min
Ratio	3:1	5:1	5:1	15:2

The two-handed, chest-encircling method for infant chest compression represents an attempt to augment blood flow through both the thoracic and the cardiac pump mechanisms. With this technique, both hands encircle the chest of an infant, while the thumbs apply sternal compressions. The encircling fingers apply diffuse thoracic force to raise intrathoracic pressure while the sternal depression by the thumbs directly compresses the heart.[80,320] Experimental models suggest that the two-thumb encircling technique generates higher blood pressures than two-finger compressions.[95] The 2000 American Heart Association guidelines recommend the two-thumb encircling over the two-finger technique.[4]

Open-Chest Cardiopulmonary Resuscitation

Open-chest CPR involves a thoracotomy. Direct compression of the heart generates blood flow. The application of this technique requires a high level of sophistication and training as well as special equipment and facilities. These requirements limit open-chest CPR to specific settings, usually in a hospital. Open-chest CPR produces cardiac output of 25% to 61% of pre-arrest values.[17,30,336] These studies and others show cardiac output two to three times greater than with conventional closed-chest CPR.[17,30,31,85,336] Increased cerebral perfusion pressure has been significant in some studies[31] but not in others.[30,85] Myocardial perfusion pressures are significantly increased compared to closed-chest CPR.[31,267] Cerebral blood flows in dogs of 150% of pre-arrest values could be produced with open-chest CPR.[147] Cross-clamping the descending aorta during open-chest CPR further increases carotid blood flow.

Survival in dogs can be improved by use of open-chest CPR following inadequate closed-chest CPR.[269] Dogs with myocardial perfusion pressure less than 30 mm Hg after 15 minutes of closed-chest external CPR received 2 to 4 minutes of either open-chest or closed-chest external CPR before attempting defibrillation. Dogs receiving open-chest CPR had significantly greater myocardial perfusion pressures and resuscitation rates.

The length of time of closed-chest CPR affects the success of subsequent open-chest CPR.[268] After 20 and 25 minutes of closed-chest CPR, the success rate of open-chest CPR dropped to 38% and 0%, respectively. This implies the benefits from open-chest CPR are time limited and early application is crucial.

There are no data to recommend the routine use of open-chest CPR in children.[6] However, the pediatric ICU is a setting where open-chest CPR could be used more often.

Postoperative cardiac patients often have a recent sternotomy and thus easier access. The use of open-chest CPR could result in better flows and allows inspection for hemopericardium. Closed-chest CPR in the immediate postoperative period may result in disruption of suture lines on the cardiac surgical repair. The use of open-chest CPR may avoid suture line rupture or allow for early recognition of this problem. In some infants with hemodynamic instability after cardiac surgery, the chest is left open initially and delayed sternal closure planned for 2 to 4 days later.[210] If cardiac arrest should occur in this setting, open-chest CPR becomes the only option. This technique also may be valuable for patients with lesions that would limit the effectiveness of conventional CPR such as critical aortic stenosis. A study in adults after cardiac surgery found a 70% survival with sternotomy versus a 20% survival with external compressions for resuscitation.[249] Tamponade, bleeding, thrombosed grafts, and arrhythmia were discovered at sternotomy in this study.

Cardiopulmonary Bypass

Cardiopulmonary bypass (CPB) represents a very effective way to restore circulation after cardiac arrest. Animal studies show that CPB increases 72-hour survival, recovery of consciousness, and preserves myocardium better than conventional CPR.[175,241] In dogs CPB results in better neurologic outcome than continued conventional CPR after a 4-minute ischemic period (neurologic outcome was dismal in both groups when the ischemic period lasted 12 minutes).[175,241] Twenty-four hour survival is possible for at least 90% of dogs after 15 or 20 minutes of cardiac arrest but only 10% of dogs after 30 minutes of arrest with CPB stabilization during defibrillation.[252] CPB decreases myocardial infarct size in a model involving coronary artery occlusion when compared to conventional CPR.[9] In most animal models, CPB facilitates resuscitation and improves success when compared to conventional CPR.

There is little experience with CPB for cardiac arrest in humans outside the operating room. Timely application of percutaneous femoral artery and vein bypass has been successful in resuscitating patients with "refractory" cardiac arrest. Unfortunately many patients who are stabilized on CPB after failing standard CPR cannot be weaned off CPB or have a low likelihood of long-term survival or of good neurologic outcome.[140,201,208,235,253] There are reports of patients with cardiac arrest in the operating room or catheterization suite who have cardiac arrest under anesthesia and fail to respond to conventional CPR but benefit from the institution of CPB. These patients are reported to have good neurologic outcomes despite over 30 minutes (even over 2 hours) of failed conventional resuscitation efforts.[172,201]

Cardiopulmonary bypass has been used for prolonged periods in children with congenital heart defects in the form of extracorporeal membrane oxygenation (ECMO). ECMO has been used as rescue therapy in children suffering cardiac arrest after cardiac surgery[86] and in children with congenital heart disease before and after cardiac surgery.[78,86,87,98,246] These studies found that 52% to 67% of the children could be weaned from the support and that 35% to 56% were survivors. The major complications were neurologic sequelae (often related to pre-ECMO events or hemorrhagic stroke on ECMO), bleeding problems on ECMO, and multi-system organ failure.[78,86,87,98,246]

Cardiopulmonary bypass requires considerable technical support and sophistication. It is impressive that it can be fully operational in less than ten minutes after request for the procedure.[140,235] Despite rapid availability and restoration of circulation the lack of effective resuscitation before institution of CPB limits the ability to preserve neurologic or cardiac function. These limitations decrease the value of CPB for patients suffering out-of-hospital cardiac arrest or requiring more than 30 minutes of conventional CPR.[64,235,318] Early studies suggest that ECMO for children with congenital heart disease and pump failure (postarrest or postcardiotomy) is beneficial when used early enough to avoid neurologic and other organ failure. Controlled studies of ECMO for cardiac support are necessary to prove this benefit.[225]

Experimental Cardiopulmonary Resuscitation Methods

Simultaneous Compression-Ventilation Cardiopulmonary Resuscitation The low efficacy of conventional CPR has led to investigations of multiple CPR modalities. These methods usually reflect attempts to enhance the contribution of the thoracic pump or cardiac pump to blood flow during CPR (Table 13-6). Simultaneous compression-ventilation CPR (SCV-CPR) is an attempt to augment conventional CPR by increasing the thoracic pump mechanism. Delivering ventilation simultaneously with every compression, (instead of interposed after every fifth compression), adds to the

Table 13-6 Contribution of Cardiac or Thoracic Pump to Various Methods of Cardiopulmonary Resuscitation

Method	Cardiac Pump	Thoracic Pump
Open-chest	++	0
High impulse	++	+
Conventional	0/+	+
Abdominal binding	0/+	++
IAC CPR*	0/+	++
SCV CPR	0/+	++
Vest CPR	0	++
Cough CPR	0	++

*Also moves blood by abdominal compression alone.
CPR, cardiopulmonary resuscitation; IAC, interposed abdominal compression; SCV, simultaneous compression ventilation.

intrathoracic pressure and should augment blood flow produced by closed-chest CPR. Several studies suggest that SCV-CPR increases the carotid blood flow when compared with conventional CPR.[15,30,52,54,139] Others confirm physiologic advantages of SCV-CPR in canine models.[160,189] In contrast SCV-CPR offers no advantage over conventional CPR in infant pigs[22] and small dogs.[14,15,266] No study has shown increased survival in humans with this technique of CPR.[166]

Abdominal Binding Researchers have used abdominal binders and military anti-shock trousers (MAST) to augment closed-chest CPR. Both methods apply continuous compression circumferentially below the diaphragm. Binders augment CPR by (1) decreasing the compliance of the diaphragm, thus maintaining intrathoracic pressure; (2) forcing blood out of the subthoracic vessels into the circulating blood volume ("autotransfusion"); and (3) increasing resistance in the sub-diaphragmatic vasculature thereby improving suprathoracic blood flow. The increase in intrathoracic pressure and blood volume leads to increased aortic pressure and carotid blood flow in both animals[160,173,223] and humans.[53,180] Unfortunately as the aortic pressure increases, the right atrial "diastolic" pressure increases to a greater extent resulting in a decrease in the coronary perfusion pressure.[223,266] This deterioration of coronary perfusion pressure coincides with a decreased generation of myocardial blood flow.[223] These techniques also decrease the cerebral perfusion pressure by transmission of the intrathoracic pressure to the intracranial vault raising the intracranial pressure.[130] Liver laceration from abdominal binder CPR is reported[139] but is no more frequent than with conventional CPR.[195,222,223,247,250] In addition, the use of abdominal binders or MAST suits to augment CPR has not increased survival in clinical studies.[195,222,266]

Abdominal Compression Interposed abdominal compression CPR (IAC-CPR) is the addition of an abdominal compression during the relaxation phase of chest compression. IAC-CPR may augment conventional CPR by (1) promoting venous blood return to the chest during the chest relaxation (abdominal compression) phase and "prime the pump," (2) increasing intrathoracic pressure adding to the duty cycle of the chest compression, and (3) compressing the aorta and sending blood retrograde to the carotid or coronary arteries.[102,247,328] Several studies show hemodynamic improvements secondary to IAC-CPR. In animals, cardiac output, cerebral and coronary blood flow improve when comparing IAC-CPR with conventional CPR in adult models[102,247,328,329] but not in an infant swine model.[100] Human studies also show an increase in aortic pressure and coronary perfusion pressure during IAC-CPR compared to conventional CPR.[16,24,55,145,330] Although one study reports a 10% aspiration rate[102] most have no aspiration or liver laceration.[16,24,205,247,262,263,328,330] Clinically IAC-CPR requires extra manpower or equipment and remains experimental. Outcome studies have mixed results with no increase in survival for pre-hospital arrests but improved survival for in-hospital arrests.[205,262,263] It is now recommended as an alternative for in-hospital, adult CPR, and so may be used in adolescents.[3a]

Vest Cardiopulmonary Resuscitation Vest CPR uses an inflatable bladder, wrapped circumferentially around the chest (resembling a blood pressure cuff) and cyclically inflated. This method of delivering chest compressions by a diffuse application of pressure has two unique characteristics. First, chest dimensions change minimally and direct cardiac compression is unlikely (a nearly pure thoracic pump technique). Second, the even distribution of pressure decreases the likelihood of trauma.

Vest CPR in dogs improves cerebral and myocardial blood flows as well as survival when compared to conventional CPR.[73,134,136,189] In a pediatric animal model of vest CPR, only a 3% permanent chest deformation occurred after 50 minutes of vest CPR[285] compared with almost 30% deformation produced by an equivalent period of conventional CPR.[275] In humans, vest CPR increases aortic systolic pressure but does not significantly increase diastolic pressure compared with conventional CPR.[312] In a preliminary study of vest CPR in victims of out-of-hospital arrest, an increased aortic and coronary perfusion pressure were demonstrated, and there was a trend toward a greater return of spontaneous circulation compared with standard CPR.[137]

The lack of metallic parts has allowed vest CPR to be used experimentally during nuclear magnetic resonance spectroscopy to study brain intracellular pH.[105] In addition, the vest has been used as an external cardiac assist device in non-arrested dogs with heart failure.[27,56] Clinically, the use of vest CPR depends on sophisticated equipment and the technique remains experimental at this time.

High-Impulse Cardiopulmonary Resuscitation High-impulse CPR refers to the application of greater than usual force during chest compression. This increase in force can be in the form of greater mass, velocity, or both. It is hypothesized that the larger impulses result in greater chest deflection causing more contact with the heart.[158] Direct cardiac compression is more likely with this form of closed-chest CPR.[157,196] High-impulse CPR can generate myocardial blood flows as high as 60% to 75% of pre-arrest values.[196] In humans, high-impulse CPR generates increased aortic pressures.[312] An outcome study in dogs compared high-impulse CPR to conventional closed-chest CPR and found no significant improvement in return of spontaneous circulation, survival, or neurologic outcome.[157]

Active Compression-Decompression Cardiopulmonary Resuscitation Active compression-decompression (ACD)–CPR requires a device that attaches to the chest and allows the rescuer to pull up on the sternum and decompress the thorax between compressions. The theoretical advantages of decompressing the chest between compressions include restoring chest wall shape, actively pulling gas into the lungs, and actively pulling blood into the intrathoracic vessels. These characteristics allow for more effect from the compression as more intrathoracic pressure can be generated and more blood ejected with the compression.

Preliminary studies in humans showed that after advanced cardiac life support failed, ACD-CPR was more effective than standard CPR at improving hemodynamic variables.[66] Following a witnessed in-hospital arrest, more patients had return of spontaneous circulation, survival at 24 hours, and had a better Glasgow coma score when they received ACD-CPR then when standard CPR was given.[67] A larger study of in-hospital cardiac arrest victims failed to show any difference in the resuscitation or outcomes between patients receiving ACD or standard CPR.[306] Several large studies of patients who suffered an out-of-hospital cardiac arrest did not find a difference in the effectiveness of ACD or standard CPR for improving the incidence of return of spontaneous circulation, hospital admission, hospital discharge, or short term neurologic outcome.[190,209,224,283,306]

Complication rates following CPR were not different following ACD-CPR or standard CPR in most studies.[190,209,283] It is interesting that the same study that showed that ACD had more complications than standard CPR (hemoptysis and sternal dislodgment) was also one of the few large studies that found ACD-CPR more effective than standard CPR for out-of-hospital arrests.[238]

Inspiratory Impedance Threshold Valve Inspiratory impedance threshold valve (ITV) describes the addition of a valve to the endotracheal tube or face mask of a patient receiving CPR. The goal is for the valve to transiently block gas exchange during the inspiratory cycle associated with the decompression phase of CPR. The belief is that this will then create a vacuum in the thorax to facilitate blood flow back to the heart.[191] The valve has been demonstrated to augment both standard CPR and ACD-CPR in adult and pediatric porcine models, with improved coronary perfusion pressures and vital organ blood flow.[168,325] A prospective, randomized, blinded, controlled trial of adults was performed where patients either received ACD-CPR or ACD-CPR plus ITV. Statistically and clinically significant improvements in maximal ETCO$_2$, diastolic blood pressure, and coronary perfusion pressure occurred in patients receiving ACD-CPR plus ITV versus those without the valve. There was also a significant decrease in the time from intubation to return of spontaneous circulation in the few patients who achieved successful resuscitation.[239] Further studies will be needed to elucidate the efficacy of ITV in pediatric resuscitation.

Phased Chest Abdominal Compression-Decompression Cardiopulmonary Resuscitation A new manual method of phased chest and abdominal compression-decompression (PCACD) cardiopulmonary resuscitation has been described.[315] PCACD-CPR resembles a combination of ACD-CPR and interposed abdominal compression CPR. It offers the theoretical advantages of both methods because chest shape is restored and blood and gas pulled into the thorax during active decompression of the chest and blood flow augmented due to the compression, and active decompression, of the abdomen. Coronary perfusion pressure, return of spontaneous circulation, short-term survival and neurologic outcome were improved in a porcine model of fibrillatory cardiac arrest resuscitated using PCACD-CPR.[315]

PHARMACOLOGY OF CARDIOPULMONARY RESUSCITATION

Epinephrine and Other Adrenergic Agonists

Redding and Pearson[251] first described the use of adrenergic agonists during CPR in 1963. These drugs, such as epinephrine, have been in use for CPR almost since the inception of closed-chest compression in 1960.[165] Redding and Pearson showed that early administration of epinephrine in a canine model of cardiac arrest improved the success rate of CPR.[251] They also demonstrated that the increase in diastolic pressure produced by the administration of adrenergic agonist drugs was responsible for the success of resuscitation.[232] They theorized that vasopressors such as epinephrine were of value because they increased systemic vascular resistance. Since that time, epinephrine continues to be the drug of choice during CPR.

Yakaitis and colleagues[347] investigated the relative importance of α- and β-adrenergic agonist actions during resuscitation. Only one in four dogs receiving both the pure β-adrenergic agonist isoproterenol and an α-adrenergic antagonist were resuscitated successfully. In contrast, all the dogs treated with both an α-adrenergic agonist drug and a β-adrenergic antagonist were resuscitated successfully. These data suggest that the α-adrenergic agonist receptor action of epinephrine is responsible for successful resuscitation following cardiac arrest.

Later studies confirmed this notion. Michael and colleagues[211] demonstrated that the effects of epinephrine during CPR are mediated by the selective vasoconstriction of peripheral vessels excluding those supplying the brain and heart. While receiving an epinephrine infusion, higher aortic vascular pressures are maintained, resulting in higher perfusion pressure to the heart and brain.[211] Despite the increase in both mean and diastolic aortic pressures, flow to other "non-vital" organs, such as the kidneys and small intestine, decreases markedly as a result of intense vasoconstriction of the vessels supplying those organs.[161,211,275]

Coronary Blood Flow

The increase in aortic diastolic pressure associated with epinephrine or other α-adrenergic agonist drugs administered during CPR is critical for maintaining coronary blood flow and improving the rate of successful resuscitation. In the beating heart, the contractile state of the myocardium is enhanced by β-adrenergic receptor agonists. During CPR these drugs may stimulate spontaneous myocardial contractions and increase the intensity of ventricular fibrillation. In the fibrillating heart the inotropic effect of β-adrenergic agonists might be deleterious by increasing intramyocardial wall pressure.[185] This increased wall pressure results in a decreased coronary perfusion pressure and a diminished myocardial blood flow. In addition, β-adrenergic stimulation could increase myocardial oxygen demand by increasing cellular metabolism and oxygen consumption. The superimposition of an increased oxygen demand on the low myocardial blood flow available during CPR could cause ischemia.

Other α-adrenergic agonist drugs have been used successfully during CPR. As expected, drugs such as methoxamine and phenylephrine cause peripheral vasoconstriction during CPR. As with epinephrine the increase in aortic diastolic pressure results in an increased coronary blood flow. However the absence of direct β-adrenergic stimulation avoids increasing oxygen uptake by the myocardium. This results in a more favorable oxygen demand-to-supply ratio in the ischemic heart. These non-epinephrine α-adrenergic agonists have been used successfully for resuscitation.[232,251,276] These drugs maintain myocardial blood flow as well as epinephrine does

during CPR.[347] Schleien and colleagues[276] found that high aortic pressures can be sustained in a canine model of CPR with the α-adrenergic agonist phenylephrine. The high levels of myocardial perfusion pressure and coronary blood flow produced were equivalent in the phenylephrine and epinephrine treated animals. This resulted in a resuscitation rate of 75% with the use of both drugs. In that study, the ratio of endocardial to epicardial blood flow did not differ between the two drug groups of animals. There continues to be debate however, about the relative merits of pure α-adrenergic agonist drugs versus epinephrine for resuscitation.[11,34,37,38,44,50,101,143,170,193,342]

Other drugs that cause peripheral vasoconstriction, such as vasopressin, have also been used successfully in both animal and in limited human studies (see below for full discussion). Even a nitric oxide synthase inhibitor, L-NAME, has been used experimentally to resuscitate piglets after ventricular fibrillation arrest by its intense vasoconstriction.[280]

Cerebral Blood Flow

During CPR, cerebral blood flow, like coronary blood flow, is dependent on peripheral vasoconstriction. Epinephrine and other α-agonist drugs produce selective vasoconstriction of non-cerebral peripheral vessels in areas of the head and scalp (i.e., tongue, facial muscle, and skin) without causing cerebral vasoconstriction in adult[211,248] and infant models of CPR.[275] The infusion of either epinephrine or phenylephrine maintained cerebral blood flow and oxygen uptake at pre-arrest levels for 20 minutes in a canine model of CPR (Figure 13-3).

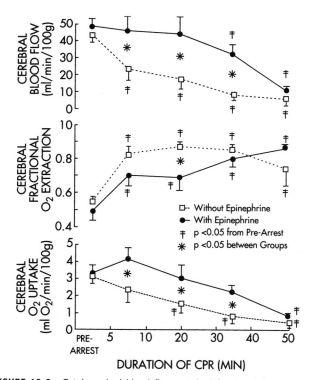

FIGURE 13-3 Total cerebral blood flow, cerebral fractional O_2 extraction, and cerebral O_2 uptake before cardiac arrest and during 50 minutes of CPR in the no epinephrine (*dashed lines*) and epinephrine (*solid line*) groups. (From Schleien CL, Dean JM, Koehler RC, et al: Effect of epinephrine on cerebral and myocardial perfusion in an infant animal preparation of cardiopulmonary resuscitation. *Circulation* 73:809–817, 1986. By permission of the American Heart Association, Inc.)

This implies that blood flow was higher than that needed to maintain adequate cerebral metabolism.[276] There were no differences in neurologic outcome 24 hours after resuscitation when either epinephrine or phenylephrine was administered 9 minutes after ventricular fibrillation.[34] Other investigators, however, found epinephrine to be more beneficial in generating vital organ blood flow.[37,38,44] This may have been due to the use of drug dosages that were not equipotent in generating vascular pressure and subsequent blood flow.

Cerebral oxygen uptake may be increased by a central β-adrenergic receptor effect if sufficient amounts of epinephrine cross the blood-brain barrier during or following resuscitation.[50,193] Additionally, epinephrine may have a vasoconstricting or vasodilating effect on cerebral vessels depending on the balance between α- and β-adrenergic effects.[342] When cerebral ischemia is very brief, epinephrine and phenylephrine have similar effects on cerebral blood flow and metabolism. In this situation the blood-brain barrier most likely is

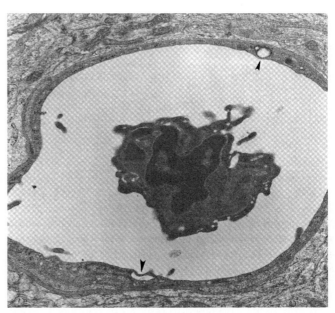

FIGURE 13-5 Transmission electron micrograph from a postarrest piglet. Luminal polymorphonuclear leucocyte within the caudate nucleus. The arrows denote endothelial vacuoles present within this microvessel. (From Schleien CL, Caceres MJ, Kuluz JW, et al: Early endothelial damage and leukocyte accumulation in piglet brains following cardiac arrest. *Acta Neuropathol* 90:582–591, 1991; with permission.)

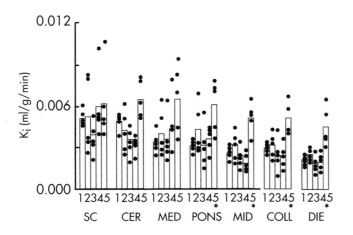

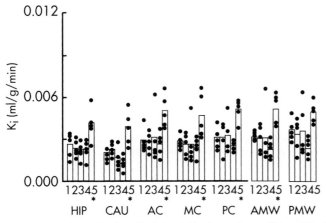

FIGURE 13-4 Mean (bars) and individual (dots) transfer coefficient (K$_i$) of α-aminoisobutyric acid for cervical spinal cord (SC), cerebellum (CER), medulla (MED), pons (PONS), midbrain (MID), superior colliculus (COLL), diencephalon (DIE), hippocampus (HIP), caudate nucleus (CAU), anterior cerebral (AC), middle cerebral (MC), and posterior cerebral (PC) artery regions, and anterior-middle (AMW) and posterior-middle (PMW) artery watershed regions. (1) control group; (2) 8 minutes ischemia and 10 minutes cardiopulmonary resuscitation; (3) 8 minutes ischemia and 40 minutes cardiopulmonary resuscitation; (4) 3 minutes after resuscitation; (5) 4 hours after resuscitation. *P < .05, different from group 1 by one-way analysis of variance and Dunnett's test. (From Schleien CL, Koehler RC, Shaffner DH, et al: Blood-brain barrier disruption after cardiopulmonary resuscitation in immature swine. *Stroke* 22:477–483, 1991.)

not disrupted.[276] Catecholamines may cross the blood-brain barrier if either mechanical disruption occurs or enzymatic barriers to vasopressors (i.e., monoamine oxidase inhibitors) are overwhelmed during tissue hypoxia.[101,170] During CPR, the blood-brain barrier may be disrupted due to the generation of large fluctuations in cerebral venous and arterial pressures during chest compressions. Also, the permeability of the barrier may increase due to the arterial pressure surge that occurs in a maximally-dilated vascular bed following resuscitation.[11] An increase in cerebral oxygen demand when cerebral blood flow is limited could affect cerebral recovery adversely. In an infant model of CPR with 8 minutes of cardiac arrest, disruption of the blood-brain barrier was present 4 hours after defibrillation (Fig. 13-4).[277] In similar protocols involving 8 minutes of cardiac arrest, endothelial vacuolization occurs in conjunction with protein extravasation through the blood-brain barrier (Fig. 13-5).[278] These theoretical effects of catecholamines on the cerebral circulation require further clarification and do not represent a contraindication to epinephrine at present. Table 13-7 displays the actions of epinephrine.

Table 13-7 Actions of Epinephrine Administration during Cardiopulmonary Resuscitation

Action	Adrenergic Effect
Decreases perfusion to nonvital organs	α
Better coronary perfusion (aortic diastolic pressure)	α
Increases intensity of ventricular fibrillation	β
Stimulates cardiac contractions	β
Intensifies cardiac contractions	β

Dosage

High doses of epinephrine improve both myocardial and cerebral blood flow in animals with cardiac arrest. Cerebral blood flow increases further in response to larger doses of epinephrine.[23,34,42] In animals, several investigators showed that high-dose epinephrine increases myocardial and subendocardial blood flow with improvement of oxygen delivery compared to oxygen consumption.[40,41,43,162] However, increased myocardial oxygen consumption and decreased left ventricular subendocardial blood flow with epinephrine are observed in fibrillating dog models.[92,185] In a swine model, high-dose epinephrine failed to increase myocardial blood flow to levels achieved with lower doses.[23] Human survival studies with high-dose epinephrine have been contradictory. In earlier studies, investigators were optimistic that higher doses of epinephrine increased aortic diastolic pressure and therefore improved the return to spontaneous circulation when compared to standard epinephrine doses. Gonzalez and colleagues[123,124] demonstrated a dose-dependent increase in aortic blood pressure in patients who failed to respond to prolonged resuscitation efforts. Likewise, Paradis and colleagues[230] demonstrated increased aortic diastolic pressure and successful resuscitation in patients failing usual ACLS protocols. In addition, they reported seven children treated successfully with 0.2 mg/kg of epinephrine, 20 times the usual dose.[119] Other investigators also reported higher aortic diastolic pressures and improvement in return of spontaneous circulation.[62,199,230] This early enthusiasm for higher doses of epinephrine was replaced by disappointment after the publication of a series of human studies failed to show improved survival from high-dose epinephrine. Stiell and colleagues[305] reported on 650 adults who suffered cardiac arrest, randomly assigned to either a standard or high-dose (7 mg) epinephrine protocol. High-dose epinephrine did not improve survival (18% vs. 23% 1-hour survival; 3% vs. 5% hospital discharge) or alter neurologic outcome. In a multicenter prospective study, Brown and colleagues reported 1280 adult patients receiving either standard (0.02 mg/kg) or high-dose (0.2 mg/kg) epinephrine following cardiac arrest.[39] Again, no differences were seen either in return to spontaneous circulation, survival to hospital discharge, or neurologic outcome between these two groups of patients. Subsequent large multi-institutional studies likewise did not show any improvement with high-dose epinephrine.[47,184,289]

High doses of epinephrine may account for some of the adverse effects following resuscitation. These result from increased myocardial oxygen consumption following resuscitation, as well as, a post-arrest hyperadrenergic state. Thus, high doses may worsen myocardial ischemia, precipitate tachyarrhythmias, hypertension, ventricular ectopy, pulmonary edema, digitalis toxicity, hypoxemia, and cardiac arrest.[6,39,279] In patients with pulmonary or systemic outflow tract obstruction or idiopathic hypertrophic subaortic stenosis, tachycardia produced by epinephrine can decrease ventricular filling and lower cardiac output post-arrest. Tang and colleagues[314] showed that epinephrine, due to a redistribution of pulmonary blood flow, induced a decrease in PaO_2 and an increase in alveolar dead space ventilation.

The Guidelines 2000 for CPR and ECC recommend a dosing interval of every 3 to 5 minutes for ongoing arrest (Table 13-8). The recommended initial resuscitation dose of epinephrine for cardiac arrest is 0.01 mg/kg (0.1 mL/kg of 1:10,000 solution) by the intravenous or intraosseous route, or 0.1 mg/kg (0.1 mL/kg of 1:1,000 solution) by the tracheal route. The same dose of epinephrine is recommended for second and subsequent doses for unresponsive asystolic and other causes of pulseless arrest, but higher doses of epinephrine (0.1 to 0.2 mg/kg; 0.1 to 0.2 mL/kg of 1:1000 solution) by any route may be considered. Other medications including pure α-agonist medications or vasopressin may be used for subsequent treatment of asystole or pulseless arrest. In a child with symptomatic bradycardia that is unresponsive to ongoing therapy with assisted ventilation and oxygenation, epinephrine may be given in a standard dose of 0.01 mg/kg (0.1 mL/kg of 1:10,000 solution) by the intravenous or intraosseous route or 0.1 mg/kg (0.1 mL/kg of 1:1000 solution) by the tracheal route.

Table 13-8 Indications for Epinephrine Administration[6]

Bradyarrhythmia with hemodynamic compromise
Asystole or pulseless arrest

Doses:

Bradycardia	0.01 mg/kg IV/IO or 0.1 mg/kg ETT repeat every 3–5 min at the same dose
Pulseless	
First dose	0.01 mg/kg IV/IO or 0.1 mg/kg ETT.
Subsequent	Consider higher doses of 0.1–0.2 mg/kg IV/IO/ETT; repeat every 3–5 min

IV, intravenous; IO, intraosseous; ETT, endotracheal tube.

Vasopressin

Vasopressin is an endogenous hormone that acts at the V_1 receptor to mediate vasoconstriction. Its other major physiologic effect of reabsorption of water in the renal tubule is by its action at the V_2 receptor. Vasopressin causes relatively selective vasoconstriction of blood vessels in the skin, skeletal muscle, intestine, and fat with less vasoconstriction of the coronary, cerebral, and renal vascular beds. This hemodynamic action results in favorable increases in blood flow to the heart and brain[181,242] and improved long-term survival compared to epinephrine in animals.[338] In both adult and pediatric porcine models with ventricular fibrillation and adult porcine models with asphyxia, the combination of vasopressin and epinephrine was more effective than either alone.[337,324] Conversely, in a pediatric porcine model of asphyxial arrest, epinephrine either alone or in combination with vasopressin was more effective than vasopressin alone in relation to left ventricular myocardial blood flow and return of spontaneous circulation.[323]

In a human study comparing the use of vasopressin and epinephrine in adults with ventricular fibrillation resistant to defibrillation, the patients receiving vasopressin along with epinephrine were more likely to survive to hospital admission and for 24 hours than those receiving epinephrine alone.[182] Vasopressin has also been used successfully in other clinical settings including adults with septic shock,[259] hemodynamic failure following heart transplant,[213] and in children with vasodilatory shock after cardiac surgery,[258] as well as all causes of vasodilatory shock in children.[303] However, there is very little data at this time on the use of vasopressin in pediatric cardiac arrest. A case series of 4 children with 6 cardiac arrests utilized vasopressin as rescue therapy after failing conventional CPR therapy with epinephrine. Two of the recipients survived longer than 24 hours and one survived to discharge. The dose used in this study was 0.4 U/kg. This retrospective case series indicates the need for future prospective studies of the efficacy of vasopressin versus epinephrine in pediatric cardiopulmonary resuscitation.[197] Vasopressin has been recommended as an alternative to epinephrine in the adult cardiac arrest protocol for patients in shock-refractory ventricular fibrillation, asystole, and pulseless electrical activity.

Sodium Bicarbonate

Clinical Effects

The use of sodium bicarbonate during CPR, although previously recommended, has not been shown to actually improve resuscitation from cardiac arrest.[125,129,298] Administration of sodium bicarbonate results in an acid-base reaction in which bicarbonate combines with hydrogen ion to form water and carbon dioxide, resulting in an elevated blood pH:

$$HCO_3^- + H^+ \rightarrow H_2CO_3 \rightarrow H_2O + CO_2$$

Because bicarbonate generates carbon dioxide, adequate alveolar ventilation must be present prior to its administration. In children, respiratory failure is the major cause of cardiac arrest. Sodium bicarbonate transiently elevates CO_2 in the blood, so that its administration during cardiac arrest may actually worsen preexisting respiratory acidosis.

Indications

Sodium bicarbonate is indicated for correction of significant metabolic acidosis especially when cardiovascular compromise is present. The typical use of sodium bicarbonate is in patients with prolonged cardiac arrest, once effective ventilation is ensured and epinephrine and chest compressions have been provided to maximize circulation. Acidosis depresses myocardial function by depressing spontaneous cardiac activity, prolonging diastolic depolarization, and depressing the electrical threshold for ventricular fibrillation, the inotropic state of the myocardium, and the cardiac responsiveness to catecholamines.[61,226,228,304] Acidosis also decreases systemic vascular resistance and blunts the vasoconstrictive response of peripheral vessels to catecholamines.[344] This vasodilation is contrary to the desire to produce vasoconstriction during CPR. In addition, pulmonary vascular resistance increases with acidosis. Rudolph and colleagues[261] observed a twofold increase in pulmonary vascular resistance in calves by lowering pH from 7.40 to 7.20 under normoxic conditions. Therefore, correction of acidosis may help in resuscitating patients who have the potential for right-to-left shunting. Sodium bicarbonate is also indicated in hyperkalemic arrest (to increase pH to drive potassium intracellularly), hypermagnesemia, tricyclic antidepressant overdose, or overdose from other sodium-channel blocking medications including cocaine, β-blockers, and diphenhydramine.[7,94,159,215] Table 13-9 covers indications for bicarbonate.

Table 13-9 Indications for Sodium Bicarbonate Administration

Hyperkalemia, hypermagnesemia
Preexisting metabolic acidosis
Long cardiopulmonary resuscitation time without blood gas availability
Pulmonary hypertensive crisis
Treatment of toxic overdoses of medications that act as sodium channel blockers; i.e., tricyclic antidepressants, cocaine, diphenhydramine, consider for β-blockers
Dose: 1 mEq/kg intravenous/intraosseous empirically, or calculated from base deficit. Ensure adequate ventilation when administering bicarbonate.

Dosage

When the $PaCO_2$ and pH are known, the dose of bicarbonate to correct the pH to 7.40 can be calculated from the formula (0.3 × weight (kg) × base deficit) = mEq bicarbonate.

Because of the possible side effects of bicarbonate and the large venous-to-arterial carbon dioxide gradient that develops during CPR, we recommend giving half the dose based on a volume of distribution of 0.6. If blood gases are not available, the initial dose is 1 mEq/kg, followed by 0.5 mEq/kg every 10 minutes of ongoing arrest.[202] Again, the importance of alveolar ventilation cannot be overemphasized, as well as the need for repeated arterial blood gas analysis.

Side Effects

The side effects due to bicarbonate administration include metabolic alkalosis, hypercapnia, hypernatremia,[345] and hyperosmolarity,[206] all of which are associated with a high mortality rate. Metabolic alkalosis causes a leftward shift of the oxyhemoglobin dissociation curve that impairs the release of oxygen from hemoglobin to tissues at a time of low cardiac output and low oxygen delivery.[32] Hypernatremia and hyperosmolarity may decrease organ perfusion by increasing interstitial edema in microvascular beds. There are many theoretical aspects of bicarbonate administration that may preclude its frequent use. It may produce a paradoxical intracellular acidosis because of the rapid entry of carbon dioxide into the cell with the slower egress of the hydrogen ion out of the cell.

A marked hypercapnic acidosis in both systemic venous and coronary sinus blood develops during cardiac arrest and may be worsened by administration of bicarbonate.[127,335] Hypercapnic acidosis in the coronary sinus may cause decreased myocardial contractility.[61,228] Falk and colleagues[107] measured the veno-arterial difference of $PaCO_2$ in five patients who received sodium bicarbonate before and after cardiac arrest. The mean veno-arterial difference ± (SD) before cardiac arrest was 4.4 ± 2.7 mm Hg and in the same patients after receiving additional sodium bicarbonate during CPR was 23.8 ± 15.1 mm Hg. In one particular patient, the difference increased from 16 to 69 mm Hg after the administration of sodium bicarbonate. In another study of 16 patients, the veno-arterial gradient for carbon dioxide was 42 mm Hg during CPR, (i.e., mean mixed venous PCO_2 of 74 mm Hg vs. a mean arterial PCO_2 of 32 mm Hg).[335]

In the central nervous system, however, intracellular acidosis probably does not occur unless overcorrection of the pH occurs. Sessler and colleagues[284] demonstrated that after administration of two doses of bicarbonate of 5 mEq/kg to neonatal rabbits recovering from hypoxic acidosis, the arterial pH increased to 7.41 and intracellular brain pH increased to prehypoxic levels. They did not observe paradoxical intracellular acidosis. Cohen and colleagues[68] showed that the intracellular brain adenosine triphosphate (ATP) concentration did not change during 70 minutes of extreme hypercarbia in rats, despite a decrease in the intracellular brain pH to 6.5. Following hypercarbia, these animals could not be distinguished from normal controls, and their brains were not morphologically different from control animals. Eleff and colleagues[105] using nuclear magnetic resonance spectroscopy to measure brain pH in dogs during CPR, showed that brain pH decreased to 6.29 after 6 minutes of ventricular fibrillation with total depletion of brain ATP (Fig. 13-6). After 6 minutes of effective CPR, the ATP level returned to 86% of pre-arrest levels, and after 35 minutes of CPR, brain pH had returned to normal despite ongoing peripheral arterial acidosis[105] Table 13-10 displays complications of bicarbonate.

Other Alkalinizing Agents

The desire to avoid the real and theoretical side effects of sodium bicarbonate has stimulated the use of several other alkalinizing agents. Unfortunately, none to date have shown real advantages over sodium bicarbonate.

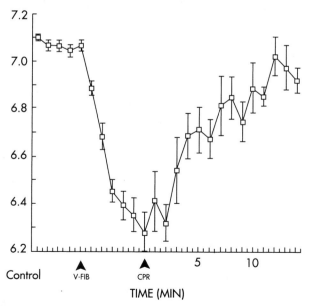

FIGURE 13-6 P magnetic resonance spectroscopy measurements of dog brain pH (pH$_i$) during vest cardiopulmonary resuscitation (CPR) after a 6-minute delay in onset of CPR from time of cardiac arrest. Arrows indicate commencement of ventricular fibrillation (V-fib) and CPR. Note the rapid decrease in pH$_i$ during the first minutes of v-fib and the slow recovery to baseline with CPR. Pre-arrest levels of cerebral blood flow were maintained throughout CPR. Data are mean standard error (n = 6). (From Eleff SM, Schleien CL, Koehler RC, et al: Brain bioenergetics during cardiopulmonary resuscitation in dogs. *Anesthesiology* 76:77–84, 1992; with permission.)

Table 13-10 Complications from Sodium Bicarbonate Administration

Metabolic alkalosis:
  Impaired O$_2$ delivery by shift of oxyhemoglobin dissociation curve
  Decreased cardiac contractility
  Decreased fibrillation threshold
  Decreased plasma K$^+$ and Ca^{++} by intracellular shift
Hypernatremia
Hyperosmolarity
Hypercapnia
Paradoxical intracellular acidosis

Carbicarb (International Medication Systems), a solution of equimolar amounts of sodium bicarbonate and sodium carbonate, works by consuming carbon dioxide and water to generate bicarbonate ion and sodium:

$$Na_2CO_3 + CO_2 + H_2O \rightarrow 2HCO_3^- + 2Na^+$$

In animal models, carbicarb administration resulted in a higher elevation of pH and less of an increase in PaCO$_2$, lactate, and serum osmolarity when compared to sodium bicarbonate use.[25,115,309]

Dichloroacetate (DCA), another alkalinizing agent, works by stimulating the activity of pyruvate dehydrogenase, which facilitates the conversion of lactate to pyruvate.[299] Initial studies showed that DCA decreased lactate concentration by half and increased bicarbonate concentration and pH when administered to humans.[301] It is also shown to improve cardiac output possibly by enhancing myocardial metabolism of lactate and carbohydrate.[300,331] Unfortunately, in a multicenter trial studying patients with lactic acidosis, DCA did not improve outcome or survival when compared to standard alkalinizing agents.[302]

Tromethamine (THAM) or tris-(hydroxymethyl) aminomethane is an organic amine that attracts and combines with hydrogen ions. It is available as a 0.3 M solution adjusted to a pH of 8.6. A dose of 3 mL/kg should raise the bicarbonate concentration by 3 mEq/L. Side effects of this drug include hyperkalemia, hypoglycemia, acute hypocarbia, and apnea. Most importantly it also acts as a peripheral vasodilator when administered during CPR, which may worsen myocardial perfusion. THAM is contraindicated in patients with renal failure.

Calcium

Clinical Effects

Indications for the administration of calcium during CPR remain limited to a few specific problems. This is primarily due to the possibility that in the setting of ischemia-reperfusion injury, calcium administration may worsen post-ischemia hypoperfusion and hasten the development of intracellular cytotoxic events that lead to cell death. Intracellular calcium overload occurs with many pathologic conditions, including ischemia, and may be a part of the final common pathway of cell death.[153,340] However, no study has shown that transient elevation of plasma calcium concentration worsens outcome from cardiac arrest.

Table 13-11 Indications for Calcium Chloride Administration

Hyperkalemia
Hypocalcemia—ionized or total
Hypermagnesemia
Calcium-channel blocker overdose
β-blocker overdose
Dose: 20 mg/kg intravenous/intraosseous, give slowly

The calcium ion is essential in myocardial excitation-contraction coupling, myocardial contractility, and enhances ventricular automaticity during asystole.[126] Therefore, calcium should be useful in the setting of asystole or pulseless electrical activity (electromechanical dissociation). Ionized hypocalcemia leads to decreased ventricular performance, peripheral vasodilation, and blunting of the hemodynamic response to catecholamines.[35,96,198,272,322] Severe ionized hypocalcemia (mean 0.67 mol/L) was present in adult patients suffering from out-of-hospital cardiac arrest[321] and in critically ill children, especially those with sepsis.[49,348] However, there is no experimental evidence for beneficial clinical effects of calcium during these clinical situations.[88,307,308]

Indications

The few firm indications for calcium use during CPR include a cardiac arrest secondary to total or ionized hypocalcemia, hyperkalemia, hypermagnesemia, or an overdose of a calcium channel blocker or a β-blocker.[7] Hypocalcemia occurs in patients with a vast array of conditions predisposing to low total body calcium stores and includes the long-term use of loop diuretics. Ionized hypocalcemia may coexist with a normal total plasma calcium concentration. This occurs in the presence of severe alkalosis, which may be seen in the intensive care unit or operating room due to iatrogenic hyperventilation. Ionized hypocalcemia also follows massive or rapid transfusion of citrated blood products in patients in the emergency or operating room areas.[89] Because calcium administration is not a first-line treatment during CPR, hypocalcemia should be considered as a cause of cardiac arrest, and if present, treated aggressively. Table 13-11 shows indications for calcium.

Dosage

The adult dose of calcium chloride is 500 mg to 1 g.[7] The pediatric dose is 20 mg/kg or 0.2 mL/kg of 10% calcium chloride solution. Calcium gluconate is as effective as calcium chloride in raising ionized calcium concentration during CPR.[141] However, at least one study suggests that calcium chloride is more effective than calcium gluconate in supporting blood pressure in the hypotensive child (see Chapter 7 on Pharmacology).[36] Calcium gluconate can be given as a dose of 100 mg/kg with a maximum dose of 2 g in children.

Side Effects

Calcium should be given slowly through a large bore, free-flowing intravenous line, preferably a central venous line.

Severe tissue necrosis can occur when calcium infiltrates into subcutaneous tissue. When administered too rapidly, calcium may cause severe bradycardia, heart block, or ventricular standstill. Care should be taken when administering calcium to children taking digoxin. Inadvertent hypercalcemia, like hypokalemia, will potentiate digoxin toxicity.

Atropine

Clinical Effects

Atropine is a parasympatholytic agent that acts by reducing vagal tone to the heart. This in turn causes an increase of the discharge rate of the sinus node, enhances atrioventricular conduction, and activates latent ectopic pacemakers.[117] Atropine has minimal effect on systemic vascular resistance, myocardial perfusion, or myocardial contractility.[118]

Indications

Atropine is indicated for treatment of asystole, pulseless electrical activity, bradycardia associated with hypotension,[122] ventricular ectopy, second- and third-degree heart block, and slow idioventricular rhythms.[273] Atropine, therefore, is potentially a useful drug in clinical states associated with excessive parasympathetic tone. Acute myocardial infarction may augment parasympathetic tone and lead to arrhythmias, including asystole, responsive to atropine. In children presenting in cardiac arrest, bradycardia or asystole is commonly the initial rhythm, so atropine may be tried in addition to epinephrine for those patients. In infants, during the perioperative period, any type of stress (i.e., laryngoscopy), may result in severe bradycardia or even asystole due to enhanced parasympathetic tone. These conditions should also be treated with atropine (Table 13-12).

Dosage

The recommended adult dose of atropine is 0.5 mg IV given every 5 minutes until a desired heart rate is obtained or to a maximum dose of 2 mg. Full vagal blockade occurs in adults receiving a dose of 2 mg. For asystole, give 1 mg IV and repeat this dose every 5 minutes if asystole persists. The pediatric dose for atropine is 0.02 mg/kg with a minimum dose of 0.15 mg and a maximum dose of 2 mg. A minimum dose is necessary because of the possible occurrence of paradoxical bradycardia resulting from a central stimulating effect on the medullary

Table 13-12 Indications for Atropine Administration[6]

Symptomatic bradycardia with atrioventricular node block
Vagal bradycardia during intubation attempts
After epinephrine for bradycardia with poor perfusion
Dose: 0.02 mg/kg IV/IO/ETT, repeat every 3 to 5 minutes at the same dose.
Minimum single dose is 0.15 mg.
Maximum single dose is 0.5 mg in a child and 1 mg in an adolescent.
Maximum total dose is 1 mg in a child and 2 mg in an adolescent.

IV, intravenous; IO, intraosseous; ETT, endotracheal tube.

vagal nuclei.[164] Atropine may be given via the intravenous, endotracheal, intraosseous, intramuscular, or subcutaneous routes. The onset of action occurs within 30 seconds, and its peak effect occurs one to two minutes following an intravenous dose.

Side Effects

Atropine should not be used in patients in whom tachycardia is undesirable. In patients following myocardial infarction or ischemia with persistent bradycardia, atropine should be used in the lowest dose possible to increase the heart rate. Tachycardia, which increases myocardial oxygen consumption and can lead to ventricular fibrillation and tachycardia, is common following large doses of atropine in these patients. In patients with pulmonary or systemic outflow tract obstruction or idiopathic hypertrophic subaortic stenosis, tachycardia can decrease ventricular filling and lower cardiac output. Electrical pacing may be a safer means of maintaining a desired heart rate in these patients.

Glucose

Presently, glucose use during CPR should be restricted to patients with documented hypoglycemia. Therefore, rapid determination of serum glucose should accompany the resuscitation. The restricted use of glucose arises because of the possible detrimental effects of hyperglycemia on the brain during ischemia. Myers and colleagues[216] first hypothesized that hyperglycemia worsens neurologic outcome following cardiac arrest. Siemkowicz and Hansen[293] confirmed this finding when they found that after ten minutes of global brain ischemia that the neurologic recovery of hyperglycemic rats was worse than in normoglycemic control animals. Hyperglycemia exaggerates ischemic neurologic injury by increasing the production of lactic acid in the brain by anaerobic metabolism. During ischemia under normoglycemic conditions, brain lactate concentration reaches a plateau. However, when hyperglycemia is present, brain lactate concentration continues to rise for the duration of the ischemic period.[294] The severity of intracellular acidosis during brain ischemia is directly proportional to the pre-ischemic plasma glucose concentration.[58] Clinical studies have shown a direct correlation between the initial serum glucose concentration and poor neurologic outcome.[12,187,243,343] Longstreth and colleagues[186] suggested that a higher admission plasma glucose concentration may be an endogenous response to severe stress and not the cause of more severe brain injury. Given the likelihood of additional ischemic events in the post-resuscitation period, it may be wise to maintain serum glucose in the normal range. Voll and colleagues[326] showed that administering insulin to hyperglycemic rats following global brain ischemia improved neurologic outcome. It is not known if active treatment of hyperglycemia improves the clinical outcome following an ischemic episode. Before any surgical procedure, when there is a possibility of an ischemic episode such as a neurosurgical procedure, tight control of the serum glucose level may be preferable.[292]

Infants and debilitated patients with low endogenous glycogen stores are prone to hypoglycemia when stressed (i.e., during surgery). In these patients, bedside monitoring of the serum glucose level is critical in the perioperative period because of the tendency for hypoglycemia. In the cardiac arrest situation, administration of glucose to the hypoglycemic patient is critical to maintain normal substrate delivery to vital organs. To treat hypoglycemia, a dose of 1 to 2 mL/kg of 50% dextrose for adults, 2 to 4 mL/kg of 25% dextrose or 5 to 10 mL/kg of 10% dextrose for children can be administered by intravenous or intraosseous line.[7] Lower doses and concentrations of glucose are recommended in infants (2 mL/kg of 10% dextrose), as they are at higher risk for hyperglycemia, hyperosmolarity, and rebound hypoglycemia.[7]

Defibrillation

Physiology

Ventricular fibrillation is a sustained burst of multiple, uncoordinated regional ventricular depolarizations and contractions that produce an ineffective cardiac output and absent myocardial blood flow. Reentrant impulses, generated within the ventricles with multiple, shifting circuits, maintain ventricular fibrillation. Several physiologic conditions lower the threshold for fibrillation including hypoxia, hypercapnia, myocardial ischemia, hypothermia, metabolic acidosis and electrolyte disturbances involving sodium, potassium, calcium, and magnesium.

When either ventricular fibrillation or ventricular tachycardia with hypotension or absent pulses is present, countershock is the treatment of choice. Drug treatment by itself cannot be relied upon to terminate ventricular fibrillation. High-voltage countershock when properly applied sends more than 2 A through the heart and can terminate ventricular fibrillation by simultaneously depolarizing and causing a sustained contraction of the myocardium. This allows spontaneous cardiac contractions to commence in a well-oxygenated environment with a normal acid base status. Modern defibrillators deliver only direct current (DC) shocks. The amount of delivered energy relates proportionally to the amount of myocardial damage produced by the countershock.[77,91] In addition, as the energy dose increases, the incidence of post-defibrillation arrhythmias increases.[77] Frequent, concentrated, high-density electric current damages the myocardium, decreases the likelihood of successful defibrillation, and leads to post-defibrillation arrhythmias.[334] These arrhythmias are thought to be associated with prolonged depolarization of the myocardial cell membrane, which increases with the intensity of the stimulus[8,150] and provides an ideal setting for reentrant arrhythmias.[8] In humans following synchronized cardioversion, the frequency of arrhythmias and the degree of ST segment displacement relate directly to the energy level.[254]

In most adult cases, energy levels of 100 to 300 J are successful when delivering external shocks with minimal delay. New biphasic defibrillators use even less energy to defibrillate.[76,281] There is no need for higher voltages ranging from 500 to 1000 J even in obese adults.[48,334] In an in-hospital group of adults, 95% were successfully defibrillated with 200 J externally, even in patients weighing more than 100 kg.[48] Another study compared the use of 175 to 320 J external shocks in 249 adult patients with ventricular fibrillation. Survival did not relate to the energy level used or the weight of the patient, which ranged up to 102 kg.[334] Others have reinforced the successful use of low energy even in large patients.[90,114] One study showed no differences in heart weight or energy per gram of heart weight in patients who ultimately had an autopsy.[155] The goal of defibrillation is to deliver a minimum of electrical energy to a critical mass of ventricular muscle and avoid an overdose of current that could further damage the heart. Depolarization of every cell of both ventricles is not necessary to terminate fibrillation. Zipes and colleagues[349] found that a critical amount of myocardial tissue must be depolarized to terminate ventricular fibrillation. Countershock terminates ventricular fibrillation most often when the shock is delivered between electrodes located at the apex of the right ventricle and the posterior base of the left ventricle, and least often when the shock is delivered between two right ventricle electrodes.

Several clinical factors affect the efficacy of ventricular defibrillation in humans. Success of defibrillation decreases with increased duration of ventricular fibrillation. Short fibrillation time is the most accurate predictor for successful defibrillation.[155,236] Defibrillatory attempts were successful in patients shocked within 8 minutes of fibrillation, whereas attempts were unsuccessful in patients shocked at a mean of 17 minutes after the onset of ventricular fibrillation.[155] Animal studies suggest that a brief period of myocardial perfusion before defibrillation improves cardiac resuscitation outcome from prolonged ventricular fibrillation.[218] Acidosis and hypoxia also decrease the success of defibrillation.[155] The temperature of the patient did not appear to alter the energy required for successful defibrillation.[313] The optimal dose of energy needed to externally defibrillate infants and children is not established conclusively, but available data suggest an initial dose of 2 J/kg.[132] Presently, if the initial dose is unsuccessful then a dose of 4 J/kg should be used on the second and subsequent attempts at defibrillation. The same doses are still recommended when the newer biphasic waveform is used in children.

Correct paddle size and position are critical to the success of defibrillation. Two paddles are used to defibrillate externally; 13 cm in diameter for adults, 8 cm for older children, and 4.5 cm for infants. The largest paddle size appropriate for the patient should be used because large size reduces the density of current flow, which reduces myocardial damage. If the entire paddle does not rest firmly on the chest wall, a current of high density will be delivered to a small contact point on the skin. The paddle should be positioned on the chest wall with most of the myocardium included between them. If for some reason, two paddles cannot be placed on the anterior chest then an alternate approach is to place one paddle anteriorly over the left precordium and the other paddle posteriorly between the scapulae. The interface between the paddle and chest wall can be electrode cream, saline, paste, soap, or moist gauze pads. The cream produces lower impedance than the paste. Precaution should be taken not to allow the substance from one paddle to touch that from the other paddle, because electric current would follow the path of least resistance. This is especially important in infants, where the distance between electrodes is very small.

When the onset of ventricular fibrillation is observed, a defibrillatory attempt should be administered as soon as possible. When the defibrillation is administered, the first three shocks should be given in succession. The most efficient way of delivering three shocks in the shortest time is to either shock through the pads or to leave the paddles on the chest for all three shocks. The only lull between shocks should be to recharge the paddles and to confirm that the rhythm is still ventricular fibrillation or ventricular tachycardia. The doses of electricity should be 2 J/kg for the first shock, 2 to 4 J/kg for the second shock and 4 J/kg for any subsequent doses. For larger children, the maximum doses should be those in the advanced cardiac life support (ACLS) protocols: 200 J, 300 J, and 360 J for all subsequent doses or lower if the biphasic defibrillator is used. If a third defibrillation attempt is unsuccessful, then continue basic life support. The sequence should follow the algorithm: shock, shock, shock, epinephrine, shock, amiodarone or lidocaine, shock, epinephrine, shock, etc. CPR should be performed after each dose of drug administration to circulate the drug before the next defibrillation. It is not necessary to increase the energy dose for each successive defibrillation attempt. On the contrary, the threshold for ventricular fibrillation often increases after CPR and the administration of resuscitation drugs. When defibrillation is unsuccessful, reversible cause of ventricular fibrillation or ventricular tachycardia should be sought and treated. These include the 4Hs and 4Ts: hypoxemia, hypovolemia, hypothermia, hyper/hypokalemia, tamponade, tension pneumothorax, toxins/poisons/drugs, and thromboembolism.

The performance of open-chest defibrillation should be used when the chest is already open during surgery or postoperatively. To perform open-chest defibrillation, a dose of 5 to 20 J of delivered energy should be used beginning with the lower energy level. Paddles, made specifically for this purpose are applied directly to the heart. Open-chest paddles have a diameter of 6 cm for adults, 4 cm for children, and 2 cm for infants. The handles should be insulated. The paddles are applied with saline-soaked pads. Place one electrode behind the left ventricle and the other over the right ventricle on the anterior surface of the heart.

Automated External Defibrillator

The recognition of the benefit of rapid defibrillation of patients in ventricular fibrillation or pulseless ventricular tachycardia has led to automated external defibrillators (AEDs) being widely available for use in public thoroughfares. The goal is to decrease the time from cardiopulmonary arrest to definitive treatment. In certain instances, it may be appropriate for these devices to be used in the hospital setting. Specifically, AEDs may be used by the first responders while awaiting the arrest team. Currently, the American Heart Association recommends the use of AEDs for children younger than 8 years old or 25 kg.[7] Because it is unclear if these devices are equivalent to manual defibrillators, the AHA presently recommends in-hospital use of defibrillators with adjustable dosage by those trained in their use.[7]

Amiodarone

Indications

Amiodarone has replaced lidocaine as the principal antiarrhythmic agent during CPR, because of its broad antiarrhythmic spectrum, fewer proarrhythmic side effects, and relatively benign hemodynamic properties.[4] Amiodarone may be effective in supraventricular tachycardias, hemodynamically stable ventricular tachycardia, or wide-complex tachycardia of uncertain origin. It is also recommended after defibrillation and epinephrine in cardiac arrest secondary to persistent ventricular tachycardia or ventricular fibrillation.

Chemistry

Amiodarone is primarily a class III antiarrhythmic, an iodinated benzofuran derivative, with a chemical structure similar to thyroxine. It is a lipophilic drug, which is highly bound to protein. It is metabolized in liver, excreted mainly in bile with little renal elimination.

Electrophysiology

Although classified mainly as a class III antiarrhythmic, its actions encompass the entire spectrum of antiarrhythmic classification. Amiodarone is a noncompetitive blocker of α- and β-adrenergic receptors.[20] Secondary to this block, amiodarone produces AV nodal suppression. This occurs as a result of prolonging the AV nodal refractory period and by slowing AV nodal conduction.[295] Amiodarone also inhibits the outward potassium current, which prolongs the QT interval,[346] thought to be its major action in acutely controlling arrhythmias. Amiodarone inhibits sodium channels resulting in slowing conduction in the ventricular myocardium resulting in a prolonged QRS duration.[203,204] This mechanism of action is more effective at higher heart rates, an important mechanism of its effectiveness in supraventricular tachycardia (SVT) and ventricular tachycardia.[204] Prolongation of the refractory periods in the atrium, ventricle, and AV node may explain the efficacy of the drug in controlling arrhythmias considered secondary to a reentry process.

Hemodynamic Effects

Due to its α-adrenergic receptor blockade, amiodarone produces vasodilation resulting in hypotension, the side effect seen most commonly with its use.[163] The drug exhibits minor negative inotropic effects, typically offset by its powerful vasodilation.[350] In patients without left ventricular dysfunction, amiodarone reduces mean arterial pressure, left ventricular end-diastolic pressure and systemic vascular resistance, and slightly increases cardiac output. Coronary vascular resistance decreases with little reflex tachycardia associated with its ability to vasodilate.[72] In patients with depressed left-ventricular function, however, significant hemodynamic deterioration has been reported.[163] Other arrhythmias observed with use of the drug include bradycardia, especially in patients with this underlying arrhythmia, and AV block.

Antiarrhythmic Effects

Amiodarone is used for a wide range of both atrial and ventricular arrhythmias in adults and children. It is effective for the treatment of life threatening and/or refractory ventricular and supraventricular arrhythmias, including atrial flutter, supraventricular tachycardia, and ventricular tachycardia. It is commonly used to treat ectopic atrial tachycardia or junctional ectopic tachycardia after cardiac surgery[110,233] and ventricular tachycardia in postoperative patients or children with underlying cardiac disease.[233,240]

Pharmacokinetics

The oral form of amiodarone is poorly absorbed, and so acute therapy by this route is impossible. Because of the drug's high lipid solubility, drug levels correlate poorly with its clinical effect. Terminal elimination is very prolonged, with a half-life lasting up to 26 to 107 days with chronic therapy.[144] After an intravenous dose, its mean half-life is 4.2 to 34.5 hours. Elimination of the drug is not dependent on either normal renal or hepatic function. It is extensively metabolized in the liver via multiple pathways. Its major degradative pathway is via de-ethylation forming N-desethylamiodarone (DEA), itself pharmacologically active. DEA is equipotent to amiodarone as a sodium-channel blocker, but less potent in its calcium-channel blocking properties. The primary route of elimination is via the bile with less than 1% excreted in the urine.

Dosage

For both supraventricular and ventricular arrhythmias, a loading infusion of 5 mg/kg IV is recommended over several minutes (for persistent pulseless ventricular tachycardia or fibrillation) to one hour, depending on the clinical need to achieve a rapid drug effect. Repeated doses of 5 mg/kg up to a maximum of 15 mg/kg per day may be used when needed for persistent arrhythmia. A continuous infusion of amiodarone 5 mcg/kg/minute then follows the loading dose.

Side Effects

The major acute side effect is related to hypotension, seen in 16% of patients, secondary to α-adrenergic receptor inhibition and proarrhythmia generation. The generation of polymorphic ventricular arrhythmias, including torsades de pointes, is due to prolongation of the QT interval.[207] This complication appears to occur less often in children than in adults. Patients with left ventricular dysfunction have a higher incidence not only of hypotension, but also congestive heart failure and acute myocardial infarction. Long-term complications include pulmonary complications such as pulmonary fibrosis, interstitial pneumonitis, and acute respiratory distress syndrome associated with a surgical procedure.[217,244] Interference with thyroid hormone metabolism leading to either hypo- or hyperthyroidism, elevated liver enzyme levels, corneal deposits, and skin discoloration have also been observed with long-term use. Neurologic abnormalities include tremors, ataxia, fatigue, headache, sleep disturbances, photosensitivity, and peripheral neuropathy, all associated with long-term use.

Lidocaine

Indications

Lidocaine has now become a second line agent (after amiodarone) in the treatment of frequent premature ventricular contractions or hemodynamically stable ventricular tachycardia. Similarly, if pulseless ventricular tachycardia or ventricular fibrillation persist after defibrillation and administration of epinephrine, lidocaine may be used as a second line adjunct after amiodarone.[4] This second line status for lidocaine recognizes that lidocaine has not been proven to lower mortality during CPR and that several toxic side effects may accompany lidocaine usage (see below).

Chemistry

Lidocaine, a class 1B antiarrhythmic, is an aromatic group 2–6 xylidine coupled to diethylglycine via an amide bond. It is a weak base with a pK_a of 7.85. Lidocaine is metabolized mainly in the liver by the microsomal enzyme system.[70] The major degradative pathway for lidocaine is by oxidative N-de-ethylation, followed by hydrolysis to 2–6 xylidine. Its minor degradative pathway is by hydroxylation of its aromatic nitrogen. Up to 10% of the drug is excreted unchanged in the urine. The percent of drug excreted unchanged increases in acidic urine. There is no biliary excretion or intestinal absorption in humans.

Electrophysiology

Lidocaine causes a decrease in automaticity and in spontaneous phase 4 depolarization for pacemaker tissue. The drug increases the ventricular fibrillation threshold and slightly increases or has no effect on the ventricular diastolic threshold for depolarization. It decreases the duration of the action potential of Purkinje fibers and ventricular muscle, while increasing the effective refractory period of these fibers. Lidocaine does not affect conduction time through the AV node or in the ventricle. By decreasing automaticity, lidocaine prevents or terminates ventricular arrhythmias due to accelerated ectopic foci. Lidocaine abolishes reentrant ventricular arrhythmias by decreasing action potential duration and conduction time of Purkinje fibers, thus reducing the nonuniformity of action. The effect on ischemic tissue where lidocaine delivery may be limited is unknown.[70]

Hemodynamic Effects

In animal models, rapid administration of intravenous lidocaine decreases stroke work, blood pressure, systemic vascular resistance[71] and left ventricular contractility,[13] and slightly increases heart rate. In healthy adults, the drug does not appear to cause any change in heart rate or blood pressure.[148,282] In patients with cardiac disease, especially in those suffering an acute myocardial infarction, excessive doses of lidocaine given by rapid infusion may lead to a decrease in cardiac function. Therefore, slow IV administration, no greater than 50 to 100 mg/minute in adults is recommended.[70]

Antiarrhythmic Effects

Lidocaine is effective in terminating ventricular premature beats (VPBs) and ventricular tachycardia in humans during general surgery, before or after cardiac surgery, following an acute myocardial infarction, and in patients with digitalis intoxication. Treatment is indicated if unifocal VPBs occur at a rate of more than five per minute. Additionally, VPBs require treatment if they occur on a normal T wave, are multifocal, or arise as runs of VPBs (ventricular tachycardia). Lidocaine is also effective in preventing and treating ventricular arrhythmias during cardiac catheterization. Infusion of lidocaine may be indicated after cardioversion from ventricular fibrillation, especially when recurrent ventricular fibrillation or tachycardia occurs. Lidocaine is not effective in the treatment of atrial or AV junctional arrhythmias. Table 13-13 lists indications for lidocaine and amiodarone.

Pharmacokinetics

After administering an intravenous dose of lidocaine the changes in plasma concentration follow a biphasic curve. The α-region, the early rapid fall in serum concentration, has an average half-life of 8 to 17 minutes. It exists due to changes in distribution of the drug within the central compartment (intravascular space) and the peripheral compartment (includes hepatic metabolism of the drug). In patients with normal liver function, the hepatic extraction ratio for lidocaine is approximately 70%. The β-region, during which there is a slower decrease in serum concentration, has an average half-life of 87 to 108 minutes. This is due to transfer of the drug from the larger peripheral compartment to the smaller central compartment.

To achieve and maintain therapeutic levels of lidocaine, a bolus dose should be given at the initiation of a constant infusion. If an infusion is begun without an initial bolus, approximately five half-lives are required to approach a plateau serum concentration.[70] Thus with a half-life of 108 minutes, a nine hour infusion would be required to reach a plateau concentration. When using a bolus administration alone, ventricular arrhythmias often return within 15 to 20 minutes because of rapid clearance from the central compartment.[148]

Lidocaine toxicity occurs most commonly in patients with severe hepatic disease or severe congestive heart failure. A decreased cardiac output results in decreased hepatic blood flow, which in turn results in decreased lidocaine clearance. During CPR, lidocaine clearance is decreased because of the

Table 13-13   Indications for Amiodarone and Lidocaine Administration[6]

Amiodarone	• Supraventricular tachycardia • Wide-complex tachycardia of uncertain origin • Persistent ventricular arrhythmia after defibrillation and epinephrine	• Dose: 5 mg/kg/ IV/IO bolus over minutes to 1 hr, repeat to max of 15 mg/kg/day. • Infusion: 5–10 mcg/kg/min
Lidocaine	• Ventricular tachyarrhythmia (not ventricular escape rhythm) • Ventricular ectopy • Raise threshold for fibrillation	• Dose: 1 mg/kg IV/IO/ETT bolus (2.5 × dose if ETT) • Infusion: 20–50 mcg/kg/min IV/IO • Reduce infusion rate if low cardiac output or liver failure is present.

IV, intravenous; IO, intraosseous; ETT, endotracheal tube.

inherent decrease in cardiac output and very low hepatic blood flow. In dogs, with use of conventional CPR to obtain a blood pressure of 20% of control values, a lidocaine bolus of 2 mg/kg IV resulted in very elevated blood and tissue concentrations. During CPR, distribution of the drug, that is usually complete in 20 minutes, was still not complete after 1 hour. In addition, lidocaine clearance and distribution may be altered due to changes in protein binding and metabolism during CPR.[59] In humans, high peak blood and tissue concentrations of lidocaine occur during CPR, with a delay in the time to peak concentration. Comparison of the peripheral and central routes of administration of lidocaine during open-chest CPR in dogs revealed no difference in time to peak serum concentration.[60]

Dosage

Patients with normal cardiac and hepatic function should receive an initial IV bolus of lidocaine of 1 mg/kg, followed by a constant IV infusion at a rate of 20 to 50 mcg/kg/minute.[7] If the arrhythmia recurs, a second IV bolus with the same dose can be given.[126] Severe diminution of cardiac output calls for a bolus of no greater than 0.75 mg/kg followed by an infusion at a rate of 10 to 20 mcg/kg/minute. Dosages should be decreased by 50% of normal in patients with hepatic disease. Patients with chronic renal disease on hemodialysis have normal lidocaine pharmacokinetics. However, since toxic metabolites may accumulate in patients receiving infusions for long periods of time, caution should be used in treating these patients. Drug interactions with lidocaine are common. Phenobarbital increases lidocaine metabolism requiring increased doses. Isoniazid and chloramphenicol decrease lidocaine metabolism, so a decreased dosage should be used. Any drug that decreases cardiac output (i.e., propranolol) will increase the serum concentration of lidocaine, while drugs, such as isoproterenol, that increase cardiac output and hepatic blood flow, will cause the serum concentration to be lower than predicted.

Side Effects

The toxic effects of lidocaine generally involve the central nervous system and include seizures, psychosis, drowsiness, paresthesias, disorientation, muscle twitching, agitation, and respiratory arrest. Treatment for seizures and psychosis consists of a benzodiazepine or a barbiturate. True allergic reactions to lidocaine are extremely rare. Cardiovascular side effects are usually seen in patients with already decreased myocardial function. Conversion of second degree heart block to complete heart block has been described.[179] Further slowing of sinus bradycardia has also been observed. These effects are infrequent and occur with large dose administration.

NEUROLOGIC OUTCOME FOLLOWING CARDIOPULMONARY RESUSCITATION

Multiple pathologic events occur in the first few minutes of cardiac arrest. Chief among these are the loss of cerebral blood flow, the loss of consciousness, the loss of brain chemical energy (ATP), and the fall in brain pH. These events are reversible if adequate blood flow is restored within 1 to

2 minutes and good recovery may be forthcoming even if cardiac arrest precedes CPR for as long as 4 to 6 minutes. While CPR remains our first response to cardiac arrest, it does not always provide cerebral blood flow that is adequate to meet metabolic needs, and therefore cerebral hypoperfusion may continue until spontaneous circulation is restored and optimized. The assessment of the duration and extent of no-perfusion and low-perfusion during a cardiac arrest and resuscitation is difficult. These difficulties in quantitating the degree of hypoperfusion suffered by a patient lead to inaccuracies in predicting a patient's likelihood of neurologic recovery. The patient who remains in a coma after apparently successful CPR poses diagnostic, therapeutic, prognostic, and ethical problems. Metabolic derangements, seizures, continued ischemia of the brainstem or of both cerebral hemispheres, and prolonged effects of sedatives or paralytics need to be considered as reversible causes of coma after a successful resuscitation. Differentiating reversible from irreversible central nervous system dysfunction is critical not only in choosing appropriate therapeutic modalities, but also in counseling the family. The remainder of this chapter will focus on the diagnostic and prognostic neurologic examination, both clinical and technological, in the patient who has suffered reversible cardiac arrest and in whom the examination may be clouded by sedative drugs.

Clinical Neurologic Examination

In the cooperative patient, the clinical neurologic examination remains the gold standard. The Glasgow Coma Scale (GCS) is widely accepted as a useful and convenient method of quantitating brainstem and cortical function and comparing it over time.[318] In the immediate post-resuscitation period, the GCS allows an hourly assessment of recovery and the opportunity to alter a therapeutic regimen. Three tests are needed to calculate the GCS score (Table 13-14). The best eye response (1 to 4 points), best motor response (1 to 6 points), and best verbal response (1 to 5 points). The maximum score is 15 and the minimum GCS value is 3. The patient is considered comatose when the GCS is 8 or less (eyes 2, motor 4, verbal 2 or E2:M4:V2). Levy and colleagues[177] reported a prospective, international study of 210 adults

Table 13-14 The Glasgow Coma Scale

Eyes	Open	Spontaneously	4
		To verbal command	3
		To pain	2
		No response	1
Motor	To verbal command	Obeys	6
	To painful stimulus	Localizes pain	5
		Withdrawal	4
		Flexion	3
		Extension	2
		No response	1
Verbal		Orientated	5
		Disorientated	4
		Inappropriate words	3
		Incomprehensible sounds	2
		No response	1

GCS score is the sum of the best response from each of the three categories. Maximum possible score = 15, minimum possible score = 3.

admitted with GCS of E2:M4:V2 or less, with anoxia as the etiology. At the end of the 24 hours, all 52 patients with no pupillary reflex died. Similarly, all patients who did not withdraw to painful stimuli or did not have roving eye movements by day 7 died. Although this study shows the predictive power of GCS, with a confidence interval of 95%, 5% of patients with these findings may be alive 5 years later.[291] No information is available to predict eventual neurologic outcome based on post-resuscitation findings in children who have required CPR for cardiac arrest.

Technological Neurologic Examination

There are few tests that allow for early prediction of which patients will emerge from coma and no tests for early prediction of rehabilitation potential. Three laboratory tests that may eventually be useful in predicting the outcome include cerebral spinal fluid (CSF) levels of creatine kinase (CK-BB) and lactate dehydrogenase (LDH 1-3) and multilevel evoked potentials. CSF enzyme levels were measured in 20 consecutive patients admitted to the adult ICU after out-of-hospital cardiac arrest.[152] Enzyme levels at 24 (creatine kinase) and 76 (LDH) hours identified all eight survivors. In a similar study, multilevel-evoked potentials were examined in 17 patients who were comatose following CPR. Evoked potentials were collected in the first 72 hours in all patients. All four patients with an intact somatosensory-evoked cerebral potential regained consciousness.[151] De Meirleir and Taylor[81] used somatosensory-evoked potentials (SEPs) to study 50 comatose children. All 27 children who died had an abnormal

initial SEP. However, there was overlap between the initial SEP score and eventual neurologic recovery. Recovery or worsening of SEPs during the first week strongly correlated with neurologic outcome. Unfortunately, neither CSF enzyme studies nor multilevel-evoked potentials could predict the degree to which the children could be rehabilitated.

Clinical Examination for Brain Death

Determination of brain death may be necessary for children who remain unresponsive despite apparently successful CPR. Depending on the locale (e.g., state law) or with adjunct testing (e.g., EEG), the neurologic examination alone is sufficient to declare brain death if the cause of coma is known, its irreversibility determined, and confounding issues such as hypothermia or the presence of sedative drugs are absent (Table 13-15). Criteria for brain death are based on the recommendations of the Ad Hoc Committee on Brain Death of The Children's Hospital in Boston.[1] Brain death is said to have occurred when cerebral and brainstem function are irreversibly absent. A clinical exam showing a lack of receptivity and responsivity is proof of absent cerebral function. Total absence of pupillary light, corneal oculocephalic, oculovestibular, oropharyngeal, and respiratory reflexes is proof of absent brainstem function. Irreversibility of absent cerebral and brainstem function is generally considered proof of brain death in the United States. Two examinations at least 6 hours apart are performed to demonstrate irreversibility. The duration between examinations may vary depending on the circumstances or possible causes. Up to 24 hours of observation may

Table 13-15 Clinical Criteria for Brain Death

Prerequisites
1. Presence of known and untreatable structural damage to the brain or irreversible systemic metabolic derangement.
2. Absence of hypothermia (core temperature over 32° C).
3. Absence of hypotension.
4. Two observations at intervals of at least 6 hours by a neurologist or neurosurgeon (who is a member of the active staff), or another physician specially trained in neurology who is approved by the neurologist-in-chief. (Many other institutions allow the critical care physician to do so.)
Note: The duration of observation has been gradually shortened. Six hours is the current usual standard, although 12–24 hours may be required if doubt exists about the cause of irreversibility of coma in adults and children, up to 3 days in premature infants or neonates.

Clinical Criteria
The following criteria should be documented in the medical record:
1. Absent brain stem function.
   a. Pupils dilated and unreactive to light.
   b. No ocular-vestibular response to 100 cc of ice water instilled in each ear separately over 30–60 seconds.
   c. Absent corneal and pharyngeal reflexes including cough on tracheal suction.
   d. The absence of respiratory movement during 5–10 minutes of apneic ventilation with 100% O_2.
Note: The patient should have a normal $PaCO_2$ at the time of apnea testing and should have apneic ventilation performed for a period of time sufficient to induce a 20 torr increase in $PaCO_2$. This usually requires 5–10 minutes.
2. Absent cerebral function:
   a. No behavioral or reflex response to painful stimuli that imply function above the level of the foramen magnum. (Note: Spinal reflexes may be preserved, and their presence does not preclude diagnosis of death.)
Note: Areflexia is common after severe brain injury. However, as the duration of absent cerebral function lengthens, it becomes more likely for spinal reflexes to reappear.

Special Cases
1. Ancillary laboratory tests: Laboratory tests are not required where the diagnosis is certain and the clinical criteria are clearly met. The EEG or imaging of blood flow can be useful diagnostic tests when there is uncertainty about either the etiology or clinical findings.
2. Therapeutic drug-induced coma: Barbiturates and hypothermia currently have a role in ameliorating damage to the brain of some severely ill patients. In the presence of therapeutic drug intoxication or hypothermia, the diagnostic and prognostic utility of the EEG diminishes. Absent cerebral blood flow as measured by imaging studies will be required in these instances and should be performed promptly when brain death is suspected.

From: The Johns Hopkins Hospital, 1998 Interdisciplinary Clinical Practice Manual.

be appropriate for toxic, metabolic, or hypoxic etiologies. The period of observation may be prolonged up to 72 hours if necessary for infants, newborns, or prematures although some view no brain death criteria in this group.[149] These examinations concentrate on the brain and ignore spinal reflexes, which often are present despite brain death. Ancillary laboratory tests (e.g., cerebral blood flow study) are required if CNS depressant drugs may be affecting the clinical examination. CNS depressants in the form of residual general anesthetics are common in the immediate postoperative period. The use of sedatives and muscle relaxants (paralysis) often used in patients with pulmonary hypertension to allow prolonged mechanical ventilation make the use of these ancillary tests important in the child who has undergone open-heart surgery.

Ancillary Tests for Brain Death

Death in the intensive care unit often involves emotional, ethical, legal, moral, and social concerns compounding the medical issues. The possibility of organ donation can further complicate matters.[79] When clinical examination alone is not satisfactory to resolve the patient's prognosis, ancillary (or confirmatory) tests are useful for diagnosis and prognosis. The additional information may influence decisions to limit, cease, or withdraw therapy.

Pharmacologic levels of anesthetics, hypothermia, metabolic abnormalities, and hemodynamic instability in postoperative patients will interfere with the clinical determination of brain death. The simplest solution is to wait for these processes to correct normally. Patients in extremis may not eliminate drugs readily, control body temperature normally, or become metabolically or hemodynamically stable. When a delay results in unacceptable stress on the family or ICU resources, ancillary tests may be helpful.

The electroencephalogram (EEG) and radionuclide cerebral flow scans are the most commonly ordered ancillary tests.[192] An invasive and less commonly used test, four-vessel angiography, represents the standard to which all other tests of brain death are compared. However, blood flow may be present to small areas of the brain in a patient who is clinically brain dead and will die of cardiovascular collapse. The presence of flow to less than 10% of the brain may be enough to refute the diagnosis of brain death.[106]

The routine use of the electroencephalogram (EEG) in the diagnosis of brain death is fraught with difficulty and controversy. When used appropriately, the EEG may be an adjunct in the diagnosis of brain death. The United States guidelines for brain death specify the entire brain, including the brainstem must fill criteria. Although individual EEG leads sample a limited portion of the brain, the full montage reflects neuronal activity over a large volume of the cerebral cortex. Additionally, the EEG machine is portable and offers little, if any, risk to the patient. Strict guidelines on how to record the EEG in suspected cerebral death have been published.[2] One of these is that maximum amplification of the signal be used (at least 2 mV/mL). Unfortunately, in the electrically noisy environment of the intensive care unit, an artifact is often amplified above the level needed to declare an EEG isoelectric (Fig. 13-7). This may in part explain a study in which 20% of all EEGs obtained for the determination of brain death were not interpretable.[45] The EEG is clearly useful when it shows cortical activity (Fig. 13-8) or is isoelectric. However, a problem occurs when a repeat EEG 24 hours later is required because of the presence of artifacts that may closely resemble cerebral activity.[1] Technical limitations of an EEG are common; a nondiagnostic EEG is not the same thing as an EEG demonstrating electrocerebral activity. It is simply nondiagnostic. In such a situation, a repeat record may be

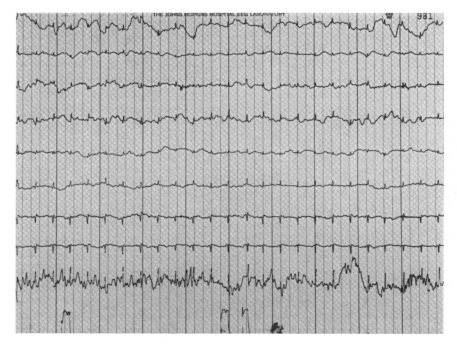

FIGURE 13-7 Isoelectric EEG from a clinically brain dead 8-month-old. Note the artifacts that mar the record. EEGs for brain death are collected at maximum gain making it difficult to obtain an absolutely flat EEG in the electrically noisy environment of the Pediatric Intensive Care Unit.

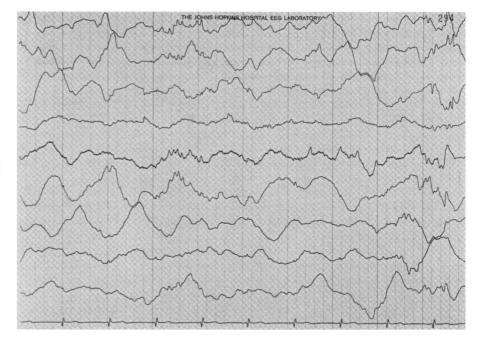

FIGURE 13-8 EEG from a deeply comatose 3-year-old child (spontaneous respirations, not clinically brain dead). The slow waves apparent on the EEG also preclude a diagnosis of brain death.

requested or a decision regarding a patient's status may be made "on other clinical grounds."[149]

Complementary tests that detect the presence of cerebral blood flow can be useful for confirming the diagnosis of brain death when the interpretation of electrical activity may have interference from patient activity (myoclonus), environmental background noise, drug administration, or metabolic abnormalities. Arterial four-vessel angiography is the definitive method to detect cerebral blood flow but recently, some less invasive measures have been described to measure cerebral blood flow which include gadolinium enhanced MRI, magnetic resonance arteriography, and intravenous digital subtraction angiography. The difficulty in transporting a critical ill child to the angiography suite or the magnetic resonance facility has led to the use of bedside radionuclide

studies such as single-photon emission computed tomography (SPECT) imaging with technetium-99m.[237] Figure 13-9 is a technetium-99m SPECT study from a 3-year-old drowning victim. Notice the filling from the Circle of Willis and the appearance of the sagittal sinus. This pattern demonstrates persistent cerebral blood flow. Contrast this with Figure 13-10 from a 3-year-old boy involved in a house fire who presented to the emergency department with ventricular fibrillation and no blood pressure. The patient responded to CPR and cardioversion and was admitted to the PICU deeply comatose (GCS E1:M1:V1) with fixed and dilated pupils. Notice filling from the external carotid system (extracranial) but bilateral absence of the arterial phase (anterior and middle cerebral artery territories), lack of visualization of the sagittal sinus during the venous phase, lack of arterial peak of cerebral

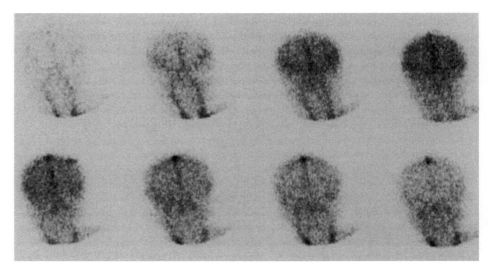

FIGURE 13-9 Technetium-99m single-photon emission computed tomography image from a 3-year-old child demonstrating blood flow to the brain as evidenced by the filling of the Circle of Willis and appearance of the sagittal sinus.

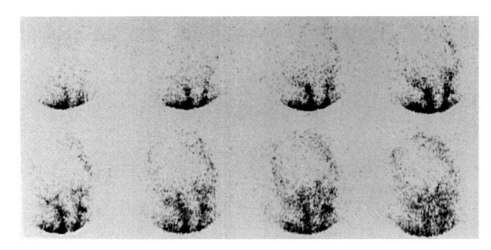

FIGURE 13-10 Technetium-99m single-photon emission computed tomography image from a 3-year-old child showing extracranial blood flow without intracranial flow. This scan is consistent with brain death.

time activity curves, and perfusion of extracranial tissues only. This scan is consistent with brain death. As with any study, threshold values and timing are important. A patient may appear clinically brain dead with no flow to the brainstem but with flow to the forebrain.[169] Therefore, these studies should be done as late as possible in the brain death workup when cerebral blood flow would not only be reduced below viability, but absent.

Transcranial Doppler (TCD) has potential use in the confirmation of brain death. A noninvasive and highly portable technique, it can be highly specific and sensitive in the hands of an experienced user.[234] In children, false-positive results are reported and care must be used to survey as much of the intracranial circulation as is possible. The presence of forward blood flow curves may be due to shunting of blood through the Circle of Willis into external arteries without cerebral perfusion.[33] These authors report that retrograde flow was specific for brain death in comatose children (retrograde flow was never seen in the survivors).[33] Reversal of diastolic flow on TCD has been seen in the presence of increased intracranial pressure. Two children have been described with reversal of diastolic cerebral blood flow and who survived after management of their increased intracranial pressure.[57] Because of its portability and lack of risks to the patient, TCD is used by some as a screen to decide when to send a patient for flow studies that have risks from contrast agents, vascular invasion, or the need to transport an unstable patient.

Ethical Considerations

Given the uncertainty in predicting awakening from a vegetative state in children who suffer cardiac arrest after cardiac surgery, the diagnosis of brain death may be necessary to determine futility of continued care. Many patients, who are in a deeply comatose state after ischemia and CPR, have multi-organ injury and die of cardiovascular collapse within a few weeks. Therefore, some would argue that brain death need never be declared since "even when the cost of care is taken into account, it is hard to justify the withdrawal of therapy for patients in medical coma simply on the basis of prognostic information available at present."[291] Bates[19] believes that it is statistically untenable to predict which comatose patient will be the rare recovery and therefore no individual (as opposed to a cohort) can be declared in an irreversible coma. Cole[69] rejects the notion of irreversibility as vague and concludes that recent medical definitions seek illegitimately to obtain the certainty of a weak construal of "irreversible" along with the freedom from moral obligation of the strong construal. The Task Force on Brain Death in Children recognized that medicine is not an exact science and that the published database is relatively small. However, they maintain that no child who has met their rigid brain death criteria has survived.[290]

The question of irreversibility of brain injury in contrast to brain death led the American Medical Association[73] to suggest that when "a patient's coma is beyond a doubt irreversible and there are adequate safeguards to confirm the accuracy of the diagnosis ... it is not unethical to discontinue means of life prolonging medical treatment." The Johns Hopkins Hospital policy on Withholding or Withdrawing Futile Life-Sustaining Medical Interventions adopted January 1992 states: "It is the policy of The Johns Hopkins Hospital that attending physicians are not required to offer life-sustaining intervention, and may refuse a request for same, if the intervention is medically futile and will not offer meaningful benefit to the patient."[149] In a study of 50 consecutive deaths in the Children's National Medical Center PICU, withdrawal of therapy, failed resuscitation, and brain death were equally represented. However, cardiac surgery patients were far more likely to die after failed CPR whereas withdrawal of therapy was more likely for patients with underlying chronic disease.[212]

References

1. Ad Hoc Committee on brain death - The Children's Hospital Boston: Determination of brain death. *J Pediatr* 10:15–19, 1987.
2. American Electroencephalographic Society: Guidelines in EEG and evoked potentials, 1986. *J Clin Neurophysiol* 1(3 suppl 1):1–152, 1986.
3. American Heart Association's guidelines for cardiopulmonary resuscitation and emergency cardiac care. *JAMA* 255:2921, 1986.
3a. American Heart Association's international emergency cardiac care and cardiopulmonary resuscitation guidelines 2000, Part 6, Section 4, Devices to assist circulation. *Circulation* 102:I105–I111, 2000.
4. American Heart Association's international emergency cardiac care and cardiopulmonary resuscitation guidelines 2000, Part 9: Pediatric basic life support. *Circulation* 102:I–253, 2000.
5. American Heart Association's guidelines for cardiopulmonary resuscitation and emergency cardiac care. *JAMA* 268:2256, 1992.

6. American Heart Association's international emergency cardiac care and cardiopulmonary resuscitation guidelines 2000, Part 10: Pediatric advanced life support. *Circulation* 102:I–291, 2000.
7. American Heart Association's PALS Provider Manual. 2002.
8. Anderson GJ, Reiser J, McAllister H, Likoff W: Electro-physiological characterization of myocardial injury induced by defibrillation during CPR. *Med Instrum* 14:54[Abstract], 1980.
9. Angelos MG, Gaddis ML, Gaddis GM, Leasure JE: Improved survival and reduced myocardial necrosis with cardiopulmonary bypass reperfusion in a canine model of coronary occlusion and cardiac arrest. *Ann Emerg Med* 19:1122–1128, 1990.
10. Anthi A, Tzelepis GE, Alivizatos P, et al: Unexpected cardiac arrest after cardiac surgery: Incidence, predisposing causes, and outcome of open chest cardiopulmonary resuscitation. *Chest* 113:15–19, 1998.
11. Arai T, Watanabe T, Nagaro T, Matsuo S: Blood-brain barrier impairment after cardiac resuscitation. *Crit Care Med* 9:444–448, 1981.
12. Ashwal S, Schneider S, Tomasi L, Thompson J: Prognostic implications of hyperglycemia and reduced cerebral blood flow in childhood near-drowning. *Neurology* 40:820–823, 1990.
13. Austen WG, Moran JM: Cardiac and peripheral vascular effects of lidocaine and procainalol. *Am J Cardiol* 16:701, 1965.
14. Babbs CF, Fitzgerald KR, Voorhees WD, Murphy RJ: High-pressure ventilation during CPR with 95% O_2:5% CO_2. *Crit Care Med* 10:505–508, 1982.
15. Babbs CF, Tacker WA, Paris RL, et al: CPR with simultaneous compression and ventilation at high airway pressure in 4 animal models. *Crit Care Med* 10:501–504, 1982.
16. Barranco F, Lesmes A, Irles JA, et al: Cardiopulmonary resuscitation with simultaneous chest and abdominal compression: comparative study in humans. *Resuscitation* 20:67–77, 1990.
17. Bartlett RL, Stewart NJ Jr, Raymond J, et al: Comparative study of three methods of resuscitation: closed-chest, open-chest manual, and direct mechanical ventricular assistance. *Ann Emerg Med* 13:773–777, 1984.
18. Barton C, Callaham M: Lack of correlation between end-tidal carbon dioxide concentrations and $PaCO_2$ in cardiac arrest. *Crit Care Med* 19:108–110, 1991.
19. Bates D: Defining prognosis in medical coma. *J Neurol Neurosurg Psychiatry* 54:569–571, 1991.
20. Bauthier J, Broekhuysen J, Charlier R, Richard J: Nature of the inhibition by amiodarone of isoproterenol-induced tachycardia in the dog. *Arch Int Pharmacodyn Ther* 219:45–51, 1976.
21. Berger S, Dhala A, Friedberg DZ: Sudden cardiac death in infants, children, and adolescents. *Pediatr Clin North Am* 46:221–234, 1999.
22. Berkowitz ID, Chantarojanasiri T, Koehler RC, et al: Blood flow during cardiopulmonary resuscitation with simultaneous compression and ventilation in infant pigs. *Pediatr Res* 26:558–564, 1989.
23. Berkowitz ID, Gervais H, Schleien CL, et al: Epinephrine dosage effects on cerebral and myocardial blood flow in an infant swine model of cardiopulmonary resuscitation. *Anesthesiology* 75:1041–1050, 1991.
24. Berryman CR, Phillips GM: Interposed abdominal compression-CPR in human subjects. *Ann Emerg Med* 13:226–229, 1984.
25. Bersin RM, Arieff AI: Improved hemodynamic function during hypoxia with Carbicarb, a new agent for the management of acidosis. *Circulation* 77:227–233, 1988.
26. Beyar R, Kishon Y, Sideman S, Dinnar U: Computer studies of systemic and regional blood flow mechanisms during cardiopulmonary resuscitation. *Med Biol Eng Comput* 22:499–506, 1984.
27. Beyar R, Halperin HR, Tsitlik JE, et al: Circulatory assistance by intrathoracic pressure variations: Optimization and mechanisms studied by a mathematical model in relation to experimental data. *Circ Res* 64:703–720, 1989.
28. Bhende MS, Thompson AE, Cook DR, Saville AL: Validity of a disposable end-tidal CO_2 detector in verifying endotracheal tube placement in infants and children. *Ann Emerg Med* 21:142–145, 1992.
29. Bhende MS, Thompson AE: Evaluation of an end-tidal CO_2 detector during pediatric cardiopulmonary resuscitation. *Pediatrics* 95:395–399, 1995.
30. Bircher N, Safar P: Comparison of standard and "new" closed-chest CPR and open-chest CPR in dogs. *Crit Care Med* 9:384–385, 1981.
31. Bircher N, Safar P, Stewart R: A comparison of standard, "MAST"-augmented, and open-chest CPR in dogs. A preliminary investigation. *Crit Care Med* 8:147–152, 1980.
32. Bishop RL, Weisfeldt ML: Sodium bicarbonate administration during cardiac arrest: Effect on arterial pH PCO_2, and osmolality. *JAMA* 235:506–509, 1976.
33. Bode H, Sauer M, Pringsheim W: Diagnosis of brain death by transcranial Doppler sonography. *Arch Dis Child* 63:1474–1478, 1988.
34. Brillman JA, Sanders AB, Otto CW, et al: Outcome of resuscitation from fibrillatory arrest using epinephrine and phenylephrine in dogs. *Crit Care Med* 13:912–913, 1985.
35. Bristow MR, Schwartz HD, Binetti G, et al: Ionized calcium and the heart: Elucidation of in vivo concentration-response relationships in the open-chest dog. *Circ Res* 41:565–574, 1977.
36. Broner CW, Stidham GL, Westenkirchner DF, Watson DC: A prospective, randomized, double-blind comparison of calcium chloride and calcium gluconate therapies for hypocalcemia in critically ill children. *J Pediatr* 115:988, 1990.
37. Brown CG, Birinyi F, Werman HA, et al: The comparative effects of epinephrine versus phenylephrine on regional cerebral blood flow during cardiopulmonary resuscitation. *Resuscitation* 14:171–183, 1986.
38. Brown CG, Davis EA, Werman HA, Hamlin RL: Methoxamine versus epinephrine on regional cerebral blood flow during cardiopulmonary resuscitation. *Crit Care Med* 15:682–686, 1987.
39. Brown CG, Martin DR, Pepe PE, et al: A comparison of standard-dose and high-dose epinephrine in cardiac arrest outside the hospital: The Multicenter High-Dose Epinephrine Study Group. *N Engl J Med* 327:1051–1055, 1992.
40. Brown CG, Taylor RB, Werman HA, et al: Myocardial oxygen delivery/consumption during cardiopulmonary resuscitation: A comparison of epinephrine and phenylephrine. *Ann Emerg Med* 17:302–308, 1988.
41. Brown CG, Taylor RB, Werman HA, et al: Effect of standard doses of epinephrine on myocardial oxygen delivery and utilization during cardiopulmonary resuscitation. *Crit Care Med* 16:536–539, 1988.
42. Brown CG, Werman HA, Davis EA, et al: Comparative effect of graded doses of epinephrine on regional brain blood flow during CPR in a swine model. *Ann Emerg Med* 15:1138–1144, 1986.
43. Brown CG, Werman HA, Davis EA, et al: The effects of graded doses of epinephrine on regional myocardial blood flow during cardiopulmonary resuscitation in swine. *Circulation* 75:491–497, 1987.
44. Brown CG, Werman HA, Davis EA, et al: The effect of high-dose phenylephrine versus epinephrine on regional cerebral blood flow during CPR. *Ann Emerg Med* 16:743–748, 1987.
45. Buchner H, Schuchardt V: Reliability of electroencephalogram in the diagnosis of brain death. *Eur Neurol* 30:138–141, 1990.
46. Callaham M, Barton C: Prediction of outcome of cardiopulmonary resuscitation from end-tidal carbon dioxide concentration. *Crit Care Med* 18:358–362, 1990.
47. Callaham M, Madsen CD, Barton CW, et al: A randomized trial of high-dose epinephrine and norepinephrine versus standard dose epinephrine in prehospital cardiac arrest. *JAMA* 268:2667–2672, 1992.
48. Campbell NP, Webb SW, Adgey AA, Pantridge JF: Transthoracic ventricular defibrillation in adults. *Br Med J* 2:1379–1381, 1977.
49. Cardenas-Rivero N, Chernow B, Stoiko MA, et al: Hypocalcaemia in critically ill children. *J Pediatr* 114:946–951, 1989.
50. Carlsson C, Hagerdal M, Kaasik AE, Siesjo BK: A catecholamine-mediated increase in cerebral oxygen uptake during immobilisation stress in rats. *Brain Res* 119:223–231, 1977.
51. Cavallaro DL, Melker RJ: Comparison of two techniques for detecting cardiac activity in infants. *Crit Care Med* 11:189–190, 1983.
52. Chandra N, Rudikoff M, Weisfeldt ML: Simultaneous chest compression and ventilation at high airway pressure during cardiopulmonary resuscitation. *Lancet* 1:175–178, 1980.
53. Chandra N, Snyder LD, Weisfeldt ML: Abdominal binding during cardiopulmonary resuscitation in man. *JAMA* 246:351–353, 1981.
54. Chandra N, Weisfeldt ML, Tsitlik J, et al: Augmentation of carotid flow during cardiopulmonary resuscitation by ventilation at high airway pressure simultaneous with chest compression. *Am J Cardiol* 48:1053–1063, 1981.
55. Chandra NC, Tsitlik JE, Halperin HR, et al: Observations of hemodynamics during human cardiopulmonary resuscitation. *Crit Care Med* 18:929–934, 1990.
56. Chandra NC, Beyar R, Halperin HR, et al: Vital organ perfusion during assisted circulation by manipulation of intrathoracic pressure. *Circulation* 84:279–286, 1991.
57. Chiu NC, Shen EY, Lee BS: Reversal of diastolic cerebral blood flow in infants without brain death. *Pediatr Neurol* 11:337–401, 1994.
58. Chopp M, Welch KM, Tidwell CD, Helpern JA: Global cerebral ischemia and intracellular pH during hyperglycemia and hypoglycemia in cats. *Stroke* 19:1383–1387, 1988.

59. Chow MS, Ronfeld RA, Hamilton RA, et al: Effect of external cardiopulmonary resuscitation on lidocaine pharmacokinetics in dogs. *J Pharmacol Exp Ther* 224:531–537, 1983.

60. Chow MS, Ronfeld RA, Ruffett D, Fieldman A: Lidocaine pharmacokinetics during cardiac arrest and external cardiopulmonary resuscitation. *Am Heart J* 102:799–801, 1981.

61. Cingolani HE, Mattiazzi AR, Blesa ES, Gonzalez NC: Contractility in isolated mammalian heart muscle after acid-base changes. *Circ Res* 26:269–278, 1970.

62. Cipolotti G, Paccagnella A, Simini G: Successful cardiopulmonary resuscitation using high doses of epinephrine. *Int J Cardiol* 33:1, 1991.

63. Clements FM, de Bruijn NP, Kisslo JA: Transesophageal echocardiographic observations in a patient undergoing closed-chest massage. *Anesthesiology* 64:826–828, 1986.

64. Cochran JB, Tecklenburg FW, Lau YR, Habib DM: Emergency cardiopulmonary bypass for cardiac arrest refractory to pediatric advanced life support. *Pediatr Emerg Care* 15:30–32, 1999.

65. Cohen JM, Chandra N, Alderson PO, et al: Timing of pulmonary and systemic blood flow during intermittent high intrathoracic pressure cardiopulmonary resuscitation in the dog. *Am J Cardiol* 49:1883–1889, 1982.

66. Cohen TJ, Tucker KJ, Lurie KG, et al: Active compression-decompression. A new method of cardiopulmonary resuscitation. Cardiopulmonary Resuscitation Working Group. *JAMA* 267:2916–2923, 1992.

67. Cohen TJ, Goldner BG, Maccaro PC, et al: A comparison of active compression-decompression cardiopulmonary resuscitation with standard cardiopulmonary resuscitation for cardiac arrests occurring in the hospital. *N Engl J Med* 329:1918–1921, 1993.

68. Cohen Y, Chang LH, Litt L, et al: Stability of brain intracellular lactate and 31P-metabolite levels at reduced intracellular pH during prolonged hypercapnia in rats. *J Cereb Blood Flow Metab* 10:277–284, 1990.

69. Cole DJ: The reversibility of death. *J Med Ethics* 18:26–30, 1992.

70. Collinsworth KA, Kalman SM, Harrison DC: The clinical pharmacology of lidocaine as an antiarrhythmic drug. *Circulation* 50:1217–1230, 1974.

71. Constantino RT, Crockett SE, Vasko JS: Cardiovascular effects and dose response relationships of lidocaine. *Circulation* 36:89, 1967.

72. Cote P, Bourassa MG, Delaye J, et al: Effects of amiodarone on cardiac and coronary hemodynamics and on myocardial metabolism in patients with coronary artery disease. *Circulation* 59:1165–1172, 1979.

73. Council on Ethical and Judicial affairs of the American Medical Association: Current opinions. Chicago American Medical Association, pp 12–13, 1986.

74. Criley JM, Blaufuss AH, Kissel GL: Cough-induced cardiac compression. Self-administered form of cardiopulmonary resuscitation. *JAMA* 236:1246–1250, 1976.

75. Criley JM, Niemann JT, Rosborough JP, Hausknecht M: Modifications of cardiopulmonary resuscitation based on the cough. *Circulation* 74:IV42–IV50, 1986.

76. Cummins RO, Hazinski MF, Kerber RE, et al: Low-energy biphasic waveform defibrillation: evidence-based review applied to emergency cardiovascular care guidelines: A statement for healthcare professionals from the American Heart Association Committee on Emergency Cardiovascular Care and the Subcommittees on Basic Life Support, Advanced Cardiac Life Support, and Pediatric Resuscitation. *Circulation* 97:1654–1667, 1998.

77. Dahl CF, Ewy GA, Warner ED, Thomas ED: Myocardial necrosis from direct current countershock. Effect of paddle electrode size and time interval between discharges. *Circulation* 50:956–961, 1974.

78. Dalton HJ, Siewers RD, Fuhrman BP, et al: Extracorporeal membrane oxygenation for cardiac rescue in children with severe myocardial dysfunction. *Crit Care Med* 21:1020–1028, 1993.

79. Darby JM, Stein K, Grenvik A, Stuart SA: Approach to management of the heartbeating "brain dead" organ donor. *JAMA* 261:2222–2228, 1989.

80. David R: Closed chest cardiac massage in the newborn infant. *Pediatrics* 81:552–554, 1988.

81. De Meirleir LJ, Taylor MJ: Prognostic utility of SEPs in comatose children. *Pediatr Neurol* 3:78–82, 1987.

82. Dean JM, Koehler RC, Schleien CL, et al: Improved blood flow during prolonged cardiopulmonary resuscitation with 30% duty cycle in infant pigs. *Circulation* 84:896–904, 1991.

83. Dean JM, Koehler RC, Schleien CL, et al: Age-related effects of compression rate and duration in cardiopulmonary resuscitation. *J Appl Physiol* 68:554–560, 1990.

84. Dean JM, Koehler RC, Schleien CL, et al: Age-related changes in chest geometry during cardiopulmonary resuscitation. *J Appl Physiol* 62:2212–2219, 1987.

85. Del Guercio LR, Feins NR, Cohn JD, et al: Comparison of blood flow during external and internal cardiac massage in man. *Circulation* 32:I171–I80, 1965.

86. del Nido PJ, Dalton HJ, Thompson AE, Siewers RD: Extracorporeal membrane oxygenator rescue in children during cardiac arrest after cardiac surgery. *Circulation* 86:II300–II304, 1992.

87. Delius RE, Bove EL, Meliones JN, et al: Use of extracorporeal life support in patients with congenital heart disease. *Crit Care Med* 20:1216–1222, 1992.

88. Dembo DH: Calcium in advanced life support. *Crit Care Med* 9:358–359, 1981.

89. Denlinger JK, Nahrwold ML, Gibbs PS, Lecky JH: Hypocalcemia during rapid blood transfusion in anaesthetized man. *Br J Anaesth* 48:995–1000, 1976.

90. DeSilva RA, Lown B: Energy requirement for defibrillation of a markedly overweight patient. *Circulation* 57:827–830, 1978.

91. DiCola VC, Freedman GS, Downing SE, Zaret BL: Myocardial uptake of technetium-99m stannous pyrophosphate following direct current transthoracic countershock. *Circulation* 54:980–986, 1976.

92. Ditchey RV, Lindenfeld J: Failure of epinephrine to improve the balance between myocardial oxygen supply and demand during closed-chest resuscitation in dogs. *Circulation* 78:382–389, 1988.

93. Ditchey RV, Winkler JV, Rhodes CA: Relative lack of coronary blood flow during closed-chest resuscitation in dogs. *Circulation* 66:297–302, 1982.

94. Donovan KD, Gerace RV, Dreyer RF: Acebutolol-induced ventricular tachycardia reversed with sodium bicarbonate. *J Toxicol Clin Toxicol* 37:481–484, 1999.

95. Dorfsman ML, Menegazzi JJ, Wadas RJ, Auble TE: Two-thumb vs. two-finger chest compression in an infant model of prolonged cardiopulmonary resuscitation. *Acad Emerg Med* 7:1077–1082, 2000.

96. Drop LJ, Scheidegger D: Plasma ionized calcium concentration: important determinant of the hemodynamic response to calcium infusion. *J Thorac Cardiovasc Surg* 79:425–431, 1980.

97. Duke T, Butt W, South M, Karl TR: Early markers of major adverse events in children after cardiac operations. *J Thorac Cardiovasc Surg* 114:1042–1052, 1997.

98. Duncan BW, Ibrahim AE, Hraska V, et al: Use of rapid-deployment extracorporeal membrane oxygenation for the resuscitation of pediatric patients with heart disease after cardiac arrest. *J Thorac Cardiovasc Surg* 116:305–311, 1998.

99. Eberle B, Dick WF, Schneider T, et al: Checking the carotid pulse check: Diagnostic accuracy of first responders in patients with and without a pulse. *Resuscitation* 33:107–116, 1996.

100. Eberle B, Schleien CL, Shaffner DH, et al: Effects of three modes of abdominal compression on vital organ blood flow in a piglet CPR model. *Anesthesiology* 73:A300, 1990.

101. Edvinsson L, Hardebo JE, MacKenzie ET, Owman C: Effect of exogenous noradrenaline on local cerebral blood flow after osmotic opening of the blood-brain barrier in the rat. *J Physiol (Lond)* 274:149–156, 1978.

102. Einagle V, Bertrand F, Wise RA, et al: Interposed abdominal compressions and carotid blood flow during cardiopulmonary resuscitation: Support for a thoracoabdominal unit. *Chest* 93:1206–1212, 1988.

103. Elam JO, Brown ES, Elder JD: Artificial respiration by mouth-to-mask method. *N Engl J Med* 250:749–754, 1954.

104. el-Banayosy A, Brehm C, Kizner L, et al: Cardiopulmonary resuscitation after cardiac surgery: A two-year study. *J Cardiothorac Vasc Anesth* 12:390–392, 1998.

105. Eleff SM, Schleien CL, Koehler RC, et al: Brain bioenergetics during cardiopulmonary resuscitation in dogs. *Anesthesiology* 76:77–84, 1992.

106. Fackler JC, Rogers MC: Is brain death really cessation of all intracranial function? *J Pediatr* 110:84–86, 1987.

107. Falk JL, Rackow EC, Weil MH: End-tidal carbon dioxide concentration during cardiopulmonary resuscitation. *N Engl J Med* 318:607–611, 1988.

108. Feneley MP, Maier GW, Gaynor JW, et al: Sequence of mitral valve motion and transmitral blood flow during manual cardiopulmonary resuscitation in dogs. *Circulation* 76:363–375, 1987.

109. Feneley MP, Maier GW, Kern KB, et al: Influence of compression rate on initial success of resuscitation and 24 hour survival after prolonged manual cardiopulmonary resuscitation in dogs. *Circulation* 77:240–250, 1988.

110. Figa FH, Gow RM, Hamilton RM, Freedom RM: Clinical efficacy and safety of intravenous amiodarone in infants and children. *Am J Cardiol* 74:573–577, 1994.

111. Fisher J, Vaghaiwalla F, Tsitlik J, et al: Determinants and clinical significance of jugular venous valve competence. *Circulation* 65:188–196, 1982.

112. Fleisher G, Delgado-Paredes C, Heyman S: Slow versus rapid closed-chest cardiac compression during cardiopulmonary resuscitation in puppies. *Crit Care Med* 15:939–943, 1987.

113. Garnett AR, Ornato JP, Gonzalez ER, Johnson EB: End-tidal carbon dioxide monitoring during cardiopulmonary resuscitation. *JAMA* 257:512–515, 1987.

114. Gascho JA, Crampton RS, Sipes JN, et al: Energy levels and patient weight in ventricular defibrillation. *JAMA* 242:1380–1384, 1979.

115. Gazmuri RJ, von Planta M, Weil MH, Rackow EC: Cardiac effects of carbon dioxide-consuming and carbon dioxide-generating buffers during cardiopulmonary resuscitation. *J Am Coll Cardiol* 15:482–490, 1990.

116. Gazmuri RJ, Weil MH, Bisera J, Rackow EC: End-tidal carbon dioxide tension as a monitor of native blood flow during resuscitation by extracorporeal circulation. *J Thorac Cardiovasc Surg* 101:984–988, 1991.

117. Gillette PC, Garson A: *Pediatric Cardiac Dysrhythmias.* New York, Grune and Stratton, 1981.

118. Gilman AG, Rall TW, Nies AS, Taylor P: *Goodman and Gilman's The Pharmacological Basis of Therapeutics.* New York, Pergamon Press, 1990.

119. Goetting MG, Paradis NA: High dose epinephrine in refractory pediatric cardiac arrest. *Crit Care Med* 17:1258–1262, 1989.

120. Goetting MG, Paradis NA: Right atrial-jugular venous pressure gradients during CPR in children. *Ann Emerg Med* 20:27–30, 1991.

121. Goetting MG, Paradis NA, Appleton TJ, et al: Aortic-carotid artery pressure differences and cephalic perfusion pressure during cardiopulmonary resuscitation in humans. *Crit Care Med* 19:1012–1017, 1991.

122. Goldberg AH: Cardiopulmonary arrest. *N Engl J Med* 290:381–385, 1974.

123. Gonzalez ER, Ornato JP, Garnett AR, et al: Dose-dependent vasopressor response to epinephrine during CPR in human beings. *Ann Emerg Med* 18:920–926, 1989.

124. Gonzalez ER, Ornato JP, Levine RL: Vasopressor effect of epinephrine with and without dopamine during cardiopulmonary resuscitation. *Drug Intell Clin Pharm* 22:868–872, 1988.

125. Graf H, Leach W, Arieff AI: Evidence for a detrimental effect of bicarbonate therapy in hypoxic lactic acidosis. *Science* 227:754–756, 1985.

126. Greenblatt DJ, Gross PL, Bolognini V: Pharmacotherapy of cardiopulmonary arrest. *Am J Hosp Pharm* 33:579–583, 1976.

127. Grundler W, Weil MH, Rackow EC: Arteriovenous carbon dioxide and pH gradients during cardiac arrest. *Circulation* 74:1071–1074, 1986.

128. Gudipati CV, Weil MH, Deshmukh HG, et al: Right atrial-jugular venous pressure gradients during experimental CPR. *Chest* 89:443s, 1986.

129. Guerci AD, Chandra N, Johnson E, et al: Failure of sodium bicarbonate to improve resuscitation from ventricular fibrillation in dogs. *Circulation* 74:IV75–IV79, 1986.

130. Guerci AD, Shi AY, Levin H, et al: Transmission of intrathoracic pressure to the intracranial space during cardiopulmonary resuscitation in dogs. *Circ Res* 56:20–30, 1985.

131. Guidelines 2000 for Cardiopulmonary Resuscitation and Emergency Cardiovascular Care. Part 6: Advanced cardiovascular life support: Section 4: Devices to assist circulation. The American Heart Association in collaboration with the International Liaison Committee on Resuscitation. *Circulation* 102:I105-I111, 2000.

132. Gutgesell HP, Tacker WA, Geddes LA, et al: Energy dose for ventricular defibrillation of children. *Pediatrics* 58:898–901, 1976.

133. Hackl W, Simon P, Mauritz W, Steinbereithner K: Echocardiographic assessment of mitral valve function during mechanical cardiopulmonary resuscitation in pigs. *Anesth Analg* 70:350–356, 1990.

134. Halperin HR, Guerci AD, Chandra N, et al: Vest inflation without simultaneous ventilation during cardiac arrest in dogs: Improved survival from prolonged cardiopulmonary resuscitation. *Circulation* 74:1407–1415, 1986.

135. Halperin HR, Tsitlik JE, Beyar R, et al: Intrathoracic pressure fluctuations move blood during CPR: Comparison of hemodynamic data with predictions from a mathematical model. *Ann Biomed Eng* 15:385–403, 1987.

136. Halperin HR, Tsitlik JE, Guerci AD, et al: Determinants of blood flow to vital organs during cardiopulmonary resuscitation in dogs. *Circulation* 73:539–550, 1986.

137. Halperin HR, Tsitlik JE, Gelfand M, et al: A preliminary study of cardiopulmonary resuscitation by circumferential compression of the chest with use of a pneumatic vest. *N Engl J Med* 329:762–768, 1993.

138. Harada Y, Fuseno H, Ohtomo T, et al: Self-administered hyperventilation cardiopulmonary resuscitation for 100s of cardiac arrest during Holter monitoring. *Chest* 99:1310–1312, 1991.

139. Harris LC, Kirimli B, Safar P: Ventilation-cardiac compression rates and ratios in cardiopulmonary resuscitation. *Anesthesiology* 28:806–813, 1967.

140. Hartz R, LoCicero J, Sanders JH Jr, et al: Clinical experience with portable cardiopulmonary bypass in cardiac arrest patients. *Ann Thorac Surg* 50:437–441, 1990.

141. Heining MP, Band DM, Linton RA: Choice of calcium salt: A comparison of the effects of calcium chloride and gluconate on plasma ionized calcium. *Anaesthesia* 39:1079–1082, 1984.

142. Higano ST, Oh JK, Ewy GA, Seward JB: The mechanism of blood flow during closed chest cardiac massage in humans: transesophageal echocardiographic observations. *Mayo Clin Proc* 65:1432–1440, 1990.

143. Holmes HR, Babbs CF, Voorhees WD, et al: Influence of adrenergic drugs upon vital organ perfusion during CPR. *Crit Care Med* 8:137–140, 1980.

144. Holt DW, Tucker GT, Jackson PR, Storey GC: Amiodarone pharmacokinetics. *Am Heart J* 106:840–847, 1983.

145. Howard M, Carrubba C, Foss F, et al: Interposed abdominal compression-CPR: its effects on parameters of coronary perfusion in human subjects. *Ann Emerg Med* 16:253–259, 1987.

146. Jackson DL, Dole WP, McGloin J, Rosenblatt JI: Total cerebral ischemia: Application of a new model system to studies of cerebral microcirculation. *Stroke* 12:66–72, 1981.

147. Jackson RE, Joyce K, Danosi SF, et al: Blood flow in the cerebral cortex during cardiac resuscitation in dogs. *Ann Emerg Med* 13:657–659, 1984.

148. Jewitt DE, Kishow Y, Thomas M: Lidocaine in the management of arrhythmias after myocardial infarction. *Circulation* 37:965, 1968.

149. *The Johns Hopkins Hospital Interdisciplinary Practice Manual.* Baltimore, Johns Hopkins University, 1998.

150. Jones JL, Lepeschkin E, Jones RE, Rush S: Response of cultured myocardial cells to countershock-type electric field stimulation. *Am J Physiol* 235:H214–H222, 1978.

151. Kano T, Shimoda O, Morioka T, et al: Evaluation of the central nervous function in resuscitated comatose patients by multilevel evoked potentials. *Resuscitation* 23:235–248, 1992.

152. Karkela J, Pasanen M, Kaukinen S, et al: Evaluation of hypoxic brain injury with spinal fluid enzymes, lactate, and pyruvate. *Crit Care Med* 20:378–386, 1992.

153. Katz AM, Reuter H: Cellular calcium and cardiac cell death. *Am J Cardiol* 44:188–190, 1979.

154. Keenan RL, Shapiro JH, Dawson K: Frequency of anesthetic cardiac arrests in infants: effect of pediatric anesthesiologists. *J Clin Anesth* 3:433–437, 1991.

155. Kerber RE, Sarnat W: Factors influencing the success of ventricular defibrillation in man. *Circulation* 60:226–230, 1979.

156. Kern KB, Carter AB, Showen RL, et al: Manual versus mechanical cardiopulmonary resuscitation in an experimental canine model. *Crit Care Med* 13:899–903, 1985.

157. Kern KB, Carter AB, Showen RL, et al: Twenty-four hour survival in a canine model of cardiac arrest comparing three methods of manual cardiopulmonary resuscitation. *J Am Coll Cardiol* 7:859–867, 1986.

158. Kernstine KH, Tyson GS, Maier GW, et al: Determinants of direct cardiac compression during external cardiac massage in intact dogs. *Crit Care Med* 10:231, 1982.

159. Kilecki PF, Curry SC: Poisoning by sodium channel blocking agents. *Crit Care Clin* 13:829–848, 1997.

160. Koehler RC, Chandra N, Guerci AD, et al: Augmentation of cerebral perfusion by simultaneous chest compression and lung inflation with abdominal binding after cardiac arrest in dogs. *Circulation* 67:266–275, 1983.

161. Koehler RC, Michael JR: Cardiopulmonary resuscitation, brain blood flow, and neurologic recovery. *Crit Care Clin* 1:205–222, 1985.

162. Koehler RC, Michael JR, Guerci AD, et al: Beneficial effect of epinephrine infusion on cerebral and myocardial blood flows during CPR. *Ann Emerg Med* 14:744–749, 1985.

163. Kosinski EJ, Albin JB, Young E, et al: Hemodynamic effects of intravenous amiodarone. *J Am Coll Cardiol* 4:565–570, 1984.

164. Kottmeier CA, Gravenstein JS: The parasympathomimetic activity of atropine and atropine methylbromide. *Anesthesiology* 29:1125–1133, 1968.

165. Kouwenhoven WB, Jude JR, Knickerbocker GG: Closed-chest cardiac massage. *JAMA* 173:1064–1067, 1960.

166. Krischer JP, Fine EG, Weisfeldt ML, et al: Comparison of prehospital conventional and simultaneous compression-ventilation cardiopulmonary resuscitation. *Crit Care Med* 17:1263–1269, 1989.

167. Kuhn C, Juchems R, Frese W: Evidence for the "cardiac pump theory" in cardiopulmonary resuscitation in man by transesophageal echocardiography. *Resuscitation* 22:275–282, 1991.

168. Langhelle A, Stromme T, Sunde K, et al: Inspiratory impedance threshold valve during CPR. *Resuscitation* 52:39–48, 2002.

169. Larar GN, Nagel JS: Technetium-99m-HMPAO cerebral perfusion scintigraphy: considerations for timely brain death declaration. *J Nucl Med* 33:2209–2211, 1992.

170. Lasbennes F, Sercombe R, Seylaz J: Monoamine oxidase activity in brain microvessels determined using natural and artificial substrates: Relevance to the blood–brain barrier. *J Cereb Blood Flow Metab* 3:521–528, 1983.

171. Lee CJ, Bullock LJ: Determining the pulse for infant CPR: Time for a change? *Mil Med* 156:190–193, 1991.

172. Lee G, Antognini JF, Gronert GA: Complete recovery after prolonged resuscitation and cardiopulmonary bypass for hyperkalemic cardiac arrest. *Anesth Analg* 79:172–174, 1994.

173. Lee HR, Wilder RJ, Downs P, et al: MAST augmentation of external cardiac compression: Role of changing intrapleural pressure. *Ann Emerg Med* 10:560–565, 1981.

174. Lee SK, Vaagenes P, Safar P, et al: Effect of cardiac arrest time on cortical cerebral blood flow generated by subsequent standard external cardiopulmonary resuscitation. *Ann Emerg Med* 13:385, 1984.

175. Levine R, Gorayeb M, Safar P, et al: Cardiopulmonary bypass after cardiac arrest and prolonged closed-chest CPR in dogs. *Ann Emerg Med* 16:620–627, 1987.

176. Levine RL, Wayne MA, Miller CC: End-tidal carbon dioxide and outcome of out-of-hospital cardiac arrest. *N Engl J Med* 337:301–306, 1997.

177. Levy DE, Bates D, Caronna JJ, et al: Prognosis in nontraumatic coma. *Ann Intern Med* 94:293–301, 1981.

178. Liberman M, Lavoie A, Mulder D, Sampalis J: Cardiopulmonary resuscitation: Errors made by pre-hospital emergency medical personnel. *Resuscitation* 42:47–55, 1999.

179. Lichstein E, Chadda KD, Gupta PK: Atrioventricular block with lidocaine therapy. *Am J Cardiol* 31:277–281, 1973.

180. Lilja GP, Long RS, Ruiz E: Augmentation of systolic blood pressure during external cardiac compression by use of the MAST suit. *Ann Emerg Med* 10:182–184, 1981.

181. Lindner KH, Prengel AW, Pfenninger EG, et al: Vasopressin improves vital organ blood flow during closed-chest cardiopulmonary resuscitation in pigs. *Circulation* 91:215–221, 1995.

182. Lindner KH, Dirks B, Strohmenger HU, et al: Randomized comparison of epinephrine and vasopressin in patients. *Lancet* 349:535–537, 1997.

183. Link MS, Wang PJ, Pandian NG, et al: An experimental model of sudden death due to low-energy chest-wall impact (commotio cordis). *N Engl J Med* 338:1805–1811, 1998.

184. Lipman J, Wilson W, Kobilski S, et al: High-dose adrenaline in adult in-hospital asystolic cardiopulmonary resuscitation: A double-blind randomized trial. *Anaesth Intensive Care* 21:192–196, 1993.

185. Livesay JJ, Follette DM, Fey KH, et al: Optimizing myocardial supply/demand balance with alpha-adrenergic drugs during cardiopulmonary resuscitation. *J Thorac Cardiovasc Surg* 76:244–251, 1978.

186. Longstreth WT Jr, Diehr P, Cobb LA, et al: Neurologic outcome and blood glucose levels during out-of-hospital cardiopulmonary resuscitation. *Neurology* 36:1186–1191, 1986.

187. Longstreth WT Jr, Inui TS: High blood glucose level on hospital admission and poor neurological recovery after cardiac arrest. *Ann Neurol* 15:59–63, 1984.

188. Luce JM, Rizk NA, Niskanen RA: Regional blood flow during cardiopulmonary resuscitation in dogs. *Crit Care Med* 12:874–878, 1984.

189. Luce JM, Ross BK, O'Quin RJ, et al: Regional blood flow during cardiopulmonary resuscitation in dogs using simultaneous and nonsimultaneous compression and ventilation. *Circulation* 67:258–265, 1983.

190. Lurie KG, Shultz JJ, Callaham ML, et al: Evaluation of active compression-decompression CPR in victims of out-of-hospital cardiac arrest. *JAMA* 271:1405–1411, 1994.

191. Lurie KG, Zielinski T, Voelckel W, et al: Augmentation of ventricular preload during treatment of cardiovascular collapse and cardiac arrest. *Crit Care Med* 30:S162–S165, 2002.

192. Lynch J, Eldadah MK: Brain-death criteria currently used by pediatric intensivists. *Clin Pediatr (Phila)* 31:457–460, 1992.

193. MacKenzie ET, McCulloch J, O'Kean M, et al: Cerebral circulation and norepinephrine: Relevance of the blood–brain barrier. *Am J Physiol* 231:483–488, 1976.

194. Mahle WT, Spray TL, Gaynor JW, Clark BJ III: Unexpected death after reconstructive surgery for hypoplastic left heart syndrome. *Ann Thorac Surg* 71:61–65, 2001.

195. Mahoney BD, Mirick MJ: Efficacy of pneumatic trousers in refractory prehospital cardiopulmonary arrest. *Ann Emerg Med* 12:8–12, 1983.

196. Maier GW, Tyson GS Jr, Olsen CO, et al: The physiology of external cardiac massage: High-impulse cardiopulmonary resuscitation. *Circulation* 70:86–101, 1984.

197. Mann K, Berg RA, Nadkarni V: Beneficial effects of vasopressin in prolonged pediatric cardiac arrest: A case series. *Resuscitation* 52:149–56, 2002.

198. Marquez J, Martin D, Virji MA, et al: Cardiovascular depression secondary to ionic hypocalcemia during hepatic transplantation in humans. *Anesthesiology* 65:457–461, 1986.

199. Martin D, Werman HA, Brown CG: Four case studies: High-dose epinephrine in cardiac arrest. *Ann Emerg Med* 19:322–326, 1990.

200. Martin GB, Gentile NT, Paradis NA, et al: Effect of epinephrine on end-tidal carbon dioxide monitoring during CPR. *Ann Emerg Med* 19:396–398, 1990.

201. Martin GB, Rivers EP, Paradis NA, et al: Emergency department cardiopulmonary bypass in the treatment of human cardiac arrest. *Chest* 113:743–751, 1998.

202. Martinez LR, Holland S, Fitzgerald J, Kountz S: pH homeostasis during cardiopulmonary resuscitation in critically ill patients. *Resuscitation* 7:109–117, 1979.

203. Mason JW: Amiodarone. *N Engl J Med* 316:455–466, 1987.

204. Mason JW, Hondeghem LM, Katzung BG: Block of inactivated sodium channels and of depolarization-induced automaticity in guinea pig papillary muscle by amiodarone. *Circ Res* 55:278–285, 1984.

205. Mateer JR, Stueven HA, Thompson BM, et al: Pre-hospital IAC-CPR versus standard CPR: Paramedic resuscitation of cardiac arrests. *Am J Emerg Med* 3:143–146, 1985.

206. Mattar JA, Weil MH, Shubin H, Stein L: Cardiac arrest in the critically ill: II: Hyperosmolal states following cardiac arrest. *Am J Med* 56:162–168, 1974.

207. Mattioni TA, Zheutlin TA, Dunnington C, Kehoe RF: The proarrhythmic effects of amiodarone. *Prog Cardiovasc Dis* 31:439–446, 1989.

208. Mattox KL, Beall AC Jr: Resuscitation of the moribund patient using portable cardiopulmonary bypass. *Ann Thorac Surg* 22:436–442, 1976.

209. Mauer D, Schneider T, Dick W, et al: Active compression-decompression resuscitation: A prospective, randomized study in a two-tiered EMS system with physicians in the field. *Resuscitation* 33:125–134, 1996.

210. McElhinney DB, Reddy VM, Parry AJ, et al: Management and outcomes of delayed sternal closure after cardiac surgery in neonates and infants. *Crit Care Med* 28:1180–1184, 2000.

211. Michael JR, Guerci AD, Koehler RC, et al: Mechanisms by which epinephrine augments cerebral and myocardial perfusion during cardiopulmonary resuscitation in dogs. *Circulation* 69:822–835, 1984.

212. Mink RB, Pollack MM: Resuscitation and withdrawal of therapy in pediatric intensive care. *Pediatrics* 89:961–963, 1992.

213. Morales DL, Gregg D, Helman DN, et al: Arginine vasopressin in the treatment of 50 patients with postcardiotomy vasodilatory shock. *Ann Thorac Surg* 69:102–106, 2000.

214. Muir JD, Randalls PB, Smith GB: End tidal carbon dioxide detector for monitoring cardiopulmonary resuscitation. *BMJ* 301:41–42, 1990.

215. Mullins ME, Pinnick RV, Terhes JM: Life threatening diphenhydramine overdose treated with charcoal hemoperfusion and hemodialysis. *Ann Emerg Med* 33:104–107, 1999.

216. Myers R: Lactic acid accumulation as a cause of brain edema and cerebral necrosis resulting from oxygen deprivation. In Korbin R, Gilleminault C (eds): *Advances in Perinatal Neurology*. New York, Spectrum, 1979, pp 84.

217. Nademanee K, Piwonka RW, Singh BN, Hershman JM: Amiodarone and thyroid function. *Prog Cardiovasc Dis* 31:427–437, 1989.
218. Niemann JT, Cairns CB, Sharma J, Lewis RJ: Treatment of prolonged ventricular fibrillation. Immediate countershock versus high-dose epinephrine and CPR preceding countershock. *Circulation* 85:281–287, 1992.
219. Niemann JT, Rosborough J, Hausknecht M, et al: Cough-CPR: Documentation of systemic perfusion in man and in an experimental model: A "window" to the mechanism of blood flow in external CPR. *Crit Care Med* 8:141–146, 1980.
220. Niemann JT, Rosborough J, Hausknecht M, et al: Blood flow without cardiac compression during closed chest CPR. *Crit Care Med* 9:380–381, 1981.
221. Niemann JT, Rosborough JP, Hausknecht M, et al: Pressure-synchronized cineangiography during experimental cardiopulmonary resuscitation. *Circulation* 64:985–991, 1981.
222. Niemann JT, Rosborough JP, Pelikan PC: Hemodynamic determinants of subdiaphragmatic venous return during closed-chest CPR in a canine cardiac arrest model. *Ann Emerg Med* 19:1232–1237, 1990.
223. Niemann JT, Rosborough JP, Ung S, Criley JM: Hemodynamic effects of continuous abdominal binding during cardiac arrest and resuscitation. *Am J Cardiol* 53:269–274, 1984.
224. Nolan J, Smith G, Evans R, et al: The United Kingdom pre-hospital study of active compression-decompression resuscitation. *Resuscitation* 37:119–125, 1998.
225. O'Rourke PP: Use of extracorporeal life support in patients with congenital heart disease: State of the art? *Crit Care Med* 20:1199–1200, 1992.
226. Orlowski JP: Cardiopulmonary resuscitation in children. *Pediatr Clin North Am* 27:495–512, 1980.
227. Ornato JP, Gonzalez ER, Garnett AR, et al: Effect of cardiopulmonary resuscitation compression rate on end-tidal carbon dioxide concentration and arterial pressure in man. *Crit Care Med* 16:241–245, 1988.
228. Pannier JL, Leusen I: Contraction characteristics of papillary muscle during changes in acid-base composition of the bathing-fluid. *Arch Int Physiol Biochim* 76:624–634, 1968.
229. Paradis NA, Martin GB, Goetting MG, et al: Simultaneous aortic, jugular bulb, and right atrial pressures during cardiopulmonary resuscitation in humans. Insights into mechanisms. *Circulation* 80:361–368, 1989.
230. Paradis NA, Martin GB, Rivers EP, et al: Coronary perfusion pressure and the return of spontaneous circulation in human cardiopulmonary resuscitation. *JAMA* 263:1106–1113, 1990.
231. Parra DA, Totapally BR, Zahn E, et al: Outcome of cardiopulmonary resuscitation in a pediatric cardiac intensive care unit. *Crit Care Med* 28:3296–3300, 2000.
232. Pearson JW, Redding JS: Influence of peripheral vascular tone on resuscitation. *Anesth Analg* 44:746, 1965.
233. Perry JC, Fenrich AL, Hulse JE, et al: Pediatric use of intravenous amiodarone: Efficacy and safety in critically ill patients from a multicenter protocol. *J Am Coll Cardiol* 27:1246–1250, 1996.
234. Petty GW, Mohr JP, Pedley TA, et al: The role of transcranial Doppler in confirming brain death: Sensitivity, specificity, and suggestions for performance and interpretation. *Neurology* 40:300–303, 1990.
235. Phillips SJ, Ballentine B, Slonine D, et al: Percutaneous initiation of cardiopulmonary bypass. *Ann Thorac Surg* 36:223–225, 1983.
236. Pionkowski RS, Thompson BM, Gruchow HW, et al: Resuscitation time in ventricular fibrillation—a prognostic indicator. *Ann Emerg Med* 12:733–738, 1983.
237. Pjura GA, Kim EE: Radionuclide evaluation of brain death. In Freeman LM, Weissman HS (eds): *Nuclear Medicine Annual 1987*. New York, Raven, 1987, pp 269–293.
238. Plaisance P, Adnet F, Vicaut E, et al: Benefit of active compression-decompression cardiopulmonary resuscitation as a prehospital advanced cardiac life support. A randomized multicenter study. *Circulation* 95:955–961, 1997.
239. Plaisance P, Lurie KG, Payen D: Inspiratory impedance during active compression-decompression cardiopulmonary resuscitation. A randomized evaluation in patients in cardiac arrest. *Circulation* 101:989–994, 2000.
240. Pongiglione G, Strasburger JF, Deal BJ, Benson DW Jr: Use of amiodarone for short-term and adjuvant therapy in young patients. *Am J Cardiol* 68:603–608, 1991.
241. Pretto E, Safar P, Saito R, et al: Cardiopulmonary bypass after prolonged cardiac arrest in dogs. *Ann Emerg Med* 16:611–619, 1987.

242. Prengel AW, Lindner KH, Keller A: Cerebral oxygenation during cardiopulmonary resuscitation with epinephrine and vasopressin in pigs. *Stroke* 27:1241–1248, 1996.
243. Pulsinelli WA, Levy DE, Sigsbee B, et al: Increased damage after ischemic stroke in patients with hyperglycemia with or without established diabetes mellitus. *Am J Med* 74:540–544, 1983.
244. Raeder EA, Podrid PJ, Lown B: Side effects and complications of amiodarone therapy. *Am Heart J* 109:975–983, 1985.
245. Raessler KL, Kern KB, Sanders AB, et al: Aortic and right atrial systolic pressures during cardiopulmonary resuscitation: A potential indicator of the mechanism of blood flow. *Am Heart J* 115:1021–1029, 1988.
246. Raithel SC, Pennington DG, Boegner E, et al: Extracorporeal membrane oxygenation in children after cardiac surgery. *Circulation* 86:II305–II310, 1992.
247. Ralston SH, Babbs CF, Niebauer MJ: Cardiopulmonary resuscitation with interposed abdominal compression in dogs. *Anesth Analg* 61:645–651, 1982.
248. Ralston SH, Voorhees WD, Babbs CF: Intrapulmonary epinephrine during prolonged cardiopulmonary resuscitation: Improved regional blood flow and resuscitation in dogs. *Ann Emerg Med* 13:79–86, 1984.
249. Raman J, Saldanha RF, Branch JM, et al: Open cardiac compression in the postoperative cardiac intensive care unit. *Anaesth Intensive Care* 17:129–135, 1989.
250. Redding JS: Abdominal compression in cardiopulmonary resuscitation. *Anesth Analg* 50:668–675, 1971.
251. Redding JS, Pearson JW: Evaluation for drugs for cardiac resuscitation. *Anesthesiology* 24:203, 1963.
252. Reich H, Angelos M, Safar P, et al: Cardiac resuscitability with cardiopulmonary bypass after increasing ventricular fibrillation times in dogs. *Ann Emerg Med* 19:887–890, 1990.
253. Reichman RT, Joyo CI, Dembitsky WP, et al: Improved patient survival after cardiac arrest using a cardiopulmonary support system. *Ann Thorac Surg* 49:101–104, 1990.
254. Resnekov L: Calcium antagonist drugs—myocardial preservation and reduced vulnerability to ventricular fibrillation during CPR. *Crit Care Med* 9:360–361, 1981.
255. Rich S, Wix HL, Shapiro EP: Clinical assessment of heart chamber size and valve motion during cardiopulmonary resuscitation by two-dimensional echocardiography. *Am Heart J* 102:368–373, 1981.
256. Rivers EP, Martin GB, Smithline H, et al: The clinical implications of continuous central venous oxygen saturation during human CPR. *Ann Emerg Med* 21:1094–1101, 1992.
257. Rogers MC, Nugent SK, Stidham GL: Effects of closed-chest cardiac massage on intracranial pressure. *Crit Care Med* 7:454–456, 1979.
258. Rosenzweig EB, Starc TJ, Chen JM, et al: Intravenous arginine-vasopressin in children with vasodilatory shock after cardiac surgery. *Circulation* 100:II182–II186, 1999.
259. Rozenfeld V, Cheng JW. The role of vasopressin in the treatment of vasodilation in shock states. *Ann Pharmacother* 34:250–254, 2000.
260. Rudikoff MT, Maughan WL, Effron M, et al: Mechanisms of blood flow during cardiopulmonary resuscitation. *Circulation* 61:345–352, 1980.
261. Rudolph AM, Yuan S: Response of the pulmonary vasculature to hypoxia and H+ ion concentration changes. *J Clin Invest* 45:399–411, 1966.
262. Sack JB, Kesselbrenner MB, Bregman D: Survival from in-hospital cardiac arrest with interposed abdominal counterpulsation during cardiopulmonary resuscitation. *JAMA* 267:379–385, 1992.
263. Sack JB, Kesselbrenner MB, Bregman D: Survival from in-hospital cardiac arrest with interposed abdominal counterpulsation during cardiopulmonary resuscitation. *JAMA* 267:379–85, 1992.
264. Safar P, Brown TC, Holtey WJ, Wilder RJ: Ventilation and circulation with closed-chest cardiac massage in man. *JAMA* 176:92–94, 1961.
265. Sanders AB, Atlas M, Ewy GA, et al: Expired PCO2 as an index of coronary perfusion pressure. *Am J Emerg Med* 3:147–149, 1985.
266. Sanders AB, Ewy GA, Alferness CA, et al: Failure of one method of simultaneous chest compression, ventilation, and abdominal binding during CPR. *Crit Care Med* 10:509–513, 1982.
267. Sanders AB, Ewy GA, Taft TV: Prognostic and therapeutic importance of the aortic diastolic pressure in resuscitation from cardiac arrest. *Crit Care Med* 12:871–873, 1984.
268. Sanders AB, Kern KB, Ewy GA: Time limitations for open-chest cardiopulmonary resuscitation from cardiac arrest. *Crit Care Med* 13:897–898, 1985.
269. Sanders AB, Kern KB, Ewy GA, et al: Improved resuscitation from cardiac arrest with open-chest massage. *Ann Emerg Med* 13:672–675, 1984.

270. Sanders AB, Kern KB, Fonken S, et al: The role of bicarbonate and fluid loading in improving resuscitation from prolonged cardiac arrest with rapid manual chest compression CPR. *Ann Emerg Med* 19:1–7, 1990.

271. Sanders AB, Kern KB, Otto CW, et al: End-tidal carbon dioxide monitoring during cardiopulmonary resuscitation. A prognostic indicator for survival. *JAMA* 262:1347–1351, 1989.

272. Scheidegger D, Drop LJ, Laver MB: Interaction between vasoactive drugs and plasma ionized calcium. *Intensive Care Med* 3:200, 1977.

273. Scheinman MM, Thorburn D, Abbott JA: Use of atropine in patients with acute myocardial infarction and sinus bradycardia. *Circulation* 52:627–633, 1975.

274. Schindler MB, Bohn D, Cox PN, et al: Outcome of out-of-hospital cardiac or respiratory arrest in children. *N Engl J Med* 335:1473–1479, 1996.

275. Schleien CL, Dean JM, Koehler RC, et al: Effect of epinephrine on cerebral and myocardial perfusion in an infant animal preparation of cardiopulmonary resuscitation. *Circulation* 73:809–817, 1986

276. Schleien CL, Koehler RC, Gervais H, et al: Organ blood flow and somatosensory evoked potentials during and after cardiopulmonary resuscitation with epinephrine or phenylephrine. *Circulation* 79:1332–1342, 1989.

277. Schleien CL, Koehler RC, Shaffner DH, et al: Blood–brain barrier disruption after cardiopulmonary resuscitation in immature swine. *Stroke* 22:477–483, 1991.

278. Schleien CL, Caceres MJ, Kuluz JW, et al: Early endothelial damage and leukocyte accumulation in piglet brains following cardiac arrest. *Acta Neuropathol* 90:582–591, 1995.

279. Schleien CL, Kuluz JW, Shaffner DH, Rogers MC: Cardiopulmonary resuscitation. In Rogers MC (ed): *Textbook of Pediatric Intensive Care.* Baltimore, Williams and Wilkins, 1992.

280. Schleien CL, Kuluz JW, Gelman B: Hemodynamic effects of nitric oxide synthase inhibition before and after cardiac arrest in infant piglets. *Am J Physiol* 274:H1378–H1385, 1998.

281. Schneider T, Martens PR, Paschen H, et al: Multicenter, randomized, controlled trail of 150-J biphasic shocks compared with 200-to 360-J monophasic shocks in the resuscitation of out-of-hospital cardiac arrest victims. Optimized Response to Cardiac Arrest (ORCA) Investigators. *Circulation* 102:1780–1787, 2000.

282. Schumacher RR, Lieberson AD, Childress RH, Williams JF Jr: Hemodynamic effects of lidocaine in patients with heart disease. *Circulation* 37:965–972, 1968.

283. Schwab TM, Callaham ML, Madsen CD, Utecht TA: A randomized clinical trial of active compression-decompression CPR vs standard CPR in out-of-hospital cardiac arrest in two cities. *JAMA* 273:1261–1268, 1995.

284. Sessler D, Mills P, Gregory G, et al: Effects of bicarbonate on arterial and brain intracellular pH in neonatal rabbits recovering from hypoxic lactic acidosis. *J Pediatr* 111:817–823, 1987.

285. Shaffner DH, Schleien CL, Koehler RC, et al: Cerebral and coronary perfusion with vest cardiopulmonary resuscitation in piglets. *Crit Care Med* 18:S243, 1990.

286. Shaffner DH, Eleff SM, Koehler RC, Traystman RJ: Effect of the no-flow interval and hypothermia on cerebral blood flow and metabolism during cardiopulmonary resuscitation in dogs. *Stroke* 29:2607–2615, 1998.

287. Shaffner DH, Eleff SM, Brambrink AM, et al: Effect of arrest time and cerebral perfusion pressure during cardiopulmonary resuscitation on cerebral blood flow, metabolism, ATP recovery, and pH in dogs. *Crit Care Med* 27:1335–1342, 1999.

288. Sharff JA, Pantley G, Noel E: Effect of time on regional organ perfusion during two methods of cardiopulmonary resuscitation. *Ann Emerg Med* 13:649–656, 1984.

289. Sherman BW, Munger MA, Foulke GE, et al: High-dose versus standard-dose epinephrine treatment of cardiac arrest after failure of standard therapy. *Pharmacotherapy* 17:252–257, 1997.

290. Shewmon DA: Commentary on guidelines for the determination of brain death in children. *Ann Neurol* 24:789–791, 1988.

291. Shewmon DA, De Giorgio CM: Early prognosis in anoxic coma. Reliability and rationale. *Neurol Clin* 7:823–843, 1989.

292. Sieber FE, Traystman RJ: Special issues: Glucose and the brain. *Crit Care Med* 20:104–114, 1992.

293. Siemkowicz E, Hansen AJ: Clinical restitution following cerebral ischemia in hypo-, normo-, and hyperglycemic rats. *Acta Neurol Scand* 58:1–8, 1978.

294. Siesjo BK: Cerebral circulation and metabolism. *J Neurosurg* 60:883–908, 1984.

295. Singh BN: Amiodarone: historical development and pharmacologic profile. *Am Heart J* 106:788–797, 1983.

296. Slonim AD, Patel KM, Ruttimann UE, Pollack MM: Cardiopulmonary resuscitation in pediatric intensive care units. *Crit Care Med* 25:1951–1955, 1997.

297. Snyder AB, Salloum LJ, Barone JE, et al: Predicting short-term outcome of cardiopulmonary resuscitation using central venous oxygen tension measurements. *Crit Care Med* 19:111–113, 1991.

298. Stacpoole PW: Lactic acidosis: The case against bicarbonate therapy. *Ann Intern Med* 105:276–279, 1986.

299. Stacpoole PW: The pharmacology of dichloroacetate. *Metabolism* 38:1124–1144, 1989.

300. Stacpoole PW, Gonzalez MG, Vlasak J, et al: Dichloroacetate derivatives. Metabolic effects and pharmacodynamics in normal rats. *Life Sci* 41:2167–2176, 1987.

301. Stacpoole PW, Lorenz AC, Thomas RG, Harman EM: Dichloroacetate in the treatment of lactic acidosis. *Ann Intern Med* 108:58–63, 1988.

302. Stacpoole PW, Wright EC, Baumgartner TG, et al: A controlled clinical trial of dichloroacetate for treatment of lactic acidosis in adults. The Dichloroacetate-Lactic Acidosis Study Group. *N Engl J Med* 327:1564–1569, 1992.

303. Starc TJ, Rosenzweig EB, Landry DW, et al: Emergency use of vasopressin in children with vasodilatory shock due to sepsis or after bypass. *Crit Care Med* 28:A71, 2001.

304. Steinhart CR, Permutt S, Gurtner GH, Traystman RJ: Beta-Adrenergic activity and cardiovascular response to severe respiratory acidosis. *Am J Physiol* 244:H46–H54, 1983.

305. Stiell IG, Hebert PC, Weitzman BN, et al: High-dose epinephrine in adult cardiac arrest. *N Engl J Med* 327:1045–1050, 1992.

306. Stiell IG, Hebert PC, Wells GA, et al: The Ontario trial of active compression-decompression cardiopulmonary resuscitation for in-hospital and prehospital cardiac arrest. *JAMA* 275:1417–1423, 1996.

307. Stueven HA, Thompson B, Aprahamian C, et al: The effectiveness of calcium chloride in refractory electromechanical dissociation. *Ann Emerg Med* 14:626–629, 1985.

308. Stueven HA, Thompson B, Aprahamian C, et al: Lack of effectiveness of calcium chloride in refractory asystole. *Ann Emerg Med* 14:630–632, 1985.

309. Sun JH, Filley GF, Hord K, et al: Carbicarb: an effective substitute for NaHCO3 for the treatment of acidosis. *Surgery* 102:835–839, 1987.

310. Suominen P, Olkkola KT, Voipio V, et al: Utstein style reporting of in-hospital paediatric cardiopulmonary resuscitation. *Resuscitation* 45:17–25, 2000.

311. Suominen P, Palo R, Sairanen H, et al: Perioperative determinants and outcome of cardiopulmonary arrest in children after heart surgery. *Eur J Cardiothorac Surg* 19:127–134, 2001.

312. Swenson RD, Weaver WD, Niskanen RA, et al: Hemodynamics in humans during conventional and experimental methods of cardiopulmonary resuscitation. *Circulation* 78:630–639, 1988.

313. Tacker WA Jr, Babbs CF, Abendschein DR, Geddes LA: Transchest defibrillation under conditions of hypothermia. *Crit Care Med* 9:390–391, 1981.

314. Tang W, Weil MH, Gazmuri RJ, et al: Pulmonary ventilation/perfusion defects induced by epinephrine during cardiopulmonary resuscitation. *Circulation* 84:2101–2107, 1991.

315. Tang W, Weil MH, Schock RB: Phased chest and abdominal compression-decompression. A new option for cardiopulmonary resuscitation. *Circulation* 95:1335–1340, 1997.

316. Taylor GJ, Rubin R, Tucker M, et al: External cardiac compression. A randomized comparison of mechanical and manual techniques. *JAMA* 240:644–646, 1978.

317. Taylor GJ, Tucker WM, Greene HL, et al: Importance of prolonged compression during cardiopulmonary resuscitation in man. *N Engl J Med* 296:1515–1517, 1977.

318. Teasdale G, Jennett B: Assessment of coma and impaired consciousness. A practical scale. *Lancet* 2:81–84, 1974.

319. Tisherman SA, Safar P, Abramson NS, et al: Feasibility of emergency cardiopulmonary bypass for resuscitation from CPR-resistant cardiac arrest: A preliminary report. *Ann Emerg Med* 20:491, 1991.

320. Todres ID, Rogers MC: Methods of external cardiac massage in the newborn infant. *J Pediatr* 86:781–782, 1975.

321. Urban P, Scheidegger D, Buchmann B, Barth D: Cardiac arrest and blood ionized calcium levels. *Ann Intern Med* 109:110–113, 1988.

322. Urban P, Scheidegger D, Buchmann B, Skarvan K: The hemodynamic effects of heparin and their relation to ionized calcium levels. *J Thorac Cardiovasc Surg* 91:303–306, 1986.

323. Voelckel WG, Lurie KG, McKnite S, et al: Comparison of epinephrine and vasopressin in a pediatric porcine model of asphyxial cardiac arrest. *Crit Care Med* 28:3777–3783, 2000.

324. Voelckel WG, Lurie KG, McKnite S, et al: Effects of epinephrine and vasopressin in a piglet model of prolonged ventricular fibrillation and cardiopulmonary resuscitation. *Crit Care Med* 30:957–962, 2002.

325. Voelckel WG, Lurie KG, Sweeney M, et al: Effects of active compression-decompression cardiopulmonary resuscitation with the inspiratory threshold valve in a young porcine model of cardiac arrest. *Pediatr Res* 51:523–27, 2002.

326. Voll CL, Auer RN: The effect of postischemic blood glucose levels on ischemic brain damage in the rat. *Ann Neurol* 24:638–646, 1988.

327. Von Seggern K, Egar M, Fuhrman BP: Cardiopulmonary resuscitation in a pediatric ICU. *Crit Care Med* 14:275–277, 1986.

328. Voorhees WD, Niebauer MJ, Babbs CF: Improved oxygen delivery during cardiopulmonary resuscitation with interposed abdominal compressions. *Ann Emerg Med* 12:128–135, 1983.

329. Walker JW, Bruestle JC, White BC, et al: Perfusion of the cerebral cortex by use of abdominal counterpulsation during cardiopulmonary resuscitation. *Am J Emerg Med* 2:391–393, 1984.

330. Ward KR, Sullivan RJ, Zelenak RR, Summer WR: A comparison of interposed abdominal compression CPR and standard CPR by monitoring end-tidal PCO2. *Ann Emerg Med* 18:831–837, 1989.

331. Wargovich TJ, MacDonald RG, Hill JA, et al: Myocardial metabolic and hemodynamic effects of dichloroacetate in coronary artery disease. *Am J Cardiol* 61:65–70, 1988.

332. Wayne MA, Levine RL, Miller CC: Use of end-tidal carbon dioxide to predict outcome in prehospital cardiac arrest. *Ann Emerg Med* 25:762–767, 1995.

333. Weale FE, Rothwell-Jackson RL: The efficiency of cardiac massage. *Lancet* 1:990–992, 1962.

334. Weaver WD, Cobb LA, Copass MK, Hallstrom AP: Ventricular defibrillation: A comparative trial using 175-J and 320-J shocks. *N Engl J Med* 307:1101–1106, 1982.

335. Weil MH, Rackow EC, Trevino R, et al: Difference in acid-base state between venous and arterial blood during cardiopulmonary resuscitation. *N Engl J Med* 315:153–156, 1986.

336. Weiser FM, Adler LN, Kuhn LA: Hemodynamic effects of closed and open chest cardiac resuscitation in normal dogs and those with acute myocardial infarction. *Am J Cardiol* 10:555–561, 1962.

337. Wenzel V, Lindner KH: Arginine vasopressin during cardiopulmonary resuscitation: Laboratory evidence, clinical experience and recommendations, and a view to the future. *Crit Care Med* 30:S157–S161, 2002.

338. Wenzel V, Lindner KH, Krismer AC, et al: Survival with full neurologic recovery and no cerebral pathology after prolonged cardiopulmonary resuscitation with vasopressin in pigs. *J Am Coll Cardiol* 35:527–533, 2000.

339. Werner JA, Greene HL, Janko CL, Cobb LA: Visualization of cardiac valve motion in man during external chest compression using two-dimensional echocardiography: Implications regarding the mechanism of blood flow. *Circulation* 63:1417–1421, 1981.

340. White BC, Winegar CD, Wilson RF, et al: Possible role of calcium blockers in cerebral resuscitation: A review of the literature and synthesis for future studies. *Crit Care Med* 11:202–207, 1983.

341. Wilder RJ, Weir D, Rush BF, Ravitch MM: Methods of coordinating ventilation and closed chest cardiac massage in the dog. *Surgery* 53:186–194, 1963.

342. Winquist RJ, Webb RC, Bohr DF: Relaxation to transmural nerve stimulation and exogenously added norepinephrine in porcine cerebral vessels: A study utilizing cerebrovascular intrinsic tone. *Circ Res* 51:769–776, 1982.

343. Woo E, Chan YW, Yu YL, Huang CY: Admission glucose level in relation to mortality and morbidity outcome in 252 stroke patients. *Stroke* 19:185–191, 1988.

344. Wood WB, Manley ES Jr, Woodbury RA: The effects of CO_2 induced respiratory acidosis on the depressor and pressor components of the dog's blood pressure to epinephrine. *J Pharmacol Exp Ther* 139:238, 1963.

345. Worthley LI: Sodium bicarbonate in cardiac arrest. *Lancet* 2:903–904, 1976.

346. Yabek SM, Kato R, Singh BN: Effects of amiodarone and its metabolite, desethylamiodarone, on the electrophysiologic properties of isolated cardiac muscle. *J Cardiovasc Pharmacol* 8:197–207, 1986.

347. Yakaitis RW, Otto CW, Blitt CD: Relative importance of alpha and beta adrenergic receptors during resuscitation. *Crit Care Med* 7:293–296, 1979.

348. Zaritsky A: Cardiopulmonary resuscitation in children. *Clin Chest Med* 8:561–571, 1987.

349. Zipes DP, Fischer J, King RM, et al: Termination of ventricular fibrillation in dogs by depolarizing a critical amount of myocardium. *Am J Cardiol* 36:37–44, 1975.

350. Zipes DP, Prystowsky EN, Heger JJ: Amiodarone: Electrophysiologic actions, pharmacokinetics and clinical effects. *J Am Coll Cardiol* 3:1059–1071, 1984.

Chapter 14

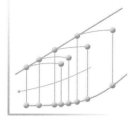

Coagulation Disorders in Congenital Heart Disease

SCOTT R. SCHULMAN, MD, FRANK H. KERN, MD,
THOMAS O. ERB, MD, and WILLIAM R. GREELEY, MD, MBA

INTRODUCTION

In 1950, Bahnson and Ziegler first observed a hemorrhagic diathesis in patients with congenital heart disease (CHD). Reviewing the first 500 patients who had undergone the Blalock-Taussig shunt, the authors remarked on the "many dilated and engorged vessels in the chest wall and mediastinum. These are often troublesome during the dissection of the mediastinal structures and probably are the main site of postoperative bleeding."[3] The authors described seven patients in whom "massive bleeding was the primary cause of death."[3] Hemorrhage was the fourth leading cause of mortality in the first group of patients to undergo the Blalock-Taussig shunt.

Two years later, in 1952, the number of patients to receive this operation had increased to 1100. In his classic article "A Hemorrhagic Disorder Occurring in Patients With Cyanotic Congenital Heart Disease," Hartmann noted that 18 patients bled to death after surgery. He remarked: "A hemorrhagic diathesis seemed to be present in most of these patients ... Typically, little or no excessive bleeding was encountered at the time of operation, but within several hours thereafter severe and uncontrollable hemorrhage began."[20] He noted that these patients had thrombocytopenia, abnormal clot retraction, low fibrinogen levels, and prolonged bleeding times and observed an association between the degree of polycythemia and the hemorrhagic diathesis.

Fifty years of progress in hematology and congenital heart disease have confirmed Hartmann's observations. Despite advances in the characterization of the hemostatic abnormalities in CHD, the precise nature of the defect remains elusive, probably due to its multifactorial nature. Preoperative hematologic screening has improved, yet perioperative hemorrhage still complicates approximately 5% of pediatric open-heart surgery.[2]

This chapter will review the process of normal coagulation in infants and children, examine the various tests of the clotting mechanism, review the alterations of hemostasis in CHD, consider the impact of cardiopulmonary bypass on hemostasis, and develop strategies for the diagnosis and management of bleeding after pediatric cardiac surgery.

THE FLUID PHASE

Coagulation factors are enzymes that circulate in an inactive form. When the coagulation mechanism is triggered, a small portion of an inactive procoagulant molecule ("factor") is cleaved off, producing an active serine protease. Serine proteases are enzymes that work by cleaving off a portion of their substrate. Cleavage of the inactive factor results in activation of that factor and is denoted by the suffix "a" after the Roman numeral (e.g., Factor XIIa). The now-active factor activates subsequent molecules in a cascade or series of chain reactions that results in the generation of thrombin. Thrombin then acts on fibrinogen to convert it to fibrin, and a stable clot is formed.

Biologic cascades, such as that described previously, are like a series of dominoes standing on end (Fig. 14-1). Once the first domino falls, a chain reaction starts. The first domino in the intrinsic arm of the coagulation cascade is factor XII. The first domino in the extrinsic branch is factor VII. Memorization of the various factor names and confusing nomenclature is less important than understanding a few general principles.

Coagulation requires a phospholipid surface. This surface can come from one of two sources. The first source is the activated platelet at the site of vascular injury. Activated platelets expose a surface phospholipid known as platelet

factor 3 (PF_3). Because PF_3 originates inside the blood vessel, the coagulation sequence that occurs on this surface is known as the intrinsic pathway. The second source of phospholipid comes from injured cells outside of the blood vessel. Tissue factor or tissue thromboplastin is the name given to this phospholipid. The extrinsic pathway of coagulation starts in damaged tissues outside of the vessel wall.

Although the bifurcation of coagulation into intrinsic and extrinsic systems is useful, the distinctions between the two are often blurred. There is a lot of interplay between the two branches of the coagulation cascade as well as between coagulation cascade reactions and platelet phase reactions. Several processes occur simultaneously.

Intrinsic Pathway

The intrinsic pathway of coagulation is so named because it occurs on a phospholipid surface that is provided by an activated platelet at sites of vascular injury. When the integrity of the blood vessel wall is violated, factor XII is exposed to collagen or connective tissue in the subendothelium. Contact of factor XII with these surfaces causes its activation. Activated factor XII (XIIa) has several substrates. XIIa catalyzes the conversion of XI to XIa. XIa in turn cleaves IX to IXa. Activated factor IX then cleaves X into Xa. However, IXa cannot do this alone. It requires the help of a cofactor, a "second activator." The second activator in this case is known as cofactor VIII. VIII is a complex molecule that is composed of two parts. One part is factor VIII, which helps IXa activate factor X. The second part is a large protein known as von Willebrand factor (vWF). Von Willebrand factor binds to a platelet membrane protein (glycoprotein Ib) and promotes platelet adhesion. Thus, factor VIII forms a complex with IXa and binds via a calcium (Ca^{++}) bridge with a phospholipid in the membrane of an activated platelet.

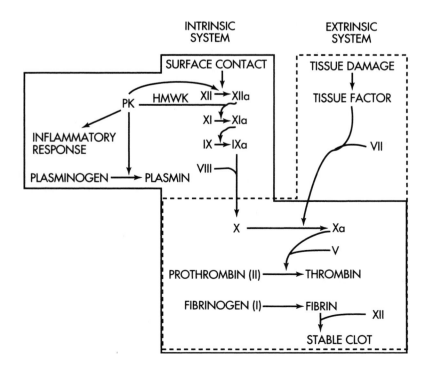

FIGURE 14-1 Scheme of blood coagulation. The suffix *a* denotes the activated factor with enzyme activity. PK, prekallikrein; HMWK, high-molecular-weight kininogen. (From Hathaway WE: Hemostasis. In Rudolph AB (ed): *Pediatrics*, 17th ed. Norwalk, CT: Appleton-Century-Crofts, 1982, pp 1110–1114.)

Reactions involving cofactors generally require phospholipid surfaces. This requirement ensures that clot forms at sites of vascular injury rather than at remote sites in the vascular tree. The need for a phospholipid surface indicates that the process of clot formation is simultaneous with and dependent upon the platelet hemostatic process.

Factor XIIa has several other actions. These include activation of both the kinin- and plasmin-generating mechanisms. This is another example of the complex interdependence of the coagulation system with other homeostatic biologic cascades. XIIa triggers not only coagulation, but also fibrinolysis, the dissolution of clot. Therefore, cardiopulmonary bypass (CPB)–induced stimulation of XIIa causes both a thrombogenic and fibrinolytic response.

Extrinsic Pathway

Tissue thromboplastin complexes with factor VII to form VIIa. VIIa proteolyses X to Xa via a Ca^{++} phospholipid bridge. The extrinsic pathway begins outside the blood vessel wall and culminates in the generation of Xa. The common pathway of coagulation begins with Xa. Cardiopulmonary bypass stimulates both the intrinsic and extrinsic pathways.

Common Pathway

Once sufficient amounts of Xa are produced, prothrombin is converted to thrombin. This conversion is facilitated by cofactor Va in concert with Ca^{++}. Thrombin then cleaves fibrinogen to fibrin. The fibrin so generated takes one of two paths. The first path is the formation of soluble fibrin (fibrin S). The second path is the formation of insoluble fibrin polymers that are cross-linked by covalent peptide bonds under the influence of factor XIIIa. This latter path results in a stable fibrin clot. Platelets are then added, and the result is a stable blood clot.

HEMOSTASIS: THE PLATELET PHASE

Primary hemostasis refers to the interaction between the blood vessel wall and the platelet. Platelets are involved in all phases of hemostasis. They form the primary hemostatic plug at sites of vascular injury. They then release vasoactive factors that produce vasoconstriction of injured blood vessels. Next, they provide a surface for certain coagulation factor reactions.

Normally, the vascular endothelial cell secretes a prostaglandin, prostacyclin. Prostacyclin prevents platelet adhesion and promotes vasodilation. Thus, prostacyclin makes the vessel nonthrombogenic. When the vascular endothelium is injured, platelets adhere to the subendothelial collagen and change shape from discoid to spherical. These activated platelets release the contents of their cytoplasmic granules, including adenosine diphosphate (ADP), serotonin, platelet factor 4, catecholamines, and thromboxane A_2. Thromboxane A_2 produces vasoconstriction and causes platelets to further aggregate, recruiting circulating platelets into the primary hemostatic plug formed at the site of vascular injury. Von Willebrand factor links the platelet to the injured endothelium via glycoprotein I_B. Fibrogen joins platelets to each other via membrane glycoproteins II_b and III_a. The need for fibrinogen is yet another example of the highly interdependent nature of the two processes of hemostasis and coagulation. Many other coagulation reactions also take place on the activated platelet membrane.

FIBRINOLYSIS

Fibrinolysis is the resolution phase of coagulation. Once a stable fibrin clot has formed and the damaged tissues have been repaired, the fibrinolytic system digests fibrin and restores normal blood flow. The key enzyme in this process is plasmin. Plasmin is formed when its inactive precursor, plasminogen, is cleaved by tissue plasminogen activator (TPA). Plasminogen activators are a heterogeneous group of proteases that are located both within the circulation and in organs as diverse as the lungs, heart, adrenal glands, and ovaries. When it is time to limit the spread of clot, TPA catalyzes the conversion of plasminogen to plasmin. Plasmin then digests the fibrin clot, which yields fibrin degradation products. Once clot lysis is complete, plasmin enters the circulation, where it is rapidly inactivated by antiplasmin, a serum protein which forms an enzyme-inhibitor complex with plasmin.

CONTROL OF COAGULATION

Several important control mechanisms limit the progression of clot and prevent complete intravascular thrombosis. Antithrombin III (AT III) is a plasma protein that binds to and inactivates thrombin. Heparin binds to AT III and accelerates the reaction between thrombin and AT III 10,000 fold. AT III also binds and inactivates other activated coagulation factors, namely, IXa, Xa, XIa, and XIIa. Protein C is another inhibitor of coagulation. It circulates in an inactive form; however, upon exposure to the endothelial-derived protein thrombomodulin and in the presence of thrombin, protein C is converted to its active form. Once activated, it inhibits cofactors V and VIII. VIII is necessary for the conversion of X to its active form, and V is necessary to help Xa convert prothrombin to thrombin. Protein C suppresses thrombin generation by inhibiting the binding of Xa to V. These cofactors function in the intrinsic and common pathways as bridges for reactions on the platelet surface. Another cofactor that enhances the binding of protein C to platelet membrane phospholipid is protein S. Protein S is a vitamin K–dependent plasma protein that enables protein C to more efficiently inhibit the binding of Xa to V.

There are other physiologic controls that limit the spread of clot. The rapid flow of blood dilutes the effective concentration of activated factors and removes them from sites of injury. Once removed, the hepatic and reticuloendothelial systems promptly and preferentially clear the activated factors from the circulation.

TESTS OF COAGULATION

Screening tests for coagulation examine each arm of the clotting pathway: intrinsic and extrinsic. Tests of the intrinsic pathway examine coagulation occurring inside the vessel; tests of the extrinsic pathway investigate coagulation occurring outside the vessel wall. The phospholipid surface upon which coagulation occurs is one basic difference between the pathways. Therefore, platelet phospholipid is used to test the intrinsic arm while tissue phospholipid is used to interrogate the extrinsic arm.

For example, to screen the intrinsic pathway, platelet phospholipid (PF_3) and Ca^{++} are added to the patient's plasma and the time to clot formation is measured. In the laboratory, a substitute for PF_3, partial thromboplastin, is used. To avoid waiting for contact activation of the intrinsic factors XII and XI, an inert surface such as kaolin or celite (diatomaceous earth) preactivates these factors and thus mimics in the test tube the contact activation that occurs when factor XII is exposed to subendothelial collagen. Preactivation gives more consistent, reproducible results. The normal activated partial thromboplastin time (aPTT) is 25 to 35 seconds. The aPTT tests both the intrinsic and common pathways, and the test will be prolonged when there is less than 30% activity of factors II, V, VIII, IX, or X.

The extrinsic and common pathways are tested by the prothrombin time. This assay involves the addition of tissue thromboplastin and Ca^{++} to patient plasma. The normal prothrombin time is 10 to 12 seconds, but varies among laboratories. Prolonged prothrombin times are seen when there is less than 30% activity of factors II, V, VII, or X, or when there is dysfibrinogenemia or hypofibrinogenemia. Note that three of the four vitamin K dependent clotting factors reside in this arm of the coagulation system.

What is the significance of vitamin K? The majority of the coagulation factors are synthesized in the liver. Factors II, VII, IX, and X undergo enzymatic transformation in the hepatocyte after synthesis. This transformation involves the addition of a carboxyl (COOH) moiety. Carboxylation is possible only with the help of vitamin K. The COOH addition allows for these factors to bind via a Ca^{++} bridge to phospholipid. Vitamin K deficient patients produce these factors, but they are nonfunctional. Vitamin K antagonists, such as warfarin, exert their anticoagulant effect by inhibiting the carboxylation step in the hepatocyte.

The international normalized ratio (INR) has been adopted in an attempt to standardize the results of the prothrombin time test. North American laboratories have traditionally used the less sensitive rabbit-brain thromboplastin in determining the prothrombin time. The World Health Organization introduced an international reference standard using the more sensitive human-brain thromboplastin. INR is defined as the prothrombin time ratio (patient/control) obtained if the international reference thromboplastin made from human brain is used to test the sample. Because the results are independent of local laboratory methods, a blood sample sent to different laboratories should yield the same INR results.

INR guides the use of the oral anticoagulant coumadin, which is required in patients at high risk for thrombosis. Among children with heart disease, this group includes patients with prosthetic heart valves and some children after Fontan surgery. Safe and effective coumadin therapy generally targets an INR range of 2 to 3. Typically, coumadin is initiated while the patient is still receiving heparin. Infants require higher doses and take longer to achieve the targeted INR range than older children.[40] Fontan patients and patients with liver disease require lower coumadin doses.

The activated clotting time (ACT) is a modification of the whole blood clotting time. It is a global measure and therefore is not a good screening test. It is useful because it is quickly accomplished at the bedside. The ACT tests the intrinsic and common pathways. It involves the addition of whole blood to a tube containing celite for maximum contact activation. The normal range is 80 to 140 seconds. This test differs from the activated partial thromboplastin time (aPTT) in that the former relies on the patient's blood as the source of PF_3 whereas the latter test eliminates the platelet variable by using cephalin as a PF_3 substitute. The ACT is performed by automated equipment and results are provided almost instantaneously. It is used in the operating room as a measure of heparin effect. Heparin, by activating antithrombin III and inhibiting factors IIa, IXa, XIa, and Xa, preferentially affects the intrinsic pathway of coagulation.

The thrombin time (TT) measures the conversion of fibrinogen to fibrin. It is independent of factor activity. TT is prolonged when the fibrinogen level is low, when there is dysfunctional fibrinogen, or in the presence of circulating inhibitors of thrombin such as activated AT III (from heparin).

TESTS OF PLATELET FUNCTION

The platelet count and the bleeding time are two commonly used tests of platelet function. Platelet count is a quantitative measure only. Normal values are 150,000 to 400,000/mm³. It tells nothing about platelet function. Platelet counts less than 20,000/mm³ are usually associated with spontaneous bleeding. Surgical bleeding occurs at counts of 40,000 to 70,000/mm³.

The bleeding time assesses platelet function as well as platelet number. This test measures the time necessary to form a stable platelet plug. The test involves a superficial skin puncture with a template. This injures the blood vessel and exposes subendothelial collagen. The blood is absorbed onto a piece of filter paper and the time until bleeding ceases is measured. Normal values range from 2 to 9 minutes. Prolongation of the bleeding time is observed when normal platelet adhesion, aggregation, and activation are impaired, when there is an abnormality of the blood vessel wall such as in connective tissue disorders like Ehlers-Danlos syndrome, or when the platelet count falls below 100,000/mm³.

Research tools used to test platelet function include quantitative measures such as clot retraction as well as quantitative molecular markers of platelet activation such as beta-thromboglobulin and platelet factor 4 levels. These tests will be discussed in the section on hemostatic abnormalities in CHD.

TESTS OF FIBRINOLYSIS

Clotted blood at 37° C should not lyse for up to 48 hours. Less than one hour is all that is needed if the fibrinolytic system is active. How does one test for fibrinolysis? A useful screening test is a fibrinogen level combined with fibrin degradation products (FDPs). If the fibrinogen level is normal and there are increased FDPs (greater than 12 g/mL), fibrinolysis is likely. The euglobulin clot lysis time (ELT) confirms fibrinolysis. The euglobulin fraction of plasma is free of inhibitors of fibrinolysis. This fraction of plasma is mixed with thrombin, and the time to clot lysis is measured. Normally the ELT is greater than 120 minutes. If the ELT is less than 120 minutes, fibrinolysis is likely.

DEVELOPMENTAL CHANGES IN HEMOSTASIS

Healthy neonates and infants up to six months of age have low levels of coagulation factors compared to adults. Coagulation factor levels reach adult values by 6 months to 1 year of age.[1] Despite low factor levels, screening tests of coagulation such as the bleeding time, prothrombin time, and activated clotting time are generally comparable to adult values.[30] How does one account for this apparent discrepancy? The inhibitors of coagulation, proteins C and S and anti-thrombin III, are all depressed in the neonatal period.[31] The presence of low factor levels that might predispose to bleeding is balanced by low levels of circulating inhibitors of coagulation, which promotes the generation of clot.

HEMOSTASIS AND COAGULATION IN CONGENITAL HEART DISEASE

Abnormalities of coagulation, hemostasis, and fibrinolysis have all been reported in CHD. The incidence of abnormalities on preoperative screening tests in CHD patients varies from 20% to 60%.[9,24] Cyanotic children, and children whose hematocrit values are greater than 60%, are most severely affected. However, acyanotic patients and newborns with CHD also manifest dysfunctional coagulation. There is no consistent pattern of abnormality. This wide range and variable presentation are likely due to the heterogeneous population that children with CHD represent. In clinical practice, preoperative laboratory assessment includes a hemoglobin and hematocrit determination along with a quantitative platelet count, a PT, and an aPTT.

Coagulation Factors

Several studies have demonstrated prolongation of the PT and aPTT in CHD.[14,42] Impaired vitamin K–dependent carboxylation appears to be a contributing factor in some patients. Low levels of factors VII and IX have been observed by some investigators. Quantitative abnormalities are even more pronounced in neonates. Factor levels are approximately 30 to 40% lower in newborns with congenital heart disease than in those neonates without structural cardiac abnormalities. One postulated cause for these low levels is impaired hepatic synthesis secondary to liver hypoperfusion. Hypofibrinogenemia (factor I) and low levels of circulating inhibitors may also play a role. Whatever the exact mechanism, children at highest risk are those with hematocrit values above 60%, cyanotic defects, left-sided obstructive lesions such as interruption of the aortic arch, and poor cardiac output.

Platelets

Children with cyanotic CHD demonstrate both quantitative and qualitative platelet defects. Thrombocytopenia occurs in approximately one third of the children.[33] Even if the absolute platelet count is normal, many of these patients have prolongation of the bleeding time.[28] Abnormal clot retraction, another qualitative test of platelet function, has also been reported. These findings suggest defects in platelet adhesion and aggregation. Quantitative functional platelet assays have demonstrated elevated levels of beta-thromboglobulin and platelet factor 4 (PF_4) in CHD patients compared to controls.[41] This observation suggests that in CHD, platelets are chronically activated and thus depleted of their vesicle contents. They exist in a functionally refractory state, unable to mount a normal response by aggregating and adhering at sites of vascular injury.

Children with noncyanotic CHD also demonstrate platelet abnormalities. These abnormalities include the loss of the von Willebrand factor (vWF) portion of the factor VIII complex.[17] The absence of a portion of vWF leads to bleeding that can be clinically significant. Although the mechanism by which children with noncyanotic CHD develop this platelet abnormality is not known, it is likely due to aberrant flow patterns or altered hemodynamics associated with the specific cardiac lesion. In most affected children studied, the vWF abnormality corrected when the cardiac defect was repaired.

Newborns with ductal-dependent pulmonary or systemic blood flow are placed on prostaglandin E (PGE_1) infusions preoperatively to maintain ductal patency. These infusions affect platelet function by preventing activation.

An occasional child will be placed on heparin preoperatively. Heparin-induced thrombocytopenia (HIT) is a rare complication of heparin therapy, occurring with an incidence of 0.5% to 5% in adult patients. The incidence in pediatric patients is presumably less. HIT is an idiosyncratic, antibody-mediated reaction that occurs within 6 to 12 days of heparin administration. The clinical features of HIT are thrombocytopenia (platelet counts typically are around 50,000/μL; however, values as low as 10,000/mm³ have been reported) and thrombosis with an increasing heparin requirement. Elevated platelet aggregation and serotonin release responses to heparin confirm the diagnosis.

Fibrinolysis

Eight percent to 40% of children with CHD demonstrate a shortened euglobulin clot lysis time on preoperative screening.[7,37] Primary fibrinolysis is a contributing factor in the coagulopathy of CHD. Perioperative inhibition of fibrinolysis produces a significant decrease in blood loss during palliative or corrective surgery for congenital heart disease.[44]

HEMOSTATIC ALTERATIONS CAUSED BY CARDIOPULMONARY BYPASS

Platelets

Cardiopulmonary bypass (CPB) is a major thrombogenic stimulus in infants and children that affects all aspects of the hemostatic system (Fig. 14-2). The major hemostatic abnormality

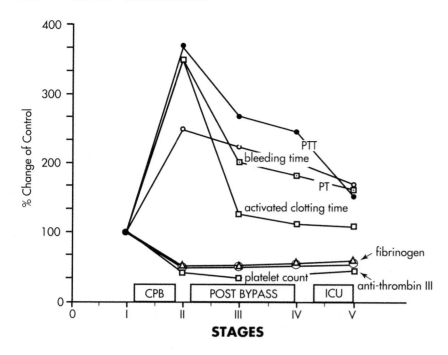

FIGURE 14-2   Plot of blood coagulation profile changes before, during, and after cardiopulmonary bypass (CPB) in 25 children. Clotting times and coagulant factors are shown as percent change from control. Stage I, baseline, before CPB; stage II, post-CPB, before protamine reversal of heparin; stage III, after protamine; stage IV, just prior to leaving the operating room; stage V, after 3 hours in the intensive care unit. PTT, partial thromboplastin time; *PT*, prothrombin time. (From Greeley WJ, Bushman GA, Kong DL, et al: Effects of cardiopulmonary bypass on eicosanoid metabolism during pediatric cardiovascular surgery. *J Thorac Cardiovasc Surg* 95:842–849, 1988.)

associated with cardiopulmonary bypass is platelet dysfunction.[8,19] Platelet abnormalities are both quantitative and qualitative. Qualitative defects are the most important. The initiation of CPB disrupts the vascular endothelium, exposing subendothelial collagen and other matrix proteins to non-endothelialized surfaces. These proteins contain regions that interact with platelets, causing platelet adherence and subsequent activation. Contact of platelets with non–prostacyclin-producing synthetic surfaces such as the oxygenator, cannulae, and bypass circuit also leads to platelet activation. Recall that activation is the process whereby the platelets undergo a shape change and as a result exposure of surface receptors. These receptors act as a plane for further platelet aggregation. Activated platelets undergo the "release reaction," which involves the extrusion of alpha granules from lysosomes within the platelet. Contents of these granules include several mediators that function to recruit additional platelets, accelerate coagulation cascade reactions, induce local vasoconstriction, and activate the complement and kinin systems. The activation of platelets produces a functionally inadequate platelet pool.

What is the clinical and laboratory evidence for platelet dysfunction during CPB? The bleeding time is significantly prolonged within minutes of initiating CPB.[45] Bleeding times of upwards of 30 minutes have been reported at bypass times of two hours. In adults, the bleeding time normalizes two to four hours after separation from CPB.

What is the biochemical evidence for platelet activation as the cause for the hemostatic defect during cardiopulmonary bypass? Greeley and colleagues[18] have shown serum thromboxane concentration increases significantly after the initiation of CPB in infants and children compared to control patients not undergoing extracorporeal circulation (Fig. 14-3). Thromboxane A_2 is a potent mediator of platelet microaggregation during CPB. Also during CPB, serum levels of platelet factor 4 (PF_4) and beta-thromboglobulin are elevated.

These peptides normally reside in the alpha granule and are secreted when platelets are activated. Alpha-granule depletion appears to be the mechanism that accounts for the qualitative platelet dysfunction seen during CPB (and hypothermia). Activated platelets are "spent." They circulate

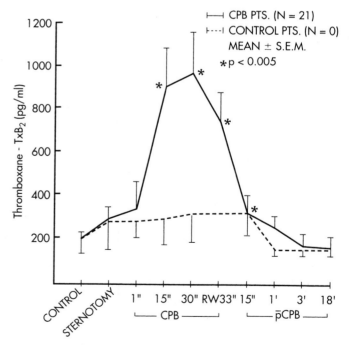

FIGURE 14-3   Thromboxane concentrations in two groups of patients. Note significantly elevated levels in group having cardiopulmonary bypass (CPB) as compared with levels in control group undergoing palliative operations without CPB. S.E.M., Standard error of the mean. (From Greeley WJ, Bushman GA, Kong DL, et al: Effects of cardiopulmonary bypass on eicosanoid metabolism during pediatric cardiovascular surgery. *J Thorac Cardiovasc Surg* 95:842–849, 1988.)

in an exhausted state, unable to respond to substances such as adenosine diphosphate (ADP) and epinephrine, which under normal circumstances induce platelet aggregation.

Whether selective alpha-granule release alone accounts for the platelet dysfunction associated with CPB is controversial. Other factors may play a role. These factors include loss of surface glycoprotein receptors, loss of dense granule contents, and the presence of circulating platelet inhibitors generated by the activation of the complement, kinin, and fibrinolytic systems.

Cardiopulmonary bypass is also associated with a quantitative disorder of platelets.[23] Hemodilution due to priming of the bypass circuit produces a 50% to 70% reduction in the number of circulating platelets in neonates and infants. This reduction is more pronounced in infants than adults, due to the disproportionately high prime volume to extracellular fluid (ECF) ratio in children. In adult patients, the platelet count decreases by only 15% to 20% with the initiation of CPB. Platelet counts in children following cardiopulmonary bypass remain significantly lower than pre-bypass values for several postoperative hours.

In summary, CPB causes platelet activation. Activated platelets are hemostatically ineffective; depleted of their contents, they are unresponsive to stimuli such as ADP and epinephrine, which, under normal circumstances, produce platelet aggregation. The qualitative and quantitative platelet abnormalities observed during CPB can persist after discontinuation of bypass and increase the potential for postoperative bleeding in children.

Coagulation Factors

The initiation of CPB is associated with a reduction in the plasma concentrations of coagulation factors. The younger the patient, the more pronounced the reduction. In neonates undergoing deep hypothermic CPB, Kern and colleagues[23] demonstrated a 50% reduction in circulating coagulation factors (Table 14-1). For example, fibrinogen levels below 1 g/L were consistently observed after discontinuation of CPB in the above series despite the addition of whole blood to the CPB prime. This decrease is due to hemodilution. Hemodilution plays a larger role in smaller patients because the priming volume of the extracorporeal circuit is significantly larger than the circulating blood volume of a neonate. In adults, factor levels remain adequate for hemostasis despite the reduced plasma concentration due to hemodilution. This may not be the case in infants and children. Recognition of the importance of supplying coagulation factors to smaller infants is reflected in the practice of priming the pump with whole blood or fresh frozen plasma rather than packed red blood cells and having whole blood available for transfusion after separation from cardiopulmonary bypass. Whole blood contains red blood cells, platelets, and coagulation factors and is a balanced product. There are several advantages to this approach: 1) the transfused blood product is from a single donor; 2) the use of a balanced product avoids depletion of red cells, which can occur with component therapy. The availability of whole blood frequently requires close cooperation with local transfusion therapy services.

Fibrinolysis

Evidence for fibrinolysis (i.e., shortened euglobulin clot lysis time, hypofibrinogenemia, elevated fibrin degradation products, and prolonged prothrombin and partial thromboplastin times) has been noted after sternotomy and initiation of CPB.[6,26] Endothelial cells secrete tissue plasminogen activator (TPA) during extracorporeal circulation.[39] TPA converts

Table 14-1 Coagulation Factor Activity and Functional Tests of Coagulation in 30 Neonates

Assay	Before CPB	1 Min on CPB	Cold CPB	Warm CPB	After Protamine	ICU
Fibrinogen (% activity)	210 ± 52	91 ± 15[a]	92 ± 19[a]	105 ± 22[a]	159 ± 58[a]	183 ± 33
Factor II (% activity)	56 ± 14	28 ± 8[a]	29 ± 9[a]	32 ± 10[a]	56 ± 14	64 ± 13[b]
Factor V (% activity)	70 ± 21	ND	ND	ND	40 ± 11[a]	48 ± 14[a]
Factor VII (% activity)	55 ± 13	26 ± 6[a]	27 ± 7[a]	29 ± 8[a]	50 ± 14[c]	63 ± 24[b]
Factor VIII (% activity)	58 ± 26	ND	ND	ND	36 ± 26[d]	73 ± 40[b]
Factor IX (% activity)	39 ± 19	24 ± 10[d]	22 ± 7[d]	33 ± 13[b]	39 ± 23	51 ± 20[b]
Factor X (% activity)	53 ± 13	31 ± 9[a]	30 ± 8[a]	33 ± 10[a]	53 ± 16	55 ± 17
Platelets (× 10⁹/L)	219 ± 57	64 ± 26[a]	65 ± 24[a]		93 ± 31[a]	161 ± 65[b]
Antithrombin III (% activity)	50 ± 17	29 ± 11[a]	28 ± 12[a]	31 ± 12[a]	51 ± 17	64 ± 21[b]
Heparin (U)	0.05 ± 0.09	0.36 ± 0.11[a]	0.39 ± 0.10[a]	0.39 ± 0.11[a]	0.08 ± 0.14	0.08 ± 0.09
ACT (sec)	167 ± 20	>700[a]	>700[a]	700[a]	148 ± 22[b]	
PT (sec)	13.4 ± 2.4	25.1 ± 3.1[a]	25.0 ± 7.1[a]	22.2 ± 5.3[a]	15.2 ± 1.6[b]	13.9 ± 1.7
PTT (sec)	58.2 ± 16.7	>90[a]	>90[a]	>90[a]	72 ± 18.8[d]	53.7 ± 14.1

CPB, Cardiopulmonary bypass; ICU, intensive care unit; ND, not detected; PT, prothrombin time; PTT, partial thromboplasin time; ACT, activated clotting time.
[a-d]Significance versus before CPB: [a]$p < 0.0001$, [b]$p < 0.05$, [c]$p < 0.01$, [d]$p < 0.002$.
From Kern FH, Morana NJ, Sears JJ, et al: Coagulation defects in neonates during cardiopulmonary bypass, *Ann Thorac Surg* 54:541–546, 1992; with permission.

plasminogen to plasmin, which degrades fibrin. However, critics of fibrinolysis as a major offender in the pathogenesis of bleeding after CPB contend that the presence of fibrin degradation products, low levels of fibrinogen, and shortened euglobulin clot lysis times are merely a reflection of non-specific factors such as hemodilution, inadequate heparin anti-coagulation, and local consumption of platelets and fibrinogen.

The exact role of fibrinolysis in the pathogenesis of post-CPB bleeding awaits further clarification. Nonetheless, inhibitors of fibrinolysis such as epsilon aminocaproic acid (EACA) and tranexamic acid have been used after open-heart surgery to decrease bleeding. Aprotinin, a serine protease inhibitor that functions at many points in the coagulation cascade including the inhibition of fibrinolysis, produces laboratory evidence of inhibition of fibrinolysis and decreased blood loss.[11]

HEMATOLOGIC MANAGEMENT DURING CARDIOPULMONARY BYPASS IN CHILDREN

Heparinization

Disruption of the vascular endothelium produces a thrombogenic surface. Normally, this surface activates the intrinsic system of coagulation. Coagulation must be blocked for cardiopulmonary bypass to proceed. Heparin produces systemic anticoagulation by binding to antithrombin III.[4]

Antithrombin III is a plasma protein that functions as a major inhibitor of coagulation. AT III binds to, and inactivates, thrombin. Heparin binds to AT III and causes the reaction between AT III and thrombin to occur at a rate 10,000 times faster than normal. The heparin–antithrombin III complex also inactivates several other activated coagulation factors including Xa, IXa, and XIa. Heparin quickly and effectively blocks the generation of fibrin with no systemic side effects. It is rapidly titratable and easily reversible.

There is a paucity of data regarding the dose-response of heparin in infants and children. It is generally believed that heparin exerts a prolonged effect in infants for two reasons: 1) the reduced metabolic capability of the infant, and 2) the exposure of the infant to more profound levels of hypothermia, which also reduces the metabolism of heparin.[22]

Heparin is administered as an intravenous bolus dose of 300 to 400 U/kg. The initial dose is empirical. It is administered before cannulation of the great vessels either by direct injection into the right atrium or through a functioning central line to assure that heparin enters the central circulation. Heparin is also added to the cardiopulmonary bypass circuit prime in a concentration equal to 2 U/mL. The most common manner of assessing the biologic effect of heparin is measurement of the activated clotting time (ACT). The ACT involves the addition of whole blood to a tube containing celite or kaolin for maximum contact activation. This activates the intrinsic and common pathways. Heparin binds to AT III and inhibits thrombin (IIa), but it also inhibits factors IXa, Xa, and XIa. The ACT is thus prolonged with systemic heparinization. However, the ACT is neither a sensitive nor a specific test of heparin effect. Hypothermia, hemodilution, and platelet abnormalities can also prolong the ACT. The aPTT is a better measure of heparin effect than the ACT. The advantage of the ACT is that it provides rapid results at the bedside, and it has therefore become the gold standard in the cardiac operating suite. An ACT of greater than 400 seconds is generally felt to prevent fibrin deposition in the extracorporeal circuit and provide adequate anticoagulation for the institution of cardiopulmonary bypass.

Recent evidence suggests that the younger the patient, the more sensitive he or she is to heparin. Neonates in the first week of life demonstrate an almost three-fold prolongation of the ACT per unit of administered heparin compared to toddlers aged three and above (Jobes, DR, unpublished data). This observation is consistent with the experimental finding that in neonates there are variable levels of both procoagulants and inhibitors in the first months of life.

In addition to the ACT, there are other methods for determining the presence of heparin. Whole blood heparin concentration can be measured either directly (by measuring heparin activity) or indirectly (by using neutralization with protamine). These methods provide for more precise protamine dosing at the conclusion of cardiopulmonary bypass because they are theoretically less influenced than the ACT by CPB-induced hypothermia and hemodilution. The direct assay has helped to provide a better understanding of the pharmacokinetics of heparin. A better in vivo test of heparin effect is obtained with protamine titration. Protamine is a polycationic alkaline molecule that combines with the negatively charged sulfated mucopolysaccharide heparin to produce a dense precipitate that is biologically inactive.

Protamine titration is both qualitative and quantitative. The qualitative test involves adding protamine in increments of 10 mcg from 0 to 50 mcg to a series of test tubes. One milliliter of blood is then added to each tube. The tubes are then observed to see which specimen clots first. If the tube containing protamine is the first to clot, heparin was present and was neutralized by the protamine. If the tube without protamine clots first, heparin was not present. The test can then be made quantitative by adding protamine in increments of 10 mcg from 0 to 50 mcg to a series of test tubes. Multiplying the concentration of protamine in the tube that clots first by the patient's blood volume yields a protamine dose that will neutralize the heparin effect. A potential drawback to this approach in infants and children is that heparin as well as whole blood or plasma is often added to the CPB prime. The addition of whole blood or plasma may actually increase factor activity and thereby impair accurate prediction of heparin effect. The Hepcon Instrument (Medtronic Blood Management, Parker, CO) is a commercially available method that uses protamine titration technology. It correlates well with laboratory-based methods of plasma heparin concentration (anti-Xa assay).

Heparin requires AT III as its substrate. Heparin resistance refers to the clinical situation in which standard heparin doses fail to produce an effect on the ACT. While low levels of AT III seem intuitively obvious as the explanation, other factors appear to play a role. These factors include ongoing active coagulation, previous heparin therapy, and drug interaction. The prospective identification of patients with heparin resistance is vital so that thrombin generation can be sufficiently suppressed during CPB. The heparin response test (HRT, International Technidyne Inc.) and the heparin dose-response test (HDR, Medtronic Blood Management, Parker, CO) are commercially available devices that aid in the detection of heparin resistance due to decreased levels of AT III. Regardless of the etiology, treatment of heparin resistance requires fresh frozen plasma (FFP). FFP contains AT III and provides the missing substrate for heparin effect.

Heparin Neutralization

Protamine is used to neutralize heparin and restore clotting activity after CPB. Analogous to the situation with heparin dosing, the dosing of protamine is often empiric. Usually 1 to 1.3 mg of protamine is administered for each 100 U of heparin given during bypass. Alternately, protamine dosage may be based on weight or on protamine titration. Protamine dosing based on heparin dose or weight typically results in an intentional protamine excess. This surfeit of protamine is felt to minimize the possibility of residual heparin causing postoperative hemorrhage. However, protamine excess can cause bleeding after CPB. Historically, it was felt that there was a wide margin of safety for protamine; doses necessary to achieve clinically significant anticoagulation were felt to be two to four times higher than doses necessary to restore normal coagulation. Recent data in adult patients have called this belief into question. Heparin neutralization that utilized doses of protamine derived from in vitro protamine titration testing resulted in lower doses of protamine and significantly reduced postoperative blood loss and transfusion requirements when compared to empiric dosing of protamine.[21] Empiric protamine dosing in children similarly results in a relative excess of protamine. Whether appropriate protamine dosing decreases blood loss and transfusion requirements in pediatric cardiovascular patients awaits further study.

Protamine dose requirements are higher in neonates younger than 1 month old compared to older infants and children. This is presumably due to the fact that heparin effect is more pronounced in neonates because of their reduced metabolic capability and their exposure to hypothermia.

Protamine frequently produces systemic hypotension in adults. Hypotension after protamine in infants and children does occur but appears to be less of a problem. It is unclear why pediatric patients are spared many of the complications of protamine therapy. When hypotension occurs it is transient and felt to be due to histamine release. Injecting the drug over 5 to 10 minutes and adequate volume replacement usually avert the fall in blood pressure in patients with a marginal cardiac output. More worrisome are anaphylactic or anaphylactoid reactions to protamine. These reactions can manifest as cutaneous flushing or protracted systemic hypotension associated with noncardiogenic pulmonary edema. A more ominous event, catastrophic pulmonary vasoconstriction (CPVC), has been reported to occur in adults at rates anywhere from 0.2% to 4% following protamine administration. CPVC reactions appear to be complement-mediated. Previous sensitization to protamine may play a role, and populations deemed by some experts to be at risk include insulin-dependent diabetics who receive protamine-containing insulin preparations and patients with cross-reacting antigens such as those with fish allergies and vasectomized men. Whatever the mechanism of these adverse reactions to protamine, infants and children appear to be spared.[16]

When quantitative protamine titration is not used to guide heparin neutralization, the end point for protamine administration is an ACT value within 10% of the baseline value obtained prior to heparinization. There are further limitations of titrating protamine effect to the ACT: thrombocytopenia, hypothermia, and hemodilution—a triumvirate frequently present after CPB—all adversely affect the ACT. Bleeding after heparin reversal is a common and difficult problem in neonates and infants.

DIAGNOSIS AND MANAGEMENT OF BLEEDING AFTER CARDIOPULMONARY BYPASS IN INFANTS AND CHILDREN

CPB alters the coagulation system through factor and platelet hemodilution and platelet dysfunction due to activation and hypothermia. These qualitative and quantitative abnormalities are greatly exaggerated in infants compared to adults. At the conclusion of CPB, infants and neonates manifest a multifactorial coagulation defect with relatively severe reductions in factor activity and platelet number and function.

Continued blood loss following heparin neutralization responds to transfusion of either platelets or coagulation factors. If fresh whole blood is not available, coagulation factors are replenished with fresh frozen plasma or cryoprecipitate. Typically, volumes of 20 mL/kg of platelets, cryoprecipitate, or fresh frozen plasma are used initially, followed by repeat dosing if bleeding persists. Some centers use thromboelastography to guide therapy.[38] Disseminated intravascular coagulopathy (DIC) screens are almost always abnormal after cardiopulmonary bypass. There is little justification for administering factors in order to correct an abnormal DIC screen in the absence of clinically significant bleeding. In addition, the time necessary to obtain DIC screen results is often prolonged. Bleeding has usually subsided or the patient has returned to the operating room for emergent reexploration to establish vascular integrity by the time DIC screen results appear.

The incidence of excessive bleeding after surgical repair of congenital heart defects is approximately 5% to 10%. Blood loss in excess of 10% of the child's circulating blood volume in any hour, or blood loss greater than 5% of the patient's blood volume per hour for more than three consecutive hours, often mandates surgical reexploration. However, differentiation between medical and surgical bleeding can be difficult. Although cyanotic, polycythemic children have the highest incidence of coagulation abnormalities on preoperative screening tests of coagulation, it is impossible to prospectively identify a population at risk for postoperative hemorrhage. In cyanotic patients who are polycythemic, preoperative phlebotomy can improve hemostasis.[43] Isovolumetric exchange with crystalloid or colloid that results in an hematocrit reduction to just below 65% has been suggested by some authors.[29] However, polycythemic children are seen with decreasing frequency in the current era of congenital heart surgery. The profile of the patient with congenital heart disease has changed. Advances in anesthetic and surgical techniques have resulted in a shift from palliative procedures to total correction in the neonatal period.[5] Palliation frequently resulted in a progressive diminution of pulmonary blood flow, which led to polycythemia, cyanosis, and coagulation abnormalities. Early total correction avoids hypoxia and the hemostatic alterations due to polycythemia and cyanosis. In place of these alterations are substituted the new hemostatic

Table 14-2 Comparison of Blood Loss in Three Groups of Children Receiving Either Very Fresh Whole Blood, Fresh Whole Blood, or Reconstituted Whole Blood

	Group I vFWB	Group II 24–48 Hrs Old	Group III Reconstituted Whole Blood
No. of subjects	52	57	52
Female	20	25	16
Male	32	32	36
Ages			
Mean ± SE (yr)	2.8 ± 0.4	3.9 ± 0.6	3.8 ± 0.8*
Range	(0–8.2)	(0–19)	(0–20)
No. <2 yr	27	30	36
No. >2 yr	25	27	16
Surgical difficulty			
Simple (no. of subjects)	11	16	9
Intermediate	12	12	12
Complex	29	29	31
Mean time ± SE on bypass (min)	86.8 ± 6.2	86.1 ± 5.8	84.2 ± 5.1†
Mean time ± SE of circulatory arrest	38.1 ± 4.3	43.6 ± 4.6	37.2 ± 3.7‡
Mean volume blood given (cm³/kg) in 24 hr	72.3 ± 9.9	75.5 ± 7.8	97.4 ± 9.6§
No. of subjects with circulatory arrest	41	42	39

*$P = 0.37$
†$P = 0.94$
‡$P = 0.51$
§$P = 0.11$

vFWB, Von Willebrand factor; SE, standard error.
From Manno CS, Hedberg KW, Kim HC, et al: Comparison of the hemostatic effects of fresh whole blood, stored whole blood, and components after open heart surgery in children, *Blood* 77:930–936, 1991; with permission.

challenges of the neonate and young infant undergoing extensive surgical repairs using cardiopulmonary bypass, hypothermia and total circulatory arrest.

The approach to hemostasis in this population should therefore reflect this multifactorial coagulation deficit. Manno and colleagues[27] have shown that the administration of fresh whole blood (less than 48 hours old) after CPB is associated with significantly less bleeding compared to component therapy (Table 14-2). The group treated with whole blood demonstrated improved platelet function as well. The additional advantage of whole blood is that it minimizes donor exposure when compared to component therapy.

Component therapy is frequently necessary when whole blood is not available. Component therapy begins with platelets, since qualitative and quantitative platelet dysfunction is a hallmark of post-CPB bleeding. Although prospective studies in adult patients utilizing random platelet transfusion after termination of CPB have failed to demonstrate any benefit,[36] platelet transfusion is warranted in the setting of thrombocytopenia and prolongation of the bleeding time with clinically significant bleeding.

Cryoprecipitate or fresh frozen plasma (FFP) is given to replenish factor deficiencies. Cryoprecipitate is preferred to FFP in some centers because it is rich in fibrinogen, and a smaller volume of cryoprecipitate is required to replenish the low fibrinogen levels seen in infants and neonates after CPB. Cryoprecipitate is often provided in 100-mL bags, which are often referred to as "units." In clinical practice, one bag per 10 kg of body weight is given after termination of cardiopulmonary bypass and protamine neutralization of heparin if medical bleeding due to hypofibrinogenemia is suspected.

The red cell mass is supported with packed red cells or washed autologous cells from the cell saver. There are no data on the optimal hematocrit after weaning from CPB.

Decisions regarding hematocrit level are individualized based on the patient's post-repair function and anatomy to optimize oxygen delivery. Children who have lesions that have been palliated or who have moderate to severe myocardial dysfunction benefit from the improved oxygen carrying capacity provided by hematocrit levels of 40%. Children with mild to moderate myocardial dysfunction tolerate hematocrit values of 30% to 35%. Hematocrit levels of 25% are usually acceptable in patients with a physiologic correction and excellent myocardial function.

BLOOD CONSERVATION DURING CONGENITAL HEART SURGERY

Current pediatric cardiac anesthetic practice should include the practice of blood conservation. An awareness of the need for blood conservation and the application of autotransfusion techniques make it possible to perform open heart surgery without blood components, even in small children. Because the transfusion of blood products is associated with numerous complications (hemolytic and febrile reactions, bacterial infection, and disease transmission, i.e., viral hepatitis, cytomegalovirus, human immunodeficiency virus, and other viruses), transfusion is to be assiduously avoided unless absolutely necessary. The decline in the quantity and quality of donor blood products has created tremendous supply difficulties for blood banks. Therefore, perioperative blood conservation should be routinely used by all members of the cardiac surgical team.

Techniques of blood conservation begin in the preoperative period. Blood conservation can be accomplished in two ways: (1) maximizing preoperative hemoglobin and hematocrit levels by nutritional support of patients, and (2) preoperatively storing the patient's own blood, to be used for later transfusion. The latter technique requires the collection of autologous blood 7–28 days before cardiac surgery and is usually limited to older children and adolescents. The most crucial measures of conserving blood occur intraoperatively. First, removal of autologous blood before CPB not only enhances blood flow during hypothermic conditions but, more importantly, decreases the number of red cells lost during surgery. Next, a surgical technique that pays meticulous attention to hemostasis during surgery will result in decreased blood loss. Another important intraoperative blood conservation technique is the use of autologous autotransfusion devices during cardiac surgery. "Cell savers" (Cell Saver—Haemonetics, Braintree, MA; BRAT-Kardiothor, Arvada, CO) for collecting, centrifuging, washing, and returning red blood cells to the patient are very effective. These blood-scavenging devices help to process red blood cells that remain in the oxygenator at the conclusion of bypass. These cell-saving techniques can yield 0.5 to 2 units of packed red blood cells per patient. Another blood-conserving technique is hemofiltration, which is used in the bypass circuit and has the ability to remove excess fluid from the circulation near or following the termination of CPB.

PHARMACOLOGIC METHODS TO REDUCE BLEEDING

There is a growing body of literature on the use of pharmacologic agents to reduce bleeding and restore hemostasis after congenital heart surgery. Since platelet activation appears to be the predominant hemostatic derangement associated with CPB, the pharmacologic prevention of activation with synthetic prostaglandins has been proposed as one strategy to decrease blood loss. In animal studies, PGI_2 decreases blood loss and prevents platelet activation.[10] In humans, there is no conclusive evidence for benefit with this approach.[13] A problem associated with prostaglandin administration is side effects: this class of drugs are potent vasodilators, and life-threatening hypotension frequently accompanies their use.

Desmopressin acetate, a synthetic vasopressin analogue whose mechanism of action, while not well understood, appears to involve VIII:vWF, has not demonstrated any benefit in decreasing blood loss during pediatric cardiovascular surgery.[35] The authors do not recommend its use in children with congenital heart disease.

In children undergoing CPB, inhibition of fibrinolysis with EACA has been shown to produce a significant reduction in blood loss compared to placebo treated controls.[44] The dose of already defined EACA is 100 to 150 mg/kg load followed by an infusion of 15 to 30 mg/kg per hour. The use of tranexamic acid (100 mg/kg bolus followed by infusion of 10 mg/kg per hour), another antifibrinolytic agent, has also significantly decreased blood loss compared to placebo treated control patients.[32]

Aprotinin is a serine protease inhibitor that binds to and inactivates the various enzymes involved in coagulation. Aprotinin has been shown to dramatically reduce blood loss in adult cardiovascular surgery.[12] In children, some groups report decreases in blood loss,[34] while others have not

demonstrated this benefit.[15] Studies where blood losses were not significantly reduced demonstrated other benefits such as the reduction in time necessary for chest closure in aprotinin treated children compared to control patients. Aprotinin also appears to attenuate CPB-induced hemostatic activation: it decreases fibrinolytic activity by reducing the formation of fibrin degradation products (Fig. 14-4). It may also decrease the inflammatory response to cardiopulmonary bypass. The loading dose of aprotinin is 30,000 kIU/kg administered over 20 to 30 minutes followed by a continuous infusion of 7000 kIU/kg per hour. An additional 30,000 kIU/kg is added to the CPB pump prime.[25]

The exact mechanism of aprotinin is not well understood. It appears to inhibit platelets, activated coagulation factors in the intrinsic pathway, and the fibrinolytic system. Side effects of aprotinin include allergic and anaphylactic reactions. Aprotinin is a heterologous protein, and prior sensitization may induce antigen-antibody–mediated responses. The incidence of these reactions is low; however, with more widespread use of aprotinin the incidence may increase. The indications for aprotinin use in pediatric cardiovascular surgery are evolving, but it appears to be of benefit in reducing postoperative blood loss.

Surgical causes of bleeding must always be considered, especially in complex repairs with lengthy suture lines such as the arterial switch operation for transposition of the great arteries. If bleeding through the chest tube exceeds 10 mL/kg in the first postoperative hour, and 5 mL/kg per hour thereafter, or if blood loss is greater than 10% of the circulating blood volume per hour despite adequate heparin neutralization and correction of hemostatic defects with the appropriate blood products, emergent surgical re-exploration may be indicated.

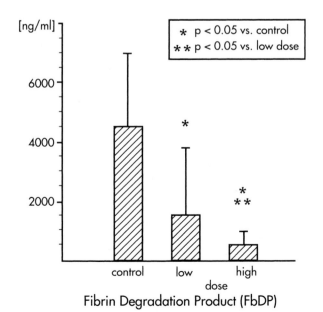

FIGURE 14-4 The influence of aprotinin on fibrinolytic activity expressed as concentration of fibrin-degradation products. (From Dietrich W, Spannagl M, Jochum M, et al: Influence of high-dose aprotinin treatment on blood loss and coagulation patterns in patients undergoing myocardial revascularization. *Anesthesiology* 73:1119–1126, 1990.)

SUMMARY

Postoperative bleeding continues to be a problem, despite two generations of progress in pediatric surgery, anesthesiology, and hematology. In this era of transfusion-acquired disease, cardiac surgery constitutes a major recipient of blood bank services. This chapter has addressed normal coagulation from a developmental perspective, highlighted pre-existing coagulation abnormalities in CHD, examined the relationship of those abnormalities to the hematologic derangement of cardiopulmonary bypass, and explored strategies for blood conservation during pediatric open-heart surgery. Newborn infant heart surgery has created a novel set of hematologic considerations that will provide new challenges and opportunities for future clinical investigation.

References

1. Andrew M, Paes B, Milner R, et al: Development of the human coagulation system in the full-term infant. *Blood* 70:165–172, 1987.
2. Arciniegas E: *Pediatric Cardiac Surgery.* Chicago, Year Book Publishing, 1985, p 51.
3. Bahnson HT, Ziegler RF: A consideration of the causes of death following operation for congenital heart disease of the cyanotic type. *Surg Gynecol Obstet* 90:68, 1950.
4. Barrowcliffe TW, Johnson EA, Thomas D: Antithrombin III and heparin. *Br Med Bull* 34:143–150, 1978.
5. Benson DW, Jr: Changing profile of congenital heart disease. *Pediatrics* 83:790–791, 1989.
6. Bick RL: Hemostasis defects associated with cardiac surgery, prosthetic devices, and other extracorporeal circuits. *Semin Thromb Hemost* 11:249–280, 1985.
7. Brodsky I, Gill DN, Lusch CJ: Fibrinolysis in congenital heart disease. Preoperative treatment with epsilon-aminocaproic acid. *Am J Clin Pathol* 51:51–57, 1969.
8. Campbell FW: The contribution of platelet dysfunction to postbypass bleeding. *J Cardiothorac Vasc Anesth* 5:8–12, 1991.
9. Colon-Otero G, Gilchrist GS, Holcomb GR, et al: Preoperative evaluation of hemostasis in patients with congenital heart disease. *Mayo Clin Proc* 62:379–385, 1987.
10. Coppe D, Sobel M, Seamans L, et al: Preservation of platelet function and number by prostacyclin during cardiopulmonary bypass. *J Thorac Cardiovasc Surg* 81:274–278, 1981.
11. Dietrich W, Mossinger HJ, Richter JA: Treatment of bleeding following CPB in neonates and infants. *Cardiology in the Young* 3:257–262, 1993.
12. Dietrich W, Spannagl M, Jochum M, et al: Influence of high-dose aprotinin treatment on blood loss and coagulation patterns in patients undergoing myocardial revascularization. *Anesthesiology* 73:1119–1126, 1990.
13. DiSesa VJ, Huval W, Lelcuk S, et al: Disadvantages of prostacyclin infusion during cardiopulmonary bypass: a double-blind study of 50 patients having coronary revascularization. *Ann Thorac Surg* 38:514–519, 1984.
14. Ekert H, Gilchrist GS, Stanton R, Hammond D: Hemostasis in cyanotic congenital heart disease. *J Pediatr* 76:221–230, 1970.
15. Elliot MJ, Allen A: Aprotinin in paediatric cardiac surgery. *Perfusion* 5(suppl):73–76, 1990.
16. Ellison N, Jobes DR: *Effective Hemostasis in Cardiac Surgery.* Philadelphia, W.B. Saunders, 1988.
17. Gill JC, Wilson AD, Endres-Brooks J, Montgomery RR: Loss of the largest von Willebrand factor multimers from the plasma of patients with congenital cardiac defects. *Blood* 67:758–761, 1986.
18. Greeley WJ, Bushman GA, Kong DL, et al: Effects of cardiopulmonary bypass on eicosanoid metabolism during pediatric cardiovascular surgery. *J Thorac Cardiovasc Surg* 95:842–849, 1988.
19. Harker LA, Malpass TW, Branson HE, et al: Mechanism of abnormal bleeding in patients undergoing cardiopulmonary bypass: acquired transient platelet dysfunction associated with selective alpha-granule release. *Blood* 56:824–834, 1980.
20. Hartmann RC: A hemorrhagic disorder occurring in patients with cyanotic congenital heart disease. *Bull Johns Hopkins Hosp* 91:49–67, 1952.
21. Jobes DR, Shaffer GW, Aitken GG: Heparin/protamine dosing guided by in vitro testing reduces blood loss and transfusion in cardiac surgery. *Anesthesiology* 77(3A):A137, 1992.
22. Jobes DR: Hemostasis, anticoagulation, reversal, and hemotherapy—How it differs between infant and adult cardiac surgical patients. *Soc Cardiovasc Anes 13th Annual Meeting Workshops* 85–92, 1992.
23. Kern FH, Morana NJ, Sears JJ, Hickey PR: Coagulation defects in neonates during cardiopulmonary bypass. *Ann Thorac Surg* 54:541–546, 1992.
24. Mahoney DH, Jr, McClain KL, Dreyer ZOE: Hematologic issues of importance for the pediatric cardiologist. In Garson A, Bricker JT, McNamara DJ (eds): *The Science and Practice of Pediatric Cardiology.* Philadelphia, Lea & Febiger, 1990, pp 2328–2349.
25. Malviya S: Monitoring and management of anticoagulation in children requiring extracorporeal circulation. *Semin Thromb Hemost* 23: 563–567, 1997.
26. Mammen EF, Koets MH, Washington BC, et al: Hemostasis changes during cardiopulmonary bypass surgery. *Semin Thromb Hemost* 11:281–292, 1985.
27. Manno CS, Hedberg KW, Kim HC, et al: Comparison of the hemostatic effects of fresh whole blood, stored whole blood, and components after open heart surgery in children. *Blood* 77:930–936, 1991.
28. Maurer HM, McCue CM, Robertson LW, Haggins JC: Correction of platelet dysfunction and bleeding in cyanotic congenital heart disease by simple red cell volume reduction. *Am J Cardiol* 35:831–835, 1975.
29. Perloff JK, Rosove MH, Child JS, Wright GB: Adults with cyanotic congenital heart disease: hematologic management. *Ann Intern Med* 109:406–413, 1988.
30. Peters M, ten Cate JW, Jansen E, Breederveld C: Coagulation and fibrinolytic factors in the first week of life in healthy infants. *J Pediatr* 106:292–295, 1985.
31. Peters M, ten Cate JW, Koo LH, Breederveld C: Persistent antithrombin III deficiency: risk factor for thromboembolic complications in neonates small for gestational age. *J Pediatr* 105:310–314, 1984.
32. Reid RW, Zimmerman AA, Laussen PC, et al: The efficacy of tranexamic acid versus placebo in decreasing blood loss in pediatric patients undergoing repeat cardiac surgery. *Anesth Analg* 84:990–996,1997.
33. Rosove MH, Hocking WG, Harwig SS, Perloff JK: Studies of beta-thromboglobulin, platelet factor 4, and fibrinopeptide A in erythrocytosis due to cyanotic congenital heart disease. *Thromb Res* 29:225–235, 1983.
34. Royston D: High-dose aprotinin therapy: a review of the first five years' experience. *J Cardiothorac Vasc Anesth* 6:76–100, 1992.
35. Seear MD, Wadsworth LD, Rogers PC, et al: The effect of desmopressin acetate (DDAVP) on postoperative blood loss after cardiac operations in children. *J Thorac Cardiovasc Surg* 98:217–219, 1989.
36. Simon TL, Akl BF, Murphy W: Controlled trial of routine administration of platelet concentrates in cardiopulmonary bypass surgery. *Ann Thorac Surg* 37:359–364, 1984.
37. Spiess BD: The contribution of fibrinolysis to postbypass bleeding. *J Cardiothorac Vasc Anesth* 5:13–17, 1991.
38. Spiess BD: Thromboelastography and cardiopulmonary bypass. *Semin Thromb Hemost* 21:24–33, 1995.
39. Stibbe J, Kluft C, Brommer EJ, et al: Enhanced fibrinolytic activity during cardiopulmonary bypass in open-heart surgery in man is caused by extrinsic (tissue-type) plasminogen activator. *Eur J Clin Invest* 14:375–382, 1984.
40. Streif W, Andrew M, Marzinotto V, et al: Analysis of warfarin therapy in pediatric patients: A prospective cohort study of 319 patients. *Blood* 94:3007–3014, 1999.
41. Suarez CR, Menendez CE, Griffin AJ, et al: Cyanotic congenital heart disease in children: hemostatic disorders and relevance of molecular markers of hemostasis. *Semin Thromb Hemost* 10:285–289, 1984.
42. Wedemeyer AL, Edson JR, Krivit W: Coagulation in cyanotic congenital heart disease. *Am J Dis Child* 124:656–660, 1972.
43. Wedemeyer AL, Lewis JH: Improvement in hemostasis following phlebotomy in cyanotic patients with heart disease. *J Pediatr* 83:46–50, 1973.
44. Williams GD, Bratton SL, Riley EC, Ramamoorthy C: Efficacy of epsilon-aminocaproic acid in children undergoing cardiac surgery. *J Cardiothorac Vasc Anesth* 13:304–308, 1999.
45. Woodman RC, Harker LA: Bleeding complications associated with cardiopulmonary bypass. *Blood* 76:1680–1697, 1990.

Chapter 15

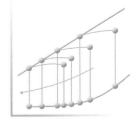

Nutrition and Metabolism in the Critically Ill Child with Cardiac Disease

AARON L. ZUCKERBERG, MD, and MAUREEN A. LEFTON-GREIF, PhD

INTRODUCTION

Nutrition is a vital consideration in children with critical heart disease for four reasons: (1) nutritional deficiency may cause heart disease; (2) congenital heart disease, particularly if associated with heart failure, may cause malnutrition, which can delay or complicate corrective surgery[147,180]; (3) although usually well tolerated, in some instances congenital heart surgery may be associated with complications

379

that lead to life-threatening metabolic and nutritional derangements; and (4) attenuation of the stress response and optimization of the metabolic and nutritional status of a child with congenital heart disease may improve outcome in the immediate postoperative period.

PROTEIN-ENERGY MALNUTRITION

Protein-energy malnutrition (PEM) is the inappropriate loss of body cell mass secondary to reduced intake or inadequate utilization of substrate. Children, especially neonates, are particularly prone to develop PEM since they have minimal metabolic reserve to combat illness. Either reduced intake or inadequate absorption may lead to caloric deprivation, which is variously labeled as *starvation, wasting,* or *marasmus.* Conversely, a hypermetabolic inflammatory process may trigger inadequate utilization of protein substrate while nonprotein caloric intake remains relatively unaffected, which is called *hypermetabolism* or *kwashiorkor.* The prevalence of PEM in hospitalized children in the United States approaches that in the underdeveloped countries, ranging from 36% to 54%.[152] The distinction between starvation and hypermetabolism is important and will affect the choice of nutritional therapy, to prevent the detrimental complications of under- or overfeeding.[110] Since PEM contributes greatly to morbidity in heart disease, it is important to understand this entity.

NUTRITIONAL DEFICIENCY AS A CAUSE OF HEART DISEASE

Starvation (Macronutrient Deficiency)

Starvation is the acute or chronic cessation of macronutrient intake without direct injury. The body responds by decreasing energy expenditure, conserving endogenous energy sources, and providing substrate to tissues (especially the central nervous system) to preserve essential function.

Cardiac Signs in Starvation

Starving children develop cardiac dysfunction. These children have low systolic blood pressures, narrow pulse pressures, and poor peripheral pulses. The cardiac silhouette is often reduced on chest radiographs. The electrocardiogram (ECG) exhibits low voltage and a shortened P-R interval. Sinus pauses occur much more frequently, especially during sleep.[72] Circulatory collapse and cardiac failure appear to be directly related to the child's weight deficit.[222] The cardiac consequences of starvation are often accentuated by vitamin and mineral deficiencies (see later, "Nutritional Syndromes in Children with Critical Heart Disease").

Metabolic Adaptations in Starvation

Because glucose is the principal energy substrate in the body and vital for the central nervous system and red blood cells, the body adapts to preserve glucose homeostasis during starvation (Fig. 15-1). Glucose is stored as glycogen in liver and muscle, but only hepatic glycogen is available for transport.

Hepatic glycogenolysis provides the first defense for glucose homeostasis during starvation. However, the hepatic glycogen supply is depleted after 24 hours in adults and sooner in infants. Thereafter, serum glucose concentration will fall, resulting in a release of the counterregulatory hormones epinephrine, cortisol, and glucagon. By stimulating proteolysis in muscle, these counterregulatory hormones provide amino acids for hepatic and renal gluconeogenesis. Increased levels of these counterregulatory hormones combined with decreased levels of insulin stimulate lipolysis and accelerate the production of ketone bodies and fatty acids, which serve as alternative fuel sources in the brain, heart, and muscle, thus reducing the need for glucose. After several days the brain adapts to the use of ketones, and the rate of muscle proteolysis declines.

Specific Micronutrient Deficiency Syndromes and Heart Disease

Iron Deficiency

Iron deficiency is a common and potentially life-threatening problem in children with cyanotic congenital heart disease. It is associated with hypercyanotic attacks ("tet spells"), cerebral thromboses, metabolic acidosis, and infection especially in the younger child.[52] The hematopoietic response to chronic hypoxia in the cyanotic patient involves both erythropoiesis and increased hemoglobin production. These adaptations maintain an oxygen delivery similar to that of acyanotic children. As the adequacy of tissue oxygen delivery is dependent on the hemoglobin concentration, and thus indirectly on iron stores, maintenance of iron sufficiency is paramount.

The iron deficient cyanotic patient may exhibit an elevated red cell count ($>6.88 \times 10^{12}$) with relatively normal hemoglobin concentration (<15 g/dL). Another clue to the presence of iron deficiency in this population comes from the fact that the hematocrit is usually greater than three times the hemoglobin level, in contrast to the usual 3:1 ratio in the iron sufficient patient. The third component of the routine blood count that points to iron deficiency in this population is a low mean corpuscular volume (MCV) reflecting the presence of a hypochromic, microcytic anemia. It is important to include inspection of the hematocrit:hemoglobin ratio and the MCV because a significant proportion of cyanotic heart disease patients with iron deficiency may have hemoglobin levels >15 g/dL.[156]

The child with critical heart disease and iron deficiency should receive iron therapy. The supplemental iron administration is usually required for over a month until the hematocrit reaches 55%. Serial hematocrits during this period are essential, because some patients will experience rapid increases in hematocrit after iron therapy and develop polycythemia (hematocrit $>60\%$). Polycythemia increases blood viscosity and also increases the risk of cerebral thromboses.

L-Carnitine Deficiency and Fatty Acid Oxidation Defects

L-Carnitine is an essential cofactor in fatty acid oxidation and energy production for myocardial contraction. This dependence on fatty acid metabolism as a source of energy is especially acute during periods of fasting when the glucose supply

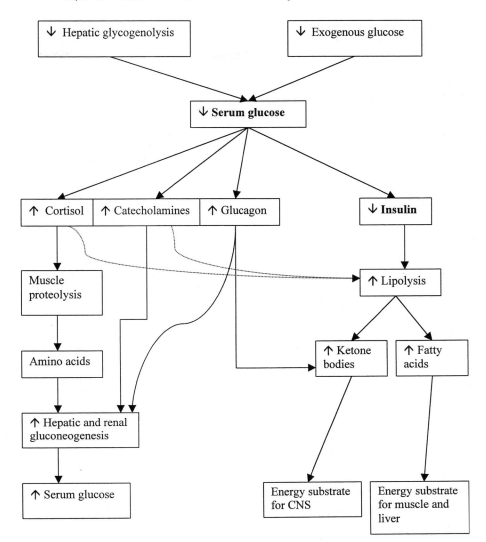

FIGURE 15-1 Metabolic and hormonal adaptation to starvation and hypoglycemia. The increased levels of counterregulatory hormones (cortisol, catecholamines, and glucagon) generate the amino acid substrate for gluconeogenesis by promoting muscle proteolysis. The decreased insulin levels aided by counterregulatory hormones generate ketones bodies and fatty acids as alternative fuels for the central nervous system, muscle, and liver, thus sparing glucose utilization.

is inadequate. For adenosine triphosphate (ATP) to be produced, free fatty acids must be transported from the cytosol across the mitochondrial membrane and into the mitochondrial matrix, where the steps of oxidative metabolism take place. L-carnitine and the enzymes carnitine acyl transferase I and carnitine acyl transferase II shuttle fatty acyl-CoA moieties into the mitochondrial matrix to provide substrate for acyl-CoA production.[189] L-carnitine is a naturally occurring substance found in red meat and dairy products. It is also synthesized in the liver from the amino acid lysine, which is a product of proteolysis in muscle.

Carnitine deficiency can be classified as either primary or secondary. *Primary carnitine deficiency* results from enzymatic defects in carnitine biosynthesis, transport, or metabolism. These autosomal recessive defects result in low plasma and tissue carnitine levels and generally present with varying combinations of cardiomyopathy, skeletal muscle weakness, or encephalopathy. Laboratory examination usually reveals hypoketotic hypoglycemia. The specific carnitine enzyme defects associated with critical heart disease are given in Table 15-1.

Secondary carnitine deficiencies are the result of excessive carnitine losses or inadequate carnitine intake or production. Inadequate carnitine production in the liver may arise in cirrhosis, in malnutrition, or after valproate therapy. Carnitine intake may be deficient with chronic total parenteral nutrition or certain vegetarian diets. Excess carnitine losses may occur with diuresis, diarrhea, or hemodialysis. In these circumstances, peripheral tissues cannot employ fatty acids as energy substrate, and the liver cannot produce ketone bodies as metabolic alternatives. Glucose therefore becomes the primary energy substrate until hepatic glucose production can no longer meet the metabolic demands. Nonketotic hypoglycemia then occurs.[193]

Since the first step in the beta-oxidation of long-chain fatty acids is catalyzed by an acyl-CoA dehydrogenase, many conditions previously classified as "primary" carnitine deficiencies are now known to be defects in the enzymes involved in the *beta-oxidation of fatty acids*. These include very long chain acyl-CoA dehydrogenase (VLCAD) deficiency, long-chain acyl-CoA, long-chain L-3-hydroxyacyl-CoA dehydrogenase (LCHAD) deficiency, or medium-chain acyl-CoA dehydrogenase (MCAD) deficiency, and glutaric acidemia type II. Patients with these enzymopathies typically have low plasma and tissue carnitine levels and an associated cardiomyopathy. The specific diagnosis is made based on the serum acylcarnitine profile and elevated urinary dicarboxylic acids. Table 15-2 lists the specific clinical findings in fatty acid oxidation defects.

Table 15-1 Carnitine Deficiency and Fatty Acid Oxidation Defects Presenting with Critical Heart Disease

Enzyme Defects Associated with Carnitine Deficiency	Features
Carnitine-acylcarnitine translocase deficiency	Life-threatening episodes in the neonatal period Cardiac arrhythmia Generalized weakness Hyperammonemia Variable hypoglycemia
Carnitine palmitoyltransferase II deficiency (hepatocardiomuscular form)	Infants or children Cardiomegaly Cardiac arrhythmia Liver disease Encephalopathy Fasting hypoketotic hypoglycemia Mild myopathy Sudden death
Primary systemic carnitine deficiency (carnitine membrane transporter deficiency) [Defect on chromosome 5q]	Dilated cardiomyopathy ECG: peaked T waves Endomyocardial biopsy: massive lipid storage and low carnitine concentration Poor response to inotropes and diuretics Dramatic response to carnitine supplementation Acute encephalopathy Hypoketotic hypoglycemia Hepatomegaly with liver steatosis Myopathy

Recurrent exacerbations of systemic carnitine deficiency or a fatty acid oxidation defect are heralded by vomiting, diarrhea, and mental status changes associated with nonketotic hypoglycemia, hyperammonemia, elevated liver transaminases, lactic acidosis, and coagulopathy.[70] The cardiac manifestations include right or biventricular hypertrophy and cardiomegaly with decreased contractility. This presentation is reminiscent of Reye syndrome with encephalopathy, shock, and weakness.

Glucose supplementation during periods of stress is the most important therapy for patients with any of the fatty acid oxidation defects. However, patients with these and other defects in the fatty oxidation cycle have been successfully treated with carnitine supplementation. An inverse correlation between survival and plasma carnitine levels has been demonstrated in cardiomyopathic patients.[198] L-carnitine supplementation in these circumstances normalizes mitochondrial

function and myocardial performance.[177] Critically ill children with carnitine deficiencies should receive adequate dietary carnitine supplementation and have their serum glucose levels monitored frequently to avoid potentially catastrophic hypoglycemia.

A *secondary carnitine deficiency* can arise from a variety of clinical situations including inadequate carnitine supply, altered hepatic function, low renal reabsorption, and poor intestinal absorption. Hyperalimentation solutions are carnitine free, and a carnitine deficiency has been documented in infants receiving hyperalimentation. Modest supplementation with 8 to 16 mg/kg/day leads to increased growth, improvement in nitrogen balance with a reduction in the triglyceride concentration, and free fatty acid to ketone body ratios.[93] Patients receiving valproate therapy are at risk for developing secondary carnitine deficiency, presumably through altered hepatic synthesis.[154] Defects in renal reabsorption of carnitine have been proposed in nearly 25% of patients with a secondary carnitine deficiency.[231] Medium-chain triglyceride (MCT) administration may alleviate the cardiac manifestations of secondary carnitine deficiency. MCTs are transported across the mitochondrial membrane independently of carnitine and are mainly oxidized. Consequently, MCTs provide a greater energy substrate than long-chain triglycerides and may minimize the consequences of a secondary carnitine deficiency.

Carnitine supplementation has been successfully utilized in children with cardiomyopathy. Winter[231] identified 51 patients with documented plasma carnitine deficiency of varied etiology, 10 of whom had evidence of a cardiomyopathy on echocardiogram. Children with total plasma carnitine values below 20 micromol/L appeared to be at higher risk than those with low free carnitine levels and elevated esterified carnitine levels. All ten children showed marked clinical and echocardiographic improvement following carnitine therapy. A multicenter retrospective study of L-carnitine supplementation in children with a cardiomyopathy as compared to an unsupplemented control group showed similar results.[94] The classification of cardiomyopathies in the treatment group was 82% dilated cardiomyopathies, 11% hypertrophic cardiomyopathies, and 6% mixed. Despite having poorer clinical functioning at baseline, children treated with L-carnitine at a mean dose of 96 mg/kg/day had one third the mortality, required fewer cardiac transplants, and demonstrated better improvement in clinical function than did the control group. A minority of patients in each group had an inferred metabolic etiology for their cardiomyopathy.[94]

Table 15-2 Clinical and Laboratory Characteristics in Various Fatty Acid Oxidation Defects

Defects	Clinical Findings						Laboratory Findings					
	CM	AR	SD	RM	HM	EC	↓Glu	↓Ket	Met Acid	↓Car	↑LFT	↑NH₃
VLCAD	✓	✓	✓	✓	±✓	✓	✓	✓	✓	✓	✓	✓
MCAD			✓		✓	✓	✓	✓		✓		✓
LCHAD	✓			✓ child	✓						✓	
GA II	✓	✓					✓	✓	✓			✓

CM, cardiomyopathy; AR, arrhythmia; SD, sudden death; RM, rhabdomyolysis; HM, hepatomegaly; EC, encephalopathy (coma, seizures); Glu, glucose; Ket, ketones; Met Acid, metabolic acidosis; Car, carnitine; LFT, liver function tests; NH₃, ammonia; VLCAD, very long-chain acyl-CoA dehydrogenase deficiency; MCAD, medium-chain acyl-CoA dehydrogenase deficiency; LCHAD, long-chain L-3-hydroxyacyl-CoA dehydrogenase deficiency; GA II, glutaric acidemia type II.

Selenium Deficiency

Ten trace elements are considered essential for the human. Infants are at increased risk for developing trace mineral deficiencies.[42,244] Of the trace elements, selenium deficiency is most likely to be associated with cardiac dysfunction.

Selenium is essential as part of the glutathione-peroxidase complex. Glutathione peroxidase together with superoxide dismutase and catalase form the cellular antioxidant defense system against free radicals and other reactive molecules, which cause lipid peroxidation and adverse interactions with intracellular macromolecules.[205] Selenium is important in maintaining muscle and nervous system integrity. Selenium is found in milk, infant formulas, meats, seafoods, cereals, and vegetables. Clinical symptoms associated with selenium deficiency include skeletal myopathy, fingernail bed abnormalities, pseudoalbinism, and red blood cell macrocytosis.[218] Selenium deficiency has been found to coexist with iodine deficiency contributing to hypothyroidism and carnitine deficiency.[171]

The cardiovascular importance of selenium deficiency is exemplified by a selenium responsive endemic cardiomyopathy, Keshan disease, which was first recognized in the selenium-deficient regions of China. It primarily affects young children and women of childbearing age and presents either acutely with cardiogenic shock or chronically as a low output state.

Autoimmune deficiency syndrome (AIDS) patients with selenium deficiency may develop dilated cardiomyopathy.[16,20] Echocardiographic evidence of cardiac disease has been documented in 66% of children with human immunodeficiency virus (HIV) infection.[104] Selenium supplementation in AIDS patients with selenium deficiency and cardiomyopathy results in normalization of left ventricular function after 3 weeks.[242] Selenium supplementation also results in enhanced lymphocyte mitogen response.[44] Overall, HIV children with low selenium levels have a more rapid progression of their disease.[40]

Patients receiving parenteral nutrition have lower blood selenium levels than enterally fed patients. The decreases in selenium appear to occur following 10 to 40 days of parenteral nutrition.[212] Serum levels appear to increase with the introduction of enteral feeds.[125] An infant with cystic fibrosis and diarrhea who developed a cardiomyopathy following institution of total parenteral nutrition has been described. Supportive interventions included the intravenous administration of 100 mcg/day of selenium, which resulted in marked improvement in cardiac function.[219] Supplements of 2 mcg/kg/day for infants and 10 to 20 mcg/day for children or 2 mcg/kg/day for repletion and 1 mcg/kg/day for maintenance have been recommended. Blood levels should be monitored to assure the adequacy and avoid the toxicity of selenium supplementation.[218]

Thiamine Deficiency

Beriberi is caused by a dietary deficiency of thiamine. Thiamine pyrophosphate, vitamin B_1, acts as a cofactor for pyruvate dehydrogenase and other enzymes involved in the pentose and tricarboxylic acid pathways. As a result, there is a reduced ability to metabolize pyruvate and lactate in the Krebs cycle. The vitamin is synthesized by a variety of plants and microorganisms. Thiamine supplementation has virtually eliminated beriberi from the Far East countries where it was historically endemic. In developed nations thiamine deficiency occurs in alcoholics and in selective diets. Childhood beriberi is seen in patients receiving unsupplemented total parenteral nutrition and in infants breast-fed by thiamine-deficient mothers.[27] Thiamine deficiency may occur in critically ill children; 12.5% of children receiving care in a PICU for more than 2 weeks and 18% of children admitted for surgical correction of complex congenital heart defects were thiamine deficient.[178]

There are three forms of beriberi heart disease. Shoshin beriberi is acute fulminant myocardial depression, on the verge of acute cardiovascular collapse. These patients are dyspneic, cyanotic, and display restlessness with an increasing metabolic acidosis. Physical exam reveals severe tachycardia, massive cardiomegaly, jugular venous distention, and hepatomegaly in the absence of peripheral edema. Although thiamine supplementation rapidly restores peripheral vascular resistance, improvement in contractility is often delayed. Thus inotropic support may be necessary during initial vitamin repletion. Acute infantile beriberi presents between the ages of 1 to 4 months in children breast-fed by thiamine-deficient mothers. Pale, irritable, edematous, and often hoarse, trivial infections can precipitate acute, life-threatening Shoshin beriberi in these babies. In the chronic form, wet beriberi, patients appear diaphoretic and edematous with sinus tachycardia, a widened pulse pressure, and a diminished arteriovenous extraction of oxygen. Skeletal muscle blood flow is increased at the expense of cerebral, hepatic, and renal perfusion.[114] The evaluation of a neonate presenting with hypotonia, a congestive cardiomyopathy, and lactic acidosis that was responsive to large supplements of thiamine suggested a defect in cellular incorporation of thiamine.[15]

Vitamin D and Calcium Deficiency

Rickets is a disease marked by deficient mineralization of the bone matrix as a result of deficiencies of calcium, phosphorus, or vitamin D. The associated hypocalcemia has been linked with a reversible cardiomyopathy in infants as well as adults.[35] Children with biochemical rickets often have evidence of cardiac dysfunction. In the most severe rickets cases, the echocardiogram may reveal a hypertrophic cardiomyopathy, as demonstrated by an increase in the ratio of the thicknesses of the intraventricular septum to the left ventricular (LV) posterior wall. These hypertrophic findings normalize following 6 months of vitamin D supplementation.[206]

Hypocalcemia, as a manifestation of hypoparathyroidism, is seen in the 22q11 deletion syndromes, DiGeorge syndrome (DGS), and velocardiofacial syndrome (Shprintzen syndrome). The incidence of this deletion is 1:4000, and it is seen in 8% of children with cleft palate and 25% of children with congenital heart defects. Of children with DGS, 60% to 90% will have hypoparathyroidism. Ten to twenty percent of these will present with hypocalcemia in the first 3 months of life; 10% of these babies will present with hypocalcemic seizures.[78,225]

Refeeding Hypophosphatemia

Children with PEM are at risk for developing refeeding hypophosphatemia. Prior to aggressive nutritional supplementation, these patients have normal serum phosphorus concentrations but their total body phosphorus is depleted. During nutritional intervention, anabolic processes increase cellular uptake of serum phosphate, usually between the second and fifth day.[146] If serum phosphate levels fall below 1 mg/dL, encephalopathy, diaphragmatic failure, dysrhythmias, acute renal failure, or hepatocellular injury may result.[90] Refeeding hypophosphatemia can be prevented by gradually increasing caloric supplementation, although aggressive nutritional support and vigilant phosphate monitoring and replenishment may be just as effective.[237]

HEART DISEASE AS A CAUSE OF MALNUTRITION

Hypermetabolism after Shock or Surgical Stress

Many events can initiate this physiological stress response including surgery, trauma, sepsis, endothelial injury, or respiratory decompensation.[111] The metabolic response to stress is very different than the one to starvation. If there is an initial hypoperfusion state, the metabolic rate decreases. Once perfusion is restored, hypermetabolism develops, which may persist for days to weeks. The hypermetabolic period is divided into catabolic and anabolic phases. However, a prolonged stress response can trigger a sustained and irreversible catabolic state.[48]

Tissue destruction during the catabolic phase causes a release of three general classes of mediators that propagate the stress response (Fig. 15-2). These include afferent and efferent neural pathways, endocrine mediators, and proinflammatory cytokines such as tumor necrosis factor α, IL-1α, IL-1β, and IL-6.[21] High levels of IL-6 and low levels of insulin-like growth factor–(IGF-1) have been associated with hypermetabolism and increased morbidity and mortality in critically ill patients.[209] End-organ effects of these catabolic mediators involve both a global increase in metabolic rate and alterations in the performance of specific organ systems. In response to tissue damage, cells migrate to the injured area in an ordered sequence to debride, control infection, catalyze wound healing, and promote angiogenesis. These cells are all metabolically dependent on glucose.

Organ system function during the stress response reflects an attempt to maximize substrate delivery. Cardiac output increases, peripheral resistance declines, capillaries leak, and new capillary beds open. Ventilation and carbon dioxide

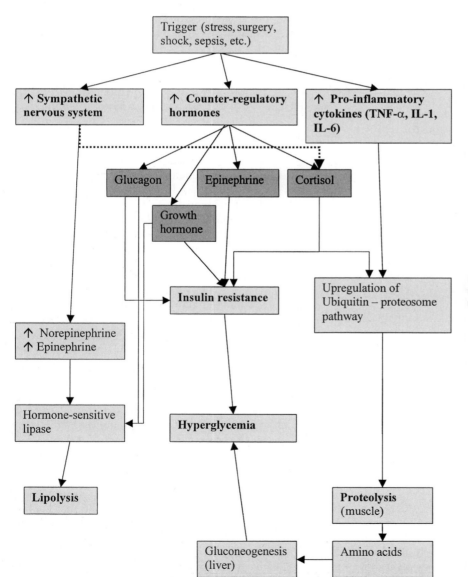

FIGURE 15-2 Metabolic, inflammatory, and neuroendocrine adaptation to stress leading to hypermetabolism.

production increase by as much as 75%. Activation of the renal mechanism leads to fluid and salt retention. Isotopic studies demonstrate fluid transfer from intracellular to extracellular compartments. This, in part, accounts for the loss of body cell mass that is the hallmark of the malnutrition.[151] Hypermetabolism increases hepatic synthesis of acute-phase reactants such as antiproteases and procoagulants and decreases the synthesis of "nonessential" substances such as albumin and other transport proteins. Gluconeogenesis increases with the utilization of substrate from smooth and skeletal muscle. The products of lipolysis provide energy to fuel these processes.

The physiological stress response appears to be under exquisite neuroendocrine axis control.[208] The postoperative increase in serum norepinepherine results from increased secretion from sympathetic nerve terminals. Spinal cord transection or regional anesthesia blocks catecholamine and vasopressin responses to injury.[96,97,201] Analgesia also is important; epidural morphine attenuates the catechol response to aortic reconstructive surgery.[34] Hume and Egdahl demonstrated that limb denervation blocks the injury-induced increase in the excretion of cortisol metabolites.[97] Thus, the nervous system appears to play a key role in mediation of the stress response.

Thyroid stimulating hormone (TSH), T4, T3, cortisol, vasopressin, glucagon, aldosterone, catecholamines, growth hormone, and the renin-angiotensin axis mediate the hypermetabolic response. Epinephrine levels rise transiently following elective surgery, but profoundly in critical illness.[34] Children have a greater early increase in epinephrine levels following trauma than adults. The adrenal cortex is more responsive to adrenocorticotropic hormone (ACTH), and cortisol is increased in most patients.[200] However, a significant minority of critically ill children including cardiac patients have low baseline cortisol levels or relative adrenal insufficiency.[142] If the data from adult studies apply to children, these patients with relative adrenal insufficiency have prolonged vasopressor dependency and higher mortality rates.[8] Vasopressin levels may increase 50-fold following surgery and remain elevated for up to 5 days.[31] Glucagon secretion is proportional to the magnitude of the insult. Glucagon may be undetectable in procedures of small magnitude but is markedly elevated following more extensive surgery or trauma, as is aldosterone.

Cytokines regulate hypermetabolism on a cellular level.[215] In particular, IL-6, tumor necrosis factor-α, and IL-1 have been implicated in the metabolic response to physiological stress.[18] Cytokine expression and effects appear to be under tight neuroendocrine control and are modulated by the hormonal response system as well.[216] An example of these interrelationships is seen in the muscle proteolysis that occurs in acute illness. Glucocorticoids, IL-1β, and corticotropin-releasing hormone–induced IL-6 release are important in the activation of the ATP-dependent ubiquitin-proteosome proteolytic pathway in muscle.[134,190]

Hyperglycemia and relative insulin resistance are important consequences of a stressed metabolism. Hepatic gluconeogenesis is increased and is not inhibited by insulin or glucose infusions. Even though global glucose utilization is increased, serum glucose levels remain elevated, and insulin levels increase. Elevated insulin levels inhibit ketosis, leaving central nervous system (CNS) tissue dependent on glucose. In most tissues, extremely high insulin levels are required to alter glucose uptake reflecting insulin resistance.[233] To achieve euglycemia, critically ill patients require five times the amount of infused insulin as do controls.[234] Hepatocyte glucose oxidation is inhibited, resulting in the conversion of partially oxidized glucose to fatty acids, leading to hepatic steatosis.[144]

Hyperglycemia and insulin resistance are common in critically ill patients.[179] This hyperglycemia has been associated with significant complications in these patients, such as increased susceptibility to serious infections, multisystem organ failure, and polyneuropathy.[138,149] In a study of over 1500 adult intensive care unit (ICU) patients, patients who were randomized to an aggressive insulin regimen targeted to maintain a blood glucose between 80 to 110 mg/dL had a more than 40% reduction in mortality as compared to those who received a conventional insulin regimen targeted to maintain blood glucose between 180 to 200 mg/dL. The aggressive insulin group also had a 43% reduction in septicemia, decreased duration of mechanical ventilation, a lower incidence of acute renal failure, and decreased stay in the ICU.[210]

Lipolysis and proteolysis are proportional to the magnitude of the physiological stress and inversely proportional to the degree of preexisting malnutrition.[5] Insulin inhibits these catabolic processes.[6] Lipolysis is mediated by an adipocyte, hormone-sensitive lipase system, which is responsive to norepinephrine, glucagon, and to a lesser degree, corticosteroids and growth hormone.

Protein breakdown, providing substrate for the synthesis of acute phase proteins and gluconeogenesis, is measured by the excretion of the nitrogenous byproducts and correlates with the change in resting energy expenditure.[100] Proteolysis is altered by catecholamines, cortisol, glucagon, IL-1, and tumor necrosis factor (TNF).[68] Protein turnover in children is increased even in mild stress, where a marked increase in protein breakdown overwhelms the increases in protein synthesis.[196] This imbalance is the result of the catabolic action of steroid hormones and catecholamines and the decreased tissue uptake of amino acids, characteristic of insulin resistance.[38] Protein turnover in critically ill children is markedly higher than that of adults or children with cancer and correlates well with the severity of their illness.[51]

Developmental Differences in the Stress Response to Surgery

The normal infant's metabolic balance is precarious. At a time when he or she has only modest reserves of carbohydrate, fat, and protein, the infant is required to support growth, thermoneutrality, and organ maturation. The infant is therefore poorly equipped to respond to the severe catabolic processes that accompany surgery or critical illness. An individual baby's outcome depends not only on the underlying disease but also on how these potentially life-threatening metabolic processes respond.

In a series of comprehensive investigations, Anand[4,5,6] and his colleagues have demonstrated that neonates mount a complex endocrine and metabolic response to surgery and critical illness. The characteristic features of the neonatal response are a hormonal surge of great magnitude but short duration. Adults undergoing similar degrees of surgical stress respond with significantly lower changes in serum hormone levels, which last up to three times as long.[160] In the immediate postoperative period, blood glucose levels are closely correlated with plasma epinephrine level and postoperative hyperglycemia is common. In contrast to adults, in whom epinephrine levels rise only in the postoperative period, neonatal epinephrine levels rise substantially during surgery. This intraoperative surge in epinephrine stimulates lipolysis, which is reflected in the significant increases in free fatty acids, glycerol, and ketone bodies noted at the end of surgery. Epinephrine not only stimulates hepatic gluconeogenesis and decreases peripheral glucose utilization; it also stimulates glucagon secretion and suppresses insulin release.[203] During the first postoperative days, catecholamine-induced fat oxidation supplies over 75% of energy requirements in children.[79] In the postoperative period, blood glucose levels are closely related to the glucagon response. Therefore, it appears that the perioperative hyperglycemic response is initiated by an epinephrine surge and maintained by glucagon secretion.

The tendency of the endocrine-metabolic interaction to favor a catabolic milieu is intimately related to the unabated stress response and can be estimated by either the insulin/glucose molar ratio or more intuitively, the insulin/glucagon ratio. A reduction in these ratios is indicative of catabolic predominance.[4] This inappropriate insulin response results in unopposed catabolism and perpetuates and exaggerates postoperative hyperglycemia.[4] The insulin/glucagon ratio is lower in babies receiving light anesthesia with unsupplemented nitrous oxide anesthetic and muscle relaxant compared to those receiving deeper anesthesia with halothane for noncardiac surgery. Catabolic predominance was confirmed by the demonstration of higher free fatty acids, ketone bodies, and urinary ratio of 3-methylhistidine to creatinine, indicative of greater degrees of lipolysis and proteolysis, respectively. Infants in the unsupplemented nitrous oxide group had significantly more postoperative complications than those who received halothane. Thus, reduction of the stress response by a more effective anesthetic technique resulted in less catabolism and improved outcome in neonates undergoing surgery.[6]

The perioperative neonatal responses of hyperglycemia, increased epinephrine, glucagon, alanine, and lactate with decreased insulin/glucagon ratio have been confirmed in newborns undergoing cardiac surgery.[4] These responses are substantially greater than those of older infants and adults undergoing cardiopulmonary bypass. The neonates who died in the postoperative period tended to have more exaggerated hormonal and metabolic responses than those who survived.[5]

These dramatic neonatal hormonal and metabolic manifestations of the stress response during cardiac surgery and in the perioperative period can be inhibited by high-dose narcotic administration. Anand and colleagues[5] randomized neonates undergoing cardiac surgery to receive either halothane and morphine followed by intermittent postoperative morphine and diazepam or high-dose sufentanil (mean dose 37 mcg/kg) followed by a 24-hour infusion of either fentanyl (8 to 10 mcg/kg/hour) or sufentanil (2 mcg/kg/hour). They demonstrated that high-dose narcotics significantly decreased these indices of stress and catabolism. Clinical outcome was significantly worse in the halothane group. Specifically, the incidences of early mortality, sepsis, disseminated intravascular coagulopathy, and persistent metabolic acidosis were higher in the halothane group.[5]

It is unclear whether the salutary effects of high-dose narcotic administration are a result of intraoperative or continuous postoperative administration of narcotics during the initial 24 hours. Other investigators have demonstrated that the postoperative stress response can be modulated by the administration of postoperative opioids and vary with the route of administration. The epidural administration of opioids has been shown to decrease cortisol, norepinephrine, and vasopressin responses more than parenteral administration.[89] These data suggest that anesthetic control of the stress response decreases catabolism and improves outcome.

Hypermetabolism in Uncorrected Congenital Heart Disease

Approximately 30% of children with congenital heart disease have increased metabolic rates with increased resting protein-energy needs compared to age matched controls.[148] Presumably, the elevated catecholamine levels increase oxygen consumption significantly. This increase in basal metabolic rate reduces the calories that usually supply growth during infancy and childhood. Even if a normal caloric intake could be assured, this would be insufficient to replenish the deficit. Often a caloric intake of 150% of normal values for age is necessary to support normal growth in this population.

MUTIFACTORIAL NUTRITIONAL SYNDROMES IN CHILDREN WITH CRITICAL HEART DISEASE

Overview

Undernutrition and growth retardation are complications of uncorrected, symptomatic congenital heart disease. The magnitude of growth failure can be astounding. Over 70% of children with cardiac disease are below the 50th percentile for height and weight 50% are below the 16th percentile for height and weight and over 35% are below the 3rd percentile for both height and weight.[147] Prolonged nutritional deficits and growth failure related to congestive heart failure may result in heightened surgical risks.[223] The etiology of undernutrition seen in children with congenital heart disease is multifactorial. Contributing factors include the increased energy expenditure of frequent infections and congestive heart failure, as well as inadequate intake and intestinal malabsorption.[183]

Controversy exists as to whether specific cardiac lesions increase this risk of undernutrition. While some studies indicate that the malnutrition risk is spread uniformly among all types of congenital heart disease,[147] others have pointed to cyanosis,[124] left-to-right shunts,[172] pulmonary hypertension,[214] or congestive heart failure[39] as having the greatest risk for malnutrition. Collectively, these data suggest that the severity of the hemodynamic compromise is an important indirect determinant of growth since it affects food intake, intestinal function, energy expenditure, and the development of hypermetabolism.[148]

Insulin and Glucose Homeostasis in Congenital Heart Disease

In children with congenital heart disease, alterations in insulin secretion and glucose homeostasis appear to be dependent on the nature of the lesion. Children with symptomatic ventricular septal defects have normal fasting glucose levels and glucose tolerance tests but lower insulin levels and surprisingly higher rates of insulin secretion, as demonstrated by higher plasma concentrations of C-peptide.[131] The higher rates of insulin secretion seen in children with congenital heart disease are a consequence of high levels of sympathetic activity, resulting in increased glucose release.[65] Conversely, children with cyanotic heart disease have *lower* fasting glucose levels, normal glucose tolerance, and insulin levels with higher rates of insulin secretion.[132] If the cyanotic infant has inadequate glucose stores, *hypoglycemia* may be the net result of the high insulin secretion rate.[9] Conversely, increases in pulmonary circulation increase *insulin clearance*, which may minimize the risk of hypoglycemia in congenital heart disease.

Growth Hormone (GH) Insensitivity

Children with congenital heart disease and malnutrition may be insensitive to growth hormone, which may partially explain growth failure in this population. Normally, GH affects metabolism in diverse ways. Its effect on protein metabolism is anabolic and leads to positive nitrogen balance. Conversely, GH has catabolic effects on fat metabolism by increasing lipolysis. The resultant increase in free fatty acids accounts for the ketogenic effect of GH. GH has an antiinsulin effect and raises serum glucose levels by increasing hepatic glucose output and decreasing glucose uptake into muscle.

GH promotes growth through its effects on cartilage and protein metabolism, which require the interaction between GH and somatomedins. Insulin growth factors (IGF) 1 and 2 constitute the main somatomedins in humans. As the name implies, these growth factors are structurally related to insulin. GH stimulates local IGF secretion in various tissues including liver, cartilage, and heart. The understanding of the mechanism by which the GH–IGF-1 interaction promotes growth is evolving. Current data suggest that GH converts stem cells into IGF responsive cells. Subsequently, local and circulating IGF stimulate growth. Insulin-like growth factor binding protein-3 (IGFBP-3), also synthesized under GH control, is the most important carrier of circulating IGF-1.[22] The GH:IGF-1:IGFBP-3 axis plays an important role in the preservation of anabolism following stress.[76]

This axis is altered in critical heart disease. Malnourished children with congenital heart disease have elevated levels of circulating GH but markedly decreased levels of IGF-1 and IGFBP-3 suggesting GH insensitivity.[19,199] Children undergoing cardiac surgery for complex congenital heart disease exhibit this GH resistance *preoperatively*. In the initial postoperative week the discrepancy between elevated GH levels and depressed IGF-1 and IGFBP-3 worsens. These GH:IGF-1:IGFBP-3 abnormalities resolve within 6 months after corrective surgery.[199] Thus it appears that critical heart disease, particularly if associated with hypoxemia or congestive heart failure, produces GH insensitivity, which may explain the growth failure in this population.

Heart Failure

Heart failure may result in poor appetite, tachypnea, vomiting, or dysphagia. Others have emphasized the importance of anorexia and early satiety in the development of this malnutritional state.[80] Feeding is often cyclical, varying with the degree of congestive heart failure. When heart failure is mild, the hungry infant overfeeds, resulting in fluid overload and impaired cardiorespiratory function. Increased patient fatigability during oral feeding then limits feeding volumes, resulting in underfeeding, as well as prolonged feeding times.[87] Persistent vomiting, thought to be a manifestation of left-to-right intracardiac shunts, which resolves following surgical correction, may be an additional contributor to inadequate intake. Underweight children with congenital heart disease have inadequate diets compared to their normalweight cohorts. With nutritional counseling, these children demonstrate a 10% weight gain from baseline over a 6-month period.[202]

Intestinal Malabsorption and Nutrient Leakage (Protein-Losing Enteropathy, Chylothorax)

Children with congenital heart disease (CHD) may accrue nutritional deficits through intestinal malabsorption or leakage of nutrients into the intestinal lumen or the pleural space. In some settings the nutrient leakage follows the malabsorption syndrome. Intestinal malabsorption may result from heart failure and is thought to be a form of intestinal lymphangiectasia. As right heart failure increases, lymphatic drainage from the gut is impeded and a functional lymphatic obstruction develops. Consequently, intestinal absorption and digestion of protein and fats are altered. Carbohydrate absorption is generally normal despite abnormal d-xylose absorption in 50% of children with congenital heart disease.[95] Fat malabsorption may occur in some patients with symptomatic congestive heart failure regardless of the underlying cardiac anomaly, but not if the heart failure has been treated effectively with diuretics.[183,207]

Small intestinal absorption of protein can be impaired in children with heart disease, particularly in patients with a single ventricle, who have undergone the Fontan operation. This *protein-losing enteropathy* (PLE) is thought to be due, in part, to increased systemic venous and mesenteric lymphatic pressure resulting in the leakage of protein in the lumen of the gut.[183] However, other factors must also play a role, because some patients develop PLE without elevated systemic venous pressure (see Chapter 5 on *Splanchnic Function* for a full discussion of PLE).

Chylothorax, a well-recognized complication of thoracic procedures, has an incidence of 0.25% to 1.9% after surgery for CHD. These chylothoraces are thought to be the result of intraoperative damage to the thoracic duct and accessory lymphatic channels.[2,117] Systemic venous hypertension can also result in chylothorax formation by impeding lymphatic duct emptying. Chylothorax should be suspected whenever a pleural effusion develops after a thoracic procedure. It is a significant complication, because large chylous effusions result in immune, nutritional, and cardiovascular derangements secondary to the loss of T lymphocytes, chylomicrons, and electrolyte-containing fluid.

If the patient has been receiving enteral nutrition including long-chain fatty acids, chyle has a creamy appearance because it contains chylomicrons and long-chain triglycerides. The diagnosis of a chylothorax is confirmed by the presence of a pleural fluid triglyceride level of >1.2 mmol/L and a total cell number of >1000 cells/μL, consisting predominantly of lymphocytes.[213] However, in the typical postoperative case of chylothorax, the child has been fasting. Therefore, the chylous effusion may appear serosanguinous without an elevated triglyceride content. Although an elevated lymphocyte count in the pleural effusion may suggest the diagnosis of chylothorax, the laboratory analysis is often nondiagnostic. The diagnosis is then made retrospectively after therapy directed at chylothorax results in resolution of the effusion.[2]

The initial management consists of tube thoracostomy for large effusions and a diet devoid of long-chain triglycerides (Fig. 15-3). Either an enteral diet containing medium-chain triglycerides or enteric rest with total parenteral nutrition

(TPN) may accomplish this dietary objective. This approach is successful in a majority of cases. Clinical improvement is defined as a decrease in effusion drainage to <10 mL/kg/day.[24] More than a third of patients receiving fat-free formulas will experience resolution of their chylothoraces within 2 weeks.[36]

Elevated central venous pressures are associated with more refractory chylothoraces.[30,117] These chylothoraces resolve slowly because of the time it takes to reach a sufficiently high intralymphatic pressure to cause lymphatic rupture.[117] Such patients require a careful hemodynamic evaluation to identify the etiology of the systemic venous hypertension. Potential causes in the surgical patient include systemic venous thrombosis, which requires anticoagulation, or pulmonary artery stenosis, which may require stent placement or surgical plasty. Chylothorax associated with postoperative pulmonary hypertension can be treated with a trial of nitric oxide (NO), which decreases right ventricular (RV) afterload and associated tricuspid regurgitation and/or augments forward flow through the pulmonary circulation.[28,137]

Somatostatin and its synthetic analogue, octreotide, have been used successfully to treat chylothorax.[106] By acting directly on splanchnic vascular receptors, octreotide reduces

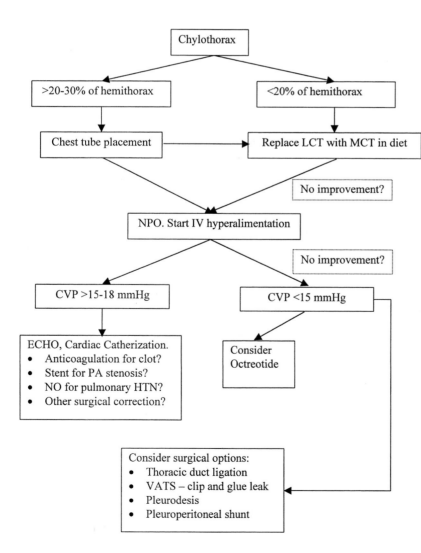

FIGURE 15-3 Management algorithm for persistent chylothorax. LCT, long-chain triglycerides; MCT, medium-chain triglycerides; NO, nitric oxide; HTN, hypertension; PA, pulmonary artery; CVP, central venous pressure; VATS, video-assisted thoracoscopic surgery.

chylomicron synthesis and transport into the lymphatic duct, thus decreasing lymphatic flow rate and limiting triglyceride loss into the pleural fluid.[13,136] Octreotide has been used both as a continuous infusion and in divided subcutaneous doses.[161] It is initiated at 10 mcg/kg/day in three divided subcutaneous doses and increased in a stepwise fashion of 5 to 10 mcg/kg/day every 3 days until chyle output decreases to minimal levels for 3 consecutive days. At this point the octreotide is weaned over the next 3 to 6 days. The dose of octreotide required to achieve total suppression of chylous effusion was reported as 20 to 40 mcg/kg/day.[47]

Patients who fail dietary and medical management of their chylothoraces require surgical interventions. Such surgical techniques include ligation of the thoracic duct, pleurodesis with talc/tetracycline or fibrin glue, video-assisted thoracoscopic surgical (VATS) identification and clipping of the site of duct leakage, or pleuroperitoneal shunting.[30,238] The VATS procedure is preceded by consumption of a meal of cream mixed with Sudan black one hour before the procedure to identify the leak site. In four of six adults with a chylothorax, the site was successfully identified, then sealed with fibrin glue and sutures or clips. The remaining two underwent pleurodesis with fibrin glue. All of these chylothoraces resolved completely by the fifth postoperative day.[73]

In two small series of children with persistent chylothorax, implantation of double valved pleuroperitoneal shunts resulted in successful resolution of their symptoms, without complications.[71,235] These shunts are removed an average of 1 to 2 months post placement. An advantage of a pleuroperitoneal shunt is to minimize the loss of chyle by facilitating its absorption by the peritoneum and allowing the formation of new lymphatic thoracic channels. The use of these shunts is limited by high right atrial pressure (>25 mm Hg) or by IVC obstruction.[24,165]

NUTRITIONAL ASSESSMENT

Anthropometrics

Anthropometric measurements provide the best estimates of muscle and fat content of the body in the clinical setting. In the absence of edema, measuring triceps and subscapular skinfold thickness assesses adipose tissue. Skeletal muscle mass can be estimated by measurements of the arm muscle circumference and is useful in assessing the depletion of lean body mass. Among a cohort of 48 consecutive children admitted for cardiac surgery, triceps skinfold thickness was < 3rd percentile in 12.5% of the cohort, and subscapular skinfold thickness was < 3rd percentile in 18.8%.[147] Mid-arm circumference and arm muscle circumference were <5th percentile in 20.1% and 16.7% of patients, respectively.[147]

The best indicator of growth failure is the change in growth rate over time. Longitudinal growth is preserved during acute short-term nutritional deprivation.[221] Therefore a low weight for height percentile suggests an acute energy imbalance, whereas a low height for age percentile indicates longstanding deficits. Many children presenting with cardiac disease weigh significantly less than normal for age in the face of appropriate height.[202] In the absence of coexisting diseases that affect body stature, the percentile of body weight indexed for length

Table 15-3 Waterlow Stages of Protein-Energy Malnutrition

Stage	WHI*	LLI†	
0	>0.9	>0.9	Normal
1	0.8–0.9	0.9–0.95	At risk
2	0.7–0.79	0.85–0.89	At risk
3	<0.7	0.85	PEM‡

*WHI, weight-height index = actual weight/50th percentile of weight for height.
†LLI, length-length index = actual length/50th percentile of length for age.
‡PEM, protein-energy malnutrition.
From Waterlow JC: Classification and definition of protein-calorie malnutrition. *BMJ* 3:566–569, 1972.

represents an appropriate measure of a child's nutritional state.[192] Waterlow's[221] classification of PEM is useful as a model for grading the degree of undernutrition (Table 15-3).

Biochemical Measurements

Nitrogen balance reflects the equilibrium between protein intake and losses. Stress produces nitrogen losses, driven by the catabolic actions of cortisol and epinephrine. Skeletal muscle breakdown provides substrate for gluconeogenesis and also releases nonessential amino acids that are excreted in the urine as urea. All patients with PEM have a negative nitrogen balance. The magnitude of the negative balance is useful in determining the process leading to the patient's malnourished state. In hypermetabolism, tissue is being catabolized for gluconeogenesis and wound repair. Acute negative nitrogen balance is the rule. Chronic starvation leads to a modestly negative nitrogen balance.[67] Drainage of proteinaceous fluids from other body cavities will further increase nitrogen loss.

Although serum protein concentrations (particularly albumin and transferrin) have been used as biochemical markers of nutritional status, these tests are neither sensitive nor specific. Albumin and transferrin do not discriminate growth-retarded children with congenital heart disease from their normal weight cohorts.[172,202] Because of a uniform water loss as well as cellular mass, isolated starvation changes plasma protein concentration only when depletion is severe. Hypermetabolism is associated with negative nitrogen balance, but hypoalbuminemia requires prolonged hypermetabolism because of the long half-life of albumin (20 days) (Table 15-4). Hypoalbuminemia in the face of a hypermetabolic state is associated with increased risk of death. The shorter half-life proteins such as retinol binding protein and prealbumin correlate better with acute changes in critically ill patients.

Table 15-4 Plasma Proteins Used for Nutritional Assessment and Their Half-Lives

Plasma Protein	$t_{1/2}$
Transferrin	8 d
Albumin	20 d
Prealbumin	2 d
Retinol-binding protein	10 hr

Predictive Methods of Energy Expenditure

An infant's caloric requirement depends on his or her basal metabolic rate, the rate of growth, and activity. In health, the daily caloric requirements decline from 115 kcal/kg at birth to 105 kcal/kg by the first birthday. Over the next 9 years, energy requirements decline to 80 kcal/kg. Following puberty, energy requirements decrease to 45 kcal/kg in teenage boys and 38 kcal/kg in teenage girls. As adipose tissue is not as metabolically active as other tissue, an undernourished infant with little or no subcutaneous fat has a higher than expected level of metabolism relative to body weight. The caloric requirements of recovering undernourished children are also increased because of active reparative anabolic processes. Fever significantly increases total energy requirements. Each degree Celsius elevation in body temperature increases caloric needs by 12%.[66]

The nutritional needs of patients in intensive care rarely conform to tabular norms, because these patients are not in a basal state. Kinney[109] has proposed the term *resting energy expenditure* (REE) for adults when they are supine and quiet or asleep and have not eaten for at least 3 hours. REE is a function of gender, age, height, and weight. However, studies of critically ill children on mechanical ventilation in whom energy expenditures were measured by indirect calorimetry reported wide differences between measured and predicted values, even after injury factors were applied.[83]

In a rigorously performed study of critically ill children, White and colleagues[227] used serial indirect calorimetry data to formulate an equation to predict energy expenditure (EE) from bedside clinical data.

$$\text{EE (kJ/day)} = (17 \times \text{age [in months]}) + (48 \times \text{weight [in kg]}) + (292 \times \text{body temperature } °C) - 9677$$

Compared to standard predictive equations, this equation correlates more closely to measured values, especially in children >2 months of age.[227] The inaccuracy of this equation in younger infants is attributed to the fact that temperature is a less reliable indicator of injury severity and the hypermetabolic component.[49]

NUTRITIONAL MANAGEMENT OF THE CARDIAC SURGICAL PATIENT

The challenges in the nutritional management of the child with critical heart disease include: (1) determining the extent of coexisting undernutrition; (2) defining the metabolic stage of development; (3) estimating the caloric requirements during critical illness; (4) appreciating the extent of exposure to catabolic, hormonal, and immunological risks that can be modulated through nutritional support; and (5) deciding the appropriate method of providing nutritional support during the critical care period.

Preoperative Nutritional Management

A nutritional evaluation should be included for all children with congenital heart disease. In children with severe undernutrition, the timing of a palliative or corrective procedure should be carefully considered. Although total correction of a longstanding nutritional deficit is unrealistic in the short term, provision of an intensive nutritional program including the use of continuous nasogastric feeds for a period of 1 to 2 weeks may restore anabolic balance. For children in whom full enteral feeding is unrealistic, TPN augmented with trophic enteral feeds may achieve many of these same salutary effects.

Nutritional formulae may be used to meet measured or calculated energy expenditure. A simple method for estimating energy requirements for weight maintenance is calculated by the following formula:

$$\text{Energy (kcal/day)} = \text{BMR} \times \text{stress factor} \times 1.25$$

Basal metabolic rate (BMR) may be derived from Table 15-5. A "stress factor" is included because the normal BMR is increased by the stress of cardiac disease. The factors associated with this stress include the manifestations of congestive heart failure such as increased myocardial work, tachypnea, salt and water retention, and ileus. The product of BMR x stress factor approximates REE. While the stress factor varies, the caloric requirements of infants with severe cardiac disease typically exceed those of normal infants by 20% to 30% (stress factor 1.2 to 1.3). The additional factor of 1.25 accounts for the 25% increase in energy requirements associated with activity. Thus, 160% of the BMR is a reasonable *first approximation* of the caloric requirements of the infant with critical heart disease.

Feeding volumes and solute composition will be dictated by heart failure and intestinal malabsorption. The protein and fat requirements for infants and children are outlined in Tables 15-6 and 15-7. With a nitrogen:calorie ratio of 1:150, the 17% calories derived from protein generally meets the recovery and growth requirements of sick infants. Although there is no recommended daily allowance for fat, it is an excellent source of calories and also provides essential fatty acids for growth. Sodium restriction to 2 to 3 mEq/kg/day should avoid exacerbation of congestive heart failure. The osmolality of enteral feeds should be <600 mosm/L to avoid the complications of vomiting, abdominal pain, and diarrhea. Predigested protein (hydrolysates) can double the osmolality of the feed and result in feeding intolerance.

Table 15-5 Mean Heights and Weights and Recommended Energy Intake in Infants and Children

Age	Weight (kg)	Height (cm)	Energy Intake (Kcal) (Range)
Infants			
0–6 mo	6	60	kg × 115 (95–145)
7–12 mo	9	71	kg × 105 (80–135)
Children			
1–3 yr	13	29	1300 (900–1800)
4–6 yr	20	112	1700 (1300–2300)
7–10 yr	28	132	2400 (1650–3300)
Males			
11–14 yr	45	157	2700 (2000–3700)
15–18 yr	66	176	2800 (2100–3900)
Females			
11–14 yr	46	157	2200 (1500–3000)
15–18 yr	55	163	2100 (1200–3000)

Table 15-6 Daily Protein Requirements in Infants and Children

Age	Protein (g)
Infants	
0–6 mo	kg × 2.2
7–12 mo	kg × 2.0
Children	
1–3 yr	23
4–6 yr	30
7–10 yr	34
Males	
11–14 yr	45
15–18 yr	56
Females	
11–14 yr	46
15–18 yr	46

Medium-chain triglycerides (MCTs) are frequently used to supplement the caloric content of enteral feeds. These fatty acids provide a high caloric density, low osmolality additive that can be absorbed and hydrolysed directly by the intestinal mucosa independent of pancreatic lipases, bile acid solubilization, and chylomicron formation. A large proportion of administered MCTs is absorbed directly into the portal circulation, bypassing the lymphatic channels that may be congested in heart failure. MCTs, are totally saturated, are devoid of the essential fatty acids, and can produce a cathartic effect.

Nutritional intervention has led to weight gain in controlled studies.[183] Complex congenital heart disease patients with poor weight gain despite calorically enriched formula feedings demonstrated improved weight gain after the implementation of continuous nasogastric feeds with the same formula supplying 137 kcal/kg/day. One study showed a 198% increase in weight gain, and another showed an average increase in daily gain of 13 g/day.[211] For the child who failed to gain weight with intermittent bolus feeds, continuous vasogastric feeding is associated with less vomiting, better absorption of nutrients, and reduced metabolic demands.[86]

In a randomized study of nutritional intervention in children with congenital heart disease complicated by congestive heart failure, the only modality that resulted in increased weight, height, and skinfold thicknesses was the implementation of 24-hour continuous nasogastric feeds. Children receiving continuous 12-hour nocturnal supplementation plus daytime oral feeds ad libitum did not reach targeted caloric intake as a consequence of decreased daytime ad-libitum feeds. Only a caloric intake approaching 150 kcal/kg/day over a 5-month period was associated with

Table 15-7 Suggested Daily Fat Requirements for Infants and Children with Cardiovascular Disease

Age	Dietary Fat (g/kg)
Infants	4–5
Children	3–4
Adolescents	2–3

significant increases in all growth parameters. A fluid intake of 165 mL/kg/day in the 24-hour continuous infusion group was not associated with worsening congestive heart failure.[176] If prolonged gastric feeding is planned, a program of oral stimulation and nonnutritive sucking is advisable to diminish the risk of food avoidance later.

Postoperative Nutritional Management

Energy Requirements

Nutritional requirements after cardiac surgery vary with age and the nature of the stress response to surgery and cardiopulmonary bypass. Limited data in infants and children following cardiac surgery suggest that their measured energy expenditure is lower than in adults.[50] In fact, Gebara and colleagues[79] showed that the resting energy expenditure (mean of 55 kcal/kg/day) of children after heart surgery is less than the predicted basal metabolic rate for normal children.

The reasons for the lower than predicted energy requirement are many. The BMR of a full-term newborn is the aggregate of the following (in kcal/kg/day): 65 kcal for maintenance metabolism, 30 kcal for growth (tissue synthesis) and energy storage, 15 kcal for physical activity, and 10 kcal for stool-related energy loss. Thermoregulation requires additional energy.[126] The infant subjected to stress responds by first decreasing tissue synthesis. Many of the children are malnourished, causing a similar reduction in growth and overall reduction in their BMR. Postoperatively, children are frequently paralyzed, sedated, mechanically ventilated, and receiving parenteral hyperalimentation in a thermoneutral environment. Of those children not paralyzed and sedated, most postoperative infants are at rest 80% to 90% of the time. Finally, metabolic measurements may not be appropriately timed to reflect the peak metabolism of the stress response.

Anand and his colleagues[5,6] in a series of studies have employed the insulin/glucose and the insulin/glucagon molar ratios to indirectly assess catabolism. The advantages of the insulin/glucose ratio are low cost, convenience, and a decreased volume of blood needed for these measurements. There are no normal values for these ratios in infants and children, and Anand focused on the changes in these ratios with interventions, such as increased anesthetic potency. Review of the data in these studies suggests that an insulin/glucose molar ratio of <16 is suggestive of catabolism, while >16 is suggestive of anabolism; an insulin/glucagon ratio of <3 is suggestive of catabolism, while >3 is suggestive of anabolism. Based on Gebara's data, infants in the immediate postoperative period utilize endogenous fat stores as the principal energy substrate, a manifestation of unopposed lipolysis and catabolism.[79]

NUTRITIONAL SUPPORT TECHNIQUES

Enteral Nutrition

Enteral nutrition is preferable. It is less costly and has fewer complications than parenteral nutrition.[59,159] Early institution of enteral feedings has been associated with lower infection rates and shorter hospital stays, compared to delayed enteral feeds, in a population of surgical ICU patients.[135] Enteral nutrients are necessary for optimal gastrointestinal function. Fasting studies in young animals show that despite maintenance of a positive nitrogen balance, total parenteral nutrition results in atrophy of the pancreas and small bowel mucosa, as well as decreased mucosal height, DNA content, intestinal brush border enzyme activity, and intestinal absorptive capacity.[82] There is an associated increase in bacterial translocation.[82] Refeeding reverses these responses.[228] The mechanisms behind the reparative response to feeding are still unclear but probably include direct intraluminal enterocyte nutrition, decreases in intestinal vascular resistance promoting enhanced intestinal perfusion, as well as the hormonal effects of feeding. Specific intraluminal substances, such as glutamine, may play a very important role in this process.[112]

Hormonal Response to Enteral Nutrition

Anabolic Hormones (Insulin, Enteroglucagon, Gastrin)

Compared with intravenous alimentation, enteral nutrition is associated with the secretion of various intestinal hormones that augment the secretion of insulin. Insulin is an important element in the growth of the infant. Infants receiving hypocaloric enteral feeds have less glucose intolerance than do those receiving total parenteral nutrition. Compared to parenteral alimentation, enteral feeds produce higher levels of gastric inhibitory polypeptide (GIP), insulin, and insulin/glucose ratios.[108] The gastrointestinal tract of the newborn is particularly vulnerable to enteral nutrient deprivation, even with adequate parenteral caloric supplementation. The changes in intestinal permeability and DNA content seen in adult animals following a 4-week fast are reproduced in neonatal rabbits starved for only 72 hours.[182]

The composition and route of feeding have major influences on the level of circulating gastrointestinal hormones and regulatory peptides. Even very small amounts of milk (12 mL/kg over 4 days) induce surges of gut hormones.[129] Maximal responses of enteroglucagon, gastrin, and GIP occur with an average intake of only 0.5 mL/kg/hour. Enteroglucagon is a trophic hormone for the small intestinal mucosa. Gastrin stimulates the growth of the gastric mucosa and exocrine pancreas, accelerates gastric acid secretion, and promotes glucose-induced insulin release.[224] Higher basal concentrations of GIP, insulin, and insulin/glucose ratio are found in infants receiving continuous gastric infusions than in those receiving intermittent bolus feedings.

Intestinal Motility Hormones (Gastrin and Motilin)

Intestinal motility increases after enteral feeding. The gastrointestinal peptides gastrin, neurotensin, and motilin modulate intestinal motor activity. Intragastric feeds result in rapidly increasing plasma levels of gastrin and motilin. Infants maintained solely on parenteral nutrition do not have similar rises in plasma levels. However, the addition of 1 mL/hour of enteral feeds results in substantially increased plasma gastrin.[85] In neonatal rats, the rise in plasma gastrin that results from feeding parallels the feeding-induced trophic changes in the gut mucosa.[122] Similar changes in plasma gastrin are seen during nasojejunal feeds.[85]

Immunologic Benefits of Enteral Nutrition

Nutrition and immune function are crosslinked at the intestinal mucosal surface. A healthy, well-maintained mucosal surface prevents bacterial translocation. Immunoglobin A (IgA) secretion provides a very specific mucosal defense system, and the regional lymphoid tissue provides the secondary defense to collect and destroy any bacteria that successfully complete a transepithelial migration. Factors that weaken this multifaceted defense include physical disruption of the mucosal barrier, alteration of the local microflora, and impaired immune defenses.[174] Interferon γ, especially under acidic conditions, and IL-4 increase intestinal epithelial permeability.[204] Clinically, shock with reduced splanchnic blood flow, parenteral nutrition, intestinal epithelial damage, and antibiotic therapy predispose the critically ill to bacterial translocation.

The endogenous microflora, unique in each section of the intestine, plays a critical role in preventing colonization with exogenous pathogenic organisms. Usually the stomach and the proximal small intestine are sterile; large populations of gram-negative organisms safely reside in the colon.[181] Antibiotic therapy and parenteral nutrition are well recognized to disrupt this normal flora. Critical illness is often associated with proximal gut overgrowth of enteric gram-negative organisms commonly found in the distal ileum. It is these organisms that are frequently responsible for nosocomial infections.[69] Gastric colonization with multiple organisms is associated with bacterial translocation and with a significant increase in postoperative complications.[133] A study in neonates found that parenteral nutrition was an independent risk factor for the development of enterobacter septicemia.[77] Nasal instrumentation alone contributes to the alteration of flora seen in critically ill children. Approximately 25% of children requiring nasotracheal intubation for greater than 5 days develop a nosocomial sinusitis. The usual pathogens in this situation are the gram-negative enteric organisms.[145,220]

The institution of enteral feedings alone can produce dramatic improvements in immune function. The bactericidal response to coagulase-negative staphylococci and tumor necrosis factor production normalized in a cohort of postoperative infants supported on parenteral nutrition when minimal enteral feeds began.[155]

Enteral nutrition is immunoprotective through a number of mechanisms. It appears that the actual composition of enteral feeds is an important factor in maintaining normal immune function. Bacterial translocation and impaired lymphocyte mitogenic responses occur in rats receiving either intravenous or orally administered TPN solution. However, the addition of fiber to oral TPN decreased bacterial translocation and restored lymphocyte mitogenic responses. Bacterial translocation was absent in those who had normal lymphocyte function.[240]

Breast milk was the first immunomodulatory diet. Breast-feeding is associated with decreased gastrointestinal and respiratory infections in the first 2 years of life. Children with cleft palate, predisposed to recurrent otitis media, who are exclusively breast-fed have a marked decrease in the incidence of middle ear effusions as compared to those receiving a cow-milk formula.[239] The protective components in breast milk include not only maternal secretory IgA and the cellular elements (macrophages, lymphocytes, and neutrophils), but oligosaccharides, iron-binding lactoferrin, and bacterial growth factors.[121] The oligosaccharide fractions of breast milk glycolipids inhibit Streptococcus pneumoniae and Haemophilus influenzae adherence to human epithelial cells.[7] By binding iron, an important growth factor for many gram-negative organisms, lactoferrin is able to decrease colonization by pathogenic gram-negative bacteria in the colon. Unique to humans, breast milk contains a stable factor, the bifidus factor, which selectively promotes the growth of Bifidobaterium bifidum.[62] The net result is a colonic ecosystem that favors the selective growth of nonpathogenic organisms.[52] Breast milk due to the bifidus factor and the presence of IL-10 confers protection against the development of necrotizing enterocolitis.[55,81]

Conditionally Essential Amino Acids in Hypermetabolism and Stress

Glutamine is the most abundant amino acid in the body. It is nonessential in normal states but has a high turnover in hypermetabolic situations. As the rate of production cannot keep up with the demands for glutamine in these circumstances, it is considered a conditionally essential amino acid during stress. Glutamine plays a pivotal role in hepatic gluconeogenesis. Along with cysteine, glutamine is a precursor for glutathione, which is important in protecting the intracellular milieu of the liver and lung from free radicals. Glutamine is important in maintaining the various functions of the mucosal cells of the intestine and is the preferred substrate for colonic cells.[115] Glutamine increases enteral blood flow and reduces bacterial translocation. Glutamine depletion results in gut atrophy and an increase in gut permeability.[184,217]

Arginine is another conditional essential amino acid. It is converted in the liver to ornithine, an important precursor in protein synthesis and collagen production during wound healing. Arginine is a potent secretogogue, stimulating growth hormone, prolactin, insulin, and glucagon secretion. Arginine enhances T cell mediated response to mitogens and interleukin-2 release following stimulation. Finally, arginine's importance in nutrition and metabolism may in part lie in its relationship to nitric oxide. Arginine is the substrate for NO-synthetase.[56] Some data suggest that nitric oxide is implicated in many gastrointestinal pathophysiological states including gastroesophageal reflux, pyloric stenosis, and the regulation of intestinal secretion.[1,32]

Route of Enteral Nutrition

The bedside decision of which type of enteral feeding to employ depends on the clinical circumstances. The awake child with intact airway protective reflexes, normal swallowing function, and normal respiratory rate should be allowed to suck or drink. This scenario applies to most cardiac surgical patients within 24 hours after extubation and removal of mediastinal tubes and transthoracic monitoring catheters. If oral feedings fail or are contraindicated, then the physician must choose between intragastric and transpyloric feedings.

Intragastric feedings via a nasogastric tube generally represent the next step if oral feedings have failed, because

nasogastric tubes are somewhat easier to position and maintain. While the data are conflicting, transpyloric feeding does not appear to have a clear-cut advantage over intragastric feeding in the prevention of aspiration or nosocomial pneumonia.[150,191]

Transpyloric feedings are clearly superior to intragastric feedings in the patient with delayed gastric emptying. Small intestinal motility and absorptive function remain intact under a variety of pathological conditions making transpyloric feedings a viable option for the majority of critically ill patients. Transpyloric tubes also minimize the consequences of impaired colonic motility, as patients can tolerate transpyloric feeds in the absence of bowel sounds.[61] Continuous transpyloric feeding in infancy affords a higher average cumulative weight gain than intermittent nasogastric feeds in some centers.[226] In the past, bedside transpyloric tube placement has met with only modest success necessitating the use of weighted, styletted feeding tubes, or a corkscrew technique.[241] Two rapid, simple, and inexpensive methods have now been described, which report success rates of >90% in bedside transpyloric feeding tube placement. One method utilizes metoclopramide, air insufflation, and positioning while the other uses just air insufflation.[45,186] The latter study was compared in a prospective randomized manner to a styletted tube insertion with adjunctive position, in which the success rate was only 44%.[186] If bedside placement fails, transpyloric tubes can be positioned under fluoroscopic guidance.

The successful placement of a transpyloric feeding tube does not ensure safe, successful enteral nutrition.[103] Nasogastric aspirates have been found to double once transpyloric enteral feeding begins. These aspirates are not refluxed feeds, but represent an increase in gastric output, which may be the result of an enteral hormonal response to the presence of feeds in the small intestine.[46] This may explain, in part, the equivalent incidence of aspiration pneumonias in transpylorically fed patients and those fed intragastrically. Transpyloric feeds are associated with accelerated small bowel transit time, more rapid gallbladder contractions, and higher levels of cholecystokinin secretion than are intragastric feeds.[118] Transpyloric feeding is successful in 90% of patients, but 10% will experience significant complications such as abdominal cramps, distention, or diarrhea, which force cessation of feeding.[157] The absolute contraindications for transpyloric feeding are intestinal obstruction, necrotizing enterocolitis, severe gastrointestinal bleeding, recent gastrointestinal surgery, and intractable diarrhea.

Maintenance of the Child Receiving Tube Feedings

Once placed, maintaining a feeding tube in its desired position can be challenging. Patients must be continuously evaluated for feeding intolerance, gastroesophageal reflux (GER), and microaspiration. As increasing gastric aspirate volume is a principal risk factor for GER, gastric residuals must be monitored regardless of feeding tube location.[143] As large-bore nasogastric tubes are associated with a higher risk of GER and prolonged duration of acid in the esophagus, it is advantageous to use as small a bore tube (10-Fr) as is practical.[153] If long-term transpyloric feedings are required, placement of a percutaneous endoscopic gastrostomy (PEG) tube with wire guided advancement under fluoroscopy into the jejunum is an excellent option.[185]

Parenteral Nutrition

Critical illness often precludes the enteral delivery of complete caloric requirements. Total parenteral nutrition is an alternative to enteral feeding when gut absorptive capacity or motility is severely disturbed. TPN solutions contain hypertonic glucose, amino acids, vitamins, and trace elements. A lipid emulsion is often administered separately. TPN is generally administered by central vein in children, because the solution's hypertonicity causes phlebitis. Since the early work by Dudrick,[63] it has been clear that under ideal circumstances TPN may supply sufficient calories to support growth. However, long-term TPN in critically ill patients is associated with a variety of complications including excess CO_2 production and difficulty in weaning from mechanical ventilation, nosocomial infection, hepatic dysfunction, and hyperglycemia in stressed patients with a decreased insulin/glucagon ratio.

Glucose is the main energy source in TPN. Glucose intolerance is associated with hyperglycemia, osmotic diuresis, and hyperosmolality. Cowett found that infants receiving glucose at a rate of 8.1 mg/kg/minute did not develop hyperglycemia, while 50% of infants receiving a rate of 11.2 mg/kg/minute did.[53] When administered in excessive amounts glucose is no longer oxidized, but rather converted to fat. Not only is this excess glucose wasted, but its conversion to fat actually inhibits fat oxidation, limiting the use of fat as an energy source. It appears that the limit for glucose oxidation is 18 g/kg/day.[102] High levels of glucose oxidation increase carbon dioxide production, which may precipitate respiratory embarrassment.

Monitoring of parenteral alimentation in the critically ill patient is based on measurements of nutrient levels in the circulation. Serum glucose levels should be monitored every time a change in glucose delivery rate takes place, when the clinical status of the patient changes significantly, or when the patient receives medications or undergoes procedures presumed to affect glucose metabolism. Sodium, potassium, magnesium, and calcium should be measured every time the rate of infusion is modified, or when required by clinical assessment. A particularly hazardous situation may arise in the cardiac patient when a reduction in diuretic dose leads to reduced urine output but potassium concentration in the TPN is not adjusted concomitantly. Plasma triglycerides should be measured on a weekly basis unless the rate of intralipid infusion has been changed.

The syndrome of TPN-induced hepatic dysfunction differs by age. Cholestasis is more common in infants. Biliary sludge and cholelithiasis are more common in older children, and steatosis is more common in adults.[173] Serum transaminases, bilirubin, and alkaline phosphatase should be measured once a week to monitor for TPN-induced complications, and ammonia should be evaluated when there is any suggestion of liver dysfunction. Ironically, children who are unable to tolerate enteral feeds are more likely to develop TPN liver disease. The reduction of enterohumoral production that accompanies enteral fasting also reduces gallbladder contractility and may cause the formation of biliary sludge. Intestinal stasis has been associated with cholestasis and the production of lithocholic acid and hepatotoxin.[23] Partial enteral feeding in conjunction with parenteral nutrition appears to be able to attenuate many of these deleterious processes and is associated with a much lower incidence of TPN-induced hepatic dysfunction.[105] The initiation of small-volume enteral feeding (12 mL/kg/d) as an adjunct to parenteral nutrition in infants results in improved feeding tolerance, earlier resumption of complete enteral nutrition, a reduction in total number of days of hyperalimentation, and a faster rise in serum gastrin and GIP levels.[182]

ORAL FEEDING, SWALLOWING, AND DYSPHAGIA IN THE CHILD WITH CONGENITAL HEART DISEASE

Etiology of Dysphagia in Children with Congenital Heart Disease

Data regarding the prevalence of feeding and swallowing problems in children with congenital heart disease are limited. Approximately 65% of parents of children with CHD recalled the presence of extensive feeding problems during infancy and early childhood.[194] An absent, poor, or weak suck has been described as a major problem in 7% to 43% of infants with CHD.[123,194] Parents attributed poor sucking and limited oral intake to fatigue and "heavy breathing."[194] Clinical presentations of feeding problems in older children with CHD include refusal to eat, frequent mealtime tantrums, general weakness, and swallowing problems. In general, feeding problems resolve with increasing age and improving medical status.

Congenital heart disease may represent one component of a genetic syndrome, some of which are strongly associated with impaired swallowing. CHARGE, VATER, the 22q11.2 deletion syndromes, and trisomy 21 all have a significant incidence of dysphagia.[37,101,139,195] Children with CHARGE may have feeding and swallowing difficulties associated with multiple cranial nerve abnormalities.[37] Some children with 22q11.2 deletion syndromes have dysphagia, nasopharyngeal reflux, hyperpharyngeal contraction, incoordination of the upper esophageal sphincter, esophageal dysmotility, and gastroesophageal reflux.[139] Children with trisomy 21 and CHD commonly have gastroesophageal reflux and dysmotility. These children remain at significant risk for gastroesophageal reflux and aspiration after operative correction of their cardiac lesion.[195]

Neurological impairment is one of the most common extracardiac complications of congenital heart disease. Many children with CHD have neurobehavioral problems even before surgery, and up to 25% of infants will have neurological dysfunction following cardiac surgery.[75,123] Chronic hypoxemia, congestive heart failure, dysrhythmias, thromboembolic events, poor perfusion states, and previous cardiac arrests are risk factors for neurologic injury.[26] Children with neurologic injuries frequently have oral-motor dysfunction, prolonged mealtimes,[110] poor weight gain, pharyngeal dysphagia with concomitant aspiration, abnormal coordination of respiration and swallowing,[230] and gastroesophageal reflux.[41,164,175] It is likely that children with CHD and neurologic deficits will have similar manifestations of dysphagia. Postoperative neurologic deficits are seen more frequently in children with acyanotic lesions.[123] For example, neurodevelopmental delay, acquired microcephaly, and poor growth are commonly seen in children following surgery for hypoplastic left heart syndrome.[166] These neurologic outcomes may be mediated in part by deep hypothermic circulatory arrest, which is employed to repair complex lesions.[64,75]

Specific Causes of Dysphagia during the Three Phases of Swallowing

The infant with dysfunctional swallowing requires a careful evaluation. Such an evaluation divides the act of swallowing into three phases—the *oral*, *pharyngeal*, and *esophageal* phases of swallowing.

During the *oral* phase, foods are processed into "swallow-ready balls" (bolus) and then transported to the back of the mouth. In infants, oral phase processing is limited to sucking fluid from a nipple. In older babies and young children, bolus formation is dependent upon the consistency of food and may require chewing skills. The airway is open during the oral phase.

Disruption of bolus formation or transfer may be seen in children who have structural defects involving the nose, nasopharynx, oral cavity, or oropharynx. The cleft palate associated with a deletion within chromosome 22q11 represents the classic example in the CATCH 22 (**C**ardiac anomaly, **A**nomalous face, **T**hymus hypoplasia/aplasia, **C**left palate, and **H**ypocalcemia) syndrome. This syndrome is not a single entity, but rather includes DiGeorge syndrome, conotruncal anomaly face syndrome, and velocardiofacial syndrome.

Children with limited endurance or those with a history of interrupted oral feeding experiences will also have a dysfunctional oral phase. Infants with CHD commonly present with a weak, poor, or uncoordinated suck. Older children may present with trouble taking a bolus from a spoon or problems with chewing. Children with underlying neurodevelopmental delay present with oral-motor problems, such as tongue thrusting or abnormal tongue posturing. Oral phase dysfunction makes feeding inefficient and may allow the bolus to prematurely enter the pharynx, putting the child at risk for aspiration.

The *pharyngeal* phase comprises of a series of integrated and complex motor events that direct and propel the bolus through the pharynx and into the esophagus, while keeping the airway protected. During this phase of swallowing, breathing stops, the larynx elevates and the vocal folds adduct, the palate elevates to approximate the posterior pharyngeal wall, and pharyngeal muscles contract to propel the bolus through a relaxed upper esophageal sphincter. The pharyngeal phase has voluntary and involuntary components.

Vocal fold paralysis and dysfunction may cause feeding problems associated with the pharyngeal phase of swallowing. Since airway protection during swallowing relies on both vocal fold closure as well as an intact pharyngeal phase, dysfunction in this phase has the highest risk of aspiration. Silent aspiration, aspiration without coughing, is a two-fold problem. The airway's primary defense mechanism does not clear aspirated material, and the presence of swallowing dysfunction is masked. Silent aspiration occurs in 40% to 97% of patients with neurogenic dysphagia[12,188]; the highest frequency occurs in children. Vocal fold paralysis compromises

airway closure during the pharyngeal phase of swallowing and may result in aspiration.[158] Presenting as stridor, breathiness, a hoarse or weak cry, and choking with feeding, surgical trauma to the left recurrent laryngeal nerve is the most common cause of vocal fold paralysis in infants 12 months or younger.[57,243] Infants who have undergone ligation of the ductus arteriosus or coarctation repair are at greatest risk.

Prolonged endotracheal intubation with or without subsequent tracheostomy is also associated with pharyngeal phase dysphagia in adults, and may be in children as well.[60] Forty-five percent of adults intubated for more than 2 days aspirated in the postextubation period, 25% overall will have silent aspiration.[120] The mechanism responsible for swallowing dysfunction post extubation is postulated to be the result of impaired proprioception from receptor dysfunction and mucosal lesions, as well as pharyngeal muscle dysfunction attributed to disuse.[58] In the absence of neurological injury, most post extubation dysphagia resolves within 96 hours of extubation, concurrent with the healing of mucosal lesions.[17]

Tachypnea alone can impair airway protection. As the respiratory rate increases, the breathing pause that usually occurs during the pharyngeal phase of swallowing is violated, and aspiration becomes more likely.[128]

The *esophageal* phase begins once the bolus passes through the upper esophageal sphincter and ends when it passes through the gastroesophageal juncture into the stomach. The esophageal phase is involuntary and the airway is open.

Esophageal dysphagia results from congenital anomalies, neurologic dysfunction, traumatic injury, and gastroesophageal reflux. Congenital anomalies including tracheoesophageal fistula and vascular rings are associated with esophageal dysphagia, as are impairments in the central nervous system that result in abnormal peristalsis.[99] Traumatic esophageal dysphagia may be the result of an increase in the use of intraoperative transesophageal echocardiogram (TEE).[88,168] These injuries include trauma from scope insertion, thermal injury, pressure necrosis, and compression of adjoining structures.[88] Injuries that occur during insertion are likely to occur at the level of the cricopharyngeus, presenting with symptoms of choking, nasopharyngeal regurgitation, or aspiration.[29]

Gastroesophageal reflux (GER) is common in infants and young children and is another cause of esophageal dysphagia. Children with CHD and syndromic anomalies, such as trisomy 21, are at increased risk for GER.[195] Patients with vascular rings and palliative shunts are also at risk for developing esophageal dysphagia and GER.[33,43] GER can be responsible for respiratory dysfunction, poor weight gain, or problematic feedings such as selective food intake or feeding refusal.[98] Furthermore, even children with intact pharyngeal swallow function may not be able to compensate and swallow safely when regurgitated materials reach the hypopharynx. Consequently, a "normal" swallowing study does not exclude the possibility of aspiration with GER.

Evaluation of Dysfunctional Swallowing

A multidisciplinary approach to the child with dysfunctional swallowing provides the best opportunity to define the pathological process. Upon completion of the history, physical examination, feeding observation, and imaging studies, the clinician should be able to identify potential causes of dysphagia, the risk of aspiration, and the practicality of oral feeding.

The history focuses on the feeding history and associated symptoms. The evaluation concentrates on the relationship between dysphagia and pulmonary symptoms, such as noisy breathing or the refusal of liquids that caused choking when the patient was younger. Apnea or laryngospasm may result from aspiration during swallowing or from GER. The most common question asked during a swallowing evaluation is whether children cough or choke during feeds. Many children with dysphagia do not cough or choke because they aspirate silently. Caregivers and practitioners are often misled into believing that a child is swallowing safely because there are no symptoms.

The physical examination focuses on an examination of the oral-motor structures and laryngeal mechanism. Observations of the oral-motor mechanism include: the presence of drooling, movement and closure of the lips and jaw, the size and shape of the tongue and its movement patterns, the height and shape of the palate, the effectiveness of velopharyngeal approximation, and the responses of oral sensory and motor system. It is important to observe an entire feeding because some children appear to do relatively well at the beginning of a feeding and become disorganized or fatigued toward the end of the meal.

The palatal gag is the most commonly assessed oral reflex. One should be cautious about eliciting a gag reflex in any child who is extremely sensitive to vagally mediated stimulation. The presence of a gag reflex does not guarantee safe swallowing.[119]

Examination of the respiratory and neurological status is important as well. Tachypnea and increased work of breathing are likely to produce problems with swallowing coordination. Oral feeding should not be initiated in infants breathing faster than 65 to 70 breaths per minute. Breathing and swallowing coordination is physiologically impossible in neonates who breathe at a rate of 80 or more breaths per minute. The child should be alert, interested in feeding, able to tolerate positioning for feeding, and able to handle bolus delivery to the stomach. If these conditions are not met, the child should not be considered ready for oral feeds.

The presence of a nonnutritive suck (NNS) is another important feeding prerequisite for infants and babies when bottle or breast-feeding is desirable. A moistened pacifier or gloved finger should stimulate a NNS. The NNS occurs at the rate of two sucks per second, whereas a nutritive suck occurs at the rate of one suck per second.[236] It is important to recognize that even a strong NNS is not a guarantee of successful oral feeding, although it is an important prerequisite for infant feeding. Strenuous efforts should be made to preserve the NNS through oral-motor stimulation whenever oral feeds are interrupted for prolonged periods of time. Some infants and babies have trouble sustaining sucking because of endurance problems. Others with a disorganized NNS may benefit from oral-motor intervention. Findings of poor oral-motor skills in children with CHD and hypotonia should prompt examiners to evaluate the possibility of central nervous system problems.[123]

Imaging studies focus on specific aspects of the swallowing process that cannot be viewed directly during the clinic or bedside assessment. These studies differ in sensitivity for detecting aspiration (Table 15-8).[127] The most common radiologic procedures used to assess pediatric dysphagia are

Table 15-8 Common Imaging Procedures for Dysfunctional Swallowing

Instrumental Procedure	Components of Swallowing Examined	Detects Aspiration Events	Origin of Aspiration Detected
Upper gastrointestinal study (UGI)	Defines anatomy and functional integrity of esophagus, stomach, and duodenum Detects esophageal strictures, ulcer disease, vascular rings, extrinsic lesions compressing the esophagus, and foreign bodies in esophagus Detects GI tract obstructions and malformation of the intestines Screens oropharyngeal function	Yes	Gross pharyngeal anomalies and concomitant aspiration GER, if contrast reaches hypopharynx Communication between esophagus and trachea
Videofluoroscopic swallow study (VFSS)	Defines anatomy and physiology of the swallowing mechanism *during* deglutition Defines "reason" for dysphagia Identifies bolus and positioning variables, and feeding strategies or maneuvers that enhance the safety of swallowing Screens esophageal function	Yes	Oropharyngeal and cervical esophageal dysfunction GER, if contrast reaches hypopharynx
Fiberoptic endoscopic evaluation of swallowing (FEES)	Views pharyngeal and laryngeal structures before and immediately following swallowing Assesses pharyngeal and laryngeal response (sensation) to direct stimulation Detects velopharyngeal insufficiency and vocal fold abnormalities	Yes	Oropharyngeal dysfunction Saliva GER, if regurgitated material reaches hypopharynx
Radionuclide imaging studies (scintigraphy)	Quantifies esophageal and gastric emptying Quantifies aspiration from saliva or GER without providing a view of the swallowing structures	Sometimes	Oropharyngeal dysfunction Saliva GER
Ultrasound (ultrasonography)	Defines oral preparatory and oral phases of deglutition Visualizes temporal relationships between movement patterns of oral and pharyngeal structures	No	

GER, gastroesophageal reflux.

Table 15-9 Differences between the Videofluoroscopic Swallow Study and Barium Swallow

Videofluoroscopic Swallow Study (VFSS)	Barium Swallow (UGI)
Examines oral cavity, pharynx, and larynx	Examines esophagus, stomach, and duodenum
Images oropharyngeal structures and does not follow the bolus	Follows the bolus through gastrointestinal tract
Controlled amounts of barium	Large amounts of barium to distend the esophagus
Set up to simulate usual or best feeding situation	Set up to examine the esophagus
Barium mixtures simulate food textures	Liquid barium
Upright or feeding position	Decubitus position

From Loughlin GM, Lefton-Greif MA: Dysfunctional swallowing and respiratory disease in children. *Adv Pediatr* 41:135–162, 1994.

the barium swallow or upper gastrointestinal study (UGI) and the videofluoroscopic swallow study (VFSS) (Table 15-9). The format of the UGI provides a screening examination of the oropharyngeal structures and therefore does not conclusively diagnose or exclude the presence of swallowing dysfunction.

The VFSS is the "gold standard" for assessing the presence of oropharyngeal dysphagia and concomitant aspiration. The design of the VFSS enables examiners to determine "not only whether the patient aspirates, but the *reason* for the aspiration, so that appropriate treatment can be initiated."[11,127] The VFSS is an appropriate procedure when a child is suspected of having pharyngeal phase dysphagia and the child is ready, willing, and able to participate in the protocol.[11] Although the VFSS provides the most comprehensive information about swallowing function and the risk of aspiration, its findings, even when normal, do not "rule out the possibility of aspiration." Individuals with normal swallowing aspirate on occasion.

MANAGEMENT OF DYSFUNCTIONAL SWALLOWING

The management goals for children with impaired swallowing are to eliminate or reduce factors contributing to airway compromise, maintain adequate nutrition, maximize the child's potential for growth and development, and facilitate positive interactions with caregivers.[10] It is likely that children with CHD will require multiple adjustments in management due to changes in their health, medical condition, and neurodevelopmental progress.

When possible, oral feeding is the desired route of nutrition. However, some children with CHD may be unable to handle any risk of aspiration because of an extremely fragile medical status or pending surgical or medical interventions. Others may not be able to support their nutrition and hydration needs by oral means alone. For children who are unable to meet their needs by oral feeding alone, three potential feeding scenarios exist:

1. Oral feedings primarily for nutrition with non-oral supplements that most frequently add fluid for hydration and calories.

2. Limited oral feedings usually meeting less than half of daily nutrition needs, and tube feedings to meet nutrition and hydration requirements.

3. Nutritional needs met via tube, with nonnutritive oral-motor stimulation that may include "tastes."[11]

Patients requiring prolonged tube feeds often will require a feeding gastrostomy tube, to avoid the complications of long-term nasogastric feeds such as sinusitis, otitis media, hypopharyngeal irritation, and tube dislocation.[25] Under most circumstances a pediatric gastroenterologist or pediatric surgeon can place a percutaneous endoscopic gastrostomy tube.[229] The contraindications to a PEG in which a child would require an open gastrostomy tube include esophageal stricture, peritonitis, massive ascites, peritoneal dialysis, portal hypertension, severe coagulopathy, and abdominal wall infection. Congenital anomalies of the gastrointestinal tract may be a relative contraindication to PEG placement. A similar caution regarding PEG exists in patients with a single ventricle and shunt-dependent pulmonary circulation, because the gastric inflation required for PEG may decrease lung volume and increase pulmonary vascular resistance. A number of studies have shown that an antireflux procedure is unnecessary for the majority of patients requiring a feeding gastrostomy who have a negative GER evaluation preoperatively.[116,162]

Some children with CHD and dysphagia may respond well to simple adjustments in their oral feeding routine that include modifications in diet, feeding position, rate of feeding, type of utensil (e.g., bottle or cup), or scheduling of meals. For example, many children with dysphagia tend to have less difficulty handling thicker liquids, particularly those children with vocal fold paralysis or neurogenic dysphagia.[12,243] However, some infants with oral-motor dysfunction or poor endurance may fatigue while drinking thicker liquids. The feeding and swallowing evaluation, including the VFSS results, should help identify modifications that are most helpful for particular children.

When possible, the best therapy for swallowing dysfunction is swallowing. Therefore feeding and swallowing teams attempt to identify any modifications that enable safe, albeit sometimes limited, oral feeding. For infants and young babies, interventions may be limited to nonnutritive stimulation to promote optimal oral-motor function and interactions with caregivers without increasing the risk of aspiration. Oral-motor and swallowing therapies promote the child's compensatory patterns (e.g., changing position or altering the consistency of foods or liquids) and strengthen the movement patterns of the swallowing structures (e.g., stimulation for nonnutritive sucking or tongue lateralization exercises for chewing).

Management of Gastroesophageal Reflux

The clinical manifestations of GER include vomiting, poor weight gain, dysphagia, abdominal or substernal pain, esophagitis, feeding intolerance, wheezing, recurrent stridor, chronic cough, recurrent pneumonia, and aspiration. GER is one of the causes of distressed behavior in infancy.[92] GER is one of the causes of apparent life-threatening events (ALTEs) in infants, found in 50% of these children once sepsis has been excluded.[140] Some children with severe GER pain develop stereotypical head and neck movements (Sandifer syndrome), which can be mistaken for seizure activity.[84] GER can be documented with an upper gastrointestinal series, an esophageal pH probe, or nuclear scintigraphy. Endoscopy and esophageal mucosal biopsies confirm the associated esophagitis. Compared to the pH probe, a UGI is neither sensitive nor specific for the diagnosis of GER. Esophageal pH monitoring remains the gold standard for the diagnosis of GER. The reflux index, the percentage of the total time that the esophageal pH is less than 4, reflects the cumulative exposure of the esophageal mucosa to acid. The mean upper limit of normal in children under 1 year of age is 11.7%. For children between 1 and 9 years of age the upper limit of normal is 5.4%. Esophageal pH probe monitoring does not detect nonacid reflux, which may occur postprandially or in children on acid suppressive regimens. The nuclear scintigraphy, also known as a milk scan, is performed by the oral ingestion of either technetium (Tc, half life of 6 hours, 1 millicurie) or indium (half life of 2.63 days, 500 microcuries) labeled formula. The patient is scanned for evidence of GER or aspiration after ingestion and then 24 hours later. Unlike the pH probe study, the milk scan can demonstrate the reflux of nonacidic gastric contents, delayed gastric emptying, and delayed GER. Evidence of aspiration, including silent aspiration, can be seen up to 24 hours after the ingestion of labeled milk, especially if indium is used as the radionuclide. Tc is useful for acute, large aspirations, while indium, because of its longer half life, is useful for silent aspiration.[141] A negative test does not exclude the possibility of aspiration on an infrequent basis.[74] As not all patients with GER have esophagitis, endoscopy with esophageal biopsies confirms the diagnosis and gives some impression of the severity of reflux.[169]

Treatment for the child with GER includes changes in formula composition, feeding positioning, acid suppression therapy, prokinetic therapy, and surgical interventions. The response to empiric therapy should be prompt, usually within 2 weeks.[163] Changes in formula are only infrequently successful at improving GER symptoms in infants.[113] The only subset of infants in whom this appears to be successful are those who have a cow milk protein allergy. In these infants elimination of cow protein resulted in a rapid improvement in symptoms. A 1- to 2-week trial of a hypoallergenic formula may be efficacious in this subset of infants. Milk-thickening has not been shown to improve reflux index but does decrease the number of episodes of vomiting.[14] GER in infants may be exacerbated when they are placed in infant seats. In children older than 1 year of age, GER seems to be reduced in the left decubitus position with elevation of the head of bed, as in adults.[91]

Pharmacological therapy for gastroesophageal reflux disease (GERD) has been directed toward (1) acid suppression and (2) enhancing esophageal peristalsis, increasing lower esophageal sphincter tone, and accelerating gastric emptying. Gastric acid suppression can be achieved with the use of histamine-2 receptor antagonists and proton pump inhibitors. Histamine-2 receptor antagonists are more efficacious for mild esophagitis than for severe esophagitis.[170] Histamine receptor antagonists may not be used as effectively as possible because of inadequate dosing.[107] A recent pharmacokinetic study of ranitidine in critically ill children suggests that adequate acid suppression can be achieved with ranitidine administered either as 1.5 mg/kg every 8 hours or as a loading dose of 0.45 mg/kg followed by a continuous infusion of 0.15 mg/kg/hour.[130] Since proton pump inhibitors require acid in the parietal cell canaliculus, concomitant administration of histamine-2 receptor antagonists with proton pump inhibitors can inhibit the latter's efficacy.[232] In children, omeprazole (40 mg per 1.73 m² surface area) and high-dose ranitidine (20 mg/kg/day) were comparable in reducing esophagitis.[54] In children refractory to histamine-2 receptor antagonists, omeprazole appears to be effective in improving esophagitis.[3] Cisapride, by releasing acetylcholine at the synapses of the myenteric plexus, is an effective prokinetic agent in the treatment of GER. However, because of an association with serious cardiac arrhythmias, cisapride has been withdrawn from the US market. The other available prokinetic agents, metoclopramide and bethanchole have not been shown to be efficacious in the treatment of GER in infants and children.[169]

Surgical fundoplication is considered when medical therapy has failed to control GER symptoms or when severe airway complications occur during treatment. Case series report that successful relief of symptoms following Nissen fundoplication occurs in 57%–92% of children. The overall complication rate is 2% to 45%. Laparoscopic fundoplication in children appears to have similar results and complication rates as compared to the open procedure, with shortened length of hospital stay. A comparison of the potential risks, benefits, and costs of prolonged medical therapy versus surgical intervention has not been well studied in children.[167,169,197]

CONCLUSIONS

Children with congenital heart disease frequently are malnourished prior to surgical intervention. The extent of undernutrition has a significant impact on the timing of surgical interventions as well as the perioperative outcome. Nutritional management is now closely linked to efforts to modulate the stress response, as well as to limit postoperative infectious and inflammatory complications. Preoperative nutritional assessment and management with immunomodulating formulas may further decrease postoperative systemic inflammatory response syndrome (SIRS). Postoperative nutritional support should be instituted early and aggressively. Enteral feedings and adequate analgesia will limit the perioperative catabolism. In light of the significant probability of postoperative dysphagia in many children with congenital heart disease, these patients may require a multidisciplinary swallowing evaluation prior to resumption of oral feeds. Gastroesophageal reflux, protein-losing enteropathy, and persistent chylothorax are significant postoperative complications with important nutritional complications in children with CHD. A staged therapeutic approach consisting of dietary changes, medical interventions, and then invasive interventions, if needed, is successful in mitigating the nutritional complications of each of these conditions in a majority of cases.

References

1. Albina JE, Reichner JS: Nitric oxide in inflammation and immunity. *New Horizons* 3:46–64, 1995.
2. Allen EM, van Heeckeren DW, Spector ML, Blumer JL: Management of nutritional and infectious complications of postoperative chylothorax in children. *J Pediatr Surg* 26:1169–1174, 1991.
3. Alliet P, Raes M, Bruneel E, Gillis P: Omeprazole in infants with cimetidine-resistant peptic esophagitis. *J Pediatr* 132:352–354, 1998.

4. Anand KJ, Brown MJ, Bloom SR, Aynsley-Green A: Studies on the hormonal regulation of fuel metabolism in the human newborn infant undergoing anaesthesia and surgery. *Horm Res* 22:115–128, 1985.

5. Anand KJ, Hansen DD, Hickey PR: Hormonal-metabolic stress responses in neonates undergoing cardiac surgery. *Anesthesiology* 73:661–670, 1990.

6. Anand KJ, Sippell WG, Aynsley-Green A: Randomised trial of fentanyl anaesthesia in preterm babies undergoing surgery: Effects on the stress response. *Lancet* 1:62–66, 1987.

7. Andersson B, Porras O, Hanson LA, et al: Inhibition of attachment of *Streptococcus pneumoniae* and *Haemophilus influenzae* by human milk and receptor oligosaccharides. *J Infect Dis* 153:232–237, 1986.

8. Annane D, Sebille V, Charpentier C, et al: Effect of treatment with low doses of hydrocortisone and fludrocortisone on mortality in patients with septic shock. *JAMA* 288:862–871, 2002.

9. Aouifi A, Neidecker J, Vedrinne C, et al: Glucose versus lactated ringer's solution during pediatric cardiac surgery. *J Cardiothorac Vasc Anesth* 11:411–414, 1997.

10. Arvedson JC, Lefton-Greif MA: Pediatric dysphagia: Complex medical, health, and developmental issues. *Semin Speech Lang* 17:257–336, 1996.

11. Arvedson JC, Lefton-Greif MA: *Pediatric Videofluoroscopic Swallow Studies: A Professional Manual with Caregiver Handouts.* San Antonio: Communication Skill Builders, 1998.

12. Arvedson J, Rogers B, Buck G, et al: Silent aspiration prominent in children with dysphagia. *Int J Pediatr Otolaryngol* 28:173–181, 1994.

13. Bac DJ, Van Hagen PM, Postema PT, et al: Octreotide for protein-losing enteropathy with intestinal lymphangiectasia. *Lancet* 345:1639, 1995.

14. Bailey DJ, Andres JM, Danek GD, Pineiro-Carrero VM: Lack of efficacy of thickened feeding as treatment for gastroesophageal reflux. *J Pediatr* 110:181–186, 1987.

15. Bakker HD, Scholte HR, Luyt-Houwen IE, et al: Neonatal cardiomyopathy and lactic acidosis responsive to thiamine. *J Inherit Metab Dis* 14:75–79, 1991.

16. Barbaro G, Lipshultz SE: The pathogenesis of HIV-associated cardiomyopathy. *Ann NY Acad Sci* 946:57–81, 2001.

17. Barquist E, Brown M, Cohn S, et al: Postextubation fiberoptic endoscopic evaluation of swallowing after prolonged endotracheal intubation: A randomized, prospective trial. *Crit Care Med* 29:1710–1713, 2001.

18. Barton BE: Il-6 like cytokines and cancer cachexia; Consequences of chronic inflammation. *Immunol Res* 23:41–58, 2001.

19. Barton JS, Hindmarsh PC, Preece MA: Serum insulin-like growth factor 1 in congenital heart disease. *Arch Dis Child* 75:162–163, 1996.

20. Baum MK, Shor-Posner G, Lai S, et al: High risk of HIV-related mortality is associated with selenium deficiency. *J Acquir Immune Defic Syndr Hum Retrovirol* 15:370–374, 1997.

21. Baumann H, Gauldie J: The acute phase response. *Immunol Today* 15:74–80, 1994.

22. Baxter RC: Insulin-like growth factor binding proteins in the human circulation. *Hormone Res* 42:140–144, 1994.

23. Beath SV, Davies P, Papadopoulou A, et al: Parenteral nutrition–related cholestasis in postsurgical neonates: Multivariate analysis of risk factors. *J Pediatr Surg* 31:604–606, 1996.

24. Beghetti M, La Scala G, Belli D: Etiology and management of pediatric chylothorax. *J Pediatr* 136:653–658, 2000.

25. Behrens R, Lang T, Muschweck H, et al: Percutaneous endosocopic gastrostomy in children and adolescents. *J Pediatr Gastreoenterol Nutr* 25:487–491, 1997.

26. Bellinger DC, Wypij D, Kuban KC, et al: Developmental and neurological status of children at 4 years of age after heart surgery with hypothermic circulatory arrest or low-flow cardiopulmonary bypass. *Circulation* 100:526–532, 1999.

27. Beriberi can complicate TPN. *Nutr Rev* 45:239–243, 1987.

28. Berkenbosch JW, Witthington DE: Management of postoperative chylothorax with nitric oxide. *Crit Care Med* 27:1022–1024, 1999.

29. Bezold LI, Pignatelli R, Altman CA, et al: Intraoperative transesophageal echocardiography in congenital heart surgery. The Texas Children's Hospital experience. *Tex Heart Inst J* 23:108–115, 1996.

30. Bond SJ, Guzzetta PC, Snyder ML, Randolph JG: Management of pediatric postoperative chylothorax. *Ann Thorac Surg* 56:469–472, 1993.

31. Bormann B, Weidler B, Dennhardt R, et al: Influence of epidural fentanyl on stress-induced elevation of plasma vasopressin (ADH) after surgery. *Anesth Analg* 62:727–732, 1983.

32. Boulant J, Fioramonti J, Dapoigny M, et al: Cholecystokinin and nitric oxide in transient lower esophageal sphincter relaxation to gastric distention in dogs. *Gastroenterology* 107:1059–1066, 1994.

33. Bove T, Demanet H, Casimir G, et al: Tracheobronchial compression of vascular origin. Review of experience in infants and children. *J Cardiovasc Surg* 42:663–666, 2001.

34. Breslow MJ, Jordan DA, Christopherson R, et al: Epidural morphine decreases postoperative hypertension by attenuating sympathetic nervous system hyperactivity. *JAMA* 261:3577–3581, 1989.

35. Brunvand L, Haga P, Tangsrud SE, Haug E: Congestive heart failure caused by vitamin D deficiency. *Acta Paediatr* 84:106–108, 1995.

36. Buttiker V, Fanconi S, Burger R: Chylothorax in children: Guidelines for diagnosis and management. *Chest* 116:682–687, 1999.

37. Byerly KA, Pauli RM: Cranial nerve abnormalities in CHARGE association. *Am J Med Genet* 45:751–757, 1993.

38. Caballero B, Wurtman RJ: Differential effects of insulin resistance on leucine and glucose kinetics in obesity. *Metabolism* 40:51–58, 1991.

39. Cameron JW, Rosenthal A, Olson AD: Malnutrition in hospitalized children with congenital heart disease. *Arch Pediatr Adolesc Med* 149:1098–1102, 1995.

40. Campa A, Shor-Posner G, Indacochea F, et al: Mortality risk in selenium-deficient HIV-positive children. *J Acquir Immune Defic Syndr Hum Retrovirol* 20:508–513, 1999.

41. Casas MJ, McPherson KA, Kenny D: Durational aspects of oral swallow in neurologically normal children and children with cerebral palsy: An ultrasound investigation. *Dysphagia* 10:155–159, 1995.

42. Chan S, Gerson B, Subramaniam S: The role of copper, molybdenum, selenium and zinc in nutrition and health. *Clin Lab Med* 18:673–685, 1998.

43. Chapotte C, Monrigal JP, Pezard P, et al: Airway compression in children due to congenital heart disease; value of flexible fiberoptic bronchoscopic assessment. *J Cardiovasc Thorac Anesth* 12:145–152, 1998.

44. Chariot P, Perchet H, Monnet I: Dilated cardiomyopathy in HIV-infected patients. *N Engl J Med* 340:732, 1999.

45. Chellis MJ, Sanders SV, Dean JM, Jackson D: Bedside transpyloric tube placement in the Pediatric Intensive Care Unit. *J Parenter Enteral Nutr* 20:88–90, 1996.

46. Chendrasekhar A: Jejunal feeding in the absence of reflux increases nasogastric output in critically ill trauma patients. *Am Surg* 62:888–889, 1996.

47. Cheung YF, Leung MP, Yip MM: Octreotide for treatment of postoperative chylothorax. *J Pediatr* 139:157–159, 2001.

48. Chroussos GP: The hypothalamic-pituitary-adrenal axis and immune-mediated inflammation. *N Engl J Med* 332:1351–1362, 1995.

49. Chwals WJ, Bistrian BR: Predicted energy expenditure in critically ill children; problems associated with increased variability. *Crit Care Med* 28:2655–2656, 2000.

50. Chwals WJ, Lally KP, Woolley MM, Mahour GH: Measured energy expenditure in critically ill infants and young children. *J Surg Res* 44:467–472, 1988.

51. Cogo PE, Carnielli VP, Rosso F, et al: Protein turnover, lipolysis and endogenous hormonal secretion in critically ill children. *Crit Care Med* 30:65–70, 2002.

52. Cook JD, Skine BS, Baynes RD: Iron deficiency: The global perspective. *Adv Exp Med Biol* 356:219, 1994.

53. Cowett RM, Oh W, Pollak A: Glucose disposal of low birth weight infants: Steady state hyperglycemia produced by constant intravenous glucose infusion. *Pediatrics* 63:389–396, 1979.

54. Cucchiara S, Minella R, Iervolino C, et al: Omeprazole and high dose ranitidine in the treatment of refractory reflux oesophagitis. *Arch Dis Child* 69:655–659, 1993.

55. Dai D, Walker WA: Protective nutrients and bacterial colonization in the immature human gut. *Adv Pediatr* 46:353–382, 1999.

56. Davies MG, Fulton GJ, Hagen PO: Clinical biology of nitric oxide. *Br J Surg* 82:1598–1610, 1995.

57. de Jong AL, Kuppersmith RB, Sulek M, Friedman EM: Vocal cord paralysis in infants and children. *Otolaryngol Clin North Am* 33:131–149, 2000.

58. de Larminat V, Montravers P, Dureuil B, Desmonts JM: Alteration in swallowing reflex after extubation in intensive care patients. *Crit Care Med* 23:486–490, 1995.

59. de Lucas C, Moreno M, Lopez-Herce J, et al: Transpyloric enteral nutrition reduces the complication rate and cost in the critically ill child. *J Pediatr Gastroenterol Nutr* 30:175–180, 2000.

60. DeVita MA, Spierer-Rundback L: Swallowing disorders in patients with prolonged orotracheal intubation or tracheostomy tubes. *Crit Care Med* 18:1328–1330, 1990.

61. Dimand RJ, Veereman-Wauters G, Braner DA: Bedside placement of pH-guided transpyloric small bowel feeding tubes in critically ill infants and small children. *J Parenter Enteral Nutr* 21:112–114, 1997.

62. Dolan SA, Boesman-Finkelstein M, Finkelstein RA: Antimicrobial activity of human milk against pediatric pathogens. *J Infect Dis* 154:722, 1986.

63. Dudrick SJ, Wilmore DW, Vars HM, Rhoads JE: Long-term total parenteral nutrition with growth, development, and positive nitrogen balance. *Surgery* 64:134–142, 1968.

64. du Plessis AJ: Cerebral hemodynamics and metabolism during infant cardiac surgery. Mechanisms of injury and strategies for protection. *J Child Neurol* 12:285–300, 1997.

65. Dzimiri N, Galal O, Moorji A, et al: Regulation of sympathetic activity in children with various congenital heart disease. *Pediatr Res* 38:55–60, 1995.

66. Eccles MP, Cole TJ, Whitehead RG: Factors influencing sleeping metabolic rate in infants. *Eur J Clin Nutr* 43:485–492, 1989.

67. Elwyn DH: Protein metabolism and requirements in the critically ill patient. *Crit Care Clin* 3:57–69, 1987.

68. Elwyn DH, Bryan-Brown CW, Shoemaker WC: Nutritional aspects of body water dislocations in postoperative and depleted patients. *Ann Surg* 182:76–85, 1975.

69. Emori TG, Gaynes RP: An overview of nosocomial infections, including the role of the microbiology laboratory. *Clin Microbiol Rev* 6:428–444, 1993.

70. Engel AG, Angelini C: Carnitine deficiency of human skeletal muscle with associated lipid storage myopathy: A new syndrome. *Science* 179:899–902, 1973.

71. Engum SA, Rescorla FJ, West KW, et al: The use of pleuroperitoneal shunts in the management of persistent chylothorax in infants. *J Pediatr Surg* 34:286–290, 1999.

72. Fagioli I, Salzarulo P, Salomon F, Ricour C: Sinus pauses in early human malnutrition during waking and sleeping. *Neuropediatrics* 14:43–46, 1983.

73. Fahimi H, Casselman FP, Mariani MA, et al: Current management of postoperative chylothorax. *Ann Thorac Surg* 71:448–450, 2001.

74. Fawcett HD, Hayden CK, Adams JC, Swischuk LE: How useful is gastroesophageal reflux scintigraphy in suspected childhood aspiration? *Pediatr Radiol* 18:311–313, 1988.

75. Ferry P: Neurological sequelae of open-heart surgery in children: An irritating question. *Am J Dis Child* 144:369–373, 1990.

76. Fleming RY, Rutan RL, Jahoor F, et al: Effect of recombinant human growth hormone on catabolic hormones and free fatty acids following thermal injury. *J Trauma* 32:698–703, 1992.

77. Fok TF, Lee CH, Wong EM, et al: Risk factors for enterobacter septicemia in a neonatal unit: Case control study. *Clin Infect Disease* 27:1204–1209, 1998.

78. Garabedian M: Hypocalcemia and chromosome 22q11 microdeletion. *Genet Couns* 10:389–394, 1999.

79. Gebara BM, Gelmini M, Sarnaik A: Oxygen consumption, energy expenditure, and substrate utilization after cardiac surgery in children. *Crit Care Med* 20:1550–1554, 1992.

80. Gingell RL, Pieroni DR, Hornung MG: Growth problems associated with congenital heart disease in infancy. In Lenventhal E (ed): *Textbook of Gastroenterology and Nutrition in Infancy*. New York, Raven Press, 1981, pp 853–860.

81. Goldman AS: Modulation of the gastrointestinal tract of infants by human milk. Interfaces and interactions. An evolutionary process. *J Nutr* 130:426s–431s, 2000.

82. Goldstein RM, Hebiguchi T, Luk GD, et al: The effects of total parenteral nutrition on gastrointestinal growth and development. *J Pediatr Surg* 20:785–791, 1985.

83. Goran MI, Broemeling L, Herndon DN, et al: Estimating energy requirements in burned children: A new approach derived from measurements of resting energy expenditure. *Am J Clin Nutr* 54:35–40, 1991.

84. Gorrotxategi P, Reguilon MJ, Arana J, et al: Gastroesophageal reflex in association with the Sandifer syndrome. *Eur J Pediatr Surg* 5:203–205, 1995.

85. Gounaris A, Anatolitou F, Costalos C, Konstantellou E: Minimal enteral feeding, nasojejunal feeding and gastrin levels in premature infants. *Acta Paediatr Scand* 79:226–227, 1990.

86. Grant J, Denne SC: Effect of intermittent versus continuous enteral feeding on energy expenditure in premature infants. *J Pediatr* 118:928–932, 1991.

87. Gremse DA, Lytle JM, Sacks AI, Balistreri WF: Characterization of failure to imbibe in infants. *Clin Pediatr* 37:305–310, 1998.

88. Greene MA, Alexander JA, Knauf DG, et al: Endoscopic evaluation of the esophagus in infants and children immediately following intraoperative use of transesophageal echocardiography. *Chest* 116:1247–1250, 1999.

89. Hakanson E, Rutberg H, Jorfeldt L, Martensson J: Effects of the extradural administration of morphine or bupivacaine on the metabolic response to upper abdominal surgery. *Br J Anaesth* 57:394–399, 1985.

90. Hall DE, Kahan B, Snitzer J: Delirium associated with hypophosphatemia in a patient with anorexia nervosa. *J Adolesc Health* 15:176–178, 1994.

91. Hamilton JW, Boisen RJ, Yamamoto DT, et al: Sleeping on a wedge diminishes exposure of the esophagus to refluxed acid. *Dig Dis Sci* 33:518–522, 1988.

92. Heine RG, Cameron DJ, Chow CW, et al: Esophagitis in distressed infants: Poor diagnostic agreement between esophageal pH monitoring and histopathologic findings. *J Pediatr* 140:14–19, 2002.

93. Helms RA, Mauer EC, Hay WW Jr, et al: Effect of intravenous L-carnitine on growth parameters and fat metabolism during parenteral nutrition in neonates. *J Parenter Enteral Nutr* 14:448–453, 1990.

94. Helton E, Darragh R, Francis P, et al: Metabolic aspects of myocardial disease and a role for L-carnitine in the treatment of childhood cardiomyopathy. *Pediatrics* 105:1260–1270, 2000.

95. Hess J, Kruizinga K, Bijleveld CM, et al: Protein-losing enteropathy after Fontan operation. *J Thorac Cardiovasc Surg* 88:606–609, 1984.

96. Hume DM: The secretion of epinephrine, norepinephrine, and corticosteroids in the adrenal venous blood of the dog following single and repeated trauma. *Surg Forum* 8:111, 1957.

97. Hume DM, Egdahl RH: The importance of the brain in the endocrine response to injury. *Ann Surg* 150:697, 1959.

98. Hyman PE: Gastroesophageal reflux: One reason why baby won't eat. *J Pediatr* 125:S103–S109, 1994.

99. Ichord RN: Neurology of deglutition. In Tuchman DN, Walter RS (eds): *Disorders of Feeding and Swallowing in Infants and Children: Pathophysiology, Diagnosis, and Treatment*. San Diego, Singular Publishing Group, 1994, pp 37–52.

100. Jackson NC, Carroll PV, Russell-Jones DL, et al: The metabolic consequences of critical illness: Acute effects on glutamine and protein metabolism. *Am J Physiol* 276:E163–E170, 1999.

101. Jaquez M, Driscoll DA, Li M, et al: Unbalanced 15;22 translocation in a patient with manifestations of DiGeorge and velocardiofacial syndrome. *Am J Med Genet* 70:6–10, 1997.

102. Jones MO, Pierro A, Hammond P, et al: Glucose utilization in the surgical newborn infant receiving total parenteral nutrition. *J Pediatr Surg* 28:1121–1125, 1993.

103. Karlowicz MG, Gowen CW: Neonatal radiology casebook. *J Perinatol* 15:432–433, 1995.

104. Kavanaugh-McHugh AL, Hutton N, Holt E, et al: Echocardiographic abnormalities in pediatric HIV infection: Prevalence and serial changes. *Int Conf AIDS* 7:282, 1991.

105. Kelly DA: Liver complications of pediatric parenteral nutrition-epidemiology. *Nutrition* 14:153–157, 1998.

106. Kelly RF, Shumway SJ: Conservative management of postoperative chylothorax using somatostatin. *Ann Thorac Surg* 69:1944–1945, 2000.

107. Khan S, Orenstein SR, Shalaby TM: The effects of increasing doses of ranitidine on intragastric pH in children. *Gastroenterology* 120:A212, 2001.

108. King KC, Oliven A, Kalhan SC: Functional enteroinsular axis in full-term newborn infants. *Pediatr Res* 25:490–495, 1989.

109. Kinney JM, Weissman C: Forms of malnutrition in stressed and unstressed patients. *Clin Chest Med* 7:19–28, 1986.

110. Klein CJ, Stanek GS, Wiles CE: Overfeeding macronutrients in critically ill adults: Metabolic complications. *J Am Diet Assoc* 98:795–806, 1998.

111. Klein S, Peters EJ, Shangraw RE, Wolfe RR: Lipolytic response to metabolic stress in critically ill patients. *Crit Care Med* 19:776–779, 1991.

112. Klimberg VS, Souba WW, Dolson DJ, et al: Prophylactic glutamine protects the intestinal mucosa from radiation injury. *Cancer* 66:62–68, 1990.

113. Kosmack SN, Shalaby TM, Farankel EA, et al: Formula changes for 100 infants with symptoms of gastroesophageal reflux disease. *J Pediatr Gastroenterol Nutr* 33:423, 2001.

114. Kozam RL, Esguerra OE, Smith JJ: Cardiovascular beriberi. *Am J Cardiol* 30:418–422, 1972.

115. Lacey JM, Wilmore DW: Is glutamine a conditionally essential amino acid? *Nutr Rev* 48:297–309, 1990.

116. Launay V, Gottrand F, Turck D, et al: Percutaneous endoscopic gastrostomy in children: Influence on gastroesophageal reflux. *Pediatrics* 97:726–728, 1996.

117. Le Coultre C, Oberhansli I, Mossaz A, et al: Postoperative chylothorax in children; differences between vascular and traumatic origin. *J Pediatr Surg* 26:519–523, 1991.

118. Ledeboer M, Masclee AA, Biemond I, Lamers CB: Effect of intragastric or intraduodenal administration of a polymeric diet on gallbladder motility, small-bowel transit time and hormone release. *Am J Gastroenterol* 93:2089–2096, 1998.

119. Leder SB: Videofluoroscopic evaluation of aspiration with visual examination of the gag reflex and velar movement. *Dysphagia* 12:21–23, 1997.

120. Leder SB, Cohn SM, Mooer BA: Fiberoptic endoscopic documentation of the high incidence of aspiration following extubation in critically ill trauma patients. *Dysphagia* 13:208–212, 1998.

121. Levy J: Immunonutrition: The pediatric experience. *Nutrition* 14:341–347, 1998.

122. Lichtenberger L, Johnson LR: Gastrin in the ontogenic development of the small intestine. *Am J Physiol* 227:390–395, 1974.

123. Limperopoulos C, Majnemer A, Shevell MI, et al: Neurologic status of newborns with congenital heart defects before open heart surgery. *Pediatrics* 103:402–408, 1999.

124. Linde LM, Dunn OJ, Schireson R, Rasof B: Growth in children with congenital heart disease. *J Pediatr* 70:413–419, 1967.

125. Litov RE, Combs GF, Jr: Selenium in pediatric nutrition. *Pediatrics* 87:339–351, 1991.

126. Lloyd DA: Energy requirements of surgical newborn infants receiving parenteral nutrition. *Nutrition* 14:101–104, 1998.

127. Logemann JA: Manual for the videofluorographic study of swallowing. 2nd ed. Austin, TX: Pro-Ed, 1993.

128. Loughlin GM, Lefton-Greif MA: Dysfunctional swallowing and respiratory disease in children. *Adv Pediatr* 41:135–162, 1994.

129. Lucas A, Bloom SR, Aynsley-Green A: Gut hormones and "minimal enteral feeding". *Acta Paediatr Scand* 75:719–723, 1986.

130. Lugo RA, Harrison AM, Cash J, et al: Pharmacokinetics and pharmacodynamics of ranitidine in critically ill children. *Crit Care Med* 29:759–764, 2001.

131. Lundell KH, Sabel KG, Eriksson BO, Mellgren G: Glucose metabolism and insulin secretion in infants with symptomatic ventricular septal defect. *Acta Paediatr Scan* 78:620–626, 1989.

132. Lundell KH, Sabel KG, Eriksson BO, Mellgren G: Glucose metabolism and insulin secretion in children with cyanotic congenital heart disease. *Acta Pediatr* 86:1082–1084, 1997.

133. MacFie J, O'Boyle C, Mitchell CJ, et al: Gut origin of sepsis: A prospective study investigating associations between bacterial translocation, gastric microflora and septic morbidity. *Gut* 45:223–228, 1999.

134. Mansoor O, Beaufrere B, Boirie Y, et al: Increased mRNA levels for components of the lysosomal, Ca²⁺-activated, and ATP-ubiquitin-dependent proteolytic pathways in skeletal muscle from head trauma patients. *Proc Natl Acad Sci USA* 93:2714–2718, 1996.

135. Marik PE, Zaloga GP: Early enteral nutrition in acutely ill patients: A systematic review. *Crit Care Med* 29: 2264–2270, 2001.

136. Markham KM, Glover JL, Welsh RJ, et al: Octreotide in the treatment of thoracic duct injuries. *Am Surg* 66:1165–1167, 2000.

137. Mavroudis C: Management of postoperative chylothorax with nitric oxide: A critical review. *Crit Care Med* 27:877, 1999.

138. McCowen KC, Malhotra A, Bistrian BR: Stress-induced hyperglycemia. *Crit Care Clin* 17:107–124, 2001.

139. McDonald-McGinn DM, LaRossa D, Goldmuntz E, et al: The 22q11.2 deletion: Screening, diagnostic workup, and outcome of results; report on 181 patients. *Genet Test* 1:99–108, 1997.

140. McMurray JS, Holinger LD: Otolaryngic manifestations in children presenting with apparent life-threatening events. *Otolaryngol Head Neck Surg* 116:575–579, 1997.

141. McVeah P, Howman-Giles P, Kemp A: Pulmonary aspiration studied by radionuclide milk scanning and barium swallow roentgenography. *Am J Dis Child* 141:917–921, 1987.

142. Menon K, Clarson C: Adrenal function in pediatric critical illness. *Pediatr Critical Care Med* 3:112–116, 2002.

143. Mentec H, Dupont H, Bocchetti M, et al: Upper digestive intolerance during enteral nutrition in critically ill patients: Frequency, risk factors, and complications. *Crit Care Med* 29:1955–1961, 2001.

144. Meszaros K, Bojta J, Bautista AP, Lang CH, Spitzer JJ: Glucose utilization by Kupffer cells, endothelial cells, and granulocytes in endotoxemic rat liver. *Am J Physiol* 260:G7–G12, 1991.

145. Mevio E, Benazzo M, Quaglieri S, Mencherini S: Sinus infection in intensive care patients. *Rhinology* 34:232–236, 1996.

146. Mezoff AG, Gremse DS, Farrell MK: Hypophosphatemia in the nutritional recovery syndrome. *Am J Dis Child* 143:1111–1112, 1989.

147. Mitchell IM, Logan RW, Pollock JCS, Jamieson MPG: Nutritional status of children with congenital heart disease. *Br Heart J* 73:277–283, 1995.

148. Mitchell IM, Davies PS, Day JM, et al: Energy expenditure in children with congenital heart disease, before and after cardiac surgery. *J Thorac Cardiovasc Surg* 107:374–380, 1994.

149. Mizock BA: Alterations in carbohydrate metabolism during stress: A review of the literature. *Am J Med* 98:75–84, 1995.

150. Montecalvo MA, Steger KA, Farber HW, et al: Nutritional outcome and pneumonia in critical care patients randomized to gastric versus jejunal tube feedings. *Crit Care Med* 20:1377–1387, 1992.

151. Moore FD: Endocrine changes after anesthesia, surgery and unanesthetized trauma in man. *Rec Prog Hormone Res* 13:511, 1957.

152. Morales E, Craig LD, MacLean WC, Jr: Dietary management of malnourished children with a new enteral feeding. *J Am Diet Assoc* 91:1233–1238, 1991.

153. Noviski N, Yehuda YB, Serour F, et al: Does the size of nasogastric tubes affect gastroesophageal reflux in children? *J Pediatr Gastroenterol Nutr* 29:448–451, 1999.

154. Ohtani Y, Endo F, Matsuda I: Carnitine deficiency and hyperammonemia associated with valproic acid therapy. *J Pediatr* 101:782–785, 1982.

155. Okada Y, Klein N, van Saene HK, Pierro A: Small volumes of enteral feedings normalise immune function in infants receiving parenteral nutrition. *J Pediatr Surg* 33:16–19, 1998.

156. Olcay L, Ozer S, Gurgey A, et al: Parameters of iron deficiency in children with cyanotic congenital heart disease. *Pediatr Cardiol* 17:150–154, 1996.

157. Panadero E, Lopez-Herce J, Caro L, et al: Transpyloric enteral feedings in critically ill children. *J Pediatr Gastroenterol Nutr* 26:43–48, 1998.

158. Perie S, Laccourreye O, Bou-Malhab F, Brasnu D: Aspiration in unilateral recurrent laryngeal nerve paralysis after surgery. *Am J Otolaryngol* 19: 18–23, 1998.

159. Pietsch JB, Ford C, Whitlock JA: Nasogastric tube feeding in children with high-risk cancer: A pilot study. *J Pediatr Hematol Oncol* 21: 111–114, 1999.

160. Platt MP, Anand KJ, Aynsley-Green A: The ontogeny of the metabolic and endocrine stress response in the human fetus, neonate and child. *Intensive Care Med* 15 Suppl 1:S44–S45, 1989.

161. Pratap U, Slavik Z, Ofoe VD, et al: Octreotide to treat postoperative chylothorax after cardiac operations in children. *Ann Thorac Surg* 72: 1740–1742, 2001.

162. Puntis JW, Thwaites R, Abel G, Stringer MD: Children with neurological disorders do not always need fundoplication concomitant with percutaneous endoscopic gastrostomy. *Dev Med Child Neurol* 42:97–99, 2000.

163. Putnam PE: GERD and crying; cause and effect or unhappy coexistence? *J Pediatr* 140:2–3, 2002.

164. Reilly S, Skuse D, Poblete X: Prevalence of feeding problems and oral motor dysfunction in children with cerebral palsy: A community survey. *J Pediatr* 129:877–882, 1996.

165. Rheuban KS, Kron IL, Carpenter MA, et al: Pleuroperitoneal shunts for refractory chylothorax after operation for congenital heart disease. *Ann Thorac Surg* 53:85–87, 1992.

166. Rogers BT, Msall ME, Buck GM, et al: Neurodevelopmental outcome of infants with hypoplastic left heart syndrome. *J Pediatr* 126:496–498, 1995.

167. Rothenberg SS: Experience with 220 consecutive laparoscopic Nissen fundoplications in infants and children. *J Pediatr Surg* 33:274–278, 1998.

168. Rousou JA, Tighe DA, Garb JL, et al: Risk of dysphagia after transesophageal echocardiography during cardiac operations. *Ann Thorac Surg* 69:486–489, 2000.

169. Rudolph CD, Mazur LJ, Liptak GS, et al: Guidelines for evaluation and treatment of gastroesophageal reflux in infants and children: Recommendations of the North American Society for Pediatric Gastroenterology and Nutrition. *J Pediatr Gastroenterol Nutr* 32:S1–S31, 2001.

170. Sabesin SM, Berlin RG, Humphries TJ, et al: Famotidine relieves symptoms of gastroesophageal reflux disease and heals erosions and ulcerations. Results of a multicenter placebo-controlled dose ranging study. *Arch Intern Med* 151:2394–2400, 1991.

171. Saito Y, Hashimoto T, Sasaki M, et al: Effect of selenium deficiency on cardiac function of individuals with severe disabilities under long-term tube feeding. *Dev Med Child Neurol* 40:743–748, 1998.

172. Salzer HR, Haschke F, Wimmer M, et al: Growth and nutritional intake of infants with congenital heart disease. *Pediatr Cardiol* 10:17–23, 1989.

173. Sax HC, Bower RH: Hepatic complications of total parenteral nutrition. *J Parenter Enteral Nutr* 12:615–618, 1988.

174. Schlegel L, Coudray-Lucas C, Barbut F, et al: Bacterial dissemination rather than translocation mediates hypermetabolic response in endotoxemic rats. *Crit Care Med* 27:1511–1516, 1999.

175. Schwarz SM, Corredor J, Fisher-Medina J, et al: Diagnosis and treatment of feeding disorders in children with developmental disabilities. *Pediatrics* 108:671–676, 2001.

176. Schwarz SM, Gewitz MH, See CC, et al: Enteral nutrition in infants with congenital heart disease and growth failure. *Pediatrics* 86:368–373, 1990.

177. Servidei S, Bertini E, DiMauro S: Hereditary metabolic cardiomyopathies. *Adv Pediatr* 41:1–32, 1994.

178. Shamir R, Dagan O, Abramovitch D, et al: Thiamine deficiency in children with congenital heart disease before and after corrective surgery. *J Parenter Enteral Nutr* 24:154–158, 2000.

179. Shangraw RE, Jahoor F, Miyoshi H, et al: Differentiation between septic and postburn insulin resistance. *Metabolism* 38:983–989, 1989.

180. Silberbach M, Shumaker D, et al: Predicting hospital charge and length of stay for congenital heart disease surgery. *Am J Cardiol* 72:958–963, 1993.

181. Simon GL, Gorbach SL: Intestinal microflora in health and disease. *Gastroenterology* 86: 174–193, 1984.

182. Slagle TA, Gross SJ: Effect of early low-volume enteral substrate on subsequent feeding tolerance in very low birth weight infants. *J Pediatr* 113:526–531, 1988.

183. Sondheimer JM, Hamilton JR: Intestinal function in infants with severe congenital heart disease. *J Pediatr* 92:572–578, 1978.

184. Souba WW: Glutamine: A key substrate for the splanchnic bed. *Ann Rev Nutr* 11:285–308, 1991.

185. Spain DA, DeWeese RC, Reynolds MA, Richardson JD: Transpyloric passage of feeding tubes in patients with head injuries does not decrease complications. *J Trauma* 39:1100–1102, 1995.

186. Spalding HK, Sullivan KJ, et al: Bedside placement of transpyloric feeding tubes in the pediatric intensive care unit using gastric insufflation. *Crit Care Med* 28:2041–2044, 2000.

187. Sperling MA: Integration of fuel homeostasis by insulin and glucagon in the newborn. *Monographs in Paediatrics* 16:39–58, 1982.

188. Splaingard ML, Hutchins B, Sulton LD, Chaudhuri G: Aspiration in rehabilitation patients: Videofluoroscopy vs bedside clinical assessment. *Arch Phys Med Rehabil* 69:637–640, 1988.

189. Stanley CA: New genetic defects in mitochondrial fatty acid oxidation and carnitine deficiency. *Adv Pediatr* 34:59–88, 1987.

190. Steinhorn DM, Kalhan S: A spoonful of sugar …? *Crit Care Med* 30:252–253, 2002.

191. Strong R, Condon S, Solinger M: Equal aspiration rates from postpylorus and intragastric-placed small-bore nasoenteric feeding tubes: A randomized, prospective study. *J Parenter Enteral Nutr* 16:59–63, 1992.

192. Taitz LS: *The Obese Child.* Boston, Blackwell Scientific Publications, 1983, pp 1–15.

193. Tein I, De Vivo DC, Bierman F, et al: Impaired skin fibroblast carnitine uptake in primary systemic carnitine deficiency manifested by childhood carnitine-responsive cardiomyopathy. *Pediatr Res* 28:247–255, 1990.

194. Thommessen M, Heiberg A, Kase BF: Feeding problems in children with congenital heart disease: The impact on energy intake and growth outcome. *Eur J Clin Nutr* 46:457–464, 1992.

195. Thompson LD, McElhinney DB, Jue KL, Hodge D: Gastroesophageal reflux after repair of atrioventricular septal defect in infants with trisomy 21: A comparison of medical and surgical therapy. *J Pediatr Surg* 34:1359–1363, 1999.

196. Tomkins AM, Garlick PJ, Schofield WN, Waterlow JC: The combined effects of infection and malnutrition on protein metabolism in children. *Clin Sci* 65:313–324, 1983.

197. Tovar JA, Olivares P, Diaz M, et al: Functional results of laparoscopic fundoplication in children. *J Pediatr Gastroenterol Nutr* 26:429–431, 1998.

198. Tripp ME, Shug AL: Plasma carnitine concentrations in cardiomyopathy patients. *Biochem Med* 32:199–206, 1984.

199. Tsai TP, Yu JM, Wu YL, et al: Change of serum growth factors in infants with isolated ventricular defect undergoing surgical repair. *Ann Thorac Surg* 73:1765–1768, 2002.

200. Udelsman R, Norton JA, Jelenich SE, et al: Responses of the hypothalamic-pituitary-adrenal and renin-angiotensin axes and the sympathetic system during controlled surgical and anesthetic stress. *J Clin Endocrinol Metab* 64:986–994, 1987.

201. Ukai M, Moran WH, Jr, Zimmermann B: The role of visceral afferent pathways on vasopressin secretion and urinary excretory patterns during surgical stress. *Ann Surg* 168:16–28, 1968.

202. Unger R, DeKleermaeker M, Gidding SS, Christoffel KK: Calories count. Improved weight gain with dietary intervention in congenital heart disease. *Am J Dis Child* 146:1078–1084, 1992.

203. Unger RH, Orci L: Glucagon and the A cell: Physiology and pathophysiology (first two parts). *N Engl J Med* 304:1518–1524, 1981.

204. Unno N, Hodin RA, Fink MP: Acidic conditions exacerbate interferon-γ induced intestinal epithelial hyperpermeability: Role for peroxynitrous acid. *Crit Care Med* 27:1429–1436, 1999.

205. Ursini F, Bindoli A: The role of selenium peroxidases in the protection against oxidative damage of membranes. *Chem Phys Lipids* 44:255–276, 1987.

206. Uysal S, Kalayci AG, Baysal K: Cardiac functions in children with Vitamin D deficiency rickets. *Pediatr Cardiol* 20:283–286, 1999.

207. Vaisman N, Leigh T, Voet H, et al: Malabsorption in infants with congenital heart disease under diuretic treatment. *Pediatr Res* 36:545–549, 1994.

208. Van den Berghe G: Novel insights into the neuroendocrinology of critical illness. *Eur J Endocrinol* 143:1–13, 2000.

209. van den Berghe G, de Zegher F, Bouillon R: Clinical review 95: Acute and prolonged critical illness as different neuroendocrine paradigms. *J Clin Endocrinol Metab* 83:1827–1834, 1998.

210. van den Berghe G, Wouters P, Weekers F, et al: Intensive insulin therapy in critically ill patients. *N Engl J Med* 345:1359–1367, 2001.

211. Vanderhoof JA, Hofschire PJ, Baluff MA, et al: Continuous enteral feedings. An important adjunct to the management of complex congenital heart disease. *Am J Dis Child* 136:825–827, 1982.

212. van Rij AM, McKenzie JM, Robinson MF, Thomson CD: Selenium and total parenteral nutrition. *J Parenter Enteral Nutr* 3:235–239, 1979.

213. van Staaten HL, Gerards LJ, Krediet TG: Chylothorax in the neonatal period. *Eur J Pediatr* 152:2–5, 1993.

214. Varan B, Tokel K, Yilmaz G: Malnutrition and growth failure in cyanotic and acyanotic congenital heart disease with and without pulmonary hypertension. *Arch Dis Child* 81:49–52, 1999.

215. Vary TC: Regulation of skeletal muscle protein turnover during sepsis. *Curr Opin Clin Nutr Metabolic Care* 1:217–224, 1998.

216. Venihaki M, Dikkes P, Carrigan A, Karalis KP: Corticotropin-releasing hormone regulates IL-6 expression during inflammation. *J Clin Invest* 108: 1159–1166, 2001.

217. Vinnars E, Hammarqvist F, von der Decken A, Wernerman J: Role of glutamine and its analogs in posttraumatic muscle protein and amino acid metabolism. *J Parenter Enteral Nutr* 14:125S–129S, 1990.

218. Vinton NE, Dahlstrom KA, Strobel CT, Ament ME: Macrocytosis and pseudoalbinism: Manifestations of selenium deficiency. *J Pediatr* 111:711–717, 1987.

219. Volk DM, Cutliff SA: Selenium deficiency and cardiomyopathy in a patient with cystic fibrosis. *J KY Med Assoc* 84:222–224, 1986.

220. Wald ER: Microbiology of acute and chronic sinusitis in children and adults. *Am J Med Sci* 316:13–20, 1998.

221. Waterlow JC: Classification and definition of protein-calorie malnutrition. *Br Med J* 3:566–569, 1972.

222. Waterlow JC, Alleyne GA: Protein malnutrition in children: Advances in knowledge in the last ten years. *Adv Protein Chem* 25:117–241, 1971.

223. Webb JG, Kiess MC, Chan-Yan CC: Malnutrition and the heart. *Can Med Assoc J* 135:753–758, 1986.

224. Weiner I, Khalil T, Thompson JC: Gastrin. In Thompson JC (ed): *Gastrointestinal Endocrinology.* New York, McGraw Hill, 1987, pp 194–212.

225. Weinzimer SA: Endocrine aspects of 22q11.2 deletion syndrome. *Genet Med* 3:19–22, 2001.

226. Wells DH, Zachman RD: Nasojejunal feedings in low–birth weight infants. *J Pediatr* 87:276–279, 1975.

227. White MS, Shepherd RW, MeEniery JA: Energy expenditure in 100 ventilated, critically ill children; improving the accuracy of predictive equations. *Crit Care Med* 28: 2307–2312, 2000.

228. Williamson RC: Intestinal adaptation (second of two parts). Mechanisms of control. *N Engl J Med* 298:1444–1450, 1978.

229. Wilson L, Oliva-Hemker M: Percutaneous endoscopic gastrostomy in small medically complex infants. *Endoscopy* 33:433–436, 2001.

230. Wilson MH: Feeding the healthy child. In Oski F (ed): *Principles and Procedures in Pediatrics*. Philadelphia, J.B. Lippincott, 1990, pp 533–552.

231. Winter SC, Szabo-Aczel S, Curry CJ, et al: Plasma carnitine deficiency. Clinical observations in 51 pediatric patients. *Am J Dis Child* 141:660–665, 1987.

232. Wolfe MM, Sachs G: Acid suppression: Optimizing therapy for gastroduodenal ulcer healing, gastroesophageal reflux disease, and stress-related erosive syndrome. *Gastroeneterology* 118:S1–S9, 2000.

233. Wolfe RR: Carbohydrate metabolism in the critically ill patient. Implications for nutritional support. *Crit Care Clin* 3:11–24, 1987.

234. Wolfe RR, Durkot MJ, Allsop JR, Burke JF: Glucose metabolism in severely burned patients. *Metabolism* 28:1031–1039, 1979.

235. Wolff AB, Silen ML, Kokoska ER, Rodgers BM: Treatment of refractory chylothorax with externalized pleuroperitoneal shunts in children. *Ann Thorac Surg* 68:1053–1057, 1999.

236. Wolff PH: The serial organization of sucking in the young infant. *Pediatrics* 42:943–956, 1968.

237. Worley G, Claerhout SJ, Combs SP: Hypophosphatemia in malnourished children during refeeding. *Clin Pediatr* 37:347–352, 1995.

238. Wurnig PN, Hollaus PH, Ohtsuka T, et al: Thoracoscopic direct clipping of the thoracic duct for chylopericardium and chylothorax. *Ann Thorac Surg* 70:1662–1665, 2000.

239. Xanthou M, Bines J, Walker WA: Human milk and intestinal host defense in newborns; an update. *Adv Pediatr* 42:171–208, 1995.

240. Xu D, Lu Q, Deitch EA: Elemental diet-induced bacterial translocation associated with systemic and intestinal immune suppression. *J Parenter Enteral Nutr* 22:37–41, 1998.

241. Zaloga GP, Roberts PR: Bedside placement of enteral feeding tubes in the intensive care unit. *Crit Care Med* 26:987–988, 1998.

242. Zazzo JF, Chalas J, Lafont A, et al: Is nonobstructive cardiomyopathy in AIDS a selenium deficiency–related disease? *J Parenter Enteral Nutr* 12:537–538, 1988.

243. Zbar RI, Smith RJ: Vocal fold paralysis in infants twelve months of age and younger. *Otolaryngol Head Neck Surg* 114:18–21, 1996.

244. Zlotkin, SH Atkinson S, Lockitch G: Trace elements in nutrition for premature infants. *Clin Perinatol* 22:223–240, 1995.

Chapter 16

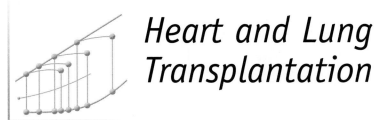

Heart and Lung Transplantation

PAUL M. KIRSHBOM, MD, J. WILLIAM GAYNOR, MD,
and THOMAS L. SPRAY, MD

INTRODUCTION

For children with advanced acquired or congenital cardiopulmonary disease, heart and lung transplantation have become important treatment alternatives.[63] Despite continued improvements in early outcomes following pediatric thoracic organ transplantation, the annual number of heart and lung transplants performed in children plateaued in 1990 and has begun to decline.[29] Donor availability continues to limit the number of transplants performed in infants and children, with as many as 15% to 30% of heart transplant candidates dying on the waiting list.[6,11] Medium- to long-term complications including chronic rejection, graft coronary vasculopathy, bronchiolitis obliterans, and the side effects of chronic immunosuppression remain serious problems, which have not been resolved by intensive research. Even with these problems, however, heart and lung transplantation improve the length and quality of life for children with end-stage cardiopulmonary disease.

INDICATIONS

Heart Transplantation

The indication for heart transplantation in children is related to the age of the child. Approximately 66% of infants younger than 1 year of age who are listed for cardiac transplantation have complex congenital heart disease, whereas the majority of older children (6 to 15 years of age) suffer from cardiomyopathies of multiple causes (Fig. 16-1). Hypoplastic left heart syndrome (HLHS) is the most frequent indication for neonatal heart transplantation with some centers utilizing transplantation as the primary therapy for this disease.[14,57] The use of transplantation as the primary therapy for HLHS is controversial, as this limits the availability of donor organs for other infants for whom there may not be alternative therapies. Other less common congenital malformations that can lead to consideration of heart transplantation include pulmonary atresia with intact ventricular septum and right ventricular dependent coronary circulation, the more complex forms of

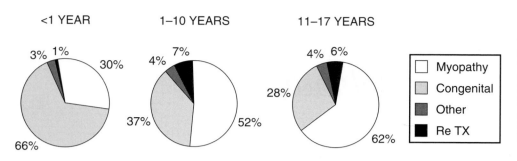

FIGURE 16-1 Indications for heart transplantation broken down by recipient age. ReTx, retransplantation. (Adapted from Boucek MM, Edwards LB, Keck BM, et al: The registry of the International Society for Heart and Lung Transplantation: Seventh Official Pediatric Report—2004. *J Heart Lung Transplant* 23:933–947, 2004; with permission from Elsevier Science.)

single ventricle, truncus arteriosus, double-outlet right ventricle, Ebstein's anomaly, unbalanced atrioventricular canal, and transposition of the great arteries.

Whereas cardiomyopathy is the second most common indication for transplantation in infants, it is the most frequent diagnosis of children requiring transplantation beyond infancy. Idiopathic dilated cardiomyopathy is the most common diagnosis followed by viral, familial, and hypertrophic cardiomyopathies. Unresectable cardiac tumors and chemotherapy-induced myocardial dysfunction are less common indications for transplantation in older children.

Despite improving outcomes after repair of complex congenital cardiac defects, some children who have undergone corrective or palliative procedures still develop end-stage cardiac disease and become candidates for transplantation. Many technical modifications have been described to overcome complex congenital anomalies and the residua of previous operations.[41,71,73]

Lung Transplantation

As with heart transplantation, the indications for pediatric lung transplantation are related to the age of the child at presentation. Infants and young children (<1 year old) most commonly present with congenital anomalies (congenital heart disease, pulmonary vein stenosis, congenital surfactant protein deficiency, and others) or pulmonary hypertension (primary or secondary) (Fig. 16-2). After the age of 1, cystic fibrosis becomes an increasingly significant problem and is the most common diagnosis in children older than 11 years of age (Fig. 16-3). Despite improvements in the treatment and prognosis of cystic fibrosis, some children develop early pulmonary dysfunction and should be considered for transplantation when they develop progressive hypercapnia or oxygen dependence, increasing frequency of hospitalizations, or poor weight gain despite adequate nutrition. Another problem that patients with cystic fibrosis face is the development of multidrug-resistant pseudomonal infections. Given the

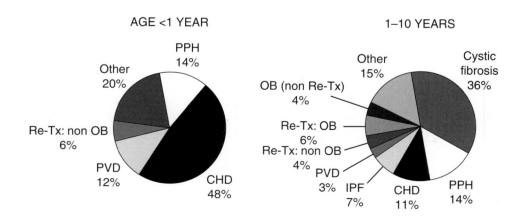

FIGURE 16-2 Indications for lung transplantation in younger recipients. CHD, congenital heart disease; IPF, idiopathic pulmonary fibrosis; PVD, pulmonary vascular disease; OB, obliterative bronchiolitis; Retx, retransplantation. (Adapted from Boucek MM, Edwards LB, Keck BM, et al: The registry of the International Society of Heart and Lung Transplantation: Seventh Official Pediatric Report—2004. *J Heart Lung Transplant* 23:933–947, 2004; with permission from Elsevier Science.)

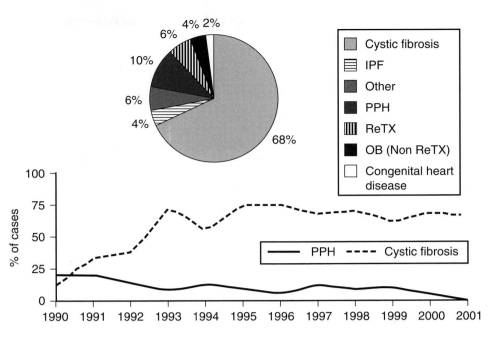

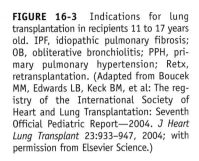

FIGURE 16-3 Indications for lung transplantation in recipients 11 to 17 years old. IPF, idiopathic pulmonary fibrosis; OB, obliterative bronchiolitis; PPH, primary pulmonary hypertension; Retx, retransplantation. (Adapted from Boucek MM, Edwards LB, Keck BM, et al: The registry of the International Society of Heart and Lung Transplantation: Seventh Official Pediatric Report—2004. *J Heart Lung Transplant* 23:933–947, 2004; with permission from Elsevier Science.)

difficulties in treating infections with these organisms in immunocompromised patients, some consideration must be given to transplant listing before development of pan-resistant strains.

Patients with primary pulmonary hypertension typically do not present for lung transplantation until adulthood; however, some children can develop rapidly worsening symptoms. Children with pulmonary hypertension due to pulmonary vein stenosis are at increased risk for sudden death while waiting for transplantation. Children with secondary pulmonary hypertension due to cardiac disease (Eisenmenger's syndrome) can be considered for bilateral lung transplantation with concomitant cardiac repair, if the cardiac defect is amenable to surgical correction, rather than combined heart-lung transplantation.[9,64]

Heart-Lung Transplantation

Though some children with Eisenmenger's syndrome have cardiac defects that are amenable to surgical repair, those with poor ventricular function, serious valvular disease, or uncorrectable cardiac anomalies must be considered for combined heart and lung transplantation. Heart-lung transplantation has been employed for patients with cystic fibrosis, occasionally with utilization of the recipient's heart for subsequent "domino" transplantation; however, the majority of institutions perform bilateral lung transplants in cystic fibrosis patients with normal cardiac function.

CONTRAINDICATIONS

Contraindications to pediatric thoracic organ transplantation include any uncontrolled medical problem that cannot be directly attributed to the organ of interest. Examples include poorly controlled diabetes mellitus, active collagen-vascular disease, hepatic or renal failure, bacterial infections outside the respiratory tract, chromosomal abnormalities or neurological dysfunction precluding a meaningful quality of life, history of medical noncompliance, and lack of family support. Even patients with end-organ dysfunction involving other organ systems may be candidates for thoracic organ transplantation if circumstances permit multiple organ transplantation. Multiple organ transplants such as heart/kidney, heart/liver, and lung/kidney or liver have been performed in children. Pulmonary infections are not considered contraindications to lung transplantation unless the organisms are resistant to all antibiotics. Down and other genetic syndromes are not contraindications to transplantation as long as the syndrome is not associated with any other contraindications and the patient's family support is capable of strict adherence to the post-transplant medical regimen. Complex congenital anomalies, including pulmonary and systemic venous abnormalities, can present technical challenges during transplantation; however, these anomalies do not constitute a contraindication in and of themselves.

Despite the technical similarities between adult and pediatric thoracic organ transplantation, it is important to remember that children are not merely small adults and that all of the contraindications to adult transplantation do not necessarily apply to children. A study from the Children's Hospital of Philadelphia confirmed that several common exclusion criteria applied to adult lung transplantation, including preoperative ventilator dependence, high-dose steroid therapy, and prior thoracotomy, had no demonstrable effect on postoperative mortality in pediatric patients.[39] A preoperative requirement of mechanical circulatory support such as extracorporeal membrane oxygenation (ECMO) is not a contraindication to transplantation as long as the patient does not develop any of the already mentioned exclusion criteria. One group of patients who require particular care are cyanotic children who have had previous thoracotomies, as they can develop considerable chest wall collaterals, which increase the risk of hemorrhage.

PREOPERATIVE MANAGEMENT

Recipient Evaluation and Management

Evaluation of a potential transplant recipient requires a multidisciplinary approach that includes cardiology, surgery, pulmonology, psychiatry, social work, and other disciplines. Medication compliance issues can be particularly difficult in adolescent patients and should be discussed with the patient and family during the preoperative evaluation. Cardiopulmonary function must be carefully evaluated with attention paid to pulmonary vascular resistance and responsiveness to pulmonary vasodilators. A transpulmonary gradient greater than 12 mm Hg or a pulmonary vascular resistance greater than 6 Wood's units that is not responsive to oxygen or other pulmonary vasodilators is a relative contraindication to heart transplantation because of the increased risk of right ventricular failure.[36]

From an infectious disease standpoint, serology for toxoplasmosis, Epstein-Barr virus, cytomegalovirus, and human immunodeficiency virus (HIV) should be obtained for all patients. Screening urine and sputum cultures as well as surveillance blood cultures also should be obtained for patients who are hospitalized. Panel reactive antibodies (PRAs) are screened to detect the presence of preformed antibodies to human lymphocyte antigens (HLAs).[78] High PRA titers suggest the need for a preoperative donor-recipient crossmatch to decrease the likelihood of hyperacute rejection. Patients with high PRA titers have been successfully transplanted with reduction of PRA levels using several different protocols including pre- and posttransplant plasmapheresis, mycophenolate mofetil, photopheresis, and intravenous immunoglobulin.[3,54,58,61,70]

Because of the limited availability of donor organs, children who are listed for thoracic organ transplantation may have to wait some time before an organ becomes available. As a result, these children are at risk for progressive cardiac or pulmonary dysfunction leading to multisystem failure. In the adult population, considerable experience has been gathered concerning the use of mechanical circulatory support as a bridge to cardiac transplantation. A variety of devices including the Heartmate, Thoratec, Novacor, Symbion, Berlin Heart, and others have been used for this purpose.[11,67] Though these devices carry with them an inherent risk of driveline infection and thromboembolic complications, patients receiving transplants after mechanical circulatory support have been reported to have posttransplant outcomes similar to those of patients receiving primary transplants.[11] The use of mechanical support as a bridge to transplant in children has been limited due to the lack of support devices of appropriate size for implantation in small children. Though there have been reports of relatively small numbers of patients bridged to transplant with paracorporeal and intracorporeal ventricular assist devices,[38,60,72] the system used most commonly in infants and children is ECMO.

ECMO has several disadvantages, including the need for continuous sedation and restriction to the intensive care unit

setting; however, availability, experience, and the widespread use of ECMO as a support device for children with respiratory failure have led to its use as a bridge to heart transplantation at many institutions.[17,19,32,37] In most cases ECMO has been required for 100 to 200 hours before transplantation,[19,32] but in one case a child was supported for 1126 hours before a heart became available for a successful transplant. One point that must be considered when ECMO is used as a bridge to either heart or lung transplantation is that ECMO frequently does not provide adequate decompression of the left ventricle, which can result in left ventricle (LV) distension and pulmonary venous hypertension. These patients may require left-sided decompression either through placement of an LV vent or creation of an atrial septal defect (ASD) to prevent secondary cardiopulmonary injury.

Children who are listed for lung transplantation are frequently critically ill with a significant percentage requiring hospitalization with or without mechanical ventilation and pressor support before donor organs become available. As a result, aggressive maneuvers may be necessary in an attempt to maintain end-organ viability and transplant candidacy for as long as possible. Over the past decade, advances in mechanical ventilation with jet and high-frequency ventilators as well as the availability of prostacyclin and nitric oxide have broadened the armamentarium available for use in these children. Despite these measures, mortality on the waiting list remains in the 19% to 25% range for infants and children.[9,31]

The use of ECMO before lung transplantation has been less common than for heart transplantation; however, there has been some experience reported in both the adult and pediatric populations. The Toronto Lung Transplant Group reported four adult patients who received pre–lung transplant ECMO support.[34,49,69] In the pediatric population, Koutlas and colleagues[39] noted two children who required pretransplant ECMO in their review of "high-risk" lung transplant recipients. Another three children who received ECMO support before lung transplantation were included in a report from the St. Louis Children's Hospital.[9] Overall the outcomes of lung transplantation after ECMO support in adults have been relatively poor with only one of the four patients reported in the literature surviving to discharge from the hospital. Of the five pediatric patients included in the reviews mentioned, two survived to discharge. Our policy when ECMO is used as a bridge for either heart or lung transplantation is to continue support until the child recovers, is successfully transplanted, or develops a contraindication to transplantation.

Donor Management

Initial donor evaluation must begin with determination of brain death. Involvement of an organ procurement agency should be initiated as soon as possible after brain death has been established to minimize the length of time between brain death and possible organ harvest. The hormonal and hemodynamic changes associated with brain death are detrimental to both cardiac and pulmonary function, so special consideration must be given to maintenance of donor organ function in the physiologically abnormal state produced by brain death.[51] Treatment with thyroxine often results in decreased inotrope requirements with salvage of some organs that might otherwise not be considered for transplantation.

Management of neurogenic shock requires volume resuscitation, but care must be employed in both the amount and type of volume administered. If possible, blood or colloids should be used and volume status should be assessed using central venous or pulmonary capillary wedge pressures. Bronchoscopy can be useful both for diagnostic and therapeutic purposes such as removal of mucous plugs, which can decrease atelectasis and improve pulmonary gas exchange.[53] Transthoracic echocardiography is usually performed on potential heart donors to rule out any intracardiac abnormalities or regional wall motion abnormality. Arterial blood gas measurement performed on potential lung donors may determine the adequacy of gas exchange, and a chest x-ray is done to rule out the possibility of pulmonary contusion or infectious infiltrate. Blood should be obtained from the potential organ donor for serologic studies to determine if there are any transmissible diseases (i.e., HIV, hepatitis, and so forth) and ABO blood typing. Even though it is important to transplant organs into ABO-compatible recipients, there is some evidence that this criterion is not absolutely necessary in neonates who have not yet developed antibodies to major blood group antigens.[74]

Given the scarcity of pediatric organs available for transplantation, many patients are considered for organ donation even if organ function is initially borderline or unacceptable. Studies have shown that aggressive donor management can significantly improve donor organ function and early post-transplant results.[53,75] There has been some interest in non-heart-beating donors for lung transplantation, but this attempt to expand the donor pool remains experimental. Because of the limited donor pool, neonatal transplant programs often accept organs from a wider geographic area, and thus with longer cold ischemic times, than an adult program would consider. de Begona[16] and colleagues have reported that longer ischemic times, even as long as 9.5 hours, do not adversely affect long-term outcomes for pediatric heart transplant recipients.

The size range of donor organs that can be accepted for pediatric heart transplants is larger than for adults. Donors up to 2.5 times the weight of the recipient can be accepted with no evidence of ill effects in most cases. Evaluations of graft growth have shown that the velocity of cardiac growth is initially slow for these oversized organs with normal growth later in life, essentially allowing the recipient to grow into the larger organ.[24] Certain children with dilated cardiomyopathy and massive cardiomegaly can tolerate organs from donors as much as three times their weight, although care must be taken to prevent atelectasis from pulmonary compression.

Another option that has increased donor organ availability for small recipients is the use of lobar transplants from adult donors into children. This technique can be applied for both brain-dead and living-related donors. Living-related lobar transplantation is a relatively new technique that provides organs for transplantation for a limited population of children. In the majority of cases children receive a lower lobe from each parent for bilateral lung transplantation. Donors have generally done well after the procedure, and early to midterm outcomes for recipients have been comparable to cadaveric transplant recipients. There have been reports that recipients of living-related lobar transplants have better pulmonary function at 2 years and experience bronchiolitis obliterans less frequently.[65]

OPERATIVE TECHNIQUES

Donor Organ Harvest

Combined thoracic and abdominal organ harvest requires the complex interaction of multiple surgical and operating room teams at several locations. From the perspective of the thoracic organ harvest team, close communication must be maintained with the implantation team or teams while coordinating activities with the abdominal harvest surgeons. As always, careful anesthesia management is critical because organ harvesting can be a protracted procedure with considerable insensible volume losses and hypothermia.

Once adequate monitoring and intravenous access has been established, a long midline incision is made, extending from the sternal notch to the pubis. A median sternotomy is performed and a sternal retractor is placed superiorly. The pericardium is incised and pericardial sutures are secured to hemostats, which allows easy access to the pleural spaces if the lungs are to be harvested. The heart is inspected to rule out undocumented injuries, atherosclerosis, or evidence of congenital anomalies. The lungs are also palpated and inspected if lung harvest is required. If the organs are felt to be acceptable, the implantation team is informed so the recipient operation can be timed appropriately.

The donor heart is mobilized in preparation for explantation. The superior vena cava (SVC) is circumferentially dissected free from surrounding tissues, exposing the azygos vein and the juncture of the innominate and jugular veins. It is often simpler to doubly ligate and divide the azygous vein at this point rather than during the explantation. After the superior venous structures have been mobilized and encircled, the inferior vena cava (IVC) is dissected free from the diaphragm and encircled with a tie or tape. The aorta must be dissected away from the pulmonary artery to allow application of the cross-clamp. At this point, the heart is covered with warm moist pads while the abdominal team completes their dissection.

It is important for the harvesting team to know the anatomy and requirements of the recipient. For patients with no anomalies or special needs, the heart can be harvested in a manner similar to adult heart transplant patients. The SVC can be divided near or just below the azygous vein, the IVC at the diaphragm, the aorta just proximal to the innominate artery takeoff, and the pulmonary artery (PA) just proximal or beyond the bifurcation (Fig. 16-4). In children with congenital heart disease, however, additional donor material may be required for reconstruction during implantation. For example, patients with hypoplastic left heart syndrome require reconstruction of the aortic arch and proximal descending aorta; thus additional aorta must be harvested for reconstruction. Patients who have had a Fontan procedure might need additional pulmonary artery to allow for PA reconstruction as well as additional length on the SVC, often including the innominate vein, for venous reconstruction. For lung harvests, the trachea is also identified and encircled between the aorta and SVC, as high as the surrounding structures allow so as to leave space above the carina.

When the abdominal team is ready, purse-string sutures are placed in the ascending aorta and, if the lungs are to be harvested, the PA just proximal to the bifurcation. Cardioplegia and pulmoplegia cannulae are inserted, de-aired,

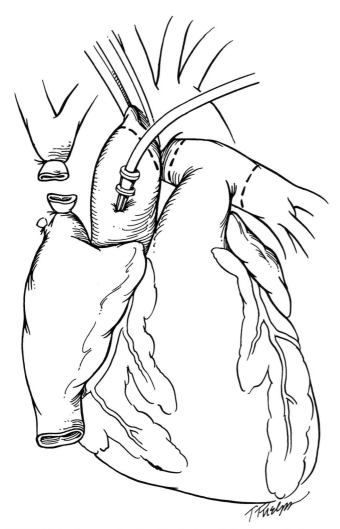

FIGURE 16-4 Donor cardiac dissection for harvest. The aorta and pulmonary artery are divided at the dotted lines.

and connected to the appropriate plegia solution. If the lungs are to be harvested, 250 to 500 mcg of prostacyclin are injected into the PA. When the systemic blood pressure begins to decrease, the SVC is ligated and the IVC is clamped at the diaphragm. The heart is allowed to empty for two to three beats before cross-clamping the aorta and initiating the plegia solutions. The IVC is incised just above the clamp to decompress the right side, and the right superior pulmonary vein is divided to decompress the left side. If the lungs are to be harvested, the left heart is vented through the left atrial appendage instead. The cardioplegia is infused using a pressure bag to maintain a pressure of 100 to 150 mm Hg while pulmoplegia is allowed to infuse to gravity. Typically, 25 mL/kg of cardioplegia and 50 mL/kg of pulmoplegia are used. The organs are immersed in slushed saline as the plegia solutions are infused. Attention must be directed to the aortic root, which must be palpated to assure an appropriate pressure, and the ventricles, which should be decompressed.

Once the plegia solutions have been infused, the heart can be excised. The IVC is transected and the apex of the heart is retracted superiorly, exposing the pulmonary veins, which

are transected in an isolated cardiac harvest (Fig. 16-5). If the lungs are needed, the left atrium is divided halfway between the entry of the pulmonary veins and the coronary sinus/left atrial appendage insertion. The SVC, aorta, and PA are divided at an appropriate level, as already described, depending on the recipient's needs. If the lungs are to be harvested, the trachea is stapled using a TA-30 stapler while the lungs are inflated to a pressure of 15 to 20 mm Hg. The lungs are dissected free from the pleural attachments and the trachea is divided above the staple line. The organs are then packed in iced plegia solution and triply bagged for transportation.

Heart Implantation

The recipient procedure is timed to minimize the cold ischemic time for the organ. If possible, the recipient team should be ready to implant the organ as soon as the organ arrives. For patients without congenital anomalies, the recipient cardiectomy is essentially the same as for adult patients. A median sternotomy is performed and the patient is placed on cardiopulmonary bypass using bicaval venous cannulation and aortic cannulation proximal to the innominate artery. The aorta is cross-clamped and the heart is removed leaving a generous cuff of aorta and PA. The atria are divided just above the atrioventricular (AV) groove.

The allograft is prepared by dissecting the aorta away from the PA and opening the left atrium by connecting the pulmonary venous ostia (Fig. 16-6). Using a running monofilament suture, the donor left atrium is then anastomosed to the recipient left atrium (Fig. 16-7). Before completion of the suture line, the left atrium is filled with cold saline to evacuate as much air as possible. The lateral wall of the donor right atrium is incised to create an appropriate opening for anastomosis to the recipient right atrial cuff (Fig. 16-8). Once the atrial suture lines are completed, the pulmonary artery and aorta are trimmed and anastomosed with running sutures (Fig. 16-9). At this point the heart is de-aired by ventilating the patient, agitating the heart, and aspirating the ventricular apex, followed by removal of the cross-clamp. The original cardioplegia site can be used as an aortic root vent or a needle can be inserted in the root for further de-airing. Many variations of the basic technique described are employed by transplant programs with equivalent success, including the use of bicaval rather than biatrial anastomosis for larger children, variation in the order of anastomoses (pulmonary artery after removal of cross-clamp, for example), and placement of a left atrial vent. For pediatric transplantation, even more than for adults, the surgeon must be flexible and able to employ different techniques as the situation demands.

Heart-Lung Implantation

En-bloc heart-lung transplantation is typically performed through a bilateral thoracosternotomy (clamshell incision) using the fourth intercostal spaces. Cardiopulmonary bypass is initiated using aortic cannulation near the innominate artery and bicaval venous cannulation. The lungs are mobilized bilaterally with care taken to protect the phrenic nerves, which are left intact on a pedicle of pericardium. The lungs are then excised by individually ligating and dividing the

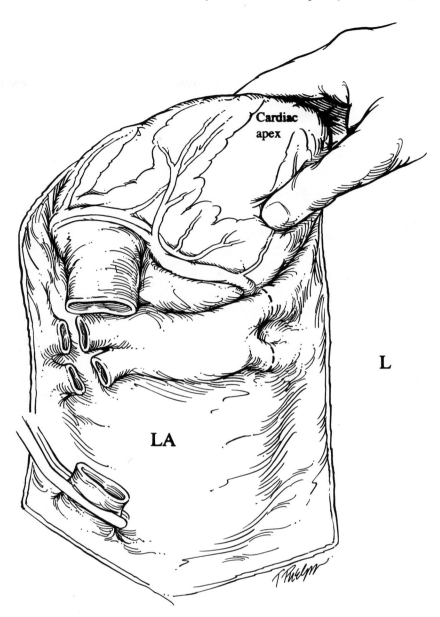

FIGURE 16-5 Cardiac harvest. The pulmonary veins are divided at the pericardium for isolated cardiac harvest. If pulmonary harvest is also necessary, the left atrium is divided to leave a cuff of atrium with the pulmonary veins. LA, left atrium.

R

L

Cardiac apex

LA

pulmonary arteries, veins, and mainstem bronchi (Fig. 16-10). The heart is excised, leaving only a cuff of aorta and right atrium. Once the heart is removed, the trachea can be mobilized in the posterior mediastinum and divided just above the carina. Extensive dissection and mobilization of the trachea should be avoided so the blood supply to that region of the airway is not compromised, which can result in the subsequent breakdown of the tracheal anastomosis.

Once this dissection is complete and adequate hemostasis has been achieved, the donor organs are placed in the mediastinum with the lungs passed behind the phrenic nerve pedicles. The trachea is anastomosed first using a combination of running suture for the membranous septum and interrupted sutures for the cartilaginous portion. The right atrium and aorta are anastomosed using running sutures, and the cross-clamp is removed after aggressive de-airing. In most cases bicaval implantation is used rather than the atrial technique so as to improve the geometry of the right atrium and decrease tricuspid regurgitation. Right atrial reimplantation is used primarily in infants and very small children to avoid the risk of caval anastomotic stricture.

Lung Implantation

Children who require bilateral sequential lung transplantation typically receive a bilateral thoracosternotomy, as described for heart-lung transplantation. The child is heparinized and cardiopulmonary bypass is initiated using aortic and right atrial cannulation. Though sequential lung transplantation without the use of cardiopulmonary bypass (CPB) is commonly used in adults and can be applied to some children, there are several advantages to the use of CPB. First, CPB makes the removal of the recipient's lungs a relatively simple, safe matter. Second, the airways can be

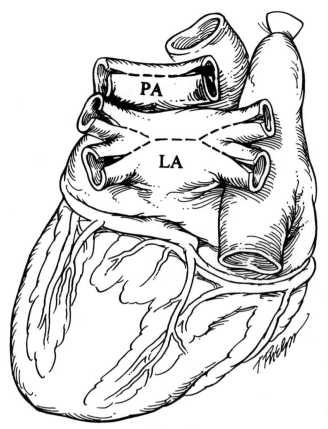

FIGURE 16-6 Cardiac harvest. The left atrial cuff is prepared by incising between the pulmonary venous orifices. The pulmonary artery (PA) bifurcation is divided. LA, left atrium.

irrigated with antibiotic solution after removal of both lungs in cases of septic lung disease. Third, the ischemic time for the second lung to be implanted is minimized if both lungs can be removed and complete exposure attained during organ transport.

When the donor lungs arrive, the lung block is wrapped in cold pads and the hilar structures are dissected. The bronchi are divided about two rings above the takeoff of the upper lobe bronchi. The pulmonary arteries are trimmed to appropriate length and the pulmonary venous confluence is divided in the midline. Typically, the left lung is implanted first, starting with the bronchial anastomosis, which is performed as close to the carina as possible. The suture technique is as described for the trachea in heart-lung transplantation. A partial occlusion clamp is placed on the recipient left atrium so as to include the upper and lower veins, which are connected to provide a large cuff of atrium for the anastomosis. This cuff is sewn to the donor pulmonary vein cuff using running absorbable suture. This clamp is left in place as the arterial anastomosis is fashioned (Fig. 16-11A). A second partial occlusion clamp is placed on the recipient PA, which is anastomosed to the donor PA with running absorbable suture. The lung is de-aired by partially unclamping the left atrium before completion of the PA anastomosis, so as to back-bleed through the lung (Fig. 16-11B).

If any cardiac repair is required in combination with the lung transplantation, this can be performed under cardioplegic arrest after the lungs have been excised. Once the repair has been completed, the aortic cross-clamp can be removed to allow myocardial reperfusion during the lung implantation.

For those patients who require only one lung, anterior thoracotomy, posterolateral thoracotomy, or unilateral thoracosternotomy can be used. CPB can be used if needed for a combined cardiac repair. The recipient pneumonectomy and lung implantation proceed as described for bilateral sequential lung transplantation.

SHORT-TERM COMPLICATIONS

The majority of heart and lung transplant patients suffer from the same types of early postoperative problems as other pediatric thoracic surgery patients, although transplant patients as a group are at increased risk for complications due to the comorbidities from which they commonly suffer. These comorbidities include congestive heart failure, malnutrition, ventilator dependence, and chronic infections in some subgroups. Hemorrhage, atelectasis, and volume shifts must be monitored and managed as with other patients. Along with these postsurgical complications are several transplant-specific issues that must be considered.

Acute Graft Dysfunction/Failure

Early dysfunction or failure of cardiac allografts has been reported to occur in between 4% and 25% of patients undergoing orthotopic heart transplantation.[23,62] The cause of acute graft dysfunction is not entirely clear and is likely multifactorial. Acute rejection certainly plays a role in some patients, whereas others show no signs of rejection. Right ventricular failure in the setting of preoperative pulmonary hypertension is the cause in other patients. Reperfusion injury superimposed likely plays a role as well. Regardless of the etiology, acute graft failure is the cause of death in approximately 30% of pediatric heart transplant patients dying within the first 30 days of surgery.[6] These patients can be markedly unstable in the operating room or they may become unstable in the early postoperative period. Significant cases of acute graft dysfunction require inotropes or ECMO for hemodynamic support. In a review of nine patients who suffered from acute thoracic organ transplant failure (four heart, three lung, and two heart-lung transplants), six required ECMO and four eventually underwent repeat transplantation.[28] One diagnosis that must be considered and either ruled out or treated quickly is acute rejection, which occurs in the majority of pediatric heart transplant patients at some point in the early postoperative period.[7] Diagnosis and treatment of rejection are discussed in a later section.

The decision regarding retransplantation in this setting has generated much discussion, and the policies of individual transplant centers vary on this point. Ethical considerations aside, some groups have reported outcomes after retransplantation that are comparable to primary transplants.[28,44]

Infection

As with adult patients, pediatric thoracic organ transplant recipients frequently experience infectious complications,

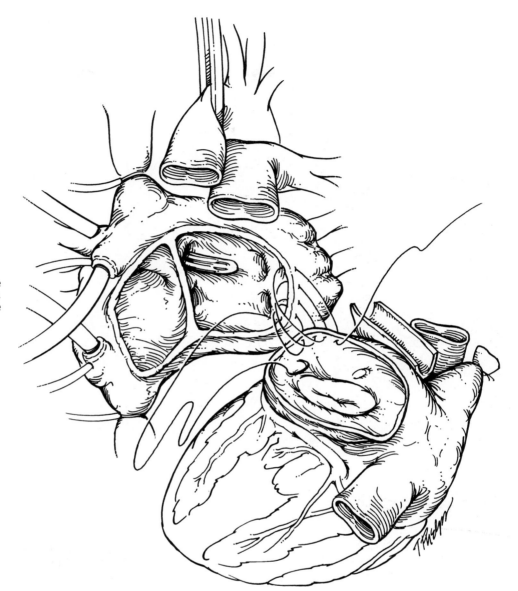

FIGURE 16-7 Cardiac implantation. The left atrial anastomosis is completed first, beginning at the base of the appendage and left superior pulmonary vein.

especially in the early postoperative period.[6,7,62,63] The high-dose immunosuppression administered immediately after surgery and during episodes of acute rejection render patients susceptible to bacterial and opportunistic viral, fungal, and parasitic infections. For example, without prophylactic treatment, the incidence of *Pneumocystis carinii* pneumonia after infant heart transplantation is 7%.[33] Because of this risk, most programs institute prophylactic trimethoprim/sulfamethoxazole, dapsone, or inhaled pentamidine (Table 16-1). Cystic fibrosis patients who undergo lung transplantation are particularly prone to bacterial pneumonias because of chronic colonization of the airways. Beyond the first 3 years posttransplant, infection becomes a less common cause of death for all groups, accounting for less than 20% of patient deaths.[6]

Cytomegalovirus (CMV) infection is a common cause of morbidity and mortality after thoracic organ transplantation. Metras and colleagues[43] reported that in a series of 49 lung transplants in 42 children, 37 patients had a significant

pulmonary infection at some point in the postoperative period. In this series, CMV pneumonitis occurred in 16 of the 42 children with only 2 survivors, with 1 survivor requiring retransplantation. CMV is also the most common viral infection identified after pediatric heart transplantation. Because CMV is such a common posttransplant problem, most programs use prophylactic ganciclovir in patients receiving either lung or heart-lung transplants; however, there is little evidence demonstrating that prophylactic ganciclovir is efficacious in this setting.[2,77]

Other viruses that can cause problems after transplantation are adenovirus, Epstein-Barr virus (EBV), and herpes. Adenoviral infections frequently cause significant graft dysfunction in patients with lung transplants.[10,28] EBV infections are less common but equally worrisome because there may be an association between EBV infection and posttransplant lymphoproliferative disorder (PTLD).[25,26] Viral infections can be particularly difficult to diagnose. One study that can be

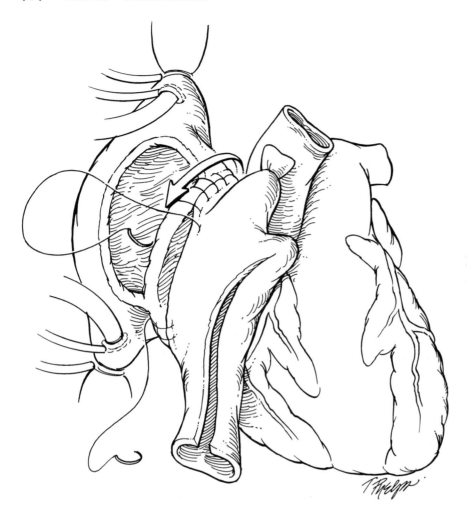

FIGURE 16-8   Cardiac implantation. The left atrial anastomosis is completed with the closure of the interatrial septum. The right atrium is prepared for biatrial implantation using a curvilinear lateral incision.

particularly useful is polymerase chain reaction (PCR) analysis of bronchoscopic alveolar lavage (BAL) fluid.[10]

Fungal infections are less common than bacterial and viral infections, but when they occur, they can be disastrous. Airway colonization by candida is common after lung transplantation, but invasive disease is rare. Invasive aspergillosis, which also occurs infrequently, is associated with an extremely poor prognosis and must be considered a relative contraindication to retransplantation.

Rejection and Immunosuppression

Between 30 days and 3 years posttransplant, the most common cause of death for heart transplant recipients is acute rejection. Beyond the third year, chronic rejection/graft coronary artery disease becomes the most common cause of death (Fig. 16-12).[6] The majority of children will suffer at least one episode of acute rejection within the first 3 years after transplantation. This fact must be balanced against the multiple complications of chronic immunosuppression, which provide incentive to minimize immunosuppressive therapy over time.

Posttransplant immunosuppression has been the topic of considerable research and discussion among transplant programs, but the majority of programs continue to use triple drug immunosuppression based on cyclosporine, azathioprine, and steroids (Tables 16-2 and 16-3). Recently, mycophenolate mofetil (CellCept) has begun to displace azathioprine as the second immunosuppressive agent. Each of these agents functions through a different mechanism and carries with it a different spectrum of complications; thus efforts have been made to minimize dosages, change to other agents, or even eliminate elements of this regimen altogether.[5,12,68]

Corticosteroids have been used as immunosuppressive agents for over 30 years, but the adverse effects of chronic steroid therapy can be particularly problematic in the pediatric transplant patient. Complications include hypertension, cushingoid appearance, hyperglycemia, and somatic growth delay. There have also been suggestions that steroid therapy may contribute to the development of graft coronary artery disease in pediatric heart transplant recipients.[56] Because of these problems, several different variations of the posttransplant steroid regimen have been evaluated. These variations include early withdrawal of steroids after induction therapy using antilymphocyte globulin or OKT3.[35,55] Other centers have weaned patients off steroids later in the posttransplant period.[12,46] These studies have shown that approximately 80% of pediatric heart transplant patients can be successfully weaned from steroids, although which patients can be successfully weaned cannot be predicted until the attempt is made.

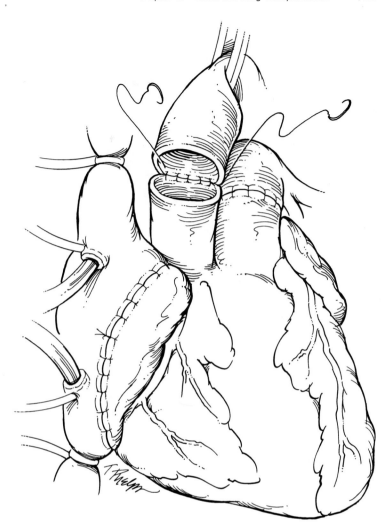

FIGURE 16-9   Cardiac implantation. The pulmonary artery and aorta are anastomosed with care taken to trim the vessels to avoid kinking or tension.

Cyclosporine revolutionized solid organ transplantation in the 1980s, and since then it has been the mainstay of immunosuppressive therapy; however, there are adverse effects associated with the use of this drug. Renal toxicity, acute tubular necrosis, hypertension, gingival hyperplasia, decreased seizure threshold, and hirsutism are the most commonly observed complications. Attempts have been made to transition patients who are experiencing persistent rejection or complications attributable to traditional triple drug therapy to a single drug regimen using the drug tacrolimus (FK506).[68] FK506 has a mechanism of action very similar to cyclosporine, as it suppresses T-cell activation and production of cytokines. Gingival hyperplasia and hirsutism are less problematic with FK506, but, like cyclosporine, FK506 decreases glomerular filtration rate and is nephrotoxic.

Many transplant programs use induction immunotherapy with antibodies directed against lymphocytes or thymocytes. Several different induction agents are available including OKT3 (a monoclonal antithymocyte preparation), ATGAM (a horse antithymocyte globulin), ALG (antilymphocyte globulin), thymoglobulin, and many others. These cytolytic therapies are typically given over the first 7 to 14 days post transplant. Patients commonly experience fever, chills, and malaise, which can be decreased by pretreatment with benadryl, solumedrol, and tylenol. Complications include lymphopenia and thrombocytopenia, which may necessitate dose reduction.

Due to the frequency of acute rejection in heart transplantation, care must be taken either to institute routine surveillance for rejection or to observe the children closely for any signs and symptoms suggestive of rejection. Clearly the gold standard for diagnosis of rejection is endomyocardial biopsy; however, in many transplant centers surveillance biopsies have not been used routinely in infants and small children because of the increased risk of cardiac perforation, the need for anesthesia, and the risk of thrombosis of access vessels. Attempts to develop reliable noninvasive methods of diagnosis for rejection have yielded mixed results. Several echocardiographic measurements, including left ventricular mass index, shortening fraction, posterior wall thickness, and septal thickness, have been used in attempts to diagnose rejection. New pericardial effusions or valvular abnormalities are also suggestive of rejection. Unfortunately, these echocardiographic findings are observer dependent and can be unreliable, particularly during the first month after transplant.[20,59] Perhaps the best available noninvasive method of surveillance

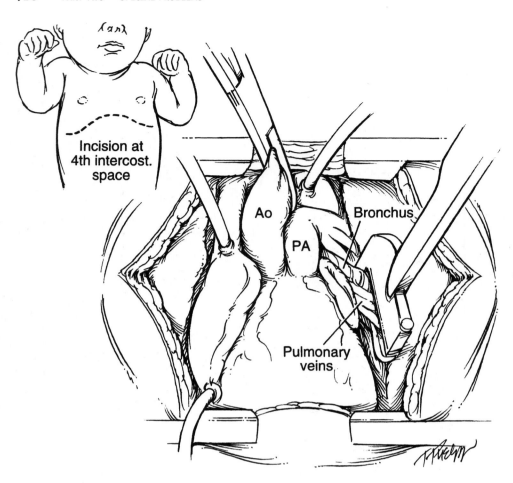

Incision at 4th intercost. space

Ao

PA

Bronchus

Pulmonary veins

FIGURE 16-10 The thoracosternotomy (clamshell) incision through the fourth intercostal space is shown in the insert. Bicaval venous cannulation is used to initiate cardiopulmonary bypass. The lungs are removed by serially dividing and ligating the pulmonary artery branches and pulmonary veins. The mainstem bronchi are stapled. Ao, aorta; PA, pulmonary artery.

for rejection is careful observation of the child for the development of signs or symptoms. Any change in appetite, decrease in energy level, fever, or increase in resting heart rate by more than 20 bpm above baseline should prompt evaluation by the transplant team to rule out rejection or infection, both of which can produce such nonspecific symptoms. If infection is ruled out, then further evaluation including endomyocardial biopsy must be performed.

Most episodes of acute rejection respond to a 3-day course of intravenous steroids. Patients with severe cases of rejection that are resistant to bolus steroid therapy typically receive OKT3, antithymocyte globulin, methotrexate, or total lymphoid irradiation, depending on the protocol of the transplant program.

Lung transplant recipients experience a similar high incidence of acute rejection in the early posttransplant period. Acute rejection can be difficult to differentiate from reperfusion injury and infection. Pulmonary function testing and routine chest radiography can be useful for surveillance beyond the early postoperative period; however, as with heart transplant, acquisition of tissue for microscopic examination is the gold standard for diagnosis of rejection. One must keep in mind that even transbronchial biopsy is not perfect because sampling errors can lead to false negative results;

therefore difficult cases may require open lung biopsy to make the final diagnosis. Acute rejection after lung transplantation is typically treated with a regimen similar to the one described previously for heart transplant rejection.

Hypertension and Renal Dysfunction

Hypertension is a common complication after thoracic organ transplantation in both the early and late postoperative periods. At 1 year and 3 years of follow-up, approximately 45% of pediatric heart transplant patients suffer from hypertension.[6] Mild renal dysfunction is common in the early postoperative period with elevation of the serum creatinine above 1.3 mg/dL. This renal dysfunction typically stabilizes and improves. Only 1.7% of patients have persistent renal dysfunction at 1 year, with another 1.7% suffering from severe dysfunction (creatinine > 2.5).[6] Both of these complications, hypertension and renal dysfunction, are felt to be due to cyclosporine and steroid therapy. Patients with significant hypertension commonly require acute treatment with nicardipine or sodium nitroprusside and conversion to chronic antihypertensive medications such as oral diltiazem. Care must be taken as these medications are instituted because of interactions with cyclosporine. In many patients,

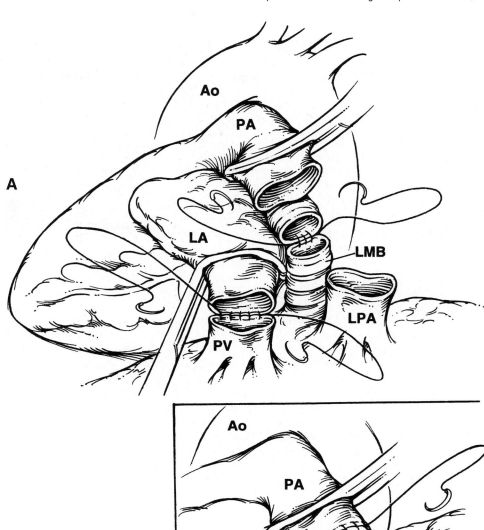

FIGURE 16-11 A, Lung implantation. Typically, the bronchus is anastomosed first, followed by the left atrial/pulmonary venous connection. **B,** The implantation is completed with the left pulmonary artery anastomosis. Ao, aorta; LA, left atrium; LMB, left mainstem bronchus; LPA, left pulmonary artery; PA, pulmonary artery; PV, pulmonary vein.

posttransplant hypertension improves over time as immunosuppressive medications are weaned.

Hyperammonemia

A rare complication that has been reported after lung and heart-lung transplantation is hyperammonemic coma. This condition, which is typically fatal, may be related to abnormal hepatic glutamine synthetase activity.[4,40] Patients initially develop altered mental status followed by progressive decline in alertness and coma. Plasma ammonia levels have been reported in the 250 to 3200 mM/L range (normal is 13 to 33 mM/L). Patients typically develop increased cerebral edema followed by herniation and death. One case report described the use of hemodialysis, intravenous sodium phenylacetate, sodium benzoate, and arginine hydrochloride, resulting in patient improvement and survival.[4]

Cardiac Denervation

The loss of cardiac innervation in heart transplant patients results in significant changes in the patient's ability to respond

Table 16-1   Infection Prophylaxis

Antibacterial prophylaxis	Perioperative cefazolin until chest tubes are removed. Chronically intubated or patients with chronic infectious lung disease receive antibiotic coverage based upon surveillance cultures.
Antiviral prophylaxis	For lung and heart-lung transplants: Ganciclovir 5 mg/kg IV twice a day × 2 weeks, then 5 mg/kg IV every day × 4 weeks. For active varicella or EBV-related lymphoproliferative disorder: Acyclovir 10 mg/kg IV three times per day × 5–7 days followed by 15–30 mg/kg/day in 4–5 divided doses × 10 days.
Antifungal prophylaxis	Nystatin for all recipients. For patients with chronic respiratory infections/cystic fibrosis: aerosolized amphotericin 5 mg in 5 mL twice a day (increase as tolerated to 20 mg twice a day in adults).
Pneumocystis carinii prophylaxis	For lung and heart-lung transplants: Bactrim (2 mg/kg PO on Monday, Wednesday, and Friday). Treat with dapsone if allergic to or intolerant of bactrim.

to inotropic medications and to stress. The donor sinoatrial (SA) node, which controls the rate of the transplanted heart, no longer receives vagal stimulation and thus tends to fire at a higher basal rate; however, stress- and exercise-induced increases in heart rate are blunted relative to normal. The loss of neuronal presynaptic uptake of catecholamines precludes the conversion of dopamine to norepinephrine, resulting in decreased cardiac response to dopamine. Norepinephrine and epinephrine, on the other hand, tend to have an accentuated inotropic effect in transplanted hearts. While the vagolytic effects of atropine are ineffective for the treatment of bradycardia, the atrioventricular node effects of digitalis are also decreased. The mechanism of action of each drug must be considered before administration in the heart transplant patient. Temporary pacing wires are frequently used in the early postoperative period to maintain an adequate heart rate and cardiac output. Permanent pacing is rarely required.

Anastomotic Complications

One of the early banes of heart-lung and lung transplantation was the bronchial or tracheal anastomosis, which was prone to anastomotic breakdown or stricture.[27] With modifications in surgical techniques, these difficulties are much less common today. Bronchial anastomotic breakdown is rare and is usually associated with prolonged mechanical ventilation or pulmonary infection, both of which can interfere with airway healing. Anastomotic stenosis occurs in about 10% to 15% of cases and can typically be treated with bronchoscopic dilatation. Recurrent stenoses may require placement of a silicone stent.

Complications involving vascular anastomoses are uncommon. Pulmonary vein stenosis can be a particularly difficult problem that presents as pulmonary hypertension with alveolar infiltrates on chest x-ray. Pulmonary artery stenosis presents as right ventricular hypertension.

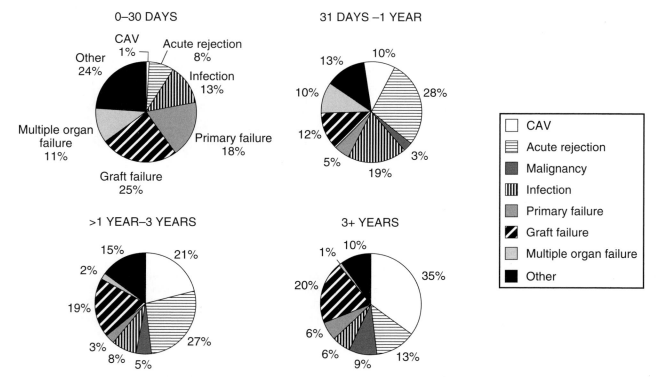

FIGURE 16-12   Causes of death in heart transplant recipients broken down by time posttransplant. (Adapted from Boucek MM, Edwards LB, Keck BM, et al: The registry of the International Society of Heart and Lung Transplantation: Seventh Official Pediatric Report—2004. *J Heart Lung Transplant* 23:933–947, 2004; with permission from Elsevier Science.)

Table 16-2   Immunosuppression Protocols

Induction Therapy	
Antithymocyte regimen	For lung and heart-lung transplants only: Thymoglobulin 1.5 mg/kg/day × 7–14 days (dose reduced to 0.75 mg/kg/day for white blood cell count < 3000 or platelet count < 75,000)
Maintenance Regimen	
Antimetabolite	Azathioprine 2–3 mg/kg/day, initial dose in operating room *or* Cellcept 15 mg/kg PO twice a day
Calcineurin inhibitor	Cyclosporine 0.25–0.5 mg/kg IV initially followed by 1.5–2.5 mg/kg/day continuous infusion to maintain serum level of 300–350 ng/mL. When taking oral medications, cyclosporine is switched to FK506 0.15–0.3 mg/kg/day.
Steroid therapy	Prednisone 1 mg/kg/day × 2 weeks (IV or PO) decreased to 0.5 mg/kg/day × 6 months followed by 0.2 mg/kg/day and finally every other day.

LONG-TERM COMPLICATIONS

Lymphoproliferative Disease

Posttransplant lymphoproliferative disease is the most commonly observed malignancy after thoracic organ transplantation. This disorder may be associated with EBV infection and has been observed after EBV seroconversion.[52] However, the role of EBV in this process remains controversial. In a study comparing the incidence of PTLD in EBV-negative recipients who received organs from EBV-positive donors, Harwood and colleagues[22] found no increase in the incidence of PTLD.

Patients who develop PTLD are treated with reduction in immunosuppression, either with or without antiviral therapy (acyclovir or foscarnet) for EBV. Since PTLD commonly develops in the oropharynx, airway, or gastrointestinal tract, local therapy may be required to treat obstructive lesions if they do not regress promptly.

Graft Coronary Artery Disease

Beyond the first year posttransplant, graft coronary artery disease becomes a progressively more significant problem. Chronic rejection/coronary artery disease is listed as the cause of death in nearly 40% of patients who die more than 3 years after transplant (see Fig. 16-12).[6] Using angiography and intracoronary ultrasound (ICUS), Dent and colleagues[18] evaluated 51 pediatric heart transplant patients a median of 3.4 years after transplant. They found a correlation between intimal thickness and time from transplant with 37% of patients exhibiting grade 2 or greater disease. The prevalence of intimal thickening was 74% in patients studied at least 5 years after transplant. Though these findings are concerning, the correlation between ICUS-determined intimal thickening and clinically significant coronary vasculopathy is not entirely clear. In this population, 4 of the 51 patients had evidence of vasculopathy on coronary angiography, with all of these patients eventually developing cardiac events, including two sudden deaths. No correlation could be identified between any factor and the development of graft coronary artery disease (CAD) other than time from transplant.

Hyperlipidemia/hypercholesterolemia is a common problem posttransplant secondary to several immunosuppressive medications and may play a role in the development of early graft vasculopathy. Patients who develop hyperlipidemia should be treated medically to control the problem. Other potential risk factors for graft vasculopathy are CMV infection and recurrent episodes of acute rejection. Graft CAD tends to be a diffuse disease that is rarely amenable to percutaneous stenting or angioplasty; thus development of graft CAD is often an indication for relisting. Unfortunately, patients who are retransplanted for graft CAD seem to be prone to redevelopment of the disease in the second graft.

Bronchiolitis Obliterans

The most significant long-term complication for lung transplant recipients is bronchiolitis obliterans or obliterative bronchiolitis (OB), which is felt to be a sequela of chronic rejection.[63] Beyond the first posttransplant year, OB/chronic rejection becomes the most common cause of death for these patients.[6] Although the etiology of OB has not been clearly delineated, several theories have been proposed, including chronic rejection,

Table 16-3   Immunosuppressive Drugs

Drug	Dosage	Levels	Complications
Azathioprine	2–3 mg/kg/day	Titrate to white blood cell level	Leukopenia, anemia, and thrombocytopenia
Corticosteroids	1 mg/kg/day initially	N/A	Hypertension, hyperglycemia, and cushingoid appearance
Cyclosporine A	1.5–2.5 mg/kg/day	300–350 ng/mL	Nephrotoxicity, hypertension, gingival hyperplasia, and hirsutism
Mycophenolate mofetil	100–2000 mg/day	N/A	Diarrhea, vomiting, and leukopenia
OKT3	2.5–10 mg/day	Titrate to white blood cell level	Fever, hypotension, pulmonary edema, and wheezing
Rapamycin	1 mg/m²	9–15 ng/mL	Hyperlipidemia, hypertension, and rash
Tacrolimus (FK506)	0.03–0.05 mg/kg/day IV initially	15–20 ng/mL	Nephrotoxicity and neurotoxicity

multiple viral infections, multiple episodes of acute rejection, airway ischemia, or a combination of these factors. It seems likely that OB represents the final result of multiple inflammatory insults, eventually leading to fibrosis and obstruction of the small airways. This syndrome occurs in between 20% and 40% of pediatric lung transplant recipients.[42,64,76]

The clinical characteristics of OB are relatively nonspecific, including progressive dyspnea, exercise intolerance, decreased breath sounds, and obstructive mechanics on spirometry studies. Patients typically do not improve with bronchodilators. Serial pulmonary mechanics can be one of the better methods available to screen patients who are old enough to cooperate with pulmonary function tests. The baseline FEV_1 is determined after the patient has recovered from the transplant. If the patient later develops symptoms, the severity of pulmonary dysfunction is staged based upon the percentage of baseline FEV_1 achievable, defined as mild (66% to 80%), moderate (51% to 65%), and severe (< 50%) bronchiolitis obliterans syndrome.[15] This staging system cannot be applied to infants and younger children, for whom clinical assessment is the best tool available.

Once OB has been diagnosed or is suspected, the only treatment that has proven beneficial is increased immunosuppression. Unfortunately, OB typically progresses despite medical therapy. Patients with progressive or severe OB may require retransplantation; however, patients who undergo retransplantation for OB seem to have a higher incidence of OB in the second graft as well.[30,50]

Gastrointestinal Disorders

Patients who have undergone thoracic organ transplantation are at increased risk for a number of gastrointestinal disorders. In a study of adult heart transplant patients, Mueller and colleagues[48] reported a 20% incidence of gastrointestinal diseases in 92 patients over a 5-year follow-up. The most common gastrointestinal problem was biliary tract disease, occurring in 17% of the affected patients, with 5% requiring cholecystectomy, followed by esophagitis (13%) and pancreatitis (10%). Cholelithiasis has been reported in 20% to 30% of heart transplant patients screened with routine ultrasonography and is felt to be due to cyclosporine-induced changes in biliary flow and bile salt metabolism.[21,66] Pediatric heart transplant patients also have an increased incidence of cholelithiasis, reported to be approximately 15% as opposed to 1% of nontransplanted children.[45] Most other gastrointestinal disorders in heart transplant patients can be attributed either to immunosuppression-associated infectious complications such as viral or fungal esophagitis or to the direct effects of steroids.

Lung transplant patients are prone to all of these complications; however, those with cystic fibrosis also suffer from additional difficulties. In a review of 70 cystic fibrosis patients who underwent lung transplantation, Minkes and colleagues[47] found that 10% required laparotomy for intestinal obstruction in the early posttransplant period. This complication has been explained by the frequency of previous laparotomies in this patient population and their viscous intestinal contents. These factors combined with postoperative narcotic use, attempts to minimize intravascular volume resulting in relative dehydration, and the use of azathioprine may impair intestinal mobility. Therapeutic efforts that can decrease the likelihood of intestinal obstruction include continuation of pancreatic enzyme supplementation, initiation of oral or nasogastric N-acetylcysteine, and correction of electrolyte and fluid abnormalities as they occur.

OUTCOMES

Heart Transplantation

Through June 2003 the registry of the International Society of Heart and Lung Transplantation included information on 5569 isolated heart transplants performed worldwide with approximately 350 to 380 new patients added per year.[6] Short- to intermediate-term survival for pediatric cardiac transplantation now approaches that seen in adults with a 1-year survival of 80% to 90% and 5-year survival of approximately 65% to 70%.[6,13,63] Mortality is highest in the early postoperative period, particularly for patients younger than 1 year; however, by 5 years posttransplant the survival curves for all children are essentially the same (Fig. 16-13).[6] Five risk factors were associated with 1-year mortality in the registry data: congenital heart disease, diagnosis other than cardiomyopathy, retransplantation, preoperative mechanical ventilation, and preoperative hospitalization.

In a review of the Pediatric Heart Transplant Study, Shaddy and colleagues[62] analyzed 191 pediatric heart transplant recipients. In this report, 1-year survival was 82% with essentially no change over the following year. Risk factors for mortality were the need for assist devices, nonidentical ABO blood types, and younger age of recipient. The most common causes of death were rejection, early graft failure, infection, and sudden death.

Lung Transplantation

As with pediatric heart transplants, the total number of pediatric lung transplants performed each year seems to have plateaued at about 60 to 80 per year.[6] In children younger than 1 year of age, the most common single indication for transplantation is congenital abnormalities followed by primary pulmonary hypertension (PPH). In older children cystic fibrosis predominates, again followed by primary pulmonary hypertension.

Early survival after pediatric lung transplantation has improved during the mid to late 1990s with 1-year survival now in the 80% range; however, long-term outcomes have not changed significantly, with 3- to 4-year survival in the 50% range (Fig. 16-14).[6] Acute graft failure and infection are the most common causes of death in the early postoperative period, with chronic rejection and bronchiolitis obliterans predominating beyond the first year.

Children who receive heart-lung transplants have long-term outcomes similar to those who receive lung transplants alone. As with the lung transplant patients, chronic rejection with bronchiolitis obliterans is the most common cause of death in the late posttransplant period.

Despite the complications that continue to cause morbidity and mortality after pediatric lung transplantation, there is ample evidence that this therapeutic modality increases both longevity and quality of life for these children, who are often

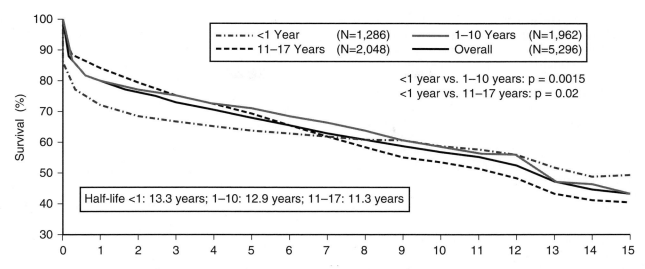

FIGURE 16-13   Pediatric heart transplantation Kaplan = Meier survival (January 1982 to June 2002). (Reprinted from Boucek MM, Edwards LB, Keck BM, et al: The registry of the International Society of Heart and Lung Transplantation: Seventh Official Pediatric Report—2004. *J Heart Lung Transplant* 23:933–947, 2004; with permission from Elsevier Science.)

critically ill before transplant.[1,8] Unfortunately, because of the prevalence of chronic rejection and bronchiolitis obliterans, lung transplantation remains essentially a palliative procedure rather than a cure for end-stage pulmonary disease. Resolution or improvement of this problem is the most important challenge facing lung transplant programs and researchers at this time.

CONCLUSION

Thoracic organ transplantation has become an accepted therapy for children and infants with end-stage cardiopulmonary disease. Significant advances in critical care, anesthesia, immunosuppression, and postoperative management have improved outcomes for these children; however, considerable

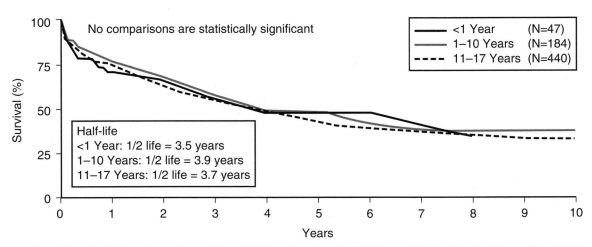

FIGURE 16-14   Actuarial survival for lung transplant recipients. (Reprinted from Boucek MM, Edwards LB, Keck BM, et al: The registry of the International Society of Heart and Lung Transplantation: Seventh Official Pediatric Report—2004. *J Heart Lung Transplant* 23:933–947, 2004; with permission from Elsevier Science.)

problems remain to be solved. There continues to be an elusive balance point between rejection and infection that is difficult to maintain, resulting in multiple episodes of acute rejection and/or multiple infections for the majority of patients. These early difficulties may then contribute to the long-term banes of thoracic organ transplantation: cardiac graft vasculopathy and bronchiolitis obliterans. Despite these difficulties, transplant waiting lists continue to grow and mortality on the waiting list remains high because of the limited supply of donor organs. Heart and lung transplantation has matured over the last decade, but there are still ample avenues for further research and improvement.

References

1. Aurora P, Whitehead B, Wade A, et al: Lung transplantation and life extension in children with cystic fibrosis. *Lancet* 354:1591–1593, 1999.
2. Bailey TC, Trulock EP, Ettinger NA, et al: Failure of prophylactic ganciclovir to prevent CMV disease in recipients of lung transplants. *J Infect Dis* 165:548–552, 1992.
3. Barr ML, Baker CJ, Schenkel FA, et al: Prophylactic photopheresis and chronic rejection: Effects on graft intimal hyperplasia in cardiac transplantation. *Clin Transplant* 14:162–166, 2000.
4. Berry GT, Bridges ND, Nathanson KL, et al: Successful use of alternate waste nitrogen agents and hemodialysis in a patient with hyperammonemic coma after heart-lung transplantation. *Arch Neurol* 56:481–484, 1999.
5. Boucek RJ Jr, Naftel D, Boucek MM, et al: Induction immunotherapy in pediatric heart transplant recipients: A multicenter study. *J Heart Lung Transplant* 18:460–469, 1999.
6. Boucek MM, Edwards LB, Keck BM, et al: The registry of the International Society of Heart and Lung Transplantation: Seventh official pediatric report–2004. *J Heart Lung Transplant* 23:933–947, 2004.
7. Braunlin EA, Canter CE, Olivari MT, et al: Rejection and infection after pediatric cardiac transplantation. *Ann Thorac Surg* 49:385, 1990.
8. Bridges ND, Mallory GB, Huddleston CB, et al: Lung transplantation in infancy and early childhood. *J Heart Lung Transplant* 15:895–902, 1996.
9. Bridges ND, Mallory GB, Huddleston CB, et al: Lung transplantation in children and young adults with cardiovascular disease. *Ann Thorac Surg* 59:813–821, 1995.
10. Bridges ND, Spray TL, Collins MH, et al: Adenovirus infection in the lung results in graft failure after lung transplantation. *J Thorac Cardiovasc Surg* 116:617–623, 1998.
11. Buz S, Drews T, Weng Y, et al: Heart transplantation after mechanical circulatory support. *Transplant Proc* 32:583–584, 2000.
12. Canter CE, Moorhead S, Saffitz JE, et al: Steroid withdrawal in the pediatric heart transplant recipient initially treated with triple immunosuppresion. *J Heart Lung Transplant* 13:74–80, 1994.
13. Chiavarelli M, de Begona JA, Vigesaa RE, et al: Heart transplantation in children. *Adv Card Surg* 3:155–174, 1992.
14. Chiavarelli M, Gundry SR, Razzouk AJ, Bailey LL: Cardiac transplantation for infants with hypoplastic left heart syndrome. *JAMA* 270:2944–2947, 1993.
15. Cooper JD, Billingham M, Egan T, et al: A working formulation for the standardization of nomenclature for clinical staging of chronic dysfunction in lung allografts. *J Heart Lung Transplant* 12:713–716, 1993.
16. de Begona JA, Gundry SR, Razzouk AJ, et al: Prolonged ischemic times in pediatric heart transplantation: Early and late results. *Transplant Proc* 25:1645–1648, 1993.
17. del Nido PJ, Armitage JM, Fricker FJ, et al: Extracorporeal membrane oxygenation support as a bridge to pediatric heart transplantation. *Circulation* 90:II66–II69, 1994.
18. Dent CL, Canter CE, Hirsch R, Balzer DT: Transplant coronary artery disease in pediatric heart transplant recipients. *J Heart Lung Transplant* 19:240–248, 2000.
19. Di Russo GB, Clark BJ, Bridges ND, et al: Prolonged extracorporeal membrane oxygenation as a bridge to cardiac transplantation. *Ann Thorac Surg* 69:925–927, 2000.
20. Gidding SS, Holzman G, Duffy CE, et al: Usefulness of left ventricular inflow Doppler in predicting rejection in pediatric cardiac transplant patients. *J Am Coll Cardiol* 19:147A, 1992.
21. Girardet RE, Rosenbloom P, Weese BM, et al: Significance of asymptomatic biliary tract disease in heart transplant recipients. *J Heart Transplant* 8:391, 1989.
22. Harwood JS, Gould FK, McMaster A, et al: Significance of Epstein-Barr virus status and post-transplant lymphoproliferative disease in pediatric thoracic transplantation. *Pediatr Transplant* 3:100–103, 1999.
23. Hauptman PJ, Aranki S, Mudge GH, et al: Early cardiac allograft failure after orthotopic heart transplantation. *Am Heart J* 127:179–186, 1994.
24. Hirsch R, Huddleston CB, Mendeloff EN, et al: Infant and donor organ growth after heart transplantation in neonates with hypoplastic left heart syndrome. *J Heart Lung Transplant* 15:1093–1100, 1996.
25. Ho M, Jaffe R, Miller G, et al: The frequency of Epstein-Barr virus infection and associated lymphoproliferative syndrome after transplantation and its manifestations in children. *Transplantation* 45:719–727, 1988.
26. Ho M, Miller G, Atchison RW: Epstein-Barr virus infections and DNA hybridisation studies in post-transplantation lymphoma and lymphoproliferative lesion: The role of primary infection. *J Infect Dis* 152:876, 1985.
27. Hoffman TM, Gaynor JW, Bridges ND, et al: Aortic homograft interposition for management of complete tracheal anastomotic disruption after heart-lung transplantation. *J Thorac Cardiovasc Surg* 121:587–588, 2001.
28. Hoffman TM, Spray TL, Gaynor JW, et al: Survival after acute graft failure in pediatric thoracic organ transplant recipients. *Pediatr Transplant* 4:112–117, 2000.
29. Hosenpud JD, Bennett LE, Keck BM, et al: The registry of the International Society of Heart and Lung Transplantation: Sixteenth Official Report–1999. *J Heart Lung Transplant* 18:611–626, 1999.
30. Huddleston CB, Mendeloff EN, Cohen AH, et al: Lung retransplantation in children. *Ann Thorac Surg* 66:199–204, 1998.
31. Huddleston CB, Sweet SC, Mallory GB, et al: Lung transplantation in very young infants. *J Thorac Cardiovasc Surg* 118:796–804, 1999.
32. Ishino K, Weng Y, Alexi-Meskishvili V, et al: Extracorporeal membrane oxygenation as a bridge to cardiac transplantation in children. *Artif Organs* 20:728–732, 1996.
33. Janner D, Bork J, Baum M, Chinnock R: *Pneumocystis carinii* pneumonia in infants after heart transplantation. *J Heart Lung Transplant* 15:758–763, 1996.
34. Jurmann MJ, Haverich A, Demertzis S, et al: Extracorporeal membrane oxygenation as a bridge to lung transplantation. *Eur J Cardiothorac Surg* 5:94–98, 1991.
35. Keogh A, Macdonald P, Harvison A, et al: Initial steroid-free versus steroid-based maintenance therapy and steroid withdrawal after heart transplantation: Two views of the steroid question. *J Heart Lung Transplant* 11:421–427, 1992.
36. Kirklin JK, Naftel DC, Kirklin JW, et al: Pulmonary vascular resistance and the risk of heart transplantation. *J Heart Lung Transplant* 7:331–336, 1988.
37. Ko WJ, Chen YS, Chou NK, et al: Extracorporeal membrane oxygenation in the perioperative period of heart transplantation. *J Formos Med Assoc* 96:83–90, 1997.
38. Konertz W, Hotz H, Schneider M, et al: Clinical experience with the MEDOS HIA-VAD system in infants and children: A preliminary report. *Ann Thorac Surg* 63:1138–1144, 1997.
39. Koutlas TC, Bridges ND, Gaynor JW, et al: Pediatric lung transplantation: Are there surgical contraindications? *Transplantation* 63:269–274, 1997.
40. Lichtenstein GR, Kaiser LR, Tuchman M, et al: Fatal hyperammonemia following orthotopic lung transplantation. *Gastroenterology* 112:236–240, 1997.
41. Menkis AH, McKenzie FN, Novick RJ, et al: Expanding applicability of transplantation after multiple prior palliative procedures. *Ann Thorac Surg* 52:722–726, 1991.
42. Metras D, Shennib H, Kreitmann B, et al: Double-lung transplantation in children: A report of 20 cases. The Joint Marseille-Montreal Lung Transplant Program. *Ann Thorac* 55:352–357, 1993.
43. Metras D, Viard L, Kreitmann B, et al: Lung infections in pediatric lung transplantation: Experience in 49 cases. *Eur J Cardiothorac Surg* 15:490–495, 1999.
44. Michler RE, Edwards NM, Hsu D, et al: Pediatric retransplantation. *J Heart Lung Transplant* 12:S319–S327, 1993.
45. Milas M, Ricketts RR, Amerson JR, Kanter K: Management of biliary tract stones in heart transplant patients. *Ann Surg* 223:747–756, 1996.
46. Miller LW, Wolford T, McBride LR, et al: Successful withdrawal of corticosteroids in heart transplantation. *J Heart Lung Transplant* 11:431–434, 1992.

47. Minkes RK, Langer JC, Skinner MA, et al: Intestinal obstruction after lung transplantation in children with cystic fibrosis. *J Pediatr Surg* 34:1489–1493, 1999.
48. Mueller XM, Tevaearai HT, Stumpe F, et al: Gastrointestinal disease following heart transplantation. *World J Surg* 23:650–656, 1999.
49. Nelems MB, Rebuck AS, Cooper JD, et al: Human lung transplantation. *Chest* 78:569–573, 1980.
50. Novick RJ, Stitt L, Schafers HJ, et al: Pulmonary retransplantation: Does the indication for operation influence postoperative lung function? *J Thorac Cardiovasc Surg* 112:1504–1514, 1996.
51. Novitsky D, Wicomb WN, Cooper DK, et al: Electrocardiographic, hemodynamic, and endocrine changes occurring during experimental brain death in the Chacma baboon. *J Heart Trans* 4:63–69, 1984.
52. Parisi F, Carotti A, Abbattista AD, et al: Intermediate and long-term results after pediatric heart transplantation: Incidence and role of pre-transplant diagnosis. *Transpl Int* 11:S493–S498, 1998.
53. Parry A, Higgins R, Wheeldon D, et al: The contribution of donor management and modified cold blood lung perfusate to post-transplant lung function. *J Heart Lung Transplant* 18:121–126, 1999.
54. Pisani BA, Mullen GM, Malinowska K, et al: Plasmapheresis with intravenous immunoglobulin G is effective in patients with elevated panel reactive antibody prior to cardiac transplantation. *J Heart Lung Transplant* 18:701–706, 1999.
55. Price GD, Olsen SL, Taylor DO, et al: Corticosteroid-free maintenance immunosuppresion after heart transplantation: Feasibility and beneficial effects. *J Heart Lung Transplant* 11:403–414, 1992.
56. Radley-Smith RC, Yacoub MH: Long-term results of pediatric heart transplantation. *J Heart Lung Transplant* 11:S277–S281, 1992.
57. Razzouk AJ, Chinnock RE, Gundry SR, et al: Transplantation as a primary treatment for hypoplastic left heart syndrome: Intermediate-term results. *Ann Thorac Surg* 62:1–8, 1996.
58. Robinson JA, Radvany RM, Mullen MG, Garrity ER: Plasmapheresis followed by intravenous immunoglobulin in presensitized patients awaiting thoracic organ transplantation. *Ther Apher* 1:147–151, 1997.
59. Santos-Ocampo SD, Sekarski TJ, Saffitz JE, et al: Echocardiographic characteristics of biopsy-proven cellular rejection in infant heart transplant recipients. *J Heart Lung Transplant* 15:25–34, 1996.
60. Scheinin SA, Radovancevic B, Parnis SM, et al: Mechanical circulatory support in children. *Eur J Cardiothorac Surg* 8:537–540, 1994.
61. Schmid C, Garritsen HS, Kelsch R, et al: Suppression of panel-reactive antibodies by treatment with mycophenolate mofetil. *J Thor Cardiovasc Surg* 46:161–162, 1998.
62. Shaddy RE, Naftel DC, Kirklin JK, et al: Outcome of cardiac transplantation in children: Survival in a contemporary multi-institutional experience. *Circulation* 94:II69–II73, 1996.
63. Spray TL: Transplantation of the heart and lungs in children. *Annu Rev Med* 45:139–148, 1994.
64. Spray TL, Mallory GB, Canter CB, Huddleston CB: Pediatric lung transplantation: Indications, techniques, and early results. *J Thorac Cardiovasc Surg* 107:990–1000, 1994.
65. Starnes VA, Woo MS, MacLaughlin EF, et al: Comparison of outcomes between living donor and cadaveric lung transplantation in children. *Ann Thorac Surg* 68:2279–2283, 1999.
66. Steck TB, Costanzo-Nordin MR, Keshavarzian A: Prevalence and management of cholelithiasis in heart transplant patients. *J Heart Lung Transplant* 10:1029, 1991.
67. Swartz MT, Votapka TV, McBride LR, et al: Risk stratification in patients bridged to cardiac transplantation. *Ann Thorac Surg* 58:1142–1145, 1994.
68. Swenson JM, Fricker FJ, Armitage JM: Immunosuppresion switch in pediatric heart transplant recipients: Cyclosporine to FK506. *J Am Coll Cardiol* 25:1183–1188, 1995.
69. Toronto Lung Transplant Group: Sequential bilateral lung transplantation for paraquat poisoning. *J Thorac Cardiovasc Surg* 89:734–742, 1984.
70. Tsau PH, Arabia FA, Toporoff B, et al: Positive panel reactive antibody titers in patients bridged to transplantation with a mechanical assist device: Risk factors and treatment. *ASAIO J* 44:M634–M637, 1998.
71. Vouhe PR, Tamisier D, Le Bidois J, et al: Pediatric cardiac transplantation for congenital heart defects: Surgical considerations and results. *Ann Thorac Surg* 56:1239–1247, 1993.
72. Warnecke H, Berdjis F, Hennig E, et al: Mechanical left ventricular support as a bridge to cardiac transplantation in childhood. *Eur J Cardiothorac Surg* 5:330–333, 1991.
73. Webber SA, Fricker FJ, Michaels M, et al: Orthotopic heart transplantation in children with congenital heart disease. *Ann Thorac Surg* 58:1664–1669, 1994.
74. West LJ, Pollock-Barziv SM, Dipchand AI, et al: ABO-incompatible heart transplantation in infants. *N Engl J Med* 344:793–800, 2001.
75. Wheeldon DR, Potter CD, Jonas M, et al: Using "unsuitable" hearts for transplantation. *Eur J Cardiothorac Surg* 8:7–9, 1994.
76. Whitehead B, Rees P, Sorensen K, et al: Incidence of obliterative bronchiolitis after heart-lung transplantation. *J Heart Lung Transplant* 12:903–908, 1993.
77. Wreghitt TG, Abel SJ, McNeil K, et al: Intravenous ganciclovir prophylaxis for cytomegalovirus in heart, heart-lung, and lung transplant recipients. *Transpl Int* 12:254–260, 1999.
78. Zales VR, Stapleton PL: Neonatal and infant heart transplantation. *Pediatr Clin North Am* 40:1023–1046, 1993.

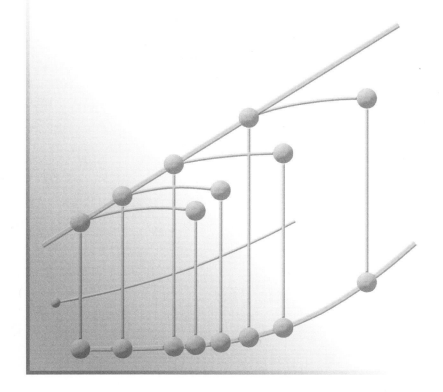

Equipment and Techniques

PART THREE

Equicure Italiano
Techniques

Chapter 17

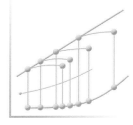

Noninvasive Diagnosis of Congenital and Acquired Pediatric Heart Disease

PHILIP J. SPEVAK, MD, and LAUREEN M. SENA, MD

INTRODUCTION

Over the past two decades, noninvasive imaging techniques have assumed the primary role in the initial diagnosis of congenital and acquired heart disease in children. The majority of children with congenital heart disease safely proceed to surgical or transcatheter treatment on the basis of noninvasive testing alone (Tables 17-1 and 17-2).[23,58,60] Echocardiography remains the primary noninvasive tool because of its excellent resolution. The examination can be performed wherever the patient is located, from the outpatient clinic to the operating room to the intensive care unit. When transthoracic acoustic windows are compromised by surgical dressings or chest tubes in the perioperative period, transesophageal echocardiography is very useful.[79,83,103]

Other noninvasive techniques including magnetic resonance imaging and computerized axial tomography are increasingly used.[34,42,50,63,96] Magnetic resonance imaging provides exquisite anatomic definition and is often helpful in imaging the aortic arch, complicated conduits, and the branch pulmonary arteries. Magnetic resonance can accurately measure right or single ventricle function and can quantify flow volumes. Images are obtained without using ionizing radiation. Computerized tomography, with the application of multidetector technology, allows for rapid acquisition with excellent spatial resolution. Computerized tomography, like magnetic resonance, is particularly well suited at demonstrating systemic or pulmonary vasculature and provides additional information in coronary artery imaging.[40]

This chapter reviews the principles and applications of these techniques from the perspective of the physician and nurse working in the intensive care unit and highlights the strengths and weakness of each imaging method.

ECHOCARDIOGRAPHY

Physical Principles

Pulse Transmission and Reflection

The clinician may wish to understand how echocardiographic images are generated.[59] In the head of an imaging transducer, piezoelectric crystals are arranged. Piezoelectric crystals have an amazing property. When physically deformed, the crystals produce small amounts of electrical energy. Conversely, when

Table 17-1　Lesions Where Noninvasive Imaging Is Generally Sufficient Before Surgical or Transcatheter Intervention

Lesion	Features to Be Identified with Noninvasive Imaging	Associated Lesions to Identify/Exclude	Indications for Cardiac Catheterization
SHUNTS			
Atrial septal defect	Type of atrial defect, size, quantification of shunt (degree of right ventricular volume overload), pulmonary artery pressure, suitability for transcatheter closure	Anomalous pulmonary venous return, pulmonary stenosis, pulmonary hypertension	Transcatheter closure commonly performed for secundum atrial septal defects. Catheterization usually unnecessary unless pulmonary hypertension or pulmonary vascular disease suspected and management depends on measure of pulmonary resistance.
Ventricular septal defect	Type, anatomic size, quantification of shunt (determined in part by left ventricular size), pulmonary artery pressure	Multiple ventricular defects, coarctation	Catheterization usually unnecessary unless pulmonary vascular obstructive disease suggests inoperability. Some defects may allow transcatheter closure.
Patent ductus arteriosus	Anatomic size, pulmonary artery pressure, quantification of shunt (determined in part by left ventricular size), arch side and branching	Coarctation of the aorta	Transcatheter closure
Complete atrioventricular canal	Size of atrial and ventricular septal defects, atrioventricular valve morphology, balance, and function	Outflow obstruction, patent ductus arteriosus	Only in rare patient where quantification of pulmonary resistance desired
CYANOTIC LESIONS			
Transposition of the great arteries	Coronary artery origins and branching, intracardiac shunts, pulmonary artery pressure. Magnetic resonance imaging useful postoperatively to assess branch pulmonary arteries, ventricular function.	Outflow obstruction, arch obstruction, septal defects	Balloon atrial septostomy when needed, usually performed in intensive care unit
Tetralogy of Fallot	Mechanism and severity of pulmonary stenosis, main pulmonary artery and branch pulmonary artery sizes, coronary artery origin and branching. Magnetic resonance imaging very useful postoperatively to image branch pulmonary arteries, quantify severity of pulmonary regurgitation, assess right ventricular function.	Multiple ventricular septal defects, aortic arch sidedness and branching	Uncommonly needed in older childhood left unrepaired and echocardiography unable to establish pertinent features. In rare cases, pulmonary balloon valvuloplasty performed to palliate and delay surgery.
Tricuspid atresia with normally related great vessels	Size of ventricular septal defect and severity of pulmonary stenosis, adequacy of foramen ovale, identification of other sources of pulmonary blood flow, branch pulmonary artery size and continuity, arch side and branching	Pulmonary stenosis, left juxtaposition of the atrial appendages	Very rare need to perform balloon atrial septostomy to enlarge foramen ovale. Minority of surgeons prefer angiogram of branch pulmonary arteries before shunt. Catheterization commonly performed before potential Glenn or Fontan operation.
Ebstein's anomaly	Morphology of tricuspid valve, severity of tricuspid regurgitation, right ventricular size and function	Pulmonary valve or branch pulmonary artery stenosis, patent ductus arteriosus, pulmonary artery pressure	Usually not necessary
Valvular pulmonary stenosis	Mechanism and severity of stenosis, tricuspid valve and right ventricular size and function, patent ductus arteriosus	Can occur with more complex heart disease including heterotaxy syndrome	Balloon dilation is now treatment of choice.
Total anomalous pulmonary venous connection	Identification of individual pulmonary veins and their size and site of return, exclusion of pulmonary venous obstruction	Can occur with other complex congenital heart disease, left heart hypoplasia	Generally not necessary and of significant risk when required to establish pulmonary venous return (potential for pulmonary hypertensive crisis)
ADMIXTURE LESIONS			
Truncus arteriosus common	Morphology and function of truncal valve, branch pulmonary size and distortion	Exclusion of multiple ventricular septal defects, ventricular hypoplasia (particularly right), aortic arch size	Generally unnecessary, rarely if pulmonary vascular obstructive disease is considered in an older infant or child

Table 17-1 Lesions Where Noninvasive Imaging Is Generally Sufficient Before Surgical or Transcatheter Intervention—Cont'd

Lesion	Features to Be Identified with Noninvasive Imaging	Associated Lesions to Identify/Exclude	Indications for Cardiac Catheterization
LEFT HEART OBSTRUCTIVE LESIONS			
Valvular aortic stenosis	Size of aortic annulus and morphology, severity of aortic obstruction, left ventricular size and function	Mitral stenosis, coarctation, left heart hypoplasia	In most cases, used as initial choice for relief of obstruction, although there is controversy concerning superiority over surgical approach
Aortic coarctation	Aortic arch anatomy and size, mechanism of aortic coarctation, aortic arch branching, left ventricular size and function. Magnetic resonance imaging or computerized axial tomography excellent when echocardiographic visualization inadequate.	Mitral and/or aortic stenosis	Generally unnecessary before surgical repair. Some favor balloon dilation versus surgical treatment.
Hypoplastic left heart syndrome	Size of atrial septal defect, tricuspid valve function, right ventricular function, nature of mitral and aortic obstruction, left ventricular size, arch morphology. Postoperatively, magnetic resonance imaging useful in examining arch and branch pulmonary arteries.	Patent ductus arteriosus, partial anomalous pulmonary venous return	Not generally needed before Norwood procedure, but performed before Glenn and before Fontan for hemodynamics and visualization of branch pulmonary arteries

electrical energy is applied to piezoelectric crystals, physical deformation occurs and ultrasound waves are generated. Ultrasound is sound in frequencies ranging from 1 to 12 MHz (million cycles per second). Exciting the crystals with electrical energy, thereby producing ultrasound, is analogous to striking a gong with a mallet and producing audible sound.

Imaging systems do not send a single pulse of electrical energy to the crystals, but multiple, very short pulses. With each electrical pulse, a pulse of acoustic energy is produced.

By pulsing the transducer repeatedly at very rapid rates, multiple acoustic pulses result. Damping materials are added to the transducer head to shorten the duration of each pulse. Short duration pulses are important in achieving excellent image resolution.

If the transducer were simply placed on the patient's chest, most of the ultrasound energy would reflect back off the skin, like light reflecting off a mirror; the ultrasound energy would never enter the patient. This is due to marked differences in

Table 17-2 Lesions Where Noninvasive Imaging Is Generally Insufficient Before Surgical or Transcatheter Intervention And Where Cardiac Catheterization Is Generally Performed

Lesion	Features to Be Identified with Noninvasive Imaging	Associated Lesions to Identify/Exclude	Indications for Cardiac Catheterization
Pulmonary atresia with intact ventricular septum	Tricuspid valve size and function, right ventricular size and function, right ventricular pressure, presence of coronary sinusoids or fistula	Coronary artery stenoses, right ventricular dependent coronary artery anatomy	Coronary artery anatomy, stenoses, presence of right ventricular dependent coronary artery distribution
Tetralogy of Fallot with pulmonary atresia	Nature of pulmonary atresia (absent main pulmonary artery versus short segment valvular pulmonary atresia), branch pulmonary artery size, coronary artery anatomy. Magnetic resonance imaging may obviate need for catheterization especially when branch pulmonary arteries good size and collaterals absent.	Multiple ventricular septal defects, aortopulmonary artery collaterals, coronary artery abnormalities, branch pulmonary artery distortion, hypoplasia, or discontinuity	Establishment of pulmonary artery supply and branch pulmonary continuity, determination of overlap between antegrade pulmonary flow and collaterals, in some cases to allow balloon dilation of stenoses, in some cases to allow embolization of aortopulmonary collaterals
Glenn or Fontan shunt	Ventricular function, valvular function	Very dependent on anatomy requiring Glenn shunt	Pulmonary artery anatomy and hemodynamics, exclusion of decompressing vertical vein from innominate vein

impedance between the transducer head and the skin. This impedance mismatch is markedly decreased by applying acoustic gel to the transducer head, thereby allowing acoustic energy to enter the patient.

For an image of the heart to be displayed, the transmitted ultrasound pulse must reach the heart and reflect back to the transducer. As the received sound deforms the piezoelectric crystals in the transducer head, energy is converted back from acoustic to electrical energy. The imaging system can then display the returning signal as an illuminated pixel on a video monitor.

Tissue properties determine how much of the acoustic energy penetrates into the tissues and how much reflects back to the transducer. Fat, for example, reflects little and transmits most energy. In contrast, bone and air reflect nearly all and transmit very little energy. This explains why it is so difficult to image the heart when there is air (e.g., pneumothorax or hyperinflated lungs) between the transducer and the heart. The air-containing structures prevent the acoustic pulses from reaching the heart, like a curtain blocking an audience's view of actors on a stage.

Signal Processing and Image Generation

Once the transducer converts the acoustic energy back into electrical energy, the imaging system performs complicated amplification and signal processing to optimize the signal-to-noise ratio. The returning signals are much weaker than the transmitted signal.

The system can accurately display a reflector's location on the monitor since the speed of sound is nearly constant through different tissue types. The distance of a reflector from the transducer is directly related to the time for sound to travel to, and from, the reflector. The imaging system calculates the distance of each reflector from the transducer using the time-distance formula:

$$D = c \times t/2$$

where D represents the distance to the target; c, the speed of ultrasound through tissue (1530 m/sec); and t, the time for the pulse of energy to travel to a reflector and back to the transducer. The longer it takes to travel to and from a reflector means that the reflector is farther away from the transducer. The process is analogous to airplanes localized with RADAR or submarines with SONAR.

Once signal amplification occurs and the distance is calculated for each reflector, other postprocessing must take place before an image is displayed on the monitor. In brief, this postprocessing involves the conversion of an electrical voltage into a gray scale value. The brightness of an illuminated pixel on the monitor correlates directly with the strength of received energy. More powerful reflectors (e.g., fibrous tissue) are represented as a brighter gray scale value (i.e., closer to white) while weaker reflectors (e.g., pericardial fluid) are represented as darker values (i.e., closer to black).

This entire process occurs at rates between 50 and 150 times per second. The system has a processing capacity, and the system operator has considerable control over how that processing power is used. Though this control is very helpful and allows image optimization, there is always the possibility that incorrect system adjustment will diminish image quality and limit diagnostic information.

Determinants of Image Resolution

Image quality is quantified by spatial and temporal resolution. *Spatial resolution* refers to two-point spatial discrimination: how closely two adjacent structures can be located and correctly resolved as two separate structures rather than incorrectly as a single reflector. Imaging systems should be able to achieve spatial resolution along the plane of the imaging beam to 0.8 mm. This means that two structures as close as 1 mm or slightly less from one another can be resolved from one another. Spatial resolution is superior along the axial plane (i.e., the plane parallel to the imaging beam) compared to the lateral plane (i.e., the plane orthogonal to the imaging probe), where spatial resolution falls to between 1 and 2 mm.

Temporal resolution refers to the ability of the system to resolve accurately the position of a moving structure in time. Though temporal resolution is unimportant in imaging a static structure like the brain (since the structure being imaged does not change position from one moment to the next), it is obviously critically important in accurately demonstrating cardiac motion. If, for example, a rapidly moving structure (e.g., a valve leaflet) moves from point A to point B and back to point A in 10 msec and the temporal resolution of the imaging system is 10 msec, the motion of the valve will not be displayed accurately. In this example, the structure will not appear to move but will appear to remain at point A. Temporal resolution is particularly important when heart rates are faster, as in the fetus or neonate. Temporal resolution as short as 8 to 10 msec can be achieved with properly configured ultrasound systems.

Transducer Selection: The Tradeoff Between Resolution and Penetration

The sonographer chooses the optimal imaging probe, weighing the requirements for spatial and temporal resolution against the requirements for tissue penetration (Figs. 17-1 and 17-2).

Tissue penetration refers to the distance an acoustic pulse can reach. Penetration is indirectly related to probe frequency and directly related to beam transmission power. Higher frequency transducers, covering frequencies between 8 and 12 MHz, provide superior spatial resolution but at the expense of lower penetration. Structures within 8 cm are typically imaged with high frequency probes. Lower frequency transducers covering frequencies between 1 and 3 MHz penetrate farther into tissue (up to 15 to 20 cm) but sacrifice spatial resolution. The sonographer tends to use the highest frequency transducer that provides adequate tissue penetration for the distance required, just as the golfer chooses the putter for short shots requiring more accuracy and the driver when shots require more power. The sonographer trades off the needs of spatial resolution against the requirements of tissue penetration.

Penetration is also directly related to transmission power. Just as a 100-watt light bulb illuminates farther than a 15-watt bulb, increased beam power allows the ultrasound beam to penetrate farther. However, acoustic power is constrained by safety limitations. Tissue warming can occur if excessively high power is used. In addition, image resolution can decrease with higher power, another tradeoff for which the sonographer must accommodate.

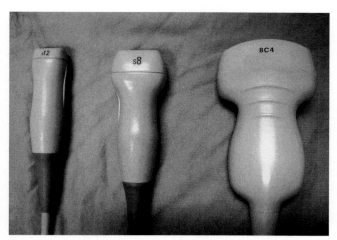

FIGURE 17-1 Transthoracic and abdominal imaging probes. The two probes on the left are phased array sector probes optimized for cardiac imaging. The smaller probe (S12), intended for neonatal imaging, is optimized to image at 12 MHz. Its smaller footprint allows the transducer to fit between narrower interspaces and shifts the acoustic focus closer to the transducer, resulting in an optimal imaging range of less than 6 to 8 cm. The 8 MHz probe (S8) in the middle has slightly inferior spatial resolution but has superior penetration. The latter is important in imaging the larger child. The probe on the right is a curvilinear probe (8C4) and is intended for fetal and abdominal imaging. The curved shape allows for a wider near field of view than the sector probes allow. When the fetus is in the near field, the wider near field of view is important.

Transducers vary in other important ways, such as location of use. Transthoracic probes acquire images from the chest wall, whereas transesophageal probes are passed from the mouth and pharynx into the esophagus or stomach. Transesophageal probes must be smaller and more flexible. Intravascular probes are mounted on catheters to allow

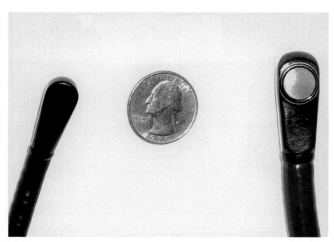

FIGURE 17-2 Transesophageal echocardiography probes. Both probes allow multiplane transesophageal imaging by electronically rotating the scan plane. The smaller probe on the left has a tip diameter 8 by 10.7 mm and is optimized for neonates and children up to approximately 20 kg. The larger probe has a tip diameter 14.9 mm and is intended for the larger child and the adult. The larger probe operates at a lower frequency, allowing for improved beam penetration but at some loss in image resolution.

intracardiac or intravascular imaging. Again, tradeoffs are present; miniaturization is achieved at the expense of some other imaging parameter, usually tissue penetration or resolution.

Harmonic Imaging

A significant improvement in image quality has been due to the application of native harmonic (also called tissue harmonic) imaging.[68,111] Traditional nonharmonic images are created by using the returning signal that is at the same frequency as the transmitted frequency. However, in practice, signals return from the patient not only at the fundamental frequency, but also at harmonics of the fundamental frequency. Harmonics are generated due to a slight nonlinear propagation of the fundamental frequency such that the peaks of the acoustic waves travel slightly faster than do the troughs of the wave. This nonlinearity results in the generation of waves at harmonics of the fundamental frequency. Using harmonic frequencies at higher frequency than the fundamental frequency can result in an improved signal-to-noise ratio and improved signal contrast. This is particularly important in patients who are hard to image, such as the obese or those with postoperative lines or tubes.

Doppler Analysis

Doppler analysis is a powerful complementary modality to two-dimensional imaging.[31] It is used primarily to quantify flow velocity and pressure gradients within the vascular system. Similar to the principles discussed concerning image generation, small packets of ultrasound energy are transmitted, but in this case to the blood pool. When ultrasound energy strikes a moving target such as the red cells, the returning signal frequency is shifted compared to the transmitted frequency. Blood flow toward the transducer shifts the returning frequency higher, whereas flow away shifts the frequency lower. This velocity causing the frequency change (referred to as the Doppler frequency shift) is characterized by the Doppler equation:

$$V = f_d \times 2c/f_o \times 1/\cos \theta$$

where V represents the velocity of the reflector (i.e., red cell); f_d, the Doppler frequency shift; c, the speed of sound in tissue; f_o, the transmitted frequency; and θ, the angle between the direction of sound propagation and the direction of motion of the reflector.

Directionality of blood flow is determined by whether the frequency shift is higher (i.e., flow toward the probe) or lower (flow away from the probe). The speed of the red cells is related to the magnitude of the frequency shift. Fast-moving targets such as flow across a stenotic valve produce a larger frequency shift. Slower moving targets such as venous flow cause less of a frequency shift. The imaging systems routinely calculate the velocity from the measured frequency shift and then display that velocity for the sonographer.

The result of Doppler interrogation is a spectral display with velocity on the Y axis and time along the X axis. The convention is to display flow away from the transducer as a positive value (i.e., above the zero baseline) and flow away from the transducer as a negative valve (i.e., below the zero baseline).

A very important relationship exists between the velocity and the pressure gradient producing this velocity. This is described by the Bernoulli equation:

$$\Delta P = 4(V_2^2 - V_1^2)$$

V_2 represents the velocity measured just distal to the site of interest, and V_1, the velocity just proximal to the site of interest. This can be used, for example, to measure the maximum instantaneous gradient across a stenotic valve (Fig. 17-3). If the velocity distal to the valve (V_2) is 4.5 m/sec and velocity just proximal (V_1) is 1.5 m/sec, then the pressure gradient resulting in this velocity increase would be:

$$\Delta P = 4\ (4.5^2 - 1.5^2)$$

or about 70 to 75 mm Hg.

Frequently V_1 is quite small, and when it is less than 1 m/sec, it can be ignored. This results in the simplified Bernoulli equation:

$$\Delta P = 4\ (V_2)^2$$

It is particularly important to include V_1 whenever the proximal velocity exceeds 1.5 m/sec. This is typically the case, for example, when measuring the gradient across an aortic coarctation. Flow accelerates around the arch normally and the velocity can reach or even exceed 1.5 m/sec. Higher velocities occur when the arch is hypoplastic. Ignoring V_1 and using only the simplified Bernoulli equation would result in an overestimate of the maximum instantaneous gradient. There are important theoretical and clinical considerations in interpreting the calculated Doppler gradient and these are discussed in the section concerning gradient assessment.

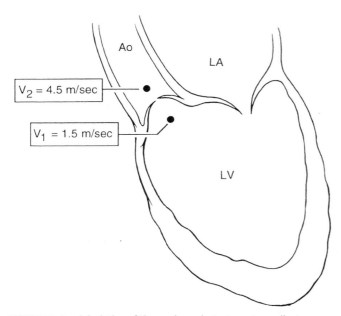

FIGURE 17-3   Calculation of the maximum instantaneous gradient across a stenotic aortic valve using the Bernoulli equation. In this example, the aortic valve is doming due to presence of severe aortic valve stenosis. Using Doppler interrogation, the velocity (V_1) is measured within the left ventricular outflow tract just proximal to the aortic valve and at V_2, just distal to the doming aortic valve leaflets. Using the Bernoulli equation, $\Delta P = 4\ (V_2^2 - V_1^2)$ where V_1 is 1.5 m/sec and V_2 is 4.5 m/sec. ΔP is 70 to 75 mm Hg. The valve gradient is a function of the orifice area and the flow across the area of interest. Ao, aorta; LA, left atrium; LV, left ventricle.

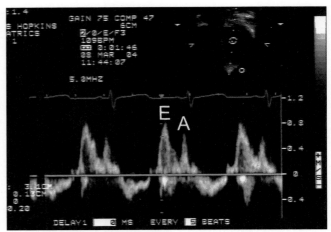

FIGURE 17-4   Pulse Doppler interrogation of the mitral valve in a healthy 3-month-old infant. Mitral valve flow is displayed as a spectral display of instantaneous velocity against time. Flow is displayed above the baseline since flow is toward the transducer. Note the scale in meters/second displayed at the right margin of the spectral display. For orientation, the gate of Doppler is displayed in the small image circled in the upper right corner. The gate is positioned just distal to the tips of the mitral valve leaflets within the left ventricle. Generally two filling waves are seen with mitral valve flow. The peak E velocity (E) occurs after mitral valve opening and the peak A velocity (A) during atrial systole. In this young infant, the E velocity is 0.8 m/sec and A velocity, 0.6 m/sec. The E/A ratio (peak E velocity/peak A velocity) is 1.3. Normal mitral and tricuspid valve velocities are displayed in Table 17-3.

There are four different methods of Doppler interrogation: pulse wave, continuous wave, high pulse repetition, and color Doppler. Each method has particular strengths and clinical applications.

Pulse Wave Doppler   This is the most frequently used Doppler technique and has the advantage of allowing velocity determination at a specific location in the heart called a gate (Figs. 17-4 and 17-5). Pulse wave Doppler can be used,

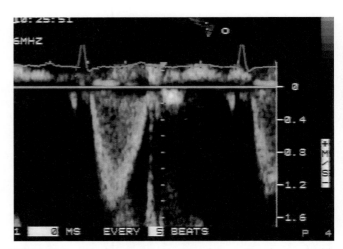

FIGURE 17-5   Pulse Doppler interrogation of the aortic valve in a healthy 9-year-old child. Aortic velocity is displayed as a spectral display of instantaneous velocity against time. In this apical four-chamber view, flow is away from the transducer so velocity is displayed below the baseline. Note the scale in meters/second displayed at the right margin of the spectral display. For orientation, the gate of pulse Doppler interrogation has been positioned just distal to the tips of the aortic valve leaflets within the ascending aorta. The maximum velocity ranges between 1.2 and 1.5 m/sec. Normal aortic valve and pulmonary valve velocities are displayed in Table 17-4.

for example, to determine the gradient across a stenotic valve or vessel stenosis or across a septal defect.

Whereas the strength of pulse wave Doppler is its ability to measure velocity at a specific location, it has a very important limitation called *aliasing*. Aliasing occurs when pulse Doppler cannot reliably calculate the speed and direction of the target. For pulse Doppler to measure flow velocity accurately, the imaging system must sample (i.e., transmit acoustic packets) at a frequency greater than twice the frequency shift produced by the flow being interrogated. When the interrogated flow velocity is quite fast, the sampling rate of the system may not be able to achieve the required sampling frequency, called the *Nyquist limit*, and if so, aliasing occurs.

Aliasing is analogous to the appearance of a spinning wheel illuminated in a dark room by a strobe light flashing at a frequency less than twice the spinning frequency. If the wheel is spinning more than twice as fast as the strobe rate, the wheel may appear to be spinning backward. If the strobe and spinning frequency are the same, the wheel may not appear to be moving at all! Aliasing becomes a clinically important limitation in cardiac imaging when blood flow is fast, such as across severely stenotic valves or vessels or restrictive ventricular septal defects.

Continuous Wave Doppler and High Pulse Repetition Doppler Fortunately, other Doppler techniques including continuous wave and high pulse repetition frequency Doppler can accurately measure these higher velocity events. They are able to do so by sampling at frequencies faster than traditional pulse Doppler interrogation (in the case of continuous wave Doppler, sampling is "nearly continuous"). Though the higher sampling rate eliminates aliasing, another problem is introduced, called *range ambiguity*.

Range ambiguity is easily understood if the reader remembers back to the strength of pulse Doppler interrogation: the ability to measure blood velocity at a specific location in the heart called a gate. When very high sampling frequencies are used with continuous wave Doppler or high pulse repetition frequency Doppler, returning signals are reaching the imaging system too fast to determine reliably the specific location from which the event is occurring (called range ambiguity). An analogy is that of a police officer using a radar gun on passing motorists. If he "fires" the gun before waiting for the last "fire" to return, he will have difficulty determining from exactly which location (car in this case) the signal is returning.

Fortunately, in clinical practice, the problem of range ambiguity in interrogating high velocity events is usually solved by applying clinical judgment and/or supplemental echocardiographic information. High velocity events occur in specific clinical situations so if locations that do make sense are suggested with continuous wave Doppler, the operator "knows" to interpret that information critically. In some situations the operator can use other information to assess for internal consistency. For example, if continuous wave Doppler suggests severe valvular pulmonary stenosis, the right ventricular pressure should be elevated. Usually, but not always, the operator can resolve range ambiguity.

Color Doppler This is a very powerful technique allowing the velocity information to be overlaid across the two-dimensional image (Fig. 17-6). Various color maps are used to encode this

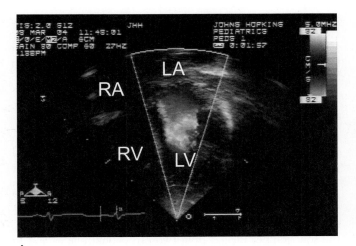

A

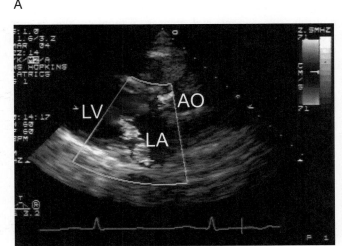

B

FIGURE 17-6 Color Doppler interrogation. **A,** Mitral valve in diastole. In this apical four-chamber view, flow across the mitral valve is demonstrated during diastole. The convention of this color map is to display flow toward the transducer (the apex of the scan triangle) as shades of yellows and red and flow away as shades of blue. The map legend in the upper right corner of the image shows that the maximum flow away (light blues) and toward (light yellows) is 82 cm/second. **B,** Parasternal long axis image showing moderate mitral regurgitation. The jet passes into the left atrium and is displayed in blue shades as flow away from the transducer. AO, aorta; LA, left atrium; LV, left ventricle; RA, right atrium; RV, right ventricle.

information, but a commonly used map displays blood flow toward the transducer in red and flow away in blue. Shades of blue are used to indicate the speed of flow away: Low velocity flow away may be a darker blue and higher velocity a lighter shade of blue. Shades of red and yellow are used to indicate the speed of flow toward the transducer: Low velocity flow toward may be a darker red and higher velocity a shade of yellow-red. Other encoding maps can display areas of turbulence, where the velocity at closely adjacent areas varies one to another in contrast to when flow is laminar.

Elements of the Normal Transthoracic Echocardiographic Examination

Those in the intensive care unit caring for patients with cardiac disease should have familiarity with the elements of a two-dimensional transthoracic echocardiogram. The three basic elements of any examination include imaging sweeps for anatomic delineation, Doppler interrogation for blood flow velocity and direction, and measurement of systolic and diastolic function.

Imaging Planes and Sweeps for Anatomic Delineation

Fan-shaped two-dimensional images are typically obtained from four acoustic windows: subcostal (just inferior to the xiphoid process), apical (~5th left intercostal space at the anterior axillary line), parasternal (2nd or 3rd left parasternal space, midclavicular line), and the suprasternal notch (Fig. 17-7).[45] Sweeps from multiple locations are important to appreciate the three-dimensional anatomy of the heart. At each location, the sonographer images from two orthogonal planes and in each plane "sweeps" through the cardiac mass, generating multiple two-dimensional images. Common scan planes are illustrated in four figures: subcostal (Fig. 17-8), apical (Fig. 17-9), parasternal (Fig. 17-10), and suprasternal notch (Fig. 17-11).

Other imaging positions are less commonly used to image particular structures: right sternal border (atrial septum) and high left parasagittal (patent ductus arteriosus). Often in the postoperative patient, bandages or chest tubes may limit imaging from some of the standard locations and nonstandard transthoracic or transesophageal windows are utilized.

The intensive care unit nurse can be helpful in repositioning the patient. Subcostal images are generally obtained with the patient lying on his or her back and sometimes with knees bent. The apical and parasternal images are obtained with the patient in left lateral decubitus position so the left lung falls posterior to the imaging plane. Suprasternal notch images are best obtained with a pillow placed behind the patient's back so the neck is hyperextended. It is also helpful to the sonographer for the lights to be dimmed so the video monitor is more easily viewed.

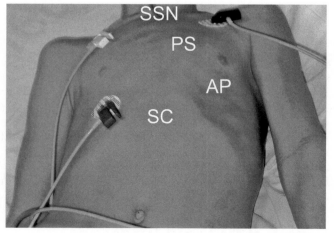

FIGURE 17-7 Orientation of scan planes in transthoracic echocardiogram. Normal scan positions. The patient is positioned with leads attached to allow electrocardiographic monitoring for timing. Four imaging positions or acoustic windows are commonly used: subcostal (SC), apical (AP), parasternal (PS), and suprasternal sternal notch (SSN).

Doppler Interrogation

Color Doppler is performed of all valves (for regurgitation or stenosis), atrial and ventricular septum (for septal defects), main pulmonary artery (for patent ductus arteriosus), and branch pulmonary arteries and aortic arch (excluding peripheral pulmonary artery stenosis and coarctation) (see Fig. 17-6). Small amounts of tricuspid and pulmonary regurgitation are common normal variants. Mild mitral regurgitation though less common is also a normal variant. A "sprung" foramen ovale, allowing a small amount of left to right flow, is also a normal variant in the child younger than 1 year of age.

Pulse Doppler is performed of each valve. The tricuspid valve and mitral valve have similar flow patterns (see Fig. 17-4). Filling generally occurs in two waves termed the E wave (during early diastolic filling of the ventricle) and the A wave (during atrial systole). Each wave has a peak velocity termed the E velocity and A velocity, respectively. In the fetus and neonate, the peak A velocity typically exceeds the peak E velocity. The E velocity typically exceeds the A velocity after 1 year of age. Normal mitral valve and tricuspid valve flow velocities are displayed in Table 17-3.[106]

Pulmonary and aortic flow velocities in healthy children are cited in Table 17-4[106] and illustrated in Figure 17-5. The normal aortic velocity exceeds that of the pulmonary velocity.[41] Accelerated flow usually indicates valve stenosis, although any condition that increases cardiac output will increase flow velocities to a mild degree. Anemia or any hyperkinetic state such as thyrotoxicosis, fever, or pain is an example.

Assessment of Systolic and Diastolic Function

Theoretical Concepts Myocardial contractility and systolic function should be distinguished from one another. Contractility is an intrinsic property of the myocardial fibers. Systolic function refers to how well the fibers shorten when loaded. Though dependent on contractility, systolic function is affected by preload and afterload. Take, for example, a hypothetical patient in the intensive care unit who becomes hypovolemic. Function would decline due to reduced preload, not because of a change in myocardial contractility. If instead the patient became quite hypertensive, function would also decrease not because of any change in contractility but because of increased afterload. Finally, consider a patient where preload and afterload remain constant, but the ventricle becomes ischemic. In this last situation, both function and contractility decrease.

Afterload is directly related to fiber wall stress at end-systole (ESWS) and can be calculated by the following equation:

$$ESWS = K * (ESP * R)/h$$

where *ESP* is end-systolic ventricular pressure; *R*, end-systole ventricular radius; and *h*, end-systolic thickness. *K* is a constant. It is important for the intensivist to understand that though afterload is related to mean arterial pressure, afterload can also be increased without an increase in arterial pressure if the ventricle is dilated or wall thickness reduced. Adriamycin cardiomyopathy is a condition in which afterload is increased due to reduced wall thickness despite normal blood pressure and heart size.

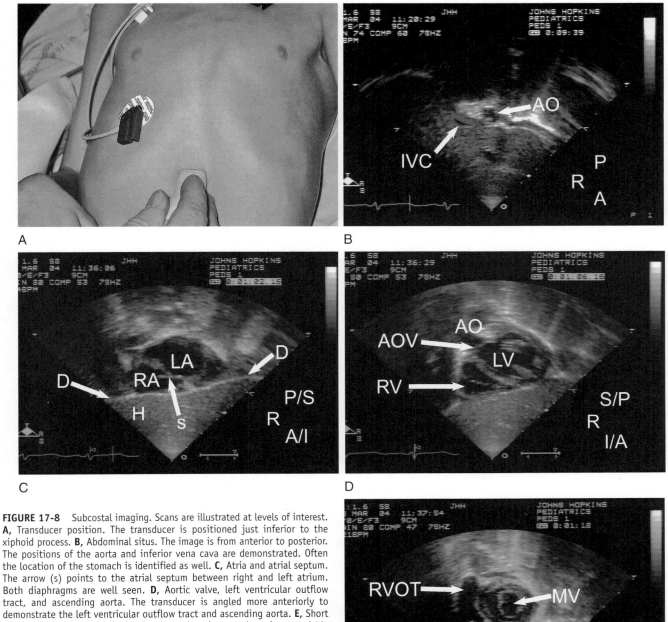

FIGURE 17-8   Subcostal imaging. Scans are illustrated at levels of interest. **A,** Transducer position. The transducer is positioned just inferior to the xiphoid process. **B,** Abdominal situs. The image is from anterior to posterior. The positions of the aorta and inferior vena cava are demonstrated. Often the location of the stomach is identified as well. **C,** Atria and atrial septum. The arrow (s) points to the atrial septum between right and left atrium. Both diaphragms are well seen. **D,** Aortic valve, left ventricular outflow tract, and ascending aorta. The transducer is angled more anteriorly to demonstrate the left ventricular outflow tract and ascending aorta. **E,** Short axis cut at level of the mitral valve. Note that the transducer is rotated 90° clockwise from images in B–D. The mitral valve is open within the left ventricle in this diastolic frame. The ventricular septum is seen between the right and left ventricle and the proximal right ventricular outflow tract with the right ventricle. A, anterior; AO, aorta; AOV, aortic valve; D, diaphragm; H, liver; I, inferior; IVC, inferior vena cava; LA, left atrium; LV, left ventricle; MV, mitral valve; P, posterior; P/S, posterior-superior; R, right; RA, right atrium; RV, right ventricle; RVOT, right ventricular outflow tract; s, atrial septum; S, superior; VS, ventricular septum.

Preload is defined as the stretch on the fibers at end-diastole. Preload is related to ventricular filling pressure but is not identical to that pressure since there is not a direct or constant relationship between filling pressure and fiber stretch. An example is the changes that occur with cardiopulmonary bypass. The changes may result in a "stiffer" ventricle so less fiber stretch occurs for the same filling pressure. Consequently, a higher filling pressure postoperatively doesn't necessarily mean that the ventricle is working at increased preload. It is important for the intensivist to remember this distinction when considering atrial pressure or mean capillary wedge pressure as a proxy for preload.

In children there is an age-dependent modulation of ventricular function with a decrease in function with age, in part related to increasing afterload.[20] The functional decrease, however, is also due to an age-dependent decrease in contractility

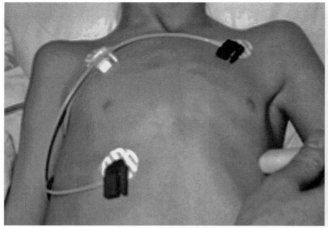

A

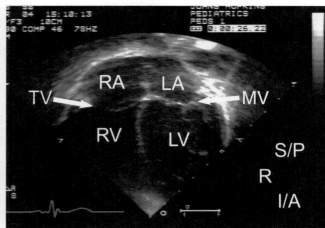

B

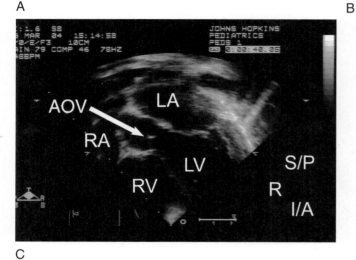

C

FIGURE 17-9 Apical imaging. Scans are illustrated at levels of interest. **A,** transducer position. The transducer is positioned at the cardiac apex usually in the fourth or fifth intercostal space along the anterior axillary line. Often the patient is positioned in the left lateral decubitus position to minimize reflection of air from the left lung. **B,** Four-chamber view. An excellent view for quickly assessing chamber size and atrioventricular valve function. The arrows point to the mitral valve and tricuspid valve. **C,** Five-chamber view. The transducer is angled anteriorly from the four-chamber view to demonstrate the aortic valve (*arrow*) and ascending aorta (just distal to the aortic valve). The other cardiac chambers are also displayed. A, anterior; AoV, aortic valve; I, inferior; LA, left atrium; LV, left ventricle; P, posterior; R, right; RA, right atrium; RV, right ventricle; S, superior.

(with higher levels of contractility seen in infants and in children in the early years of life).

Diastolic function relates to the ability of the heart to relax and is an energy-consuming process. The importance of diastole is being increasingly recognized, in part because there is an improved theoretical understanding of diastole and because there are improved noninvasive tools for measuring diastolic function. Diastole has three phases: passive filling, diastasis, and atrial systole (sometimes called active filling). The timing and rate of ventricular filling are related to filling pressure, diastolic function, and pericardial constraint.

Clinical Assessment of Systolic Function. Global systolic function is most commonly assessed in the intensive care unit using measures of ejection performance such as ejection fraction or shortening fraction. Ejection fraction is the percent change in end-diastolic volume:

$$\frac{(\text{End-diastolic volume} - \text{end-systolic volume})}{\text{end-diastolic volume}} \times 100$$

Volumes are most accurately measured using a biplane rather than single plane method. Normative ranges for ventricular volumes are available for children[22,114] with normal left ventricular ejection fraction reported as 60.3% ± 6.7%.[11] Frequently apical views are used to assess ejection fraction,

but it is possible to measure ejection fraction from other acoustic windows.

Often, rather than using ejection fraction, shortening fraction is measured. Shortening fraction, or percent change in ventricular diameter, is calculated using the following formula:

$$\frac{(\text{End-diastolic dimension} - \text{end-systolic dimension})}{\text{end-diastolic dimension}} \times 100$$

The shortening fraction is easy to measure and is a useful measure of systolic function when ventricular geometry is normal (Fig. 17-12). Normal values for shortening fraction range from approximately 29% to 41%,[20,99] with the higher range in neonates and younger children. When the normal left ventricular shape is altered, biplane methods such as ejection fraction provide a more accurate measure of systolic function. In addition, some studies have demonstrated considerable interobserver variability in the measurement.

As mentioned, both ejection fraction and shortening fraction are load dependent, and their interpretation must consider loading conditions. In addition, both are measures of global function. Any measure of systolic function must also consider whether there are regional wall motion abnormalities. Wall motion abnormalities in children are more commonly seen postoperatively after surgical incisions or placement of patches, with coronary artery abnormalities

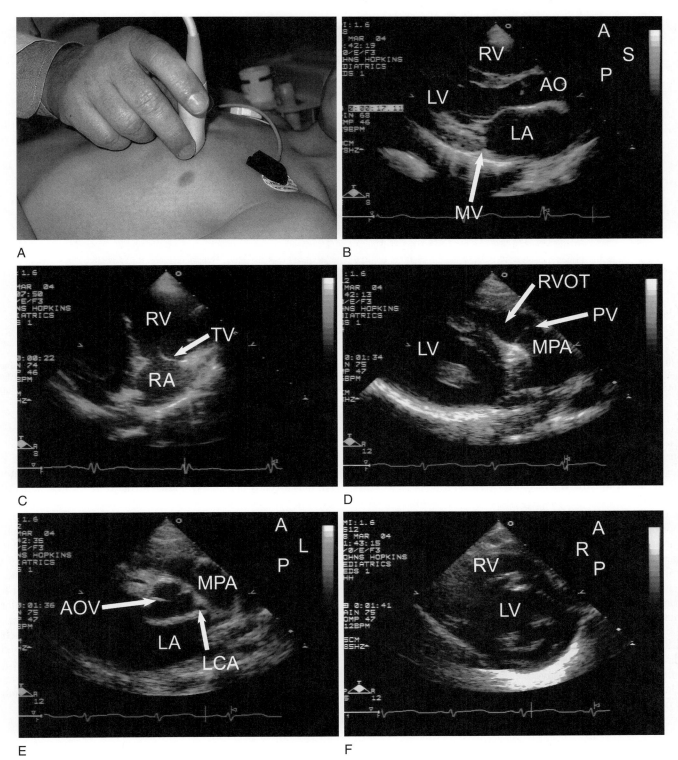

FIGURE 17-10 Parasternal imaging planes. Scans are illustrated at levels of interest. **A,** Transducer position. The transducer is positioned in the second or third intercostal space in the midclavicular line. Left lung interference is often minimized by positioning the patient in the left lateral decubitus position. **B,** Long axis view at level of aorta. Demonstrates the left atrium and ventricle, aortic valve, mitral valve, and ascending aorta. **C,** Long axis view angled to the tricuspid valve. Tricuspid valve inflow, right atrium, and right ventricle are demonstrated. **D,** Long axis view angled to the left to the pulmonary valve. The right ventricular outflow tract, pulmonary valve, and main pulmonary artery are displayed. **E,** Short axis view at the aortic valve. The transducer is rotated to display the heart in its short axis. This view displays aortic valve morphology, the proximal coronary arteries, pulmonary valve, and main pulmonary artery well. **F,** Short axis at ventricular level. Sweeping inferiorly from the aortic valve, a short axis view of both ventricles is displayed. This is a standard view for assessing left ventricular function. The mitral valve is seen within the left ventricle. A, anterior; AO, aorta; AOV, aortic valve; L, left; LA, left atrium; LCA, left main coronary artery; LV, left ventricle; MPA, main pulmonary artery; P, posterior; PV, pulmonary valve; R, right; RA, right atrium; RV, right ventricle; RVOT, right ventricular outflow tract; S, superior; TV, tricuspid valve.

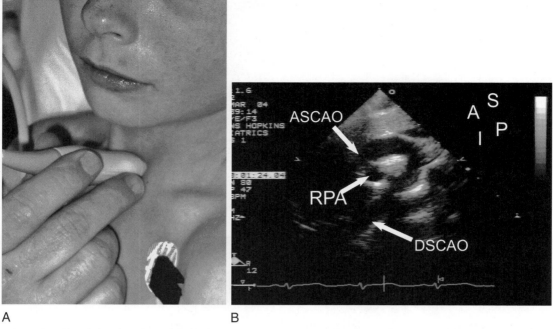

FIGURE 17-11   Suprasternal notch imaging plane. **A,** Transducer position. The transducer is positioned in the suprasternal notch. **B,** Aortic arch view. The aortic arch is seen in a long axis view. The right pulmonary artery is displayed posterior to the ascending aorta. The arch can be imaged in short axis by rotating the transducer 90°. A, anterior; ASCAO, ascending aorta; DSCAO, descending aorta; I, inferior; P, posterior; RPA, right pulmonary artery; S, superior.

or with cardiomyopathy.[92,93] The neonate has regional wall motion abnormalities with systolic septal flattening persisting until day 5, making fractional shortening a less consistently reliable measure of systolic function.[94] Techniques such as wall stress analysis have been used to measure contractility noninvasively[16-19] but are less commonly applied in the intensive care unit than in the outpatient area, as the necessary views are difficult to obtain due to interference by surgical dressings and tubes.

Other measures including dP/dT and the myocardial performance index have been described, and the interested reader is referred to other sources for more information.[25,27-29]

Clinical Assessment of Diastolic Function   The assessment of diastolic function is best evaluated using tissue Doppler analysis of the atrioventricular valve annular motion. The atrioventricular annulus moves away from the cardiac apex during diastole. Therefore when viewed from the apical four-chamber view,

diastolic motion is away from the transducer. Similar to the E and A waves of mitral valve inflow, the atrioventricular annuli display an early diastolic (E') and late diastolic (A') motion. An example of normal mitral valve annular motion is displayed in Figure 17-13 and normal values are displayed in Table 17-5.[26] Annular motion varies significantly with age, with increasing E' and E/E' in the older child as compared to the infant.

There are three clinical stages of diastolic dysfunction.[37,54] The intensivist should be familiar with these stages. In mild diastolic dysfunction (stage 1, also called impaired relaxation), left ventricular relaxation is abnormal, but left ventricular filling pressure and compliance are still nearly normal. There is increased reliance on atrial systole to achieve left ventricular filling. Impaired relaxation is manifest by decreased early mitral inflow (E) and mitral annular velocities (E'), increased late mitral inflow (A) and mitral annular velocities (A'), and so-called reversed E/A and E'/A' ratios (in which these ratios are less than one).

Table 17-3   Mitral and Tricuspid Valve Flow Velocities in Healthy Children

	Peak E Velocity	Peak A Velocity	E/A Ratio
Mitral valve	0.9 ± 0.11 m/sec	0.49 ± 0.08 m/sec	1.9 ± 0.4
Tricuspid valve	0.6 ± 0.10 m/sec	0.40 ± 0.10 m/sec	1.6 ± 0.5

In healthy neonates and fetuses, the peak A velocity typically exceeds the peak E velocity. Values are displayed as mean ± one standard deviation from the mean. *m/sec,* meters per second.
From Snyder AR, Serwer GA, Ritter SB: The normal echocardiographic examination. In *Echocardiography in Pediatric Heart Disease.* St. Louis, Mosby, 1997:22–75.

Table 17-4 Aortic and Pulmonary Valve Flow Velocities in Healthy Children

	Peak Velocity	Mean Velocity
Aortic valve (adult)	1.35 ± 0.18 m/sec	
Aortic valve (child)	1.50 ± 0.15 m/sec	0.28 ± 0.05 m/sec
Pulmonary valve (child)	0.90 ± 0.10 m/sec	
Pulmonary valve (newborn)	0.80 ± 0.12 m/sec	

Values are displayed as mean ± one standard deviation from the mean. m/sec, meters per second.

From Snyder AR, Serwer GA, Ritter SB: The normal echocardiographic examination. In *Echocardiography in Pediatric Heart Disease.* St. Louis, Mosby, 1997:22–75.

With worsening diastolic dysfunction (stage 2, also called pseudonormalization or moderate diastolic dysfunction), left ventricular compliance is abnormal, and this results in elevated left ventricular end-diastolic pressure. Now the E/A ratio normalizes while the E′/A′ ratio remains abnormal. The E/A ratio is preload dependent whereas the E′/A′ is relatively less so. With stage 3, or severe diastolic dysfunction (termed *restrictive pattern*), there is even worse ventricular compliance and even more elevated filling pressure. This stage is recognized by markedly elevated E and E′, and elevated E/A and E/E′ ratios. Stage 3 has been further differentiated into reversible and irreversible patterns based on the response to Valsalva maneuver. The irreversible pattern has a worse prognosis.

The E/E′ ratio is useful in estimating left ventricular end-diastolic pressure. Since E, mitral inflow velocity, is preload dependent; and E′, mitral annular velocity, is not preload dependent, the ratio increases with increased filling pressure. In an adult population[74]:

$$PCWP = 1.24 \ E/E' + 1.9 \ mm \ Hg$$

where *PCWP* represents pulmonary capillary wedge pressure or left ventricular end-diastolic pressure. Tissue Doppler of

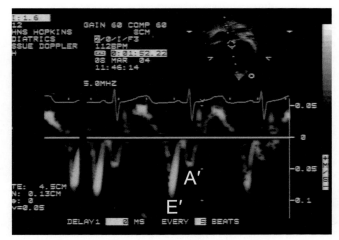

FIGURE 17-13 Pulse tissue Doppler analysis of mitral annular motion in a healthy infant. Flow is below the baseline since the mitral valve annulus moves away from the transducer in this apical view. The early diastolic velocity (E′) is larger (9 cm/sec) than the velocity during atrial systole (A′ equals 4 cm/sec). Note that the motion of the mitral valve annulus is in the opposite direction to mitral valve inflow (flow is toward the apex during diastole).

mitral valve annular motion is increasingly being reported to detect diastolic dysfunction even in early or in subclinical disease states.[71–73,118]

Application of Echocardiography to Other Clinical Problems

Gradient Assessment

As discussed previously, the modified Bernoulli equation can be used to assess the maximum instantaneous gradient across a stenotic valve (see Fig. 17-3). It is important to understand how this Doppler-derived measurement is different from the peak-to-peak gradient typically measured in the catheterization laboratory.

Again using the example of aortic valve stenosis, the Doppler-derived maximum instantaneous gradient measures the maximum gradient at any instant in time between the left ventricular pressure and the aortic pressure. In the catheterization laboratory, peak-to-peak gradient is typically reported: the difference between the peak left ventricular pressure and the peak aortic pressure. Since peak left ventricular pressure and peak aortic pressure do not occur at the same instant in time, it is unlikely that the maximum

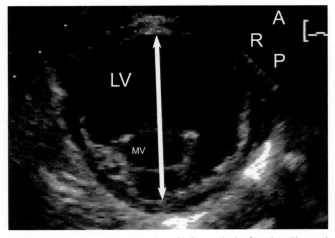

FIGURE 17-12 M-mode examination of left ventricular function. Short axis view of the left ventricle obtained in the parasternal short axis view. The mitral valve (MV) is open within the left ventricle (LV) in this diastolic frame. The long arrow demonstrates the left ventricular endocardial dimension. By using the equivalent view in systole, the shortening fraction (or percent change in short axis diameter) can be calculated. This ventricle is dilated with increased dimension to wall thickness ratio. A, anterior; P, posterior; R, right.

Table 17-5 Mitral and Tricuspid Annular Tissue Doppler in Health Children

	E′	A′	E/E′
Lateral mitral	16.0–17.1	6.2–6.6	5.9–6.4
Medial mitral	12.2–13.0	5.9–6.3	7.5–8.0
Tricuspid	15.6–16.7	9.9–10.5	3.6–4.0

From Eidem BW, McMahon CJ, Cohen RR, Wu J, Finkelshteyn I, Kovalchin JP, Ayres NA, Bezold LI, O'Brian Smith E, Pignatelli RH: Impact of cardiac growth on Doppler tissue imaging velocities: A study in healthy children. *J Am Soc Echocardiogr* 2004;17:212–221.

instantaneous gradient will be identical to the peak-to-peak gradient. One can calculate a maximum instantaneous gradient in the catheterization laboratory by simultaneously measuring left ventricular pressure and aortic pressure. One can then compare the maximum instantaneous gradient that is derived with Doppler to that which is measured in the catheterization laboratory.

There is a good but imperfect correlation between the Doppler-derived maximum instantaneous gradient and the catheterization-derived peak-to-peak gradient.[4] At higher gradients, the Doppler maximum instantaneous gradient may exceed the catheter peak-to-peak gradient but correlates better with the catheter peak instantaneous gradient. Doppler mean gradient correlates well with catheter mean gradient across a broad range of gradients. One of the most important explanations for the differences between Doppler- and catheterization-derived maximum instantaneous gradients is related to pressure recovery. Immediately after a stenotic lesion, energy is converted back to pressure from kinetic energy. In the case of aortic stenosis, the pressure in the ascending aorta is therefore higher, compared to just distal to the stenotic leaflets. The catheter measurement of ascending aortic pressure is likely at the point where pressure recovery has occurred. Some have attempted to account for pressure recovery by correcting the Doppler-derived maximum instantaneous gradient to result in a better predictor of the catheter-based peak-to-peak gradient.[6,13,35,36]

Determination of Pulmonary Artery Pressure

In many situations in the intensive care unit, determination of pulmonary artery pressure is important. Echocardiography and Doppler provide several qualitative and quantitative measures of pulmonary artery pressure.

A qualitative measure of pulmonary artery hypertension is the position of the interventricular septum during systole. Normally, the septum is concave toward the left ventricle since right ventricular pressure is significantly less than left ventricular systolic pressure. When right ventricular pressure is greater than or equal to one-half left ventricular pressure, the septal configuration changes. The septum becomes "flat" or without the normal curvature.[56] This is illustrated in Figure 17-14 in a patient with a large ventricular septal defect. In the absence of significant pulmonary stenosis, one then also knows that pulmonary artery pressure is at least one-half systemic level as well.

In some patients there are other techniques available to quantify right ventricular or pulmonary artery pressure. If a ventricular septal defect is present, as in Figure 17-14, one can calculate right ventricular pressure using the velocity of blood flow across the septal defect.[62] In this example, the velocity is only 1 m/sec. One applies the Bernoulli equation described previously to calculate the pressure gradient between right ventricular pressure (RVP) and left ventricular pressure (LVP) resulting in this velocity:

$$\Delta RVP - LVP = 4 * (\text{velocity across ventricular septal defect})$$
$$= 4 \text{ mm Hg}$$

One subtracts this (significant) gradient from estimated left ventricular pressure to estimate right ventricular pressure,

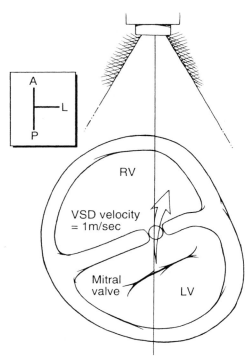

FIGURE 17-14 Estimation of right ventricular pressure in patient with large ventricular septal defect. Note in this systolic frame that the ventricular septum is flat (or neutral) in position without curvature into either ventricle. This occurs when right ventricular pressure is at least one-half left ventricular pressure. One can derive a quantitative measure of right ventricular pressure by measuring the velocity of the ventricular septal defect gradient using Doppler and then calculating the pressure difference between right and left ventricles. In this case estimated RV pressure is systemic in the absence of any significant gradient between the ventricles. A, anterior; L, left; LV, left ventricle; P, posterior; RV, right ventricle; VSD, ventricular septal defect.

which in this case is systemic. The left ventricular pressure is estimated from the systemic systolic blood pressure. Left ventricular pressure and systemic pressure are the same when there is no significant valvular aortic stenosis. When aortic stenosis is present, one adds the gradient across the aortic valve to the systemic systolic pressure to estimate left ventricular pressure.

When tricuspid regurgitation is present, one can use Doppler interrogation to measure the velocity of the tricuspid regurgitation jet and then calculate the pressure gradient resulting in this velocity.[8,30,104] As illustrated in Figure 17-15, the velocity of tricuspid regurgitation is 4 m/sec. Using the Bernoulli equation, the pressure gradient between right ventricle and right atrium is:

$$\Delta RV - RA = 4 * (\text{tricuspid regurgitation velocity})^2$$
$$= 4 * 4^2 = 64 \text{ mm Hg}$$

By adding 64 mm Hg to the estimated right atrial pressure during systole, one can estimate right ventricular pressure. One can then subtract any gradient across the pulmonary valve to estimate the pulmonary artery pressure.[30]

Finally, if a patent ductus arteriosus is present, the pulmonary artery pressure can be estimated from the velocity across the ductus arteriosus. In Figure 17-16, the ductus is restrictive, resulting in a flow jet of 4 m/sec. Again, one can use

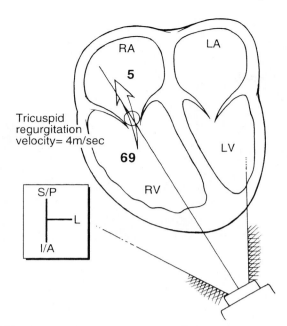

FIGURE 17-15   Estimation of right ventricular pressure from the velocity of tricuspid regurgitation. The velocity of tricuspid regurgitation is 4 m/sec. Using the Bernoulli equation the pressure gradient between right atrium and right ventricle is 64 mm Hg. Adding this gradient to the right atrial pressure, one can estimate right ventricular pressure. Estimated right ventricular pressure is 69 mm Hg. RA, right atrium; I/A, inferior-anterior; L, left; LA, left atrium; LV, left ventricle; RV, right ventricle S/P, superior-posterior.

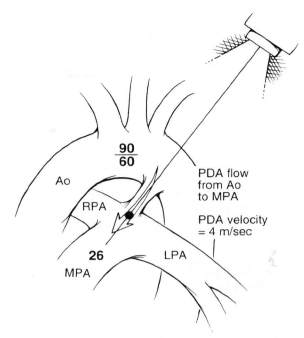

FIGURE 17-16   Estimation of pulmonary artery pressure from the velocity across the ductus arteriosus. The velocity across the ductus is 4 m/sec. Therefore the pressure gradient is 64 mm Hg. The pulmonary artery pressure is therefore 64 mm Hg less than the systolic aortic pressure of 90 mm Hg. Estimated pulmonary artery pressure (26 mm Hg) is therefore normal. Ao, aorta; LPA, left pulmonary artery; MPA, main pulmonary artery; PDA, patent ductus arteriosus; RPA, right pulmonary artery.

the Bernoulli equation to calculate the pressure gradient across the ductus between the aorta (Ao) and pulmonary artery (PA):

$$\Delta Ao - PA = 4 * (\text{ductus arteriosus velocity})^2$$
$$= 4 * 4^2 = 64 \text{ mm Hg}$$

By subtracting this systolic gradient from the systemic systolic blood pressure, one can estimate the pulmonary artery pressure.

One can also estimate the diastolic pulmonary artery pressure in the presence of pulmonary regurgitation. The velocity of pulmonary regurgitation is measured across the pulmonary valve at end-diastole, and the Bernoulli equation is used to calculate the pressure gradient between pulmonary artery diastolic pressure and right ventricular diastolic pressure. A high velocity jet suggests that the pulmonary artery diastolic pressure is elevated.

Echocardiographic Guidance of Procedures in the Intensive Care Unit

Balloon Atrial Septostomy

In transposition of the great arteries, balloon atrial septostomy can increase the oxygen saturation by allowing for greater intracardiac mixing. This potentially lifesaving procedure, first described by William Rashkin, was initially performed under fluoroscopy.[84,85,116] Several studies have shown more recently that the procedure can be performed safely and with equal efficacy in the intensive care unit under echocardiographic guidance, thereby avoiding patient transfer to the catheterization laboratory.[56,57,66] Hospital charges may also be lower when the balloon atrial septostomy is performed at the patient bedside.[119]

Imaging during the procedure is possible from either the apical or low parasternal acoustic windows. This allows the cardiologist performing the septostomy to work from either the umbilicus or the femoral vein without interference by the echocardiographer. Alternatively, balloon atrial septostomy can be performed under transesophageal echocardiographic guidance.[57]

Images from a balloon atrial septostomy are illustrated in Figure 17-17. As the catheter enters the right atrium, the echocardiographer may be able to help guide the positioning of the catheter in the left atrium. The catheter should be positioned well into the left atrium but not with the tip so far as to be in the left atrial appendage or touching the lateral wall. If the catheter is positioned too far within the left atrium, balloon inflation could tear the atrial wall. As the balloon is inflated, it should be noted to be free within the left atrium before the septostomy pull is performed. If the balloon is not free or is overinflated, atrial wall avulsion can occur with the pull. After the septostomy is performed, but before the catheter is removed, the echocardiographer should determine that the defect created is adequate (generally at least 4 mm) and that the defect margins are clear. Once the procedure is completed, the heart should be scanned to exclude any iatrogenic damage to the mitral valve or tricuspid valve or the inferior vena cava. Pericardial effusion should be excluded.

Pericardiocentesis

Two-dimensional imaging is excellent for the visualization of pericardial effusion. The amount of fluid and its distribution should be imaged from multiple imaging windows and planes.

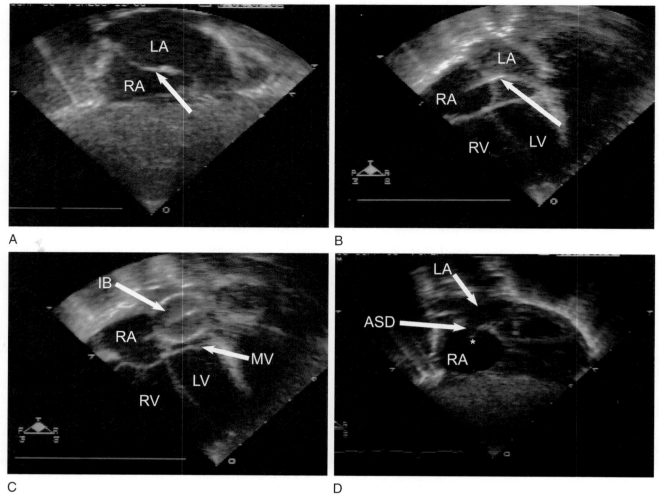

FIGURE 17-17   Echocardiographic visualization for balloon atrial septostomy. **A,** Before septostomy. Subxiphoid view before patient is prepared and draped showing intact atrial septum. **B,** Catheter across into the left atrium, balloon not yet inflated. Note that the catheter tip extends to the left atrial wall. Before balloon inflation, the catheter should be pulled back so that the balloon is inflated within the left atrium and not within the left atrial appendage. **C,** Balloon inflated within the left atrium. The balloon should not cross the mitral valve and be free within the left atrium before the septostomy is performed. If the balloon is overinflated and not free, it is possible to avulse the left atrial wall during septostomy. **D,** Atrial septal defect after septostomy. Note the torn edges of the defect. An adequate septostomy should create a defect with clear margins that is at least 4 mm in diameter. ASD, atrial septal defect; IB, inflated balloon; LA, left atrium; LV, left ventricle; MV, mitral valve; RA, right atrium; RV, right ventricle.

One should determine if the effusion is loculated or not, and whether it is circumferential or not. Noncircumferential effusions are generally small.

There are several echocardiographic signs of pericardial tamponade. When the pericardial pressure exceeds right atrial pressure, there will be a diastolic free wall collapse of the right atrial free wall. One may see a similar finding of the right ventricular free wall. There are also changes in the Doppler inflow patterns of the atrial ventricular valves with pericardial tamponade. A sensitive finding is more than a 25% variation in peak inflow velocity during inspiration versus expiration. With increasing degrees of tamponade, there will be more variability in inflow velocity with the respiratory cycle.

Pericardiocentesis can be performed under echocardiographic guidance, again obviating the transfer of the patient to the catheterization laboratory. Generally, pericardiocentesis is performed from a subcostal or, less commonly, an apical approach. Before the procedure, images are obtained to measure the distance from the needle entry site to the proximal edge of pericardial fluid. One also measures the rim of pericardial fluid. In general, fluid collections with rims less than 5 mm in dimension are difficult to tap, whereas those greater than 10 mm are generally relatively easy to drain. One can anticipate the appropriate angle of entry for the needle by considering the angle of the transducer at the appropriate plane (Fig. 17-18).

Line Displacement or Dislodgement   When chest radiograph cannot adequately demonstrate the position of intravascular catheters, ultrasound is quite good at doing so. One can also assess the presence of thrombus or vegetation on the line, but when a mass is identified, it may not be possible to distinguish one from the other echocardiographically. In some cases, a line may dislodge and be in the pericardial or pleural space. When such a question arises, injection of a small amount of saline through the catheter, resulting in a contrast injection, is quite useful in demonstrating the position of the catheter. If contrast is seen in the pericardial space, then the catheter must have some communication with that cavity.

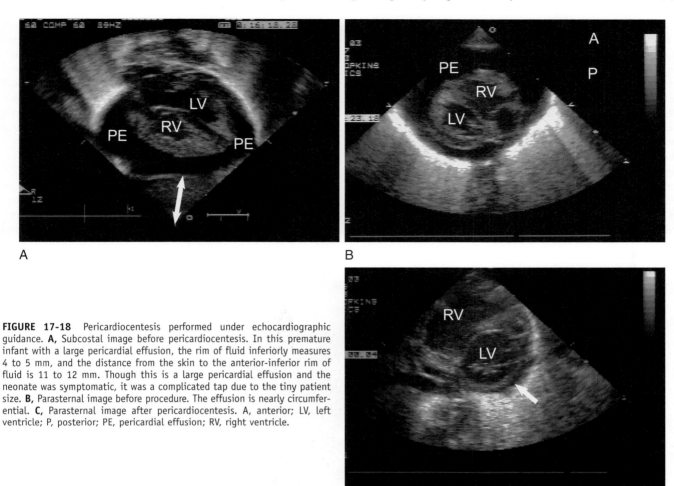

FIGURE 17-18 Pericardiocentesis performed under echocardiographic guidance. **A,** Subcostal image before pericardiocentesis. In this premature infant with a large pericardial effusion, the rim of fluid inferiorly measures 4 to 5 mm, and the distance from the skin to the anterior-inferior rim of fluid is 11 to 12 mm. Though this is a large pericardial effusion and the neonate was symptomatic, it was a complicated tap due to the tiny patient size. **B,** Parasternal image before procedure. The effusion is nearly circumferential. **C,** Parasternal image after pericardiocentesis. A, anterior; LV, left ventricle; P, posterior; PE, pericardial effusion; RV, right ventricle.

Correspondingly, if contrast is seen in the pleural space, the catheter has extravasated into the chest.

Transesophageal and Intraoperative Echocardiography

Transesophageal probes are available for patients as small as 2 to 2.5 kg. Though single-plane probes exist, most imaging today is performed with multiplane probes and less commonly biplane probes. Single-plane imaging is inadequate for assessing outflow tract pathology.[97] Multiplane imaging when possible is likely to improve imaging over biplane imaging but may not be possible in some smaller patients.[105]

Besides the electronic control of the imaging plane, the operator can mechanically flex or extend the probe tip and shift the probe from right to left. The mechanical steering allows the operator to achieve nearly any plane desired. Occasionally, contact with the esophagus or stomach is poor or image quality obscured by adjacent nasogastric tubes.

Indications

The most frequent indication for transesophageal echocardiography is in the operating room or in the perioperative period. The transesophageal approach does not compromise the operative field and images are not obscured by chest tubes and dressings as with transthoracic imaging. Transesophageal echocardiography is also sometimes helpful in the outpatient setting in larger children or young adults where acoustic windows are limited. However, magnetic resonance imaging is frequently used as an alternative modality for this group of patients. Finally, transesophageal echocardiography is useful in the guidance of interventional catheterization procedures, such as the closure of atrial septal defect, or in the assistance of balloon atrial septostomy. There is also increasing experience with intracardiac probes as an alternative technique for guiding interventional procedures.[5,21,95]

MAGNETIC RESONANCE IMAGING

Technological advances including the development of more rapid imaging sequences with improved resolution have expanded considerably the role of magnetic resonance imaging in the anatomical and functional evaluation of congenital and acquired pediatric heart disease. A thorough knowledge of the strengths and limitations of each imaging modality is critical in optimizing the evaluation of the patient with heart disease.

As noted previously in this chapter, noninvasive evaluation of congenital heart disease usually begins with echocardiography. In a subset of patients with limited acoustic windows or with questions poorly addressed with echocardiography, magnetic resonance imaging can play an important complementary role. With the large field of view and the ability to image in multiple planes, magnetic resonance can evaluate the cardiac chambers, the pulmonary arteries, and aorta, and provide information about the tracheobronchial tree and situs abnormalities (Fig. 17-19).[51] Magnetic resonance can add important information in delineating venous anatomy[38] and surgically created intracardiac conduits or baffles,[61,113] which can be difficult to evaluate by echocardiography, particularly in older patients.[117] Magnetic resonance imaging has certain advantages compared to angiography: It is noninvasive, does not involve ionizing radiation,

and does not use iodinated contrast with the inherent risks of renal compromise and allergic reaction. Gadolinium-based contrast agents used for magnetic resonance angiography have significantly less risk of allergic reaction and no risk of renal injury. Patients with pacemakers, other implantable electrical stimulators, or ventricular assist devices are currently not typically evaluated with magnetic resonance imaging, but research is in progress that may allow magnetic resonance imaging of patients with pacemakers.

Examination Preparation

In order to select the appropriate imaging planes and sequences, the specific indications for the magnetic resonance examination and pertinent clinical information need to be identified

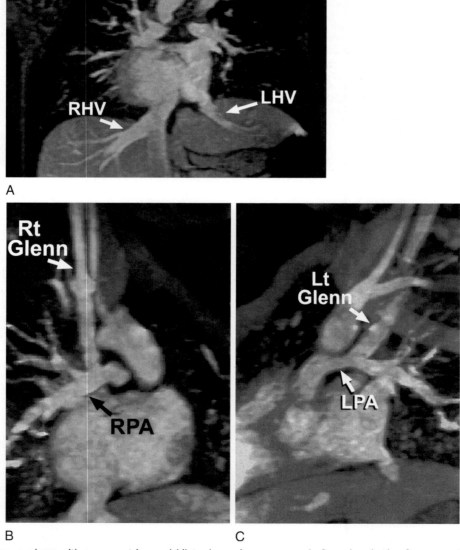

FIGURE 17-19 Heterotaxy syndrome with common atrium and bilateral superior vena cava. **A,** Coronal projection from magnetic resonance angiography demonstrates separate entrance of the right hepatic vein (RHV) and left hepatic vein (LHV) into a common atrium. Oblique coronal projections demonstrate right (**B**) and left (**C**) Glenn shunts to the pulmonary arteries (RPA and LPA).

before the examination. The imaging protocol will often vary depending on the type of anatomic or functional information needed to answer the clinical question.

Children younger than 5 to 8 years of age usually require sedation and often need the assistance of anesthesiologists, if patients are cyanotic or more acutely ill at the time of the examination. Older children and adults may need light sedation or an anxiolytic. Since some examinations are quite lengthy, it is useful to have the patient void before entering the scanner. Pulse oximetry is used to monitor sedated patients, and a nurse experienced in patient sedation and monitoring is present. With currently available machines, successful cardiac magnetic resonance imaging requires electrocardiographic gating during image acquisition to suppress cardiac motion. The electrocardiographic tracing can be used to calculate the patient's heart rate and demonstrate changes in cardiac rhythm, but it cannot be used for diagnostic electrocardiographic purposes since the magnetic resonance signal alters the electrocardiographic signal. Some arrhythmias limit electrocardiographic gating, requiring more rapid acquisition pulse sequences.

Pulse Sequences

Several pulse sequences are currently used in cardiac MR imaging. With conventional spin echo (CSE), flowing blood in cardiac chambers and vessels appears black (signal void) (Fig. 17-20A). CSE images have excellent contrast resolution, and multiple slices are acquired at a single point in the cardiac cycle for morphologic assessment.

Gradient echo (GRE) images display the blood pool as white (Fig. 17-20B). Data are obtained throughout the cardiac cycle and displayed in a cine format. On these dynamic "white blood" cine images, turbulent blood flow through areas of blood vessel or valvular stenosis or regurgitation results in a signal void

(Fig. 17-20C).[102] More recent technology has produced higher gradient strengths and allowed the development of steady state free precession (SSFP) techniques. This has resulted in improved contrast and allows scans to be completed more quickly. Three-dimensional sequences can be acquired in some patients with a single breath-hold, which has significantly shortened scanning times, of much import when imaging children.[46] More commonly, two-dimensional sequences are used whereby imaging at multiple locations is performed throughout the cardiac cycle. The cine format allows for dynamic evaluation of flow throughout the cardiac cycle in systole and diastole and provides quantitative information about regional and global ventricular function including ventricular mass, volume, stroke volume, ejection fraction, and cardiac index.[33] The measurement of these parameters with magnetic resonance imaging is more accurate than alternative imaging modalities that rely on single-plane data or even limited multiplane data. This is a distinct advantage in congenital heart malformations when ventricular morphology is variable.

Phase contrast (PC) magnetic resonance is another sequence used to quantify blood velocity and volume and displays the information as a cine format like GRE and SSFP techniques. PC is used to quantify cardiac shunts, flow gradients across stenoses, and the volume of valvular regurgitation.[70,87,89] In stenotic lesions, dark flow jets can be visualized at sites of pressure gradients and the severity quantified using the Bernoulli equation as in echocardiography.[51] When protons in the blood pool are in motion, they acquire a phase shift when passed through a special gradient. The phase shift is proportional to the velocity of blood flow, and both flow direction and peak flow velocity in the vessel can be measured (Fig. 17-21).[70] Since the velocity of blood flow is measured across the entire vessel area, PC magnetic resonance is likely more accurate

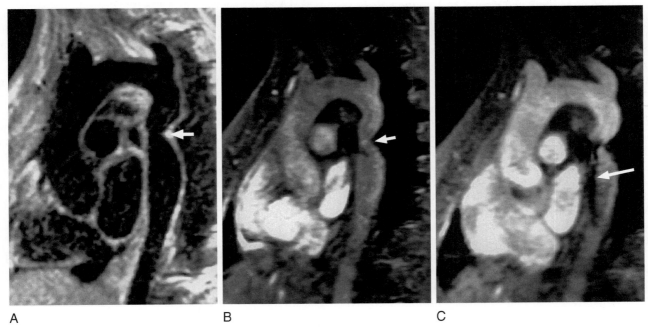

| A | B | C |

FIGURE 17-20   Coarctation of the aorta. **A,** Oblique sagittal conventional spin echo image. **B,** Oblique sagittal gradient echo image. Focal narrowing of the aortic isthmus (*arrow*) with poststenotic dilation. **C,** Fast gradient echo cine image during systole demonstrates turbulent jet (*large arrow*) indicating significant stenosis at the level of coarctation.

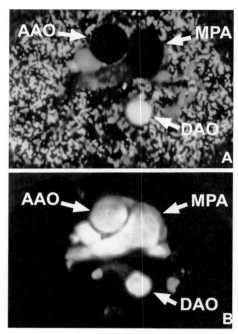

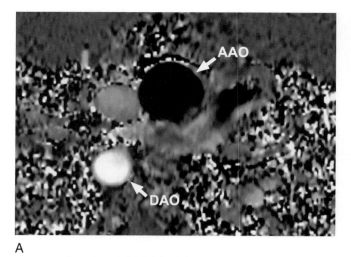

A

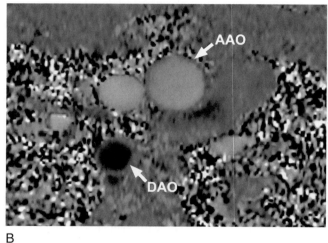

B

FIGURE 17-21 Use of velocity mapping techniques. **A,** Axial phase contrast, and **B,** Gradient echo image. Both images are obtained during systole, and the imaging planes are perpendicular to the ascending and descending aorta. Flow is demonstrated on the phase contrast image **(A)** depicted as black with blood flow toward the head in the ascending aorta and main pulmonary artery but in the opposite direction (displayed as white) in the descending aorta. In the gradient echo image, flow, in no matter what direction, is displayed as white (i.e., nondirectional display). AAO, ascending aorta; DAO, descending aorta; MPA, main pulmonary artery.

FIGURE 17-22 Truncal valve regurgitation status post repair with axial phase contrast images. **A,** Systolic frame. Flow toward the feet in the descending aorta (depicted as white) and toward the head (black) in the ascending aorta. **B,** Diastolic frame shows reversal with black (descending aorta) and white (ascending aorta) due to truncal valve regurgitation. AAO, ascending aorta; DAO, descending aorta.

than flow measurements obtained using Doppler echocardiography, which assumes that the velocity is uniform over the entire cross-sectional area of the vessel. In addition, PC magnetic resonance allows flow quantification in vessels that may be difficult to interrogate by Doppler, such as the pulmonary arteries. This can allow the noninvasive calculation of the pulmonary to systemic flow ratio ($Q_p:Q_s$).[80] Similarly, PC magnetic resonance can be used to assess the severity of valvular regurgitation (Fig. 17-22). Using an approach similar to Doppler echocardiography, the peak flow velocities can be measured across stenotic lesions in native vessels or valves or surgically placed conduits. The peak instantaneous pressure gradients can then be estimated using the modified Bernoulli equation: maximum instantaneous gradient = $4V^2$, where V^2 is the maximum instantaneous velocity. Pressure gradients measured with this technique correlate well with Doppler echocardiography data,[24,55,61] but more extensive validation studies and technical improvements are needed.

Magnetic resonance angiography has gained widespread acceptance and is a three-dimensional fast spoiled GRE sequence after administration of gadolinium.[82] This sequence has the ability to illustrate a large area of cardiac anatomy in a short imaging time, requiring only 20 seconds for one acquisition and can be performed in a single breath-hold. A longer acquisition is required in patients who are unable to breath-hold. Information about overall cardiac and extracardiac anatomy is easily displayed in multiple projections using post-processing techniques.[52] Vessels of interest can be isolated from the overall vascular anatomy and then displayed in

a similar manner to conventional angiographic images. Contrast-enhanced three-dimensional magnetic resonance angiography is very versatile. It can be used for preoperative evaluation of coarctation and vascular rings[48] as well as more complex congenital heart disease such as pulmonary atresia and anomalous pulmonary venous connection (Fig. 17-23). Postsurgical evaluation of patency of intracardiac baffles and conduits as well as bidirectional Glenn and Fontan anastomoses are well delineated with this technique (see Fig. 17-19).[75]

Applications of Magnetic Resonance Imaging

Vascular Rings and Slings

The most common types of vascular anomalies to cause symptomatic tracheal and esophageal compression are right aortic arch with aberrant left subclavian, double aortic arch, and pulmonary sling. In infants and children, respiratory problems that are produced from these anomalies vary from

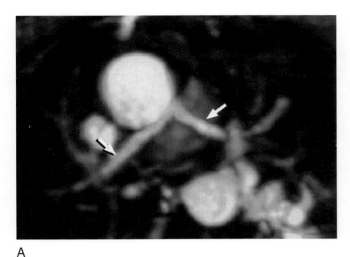

A

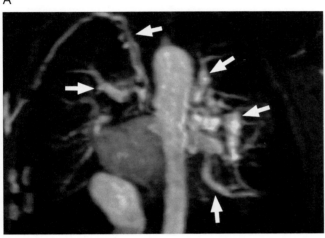

B

FIGURE 17-23 Tetralogy of Fallot with pulmonary atresia. **A,** Axial and **B,** coronal images from a three-dimensional magnetic resonance angiography demonstrate diminutive right and left pulmonary arteries (arrows in A) and multiple aortopulmonary collateral vessels from the descending aorta (arrows in B).

wheezing to frank respiratory failure. If the vascular ring exhibits less compression, it may be diagnosed in the older child with esophageal compression as the primary cause of symptoms. With the double aortic arch, the right arch is more often dominant and cephalic in location as compared with the left arch. However, the left arch is occasionally dominant and one of the arches may be atretic or have an associated coarctation.

An initial workup with a barium esophagram can demonstrate impressions on the esophagus suggesting that a ring is present. With improvements in cross-sectional imaging in recent years, both computerized tomography and magnetic resonance imaging have been utilized to depict the arch anatomy more precisely. These techniques may help guide the subsequent surgical approach, which is particularly important due to the possibility of a coarctation or more complex anatomic variant that may be accessible via the standard left thoracotomy.[67] Helical computerized tomography with iodinated contrast can be performed very quickly without sedation in the neonate with significant respiratory distress. Both computerized tomography and magnetic resonance provide

multiplane images and characterize the anomalous vasculature and the extent of airway compression (Fig. 17-24). It is generally accepted that the high association of vascular rings with intracardiac anomalies warrants evaluation with echocardiography, particularly in the neonate. Echocardiography tends to be the examination of choice for initial evaluation, as it may adequately assess the anomalous vasculature as well. Imaging with magnetic resonance or computerized tomography may be performed when echocardiography is inadequate or in the older child. The preference of magnetic resonance versus computerized tomography depends on the clinical condition of the patient, availability of equipment, and experience of the imager. Although both techniques have three-dimensional imaging capabilities, contrast-enhanced magnetic resonance angiography tends to be preferred over computerized tomography, particularly for evaluation of associated coarctation or more complex anatomic variants.

Pulmonary sling or aberrant left pulmonary artery is a congenital anomaly in which the left pulmonary artery arises from the right pulmonary artery (Fig. 17-25). As the left pulmonary artery courses to the left, it often compresses the right main stem bronchus and then passes between the trachea and esophagus. Although not technically a vascular ring, this anomaly can cause significant respiratory compromise in the newborn period. Two subgroups of patients with pulmonary artery sling have been described.[7] The first group presents with wheezing and cyanosis in association with hyperinflation of the right lung. The other group has associated tracheal and right mainstem stenosis due to complete cartilaginous rings (the "ringsling" complex).[114] Imaging in multiple planes demonstrates the aberrant left pulmonary artery and the airway abnormality. Since these patients have more of an intrinsic airway abnormality, prognosis after reimplantation of the pulmonary artery alone has been poor. Attempts to correct the tracheal stenosis have had varied success.

Aortic Disease

The Marfan syndrome and type IV Ehlers-Danlos syndrome are connective tissue disorders that can have cardiovascular manifestations (see Chapter 47). Both are associated with cystic medial necrosis of the aortic wall, which has a characteristic appearance on magnetic resonance imaging, with dilation of the aortic root and proximal ascending aorta and effacement of the sinotubular junction (Fig. 17-26). The dilation of the aortic root can be associated with aortic regurgitation. Magnetic resonance imaging is quite useful in following the aortic size and in excluding dissection. The size and the extent of the aortic aneurysm can be accurately delineated with CSE, fast cine GRE or SSFP, and three-dimensional gadolinium-enhanced angiography.[12] Fast cine GRE, SSFP, or PC magnetic resonance imaging can be performed to assess for the severity of regurgitation.[39,49]

More serious complications of Marfan or Ehlers-Danlos syndrome include dissection and rupture of the ascending aorta. Transesophageal echocardiography (TEE), computerized tomography, or magnetic resonance imaging should be performed urgently if dissection is suspected. Patients can develop acute severe aortic valve regurgitation and the dissection can involve the coronary arteries or arch branch vessels, resulting in myocardial or cerebral ischemia. If the

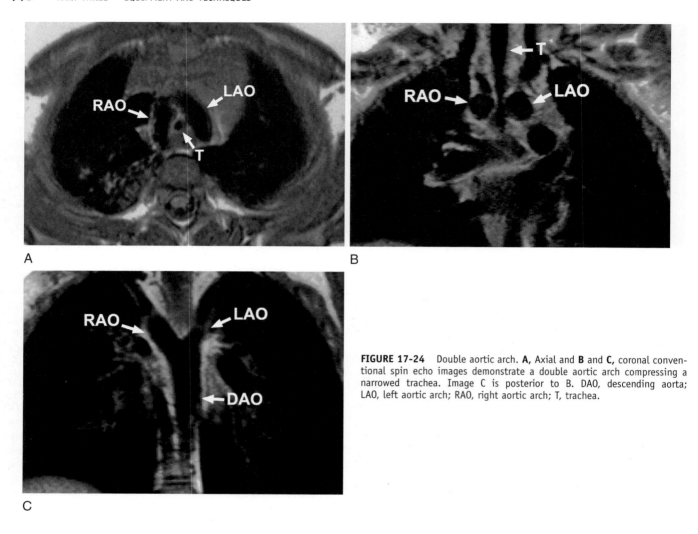

FIGURE 17-24   Double aortic arch. **A,** Axial and **B** and **C,** coronal conventional spin echo images demonstrate a double aortic arch compressing a narrowed trachea. Image C is posterior to B. DAO, descending aorta; LAO, left aortic arch; RAO, right aortic arch; T, trachea.

aortic rupture extends into the pericardium, hemopericardium with tamponade can occur. Magnetic resonance imaging is highly sensitive and specific for the detection and characterization of the extent and orientation of the intimal flap, delineation of the true and false lumen, intramural hematoma, and involvement of the arch and coronary arteries. Comparison studies of magnetic resonance imaging and transesophageal echocardiography evaluation of aortic dissection have demonstrated similar high sensitivities (98% to 100%); however, magnetic resonance imaging has significantly higher specificity (98% to 100%) than transesophageal echocardiography (68% to 77%) in high-risk populations.[76,77] Other predisposing conditions that may be associated with aortic dissection in children include Turner's syndrome, bicommissural aortic valve, prior surgical repair, and balloon dilation of coarctation.

Coarctation of the Aorta

Coarctation is defined as a narrowing of the proximal descending aorta in the juxtaductal region (see Chapter 27). Coarctation is frequently associated with arch hypoplasia. Magnetic resonance demonstrates well discrete narrowing of the aorta distal to the left subclavian artery with a prominent posterior shelf as well as hypoplasia of the more proximal arch in the

diffuse form. Both CSE and GRE sequences delineate the site, extent, and anatomic severity of the stenosis, as well as the involvement of arch vessels and degree of poststenotic dilation (see Fig. 17-20). PC magnetic resonance imaging can demonstrate a jet of turbulent flow in the descending aorta from the site of narrowing. The length of this jet has been correlated with the severity of the stenosis.[90] Measurement of the peak velocity at the level of stenosis can be used to estimate the hemodynamic gradient, and close correlation has been observed between values obtained with PC magnetic resonance imaging and Doppler echocardiography.[69]

Assessment of collateral blood flow to the descending aorta with magnetic resonance imaging is important for preoperative evaluation because cross-clamping the aorta with insufficient collateral circulation may result in spinal cord ischemia. In addition, quantification of the collateral blood flow can be used to assess the significance of the degree of luminal narrowing visualized morphologically. Collateral vessels are well visualized on three-dimensional magnetic resonance angiographic (MRA) images after gadolinium administration (Fig. 17-27). PC magnetic resonance imaging can be used to quantify the contribution of collateral circulation. Blood flow is measured within the descending aorta from just below the level of coarctation and from the level of the diaphragm. The difference in blood flow at these levels is felt to represent the collateral circulation from the

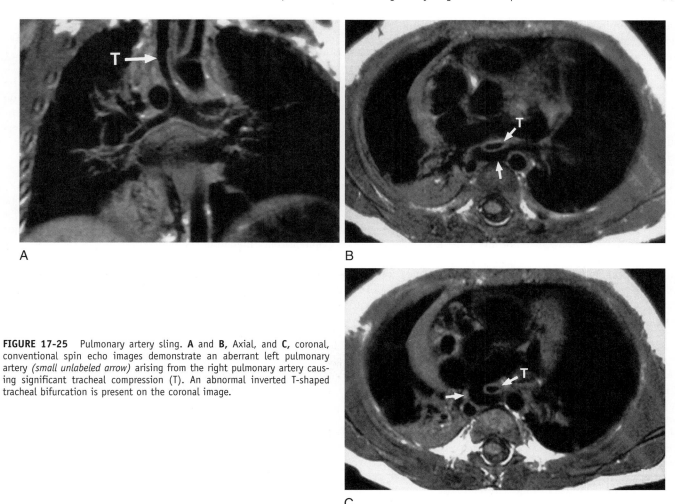

FIGURE 17-25   Pulmonary artery sling. **A** and **B**, Axial, and **C**, coronal, conventional spin echo images demonstrate an aberrant left pulmonary artery *(small unlabeled arrow)* arising from the right pulmonary artery causing significant tracheal compression (T). An abnormal inverted T-shaped tracheal bifurcation is present on the coronal image.

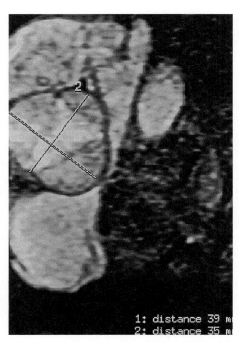

FIGURE 17-26   The Marfan syndrome. Oblique gradient echo image perpendicular to the root of the aorta demonstrates dilation of the sinus of Valsalva. Measurements are made in two orthogonal planes.

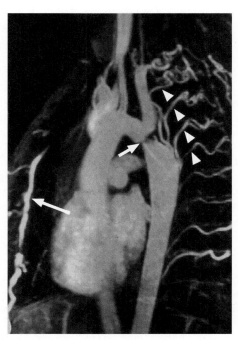

FIGURE 17-27   Coarctation of the aorta. Focal narrowing of the aortic isthmus (*small arrow*). Multiple intercostal collateral arteries (*arrowheads*) supply the descending aorta. A dilated internal mammary artery (*large arrow*) is also present.

intercostal arteries. An 8% decrease in flow between these two levels is seen in normal individuals, whereas patients with hemodynamically significant coarctation have an average increase in flow of 80%.[108] By assessing the contribution to total flow by the collateral circulation, this technique provides a noninvasive measurement of the severity of anatomic and physiologic obstruction at the level of the coarctation.

Magnetic resonance imaging is a valuable method for follow-up of postsurgical repair or balloon angioplasty of coarctation. Magnetic resonance imaging can demonstrate restenosis, dissection, and false aneurysm formation,[32,115] which can be difficult to visualize by echocardiography due to more limited field of view, particularly if the aorta is very tortuous (Fig. 17-28). Magnetic resonance imaging can view the entire arch within a single plane and more easily depict tortuosity, especially with three-dimensional imaging techniques. Patients who have had repair of coarctation using prosthetic patches are at risk for developing aneurysms at the repair site,[12] which are well visualized on magnetic resonance.

Pulmonary Arteries

The evaluation of the pulmonary arteries in childhood congenital heart disease, especially in patients with right ventricular outflow tract obstructive lesions, has become a major application of magnetic resonance. Accurate assessment of the presence, caliber, and confluence of the pulmonary arteries is essential for appropriate surgical correction or palliation (Fig. 17-29). Although angiography continues to be regarded as the gold standard for imaging the pulmonary arteries, dilution of contrast by unopacified blood from shunts or collaterals as well as obstruction to the right ventricular outflow tract obstruction may impair visualization of small caliber pulmonary arteries.[81] Magnetic resonance can identify central pulmonary arteries that are not visualized by angiography.[109] Echocardiography also has limitations in delineating the morphology of the distal main pulmonary arteries, particularly in older patients.[47] CSE and GRE imaging techniques accurately depict the main pulmonary arteries, and three-dimensional gadolinium-enhanced magnetic resonance angiography is performed to evaluate the hilar and intrapulmonary segments as well as possible aortopulmonary collateral vessels (Fig. 17-30). The aortopulmonary collateral vessels may originate from the descending aorta, the brachiocephalic arteries, or the abdominal aorta (they often have a markedly tortuous course and an asymmetric distribution within the lungs, so true pulmonary arteries, aortopulmonary collaterals, or both may supply some segments). The three-dimensional capability of magnetic resonance angiography is useful for accurate preoperative delineation of the collateral circulation.[109]

Pulmonary Veins

Magnetic resonance has been shown to provide as good or better visualization in the diagnosis of pulmonary vein stenosis and anomalous pulmonary venous connections compared with both echocardiography and angiography (Fig. 17-31).[15,65] Assessment of the normal pulmonary veins can be difficult by echocardiography due to their posterior location. Axial CSE and three-dimensional gadolinium-enhanced magnetic resonance images can demonstrate the pulmonary veins entering into the left atrium in the majority of patients with normal pulmonary venous connections and are even more accurate in delineating abnormal pulmonary venous connections. Anomalous pulmonary veins may return to systemic veins above the heart (innominate, subclavian veins, or SVC), directly to the right atrium or coronary sinus, or below the heart to the IVC or portal vein. Magnetic resonance imaging can depict total or partial anomalous pulmonary venous connection,[15,112] cor triatriatum, and pulmonary venous stenosis after surgical redirection (Fig. 17-32).[98]

Postoperative Assessment

The evaluation of surgical results and possible complications involving palliative shunts, conduits, and intracardiac baffles and the patency of the pulmonary arteries has become a major application of magnetic resonance, imaging in cyanotic congenital heart disease. Magnetic resonance imaging is most often utilized if a full evaluation of the postoperative cardiac status is limited on echocardiography due to artifacts from prosthetic patch materials; calcification of homografts, baffles, or conduits; or limitations of field of view. In addition, suspected tracheal and esophageal compression by surgically constructed structures, especially pulmonary arterial conduits[22] and the reconstructed aortic arch post Norwood procedure for hypoplastic left heart syndrome,[1] is more easily demonstrated on magnetic resonance imaging.

Extracardiac conduits are prosthetic or homograft tubes used to create venoarterial, ventriculoarterial, and arterioarterial connections when the structures to be connected are too far away from each other to allow a direct anastomosis. There are different mechanisms of conduit obstruction: formation of a thick endothelial peal, scarring at sites of anastomosis, and kinking of the conduit associated with growth of structures at either end. Magnetic resonance imaging allows more complete visualization of conduits in their entirety than echocardiography or angiography due to a wide field of view and three-dimensional imaging capability (Fig. 17-33).[10] Right ventricular to pulmonary artery conduits are used in tetralogy of Fallot with pulmonary atresia or, in a small subset of patients, tetralogy of Fallot (severe pulmonary stenosis or anomalies of the coronary arteries limiting safe access to the right ventricular outflow tract). Echocardiographic evaluation can be difficult due to the substernal location of these conduits, and magnetic resonance imaging can be used for evaluation of possible conduit obstruction (Fig. 17-34).

Most patients with tetralogy of Fallot are repaired via infundibulotomy and patch widening of the right ventricular outflow tract. The reconstructed outflow tract can become narrowed, or a pseudoaneurysm can develop (Fig. 17-35). In addition, pulmonary regurgitation is an extremely common complication after repair of tetralogy of Fallot when a transannular patch is used. The pulmonary regurgitation can become quite severe, leading to significant volume overload and dysfunction of the right ventricle.[78,86] Magnetic resonance imaging has been found to be more accurate in quantifying right ventricular volumes and function and pulmonary regurgitation than echocardiography[44] and is now used in some centers for the routine follow-up of patients with tetralogy of Fallot (Fig. 17-36).

Intracardiac baffles are used to redirect venous blood flow through the heart in transposition of the great arteries in the Mustard or Senning operations and to redirect systemic

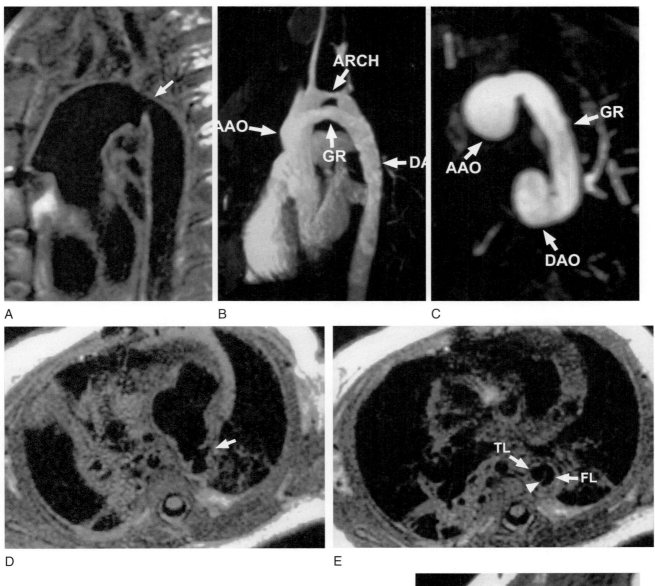

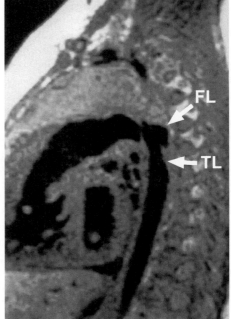

FIGURE 17-28   Recurrent coarctation status post surgery. Images from different patients. **A,** Conventional spin echo oblique sagittal image demonstrates residual coarctation (*arrow*) after reconstruction of the aortic arch for hypoplastic left heart syndrome. **B** and **C,** Sagittal and axial images from a magnetic resonance angiography demonstrating a jump graft (GR) from the ascending (AAO) to descending (DA and DAO) aorta for severe hypoplasia of the aortic arch (ARCH). **D, E,** and **F,** Dissection after balloon angioplasty for coarctation. Axial (D,E) and oblique sagittal (F) conventional spin echo images show irregularity of the aortic isthmus (*small arrow in D*) and a dissection flap (*arrowhead in E*) separating true (TL) and false (FL) lumen.

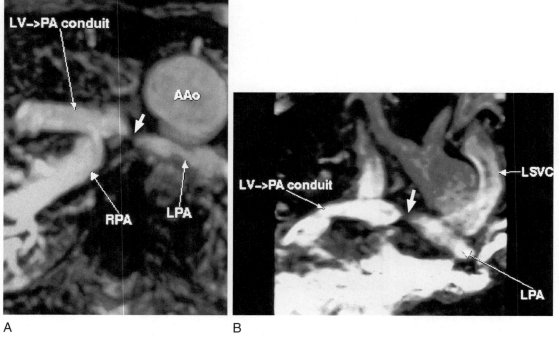

FIGURE 17-29   Heterotaxy with discontinuous pulmonary arteries status post left ventricle to pulmonary artery conduit (LV-PA conduit) and left superior vena cava to left pulmonary artery Glenn anastomosis. Axial (**A**) and coronal (**B**) projections from a magnetic resonance angiography clearly demonstrate discontinuity of the left (LPA) and right (RPA) pulmonary arteries (*unlabeled arrow in A and B*), which are in close proximity to allow subsequent surgical connection. Left superior vena cava (LSVC) seen best in B. AAo, ascending aorta.

venous blood in the Fontan procedure for functionally univentricular hearts. In the Mustard or Senning operation, systemic venous blood is redirected to the mitral valve. The pulmonary venous blood is redirected to the tricuspid valve. Both systemic and pulmonary venous pathways have the potential for obstruction, which can be assessed by magnetic resonance (Fig. 17-37).[91,100,110]

In an older variant of the Fontan operation, an anastomosis between the superior vena cava and the pulmonary artery was performed. More recently, an intracaval baffle or an external conduit is created to direct systemic venous return from the inferior vena cava to the pulmonary artery (see Chapter 41). Possible complications include pulmonary venous obstruction due to extrinsic compression by the adjacent baffle or enlarged cardiac structures (Fig. 17-38), pulmonary artery obstruction at the level of anastomosis, and systemic venous obstruction connecting to the right atrium outside the baffle, most commonly, the hepatic veins. Imaging evaluation is directed to establish patency of the lateral tunnel and the superior vena cava to pulmonary artery anastomosis. In the past the right atrium was incorporated into the systemic venous to pulmonary artery connection, and not infrequently patients would develop intraatrial thrombus due to stasis; this complication can also be evaluated with magnetic resonance imaging (Fig. 17-39).[101] Pulmonary artery obstruction after the Fontan operation can arise due to preexisting pulmonary artery distortion from a prior BT shunt or compression by a large reconstructed aortic arch post Norwood procedure for hypoplastic left heart syndrome, which tends to affect the left pulmonary artery preferentially. Conventional spin echo magnetic resonance imaging or three-dimensional magnetic resonance angiography is performed to assess for areas of narrowing together with PC magnetic resonance imaging to measure the flow distribution through the pulmonary arteries to both lungs.[14,53,88]

In patients with transposition of the great arteries with ventricular septal defect and pulmonary stenosis, the Rastelli operation consists of a baffle within the right ventricle to divert left ventricular blood passing through the ventricular septal defect to the aorta (see Chapter 33). The pulmonary artery is divided from the aorta and connected to a conduit from the right ventricle. Magnetic resonance imaging can be used to assess for obstruction of the baffle as well as the right ventricle to pulmonary artery conduit and the branch pulmonary arteries (Fig. 17-40). After the arterial switch or Jatene operation for transposition of the great arteries, magnetic resonance can be used for evaluation of the aortic and pulmonary anastomosis, as well as the branch pulmonary arteries, which are draped on either side of the aorta (Fig. 17-41).[9,43]

Constrictive pericarditis results from progressive pericardial fibrosis, which can lead to impaired ventricular diastolic filling. In children the most common etiologies are from viral or tuberculosis infection. Conventional spin echo magnetic resonance imaging is accepted as an accurate technique for evaluation of the pericardium, and pericardial thickening greater than 4 mm on magnetic resonance imaging is diagnostic of constrictive pericarditis in the setting of raised filling pressures and dilation of the atria, inferior vena cava, and hepatic veins.[107] The differentiation of constrictive pericarditis from restrictive cardiomyopathy is critical, as both entities can present with impaired ventricular filling at catheterization, and constrictive pericarditis requires surgical resection of the pericardium for treatment. The presence of pericardial thickening on magnetic resonance imaging has been found to be an important feature distinguishing constrictive pericarditis from restrictive cardiomyopathy (Fig. 17-42).[64]

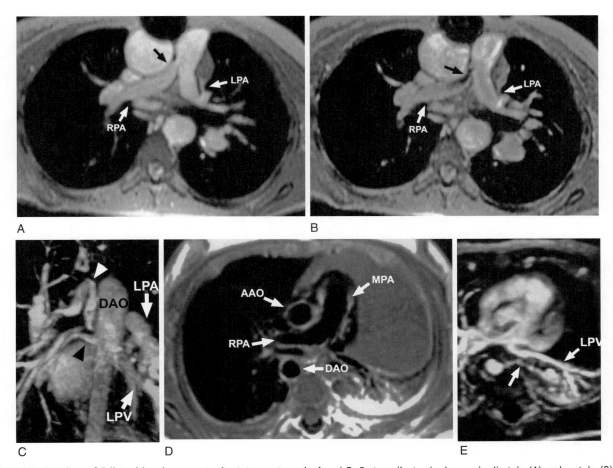

FIGURE 17-30 Tetralogy of Fallot with pulmonary atresia status post repair. **A** and **B,** Fast gradient echo images in diastole (A) and systole (B) demonstrate a focal stenosis with turbulent jet in systole (*black arrow*) of the proximal right pulmonary artery (RPA). **C,** Coronal projection from a magnetic resonance angiography of the same patient demonstrates large collateral vessels from the descending aorta (DAO) (*arrowheads*) supplying the right lung. **D,** Left pulmonary artery (LPA) atresia. Axial conventional spin echo image demonstrates a single RPA arising from the main pulmonary artery (MPA). There is a right aortic arch with the ascending aorta (AAO) to the left of the DAO. **E,** Axial projection from magnetic resonance angiography. Collateral vessel (*unlabeled arrow*) from the DAO supplying the left lung. LPV, left pulmonary vein.

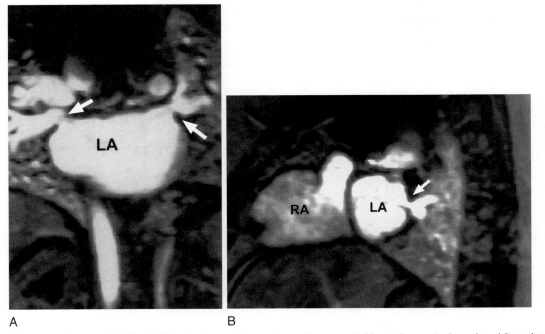

FIGURE 17-31 Pulmonary vein stenosis. Patient with heterotaxy syndrome and complex congenital heart disease. **A,** Coronal, and **B,** sagittal. Fast gradient echo images demonstrate focal stenosis of the right and left pulmonary veins (*arrows*). LA, left atrium; RA, right atrium.

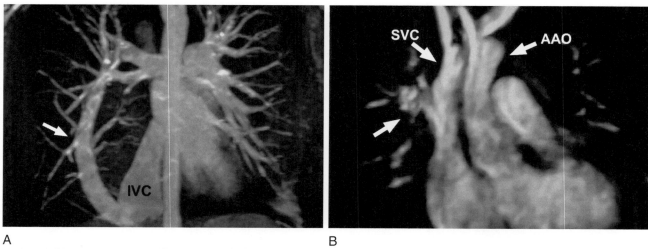

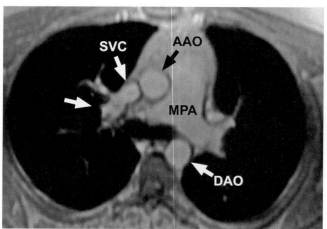

FIGURE 17-32 Partial anomalous pulmonary venous return (PAPVR). Scimitar syndrome. **A**, Coronal projection from a magnetic resonance angiography demonstrates a large vein (*arrow*) from the right lung draining the entire right pulmonary venous system to the inferior vena cava (IVC). **B** and **C**, Partial anomalous pulmonary venous return to the superior vena cava (SVC). Coronal magnetic resonance angiography (B) and axial fast gradient echo image (C) demonstrate the right upper pulmonary vein (*arrow*) draining to the SVC. The main pulmonary artery (MPA) is enlarged due to the left to right shunt. AAO, ascending aorta; DAO, descending aorta.

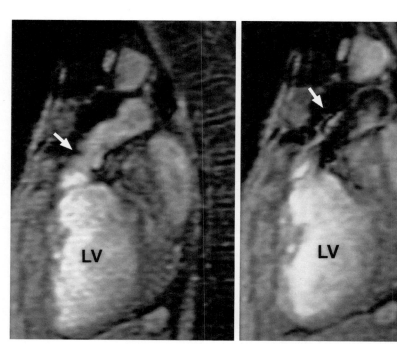

FIGURE 17-33 Conduit obstruction. {I,D,D} double outlet right ventricle status post left ventricle to pulmonary artery conduit. Sagittal fast gradient echo images in diastole (**A**) and systole (**B**) demonstrate focal narrowing of the proximal conduit (*arrow in A*) and turbulent flow causing dephasing (*arrow in B*) due to significant stenosis. Dephasing causes the turbulent area to appear black. LV, left ventricle.

FIGURE 17-34 Tetralogy of Fallot status post right ventricle to pulmonary artery (RV-PA) conduit now with obstruction. **A,** Oblique sagittal, and **B,** axial, magnetic resonance angiography images demonstrate flow within a stent (ST) in an RV-PA conduit with proximal stenosis (arrow *in A*) and stenosis of both proximal branch pulmonary arteries (seen best in B). The stent is positioned in the distal conduit where the (white) flow column is narrowed. AAO, ascending aorta; DAO, descending aorta; LPA, left pulmonary artery; LV, left ventricle; RPA, right pulmonary artery; RV, right ventricle.

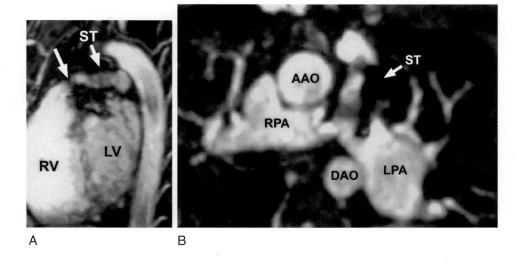

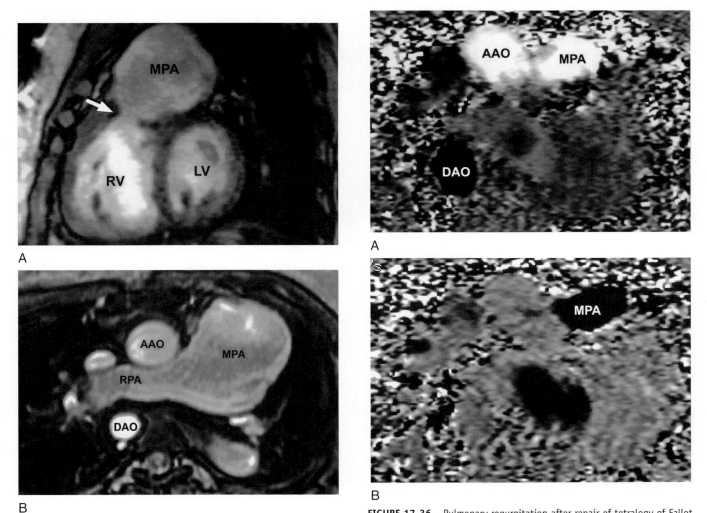

FIGURE 17-35 Tetralogy of Fallot status post right ventricular outflow tract augmentation now with severe obstruction. **A,** Sagittal, and **B,** axial, fast gradient echo images demonstrate severe narrowing of the right ventricular outflow tract (arrow *in A*) and associated poststenotic dilation of the main pulmonary artery. AAO, ascending aorta; DAO, descending aorta; LV, left ventricle; RPA, right pulmonary artery; RV, right ventricle.

FIGURE 17-36 Pulmonary regurgitation after repair of tetralogy of Fallot. **A,** Systolic frame. Phase contrast images perpendicular to the main pulmonary artery (MPA) demonstrate forward flow (*white in A*) in systole in both the MPA and ascending aorta (AAO). Flow in the descending aorta (DAO) is black since it is in the opposite direction compared to flow in the ascending aorta. **B,** Diastolic frame. Note that flow in the MPA is black with reversal of flow due to pulmonary regurgitation.

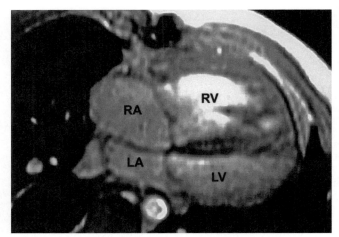

A

FIGURE 17-37 Transposition of the great arteries status post Senning repair. **A,** Four-chamber fast gradient echo image demonstrates a hypertrophied systemic right ventricle. **B,** Coronal magnetic resonance angiography demonstrates the systemic venous pathway to the left atrium. **C,** Sagittal magnetic resonance angiography demonstrates the pulmonary venous pathway to the right atrium. IVC, inferior vena cava; LA, left atrium; LV, left ventricle; MPV, common or main pulmonary vein; RA, right atrium; RV, right ventricle; SVC, superior vena cava.

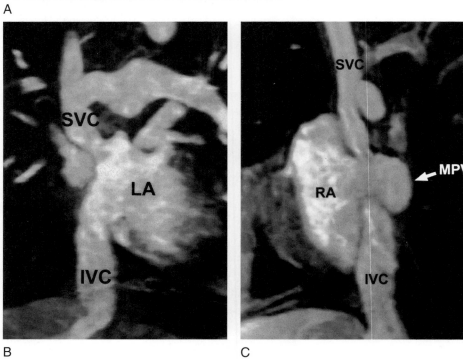

B

C

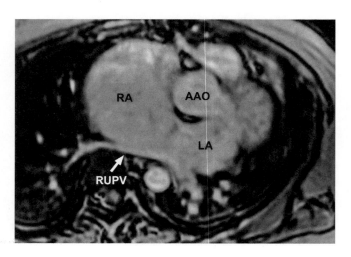

FIGURE 17-38 Pulmonary venous obstruction status post Fontan for tricuspid atresia. Axial fast gradient echo image demonstrates a dilated right atrium (RA) causing compression of the right upper pulmonary vein (RUPV) as it enters the left atrium (LA). AAO, ascending aorta.

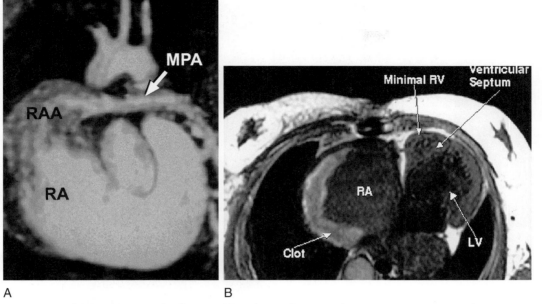

A   B

FIGURE 17-39 Thrombosis complicating Fontan procedure for tricuspid atresia. **A,** Oblique sagittal magnetic resonance angiography demonstrates a surgically created anastomosis between the right atrial appendage (RAA) and the main pulmonary artery (MPA). **B,** Axial conventional spin echo image demonstrates a layer of increased signal intensity lining the wall of the dilated right atrium consistent with adherent thrombus (Clot). LV, left ventricle; RA, right atrium; RV, right ventricle.

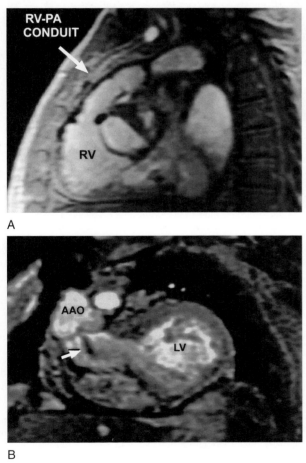

A

B

FIGURE 17-40 Transposition of the great arteries with ventricular septal defect and pulmonary stenosis status post Rastelli. **A,** Sagittal fast gradient echo demonstrates a right ventricle (RV) to pulmonary artery (PA) conduit. **B,** Coronal fast gradient echo in diastole shows left ventricle (LV) to ascending aorta (AAO) pathway through the ventricular septal defect. There is turbulent flow jet from aortic regurgitation (*arrow pointing to black flow jet*).

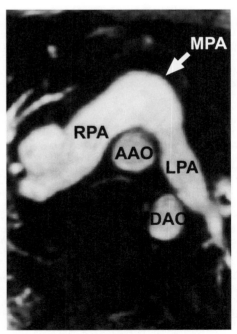

FIGURE 17-41 Transposition of the great arteries status post arterial switch. Axial fast gradient echo image demonstrates an anterior main pulmonary artery (MPA) with branch pulmonary arteries (RPA and LPA) draped on either side of the ascending aorta (AAO). DAO, descending aorta.

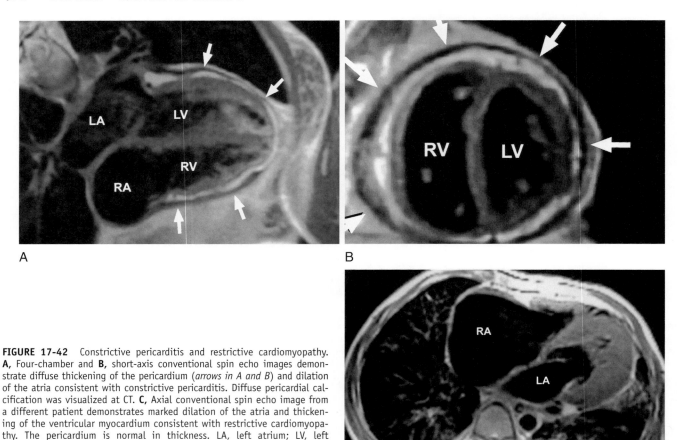

FIGURE 17-42 Constrictive pericarditis and restrictive cardiomyopathy. **A,** Four-chamber and **B,** short-axis conventional spin echo images demonstrate diffuse thickening of the pericardium (*arrows in A and B*) and dilation of the atria consistent with constrictive pericarditis. Diffuse pericardial calcification was visualized at CT. **C,** Axial conventional spin echo image from a different patient demonstrates marked dilation of the atria and thickening of the ventricular myocardium consistent with restrictive cardiomyopathy. The pericardium is normal in thickness. LA, left atrium; LV, left ventricle; RA, right atrium; RV, right ventricle.

References

1. al Ali F, Higgins CB, Gooding CA: MRI of tracheal and esophageal compression following surgery for congenital heart disease. *J Comput Assist Tomogr* 18:39–42, 1994.
2. Allan LD, Leanage R, Wainwright R, et al: Balloon atrial septostomy under two-dimensional echocardiographic control. *Br Heart J* 47:41–43, 1982.
3. Baker EJ, Allan LD, Tynan MJ, et al: Balloon atrial septostomy in the neonatal intensive care unit. *Br Heart J* 51:377–378, 1984.
4. Barker PC, Ensing G, Ludomirsky A, et al: Comparison of simultaneous invasive and noninvasive measurements of pressure gradients in congenital aortic valve stenosis. *J Am Soc Echocardiogr* 15:1496–1502, 2002.
5. Bartel T, Muller S, Caspari G, Erbel R: Intracardiac and intraluminal echocardiography: Indications and standard approaches. *Ultrasound Med Biol* 28:997–1003, 2002.
6. Baumgartner H, Stefenelli T, Niederberger J, et al: "Overestimation" of catheter gradients by Doppler ultrasound in patients with aortic stenosis: A predictable manifestation of pressure recovery. *J Am Coll Cardiol* 33: 1655–1661, 1999.
7. Berdon WE, Baker DH, Wung JT, et al: Complete cartilage-ring tracheal stenosis associated with anomalous left pulmonary artery: The ring-sling complex. *Radiology* 152:57–64, 1984.
8. Berger M, Haimowitz A, Van Tosh A, et al: Quantitative assessment of pulmonary hypertension in patients with tricuspid regurgitation using continuous wave Doppler ultrasound. *J Am Coll Cardiol* 6:359–365, 1985.
9. Blakenberg F, Rhee J, Hardy C, et al: MRI vs echocardiography in the evaluation of the Jatene procedure. *J Comput Assist Tomogr* 18: 749–754, 1994.
10. Bornemeier RA, Weinberg PM, Fogel MA: Angiographic, echocardiographic, and three-dimensional magnetic resonance imaging of extracardiac conduits in congenital heart disease. *Am J Cardiol* 78:713–717, 1996.
11. Brangenberg R, Burger A, Romer U, et al: Echocardiographic assessment of left ventricular size and function in normal children from infancy to adolescence: Acoustic quantification in comparison with traditional echocardiographic techniques. *Pediatr Cardiol* 23:394–402, 2002.
12. Bromberg BI, Beekman RH, Rocchini AP, et al: Aortic aneurysm after patch aortoplasty repair of coarctation: A prospective analysis of prevalence, screening tests and risks. *J Am Coll Cardiol* 14:734–741, 1989.
13. Cape EG, Jones M, Yamada I, et al: Turbulent/viscous interactions control Doppler/catheter pressure discrepancies in aortic stenosis: The role of the Reynolds number. *Circulation* 94:2975–2981, 1996.
14. Caputo GR, Kondo C, Masui T, et al: Right and left lung perfusion: In vitro and in vivo validation with oblique-angle, velocity-encoded cine MR imaging. *Radiology* 180:693–698, 1991.
15. Choe YH, Lee HJ, Kim HS, et al: MRI of total anomalous pulmonary venous connections. *J Comput Assist Tomogr* 18:243–249, 1994.
16. Colan SD, Borow KM, MacPherson D, Sanders SP: Use of the indirect axillary pulse tracing for noninvasive determination of ejection time, upstroke time, and left ventricular wall stress throughout ejection in infants and young children. *Am J Cardiol* 53:1154–1158, 1984.
17. Colan SD, Borow KM, Neumann A: Use of the calibrated carotid pulse tracing for calculation of left ventricular pressure and wall stress throughout ejection. *Am Heart J* 109:1306–1310, 1985.
18. Colan SD, Borow KM, Neumann A: Left ventricular end-systolic wall stress-velocity of fiber shortening relation: A load-independent index of myocardial contractility. *J Am Coll Cardiol* 4:715–724, 1984.

19. Colan SD, Fujii A, Borow KM, et al: Noninvasive determination of systolic, diastolic and end-systolic blood pressure in neonates, infants and young children: Comparison with central aortic pressure measurements. *Am J Cardiol* 52:867–870, 1983.

20. Colan SD, Parness IA, Spevak PJ, Sanders SP: Developmental modulation of myocardial mechanics: Age- and growth-related alterations in afterload and contractility. *J Am Coll Cardiol* 19:619–629, 1992.

21. Dairywala IT, Li P, Liu Z, et al: Catheter-based interventions guided solely by a new phased-array intracardiac imaging catheter: in vivo experimental studies. *J Am Soc Echocardiogr* 15:150–158, 2002.

22. Donnelly LF, Strife JL, Bailey WW: Extrinsic airway compression secondary to pulmonary arterial conduits: MR findings. *Pediatr Radiol* 27: 268–270, 1997.

23. d'Orsogna L, Sandor GG, Patterson MW, et al: Influence of echocardiography in preoperative cardiac catheterization in congenital heart disease. *Int J Cardiol* 24:19–26, 1989.

24. Eichenberger AC, Jenni R, von Schulthess GK: Aortic valve pressure gradients in patients with aortic valve stenosis: Quantification with velocity-encoded cine MR imaging. *AJR Am J Roentgenol* 160:971–977, 1993.

25. Eidem BW, Cetta F, Webb JL, et al: Early detection of cardiac dysfunction: Use of the myocardial performance index in patients with anorexia nervosa. *J Adolesc Health* 29:267–270, 2001.

26. Eidem BW, McMahon CJ, Cohen RR, et al: Impact of cardiac growth on Doppler tissue imaging velocities: A study in healthy children. *J Am Soc Echocardiogr* 17:212–221, 2004.

27. Eidem BW, O'Leary PW: The potential impact of alteration in preload on the myocardial performance index (MPI). *J Am Soc Echocardiogr* 13: 644, 2000.

28. Eidem BW, O'Leary PW, Tei C, Seward JB: Usefulness of the myocardial performance index for assessing right ventricular function in congenital heart disease. *Am J Cardiol* 86:654–658, 2000.

29. Eidem BW, Sapp BG, Suarez CR, Cetta F: Usefulness of the myocardial performance index for early detection of anthracycline-induced cardiotoxicity in children. *Am J Cardiol* 87:1120–1122, A9, 2001.

30. Ensing G, Seward J, Darragh R, Caldwell R: Feasibility of generating hemodynamic pressure curves from noninvasive Doppler echocardiographic signals. *J Am Coll Cardiol* 23:434–442, 1994.

31. Evans DH, McDicken WN: *Doppler Ultrasound: Physics, Instrumental, and Clinical Applications.* West Sussex, UK: John Wiley & Sons, 2000.

32. Fawzy ME, von Sinner W, Rifai A, et al: Magnetic resonance imaging compared with angiography in the evaluation of intermediate-term result of coarctation balloon angioplasty. *Am Heart J* 126:1380–1384, 1993.

33. Fogel MA: Assessment of cardiac function by magnetic resonance imaging. *Pediatr Cardiol* 21:59–69, 2000.

34. Fogel MA, Hubbard AM, Fellows KE, Weinberg PM: MRI for physiology and function in congenital heart disease: Functional assessment of the heart preoperatively and postoperatively. *Semin Roentgenol* 33:239–251, 1998.

35. Garcia D, Dumesnil JG, Durand LG, et al: Discrepancies between catheter and Doppler estimates of valve effective orifice area can be predicted from the pressure recovery phenomenon: Practical implications with regard to quantification of aortic stenosis severity. *J Am Coll Cardiol* 41: 435–442, 2003.

36. Garcia D, Pibarot P, Dumesnil JG, et al: Assessment of aortic valve stenosis severity: A new index based on the energy loss concept. *Circulation* 101:765–771, 2000.

37. Garcia MJ, Thomas JD, Klein AL: New Doppler echocardiographic applications for the study of diastolic function. *J Am Coll Cardiol* 32: 865–875, 1998.

38. Geva T, Vick GW III, Wendt RE, Rokey R: Role of spin echo and cine magnetic resonance imaging in presurgical planning of heterotaxy syndrome: Comparison with echocardiography and catheterization. *Circulation* 90:348–356, 1994.

39. Globits S, Frank H, Mayr H, et al: Quantitative assessment of aortic regurgitation by magnetic resonance imaging. *Eur Heart J* 13:78–83, 1992.

40. Goo HW, Park IS, Ko JK, et al: CT of congenital heart disease: Normal anatomy and typical pathologic conditions. *Radiographics* 23 Spec No:S147–S165, 2003.

41. Grenadier E, Oliveira Lima C, Allen HD, et al: Normal intracardiac and great vessel Doppler flow velocities in infants and children. *J Am Coll Cardiol* 4:343–350, 1984.

42. Haramati LB, Glickstein JS, Issenberg HJ, et al: MR imaging and CT of vascular anomalies and connections in patients with congenital heart disease: Significance in surgical planning. *Radiographics* 22:337–347, 2002.

43. Hardy CE, Helton GJ, Kondo C, et al: Usefulness of magnetic resonance imaging for evaluating great-vessel anatomy after arterial switch operation for D-transposition of the great arteries. *Am Heart J* 128:326–332, 1994.

44. Helbing WA, Bosch HG, Maliepaard C, et al: Comparison of echocardiographic methods with magnetic resonance imaging for assessment of right ventricular function in children. *Am J Cardiol* 76:589–594, 1995.

45. Henry WL, DeMaria A, Gramiak R, et al: Report of the American Society of Echocardiography Committee on Nomenclature and Standards in Two-dimensional Echocardiography. *Circulation* 62:212–217, 1980.

46. Hernandez RJ, Aisen AM, Foo TK, Beekman RH: Thoracic cardiovascular anomalies in children: Evaluation with a fast gradient-recalled-echo sequence with cardiac-triggered segmented acquisition. *Radiology* 188:775–780, 1993.

47. Hiraishi S, Misawa H, Hirota H, et al: Noninvasive quantitative evaluation of the morphology of the major pulmonary artery branches in cyanotic congenital heart disease: Angiocardiographic and echocardiographic correlative study. *Circulation* 89:1306–1316, 1994.

48. Ho VB, Prince MR: Thoracic MR aortography: Imaging techniques and strategies. *Radiographics* 18:287–309, 1998.

49. Honda N, Machida K, Hashimoto M, et al: Aortic regurgitation: Quantitation with MR imaging velocity mapping. *Radiology* 186: 189–194, 1993.

50. Hong YK, Park YW, Ryu SJ, et al: Efficacy of MRI in complicated congenital heart disease with visceral heterotaxy syndrome. *J Comput Assist Tomogr* 24:671–682, 2000.

51. Hoppe UC, Dederichs B, Deutsch HJ, et al: Congenital heart disease in adults and adolescents: Comparative value of transthoracic and transesophageal echocardiography and MR imaging. *Radiology* 199: 669–677, 1996.

52. Keller PJ, Drayer BP, Fram EK, et al: MR angiography with two-dimensional acquisition and three-dimensional display: Work in progress. *Radiology* 173:527–532, 1989.

53. Kersting-Sommerhoff BA, Seelos KC, Hardy C, et al: Evaluation of surgical procedures for cyanotic congenital heart disease by using MR imaging. *AJR Am J Roentgenol* 155:259–266, 1990.

54. Khouri SJ, Maly GT, Suh DD, Walsh TE: A practical approach to the echocardiographic evaluation of diastolic function. *J Am Soc Echocardiogr* 17:290–297, 2004.

55. Kilner PJ, Firmin DN, Rees RS, et al: Valve and great vessel stenosis: Assessment with MR jet velocity mapping. *Radiology* 178:229–235, 1991.

56. King ME, Braun H, Goldblatt A, et al: Interventricular septal configuration as a predictor of right ventricular systolic hypertension in children: A cross-sectional echocardiographic study. *Circulation* 68:68–75, 1983.

57. Kipel G, Arnon R, Ritter SB: Transesophageal echocardiographic guidance of balloon atrial septostomy. *J Am Soc Echocardiogr* 4:631–635, 1991.

58. Krabill KA, Ring WS, Foker JE, et al: Echocardiographic versus cardiac catheterization diagnosis of infants with congenital heart disease requiring cardiac surgery. *Am J Cardiol* 60:351–354, 1987.

59. Kremkau FW: *Diagnostic Ultrasound: Principles and Instruments,* 6th ed. Philadelphia, WB Saunders, 2002.

60. Marino B, Corno A, Carotti A, et al: Pediatric cardiac surgery guided by echocardiography: Established indications and new trends. *Scand J Thorac Cardiovasc Surg* 24:197–201, 1990.

61. Martinez JE, Mohiaddin RH, Kilner PJ, et al: Obstruction in extracardiac ventriculopulmonary conduits: Value of nuclear magnetic resonance imaging with velocity mapping and Doppler echocardiography. *J Am Coll Cardiol* 20:338–344, 1992.

62. Marx GR, Allen HD, Goldberg SJ: Doppler echocardiographic estimation of systolic pulmonary artery pressure in pediatric patients with interventricular communications. *J Am Coll Cardiol* 6:1132–1137, 1985.

63. Marx GR, Geva T: MRI and echocardiography in children: How do they compare? *Semin Roentgenol* 33:281–292, 1998.

64. Masui T, Finck S, Higgins CB: Constrictive pericarditis and restrictive cardiomyopathy: Evaluation with MR imaging. *Radiology* 182:369–373, 1992.

65. Masui T, Seelos KC, Kersting-Sommerhoff BA, Higgins CB: Abnormalities of the pulmonary veins: Evaluation with MR imaging and comparison with cardiac angiography and echocardiography. *Radiology* 181:645–649, 1991.

66. Matsunaga S, Suzuki K, Ichinose E, et al: Application of two dimensional echocardiography for the intracardiac manipulation: The evaluation of atrial septal movement before and after balloon atrial septostomy. (author's transl) *J Cardiogr* 11:217–224, 1981.

67. McFaul R, Millard P, Nowicki E: Vascular rings necessitating right thoracotomy. *J Thorac Cardiovasc Surg* 82:306–309, 1981.

68. McMahon CJ, Fraley JK, Kovalchin JP: Use of tissue harmonic imaging in pediatric echocardiography. *Cardiol Young* 11:562–564, 2001.

69. Mohiaddin RH, Kilner PJ, Rees S, Longmore DB: Magnetic resonance volume flow and jet velocity mapping in aortic coarctation. *J Am Coll Cardiol* 22:1515–1521, 1993.

70. Mostbeck GH, Caputo GR, Higgins CB: MR measurement of blood flow in the cardiovascular system. *AJR Am J Roentgenol* 159:453–461, 1992.

71. Nagueh SF, Kopelen HA, Lim DS, et al: Tissue Doppler imaging consistently detects myocardial contraction and relaxation abnormalities, irrespective of cardiac hypertrophy, in a transgenic rabbit model of human hypertrophic cardiomyopathy. *Circulation* 102:1346–1350, 2000.

72. Nagueh SF, Lakkis NM, Middleton KJ, et al: Doppler estimation of left ventricular filling pressures in patients with hypertrophic cardiomyopathy. *Circulation* 99:254–261, 1999.

73. Nagueh SF, McFalls J, Meyer D, et al: Tissue Doppler imaging predicts the development of hypertrophic cardiomyopathy in subjects with subclinical disease. *Circulation* 108:395–398, 2003.

74. Nagueh SF, Middleton KJ, Kopelen HA, et al: Doppler tissue imaging: A noninvasive technique for evaluation of left ventricular relaxation and estimation of filling pressures. *J Am Coll Cardiol* 30:1527–1533, 1997.

75. Nienaber CA, Rehders TC, Fratz S: Detection and assessment of congenital heart disease with magnetic resonance techniques. *J Cardiovasc Magn Reson* 1:169–184, 1999.

76. Nienaber CA, von Kodolitsch Y, Brockhoff CJ, et al: Comparison of conventional and transesophageal echocardiography with magnetic resonance imaging for anatomical mapping of thoracic aortic dissection: A dual noninvasive imaging study with anatomical and/or angiographic validation. *Int J Card Imaging* 10:1–14, 1994.

77. Nienaber CA, von Kodolitsch Y, Nicolas V, et al: The diagnosis of thoracic aortic dissection by noninvasive imaging procedures. *N Engl J Med* 328:1–9, 1993.

78. Niezen RA, Helbing WA, van der Wall EE, et al: Biventricular systolic function and mass studied with MR imaging in children with pulmonary regurgitation after repair for tetralogy of Fallot. *Radiology* 201:135–140, 1996.

79. O'Leary PW, Hagler DJ, Seward JB, et al: Biplane intraoperative transesophageal echocardiography in congenital heart disease. *Mayo Clin Proc* 70:317–326, 1995.

80. Powell AJ, Geva T: Blood flow measurement by magnetic resonance imaging in congenital heart disease. *Pediatr Cardiol* 21:47–58.

81. Presbitero P, Bull C, Haworth SG, de Leval MR: Absent or occult pulmonary artery. *Br Heart J* 52:178–185, 1984.

82. Prince MR, Yucel EK, Kaufman JA, et al: Dynamic gadolinium-enhanced three-dimensional abdominal MR arteriography. *J Magn Reson Imaging* 3:877–881, 1993.

83. Randolph GR, Hagler DJ, Connolly HM, et al: Intraoperative transesophageal echocardiography during surgery for congenital heart defects. *J Thorac Cardiovasc Surg* 124:1176–1182, 2002.

84. Rashkind WJ, Miller WW: Transposition of the great arteries. Results of palliation by balloon atrioseptostomy in thirty-one infants. *Circulation* 38:453–462, 1968.

85. Rashkind WJ, Miller WW: Creation of an atrial septal defect without thoracotomy: A palliative approach to complete transposition of the great arteries. *JAMA* 196:991–992, 1966.

86. Rebergen SA, Chin JG, Ottenkamp J, et al: Pulmonary regurgitation in the late postoperative follow-up of tetralogy of Fallot: Volumetric quantitation by nuclear magnetic resonance velocity mapping. *Circulation* 88:2257–2266, 1993.

87. Rebergen SA, Niezen RA, Helbing WA, et al: Cine gradient-echo MR imaging and MR velocity mapping in the evaluation of congenital heart disease. *Radiographics* 16:467–481, 1996.

88. Rebergen SA, Ottenkamp J, Doornbos J, et al: Postoperative pulmonary flow dynamics after Fontan surgery: Assessment with nuclear magnetic resonance velocity mapping. *J Am Coll Cardiol* 21:123–131, 1993.

89. Rebergen SA, van der Wall EE, Doornbos J, de Roos A: Magnetic resonance measurement of velocity and flow: Technique, validation, and cardiovascular applications. *Am Heart J* 126:1439–1456, 1993.

90. Rees S, Somerville J, Ward C, et al: Coarctation of the aorta: MR imaging in late postoperative assessment. *Radiology* 173:499–502, 1989.

91. Rees S, Somerville J, Warnes C, et al: Comparison of magnetic resonance imaging with echocardiography and radionuclide angiography in assessing cardiac function and anatomy following Mustard's operation for transposition of the great arteries. *Am J Cardiol* 61:1316–1322, 1988.

92. Ren JF, Marchlinski FE, Callans DJ, Herrmann HC: Clinical use of AcuNav diagnostic ultrasound catheter imaging during left heart radiofrequency ablation and transcatheter closure procedures. *J Am Soc Echocardiogr* 15:1301–1308, 2002.

93. Rein AJ, Colan SD, Parness IA, Sanders SP: Regional and global left ventricular function in infants with anomalous origin of the left coronary artery from the pulmonary trunk: Preoperative and postoperative assessment. *Circulation* 75:115–123, 1987.

94. Rein AJ, Lewis N, Sapoznikov D, et al: Quantitation of regional ventricular asynergy using real-time two-dimensional echocardiography. *Isr J Med Sci* 18:457–461, 1982.

95. Rein AJ, Sanders SP, Colan SD, et al: Left ventricular mechanics in the normal newborn. *Circulation* 76:1029–1036, 1987.

96. Roest AA, Helbing WA, van der Wall EE, de Roos A: Postoperative evaluation of congenital heart disease by magnetic resonance imaging. *J Magn Reson Imaging* 10:656–666, 1999.

97. Rosenfeld HM, Gentles TL, Wernovsky G, et al: Utility of intraoperative transesophageal echocardiography in the assessment of residual cardiac defects. *Pediatr Cardiol* 19:346–351, 1998.

98. Ross RD, Bisset GS III, Meyer RA, et al: Magnetic resonance imaging for diagnosis of pulmonary vein stenosis after "correction" of total anomalous pulmonary venous connection. *Am J Cardiol* 60:1199–1201, 1987.

99. Rowland DG, Gutgesell HP: Noninvasive assessment of myocardial contractility, preload, and afterload in healthy newborn infants. *Am J Cardiol* 75:818–821, 1995.

100. Sampson C, Kilner PJ, Hirsch R, et al: Venoatrial pathways after the Mustard operation for transposition of the great arteries: Anatomic and functional MR imaging. *Radiology* 193:211–217, 1994.

101. Sampson C, Martinez J, Rees S, et al: Evaluation of Fontan's operation by magnetic resonance imaging. *Am J Cardiol* 65:819–821, 1990.

102. Sechtem U, Pflugfelder PW, White RD, et al: Cine MR imaging: Potential for the evaluation of cardiovascular function. *AJR Am J Roentgenol* 148:239–246, 1987.

103. Siwik ES, Spector ML, Patel CR, Zahka KG: Costs and cost-effectiveness of routine transesophageal echocardiography in congenital heart surgery. *Am Heart J* 138:771–776, 1999.

104. Skinner JR, Boys RJ, Hunter S, Hey EN: Noninvasive assessment of pulmonary arterial pressure in healthy neonates. *Arch Dis Child* 66:386–390, 1991.

105. Sloth E, Hasenkam JM, Sorensen KE, et al: Pediatric multiplane transesophageal echocardiography in congenital heart disease: New possibilities with a miniaturized probe. *J Am Soc Echocardiogr* 9:622–628, 1996.

106. Snyder AR, Serwer GA, Ritter SB: The normal echocardiographic examination. In *Echocardiography in Pediatric Heart Disease*. St. Louis, Mosby, 1997, pp 22–75.

107. Soulen RL, Stark DD, Higgins CB: Magnetic resonance imaging of constrictive pericardial disease. *Am J Cardiol* 55:480–484, 1985.

108. Steffens JC, Bourne MW, Sakuma H, et al: Quantification of collateral blood flow in coarctation of the aorta by velocity encoded cine magnetic resonance imaging. *Circulation* 90:937–943, 1994.

109. Strouse PJ, Hernandez RJ, Beekman RH III: Assessment of central pulmonary arteries in patients with obstructive lesions of the right ventricle: Comparison of MR imaging and cineangiography. *AJR Am J Roentgenol* 167:1175–1183, 1996.

110. Theissen P, Kaemmerer H, Sechtem U, et al: Magnetic resonance imaging of cardiac function and morphology in patients with transposition of the great arteries following Mustard procedure. *Thorac Cardiovasc Surg* 39 Suppl 3:221–224, 1991.

111. Thomas JD, Rubin DN: Tissue harmonic imaging: Why does it work? *J Am Soc Echocardiogr* 11:803–808, 1998.

112. Vesely TM, Julsrud PR, Brown JJ, Hagler DJ: MR imaging of partial anomalous pulmonary venous connections. *J Comput Assist Tomogr* 15:752–756, 1991.

113. Vick GW III, Rokey R, Huhta JC, et al: Nuclear magnetic resonance imaging of the pulmonary arteries, subpulmonary region, and aorticopulmonary shunts: A comparative study with two-dimensional echocardiography and angiography. *Am Heart J* 119:1103–1110, 1990.

114. Vogel M, Staller W, Buhlmeyer K: Left ventricular myocardial mass determined by cross-sectional echocardiography in normal

newborns, infants, and children. *Pediatr Cardiol* 12:143–149, 1991.

115. von Schulthess GK, Higashino SM, Higgins SS, et al: Coarctation of the aorta: MR imaging. *Radiology* 158:469–474, 1986.

116. Watson H, Rashkind WJ: Creation of atrial septal defects by balloon catheter in babies with transposition of the great arteries. *Lancet* 1: 403–405, 1967.

117. Weinberg PM, Fogel MA: Cardiac MR imaging in congenital heart disease. *Cardiol Clin* 16:315–348, 1998.

118. Yamada H, Goh PP, Sun JP, et al: Prevalence of left ventricular diastolic dysfunction by Doppler echocardiography: Clinical application of the Canadian consensus guidelines. *J Am Soc Echocardiogr* 15:1238–1244, 2002.

119. Zellers TM, Dixon K, Moake L, et al: Bedside balloon atrial septostomy is safe, efficacious, and cost-effective compared with septostomy performed in the cardiac catheterization laboratory. *Am J Cardiol* 89: 613–615, 2002.

Chapter 18

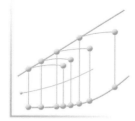

Diagnostic and Therapeutic Cardiac Catheterization

MARTIN P. O'LAUGHLIN, MD, PC, and RICHARD E. RINGEL, MD

INTRODUCTION

Over the past decade, the improving resolution of echo-cardiographic and magnetic resonance imaging along with the utilization of transesophageal echocardiography has greatly reduced the diagnostic role of cardiac catheterization. During the same period, however, the role of cardiac catheterization as an adjunct or therapeutic alternative to cardiac surgery has been expanding. Catheterization-based interventions are frequently critical in preparing marginal candidates for complex surgical procedures or for palliating patients with unresolved problems in the postoperative period. Hemodynamic assessment of infants and children with congenital heart disease is occasionally required preoperatively to determine surgical candidacy and postoperatively to assess the hemodynamic response to surgical intervention.

Catheter-based techniques also have a role in the diagnosis and therapy of children with acquired heart disease. This chapter reviews these and other issues and discusses the practical management of critically ill infants and children undergoing catheterization. In addition, the role of catheterization and catheter techniques in the postoperative care of patients with congenital heart disease is discussed.

THERAPEUTIC CATHETERIZATION AS AN ALTERNATIVE TO SURGERY

Dr. William Rashkind[49] ushered in the era of therapeutic cardiac catheterization in 1966 with the performance of

463

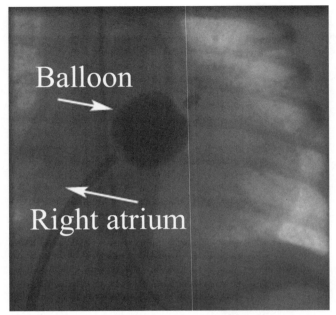

FIGURE 18-1   Posteroanterior cineangiographic frame of a patient undergoing a balloon atrial septostomy. The inflated balloon is in the left atrium, ready to be pulled back into the right atrium.

the first balloon atrial septostomy for management of infants with transposition of the great arteries (Fig. 18-1). At that time no surgical alternative existed and the creation of a large atrial communication served as a palliative procedure to allow enough intracardiac mixing to produce arterial oxygen concentrations compatible with life and thereby delay surgery until the child became older and larger. In the modern era, balloon septostomy is used more frequently as an adjunct to surgical repair (see discussion to follow). Nevertheless this technique led the way for development of an array of procedures that now can replace cardiac surgery.

Critical Pulmonary Valve Stenosis

The use of balloon dilation catheters to relieve pulmonary valve stenosis was first described for use in older children, but with the miniaturization of these catheters, the technique is applicable to critically ill infants as small as 1 kg. Balloon pulmonary valvotomy has now essentially replaced surgery as the first-line technique for this disorder once the diagnosis is established echocardiographically.

In neonates the indication for dilation is severe or critical valve stenosis, where there is significant hypoxemia due to right-to-left atrial shunting through a patent foramen ovale. Rarely, neonates may show signs of right heart failure when the foramen is restrictive. When there is reduced transpulmonary valve flow, Doppler gradients cannot be relied on alone to establish the severity of obstruction. Reduced antegrade pulmonary blood flow occurs when the right ventricle is hypertrophied and has decreased compliance or if the pulmonary vascular resistance is elevated. Finally, in neonates with severe (not critical) pulmonary valve stenosis, it may be necessary to allow closure of the ductus arteriosus and/or for the pulmonary vascular resistance to fall to be certain of the severity of pulmonary stenosis.

In older infants and children, a Doppler-derived peak instantaneous gradient of at least 50 mm Hg is considered an indication for intervention.

In neonates, balloon valvotomy should be performed soon after the diagnosis of critical valvular pulmonary stenosis is made. Patients are electively intubated before catheterization and prostaglandin E_1 infused to maintain ductal patency. A patent ductus has two benefits: First, the flexible guide wire used to position the balloon catheter across the stenotic valve can be advanced across the ductus into the descending aorta, thereby allowing better stabilization of the catheter; second, the ductus provides an additional route for pulmonary blood flow during the procedure, which may improve patient stability.

Catheterization is usually performed via the femoral vein. Entry to the right ventricle via the umbilical vein is difficult and usually not used even when umbilical venous access is available. After right heart hemodynamic measurements are made, the pulmonary valve annulus is measured from the right ventriculogram and compared to the measurement from echocardiography. Usually the measurements are similar. A diagnostic catheter is used in conjunction with flexible guide wires to cross the pulmonary valve. The diagnostic catheter is exchanged for the balloon dilation catheter. Depending on the severity of the stenosis, an inflated balloon size equal to the annulus size is selected for the first valvotomy, or in severe situations, the valve may need to be predilated with a smaller balloon (3 or 4 mm diameter) just to enable passage of the appropriate-sized valvotomy catheter. After the valvotomy is performed, hemodynamic measurements and angiography are repeated (Fig. 18-2). If the result is inadequate, redilation with balloon sizes up to a maximum diameter of 1.3 times the annulus diameter can be performed.

Prostaglandin E_1 infusion may be needed after successful valvuloplasty until right ventricular compliance improves and allows sufficient antegrade pulmonary blood flow to maintain acceptable systemic oxygen saturation. Ductal patency may be needed in some patients for days after successful valvotomy. Infrequently, when there is very severe tricuspid valve or right ventricular hypoplasia, a modified Blalock-Taussig shunt may be needed.

Effective gradient relief is achieved in approximately 90% of neonates. Success rates are lower in infants with dysplastic valves, sometimes occurring as part of Noonan's syndrome. Complications are unusual but include femoral venous thrombosis and, very rarely, right ventricular free wall or pulmonary arterial/annular perforation. In those with restenosis, repeat dilation can be performed, but in a subset, surgical right ventricular outflow tract enlargement and/or pulmonary valvotomy may be needed.[16,17,28,39,45] Among neonates with successful initial gradient relief, approximately 85% will not require additional surgical or catheter intervention.

Pulmonary Valve Atresia with Intact Ventricular Septum

Infants with pulmonary valve atresia and intact ventricular septum should have coronary arteriography to identify the subset of patients with right ventricular dependent coronary circulation. The initial management and preparation for the catheterization laboratory are the same as for infants with critical pulmonary valve stenosis.

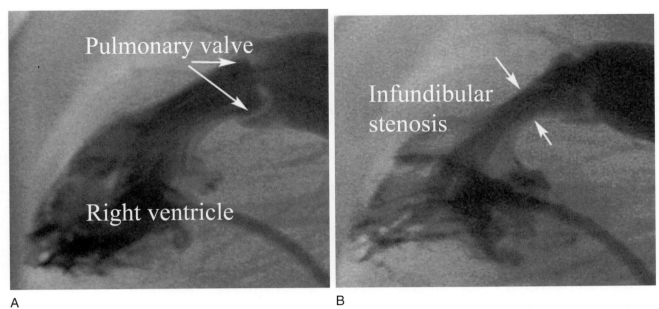

A   B

FIGURE 18-2   A, Predilation lateral cineangiographic frame in a patient with severe pulmonary valve stenosis. The injection is in the right ventricle, and the thickened doming pulmonary valve is seen *(arrows)*. There was a 70 mm Hg peak-to-peak systolic gradient from the right ventricle to the main pulmonary artery. **B,** After balloon dilation of the pulmonary valve, there is an increased diameter of the flow orifice at the pulmonary valve. The right ventricular pressure fell to 45 mm Hg, with a 25 mm Hg systolic gradient across the infundibular stenosis *(arrows)*. This hypertrophic infundibular stenosis resolved without treatment.

When pulmonary atresia with an intact ventricular septum develops in later fetal life, the infundibulum may be better expanded and the atresia, membranous. In this subset alone, some have used catheter-based intervention to relieve the obstruction, decompress the right ventricle, and avoid an extensive surgical procedure. Only those neonates with pulmonary atresia and well-formed right ventricular outflow tracts are candidates for interventional catheterization.

Use of catheter-based techniques for this type of pulmonary atresia has been controversial but may be gaining wider acceptance. Among selected patients with pulmonary atresia with intact septum taken to the catheterization laboratory, valve perforation and dilation has been accomplished in approximately 80%, but this usually has not been the only procedure required. Approximately 65% have undergone subsequent procedures.[1,48] Some patients may require prolonged administration of prostaglandin E₁, repeat balloon valvuloplasty, or subsequent placement of a modified Blalock-Taussig shunt. Between 6% and 40% of those who have transcatheter valve perforation later have surgical right ventricular outflow tract reconstruction. Stent implantation also has been used to maintain patency of the dilated right ventricular outflow tract. A successful outcome, resulting in a biventricular circulation, appears to depend primarily upon the tricuspid valve and pulmonary valve annular diameters and the right ventricular size.[7,48]

One of three techniques can be used to perforate the pulmonary valve. All require the positioning of an angled catheter within the right ventricular infundibulum with the tip apposed to the atretic pulmonary valve. The simplest, but least effective, is the passage of the stiff end of an ultrafine "coronary" guide wire through the catheter. The stiff end of the wire is then used to puncture the valve, after which the

wire is removed and a floppy wire used to cross the valve (Fig. 18-3). Alternatively, laser-tipped or radiofrequency guide wires have been used to "burn" a small hole in the valve and thus allow passage of guide wires and balloon catheters to perform the valvotomy.

Tetralogy of Fallot

Neonates with tetralogy of Fallot presenting with severe cyanosis are initially stabilized with prostaglandin E₁ to provide adequate pulmonary blood flow and systemic oxygenation. Surgical management varies among institutions, with some centers palliating by placing a systemic-to-pulmonary arterial shunt and others performing a complete repair at presentation.

Certain anatomic features may complicate early repair. Origin of the left anterior descending coronary artery from the right coronary artery can in some cases motivate the placement of a right ventricle–to–pulmonary artery conduit to relieve right ventricular outflow tract obstruction. Hypoplasia of the pulmonary arteries may also complicate or preclude a single-stage total correction.

Some have used balloon pulmonary valvotomy to increase effective pulmonary blood flow and thereby reduce cyanosis.[40,42] Although improved growth of the pulmonary annulus and the branch pulmonary arteries has been reported,[15,40,42] this is not a universal finding.[19] Whether this approach reduces the need for transannular patching of the right ventricle outflow tract at the time of surgical repair remains uncertain.[3] This technique, when used in conjunction with balloon dilation of the branch pulmonary arteries, may be most useful in infants with severely diminutive pulmonary arteries.[23]

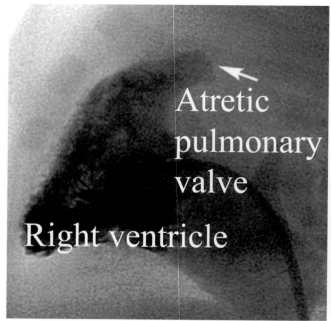

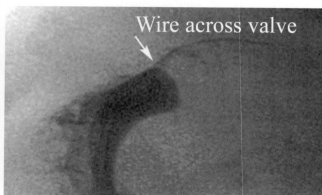

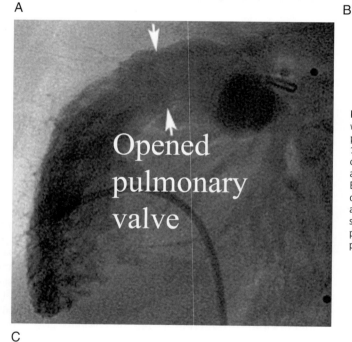

FIGURE 18-3 **A,** Lateral view of a right ventricular injection in a patient with pulmonary valve atresia and intact ventricular septum. The atretic pulmonary valve level is seen *(arrow)*. The right ventricular pressure was 105 mm Hg systolic, more than twice the systemic arterial systolic pressure of 51 mm Hg. **B,** The atretic pulmonary valve plate has been perforated with a guide wire, and the wire is seen in position across the valve *(arrow)*. Balloon dilation followed. **C,** Four months after the perforation and dilation of the atretic pulmonary valve, right ventricular injection demonstrates a widely patent pulmonary valve *(arrows)*. There was less than one-half systemic right ventricular systolic pressure, and there was an 11 mm Hg peak-to-peak gradient across the right ventricular outflow tract and pulmonary valve.

Critical Aortic Valve Stenosis

Critical aortic valve stenosis is usually diagnosed in neonates when they present with systolic murmur and reduced systemic output. This frequently occurs around the time of closure of the ductus arteriosus. In some cases of aortic valve stenosis there is associated left heart hypoplasia. Determination of the adequacy of the left ventricle is crucial in deciding whether to pursue biventricular management including balloon aortic valvuloplasty or single ventricle management, as with hypoplastic left heart syndrome. A scoring system based on aortic root and mitral valve annular diameter, left ventricular length, and left ventricular mass has been developed for this purpose.[37] Another means of assessing left heart adequacy is the demonstration of antegrade systolic flow into the ascending aorta and transverse arch using color and pulsed Doppler. If there is retrograde blood flow from the ductus arteriosus back to the aortic root, there is little chance that the left side of the heart can sustain adequate systemic output.[22]

Depressed left ventricular function due to a poorly opening aortic valve represents an indication for balloon angioplasty if the left heart is otherwise adequate. Unlike in older infants and children with aortic valve stenosis, the peak instantaneous pressure gradient may not reflect the severity of obstruction when left ventricular stroke volume is reduced.

Prostaglandin E_1 infusion to maintain ductal patency and elective intubation are generally recommended before the catheterization. Insertion of umbilical venous and arterial catheters is often helpful for pressure monitoring, blood sampling, or providing catheter access.

Cardiac catheterization is performed via either the femoral or umbilical vessels. After hemodynamic measurements, left ventricular angiography is usually performed to assess left ventricular size and function as well as the left ventricular outflow tract and annular diameters.

The preferred route for dilation is debated. Alternatives include a retrograde approach from either the umbilical, femoral, or carotid arteries; or an antegrade approach via the umbilical or femoral veins. Access via the umbilical artery is attractive to avoid the risk of femoral or carotid artery injury or occlusion. However, the course of the umbilical artery may complicate this approach, and for this reason many interventional cardiologists still prefer the femoral artery approach. Given the technological advances in balloon catheter development, catheters generally fit through 3 or 4 French sheaths, and with careful attention severe injury of the femoral artery is now rare. However, femoral artery occlusion has been reported in up to 30% to 65% of infants.[6,21]

The carotid artery has been used as an alternative site of arterial access.[8,25] The right carotid artery is exposed via cutdown, and the anterior wall opened. The vessel is dilated and a 4 or 5 French sheath is inserted through the opening. A soft tipped guide wire is then used to cross the aortic valve. Given the straight course from the right carotid toward the ascending aorta, crossing the valve is often easier than from the femoral or umbilical artery approach.

Once the guide wire has crossed the aortic valve by any of these approaches, the balloon catheter is positioned across the annulus. Generally, a balloon sized 1 mm smaller than the angiographically measured diameter of the aortic annulus is selected for initial dilation. Pressure measurements and aortography are repeated, and if aortic insufficiency is either absent or mild, but significant pressure gradient remains, then a second balloon either equal to the aortic annulus or at most 1 mm larger than the diameter of the aortic annulus can be selected for repeat valvotomy. Aortography is repeated after dilation to evaluate the degree of valvular insufficiency as well as to look for injury to the aortic root or ascending aorta. The risk of increased aortic regurgitation or a tear of the left ventricular outflow tract increases with oversized balloons.

The antegrade approach to balloon aortic valvotomy offers yet another option. Either a preshaped "coronary" catheter or a balloon-tipped "wedge" catheter is advanced from the umbilical or femoral vein through the right atrium and across the foramen ovale into the left atrium. The catheter is then manipulated through the mitral valve and gently looped within the left ventricle. With the use of a soft-tipped flexible guide wire, the aortic valve is crossed and the guide wire advanced so that the tip of the wire advances around the aortic arch and down into the abdominal aorta. This technique avoids injury to systemic arteries and can help sometimes in crossing severely stenosed aortic valves that cannot be crossed in the retrograde fashion.[26]

Critical neonatal aortic valve stenosis presents a difficult management issue. Regardless of whether the initial palliation is performed surgically or by one of the previously described catheter techniques, mortality is 10% to 20% and is similar for surgical and nonsurgical approaches.[6,11,13,26] Apart from the mortality risk, each of the techniques carries its own morbidity. Umbilical arterial access often takes longer than the other approaches and can expose the baby to a longer period of instability as well as the risk of sepsis related to manipulation of the difficult-to-sterilize umbilical stump. Femoral artery access carries a risk of arterial thrombosis, which generally requires thrombolytic therapy. If that treatment is unsuccessful, there may be reduced access for future aortic intervention, and leg-length discrepancy may develop. When the carotid artery is used for arterial access, residual stenosis or even total occlusion remains a risk for neonates. Finally, the antegrade valvotomy technique has a small risk of inducing serious ventricular arrhythmia or producing mitral regurgitation from a tear of the mitral valve.[26] Any of the techniques has the potential for producing aortic annulus rupture, coronary artery injury, or severe aortic valve insufficiency.

A majority of interventions for critical neonatal aortic stenosis are successful, greatly reducing the transvalvuvar pressure gradient, improving left ventricular function, and creating either no or only mild aortic valve insufficiency.[6,8,11,13,25,26] For those in whom the procedure is successful, repeat valvotomy may still be required in as many as 30% within the next 4 months.[6] For the majority of patients balloon dilation of aortic valve stenosis in the neonatal period can be a lifesaving procedure and the first step in the long-term management of a very difficult congenital cardiac anomaly.

Neonatal Coarctation of the Aorta

Neonates with coarctation of the aorta can present with cardiovascular collapse and a sepsis-like picture in the first 10 days of life as the ductus closes. Acidosis from decreasing systemic blood flow, in addition to the sudden imposition of increased afterload, can cause left ventricular dysfunction and heart failure. The diagnosis of coarctation is made from the clinical recognition of decreased lower extremity pulses and blood pressure and is confirmed by echocardiographic imaging. There is no doubt that relief of the aortic obstruction is required, but whether there is a role for catheter-based intervention remains controversial.[12,35,36]

Both surgical repair and balloon dilation of aortic coarctation are highly successful at acutely relieving the blood pressure gradient and heart failure produced by severe obstruction. Both are associated with acceptably low levels of morbidity and mortality, but balloon dilation of native coarctation is less successful in accomplishing long-term stenosis relief. Recurrence of obstruction within the first 6 to 12 months of life is common.[9,33] Balloon dilation of infantile coarctation is associated with a risk of femoral artery injury, which may limit femoral arterial access for future interventional procedures. Most centers have abandoned balloon dilation as the first-line management of critical neonatal coarctation of the aorta. However, the technique is favored by some for the treatment of toddlers and children with aortic coarctation and should be considered for individual neonates thought to be at increased surgical risk.

CARDIAC CATHETERIZATION IN PREPARATION FOR CARDIAC SURGERY

As noted in the chapter opening, the role of diagnostic catheterization to define intracardiac anatomy has been decreasing steadily and for the most part has been replaced by echocardiography and magnetic resonance imaging. Many centers no longer have routine indications for preoperative catheterizations, but in individual circumstances and for particularly complex lesions, ventriculography can provide the surgeon with an additional perspective of the intracardiac relationships to aid in operative management. However, the predominant roles for cardiac catheterization in the preoperative management of children with congenital heart disease are to assess cardiopulmonary hemodynamic status, obtain angiographic images of the pulmonary vascular bed, identify the presence of abnormal arterial or venous connections, and prepare the patient for surgery with therapeutic catheterization techniques.

Assessment of Hemodynamic Status

Measurement of pulmonary-to-systemic blood flow ratio and measurement of pulmonary arterial pressure have long been used as criteria to decide which infants should undergo surgical correction of their ventricular septal defects. Criteria such as a pulmonary-to-systemic flow ratio of 2:1 or greater and pulmonary-to-systemic arterial systolic pressure ratio of greater than or equal to 0.75 have been employed. In the current era, catheterization is rarely needed to make this determination, as echocardiography in conjunction with clinical judgment now suffice to make this decision. However, the toddler or school-age child with cardiomegaly or poor growth parameters and a moderate-size ventricular septal defect still occasionally confronts the pediatric cardiologist. For these patients cardiac catheterization may be helpful in confirming the presence of a left-to-right shunt significant enough to warrant surgical closure.

Cardiac catheterization–derived calculation of pulmonary vascular resistance has been used to help estimate the risk for surgical correction of ventricular septal defects. The response of pulmonary vascular resistance to pulmonary vasodilator agents has also been used as a test for operability, but these calculations are less than perfect predictors of survival.[24,30,31] There are both theoretical and practical limitations to calculations of pulmonary vascular resistance that limit their accuracy at predicting successful outcome.[4]

Pulmonary vascular resistance is usually described in mm Hg per liter/minute/m^2 (indexed Wood units). This measurement is obtained from the mean pulmonary arterial pressure minus the mean left atrial pressure divided by the pulmonary blood flow indexed to body surface area. Perhaps the largest source of error in this calculation comes from calculation of pulmonary blood flow. Thermodilution techniques cannot be used in patients with cardiac shunts and thus the Fick calculation (oxygen consumption divided by pulmonary venous oxygen content minus pulmonary arterial oxygen content) must be employed to estimate pulmonary blood flow. Errors enter this equation primarily from the measurement of oxygen consumption. Even though many catheterization laboratories employ equipment to measure directly arterial oxygen consumption, the most commonly used apparatus cannot be employed with children on oxygen supplementation or mechanical ventilation. In those circumstances an estimated value must be used based on age and weight. Such estimates can introduce a substantial error into the calculated value. Two indexed Wood units represent the upper limits of normal for pulmonary vascular resistance in infants and children. However, uncomplicated Fontan palliation can be accomplished in children whose calculated resistance is as high as 3 to 4 indexed Wood units. Another way of representing pulmonary vascular resistance is as a ratio to systemic vascular resistance. When the resistance estimate is presented as a ratio, oxygen consumption is no longer a necessary part of the equation, and thus the error introduced by estimated consumption values is eliminated. Pulmonary-to-systemic vascular resistance ratios in infants and children are typically less than 0.1 and are considered elevated when greater than 0.25.

If pulmonary vascular resistance remains greater than 7 to 8 Wood units $\times$ m^2 even after administration of pulmonary vasodilators such as oxygen, isoproterenol, or nitric oxide, then after septal defect closure there is an increased postoperative probability of pulmonary hypertension due to pulmonary vascular disease.[4,30,31] Patients with pulmonary-to-systemic vascular resistance ratios > 0.75 are unlikely to respond to pulmonary vasodilator therapy with isoproterenol.[31]

Successful Fontan palliation depends importantly on low pulmonary vascular resistance, and therefore before the Fontan, cardiac catheterization with measurement of mean pulmonary arterial pressure and estimation of pulmonary vascular resistance is indicated. Pulmonary arterial pressure often can be measured directly by passing a catheter through a modified Blalock-Taussig shunt or into a banded pulmonary artery. However, in certain circumstances this may not be technically feasible. In those situations measurement of pulmonary venous wedge pressure gives a reasonable estimate of mean pulmonary arterial pressure, if the mean pulmonary arterial pressure is less than 20 mm Hg.

The originally strict Fontan criteria of Choussat and colleagues[5] have been relaxed over the years and now differ among cardiac centers worldwide.[27,43] However, preoperative mean pulmonary arterial pressures in excess of 15 mm Hg, ventricular end-diastolic pressure greater than 12 mm Hg, and/or pulmonary vascular resistance above 3 to 4 Wood units $\times$ m^2 appear to predict poorer postoperative outcome.

Imaging of the Pulmonary Vascular Bed

Preoperative contrast ventriculography is no longer routinely required before open-heart surgical repair of most congenital cardiac defects. Occasionally, when there are questions as to the adequacy of ventricular size or the relationship of the great arteries to the ventricles (as in some cases of double outlet right ventricle), ventriculography can provide another anatomic perspective that can be crucial in surgical planning. Imaging of the pulmonary bed is usually required, however, before right ventricular outflow tract reconstruction of tetralogy of Fallot/pulmonary atresia. Likewise, definition of pulmonary arterial anatomy is needed before progressing from a systemic arterial shunt dependent pulmonary circulation such as hypoplastic left heart status post Norwood stage I palliation to either a bidirectional cavopulmonary (Glenn) shunt or a total cavopulmonary (Fontan) connection.

Definition of pulmonary arterial anatomy and aortic-to-pulmonary arterial connections has become an essential part of preoperative cardiac catheterization for a range of cardiac conditions. One half of neonates with tetralogy of Fallot and pulmonary trunk atresia exhibit discrete pulmonary artery stenoses and another third display diffuse hypoplasia. Pulmonary blood flow is entirely dependent on multiple aortopulmonary collateral arteries in 38% of patients.[18] Before a surgical plan can be generated, the size, location, confluence, and distribution of pulmonary arteries must be mapped in relationship to any significant aortopulmonary collateral arteries. Cineangiography well defines the anatomy and relationships. Balloon occlusion aortography and selective arteriography are often needed to identify the true pulmonary arteries and their confluence. Some have recently suggested an additional role for magnetic resonance angiography in visualization of the pulmonary artery bed.

If confluent pulmonary arteries cannot be identified via arteriography, then pulmonary venous wedge angiography may be helpful. In this technique an end hole catheter is advanced from a systemic vein, across the foramen ovale, through the left atrium, and into a pulmonary vein. The catheter is wedged into a distal branch, after which contrast is injected into the pulmonary bed and flushed through with heparinized solution. In this way contrast is "forced" retrograde through the capillary bed and arterioles into the segmental pulmonary arteries. If central pulmonary arteries are present but have little or no antegrade flow, they will be opacified by this technique.

Multiple angiograms are used preoperatively to construct a map of the pulmonary arterial circulation, which the surgeon can use to plan an approach that combines the various arterial vessels feeding the pulmonary bed (unifocalization) for connection to the right ventricular outflow tract. After surgical rehabilitation has been initiated, angiography is needed to define the patency of these arteries. Some lung segments may be supplied both by true pulmonary arteries as well as by collaterals. Since the ultimate goal is to rehabilitate the true pulmonary arteries, eliminating competition from overlapping collateral arteries can facilitate their normal growth, and coil embolization techniques play an important role in the effective palliation of tetralogy of Fallot and pulmonary atresia. Discrete stenoses are common in the proximal and even distal pulmonary arterial tree.[18] Often these stenoses need to be balloon dilated before final repair.

Preoperative catheterization for patients with tetralogy of Fallot without pulmonary atresia is usually unnecessary. Proximal coronary artery anatomy and additional ventricular septal defects can usually be identified echocardiographically in infants with tetralogy of Fallot. In many centers, catheterization is reserved for situations in which echocardiography is not definitive or there is concern about the adequacy of the pulmonary arterial tree. Although diffuse hypoplasia of the pulmonary tree is uncommon, as many as 30% of patients can have discrete pulmonary arterial stenoses, more commonly seen in the left pulmonary artery.[18] When initial palliation for an infant with tetralogy of Fallot has included a modified

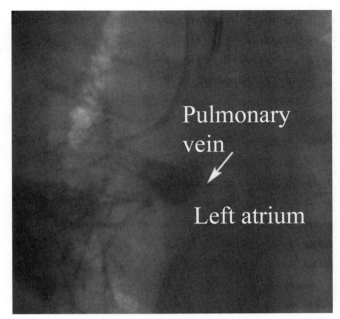

FIGURE 18-4   In this patient, a severely stenotic right pulmonary vein is seen. The orifice into the left atrium is pinhole sized *(arrow)*. The pulmonary vein was filled with contrast only by means of a pulmonary artery wedge angiogram, in which the contrast material was injected directly into a distal pulmonary artery and followed with flush solution. This technique allowed filling of the highly stenotic pulmonary vein, which otherwise was not well seen. The patient had repair of the pulmonary vein stenosis as an urgent procedure.

Blalock-Taussig shunt, visualization of the pulmonary arterial tree is necessary before complete repair to demonstrate whether stenosis has developed at the shunt insertion site or elsewhere in the pulmonary arteries. Sometimes catheterization is needed for this visualization.

Pulmonary vein stenosis can be diagnosed (and in very rare instances successfully treated) at cardiac catheterization. A measurement of a pressure gradient across the stenosis is important, although care must be taken to recognize partial or total occlusion of the pulmonary vein by the catheter. If the pulmonary veins cannot be entered, then a pulmonary artery wedge angiogram as described previously may be used to delineate the pulmonary veins in certain cases (Fig. 18-4).

Identification of Abnormal Vascular Connections

Pulmonary artery distortion is considered a major risk factor for Fontan palliation. Therefore identification of such stenoses plays a critical role in preparing a patient for bidirectional cavopulmonary connection or for a total cavopulmonary anastomosis. Likewise, venoatrial connections, typically from the innominate vein to a left pulmonary vein, can produce significant cyanosis after these palliations, and thus contrast injection into the innominate vein is routinely performed during preoperative catheterization. Finally, aortopulmonary collateral arteries are commonly found in patients with single ventricle physiology, particularly in association with pulmonary hypoperfusion and the prior placement of systemic-to-pulmonary arterial shunts.[34]

Interventional Catheterization to Prepare for Congenital Heart Surgery

Ancillary problems, identified by preoperative echocardiography or catheterization, are predominantly managed in the operating room. However, there are a number of interventional catheterization procedures that can be performed in advance of surgery to either reduce surgical risk or improve postoperative results.

Atrial Septostomy

Balloon atrial septostomy is used to improve systemic oxygenation in profoundly cyanotic infants with transposition of the great arteries when mixing is inadequate. Septostomy can be performed at the bedside with echocardiographic guidance or in the catheterization laboratory under fluoroscopy. A balloon atrial septostomy catheter can be guided from the umbilical vein, through the ductus venosus into the right atrium and across the foramen ovale into the left atrium. When the ductus venosus has closed, then access may be obtained via the femoral vein. The technique has low morbidity and mortality and results are generally good with an immediate increase in preductal and postductal arterial oxygen saturation.

In severe mitral stenosis or atresia, alone or as part of hypoplastic left heart syndrome, premature closure of the foramen ovale can result in severe left atrial hypertension and associated pulmonary artery hypertension and lymphangiectasia.[46] Emergent decompression of the left atrium is necessary to lower pulmonary vascular resistance and improve oxygenation and cardiac output in these infants before surgical palliation. Balloon atrial septostomy is generally not effective, but static dilation of the atrial septum is performed with progressively larger balloon dilation catheters and can achieve short-term relief of the left atrial hypertension. If the septum has become particularly thick, balloon dilation may need to be preceded by blade septostomy.

Balloon atrial septostomy is rarely required in infants with tricuspid atresia. In some patients, the foramen is restrictive and balloon septostomy may be helpful in enlarging the foramen. Often septostomy is ineffective and surgical septectomy may be required.

Preoperative Closure of Aortopulmonary Collateral Arteries

Aortopulmonary collateral arteries are common in some patients with tetralogy of Fallot with pulmonary atresia, and embolization of collaterals is performed to eliminate sources of pulmonary overcirculation and to encourage growth of true pulmonary arteries supplying flow to lung segments with dual supply.[34]

Elimination of collateral vessels is also important in preparing infants and children for the bidirectional Glenn or Fontan procedures. Aortopulmonary collaterals are more common in patients with bidirectional Glenn or Fontan procedure, particularly those who have also had previous Blalock-Taussig shunts.[46] The collateral arteries represent a volume load for the ventricle and may "steal" blood flow away from the cerebral circulation during periods of low-flow cardiopulmonary bypass (Fig. 18-5). Significant collateral

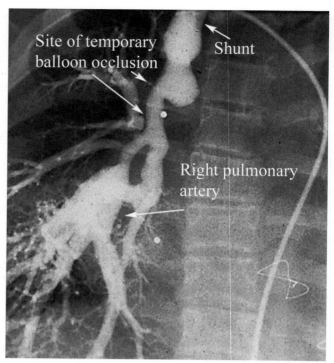

FIGURE 18-5 Cineangiographic frame from a teenage girl with tetralogy of Fallot with pulmonary atresia, who was undergoing aortic valve and ascending aorta replacement for severe aortic regurgitation. The right Blalock-Taussig shunt was felt to pose a danger of cerebral steal during the operation. The morning of the operation, the patient was brought into the catheterization laboratory. A wire was placed across the shunt into the distal right pulmonary artery, and a balloon dilation catheter was positioned across the site of temporary balloon occlusion. When the patient was in the operating room and undergoing cardiopulmonary bypass, the balloon was inflated, and it remained at inflation pressure throughout the period of aortic repair. This decreased the risk of cerebral steal and reduced the pulmonary venous return to the operative field as well.

flow has been associated with a longer duration of pleural effusion after either bidirectional cavopulmonary shunting or Fontan completion.[41] Thus before either procedure, identification and elimination of significant collaterals must be carried out (Fig. 18-6).[29,41]

Closure of Venous Decompressing Channels

After bidirectional cavopulmonary shunt or Fontan palliation, central venous pressure rises and previously unimportant channels can develop, allowing systemic venous return to bypass the lung (i.e., a right-to-left shunt). It is routine to identify and embolize significant venoatrial connections before these procedures, and after these procedures in patients who have worsening cyanosis.

The technique for coil embolization has been described in detail[34] and most commonly involves using a Gianturco coil, a stainless steel spring onto which is woven polyester fibers. These coils come in a variety of diameters and lengths and can be delivered through 4 French arterial or venous catheters, as needed. For very small infants or to embolize very small collateral arteries or veins, platinum microcoils are available for delivery through 3 French catheter systems.

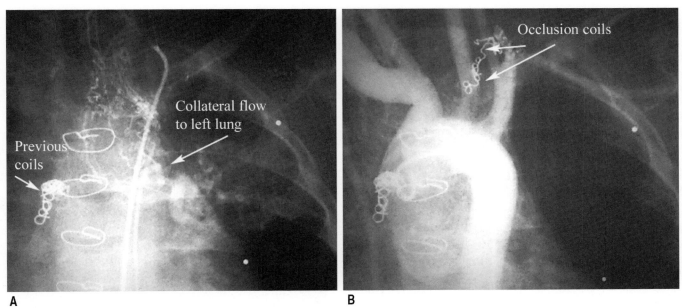

FIGURE 18-6 **A,** Cineangiographic frame from a patient with multiple aortopulmonary collaterals. Previous coils are seen in place in the right pulmonary artery distribution. There remains significant flow to the left pulmonary artery via the collateral *(long arrow)*. **B,** A number of occlusion coils *(arrows)* have been placed in the collateral, which rises from the left vertebral artery. No additional flow is seen into the left pulmonary artery via the collateral.

Preoperative or Intraoperative Dilation of Pulmonary Arteries

When there are stenoses in the pulmonary arteries, which might prove difficult for the surgeon to treat in the operating room, balloon dilation or stenting may be required before surgery. Cardiac catheterization allows one to define the exact level of stenosis and to position a balloon dilation catheter or stent across the affected area.

Pulmonary artery stenoses, even proximal ones, may be difficult or impossible to treat with surgical patch angioplasty. Implantation of intravascular stents in the cardiac catheterization laboratory has been used successfully to treat branch pulmonary artery stenoses before surgery. However, in some cases the course of the catheter and sheath to the stenoses, or the patient's size or vascular access, makes implantation difficult or impossible in the catheterization laboratory. In rare cases, balloon stenting in the operating room has been used for treatment of some pulmonary artery stenoses. In this technique, the stent is chosen, usually from preoperative cardiac catheterization measurements, and mounted on an appropriate balloon. After the patient is supported on cardiopulmonary bypass, the main pulmonary artery or conduit is opened, and the orifices of the branch pulmonary arteries are identified. The surgeon places the stent/balloon apparatus into position so the proximal end of the stent is visible in the main pulmonary artery, and the balloon is inflated. The stent expands and holds open the artery. The placement takes only a few minutes, and the strategy dramatically reduces the time required for branch pulmonary artery angioplasty.[32]

CARDIAC CATHETERIZATION AFTER CARDIAC SURGERY

Postoperative cardiac catheterization may be indicated in a postoperative patient who is doing poorly and for whom the clinical findings and noninvasive imaging results provide insufficient physiologic or anatomic information to guide management or for whom the problem can be improved by interventional catheterization. Such circumstances are discussed in the following sections.

Residual Right Ventricular Outflow Tract Obstruction

After repair of tetralogy of Fallot or of other defects that require right ventricular–to–pulmonary artery conduits, residual right ventricular outflow tract or conduit obstruction might be known or suspected by echocardiography. There may still be insufficient information available to decide whether to return to the operating room or what intervention is needed. If only accurate measurement of right ventricular pressure is needed, this can be performed in some cases with a pullback of a pulmonary artery catheter placed at the time of the original operation. If an intracardiac line was not placed and simply right ventricular pressure is needed, a flow-directed catheter can be passed in the intensive care unit. Otherwise the patient is transported to the catheterization laboratory for investigation. It is unusual for residual obstruction that is immediately present postoperatively to be amenable to balloon dilation or stent implantation. Usually, reoperation is needed if sufficient obstruction is present to require intervention.

Residual Left-to-Right Shunt after Intracardiac Repairs

It is unusual for the patient to leave the operating room with a significant residual shunt in the era of intraoperative transesophageal echocardiography. Significant residual defects usually result in going back on cardiopulmonary bypass to close them. Rarely, residual ventricular septal defects represent additional defects not diagnosed preoperatively.

If one requires a physiologic quantification of the size of a residual shunt, the surgeon can introduce a pulmonary artery catheter. Pulmonary artery saturations in excess of 80%, when the patient is receiving less than 40% inspired oxygen concentration, probably indicate a residual Q_p/Q_s ratio of 2:1 or greater. Again, if there is no indwelling pulmonary arterial catheter, then a flow-directed catheter may be inserted at the bedside or a formal cardiac catheterization performed. In some cases catheter-delivered device occlusion of residual muscular defects may be indicated.

Hypoxemia after Systemic Arterial Shunt Procedures

Unexpected hypoxemia after cardiac surgery can be due to multiple causes, cardiac and noncardiac, and cardiac catheterization is sometimes needed to identify the cause and potential treatment. When, for example, the preoperative anatomy involves severe pulmonary stenosis or atresia and a Blalock-Taussig shunt is placed, postoperative cyanosis could be due to shunt malfunction. The patency of such shunts can usually be determined echocardiographically; however, the sensitivity of echocardiography is often insufficient to determine if there is clinically significant narrowing of the shunt or distortion of the branch pulmonary arteries.

Angiography remains an excellent means to identify shunt or branch pulmonary artery narrowing and pulmonary venous desaturation. Injecting contrast through an arterial catheter near the shunt takeoff achieves optimal imaging. Angiography has the advantage of clearly imaging the insertion of the shunt and the branch pulmonary arteries. Very rarely, if a small patient cannot be moved from the pediatric intensive care unit, radial, brachial, or umbilical artery contrast injection (Fig. 18-7) may demonstrate some features of the anatomy.[2,47]

Systemic Venous-to-Pulmonary Artery Shunts

Systemic venous-to-pulmonary artery shunts or anastomoses are another form of palliation for cyanotic congenital heart disease; they allow systemic venous blood to be diverted directly into the pulmonary bed. They avoid the volume load inherent in the systemic arterial shunts such as the Blalock-Taussig shunt. The connection between the superior vena cava and the right pulmonary artery was first described by Dr. William Glenn in 1955[14] but has been modified to what is termed the bidirectional Glenn. Branch pulmonary artery continuity is maintained and the superior vena cava is connected to the right pulmonary artery, allowing flow to travel to both branch pulmonary arteries.

Potential postoperative problems after the bidirectional Glenn include unexpected hypoxemia or elevated pressure in the superior vena cava. The success of this procedure depends on undistorted branch pulmonary arteries and low pulmonary resistance. In the immediate postoperative period, echocardiography may not adequately image the caval anastomosis and branch pulmonary arteries, and angiography is quite useful. When the catheter is introduced into the superior vena cava, pressure is recorded and a venous saturation obtained (which reflects cardiac output). In most cases when this is needed, the patient is taken to the catheterization laboratory. However, in some situations, single-frame bedside venograms

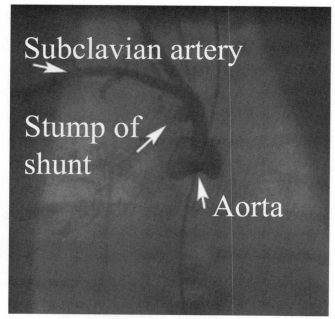

FIGURE 18-7 Countercurrent aortography: A small amount of contrast has been injected into the right radial artery via the radial arterial line in this patient in whom shunt occlusion was suspected. The subclavian artery, the right common carotid, and part of the transverse aorta fill with contrast. The origin or "stump" of the shunt is seen, without flow to the pulmonary arteries. This shunt occlusion is demonstrated without the need for placement of a catheter in the femoral artery.

are performed. A hand injection of contrast is performed via an angiographic or end-hole catheter. The usual dose is 1 mL/kg, and the contrast is given as quickly as possible. During the injection or at the instant it is finished, the radiology technician is asked to trigger the exposure. This will often give a quite serviceable image of a bidirectional cavopulmonary shunt, or even a portion of a Fontan circuit (Fig. 18-8). Results of local infusion treatment of thrombosis may be able to be recorded by the same radiographic technique, with injection through the infusion catheter itself (Fig. 18-9). This technique has the advantage of being performed at the bedside but does not allow exclusion of venous decompressing veins in the patient who is unexpectedly hypoxemic. A formal catheterization provides additional hemodynamic information and superior angiography, and can allow for balloon angioplasty if appropriate. Interventional catheterization options are limited in the early postoperative period at recent anastomotic sites.

Fenestrated Fontan Baffles

As discussed in Chapter 39, there are different methods of performing the Fontan operation. The major distinction is between the method using an external conduit and an alternative method using an intracaval baffle. The latter is in some cases fenestrated. The surgically created 4 to 5 mm fenestration allows a portion of the systemic venous return to escape or "pop off" to the left atrium. The right-to-left shunt allows for decompression of the right-sided pathway, and this may decrease the incidence of low cardiac output, ascites, pleural effusions, and peripheral edema.

If a patient has normal systemic arterial oxygen saturation, elevated caval pressures, and low cardiac output early after

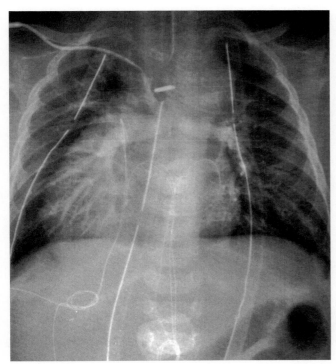

FIGURE 18-8 Bedside venogram in a postoperative patient. This child has dextrocardia, as visible on the chest radiograph. Chest tubes are in position. Function and adequacy of a new bidirectional cavopulmonary anastomosis were questioned. Via a right subclavian intravenous line, 0.5 to 1 mL/kg of contrast was injected briskly. When the end of the injection was near, a single chest radiograph was taken. After development of the chest radiograph, it was noted that the contrast from the subclavian line flowed into the anastomosis and filled the right pulmonary artery and left pulmonary artery. This enabled confirmation of the patency of the anastomosis without requiring the patient to be transported for cardiac catheterization.

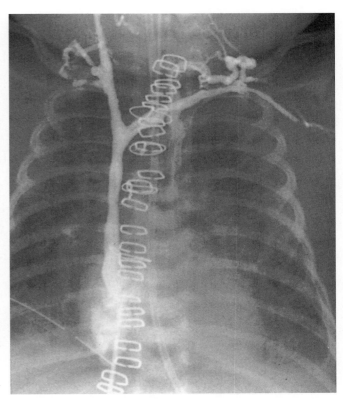

FIGURE 18-9 Anteroposterior still-frame cineangiogram of a superior vena cava after thrombolysis. A 4 French catheter had been left in the left innominate vein for urokinase infusion. Posttreatment angiography was performed at the bedside and demonstrated patency of the left innominate vein, the right internal jugular vein, and the superior vena cava. After this information was obtained, the urokinase was discontinued, and it was possible to remove the catheter.

fenestrated Fontan repair, one should suspect that the fenestration might have closed spontaneously. A patent fenestration will often be visible with color Doppler or venous contrast injection. In the patient compromised with a closed fenestration, consideration should be given to attempting to reopen the surgically placed fenestration in the cardiac catheterization laboratory. Sometimes the previous fenestration may be able to be located with a catheter and mechanically probed to reopen it. In other cases, a transseptal puncture between the lateral tunnel and the atrium may be necessary to allow placement of the transseptal sheath. Once access to the left atrium is achieved, then the pathway or fenestration can be dilated with a balloon dilation catheter placed over a wire. The balloon is centered on the septum (which may be tagged with contrast through the long needle, if necessary) and then inflated. To establish a lasting fenestration of 3 to 5 mm, a balloon size of some 6 to 10 mm may be necessary. It is suggested that one start with the smaller range of balloon, then check the appearance of the fenestration and the patient's systemic arterial oxygen saturation at each step before increasing the diameter of the dilation balloon. Sometimes it has been necessary to stent the atrial septum in order for the fenestration to stay open for any period of time postoperatively. It is reasonable to try balloon dilation alone first, then to consider placement of a stent if the fenestration

closes spontaneously again and if it is required for the clinical care of the patient.

An alternative clinical problem in the patient with a fenestrated Fontan is intractable hypoxemia. In some situations the physiology may be improved by closing the fenestration. A number of different catheter-delivered devices have been used with excellent success. Currently, the CardioSEAL device (Nitinol Medical Technologies, Boston, Massachusetts) has a United States Food and Drug Administration Humanitarian Device Exemption approval for this use. In this technique the fenestration to be closed is crossed with a catheter and wire. A long sheath is placed and through it a double umbrella device is introduced and opened so that one umbrella is on each side of the atrial septum or tunnel wall. The device covers the fenestration from either side and is held in place by the spring action of the two opposing umbrellas. It then is released from the delivery catheter and implanted permanently.

Closure of Collateral Veins to the Left Atrium after Glenn or Fontan Surgery

As discussed previously, unexpected hypoxemia after bidirectional cavopulmonary surgery or after a nonfenestrated Fontan palliation can be due to decompressing systemic veins

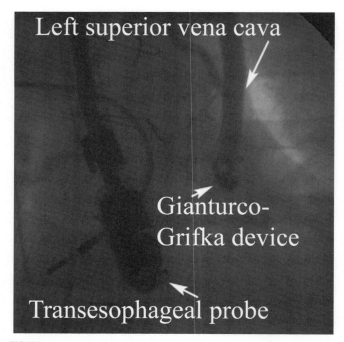

FIGURE 18-10 In this postoperative patient, a left superior vena cava draining to the coronary sinus on the left atrial side of the lateral tunnel was contributing to cyanosis. A Gianturco-Grifka vascular occlusion device was placed in the mid to lower portion of the left superior vena cava *(short arrow)*. This resulted in complete occlusion and resolution of cyanosis.

to the pulmonary veins or left atrium. These communications, when they cause significant systemic arterial desaturation, can be closed using vascular occlusion devices such as Gianturco coils or the Gianturco-Grifka sack (Cook, Bloomington, Indiana) (Fig. 18-10).

In some patients with heterotaxy and Fontan-type repairs, one or more hepatic veins may inadvertently drain to the left-sided circulation (usually the floor of the common atrium) and not be incorporated in the Fontan baffle. They may require occlusion to eliminate a significant right-to-left shunt. In one case, a Spider inferior vena cava filter (Cook, Bloomington, Indiana) was placed first in the hepatic vein. Then multiple Gianturco coils were packed proximally in the vein to effect occlusion (Fig. 18-11).

USE OF INTRACARDIAC MONITORING LINES

As suggested previously, intracardiac monitoring lines placed in the operating room may be very helpful in the postoperative management of patients with congenital heart disease. Right and left atrial lines allow an accurate determination of filling pressure and a secure route for administration of medicines and fluids as well. Mixed venous saturation inversely correlates with cardiac output. The pulmonary artery saturation provides the best-mixed venous sample when there is no left-to-right shunt. Otherwise, superior vena cava saturation

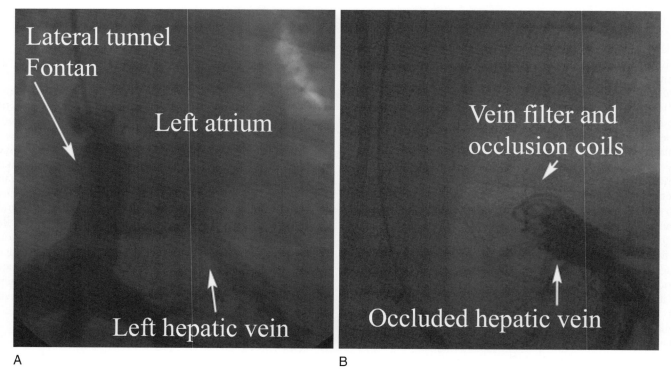

A   B

FIGURE 18-11 **A,** In this postoperative patient, a lateral tunnel Fontan has been completed. However, a left hepatic vein *(short arrow)* continued to fill through the hepatic venous system and empty into the left atrium, causing severe cyanosis. **B,** An inferior vena caval filter (Spider, Cook, Bloomington, Indiana) was placed via a transhepatic vein approach in the distal hepatic vein just caudad to the left atrium. Through that transhepatic sheath, vascular occlusion coils were positioned, held in place by the vein filter. This resulted in occlusion of the hepatic vein *(long arrow)* and resolution of cyanosis.

is usually the next best choice, since right atrial blood is frequently heterogeneous in oxygen saturation, given the differences in saturation among the superior vena cava, the inferior vena cava, and the coronary sinus.

Pulmonary artery catheters allow the measurement of pulmonary artery pressure and along with the left atrial (LA) pressure allow one to estimate the pulmonary vascular resistance (PVR):

$$PVR = (\text{mean PA pressure} - \text{mean LA pressure})/Q_p$$

where Q_p represents pulmonary blood flow. Q_p is estimated by using the Fick equation or, less frequently, thermodilution measurements. Using the Fick equation,

$$Q_p = VO_2/(C_{pv} - C_{pa})$$

where VO_2 is oxygen consumption, C_{pv} equals the oxygen content in pulmonary venous blood, and C_{pa} is the oxygen content in pulmonary artery blood. Oxygen content of any sample is:

$$1.34 \text{ mL } (O_2/g \text{ per dL Hb}) * Hb \text{ (g per dL)}$$
$$* \text{ oxygen saturation of the sample} * 10$$

Left atrial saturation can be assumed to be the same as the pulmonary venous saturation if there is no right-to-left atrial shunt. One generally uses an assumed oxygen consumption for the patient's age and heart rate.

The cardiac output (Q_s) can also be estimated from the Fick equation as:

$$Q_s = VO_2/(C_{sa} - C_{mv})$$

where C_{sa} is the oxygen content of systemic arterial blood and C_{mv} is the oxygen content of mixed venous blood. If a right atrial line is in place, then along with the arterial line one can calculate the systemic vascular resistance.

When intracardiac lines are used, extreme care must be taken to check that the zero levels are set and the pressure transducers are properly calibrated and positioned at the patient's mid-chest level. Pressure waveforms must be observed and appropriate for the chambers or vessels being recorded. One must be careful not to introduce air into the intracardiac lines and to be aware of the small incidence of significant bleeding after removal of intracardiac lines, particularly the pulmonary artery line in a patient with pulmonary artery hypertension. Judicious use of the intracardiac and arterial monitoring lines is extremely useful in understanding the postoperative physiology and may obviate the need to go to a catheterization laboratory for diagnosis.

PERCUTANEOUS DRAINAGE OF PERICARDIAL OR PLEURAL EFFUSIONS

Pericardial effusions are readily diagnosed with two-dimensional echocardiography (Fig. 18-12A). Global tamponade results in certain findings including diastolic collapse of the right atrial and right ventricular walls and accentuated respiratory variation in mitral valve inflow. A respiratory variation of greater than 15% to 20% in the mitral valve Doppler E wave, in the absence of severe respiratory disease, indicates a hemodynamically significant effusion (Fig. 18-12B). These methods for evaluating the hemodynamic significance of effusion do not consistently apply in the postoperative period

when the effusions are loculated or in some cases of single ventricle physiology.

Once a pericardial effusion is found, pericardiocentesis is performed under echocardiographic guidance.[38,44] The needle and wires introduced are hyperechoic in the pericardial space. Little or no pericardial fluid is usually left at the end of the procedure. Pleural effusions are drained using either surgically placed thoracostomy tubes or percutaneously placed "pericardiocentesis" pigtail catheters.

DECOMPRESSION OF THE LEFT ATRIUM IN PATIENTS ON EXTRACORPOREAL MEMBRANE OXYGENATION

When a patient is supported by extracorporeal membrane oxygenation while being treated for severe left ventricular dysfunction, the left ventricle may not be able to eject enough blood volume to decompress the left atrium. This can result in pulmonary edema and subendocardial ischemia. In such cases, consideration should be given to bedside transseptal balloon dilation atrial septostomy for decompression of the left atrium. In one such case in the intensive care unit, a transseptal sheath and dilator were advanced over their long needle using transesophageal echocardiographic guidance into the markedly enlarged left atrium. After the sheath was across the septum, a 12-mm and then a 20-mm balloon were inflated creating a 12 by 9 mm defect and reducing the mean left atrial pressure from 65 to 30 mm Hg. The frothy pulmonary edema resolved promptly, and the patient stabilized.[20] The procedure has also been described for blade and balloon atrial septostomy.

THERAPY FOR ACQUIRED HEART DISEASE

Catheter Embolus Retrieval

Rarely, indwelling venous catheters break off from their hubs or are sheared off as they are removed. The distal fragment may then embolize and become entangled within the right ventricle or enter the pulmonary artery. Leaving an intracardiac foreign body in place risks perforation or infection, and it is recommended that it be removed. Transcatheter retrieval is performed using a long sheath guided by means of a catheter until the sheath is next to the foreign body to be removed. Then the guide catheter is removed and a retrieval or snare catheter is introduced through the sheath and against or around the foreign body. While the foreign body is held firmly by the retrieval catheter, the catheter and foreign body are drawn back into the sheath and the entire apparatus removed from the patient. This eliminates the need for even a femoral venous cutdown, since the foreign body is withdrawn from the body while completely within the sheath.

Local Thrombolytic Therapy

Vascular thromboses may complicate postoperative recovery in patients with congenital heart disease. Superior vena cava syndrome has been reported after open-heart surgery, and it can be particularly devastating in neonatal patients.

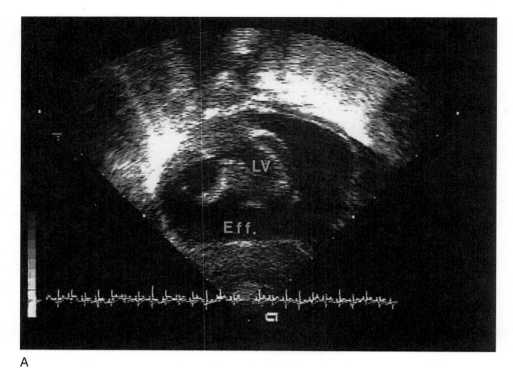

A

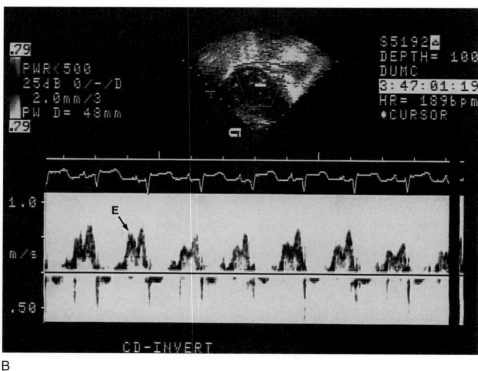

B

FIGURE 18-12 A, Subcostal view of an infant with a large pericardial effusion (Eff). The pericardial effusion encompasses the heart in this patient. LV, left ventricle. **B,** Mitral valve Doppler inflow in the same patient with a large pericardial effusion. Note the large variation in the early filling velocity (E wave) that occurs with respiration. This is indicative of impending tamponade.

Catheter disruption of thrombus, balloon dilation of venous structures, and even stent implantation in occluded venae cavae have been used to treat such blockages.[10] In the authors' recent experience, a patient developed protein-losing enteropathy almost 3 years after successful Fontan surgery, secondary to thrombotic occlusion of the entire left pulmonary artery. Systemic or local treatment with thrombolytic medicines has been applied in such cases, and this post-Fontan patient had complete resolution of the thrombus after 12 hours of treatment with tissue plasminogen activator through a catheter placed straddling the thrombosed segment.

Temporary or Permanent Pacing

After some types of open-heart surgery, especially repair of atrioventricular canal or subaortic stenosis, there is a risk of

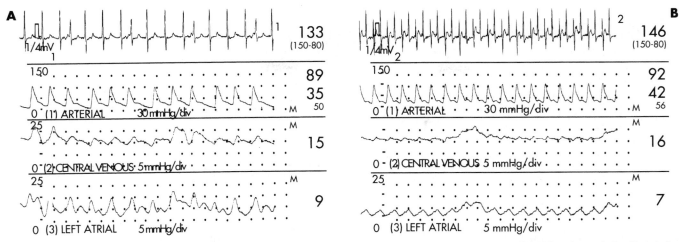

FIGURE 18-13 *A,* Monitor screen for a patient after repair of tetralogy of Fallot. Rhythm shows junctional tachycardia with atrioventricular dissociation, and the left atrial tracing shows exaggerated v waves. There is absence of effective atrial augmentation of cardiac output. *B,* With atrial pacing at a rate of 146 bpm, there is an increase in the systolic blood pressure. The arterial waveforms are regular, and the left atrial waveform shows a more normal v wave.

temporary or permanent complete atrioventricular block. Using temporary pericardial pacing wires in the operating room initially treats this problem. Should the pacing thresholds of the temporary wires be unacceptably high or not be effective for other reasons, then one can acutely administer isoproterenol or epinephrine and use a transcutaneous pacemaker. At this point a temporary ventricular pacemaker might be required, and a catheter pacing wire is placed via the jugular or subclavian (occasionally femoral) vein into the right ventricular apex. This technique is similar to placement of a Swan-Ganz catheter, except that the destination is the right ventricle rather than the pulmonary artery and that there is no pressure lumen for checking placement. Proper placement may be confirmed by echocardiographic localization of the tip of the catheter, by chest radiograph, and by restoration of the paced rhythm and resolution of the bradycardia.

Certain postoperative cardiac rhythms may be able to be diagnosed or treated with the use of the temporary pacing wires. Atrial lead electrocardiograms may show the relationship of atrial to ventricular depolarizations not visible from surface leads. One performs a standard rhythm strip showing leads I, II, and III, with the epicardial atrial pacing wire ends attached temporarily to the cables for leads aVR and aVL. Oftentimes, leads I and II show prominent atrial electrograms while lead III shows a surface tracing for mapping the QRS. The atrial leads may be used to pace the atrium in order to overdrive atrial flutter or to capture the atrium and restore atrioventricular synchrony in cases of junctional tachycardia (Fig. 18-13).

CONCLUSION

Principles and techniques from the cardiac catheterization laboratory may be used before, during, or after surgery to assist with the recovery and well-being of children in the pediatric cardiac intensive care unit. New techniques and applications continue to be invented, modified, and adapted for use in the laboratory, in the operating room, and at the bedside, especially in the area of interventional catheterization.

References

1. Alwi M, Geetha K, Bilkis AA, et al: Pulmonary atresia with intact ventricular septum percutaneous radiofrequency-assisted valvotomy and balloon dilation versus surgical valvotomy and Blalock-Taussig shunt. *J Am Coll Cardiol* 35:468–476, 2000.
2. Anjos R, Kakadekar A, Murdoch I, et al: Countercurrent aortography: An alternative to cardiac catheterization in infancy. *Pediatr Cardiol* 13:10–13, 1992.
3. Battistessa SA, Robles A, Jackson M, et al: Operative findings after percutaneous pulmonary balloon dilation of the right ventricular outflow tract in tetralogy of Fallot. *Br Heart J* 64:321–324, 1990.
4. Berger RM: Possibilities and impossibilities in the evaluation of pulmonary vascular disease in congenital heart defects. *Eur Heart J* 21:17–27, 2000.
5. Choussat A, Fontan F, et al: Selection criteria for Fontan procedure. In Anderson RH, Shinebourne EA (eds): *Paediatric Cardiology.* Edinburgh, Churchill Livingstone, 1977, p 559.
6. Egito ES, Moore P, O'Sullivan J, et al: Transvascular balloon dilation for neonatal critical aortic stenosis: Early and midterm results. *J Am Coll Cardiol* 29:442–447, 1997.
7. Fedderly RT, Lloyd TR, Mendelsohn AM, Beekman RH: Determinants of successful balloon valvotomy in infants with critical pulmonary stenosis or membranous pulmonary atresia with intact ventricular septum. *J Am Coll Cardiol* 25:460–465, 1995.
8. Fischer DR, Ettedgui JA, Park SC, et al: Carotid artery approach for balloon dilation of aortic valve stenosis in the neonate: A preliminary report. *J Am Coll Cardiol* 15:1633–1636, 1990.
9. Fletcher SE, Nihill MR, Grifka RG, et al: Balloon angioplasty of native coarctation of the aorta: Midterm follow-up and prognostic factors. *J Am Coll Cardiol* 25:730–734, 1995.
10. Frias PA, Johns JA, Drinkwater DC, Doyle TP: Percutaneous stent placement as treatment for an infant with superior vena cava syndrome. *Catheter Cardiovasc Interv* 52:355–358, 2001.
11. Gatzoulis MA, Rigby ML, Shinebourne EA, Redington AN: Contemporary results of balloon valvuloplasty and surgical valvotomy for congenital aortic stenosis. *Arch Dis Child* 73:66–69, 1995.
12. Gibbs JL: Treatment options for coarctation of the aorta. *Heart* 84:11–13, 2000.
13. Gildein HP, Kleinert S, Weintraub RG, et al: Surgical commissurotomy of the aortic valve: Outcome of open valvotomy in neonates with critical aortic stenosis. *Am Heart J* 131:754–759, 1996.

14. Glenn WWL: Circulatory bypass of the right side of the heart. IV. Shunt between superior vena cava and distal right pulmonary artery: Report of clinical application. N Engl J Med 259:119, 1955.

15. Godart F, Rey C, Prat A, et al: Early and late results and the effects on pulmonary arteries of balloon dilation of the right ventricular outflow tract in tetralogy of Fallot. Eur Heart J 19:595–600, 1998.

16. Gournay V, Piechaud JF, Delogu A, et al: Balloon valvotomy for critical stenosis or atresia of pulmonary valve in newborns. J Am Coll Cardiol 26:1725–1731, 1995.

17. Hanley FL, Sade RM, Freedom RM, et al: Outcomes in critically ill neonates with pulmonary stenosis and intact ventricular septum: A multiinstitutional study. Congenital Heart Surgeons Society. J Am Coll Cardiol 22:183–192, 1993.

18. Harikrishnan S, Tharakan J, Titus T, et al: Central pulmonary artery anatomy in right ventricular outflow tract obstructions. Int J Cardiol 73:225–230, 2000.

19. Heusch A, Tannous A, Krogmann ON, Bourgeois M: Balloon valvoplasty in infants with tetralogy of Fallot: Effects on oxygen saturation and growth of the pulmonary arteries. Cardiol Young 9:17–23, 1999.

20. Johnston TA, Jaggers J, McGovern JJ, O'Laughlin MP: Bedside transseptal balloon dilation atrial septostomy for decompression of the left heart during extracorporeal membrane oxygenation. Catheter Cardiovasc Interv 46:197–199, 1999.

21. Kocis KC, Snider AR, Vermilion RP, Beekman RH: Two-dimensional and Doppler ultrasound evaluation of femoral arteries in infants after cardiac catheterization. Am J Cardiol 75:642–645, 1995.

22. Kovalchin JP, Brook MM, Rosenthal GL, et al: Echocardiographic hemodynamic and morphometric predictors of survival after two-ventricle repair in infants with critical aortic stenosis. J Am Coll Cardiol 32:237–244, 1998.

23. Kreutzer J, Perry SB, Jonas RA, et al: Tetralogy of Fallot with diminutive pulmonary arteries: Preoperative pulmonary valve dilation and transcatheter rehabilitation of pulmonary arteries. J Am Coll Cardiol 27:1741–1747, 1996.

24. Lock JE, Einzig S, Bass JL, Moller JH: The pulmonary vascular response to oxygen and its influence on operative results in children with ventricular septal defect. Pediatr Cardiol 3:41–46, 1982.

25. Maeno Y, Akagi T, Hashino K, et al: Carotid artery approach to balloon aortic valvuloplasty in infants with critical aortic valve stenosis. Pediatr Cardiol 18:288–291, 1997.

26. Magee AG, Nykanen D, McCrindle BW, et al: Balloon dilation of severe aortic stenosis in the neonate: Comparison of anterograde and retrograde catheter approaches. J Am Coll Cardiol 30:1061–1066, 1997.

27. Mair DD, Puga FJ, Danielson GK: The Fontan procedure for tricuspid atresia: Early and late results of a 25-year experience with 216 patients. J Am Coll Cardiol 37:933–939, 2001.

28. McCrindle BW: Independent predictors of long-term results after balloon pulmonary valvuloplasty. Valvuloplasty and Angioplasty of Congenital Anomalies (VACA) Registry Investigators. Circulation 89:1751–1759, 1994.

29. McElhinney DB, Reddy VM, Tworetzky W, et al: Incidence and implications of systemic to pulmonary collaterals after bidirectional cavopulmonary anastomosis. Ann Thorac Surg 69:1222–1228, 2000.

30. Moller JH, Patton C, Varco RL, Lillehei CW: Late results (30 to 35 years) after operative closure of isolated ventricular septal defect from 1954 to 1960. Am J Cardiol 68:1491–1497, 1991.

31. Neutze JM, Ishikawa T, Clarkson PM, et al: Assessment and follow-up of patients with ventricular septal defect and elevated pulmonary vascular resistance. Am J Cardiol 63:327–331, 1989.

32. O'Laughlin MP: Catheterization treatment of stenosis and hypoplasia of pulmonary arteries. Pediatr Cardiol 19:48–56, 1998.

33. Ovaert C, McCrindle BW, Nykanen D, et al: Balloon angioplasty of native coarctation: Clinical outcomes and predictors of success. J Am Coll Cardiol 35:988–996, 2000.

34. Perry SB, Radtke W, Fellows KE, et al: Coil embolization to occlude aortopulmonary collateral vessels and shunts in patients with congenital heart disease. J Am Coll Cardiol 13:100–108, 1989.

35. Qureshi SA, Rosenthal E, Tynan M: Should balloon angioplasty be used instead of surgery for native aortic coarctation? Heart 77:86–87, 1997.

36. Rao PS: Should balloon angioplasty be used instead of surgery for native aortic coarctation? Br Heart J 74:578–579, 1995.

37. Rhodes LA, Colan SD, Perry SB, et al: Predictors of survival in neonates with critical aortic stenosis. Circulation 84:2325–2335, 1995.

38. Sanders WH, Lampmann LE: Percutaneous ultrasound-guided management of pericardial fluid. Eur J Radiol 12:147–149, 1991.

39. Santoro G, Formigari R, Di Carlo D, et al: Midterm outcome after pulmonary balloon valvuloplasty in patients younger than one year of age. Am J Cardiol 75:637–639, 1995.

40. Sluysmans T, Neven B, Rubay J, et al: Early balloon dilation of the pulmonary valve in infants with tetralogy of Fallot: Risks and benefits. Circulation 91:1506–1511, 1995.

41. Spicer RL, Uzark KC, Moore JW, et al: Aortopulmonary collateral vessels and prolonged pleural effusions after modified Fontan procedures. Am Heart J 131:1164–1168, 1996.

42. Sreeram N, Saleem M, Jackson M, et al: Results of balloon pulmonary valvuloplasty as a palliative procedure in tetralogy of Fallot. J Am Coll Cardiol 18:159–165, 1991.

43. Stamm C, Friehs I, Mayer JE Jr, et al: Long-term results of the lateral tunnel Fontan operation. J Thorac Cardiovasc Surg 121:28–41, 2001.

44. Taavitsainen M, Bondestam S, Mankinen P, et al: Ultrasound guidance for pericardiocentesis. Acta Radiol 32:9–11, 1991.

45. Tabatabaei H, Boutin C, Nykanen DG, et al: Morphologic and hemodynamic consequences after percutaneous balloon valvotomy for neonatal pulmonary stenosis: Medium-term follow-up. J Am Coll Cardiol 27:473–478, 1996.

46. Triedman JK, Bridges ND, Mayer JE Jr, Lock JE: Prevalence and risk factors for aortopulmonary collateral vessels after Fontan and bidirectional Glenn procedures. J Am Coll Cardiol 22:207–215, 1993.

47. Ueda K, Saito A, Nakano H: Aortography by countercurrent injection via the radial artery in infants with congenital heart disease. Pediatr Cardiol 2:231–236, 1982.

48. Wang JK, Wu MH, Chang CI, et al: Outcomes of transcatheter valvotomy in patients with pulmonary atresia and intact ventricular septum. Am J Cardiol 84:1055–1060, 1999.

49. Watson H, Rashkind WJ: Creation of atrial septal defects by balloon catheter in babies with transposition of the great arteries. Lancet 1:403–405, 1967.

Chapter 19

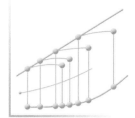

Perioperative Monitoring

LAURA A. HASTINGS, MD, EUGENIE S. HEITMILLER, MD,
and DANIEL NYHAN, MD

INTRODUCTION

Children undergoing cardiac surgery require both basic non-invasive and more extensive invasive monitoring for proper perioperative care.[93,149] These monitors are common to the operating room (OR) and intensive care unit (ICU). Basic monitoring for all patients includes heart and breath sounds, electrocardiogram (ECG), noninvasive blood pressure measurement, pulse oximetry, capnography, and temperature. The use of invasive monitoring depends on the patient's clinical status as well as the proposed operative procedure and includes monitoring of urinary output with a bladder catheter and monitoring of arterial blood pressure, central venous pressure (CVP), and pulmonary artery pressure with catheters. Left atrial catheters may be inserted by the surgeon intraoperatively. With progress in technology, more extensive cardiorespiratory monitoring has become available, including intraoperative echocardiography (transesophageal and epicardial), noninvasive cardiac output determinations, continuous mixed venous saturation, and online measurements of arterial blood gases, glucose, and hemoglobin. Monitoring of the central nervous system with evoked potentials, electroencephalography, transcranial Doppler, and cerebral oximetry is also being increasingly used.

ELECTROCARDIOGRAPHIC MONITORING

The electrocardiogram is indicated for all children with critical heart disease in the perioperative period to detect arrhythmias, ischemia, conduction defects, and electrolyte disturbances.[106] It displays the electric forces produced by the atria and ventricles during the cardiac cycle. Measurements include either a three-, four- or five-electrode system.

The best use of ECG information is critically dependent on correct lead placement and the ability to interpret the information in light of the developmental differences of the ECG in children at different ages. Lead placement is predicated on an understanding of normal cardiac electrophysiology; this is important because incorrect placement may result in abnormal waveforms.

The three-electrode system uses electrodes on the right arm, left arm, and left leg, examining leads I, II, and III. These are bipolar leads whereby the potential between two points, a positive and a negative electrode, is measured. Augmented leads are an expansion of the three-electrode system, with one lead set as an exploring electrode (positive terminal) and the remaining two leads connected and set at zero potential. These are therefore referred to as unipolar limb leads, whereby the exploring electrode is placed on one limb and labeled accordingly: aVR, right arm; aVL, left arm; and aVF, left leg. This unipolar lead system produces larger or "augmented" deflections labeled by the prefix "a." Thus six frontal plane axes can be obtained from three leads.

The five-electrode system is most often used during cardiac surgery, utilizing one electrode on each extremity and one precordial lead, so the leads of the entire limb act as a common ground for the precordial unipolar lead. The precordial lead is usually placed in the V_5 position. The advantage to having the precordial lead monitored simultaneously lies in the enhanced ability to detect ischemic events utilizing ST-segment trending. An adult study identified leads V5 and III as the most sensitive pair for identifying ischemia during cardiac surgery.[67]

The ECG recording by standard convention is calibrated with a 1-mV deflection equaling 10 mm on the strip chart recorder and with the paper speed set to 25 mm/sec. The skin where the electrode is placed should be clean and lightly abraded to remove the stratum corneum, which is a source of electric resistance. The electrodes must be moist and not outdated. Practically, ECG leads on infants can be placed on the right and left shoulders and right and left side of the abdomen.

ST-Segment and Arrhythmia Analysis

ECG monitors are available that have the capacity to detect ST-segment changes and provide trend analysis. These monitors have microprocessors that allow processing of ECG signals and measurement of ST-segment elevation or depression. The ST-segment changes can be continuously displayed on the monitor.

The normal ST segment in a child is usually isoelectric, but elevation or depression of the ST segment of up to 1 mm in the limb leads and up to 2 mm in the precordial leads may not be abnormal.[29] In the operating room, ST-segment changes can be seen with acute hypoxia or an embolic event such as air to the coronary arteries that leads to myocardial ischemia. Continuous automated ST-segment trend devices (ST trend monitors) are available to facilitate perioperative ischemia detection. Compared to Holter recordings for ischemia, the overall sensitivity and specificity of ST trend monitors were 74% and 73%, respectively.[85]

T-wave amplitude changes are associated with a variety of conditions in children undergoing cardiac surgery. Tall, peaked T waves accompany hyperkalemia and left ventricular hypertrophy. Flat or very low T waves may occur in normal newborns as well as in conditions including hypokalemia, hypothyroidism, digitalis use, pericarditis, myocarditis, and ischemia (Table 19-1). Hypokalemia is also associated with prominent U waves. Hypocalcemia is associated with a prolonged ST-segment duration, a prolonged QTc interval, and a normal T-wave duration. Hypercalcemia exhibits the opposite changes, with a shortened ST segment and QTc and a normal T-wave duration.

Arrhythmia analysis is available with most modern ECG monitoring equipment. Arrhythmias, particularly premature ventricular beats and ventricular tachycardia, can occur during surgery in children with or without heart disease. The incidence of these ventricular arrhythmias is reported to be significantly higher with the use of halothane when compared

Table 19-1 Common Causes of ECG Changes

T waves	Peaked	Hyperkalemia, left ventricular hypertrophy
	Flattened	Normal newborns, hypokalemia, hypothyroidism, digitalis use, pericarditis, myocarditis, ischemia
U waves	Prominent	Hypokalemia
ST segment	Prolonged	Hypocalcemia
	Shortened	Hypercalcemia
QTc interval	Prolonged	Hypocalcemia
	Shortened	Hypercalcemia

A **B**

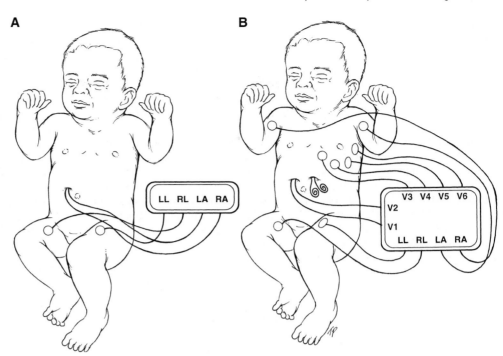

FIGURE 19-1 Lead placement for atrial electrocardiogram. **A,** A method for recording a bipolar atrial electrogram involves connecting the atrial leads to the right arm (RA) and left arm (LA) leads leaving the leg leads connected to the right and left legs (RL and LL). The atrial impulse is very prominent in lead aVF and observable, but less prominent, in the other limb leads. **B,** An alternate method for recording a unipolar atrial electrogram from temporary epicardial wires. This setup requires normal attachment of limb leads to establish a central Wilson terminus (plus V3). One atrial wire is connected to V1, the other to V2, and a V1-V2-V3 montage is recorded. Two unipolar atrial electrograms with large amplitude (far-field) ventricular electrograms will appear as V1 and V2.

with isoflurane[34] or sevoflurane.[19,143] Arrhythmias are also more commonly seen with hypercapnia and light planes of anesthesia.[117] An ominous sign in children is sinus bradycardia, which is a sensitive indicator of hypoxemia and carries an 8% risk of death.[73] Arrhythmias can also be seen transiently with surgical manipulation of the heart.

Arrhythmias can be evaluated in pediatric cardiac surgical patients in the perioperative period utilizing the temporary atrial epicardial electrodes that are placed during cardiac surgery (Fig. 19-1). Studies have demonstrated that using the atrial electrodes is safe and improves the ability to diagnose atrioventricular conduction disturbances and narrow QRS tachycardias.[63,147] The great advantage of the atrial electrocardiogram over the standard surface ECG is the ability to clearly identify atrial activity when P-waves on the surface ECG may have been buried in the QRS or T-wave.

ECG Artifacts

Artifacts can occur if lead wires are loose, broken, or twisted on themselves, if leads are crossed with other monitoring cables, or if leads are placed on bony prominences. ECG artifact and interference may also be due to patient movement or to the use of other equipment in the operating room. If the equipment is not properly grounded, 60-Hz alternating current can produce interference. Electrocautery is a major source of interference because it produces high-frequency electrical activity that often completely obliterates the ECG. The cardiopulmonary bypass (CPB) pump is another source of interference that can result in the ECG appearing as ventricular tachycardia or fibrillation.[76]

Risks of ECG Monitoring

The major risks of ECG monitoring in the operating room are burns and electric shock. Burns can potentially occur when

electrocautery and ECG monitoring are used simultaneously. The electrocautery delivers high-frequency electric energy that has a high current density at the point of contact with the patient; this allows the device to burn or cut tissue. A grounding pad placed against the skin of the patient allows the current to return to the electrocautery machine. If the grounding pad is not properly placed, it is possible for current to flow to ground via the ECG electrodes. A burn can result because the small surface area of the ECG electrodes allows a high current density at that point.

The risk of electric shock is small with properly maintained modern electric equipment. For electric shock to occur, the patient must be in contact with an electric current and with something that is grounded, thereby completing an electric circuit.[74] If the current is in the range of 100 mA, macroshock occurs, which can cause the heart to fibrillate. A much smaller amount of leakage current, known as microshock, can also cause fibrillation if a patient has current applied directly to the heart via implanted pacemaker wires, or an electrolyte-filled intracardiac catheter. In this situation, as little as 10 μA of leakage current can cause the heart to fibrillate.

NONINVASIVE METHODS OF BLOOD PRESSURE MEASUREMENT

Noninvasive methods measure blood pressure indirectly and employ an occlusive cuff around an arm or a leg. To measure the blood pressure accurately, it is imperative to use an appropriately sized blood pressure cuff. The American Heart Association recommends a cuff for which inflatable bladder width is 40% the circumference of the midpoint of the limb, or 20% greater than the diameter of the extremity. The length of the bladder should be twice the recommended width.[78] For children, choosing the largest cuff that fits the child's arm can minimize errors. A cuff that is too large underestimates blood pressure; one that is too small overestimates it. Marks and Groch[90] studied 50 patients and found that adjusting the cuff width to 40% of the arm's circumference overestimated the blood pressure for most arms, with notably high errors for small arms. The optimum cuff width was found to be proportional to the logarithm of the arm's circumference.[90]

Cuff placement is also very important. An incorrectly placed cuff may give inaccurate information or may with prolonged use directly compress a nerve, resulting in a neuropathy. In infants a thigh or calf cuff may be used if the upper arm cuff interferes with peripheral venous catheter flow or if descending aortic pressure is to be monitored, as in children having undergone an aortic coarctation repair. Systolic pressures in the calf are approximately the same as in the arm in preterm infants until 1 week of age, when the calf pressure is lower.[82] The systolic pressure in the calf remains lower than in the arm (1 to 3 mm Hg) from birth until 6 months of age. Then the calf pressure begins to exceed arm pressure in infants older than 6 months of age.[33] In older children and adults, the systolic thigh blood pressure is normally higher than in the arm, but diastolic pressures are usually about the same.[125]

The classic method of noninvasive blood pressure measurement is the detection of Korotkoff's sounds with a stethoscope (Fig. 19-2). The cuff must be inflated above the systolic pressure and is then deflated slowly (2 to 3 mm Hg per second or 2 mm Hg per heartbeat). As the cuff pressure falls below the systolic pressure, the arterial wall is partially opened, allowing turbulent flow to pass. This turbulent flow is audible through the stethoscope. The first sound defines the systolic pressure. As the cuff pressure falls below diastolic pressure, the Korotkoff's sounds disappear because the obstruction to

flow by the cuff is eliminated. In some patients the sounds never totally disappear, and in these the diastolic pressure is taken as the point of fading or dampening of the sounds, rather than their disappearance.

If a stethoscope is not available or if the sounds are difficult to hear, as is often the case in infants, the systolic pressure may be determined using palpation, ultrasonic flow probes, or the pulse oximeter. Riva-Rocci described the palpation method in 1896, which involved placing a cuff around the arm, filling it with air until the radial pulse disappeared, and then slowly deflating the cuff until the pulse reappeared. The two readings were averaged and the result was taken as the systolic pressure. Diastolic pressure cannot be determined by this method.

Ultrasonic blood flow detectors, also called Doppler flow probes, are very accurate in detecting the systolic pressure. The detector is placed over the artery distal to the blood pressure cuff, which is slowly deflated. The pressure at which the characteristic swishing sound of arterial blood flow is first heard is the systolic blood pressure. The pulse oximeter can be used to monitor systolic blood pressure in a similar fashion. As the cuff is slowly deflated, a sudden oscillation in the output of the blood flow detector of the pulse oximeter correlates with the systolic pressure. This method was found to correlate with Doppler ultrasonography ($r=0.996$) and arterial cannulation ($r=0.88$).[135] However, movement of the detector or constriction of the blood vessels beneath the detector can result in erroneous measurements.

How well do noninvasive methods correlate with invasive (direct) methods of blood pressure measurement? Many studies have been carried out to examine this question. It seems that the best correlation results when the systolic pressure, determined noninvasively by the Riva-Rocci palpation method, is

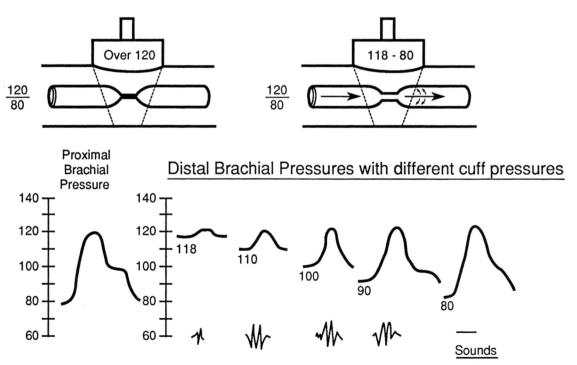

FIGURE 19-2 Noninvasive blood pressure measurement with a blood pressure cuff and Korotkoff's sounds. (From Abel FL, McCutcheon EF: *Cardiovascular Function: Principles and Application.* Boston, Little, Brown, 1979, p 231; with permission.)

Table 19-2 Differences ($\Delta P = P_{monitor} - P_{ref}$) for the Three Monitors Tested

Manufacturer	ΔP_{sys} (mm Hg)	ΔP_{dias} (mm Hg)	ΔP_{MAP} (mm Hg)	n
Dinamap 8100	0.0 ± 4.2	-3.7 ± 4.5	-3.6 ± 3.5	150
Hewlett-Packard M-1008B	-4.1 ± 6.0	-20.6 ± 7.3	-14.7 ± 6.2	150
SpaceLabs M-90 426	-1.7 ± 3.5	-4.2 ± 3.8	-2.9 ± 2.3	150

Values are expressed as means $\pm$ SD. n, number of differences; ΔP, NIBP monitor value; P_{sys}, systemic blood pressure; P_{bias}, diastolic blood pressure; P_{MAP}, mean arterial blood pressure.
From Papadopoulos G, Miede S, Elisaf F: Assessment of the performances of three oscillometric blood pressure monitors for neonates using a simulator. *Blood Press Monit* 4:27–33, 1999; with permission.

compared with the pressure measured by the return-to-flow method with an arterial catheter. This is performed by placing a blood pressure cuff on the same arm as the radial artery catheter and inflating it until the pulsatile trace disappears. The air is then slowly released and the pressure at which the first pulsatile trace reappears on the arterial tracing is the systolic blood pressure.[22]

Automated Methods

The development of automated sphygmomanometers has largely replaced the use of the stethoscope and cuff in the OR and ICU. The oscillometric method detects variations in the pressure within a blood pressure cuff during deflation. Pressure is increased in the cuff until no oscillations are seen; pressure is then decreased until oscillations in the pressure are noted. This point is at or near the systolic pressure. As the pressure decreases, the oscillations reach a maximum and begin to decrease. The mean arterial pressure is associated with the point of maximal oscillation. The diastolic pressure is then calculated from the systolic pressure and the mean arterial pressure. This oscillatory method is effective in hypotensive patients.

Studies assessing the accuracy of automated devices have shown variable results when compared to either direct or auscultatory methods of measuring arterial blood pressure. In general the automated oscillometric methods underestimate systolic pressure and overestimate diastolic pressure when compared with the direct method of measuring arterial blood pressure in critically ill patients.[23,98] In noncritically ill patients the oscillatory blood pressure devices meet the standards defined by the Association for the Advancement of Medical Instrumentation.

When compared with the auscultatory method, oscillometric devices overestimate the systolic pressure and slightly underestimate the diastolic pressure in children.[86] When measurement of systolic pressure obtained using the oscillometric method was compared with using the mercury sphygmomanometer, the oscillometric method resulted in a measurement 5 mm Hg higher. The difference between the two measuring techniques was less for older subjects (older than age 22 years) than with the younger subjects (age 11 to 22 years). The authors suggested the difference may be linked to the different effects of age-dependent arterial remodeling on the two measurement techniques.[21]

There appear to be differences in accuracy among the different brands of automated blood pressure devices, whereby the Hewlett-Packard M-1008B significantly underestimates the *diastolic and mean* arterial blood pressure when compared to the others (Table 19-2).[100] Utilizing a simulator, three

oscillometric blood pressure devices were compared: Dinamap 8100, SpaceLabs M-90 426, and Hewlett-Packard M-1008B. If there are large changes in blood pressure over a short time, the readings may not be accurate and the blood pressure in patients with severe arrhythmias may not be accurately measured. A noninvasive continuous blood pressure measurement device, NCAT N-500, that uses tonometry for its continuous measurement and intermittent oscillometric blood pressure measurement for calibration has been shown to have clinically unacceptable accuracy.[41] Noninvasive continuous blood pressure monitoring such as tonometry has not been utilized for pediatric cardiac surgery; however, future advances could change that.

Complications of Noninvasive Monitoring

Automated methods of noninvasive blood pressure monitoring have become standard practice in the OR and ICU because they are relatively safe, generally reliable, and easy to use. However, if the cuff is inflated too frequently or for a prolonged time, skin avulsion and venostasis can result.[12] In addition, ulnar neuropathies have been reported to result from a poorly positioned cuff.[134]

INTRAVASCULAR PRESSURE MONITORING

Monitoring of intravascular pressure, whether arterial or venous, requires an understanding of the equipment used. Current clinical practice typically employs an end-hole catheter inserted into a vessel, with the catheter connected to a pressure transducer by a coupling system and the transducer connected to a monitor through a preamplifier module. Certain aspects of this catheter-transducer-monitor system are common to all types of pressure monitoring. The catheters vary with the vessel being catheterized (systemic artery versus pulmonary artery versus central venous) and are discussed in their respective sections of this chapter. This section addresses the intrinsic workings of the pressure measuring equipment most commonly used in the OR and ICU.

Transducers

The transducer is the device that translates pressure into an electric signal that can then be processed into a waveform or numerical display. The classic resistive transducer consists of a pair of resistors incorporated into a circuit on the arms of a Wheatstone bridge. It has a stiff, low-compliance, pressure-sensing diaphragm that can bend and create a small volume change in response to a pressure change.[18] The volume change is applied to a wire inside the transducer that receives electric current from a preamplifier. The volume change alters the electrical resistance of the wire either by applying a stretch force that changes the length and cross-sectional area of that wire, thereby increasing the electrical resistance, or by allowing the wire to contract, decreasing the electrical resistance. The electric current from the transducer is then returned to the preamplifier, which converts the change in electrical resistance (pressure) into an electrical signal that can then be displayed by the monitor.

Currently manufactured transducers use semiconductor technology with silicon crystals that are similar to wires in that they change resistance in linear proportion to applied pressure. The modern disposable transducers have a silicon diaphragm into which resistive elements have been etched. They can be miniaturized for direct insertion into small arterial vessels. Disposable transducers are widely used and have essentially replaced nondisposable transducers in clinical practice. The disposable external transducers are accurate and durable and can be repeatedly recalibrated during long-term use.[8] Intravascular (catheter tip) transducers have the advantage of being directly inserted into the arterial tree; however, they are very expensive and have not been used for long-term monitoring because of baseline drift. Newer catheter-tip transducers are being developed to overcome the problem of baseline drift.[77]

Coupling System

The coupling system consists of fluid-filled extension tubing, a stopcock for blood sampling and balancing the transducer to atmospheric pressure, and a continuous infusion device to flush blood and air from the catheter and transducer. The solution in the coupling system should contain heparin to reduce the incidence of catheter thrombosis. Continuous flush devices containing a heparinized solution at 1 U/mL through radial artery catheters prolong the duration of patency and decrease risk of clot formation.[108] An adult study of 108 patients found greater accuracy of blood pressure with a continuous heparinized flush (2 U/mL saline).[81]

The stopcock is required to open the transducer for balancing to atmospheric pressure or to withdraw blood. Unfortunately, it is also an entry port into the circulation for bacteria, air bubbles, and clots. Therefore meticulous care is required to prevent inadvertent entry of air bubbles or embolic material, especially in patients with intracardiac or intravascular shunts.

Natural Frequency and Damping Characteristics of the Pressure Monitoring System

The extension tubing that connects the intravascular catheter to the transducer is a major source of resonance or "ringing" artifact in response to rapidly changing components of the pressure waveform. The catheter-tubing apparatus can lower the natural frequency of the system into a range where the harmonic content of the pulse-pressure wave causes the system to oscillate.

The natural frequency, fn, at which a catheter-tubing system tends to "ring" is described as follows:[51]

$$fn = \frac{1}{2} \frac{D^2}{4pL} \times \frac{P}{V}$$

where:
D = diameter
p = density of solution
L = length
P/V = compliance.

To keep the natural frequency of a pressure monitoring system higher than the frequencies in the arterial pulse-pressure wave, the diameter of the catheter and tubing should be maximized and the length and compliance minimized.[14] However, in certain situations the length of the extension tube may need to be greater than optimal in order to reach the patient. The length of the tubing is inversely proportional to the natural frequency, so the longer the tubing, the lower is the natural frequency and the more likely the system is to resonate, or "ring," with the pulse-pressure wave. This results in systolic overshoot. Shinozaki and colleagues[123] showed that the systolic pressure was augmented 7.2% with 3 feet of extension tubing, 9.2% with 6 feet, and 31.3% with 8 feet.

Another factor that can produce "ringing" or hyperresonance in the coupling system is the presence of small bubbles. Shinozaki[123] and colleagues found that adding 0.05 to 0.25 mL of air to the catheter tubing system augmented the systolic pressure by 40 mm Hg (from 150 to 190 mm Hg), whereas diastolic and mean pressure changed by no more than 3 mm Hg.[123]

Damping is the opposite of resonance. It is the tendency of an oscillation to die down.[14] At a maximal damping coefficient of 1.0 there would be no resonance and only arterial pressure would be displayed (i.e., 100% of the system's frequencies would be recorded accurately). Optimal damping occurs in the range of 0.6 to 0.7, where only 5% overshoot exists and there is rapid return to the actual pressure value. Most catheter-tubing systems are underdamped (0.2 or less).[14] This means that only frequencies equal to 20% of the system's resonating frequencies are recorded accurately. Thus, for example, if a system has a natural frequency of 30 Hz and a damping coefficient of 0.2, only events up to 6 Hz are recorded accurately without "ringing."

An underdamped system results in overshoot of the actual systolic pressure. This can be identified as a tall, narrowly peaked waveform with a notch in the arterial tracing immediately after the systolic pressure. Some systems can correct this by electronic damping with a filter switch on the amplifier. Motion of the catheter within a vessel or a chamber, known as catheter *whip* or *fling,* can also result in oscillation of the pressure tracing with a large pressure swing (Table 19-3). This is commonly seen with pulmonary artery catheters.

Table 19-3 Causes of Artificial Systolic Overshoot (Monitoring System Resonance "Ring")

Catheter in distal artery
Long extension tubing
Small bubbles
Underdamping of system
Catheter motion in vessel ("whip or fling")

Overdamping occurs as a result of compliant catheters and tubing as well as gross air bubbles or blood in the system. Air is very compressible and thus decreases the response of the system, which leads to increased damping. A damped pressure tracing may also be caused by a partial clot or piece of tissue in the catheter. With overdamping, the displayed arterial waveform will have a slow upstroke, a poorly defined dicrotic notch, and a narrow pulse pressure. The displayed systolic pressure may be significantly less than the actual pressure and could result in unwarranted changes in clinical management based on erroneous data. This situation can often be avoided by a continuous flush system whereby an appropriate filter is used and air is carefully removed from the drip chamber of the tubing.

A bedside method for determining the natural frequency and damping of a pressure monitoring system entails flushing the catheter so that a square wave pulse of 300 mm Hg is applied to the system. After the system is flushed, resonant waves can be observed in the pulse-pressure contour, and the natural frequency of the system can be calculated by dividing the paper speed (mm/sec) by the number of millimeters between resonant peaks (Fig. 19-3).[14] The damping coefficient

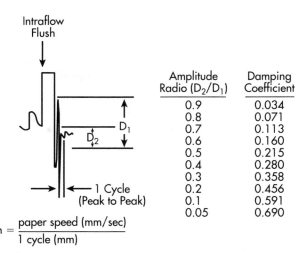

Amplitude Radio (D_2/D_1)	Damping Coefficient
0.9	0.034
0.8	0.071
0.7	0.113
0.6	0.160
0.5	0.215
0.4	0.280
0.3	0.358
0.2	0.456
0.1	0.591
0.05	0.690

$$fn = \frac{\text{paper speed (mm/sec)}}{1 \text{ cycle (mm)}}$$

FIGURE 19-4 Calculation of the natural frequency *(fn)* and damping coefficient of an arterial pressure monitoring system. The waveforms induced by an Intraflow flush are analyzed in terms of the time between cycles and the height of the induced resonant waves. (From Bedford RF: Invasive blood pressure monitoring. In Blitt CD [ed]: *Monitoring in Anesthesia and Critical Care Medicine.* New York, Churchill Livingstone, 1990, p 110; with permission.)

can be calculated from the relative heights of the resonant waves (D_2/D_1) and applying the table in Figure 19-4.[14]

Zero Adjustment and Calibration

Change in the zero position of the transducer is a source of measurement error that would not necessarily change the waveform but would read out erroneous values. Deviations from the conventional reference level of the transducer at the midaxillary line produce falsely high values if the transducer is set lower than the reference level, or falsely low values if the transducer is set higher than the reference level. The transducer level has the greatest effect on measurements of low-pressure systems (e.g., CVP, left atrial pressure), although the effect on arterial pressure is also important. For every 15 cm that the patient moves above the level of the transducer, the systemic arterial pressure readout will increase by 10 mm Hg.[14]

Blood pressure is measured relative to atmospheric pressure because the atmosphere has an equal effect on both the blood pressure and the transducer.[14] The electronic zero is set by opening the transducer to atmospheric pressure via the stopcock. The level at which the transducer is usually maintained for cardiac patients in the supine position is the midaxillary line, the level of the left ventricle. For noncardiac surgery the pressure of interest is sometimes different (e.g., cranial), changing the location of the transducer.

Problems and Complications Due to Equipment

It cannot be emphasized enough that accurate intravascular measurements are critical to proper patient management. There are several well-known causes of inaccurate measurement. One of the most common is catheter obstruction due to compression, kinking, or clot formation. Leaks can occur in the pressure tubing or at connection points. Air bubbles anywhere in the system will result in inaccurate measurements. Transducer malfunction

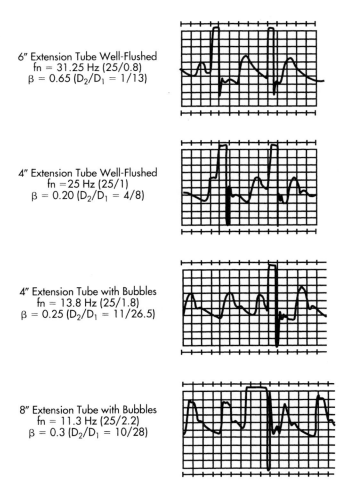

6" Extension Tube Well-Flushed
fn = 31.25 Hz (25/0.8)
β = 0.65 (D_2/D_1 = 1/13)

4" Extension Tube Well-Flushed
fn = 25 Hz (25/1)
β = 0.20 (D_2/D_1 = 4/8)

4" Extension Tube with Bubbles
fn = 13.8 Hz (25/1.8)
β = 0.25 (D_2/D_1 = 11/26.5)

8" Extension Tube with Bubbles
fn = 11.3 Hz (25/2.2)
β = 0.3 (D_2/D_1 = 10/28)

FIGURE 19-3 Calculated values of the natural frequency *(fn)* and damping coefficient *(β)* for an arterial pressure monitoring system. Longer extension tubing and air bubbles tend to lower fn. Short extension tubing and no air bubbles result in the highest fn. (From Bedford RF: Invasive blood pressure monitoring. In Blitt CD [ed]: *Monitoring in Anesthesia and Critical Care Medicine.* New York, Churchill Livingstone, 1990, p 112; with permission.)

can occur from faulty wiring or cable defects.[107] Drift in the measurement mandates evaluation for malfunction at all levels of the system.

INVASIVE METHODS OF ARTERIAL BLOOD PRESSURE MEASUREMENT

Both noninvasive and invasive blood pressure measurements are used in children undergoing cardiac surgery. Although an intra-arterial catheter is standard monitoring in cardiac patients, a noninvasive technique is used to measure the blood pressure upon arrival at the OR or ICU, and the occlusive cuff remains on the patient in case the intra-arterial catheter or monitor fails.

Arterial cannulation allows the continuous monitoring of arterial pressure and provides access for arterial blood sampling. The arterial pressure tracing is a particularly useful monitor in the OR because electrocautery often causes interference that interrupts the ECG but not the arterial pressure waveform. Thus the heart continues to be monitored and rhythm disturbances may be seen by changes in the arterial waveform.

Normal arterial blood pressure varies with a child's age. Blood pressure is lower in infants and increases to adult values by adolescence (Fig. 19-5).[62]

Catheters

The most commonly used technique for peripheral artery catheterization is the catheter-over-needle, first described by Barr in 1961.[9] Catheters are manufactured from a variety of materials, including Teflon, polypropylene, polyvinyl chloride, and polyethylene. Polypropylene catheters are stiffer and are more prone to thrombus formation in radial arteries than are Teflon catheters.[17,38,43]

The size of the catheter is important for optimal monitoring and patient safety. An important factor for the development of thrombosis is the size of the catheter relative to the

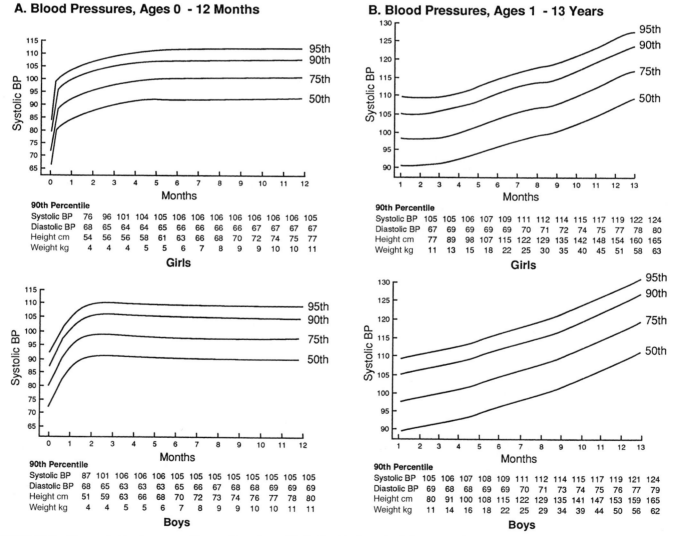

FIGURE 19-5   Changes in blood pressure with age. (From Horan MJ, Sinaiko AR: Synopsis of the Report of the Second Task Force on Blood Pressure Control in Children. *Hypertension* 10:115–121, 1987; with permission.)

size of the vessel; the smaller the catheter size, the lower is the incidence of thrombosis.[16] This has been shown in adults whereby with the same-sized catheter, women have a higher incidence of thrombosis than men, presumably because of the smaller diameter of the vessel. In adults a 30% incidence of thrombosis has been reported when 20-gauge catheters are left in for 7 to 10 days.[15,26] In newborns the incidence of radial artery occlusion has been reported to be as high as 63%, not related to birth weight, gestational age, or duration of cannulation. In all infants, blood flow in the radial artery resumed within 1 month after removal of the catheter.[57] A 24-gauge catheter can be used in small infants to monitor blood pressure but may not be reliable for withdrawing blood samples.

The small-sized catheters used in children also tend to kink more easily than the larger catheters used in adults. A study in adults showed that 20% of 20-gauge catheters kink within 24 hours of insertion.[16] Methods of unkinking a catheter include rotating it through a 180-degree arc or applying distal traction and withdrawing it slightly. The often-used method of hyperextending the wrist is thought to be associated with median nerve injury.[14] Alternatively, the catheter may be exchanged using a sterile Seldinger technique.

Radial Artery Cannulation

The radial artery is the most frequently used site for arterial cannulation because it is easy to access and there is a very low complication rate at this site when the catheter is properly inserted and maintained. The decision to place the radial artery catheter on the right or left depends on whether the blood flow to the arm is expected to be interrupted. For example, the arterial catheter is placed in the right arm if the left subclavian artery is to be used as a flap for aortic coarctation repair. The arterial catheter is placed in the left arm if the right subclavian artery is to be used for an arterial-to-pulmonary shunt. In patients with right-to-left shunting through a patent ductus arteriosus, the right radial artery represents the blood oxygen saturation and pressure to the brain, since the right subclavian and common carotid arteries arise from the aorta proximal to the ductus arteriosus. In this case a right radial artery catheter would be indicated. If there are no other reasons to use one hand rather than the other, in children old enough to determine handedness, the left radial artery is used in right-handed patients, and vice versa.

Collateral blood flow to the hand may be assessed by Allen's test before inserting a catheter.[2] This is performed in older children by applying pressure over the area of the radial and ulnar arteries at the wrist and having the patient squeeze the hand several times until the blood is exsanguinated. The pressure is then released from the ulnar artery, and the time until the nailbed capillaries refill is measured. Collateral flow is considered normal if the refill time is 5 seconds.[16] In young children and infants, this test requires two persons, one to compress the arteries and one to compress the patient's hand approximately 10 times. When the ulnar compression is released, normal color should appear in the hand within 5 seconds. The predictive value of Allen's test is questionable. Marshall[91] and Sellden[122] reported large series of children who underwent arterial catheterization without a preliminary Allen's test and had no complications. Mangano and Hickey[89]

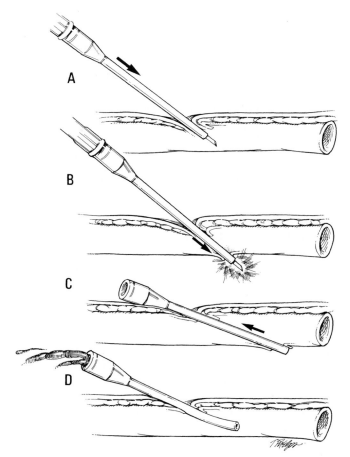

FIGURE 19-6 Radial artery cannulation. **A,** The catheter-over-needle unit is inserted into the artery. When arterial blood flow is seen in the needle hub, the catheter may be advanced over the needle into the artery. Another technique is to advance the catheter and needle farther until blood flow ceases, thereby transfixing the artery **(B)**, then remove the needle **(C)**, and withdraw the catheter until blood flow is seen. The catheter is then advanced into the artery **(D)**.

reported a case of hand ischemia requiring amputation in an adult patient with normal Allen's test results. Collateral flow to the hand can also be assessed without the need of patient cooperation by Doppler ultrasonography (probe placed over the lateral aspect of the superficial palmar arch) and pulse oximetry (probe placed on the thumb)[104] and by digital blood pressure monitor.[48]

The steps for radial artery catheter placement are as follows, illustrated in Figure 19-6. Dorsiflex the wrist. It is easiest to immobilize the wrist with an armboard and tape. Identify the artery and its course. Wearing sterile gloves, prepare the skin over the artery with an iodine-containing solution and alcohol (providing there are no allergies to either substance). If the patient is awake, anesthetize the skin with 0.5 to 1% lidocaine, using a 25- or 30-gauge needle to produce a skin wheal over the radial artery. Then inject a small amount of anesthetic below the skin so the area is anesthetized but the vessel is not disturbed. Use a needle to break the skin at the point where the catheter is to be inserted. Insert a catheter-over-needle unit over the radial artery. At this point, several techniques may be used:

1. Advance the needle and catheter until arterial blood flow is seen. After advancing both the needle and catheter into the artery a small distance, keep the needle stationary and slide the catheter over the needle into the artery.
2. Advance the needle and catheter until arterial blood flow is seen. Continue to advance the needle and catheter until blood flow stops, pull the needle and catheter back until blood flow returns, then advance the catheter over the needle into the artery.
3. Advance the needle and catheter until blood flow stops, remove the needle, then slowly pull the catheter back until blood flow is seen through the catheter and advance the catheter into the artery.
4. Use the same technique as in number 3, but before pulling back the catheter, attach a syringe with heparinized saline. While pulling back the catheter, apply gentle aspiration to the syringe until blood flow returns. Flush the catheter while advancing it into the vessel.

If it is difficult to advance the catheter at a particular point in spite of good arterial blood flow, bring the catheter back to the point of good blood flow, advance sterile flexible wire through the catheter, and pass the catheter over the wire. This technique is worth trying in cases in which arterial cannulation is particularly difficult. In patients with weak or nonpalpable pulses, the artery can be located by a Doppler flow probe. The catheter is guided by the tone changes in the Doppler signal as the artery is compressed. Doppler probes able to fit in a 22-gauge needle can facilitate catheter placement.[26]

Surgical cutdown may be required in patients who have undergone repeated arterial catheterizations. A surgical cutdown may be pursued early if a low probability of success with percutaneous placement is suspected (Fig. 19-7). Prior surgical cutdown does not preclude placement of a percutaneous or surgically placed arterial line provided a pulse is present. Antegrade cannulation of the radial artery by cutdown technique can also be used if the standard retrograde technique is unsuccessful.[113]

Alternative Sites for Arterial Catheterization

Other sites for arterial cannulation include the femoral, axillary, dorsalis pedis, and posterior tibial arteries. In newborns the umbilical artery can be cannulated, provided an adequate stump remains. Catheters can be placed "high" at T6–T9 or low at L3–L5. Green[55] found conflicting accounts over the benefits of high versus low lines, whereas Barrington[10] searched randomized controlled trials and concluded that evidence was lacking to support the use of low lines and that high lines should be used exclusively. The femoral artery is a frequently used cannulation site in children and provides reliable blood pressure measurements. Its use may be limited in patients who have had multiple cardiac catheterizations via the femoral vessels. For patients who will require multiple catheterizations in the future, one may try to save the femoral vessels for the cardiologists if feasible. The dorsalis pedis and posterior tibial arteries are not commonly used because they are often unreliable after CPB and in the immediate postoperative period owing to peripheral vasoconstriction and decreased perfusion.

Waveform Interpretation

When central arterial pressures are used (e.g., femoral, axillary), much information can be derived from the pressure waveform. The upstroke of the arterial waveform provides information about cardiac contractility. If the rate of rise of the pressure wave is rapid, the contractile state is probably good. A slow upstroke can be a sign of poor contractility but is also associated with aortic stenosis and peripheral vasoconstriction.

The position of the dicrotic notch is associated with changes in vascular resistance. A dicrotic notch that is high on the downslope of the arterial pressure trace may occur with increased systemic vascular resistance, whereas low resistance would be indicated by a low-placed dicrotic notch. The stroke volume can be correlated with the area under the systolic portion of the pressure curve. The left ventricular end-systolic pressure can be estimated by the aortic dicrotic notch pressure. These indices of cardiac contractility are

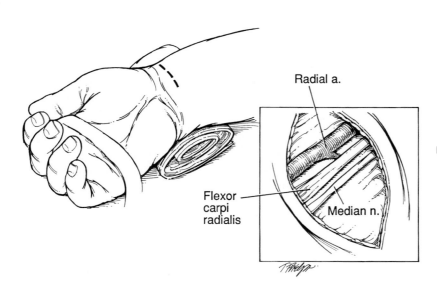

Radial a.

Flexor carpi radialis

Median n.

FIGURE 19-7 Surgical cutdown for radial artery cannulation.

reliable with central aortic catheters. When aortic and radial artery measurements are compared (in adults), the difference between the central and peripheral dicrotic notch pressures is approximately 8 mm Hg, the aortic pressure being higher.[35] Therefore, in order to use the radial artery pressure waveform to construct a calculated end-systolic pressure, 8 mm Hg should be added to the notch pressure.

In contrast to the dicrotic notch pressure, which decreases with the more distally placed arterial catheter, the peak systolic pressure is higher in the more distal arteries. The peak systolic pressure in the radial artery is reported to be 8 to 9 mm Hg higher than in the ascending aorta.[35] This is due to the wave-reflection phenomenon. As the pressure wave passes down the arterial tree, it is modified by arterial narrowing, loss of arterial elastic tissue, and the addition of reflected waves until it reaches the distal catheter.

Changes in pulse pressure (the difference between systolic and diastolic pressure) can provide very useful information. Pericardial tamponade is associated with a narrow pulse pressure on the arterial waveform. Aortic insufficiency is associated with a low diastolic pressure, resulting in a wide pulse pressure.

Hypovolemia is often accompanied by a respiratory variation in the arterial pressure trace whereby the blood pressure decreases with positive-pressure ventilation (PPV). This decrease occurs because positive intrathoracic pressure reduces the venous return to the heart, which can be very pronounced in hypovolemic patients.

Radial artery pressures may be inaccurate during the peribypass period.[40,114] This is most likely due to changes in peripheral vascular resistance. Both vasoconstriction and vasodilation have been considered as causes of this condition. The difference has been noted on initiation of cardiopulmonary bypass.[27] The pressure gradient was unaffected by sodium nitroprusside or phenylephrine during cardiopulmonary bypass.[114]

Complications of Invasive Monitoring

Monitoring blood pressure via an arterial catheter in a child undergoing cardiac surgery is considered a standard of care and is a safe procedure in most cases. However, serious complications have been associated with arterial catheters,[30,122] including bleeding, infection, vascular compromise, nerve damage, and accidental injection. Development of arteriovenous fistula, carpal tunnel syndrome,[133] and radial artery aneurysm[20] have been reported as late sequelae.

Bleeding due to line placement is usually not a problem in the absence of coagulopathy, but a hematoma may result after the catheter is removed or after several unsuccessful attempts. Hematoma formation at the site of radial artery cannulation has been reported to be associated with a greater incidence of vascular occlusion.[25] However, recanalization occurs within 1 month of removal of the catheters in most patients; permanent obstruction is rare.[57] Significant hemorrhage may occur if the catheter and tubing become disconnected. Pediatric intravenous T connectors without Leur-Lok are prone to disconnect and should be used with caution, if at all, when the cannula site is not visible. Proper use of Luer-Lok tubing prevents such disconnection.

The risk of infection due to arterial catheters has been reported to be very low. In children the risk of bacteremia from an arterial catheter was essentially nonexistent in the first 48 hours.[49]

The incidence of thrombosis and diminished blood flow has been found to be high, but studies have shown this not to be clinically significant in most cases associated with radial artery cannulation.[57] However, loss of extremities from umbilical and femoral arterial catheters has been reported.[138] Kocis and colleagues[79] studied 30 children who had a femoral artery catheter placed for perioperative monitoring and found a 7% incidence of femoral artery complications by clinical criteria. By ultrasound, 20% of the patients had complete femoral obstruction and 3% had partial femoral artery obstruction. Distal vascular insufficiency associated with femoral artery placement correlated significantly with younger age[52] and resolved after removal of the catheter. Vasospasm may be seen after the catheter is removed but is usually transient. Catheterization of both the femoral artery and vein in the same extremity may lead to limb ischemia in patients likely to experience low-flow states; infants appear to be at greatest risk in this regard.

The axillary artery also provides a centrally located catheter. Because of its position close to the aortic arch, there is an increased risk of cerebral embolus from air or debris when the catheter is flushed; however, embolus can occur with arterial cannulation of any site.[30] In a study of 96 arterial catheters, Norwood and colleagues[97] found the axillary site to have the highest risk of infection. The brachial artery is easily accessible but is rarely used because it is a peripheral "end artery" without collateral flow. Thrombosis of this vessel would remove the blood supply to the forearm and hand and risk potential loss of the entire hand.

Retrograde flow has been shown to occur during routine flushing of both peripheral and umbilical artery catheters.[30] This can result in flushing of air bubbles and debris into major vascular systems, including the carotid and superior mesenteric arteries. This can be prevented in infants by flushing small volumes over several seconds. Blanching of the forearm can be seen with radial artery flushing. Frequent flushes with large volumes may result in skin and muscle damage of the forearm.[133]

CENTRAL VENOUS PRESSURE

Central venous pressure (CVP) monitoring is indicated for children undergoing cardiovascular surgery or surgical procedures that use CPB or are associated with large blood losses or fluid shifts, and for children who require vasoactive drugs, parenteral hyperalimentation, or venous access (owing to inadequate peripheral veins).

Insertion Sites and Techniques

CVP catheters can be placed via the external or internal jugular, subclavian, axillary,[92] basilic, femoral,[141] or umbilical vein of a newborn. They may also be placed directly intraoperatively by the cardiac surgeon. The internal and external jugular veins are most often used for cardiac surgery and are discussed subsequently. A subclavian catheter may be used less frequently in cardiac surgery because of the following reasons: (1) it is likely to be in the surgical field and cannot be reached by the anesthesiologist during surgery; (2) it may kink when the chest retractor is placed; (3) it carries the highest risk of pneumothorax of any approach; and (4) other vascular structures such as the subclavian artery and, on the left, the thoracic duct may be injured. It is, however, the central venous site of choice according to the Centers for Disease Control and Prevention (CDC) recommendations in terms of infection rates. Kinking with the chest retractor can frequently be avoided by securing the hub in an inferior position. The basilic vein has the advantage of having a low rate of complications, but the success rate of central placement is low. However, because the arms are tucked at the patient's sides during cardiac surgery, a catheter in a basilic or axillary vein would be inaccessible to the anesthesiologist.

CVP catheters are usually placed in children after the induction of anesthesia and tracheal intubation. Before placement of a CVP catheter, the ECG must be monitored, because arrhythmias may be induced with the wires or catheters as they enter the heart. Patients are placed in the Trendelenburg position if they will tolerate this; alternatively, the legs may be raised with the patient flat or in a slight head-up position. This positioning distends the internal jugular veins and decreases the risk of air embolism. The area is prepared with an iodine-containing solution (assuming there is no allergy to iodine; otherwise, alcohol is used) and draped with sterile towels. If the patient is not anesthetized, 0.5% to 1% lidocaine is used for local anesthesia. A small needle (25 or 22 gauge) is often used to locate the vein (Fig. 19-8). When venous blood is freely aspirated, a wire is placed through the needle, and the needle is removed leaving the wire in place (Seldinger technique). Ultrasound guidance may be used to place these catheters.[109,142] Transesophageal echocardiography can be used to guide or check placement of a venous catheter.[5]

The size of catheter to be used is related to the size of the child. A rough guideline is to use a 3 French (Fr) catheter in infants weighing less than 3 kg, a 4 Fr in children less than 10 kg, a 5 Fr in those of 10 to 20 kg, and a 6 Fr in those more than 20 kg. In larger children, if two catheters are to be placed, the second needle insertion is performed before inserting the catheter over the wire, because catheter shearing and embolization can occur if the needle inadvertently cuts into the first catheter. After the catheter is placed over the wire, placement in the vein is confirmed by the lack of pulsatile flow and by measuring the pressure waveforms. The color and pressure of the venous blood may be altered by intracardiac lesions. Significant left-to-right shunting may cause the venous blood to appear redder; right-to-left shunting can cause the venous blood to be darker and the arterial blood to be the color of "normal" venous blood. The chest radiograph serves as another important means to confirm correct placement of the CVP catheter. Necessary, but not sufficient, radiologic criteria for ideal placement in the superior vena cava or right atrium include (1) catheter tip to the right of the spine and (2) distal portion of the catheter coursing inside of and parallel to the lumen of the superior vena cava or right atrium (as opposed to pointing at the wall).

Waveform Interpretation

The normal CVP trace has three positive waves, *a*, *c*, and *v*, and two negative waves, *x* and *y* (Fig. 19-9). The *a* wave is

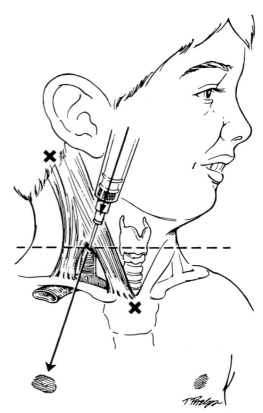

FIGURE 19-8 Internal jugular cannulation. Head turned to the opposite side. Needle puncture at the apex of the triangle formed by the heads of the sternocleidomastoid muscle (midway between the sternal notch and the mastoid process). Needle aimed at the ipsilateral nipple. (From Schleien CL: Cardiopulmonary resuscitation. In Nichols DG, Yaster M, Lappe DG, Buck JR [eds]: *Golden Hour: The Handbook of Advanced Pediatric Life Support.* St. Louis, Mosby–Year Book, 1991, p 124; with permission.)

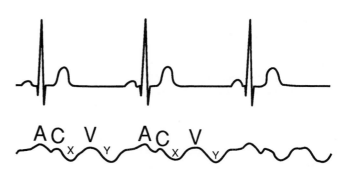

FIGURE 19-9 Central venous pressure trace with corresponding electrocardiogram (ECG). The a wave is produced by atrial contraction, occurring after the P wave on the ECG. The c wave is produced by bulging of the tricuspid valve upward into the right atrium after valve closure. The x descent is caused by the tricuspid valve being pulled away from the right atrium by the contracting ventricle during systole. The v wave occurs before the opening of the tricuspid valve and is the result of a rapid late systolic filling of the atrium. The y descent occurs as the tricuspid valve opens and blood enters the ventricle. (From O'Rourke RA: The measurement of systemic blood pressure: Normal and abnormal pulsations of the arteries and veins. In Hurst JW (ed): *The Heart.* New York, McGraw-Hill, 1990, p 159; with permission.)

Table 19-4 Characteristics of Abnormal Central Venous Pressure Trace

Wave	Physiology	Associated Disease
"Cannon" a	Right atrium contracts against obstructed tricuspid valve	Tricuspid stenosis Right atrial myxoma Complete heart block
	Resistance to right ventricular filling	Pulmonary hypertension Pulmonary stenosis
Absent a	No effective atrial contraction	Atrial fibrillation
"Giant" v	Right ventricular pressure transmitted to right atrium	Tricuspid regurgitation

caused by atrial contraction, the c wave by ventricular contraction against a closed tricuspid valve, and the v wave by atrial filling. The v wave is normally lower in amplitude than the a wave, but in the presence of an atrial septal defect the higher left atrial pressure may be transmitted to the right atrium during atrial filling, causing the a and v waves to be equal in amplitude. Characteristics of an abnormal CVP trace are summarized in Table 19-4.

Right and left atrial pressures, in the presence of normal tricuspid and mitral valve function, reflect their respective ventricular end-diastolic pressures. Ventricular end-diastolic pressure is determined by ventricular compliance (the relationship between volume and pressure), afterload, and function. High filling pressures may reflect poor function and not intravascular volume. Thus, after cardiac bypass and surgery, which impair ventricular function, the filling pressures, for given intravascular volume and output, must be higher. Changing filling pressures may reflect changes in cardiac function. Increasing left atrial pressures in the postoperative period may indicate deteriorating left ventricular function, whereas falling pressures with adequate perfusion are generally more encouraging. The temptation to equate filling pressures with volume must be resisted. As with all monitored parameters, interpretation of these pressures requires a thorough understanding of the child's clinical condition.

Normal values for CVP in infants are difficult to define. Spontaneously breathing healthy babies generally have CVP values from −2 to +4 mm Hg. In infants with congenital heart disease (CHD), the values are in the range of 4 to 8 mm Hg. Infants ventilated for respiratory disease have values of 2 to 6 mm Hg and often do not tolerate values less than 3 mm Hg. CVP measurements above 8 mm Hg are often associated with myocardial dysfunction or high intrathoracic pressure, such as with pneumothorax.[129] Pressures measured at end expiration from femoral catheters positioned in the inferior vena cava give accurate CVP values.[87] It should be noted that measurements from catheters placed in the subclavian or internal jugular veins in patients with cavopulmonary (Glenn) shunts will reflect the pulmonary artery pressure.

Artifacts and Errors in Measurement

The transducer position, which is particularly important for accurate measurement of CVP, is conventionally at the level of the right atrium, the midaxillary line. If the patient's position changes, measurements that are erroneously high (if the transducer is too low) or low (if the transducer is too high)

will result. Because changes in the CVP of just a few millimeters of mercury can be a significant finding, one must be vigilant to keep the transducer level in the correct position and accurately zeroed. It is also necessary to check the pressure waveform. The catheter may be long enough to pass through the tricuspid valve into the right ventricle in some patients, or the waveform may be overdamped if the catheter is against the chamber wall or if blood or air bubbles are in the tubing.

Complications

The most common complication of internal jugular vein catheterization is inadvertent carotid artery puncture. The use of ultrasound guidance for internal jugular cannulation decreased the frequency of carotid artery puncture from 25% to 0% in 95 infants.[142] Other complications of insertion include local hematoma, air embolism, catheter malposition (resulting in infiltration or extravasation of drugs and fluid into neck tissue, mediastinum, or pericardial or pleural cavities), pneumothorax, hemothorax, and Horner's syndrome. Trauma to the thoracic duct (with left-sided attempts), trauma to the brachial plexus, and subclavian artery puncture can occur. There appear to be fewer complications after ultrasound-guided internal jugular and subclavian venous catheter placement.

Failure to cannulate the vessel is also a complication of jugular cannulation. The small vessels in close proximity to one another make small children particularly challenging. One study found the rate of successful cannulation of the internal jugular vein to be significantly decreased in children younger than 3 months of age and weighing less than 4.0 kg.[60] The success rate tends to correlate with the experience of the person doing the procedure.[133]

Some patients may have a higher risk of insertion complications because of preexisting clinical conditions, such as contralateral diaphragmatic dysfunction; congenital abnormalities, including short or webbed necks; or previous internal jugular catheterizations. Complications related to indwelling catheters include infection, thrombophlebitis, superior vena cava thrombosis, and intracardiac thrombus formation.

The risk of infection related to internal jugular vein catheterization has been reported to be 11% in children, and the risk of catheter-related septicemia 0.5% to 1.0%. The incidence of having positive catheter-tip cultures without complications related to culture positivity has been reported to be 5%.[36] In situ time and open-heart surgery in infants younger than 1 year of age have proved to be the most significant independent risk factors for a positive tip culture. The safe in situ time has been reported to be 3 days for infants and 6 days for older children.[36]

PULMONARY ARTERY PRESSURE

Percutaneous pulmonary artery catheterization is frequently used in adults undergoing cardiac surgery but is less common in children and very infrequent in infants. The reasons include difficulty in gaining access, based on both size and variable anatomy, and doubts regarding the accuracy of the data obtained. In neonates and small infants a transthoracic pulmonary artery catheter can be placed directly after repair by the surgeon for postoperative monitoring.

Pulmonary Artery Catheters

Balloon-tipped, thermodilution pulmonary artery catheters are available in sizes 4 and 5 Fr for children weighing 10 to 18 kg, and 6 and 7 Fr for children weighing more than 18 kg. Children who weigh less than 10 kg can be monitored with 2 and 3 Fr double-lumen catheters that consist of a distal port and a thermistor.

Pulmonary artery catheters can be placed via the external or internal jugular veins or the femoral vein. They are placed through an introducer, which is approximately one half to one whole size larger than the catheter, depending on the manufacturer's design.

Waveform Interpretation and Hemodynamic Measurements

Accurate interpretation of pulmonary artery catheter data often depends on the location of the catheter tip, the patient's pulmonary status, and the presence of hypovolemia. To obtain accurate pulmonary catheter measurements, the catheter tip must be in an area where the pulmonary artery blood pressure is greater than the pulmonary venous blood pressure or the pulmonary alveolar pressure. Identification of the catheter tip at the level of the left atrium on a lateral chest radiograph fulfills these requirements. West and colleagues[144] described three zones of the lung, illustrated in Figure 19-10. If the catheter tip is in zone I, the alveolar pressure will be greater than the pulmonary artery or pulmonary venous pressure, so airway pressure will be transmitted to the catheter, and the resulting waveform will be significantly affected by changes in ventilation.

Hypovolemic patients often have low pulmonary artery and pulmonary venous pressures. If, in addition to the hypovolemia, the alveolar pressure is high, the alveolar pressure will be transmitted to the pulmonary artery catheter and erroneously high filling pressures will be measured. This scenario is often seen in hypovolemic patients who are receiving greater than 10 cm H_2O of positive end-expiratory pressure (PEEP).

Because the pulmonary artery pressure can be greatly affected by airway pressure, hemodynamic measurement should be made at end expiration whether the patient is spontaneously breathing or mechanically ventilated. If a patient is spontaneously breathing, but the breathing is labored or obstructed, a large negative intrapleural pressure can be generated during inspiration, which can then be transmitted to the pulmonary circulation and cause negative filling pressures. If the patient is receiving positive-pressure ventilation, the positive pressure can be transmitted, resulting in falsely high pulmonary artery pressure measurements.

The normal pulmonary artery waveforms seen during the insertion of the catheter are illustrated in Figure 19-11. After the catheter is passed through the length of the introducer, the catheter balloon is inflated and the catheter is advanced until the right atrial pressure is obtained. In patients with an intracardiac defect and a left-to-right shunt (e.g., those with atrial or ventricular septal defect), the catheter should not be passed beyond the introducer until after surgical repair, to avoid the risk of thrombus formation on the catheter and emboli to the systemic circulation. Having the patient in a slight head-up (reverse Trendelenburg) and right lateral tilt position often facilitates catheter flotation. After the catheter crosses the tricuspid valve, a sudden increase in systolic pressure is seen as it enters the right ventricle. The diastolic pressure is low in both the right atrial and ventricular chambers. When the catheter passes the pulmonic valve and enters the pulmonary artery, the diastolic pressure increases with little change in the systolic pressure. As the catheter is slowly advanced from this point, the pulmonary capillary wedge pressure (PCWP) is obtained when the mean pressure drops and the tracing is atrial in appearance. The balloon should then be deflated and the pulmonary artery waveform should reappear. If not, the catheter may be overwedged and

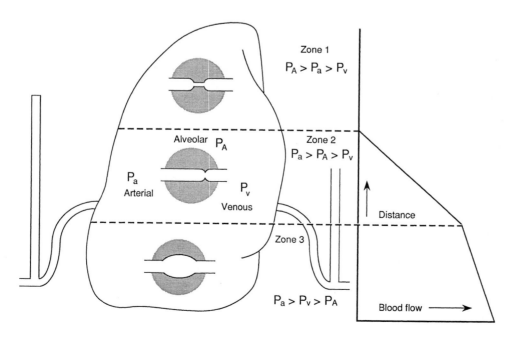

FIGURE 19-10 Three zones of the lung, showing the uneven distribution of blood flow in the lung based on pressures affecting the capillaries. P_A, Pulmonary alveolar pressure; P_a, pulmonary artery pressure; P_v, pulmonary venous pressure. (From West JB, Dollery CT, Naimark A: Distribution of blood flow in isolated lung: Relation to vascular and alveolar pressures. *J Appl Physiol* 19:713, 1964; with permission.)

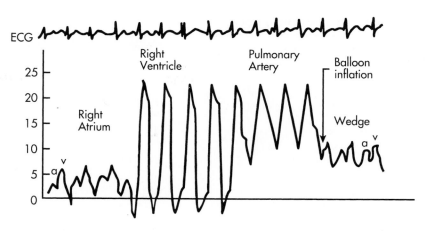

FIGURE 19-11 Normal pressure waveforms obtained during pulmonary artery catheter insertion. With the balloon inflated, the catheter passes from the right atrium to the right ventricle, seen as a sudden increase in systolic pressure. As the catheter enters the pulmonary artery, diastolic pressure suddenly increases. When the catheter reaches the pulmonary capillary wedge position, mean pressure decreases and an atrial waveform is obtained. ECG, electrocardiogram.

need to be pulled back. The length the catheter is inserted depends on the patient's size and the site of insertion (internal jugular versus femoral vein). In small children the distance between the tip of the catheter and the CVP port may be longer than the distance between the pulmonary artery and a right internal jugular insertion site. This would allow entrainment of air through the CVP port. The clinician should exercise caution in choosing the insertion site such that the CVP port is inside the body. A sterile sheath placed over the catheter allows the catheter to be repositioned at a later time if necessary. The catheter can also be placed with the assistance of fluoroscopy.[65]

The pulmonary capillary wedge waveforms give information about the left side of the heart, as CVP gives information about the right heart. The presence of a large *v* wave can indicate mitral regurgitation or a decrease in ventricular compliance (Fig. 19-12). Large or "cannon" *a* waves occur with nodal rhythm and complete heart block.

Intracardiac Measurements

Pulmonary artery catheters directly measure right atrial pressure (proximal port), pulmonary artery pressure (distal port), pulmonary capillary wedge pressure (from the distal port

when the balloon is inflated), cardiac output, and blood temperature (using the wiring to the thermistor). Normal intracardiac pressures and oxygen saturations are shown schematically in Figure 19-13. From these parameters, indices of both hemodynamic function (Table 19-5) and respiratory function (Table 19-6) can be derived. With this information, volume status, ventricular function, and the presence of pulmonary hypertension can be assessed. Interpretation of abnormal values is shown in Table 19-7.

Pulmonary artery catheters directly measure cardiac output using the thermodilution technique. This and other methods of cardiac output measurements are discussed later in this chapter.

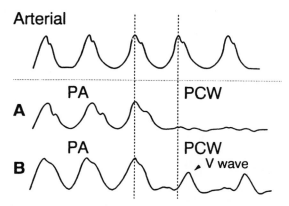

FIGURE 19-12 The relationship of a systemic arterial waveform, a pulmonary artery (PA) waveform, and a pulmonary capillary wedge (PCW) waveform in the normal patient **(A)** and in the presence of a *v* wave **(B)**. (From Reich DL, Kaplan JA: Hemodynamic monitoring. In Kaplan JA [ed]: *Cardiac Anesthesia*. Philadelphia, WB Saunders, 1993, p 276; with permission.)

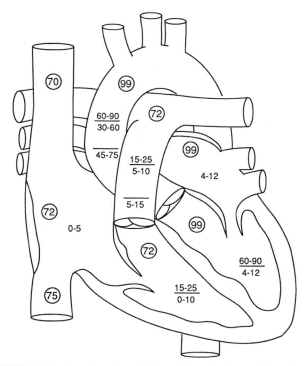

FIGURE 19-13 Normal cardiac catheterization values in an infant. Oxygen saturation numbers are circled. Systolic, diastolic, and mean pressures are expressed as ranges.

Table 19-5 Hemodynamic Values Derived from Pulmonary Artery Catheter

Derived Value	Formula	Normal Range
Cardiac index (CI)	$\dfrac{CO}{BSA}$	$3-4.2$ L $\cdot$ min^{-1} $\cdot$ m^{-2}
Stroke volume (SV)	$\dfrac{CO}{HR} \times 1000$	1 mL $\cdot$ kg^{-1} $\cdot$ beat^{-1}
Stroke volume index (SVI)	$\dfrac{CI}{HR} \times 1000$	$40-60$ mL $\cdot$ m^{-2} $\cdot$ beat^{-1}
Systemic vascular resistance index	$\dfrac{MAP - CVP}{CI} \times 80$	$700-1600$ dynes $\cdot$ sec $\cdot$ cm^{-5} $\cdot$ m^{-2}
Systemic vascular resistance index (R_s) (Wood units/m²)	$\dfrac{MAP - CVP}{Q_s/BSA}$	$9-12$ mm Hg $\cdot$ min $\cdot$ L^{-1} $\cdot$ m^{-2} (infants) $13-18$ mm Hg $\cdot$ min $\cdot$ L^{-1} $\cdot$ m^{-2} (children)
Pulmonary vascular resistance index	$\dfrac{MPAP - PCWP}{CI} \times 80$	$20-130$ dynes $\cdot$ sec $\cdot$ cm^{-5} $\cdot$ m^{-2}
Pulmonary vascular resistance index (R_p) (Wood units/m²)	$\dfrac{MPAP - PCWP}{Q_p/BSA}$	< 2 mm Hg $\cdot$ min $\cdot$ L^{-1} $\cdot$ m^{-2}
R_p/R_s		< 0.1
Left ventricular stroke work index (LVSWI)	$(MAP - PCWP) \times SVI \times 0.0136$	$45-60$ g $\cdot$ m $\cdot$ m^{-2} $\cdot$ beat^{-1}
Right ventricular stroke work index (RVSWI)	$(MPAP - CVP) \times SVI \times 0.0136$	$5-10$ g $\cdot$ m $\cdot$ m^{-2} $\cdot$ beat^{-1}

CO, Cardiac output; BSA, body surface area; HR, heart rate; MAP, mean arterial pressure; CVP, central venous pressure; MPAP, mean pulmonary artery pressure; PCWP, pulmonary capillary wedge pressure; Q_s, systemic blood flow; Q_p, pulmonary blood flow.

Table 19-6 Derived Indices of Respiratory Function

$\dot{Q}s/\dot{Q}t = \dfrac{CCO_2 - CaO_2}{CCO_2 - CVO_2}$ (normal $<5\%$)

$A-aO_2 = PAO_2 - PaO_2$ (normal <9 mmHg if $FiO_2 = 0.21$)
$\quad\quad\quad$ (<34 mmHg if $FiO_2 = 1.0$)

$\dot{V}O_2 = CI(CaO_2 - CvO_2) \times 10$ (normal $= 140-160$ ml $\cdot$ min $\cdot$ m^{-2})

$DO_2 = CI(CaO_2) \times 10$ (normal $= 400-600$ ml $\cdot$ min $\cdot$ m^{-2})

where:
$A-aO_2$ = alveolar-arterial O_2 gradient
CaO_2 = arterial O_2 content (Hgb $\times 1.39 \times SaO_2$) + (PaO$_2 \times 0.0031$)
$Ca-VO_2$ = arteriovenous O_2 content difference
CcO_2 = capillary O_2 content (Hgb $\times 1.39^*$) + [$FiO_2 \times 713$ - (PaCO$_2$)] $\times 0.0031$
CO = cardiac output
$C\bar{v}O_2$ = mixed venous O_2 content (Hgb $\times 1.39 \times S\bar{v}O_2$) + ($\bar{V}PO_2 \times 0.0031$)
DO_2 = tissue oxygen delivery
PaO_2 = arterial O_2 tension
PAO_2 = alveolar O_2 tension (P$_B^\dagger$ - 47)(FiO$_2$) - (PACO$_2$/R)
$P\bar{v}O_2$ = mixed venous oxygen tension
$\dot{Q}s/\dot{Q}t$ = intrapulmonary shunt
SaO_2 = arterial oxygen saturation
$S\bar{v}O_2$ = mixed venous oxygen saturation
VO_2 = minute O_2 consumption

*Assumes $FiO_2 <0.35$ ($SaO_2 = 100\%$)
†Assumes barometric pressure (P_B) = 760 mm Hg and respiratory quotient (R) = 1.

Mixed venous oxygen saturation can be measured by drawing a blood sample from the pulmonary artery (distal) port of the pulmonary artery catheter. It is important that the balloon is deflated and the catheter not be in a wedged position when the sample is drawn; otherwise an arterialized pulmonary venous sample will be obtained rather than a mixed venous pulmonary artery sample. The mixed venous oxygen saturation (SvO_2) reflects the adequacy of perfusion and can be used to diagnose the presence of left-to-right intracardiac shunts or decreased oxygen delivery. Under normal circumstances, SvO_2 is 75% been compared with an arterial oxygen saturation (SaO_2) of 95% to 100%. SvO_2 varies directly with hemoglobin, cardiac output, and arterial O_2 saturation, and indirectly with metabolic rate. When SvO_2 falls, hemoglobin, cardiac output, and arterial oxygen saturation should be directly measured. If these indices are stable, it suggests that the metabolic rate may have significantly increased. This can occur, for example, in the postoperative period when a hypothermic patient begins shivering as the muscle paralysis wears off. Conversely, when hemoglobin, cardiac output, or arterial oxygen saturation has fallen sufficiently to produce an SvO_2 less than 65%, adequate tissue oxygen delivery is

Table 19-7 Interpretation of Abnormal Hemodynamic Values

	CVP	PCWP	SVR	CI	Comment
Hypovolemia	↓	↓	↑	↓	Confirm diagnosis with fluid challenge
Cardiogenic shock	↑	↑	↑	↓	PCWP is low in isolated right heart failure
Septic shock	↓	↓	↓ or ↑	variable	EF is decreased; SV and CO are maintained by LV dilation and increased HR; mixed venous O_2 saturation may be high
Tamponade	↑	↑	↑	↓	Equalization of diastolic pressures

CI, cardiac index; CO, cardiac output; CVP, central venous pressure; EF, ejection fraction; HR, heart rate; LV, left ventricular; PCWP, pulmonary capillary wedge pressure; SV, stroke volume; SVR, systemic vascular resistance.

threatened and the abnormal variable should be corrected. SvO_2 is more difficult to interpret under conditions of intracardiac shunts, peripheral shunts, sepsis, cirrhosis, and cyanide poisoning. Vedrinne and colleagues[140] found continuous oxygen saturation in mixed venous blood to be useful in 57% of adult patients, and identified independent preoperative risk factors associated with its usefulness.

Complications of Insertion

The complications of passing the flow-directed percutaneous pulmonary artery catheter include arrhythmias, the development of right bundle branch or complete heart block, pulmonary artery rupture, pulmonary infarction, air embolus, catheter knotting or kinking, and valvular damage. Arrhythmias can be precipitated by the catheter touching the atrium or ventricle. This is more likely to happen if the balloon is not inflated or if the catheter coils in the right ventricle. Administration of lidocaine may help decrease ventricular arrhythmias. The development of a right bundle branch or complete heart block has been reported during passage of the pulmonary artery catheter through the right ventricle. In older children with preexisting left bundle branch block, a pulmonary artery catheter with pacing capability can be used to pace the heart if complete heart block develops.

Knotting or kinking of the catheter can occur if an excessive amount of catheter is passed into the heart in an attempt to enter the pulmonary artery or to wedge the catheter.[133] The catheter can curl and develop a knot. This is more likely in patients with large atrial and/or ventricular cavities as well as in low-flow states. Damage to tricuspid or pulmonary valves can occur if the catheter is pulled back through a closed valve while the balloon is inflated. For this reason it is important to be vigilant about allowing the balloon to deflate before withdrawing the catheter. The catheter may also migrate to an aberrant area due to abnormal anatomy. This can have profound effects on the validity of the pressure tracings and the cardiac outputs.

Complications of Indwelling Catheters

Even with successful, uncomplicated insertion, complications may develop later with an indwelling pulmonary artery catheter. Intracardiac thrombus formation can occur if a thrombus forms from the tip of the catheter. The thrombus can then embolize to the pulmonary artery or lead to thrombocytopenia. Postoperative thrombocytopenia was seen in 29 of 54 children with percutaneous pulmonary artery catheters without clot noted; although this was not different from 48% of 57 patients who did not have catheters during the same time period.[65]

Pulmonary artery rupture can occur if the balloon is inflated in a small or diseased pulmonary arterial branch, causing the vessel to tear; patients with pulmonary hypertension are at greater risk for this complication. Patients will immediately develop hemoptysis or blood via the endotracheal tube. Depending on the severity of the bleeding, therapy ranges from conservative support to the use of a double-lumen endotracheal tube to protect the normal lung, which is possible only in larger children. Selective, one-lung ventilation can be transiently accomplished by placing the endotracheal tube in the bronchus of the normal lung. In some cases, surgery may be required for massive hemorrhage. Pulmonary infarction can occur if the catheter is allowed to remain in the wedge position for an extended period.

Air embolus can be introduced by attempts to inflate a ruptured balloon or by inadvertent introduction of air through one of the catheter ports. This is particularly important to watch for in patients with low right atrial pressure or who generate large negative inspiratory pressures. If these patients are in the sitting position and the introducer or a catheter port is open to air, entrainment of air can occur during inspiration.

For patients undergoing heart surgery, a pulmonary artery catheter can be inadvertently sutured into the heart.[120] This is most likely to happen after CPB when the pulmonary artery vent is removed and the insertion site is sutured closed. This is best prevented by ensuring mobility before closure of the chest.

Removal of a transthoracic pulmonary artery line can be associated with bleeding at the insertion site. This may be enough to obstruct flow to the pulmonary artery and cause an arrest. Before removing a pulmonary artery line, blood for transfusion and a thoracic surgeon for emergency thoracotomy should be available.

LEFT ATRIAL PRESSURE

Direct measurement of left atrial pressure is indicated when pulmonary artery catheter monitoring is technically difficult or when the patient's anatomy or clinical condition makes the use of a pulmonary artery catheter impossible. Such conditions exist with tricuspid stenosis or atresia, pulmonary stenosis or atresia, severe pulmonary hypertension, and right heart failure. Infants with pulmonary hypertension may benefit from simultaneous measurement of pulmonary artery and left atrial pressures via transthoracic lines. The mean left atrial pressure is used as an indication of the left ventricular end-diastolic pressure, provided the mitral valve is normal. The catheter can be placed through a purse-string suture in the right superior pulmonary vein and guided into the left atrium.

The left atrial pressure waveform has a, c, and v waves similar to the waveform from the right atrium and pulmonary capillary wedge tracing. Left atrial pressure measured directly is more accurate than pulmonary capillary wedge pressure because it is not affected by the lungs. It is important to note that the left atrial catheter must be placed surgically and has the serious disadvantage of being a possible site for air entry into the left side of the heart. The consequences of air or clot embolism on the left (systemic) circulation may be profound, with potential neurologic or coronary vascular occlusion and possibly devastating consequences. Bleeding can also occur with removal of the left atrial line. Data obtained from a percutaneous left atrial line can be used to interpret the clinical situation. Low left atrial pressure, particularly with low right atrial pressure (CVP), is suggestive of volume depletion, whereas high left atrial pressure is suggestive of left ventricular dysfunction, volume overload, tamponade, or mitral valve regurgitation.

CARDIAC OUTPUT

Cardiac output is defined as the amount of blood ejected by the left ventricle in 1 minute; it is equal to the heart rate multiplied by the stroke volume. In neonates, cardiac output is normally 400 to 500 mL/kg/min because of residual left-to-right shunts (patent foramen ovale, patent ductus arteriosus). In normal infants these shunts close after the first week of life, and the cardiac output falls to 150 to 300 mL/kg/min. As cardiac output falls, an increase in peripheral vasoconstriction occurs to produce the gradual rise in blood pressure with age. Premature infants have a relatively higher cardiac output than full-term babies with a cardiac index of 5.5 L/min/m^2.[59]

It is self-evident that the ability to measure cardiac output is important for the clinical management of cardiac surgery patients. Although several methods are available for measuring cardiac output, the indicator dilution technique is the most widely used for neonates, infants, and children with congenital heart lesions. This section discusses the indicator-dilution technique in which either oxygen, cold injectate (thermodilution), or green dye is used as the indicator, as well as Doppler flow probes to measure cardiac output. The thermodilution, green dye, and Fick methods for measuring cardiac output are, for the most part, equally accurate when carried out properly.[132,145]

Fick Method

The Fick method can be used to measure either pulmonary or systemic blood flow. According to the Fick principle, cardiac output is equal to the oxygen consumption divided by the arteriovenous oxygen difference. Thus, for pulmonary blood flow (Q_p), the oxygen uptake by the lungs is divided by the difference between the pulmonary venous and pulmonary arterial oxygen content. For systemic blood flow (Q_s), the oxygen consumption is divided by the difference between the arterial and mixed venous oxygen content. This knowledge of systemic and pulmonary blood flows makes it possible to calculate the amount of intracardiac shunt, Q_p/Q_s:

$$Q_p / Q_s = \frac{SO_2(Ao) - SO_2(RA)}{SO_2(PV) - SO_2(PA)}$$

where
  SO_2 = oxygen saturation
  Ao = aorta
  RA = right atrium
  PV = pulmonary vein
  PA = pulmonary artery

This principle is the basis for monitoring mixed venous oxygen saturation (SvO_2) as an indicator of cardiac output. Oxygen consumption is, in general, between 140 and 160 mL/min/m^2. Thus, if arterial saturation is stable, a fall in SvO_2 indicates decreased cardiac output.

Dye Dilution

The dye dilution technique uses indocyanine green (also known as Cardio-Green or green dye) because it is nontoxic, is rapidly removed from the circulation by the liver, and has a half-life in the circulation of about 10 minutes. It has a peak absorption wavelength at 805 nm, which is near the point at which the absorption of light by oxygenated and reduced hemoglobin is identical, so changes in blood oxygen concentrations will not affect the cardiac output determination.

The technique requires a central vein and an arterial catheter. The dye solution is injected rapidly into the CVP catheter, and continuous sampling of arterial blood from the arterial catheter (withdrawn at a constant rate by a syringe in a calibrated pump) is begun. The blood passes through a densitometer, and the change in indicator concentration is measured over time, generating a dye concentration versus time curve. The area under the curve is calculated, and the cardiac output is computed by the Stewart-Hamilton equation[58] whereby cardiac output is equal to the amount of injected indicator divided by the area under the curve:

$$\text{Indicator dye cardiac output} = Q =$$

$$\frac{60 \times i}{A \times CF} = \frac{60 \times i}{C \times t}$$

where
  i = amount of dye injected (mg)
  A = area of first pass of green dye curve measured in millimeters deflection multiplied by duration of first pass in seconds
  CF = calibration factor of standard measured in milligrams green dye per liter per millimeter deflection
  C = mean concentration of dye under the curve (mg/L)
  t = duration of curve (sec)

In the presence of a shunt the normal cardiac output curve is distorted (Fig. 19-14). Right-to-left shunting results in an early-appearing hump on the buildup slope due to dye that has bypassed the pulmonary vasculature. Left-to-right shunting results in a decreased peak concentration of dye, a prolonged disappearance time, and a slow return to baseline with a loss of the recirculation peak. The daily maximum dye dose is 2 mg/kg.[133] Repeated measurements may result in a significant amount of blood loss. Dye dilution combined with pulse dye densitometry, based on the principles of pulse oximetry, compared favorably with thermodilution in 22 adults.[64]

Thermodilution

The thermodilution technique for measuring cardiac output is performed using a pulmonary artery catheter or a thermistor in the pulmonary artery. It has proved accurate and reproducible in children with valvular stenosis, cardiomyopathy, or corrected intracardiac shunts.[46]

After a stable baseline blood temperature is measured, a known volume of saline or 5% dextrose in water (D$_5$W), either iced or at room temperature with the appropriate constant entered into the computer, is injected into the right atrium. Cardiac output is calculated by application of the dye dilution principle, which was initially described for the dye injection method of cardiac output determination.[58] For thermodilution the equation is modified to take into account the change in blood temperature:

$$Q = \frac{V(T_B - T_I)K_1 K_2}{\int_0^\infty T_B(t)\,dt}$$

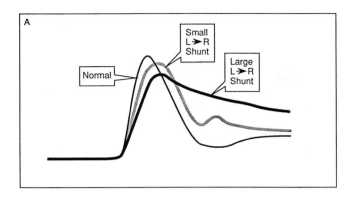

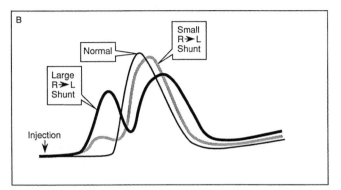

FIGURE 19-14 Examples of cardiac output curves obtained by the dye dilution method in normal, left-to-right (**A**), and right-to-left (**B**) shunt. In **A**, the normal recirculation curve can be seen. The effect of a small left-to-right shunt is decreased peak height and apparent "early" recirculation. A large left-to-right shunt shows slurring of the dye peak with no second peak. In **B**, a small right-to-left shunt has an early peak as contrast material rapidly enters the systemic circulation. This pattern is more pronounced with a large right-to-left shunt.

where

Q = cardiac output
V = volume injected
T_B = blood temperature
T_I = injectate temperature
K_1 = empiric factor used to correct for injectate warming, which is specific for catheter size (e.g., for 7 Fr catheters, $K_1 = 0.825$) and adjusts units to L/min
K_2 = computational constant for the specific gravity and specific heat of the blood and the injectate (D_5W), the product of which equals approximately 1.08
$T_B(t)dt$ = the change in blood temperature as a function of time (the area under the curve)

Thus the change in blood temperature over time is inversely proportional to the cardiac output.

To obtain accurate cardiac output measurements, several technical factors must be considered. First, the catheter thermistor must be freely floating in the pulmonary artery. If the thermistor is up against the vessel wall, it will not be in contact with the injectate, and the change in blood temperature will not be accurately measured. Second, the injectate volume and temperature must correspond to the settings on the cardiac output computer. If the injectate is too warm or the volume is too small, the cardiac output as computed will be erroneously high. Conversely, the use of injectate temperatures cooler than or volumes greater than those programmed into the computer will yield falsely low cardiac output readings.

A rapid injection rate (4 seconds or less) is also important for accurate measurement.

The presence of either a left-to-right or right-to-left shunt will result in erroneous cardiac output measurements. The pulmonary artery catheter measures only right heart cardiac output and reflects left heart output only if the two are equal, that is, in the absence of shunts. Tibby and colleagues[136] studied femoral artery thermodilution in 24 children and found good correlation with Fick-derived cardiac output measurements.

Flow Probes

Noninvasive methods to determine cardiac output have been studied extensively. Cardiac output is equal to the product of the blood flow velocity in a vessel and the vessel's cross-sectional area. Ultrasonography can be used to measure ascending aortic blood flow velocity by the Doppler technique. The ultrasound waves can be emitted and detected via transthoracic transducers,[121,146] esophageal transducers,[94] transducers mounted on the tip of an endotracheal tube,[124] or miniaturized flow probes implanted directly onto the ascending aorta.[47,72,84] The diameter of the aorta is measured by two-dimensional echocardiography (during systole), and the cross-sectional area is calculated. The cardiac output calculated is a left heart output without coronary blood flow, since the measurement is made above the takeoff of the coronary arteries. It will therefore be less than the cardiac output measured by the indicator dilution technique.

The Doppler method of determining cardiac output is subject to measurement inaccuracies at several points. They include the following: incorrect determination of vessel diameter, incorrect determination of the mean velocity by measuring only one point within the vessel, or a beam angle greater than 20 degrees to the axis of blood flow. Abnormal aortic anatomy can have variable effects. Disease of the aortic valve or other conditions that produce turbulence in the ascending aorta may alter the accuracy of the Doppler measurement, which assumes laminar flow.

Several sites have been studied to determine cardiac output. A transthoracic ultrasound transducer placed in the suprasternal notch and directed toward the ascending aorta is a noninvasive method of measuring aortic blood flow velocity.[102,146] The pulsed Doppler technique has been shown to have a good correlation with the Fick method for calculating cardiac output in children,[3] and the dual-beam Doppler technique had acceptable agreement with thermodilution-measured cardiac output in critically ill infants.[71,146] However, this method is used for diagnostic purposes rather than monitoring purposes in the OR setting with patients undergoing median sternotomy, because it requires intermittent placement of a sterile probe directly on the heart.

Transesophageal echocardiography probes with continuous-wave Doppler capability are now commercially available in sizes suitable for use in infants and small children. Muhiudeen and colleagues[94] studied 35 adult patients undergoing major cardiac or vascular surgery and found only a modest correlation between cardiac outputs from transesophageal echocardiography (TEE) pulsed Doppler and thermodilution. Tibby and colleagues[137] studied 100 children 4 days of age to 18 years who were ventilated in the ICU and evaluated transesophageal Doppler ultrasonography as a means of deriving cardiac output. In comparison with femoral artery thermodilution, they found a good correlation. Cardiac output was determined using an equation that factored in the patient's height squared. Notably, this technique looks at descending aortic flow and does not consider great vessel flow. Transtracheal Doppler cardiac output measurements do not correlate well with thermodilution cardiac output in adults.[124] In children, despite new technology, positioning can be difficult and interpretation of data requires experience.[103]

A more invasive method of measuring cardiac output entails intraoperatively attaching a miniature ultrasound probe to the adventitia of the ascending aorta. This probe is connected to monitoring equipment by wires that exit the chest wall through a small stab wound.[72,84] The aortic diameter measurements are made intraoperatively by ultrasound. Flow probes allow continuous monitoring of cardiac output in the postoperative period. The probe is removed by gentle traction. Lequier and colleagues[84] studied 11 children after surgical repair of congenital heart disease and found good correlation with Doppler echocardiographic determinations of cardiac output. The probe measurements accurately reflected the condition of the patients, and there were no complications (bleeding, infection, or problems removing the probe).

Bioimpedance Cardiac Output

Measurement of cardiac output by thoracic impedance is based on an empiric equation for calculation of left ventricular stroke volume described by Kubicek and colleagues[80] in 1966. An alternating current of low amplitude and high frequency is introduced and simultaneously sensed by two sets of electrodes placed around the neck and lower thorax. Changes in thoracic impedance occur with respiration and pulsatile blood flow. Only the cardiac-induced pulsatile component is analyzed when measuring cardiac output. The correlation between thoracic impedance and thermodilution cardiac output is reported to be good by some,[24,130] but not all,[11] reports. In children less than 125 cm in length, the measured thoracic length did not result in accurate bioimpedance cardiac output measurements.[66] In addition, intracardiac shunts interfere with measurements.

INTRAOPERATIVE ECHOCARDIOGRAPHY

Transesophageal echocardiography and epicardial echocardiography are both used in the OR. The miniaturization of TEE probes and advances in technology have resulted in significant increases in use for both diagnosis and monitoring. Previously, limited views were available with TEE. However, biplane and omniplane probes are now available. TEE can be used as a continuous monitor of structure and function. Intraoperative echocardiography is indicated during repair of congenital heart defects in which residual shunts, outflow tract obstruction, valve regurgitation, or stenosis is suspected. It is also used to evaluate ventricular function.[50,139] Siwik and associates[127] studied 63 children undergoing complex intracardiac repairs and found that TEE altered the surgical therapy in 3% of the cases. Rosenfeld and colleagues[118] evaluated the accuracy of intraoperative TEE in 86 children and found the accuracy varied with different lesions. TEE overestimated the severity of right ventricular outflow tract obstruction in

13% of the cases compared with directly measured operative and postoperative pressure gradients. TEE was shown to be a reliable predictor of postoperative ventricular septal defects, aortic and mitral regurgitation, and mitral stenosis.[118] Complications with TEE are infrequent. Although TEE has been shown not to interfere with mechanical ventilation in infants weighing 2 to 5 kg, ventilation should be monitored continuously.[4] The probe should be manipulated carefully to avoid undesired extubation. Abnormalities were noted in the esophagus of 64% of 50 patients after TEE, more commonly in smaller patients (<9 kg). No long-term feeding issues were noted.[56] See Chapter 17 for a full description of echocardiography techniques and uses.

PULSE OXIMETRY

Pulse oximetry is monitored continuously in all critically ill patients. The pulse oximeter measures arterial oxygen saturation (SaO_2) from the pulsatile delivery of oxygenated blood. It is a continuous, noninvasive monitor of oxygenation that can readily detect reductions in oxygenation due to pulmonary complications or to inadequate perfusion. It has been found to be superior to either the capnograph or clinical judgment in providing early warning of desaturation events.[32]

The pulse oximeter probe is usually placed on the fingers, toes, or earlobes or over the nose. In small infants it can be placed across the hand or the foot. Studies have shown that accurate measurements are also obtained when the sensor is placed on the tongue or cheek.[31,112] Reynolds and associates[112] showed that cheek and tongue sensors detected both desaturation and resaturation earlier than peripherally placed sensors.

Pulse oximetry works on the principle of infrared absorbance of blood at two wavelengths (660 nm and 940 nm) as it passes through the capillary bed. Microprocessors subtract the nonpulsatile absorption from the signal. Since the pulse oximeters analyze two wavelengths, only two forms of hemoglobin are assayed: oxyhemoglobin and reduced hemoglobin. The saturation is calculated as [oxyhemoglobin]/[reduced+oxyhemoglobin]. Falsely high saturations occur when carboxyhemoglobin or methemoglobin is present. Co-oximetry can distinguish these dyshemoglobins because multiple wavelengths are used.

Pulse oximetry readings of SaO_2 are considered accurate and reliable in the range of 90% to 100%. However, several studies have shown that at low levels of saturation (SaO_2 below 80%), pulse oximetry is not as accurate as at higher saturations and overestimates the true value (Fig. 19-15).[119] The higher hemoglobin level of children with cyanotic heart disease does not appear to be responsible for the inaccuracy.[119] Clinicians must keep this fact in mind when using pulse oximetry to estimate the adequacy of pulmonary blood flow in infants with single ventricle and (Blalock-Taussig) shunt-dependent pulmonary blood flow.

The reliability of oximetry in children being rewarmed after hypothermic CPB was examined by Macnab and colleagues,[88] who compared pulse oximeter readings using the Ohmeda Biox 3700 with simultaneous hemoximeter (OSM-2, Radiometer) readings. They found the pulse oximeter tested to be reliable in these children with core temperatures as low as 31° C.

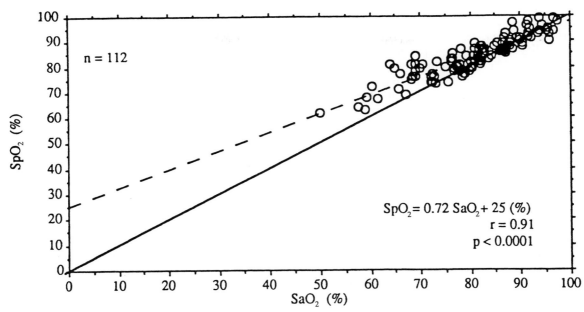

FIGURE 19-15   Comparison of arterial oxygen saturations measured with the pulse oximeter (SpO_2) and CO-oximeter (SaO_2). The *solid line* is the line of identity; the *dashed line* represents linear regression of 112 simultaneous measurements. At SaO_2 <80%, pulse oximetry overestimates true systemic arterial O_2 saturation in patients with cyanotic heart disease. (From Schmitt HJ, Schuetz WH, Proeschel PA, Jaklin C: Accuracy of pulse oximetry in children with congenital heart disease. *J Thorac Cardiovasc Anesth* 7:61–65, 1993; with permission.)

Other causes of inaccurate pulse oximeter readings include the use of intravenous methylene blue, extraneous operating room lights or infrared lights, patient movement, and electrocautery. Complications of pulse oximetry stem from the use of the finger clamp design of oximeter probe, which has been reported to cause ischemic finger injury.[28] The advantages, however, far outweigh the disadvantages, and the pulse oximeter is considered an essential monitor in the management of patients undergoing cardiac surgery.

CENTRAL NERVOUS SYSTEM MONITORING

Evaluation of the central nervous system is a natural interest during and after cardiac surgery. Indications of inadequate brain protection, perfusion, or oxygen delivery can hasten appropriate therapy. Austin and colleagues[7] did a retrospective cohort study of the potential benefit of interventions based on intraoperative neurophysiologic monitoring in pediatric patients undergoing the repair of congenital cardiac abnormalities. Specifically, they evaluated the impact of electroencephalography (EEG), transcranial Doppler (TCD) ultrasonic measurement of middle cerebral artery blood flow velocity, and transcranial near-infrared cerebral oximetry on postoperative neurologic sequelae and length of stay. Significant changes in brain perfusion or metabolism were noted in 70% of the 250 patients, with 74% of those changes resulting in alterations in management. This retrospective study showed a reduction in length of stay and neurologic sequelae with the use of these types of monitoring.

Although quite bulky in the operating room, EEG can demonstrate electrical activity associated with cerebral metabolism in patients undergoing deep hypothermia or total

circulatory arrest. A nonisoelectric EEG suggests inadequate brain protection in these conditions and may prompt additional therapy such as additional cooling or a barbiturate. In the Boston transposition study, EEG seizures during the perioperative period were found in 20% of the infants, compared to clinical seizures in 6% of the infants.[61]

Transcranial Doppler is a noninvasive, continuous monitor that demonstrates changes in velocity and blood flow (assuming constant artery diameter) in the cerebral arteries[116] as well as the detection of emboli.[115] It is limited by difficulty in reproducibility and by inaccurate signals with patient movement. Variation with operators also has a large influence on the results.

In the quest to balance the oxygen supply and demand to the brain, oxygen utilization can be assessed by jugular bulb saturations or regional cerebral oxygen saturations.[37] Correlation between jugular bulb saturations and cerebral oximetry by infrared spectroscopy was better in infants ($r = 0.85$) than children ($r = 0.57$).[37] Near-infrared spectroscopy (NIRS) can be used to monitor cerebrovascular hemoglobin oxygen saturations. It is portable and noninvasive and is influenced by cerebral blood flow, blood oxygen saturation, and the rate of cerebral oxygen consumption.[83] However, it has not been proven to be a reliable intraoperative monitor during congenital heart surgery.[96]

ACID-BASE MANAGEMENT

Many of the pediatric cardiac surgical procedures performed with the aid of CPB utilize hypothermia with the objective of decreasing tissue oxygen demands. The most extreme application of this maneuver is seen during total circulatory arrest when the patient's temperature may be decreased to less than

20° C (deep hypothermic circulatory arrest [DHCA]). A specific approach to acid-base management during hypothermia is not universally accepted. This likely reflects the multiple variables (including the specific approach to acid-base management) that may influence a predetermined measured parameter, rendering it difficult to determine the significance of any specific variable in a clinical setting. There is now considerable evidence (biochemical, comparative physiologic) to suggest that there may be a preferred method of acid-base management in homeothermic tissue subjected to the pathophysiologic condition of hypothermia. However, definitive clinical recommendations remain elusive. Acid-base management during hypothermia requires an understanding of (1) the influence of temperature on the pH of neutrality of H_2O (pNH$_2$O), the pKa of physiologically important buffer systems (e.g., imidazole), and the solubility and partial pressure of blood gases (e.g., carbon dioxide); (2) the differing acid-base control mechanisms in homeotherms (endotherms), ectotherms, and hibernators; (3) the rationale for the "alphastat" approach to acid-base management; and (4) the available laboratory and clinical data.

Influence of Temperature on pNH$_2$O, pKa, and Partial Pressure of Blood Gases

This is best understood by considering two H_2O molecules (Fig. 19-16). In an aqueous medium, there is a finite tendency for the hydrogen atom to break its covalent bond with the oxygen atom of its native water molecule and form a covalent bond with the oxygen atom of the adjacent water molecule. This results in the formation of a hydronium (H_3O^+) ion (although often incorrectly referred to as a hydrogen [H^+] ion) and a hydroxyl (OH^-) ion (see Fig. 19-16). There will always be an equal number of H_3O^+ and OH^- ions formed; thus there will always be a state of electric neutrality. If, at 25°C, one actually measures (via conductivity experiments) the number of H_3O^+ ions (and thus by inference the number of OH^- ions) present, one finds that there are 1×10^{-7} H_3O^+ ions per liter of aqueous solution. The negative logarithm (i.e., the pH) of $1 \times 10^{-7} = 7.0$. Hence the pH of neutrality (equal numbers of positive and negative charges) of water (pNH$_2$O) at 25°C is 7.0 pH units. If one facilitates the formation of H_3O^+ (and OH^-) ions (e.g., by increasing the thermal energy available, i.e., increasing the temperature), the pH will decrease; however, the state of electrical neutrality is preserved. The converse occurs with a decrease in temperature. Thus there is an inverse relationship between pNH$_2$O and temperature:

$$pNH_2O \propto \frac{1}{T}$$

where T = temperature.

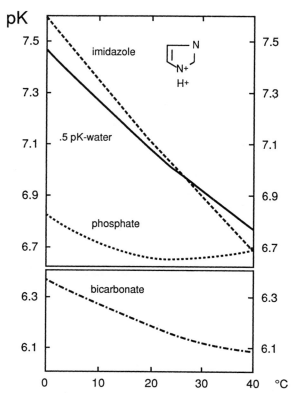

FIGURE 19-17 Changes in the dissociation constant, pK of CO_2-bicarbonate, phosphate, and imidazole with temperature. The 0.5 pK of water, or neutrality, is also shown. (From Rahn H, Reeves RB, Howell BJ: Hydrogen ion regulation, temperature, and evolution. *Am Rev Respir Dis* 112:165–172, 1975; with permission.)

Influence of Temperature on pKa of Buffers

The concepts just discussed can be extended to any acid and its conjugate base, including buffer systems, because buffers by definition are weak acids and bases. A buffer is most likely to exert an important physiologic role if it has a pKa near the intracellular pH. Histidine (a basic amino acid) is an important component of proteins and enzymes, and its imidazole ring is recognized as the single most important intracellular buffer. Imidazole has a pKa of 6.8. However, as with pNH$_2$O, there is an inverse relationship between the pKa of imidazole and temperature (Fig. 19-17).

INFLUENCE OF TEMPERATURE ON PARTIAL PRESSURE OF BLOOD GASES

There is a direct relationship between temperature and the partial pressure of blood gases (oxygen and carbon dioxide). The partial pressure of carbon dioxide decreases with a decrease

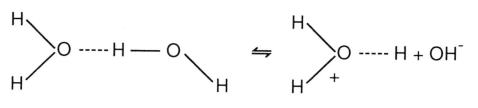

FIGURE 19-16 Ionization of water. A hydrogen atom breaks its covalent bond from one water molecule and attaches to another, resulting in the formation of one positive charge (hydronium/hydrogen ion) and one negative charge (hydroxyl ion).

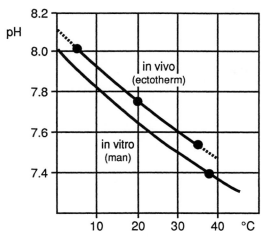

FIGURE 19-18 The pH values of human blood when removed at 37° C and cooled or warmed in vitro, compared with the similar in vivo behavior of an ectotherm acclimated to various body temperatures. (From Rahn H, Reeves RB, Howell BJ: Hydrogen ion regulation, temperature, and evolution. *Am Rev Respir Dis* 112:165–172, 1975; with permission.)

in temperature for a number of reasons, including (1) an increase in gas solubility with a decrease in temperature and (2) changes in the pKa of the carbamino and bicarbonate systems with temperature.

Acid-Base Control in Ectotherms, Hibernators, and Mammalian (Homeothermic) Blood during Hypothermia

The influence of temperature on the pH and PCO_2 of ectotherms is shown in Figures 19-18 and 19-19, respectively. The pH and PCO_2 increase and decrease, respectively, with a decrease in temperature in a manner predicted from basic physiologic principles (see previous discussion and Table 19-8). Also illustrated in Figures 19-18 and 19-19 is the behavior of human blood under in vitro conditions; it can be seen that human blood behaves qualitatively and quantitatively similarly to the behavior observed in vivo in ectotherms.

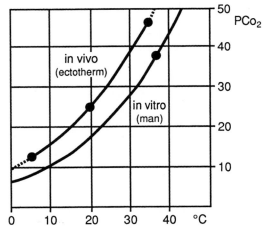

FIGURE 19-19 PCO_2 values of human blood when removed at 37° C and cooled or warmed in vitro, compared with the similar in vivo behavior of an ectotherm acclimated to various body temperatures. (From Rahn H, Reeves RB, Howell BJ: Hydrogen ion regulation, temperature, and evolution. *Am Rev Respir Dis* 112:165–172, 1975; with permission.)

Table 19-8 Differences between Alpha–Stat and pH–Stat ABG Measurements

	Normothermia	Hypothermia–pH-Stat	Hypothermia–Alpha-Stat
pH	7.4	7.4	>7.4
PCO$_2$ (mm Hg)	40	40	<40

The decrease in PCO_2 with temperature in conjunction with the leftward shift in the CO_2 dissociation curve has the net effect of maintaining the total CO_2 content as a constant (Fig. 19-20).

Rationale Behind "Alpha-Stat"

Imidazole is an important intracellular buffer because it is a building block for proteins and enzymes and because it has a pKa (at 37° C) of 6.8 (close to intracellular pH). Alpha (α) is the term used to define the degree of dissociation of imidazole. Specifically, it is defined as the ratio of unprotonated to total imidazole (e.g., in an alkaline environment, all the imidazole buffer is unprotonated and its alpha number will be 1.0). In the region of "normal" intracellular pH, imidazole exists in both proton donor and proton acceptor forms; that is, it has an alpha number between 0 and 1.0. Moreover its precise alpha number will be profoundly influenced by even small changes in pH, because at intracellular pH it is on the steep part of its dissociation curve (see Fig. 19-20).

In addition to the ambient pH changing the alpha number of imidazole at any specific temperature, changes in temperature per se change not only the ambient pH but the pKa of the imidazole buffer system (see previous discussion). In homeothermic tissue subjected to hypothermia in vitro, the

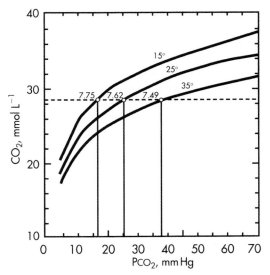

FIGURE 19-20 Carbon dioxide (CO_2) dissociation curves of oxygenated blood of the turtle, *Pseudemys scripta*, at three temperatures. Arterial pH and associated PCO_2 values observed in intact animals are shown. Note that the total CO_2 content of blood is maintained at a constant level. PCO$_2$, partial pressure of carbon dioxide. (From White RN, Weinstein Y: Carbon dioxide transport and acid-base balance during hypothermia. In Utley JR [ed]: *Pathophysiology and Techniques of Cardiopulmonary Bypass.* Baltimore, Williams and Wilkins, 1983; with permission.)

pNH_2O, the pKa of imidazole, and tissue pH change in a qualitatively and quantitatively similar manner, so the tendency for imidazole to remain protonated or unprotonated remains constant. Hence the alpha number of imidazole remains constant (alpha-stat condition). If, in contrast, during hypothermia the pH is kept constant (e.g., indirectly by keeping blood pH constant, pH-stat), the alpha number of imidazole is altered and thus potentially the function of proteins and enzymes of which it is an important component is altered as well. Indeed there is evidence that several enzymes do in fact exhibit this phenomenon.[148] This is probably the result of improved metabolic suppression/recovery with alpha-stat. See Chapter 20 on "Cardiopulmonary Bypass" for further discussion of alpha-stat versus pH-stat blood gas management strategies during hypothermia.

Laboratory and Clinical Information

As stated at the outset, there is no universally accepted method of acid-base management during hypothermia. However, there is increasing (though not necessarily definitive) laboratory and clinical information indicating that the alpha-stat method of acid-base management may be preferred during hypothermia (at least in adults).

Studies of the distribution of radiolabeled chloride across the red blood cell membrane, and the resultant hematocrit level, indicate that chlorine distribution and red blood cell volume are maintained stable if the pH is allowed to increase with a decrease in temperature.[110] In vitro studies of myocardium indicate the deleterious effects of respiratory acidosis (pH = 7.4 and PCO_2 = 40 representing increasing levels of respiratory acidosis as the temperature drops below 37° C) on myocardial function.[105] In contrast other workers[126] failed to show an influence of pH (irrespective of temperature) in isolated blood perfused left ventricles; however, the temperature range was modest (37° C to 27° C). In a controlled laboratory study, Becker and coworkers[13] compared the alpha- and pH-stat methods of acid-base management during hypothermia. Their results indicate a preferred influence of alpha-stat on total and regional cerebral blood flow, electric and mechanical heart function, regional organ blood flow, and myocardial and regional lactate metabolism.

The more recently available clinical data indicating a preferred method of acid-base management during hypothermia are potentially confusing. This is partly related to the differential results in adults versus children. Indeed this observation likely reflects the differing mechanisms underlying neurological injury during cardiac surgery procedures in these two groups. In adults neurological injury is usually secondary to thromboembolic phenomena, whereas in children relative hypoperfusion predominates as a mechanism of injury. Other factors should also be considered when interpreting studies comparing pH-stat and alpha-stat. These include the following:

1. The influence of age on cerebral vasoreactivity. It has been clearly demonstrated that the cerebrovascular response to CO_2 is blunted in infants younger than 1 year of age.[75]
2. Deep hypothermia, per se, also blunts the cerebrovascular response to CO_2.
3. During moderate hypothermia, an alpha-stat approach preserves, but a pH approach blunts, cerebral autoregulation.[53,68,69]

4. Deep hypothermia blunts cerebral autoregulation irrespective of pH management.[54]
5. The differential influence of a pH-stat strategy versus an alpha-stat strategy on cerebral blood flow and thus on the disposition to cooling of deep cerebral structures, and metabolic suppression/recovery (as assessed by cerebral metabolic rate for oxygen [$CMRO_2$]). A pH-stat approach promotes cerebral blood flow and brain cooling. An alpha-stat approach improves metabolic suppression/recovery compared to a pH-stat approach.
6. The relationship between the pH outside versus inside the cell, and the ability/inability of cell membranes to preserve this transmembrane gradient under the prevailing conditions.

Regarding adults, three studies[95,101,131] have looked at neurological outcome and have clearly shown that neurological outcome is improved in patients who are managed with an alpha-stat approach, compared to those managed with a pH-stat approach. However, the data in children are less clear. One small clinical study suggests that a pH-stat approach is preferable.[45] Thus one is left to look also at animal studies and nonoutcome variables, for example, cerebral blood flow and $CMRO_2$, to try to determine the best approach in children. Taken together, these studies would support an approach that promotes efficient cooling of all cerebral structures, including deep cerebral structures (i.e., a pH-stat approach) and efficient arrest and recovery of metabolic mechanisms (i.e., an alpha-stat approach).[6,179] This has prompted some to recommend a crossover strategy (perhaps especially if profound hypothermia is used) utilizing a pH-stat approach management strategy while cooling and, once cooled, changing to an alpha-stat approach.[39,75] (See Chapter 20 for discussion of combined alpha-stat and pH-stat approach.)

RESPIRATORY GAS AND ANESTHETIC MONITORING

Capnography is the continuous display of the instantaneous carbon dioxide concentration in the breathing circuit. It is indicated in all intubated, mechanically ventilated patients. Capnography has become essential in providing immediate, accurate evidence of successful (or unsuccessful) endotracheal intubation. The display can validate the numeric result as well as provide information. Decrease in end-tidal CO_2 ($ETCO_2$) can be associated with circuit malfunction (disconnect or obstruction), acute or chronic air trapping diseases, pulmonary embolism, poor cardiac output, shunt, or overventilation. Increases in $ETCO_2$ can occur with hypoventilation, endobronchial intubation, increases in temperature, or early signs of malignant hyperthermia. The usual difference between $PaCO_2$ and $ETCO_2$ is 3 to 5 mm Hg.[42]

Normally, one third (30%) of each breath takes no part in gas exchange and is dead space ventilation. The presence of an endotracheal tube increases the total dead space to 46%, and patients with controlled breathing using a mask have a dead space of 64%.[70] The effects of increased dead space can usually be corrected by increasing the respiratory minute volume. The total dead space normally increases with age. If the end-tidal CO_2 is lower than the $PaCO_2$, this is evidence of dead space ventilation, which may be due to decreased pulmonary blood flow from right-to-left shunts, hypotension, excessive airway pressure with increased zone 1 ventilation, or pulmonary embolus.

TEMPERATURE

Temperature is measured at several sites in patients undergoing cardiac surgery. The most commonly used sites in the operating room include the pulmonary artery (via pulmonary artery catheter thermistor), nasopharynx, esophagus, rectum, skin, and bladder (via the urinary catheter). An accurate core temperature can also be measured by a probe placed at the tympanic membrane. In general the core temperature represents the temperature of the vital organs. Peripheral temperature is measured by rectal and skin temperature probes.

During cardiopulmonary bypass, the temperature of the heat exchanger is measured in the pump arterial line. This represents the lowest temperature during cooling and the highest during rewarming. The pump venous line temperature (blood returning from the patient) represents the general core temperature during CPB.

When there are rapid changes in blood temperature during CPB, a gradient will exist between the core and peripheral temperatures. This occurs because the vessel-rich organs receive a greater proportion of the blood flow, so at the time CPB is discontinued the core temperature may be 2° C to 5° C higher than the rectal or skin temperature. The core heat then dissipates to the cooler periphery, so the temperature upon arrival at the ICU is often closer to the lower peripheral temperature at the time CPB was discontinued. For mild hypothermia (rectal temperature approximately 36.0° C) gradual spontaneous warming in the ICU is satisfactory. More profoundly hypothermic patients (rectal temperature less than 35.5° C) are warmed with a convection blanket or a radiant warmer.

URINARY OUTPUT

Urinary output is measured in all patients undergoing cardiac surgery. An acceptable output (0.5 to 1 mL/kg/hr) is under most circumstances a reliable indication of adequate renal perfusion, and thus cardiac output and blood volume. A decrease in urinary output (oliguria) can occur in patients during cardiac surgery owing to hypothermia, total circulatory arrest, low cardiac output, or lack of pulsatile flow during CPB. When the patient is rewarmed and pulsatile flow restored, urinary output returns to normal in most cases. The volatile anesthetics are known to depress renal function, but the effects are transient and reversible after these agents are discontinued. Some institutions include mannitol in the CPB prime. This may produce a diuresis for several hours after surgery. Conversely, oliguria during the first 24 to 48 hours after cardiac surgery may occur even in the presence of normal cardiac output. Such oliguria presumably reflects the transient ischemia or inflammatory injury to the kidney that occurred during CPB. Diuretic administration (typically furosemide) counteracts the salt and water retention and resulting edema that arise during the oliguric phase of the postoperative course.

Hemolysis may occur during CPB and is usually treated with additional diuretics and fluid to avoid damage to renal tubules. If the urine is allowed to become concentrated in the face of hemolysis, hematin precipitation can occur within the renal tubules, and the patient is at risk of acute renal failure. If hemolysis develops subsequent to a blood transfusion, the possibility of a transfusion reaction must be ruled out.

CONCLUSION

Integration of the information obtained from sophisticated monitoring improves and supplements clinical judgment. No single parameter can be correctly understood in isolation. Poor capillary refill, poor pulses, cold extremities, and poor urinary output paint a grim picture regardless of the blood pressure or normal "filling" pressures. An understanding of the patterns of hemodynamic response is necessary to interpret the information obtained by perioperative monitoring. The clinical setting and the results of clinical examination of the child must be known to interpret data obtained during monitoring.

References

1. Abel FL, McCutcheon EF: *Cardiovascular Function: Principles and Application.* Boston, Little, Brown, 1979.
2. Allen EV: Thromboangiitis obliterans: Methods of diagnosis of chronic occlusive arterial lesions distal to the wrist with illustrated cases. *Am J Med Sci* 178:237, 1929.
3. Alverson DC, Eldridge M, Dillon T, et al: Noninvasive pulsed Doppler determination of cardiac output in neonates and children. *J Pediatr* 101:46–50, 1982.
4. Andropoulos DB, Ayres NA, Stayer SA, et al: The effect of transesophageal echocardiography on ventilation in small infants undergoing cardiac surgery. *Anesth Analg* 90:47–49, 2000.
5. Andropoulos DB, Stayer SA, Bent ST, et al: A controlled study of transesophageal echocardiography to guide central venous catheter placement in congenital heart surgery patients. *Anesth Analg* 89:65–70, 1999.
6. Aoki M, Nomura F, Stromski ME, et al: Effects of pH on brain energetics after hypothermic circulatory arrest. *Ann Thorac Surg* 55:1093–1103, 1993.
7. Austin EH III, Edmond HL Jr, Auden SM, et al: Benefit of neurophysiologic monitoring for pediatric cardiac surgery. *J Thorac Cardiovasc Surg* 114:707–715, 1997.
8. Bailey RH, Bauer JH, Yanos J: Accuracy of disposable blood pressure transducers used in the critical care setting. *Crit Care Med* 23:187–192, 1995.
9. Barr PO: Percutaneous puncture of the radial artery with a multipurpose Teflon catheter for indwelling use. *Acta Physiol Scand* 51:343, 1961.
10. Barrington KJ: Umbilical artery catheters in the newborn: Effects on position of the catheter tip. *Cochrane Database Syst Rev* CD000505, 2000.
11. Barry BN, Mallick A, Bodenham AR, Vucevic M: Lack of agreement between bioimpedance and continuous thermodilution measurement of cardiac output in intensive care unit patients. *Crit Care* 1:71–74, 1997.
12. Bause GS, Weintraub AC, Tanner GE: Skin avulsion during oscillometry. *J Clin Monit* 2:262–263, 1986.
13. Becker H, Vinten-Johansen J, Buckberg GD, et al: Myocardial damage caused by keeping pH 7.40 during systemic deep hypothermia. *J Thorac Cardiovasc Surg* 82:810–821, 1981.
14. Bedford RF: Invasive blood pressure monitoring. In Blitt CD (ed): *Monitoring in Anesthesia and Critical Care Medicine.* New York, Churchill Livingstone, 1990.
15. Bedford RF: Long-term radial artery cannulation: Effects on subsequent vessel function. *Crit Care Med* 6:64–67, 1978.
16. Bedford RF: Radial arterial function following percutaneous cannulation with 18- and 20-gauge catheters. *Anesthesiology* 47:37–39, 1977.
17. Bedford RF, Major MC: Percutaneous radial-artery cannulation: Increased safety using Teflon catheters. *Anesthesiology* 42:219–222, 1975.
18. Bedford RF, Shah NK: Blood pressure monitoring: Invasive and noninvasive. In Blitt CD, Hines RL (ed): *Monitoring in Anesthesia and Critical Care Medicine:* New York, Churchill Livingstone, 1995, 3rd ed, pp 95–130.

19. Blayney MR, Malins AF, Cooper GM: Cardiac arrythmias in children during outpatient general anaesthesia for dentistry: A prospective randomised trial. *Lancet* 354:1864–1866, 1999.

20. Bridge PM, Lerhaupt K, Armstrong MB: Recurrent radial artery aneurysm in a five-month-old infant. *J Natl Med Assoc* 92:309–311, 2000.

21. Brinton TJ, Walls ED, Yajnik AK, Chio S: Age-based differences between mercury sphygmomanometer and pulse dynamic blood pressure measurements. *Blood Press Monit* 3:125–129, 1998.

22. Bruner JM, Krenis LJ, Kunsman JM, Sherman AP: Comparison of direct and indirect methods of measuring arterial blood pressure, part III. *Med Instrum* 15:182–188, 1981.

23. Bur A, Hirschl MM, Herkner H, et al: Accuracy of oscillometric blood pressure measurement according to the relation between cuff size and upper-arm circumference in critically ill patients. *Crit Care Med* 28:371–376, 2000.

24. Castor G, Molter G, Helms J, et al: Determination of cardiac output during positive end-expiratory pressure: Noninvasive electrical bioimpedance compared with standard thermodilution. *Crit Care Med* 18:544–546, 1990.

25. Cederholm I, Sorensen J, Carlsson C: Thrombosis following percutaneous radial artery cannulation. *Acta Anaesthesiol Scand* 30:227–230, 1986.

26. Cetta F, Graham LC, Eidem BW: Gaining vascular access in pediatric patients: Use of the P.D. Access Doppler needle. *Catheter Cardiovasc Interv* 51:61–64, 2000.

27. Chauhan S, Saxena N, Mehrotra S, et al: Femoral artery pressures are more reliable than radial artery pressures on initiation of cardiopulmonary bypass. *J Cardiothorac Vasc Anesth* 14:274–276, 2000.

28. Chemello PD, Nelson SR, Wolford LM: Finger injury resulting from pulse oximeter probe during orthognathic surgery. *Oral Surg Oral Med Oral Pathol* 69:161–163, 1990.

29. Chiang LK, Dunn, AE: Cardiology. In Siberry GK, Iannone R (eds): *The Harriet Lane Handbook*, 15th ed. St. Louis, Mosby, 2000, p 141.

30. Cilley RE: Arterial access in infants and children. *Semin Pediatr Surg* 1:174–180, 1992.

31. Cote CJ, Daniels AL, Connolly M, et al: Tongue oximetry in children with extensive thermal injury: Comparison with peripheral oximetry. *Can J Anaesth* 39:454–457, 1992.

32. Cote CJ, Rolf N, Liu LM, et al: A single-blind study of combined pulse oximetry and capnography in children. *Anesthesiology* 74:980–987, 1991.

33. Crapanzano MS, Strong WB, Newman IR, et al: Calf blood pressure: Clinical implications and correlations with arm blood pressure in infants and young children. *Pediatrics* 97:220–224, 1996.

34. Cripps TP, Edmondson RS: Isoflurane for anesthesia in the dental chair: A comparison of the incidence of cardiac dysrhythmias during anaesthesia with halothane and isoflurane. *Anaesthesia* 42:189–191, 1987.

35. Dahlgren G, Veintemilla F, Settergren G, Liska J: Left ventricular end-systolic pressure estimated from measurements in a peripheral artery. *J Cardiothorac Vasc Anesth* 5:551–553, 1991.

36. Damen J: Positive bacterial cultures and related risk factors associated with percutaneous internal jugular vein catheterization in pediatric cardiac patients. *Anesthesiology* 66:558–562, 1987.

37. Daubeney PE, Pilkington SN, Janke E, et al: Cerebral oxygenation measured by near-intrared spectroscopy: Comparison with jugular bulb oximetry. *Ann Thorac Surg* 61:930–934, 1996.

38. Davis FM, Stewart JM: Radial artery cannulation: A prospective study in patients undergoing cardiothoracic surgery. *Br J Anaesth* 52:41–47, 1980.

39. Davies LK: Cardiopulmonary bypass in infants and children: How is it different? *J Cardiothorac Vasc Anesth* 13:330–345, 1999.

40. De Hert SG, Vermeyen M, Moens MM, et al: Central-to-peripheral arterial-pressure gradient during cardiopulmonary bypass: Relation to pre- and intra-operative data and effects of vasoactive agents. *Acta Anaesthesiol Scand* 38:479–485, 1994.

41. De Jong JR, Ros HH, De Lange JJ: Noninvasive continuous blood pressure measurement during anaesthesia: A clinical evaluation of a method commonly used in measuring devices. *Int J Clin Monit Comput* 12:1–10, 1995.

42. Desiderio DP: Intraoperative monitoring. *Chest Surg Clin N Am* 7:721–733, 1997.

43. Downs JB, Rackstein AD, Klein EF Jr, Hawkins IF Jr: Hazards of radial-artery catheterization. *Anesthesiology* 38:283–286, 1973.

44. Dumas C, Wahr JA, Tremper KK: Clinical evaluation of a prototype motion artifact resistant pulse oximeter in the recovery room. *Anesth Analg* 83:269–272, 1996.

45. DuPlessis AJ, Jonas RA, Wypij D, et al: Perioperative effects of alpha-stat versus pH-stat strategies for deep hypothermic cardiopulmonary bypass in infants. *J Thorac Cardiovasc Surg* 114:990–1001, 1997.

46. Freed MD, Keane JF: Cardiac output measured by thermodilution in infants and children. *J Pediatr* 92:39–42, 1978.

47. Fratacci MD, Payen D, Beloucif S, Laborde F: Doppler cardiac-output and left-ventricular performance after cardiac surgery: Pulsed Doppler ascending aorta and pulmonary blood flows and left-ventricular function using implanted microprobes. *Chest* 101:380–386, 1992.

48. Fuhrman TM, Reilley TE, Pippin WD: Comparison of digital blood pressure, plethysmography, and the modified Allen's test as means of evaluating the collateral circulation to the hand. *Anaesthesia* 47:959–961, 1992.

49. Furfaro S, Gauthier M, Lacroix J, et al: Arterial catheter-related infections in children: A 1-year cohort analysis. *Am J Dis Child* 145:1037–1043, 1991.

50. Fyfe DA, Ritter SB, Snider AR, et al: Guidelines for transesophageal echocardiography in children. *J Am Soc Echocardiogr* 5:640–644, 1992.

51. Gravenstein JS, Paulus DA: *Monitoring Practice in Clinical Anesthesia*. Philadelphia, JB Lippincott, 1982.

52. Graves PW, Davis AL, Maggi JC, Nussbaum E: Femoral artery cannulation for monitoring in critically ill children: Prospective study. *Crit Care Med* 18:1363–1366, 1990.

53. Greeley WJ, Ungerleider RM, Kern FH, et al: Effects of cardiopulmonary bypass on cerebral blood flow in neonates, infants, and children. *Circulation* 80:I209–I215, 1989.

54. Greeley WJ, Ungerleider RM, Smith LR, Reves JG: The effects of deep hypothermic cardiopulmonary bypass and total circulatory arrest on cerebral blood flow in infants and children. *J Thorac Cardiovasc Surg* 97:737–745, 1989.

55. Green C, Yohannan MD: Umbilical arterial and venous catheters: Placement, use, and complications. *Neonatal Netw* 17:23–28, 1998.

56. Greene MA, Alexander JA, Knauf DG, et al: Endoscopic evaluation of the esophagus in infants and children immediately following intraoperative use of transesophageal echocardiography. *Chest* 116:1247–1250, 1999.

57. Hack WW, Vos A, van der Lei J, Okken A: Incidence and duration of total occlusion of the radial artery in newborn infants after catheter removal. *Eur J Pediatr* 149:275–277, 1990.

58. Hamilton WF, Riley RL, Ahyah AM, et al: Comparison of the Fick and dye injection methods of measuring the cardiac output in man. *Am J Physiol* 153:309, 1948.

59. Hatch DJ, Sumner E: *Neonatal Anesthesia*. Chicago, Mosby–Year Book, 1981.

60. Hayashi Y, Uchida O, Takaki O, et al: Internal jugular vein catheterization in infants undergoing cardiovascular surgery: An analysis of the factors influencing successful catheterization. *Anesth Analg* 74:688–693, 1992.

61. Helmers SL, Wypij D, Constantinou JE, et al: Perioperative electroencephalographic seizures in infants undergoing repair of complex congenital heart defects. *Electroencephalogr Clin Neurophysiol* 102:27–36, 1997.

62. Horan MJ, Sinaiko AR: Synopsis of the report of the Second Task Force on Blood Pressure Control in Children. *Hypertension* 10:115–121, 1987.

63. Humas RA, Porter CJ, Puga FJ, et al: Utility of temporary atrial epicardial electrodes in postoperative pediatric cardiac patients. *Mayo Clin Proc* 64:516–521, 1989.

64. Imai T, Takahashi K, Fukura H, Morishita Y: Measurement of cardiac output by pulse dye densitometry using indocyanine green: A comparison with the thermodilution method. *Anesthesiology* 87:816–822, 1997.

65. Introna RPS, Martin DC, Pruett JK, et al: Percutaneous pulmonary artery catheterization in pediatric cardiovascular anesthesia: Insertion techniques and use. *Anesth Analg* 70:562–566, 1990.

66. Introna RP, Pruett JK, Crumrine RC, Cuadrado AR: Use of transthoracic bioimpedance to determine cardiac output in pediatric patients. *Crit Care Med* 16:1101–1105, 1988.

67. Jain U: An electrocardiographic lead system for coronary artery bypass surgery. *J Clin Anesth* 8:19–24, 1996.

68. Johnsson P, Messeter K, Ryding E, et al: Cerebral vasoreactivity to carbon dioxide during cardiopulmonary perfusion at normothermia and hypothermia. *Ann Thorac Surg* 48:769–775, 1989.

69. Johnsson P, Messeter K, Ryding E, et al: Cerebral blood flow and autoregulation during hypothermic cardiopulmonary bypass. *Ann Thorac Surg* 43:386–390, 1987.

70. Kain ML, Panday J, Nunn JF: The effect of intubation on the dead space during halothane anaesthesia. *Br J Anaesth* 41:94–103, 1969.

71. Kapusta L, Hopman JC, Daniels O: The agreement between pulmonary and systemic blood flow measurements in babies by dual beam Doppler echocardiography. *Eur Heart J* 12:112–116, 1991.

72. Keagy BA, Wilcox BR, Lucas CL, et al: Constant postoperative monitoring of cardiac output after correction of congenital heart defects. *J Thorac Cardiovasc Surg* 93:658–664, 1987.

73. Keenan RL, Shapiro JH, Kane FR, Simpson PM: Bradycardia during anesthesia in infants. An epidemiologic study. *Anesthesiology* 80:976–982, 1994.

74. Kennedy DJ, Royster RL: Electrocardiographic monitoring for arrhythmias. In Blitt CD, Hines RL (eds): *Monitoring in Anesthesia and Critical Care Medicine*, 3rd ed. New York, Churchill Livingstone, 1995, p 153.

75. Kern FH, Ungerleider RM, Quill TJ, et al: Cerebral blood flow response to changes in arterial carbon dioxide tension during hypothermic cardiopulmonary bypass in children. *J Thorac Cardiovasc Surg* 101:618–622, 1991.

76. Khambatta HJ, Stone JG, Wald A, Mongero LB: Electrocardiographic artifacts during cardiopulmonary bypass. *Anesth Analg* 71:88–91, 1990.

77. Kinefuchi Y, Fukuyama H, Suzuki T, et al: Development of a new catheter-tip pressure transducer. *Tokai J Exp Clin Med* 24:85–92, 1999.

78. Kirkendall WM, Feinleib M, Freis ED, Mark AL: Recommendations for human blood pressure determination by sphygmomanometers. Subcommittee of the AHA Postgraduate Education Committee. *Circulation* 62:1146A–1155A, 1980.

79. Kocis KC, Vermilion RP, Callow LB, et al: Complications of femoral artery cannulation for perioperative monitoring in children. *J Thorac Cardiovasc Surg* 112:1399–1400, 1996.

80. Kubicek WG, Karnegis JN, Patterson RP, et al: Development and evaluation of an impedance cardiac output system. *Aerosp Med* 37:1208–1212, 1966.

81. Kulkarni M, Elsner C, Ouellet D, Zeldin R: Heparinized saline versus normal saline in maintaining patency of the radial artery catheter. *Can J Surg* 37:37–42, 1994.

82. Kunk R, McCain GC: Comparison of upper arm and calf oscillometric blood pressure measurement in preterm infants. *J Perinatol* 16:89–92, 1996.

83. Kurth CD, Steven JM, Nicholson SC: Cerebral oxygenation during pediatric cardiac surgery using deep hypothermic circulatory arrest. *Anesthesiology* 82:74–82, 1995.

84. Lequier LL, Leonard SR, Nikaidoh H, et al: Extravascular Doppler measurement of cardiac output in infants and children after operations for congenital heart disease. *J Thorac Cardiovasc Surg* 117:1223–1225, 1999.

85. Leung JM, Voskanian A, Bellows WH, Pastor D: Automated electrocardiograph ST segment trending monitors: Accuracy in detecting myocardial ischemia. *Anesth Analg* 87:4–10, 1998.

86. Ling J, Ohara Y, Orime Y, et al: Clinical evaluatioin of the oscillometric blood pressure monitor in adults and children based on the 1992 AAMI SP-0 standards. *J Clin Monit* 11:123–130, 1995.

87. Lloyd TR, Donnerstein RL, Berg RA: Accuracy of central venous pressure measurement from the abdominal inferior vena cava. *Pediatrics* 89:506–508, 1992.

88. Macnab AJ, Baker-Brown G, Anderson EE: Oximetry in children recovering from deep hypothermia for cardiac surgery. *Crit Care Med* 18:1066–1069, 1990.

89. Mangano DT, Hickey RF: Ischemic injury following uncomplicated radial artery catheterization. *Anesth Analg* 58:55–57, 1979.

90. Marks LA, Groch A: Optimizing cuff width for noninvasive measurement of blood pressure. *Blood Press Monit* 5:151–152, 2000.

91. Marshall AG, Erwin DC, Wyse RK, Hatch DJ: Percutaneous arterial cannulation in children. Concurrent and subsequent adequacy of blood flow at the wrist. *Anaesthesia* 39:27–31, 1984.

92. Metz RI, Lucking SE, Chaten FC, et al: Percutaneous catheterization of the axillary vein in intants and children. *Pediatrics* 85:531–533, 1990.

93. Millar CL, Burrows FA: Invasive monitoring in the pediatric patient. *Int Anesthesiol Clin* 30:91–108, 1992.

94. Muhiudeen IA, Kuecherer HF, Lee E, et al: Intraoperative estimation of cardiac output by transesophageal pulsed Doppler echocardiography. *Anesthesiology* 74:9–14, 1991.

95. Murkin JM, Martzke JS, Buchan AM, et al: A randomized study of the influence of perfusion technique and pH management strategy in 316 patients undergoing coronary artery bypass surgery. II. Neurologic and cognitive outcomes. *J Thorac Cardiovasc Surg* 110:349–362, 1995.

96. Nollert G, Shin'oka T, Jonas RA: Near-infrared spectrophotometry of the brain in cardiovascular surgery. *Thorac Cardiovasc Surg* 46:167–175, 1998.

97. Norwood SH, Cormier B, McMahon NG, et al: Prospective study of catheter-related infection during prolonged arterial catheterization. *Crit Care Med* 16:836–839, 1988.

98. Ochiari H, Miyazaki N, Miyata T, et al: Assessment of the accuracy of indirect blood pressure measurements. *Jpn Heart J* 38:393–407, 1997.

99. O'Rourke RA: The measurement of systemic blood pressure: Normal and abnormal pulsations of the arteries and veins. In Hurst JW (ed): *The Heart*. New York, McGraw-Hill, 1990, pp 149–162.

100. Papadopoulos G, Miede S, Elisaf M: Assessment of the performances of three oscillometric blood pressure monitors for neonates using a simulator. *Blood Press Monit* 4:27–33, 1999.

101. Patel RL, Turtle MR, Chambers DJ, et al: Alpha-stat acid-base regulation during cardiopulmonary bypass improves neuropsychologic outcome in patients undergoing coronary artery bypass grafting. *J Thorac Cardiovasc Surg* 111:1267–1279, 1996.

102. Perrino AC Jr: Cardiac output monitoring by echocardiography: Should we pass on Swan-Ganz catheters? *Yale J Biol Med* 66:397–413, 1993.

103. Peterson RJ, Kissoon N, Bayne EJ, et al: Transtracheal Doppler in infants and small children following surgery for congenital heart disease: Rational use of an improved technology. *Crit Care Med* 22:1294–1300, 1994.

104. Pillow K, Herrick IA: Pulse oximetry compared with Doppler ultrasound for assessment of collateral blood flow to the hand. *Anaesthesia* 46:388–390, 1991.

105. Poole-Wilson PA, Langer GA: Effect of pH on ionic exchange and function in rat and rabbit myocardium. *Am J Physiol* 229:570–581, 1975.

106. Pratila M, Pratilas V: Electrophysiologic effects of anesthetic agents. In Thys DM, Kaplan JA (eds): *The ECG in Anesthesia and Critical Care*. New York, Churchill Livingstone, 1987.

107. Raines DE, Hogue CW Jr, Wickens C, et al: Artifactual hypertension due to transducer cable malfunction. *Anesthesiology* 74:1149–1151, 1991.

108. Randolph AG, Cook DC, Gonzales CA, Andrew M: Benefit of heparin in peripheral venous and arterial catheters: Systematic review and meta-analysis of randomized controlled trials. *BMJ* 316:969–975, 1998.

109. Randolph AG, Cook DJ, Gonzales CA, Pribble CG: Ultrasound guidance for placement of central venous catheters: A meta-analysis of the literature. *Crit Care Med* 24:2053–2058, 1996.

110. Reeves RB: Temperature-induced changes in blood acid-base status: pH and PCO_2 in a binary buffer. *J Appl Physiol* 40:752–761, 1976.

111. Reich DL, Kaplan JA: Hemodynamic monitoring. In Kaplan JA (ed): *Cardiac Anesthesia*. Philadelphia, WB Saunders, 1993, pp 261–298.

112. Reynolds LM, Nicolson SC, Steven JM, et al: Influence of sensor site location on pulse oximetry kinetics in children. *Anesth Analg* 76:751–754, 1993.

113. Rhee KH, Berg RA: Antegrade cannulation of radial artery in infants and children. *Chest* 107:182–184, 1995.

114. Rich GF, Lubanski RE, McLoughlin TM: Differences between aortic and radial artery pressure associated with cardiopulmonary bypass. *Anesthesiology* 77:63–66, 1992.

115. Ringelstein EB, Droste DW, Babikian VL, et al: Consensus on microembolus detection by TCD. International Consensus Group on Microembolus Detection. *Stroke* 29:725–729, 1998.

116. Rodriguez RA, Hosking MC, Duncan WJ, et al: Cerebral blood flow velocities monitored by transcranial Doppler during cardiac catheterizations in children. *Cathet Cardiovasc Diagn* 43:282–290, 1998.

117. Rolf N, Cote CJ: Persistent cardiac arrhythmias in pediatric patients: Effects of age, expired carbon dioxide values, depth of anesthesia, and airway management. *Anesth Analg* 73:720–724, 1991.

118. Rosenfeld HM, Gentles TL, Wernovsky G, et al: Utility of intraoperative transesophageal echocardiography in the assessment of residual cardiac defects. *Pediatr Cardiol* 19:346–351, 1998.

119. Schmitt HJ, Schuetz WH, Proeschel PA, Jaklin C: Accuracy of pulse oximetry in children with cyanotic congenital heart disease. *J Cardiothorac Vasc Anesth* 7:61–65, 1993.

120. Schwartz KV, Garcia FG: Entanglement of Swan-Ganz catheter around an intracardiac structure. *JAMA* 237:1198–1199, 1977.

121. Seear MD, d'Orsogna L, Sandor GG, et al: Doppler-derived mean aortic flow velocity in children: An alternative to cardiac index. *Pediatr Cardiol* 12:197–200, 1991.

122. Sellden H, Nilsson K, Larsson LE, Ekstrom-Jobal B: Radial arterial catheters in children and neonates: A prospective study. *Crit Care Med* 15:1106–1109, 1987.

123. Shinozaki T, Deane RS, Mazuzan JE: The dynamic responses of liquid-filled catheter systems for direct measurements of blood pressure. *Anesthesiology* 53:498–504, 1980.

124. Siegel LC, Fitzgerald DC, Engstrom RH: Simultaneous intraoperative measurement of cardiac output by thermodilution and transtracheal Doppler. *Anesthesiology* 74:664–669, 1991.

125. Simpson JA, Jamieson G, Dickhaus DW, Grover RF: Effect of size of cuff bladder on accuracy of measurement of indirect blood pressure. *Am Heart J* 70:206, 1965.

126. Sinet M, Muffat-Joly M, Bendaace T, Pocidalo JJ: Maintaining blood pH at 7.4 during hypothermia has no significant effect on work of the isolated rat heart. *Anesthesiology* 62:582–587, 1985.

127. Siwik ES, Spector ML, Patel CR, Zahka KG: Costs and cost-effectiveness of routine transesophageal echocardiography in congenital heart surgery. *Am Heart J* 138:771–776, 1999.

128. Skaryak LA, Chai PJ, Kern FH, et al: Blood gas management and degree of cooling: Effects on cerebral metabolism before and after circulatory arrest. *J Thorac Cardiovasc Surg* 110:1649–1657, 1995.

129. Skinner JR, Milligan DW, Hunter S, Hey EN: Central venous pressure in the ventilated neonate. *Arch Dis Child* 67:374–377, 1992.

130. Spinale FG, Smith AC, Crawford FA: Relationship of bioimpedance to thermodilution and echocardiographic measurements of cardiac function. *Crit Care Med* 18:414–418, 1990.

131. Stephan H, Weyland A, Kazmaier S, et al: Acid-base management during hypothermic cardiopulmonary bypass does not affect cerebral metabolism but does affect blood flow and neurological outcome. *Br J Anaesth* 69:51–57, 1992.

132. Stetz CW, Miller RG, Kelly GE, Raffin TA: Reliability of the thermodilution method in the determination of cardiac output in clinical practice. *Am Rev Respir Dis* 126:1001–1004, 1982.

133. Steven JM, Nicolson SC: Monitoring the pediatric patient. In Blitt CD, Hines RL (eds): *Monitoring in Anesthesia and Critical Care Medicine*, 3rd ed. New York, Churchill Livingstone, 1995, pp 677–726.

134. Sy WP: Ulnar nerve palsy possibly related to use of automatically cycled blood pressure cuff. *Anesth Analg* 60:687–688, 1981.

135. Talke P, Nichols RJ Jr, Traber DL: Does measurement of systolic blood pressure with a pulse oximeter correlate with conventional methods? *J Clin Monit* 6:5–9, 1990.

136. Tibby SM, Hatherill M, Marsh MJ, et al: Clinical validation of cardiac output measurements using femoral artery thermodilution with direct Fick in ventilated children and infants. *Intensive Care Med* 23:987–991, 1997.

137. Tibby SM, Hatherill M, Murdoch IA: Use of transesophageal Doppler ultrasonography in ventilated pediatric patients: Derivation of cardiac output. *Crit Care Med* 28:2045–2050, 2000.

138. Tyson JE, deSa DJ, Moore S: Thromboatheromatous complications of umbilical arterial catheterization in the newborn period: Clinicopathological study. *Arch Dis Child* 51:744–754, 1976.

139. Ungerleider RM, Greeley WJ, Sheikh KH, et al: Routine use of intraoperative epicardial echocardiography and Doppler color flow imaging to guide and evaluate repair of congenital heart lesions: A prospective study. *J Thorac Cardiovasc Surg* 100:297–309, 1990.

140. Vedrinne C, Bastien O, DeVarax R, et al: Predictive factors for usefulness of fiberoptic pulmonary artery catheter for continuous oxygen saturation in mixed venous blood monitoring in cardiac surgery. *Anesth Analg* 85:2–10, 1997.

141. Venkataraman ST, Thompson AE, Orr RA: Femoral vascular catheterization in critically ill infants and children. *Clin Pediatr* 36:311–319, 1997.

142. Verghese ST, McGill WA, Patel RI, et al: Ultrasound-guided internal jugular venous cannulation in infants: A prospective comparison with the traditional palpation method. *Anesthesiology* 91:71–77, 1999.

143. Viitanen H, Baer G, Koivu H, Annila P: The hemodynamic and Holter-electrocardiogram changes during halothane and sevoflurane anesthesia for adenoidectomy in children aged 1 to 3 years. *Anesthes Analg* 87:1423–1425, 1999.

144. West JB, Dollery CT, Naimark A: Distribution of blood flow in isolated lung: Relation to vascular and alveolar pressures. *J Appl Physiol* 19:713, 1964.

145. Wippermann CF, Huth RG, Schmidt FX, et al: Continuous measurement of cardiac output by the Fick principle in infants and children: Comparison with the thermodilution method. *Intensive Care Med* 22:467–471, 1996.

146. Wippermann CF, Schranz D, Huth R, et al: Determination of cardiac output by an angle and diameter independent dual beam Doppler technique in critically ill infants. *Br Heart J* 67:180–184, 1992.

147. Yabek SM, Akl BF, Berman W Jr, et al: Use of atrial epicardial electrodes to diagnose and treat postoperative arrhythmias in children. *Am J Cardiol* 46:285–289, 1980.

148. Yancy PH, Somero GN: Temperature dependence of intracellular pH: Its role in the conservation of pyruvate Km values of vertebrate lactate dehydrogenase. *J Comp Physiol* 125:129, 1978.

149. Yemen TA: Noninvasive monitoring in the pediatric patient. *Int Anesthesiol Clin* 30:77–90, 1992.

Chapter 20

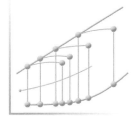

Cardiopulmonary Bypass in Infants and Children

JAMES JAGGERS, MD, and ROSS M. UNGERLEIDER, MD

INTRODUCTION

The idea of coupling extracorporeal circulation and oxygenation and surgical repair of the heart originated with Dr. John Gibbon Jr. Inspired by the tragic death of a pregnant woman from a pulmonary embolus, Gibbon was the first to establish the feasibility of artificially supported circulation during temporary occlusion of the pulmonary artery. In 1953 he used extracorporeal circulation successfully in a young woman, Celia Bavole, to facilitate open cardiac repair of an atrial septal defect.[58] Despite this one success, however, Dr. Gibbon lost several other patients and he abandoned this technique. In fact, aside from Dr. Gibbon's one successful procedure, early experience with the clinical use of cardiopulmonary bypass was uniformly dismal and most surgical groups continued to seek alternative methods to correct heart defects (Table 20-1). In 1954 Lillehei and associates began using the technique of controlled cross-circulation using a compatible adult as the pump-oxygenator to repair congenital heart defects. Over a period of 16 months, 47 patients were operated on and 28 survived.[109,110] This really began the remarkable era of heart surgery. For the first time, surgeons were able to repair intracardiac defects with the luxury of time as the patient's body was provided with nutrient perfusion by an exogenous (albeit human) pump/oxygenator. Nevertheless, the use of other humans as pump oxygenators carried impractical risks. Further investigation led to the development of safer extracorporeal circuits. The addition of heat exchangers allowed core cooling and rewarming of internal organs in a way that surface cooling could not, and this allowed pump flow rates to be decreased and prolonged the period of safe operation. Bigelow first demonstrated the application of hypothermia to cardiac surgery in 1950. He showed that dogs cooled to 20°C could survive a 15-minute period of total circulatory arrest.[15] In 1952, Lewis and Taufic were the first to apply hypothermia and inflow occlusion for repair of atrial septal defect in humans.[108,176]

Although the mechanism of the propulsion with the roller pump has not changed, the mechanisms of oxygenation have undergone an evolution. Gibbon's first oxygenator was a rotating film oxygenator. Kirklin's group adopted the stationary film oxygenator that was developed with technical support from IBM.[92] Bubble oxygenators were developed in the late 1950s and were mass-produced in the 1960s. This revolutionized the field of cardiac surgery. Membrane oxygenators utilizing thin sheets of permeable Teflon were developed and had some advantages over bubble oxygenators. However, the rapid expansion of cardiac surgery in the 1960s required a preassembled, sterile, and disposable oxygenator, and the membrane oxygenator was far from ready. The advent of coronary

Table 20-1 Open-Heart Surgery with Total Cardiopulmonary Bypass: Results of All Reported Cases 1951–1954 (Before cross-circulation, 3/26/54)

Surgeon	Number of Patients	Oxygenator Type	Year	Number of Survivals	Number of Deaths
Dennis	2	Film	1951	0	2
Helmsworth	1	Bubble	1952	0	1
Gibbon	6	Film	1953	1 (ASD repair)	5
Dodrill	1	Autogenous	1953	0	1
Mustard	5	Monkey lungs	1951–1953	0	5
Clowes	3	Bubble	1953	0	3
Total	18			1 (5.5%)	17 (94.5%)

ASD, atrial septal defect.

and valve surgery in the 1960s corresponded to the use of mass-produced bubble oxygenators. By the 1970s, many centers were switching to membrane oxygenators because of increased safety and fewer complications with longer exposure time. With the advancement of gas-permeable, extraluminal flow oxygenator fibers, the production of bubble oxygenators has all but disappeared in the United States.

Advances in the techniques of surgery and perioperative care have extended the limits of patients being exposed to cardiopulmonary bypass (CPB) at both ends of the age spectrum. Miniaturization of some of the elements of the cardiopulmonary bypass circuit has made neonatal heart surgery safer and more efficient. The next great advances will be in the modulation of the systemic inflammatory response and injury from cardiopulmonary bypass. In this chapter, we review the basic physiology of CPB, the systemic inflammatory effects of CPB, strategies employed in the application of CPB (including the use of deep hypothermic circulatory arrest), and our current recommendations for how best to manage the use of CPB in infants and children.

CARDIOPULMONARY BYPASS FOR INFANTS VERSUS ADULTS

There are numerous differences between infants and adults that affect their response to CPB and which must be accounted for in CPB management strategies (Table 20-2). Procedures performed on infants and children may require extremes of temperature, hemodilution, and perfusion flow rates. Certain anatomic features, such as the presence of large aortopulmonary collaterals or interrupted aortic arch, require alteration of bypass strategies and/or cannulation techniques. Circuit capacity

Table 20-2 Differences between Infants and Adults that Affect Their Response to CPB

Smaller circulating blood volume
Higher oxygen consumption rate
Reactive pulmonary vascular bed
Presence of intracardiac and extracardiac shunting
Immature organ systems
Altered thermoregulation
Poor tolerance to microemboli

cannot currently be reduced proportionate to patient size. Therefore significant hemodilution in neonates and small infants is unavoidable. In addition to the decrease in hematocrit associated with hemodilution, clotting factors and plasma proteins are also significantly diluted, resulting in dilutional coagulopathy. Other organ systems in neonates and infants are not mature. For example, the production of vitamin K dependent clotting factors by the liver is diminished. Neonates and infants require much higher flow rates per body surface area to meet metabolic demands. Neonates are often perfused at flow rates up to 200 mL/kg/minute. As temperature is reduced, flow rates can be decreased. This has the benefit of producing less blood in a small and complicated surgical field. Small children also have impaired thermoregulation that requires significant attention to temperature monitoring. Furthermore, in some instances, patients are cooled to profoundly hypothermic temperatures (e.g., 15°C to 18°C) and the pump is then turned off (deep hypothermic circulatory arrest). This provides the surgeon with the opportunity to remove the cannulae from the patient and to perform a precise repair in an operative field unencumbered by blood, cannulae, or other apparatus related to CPB. When CPB is resumed, patients are rewarmed to their normal temperature.

The period of time from 6 months' gestation to 6 months post term is a critical time in the development of the brain's cortical connections, which result in perceptual and cognitive functions.[141] Also in neonates and young infants, there is a process called "plasticity," which is the potential for remodeling in response to environmental stimuli.[128] In general the immature brain tolerates oxygen deprivation better than the mature brain. This supports the clinical observations that infants tolerate longer periods of deep hypothermic circulatory arrest (DHCA) better than older children or adult patients. The lungs are also immature at birth, and lung development proceeds up to about 8 years of age.[168] At birth, the number of alveoli present is approximately one tenth of what it is in the adult. The lungs of the neonate are quite fragile and have increased potential for pulmonary edema and hypertension.[90] The kidneys of neonates and infants have high vascular resistance with preferential blood flow away from the outer cortex. Sodium reabsorption and excretion, concentrating and diluting mechanisms, and acid-base balance capacity are limited. These characteristics must be taken into account in the management of CPB in infants. Finally, the immune system of the neonate is immature.

Complement generation is impaired and neonatal mononuclear cells are dysfunctional.[89] These differences and many more make CPB in the infant and neonate a specialized endeavor that requires great attention to detail and the ability to adapt to unexpected situations.

PHYSIOLOGY OF CARDIOPULMONARY BYPASS

Improvements in technology have reduced the morbidity associated with cardiopulmonary bypass. The safe conduct of CPB in the neonate and infant requires a comprehensive understanding of the physiologic alterations associated with CPB. These variables include circuit design, hemodilution, choice of cannulae, degree of hypothermia, acid-base strategies, and selected flow rates (including selection of low-flow or "no-flow" deep hypothermic circulatory arrest).[157]

Hypothermia

The principle clinical effect of hypothermia is the reduction in metabolic rate and molecular movement. As the temperature is lowered, both basal and functional cellular metabolism are reduced and the rate of adenosine triphosphate (ATP) consumption is decreased. Whole-body oxygen consumption decreases directly with body temperature (Fig. 20-1). According to Arrhenius's equation, the logarithmic rate of chemical reactions is inversely proportional to the reciprocal of the absolute temperature. The multiple by which the reaction rate decreases for every 10°C is termed the Q^{10}.

Reanalysis of published data suggests a Q^{10} of 3.65 for infants compared to approximately 2.6 for adults.[65] This higher Q^{10} for infants suggests greater metabolic suppression related to hypothermia, which might enable these patients to tolerate longer periods of "imperfect" perfusion or ischemia. In patients on CPB, as the temperature of the patient decreases, the oxygen consumption becomes independent of the flow rate. This is the basis for which minimal pump flow rates (MPFR)—the minimal flow necessary to meet metabolic demands—can be predicted.[86]

There are several advantages to the use of hypothermia in conjunction with CPB. Hypothermia facilitates surgical exposure by allowing decreases in flow rate, which result in less blood returning to the heart through collateral vessels. Systemic hypothermia also decreases the rate of myocardial rewarming between cardioplegia applications. The use of hypothermia is mandatory for brain protection when prolonged periods of circulatory arrest are utilized. Hypothermia also affords some protection to other organs during periods of CPB and low-flow states. Cerebral blood flow is preserved through a wide range of blood pressures in both adults and children at moderate to normothermic conditions. (Figs. 20-2 and 20-3). At deep hypothermic conditions (18°C to 22°C) this autoregulation of cerebral blood flow is lost and cerebral blood flow seems to be more directly correlated with mean arterial pressure (Fig. 20-4). At deep hypothermia, cellular metabolism is so low and membrane fluidity is reduced to such a large extent that cellular basal metabolic needs and cellular membrane integrity can be maintained for a relatively long period of time, and this is probably why the clinical outcomes following periods of DHCA seem to be

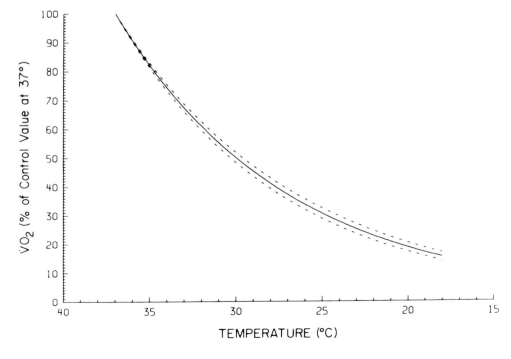

FIGURE 20-1 Whole body oxygen consumption as a function of body temperature. (From Bigelow WG, Callaghan JC, Hopps JA: General hypothermia for experimental intracardiac surgery: The use of electrophrenic respirations, an artificial pacemaker for cardiac standstill, and radio frequency rewarming in general hypothermia. *Ann Surg* 132:531–539, 1950; with permission.)

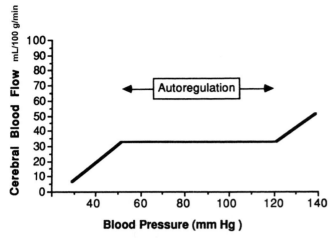

FIGURE 20-2 Cerebral blood flow is preserved through a wide range of systolic blood pressures in the normal adult. (From Venn GE: Cerebral vascular autoregulation during cardiopulmonary bypass. *Perfusion* 4:105, 1989; with permission.)

unaffected by arrest durations below 45 minutes at 18°C.[194] (Fig. 20-5).

Although hypothermia ameliorates the hypoxia-induced depression of cellular ATP content and membrane injury, there is evidence to suggest that hypothermia and hypoxia result in a significant increase in intracellular calcium and sodium during subsequent reperfusion.[132] This has important implications for the management of oxygenation during resumption of CPB after hypothermic circulatory arrest. In the heart, the contribution of hypothermia to lowering basal metabolic rate is relatively small compared to the effects of stopping electromechanical work. A sudden decrease in perfusion temperature appears to result in a marked increase in the resting tension of the myocardium. This is referred to as a "rapid cooling contracture."[145] This may be due to a sudden release of intracellular calcium stores within the sarcoplasmic reticulum. This cold-induced increase in resting myocardial tone may lead to impaired recovery of systolic and diastolic function

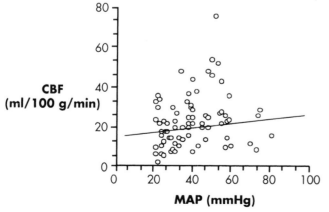

FIGURE 20-3 At moderate hypothermia, (25°C) cerebral blood flow (CBF) is independent of mean arterial pressure (MAP). Data from human infants based on Xenon clearance methodology. (From Greeley WJ, Kern FH, Ungerleider RM, Boyd JL III, et al: The effect of hypothermic cardiopulmonary bypass and total circulatory arrest on cerebral metabolism in neonates, infants, and children. *J Thorac Cardiovasc Surg* 101:783–794, 1991; with permission.)

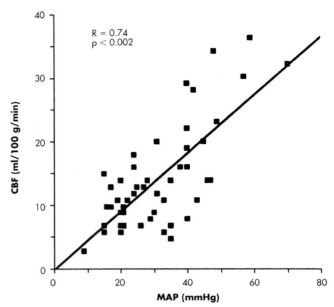

FIGURE 20-4 Data obtained from the human infant demonstrates that cerebral autoregulation is lost at deep hypothermic temperatures (<22° C) with cerebral blood flow (CBF) related in a linear manner to mean arterial pressure (MAP). (From Greeley WJ, Kern FH, Ungerleider RM, Boyd JL III, et al: The effect of hypothermic cardiopulmonary bypass and total circulatory arrest on cerebral metabolism in neonates, infants, and children. *J Thorac Cardiovasc Surg* 101:783–794, 1991; with permission.)

after reperfusion. This has led some groups to avoid cold perfusion of the heart before the aortic cross-clamp is applied and to use warm induction cardioplegia when possible.[145,191] Lowering of the serum ionized calcium levels with citrate may ameliorate some of the adverse effects of hypothermic cardiac perfusion.[5] Hypocalcemic prime solutions commonly used today do not seem to result in rapid cooling and cold induction of ischemia.[72]

The adverse effects of rapid cooling have been demonstrated experimentally in the kidneys, liver, and lungs as well. Clinically there are many variables involved, however, and there does not appear to be readily apparent injury to the patient from rapid cooling on CPB. It does appear that the neonate is able to tolerate the stress of profound hypothermia without difficulty. This has previously been attributed to a greater glycolytic activity and higher glycogen reserves in the neonate. However, neonates may also possess differential ionic channel density or have different membrane function when compared to older subjects. These theories remain speculative.

The degree of hypothermia selected is dependent on the needs for reduced flow to enhance surgical repair and the expected duration of aortic cross-clamp and cardiac ischemia. Three distinct methods of CPB are used: (1) mild hypothermia (30° C to 34° C), (2) moderate hypothermia (25°C to 30°C), or (3) deep hypothermia (15°C to 22° C). Deep hypothermia is often used when periods of low flow or circulatory arrest (DHCA) is desired. The technique selected is based on (1) the required surgical conditions, (2) the patient size, (3) the type and expected duration of the operation, and 4) the potential physiologic impact on the patient. Mild and moderate hypothermic CPB are the principal methods of bypass employed for older children and adolescents. Mild hypothermia may also

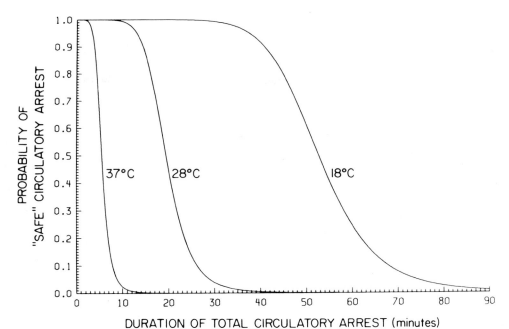

FIGURE 20-5 The probability of safe circulatory arrest is related to the duration of arrest and the temperature at which it occurs. (From Kirklin JW, Barratt-Boyes BG [eds]: *Cardiac Surgery*, 2d ed. New York, Churchill Livingstone, 1993, p 1779; with permission.)

be chosen for less demanding cardiac repairs in infants, such as an atrial septal defect (ASD), ventricular septal defect (VSD), or uncomplicated atrioventricular septal defect (AVSD). More complex procedures such as a pulmonary autograft aortic valve replacement might lead to selection of moderate hypothermia to help maintain adequate cardiac protection during a longer aortic cross-clamp period. Recommendations for optimal pump flow rates for children are based on the body surface area and maintaining efficient organ perfusion as determined by arterial blood gases, acid-base balance, and whole-body oxygen consumption during cardiopulmonary bypass. Normothermic flow rates for children are based on body weight (Table 20-3). At hypothermic temperatures, metabolism is reduced, and therefore pump flow rates may be reduced accordingly (Table 20-4).

Deep hypothermic cardiopulmonary bypass is generally reserved for neonates and infants requiring complex cardiac repairs. However, certain older children with complex cardiac disease or aortic arch anomalies may benefit from a short period of circulatory arrest. For the most part, deep hypothermia is selected to allow the surgeon to operate under conditions of low-flow CPB (as in repairing the pulmonary arteries of patients with substantial aortopulmonary collateral flow) or deep hypothermic circulatory arrest (as when repairing the aortic arch). Low pump flows improve the operating conditions for

the surgeon by providing a near bloodless field and better visualization of critical portions of the repair at selected times during the procedure. When DHCA is employed for the intracardiac portion of the repair, venous return can be accomplished with a single atrial cannula. This has the advantage of providing optimal venous return and complete decompression of the heart. During deep hypothermic circulatory arrest, the surgeon can remove the atrial and/or aortic cannula. Utilizing this technique, surgical repair may be more precise because of the bloodless and cannula-free operative field. As the temperature of the patient decreases, the oxygen consumption becomes independent of the flow rate. This is the basis for which minimal pump flow rates may be decreased related to the degree of hypothermia based on the equation[86]:

$$MPFR(T) = e^{0.1171(T-37°)} \cdot (100mL \cdot kg^{-1} \cdot min^{-1}) \text{ where:}$$

MPFR(T) = minimal pump flow rate at temperature (T)
$100mL \cdot kg^{-1} \cdot min^{-1}$ = normothermic pump flow rate
$e^{0.1171(T-37°C)}$ = CMRO₂ (cerebral metabolic rate for oxygen) at temperature T °C[i]

Table 20-4 Predicted Minimal Pump Flow Rates (MPFRs)

Temperature	CMRO₂ (mL/100 g/min)	Predicted MPFR (mL·kg⁻¹·min⁻¹)
37	1.48	100
32	0.823	56
30	0.654	44
28	0.513	34
25	0.362	24
20	0.201	14
18	0.159	11
15	0.112	8

From Kern FH, Ungerleider RM, Reves JG, et al: The effects of altering pump flow rate on cerebral blood flow and metabolism in neonates, infants, and children. *Ann Thorac Surg* 57:1366–1372, 1993; with permission.

Table 20-3 Recommended Pump Flow Rates for Normothermic Cardiopulmonary Bypass

Patient Weight (kg)	Pump Flow Rate (mL/kg/min)
<3	150–200
3–10	125–175
10–15	120–150
15–30	100–120
30–50	75–100
>50	50–75

Although hypothermia ameliorates the hypoxia-induced depression of cellular ATP content and membrane injury, there is evidence to suggest that hypothermia and hypoxia result in a significant increase in intracellular calcium and sodium with subsequent reperfusion.[132] This has important implications for the management of oxygenation during resumption of CPB after hypothermic circulatory arrest. Hypothermia preserves organ function by maintaining cellular ATP stores despite reduced oxygen delivery, reducing excitatory neurotransmitter release, and preventing calcium entry into the cell. In summary, some element of hypothermia is usually necessary and beneficial in the management of CPB in neonates and infants. Hypothermia helps to preserve organ function during ischemia, aids in the operative exposure, and increases the safety of CPB.

Recently, a few groups have reported excellent results using normothermic CPB for infants. This technique, however, has not yet gained widespread acceptance.

Pulsatile Versus Nonpulsatile Flow

The desirability of pulsatile perfusion has been contemplated and studied since the introduction of extracorporeal circulation in the 1950s. Hundreds of experiments have been performed to try to prove that pulsatile perfusion is preferable to the more commonly employed nonpulsatile or laminar flow perfusion. The inability to reproduce normal physiologic pulsatile blood flow, as well as the additional complexity of these systems, led to the adoption of laminar flow systems. In some studies, the use of pulsatile perfusion results in a decrease in systemic vascular resistance after CPB and an increase in cardiac index in adult patients.[167] Others have found that nitric oxide, a potent vasodilator produced from cultured endothelial cells, is increased with pulsatile flow as compared to laminar flow.[134] This may be important at the microcirculatory level. This may affect vascular endothelial function, thrombogenicity, and overall vascular tone. Many have reported beneficial hemodynamic effects of pulsatile perfusion with reduction in the need for inotropes and intra-aortic balloon pump therapy.[23] It appears that the major benefit of pulsatile perfusion is associated with the reduction in post-CPB vasoconstriction and resultant improvement in cardiac index.[167] There is also evidence that pulsatile perfusion improves splanchnic perfusion when compared to nonpulsatile perfusion.[55,112] In our own experience with a neonatal porcine model of cardiopulmonary bypass and circulatory arrest, we found that there was no difference in cerebral blood flow either before or after an arrest period when comparing pulsatile to nonpulsatile perfusion. There was an improvement in the pre-arrest period and post arrest on renal blood flow and myocardial blood flow.[112,173,174] The availability of effective pulsatile pumps is limited and the clinical superiority is yet to be proven.

Strategies for CO_2 Management: Alpha-Stat and pH-Stat

The role of CO_2 management in CPB has been studied extensively in animals and adult patients. Based on the effect of CO_2 on arterial and intracellular pH at hypothermic temperatures, two divergent blood gas management strategies have been championed: Alpha-stat (temperature uncorrected) and pH-stat (temperature corrected).[4,33,79,132,151,161,162,183]

Alpha-stat strategy maintains a pH of 7.40 measured without mathematical correction for the effects of temperature, whereas pH-stat uses a mathematical correction for the effects of temperature on pH. With temperature corrected measurements, blood pH becomes increasingly alkalotic as the blood cools. To correct for this alkalotic "pH," CO_2 is added to maintain a temperature corrected pH of 7.40 (pH-stat). The addition of CO_2, however, lowers intracellular pH (pHi) resulting in an imbalance between H^+ and OH^- ions, that is, the loss of electrochemical neutrality. Intracellular enzymatic function is dependent on maintaining a normal pHi, and therefore cellular enzyme function may be impaired using pH stat. An acidotic pHi is problematic because at hypothermic temperatures the normal buffering systems (NH_3^-, HCO_3^-) become ineffective. At hypothermia, buffering capacity is limited to negative charges of the amino acids composing intracellular proteins. The amino acid histidine is the most important buffer at hypothermia because it contains an alpha-imidazole ring with many negatively charged moieties that can buffer H^+ ions. The reason uncorrected blood gas measurement is called alpha-stat is in reference to the alpha-imidazole ring of histidine. The principal advantage of alpha-stat strategy therefore is preserving intracellular electrochemical neutrality, maintaining appropriate intracellular pH (pHi), and improving the efficiency of intracellular enzymatic function.[163]

During moderate hypothermia selecting one blood gas management strategy over the other appears less critical because brain intracellular pH differences are small.[9,166] During deep hypothermia with or without DHCA, the addition of CO_2 during active brain cooling could potentially improve the distribution of the cold perfusate to deep brain structures. Recent evidence suggests that pH-stat management enhances the distribution of extracorporeal perfusate to the brain and may help cool the brain more thoroughly and rapidly.[161,187] Although improved cooling was demonstrated in these studies, metabolic recovery after circulatory arrest was shown to be impaired, suggesting that the acid load induced by pH-stat had a negative effect on enzymatic function after cerebral rewarming.[79]

In an effort to retain the benefits of pH-stat on cooling and eliminate its negative effects on enzymatic function, our group has suggested a combined blood gas management strategy using pH-stat and alpha-stat in succession. A group of neonatal pigs that underwent initial cooling with pH-stat, followed by switching to alpha-stat before DHCA, demonstrated improved metabolic suppression over alpha-stat alone as well as a significant enhancement in metabolic recovery after rewarming. This suggests that initial cooling with pH-stat, followed by a switch to alpha-stat to normalize the pH in the brain before ischemic arrest, may be an alternative and effective approach. Other factors that may result in maldistribution of pump flow away from the cerebral circulation and contribute to inefficient cerebral cooling include anatomic variants (large aortopulmonary collaterals)[97,192] or technical problems (aortic and venous cannulae misplacements).[87] Cyanotic patients with known aortopulmonary collaterals may benefit from the cerebral vasodilation of pH-stat during early cooling.[94] Once cool, however, if DHCA or deep hypothermia with low flow is planned, converting to an alpha-stat strategy may help preserve intracellular brain pH and improve neurologic outcome after the procedure.

Myocardial Protection

Neonatal repair is the preferred approach to many congenital heart defects. As the complexity of and time required for repair increase, the need for effective and optimal myocardial protection increase, also. There is some laboratory evidence that the immature myocardium has different structural and functional characteristics than the adult myocardium.[16] The immature heart is less compliant and this results in a very limited range of the Starling curve. The normal neonatal heart is operating at maximal saturation of adrenergic stimulation, and there is an exaggerated negative inotropic response to anesthetic agents and therefore a requirement for greater doses of inotropic agents when they are needed.[21] The immature myocardium relies heavily on glucose as its major substrate and also has a greater reliance on extracellular calcium for calcium-mediated excitation contraction coupling.[20,148] It is widely accepted that the immature heart has a greater tolerance to ischemia than the adult or mature heart. However, most of this laboratory data has been obtained with normal hearts. It is unclear what the ischemic tolerance is when there are preexisting conditions such as cyanosis, hypertrophy, or acidosis. Many of these conditions may be present in neonates and infants who require surgical correction of their heart defect and may compromise myocardial protection. Infants and children with chronic cyanosis, as a result of inadequate pulmonary blood flow, often have increased bronchial collateral flow. This increased blood return to the left heart can result in insufficient myocardial protection by warming the heart and washing out cardioplegia.[74] Hypertrophied ventricles may also have inadequate myocardial protection and subendocardial ischemia during prolonged arrest periods.

Hypothermia remains the most important factor for successful myocardial protection in infants.[35] Electromechanical arrest, ventricular decompression, and hypothermia all work together to decrease the myocardial oxygen consumption. Topically applied iced saline may be helpful; however, it often interferes with the operative procedure and may result in phrenic nerve palsy. Therefore, many groups use topical cooling intermittently. Typically cardioplegia is delivered through a catheter or needle in the aortic root after the cross-clamp has been applied. Retrograde cardioplegia delivery has received significant attention and is gaining in popularity in neonates. It is particularly useful in neonates requiring prolonged aortic crossclamp time and in whom delivery of cardioplegia into the aortic root may not be possible (e.g., aortic valve replacement, arterial switch operation, etc.). Blood cardioplegia may be superior to crystalloid cardioplegia especially for longer (> 1 hr) myocardial ischemic time.[35]

Typically, cardioplegia solutions should have a calcium concentration that is below the serum concentration.[7] Despite the potential for excessive calcium influx secondary to hyperkalemic-induced membrane depolarization, potassium remains the most widely used cardiac arresting agent in all of cardiac surgery. Magnesium helps to maintain that negative resting membrane potential and also inhibits sarcolemmal calcium influx.[100] The addition of magnesium to blood cardioplegia results in significantly improved functional recovery. Magnesium enrichment of hypocalcemic cardioplegic solutions can result in near complete functional recovery, but even high-dose magnesium supplementation cannot reverse dysfunction in severely stressed hearts that receive normocalcemic cardioplegia.[101] Typically, an initiating dose of 30 mL/kg cardioplegia solution at 4° C is delivered. Although there is no conclusive evidence either to support or refute the practice, many surgeons will use multiple doses of cardioplegia at approximately 20- to 30-minute intervals during the ischemic period. This practice may be helpful when there are significant bronchial collaterals, or in operations performed using mild or moderate hypothermia, both of which may result in premature warming of the heart.

In certain operations on the right side of the heart in which the septa are intact, that is, tricuspid valve repair or pulmonary valve repair or replacement, a technique referred to as "empty beating" may be employed, in which case little myocardial ischemia occurs and a cross-clamp is not employed. This is a reasonable technique as long as there is no communication between the right and left sides of the heart through which air can pass and result in air embolus to the systemic circulation. Mild hypothermia with fibrillatory arrest can be used in operations on the right side of the heart, especially when a significant intracardiac communication exists, such as an atrial septal defect. This technique is not recommended when there is significant aortic valve regurgitation because severe left ventricular distention will occur.

Intramyocardial air has also been suggested as a contributing factor for myocardial dysfunction after pediatric cardiac surgery.[10,66] In 4% of 350 consecutive pediatric patients undergoing repair of congenital cardiac defects, intramyocardial air was detected in the immediate post-bypass period using intraoperative echocardiography, despite aggressive "de-airing" maneuvers before removing the aortic cross-clamp.[66] Echocardiographic imaging demonstrated increased echogenic areas localized to the right ventricular free wall and along the inferior portion of the intraventricular septum. Hemodynamic instability was apparent in some of these patients, but in many cases the intramyocardial air produced no clinical signs. None of the patients had clinical evidence of air embolism to other organs (e.g., brain). The distribution of air was localized to the area supplied by the right coronary artery. The right coronary artery is a likely source for embolization of retained left ventricular air because of the location of the ostium of the right coronary artery on the anterior aspect of the aorta. Therefore, residual left ventricular air is more likely to enter the right coronary artery and result in right ventricular ischemia and dysfunction except in patients undergoing an arterial switch procedure for D-transposition in which the left coronary artery and left ventricle may be involved. The aortic cross-clamp is left in place and the cardioplegia needle is used to vent air from the left ventricle. Therapy for myocardial air embolism is directed at increasing perfusion pressure to propel air through the arterioles and capillary bed. Dramatic hemodynamic and echocardiographic improvements have been demonstrated in patients with intramyocardial air after the administration of phenylephrine or reperfusing the heart with high pump flow rates and high perfusion pressures on CPB.[66] Some groups "blow" carbon dioxide (CO_2) over the operative field to limit the risk of significant air embolus.

Endocrine Response to CPB

CPB is associated with tremendous increases in native catecholamines, particularly epinephrine and norepinephrine.

This is due partly to surgical stress, but also to peripheral vaso-constriction with relative ischemia, lack of pulsatile blood flow, and acidosis.[112,114] This elevation of catecholamines extends into the postoperative period.[47] It seems that the initial increases in catecholamine levels fall considerably upon reperfusion of the lungs. This is probably related to the uptake and metabolism of the catecholamines in the lungs. When the lungs are excluded from the circulation (total CPB), there is significant accumulation of norepinephrine. Hypothermia also has the effect of raising the serum catecholamine levels not only by increasing production, but also by the down-regulation of catecholamine receptors and decreasing the metabolism. Circulatory arrest also results in increases of catecholamines, but it is likely the rewarming, reperfusion phase of circulatory arrest that is most associated with catecholamine surge.[172,193] Catecholamine levels tend to fall rapidly once normothermia is achieved and bypass discontinued. It is clear that the level of anesthesia has a great influence on the surge of catecholamines associated with CPB and surgery. The anesthetic management of neonates has been shaped largely based on the findings of Anand and Hickey.[2] High-dose narcotic induction and maintenance can result in reduction of catecholamine and reduce postoperative complications. However, there is a rise in serum cortisol after induction of anesthesia and surgery. After the onset of CPB, the cortisol levels fall secondary to hemodilution. After CPB, the level again begins to rise and this continues for 24 hours, after which it gradually falls to normal. The effect of ultrafiltration on the levels of glucocorticoids is not known.

It appears that hypothermia and CPB result in a decrease in the level of insulin as well as decreased peripheral response to the insulin. The net result is an increase in the serum glucose level. The level of insulin increases after reperfusion and rewarming.[142] Glucagon and human growth hormone are released as part of the general stress response. Growth hormone is an anabolic hormone that tends to rise in both adults and children during and after CPB. There are a few studies that show an increase in glucagon during the CPB period and there is clearly a gradual rise in glucagon levels after surgery that peaks at about 6 hours.[89]

Thyroid hormones decrease during the CPB period and into the first several days after surgery.[32,125] The reasons for this include hemodilution, decrease in thyroid binding globulin, and increased glucocorticoid levels. The lowest levels of thyroid hormones seem to be associated with poor outcome. For this reason, triiodothyronine administered intravenously after CPB can be a useful inotropic agent.

Renal Response

Renal dysfunction is an important cause of morbidity and mortality after CPB. The general stress of surgery results in decreased renal blood flow and glomerular filtration rate (GFR) secondary to central nervous system influences. There is also an increase in vasopressin release, which results in fluid accumulation. Cortical blood flow within the kidney is decreased in favor of medullary blood flow. The elevation of vasopressin may last for 48 to 72 hours after surgery.[139] There is also an activation of the renin-angiotensin system with increased aldosterone production and fractional excretion of potassium. Hypothermia has been shown to decrease renal perfusion.[112,183] The duration of CPB is a risk factor for

injury as are preoperative renal dysfunction and heart failure. It is not uncommon for temporary oliguric renal dysfunction to occur after neonatal heart surgery and generally improve by 24 to 48 hours after surgery. Routine placement of peritoneal dialysis catheters at the time of cardiac surgery has been recommended by some for the high-risk infant. However, once peritoneal dialysis is instituted after cardiac surgery, it has been our experience that native urinary output diminishes, related in part to decreases in glomerular filtration rate from reduced cardiac output, and we worry that this may further impair or delay recovery of renal function. Since renal function generally returns to normal as cardiac function and systemic perfusion improve in the first 24 to 48 hours of post-bypass convalescence, the use of peritoneal dialysis after neonatal heart surgery should be reserved for those infants with severely impaired renal function beyond the immediate postoperative period.

Pulmonary Dysfunction

Pulmonary injury can be manifest in several ways, since the lungs have both a parenchymal and a vascular component. Parenchymal effects of CPB are reflected by alterations in pulmonary compliance most commonly related to an increase in lung water. The impact of this on the patient is a diminished ability of the lungs to perform their function in gas exchange which may result in a requirement for increased ventilatory support. Vascular effects are manifested by changes in pulmonary vascular resistance, which in turn affects function of the right ventricle. The lungs are in a unique position in the circulation and may be vulnerable to different mechanisms of injury.

There are multiple specialized cells within the lung, including many cells of inflammation. The lung is an important source and target of the inflammatory response to CPB. Part of the pulmonary derangement that occurs is related to the inflammatory response from CPB (see the following). This is manifest as decreased functional residual capacity (FRC), compliance, and gas exchange as well as increased pulmonary vascular resistance and pulmonary artery pressure.[119]

Inflammation is not the only factor that produces impairment of pulmonary function from CPB. When patients are placed on bypass, the lungs have a sudden and significant decrease in antegrade flow via the pulmonary artery. During "total" bypass, the lungs only receive "nutrient" flow from their bronchial supply. This relative ischemia of the lungs, in addition to the inflammatory effect of CPB may result in significant clinical pulmonary dysfunction.[30] It seems that low-flow cardiopulmonary bypass produces worse pulmonary injury than circulatory arrest,[159,190] suggesting that the interaction between the inflammatory and ischemic components is complex. Both the inflammatory and ischemic factors produce damage to the pulmonary endothelium[30,93,95,96] and this leads to increases in post-CPB pulmonary vascular resistance and pulmonary artery pressure, both of which can have significant implications in neonates and small infants, especially after certain types of procedures, such as a Norwood procedure for hypoplastic left heart syndrome.

A number of suggestions have been made for limiting this pulmonary dysfunction. Some intriguing work with Perflubron (liquid ventilation) infused into the lungs before bypass demonstrate that the anti-inflammatory and oxygen-carrying capabilities of this compound can have a dramatic effect on postbypass pulmonary parenchymal and vascular function.[28,31] The use of steroids may lessen the inflammatory response to CPB. Steroids given before exposure to CPB reduce lung water accumulation, improve post-CPB pulmonary compliance, and limit post-CPB pulmonary hypertension.[111] Modified ultrafiltration after CPB seems to improve pulmonary function immediately compared to function in patients who do not undergo ultrafiltration.[8,46,80,99,119,130,131,175,186] All of this suggests that some significant advances can be made with respect to the pulmonary response to cardiopulmonary bypass.

Neurologic Injury

The very real incidence of neurologic injury (10% to 25% of patients in some series)[49-51,89] after infant cardiac repair has stimulated intensive investigation into the effects of CPB on the brain. Clearly, the neonate or infant with congenital heart disease constitutes a patient at risk for neurologic impairment. This risk seems to have three elements: (1) pre-existing risk associated with various congenital heart lesions, (2) injury induced by CPB and the various CPB strategies that can be employed by the surgical team, and (3) injury sustained during the "vulnerable" period after exposure to CPB. When neurologic injury is manifest in a patient after CPB, it is often difficult to ascertain which of these elements played the most prominent role, and indeed it is often the combination of all three in some measure that relates to clinically apparent neurologic injury.

The risk for abnormal neurologic development, even without exposure to CPB or without repair of the lesion, ranges from 2% to 10% for a variety of congenital heart lesions. This may relate to abnormal cerebral perfusion patterns or to actual associated structural anomalies within the brain. Certain cardiac defects associated with syndromes (i.e., atrioventricular septal defects and trisomy 21) have an even higher incidence of abnormal brain development irrespective of whether the patient is exposed to cardiopulmonary bypass. The natural history of neurologic development without cardiac surgery is not known and is unlikely ever to be known for several serious and life-threatening congenital cardiac lesions. Nevertheless, there are data generated by our group, as well as by others, that cerebral flow patterns are extremely abnormal in these infants before they are placed on CPB. Finally, the condition of infants at the time of presentation greatly affects their neurologic outcome.[62] From all of this it can be easily appreciated that patients with congenital heart disease comprise a group that has an inherently high risk for neurologic abnormality after cardiac surgery.

The physiology of CPB produces many "alterations" that might relate to neurologic injury. During CPB, microembolic events commonly occur and can contribute to end-organ injury.[33] Alteration in cerebral blood flow can be demonstrated by middle cerebral artery transcranial Doppler, retinal angiography, echocardiography, and infrared spectroscopy, although none of these methods have been clearly shown to be clinically beneficial. Direct evidence of air embolism is visualization of air in the coronary vessels, electrocardiographic changes of ST-segment elevation, and blanching of the skin of the head.[19,42,66] Neurologic events have been correlated with the presence of focal dilatations of the microvasculature or very small aneurysms in terminal arterioles and

capillaries within the cerebral circulation. The use of membrane oxygenators, arterial filters, and adequate heparinization (ACT [activated clotting time] > 400 sec) for CPB decreases the number of microemboli and may reduce the incidence of embolic events during CPB.[18,155,195] Yet despite these methods, air embolism remains an important factor in postoperative neurologic dysfunction.

During pediatric cardiopulmonary bypass, the frequency in which the left side of the circulation is exposed to air increases the likelihood of systemic air embolization. In a report of perioperative neurologic effects in neonates undergoing the arterial switch operation for transposition of the great arteries, the presence of a VSD was associated with an increased incidence of postoperative seizure activity.[133] Although this could be related to longer periods of DHCA, the data could also suggest a higher incidence of air embolism as an etiology for neurologic dysfunction. When recognized, cerebral air embolism can be treated by attempts to reduce gas bubble size by reestablishing hypothermic CPB or through the use of hyperbaric oxygen therapy in the early postoperative period.[6] Major cerebral air embolism has also been treated with retrograde cerebral perfusion in adult patients, although experience with this modality in children is limited. Both hypothermia and hyperbaric therapy reduce the size of gaseous microbubbles and allow them to pass through the arterial and capillary beds, resulting in reduced ischemia.

HYPOTHERMIC INJURY TO THE BRAIN

Early experience with deep hypothermia suggested that using extremely low temperatures (esophageal temperatures of less than 10° C) resulted in a dramatic increase in neurologic and pulmonary injury. Neurologic sequelae, especially choreoathetosis, were commonly reported.[24,41,45] Neuropathologic examination of the brain of animals undergoing profound levels of hypothermia revealed microvascular lesions compatible with the no-reflow phenomenon.[135,169] Similar histologic brain lesions were observed in children who died after cardiac surgery using circulatory arrest.[17] These early reports diminished the enthusiasm for profound levels of hypothermia and most institutions limited hypothermic temperatures to 18°C to 20°C.

More recent, and probably more accurate, information suggests that some of these early fears are unfounded. Profound hypothermia does not seem to create cerebral injury[59,161] and in fact may correlate with improved cerebral protection during periods of DHCA. However, risk for injury may be affected by the type of blood gas management strategy used during DHCA (pH-stat versus alpha-stat), the duration of the time spent cooling, the duration of the period of DHCA, or the presence of significant aortopulmonary collaterals.*

The lower limit at which hypothermia causes significant end-organ damage is not known. Current clinical practices suggest however that temperatures of 15°C and below are probably no worse than temperatures of 18°C to 20°C, as long as appropriate hemodilution is used. It seems clear that at hypothermic temperatures (<22°C) autoregulation of cerebral blood flow is lost and decreases in a linear fashion with decreases in mean arterial pressure.[65]

---

*See references 11,84,94,97,104,116,135,161,162

It is now well recognized that cerebral blood flow decreases in a linear relationship to decreasing temperature whereas cerebral metabolism is reduced exponentially as temperature is decreased (Fig. 20-6). This provides most of the cerebral protection afforded to the brain by cooling, since cerebral metabolic needs for oxygen are significantly lowered and cerebral blood flow becomes "luxurious." Nevertheless, cerebral metabolism persists, even at very low temperatures, and the brain is therefore susceptible to ischemic injury despite hypothermia if cerebral blood flow is eliminated (e.g., DHCA) for prolonged periods of time. It is possible to predict the amount of cerebral blood flow required to support cerebral metabolic needs at decreasing temperatures and this is the rationale behind continuous low perfusion CPB (Table 20-3).[65,86,166]

Cerebral blood flow is regulated by several adjustable parameters. Although cerebral blood flow seems to be "autoregulated" at normothermic and moderately hypothermic temperatures,[36] autoregulation is lost at temperatures below 22°C[65,67-69] and cerebral flow is more dependent on mean arterial pressure. Fortunately, at these cold temperatures the brain needs very little blood flow.[86] The acid-base strategy employed during cooling also affects cerebral blood flow and metabolism. Alpha-stat is a more commonly used method, but there has recently been enthusiasm in some centers for more routine use of pH-stat strategies.[4,79] pH-stat requires addition of CO_2 to the circuit during cooling so the blood gases are "corrected" for the alkalosis that occurs with hypothermia. CO_2 is a potent cerebral vasodilator and addition of CO_2 to the circuit significantly increases blood flow to the brain.[88,161] Although this might promote more homogeneous cerebral cooling, the addition of CO_2, especially at temperatures below 15°C, creates significant acidosis (pH <6.9) in the circulating blood as well as at the cellular level. This acidosis at the time of circulatory arrest may be the reason for substantial impairment in cerebral metabolic recovery in animals subjected to these conditions experimentally.[161] However, if pH-stat is used for cooling and then the CO_2 is removed from the circuit (the patient is returned to alpha-stat blood gas management for a few minutes before establishing DHCA), the acidotic effects of pH-stat with respect to cerebral metabolic recovery may be alleviated.[162] Recent work suggests that hyperoxygenation on CPB in combination with pH-stat cooling can produce enhanced cerebral protection and extend the "safe period" of DHCA.

One group of patients that seems to be at increased risk for neurologic injury, and especially for choreoathetosis, is the group with significant aortopulmonary collaterals (such as older, cyanotic patients).[44,192] This has been demonstrated in an elegant experimental model by Kirshbom,[97] who also demonstrated how utilization of pH-stat cooling protected the brains of these particular animals.[94] It is important to note, however, that neither alpha-stat nor pH-stat strategies protect the brain from significant structural or metabolic derangement after prolonged periods (60 minutes) of DHCA, with either strategy associated with indistinguishable damage.[104]

There may be some relatively simple interventions that can limit injury from DHCA. Intravenous methylprednisolone (10 mg/kg) given at least 8 hours before CPB exposure significantly improves cerebral metabolic recovery and renal function recovery after DHCA.[102] There is also evidence that aprotinin,[3] thromboxane A2 receptor blockade,[170] platelet activating factor inhibitors,[105] or free radical scavengers[103] might improve cerebral recovery after DHCA, but none of the above, except for aprotinin or steroid is currently clinically useful. Recognition of high-risk groups (severe cyanosis, substantial aortopulmonary collaterals) might prompt utilization of pH-stat cooling, and in light of recent clinical work it might be warranted to use hyperoxygenation if a period of circulatory arrest is planned. It may also be helpful to switch to alpha-stat before inducing DHCA. It is important to cool for an adequate duration prior to using DHCA. Some authorities suggest that cooling duration be around 20 minutes. However, cooling duration needs to be considered as only one element in preparing the patient for DHCA and exists against a complex "backdrop" that includes target temperature, pH strategy used for cooling, hematocrit, patient's individual and unique biologic risk for DHCA, and, probably most importantly, the duration of uninterrupted circulatory arrest prior to cerebral reperfusion. In general, long periods of uninterrupted circulatory arrest at "warmer" temperatures would benefit from a longer duration of pre-arrest cooling. Patients cooled for less time have a higher likelihood of brain injury,[11,64,65,75,84] and if jugular venous oxygen saturations can be measured, it is probably unwise to use prolonged periods of DHCA if jugular venous oxygen saturations remain below 95%.[65,84] If continuous low-flow cardiopulmonary bypass can be used, this might be better for cerebral protection although the effects of continuous low-flow perfusion on the lung as well as on the microvasculature might be deleterious compared to DHCA.[159,190]

DHCA should only be used for the period of time necessary to benefit from its advantages, since brain injury does seem to relate to the duration of the arrest period.[48,54,64,116,189] The effect of 60 minutes of DHCA on the brain's microvasculature can be seen in Figure 20-7. There is typically loss of normal architecture, extraluminal edema and protein deposition, leukocyte accumulation, and vacuolization of surrounding neuron cytoplasm. Perhaps the most exciting and practical information for the surgical team was provided by Langley and by Mault[104,117] who separately demonstrated that periods of DHCA up to 60 minutes can be associated with absolutely normal recovery of cerebral metabolism as well as preservation of neural microarchitecture if the brain is perfused from the pump for 1 minute (25 to 50 mL/kg/minute) every 15 to 20 minutes (Fig. 20-8). This means that sequential periods of DHCA can be utilized

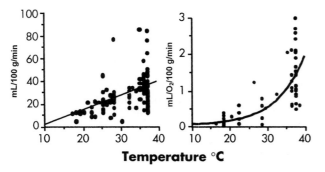

CBF vs Temperature   CMRO2 vs Temperature

FIGURE 20-6 Cerebral blood flow (CBF) decreases in a linear relationship to decreasing temperature whereas cerebral metabolism is reduced exponentially as temperature is decreased.

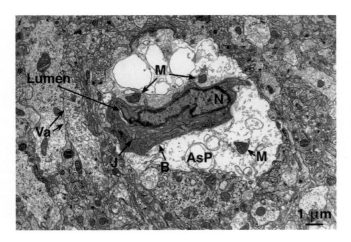

FIGURE 20-7 Electron micrograph of brain arteriole after 60 minutes of DHCA and reperfusion and rewarming to 37° C. There is loss of normal gap junction architecture and extravasation of protein and fluid into the periarteriolar tissue. There is also infiltration of the area with mononuclear cells. This loss of normal architecture is consistent with the no-reflow phenomena. AsP, astrocyte foot process; B, basal lamina; J, junctional complex; M, mitochondria; Va, vacuole.

as long as they are not prolonged beyond 15 to 20 minutes. If the brain is perfused between periods of DHCA, the duration of the DHCA periods may not be additive.[118] Similar findings have been alluded to by Miura[126] and Robbins.[146]

Even when planning aortic arch reconstruction, such as with a Norwood procedure, it is possible to provide intermittent or continuous low-flow cerebral perfusion by first placing the proximal shunt on the innominate artery and then by moving the arterial cannula to the shunt.[140] During the period of DHCA, the head should be packed in ice.[116] Although little can be done during reperfusion to improve cerebral recovery,[64] use of modified ultrafiltration after weaning from CPB may improve recovery of cerebral metabolism.[160,175] After DHCA, cardiac output and cerebral oxygen delivery should be maintained, since this is the period when the brain is most "vulnerable" to injury.[121,122] There is also information that the brain might be better protected after DHCA if the patient is removed from CPB at rectal temperatures of 34°C as opposed to 36°C or warmer.[158]

The most recent data regarding DHCA versus continuous flow hypothermic CPB suggests that at 8 year follow-up, there are no significant differences between groups.[12,178,194] Both groups are impaired compared to normal, but it is difficult to impugn DHCA as a cause of long-term neurologic outcome as it compares to continuous low flow. The patients exposed

to DHCA seem to have more issues with motor skills whereas those exposed as infants to primarily hypothermic low-flow strategies have more problems with attention deficit and other learning disabilities. Even more intriguing are the data reported by the group from Children's Hospital of Philadelphia suggesting that neonates may be at risk for CPB, regardless of which strategy is used.[56] It is certainly clear that neurodevelopmental outcome for infants who undergo repair of congenital heart disease is multifactorial and only relates in part to the CPB strategies that are used. There are numerous other issues that involve preoperative risk factors, genetic predisposition, postoperative factors, and many more that are also important and that need to be considered when evaluating the impact of CPB strategies on long-term neurologic outcome.[57, 178]

THE SYSTEMIC INFLAMMATORY RESPONSE

The systemic inflammatory response to CPB is indeed multifaceted. It involves a complex interaction of many systems and cellular elements in the body, all of which are normal teleological responses to noxious stimuli. It is important to consider the biochemical events and pathways not individually, but as a complex interaction with regulatory and counter-regulatory effects. With the exposure of the blood to foreign surfaces of

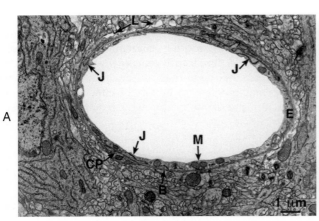
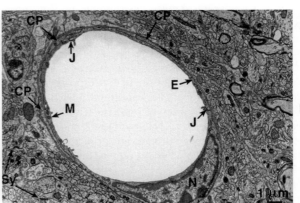

FIGURE 20-8 Electron micrographs of cerebral architecture **(A)** before and **(B)** after 60 minutes of DHCA with intermittent reperfusion periods every 15 minutes at 25 mL/kg/min. There is no alteration in architecture when intermittent perfusion is employed. CP, small cellular projection; E, endothelial layer; J, junctional complex; M, mitochondria.

the circuit and oxygenator, the initiating event appears to be contact activation of the blood elements. Other factors including tissue ischemia and reperfusion, hypotension with non-pulsatile perfusion, relative anemia, blood product administration, and heparin and protamine administration may also play a role in the inflammatory response to CPB. One of the initial responses is complement activation.[164] The complement system is composed of more than 30 different proteins. It appears that the alternate pathway of activation is the most important in CPB. This results in the formation of C3a and C5a,[89] which are important anaphylotoxins, chemotactic agents for neutrophils, and inflammatory mediators. C5a formation results in the production of other cytokines and activation of cellular elements such as macrophages and platelets. Complement also has intrinsic lytic properties.[27,91,127,154]

The next major step in the process is neutrophil activation and the neutrophil-endothelial cell interaction. This step can result in direct tissue injury as well as elaboration of many toxic substances including other cytokines. Neutrophils probably play a major role in the ischemia-reperfusion injury associated with pulmonary and neurologic injury. Complement activation also results in the elaboration of many different cytokines from monocytes, macrophages, and endothelial cells. These cytokines mediate many of the inflammatory reactions, some regulatory (TnF, IL1, IL6, IL8, and LPS)[52] and some counter-regulatory (IL4 and IL10). These cytokines have been associated with CPB and will increase with bypass duration.[165]

Cardiopulmonary bypass is also a very procoagulant stimulus. Heparin inhibits the formation of clot; however, it does not prevent the expression of tissue factor on endothelial cell. The expression of tissue factor on the endothelial cell surface is central to the extrinsic system of coagulation. Tissue factor results in the production of thrombin, which by itself has significant inflammatory and thrombotic properties.[22] It appears that initially after CPB there is a relative thrombolytic state. However, shortly thereafter, a hypercoagulable state prevails.[78] In infants undergoing open cardiac surgery, there may be ongoing inflammatory stimulus for tissue factor activation that extends into the postoperative period.[78] Arachadonic acid pathway activation also occurs in cells that are irritated or ischemic, especially in the lung. This results in production of thromboxanes, leukotrienes, and prostaglandin. Endothelial injury results in altered microcirculatory function, which is responsible for elevations in pulmonary, cerebral, and systemic vascular resistances, a common finding after hypothermic CPB. Endothelial injury impairs release of important vasodilators such as nitric oxide and prostacyclin, and promotes release of vasoconstrictors such as thromboxane A_2 and endothelin (also known to have inotropic effects in the myocardium).[25,29,53] In addition to these properties the endothelial surface (pulmonary endothelium in particular) is responsible for the metabolism of vasoconstrictors such as angiotensin, catecholamines, and eicosanoids.[188] Injured endothelium, by virtue of reduced production of nitric oxide and impaired metabolism of mediators of vasodilatation, promotes vasoconstriction.[30,93,96,188] Endothelial cells also play an important regulatory role in water and solute transport. Abnormalities in endothelial function promote increased capillary permeability and increases in interstitial edema.[153]

The worst responses to the inflammatory insult are at the extremes of age; the very young and the very old. In infants

and neonates, the response is characterized by post-bypass adult respiratory distress syndrome (ARDS), pulmonary hypertension, total body edema, coagulation abnormalities, myocardial dysfunction, and hemodynamic instability. These adverse sequelae translate into prolonged ventilation, prolonged inotropic support, renal dysfunction, bleeding and later thrombosis, and inability to close the chest in the operating room, and potentially the need for post-cardiotomy mechanical support. In particular, the pulmonary injury seems to be quite profound and is a major source of morbidity. Injury to the lungs results in increased pulmonary vascular resistance and loss of endothelial dependent pulmonary vasorelaxation. This is likely a neutrophil-mediated injury secondary to ischemia-reperfusion.

Potential areas of therapeutic intervention include heparin bonded circuits to prevent contact activation, circuit miniaturization to reduce priming volumes and oxygenator exposure, the use of deep hypothermic circulatory arrest versus low-flow bypass (which seems to limit duration of CPB exposure time and is associated with less post-bypass edema),[54,190] anticytokines or antiadhesion molecule therapy, simple leukocyte depletion, serine protease inhibition (aprotinin), modified ultrafiltration, and anti-inflammatory agents.

Corticosteroids have been used for many years with cardiopulmonary bypass. Steroids affect the inflammatory process at many levels. They may reduce complement activation and decrease complement-mediated neutrophil adhesion and degranulation. They may act as an inhibitor of some cytokine release and a promoter of others. They decrease the production of acute phase reactants and decrease production of antibody. The more powerful effects of steroids act through inhibition of the signal transduction pathways within the cell. This results in decreased production of mRNA for protein synthesis of inflammatory mediators and cellular products of inflammation. Since some of this process takes time, it is not surprising that high-dose steroids given several hours before exposure to CPB produce more significant reduction in the inflammatory response than when steroids are given in the pump prime (immediately upon exposure to CPB) or not at all.[111] Because of interest in this area and the advances in the areas of molecular biology, the entire process of the whole-body inflammatory response seems considerably more complex than it did several years ago. Once the molecular mechanisms of inflammation are unraveled, improved outcomes for the most complex of congenital cardiac defects can be realized.

Recent information generated from our laboratory in Oregon demonstrates that removing blood from the prime for neonatal CPB significantly reduces the inflammatory response. Miniaturized circuits that can enable the use of asanguious prime may produce an important effect on the outcome for neonates and small infants who require CPB for repair of their cardiac defect.[81,82]

THE EXTRACORPOREAL CIRCUIT

Prime

The trend in modern pediatric bypass equipment is to reduce the size of the extracorporeal circuit in order to reduce the prime volume. The priming volume may actually exceed the blood volume of a neonate by as much as 200% to 300%. This is in contrast to an adult CPB patient for whom the priming volume accounts for only 25% to 33% of the patient's blood volume. High priming volume can produce a low (<15%) hematocrit on CPB in small infants. This mandates the use of donor blood in the prime. What constitutes the lowest acceptable hematocrit is debated, but it is generally considered to be between 15% and 20%. The use of donor blood has several disadvantages including viral particle transmission; complement activation; transfusion reaction; lactate, potassium, and glucose infusion; and CPD (citrate-phosphate-dextrose) infusion.[143,152] Hemodilution during CPB reduces plasma proteins and clotting factors, decreases colloid osmotic pressure (resulting in enhanced interstitial edema), produces electrolyte imbalances, results in release of stress hormones, and activates inflammatory mediators. For these reasons, priming volumes should be kept to a minimum and transfusions avoided as much as is possible.

Blood viscosity increases as temperature is lowered. Blood flow through microcirculation is impaired by the combination of hypothermia, high hematocrits, and the nonpulsatile flow.[183] The optimal level of hemodilution during pediatric cardiopulmonary bypass is based on providing adequate oxygen delivery at hypothermic temperatures and during rewarming. Hematocrits as low as 10% appear to provide adequate oxygen delivery during hypothermic CPB. During rewarming, however, when the oxygen demand rises, such a low hematocrit may be insufficient to meet the body's recovering metabolic needs.[73,83,107] Cerebral oxygen delivery is an especially important consideration since cerebral autoregulation is impaired at deep hypothermic temperatures in infants[65] and after deep hypothermic circulatory arrest. In neonates undergoing deep hypothermic CPB (15°C to 20°C), a hematocrit of 20 ± 2% is generally targeted. Some groups are currently advocating a significantly higher hematocrit to approximately 35% to 40% while on hypothermic CPB because of potentially improved neurologic outcomes.[70] The necessary hematocrit level varies depending on the degree of hypothermia. Levels as low as 12% to 14% may be well tolerated at 18°C.[34] Because these data were obtained from adult dogs, it is unclear how this may relate to a neonate or infant.

The following formula estimates the amount of red blood cells that must be added to achieve target hematocrit of 20%:

$$\text{Added RBCs (mL)} = (\text{BVpt} + \text{TPV})(\text{Hct Desired}) - (\text{BVpt})(\text{Hct pt})$$

where added RBCs = mL of packed red blood cells added to the prime volume, BVpt = patient's blood volume (80% to 85% of body weight in infants), TPV = total priming volume, Hct desired = the desired hematocrit on CPB, and Hct pt = starting hematocrit of the patient.

Most institutions use packed red blood cells in their priming solutions. However, some institutions substitute whole blood. Whole blood can aid in maintaining colloid oncotic pressure and increasing the level of circulating clotting factors. The disadvantage of a whole-blood prime is a much higher glucose content in the priming solution. Hyperglycemia is a risk factor for neurologic injury in the presence of cerebral ischemia. Whole blood may also be used after CPB. This preserves much of the clotting factor and platelet functions of the donor blood as well as increases

the hematocrit. Fresh whole blood has the added advantage of being beneficial for hemostasis. The addition of packed red blood cells to the prime can result in high lactate and potassium levels in the prime, depending on the age of the donor cells. A technique of ultrafiltering the blood before it reaches the prime can be useful in removing these by-products.

The addition of colloid to the prime increases the protein content and therefore the oncotic pressure of the perfusate. This may prevent some of the capillary leak of fluid and result in improved organ function after CPB. Alternatively, whole blood may be used as part of the priming solution. Reduction in plasma protein concentration has been shown experimentally to impair lymphatic flow and alter pulmonary function by increasing capillary leak. Although adult studies have not demonstrated any advantage to adding albumin to pump prime, one study has suggested that maintaining normal colloid osmotic pressure may improve survival in infants undergoing CPB.[71,115]

Pediatric priming solutions contain variable levels of electrolytes, buffer (sodium bicarbonate or THAM), calcium, glucose, and lactate. Electrolytes, glucose, and lactate levels may be quite high if the prime includes large amounts of stored CPD (citrate-phosphate-dextrose) blood, or quite low if a minimal amount of bank blood is added. Calcium levels are generally very low in priming solutions and this may account for the rapid slowing of the heart with the initiation of bypass. Low calcium primes are generally preferred because of the potentially deleterious effects of ionized calcium during periods of ischemic arrest.[145] Buffer is added to maintain a physiologic pH. Controversial supplementary additives included in pediatric priming solutions include mannitol and steroids. Mannitol is added to promote an osmotic diuresis and to scavenge oxygen free radicals from the circulation. Steroids are added to reduce ion shifts during periods of ischemia and to reduce the inflammatory response, capillary leak, and secondary injury after a period of ischemia.

Oxygenators

In the pediatric population, oxygenators must provide efficient gas exchange over a wide range of temperatures (10°C to 40°C), pump flow rates (0 to 200 mL/kg/min), hematocrit (15% to 30%), line pressures, and gas flow rates. Both bubble and membrane oxygenators can achieve effective gas exchange under these diverse conditions. Bubble oxygenators allow fresh gas in the form of microbubbles to mix directly with circulating blood in an oxygenating column. The direct interface of blood and gas is traumatic to blood cellular elements, causing increased red blood cell hemolysis, platelet microaggregation, complement activation, and release of mediators of the inflammatory response.[120,150,184] These undesirable effects are minimized with the use of membrane oxygenators.

The membrane oxygenator acts as a synthetic alveolar-capillary membrane, where a direct interface between the blood and fresh gas is minimized or absent. Most membrane oxygenators used for cardiopulmonary bypass are composed of microporous hollow fibers. A microporous membrane contains pores of 3 to 5 microns in size, which allow a minimal contact between the blood and gas. The advantage of micropores is improved gas exchange with a smaller total membrane surface area. The disadvantage is that if negative pressure develops on the blood side of the membrane, gas emboli can be entrained into the blood and result in gas embolization in the arterial blood of the patient. Newer microporous hollow fiber oxygenators require very low prime volumes (50 to 140 mL). Newer devices such as the Cobe Micro and Dideco Lilliput have been designed to be exclusive neonatal oxygenators. The heat exchanger–oxygenator module requires a priming volume of just 60 mL and the device includes a volume control reservoir system with a maximum priming volume of 90 mL. Despite the low oxygenator priming volumes, flow rates of 800 mL/minute are achieved. This would allow perfusion flow rates of 150 mL/kg in neonates and young infants up to 5.3 kg. In conjunction with reduced tubing length and more thoughtful system designs, total prime volumes of 250 mL may be achievable using the Cobe and Lilliput devices.[120]

A third type of membrane oxygenator is composed of nonporous silicone and is arranged in folded sheets. Nonporous silicone membrane oxygenators are more expensive and require a larger surface area for gas exchange than microporous membrane devices do. Silicone membrane devices provide no clear advantage for short-term perfusion, but are the only membrane oxygenators recommended for long-term perfusion such as extracorporeal membrane oxygenation (ECMO) support.

Pumps

There are two types of pumps currently used for CPB: roller pumps and centrifugal pumps. Roller pumps are the most widely used in pediatric perfusion. Roller pumps consist of two rollers that are oriented 180 degrees from each other. They provide continuous blood flow by partially occluding the tubing between the roller and the pump casing. Blood is displaced in a forward direction by the roller, causing continuous, nonpulsatile flow. The second roller acts as a valve to minimize backflow. The rollers are never totally occlusive because that would encourage hemolysis. Ideally, the occlusion for each roller should be set independent of the other. This is especially true in neonatal and infant perfusion where maladjustment in occlusion can result in a higher percentage error in estimating pump flow rate and increased red cell hemolysis.

Centrifugal pumps are newer devices, which have gained increasing interest because of experience gained in extracorporeal membrane oxygenation (ECMO) and ventricular assist devices. Flow is maintained by the entrainment of blood against spinning impellers (curved blades) or by creating a vortex utilizing a centrifugal cone. The advantages of centrifugal pumps include a reduced priming volume, less damage to formed blood elements, and the concept that vortex design may assist in air removal.[76] These pumps are also capable of producing pulsatile blood flow, which may improve flow in the microcirculation.

Tubing

Tubing size should be kept as small as possible to reduce prime volume, but must be large enough to achieve effective flow rates and low line pressure. Both the length and the diameter of the tubing contribute to prime volume. In neonates, 3/16-inch tubing is used for the arterial and 1/4-inch tubing for the venous limbs of the circuit. Tube length is kept as short as possible by positioning the pump close to the surgical field. Quarter-inch tubing requires approximately 30 mL of volume per meter of tube length. A 3.5-kg newborn, for example, has a blood volume of approximately 300 mL. Each meter of tubing therefore requires an increase in prime volume equal to 10% of the newborn's circulating blood volume. Moving the pump heads closer to the patient and using vacuum-assisted venous drainage (VAVD) rather than gravity-controlled venous drainage can significantly reduce tubing length and priming volume. Tubing diameter for the circuit should be chosen to provide the maximal flow with a minimum of volume in the prime.

More recently, some groups have been advocating the use of 3/16-inch tubing for the venous side. This can be accomplished when accompanied with VAVD and allows for further reductions in prime volume.[81,82]

Initiation of CPB

Once CPB begins it is essential to observe the heart. Ineffective venous drainage can rapidly result in ventricular distention. This is especially true in infants and neonates where ventricular compliance is low and the heart is relatively intolerant of excessive preload augmentation due to a flat Starling curve. If distention occurs, pump flow must be reduced and the venous cannula repositioned. Distention is also common in patients with ventricular level shunts who have separate caval cannulation. Once the patient is placed on CPB, pulmonary resistance drops enormously, all blood in the heart (including collateral return) stays in the pulmonary circulation, and the systemic return to the cannulae becomes problematic. These patients may require left atrial decompression. If the repair is going to take place under deep hypothermic circulatory arrest, CPB is used as a cooling vehicle. The repair occurs during the arrest period. Venous cannulation can therefore be simplified. A large single venous cannula is placed in the right atrium to achieve effective venous drainage. With improvements in the understanding of how best to protect patients during "controlled" periods of DHCA, complex venous anatomy becomes a very strong indication for utilizing a DHCA strategy. Once cooled, the cannulae are removed and surgery proceeds in a cannula-free field. Some groups have advocated collecting 20 mL/kg of whole blood from the patient immediately after institution of CPB, to be infused after the completion of the repair and when the patient has been weaned from CPB. This in theory returns functional platelets and clotting factors back to the patient and aids in hemostasis and stability. More recently, many centers are advocating a system of assisted venous drainage in which negative pressure is applied to the venous reservoir and blood is actively evacuated from the atria. This may allow for decreasing priming volumes and reducing the sizes of venous cannulae.[106] The immediate effects of negative pressure on blood components have not, however, been fully explored.

ANTICOAGULATION AND BLEEDING MANAGEMENT

Maintaining anticoagulation during CPB is crucial. Many methods of anticoagulation monitoring have been utilized. The activated clotting time (ACT) has been the standard because of reproducibility and ease of use. The amount of heparin to be delivered has been based on the patient's weight in kilograms and a dose response curve as described by Bull and colleagues.[26] This very simple approach is used by many centers; however, it does not take into account the patient's blood volume, the effects of hypothermia and hemodilution, and preexisting heparin therapy. Another approach is to measure heparin levels directly with the HEPCON device (Heparin Management System, Medtronic, Minneapolis, Minn.). With this method, a dose response curve is calculated with a 2-mL sample of blood. Both heparin and protamine doses are calculated based on the patient's blood volume. In infants and neonates, most centers add blood to the circuit prime and consequently add heparin as well. Adequate anticoagulation is crucial, otherwise intravascular coagulation, thrombosis, consumption of clotting factors, and oxygenator dysfunction may occur. Several CPB-related bleeding complications are related to heparin. These include AT-III deficiency, heparin-induced thrombocytopenia, and inadequate heparin neutralization. Healthy newborns have only half as much AT-III concentration as adults. Using a standard dose of heparin may result in inadequate anticoagulation and intravascular coagulation. Administration of fresh frozen plasma or recombinant AT-III easily remedies this problem.

It has recently become apparent that the incidence of Heparin Induced Thrombocytopenia and Thrombosis (HITT) is similar in children as it is in adults (approximately 1% of patients).[1] This problem can have lethal complications unless recognized early in the postoperative period. This event is often heralded by thrombocytopenia, and a drop in the platelet count during the post-operative convalescence should suggest to the intensive care team the need to get a HITT assay, and to remove heparin from all intravenous lines. Patients who are found to have HITT require anticoagulation (usually with argantroban) to protect them from thrombosis. There has also been an interesting correlation recognized between aortic valve disease and platelet function disorders (such as von Willebrand's disease) and this should be investigated preoperatively in patients with aortic valve pathology.

There are many reasons for abnormal coagulation in the perioperative period and it is clearly beyond the scope of this chapter to address this in detail (see Chapter 14). There are, however, a few important points that should be emphasized. First, coagulation factors are decreased upon CPB and into the postoperative period. Hemodilution is responsible for some of this decrease; however ongoing activation of the extrinsic clotting system during bypass results in consumption of factors. Second, there is a qualitative and quantitative platelet defect. This platelet activation results from initial contact activation with the artificial surfaces of the circuit and oxygenator. The ongoing production of thrombin also results in significant activation of platelets. There are few studies addressing the use of heparin in infant heart surgery. Much of what we practice is extrapolated from adult literature. Excess anticoagulation can result in excessive bleeding and risk of intracranial hemorrhage. Too little heparin can result in ongoing intravascular coagulation and circuit/oxygenator malfunction. Young children seem to require higher doses of heparin to maintain activated clotting times of 350 to 450 seconds. It is important to realize that activated clotting time (ACT) levels are highly variable and do not correlate with actual heparin levels.

Newer anticoagulants are being examined in adult populations, but few studies in children have been done.

WEANING FROM CPB

When weaning from CPB, the heart is allowed to fill by partially clamping the venous return line and reducing the arterial inflow until adequate blood volume is achieved. It is important that the anesthesiologist resumes ventilation. Blood volume is assessed by direct visualization of the heart and by measuring right atrial or left atrial filling pressures. When filling pressures are adequate the venous cannula is clamped and the arterial inflow is stopped. The arterial cannula is left in place so that a slow infusion of residual pump blood can be used to optimize filling pressures. Myocardial function is assessed by direct cardiac visualization, intracardiac monitoring, and intraoperative echocardiography.[14,66,177,179-181] In corrected physiology the pulse oximeter can also be used as a crude measure of cardiac output. Low saturations or the inability of the oximeter probe to register a pulse may be a sign of very low output and high systemic resistance.[156]

After the repair of complex congenital heart defects the anesthesiologist and surgeon may have difficulty weaning patients from cardiopulmonary bypass. Under these circumstances a distinction must be made among: (1) a poor surgical result with a residual defect requiring re-repair or a residual defect that cannot be repaired and which describes the lesion as being "inoperable," (2) pulmonary artery hypertension, and/or (3) right or left ventricular dysfunction. Two methods of evaluation are used in the operating room. First, an intraoperative "cardiac catheterization" can be performed to assess isolated pressure measurements from the various chambers of the heart. Catheter measurements in various chambers and at various locations can help uncover residual pressure gradients across valves, repaired sites of stenosis, and conduits. Furthermore, blood samples can be obtained and analyzed for oxygen saturation data to look for residual shunts. Transthoracic monitoring catheters in the left atrium, right atrium, and/or pulmonary artery can be quite helpful in weaning from bypass and into the postoperative period.[61]

In addition intraoperative echocardiography with Doppler color flow has been used to provide an intraoperative "picture" of structural or functional abnormalities that might exist. If structural abnormalities are found, the patient can be replaced on CPB and residual defects can be repaired before leaving the operating room. Leaving the operating room with a significant residual structural defect adversely affects survival, and increases patient morbidity and cost.[14,179-181] With the introduction of improved probes, transesophageal echocardiography (TEE) can now be employed in babies as small as 2 kg. This has the advantage of being less obtrusive to the surgical team and enables accurate preoperative and postoperative evaluations without delaying the operation.[14] Functional problems can also be identified by echocardiography. Once diagnosed, therapy can be directed to the specific problem.

Left ventricular dysfunction can be treated by optimizing preload and heart rate, increasing coronary perfusion pressure, correcting ionized calcium levels, and adding inotropic support. Inotropic support is usually begun with calcium chloride supplementation (10 mg/kg) and dopamine or dobutamine (5 to 15 mcg/kg/min). If function remains poor, a second drug is usually added. For left ventricular dysfunction, a more potent inotrope is generally begun, such as epinephrine at a dose of 0.05 to 0.1 mcg/kg/minute and titrated to effect. Milrinone, a phosphodiesterase inhibitor, has fewer side effects and is easy to titrate safely. This combination of milrinone and epinephrine is very effective for left ventricular dysfunction because it addresses left ventricular contractility through non-beta receptor mediated mechanisms (epinephrine-alpha receptor, milrinone-phosphodiesterase inhibition), an important approach after pediatric CPB. The addition of milrinone during rewarming period is also helpful in increasing peripheral perfusion and decreasing systemic vascular resistance. If very high doses of inotrope are required to wean from CPB, mechanical circulatory support with extracorporeal membrane oxygenation (ECMO) or a left ventricular assist device (LVAD) should be considered.

Pulmonary artery hypertension is a common problem after CPB in children. It is treated with ventilatory manipulations. The goal is to reduce pulmonary vascular resistance by regulating $PaCO_2$, pH, PAO_2 (alveolar), PaO_2 (arterial), and lung volumes. Arterial pH is a potent mediator of pulmonary vascular resistance (PVR) especially in the newborn.[43] Maintaining a mildly alkolotic pH by manipulating $PaCO_2$ or serum bicarbonate is effective in modulating PVR.[113,129] Increases in both the arteriolar (PaO_2) and the alveolar (PAO_2) partial pressure of oxygen decrease PVR.[149] Since increasing FiO_2 reduces PVR in patients with intracardiac shunts, one can infer a direct pulmonary vasodilatory effect of the alveolar rather than arterial PO_2. Adjusting lung volumes through ventilatory mechanics also plays a major role in controlling pulmonary vascular resistance. After CPB, total lung water is increased, lung compliance is reduced, and closing capacity exceeds functional residual capacity. Airway closure occurs before end exhalation, producing areas of lung that are perfused but underventilated. These segments of lung become increasingly hypoxemic and secondary hypoxic vasoconstriction occurs. The result is elevated PVR and reduced pulmonary blood flow.

Nitric oxide (NO) is an endothelium-derived vasodilator that can be administered as an inhaled gas. Although a nonselective smooth muscle vasodilator, NO is rapidly inactivated by hemoglobin and therefore when administered via an inhaled route, the systemic circulation is protected from its vasodilating properties. Reduction in pulmonary vascular resistance has been demonstrated in adult patients with mitral valve stenosis and in children with reactive pulmonary hypertension after congenital heart surgery.[147]

If right ventricular dysfunction and pulmonary artery hypertension persist, cardiac output can be augmented by creating a small atrial septal defect (ASD) or by leaving a residual persistent foramen ovale to allow blood to shunt at the atrial level. This approach improves left ventricular filling, augments cardiac output, and improves oxygen delivery to tissue. Finally, leaving the chest open allows the right ventricle to obtain a larger end-diastolic dimension, thereby improving diastolic filling and right ventricular stroke volume. This may occasionally be necessary in neonates and infants with right heart dysfunction after weaning from CPB. This also prevents the effects of decreased chest wall compliance and mediastinal swelling on pulmonary and cardiac mechanics. If these methods fail, consideration for mechanical circulatory support should be considered.

MODIFIED ULTRAFILTRATION

There can be a significant accumulation of total body water during even routine open cardiac procedures. This edema is distributed not only in the periphery, but also in vital areas such as the brain, heart, gut, and lungs. This increase in total body water can be partially controlled by limiting the excess crystalloid given with the pump prime and also by removing this fluid by various means during or after CPB. Various techniques include peritoneal dialysis, aggressive diuresis, conventional (on pump) ultrafiltration and post-CPB (modified) ultrafiltration.[46,60,137] The technique of modified ultrafiltration is performed in the immediate post-bypass period. Most commonly, blood is removed from the aortic cannula, passed through a hemofilter, and then returned as oxygenated, hemoconcentrated, and ultrafiltered blood to the cannula in the right atrium. Modified ultrafiltration has the advantage of filtering only the patient's extracellular blood volume and not the CPB circuit. This results in greater hemoconcentration.[175] Both conventional and modified ultrafiltration have been shown to remove inflammatory mediators from the circulation.[124] However, modified ultrafiltration may be more effective in hemoconcentrating the patient's blood and in improving ventricular functional recovery.[37,131] Most complications with MUF are minor and seem to disappear as the team acquires experience with the technique.[40] Figure 20-9 displays one of the commonly used schema for modified ultrafiltration.

POST-CARDIOTOMY MECHANICAL SUPPORT

Occasionally, despite a technically successful operation, myocardial dysfunction precludes separation from CPB. In this situation, the choices for support in the infant are limited. The intra-aortic balloon pump is the most widely used device for adults. The use of this device is clearly limited because of size in the small child. Also, the biggest advantage of this device is that it improves coronary artery perfusion. This is seldom a significant problem in the child. In fact cardiac output is augmented only by about 15%. This device has been used in children as young as 5 years of age, but because of the risks of femoral artery injury and the difficulty the device has in synchronizing to higher heart rates its use in children is limited. Extracorporeal membrane oxygenation (ECMO) and ventricular assist device (VAD) are the other more commonly used options in children (see Chapter 21). The large experience with ECMO in the neonatal pulmonary dysfunction population has made ECMO the primary mode of support in most centers, but VAD may be quite useful and appropriate for certain patients.[38]

The indications for mechanical support vary significantly among surgeons and institutions, depending on the availability

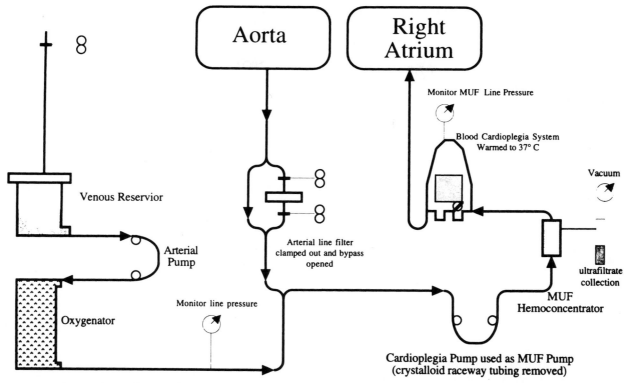

FIGURE 20-9 A schematic for modified ultrafiltration (MUF) in which the cardioplegia warmer is used to prevent patient cooling during the ultrafiltration process. (From Darling E, Nanry K, Shearer I, Kaemmer D, Lawson S: Techniques of paediatric modified ultrafiltration: 1996 survey results. *Perfusion* 13:93–103, 1998; with permission.)

and familiarity of the support devices. In general, cardiac and pulmonary dysfunction should be reversible and there should be no significant residual defects. One should optimize medical management based on physiologic data. It is important to note that there should likely be different thresholds for initiation of support depending on the specific lesion. For example, patients undergoing repair of complex arch reconstruction with single ventricle physiology are likely to be less stable a few hours after surgery. If a patient requires high doses of inotrope in the operating room in order to wean from CPB, strong consideration should be given to initiating post-cardiotomy support before leaving the operating room. In patients that have both pulmonary and cardiac dysfunction, we favor ECMO support. If, however, the pulmonary status is adequate, VAD may be preferable because one can avoid high levels of anticoagulation and the inflammatory insult associated with the addition of an oxygenator to the circuit. If VAD is initiated and pulmonary status deteriorates or right ventricular function deteriorates, then an oxygenator can be spliced into the circuit very quickly. When VAD is used in patients with single ventricle palliation and an aortopulmonary shunt, the shunt must be left open in order for oxygenation to occur. When ECMO is initiated in these same patients, we have elected to leave the shunt patent to perfuse the lungs and the flow rate is simply maintained at two to three times normal. This requires increased flow rates

in order to perfuse both the pulmonary and systemic circulation. This strategy ensures antegrade pulmonary blood flow and limits the risk of damaging the shunt, which may lead to thrombosis of the shunt.[77] There is recent evidence that routine use of VAD following Norwood operation may lead to improved neurologic outcomes, possibly due to the vulnerability of the hypoxemic brain (by definition, all patients are hypoxemic following the Norwood Procedure), after exposure to CPB.[171,182]

The most common complications related to mechanical device support are bleeding and embolism. Surgical bleeding should be ruled out early and coagulopathy treated completely and quickly. Neurologic events, either bleeding or embolic, are not uncommon and are relative contraindications for the initiation and maintenance of support. We have found that 60% of patients that have required post-cardiotomy support with either VAD or ECMO can be successfully discharged from the hospital.[77]

CONCLUSION

Cardiopulmonary bypass and extracorporeal support have evolved from the futuristic vision of surgical pioneers to safe and efficient means of support for infants and children undergoing complex cardiac procedures. CPB in infants and neonates poses many challenges and should be undertaken in centers specializing in the care of infants with congenital heart disease. The physiology of CPB and hypothermia has been gradually elucidated, pathophysiologic effects determined, and therapies addressed. Our technical ability to address surgically the most complex of problems has improved over the last decade with reduction in mortality rates to less than 5% for most complex lesions. CPB is still responsible for significant morbidity. Miniaturization of bypass circuitry, modulation of the inflammatory response, advancement of technology, and improvement in techniques of perfusion will maximize the safety of extracorporeal circulation and provide the next major step in producing better outcomes.

References

1. Alsoufi B, Boshkov LK, Kirby A, et al: Heparin-induced thrombocytopenia (HIT) in pediatric cardiac surgery: An emerging cause of morbidity and mortality. In Jonas R (ed): *Seminars in Thoracic and Cardiovascular Surgery*. Philadelphia, WB Saunders, 2004, pp 155–171.
2. Anand KJ, Hickey PR: Halothane-morphine compared with high dose sufentanil for anesthesia and postoperative analgesia in neonatal cardiac surgery. *N Engl J Med* 326:1–9, 1992.
3. Aoki M, Jonas RA, Nomura F, et al: Effects of aprotinin on acute recovery of cerebral metabolism in piglets after hypothermic circulatory arrest. *Ann Thorac Surg* 58:146–153, 1994.
4. Aoki M, Nomura F, Stromski ME, et al: Effects of pH on brain energetics after hypothermic circulatory arrest. *Ann Thorac Surg* 55:1093–1103, 1993.
5. Aoki M, Nomura F, Kawata H, Mayer JE Jr: The effect of calcium and preischemic hypothermia on recovery of myocardia after cardioplegic ischemia in neonatal lambs. *J Thorac Cardiovasc Surg* 105:207–212, 1993.
6. Armon C, Deschamps C, Adkinson C, et al: Hyperbaric treatment of cerebral air embolism sustained during an open-heart surgical procedure. *Mayo Clin Proc* 66:565–571, 1991.
7. Baker E, Olinger G, Baker J: Calcium content of St. Thomas II cardioplegic solution damages ischemic immature myocardium. *Ann Thorac Surg* 52:993–999, 1991.
8. Bando K, Vijay P, Turrentine MW, et al: Dilutional and modified ultrafiltration reduces pulmonary hypertension after operations for congenital heart disease: A prospective randomized study. *J Thorac Cardiovasc Surg* 115:517–525, 1998.
9. Bashein G, Townes BD, Nessly ML, et al: A randomized study of carbon dioxide management during hypothermic cardiopulmonary bypass. *Anesthesiology* 72:7–15, 1990.
10. Bell C, Rimar S, Barash P: ST-segment changes consistent with myocardial ischemia in the neonate: A report of three cases. *Anesthesiology* 71:601–604, 1989.
11. Bellinger DC, Jonas RA, Rappaport LA, et al: Developmental and neurologic status of children after heart surgery with hypothermic circulatory arrest or low-flow cardiopulmonary bypass. *N Engl J Med* 332:549–555, 1995.
12. Bellinger DC, Wypij D, du Plessis AJ, et al: Neurodevelopmental status at eight years in children with dextro-transposition of the great arteries: The Boston Circulatory Arrest Trial. *J Thorac Cardiovasc Surg* 126:1385–1396, 2003.
13. Bellinger DC, et al: Rapid cooling of infants on cardiopulmonary bypass adversely affects later cognitive function. *Circulation* 78:A358, 1988.
14. Bengur AR, Li JS, Herlong JR, et al: Intraoperative transesophageal echocardiography in congenital heart disease. *Semin Thorac Cardiovasc Surg* 10:255–264, 1998.
15. Bigelow WG, Callaghan JC, Hopps JA: General hypothermia for experimental intracardiac surgery: The use of electrophrenic respirations, an artificial pacemaker for cardiac standstill, and radio frequency rewarming in general hypothermia. *Ann Surg* 132:531–539, 1950.
16. Billingsley A, Laks H, Haas G: Myocardial protection in children. In Baue A, Geha A, Hammond G (eds): *Glenn's Textbook of Cardiovascular Surgery*. East Norwalk, Conn., Appleton Lange, 1991.
17. Bjork, VO, Hultquist G: Contraindications to profound hypothermia. *J Thorac Cardiovasc Surg* 44:1–9, 1962.
18. Blauth C, Smith P, Newman S, et al: Retinal microembolism and neuropsychiatric deficit following clinical cardiopulmonary bypass: Comparison of a membrane and a bubble oxygenator. *Eur J Cardiothorac Surg* 3:135–138, 1989.
19. Blauth CI, Arnold JV, Schulenberg WE, et al: Cerebral microembolism during cardiopulmonary bypass: Retinal microvascular studies in vivo with fluorescein angiography. *J Thorac Cardiovasc Surg* 95:668–676, 1988.
20. Boucek RJ, Shelton M, Artman M, et al: Comparative effects of verapamil, nifedipine, and diltiazem on contractile function in the isolated immature and adult rabbit heart. *Pediatr Res* 18:948–952, 1984.
21. Boudreaux JP, Schieber RA, Cook DR: Hemodynamic effects of halothane in the newborn piglet. *Anesth Analg* 63:731–737, 1984.
22. Boyle EM Jr, Verrier ED, Spiess BD: Endothelial cell injury in cardiovascular surgery: The procoagulant response. *Ann Thorac Surg* 62:1549–1557, 1996.
23. Bregman D, Bowman FO Jr, Parodi EN, et al: An improved method of myocardial protection with pulsation during cardiopulmonary bypass. *Circulation* 56:II157–160, 1977.
24. Brunberg JA, Doty DB, Reilly EL: Choreoathetosis in infants following cardiac surgery with deep hypothermia and circulatory arrest. *J Pediatr* 84:232–235, 1974.
25. Bui KC, Hammerman C, Hirschl RB, et al: Plasma prostanoids in neonates with pulmonary hypertension treated with conventional therapy and with extracorporeal membrane oxygenation. *J Thorac Cardiovasc Surg* 101:973–983, 1991.
26. Bull BS, Huse WM, Brauer FS, Korpman RA: Heparin therapy during extracorporeal circulation II: Use of a dose response curve to individualize heparin and protamine dosage. *J Thorac Cardiovasc Surg* 69:685–689, 1975.
27. Butler J, Rocker GM, Westaby S: Inflammatory responses to cardiopulmonary bypass. *Ann Thorac Surg* 55:552–559, 1993.
28. Cannon ML, Cheifetz IM, Craig DM, et al: Optimizing liquid ventilation as a lung protection strategy for neonatal cardiopulmonary bypass: Full functional residual capacity dosing is more effective than half functional residual capacity dosing. *Crit Care Med* 27:1140–1146, 1999.
29. Cave AC, Manche A, Derias NW, Hearse DJ: Thromboxane A2 mediates pulmonary hypertension after cardiopulmonary bypass in the rabbit. *J Thorac Cardiovasc Surg* 106:959–967, 1993.
30. Chai PJ, Williamson JA, Lodge AJ, et al: Effects of ischemia on pulmonary dysfunction after cardiopulmonary bypass. *Ann Thorac Surg* 67:731–735, 1999.
31. Cheifetz IM, Cannon ML, Craig DM, et al: Liquid ventilation improves pulmonary function and cardiac output in a neonatal swine model of cardiopulmonary bypass. *J Thorac Cardiovasc Surg* 115:528–535, 1998.
32. Chu SH, Huang TS, Hsu RB, et al: Thyroid hormone changes after cardiovascular surgery and the clinical implications. *Ann Thorac Surg* 52:791–796, 1991.
33. Clark RE, Dietz DR, Miller JG: Continuous detection of microemboli during cardiopulmonary bypass in animals and man. *Circulation* 54:III74–178, 1976.
34. Cook DJ, Orszulak TA, Daly RC: Minimum hematocrits at differing cardiopulmonary bypass temperatures in dogs. *Circulation* 98:II170–175, 1998.
35. Corno AF, Bethencourt DM, Laks H, et al: Myocardial protection in the neonatal heart: A comparision of topical hypothermia and crystalloid and blood cardioplegia solutions. *J Thorac Cardiovasc Surg* 93:163–172, 1987.
36. Croughwell N, Smith LR, Quill T, et al: The effect of temperature on cerebral metabolism and blood flow in adults during cardiopulmonary bypass. *J Thorac Cardiovasc Surg* 103:549–554, 1992.
37. Daggett CW, Lodge AJ, Scarborough JE, et al: Modified ultrafiltration versus conventional ultrafiltration: A randomized prospective study in neonatal piglets. *J Thorac Cardiovasc Surg* 115:336–342, 1998.
38. Darling EM, Kaemmer D, Lawson DS, et al: Use of ECMO without the oxygenator to provide ventricular support after Norwood Stage I procedures. *Ann Thorac Surg* 71:735–736, 2001.
39. Darling E, Nanry K, Shearer I, et al: Techniques of paediatric modified ultrafiltration: 1996 survey results. *Perfusion* 13:93–103, 1998.
40. Darling EM, Shearer R, Katherine N, et al: Modified ultrafiltration in pediatric cardiopulmonary bypass. *J Extra-Corporeal Technology* 26:205–209, 1994.

41. DeLeon S, Ilbawi M, Arcilla R, et al: Choreoathetosis after deep hypothermia without circulatory arrest. *Ann Thorac Surg* 50:714–719, 1990.
42. Deverall PB, Padayachee TS, Parsons S, et al: Ultrasound detection of microemboli in the middle cerebral artery during cardiopulmonary bypass surgery. *Eur J Cardiothorac Surg* 2:256–260, 1988.
43. Drummond WH, Gregory GA, Heymann MA, Phibbs RA: The independent effects of hyperventilation, tolazoline, and dopamine in infants with persistant pulmonary hypertension. *J Pediatr* 98:603–611, 1981.
44. du Plessis AJ, Treves ST, Hickey PR, et al: Regional cerebral perfusion abnormalities after cardiac operations: Single photon emission computed tomography (SPECT) findings in children with postoperative movement disorders. *J Thorac Cardiovasc Surg* 107:1036–1043, 1994.
45. Egerton N, Egerton WS, Kay JH: Neurologic changes following profound hypothermia. *Ann Surg* 157:366–373, 1962.
46. Elliott MJ: Ultrafiltration and modified ultrafiltration in pediatric open heart operations. *Ann Thorac Surg* 56:1518–1522, 1993.
47. Engelman RM, Haag B, Lemeshow S, et al: Mechanism of plasma catecholamine increases during coronary artery bypass and valve procedures. *J Thorac Cardiovasc Surg* 86:608–615, 1983.
48. Fallon P, Roberts I, Kirkham FJ, et al: Cerebral hemodynamics during cardiopulmonary bypass in children using near-infrared spectroscopy. *Ann Thorac Surg* 56:1473–1477, 1993.
49. Ferry PC: Neurologic sequelae of open-heart surgery in children: An "irritating question." *Am J Dis Child* 144:369–373, 1990.
50. Ferry PC: Neurologic sequelae of cardiac surgery in children. *Am J Dis Child* 141:309–312, 1987.
51. Fessatidis IT, Thomas VL, Shore DF, et al: Brain damage after profoundly hypothermic circulatory arrest: Correlations between neurophysiologic and neuropathologic findings. An experimental study in vertebrates. *J Thorac Cardiovasc Surg* 106:32–41, 1993.
52. Finn A, Naik S, Klein N, et al: Interleukin-8 release and neutrophil degranulation after pediatric cardiopulmonary bypass. *J Thorac Cardiovasc Surg* 105:234–241, 1993.
53. Finn A, Dreyer WJ: Neutrophil adhesion and the inflammatory response induced by cardiopulmonary bypass. *Cardiol Young* 3:244–250, 1993.
54. Fisk GC, Wright JS, Hicks RG, et al: The influence of duration of circulatory arrest at 20 degrees C on cerebral changes. *Anaesth Intensive Care* 4:126–134, 1976.
55. Gaer JA, Shaw AD, Wild R, et al: Effect of cardiopulmonary bypass on gastrointestinal perfusion and function. *Ann Thorac Surg* 57:371–375, 1994.
56. Galli KK, Zimmerman RA, Jarvik GP, et al: Periventricular leukomalacia is common following neonatal cardiac surgery. *J Thorac Cardiovasc Surg* 127:692–704, 2004.
57. Gaynor JW, Gerdes M, Zackai EH, et al: Apolipoprotein E genotype and neurodevelopmental sequelae of infant cardiac surgery. *J Thorac Cardiovasc Surg* 126:1736–1745, 2003.
58. Gibbon JH: Application of mechanical heart lung apparatus to cardiac surgery. *Minn Med* 37:171, 1954.
59. Gillinov AM, Redmond JM, Zehr KJ, et al: Superior cerebral protection with profound hypothermia during circulatory arrest. *Ann Thorac Surg* 55:1432–1439, 1993.
60. Giuffre RM, Tam KH, Williams WW, Freedom RM: Acute renal failure complicating pediatric cardiac surgery: A comparison of survivors and non-survivors following acute peritoneal bypass. *Pediatr Cardiol* 13:208–213, 1992.
61. Gold JP, Jonas RA, Lang P, et al: Transthoracic intracardiac monitoring lines in pediatric surgical patients: A ten-year experience. *Ann Thorac Surg* 42:185–191, 1986.
62. Grayck EN, Meliones JN, Kern FH, et al: Elevated serum lactate correlates with intracranial hemorrhage in neonates treated with extracorporeal life support. *Pediatrics* 96:914–917, 1995.
63. Greeley WJ, et al: Mechanisms of injury and methods of protection of the brain during cardiac surgery in neonates and infants. *Cardiol Young* 3:317–330, 1993.
64. Greeley WJ, Bracey VA, Ungerleider RM, et al: Recovery of cerebral metabolism and mitochrondrial oxidation state is delayed after hypothermic circulatory arrest. *Circulation* 84:III400–406, 1991.
65. Greeley WJ, Kern FH, Ungerleider RM, et al: The effect of hypothermic cardiopulmonary bypass and total circulatory arrest on cerebral metabolism in neonates, infants, and children. *J Thorac Cardiovasc Surg* 101:783–794, 1991.
66. Greeley WJ, Kern FH, Ungerleider RM, Kisslo JA: Intramyocardial air causes right ventricular dysfunction after repair of congenital heart lesions. *Anesthesiology* 73:1042–1046, 1990.
67. Greeley WJ, Ungerleider RM, Smith LR, Reves JG: The effects of deep hypothermic cardiopulmonary bypass and total circulatory arrest on cerebral blood flow in infants and children. *J Thorac Cardiovasc Surg* 97:737–745, 1989.
68. Greeley WJ, Ungerleider RM, Kern FH, et al: Effects of cardiopulmonary bypass on cerebral blood flow in neonates, infants, and children. *Circulation* 80:I209–215, 1989.
69. Greeley W, Ungerleider R, Smith LR, Reves J: Cardiopulmonary bypass alters cerebral blood flow in infants and children during and after cardiovascular surgery. *Circulation* 78:II356–363, 1988.
70. Gruber EM, Jonas RA, Newburger JW, et al: The effect of hematocrit on cerebral blood flow velocity in neonates and infants undergoing deep hypothermic cardiopulmonary bypass. *Anesth Analg* 89:322–327, 1999.
71. Haneda K, Sato S, Ishizawa E, Horiuchi T: The importance of colloid oncotic pressure during open heart surgery in infants. *Tohoku J Exp Med* 147:65–71, 1985.
72. Heinle JS, Lodge AJ, Mault JR, et al: Myocardial function is normal after rapid cooling of the in vivo neonatal heart. *Ann Thorac Surg* 57:326–333, 1994.
73. Henling CE, Carmichael MJ, Keats AS, Cooley DA: Cardiac operation for congenital heart disease in children of Jehovah's Witnesses. *J Thorac Cardiovasc Surg* 89:914–920, 1985.
74. Hetzer R, Warnecke H, Wittrock H, et al: Extracoronary collateral myocardial blood flow during cardioplegic arrest. *J Thorac Cardiovasc Surg* 28:191–196, 1980.
75. Hindman BJ, Dexter F, Cutkomp J, et al: Brain blood flow and metabolism do not decrease at stable brain temperature during cardiopulmonary bypass in rabbits. *Anesthesiology* 77:342–350, 1992.
76. Horton AM, Wutt W: Pump-induced haemolysis: Is the constrained vortex pump better or worse than the roller pump? *Perfusion* 7:103–108, 1992.
77. Jaggers JJ, Forbess JM, Shah AS, et al: Extracorporeal membrane oxygenation for infant postcardiotomy support: Significance of shunt management. *Ann Thorac Surg* 69:1476–1483, 2000.
78. Jaggers JJ, Neal MC, Smith PK, et al: Infant cardiopulmonary bypass: A procoagulant state. *Ann Thorac Surg* 68:513–520, 1999.
79. Jonas RA, Bellinger DC, Rappaport LA, et al: Relation of pH strategy and developmental outcome after hypothermic circulatory arrest. *J Thorac Cardiovasc Surg* 106:362–368, 1993.
80. Journois D, Pouard P, Greeley WJ, et al: Hemofiltration during cardiopulmonary bypass in pediatric cardiac surgery. Effects on hemostasis, cytokines, and complement components. *Anesthesiology* 81:1181–1189, 1994.
81. Karamlou T, Hickey E, Silliman CC, et al: Reducing risk in infant cardiopulmonary bypass: The use of a miniaturized circuit and a crystalloid prime improves cardiopulmonary function and increases cerebral blood flow. *Pediatric Cardiac Surgery Annual* 2005.
82. Karamlou T, Schultz J, Shen I, Ungerleider RM: Use of a miniaturized circuit and an asanguineous prime to reduce organ dysfunction following infant cardiopulmonary bypass. *Ann Thorac Surg* 2005.
83. Kawashima Y, Yamamoto Z, Manabe H: Safe limits of hemodilution in cardiopulmonary bypass. *Surgery* 76:391–397, 1974.
84. Kern FH, Ungerleider RM, Schulman SR, et al: Comparing two strategies of cardiopulmonary bypass cooling on jugular venous oxygen saturation in neonates and infants. *Ann Thorac Surg* 60:1198–1202, 1995.
85. Kern FH, Greeley WJ, Ungerleider RM: Cardiopulmonary bypass. In Nichols DG, Cameron DE, Greeley, WH, et al (eds): *Critical Heart Disease in Infants and Children.* St. Louis, Mosby, 1995, pp 497–530.
86. Kern FH, Ungerleider RM, Reves JG, et al: Effect of altering pump flow rate on cerebral blood flow and metabolism in infants and children. *Ann Thorac Surg* 56:1366–1372, 1993.
87. Kern FH, Jonas RA, Mayer JE Jr, et al: Temperature monitoring during infant CPB: Does it predict efficient brain cooling? *Ann Thorac Surg* 54:749–754, 1992.
88. Kern FH, Ungerleider RM, Quill TJ, et al: Cerebral blood flow response to changes in arterial carbon dioxide tension during hypothermic cardiopulmonary bypass in children. *J Thorac Cardiovasc Surg* 101:618–622, 1991.
89. Kirklin JW, Barratt-Boyes BG (eds): *Cardiac Surgery,* 2nd ed. New York, Churchill Livingstone, p. 1779, 1993.
90. Kirklin JK, Kirklin JW, Pacifico AD: Deep hypothermia and total circulatory arrest. In Arcinegas E (ed): *Pediatric Cardiac Surgery.* Chicago, Year Book Medical Publishers, 1985.

91. Kirklin JK, Westaby S, Blackstone EH, et al: Complement and the damaging effects of cardiopulmonary bypass. *J Thorac Cardiovasc Surg* 86:845–857, 1983.

92. Kirklin JA, Dushane JW, Wood EH: Intracardiac surgery with the aid of a mechanical pump oxygenator system: Report of eight cases. *Proc Mayo Clinic* 30:201–206, 1955.

93. Kirshbom PM, Page SO, Jacobs MT, et al: Cardiopulmonary bypass and circulatory arrest increase endothelin-1 production and receptor expression in the lung. *J Thorac Cardiovasc Surg* 113:777–783, 1997.

94. Kirshbom PM, Skaryak LR, DiBernardo LR, et al: pH-stat cooling improves cerebral metabolic recovery after circulatory arrest in a piglet model of aortopulmonary collaterals. *J Thorac Cardiovasc Surg* 111:147–157, 1996.

95. Kirshbom PM, Jacobs MT, Tsui SS, et al: Effects of cardiopulmonary bypass and circulatory arrest on endothelium-dependent vasodilation in the lung. *J Thorac Cardiovasc Surg* 111:1248–1256, 1996.

96. Kirshbom PM, Tsui SS, DiBernardo LR, et al: Blockade of endothelin-converting enzyme reduces pulmonary hypertension after cardiopulmonary bypass and circulatory arrest. *Surgery* 118:440–445, 1995.

97. Kirshbom PM, Skaryak LA, DiBernardo LR, et al: Effects of aortopulmonary collaterals on cerebral cooling and cerebral metabolic recovery after circulatory arrest. *Circulation* 92:II490–494, 1995.

98. Kirshbom PM, et al: Aortopulmonary collaterals decrease the rate of cerebral cooling and alter regional cerebral perfusion during cardiopulmonary bypass. *Surgical Forum* 45:258–259, 1994.

99. Koutlas TC, Gaynor JW, Nicolson SC, et al: Modified ultrafiltration reduces postoperative morbidity after cavopulmonary connection. *Ann Thorac Surg* 64:37–42, 1997.

100. Kraft LF, Katholi RE, Woods WT, James TN: Attenuaion by magnesium of the electrophysiologic effects of hyperkalemia on human and canine heart cells. *Am J Cardiol* 45:1189–1195, 1980.

101. Kronon MT, Allen BS, Hernan J, et al: Superiority of magnesium cardioplegia in neonatal myocardial protection. *Ann Thorac Surg* 68:2285–2291, 1999.

102. Langley SM, Chai PJ, Jaggers JJ, Ungerleider RM: Preoperative high-dose methylprednisolone attenuates the cerebral response to deep hypothermic arrest. *Eur J Cardiothorac Surg* 17:279–286, 2000.

103. Langley SM, Chai PJ, Jaggers JJ, Ungerleider RM: The free radical spin trap alpha-phenyl-tertbutyl nitrone attenuates the cerebral response to deep hypothermic ischemia. *J Thorac Cardiovasc Surg* 119:305–313, 2000.

104. Langley SM, Chai PJ, Miller SE, et al: Intermittent perfusion protects the brain during deep hypothermic circulatory arrest. *Ann Thorac Surg* 68:4–13, 1999.

105. Langley SM, Chai PJ, Jaggers JJ, Ungerleider RM: Platelet activating factor antagonism improves cerebral recovery after circulatory arrest. *Ann Thorac Surg* 68:1578–1584, 1999.

106. Lau CL, Posther KE, Stephenson GR, et al: Mini-circuit cardiopulmonary bypass with vacuum assisted venous drainage: Feasibility of an asanguinous prime in the neonate. *Perfusion* 14:389–396, 1999.

107. Leone BJ, et al: Effects of hemodilution and anesthesia on regional function of compromised myocardium. *Anesthesiology* 73:A596, 1990.

108. Lewis FJ, Taufic M: Closure of atrial septal defects with the aid of hypothermia: Experimental accomplishments and the report of the one successful case. *Surgery* 33:52, 1953.

109. Lillehei CW, Cohen M, Warden HE: Direct vision intracardiac surgery by means of controlled cross-circulation or continuous arterial reservoir perfusion for correction of ventricular septal defects, atrioventricularis communis, isolated infundibular pulmonic stenosis, and tetralogy of Fallot. Proceeding of the Henry Ford Symposium. In Lam CR (ed): Philadelphia, WB Saunders, 1955, pp 371–392.

110. Lillehei CW, Varco RL, Cohen M, et al: The first open heart repairs of ventricular septal defect, atrioventricular communis, and tetralogy of Fallot using extracorporeal circulation by cross-circulation: A 30-year follow-up. *Ann Thorac Surg* 41:4–21, 1986.

111. Lodge AJ, Undar A, Daggett CW, et al: Methylprednisolone reduces the inflammatory response to cardiopulmonary bypass in neonatal piglets: Timing of dose is important. *J Thorac Cardiovasc Surg* 117:515–522, 1999.

112. Lodge AJ, Undar A, Daggett CW, et al: Regional blood flow during pulsatile cardiopulmonary bypass and after circulatory arrest in an infant model. *Ann Thorac Surg* 63:1243–1250, 1997.

113. Lyrene RK, Welch KA, Godoy G, Philips JB III: Alkalosis attenuates hypoxic pulmonary vasoconstriction in neonatal lambs. *Pediatr Res* 19:1268–1271, 1985.

114. Malm JR, Manger WM, Sullivan SF, Papper EM, Nahas GG: The effect of acidosis on sympatho-adrenal stimulation: Particular reference to cardiopulmonary bypass. *JAMA* 197:121–125, 1966.

115. Marelli D, Paul A, Samson CP: Does the addition of albumin to the prime solution in cardiopulmonary bypass affect the clinical outcome? *J Thorac Cardiovasc Surg* 98:751–756, 1989.

116. Mault JR, Ohtake S, Klingensmith ME, et al: Cerebral metabolism and circulatory arrest: effects of duration and strategies for protection. *Ann Thorac Surg* 55:57–63, 1993.

117. Mault JR, Ungerleider RM: Intermittent perfusion during hypothermic circulatory arrest: A new and effective technique for cerebral protection. *Surgical Forum* 43:314–316, 1992.

118. Mault JR, Whitaker EG, Heinle JS, et al: Cerebral metabolic effects of sequential periods of hypothermic circulatory arrest: Effects of a second period of circulatory arrest on the brain. *Ann Thorac Surg* 57:96–100, 1994.

119. Meliones JN, Gaynor JW, Wilson BG, et al: Modified ultrafiltration reduces airway pressures and improves lung compliance after congenital heart surgery. *J Am Col Cardiol* 25:271A, 1995.

120. Menghini A: Oxygenator design: A global approach. *Perfusion* 8:87–92, 1993.

121. Mezrow CK, Gandsas A, Sadeghi AM, et al: Metabolic correlates of neurologic and behavioral injury after prolonged hypothermic circulatory arrest. *J Thorac Cardiovasc Surg* 109:959–975, 1995.

122. Mezrow CK, Sadeghi AM, Gandsas A, et al: Cerebral effects of low-flow cardiopulmonary bypass and hypothermic circulatory arrest. *Ann Thorac Surg* 57:532–539, 1994.

123. Mezrow CK, et al: A vulnerable interval for cerebral injury: Comparison of hypothermic circulatory arrest and low flow cardiopulmonary bypass. *Cardiol Young* 3:287–298, 1993.

124. Millar AB, Armstrong L, van der Linden J, et al: Cytokine production and hemofiltration in children undergoing cardiopulmonary bypass. *Ann Thor Surg* 56:1499–1502, 1993.

125. Mitchell IM, Pollock JC, Jamieson MP, et al: The effects of cardiopulmonary bypass on thyroid function in infants weighing less than five kilograms. *J Thorac Cardiovasc Surg* 103:800–805, 1992.

126. Miura T, Laussen P, Lidov HG, et al: Intermittent whole-body perfusion with "somatoplegia" versus blood perfusate to extend duration of circulatory arrest. *Circulation* 94:II56–62, 1996.

127. Moat NE, Shore DF, Evans TW: Organ dysfunction and cardiopulmonary bypass: The role of complement and regulatory proteins. *Eur J Cardiothorac Surg* 7:563–573, 1993.

128. Moore RY: Normal development of the nervous system: Prenatal and perinatal factors associated with brain disorders. *NIH Publications* 33–51, 1985.

129. Morray JP, Lynn AM, Mansfield PB: Effects of pH and PCO_2 on pulmonary and sustemic hemodynamics after surgery in children with congenital heart disease and pulmonary hypertension. *J Pediatr* 113:474–479, 1988.

130. Naik SK, Elliott MJ: Ultrafiltration and paediatric cardiopulmonary bypass. *Perfusion* 8:101–112, 1993.

131. Naik SK, Knight A, Elliott MJ: A prospective randomized study of a modified technique of ultrafiltration during pediatric open heart surgery. *Circulation* 84:III422–431, 1991.

132. Navas JP, Anderson W, Marsh JD: Hypothermia increases calcium content of hypoxic myocytes. *Am J Physiol* 259:H333–339, 1990.

133. Newburger JW, Jonas RA, Wernovsky G, et al: A comparison of the perioperative neurologic effects of hypothermic circulatory arrest versus low-flow cardiopulmonary bypass in infant heart surgery. *N Engl J Med* 329:1057–1064, 1993.

134. Noris M, Morigi M, Donadelli R, et al: Nitric oxide synthesis by cultured endothelial cells is modulated by flow conditions. *Circ Res* 76:536–543, 1995.

135. Norwood WI, Norwood CR, Castaneda AR: Cerebral anoxia: Effect of deep hypothermia and pH. *Surgery* 86:203–210, 1979.

136. Orenstein JM, Sato N, Aaron B, et al: Microemboli observed in deaths following cardiac surgery. *Hum Pathol* 13:1082–1090, 1982.

137. Paret G, Cohen AJ, Bohn DJ: Continuous arterio-venous hemofiltration after cardiac operation in infants and children. *J Thorac Cardiovasc Surg* 1225–1230, 1992.

138. Pearson DT, et al: A clinical evaluation of the performance characteristics of one membrane and five bubble oxygenators: Haemocompatibility studies. *Perfusion* 1:81–98, 1986.

139. Philbin DM, Levine FH, Emerson CW, et al: Plasma vasopressin levels and urinary flow during cardiopulmonary bypass in patients with valvular heart disease. *J Thorac Cardiovasc Surg* 78:779–783, 1979.

140. Pigula FA, Nemoto EM, Griffith BP, Siewers RD: Regional low-flow perfusion provides cerebral circulatory support during neonatal aortic arch reconstruction. *J Thorac Cardiovasc Surg* 119:331–339, 2000.

141. Purpura, D: Normal and aberrant neuronal development in the cerebral cortex of the human fetus and young infant. In Brazier MAB (ed): *Growth and Development of the Brain: Nutritional, Genetic, and Environmental Factors.* New York, Raven Press, 1975, pp 33–49.

142. Ratcliffe JM, Wyse RK, Hunter S, et al: The role of priming fluid in the metabolic response to cardiopulmonary bypass in children less than 15 kg of body weight undergoing open heart surgery. *Thorac Cardiovasc Surg* 36:65–74, 1988.

143. Ratcliffe JM, Elliott MJ, Wyse RK, et al: The metabolic load of stored blood: Implications for major transfusions in infants. *Arch Dis Child* 61:1208–1214, 1986.

144. Rebeyka I, Diaz R, Waddell J: Magnesium based blood cardioplegia in a neonatal heart model. *Circulation* 86:I–630, 1992.

145. Rebeyka IM, Hanan SA, Borges MR, et al: Rapid cooling contracture of the myocardium: The adverse effect of pre-arrest cardiac hypothermia. *J Thorac Cardiovasc Surg* 100:240–249, 1990.

146. Robbins RC, Balaban RS, Swain JA: Intermittent hypothermic asanguineous cerebral perfusion (cerebroplegia) protects the brain during prolonged circulatory arrest. *J Thorac Cardiovasc Surg* 99:878–884, 1990.

147. Roberts JD Jr, Chen TY, Kawai N, et al: Inhaled nitric oxide reverses pulmonary vasoconstriction in the hypoxic and acidotic newborn lamb. *Circ Res* 72:246–254, 1993.

148. Rolph T, Jones C: Regulation of glycolytic flux in the heart of the fetal guinea pig. *J Dev Physiol* 5:31–39, 1983.

149. Rudolph AM, Yuan S: Response of the pulmonary vasculature to hypoxia and H+ ion concentration changes. *J Clin Invest* 45:399, 1966.

150. Sade RM, Bartles DM, Dearing JP, Campbell LJ, Loadholt CB: A prospective randomized study of membrane versus bubble oxygenators in children. *Ann Thorac Surg* 29:502–511, 1980.

151. Sakai TH, Kurihara S: Rapid cooling contracture of toad cardiac muscle. *Japan J Physiol* 365:131–146, 1974.

152. Salama A, Mueller-Eckhardt C: Delayed hemolytic transfusion reactions: Evidence for complement activation involving allogenic autologous red cells. *Transfusion* 214:188–193, 1984.

153. Seghaye MC, Grabitz RG, Duchateau J, et al: Inflammatory reaction and capillary leak syndrome related to cardiopulmonary bypass in neonates undergoing cardiac operations. *J Thorac Cardiovasc Surg* 112:687–697, 1996.

154. Seghaye MC, Duchateau J, Grabitz RG, et al: Complement, leukocytes, and leukocyte elastase in full term neonates undergoing cardiac operations. *J Thorac Cardiovasc Surg* 108:29–36, 1994.

155. Semb BK, Pedersen T, Hatteland K, et al: Doppler ultrasound estimation of bubble removal by various arterial line filters during extracorporeal circulation. *Scand J Thorac Cardiovasc Surg* 16:55–62, 1982.

156. Severinghaus JW, Spellman MJ Jr: Pulse oximeter failure thresholds in hypotension and vasoconstriction. *Anesthesiology* 73:532–537, 1990.

157. Shen I, Giacomuzzi C, Ungerleider RM: Current strategies for optimizing the use of cardiopulmonary bypass in neonates and infants. *Ann Thorac Surg* 75:S729-734, 2003.

158. Shum-Tim D, Nagashima M, Shinoka T, et al: Postischemic hyperthermia exacerbates neurologic injury after deep hypothermic circulatory arrest. *J Thorac Cardiovasc Surg* 116:780–792, 1998.

159. Skaryak LA, Lodge AJ, Kirshbom PM, et al: Low-flow cardiopulmonary bypass produces greater pulmonary dysfunction than circulatory arrest. *Ann Thorac Surg* 62:1284–1288, 1996.

160. Skaryak LA, Kirshbom PM, DiBernardo LR, et al: Modified ultrafiltration improves cerebral metabolic recovery after circulatory arrest. *J Thorac Cardiovasc Surg* 109:744–752, 1995.

161. Skaryak LA, Chai PJ, Kern FH, et al: Blood gas management and degree of cooling: effects on cerebral metabolism before and after circulatory arrest. *J Thorac Cardiovasc Surg* 110:1649–1657, 1995.

162. Skaryak LA, et al: Combining alpha-stat and pH-stat blood gas strategies during cooling prior to circulatory arrest provides optimal recovery of cerebral metabolism. Presented at the American Heart Association 66th scientific session, November 1993.

163. Somero GN, White FN: Enzymatic consequences under alpha-stat regulation. In Rahn H, Prakash O (eds): *Acid Base Regulation and Body Temperature.* Boston, Nijhoff, 1985, pp 55–80.

164. Sonntag J, Dahnert I, Stiller B, et al: Complement and contact activation during cardiovascular operations in infants. *Ann Thorac Surg* 65:525–531, 1998.

165. Steinberg JB, Kapelanski DP, Olson JD, Weiler JM: Cytokine and complement levels in patients undergoing cardiopulmonary bypass. *J Thorac Cardiovasc Surg* 106:1008–1016, 1993.

166. Swain JA, McDonald TJ Jr, Griffith PK, et al: Low flow hypothermic cardiopulmonary bypass protects the brain. *J Thorac Cardiovasc Surg* 102:76–83, 1991.

167. Taylor KM: Cardiopulmonary bypass. In Taylor KM (ed): *Cardiopulmonary Bypass.* London, Chapman and Hall Medical, 1986.

168. Thurlbeck WM, Angus GE: Growth and aging of the normal human lung. *Chest* 67:3S–6S, 1975.

169. Treasure T, Naftel DC, Conger KA, et al: The effect of hypothermic circulatory arrest on cerebral function, morphology, and biochemistry. *J Thorac Cardiovasc Surg* 86:761–770, 1983.

170. Tsui SS, Kirshbom PM, Davies MJ, et al: Thromboxane A2-receptor blockade improves cerebral protection for deep hypothermic circulatory arrest. *Eur J Cardiothorac Surg* 12:228–235, 1997.

171. Tsui S, Schultz J, Shen I, Ungerleider RM: Postoperative hypoxemia exacerbates potential brain injury after deep hypothermic circulatory arrest. *Ann Thorac Surg* 78:188–196, 2003.

172. Turley K, Roizen M, Vlahakes GJ, et al: Catecholamine response to profound hypothermia and circulatory arrest in infants. *Circulation* 62:I175–179, 1980.

173. Undar A, Lodge AJ, Daggett CW, et al: Error associated with the choice of an aortic cannula in measuring regional cerebral blood flow with microspheres during pulsatile CPB in a neonatal piglet model. *ASAIO J* 43:M482–486, 1997.

174. Undar A, Lodge AJ, Runge TM, et al: Design and performance of a physiologic pulsatile flow neonate-infant cardiopulmonary bypass system. *ASAIO J* 42:M580–583, 1996.

175. Ungerleider RM: Effects of cardiopulmonary bypass and use of modified ultrafiltration. *Ann Thorac Surg* 65:S35–S59, 1998.

176. Ungerleider RM: Congenital heart disease. In Sabiston DC Jr (ed): *Atlas of Cardiothoracic Surgery.* Philadelphia, WB Saunders, 1995, pp 255–377.

177. Ungerleider RM: Decision making in pediatric cardiac surgery using intraoperative echo. *Int J Card Imaging* 4:33–35, 1989.

178. Ungerleider RM, Gaynor JW. The Boston Circulatory Arrest Study: An analysis. *J Thorac Cardiovasc Surg* 127:1256-1261, 2004.

179. Ungerleider RM, Greeley WJ, Kanter RJ, Kisslo JA: The learning curve for intraoperative echocardiography during congenital heart surgery. *Ann Thorac Surg* 54:691–698, 1992.

180. Ungerleider RM, Greeley WJ, Sheikh KH, et al: The use of intraoperative echo with Doppler color flow imaging to predict outcome after repair of congenital cardiac defects. *Ann Surg* 210:526–533, 1989.

181. Ungerleider RM, Kisslo JA, Greeley WJ, et al: Intraoperative echocardiography during congenital heart operations: Experience from 1,000 cases. *Ann Thorac Surg* 60:S539–542, 1995.

182. Ungerleider RM, Shen I, Yeh T, et al: Routine mechanical ventricular assist following the Norwood procedure—improved neurologic outcome and excellent hospital survival. *Ann Thorac Surg* 77:18–22, 2004.

183. Utley JR, Wachtel C, Cain RB, et al: Effects of hypothermia, hemodilution and pump oxygenation on organ water content, blood flow and oxygen delivery and renal function. *Ann Thorac Surg* 31:121–133, 1981.

184. van Oeveren W, Kazatchkine MD, Descamps-Latscha B, et al: Deleterious effects of cardiopulmonary bypass: A prospective study of bubble versus membrane oxygenators. *J Thorac Cardiovasc Surg* 89:888–899, 1985.

185. Venn GE: Cerebral vascular autoregulation during cardiopulmonary bypass. *Perfusion* 4:105, 1989.

186. Wang MJ, Chiu IS, Hsu CM, et al: Efficacy of ultrafiltration in removing inflammatory mediators during pediatric cardiac operations. *Ann Thorac Surg* 61:651–656, 1996.

187. Watanabe T, Orita H, Kobayashi M, Washio M: Brain tissue pH oxygen tension and carbon dioxide tension in profoundly hypothermic cardiopulmonary bypass. *J Thorac Cardiovasc Surg* 97:396–401, 1989.

188. Watkins L Jr, Lucas SK, Gardner TJ, et al: Angiotensin II levels during cardiopulmonary bypass: A comparison of pulsatile and nonpulsatile flow. *Surg Forum* 30:229–230, 1979.

189. Wells FC, Coghill S, Caplan HL, Lincoln C: Duration of circulatory arrest does influence the psychological development of children after cardiac operation in early life. *J Thorac Cardiovasc Surg* 86:823–831, 1983.

190. Wernovsky G, Wypij D, Jonas RA, et al: Postoperative course and hemodynamic profile after the arterial switch operation in neonates and infants: A comparison of low-flow cardiopulmonary bypass and circulatory arrest. *Circulation* 92:2226–2235, 1995.

191. Williams WG, Rebeyka IM, Tibshirani RJ, et al: Warm induction blood cardioplegia in the infant, a technique to avoid rapid cooling myocardial contracture. *J Thorac Cardiovasc Surg* 100:896–901, 1990.

192. Wong PC, Barlow CF, Hickey PR, et al: Factors associated with choreoathetosis after cardiopulmonary bypass in children with congenital heart disease. *Circulation* 86:II118–126, 1992.

193. Wood M, Shang DG, Wood AJ: The sympathetic response to profound hypothermia and circulatory arrest in infants. *Can Anaesth Soc J* 27:125–131, 1980.

194. Wypij D, Newburger JW, Rappaport LA, et al: The effect of duration of deep hypothermic circulatory arrest in infant heart surgery on late neurodevelopment: The Boston Circulatory Arrest Trial. *J Thorac Cardiovasc Surg* 126:1397-1403, 2003.

195. Young JA, Kisker CT, Doty DB: Adequate anticoagulation during cardiopulmonary bypass determined by activated clotting time and the appearance of fibrin monomer. *Ann Thorac Surg* 26:231–240, 1978.

Chapter 21

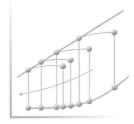

Mechanical Circulatory Support in Infants and Children

TOM R. KARL, MD, MS, PAUL M. KIRSHBOM, MD,
and STEPHEN B. HORTON, PhD, CCP (Aus), CCP (USA)

INTRODUCTION

The development of cardiopulmonary bypass (CPB) technology ushered in the modern era of cardiac surgery. In addition, it has permitted advances in the related technologies of the ventricular assist device (VAD) and extracorporeal membrane oxygenation (ECMO), which can support the failing circulation outside of the operating room (Table 21-1).

In 1971 DeBakey reported the first successful ventricular assist device.[17] The basic concept required drainage of left or right heart blood into a pumping chamber followed by ejection of the blood into the aorta (left ventricular assist device [LVAD]) or pulmonary artery (right ventricular assist device [RVAD]), respectively. The ensuing 30 years have produced a steady refinement in indications and technique. The increasingly favorable results in adults have made VAD an accepted treatment for myocardial failure until either recovery of native heart function or transplantation occurs.

ECMO differs from VAD because of the inclusion of a device for gas exchange (the membrane oxygenator) into the circuit. This design feature allowed the early developers of ECMO to focus on respiratory support rather than cardiovascular support.[66] In the 1970s Bartlett[4] reported the first neonatal ECMO survivor and Zapol[67] reported the failure of ECMO to improve survival from adult respiratory distress syndrome. Despite the early focus on respiratory failure, the design of the standard venoarterial (VA) ECMO circuit, in which systemic venous blood drains from the right atrium into the circuit and is then pumped through an oxygenator and heat exchanger back into the aorta, has made ECMO an important tool for supporting the failing heart. In fact the

Table 21-1   Design and Management Aspects of Various Mechanical Circulatory Assist Devices

	CPB	VAD (Centrifugal)	ECMO (Roller head)
Cannulation sites	Chest	Chest	Chest or cervical or femoral
Initial blood flow rates	100% calculated CO	Pt with 2 ventricles: 75–100% calculated CO	Pt with 2 ventricles: 75–100% calculated CO
		Pt with single ventricle: 150% calculated CO	Pt with single ventricle: 150% calculated CO
Gas exchange source	Oxygenator only	Lungs	Lungs and oxygenator
Blood reservoir (bladder)	Large	None	Small
ACT at >50% calculated CO (Hemotec)	>350 seconds	160–180 seconds (nonheparin bonded circuit) 140–150 seconds (heparin bonded circuit)	160–180 seconds (nonheparin bonded circuit) 140–150 seconds (heparin bonded circuit)
Ventilator strategy	None (if no cardiac ejection)	Full ventilatory support for adequate ABG Usually lower PEEP (4 cm H$_2$O) to promote venous return	Ventilatory support varies depending on ECMO flow rate and lung function Usually higher PEEP ($\leq$10 cm H$_2$O) to maintain ideal lung volume
Duration of support	Hours	1–14 days	1–21 days

Maximum CO calculated at 200 mL/kg/min in the infant: ABG, arterial blood gas; ACT, activated clotting time; CO, cardiac output; CPB, cardiopulmonary bypass; PEEP, positive end-expiratory pressure.

majority of the world experience with extracorporeal life support for cardiac failure in children has been with ECMO, as detailed in the annual Extracorporeal Life Support Organization (ELSO) reports.[8,11]

In contrast VAD systems have only recently been introduced for children. In the last decade, many new VAD systems have been designed, some suitable for neonates. However, the experience with VAD support of smaller children (<20 kg) remains limited to date. This is partly due to technical considerations such as cannulation and space problems. In addition low flow rates in small patients may create a diathesis for thromboembolic complications when adult-sized systems are applied in this population.[30] Finally, a general impression that children with complex congenital heart disease would not tolerate univentricular support without an oxygenator in the circuit has led many pediatric cardiac teams to prefer ECMO over VAD. The unavailability of implantable ventricular assist devices for small children in some parts of the world has reinforced the preference for ECMO.[26] Our own experience does not completely support this concept and an increasing body of literature suggests an advantage of VAD over ECMO in certain circumstances.[10,36,38,39,63] This chapter compares VAD with ECMO for circulatory support in children based primarily on our experience at the Royal Children's Hospital in Melbourne and the Children's Hospital of Philadelphia.[10,36,38,39,40,61]

GENERAL INDICATIONS AND CONTRAINDICATIONS

As with any other labor-intensive, invasive, and potentially hazardous therapy, mechanical circulatory assistance requires careful prospective definition of the indication, duration, and desired end point. The specific goals may vary with the clinical scenarios described as follows.

Postoperative Support

Failure to wean a patient from cardiopulmonary bypass (CPB) has been the most common indication for circulatory support at our institutions. The need for sustained mechanical circulatory support after heart surgery has arisen when, despite optimization of blood volume, ventilation, acid-base balance, and vasoactive/inotropic drug support, native cardiac output was insufficient to terminate CPB. A small subset had refractory low cardiac output within 24 hours of apparently satisfactory weaning from CPB.

The cardiac team must carefully weigh the risks, benefits, and timing of long-term mechanical support. Because residual cardiac defects can cause low cardiac output, technical failure of the operation should be ruled out before commencement of VAD or ECMO. In practice this may be quite difficult.[65] Transesophageal echocardiography, as well as direct cardiac chamber pressure and oxygen saturation measurements, may assist in diagnosing residual cardiac defects. An intraoperative review of preoperative data and imaging can also be helpful. Once the team has fully considered the precise anatomical and physiologic diagnosis, then prognostic, social, and ethical considerations must be weighed before instituting long-term mechanical circulatory support. If recovery of native heart function is unlikely, then the realistic prospects for heart transplantation should be weighed before committing to VAD or ECMO. Social factors deserve attention, including an assessment of the potential emotional impact on the family of a sudden, unexpected intraoperative death versus a prolonged intensive care unit (ICU) death. Finally, one must consider which type of support is best for a given patient.

There are numerous *relative* contraindications to the use of VAD and ECMO. Examples include intracranial hemorrhage, neurologic impairment, multiorgan system failure, uncontrolled sepsis, severe coagulopathy, prolonged cardiac arrest, and the presence of a univentricular circulation. In practice, though all relevant, most of these features are difficult or impossible to assess accurately in a child urgently needing placement of a support device, especially intraoperatively. Furthermore, there is only a limited ability to estimate the recovery potential of the critically ill child with circulatory failure. ECMO has also been employed in a small series of noncardiac patients, specifically for the treatment of multiorgan system failure, with a 50% survival.[23] Therefore in institutions capable of offering circulatory support, almost any child accepted for open heart surgery will also be a candidate for VAD or ECMO should the need arise. Other types of patients must be assessed on an individual basis.

The general aim of postoperative centrifugal pump VAD and ECMO support is recovery of the child within a few days. In our units, the typical limit would be 5 days. Similarly, other groups have suggested increased probability of death, if separation from mechanical support cannot be accomplished within 3 days[50] or 6 days.[1]

Support for Nonsurgical Conditions

Less commonly, we have supported children for circulatory failure due to nonsurgical conditions. This population includes children with acute myocarditis, sepsis syndrome, cardiac trauma, and posttransplantation rejection. As a group these patients present with low cardiac output, refractory arrhythmias, or both. The acute fulminant myocarditis and sepsis groups typically comprise children with structurally normal hearts, who were well prior to the onset of the infection. Patients with overwhelming sepsis may expect complete recovery of circulatory function provided the medical team can clear the infection, prevent multiorgan dysfunction, and avoid technical complications of the support procedure. The septic process often includes pneumonia and respiratory failure. Therefore ECMO is often the procedure of choice to support the septic patient with refractory circulatory failure.

A patient with acute fulminant myocarditis may benefit especially from mechanical circulatory assistance, if it allows or even promotes myocardial recovery and avoids the need for transplantation. The clinical picture on presentation often entails worsening cardiogenic shock with increasing inotrope requirements, which in turn exacerbate ventricular dysrhythmias. Surprisingly, this patient population appears to have a better long-term outcome than nonfulminant myocarditis, if the patient can be supported through the acute phase.[45,49] Mechanical circulatory assistance may aid in myocardial healing by allowing ventricular rest and unloading. VAD may be preferable to ECMO in this setting because it unloads the left ventricle completely, which may lead to "rapid reverse remodeling" of the ventricle.[21] The possibility of recovery combined with the scarcity of donor organs has led to prolonged circulatory support of up to several months. There is a small subset of children with acute myocarditis who may recover (without transplantation) after prolonged VAD support.[48] For planned long-term support, centrifugal pump VAD or ECMO is probably not the best choice of device, although in many intensive care units a better system is not yet available. Hetzer and colleagues have reported successful support in children of all ages using a pneumatic paracorporeal VAD for as long as 98 days.[31]

Cardiomyopathy becomes an indication for ECMO or VAD when decompensation leads to oliguria, azotemia, metabolic acidosis, increased arteriovenous oxygen saturation gradient (>40%), or increasing requirements for two or more inotropes. Although recovery of adequate native heart function is possible in rare instances, most of these patients will receive ECMO or VAD as a bridge to transplantation. Though ECMO has the advantage of allowing emergency extrathoracic cannulation in the ICU, it has the disadvantage of not fully unloading the poorly ejecting left heart unless atrial septostomy (or septectomy) is performed or a separate decompression cannula is placed in the left atrium. In contrast VAD unloads the left heart more completely as described previously for myocarditis.

In selected cases there may be an option for a bridge to transplantation, with or without interim conversion to a pulsatile paracorporeal support system designed for longer term use (see subsequent discussion).[3,18,41,42,43,48] The pulsatile VAD systems are usually driven by a pneumatic pump and have the advantage of allowing extubation, mobilization, and feeding of some patients.[46] For patients weighing less than 20 kg, 2 weeks would be considered to be the maximum realistic projected duration of support in our own units when bridge to transplantation is the goal, although again one sees exceptions in clinical practice.[19,41] Pediatric experience with extracorporeal support as a bridge to transplantation has lagged well behind that in adults. Patients supported specifically for bridging (i.e., those felt to have irreversible cardiac dysfunction) must prospectively meet institutional criteria for transplantation.[48] Issues such as size, blood group, and donor availability should be taken into consideration. Typically, this group would include patients with acute myocarditis, cardiomyopathy, inoperable end-stage congenital heart disease, or failure of a previous transplant.

The contraindications to mechanical support for nonsurgical conditions are similar to those for surgical conditions. The major difference between the two scenarios lies in the ability to perform a detailed neurological assessment for the nonsurgical patient in the intensive care unit. Clear-cut evidence of significant neurological injury would contraindicate mechanical support at most centers.

Post–Cardiac Arrest Support

There is now considerable experience with the use of mechanical support after cardiac arrest. Because neurologic outcome is a primary concern, the prearrest neurologic condition and the duration of the arrest and resuscitation (ischemic time) largely determine the outcome of postarrest mechanical circulatory support. Recovery of cardiac function can occur well beyond the point of severe brain damage, but the upper limit is unknown. We have initiated either VAD or ECMO support during prolonged (1 hour) cardiac arrests with good quality survival. If VAD is instituted for a postoperative cardiac arrest (i.e., outside the operating room), then CPB or ECMO may be required initially, but in some cases we have been able to place asystolic postoperative patients undergoing open cardiac massage directly onto LVAD, with a successful outcome.

In the Pittsburgh experience, 11 of 17 patients with cardiac arrest (6 of 11 of whom had more than 15 minutes of cardiac massage) survived to discharge after ECMO support.[18] The results at Children's Hospital of Philadelphia have been similar, as 7 of the 11 patients placed on ECMO after a cardiac arrest and listed for transplant were either successfully weaned from ECMO (n=2) or survived to transplant (n=5).[41] A review of the ELSO registry from 1989 to 1995 by Doski and colleagues[20] revealed that 13% of patients (839 of 6335) supported with ECMO during that period suffered a pre-ECMO cardiac arrest. Overall survival for these children was 60.8% versus 81.6% for those who did not require CPR before ECMO ($P < 0.001$). Analysis of 112 survivors of postarrest ECMO showed that 63% had no apparent neurologic impairment whereas only 4% were graded as severely impaired.[20] Aharon and colleagues[1] noted that cardiopulmonary arrest before ECMO affected outcome adversely only when the CPR time was prolonged for more than 45 minutes. Clearly, we have been obliged to reevaluate the issue of acceptable resuscitation times for children in the era of circulatory support.

THE VENTRICULAR ASSIST DEVICE

Equipment

The ventricular assist device (VAD) circuit at the Royal Children's Hospital formerly consisted of a centrifugal pump head (BioMedicus, Eden Prairie, Minn., USA) mounted on a flexible drive cable (Fig. 21-1). More recently, they have switched to a Quadroxx D and Jostra system. The system monitors inlet pressure, outlet pressure, and arterial flow. Mounting the pump head directly onto the patient's bed minimizes the tubing length. We and others have tended to employ heparin-bonded circuits in recent years, which may improve biocompatibility and decrease thrombus formation.

The important component inside the centrifugal pump head is an impeller consisting of rotator cones or vanes, which upon rotation create a constrained vortex. The impeller is coupled electromagnetically to the drive console,

so that the operator can set the rotational speed of the pump. Rotation of the cones creates a pressure differential with subatmospheric pressure at the tip of the cone establishing suction in the venous cannula (Fig. 21-2) and positive pressure at the outlet (arterial cannula). This contrasts with the ECMO roller pump where venous inflow is passive and dependent on gravity. Because there are no valves or diaphragms, the flow is nonpulsatile. Hemolysis may develop unless this inlet pressure is maintained above −20 mm Hg. The absence of an oxygenator in the VAD circuit reduces trauma to blood cells and eliminates a common site for thrombus formation. This decreases the need for anticoagulation, which is especially helpful when VAD support is initiated intraoperatively.

Physiology of Blood Flow during Mechanical Support

The centrifugal pump output (flow) depends on preload and afterload in addition to rotational speed of the pump. A reduction in preload from inlet obstruction or any other cause decreases pump output. Continued rotation of the pump creates a more negative inlet pressure. If the inlet pressure falls below −20 mm Hg, excessive hemolysis may result. Therefore the operator must either lower pump speed (rpm) to raise inlet pressure (i.e., render it less "negative" or less subatmospheric) or increase venous return by other means such as adding volume to the circuit. Conversely, a significant reduction in afterload automatically results in an

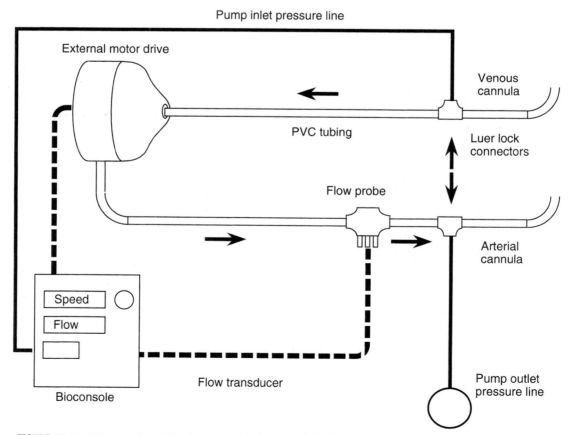

FIGURE 21-1   Schematic of centrifugal pump ventricular assist device (VAD) circuit used at the Royal Children's Hospital.

Centrifugal Pump VAD

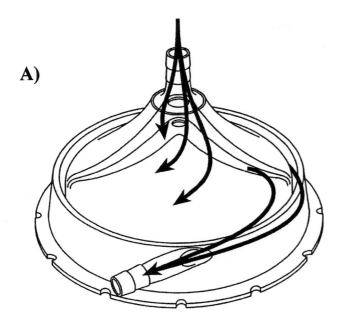

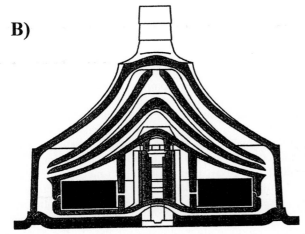

FIGURE 21-2 BioMedicus centrifugal pump, intact **(A)** and cutaway **(B)** views. Blood enters at the apex of the cone, and energy is implanted by the (constrained) vortex created by spinning cones along the vertical axis. Blood is ejected tangentially at the base of the cone. Mechanical energy is transferred to the cones by a spinning external magnet coupled to a second magnet inside the cone. VAD, ventricular assist device.

increase in flow without any change in rotational speed of the pump. Thus there is no way to determine a priori the flow from the rotational speed of the pump, and a flow probe is necessary. The most efficient (and least hemolytic) settings for a centrifugal pump occur at the lowest pump speed for a given flow.

In contrast, pump output during roller head ECMO depends solely (within certain limits) on the displacement volume and the speed (rpm) of the pump. Diminished preload in a roller pump would generate a subatmospheric pressure, which could cause collapse of the pump tubing. The bladder in the roller pump circuit contains a reservoir for blood, which is added to the circuit volume and thereby reduces the

risk of sudden collapse of the pump tubing. Pump output of the roller pump remains constant until contraction of the bladder triggers an alarm and intermittent cessation of the roller pump rotation. Diminished afterload leads to hypotension unless roller pump speed is increased. Outlet (arterial cannula) obstruction during roller head ECMO risks overpressurization and rupture of the tubing.

Table 21-2 illustrates the differences between centrifugal pump VAD and roller pump ECMO. Our investigations indicate that proper use of a centrifugal pump circuit results in less hemolysis than in the roller pump circuit.[32] Other advantages of the centrifugal pump include a reduced risk of air embolism and an reduced risk of tubing rupture. The battery backup makes the pump convenient for transport of the patient and device during a period of assist. Most important, the centrifugal pump allows fine-tuning of the peripheral circulation before and during weaning, as it is responsive (flow at a given pressure) to the patient's intravascular volume and resistance. Biventricular assist is also possible with a centrifugal pump, and we have rarely employed right atrial/pulmonary arterial plus left atrial/aortic cannulation, using two pump heads adjusted for approximately 1:0.7 flow ratio. This set up is technically cumbersome in a small child because it requires four cannulas. We would normally prefer ECMO in such a situation.

Specific Indications and Scenarios

Isolated Left Ventricular Failure in Patients with Biventricular Circulation

Short-term circulatory support has been particularly effective for postoperative patients with anomalous origin of the left coronary artery from the pulmonary artery (ALCAPA),[9] transposition of the great arteries (TGA) after arterial switch,[16] and donor heart dysfunction after transplantation. Our patients with ALCAPA and TGA as a group had a 0.91 (CL = 0.59 to 1.0) overall survival probability (P = 0.002). The unifying thread in such cases is undoubtedly the presence of two anatomically normal ventricles, with one being temporarily (but critically) impaired. Conversely, patients whose cardiac abnormalities bear a poor prognosis without VAD (left heart obstructive syndromes, complex univentricular hearts) may do poorly after VAD support.

The Univentricular Circulation

The use of VAD in patients with a univentricular circulation is currently a point of controversy. We (and others) have successfully supported patients with VAD after the Norwood operation for hypoplastic left heart syndrome as well as after bidirectional cavopulmonary shunts performed as part of the treatment of other complex univentricular variants. In such cases, higher than normal flows (~1.5 X calculated) may be required, since the assist device provides both pulmonary and systemic output. In our own practice, Blalock shunts have been left open during VAD (as well as ECMO) support in such cases. Jaggers and colleagues[34] have suggested improved survival rates when the Blalock shunt is left open during ECMO support of patients with univentricular physiology. Ungerleider and colleagues have suggested that VAD support following the Norwood procedure, with oxygenation provided by the lungs

Table 21-2 Comparison of Indications, Technical Features, Blood Flow Physiology, and Complications of ECMO and VAD

	ECMO (Roller pump)	VAD (Centrifugal pump)
Indications		
Severe pulmonary hypertension	Preferred	Possible
Postoperative univentricular failure	Possible	Preferred
Postoperative biventricular failure	Preferred	Possible (BiVAD)
Isolated LV failure (e.g., ALCAPA, TGA)	Possible	Preferred
Myocarditis/cardiomyopathy	Possible	Preferred
Technical Features		
Number of cannulas for biventricular support	2	4
Pump	Positive displacement, occlusive	Kinetic, vacuum effect, nonocclusive
Oxygenator	Yes	No
Venous reservoir (bladder)	Yes	No
Physiology		
Left heart unloading	Incomplete	More complete (with LVAD)
Flow (L/min)	Predictable; Flow = displacement volume x rpm	Less predictable; Flow dependent on rpm, preload, and afterload
Inlet (venous) obstruction	Constant flow until reservoir (partially) drained	Decreased flow
Outlet (arterial) obstruction	Constant flow until pressure alarm or tubing rupture	Decreased flow
Risks/Complications		
Cavitation/air embolism	++	+/−
Hemolysis	++	+
Retrograde flow	0	+
Tubing rupture	+	0

ALCAPA, anomalous left coronary artery from the pulmonary artery; SV, stroke volume; TGA, transposition of the great arteries.

through the open BT shunt, can improve survival and improve neurologic outcomes. The use of VAD to augment cardiac output in hypoxemic infants (e.g., Norwood patients) recovering from surgery is intriguing, especially since research indicates that patients may be more vulnerable to brain injury when cardiac output (and cerebral oxygen delivery) is impaired.[62]

Borderline Pulmonary Hypertension or Right Ventricular Dysfunction

Mild cases of pulmonary hypertension may respond to a left ventricular assist device (LVAD) alone. The decrease in left atrial pressure usually seen with LVAD may dramatically improve pulmonary hypertension and right ventricular dysfunction in borderline cases, especially with concurrent use of nitric oxide. Right ventricular function is sensitive to left ventricular function in a number of ways. By unloading the left ventricle with VAD, right ventricular filling is improved and the decrease in chamber size and septal shift may improve tricuspid valve function as well.[53] Therefore each case must be assessed on its own merits, and we prefer to employ the simplest effective level of support (i.e., VAD rather than ECMO) whenever possible.

Hemodynamic Assessment

Careful assessment and individual judgment are needed before attempting VAD support in certain patients. For example, patients with global right ventricular and left ventricular failure will probably require ECMO or a biventricular assist device (BiVAD) to achieve hemodynamic stability. The same could be said for patients with severe pulmonary hypertension or pulmonary dysfunction complicating their clinical picture.

In order to assess the prospects for VAD rather than ECMO intraoperatively, a venous cannula is placed in the left atrium, then the right atrial or caval cannula used for CPB is clamped. This system is used to assess the effect of partial left heart bypass. Right atrial and pulmonary artery pressure, as well as right ventricular function, are observed at 150 mL/kg/min pump flow. If all are satisfactory (right atrial pressure <12 mm Hg, pulmonary artery systolic pressure <1/2 systemic, no right ventricular dilation), then the patient is ventilated normally while gas exchange in the oxygenator is temporarily interrupted. If pCO_2, pO_2, acid-base status, and hemodynamics remain acceptable, the patient is recannulated for VAD. Otherwise, conversion to ECMO (or possibly biVAD) will probably be a better strategy.

VAD Cannulation and Initial Management

Intraoperative placement of VAD after failure to wean from CPB represents the most common scenario for instituting VAD. In this circumstance, cannulation is usually transmediastinal, using the left atrial appendage or left atrial body (at the right superior pulmonary vein junction) for drainage, and the ascending aorta for arterial return. For children with a univentricular circulation, the right atrial appendage and ascending aorta can be used. We employ standard or heparin-bonded CPB cannulas designed to carry 150 mL/kg/min flow. Purse string sutures and tourniquets secure the cannulas in the same way as for CPB. The tourniquets are held fast with vascular clips and left inside the mediastinum.

Upon initiation of VAD, the flow rates are increased quickly from minimum levels to 150 mL/kg/min. Once hemodynamic stability returns, flow is reduced to 70% of calculated resting cardiac output. In order to diminish the risk of stasis and thrombus formation, we allow for some cardiac ejection if possible by maintaining the left atrial pressure of 3 to 4 mm Hg. Heparin can be reversed with protamine, and hemostasis can be secured as for other CPB cases. However, administration of protamine to patients supported with a heparin-bonded circuit may neutralize some of the advantages of coating, and could result in a significantly greater heparin requirement or the potential for thrombus formation during VAD support.[3] When hemostasis has been secured (often a prolonged exercise), the skin is closed, with cannulas exiting at either pole of the wound. Alternately, a polytetrafluorethane (PTFE) membrane is sutured to the skin edges, leaving the sternum open in either case.

Critical Care Management during VAD Support

During VAD support, patients are sedated and fully ventilated. Inotropes are minimized to the level required to maintain adequate right heart function, based on central venous pressure, oxygenation, and echocardiographic assessment. Arterial pressure, VAD inlet/outlet pressure, right and left atrial pressure, total flow, and activated clotting time (ACT) are recorded hourly. When postoperative bleeding subsides, systemic heparin anticoagulation is begun (approximately 20 IU/kg/hour), keeping the activated clotting time around 140 to 150 seconds.

Two different systems are commercially available for ACT measurement, employing either diatomaceous earth (Hemochron, International Technidyne Corporation, Edison, N.J., USA) or kaolin (Hemotec, Medtronic, Parker, Col., USA). We have found the Hemotec method advantageous, as it requires only 0.2 mL of blood per sample to yield reproducible results. The Hemochron ACT is, on average, 1.1 times that obtained with Hemotec equipment in our experience.

With heparin bonding, the system can theoretically be operated without heparin or at reduced doses in situations of high flow in larger patients. However, clots may form in heparin-bonded circuits with or without anticoagulation, and this risk of thrombosis must constantly be weighed against the risk of bleeding.[12]

Inhaled nitric oxide is an effective and inexpensive treatment for pulmonary hypertension, and is also useful for support of the right heart during low cardiac output states requiring LVAD support. Even if pulmonary artery pressure is normal, some patients may benefit hemodynamically, with improved left atrial filling. A secondary benefit may be an improvement in ventilation/perfusion mismatch in selected patients with pulmonary dysfunction. Methemoglobinemia and NO_2 toxicity are rare in clinical practice, especially at doses less than 20 ppm.

Normothermia is maintained during VAD with a heating/cooling blanket and the heat generated by the centrifugal pump head itself. Peritoneal dialysis or venovenous hemofiltration can be used to remove excess interstitial fluid or correct fluid and electrolyte abnormalities. Vasodilators, parenteral nutrition, and antibiotics are also administered as needed.

In general the measures used for metabolic support are much the same as those required for other critically ill cardiac patients not being supported with VAD.

Daily plasma-free hemoglobin should remain below 60 mg/dL. An elevated hemoglobin level, especially in conjunction with noise or vibrations in the pump head, may indicate imminent mechanical failure. Under these circumstances the pump head can be easily changed with only a very brief period off VAD. In any case the pump head is changed routinely after 7 days. We will replace a pump head earlier in the presence of signs of impending failure. The median pump head life has been 71.5 hours (range 0.5 to 480) hours in our experience. Table 21-3 lists a number of technical problems related to centrifugal pump VAD in children.

Weaning from VAD

The return of a pulsatile systemic arterial pressure trace at full flow represents the first sign that ventricular function may be improving sufficiently to attempt weaning from VAD or ECMO. Transesophageal echocardiogram aids in the assessment by demonstrating improved ventricular contractility and a Starling response to volume loading. We employ gradual flow reduction as the left ventricle begins to eject, down to a pump speed of 1800 to 2000 rpm or a minimum total flow of 150 mL/min. Normal ventilation and low-dose inotropic support are maintained. Temporary augmentation of heparin is generally required at low flows. If non-heparin-bonded tubing is used, the target ACT is increased to 200 to 220 seconds. The cannulas may be heparin flushed (5 IU/mL saline) to test the hemodynamics and pulmonary function with pump support discontinued. Decannulation is generally performed in an operating room, with concurrent sternal closure whenever possible.

EXTRACORPOREAL MEMBRANE OXYGENATION (ECMO)

Equipment

Our ECMO circuits employ a closed venoarterial (VA) circuit and may incorporate either a centrifugal pump (Royal Children's Hospital, Fig. 21-3) or a roller head pump (Children's Hospital of Philadelphia).[10,26] Venous blood drains by gravity into a distensible reservoir and is then pumped through a membrane oxygenator for O_2 and CO_2 exchange. The oxygenated blood then passes through a countercurrent heat exchanger, where it is warmed to the desired temperature before emptying from the arterial cannula into the aorta. Recently, we have employed a heparin-bonded circuit in selected cases. Inlet (venous) pressure and oxygen saturation as well as outlet (postmembrane) pressure and blood temperature are monitored continuously. Also a hollow fiber oxygenator can be employed, which from a purely technical point of view is not ECMO (i.e., no membrane). Hollow fiber oxygenators are easy to prime and very effective, but have a shorter useful life than membrane oxygenators. More recently, a Quadroxx D oxygenator has been used for 7 weeks at RCH.

Table 21-3 Common Technical Problems Encountered with Centrifugal Pump VAD in Children and Possible Solutions

Problem	Comments and Possible Solutions

1. High arterial outlet pressure:
  a) Acute
    1. Cannula position has changed
    2. Thrombus partly obstructing cannula
    3. LV ejection above support provided by pump (equivalent of increased vascular resistance)
  b) Chronic
    1. Flow too high for selected cannula
	1. Adjust cannula position.
	2. Recannulate, adjust ACT as required.
	3. Consider weaning with flow reduction; vasodilator therapy.
	
	1. Recannulate with larger cannula.

2. Low (subatmospheric) inlet pressure:
  a) Acute
    1. Cannula position has changed
    2. Thrombus partially obstructing cannula
    3. Atrial wall collapsed around cannula
 	
    4. Hypovolemia
  b) Chronic
    1. Flow too high for selected cannula
    2. Failing RV, poor LA filling
	1. Adjust cannula position.
	2. Recannulate, adjust ACT as required.
	3. Reduce flow temporarily (by decreasing rpm) then slowly return to normal flow.
	4. Infuse volume expander.
	
	1. Recannulate with larger cannula.
	2. Pulmonary vasodilators, inotropes; consider RVAD or ECMO.

3. Inability to achieve nominal flow:
  a) Any combination of circumstances outlined in 1 and 2
  b) Cardiac tamponade
	a) See 1 and 2.
	b) Exploration, hemostasis, drainage.

4. Excessive hemolysis:
  a) Low inlet pressure (<−20 mm Hg)
  b) Thrombus in pump head (especially if pump head is noisy)
  c) Venous cannula too small (especially if inlet pressure is low)
	a) See 2.
	b) Change pump head, adjust ACT as required.
	c) Recannulate with larger cannula.

5. Inconsistent ACT readings:
  a) Incorrect preparation of kaolin suspension
  b) Incorrect preparation of cuvettes
 	
  c) Sensor contaminated with blood
 	
  d) Concurrent platelet infusion
  e) Ongoing variation in heparin metabolism
	a) Kaolin suspension should be mixed just prior to use.
	b) Cuvettes should be stored at 2–25° C, and warmed to 37° C just before use.
	c) Clean sensor with H_2O_2. Check to see that blood has actually clotted when ACT reading is made.
	d) Increase heparin dosage by 10% during platelet infusion.
	e) Adjust heparin dose.

6. Air in VAD circuit:
  a) Air entrainment around insertion site (if inlet pressure is subatmospheric)
 	
  b) Open or faulty tap or connector in system
  c) Crack in pump housing
  d) Acute inlet obstruction with very low pressure
	a) Reduce support to increase filling pressure in LA. Infuse volume expander, revise cannulation suture to obtain a seal. Positioning the outlet at 5 o'clock will create a bubble trap to sequester gross air, although small bubbles can still embolize.
	b) Change or close connectors or taps; de-air (venous side).
	c) Change pump head.
	d) See 2a. Under these circumstances, gas can be drawn out of solution in venous limb of circuit.

7. Noisy pump head: a) Thrombus in pump head	a) Thrombus on wall of cone or bearing causes cone to spin eccentrically. Hemolysis often occurs concurrently. Pump head should be changed.

ACT, activated clotting time; LA, left atrium; LV, left ventricle; RV, right ventricle; RVAD, right ventricular assist device.

The Physiology of Blood Flow and Oxygenation

The Biventricular Circulation

ECMO patients may have some combination of biventricular failure, severe pulmonary hypertension, or coexisting pulmonary parenchymal disease. The total systemic arterial blood flow is the sum of ECMO pump output and left heart output. ECMO pump output is increased to maintain adequate mean arterial pressure (>40 mm Hg for the infant) and mixed venous oxygen saturation ($SvO_2 > 60\%$), bearing in mind that SvO_2 may be elevated by a left-to-right shunt at the atrial level.

The systemic arterial oxygen saturation equals the weighted average of ECMO pump blood and the left heart blood oxygen saturations. Thus early in the course, when left heart and pulmonary function are most compromised, ECMO pump flow is the predominant (or sole) determinant of systemic arterial flow and oxygen saturation (SaO_2). The poorly ejecting left heart must be decompressed as described subsequently. Air can be added to the gas mixture in the oxygenator in order to avoid hyperoxia. Later in the course, left heart blood assumes a greater proportion of systemic arterial blood flow as reflected in an improving arterial wave contour on the monitor. If left heart function improves before pulmonary function, the SaO_2 will decrease and the

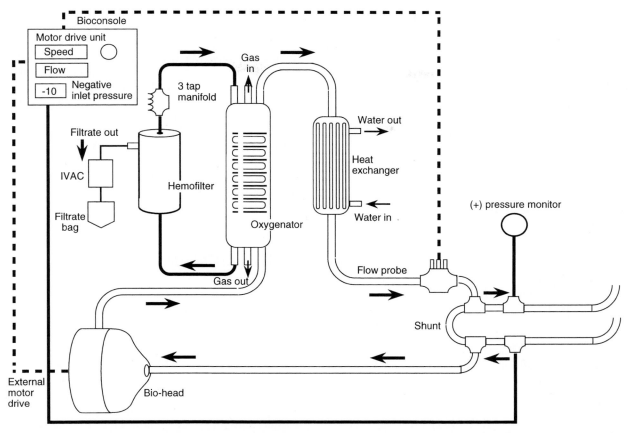

FIGURE 21-3   Schematic of centrifugal pump ECMO circuit used at the Royal Children's Hospital. *ECMO,* extracorporeal membrane oxygenation.

oxygen concentration in the membrane oxygenator and the ventilator must be increased to return SaO$_2$ to a desired level. If pulmonary function is normal, then ECMO flow rates are reduced and ventilator support is increased. Since coronary hypoxemia is a risk of improving left heart function, the electrocardiogram (ECG) pattern must be monitored closely.

The Univentricular Circulation

ECMO has been used effectively to support patients with a single ventricle, most frequently after the Norwood operation for hypoplastic left heart syndrome. The mixed systemic and pulmonary venous blood drains into the right atrial cannula and is pumped into the aorta. Although rarely a problem after the Norwood operation, any restriction to flow at the atrial level is corrected with septostomy or septectomy. The Blalock shunt, if present, remains patent. ECMO flow is higher than in a patient with biventricular physiology in order to supply both the systemic and pulmonary circulations. The goals in this setting are to maintain adequate total O$_2$ delivery to end organs and avoid pulmonary overcirculation. Fortunately, standard sized shunts (3.5–4 mm) usually provide enough limitation to pulmonary blood flow that increasing VAD flow rate mostly augments systemic perfusion. Because the lungs are used as the "oxygenator," FiO$_2$ and respiratory rate are adjusted to porvide adequate oxygenation and ventilation. Initial results with this application of VAD following the Norwood procedure have been encouraging.[63]

Special considerations apply to the patient with a bidirectional cavopulmonary shunt. Because access to the right atrium from the internal jugular vein is not possible, these patients are not good candidates for cervical cannulation. A better approach may be transthoracic cannulation with placement of a venous cannula in the common atrium.

ECMO Cannulation and Initial Management

Cannulation technique depends on the circumstances at the time of initiating support. For patients who cannot be separated from CPB, the ascending aortic cannula used for CPB can be left in situ, and a second cannula placed in the right atrial appendage. Both cannulas should support 150 mL/kg/min flow with a pump inlet pressure of >20 mm Hg (for centrifugal pump ECMO) and an outlet pressure of <200 mm Hg.

In using ECMO for patients with minimal left ventricular ejection, left atrial or left ventricular decompression may be necessary to provide optimal cardiac support and to prevent hemorrhagic pulmonary edema.[18,29] A second venous cannula can be placed in the left atrial appendage or right superior pulmonary vein if further decompression is required to cope with the collateral return to the left side imposed by ECMO. This can also be accomplished via balloon or blade septostomy in some patients.[2,29] Direct skin (or PTFE membrane to skin) closure is generally used, with cannulas exiting through the upper and lower poles of the wound. Patients cannulated independent of a transsternal procedure generally undergo right cervical cannulation of the carotid artery and internal jugular vein.[37] Permanent ligation of a carotid artery distal to the arterial cannula is unnecessary. With our current technique, reconstruction of the cervical vessels after decannulation has resulted in good long-term patency.[37] Follow-up studies have not resolved the question of whether reconstruction or ligation of the carotid artery yields better long-term neurologic outcome, although intuitively it seems difficult to justify permanent ligation of a major branch of the aorta when reconstruction can be easily performed.

Critical Care Management during ECMO Support

Patients on ECMO are managed in the ICU by a specialist team including an ECMO nurse or therapist, cardiac surgeons, intensivists, and perfusionists. Sedation and paralysis are generally required, along with antibiotics and parenteral nutrition. If cervical cannulation was used, paralysis can usually be cautiously discontinued to permit periodic neurologic assessments. Most of the principles outlined in the VAD strategy apply here to ECMO patients as well. Flows on ECMO are initially 120 to 150 mL/kg/min, but sometimes higher in septic patients. Serum lactate is a useful guide to adequacy of flow. Heparin is infused to maintain an ACT of 160 to 180 seconds for non-heparin-bonded or 140 to 150 seconds for heparin-bonded circuits while the patient is receiving ECMO flows of greater than 50% calculated cardiac output. Inlet pressure should be kept on the positive side of −20 mm Hg via appropriate cannula position and attention to patient blood volume status, as for VAD patients. Platelet counts are maintained at greater than 75,000/mm^3 and epsilon-amino caproic acid (Amicar) is given by continuous infusion if there is any significant postsurgical bleeding. We routinely employ continuous hemofiltration via a shunt placed in parallel with the oxygenator, at 10 to 30 mL/min flow (see Fig. 21-3). A volumetric pump, placed in series with the ultrafiltrate collection line, can control the volume of fluid removed (see Chapter 4). Ventilator support is reduced to provide the lowest cardiac filling pressures, but must be increased as cardiac ejection improves to prevent coronary hypoxemia. Many of the problems and solutions noted for centrifugal VAD also apply to the centrifugal ECMO circuit; however, some more complex issues may arise due to the presence of the oxygenator. Table 21-4 presents a guide for troubleshooting ECMO problems.

The circuit and management techniques at the Children's Hospital of Philadelphia are similar to Royal Children's Hospital except for the use of a roller pump rather than a centrifugal pump system. Membrane oxygenators with non-heparin-bonded circuits are standard. Heparin infusion is titrated to maintain the ACT between 180 and 200 seconds for the majority of patients.

Weaning from ECMO

The weaning process from ECMO is similar to that described for VAD. However, with ECMO the stepwise weaning process usually culminates in complete termination of support while blood continues to circulate across the opened bridge in the circuit (see Fig. 21-3). This allows a brief trial without any ECMO support while the cannulas remain in situ. Because prolonged ECMO support increases the risk of clot formation in the circuit, these trials off ECMO with cannulas in situ should last no longer than 20 to 30 minutes if ECMO support has extended beyond 1 to 2 weeks. Similarly, flushing the cannulas is avoided during weaning if support has been prolonged or if fibrin strands are visible in the arterial cannula. Patients with transthoracic cannulation are decannulated in the operating room with subsequent sternal closure. Patients cannulated in the neck are usually decannulated in the ICU.

ECMO AS A BRIDGE TO TRANSPLANTATION

There have been several reports concerning the use of ECMO as a bridge to transplant, even for postoperative patients whose initial plan was intracardiac repair.[14,18] At Children's Hospital of Philadelphia, 31 patients were supported with ECMO and concurrently listed for primary heart transplantation between 1994 and 2000. Of these 31 patients, 6 recovered cardiac function, were successfully weaned, and survived to discharge after a median ECMO duration of 4.2 days (range 1.4 to 7.9). Of the remaining 25 patients, 12 were successfully bridged to transplant. Thus 18 of the 31 patients (0.58, CL = 0.40 to 0.76) were either bridged to recovery or transplant. Overall, 15 of 31 patients (0.48, CL = 0.30 to 0.67) survived to discharge.[41]

Four of the patients who were successfully bridged to transplant required more than 500 hours of ECMO support before an organ became available. In fact, of the eight patients on the waiting list for more than 250 hours on ECMO, seven survived to transplantation. These results suggest that there should be no arbitrary time cutoff for mechanical support, as long as patients do not develop complications that render them unsuitable for transplantation. Analysis of survival after heart transplantation in this group has shown that there is no difference between patients who had a transplant after ECMO support (n = 12) and those who did not require ECMO (n = 48). Twelve-month actuarial survival for the ECMO group was 83% as opposed to 73% for the non-ECMO group.[41]

The results for patients placed on ECMO as a bridge to lung or heart-lung transplantation have not been as favorable as those of the heart transplant group. Of the 14 patients in the lung/heart-lung group, only 1 was successfully weaned from ECMO and 1 other survived to transplant. This result occurred despite an average ECMO duration of 455 hours, suggesting that donor organ scarcity is the limiting factor for these patients, rather than an inability to provide mechanical support.

The question of when transplantation is a better option than continued extracorporeal support in a postoperative patient continues to challenge our judgment. At present the majority of cardiac extracorporeal support in children is performed with a view to myocardial recovery. The usefulness of centrifugal pump VAD and ECMO as a bridge to transplant

Table 21-4 Common Technical Problems Encountered with Centrifugal Pump ECMO in Children and Possible Solutions

Problem	Comments and Possible Solutions
1. Air in venous side of circuit (up to pump head): sources include IV cannulas, connectors, pressure monitoring line and taps	a) Clamp arterial cannula and shunt, stop pump, ventilate patients, and attempt to maintain cardiac output. b) De-air with syringe via pump inlet pressure line.
2. Air in oxygenator: caused by membrane rupture, excess gas flow to blood flow ratio, air in venous line or pump head, entrainment from connectors or oxygenator shunt line infusions	a) Clamp ECMO lines between pump head and oxygenator, stop pump, ventilate patient, and attempt to maintain cardiac output. b) De-air with syringe via tap in shunt manifold. c) Reinstitute ECMO after securing point of air entry or adjusting gas flow; may require circuit change for oxygenator failure (see 6).
3. Air in arterial side of circuit (and patient): causes include membrane rupture (obstructed gas outlet port), entrainment from connectors or hemofilter, and major venous emboli	a) Clamp arterial cannula and shunt, stop pump, ventilate patient, and attempt to maintain cardiac output. b) Place patient head down. c) Replace blood volume. d) De-air arterial cannula with syringe, then clamp line. e) De-air circuit by aspirating via arterial cannula tap and/or oxygenator manifold. f) Secure air entry site or replace oxygenator if necessary. g) Reinstitute ECMO.
4. ↓ $HbSO_2$ (patient) a) Decreased flow b) Anemia c) Inadequate FiO_2 or ventilation d) Excessive shunt flow e) Pneumothorax f) Oxygenator failure (indicated by ↓ pre to post oxygenator pO_2 gradient)	a) Adjust flow. b) Transfuse red cells. c) ↑ ventilator FiO_2, optimize ventilation. d) Restrict shunt flow. e) X-ray, chest drain. f) ↑ Oxygenator FiO_2. If ineffective, replace oxygenator (see 6).
5. ↑ pCO_2 (patient) a) Inadequate ventilation of patient b) Pneumothorax c) Oxygenator failure (indicated by ↓ pre to post oxygenator pCO_2 gradient)	a) Optimize ventilation. b) X-ray, chest drain. c) ↑ Gas sweep. If ineffective, replace oxygenator (see 6).
6. Oxygenator failure a) Inadequate anticoagulation b) Inadequate flow through oxygenator (high preoxygenator pressure indicates obstruction) c) Membrane rupture or perforation d) Plasma leak (hollow fiber oxygenator)	a) Clamp arterial cannula, stop pump. b) Support patient with ventilation, inotropes, and fluids as required. c) New oxygenator and circuit can be connected across bridge in old circuit. De-air and recommence ECMO. d) Correct associated coagulation problems. e) Maintain adequate flow through oxygenator by high patient or shunt flow.

depends heavily on the availability of suitable donor hearts, a major problem in many parts of the world.

OUTCOME OF VAD AND ECMO IN CHILDREN

From 1989 to 1998, we supported 53 infants and children with centrifugal pump VAD at the Royal Children's Hospital (RCH). This figure represents approximately 1.2% of our cardiopulmonary bypass cases during that time period. The median age of supported patients was 3.5 months (2 days to 19 years) and the median weight was 4 kg (1.9 to 70). The diagnoses and operative procedures crossed the spectrum of congenital and acquired heart disease in children. Operations preceding VAD support included the Norwood procedure (n=10), mitral valve replacement (n=2), aortic root procedures (n=8), arterial switch (n=8), repair of supra-aortic stenosis (n=3), heart or heart lung transplant (n=3), ALCAPA repair (n=5), cavopulmonary connection (n=3),

and others. Of the 53 children supported, 38 were weaned from VAD (0.72, CL=0.57 to 0.83) and 24 were ultimately discharged from the hospital (0.46, CL=0.31 to 0.61). Postweaning deaths generally reflected continued cardiac problems rather than morbidity specifically attributable to the VAD. Age, weight, timing of support (intraoperative versus postoperative), cyanosis, and the presence of a mechanical valve were not associated with incremental risk ($p > 0.05$ for all). The need for dialysis or ultrafiltration has been identified in other published series as a risk factor for death.[54] At the Royal Children's Hospital, however, both dialysis and ultrafiltration are used routinely (as needed) during both VAD and ECMO and have not emerged as independent risk factors. Taking initiation of VAD as day zero, Kaplan-Meier survival at 1 year for all the VAD patients was 0.44 (CL=0.31 to 0.58), suggesting a sharp decline in hazard function at the point of hospital discharge.

The median support time was 75 hours (range 19 to 428) for patients who could be weaned from VAD. For patients ultimately not weanable, it was 79.5 hours (range 2 to 114).

For those discharged, the median support time was 71.5 hours (range 38 to 144), and for patients not discharged the median time was 88 hours (range 2 to 428). Thus, analyzed in various ways, VAD time was similar for survivors and nonsurvivors ($P = 0.69$). The interpretation of support time data is possibly confounded by the fact that VAD was electively terminated in some children who showed no signs of ventricular recovery after 72 hours, in the absence of a realistic transplant option.

The VAD group of particular interest to us consists of children weighing less than 6 kg, whose options for support are perhaps more limited and who have presented the greatest technical challenge. It has been suggested that many of these patients are suitable only for ECMO.[36] At the Royal Children's Hospital, we analyzed a subset of 34 patients, ages 2 to 258 days (median 60 days) and weight 1.9 kg to 5.9 kg (median 3.7 kg). Twenty-four were unweanable from cardiopulmonary bypass, and 10 required support in the intensive care unit for postoperative refractory low cardiac output. Weaning and decannulation were performed in 22 of 34 (0.63, CL=0.45 to 0.78), similarly to the patients weighing more than 6 kg ($p=0.07$). One-year Kaplan-Meier survival was 0.31 (CL=0.17 to 0.47), most deaths being due to irreversible cardiac disease. Within the less than 6 kg group, neither age, weight, VAD duration, cardiopulmonary bypass duration, cross-clamp duration, nor the presence of univentricular anatomy proved useful in prediction of discharge from the hospital ($P > 0.05$).[61] The smallest patient in our series was a 19-day-old, 1.9-kg baby with Taussig-Bing anomaly and aortic arch obstruction, who was placed on VAD postoperatively during a prolonged cardiac arrest, surviving with no neurologic sequelae.

Complications were frequent in VAD patients of all ages, as has been the case in most reported series. Bleeding requiring exploration occurred in 15 patients. Three patients had sepsis with clinical signs and positive blood cultures, and positive blood cultures without clinical signs were found in another 5 patients. Transient neurologic defects were noted in 3 survivors, and 2 have had persistent mild neurologic complications. There have been no permanent renal sequelae. Mechanical complications were also frequent (20 patients), but usually manageable with appropriate surveillance and intervention. Included were pump head failure, cracked connectors, kinked cannulas, and air or clots in the circuit. Only 4 patients required an emergency circuit change as the primary intervention. The true incidence of all complications is underestimated, since assessment was incomplete in the nonsurvivors.

During the same time frame as the Royal Children's Hospital VAD experience discussed, 40 children with cardiac or combined cardiopulmonary failure (not necessarily related to surgery) were supported with centrifugal pump ECMO.[40] Indications included failure to be weaned from cardiopulmonary bypass (n=12), sepsis syndrome (n=9), trauma/cardiomyopathy/myocarditis (n=6), cardiopulmonary dysfunction not related to surgery (n=6), and postoperative low cardiac output/arrest (n=7). This analysis excludes children supported at the Royal Children's Hospital solely for pulmonary indications. Of the ECMO patients, 19 were weaned, 3 were bridged to transplant, and 19 were eventually discharged. Thus, although the weaning probability was better with VAD (0.71 vs. 0.48, $P=0.014$), the discharge probability was similar with VAD and ECMO (0.46 vs. 0.48, $P=1.0$). In interpreting these results one must consider that most of the VAD patients could have been supported with ECMO, but the reverse would not generally apply. The ELSO results for ECMO are similar, and have been recently tabulated to July 2002. Of 19,889 patients supported to date by reporting centers, 4081 (21%) were in the "cardiac" category. Within this group, 3179 had cardiac surgery before support, 272 had a transplant related indication, 131 had myocarditis, and 300 had other cardiomyopathies. Overall survival to discharge among the 4081 children supported was 38% for neonates and 41% for pediatric patients (1 month to 18 years old). The survival probabilities for the various subgroups were: 37% for postoperative patients not bridged to transplant, 44% for postoperative patients bridged to transplant, 43% for heart transplant, 59% for myocarditis, and 47% for cardiomyopathy. If one looks at the results of ECMO in children stratified by indications, one finds that to date they have been significantly better for pulmonary support than for cardiac support (survival probability 0.75 vs. 0.42, $P = 0.0001$). The most frequent complications related to the ECMO circuit (primarily roller pump) were oxygenator failure, cannula problems, tubing rupture, and pump malfunction (1% to 6% of patients). The most frequently occurring patient events were hemorrhage, arrhythmia, and renal insufficiency (16% to 28% of patients). Inotropes were required in 59% of patients during ECMO support.

Results of VAD and ECMO support have been remarkably similar across a number of published series,[3,12,22,35,42,56,68] suggesting that the patient population supported probably exerts more influence than the technique of support. Ibrahim and colleagues assessed the long-term outcome (median follow-up 42 months) of 35 children who survived either VAD or ECMO support.[33] They found 80% of the patients enjoyed good or excellent general health with an NYHA class I or II cardiac status in 90%. However, neurologic impairment was more common in the ECMO group than in VAD patients (62% vs. 20%), reflecting a combination of factors among ECMO patients including younger age, complex cyanotic lesions, hypothermic circulatory arrest, the greater complexity of the ECMO circuit, and the need for anticoagulation during ECMO.[33]

At least for postoperative patients, a common feature in these series is that patients who are likely to recover tend to do so within the first few days. Beyond 2 weeks, complications of VAD such as sepsis and multiorgan system failure may supervene. A key question is whether or not paracorporeal pulsatile systems designed for longer term support and patient mobilization will allow cardiac recovery to occur over a longer time span, or allow more patients to survive in a good enough condition to undergo successful transplantation should a heart donor become available (see subsequent discussion).

Results with short-term VAD and ECMO in our own units and most others reflect a policy of expanding the indications to include nearly all cardiac surgical patients who are not expected to survive without support. Whether this strategy is appropriate or not is a decision to be taken by each team in the context of local resources and philosophy. To most of us, a 30% to 40% long-term survival probability would immediately justify the effort and expense, especially if the child might have minimal or no disability. Thus improvements in the technical aspects, safety, and efficacy of centrifugal pump VAD may be obscured to a degree by the liberalization of indications for its use.

VAD VERSUS ECMO FOR CHILDREN

Due to severe right heart failure, pulmonary problems, or complexity of the cardiac anatomy, some patients can be supported only with ECMO. However, in many children, even those with complex congenital heart disease (CHD), either type of system may be suitable. Previous institutional experience with neonatal ECMO for isolated pulmonary problems will have a strong influence on the choice of support systems, due to availability of equipment and trained personnel. One might consider the following points in decision-making regarding centrifugal pump VAD versus ECMO.

Simplicity

VAD is straightforward in concept and design and requires little technical attention after insertion. Only a few minutes are required to set up and prime the circuit, providing an advantage in the cardiac arrest situation. ECMO is generally more complex to set up, prime, and de-bubble. Although certain techniques can be employed to simplify ECMO system preparation (discussion to follow), average setup time is still considerably longer in most cases. ECMO support can be established in some patients with peripheral closed chest cannulation, which is generally not possible with VAD in small children. The potential for complete left ventricular support with ECMO may be limited without the addition of a left ventricular vent, which complicates the system considerably and may increase the risk of complications.

ECMO Rapid Deployment

Several institutions that use ECMO as the primary mechanical support device for emergent circulatory support have developed rapid deployment strategies to decrease the time required to initiate ECMO support. At Children's Hospital of Philadelphia, two ECMO circuits (one for infants and the other for older children) are kept primed with crystalloid, sterile, and ready for use at all times, decreasing preparation time for emergent applications to 10 to 15 minutes. Larger children can be placed on ECMO with the crystalloid prime alone until crossmatched blood is available. Smaller children and infants often require O- blood, which is kept available at all times, to avoid excessive hemodilution during emergent initiation of ECMO.

Oxygenation

ECMO potentially provides pulmonary as well as cardiac support, although during periods of cardiac ejection the coronaries may be perfused with blood having a hemoglobin saturation closer to the left atrial level than to that of the oxygenator outlet. Therefore there is a potential for myocardial ischemia if pulmonary function is severely impaired. The oxygenator itself may contribute to this problem. Patients supported with VAD are totally dependent on the lungs for gas exchange, but pO_2 tends to remain uniform throughout the arterial circulation, barring residual intracardiac shunts at ventricular level in patients with significant cardiac ejection. If an interatrial communication is present in the LVAD patient, significant right-to-left shunting (consequent to the low left atrial pressure) can cause uniform and significant arterial desaturation.

Anticoagulation and Blood Elements

LVAD requires little anticoagulation, especially at higher flows. An important factor is that one can administer protamine and completely reverse anticoagulation before closure of the chest after intraoperative placement. By comparison, ECMO requires higher levels of anticoagulation, even with a heparin-bonded circuit. Also, the presence of the oxygenator results in more platelet damage, platelet consumption, and hemolysis, even when the centrifugal pump is used. The data from the Royal Children's Hospital suggest that there was a lower blood and platelet transfusion requirement for VAD than for ECMO ($P < 0.06$). The exact safe level of anticoagulation for either circuit may be difficult to establish, and an approach based on individual patient and circuit factors is required.

Measurable improvement in the results of extracorporeal circulatory support with the use of heparin-bonded systems probably has not yet been realized. The heparin-bonded process involves end-point covalent bonding of fragmented heparin molecules to the circuit components, including oxygenator, tubing, pump head, cannulas, and all connectors.[6] The bioactive surface covalently binds the polysaccharide containing the active sequence of heparin, through end-point attachment, which is said to provide a uniform degree of thromboresistance. There is a need for continuous movement of blood over the surfaces of the circuit for the heparin-bonding process to be effective. Theoretically, there is a risk of increased thrombogenicity in patients with antithrombin III deficiency. Heparin-coated circuits may reduce the heparin requirement for both VAD and ECMO, but in small children the prospects for either type of support without heparin are still poor.[52,58] Accumulating experience at the Royal Children's Hospital and elsewhere would suggest that postoperative bleeding is less with the heparin-bonded system for cardiac extracorporeal life support (ECLS). Thus the indications for ECMO and VAD may ultimately be extended to patients with hemorrhage, coagulopathy, and acute respiratory distress syndrome from trauma.[57] This system is obviously attractive for intraoperative conversion of CPB to ECMO or VAD. However, even with a fully bonded circuit and moderate heparin doses, the problem of thrombus formation in the tubing and pump head has not been eliminated.[5]

The heparin-bonded circuit may have the advantage of improved biocompatibility.[25,55,59] Recent studies in humans would suggest that serum concentrations of various inflammatory mediators during support are reduced with heparin-bonded circuits (using low-dose heparin) as compared to non-bonded circuits with higher dose heparin. Also, in animals, CPB-induced pulmonary injury appears to be less severe with heparin-bonded than non-bonded circuits.[55] Heparin coating reduces complement activation during cardiopulmonary bypass.[51,64] There is also a tendency toward reduced thrombin activation[44,64] and granule release by neutrophils.[7,64] The clinical significance of these findings has perhaps not been fully demonstrated, especially relating to VAD and ECMO.

The main disadvantage of commercially available heparin-bonded oxygenators is that heparin cannot be bonded to the silicone polymers used in membranes, so hollow fiber oxygenators are required. Hollow fiber oxygenators are subject to serum leakage with prolonged usage, and therefore are less suitable for long-term support. Whether or not the improved biocompatibility and decreased lung injury can offset this disadvantage is currently under study. In clinical practice, we have employed heparin-bonded circuits for up to 8 days, although the median time span is closer to 48 hours. This is in contrast to the non-heparin-bonded membrane, which has a median ECMO life of approximately 5 days.

COST

At the Royal Children's Hospital, LVAD adds $500 per day to the patient's hospital costs versus $2000 per day for ECMO. We currently employ two nurses per patient (an ECMO specialist and the patient's regular ICU nurse) during ECMO support, but only one for management of both the VAD system and the patient. In either case, a perfusionist, cardiac surgeon, and intensivist are available for assistance in troubleshooting the system and for patient management problems.

LONG-TERM SUPPORT

Neither the centrifugal pump VAD nor ECMO system is eminently suitable for long-term support in children. The limiting factor for both systems is usually the development of sepsis. Though the longest successful VAD and ECMO supports at the Royal Children's Hospital have been 144

and 120 hours, respectively, there have been reports of successful transplantation after prolonged support, even up to 1126 hours.[19] A major limitation of these systems is the inability to wean most patients from ventilator support during centrifugal pump VAD and ECMO, mobilize them, and make them independent of ICU care. This experience compares unfavorably to that with adults, in whom patient extubation and mobilization can often be accomplished using intracorporeal or paracorporeal devices. Chronic support (>30 days) is possible in the latter group, either by way of recovery or bridge to transplant, and some patients can even be discharged from the hospital before (or as an alternative to) transplantation.[24,48] In either case the rehabilitation and improvement in end organ function can be dramatic. To date this degree of mobilization has not been possible with small children, even with implantable devices designed for chronic support.

OTHER SUPPORT SYSTEMS

The future of centrifugal pump VAD might be considered uncertain in light of recent advancements with paracorporeal or totally implantable pulsatile systems. The importance of pulsatile flow has been debated for many years, but the real issue is suitability for safe longer term support. Examples of systems that may be suitable for children or in some cases infants include the following: Berlin Heart,[48] the Medos/HIA assist[3] (both in clinical use in Europe), the Toyoba and Zeon pumps[60] (in clinical use in Japan), the Thoratec VAD (Thoratec Laboratories Corporation, Berkeley, Calif., USA)

Table 21-5   Extracorporeal Support Device that Have Been Used Clincially in Children

Device	Technical Features	Type of Support	Pediatric Application	Availability	Anticoagulation
Intra-aortic balloon pump (Datascope, Paramus, N.J., USA)	Thoracic aortic occlusion in diastole maintains proximal perfusion pressure, with afterload reduction in systole as balloon deflates. Transfemoral or transaortic insertion.	Left heart assist for patients with borderline cardiac output who do not have severe LV dysfunction	Limited, due to size constraints. Most effective with m-mode echo timing. Has been used in infants and older children. Short-term assist.	Worldwide	Various (antiplatelet, heparin, dextran)
Hemopump (DLP, Medtronic, Grand Rapids, Mich., USA)	Axial flow pump, transaortic valve positioning required, external console, percutaneous drive cable. 14F, 21F, & 24F pumps.	Nonpulsatile, left-sided, maximal flow 3.5 L/min. Short-term assist.	Limited, due to requirements of insertion technique. Short-term assist.	Europe (investigated in USA)	Systemic heparinization
Centrifugal pump (BioMedicus, Eden Prairie, Minn., USA)	Constrained vortex pump, external power console, and pump	Left, right, or biVAD nonpulsatile, short-term assist	Suitable for patients of all weights and ages. Short-term assist.	Worldwide	Systemic heparinization (see text)
ECMO (various devices in use)	External pump (roller or centrifugal) and power supply, with membrane (or hollow fiber) oxygenator, in closed circuit	Nonpulsatile support of heart and lungs. May require left heart venting for adequate support.	Suitable for patients of all weights and ages. Short-term assist.	Worldwide (in various formats)	Systemic heparin (see text)
Berlin Heart and Medos/HIA heart assist system	Pneumatic paracorporeal VAD, with compressible polyurethane ventricles and inlet/outlet valves.	Pulsatile support as LVAD, RVAD, or biVAD	Suitable for all patients down to neonatal age. May be suitable for long-term support.	Europe	Systemic heparinization

biVAD, biventricular assist device; LVAD, left ventricular assist device; RVAD, right ventricular assist device.

(in clinical use worldwide, including some limited application for patients <20 kg), the University of Pittsburgh mini-centrifugal pump (not yet in clinical use),[47] the Pierce-Donachy pediatric system (not yet in clinical use),[13] the Jarvik 2000 (Jarvik Research, New York City), and others.[28] Certainly these devices will play an important role in establishment of long-term support for recovery for bridging to transplantation. Also, there are a number of devices available for children weighing more than 50 to 60 kg (flow >2.5 to 3 L/min), who from a technical point of view could be considered similar to adults. For short-term support, however, the role of these devices remains controversial. The costs involved at the time of this writing for the clinically available systems are substantially greater than centrifugal pump VAD, both for the driving system and the disposable equipment required per ventricle per patient. Some of the devices that have been employed clinically in children are listed in Table 21-5. We believe that for most cardiac surgical units, especially those not actively involved with transplantation, the simplicity, availability, cost effectiveness, and good outcome (in selected cases) would ensure the place of centrifugal pump VAD and ECMO in our surgical armamentarium for the foreseeable future.

Acknowledgments

Many individuals at the RCH and Children's Hospital of Philadelphia have contributed to the clinical work summarized herein, including perfusion, intensive care unit, anesthesia, blood bank, and cardiology staff members.

References

1. Aharon AS, Drinkwater DC Jr, Churchwell KB, et al: Extracorporeal membrane oxygenation in children after repair of congenital cardiac lesions. *Ann Thorac Surg* 72:2095–2101, 2001.
2. Alexi-Meskishvili V, Weng Y, Uhlemann F, et al: Prolonged open sternotomy after pediatric open heart operations: Experience with 1134 patients. *Ann Thorac Surg* 59:379–383, 1995.
3. Ashton RC Jr, Oz MC, Michler RE, et al: Left ventricular assist device options in pediatric patients. *ASAIO J* 41:M277–M280, 1995.
4. Bartlett RH, Gazzaniga AB, Huxtable RF, et al: Extracorporeal circulation (ECMO) in neonatal respiratory failure. *J Thorac Cardiovasc Surg* 74:826–833, 1977.
5. Bianchi JJ, Swartz MT, Raithel SC, et al: Initial clinical experience with centrifugal pumps coated with the Carmeda process. *ASAIO J* 38:143–146, 1992.
6. Bindslev L, Bohm C, Jolin A, et al: Extracorporeal carbon dioxide removal performed with surface-heparinized equipment in patients with ARDS. *Acta Anaesthesiol Scand* 95:125–130, 1991.
7. Borowiec J, Thelin S, Bagge L, et al: Heparin-coated circuits reduce activation of granulocytes during cardiopulmonary bypass: A clinical study. *J Thorac Cardiovasc Surg* 104:642–647, 1992.
8. Butt W, Karl T, Horton A, et al: Experience with extracorporeal membrane oxygenation in children more than 1 month old. *Anaesth Intensive Care* 20:308–310, 1992.
9. Cochrane AD, Coleman DM, Davis AM, et al: Excellent long-term functional outcome after surgery for ALCAPA. *J Thorac Cardiovasc Surg* 117:332–342, 1999.
10. Cochrane AD, Horton AM, Butt WW, et al: Neonatal and pediatric extracorporeal membrane oxygenation. *Austral As J Cardiac Thorac Surg* 1:17–22, 1992.
11. Conrad SA, Rycus PT: Extracorporeal life support 1997. *ASAIO J* 44:848–852, 1998.
12. Costa RJ, Chard RB, Nunn GR, Cartmill TB: Ventricular assist devices in pediatric cardiac surgery. *Ann Thorac Surg* 60:S536–S538, 1995.
13. Daily BB, Pettitt TW, Sutera SP, Pierce WS: Pierce-Donach pediatric VAD: Progress in development. *Ann Thorac Surg* 61:437–443, 1996.

14. Dalton HJ, Siewers RD, Fuhrman BP, et al: Extracorporeal membrane oxygenation for cardiac rescue in children with severe myocardial dysfunction. *Crit Care Med* 21:1020–1028, 1993.
15. Darling EM, Kaemmer D, Lawson DS, et al: Use of ECMO without the oxygenator to provide ventricular support after Norwood stage I procedures. *Ann Thorac Surg* 71:735–736, 2001.
16. Davis A, Wilkinson JL, Karl TR, Mee RBB: Arterial switch for TGA. IVS after 21 days of life. *J Thorac Cardiovasc Surg* 106:111–115, 1993.
17. DeBakey ME: Left ventricular bypass for cardiac assistance: Clinical experience. *Am J Cardiol* 27:3–11, 1971.
18. del Nido PJ, Armitage JM, Fricker FJ, et al: Extracorporeal membrane oxygenation support as a bridge to pediatric heart transplantation. *Circulation* 90(5-2):II66–II69, 1994.
19. Di Russo GB, Clark BJ, Bridges ND, et al: Prolonged extracorporeal membrane oxygenation as a bridge to cardiac transplantation. *Ann Thorac Surg* 69:925–927, 2000.
20. Doski JJ, Butler TJ, Louder DS, et al: Outcome of infants requiring cardiopulmonary resuscitation before extracorporeal membrane oxygenation. *J Pediatr Surg* 32(9):1318–1321, 1997.
21. Duncan BW, Bohn DJ, Atz AM, et al: Mechanical circulatory support for the treatment of children with acute fulminant myocarditis. *J Thorac Cardiovasc Surg* 122:440–448, 2001.
22. Duncan BW, Hraska V, Jonas RA, et al: Mechanical circulatory support in children with cardiac disease. *J Thorac Cardiovasc Surg* 117:529–542, 1999.
23. Farmer DL, Cullen ML, Philippart AI, et al: Extracorporeal membrane oxygenation as salvage in pediatric surgical emergencies. *J Pediatr Surg* 30:347–348, 1995.
24. Fey O, El-Banayosy A, Arosuglu L, et al: Out-of-hospital experience in patients with implantable mechanical circulatory support: Present and future trends. *Eur J Cardio Thorac Surg* 11:S51–S53, 1997.
25. Fosse E, Moen O, Johnson E, et al: Reduced complement and granulocyte activation with heparin-coated cardiopulmonary bypass. *Ann Thorac Surg* 58:472–477, 1994.
26. Frazier EA, Faulkner SC, Seib PM, et al: Prolonged extracorporeal life support for bridging to transplant: Technical and mechanical considerations. *Perfusion* 12:93–98, 1997.
27. Frazier EA, Faulkner SC, Seib PM, et al: Extracorporeal membrane oxygenation life support: A new approach. *Perfusion* 8:239–247, 1993.
28. Goldstein DJ, Oz MC (eds): *Cardiac Assist Devices*. Arkmonk, NY, Futura, 2000.
29. Hausdorf G, Loebe M: Treatment of low cardiac output syndrome in newborn infants and children. *Zeitschrift fur Kardiologie* 83:91–100, 1994.
30. Herwig V, Severin M, Waldenberger FR, Konertz W: MEDOS/HIA-assist system: First experiences with mechanical circulatory support in infants and children. *Int J Artif Organs* 20:692–694, 1997.
31. Hetzer R, Loebe M, Potapov EV: Circulatory support with pneumatic paracorporeal ventricular assist device in infants and children. *Ann Thorac Surg* 65:1498–1506, 1998.
32. Horton AM, Butt WW: Pump-induced hemolysis: Is the constrained vortex pump better or worse than the roller pump? *Perfusion* 7:103–108, 1992.
33. Ibrahim AE, Duncan BW, Blume ED, Jonas RA: Long-term follow-up of pediatrics patients requiring mechanical circulatory support. *Ann Thorac Surg* 69:186–192, 2000.
34. Jaggers JJ, Forbess JM, Shah AS, et al: Extracorporeal membrane oxygenation for infant postcardiotomy support: Significance of shunt management. *Ann Thorac Surg* 69:1476–1483, 2000.
35. Kanter KR, Pennington G, Weber TR, et al: Extracorporeal membrane oxygenation for postoperative cardiac support in children. *J Thorac Cardiovasc Surg* 93:27–35, 1987.
36. Karl TR: Extracorporeal circulatory support in infants and children. *Semin Thorac Cardiovasc Surg* 6:154–160, 1994.
37. Karl TR, Iyer KS, Mee RBB: Infant ECMO cannulation technique allowing preservation of carotid and jugular vessels. *Ann Thorac Surg* 50:105–109, 1990.
38. Karl TR, Horton SB, Mee RBB: Left heart assist for ischemic postoperative ventricular dysfunction in an infant with anomalous left coronary artery. *J Card Surg* 4:352–354, 1989.
39. Karl TR, Horton SB, Sano S, Mee RBB: Centrifugal pump left heart assist in pediatric cardiac surgery: Indications, techniques, and results. *J Thorac Cardiovasc Surg* 102:624–630, 1991.
40. Karl TR: Circulatory support in children. In Hetzer R, Hennig E, Loebe M (eds): *Mechanical Circulatory Support*. Berlin, Springer, 1997, pp 7–20.

41. Kirshbom PM, Bridges ND, Myung RJ, et al: Use of extracorporeal membrane oxygenation in pediatric thoracic organ transplantation. *J Thorac Cardiovasc Surg* 123:130–136, 2002.

42. Konertz W, Reul H: Mechanical circulatory support in children. *Int J Artif Organs* 20:657–658, 1997.

43. Konertz W, Hotz H, Schneider M, et al: Clinical expertise with the MEDOS HIA-VAD system in infants and children. *Ann Thorac Surg* 63:1138–1144, 1997.

44. Larsson R, Larm O, Olsson P: The search for thromboresistance using immobilized heparin: Blood in contact with natural and artificial surfaces. *Ann N Y Acad Sci* 516:102–115, 1987.

45. Lee KJ, McCrindle BW, Bohn DJ, et al: Clinical outcomes of acute myocarditis in childhood. *Heart* 82:226–233, 1999.

46. Levi D, Marelli D, Plunkett M, et al: Use of assist devices and ECMO to bridge pediatric patients with cardiomyopathy to transplantation. *J Heart Lung Transplant* 21:760–770, 2002.

47. Litwak P, Butler KC, Thomas DC, et al: Development and initial testing of a pediatric centrifugal blood pump. *Ann Thorac Surg* 61:448–451, 1996.

48. Loebe M, Hennig E, Muller J, et al: Long-term mechanical circulatory support as a bridge to transplantation, for recovery from cardiomyopathy, and for permanent replacement. *Eur J Cardio Thorac Surg* 11:S18–S24, 1997.

49. McCarthy RE III, Boehmer JP, Hruban RH, et al: Long-term outcome of fulminant myocarditis compared with acute (nonfulminant) myocarditis. *N Engl J Med* 342:690–695, 2000.

50. Mehta U, Laks H, Sadeghi A, et al: Extracorporeal membrane oxygenation for cardiac support in pediatric patients. *Am Surg* 66:879–886, 2000.

51. Mollnes TE, Videm V, Gotze O, et al: Formation of C5a during cardiopulmonary bypass: Inhibition by precoating with heparin. *Ann Thorac Surg* 52:92–97, 1991.

52. Muehrcke DD, McCarthy PM, Stewart RW, et al: Extracorporeal membrane oxygenation for postcardiotomy shock. *Ann Thorac Surg* 61:684–691, 1996.

53. Pavie A, Leger P: Physiology of univentricular versus biventricular support. *Ann Thorac Surg* 347–349, 1996.

54. Pennington DG, Swartz MT: Circulatory support in infants and children. *Ann Thorac Surg* 55:233–237, 1993.

55. Redmond JM, Gillinov AM, Stuart RS, et al: Heparin-coated bypass circuits reduce pulmonary injury. *Ann Thorac Surg* 56:474–478, 1993.

56. Rogers AJ, Trento A, Siewers RD, et al: Extracorporeal membrane oxygenation for postcardiotomy shock in children. *Ann Thorac Surg* 47:903–906, 1989.

57. Rossaint R, Slama K, Lewandowski K, et al: Extracorporeal lung assist with heparin-coated systems. *Int J Artif Organs* 15:29–34, 1992.

58. Schreurs HH, Wijers MJ, Gu YJ: Heparin-coated bypass circuits: Effects on inflammatory response in pediatric cardiac operations. *Ann Thorac Surg* 66:166–171, 1998.

59. Shigemitsu O, Hadama T, Takasaki H, et al: Biocompatibility of a heparin-bonded membrane oxygenator (Carmeda MAXIMA) during the first 90 minutes of cardiopulmonary bypass: Clinical comparison with the conventional system. *Artif Organs* 18:963–971, 1994.

60. Takano H, Nakatani T: Ventricular assist systems: Experience in Japan with Yoyobo pump and Zeon pump. *Ann Thorac Surg* 61:317–322, 1996.

61. Thuys CA, Mullaly RJ, Horton SB, et al: Centrifugal ventricular assist in children under 6 kg. *Eur J Cardio Thorac Surg* 13:130–134, 1998.

62. Tsui SS, Scholtz JM, Shen I, Ungerleider RM: Postoperative hypoxemia exacerbates potential brain injury after deep hypothermic circulatory arrest. *Ann Thorac Surg* 78:188–196, 2004.

63. Ungerleider RM, Shen I, Yeh T, et al: Routine mechanical ventricular assist following the Norwood procedure: Improved neurologic outcome and excellent hospital survival. *Ann Thorac Surg* 77:18–22, 2004.

64. Videm V, Mollnes TE, Garred P, Svennivig JL: Biocompatibility of extracorporeal circulation: In vitro comparison of heparin-coated and uncoated oxygenator circuits. *J Thorac Cardiovasc Surg* 101:654–660, 1991.

65. Warnecke H, Berdjis F, Hennig E, et al: Mechanical left ventricular support as a bridge to cardiac transplantation in childhood. *Eur J Cardio Thorac Surg* 5:330–333, 1991.

66. Zapol W, Pontoppidan H, McCullough N, et al: Clinical membrane lung support for acute respiratory insufficiency. *Trans Am Soc Artif Intern Organs* 18:553–560, 1972.

67. Zapol WM, Snider MT, Hill JD, et al: Extracorporeal membrane oxygenation in severe acute respiratory failure: A randomized prospective study. *JAMA* 242:2193–2196, 1979.

68. Ziomek S, Harrell JE Jr, Fasules JW, et al: Extracorporeal membrane oxygenation for cardiac failure after congenital heart operation. *Ann Thorac Surg* 54:861–868, 1992.

Chapter 22

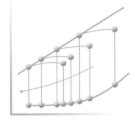

Nursing Care of the Child with Congenital Heart Disease

PATRICIA A. KANE, MSN, CPNP,
COLEEN ELIZABETH MILLER, RN, MS, PNP,
JUDITH A. ASCENZI, RN, MSN, and
DOROTHY G. LAPPE, RN, MS, MBA

INTRODUCTION

Nurses play a critical role in the life of the child with congenital heart disease (CHD) and their families. This chapter describes the advanced skills and knowledge needed by nurses who care for the child with congenital heart disease, discusses the various complex and challenging roles and responsibilities of the pediatric cardiac nurse, explores the psychosocial impact of congenital heart disease on children and families, and discusses the nurse's role in assisting family adaptation at each phase of the illness and treatment.

PEDIATRIC CARDIAC NURSING SKILLS AND KNOWLEDGE

Development of Advanced Pediatric Cardiovascular Curriculum

The care of infants and children with congenital heart disease is complex and challenging. A solid knowledge base facilitates the delivery of quality care by the pediatric critical care nurse. The bedside nurse needs to demonstrate advanced clinical judgment and reasoning skills to provide care for these complex, critically ill children.

A systematic, comprehensive curriculum addressing issues specific to the child with congenital heart disease enhances the skills and competency of an experienced intensive care unit (ICU) nurse. The curriculum is presented in various formats including lectures, workshops, self-learning activities, and one-to-one preceptor opportunities. The goals of the program are for the learner to be able to: (1) describe common congenital heart defects and surgical interventions, (2) perform a safe admission of a child to the intensive care unit after cardiac surgery, (3) identify potential postoperative complications, and (4) demonstrate appropriate nursing interventions (Table 22-1).

Educational activities are also extended to the nurses who will continue the plan of care after transfer from the ICU. In addition to general information on congenital heart

Table 22-1   Advanced Pediatric Cardiac Core Curriculum

Congenital Heart Defects and Surgical Interventions
Atrial septal defect
Ventricular septal defect
Atrioventricular septal defects
Pulmonary stenosis
Aortic stenosis
Coarctation of the aorta
Tetralogy of Fallot
Transposition of the great arteries
Tricuspid atresia
Total anomalous pulmonary venous return
Truncus arteriosus
Hypoplastic left heart syndrome
Cardiopulmonary Bypass
Routine Postoperative Care
Pharmacology
Complications
Low cardiac output
Excessive bleeding/tamponade
Acute renal failure
Electrolyte imbalances
Arrhythmias
Pulmonary hypertension
Neurologic deficits
Infection
Advanced Technical Skills
Cardioversion/defibrillation
Open thoracotomy tray
Pacemakers

Table 22-2   Basic Intensive Care Unit Bedside Equipment

Cardiac monitor
Noninvasive blood pressure monitor
Resuscitation bag and appropriate-sized mask
Suction equipment and catheters
Infusion pumps, syringe pumps
External pacemaker
Diapers, personal care items

disease and surgical procedures, other topics include routine postoperative care, common late complications, and routine discharge instructions. Early recognition and prompt treatment of potential complications greatly affect outcome and length of hospital stay.

The Nurse's Role: Preoperative Care

In the current health care era, most children receive preoperative evaluations in the outpatient setting. However, neonates with ductal dependent cardiac defects require immediate care in an ICU. As congenital cardiac diagnoses are increasingly made in utero, the delivery of a child with a ductal dependent cardiac lesion can be planned prior to the baby's birth. Arrangements for the infant to be delivered in the hospital where the baby's cardiac care will be delivered eliminate potentially dangerous transfers and separation from parents. Early diagnosis allows the parents to inform family members and make arrangements for the child's hospitalization. Unfortunately, some infants are not diagnosed until after birth and therefore require emergent transfer to an ICU. This may create a great deal of anxiety for the family and require extensive communication and planning if the mother is hospitalized elsewhere.

The goals for preoperative ICU care consist of maintaining hemodynamic stability and preventing infection. Most children needing an ICU as a neonate require prostaglandins to maintain ductal patency prior to surgery or hemodynamic support in the form of inotropes and mechanical ventilation due to severe cardiorespiratory compromise. The ICU nurse

plays a pivotal role in providing family-centered care during this extremely stressful time.

The Nurse's Role: Admission of the Child to the ICU Following Surgery

The ICU nurse makes preparations to ensure the delivery of safe, efficient, individualized care to the child and family while the child is in the operating room (OR). By reviewing clinical data and the proposed surgical plan,[26] the nurse can anticipate the postoperative care and potential complications. The ICU bedside should be prepared with necessary equipment to allow the nurse to deliver care without leaving the bedside; this preparation should be done while the child is in the operating room. Table 22-2 provides a list of routine bedside supplies. Emergency equipment listed in Table 22-3 should be immediately available in the unit and brought to the child's bedside as needed.

The admitting ICU nurse and the circulating nurse in the operating room will communicate during the procedure and prior to the child's arrival to the ICU. This communication includes information about the surgical procedure performed, cardiopulmonary bypass (CPB) time, aortic cross-clamp time, circulatory arrest time, hemodynamic status after separation from bypass, monitoring lines and tubes, vasoactive infusions, as well as any complications. After receiving this report, the admitting nurse makes final preparations for admission of the child to the ICU. For example, a long CPB or aortic cross-clamp time may indicate that the patient will require important hemodynamic support while the heart recovers, usually in the form of inotropic agents (which require infusion pumps to be available) and possibly the need for postoperative extracorporeal membrane oxygenation (ECMO), for which the nurse can prepare by alerting the ICU staff to this possibility. The use of circulatory arrest may make it less likely that the patient will be extubated early and the nurse can prepare

Table 22-3   Emergency Equipment

Electrocardiogram machine
Defibrillator with internal and external paddles in neonatal, pediatric, and adult sizes
Thoracotomy tray with infant-, child-, and adult-sized rib spreaders
Chest tube insertion tray
Transcutaneous, transthoracic, and transmyocardial pacing catheters
Atrioventricular sequential pacemaker
Emergency medications

for more prolonged mechanical ventilation. In all cases, the practice patterns of each institution help predict the types of care that will be needed for specific patients.

The cardiac OR, ICU nurses, or the cardiovascular nurse practitioner will provide periodic updates to the family while the child is in the operating room. Communication during the procedure has been demonstrated to significantly relieve parental anxiety. The goal of the admission process to the ICU is to ensure safe transfer of care from the cardiac anesthesiology team to the ICU postoperative team. An admission protocol is useful to guarantee a safe, efficient admission each time, regardless of individual personnel involved in the process. The priorities for admission are listed in the Table 22-4.

The personnel at the bedside should be limited to those required for direct patient care responsibilities, including the cardiac anesthesiologist, surgeon, intensive care physician, respiratory therapist, and two ICU nurses. The anesthesiologist is responsible for overseeing care during the transition from the OR to the ICU.

A minimum of two nurses is required to admit a post–cardiopulmonary bypass patient to the intensive care unit. Each ICU nurse assumes a predetermined role in order for the child's arrival and admission to the critical care unit to be accomplished smoothly and safely.[15] The first nurse, usually the nurse assigned to care for the patient, performs a baseline physical assessment. The second nurse is responsible for managing drainage tubes and hemodynamic monitors. A respiratory therapist and the critical care physicians are also present at the time of the patient's arrival at the intensive care unit.

When the child returns from the operating room, the priorities of assessment for the bedside nurse follow the ABC's—airway, breathing, and circulation. Initial assessment of the child who is intubated and receiving hand ventilation includes determining if endotracheal tube is patent and appropriately positioned, and ventilation is adequate. In collaboration with the anesthesiologist, the respiratory therapist establishes appropriate ventilator setting and attaches the patient to the ventilator. If the child is extubated, assessment focuses on the patency of the airway and the child's spontaneous respiratory effort.

Once adequate ventilation has been established, the primary nurse assesses the child's cardiovascular function. This provides a baseline to guide the delivery of care throughout the postoperative recovery period. The nurse at the bedside performs a full cardiovascular assessment every 15 minutes until the child is hemodynamically stable. Once stability has been achieved, the nurse should perform a cardiovascular assessment every hour. The cardiovascular assessment includes measuring vital signs, assessing cardiac rhythm, evaluating peripheral pulses and perfusion, calculating accurate intake and output assessment, and monitoing the child's neurologic status.

The second nurse at the bedside transfers monitoring lines from the transport monitor to the ICU monitor. The use of a transport monitor compatible with the ICU monitors simplifies this procedure and eliminates interruption of monitoring vital signs. This nurse also regulates and labels intravascular infusion lines and drainage systems including chest tubes, urinary catheters, and nasogastric tube. This nurse then obtains admission blood work consisting of complete blood count, chemistry panel, arterial blood gas, and coagulation panel. Performing these tasks in a sequential fashion promotes order during the admission process and allows completion of these vital tasks in an expeditious fashion.

Parameters for acceptable vital signs are identified and care is transferred to the ICU team. Additional discussions with the ICU staff before the surgical team departs include plans for extubation and plans for pain management.

A chest radiograph is obtained on admission to document endotracheal tube position and lung expansion as well as to record position of monitoring lines and drainage tubes. The bedside nurse plays an important role in monitoring the child's airway and protecting against accidental extubation while positioning the child for the chest x-ray. Positioning the child in a consistent, supine position and moving wires and tubing out of the x-ray field facilitates the interpretation of the film and decreases the need to repeat x-rays. Specific unit procedures aid this process so that a change in caregivers does not affect the quality of the chest x-ray.

The Nurse's Role: Routine Postoperative ICU Nursing Care for the Child after Cardiac Surgery

Immediate postoperative care of the child recovering from cardiovascular surgery is aimed at monitoring vital signs and identifying and treating potential life-threatening complications.[11] The ICU bedside nurse is the most consistent caregiver during this time.[19] Ongoing serial nursing assessments identify subtle changes in the child's condition. The nurse needs to be capable of distinguishing between normal convalescent changes requiring only further monitoring and abnormal changes requiring increased support, monitoring, and additional therapy. Rapid, effective responses to changes influence the treatment and recovery of the child.

The bedside ICU nurse actively participates in clinical rounds to review the child's surgical repair (definitive or palliative procedure) and establish the plan of care. The type of cardiac defect, surgical procedure, and the child's age and weight influence the postoperative course. Healthy children admitted to the hospital for elective surgical repair have a more predictable, shorter hospital course than does a critically ill neonate undergoing urgent surgery. Most centers utilize critical pathways to streamline care for predictable patients after cardiac surgery.[29] Critical pathways along with nursing care plans (Table 22-5) aid in delivering consistent, cost-effective care.

Table 22-4 Pediatric Cardiac Surgical Admission Protocol

1. Mechanical ventilation and/or oxygen therapy initiated
2. Monitoring transferred to PICU monitor
3. Chest tube(s) attached to suction
4. Infusion lines transferred, regulated, labeled
5. Pacemaker checked
6. Foley drained
7. Nasogastric tube inserted and attached to drainage system
8. Admission blood work obtained
9. Chest radiograph ordered

Table 22-5   Interventions for Postoperative Care after Cardiac Surgery

Problem	Patient-specific Intervention
Hypoxia	1. Assess respiratory status every 15 min until stable, then q1 hrs 2. Monitor rate and depth of respirations 3. Monitor presence and quality of breath sounds 4. Assess color of mucous membranes and lips 5. Obtain arterial blood gases as ordered and prn with changes in patient's condition 6. Turn every 2 hrs unless contraindicated by hemodynamic instability
Respiratory distress	1. Assess breath sounds before and after suctioning 2. Maintain patency of artificial airway 3. Two-person suctioning for patient with pulmonary hypertension or hemodynamic instability
Decreased cardiac output	1. Cardiovascular assessment every hour and with changes 2. Vital signs every 15 min until stable 3. Measure four-extremity blood pressure on admission 4. Record accurate intake and output 5. Measure chest tube drainage every hour, replace output as ordered 6. Check external pacemaker settings 7. Six-lead ECG on admission and every morning 8. Laboratory studies as ordered
Neurologic deficit	1. Assess neurologic status q4 hrs and with changes 2. Provide age-appropriate diversional activity as tolerated 3. Plan care to allow uninterrupted periods of rest 4. Minimize noxious effects of PICU environment
Decreased urine output	1. Record accurate intake and output every hour 2. Obtain electrolytes as ordered 3. Institute peritoneal dialysis or continuous arteriovenous hemofiltration as ordered 4. Daily weights on same scale, with same clothing
Pain	1. Pain management per pain service 2. Provide incisional site splinting as necessary 3. Provide diversional activities
Infection	1. Suture line care every day and as needed 2. Invasive site care every day 3. Monitor temperature every hour for 24 hrs, then every 2 hrs, if afebrile 4. Get patient out of bed as soon as possible
Parental stress	1. Encourage parents to express feelings related to child's illness, hospital experience, and current fears 2. Provide information to assist parents in their basic needs 3. Encourage parents to establish their parent role in PICU through participation in child's care 4. Invite participation in parent support group 5. Provide parents with information about stress, adjustment, and parenting roles*
Child/parent education	1. Arrange preoperative PICU tour 2. Provide information about child's condition 3. Prepare parent for child's transition from PICU

ECG, electrocardiogram; PICU, pediatric intensive care unit.
*Visconti KJ, Sandino KJ, Rappaport LA, et al: Influence of parental stress on the behavioral adjustment of children with transposition of the great arteries. *J Dev Behav Pediatr* 23:314–321, 2002.

Hemodynamic Stability

Monitoring the child for signs and symptoms of adequate cardiac output is a primary objective during the first 24 to 48 hours after surgery. Perfusion that is inadequate to meet the body's oxygen demands will usually present with acidosis. However, perfusion that meets oxygen demands in a sedated patient can still be impaired and it is important to recognize the patients whose cardiac output is marginal and in whom a slight increase in systemic oxygen demand (such as by fever, work of breathing, or sepsis) might create a scenario of inadequate perfusion. Adequate systemic perfusion requires an age-appropriate heart rate for the child's clinical condition, adequate preload or intravascular volume, good myocardial function, and appropriate afterload.[11] Residual cardiac disease, decreased cardiac contractility, and alteration of preload and afterload may alter these parameters, resulting in poor cardiac output. Vital signs including oxygen saturation, intracardiac pressure, toe temperature, chest tube drainage, and urine output are carefully monitored and recorded at least every hour for the first 24 hours after surgery.

Unexpected residual cardiac disease has become rare in the era of intraoperative transesophageal echocardiography (TEE).[2] Intraoperative TEE after the surgical repair gives the surgeon information regarding cardiac function and anatomy before separation from cardiopulmonary bypass. If significant residual lesions (intracardiac shunts, obstruction to flow, valve regurgitation) exist, the surgeon corrects the remaining problem before leaving the operating room. The use of TEE has significantly decreased the need to return to the operating room for reoperation in the immediate postoperative period.

Inadequate intravascular volume as measured by right atrial pressure, left atrial pressure, and blood pressure can result from hemorrhage, inadequate fluid administration, fluid leaking into the third space, and excessive diuresis. Postoperative bleeding can occur from cannulation sites, suture lines, or postbypass coagulopathy. A long cardiopulmonary bypass run leads to platelet dysfunction and diffuse capillary leak. Packed red blood cells, platelets, and fresh frozen plasma should be readily available for replacement due to grossly abnormal coagulation laboratory values or prolonged and excessive bleeding.

Despite ongoing improvements in perfusion techniques, the use of cardiopulmonary bypass continues to be associated with postoperative morbidity. Cardiopulmonary bypass affects both intravascular volume and cardiac contractility. The use of an external circuit for circulation and oxygenation has been shown to result in the stimulation of an inflammatory response and subsequent capillary leak. This inflammatory response syndrome results in injury to multiple body systems including the lungs, systemic vasculature, and myocardium. The systemic effects of the CPB inflammatory syndrome may result in substantial increase in intravascular permeability with fluid moving into the tissues, resulting in decreased intravascular volume. The use of methylprednisolone at 6 hours and 12 hours before surgery may reduce the inflammatory injury seen after cardiopulmonary bypass.[20] Close monitoring of the child's vital signs, perfusion, and urine output is essential to ensure that fluid shifting into the third space is not resulting in hypotension and poor end organ perfusion.

Decreased cardiac output in the postoperative period may be due to the surgical procedure, hypoxemia, acidosis, electrolyte imbalances, prolonged bypass time, or arrhythmias. Treatment options include fluid boluses, vasoactive infusions, temporary pacing and/or mechanical support (see Chapters 7, 8, and 21).

Hypoxemia and acidosis are identified by routine arterial blood gas monitoring. Knowledge of the surgical procedure performed is essential to determine the expected oxygen saturation for a patient. Patients with uncorrected single ventricle physiology (e.g., those with shunts or Glenn anastomoses) will be hypoxemic because they have mixing lesions and oxygen saturations in the 80% range may be normal and expected, whereas patients with corrected circulation and normal lungs should be expected to have saturations above 90%. Inadequate cardiac output will result in poor oxygen delivery to tissues and metabolic acidosis. Serial lactic acid measurement provides information regarding the adequacy of perfusion.[16] Persistently elevated lactic acid levels are a marker for poor outcome after cardiac surgery. Mixed venous saturation (SvO_2) monitoring also provides information regarding oxygen delivery and utilization. Low mixed venous saturations may indicate a residual right-to-left cardiac shunt or decreased cardiac output. Continuous noninvasive monitoring provides trends in the patient's perfusion. Commonly, patients have continuous pulse oximetry and cerebral infrared spectroscopy monitoring in the early postoperative period. Analyzing laboratory data and monitoring trends must be done in conjunction with physical examinations.

Monitoring Lines Intracardiac monitoring lines placed either percutaneously or transthoracically, provide valuable information regarding cardiac function, intravascular volume, and afterload in the immediate postoperative period. Left atrial catheters are placed at the junction of the left atria and upper pulmonary vein, and pulmonary catheters are placed in the main pulmonary artery.[9] The surgeon places transthoracic lines in the operating room based on protocol, the child's physiology, and anticipated postoperative course. Right-sided lines may be used for infusions in the absence of other central lines and any residual right-to-left shunt. Left-sided transthoracic lines are not used routinely to infuse fluids or medications due to increased risk of introducing air or particulate matter emboli into the arterial circulation.

If the child has had obstruction to pulmonary blood flow, as in tetralogy of Fallot or pulmonic stenosis, the ICU nurse can anticipate a right-sided pressure line to assess preload and adequacy of right ventricular function. Conversely, with left-sided obstructive lesions, as with aortic stenosis and hypoplastic left heart syndrome, the ICU nurse can anticipate a left atrial line to assess mitral valve and left ventricular function after repair. Chest tubes generally remain in place until transthoracic lines are removed, due to potential bleeding after catheter removal.

Arterial lines are utilized in the postoperative period for direct blood pressure monitoring and easy blood gas sampling. Common sites for arterial lines in children include the radial, femoral, and umbilical arteries. Left radial arterial lines are not used for infants undergoing subclavian flap repair for coarctation of the aorta, due to the surgical repair. Arterial blood pressures are correlated with noninvasive blood pressure monitoring whenever there is a question regarding the accuracy of the arterial line. A poor waveform on the monitor or the inability to withdraw blood from the catheter may give false recordings. The ICU nurse troubleshoots the monitoring issues to determine accurate patient data. Nonfunctioning arterial lines are rewired, replaced, or removed. Depending on ICU protocols, umbilical artery catheters are removed before initiating feeding, to ensure stable gastrointestinal perfusion.

Central venous pressures are measured and recorded in the postoperative period. Common cannulation sites include internal and external jugular veins, femoral veins, and umbilical veins. Central venous lines often have several lumens that allow for the administration of multiple medications and fluids while monitoring venous pressures. Central venous pressure readings provide valuable information regarding intravascular volume and right ventricular compliance.

Careful assembly of the transducers, tubing, and stopcocks is essential to prevent contamination and incomplete priming of the tubing resulting in entrapped air. Air within the closed system will alter the accuracy of the monitoring system and may result in an embolic event. Ensuring that precise information is obtained from the transducers depends on the accuracy of leveling and calibrating the system. The ICU nurse routinely calibrates and levels the transducers at change of shift and after a change in the patient's position.

Arrhythmias After open-heart surgery, all patients have temporary pacing wires, which were placed in the operating room. Both atrial and ventricular pacing wires are placed to allow for atrioventricular (AV) sequential pacing if needed. Ideally, the wires are tested in the operating room. The ICU nurse should be knowledgeable about the temporary pacing equipment and be able to troubleshoot problems. Any child with documented or high probability of a conduction disturbance is automatically connected to the temporary pacemaker.

Dysrhythmias in the immediate postoperative period may have a significant impact on cardiac output due to loss of atrioventricular synchrony (junctional ectopic tachycardia, heart block) or inadequate filling time (supraventricular tachycardia). These dysrhythmias may result from electrolyte imbalances, intracardiac monitoring lines, tissue swelling, or surgical injury to the conduction system. Less commonly, they result from congenital abnormalities of the conduction system associated with structural defects and myocardial disease secondary to poor postoperative perfusion.[17] The most common types of difficult rhythm problems after open-heart surgery include supraventricular tachycardia (SVT), junctional ectopic tachycardia (JET), and atrioventricular block.

SVT usually occurs as junctional ectopic tachycardia (JET), which can produce heart rates in infants in excess of 180 (and as high as 240) beats per minute. Suspicion for JET should be entertained whenever an infant exhibits this degree of tachycardia. JET is particularly frequent after repair of tetralogy of Fallot and repair of atrioventricular septal defects, and extreme tachycardia following these procedures should raise concern for JET. The diagnosis is often easy to make by looking at the tracing of the atrial lines and observing the presence of cannon A waves—which would not be present in sinus tachycardia. A cardiologist can assist in the diagnosis by evaluating an atrial electrogram, which can be obtained from the atrial pacing leads. If the patient is hemodynamically stable, treatment can be provided by gently cooling the patient (with an ambient temperature blanket) to 35 degrees centigrade, which will slow the junctional rate and allow atrial pacing at a slightly faster rate to restore atrioventricular synchrony. If the patient is hemodynamically unstable, cooling may increase afterload and exacerbate the hemodynamic instability. In these cases, pharmacologic intervention (currently, amiodarone is the recommended agent) may be necessary. In extreme cases, the infant may need mechanical circulatory assist (ECMO) to support the hemodynamics until the heart rate stabilizes. JET is usually self-limited and will resolve in 1 to 3 days.

Surgically induced permanent atrioventricular block occurs in up to 3% of postoperative patients. Surgical repairs with the highest risk of trauma to the atrioventricular node include resection of subaortic stenosis, aortic valve replacement procedures, VSD closure especially in patients with atrioventricular discordance (L-TGA), mitral valve replacement and repair of atrioventricular septal defects. Surgical heart block is usually observed in the operating room, however, it may not present until the postoperative period.[17] Patients require the use of a temporary pacemaker until normal sinus rhythm returns or a permanent pacemaker is placed. The recovery waiting time before proceeding to permanent pacemaker is broadly accepted as 7 to 14 days. Children who have recovery from complete heart block are at risk for late atrioventricular conduction abnormalities.[35]

Excessive Bleeding and Cardiac Tamponade After surgery, chest tubes are placed in the pleural and mediastinal spaces. Chest tubes facilitate drainage of blood and serous fluid and are assessed frequently for patency and amount of drainage. Heparin used during cardiopulmonary bypass is partially reversed with protamine in the operating room. The process of returning to a noncoagulopathic state may take longer than 8 hours, particularly in the neonate with immature liver function. Drainage in excess of 5mL/kg/hour is reported to the surgical team. Drainage from the chest tubes typically changes from bloody to serosanguinous in the first few hours after surgery. Once the chest drainage has diminished, the chest tubes are removed.

A sudden cessation of drainage from previously draining chest tubes coupled with decreasing systemic perfusion and rising right or left atrial (RA, LA) pressures is regarded with a high degree of suspicion for cardiac tamponade. Blocked chest tubes prevent adequate drainage of fluid from the pericardial space. Cardiac output is impaired due to fluid accumulation around the heart, which interferes with diastolic filling and systolic ejection. Signs of cardiac tamponade include hypotension, tachycardia, narrowing pulse pressure, and elevated right atrial and left atrial filling pressures. Pulses paradoxus, a fall in systolic blood pressure by 8 to 10 mm Hg during inspiration, is a classic sign but may be difficult to appreciate in a child with tachycardia and hypotension. Other signs may include muffled heart sounds and decreased voltage on the surface electrocardiogram (ECG). Echocardiography in the ICU can demonstrate whether or not there is substantial fluid around the heart and can even, in some cases, show compression of cardiac chambers by the fluid—which would be very suggestive of tamponade. Clearing occluded chest tubes or opening the chest will rapidly restore hemodynamic stability.

Extracorporeal Membrane Oxygenation When a child's cardiac function is inadequate to sustain sufficient cardiac output after surgery, extracorporeal membrane oxygenation (ECMO) or ventricular assist device may be required. If unable to wean from cardiopulmonary bypass in the operating room, the child may be placed on mechanical assistance in the operating room or during the first hours after surgery in the ICU. Indications for the use of ECMO after cardiac surgery include poor systemic perfusion despite high-dose vasoactive infusions, hypotension, cardiac index less than 2.0 L/m^2/minute for 3 hours, base deficit greater than 5 mEq/L for 3 hours, or oliguria less than 0.5 mL/kg/hour.[6] The bedside ICU nurse plays a crucial role in the early identification and communication of alarming hemodynamic trends.

Delayed Sternal Closure Complicated surgical procedures associated with long cardiopulmonary bypass times may result in myocardial swelling that prohibits immediate sternal closure. The child's sternum is left open to facilitate maximal myocardial function. When the sternum is left open, a surgical material is sewn to the skin and creates a continuous barrier with the skin. The risk of infection is increased and sterile technique must be followed for procedures done near the surgical incision. Caution is taken to avoid any pressure to the open chest. A sign placed at the child's bedside warning that the sternum is open helps inform all members of the health care team. In the event of cardiac arrest, the eshmark can be removed to facilitate internal cardiac massage using sterile gloves. As long as the sternum is open, the child remains intubated and ventilated and either heavily sedated or paralyzed and sedated with vecuronium (0.1 mg/kg/dose) and continuous fentanyl infusion (1 to 2 mcg/kg/hour) to prevent movement. The surgeon will attempt sternal closure as soon as the child is hemodynamically stable and has achieved successful diuresis. This is commonly performed in the ICU and does not always require a return transport to the operating room. The anesthesiologist delivers adequate pain medication, monitors vital signs and arterial blood gases, and adjusts the ventilator to maintain adequate oxygenation throughout the procedure. Closing the sternum may create changes in the patient's ventilatory management due to alteration in pulmonary compliance.[22] When sternal closure results in elevation of the central venous pressure (CVP), it is sometimes necessary to leave the chest open for a short while longer to allow for more diuresis. Closing the sternum in these circumstances can inhibit fluid mobilization and diuresis. It is helpful for the nursing staff to point out hemodynamic changes (such as elevation in the CVP or decreases in the blood pressure) to the surgeon when the sternum is closed in the ICU so that these alterations can be included in the decision-making process regarding whether to proceed with the procedure. After successful sternal closure, plans focus on weaning ventilatory support, extubating, and monitoring for signs of sternal wound infection.

Respiratory Status and Pleural Effusions

Many postoperative cardiovascular patients remain intubated and mechanically ventilated after surgery. Meticulous attention to maintaining airway patency is essential to prevent hypoxemia. A subset of postoperative patients poses a significant challenge in maintaining adequate oxygenation, normal pulmonary artery pressures, and systemic perfusion during routine endotracheal suctioning. Children with elevated pulmonary artery pressures are at risk for developing an acute pulmonary hypertensive crisis during endotracheal tube (ETT) suctioning if adequate oxygenation is not maintained. Suctioning strategies for children at risk for developing pulmonary hypertension should include sedation, hyperoxygenation before suctioning, and suctioning conducted by two care providers to minimize time off the ventilator.
Pleural effusions may interfere with weaning from ventilatory support or necessitate reintubation in the previously extubated child. Small to moderate pleural effusions can be treated with aggressive diuresis; however, large effusions, and especially large effusions that result in hemodynamic changes, require drainage. Children with elevated venous pressures are at higher risk for developing pleural effusions. Serial respiratory assessments and chest x-rays are needed to monitor the size of pleural effusions and response to therapy.

Chest tubes are commonly removed within 24 to 48 hours after surgery. It is essential to provide adequate pain management before chest tube removal. The use of narcotics, non-narcotic analgesia, and distraction techniques are efficacious and synergistic. After chest tube removal, the ICU nurse assesses the child's respiratory status and effort. Potential problems associated with removal of chest tubes include pneumothorax and lung collapse. Chest tube sutures are commonly left in situ for 5 to 7 days and are often removed at the first follow-up visit after the site has adequately healed.

Electrolyte Imbalances

Normal levels of sodium, potassium, calcium, and magnesium are essential for excitable membrane function and effective myocardial contraction. A full serum chemistry blood panel including magnesium should be obtained with the postoperative admission blood work. Hypokalemia resulting from an increase in intravascular water, treatment of acidosis, and use of diuretic therapy may result in conduction and rhythm disturbances. Hyperkalemia resulting from impaired renal function (acute tubular necrosis) or administering excessive doses of potassium chloride is also detrimental to the cardiac system.

Calcium is essential for adequate cardiac contractility. A decreased ionized calcium level has been demonstrated after CPB. In young infants, hypocalcemia is more likely to develop due to the lack of adequate calcium reserves in the sarcoplasmic reticulum. Calcium stores increase with age and

muscle mass, therefore making it less of a postoperative problem in older children. Hypocalcemia may also result from multiple blood transfusions.

Hypomagnesia may occur after bypass and intense diuresis. Cardiovascular effects of decreased magnesium include depressed myocardial contractility, arrhythmias, and increased sensitivity to digoxin. Low magnesium levels have been shown to be associated with an increased incidence of junctional ectopic tachycardia in the immediate postoperative period.[8]

Altered Neurologic Status

There is potential for serious neurologic complications after CPB. The ICU nurse performs a comprehensive neurologic examination soon after admission to assess pupillary response and movement of all extremities. As the child emerges from anesthesia, the neurologic examination includes the child's responses. Cerebral protection during cardiopulmonary bypass has become very sophisticated during the past decade resulting in few adverse neurologic events.[12] Repair of coarctation of the aorta requires special attention to the movement of the lower extremities due to the risk of interrupted perfusion to the spinal cord subsequent to clamping of the aorta. An extremely small percentage (0.4%, or 1/250) of these patients can have lower extremity paralysis following surgery and although this cannot be altered by postoperative ICU care, recognition of this possibility (or more often, elimination of this as a possibility by observing movement in the lower extremities as the child recovers) provides important information to the other members of the health care team as well as to anxious family members. Infants and children undergoing surgery that requires circulatory arrest warrant extra attention to monitor their neurologic status. The presence of seizures in the postoperative period following neonatal CPB can be a harbinger of brain injury, and should be rapidly investigated and treated with anticonvulsant therapy. The occurrence of major, hemispheric stroke is uncommon following infant cardiac surgery, but should be considered if the child demonstrates major focal findings suggestive of this diagnosis.

Infection

Broad-spectrum antibiotics are started intraoperatively to prevent infection. Antibiotics are continued during the immediate ICU recovery phase until central lines and drainage tubes are removed. Early signs of infection including fever, elevated white blood cell count, thrombocytopenia, elevated CRP, and wound drainage warrant careful monitoring and cultures. Good hand washing and timely removal of central monitoring lines and tubes decrease the incidence of infection.

Acute Renal Failure

Impaired renal function after cardiac surgery results in decreased urine output, increased water weight gain, and elevated serum creatinine, blood urea nitrogen, and potassium values. Urine output is closely monitored during the immediate postoperative period with expected urine output equal to 1 mL/kg/hour. Decreased urine output associated with low filling pressures (left atrial and central venous pressures) is challenged with 5 to 10 mL/kg fluid boluses. Decreased urine output associated with normal or elevated filling pressures is treated with intravenous diuretics. Because excessive fluid overload delays extubation, increases the risk of infection, and prolongs the ICU recovery time, more aggressive therapy including peritoneal dialysis is pursued. Critically ill newborns and infants undergoing complex surgery may have temporary peritoneal dialysis catheters placed in the OR during surgery; if not used during the first 24 hours, they are promptly removed.

Accurate intake and output records are calculated and children are weighed daily to assess weight gain or loss compared to their preoperative weight. Diuretics are used until the child returns to his or her baseline weight.

Pain Management and Sedation

Pediatric pain teams assist in the management of pain and sedation after surgery. Infants and children who will remain intubated overnight receive a combination of intravenous narcotics (fentanyl, morphine, hydromorphone) and sedatives (midazolam hydrochloride, lorazepam) to keep them comfortable. Sedation medicines are held before extubation to facilitate wakefulness and adequate respiratory effort. To gain cooperation and alleviate the pain and discomfort associated with chest tube, transthoracic line, and pacemaker wire removal, patients are treated with fentanyl (1 to 2 mcg/kg/dose). Pain medications are titrated to attain an adequate level of pain management and alertness with acceptable hemodynamic parameters.

Infants and children who have required extensive use of narcotics and benzodiazepines may experience withdrawal if medications are abruptly discontinued. Signs and symptoms include jitteriness, insomnia, seizures, diarrhea, diaphoresis, agitation, nausea and vomiting, tachycardia, and hypertension. A slow wean over 5 to 10 days by decreasing the total daily dose by 10% to 20% and increasing the time intervals between doses will alleviate trouble with withdrawal behaviors.

Transfer to the General Care Unit

Transfer of the child from the ICU to the general pediatric care unit is a milestone in the child's physical recovery from surgery. Older children undergoing relatively simple procedures spend 1 night in the ICU. Most monitoring lines and drainage tubes are removed the morning after surgery and the child encouraged to ambulate with assistance. Transfer to an intermediate care unit or less intensive care setting is appropriate. Neonates and infants undergoing complex procedures typically have longer ICU stays.

Transfer orders include instructions to monitor vital signs every 4 hours, wean supplemental oxygen, record intake and output measurements and daily weights, advance the diet as tolerated, and encourage activity out of bed.

The Nurse's Role: Preparation for Discharge Home

Discharge plans and needs depend on the age of the child, the congenital heart defect, and surgical procedure, as well as consideration of any coexisting medical problems.

Routine discharge instructions include information about bathing, activity restrictions, diet, medications, suture line care, and follow-up appointments. Children can usually resume their usual bathing or showering routine 1 week after surgery. Newborns are generally ready for tub bathing after the umbilical cord has fallen off. If there is delayed wound-healing, parents are instructed to sponge-bathe the child until the wound is healed.

Babies and young children generally do not need formal activity restrictions. They move around freely and rest when they feel tired or hurt. Caregivers are instructed not to pick babies up by grabbing them under the arms but rather to provide support under the buttocks and the back of the baby's head when lifting. Many infants and toddlers are ready to return to a day care setting about 2 to 3 weeks after surgery.

School-age children and adolescents need more structured information. Median sternotomy incisions require 6 to 8 weeks for complete bone healing. During this time, children are instructed to avoid strenuous activities including bike riding, roller-blading, skateboarding, diving, climbing, weight-lifting, and any activity likely to result in chest wall trauma. They are usually ready to return to school starting with half days and gradually working up to full days about 3 weeks after surgery. They should not participate in sports or physical education classes for 6 to 8 weeks. With these general guidelines, parents work with personnel in the school system to institute home schooling or tutoring to keep the children current with their school activities. A small group of children who require a lengthier recovery period will need individualized activity restrictions and guidelines on when to return to school.

Diet

Before discharge, children need to tolerate a sufficient amount of oral fluids. Many children do not regain their "usual" appetite for 1 to 2 weeks after surgery. Narcotics can alter wakefulness and interest in eating as well as interfere with the gastrointestinal system, causing nausea, vomiting, and constipation. A balance between pain control and comfort needs to be established before most children are interested in eating. For children who are picky eaters, families are encouraged to bring in food and treats from home. Most children will not have dietary restrictions.

Pediatric nutritionists follow and meet with children and families who require special dietary instructions. Children taking warfarin (Coumadin) are given information regarding foods high or low in vitamin K that interact with blood-thinning medication. Children who have been treated for a chylothorax will be instructed on a low- or no-fat diet to prevent the reaccumulation of pleural fluid. Fatty foods are slowly reintroduced into the diet while monitoring serial chest x-rays to observe for pleural effusions.

Critically ill newborns and infants who have had a prolonged or difficult postoperative period may have trouble nipple feeding. Newborns denied oral feeds for weeks after birth need time and encouragement to learn to coordinate their suck and swallow before they are successful oral feeders. These infants may need temporary supplemental or complete nasogastric tube feeding and high calorie formula to demonstrate weight gain. Because high calorie formula may lead to feeding intolerance including emesis and/or diarrhea, infants are observed for 24 to 48 hours on specialty formula before discharge. Increased calorie formula other than 24 calories per ounce is not commercially available; therefore the family is given the recipe to prepare the formula at home.

Pediatric nutritionists and occupational therapists work with the team to develop a feeding regimen that may include a combination of bottle-feeding and tube feeding. A typical regimen may include four bolus feeds during the day with orders to allow the baby to attempt bottle-feeding for 15 to 20 minutes and then to gavage feed the remainder of the feeding. At nighttime, the baby may receive continuous nasogastric feeds for 8 to 10 hours. As the baby recovers from surgery and with continued help from occupational therapy, the baby is eventually weaned off tube feedings. The caloric density of the formula is decreased and the volume of feeds increased as the baby makes appropriate weight gain.

Injury to the recurrent laryngeal nerve during surgery resulting in temporary vocal cord paresis puts the infant at risk for aspiration with oral feeds. Any infant with a hoarse or inaudible cry, coughing, or oxygen desaturations during nipple feeding is evaluated before discharge by an otolaryngologist. If the evaluation demonstrates decreased vocal cord movement, the infant is either reassessed with thickened oral feeds or started on nasogastric tube feeds until recovery occurs.

Medications

In the immediate postoperative period, children are given intravenous (IV) narcotics for pain management. As recovery progresses, the IV medication is converted to an oral form (liquid or pill). By the time of discharge, many children have transitioned to acetaminophen or ibuprofen for pain control. Older children and adolescents may need extra days of oral narcotics such as oxycodone or codeine.

Diuretics are used in the postoperative period to remove excess fluid. Many children are discharged home on daily or twice-daily diuretics (furosemide [Lasix], spironolactone [Aldactone], chlorothiazide [Diuril]). Diuretics are not given immediately before bedtime to avoid bedwetting accidents or frequent trips to the bathroom throughout the night.

Other medications that may be needed after surgery include digoxin, ACE (angiotensin converting enzyme) inhibitors, beta-blockers, anticoagulants, and antiarrhythmia agents. Attention is given to the scheduling of medications. While in the hospital a 24-hour awake caregiver is routine. A home medication schedule should allow the parent and child to sleep through the night. When feasible, children should be on daily or twice-daily medication dosing so they do not need to take medication to school or day care.

Parents who need to give multiple medications benefit from a printed schedule to post in a convenient area in the house (refrigerator, bathroom) to remind them when and what medications to give to their child.

Oxygen

Before discharge, most children are weaned off supplemental oxygen. A small group of children require oxygen beyond the immediate postoperative period. If the child has met all other discharge criteria except for weaning to room air with acceptable oxygen saturations, arrangements are made for home oxygen therapy. A portable oxygen unit is delivered to the hospital to accompany the child home and a larger oxygen unit setup in the home.

Depending on the situation, some children are sent home on a constant level of oxygen and are weaned off oxygen during a routine clinic visit 1 to 2 weeks after discharge. For the more fragile child requiring home oxygen, a pulse oximeter is used in the home to regulate the amount of oxygen needed to maintain a target saturation. Respiratory therapists and pediatric nurses providing home care assist the family in the use of the home oxygen system.

Wound Care

In most cases, postoperative dressings are removed the second day after surgery. Most incisions require little care. While in the hospital, the wound is painted daily with a povidone-iodine liquid or covered with a topical skin adhesive. For the wound with minimal drainage or partial separation, care consists of twice-daily cleaning with sterile saline solution and covering with a dry sterile gauze dressing. For significant wound dehiscence or superficial infection, the area may require twice-daily wet-to-dry dressing changes and oral antibiotics. Treatment for extensive wound infection or dehiscence requires IV antibiotics, surgical debridement, and closure in the operating room. Most incisional sutures are absorbable and do not require removal. Sternal wires rarely create problems necessitating removal. Chest tube stitches are ready for removal 5 to 7 days after chest tube removal.

Home Care

With shorter hospital stays, home care nurses are vital to the ongoing recovery process. They assess the child and reinforce teaching started in the hospital. Skilled pediatric home care nurses monitor the child's cardiopulmonary status, measure oxygen saturations, check weight gain, review medications, and watch for signs of potential postoperative complications. Home care nurses help the family to problem-solve issues in setting up the house to meet the needs of the recovering child. They communicate their findings either to the primary caregiver or the pediatric cardiology team as indicated in the home care discharge orders.

At the time of discharge, family members are instructed to monitor their child for signs of potential complications. Low-grade fevers (less than 101° F) can be treated with acetaminophen or ibuprofen. A reoccurring low-grade fever or temperature higher than 101° F requires physician screening for possible signs of infection. Any redness, swelling, drainage, or opening of the wound should also prompt the parent to call the physician. Other general indications to notify a physician may include persistent vomiting, nausea, diarrhea, belly pain, difficulty breathing, or irritability. Families and pediatricians are instructed to defer routine immunizations to 4 to 6 weeks after cardiac surgery.

On the day of discharge, an appointment is made for the child to be seen by the primary caregiver within 2 to 3 days after discharge. A telephone report is given to the primary care physician and/or a copy of the hospital discharge summary is faxed to the office. An appointment is made for the child to be seen in the pediatric cardiology clinic 10 to 14 days or sooner after discharge, depending on individual needs.

For infants and young children with ongoing medical needs beyond the typical postoperative phase, an early intervention program may be beneficial to assist with their recovery and development.

The Pediatric Nurse Practitioner's Role in the Care of the Child with Congenital Heart Disease

Nursing is vital to the care of the child with congenital heart defect; there are multiple roles and responsibilities to be fulfilled. The educational preparation of the nurse intervening varies between institutions. The most critical factor is that the institution considers the unique talents of the nurse and develops a team so that the members complement each other in providing comprehensive care. Depending on the institution and the size of the pediatric cardiac program, the roles and responsibilities of pediatric cardiac nurses vary.

The pediatric nurse practitioner (PNP) is an essential member of the inpatient team. She meets with the child and family during the initial phase of diagnosis and assessment and facilitates the scheduling of tests (ECG, echocardiogram, cardiac catheterization, magnetic resonance imaging [MRI]). With the pediatric cardiologist and cardiac surgeon, the PNP prepares and educates the family and health care team for the upcoming surgery. Since most children are admitted to the hospital on the same day as their surgery, the PNP may see the child a few days before surgery to evaluate for any intercurrent illness, to perform the history and physical and to provide eating and drinking instructions to the parents. On the day of surgery, the PNP writes the postoperative orders, communicates with the admitting ICU nurse and physician team, and monitors the child's admission from the OR to the ICU. During the child's ICU stay, the PNP monitors the child's progress, identifies potential problems, and prepares for transfer to the general care unit. Once the child has been transferred out of the ICU, the PNP works with the cardiology team to ready the child and family for discharge. Under the guidance of the PNP, the bedside nurse teaches the family about home care needs and reviews discharge instructions and medications. The PNP communicates with the primary care physician, arranges for home care nursing, and orders medical equipment as needed.

In addition to daily clinical rounds, the PNP conducts informal bedside and formal classroom/conference teaching, mentors graduate nursing students, and participates in the nursing department committee activities.

PSYCHOSOCIAL IMPACT OF CONGENITAL HEART DISEASE IN THE CHILD

Initial Presentation and Diagnosis

The diagnosis of congenital heart disease imposes significant changes and adjustments to family life.[1] Parental expectations and hopes for a healthy child are altered by the presence of heart disease. The severity of illness, the timing of the diagnosis, the presentation leading to the diagnosis, previous experiences with illness, and individual and family adaptation skills affect the family's responses to the child. The nurse plays an important role in the family's adaptation through each stage of the child's care by providing education, educational material, and support dependent on the family's needs.

Advances in medical technology have increased the prenatal diagnosis of CHD. If a prenatal diagnosis is made describing a critical congenital heart defect, the pregnancy is closely monitored and plans made to deliver at an institution where appropriate support is available for the baby. Maternal anxiety is typically increased when the diagnosis of CHD is made by fetal echocardiography.[28] Support and information provided to the parents is crucial at this point.

If not diagnosed prenatally, serious CHD is usually detected during the first few weeks to months of life. Presentation in the neonatal period varies greatly. Symptoms that may lead to diagnosis include tachypnea with feeding intolerance, a murmur noted on a routine well-baby examination, cyanosis, and/or complete cardiovascular collapse. These differences in symptoms may influence the severity of the child's physiologic state but have little influence on parental reactions to the diagnosis. Three issues typically confront the family of an ill infant: (1) fear of loss and the unknown, (2) grief, and (3) guilt. Each family member individually prepares for what is to come. Frequently, parents do not communicate their feelings with each other and may need help acknowledging and communicating their feelings. During the initial workup, denial is the strongest coping mechanism.

The final diagnosis of the child's heart defect presents a new reality and summons the family's previous coping mechanisms. At this time, parents experience grief for the loss of their expected normal child. This mourning is necessary for them to accept the imperfect child. The family will cope only as well as each of its members do. Each family member needs to express individual feelings before the family unit is able to cope. Mothers often express guilt as an overwhelming emotion, whereas fathers frequently suffer loss of self-esteem over the birth of an imperfect child.[11] The family's ability to cope at this time is related to other factors, including the severity of illness; the suddenness of diagnosis and treatment; the meaning of the diagnosis to each individual member; the effect of the diagnosis on the family, including financial and lifestyle changes; and the presence and effect of support systems.

Staff interventions that aid coping at the time of diagnosis include provision of honest information about the child's condition and plan of care, establishment of support systems, and permission to establish and maintain the parenting role. At this time, parents typically seek general knowledge about CHD and specific details about their child with CHD. General questions parents need to have answered, whether they verbalize the questions or are afraid to ask, include: What causes CHD? What did I do wrong? What is our risk for having another child with CHD? Will our child survive? Specific questions parents may ask about their child include: What medical care will be provided to my child, including the need for doctor's appointments, medications, and additional testing? What signs do I look for in my child at home? Will my child be restricted in activities? Does my child need surgery? What can we expect now and in the future for my child? Answers to these questions need to be reiterated frequently to provide reassurance to family members. Another potential source of parental stress is the financial burden resulting from hospitalization, future health care costs, missed work days, and potential change in day care needs. Health insurance coverage should be examined to ensure optimal coverage.

After diagnosis, anger is a common parental response. This anger may be expressed toward God for letting this happen to their child, society for creating an imperfect world, the medical staff for making the diagnosis, themselves for giving birth to an impaired child, and the child for not being perfect. Guilt often accompanies this anger. Interventions by the health care team need to focus on the implications of these feelings. Time spent understanding the parents' perceptions of the child's illness is imperative for proper family functioning. Successful coping is contingent on parents' beliefs of what is wrong and the resultant consequences of their perceived diagnosis. Open, honest communication about the child's condition needs to be repeated to allow absorption and acceptance of facts in the face of stress.

Parent groups can be an additional source of support for families.[4,11,18] Parents who share similar experiences and solutions are able to help others. These groups allow family members to validate their thoughts and feelings in attempts to adjust to changes resulting from caring for their child with CHD. Parent support groups aid families through individual meetings during particularly stressful times. A parent is called on to help families at the time of a child's diagnosis, before diagnostic testing, before surgical treatment, at the time of discharge from the hospital, and during times of need after hospitalization. The supporting parents, drawing on their own experiences, are sensitive to other families faced with similar, familiar concerns. In addition to individual meetings with families, group support meetings provide ongoing discussion of issues that confront families over time. Parents find these meetings worthwhile at significant times in the child's life. Meetings usually concentrate on life experiences rather than focus on medical details. Typical discussions concentrate on children playing with other children, starting school, and engaging in sport activities; sibling reactions; and acceptance by family members, teachers, friends, and neighbors. By participating in these groups, parents benefit from receiving guidance and support in addition to the rewards gained by helping others.[23]

If CHD is not detected during early childhood, a preschool or pre-sports physical examination is another period when it is identified. Typically, cardiac lesions diagnosed at this time are usually not life threatening. However, CHD diagnosed at this time needs to be evaluated and treated in order to maintain good future health. Since the age of the child at the time of elective cardiac surgery or catheter intervention does not influence the course of psychological distress of parents or the styles of coping used by the parents, nursing interventions should be aimed at education and support of the child and family.[30]

Medical-Surgical Plan

After diagnosis, a strategy is proposed by a multidisciplinary group, including pediatric cardiac surgeons, pediatric cardiologists, anesthesiologists, nurses, and social workers outlining the medical and surgical care plan. The decision to perform surgery presents another crisis point for the child and family. A host of emotions accompany this time, including relief that the decision is made, fear of the unknown, anxiety over the outcome of surgery, and anticipation of changes in family life after surgery. At this time an enormous amount of information is presented to the family. Despite efforts to answer all parental questions, there are topics that parents find difficult to discuss.[5] The staff must be aware of these issues and willing to explore them with family members.

Surgery on a child's heart inflicts fear and apprehension in family members.[14] Parents of a critically ill infant will be absorbed with thoughts of their child's survival,[24] whereas parents of an asymptomatic, healthy child may actually have a more difficult time accepting the diagnosis and surgical plan. Nursing interventions at this time need to focus on each family individually. The team should take cues from the family regarding the timing for preparation and the depth of information given at this time. Honest information about what to expect during and after surgery should be the central theme of interventions.

Developmental Needs of Children

The developmental characteristics of children must be taken into account by staff members as they respond to their physical needs (Table 22-6).[3,21] The essential task during infancy involves the development of a trusting relationship,[21] and the infant and parents must participate in the bonding process. Denial and disappointment over the birth of a child with a congenital defect may affect this process. Infants with CHD may be less securely attached to their mothers than those without a major health problem.[18] Therefore efforts to enhance mother-child bonding will influence the infant's relationship with the mother. Fathers are essential to the child's sense of trust and must be included in the process of care and recovery. Staff should encourage parents to interact in the care of their infant by wiping away tears, talking, singing, soothing, rocking, changing diapers, or holding the baby. Appropriate sensory experiences are fulfilled when familiar toys are placed within the infant's view or reach, musical toys are used, and the child is touched or cuddled. Noxious stimuli should be controlled if possible. Sufficient lighting in the ICU allows adequate observation and assessment of the child; however, glaring lights should be avoided. Nursing care should be planned to provide uninterrupted sleep periods; a day-night sequence is useful. Reduction of loud noises as much as possible fosters the short sleep cycles in the ICU. Quiet, gentle, loving care at the bedside should focus on the child. The staff should avoid conversations about their personal or social lives, work schedules, or work operations at the child's bedside.

Toddlers' developmental needs include autonomy, exploration, and security.[3] During times of stress, they demonstrate signs of regression. Their relationship with parents is intense; separation anxiety occurs in their absence. Nursing interventions for toddlers in the ICU include promotion of the parent-child relationship. Parents are encouraged to visit often and participate in the child's care, including bathing, holding, and soothing during and after painful procedures. During the parents' absence, family pictures and tape recordings maintain the child's family contact. Routine care delivered by consistent caregivers adds to the toddler's sense of security. Choices should not be offered if there are none. The child should be encouraged to participate in care activities, and allowed to express fear and anger by crying during painful procedures. Children should not be told that "it does not hurt," because it usually does; that "it is okay," because to them it is not; and "just once" because, most often, this is not the case.

Table 22-6 Interventions to Care for Developmental Needs of Hospitalized Children

Age	Developmental Task	Effects of Hospitalization	Nursing Interventions
Infant	Develop sense of trust	Separation from parents is stressful. Hospital's strange environment, including sights, sounds, and smells, produces anxiety. Disruption of routines results in distrust.	Provide consistent caregivers. Decrease separation from parents. Tape family pictures to child's crib. Provide comforting, familiar environment, including blankets and toys from home. Promote uninterrupted periods of rest while avoiding overstimulation by performing all tasks at one time.
Toddler	Develop autonomy	Frightened by strange environment Perceives illness and hospitalization as punishment for bad behavior	Minimize separation from parents. Involve family in procedures. Provide consistent caregivers to decrease number of people toddler must adapt to, thereby increasing child's sense of trust. Allow as much movement as possible, using loose restraints only if necessary. Encourage hospital play. Acknowledge child's feelings while providing appropriate means to deal with them. Include familiar toys at bedside. Provide constant reassurance.
Preschool age	Develop initiative and autonomy	Difficulty separating reality from fantasy Fears unknown Frightened of bodily injury Threatened by procedures	Provide reassurance about healing and getting better. Provide appropriate choices in care. Support family if child engages in regressive behavior. Encourage hospital play for child to act out aggressions; allow child to assume role of nurse or doctor.
School-age	Develop sense of industry and accomplishment	Loss of control produces anxiety. Concerned with privacy and modesty Fears of bodily mutilation and injury are prevalent.	Tell child what is going to occur. Provide time for explanations about procedures.* Repeat explanations frequently. Reduce stimuli. Provide periods of undisturbed sleep. Respect child's privacy. Provide realistic choices that children can make, i.e., do not ask if they want blood drawn, but allow them to choose from which finger or site to have blood drawn.
Adolescent	Develop sense of identity	Fears loss of control Anxious about loss of identity, separation from peer group Apprehensive about changes in body image	Provide privacy to teenager. With teen's approval, facilitate contact with peers. Involve adolescent in decision making. Verify understanding of perceptions of illness, procedures, and hospitalization.† Provide time for favorite activities.

*Purcell C: Preparation of school-age children and their parents for intensive care following cardiac surgery. *Intensive Crit Care Nurs* 6:218–225, 1996.
†Velldtman GR, Matley SL, Kendall L, et al: Illness understanding in children and adolescents with heart disease. *Heart* 84:395–397, 2000.

Preschool children are involved with discovery and initiative.[26] They are egocentric, seeing the world from their viewpoint. The preschool child interprets events in response to good or bad behavior; illness and surgery are therefore seen as punishments.[21] Staff should reassure the child by saying "this is not your fault." Strategies to promote preschoolers' sense of psychological well-being include preparing them for procedures shortly before carrying them out; explaining who you are, what you are going to do, what the purpose of the procedure is, and what it will feel like, and providing opportunities for them to make choices. Engaging children in therapeutic play allows expressions of aggression and fear.[26] Preschoolers should be given permission to scream or cry during painful procedures, and again be assured that what is happening is not their fault.

School-age children are achieving a sense of industry.[3] The socialization process associated with attending school aids in this accomplishment. This is an age when peer approval and acceptance is essential. Separation from family members is easier.[21] Interventions guided toward school-age children in the ICU include encouragement of visitors, provision of

privacy, and honest explanations regarding procedures, including what will be done, the effects on body parts, and associated pain. The school-age child is inquisitive about the environment, and should if possible be protected from scenes involving other patients.

The major developmental task of adolescence is to develop a sense of identity.[31] The importance of body image to the teenager contributes to self-conscious behavior related to appearance, and the imperfections imposed by CHD and cardiac surgical repair. Relationships with and acceptance by peers are critical. Privacy is important to the teenager and should be provided in the ICU. Honest communication regarding the physical consequences of surgery, a forum to express fears, and contact with peers during the hospitalization will aid the adolescent patient in recovery after surgery for repair of CHD.

FAMILY-CENTERED CARE

Medical and surgical treatments of CHD have been addressed throughout this textbook. The child with CHD must be viewed as an individual as well as a member of a family unit, whose illness affects all members. Knowledgeable, trusting, calm, and secure parents are the child's best support. Therefore the care of the child must extend to include care of all family members. In addition to delivering high technological care, the ICU staff must understand and respond to the psychological needs of the child and family, and deliver care to meet those needs.[7]

Involving families in the care of children is the underpinning of quality pediatric health care.[27] Parents' participation in the postoperative care of the child in the ICU is an essential part of recovery. A tour of the ICU before the child's admission introduces the family to the environment. It is helpful for the child and parents to see the ICU milieu before they experience these sights with the child in the ICU bed. The nurse conducting the tour should take cues from the family and offer information that they want to hear. Explanations about why the child will be in the ICU and what will happen during this hospital stay are the highlights of this preoperative education. The family should be introduced to familiar ICU sights and sounds, and reassured that a nurse will be present at all times and will provide explanations about the care delivered.

Despite preoperative preparation, the family experiences a wide array of emotions during their first visit to their child in the ICU. A combination of emotions are present and often displayed, including, but not limited to, relief, joy, anxiety, caring, distrust, hostility, and fear. This first visit should take place as soon as possible after admission, and usually can happen within the first hour after surgery. Before this first visit, the child should be clean and covered and the bedside organized. Ideally, the ICU nurse should greet the family outside the child's room, provide a brief description of the child's appearance, and enter the room with the family. Brief explanations of the use and purpose of each device aid parents' adjustment to the sight of their pale, motionless, seemingly lifeless child surrounded by a maze of monitors, wires, and tubes. The family may be overwhelmed at first by the appearance of their child, but should be encouraged and assisted in touching and speaking to the child in an effort to restore their parenting roles. Parents cope with this visit by proceeding at their own pace; the nurse should respond to the family member's reactions and encourage a short first visit. The ICU nurse plays a pivotal role in identifying and alleviating parental fears at this time by encouraging parents to ask questions and express their fears and anxieties. A liberal visiting policy for the parents is crucial.

Subsequent visits become less difficult as the family becomes more familiar with the ICU environment and staff. Parents should be encouraged to visit frequently.[13] However, personal needs must be considered despite the parents' desire to stay at their child's bedside 24 hours per day. The staff influence parental decisions through the development of a trusting and caring relationship. Parents are more willing and able to leave their child if they know they will be contacted when changes occur in their child's condition and are encouraged to call whenever they wish.[34] It is important that parents receive the staff's approval and support in considering their own needs. The staff should encourage parents to eat, rest, shower, and talk to each other and other children during their child's hospital stay. When the parents' daily living needs are included

as part of the total orientation to the intensive care environment, the message about care of the family unit is delivered.

Parental involvement in the child's care benefits both child and parents. The extent of involvement depends on the child's condition. A critically ill child profits from the presence of the family through emotional and physical support. Through touching, holding, talking, and reading, family members provide emotional support. Encouragement by the staff to join in these activities allows the family to take an active role in the child's recovery. Parents may take part in their child's physical care by bathing, dressing, and feeding him or her. Participation in these tasks maintains the parenting role in the ICU setting. Parents' responses to their child's stay in the ICU are influenced by communication with staff members. Honest, current, and accurate communication strengthens the relationship between family and staff. Parental adaptation to their child's ICU admission contributes to the recovery of both child and family.

Transfer of the child from the ICU to the general pediatric care unit is usually accompanied by various parental responses. Although excited and relieved that their child is well enough to leave the ICU, many families feel frightened for their child and themselves. The child now requires less intense nursing care, and the nursing, medical, and surgical teams once always near the child's bedside are now less visible. Preparing and reassuring the child and family that these factors are positive signs will help abate parental fear and anxiety. This transition is smoother when explanations about the child's condition, needs for care on the general care unit, and expectations for care on the pediatric floor are made. For children who had an extended ICU stay, a visit to the general care unit may ease transition from the ICU to the floor. The staff's awareness of these characteristic responses and willingness to discuss the parents' feelings will facilitate the transfer process.

The impact of CHD on the child and family continues after surgical correction of the lesion. Adjustments must be made to accept the "new" child into the family. A second mourning period often accompanies this change. Families experience grief over the loss of a perfect child after the diagnosis of CHD. In order to accept the child with repaired CHD, family members must mourn the loss of their previously imperfect child. Difficulties with acceptance of the child after corrective surgery lead to continued overprotection of the child by family members and result in problems of psychological adjustment and adaptation. Strategies to assist parents during this time include: (1) providing information about the child's recovery and restrictions, (2) acknowledgment of the second mourning phase, (3) referral to parent groups, and (4) attention to the family's emotional support.

At first, families may find it difficult to allow the child whom they regarded as ill with cardiac problems before surgical correction to assume the role of a healthy, normal child. Children are often best able to gauge their own abilities and limitations. Encouraging family members to allow the child to adapt to new or familiar activities is crucial.[5] Most children recover rapidly from heart surgery and are ready to return to active play, day care, or school in just a few weeks. The family's ability to encourage normal activities and to allow the child to participate at his or her own pace will enhance the child's recovery and adjustment after surgical repair of the CHD.

References

1. Apley J, Barbour RF, Westmacott I: Impact of congenital heart disease on the family: Preliminary report. *BMJ* 1:103–105, 1967.
2. Bengur AR, Li JS, Herlong JR, et al: Intraoperative transesophageal echocardiography in congenital heart disease. *Semin Thorac Cardiovasc Surg* 10:255–264, 1998.
3. Bowen J: Helping children and their families cope with congenital heart disease. *Crit Care Quart* 8:65–70, 1985.
4. Brown DG, Glazer H, Higgins M: Group intervention: A psychosocial and educational approach to open heart surgery patients and their families. *Soc Work Health Care* 9:47–59, 1983.
5. Carey LK, Nicholson BC, Fox RA: Maternal factors related to parenting young children with congenital heart disease. *J Pediatr Nurs* 17: 174–183, 2002.
6. Delius RE, Caldarone C: Mechanical support of the pediatric cardiac patient. *Semin Thorac Cardiovasc Surg Pediatr Card Surg Ann* 3:179–185, 2000.
7. DeMaso DR, Beardslee WR, Silbert AR, Fyler DC: Psychological functioning in children with cyanotic heart defects. *J Dev Behav Pediatr* 11:289–294, 1990.
8. Dorman BH, Sade RM, Burnette JS, et al: Magnesium supplementation in the prevention of arrhythmias in pediatric patients undergoing surgery for congenital heart defects. *Am Heart J* 139:522–528, 2000.
9. Flori HR, Johnson LD, Hanley FL, Fineman JR: Transthoracic intracardiac catheters in pediatric patients recovering from congenital heart defect surgery: Associated complications and outcomes. *Crit Care Med* 28:2997–3001, 2000.
10. Goldberg S, Simmons RJ, Newman J, et al: Congenital heart disease, parental stress, and infant-mother relationships. *J Pediatr* 119:661–666, 1991.
11. Hazinski MF: Cardiovascular disorders. In Hazinski MF (ed): *Nursing Care of the Critically Ill Child*. St Louis, Mosby-Year Book, 1992, pp 117–394.
12. Jaggers J, Ungerleider RM: Cardiopulmonary bypass in infants and children. *Semin Thorac Cardiovasc Surg Pediatr Card Surg Annu* 3:82–109, 2000.
13. Jensen CA: Nursing care of a child following an arterial switch procedure for transposition of the great arteries. *Crit Care Nurse* 12:51–57, 1992.
14. Kashani IA, Higgins SS: Counseling strategies for families of children with heart disease. *Pediatr Nurs* 12:38–40, 1986.
15. Lappe DG, Beers MC, Hesterberg M: Pediatric intensive care nursing. In Rogers MC (ed): *Textbook of Pediatric Intensive Care*. Baltimore, Williams and Wilkins, 1992, pp 1588–1610.
16. Laussen P: Neonates with congenital heart disease. *Curr Opin Pediatr* 13:220–226, 2001.
17. LeRoy S: Clinical dysrhythmias after surgical repair of congenital heart disease. *AACN Clin Issues* 12:87–99, 2001.
18. Linde LM: Psychiatric aspects of congenital heart disease. *Psychiatr Clin North Am* 5:399–406, 1982.
19. Lloyd P: Postoperative nursing care following open heart surgery in children. *Nurs Clin North Am* 5:399–401, 1970.
20. Lodge AJ, Chai PJ, Daggett CW, et al: Methylprednisolone reduces the inflammatory response to cardiopulmonary bypass in neonatal piglets: Timing of dose is important. *J Thorac Cardiovasc Surg* 117:515–522, 1999.
21. Loeffel M: Developmental considerations of infants and children with congenital heart disease. *Heart Lung* 14:214–217, 1985.
22. Main E, Elliott MJ, Schindler M, Stocks J: Effect of delayed sternal closure after cardiac surgery on respiratory function in ventilated infants. *Crit Care Med* 29:1798–1802, 2001.
23. Maurer S, Kramer GF: *A Parent's Guide to Children's Congenital Heart Defects: What They Are, How to Treat Them, How to Cope with Them*. Three Rivers, Mich.,Three Rivers Press, 2001.
24. Miles MS, Mattioli L, Diehl AM: Parent counseling: Psychological support of parents of children with critical heart disease. *J Kans Med Soc* 78: 134–136, 151, 1977.
25. Purcell C: Preparation of school-age children and their parents for intensive care following cardiac surgery. *Intensive Crit Care Nurs* 12:218–225, 1996.
26. Rushton CH: Preparing children and families for cardiac surgery: Nursing interventions. *Issues Compr Pediatr Nurs* 6:235–248, 1983.
27. Rushton CH: Family-centered care in the critical care setting: Myth or reality? *Child Health Care* 19:68–78, 1990.
28. Sklansky M, Tang A, Levy D, et al: Maternal psychological impact of fetal echocardiography. *J Am Soc Echocardiogr* 15:159–166, 2002.
29. Turley K, Tyndall M, Turley K, et al: Radical outcome method: A new approach to critical pathways in congenital heart disease. *Circulation* 92:II245–249, 1995.
30. Utens EM, Versluis-Den Bieman HJ, et al: Does age at the time of elective cardiac surgery or catheter intervention in children influence the longitudinal development of psychological distress and styles of coping of parents? *Cardiol Young* 12:524–530, 2002.
31. Uzark K: Counseling adolescents with congenital heart disease. *J Cardiovasc Nurs* 6:65–73, 1992.
32. Veldtman GR, Matley SL, Kendall L, et al: Illness understanding in children and adolescents with heart disease. *Heart* 84:395–397, 2000.
33. Visconti KJ, Saudino KJ, Rappaport LA, et al: Influence of parental stress and social support on the behavioral adjustment of children with transposition of the great arteries. *J Dev Behav Pediatr* 23:314–321, 2002.
34. Ward CR, Constancia PE, Kern L: Nursing interventions for families of cardiac surgery patients. *J Cardiovasc Nurs* 5:34–42, 1990.
35. Weindling SN, Saul JP, Gamble WJ, et al: Duration of complete atrioventricularblock after congenital heart surgery. *Am J Cardiol* 82:525–527, 1998.

PART FOUR

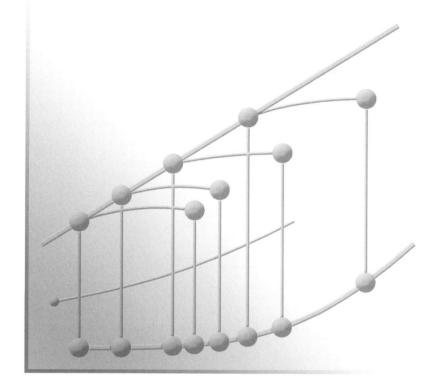

Congenital Heart Defects

Chapter 23

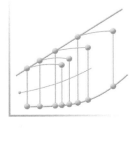

Perioperative Management of Patients with Congenital Heart Disease: A Multidisciplinary Approach

LAURA IBSEN, MD, IRVING SHEN, MD, and ROSS M. UNGERLEIDER, MD

BASIC PRINCIPLES

The perioperative care of the infant, child, and adult with congenital heart disease (CHD) requires a coordinated, multidisciplinary approach to patient care that emphasizes teamwork and the unique contributions of all those involved in the continuum of patient care: pediatric cardiologist, pediatric cardiac surgeon, pediatric intensivist, pediatric cardiovascular anesthesiologist, perfusionist, pediatric nurses, advanced practice nurses, physician's assistants, respiratory therapists, child life therapists, and family members. Each member of the team brings unique knowledge and perspective to the care of the patient, and recognizing and integrating all members of the team in the ongoing care of the patient are essential in providing optimal care for these patients. The presence of trainees from medicine, nursing, respiratory therapy, or other disciplines adds to the size and complexity of the team caring for the patient, and the roles and responsibilities of these individuals must be explicitly acknowledged.

Perioperative care encompasses both pre- and postoperative care of the patient with congenital heart disease. Although many infants and children with congenital heart defects are managed as outpatients until their repairs, some infants or older children with severely abnormal physiology require stabilization and critical care before surgery. Many of the basic principles of cardiac intensive care apply to both pre- and postoperative care and are considered in this chapter. In addition to supportive care and stabilization, preoperative management includes thorough evaluation of the anatomy and physiology of the heart and the physiologic status of the patient as a whole so that appropriately planned and timed surgery can take place.

Basic principles of pediatric critical medical and nursing care remain relevant in the pediatric congenital cardiac patient. Pediatric cardiac patients are cared for in specialized cardiac intensive care units and in multidisciplinary intensive care units. There are some data that institutions that perform more surgeries have improved outcomes.[50] Regardless of the focus of the unit, a commitment to ongoing education and training of all those involved in the care of the cardiac surgical patient, as well as a collaborative and supportive environment, is essential. We feel strongly that a unit dedicated to the care of infants and children is best able to care for these patients.

GENERAL PRINCIPLES OF OXYGEN DELIVERY AND UTILIZATION

The major goal in caring for all infants and children with cardiac disease is to ensure adequate tissue oxygen delivery. The primary function of the heart is to provide adequate blood flow (cardiac output) to the organism to preserve organ function. The amount of blood flow required is dependent on tissue oxygen demand and blood oxygen supply. Conditions that increase demand, such as increased metabolism from fever or infection, or that decrease supply, such as hypoxemia or anemia, can affect the amount of cardiac output required to sustain normal organ function. Patients with heart defects may have difficulty providing adequate cardiac output if they have inefficient pump function (e.g., intra- or extracardiac shunts, valvular insufficiency, arrhythmias) or depressed pump function (e.g., diminished ventricular contractility). Furthermore, conditions of the vasculature that the heart is pumping into, such as hypovolemia or increased peripheral vascular resistance, can affect the ability of the heart to generate adequate cardiac output. For health care providers to manage effectively patients who may be experiencing several of these issues, it is critical that the providers understand some of the basic calculations that describe adequacy of cardiac output and tissue oxygen delivery.

Oxygen delivery (DO_2) is described by the following equation: $DO_2 = Q_s(CaO_2)$, where Q_s is the systemic cardiac output and CaO_2 is arterial O_2 content. In turn, CaO_2 (mL/dL) = Hgb (g/dL) $\cdot$ SaO_2 $\cdot$ 1.34 (mL/g) + PaO_2 (mm Hg) $\cdot$ 0.003 (mL/dL/mm Hg), where Hgb is the hemoglobin concentration, SaO_2 is the arterial O_2 saturation, and PaO_2 is the arterial O_2 tension. Oxygen utilization (VO_2) is $Q_s(CaO_2 - CvO_2)$, where CvO_2 is the mixed venous oxygen content. Oxygen delivery is therefore primarily dependent on systemic cardiac output, hemoglobin concentration, and oxygen saturation. Dissolved oxygen (PaO_2) makes only a very small contribution to oxygen delivery.

Ventricular output (Q) is directly related to heart rate and stroke volume. Stroke volume is dependent on preload, afterload, and myocardial contractility. Both pulmonary blood flow (Q_p) and systemic blood flow (Q_s) are determined by these fundamental forces. In the patient with two ventricles, ventricular interdependence, or the effect of one ventricle on the other, may play a role in pulmonary or systemic blood flow. In some situations, including the postoperative state, the pericardium and restriction due to the pericardial space may also play a role in ventricular output by altering preload.

When evaluating the loading conditions of the heart and myocardial contractility, it is important to consider the two ventricles independently as well as their effect on one another. In previously healthy pediatric patients without heart disease, right atrial filling pressures are commonly assumed to reflect the loading conditions of the left as well as the right ventricle. In the patient with congenital heart disease, this is frequently not true. Preexisting lesions and the effects of surgery may affect the two ventricles differently. For example, the presence of a right ventricular outflow tract obstruction will lead to hypertrophy of the right ventricle. That right ventricle will be noncompliant, and the right atrial pressure may therefore not accurately reflect the adequacy of left ventricular filling.

Oxygen content (CaO_2) is primarily a function of hemoglobin concentration and arterial oxygen saturation. Thus patients who are chronically hypoxemic can improve oxygen delivery at any given cardiac output by maintaining a high hemoglobin concentration. Arterial oxygen saturation may be affected by inspired oxygen content (when there is parenchymal lung disease), by mixed venous oxygen content of blood (if there is mixing of systemic and pulmonary venous return), by pulmonary abnormalities, and by the presence of a right-to-left intracardiac shunt. Low mixed venous oxygen content contributes to desaturation and suggests increased oxygen extraction due to inadequate oxygen delivery, which in turn is due either to systemic cardiac output inadequate to meet metabolic needs or to inadequate hemoglobin concentration.

In the patient with a large intracardiac shunt, cardiac output, shunt fraction (Q_p:Q_s), and arterial oxygen content are also affected by the relative resistances of the downstream circuits. In the case of an atrial septal defect (ASD), the downstream circuits are the ventricles and the amount and direction of shunt flow depend on the resistance of the ventricles to filling with blood. Ventricular resistance is defined as *compliance* and is measured by $\Delta P/\Delta V$ (change in pressure/change in volume). A compliant cardiac chamber will have very little change in filling pressure for large increments of filling volume. Poorly compliant chambers may exhibit significant increases in filling pressure for relatively small amounts of additional volume. In the case of an ASD, shunt flow is usually left to right because the right ventricle is usually more compliant (distensible) than the left ventricle. However, in newborn infants with ASDs, the right ventricle may be relatively stiff, or noncompliant, and the direction of shunt flow in an infant with an ASD and a poorly compliant right ventricle may be right to left and this will result in some arterial oxygen desaturation, often referred to as cyanosis of the newborn. For ventricular septal defects (VSDs) and extracardiac shunts, the downstream chambers are the systemic and pulmonary vasculature. In most cases the pulmonary vascular resistance is substantially less than systemic vascular resistance and shunt flow will be toward the pulmonary circuit. However, factors can increase pulmonary vascular resistance (hypoxemia, hypercarbia, pneumonia) or decrease systemic resistance (sepsis) and this could result in a right-to-left shunt and systemic arterial oxygen desaturation. Anatomic narrowing of the pulmonary outflow tract in association with a large VSD (as is seen in tetralogy of Fallot or in single ventricle with pulmonary stenosis) can result in a substantial shunt toward the less resistant systemic outflow tract and can produce marked systemic oxygen desaturation. Furthermore, patients with certain conditions that result in complete mixing of pulmonary and systemic venous return before cardiac ejection (such as single ventricle, total anomalous pulmonary venous return [TAPVR], pulmonary atresia with VSD, or truncus arteriosus) will present with hypoxemia that will not respond to oxygen and will need adequate hemoglobin and an increased cardiac output to meet tissue oxygen demand.

A thorough understanding of these fundamental principles of cardiac output and oxygen delivery is essential to provide proper perioperative care to the patient with congenital heart disease.

GENERAL PRINCIPLES OF ANATOMY AND PATHOPHYSIOLOGY AFFECTING PREOPERATIVE AND POSTOPERATIVE MANAGEMENT

An understanding of the anatomy and pathophysiology of the congenital cardiac lesion under consideration allows one to determine the preoperative care or resuscitation needed and to predict the expected postoperative recovery.

Acyanotic Heart Disease

Children with acyanotic heart disease may have one (or more) of three basic defects: (1) left-to-right shunts (e.g., atrial septal defect, ventricular septal defect); (2) defects of ventricular inflow or outflow (e.g., mitral stenosis, aortic valve disease, aortic coarctation); and (3) primary myocardial dysfunction (e.g., cardiomyopathy) (Table 23-1). These lesions may lead to decreased systemic oxygen delivery by causing maldistribution of flow with excessive pulmonary blood flow (Q_p) and diminished systemic blood flow (Q_s) ($Q_p:Q_s>1$), by impairing oxygenation of blood in the lungs caused by increased intra- and extravascular lung water, and by decreasing ejection of blood from the systemic ventricle.

Maldistribution of Flow: $Q_p:Q_s > 1$

In infants with left-to-right shunts, pulmonary blood flow (Q_p) increases as pulmonary vascular resistance (R_p) decreases from the high levels present perinatally.[25,86] If Q_p is sufficiently increased, pulmonary artery pressure may also increase, particularly with left-to-right shunts distal to the tricuspid valve, such as a large VSD or aortopulmonary window. As pulmonary flow increases, left ventricular volume overload may occur with cardiac failure, decreased systemic output, pulmonary congestion, and edema. Over time, increased Q_p

Table 23-1 Mechanism of Decreased Systemic O_2 Delivery in Various Types of Acyanotic Heart Disease

Mechanism	ACYANOTIC LESION CATEGORY		
	Left-to-Right Shunt	Inflow/Outflow Obstruction	Myocardial Dysfunction
Decreased contractility		*	*
Pulmonary edema and V/Q mismatch	*	*	*
Maldistribution of flow ($Q_p:Q_s>1$)	*		

V/Q, ventilation/perfusion.

Table 23-2 Correlation of Preoperative Pulmonary Vascular Morphometric Changes with Variations in Pulmonary Blood Flow (Q_p), Pressure (P_{pa}), and Resistance (R_p)

Grade	Morphometrics	Catheterization Data
A and B (mild)	Neomuscularization ↑ medial thickness: <1.5 × normal (A) 1.5–2 × normal (B — mild)	↑ Q_p Normal P_{pa} at rest
B (severe)	Neomuscularization ↑ medial thickness: >2 × normal	↑ Q_p ↑ P_{pa} (≈ half systemic) Normal R_p
C	Same as B (severe) ↓ arterial number (relative to alveoli) and usually ↓ arterial size	↑ P_{pa} ↑ R_p (>3.5 U/m²)

Upward arrow, increases; *downward arrow*, decreases.
From Rabinovitch M, Haworth SG, Castaneda AR, et al: Lung biopsy in congenital heart disease: A morphometric approach to pulmonary vascular disease. *Circulation* 58:1107–1122, 1978.

leads to a series of pulmonary microvascular changes that first produce reversible pulmonary vasoconstriction and later fixed pulmonary vascular disease (see Chapter 3). As R_p increases over time, Q_p decreases (Table 23-2). The primary determinant of pulmonary blood flow is pulmonary vascular resistance. In patients with increased and reactive R_p, left ventricle (LV) function may be normal but oxygen delivery may be limited by decreased right ventricle (RV) output or by the development of intracardiac right-to-left shunting. If pulmonary pressures exceed systemic pressures, right-to-left shunting predominates and the patient becomes cyanotic. Depending on the type and size of the lesion, pulmonary overcirculation that remains uncorrected may lead to pulmonary vascular obstructive disease as early as 6 months of age. This increase in R_p occurs more commonly when the shunt is at the ventricular (VSD) or great vessel (e.g., truncus arteriosus) level than at the atrial level (ASD).

Pulmonary overcirculation can lead to congestive heart failure through several mechanisms. Increased Q_p leads to left (systemic) ventricular volume overload and raises left ventricular end-diastolic, left atrial, and pulmonary venous pressures. The increases in pulmonary artery and pulmonary venous pressures raise the pulmonary hydrostatic pressure gradient, and these promote transudation of fluid into the interstitial space and ultimately lead to alveolar edema. Right ventricular volume (from shunts at the atrial or ventricular level), end-diastolic pressure, and hence right atrial and systemic venous pressures are also elevated. Venous return may be decreased. High systemic venous pressure contributes to interstitial edema and may lead to decreased organ perfusion. The maldistribution of flow with reduced Q_s is accompanied by a reduction in renal blood flow and resultant stimulation of the renin-angiotensin system[16] (see Chapter 4). Fluid accumulation is aggravated by sodium and water retention by the kidney.

Pulmonary edema reduces CaO_2 through increased intrapulmonary shunting in the lungs (ventilation/perfusion [V/Q] mismatch). In addition to pulmonary overcirculation, other causes of pulmonary edema in patients with acyanotic heart disease include left ventricular inflow or outflow obstruction and diastolic dysfunction of the left ventricle. These children demonstrate an increased respiratory rate, diffuse rales, and increased work of breathing. The chest x-ray demonstrates diffuse interstitial and alveolar infiltrates.

Myocardial Dysfunction

Diastolic and to a lesser extent systolic dysfunction decrease oxygen delivery in patients with cardiomyopathy.[51] Diastolic dysfunction raises left ventricular end-diastolic pressure (LVEDP) and pulmonary venous pressures, ultimately leading to pulmonary edema. Systolic dysfunction decreases ejection fraction and systemic output. Cardiomyopathy represents the primary defect in a variety of heritable and inflammatory heart diseases (see Chapters 44 and 47). Patients with structural congenital heart defects may also develop myopathic changes in the heart. Graham[33] has shown that cardiomyopathy may be produced by volume or pressure overload, depending on the type of defect (Table 23-3). The myopathic changes are important both pre- and postoperatively.

Cyanotic Heart Disease

Children with cyanotic heart disease have a right-to-left shunt and therefore always demonstrate systemic arterial desaturation. As with acyanotic heart disease, there may

Table 23-3 Examples of Ventricular Dysfunction in Acyanotic Congenital Heart Lesions with Volume and/or Pressure Overload

Defect	Preoperative LV	Preoperative RV	Predicted Long-term Postoperative Function
VOLUME OVERLOAD			
Large VSD	↑↑ dilation, hypertrophy ↓ contractility	↑ Dilation	N if operated on before 2 yr
Large ASD	(Low) normal volume, N mass, N contractility	↑↑ Dilation ↓ compliance N contractility	N if operated on before 5 yr
PRESSURE OVERLOAD			
Aortic Stenosis	*Infant* ↓, N, or ↑ volume, no hypertrophy ↓ contractility	N	N unless LV is hypoplastic (<50% normal volume) AS or AI recurs
	Child (Low) normal volume, hypertrophy N contractility		
Infant CoA	↓ or N volume, variable hypertrophy ↓↓ contractility	↑↑ volume ↓ or N contractility	Normal

Upward arrow, increases; *downward arrow*, decreases; AI, aortic insufficiency; AS, aortic stenosis; ASD, atrial septal defect; CoA, coarctation of the aorta exhibits pressure overload to the left ventricle (LV) and volume overload to the right ventricle (RV) because of left-to-right shunt at the atrial level; N, normal; VSD, ventricular septal defect.
Data from references 22, 34, 37, 48.

be some combination of shunt, obstruction, and myopathic changes, all of which must be considered. Infants with cyanotic heart disease may be divided into two physiologically distinct groups, those with decreased pulmonary blood flow and those with increased pulmonary blood flow.

Ductal Dependent Pulmonary Blood Flow (Decreased Pulmonary Blood Flow)

These patients have decreased systemic venous blood entering the pulmonary circulation. Patients in this group may have obstruction to flow from the pulmonary ventricle either at the outlet (e.g., tetralogy of Fallot, pulmonary atresia) or at the inlet (e.g., tricuspid atresia). Patients whose pulmonary blood flow is dependent on a patent ductus arteriosus may present with severe hypoxemia and acidosis as the ductus closes (usually within hours to days of birth). With decreased Q_p and the obligatory presence of an atrial or ventricular septal defect (to "decompress" the systemic venous return to the systemic side of the circulation), the blood in the systemic ventricle consists of desaturated systemic venous blood (via the septal defect) and a smaller volume of saturated pulmonary blood ($Q_p:Q_s < 1$). The decreased Q_p results in decreased oxygen uptake from the lungs and thus decreased systemic oxygen delivery. In the initial stages, Q_s may be normal. If systemic oxygen delivery remains inadequate, anaerobic metabolism and myocardial dysfunction develop, resulting in a further reduction in oxygen delivery. The end result can be severe hypoxemia and acidosis. Patients with decreased Q_p require a stable source of pulmonary blood flow and a high hemoglobin concentration (>14 mg/dL) to maximize oxygen content (CaO_2) and oxygen delivery (DO_2).

Ductal Dependent Systemic Blood Flow (Increased Pulmonary Blood Flow)

Patients with ductal dependent systemic blood flow have increased pulmonary blood flow but decreased systemic blood flow due to obstruction of systemic output, which can occur at a variety of locations.[39,72,73] These infants may have acceptable arterial saturation but develop decreased oxygen delivery as a result of decreased systemic output (i.e., hypoplastic left heart syndrome, interrupted aortic arch, neonatal coarctation of the aorta). Patients may present with profound shock due to dramatic reduction in systemic perfusion and oxygen delivery as their ductus begins to close. Systemic blood flow in patients with severe left ventricular outflow obstruction is dependent on flow through a patent ductus arteriosus into the aorta distal to the obstruction.

PREOPERATIVE STABILIZATION, SURGICAL PLANNING

The degree to which infants and children require preoperative stabilization depends on the nature and severity of the lesion, the degree to which the lesion has affected the myocardial function, and the presence of other organ system involvement. Many of the concepts involved in preoperative stabilization are applicable to postoperative care.

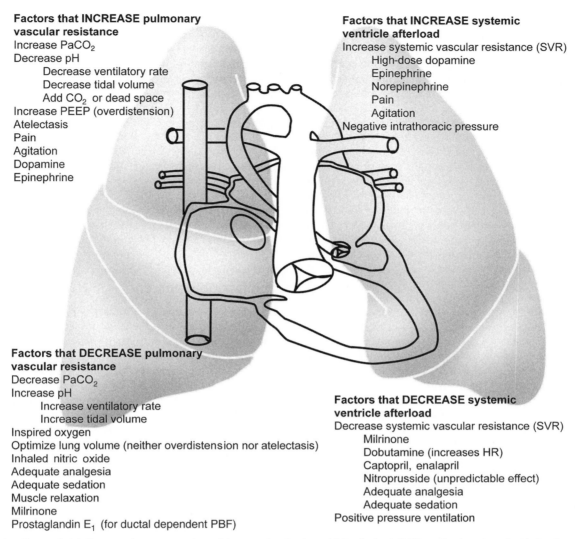

Factors that INCREASE pulmonary vascular resistance
Increase $PaCO_2$
Decrease pH
  Decrease ventilatory rate
  Decrease tidal volume
  Add CO_2 or dead space
Increase PEEP (overdistension)
Atelectasis
Pain
Agitation
Dopamine
Epinephrine

Factors that INCREASE systemic ventricle afterload
Increase systemic vascular resistance (SVR)
  High-dose dopamine
  Epinephrine
  Norepinephrine
  Pain
  Agitation
Negative intrathoracic pressure

Factors that DECREASE pulmonary vascular resistance
Decrease $PaCO_2$
Increase pH
  Increase ventilatory rate
  Increase tidal volume
Inspired oxygen
Optimize lung volume (neither overdistension nor atelectasis)
Inhaled nitric oxide
Adequate analgesia
Adequate sedation
Muscle relaxation
Milrinone
Prostaglandin E_1 (for ductal dependent PBF)

Factors that DECREASE systemic ventricle afterload
Decrease systemic vascular resistance (SVR)
  Milrinone
  Dobutamine (increases HR)
  Captopril, enalapril
  Nitroprusside (unpredictable effect)
  Adequate analgesia
  Adequate sedation
Positive pressure ventilation

FIGURE 23-1   Factors that influence pulmonary vascular resistance and systemic ventricle afterload. $PaCO_2$, systemic carbon dioxide tension; PBF, pulmonary blood flow; PEEP, positive end-expiratory pressure; HR, heart rate.

Preoperative stabilization of the ill infant or child focuses on establishing adequate oxygen delivery through manipulation of total cardiac output, Q_p, Q_s, hemoglobin concentration, and oxygen saturation. Additionally, any abnormalities of other organ systems, such as pneumonia, renal insufficiency, or seizures, must be evaluated and corrected if possible.

Manipulation of Q_p and Q_s and the balance between the pulmonary and systemic circulations is achieved by manipulation of the preload, afterload, and inotropic state of the right and left ventricles (Fig. 23-1). Pulmonary vascular resistance is affected by pH, alveolar pO_2 (partial pressure of oxygen), lung volume (atelectasis or overdistension), noxious stimuli, hematocrit, and many medications. The patient with excessive pulmonary blood flow and consequent low systemic oxygen delivery can be managed with maneuvers to increase pulmonary vascular resistance (R_p), which will lead to decreased Q_p and increased Q_s. In the patient with ductal dependent pulmonary or systemic blood flow, the balance of pulmonary and systemic flow can be manipulated by manipulation of pulmonary vascular resistance or the systemic

vascular resistance if needed. In these patients it is important to maintain ductal patency with the infusion of prostaglandin E_1 (PGE_1).

Afterload reduction may improve myocardial function by decreasing ventricular wall tension, thus improving stroke volume and decreasing myocardial oxygen consumption. Systemic vascular resistance can be lowered by agents that vasodilate (milrinone, dobutamine) and by avoiding agents that raise systemic vascular resistance (SVR) (high-dose dopamine, epinephrine, norepinephrine) or situations that raise SVR (pain, agitation). Patients with left-to-right shunts and LV volume overload show improved LV function after cautious reduction of elevated systemic afterload. Congestive heart failure (CHF) in infants with VSD is associated with stimulation of the renin-angiotensin system. Angiotensin converting enzyme (ACE) inhibition with captopril or enalapril reduces systemic vascular resistance (R_s), decreases Q_p:Q_s, and increases LV output in a dose-dependent manner.[13] Potent intravenous vasodilators such as nitroprusside have unpredictable effects on R_p/R_s and therefore on Q_p:Q_s and should generally be avoided in infants with left-to-right shunts and volume overload.[8]

Children with left ventricular outflow obstruction and pressure overload such as severe aortic stenosis may have massively increased, fixed afterload. Vasodilator administration will not increase Q_s, but rather may cause shock, myocardial ischemia, or life-threatening arrhythmias. In this situation, afterload reduction is accomplished by relief of the fixed obstruction by surgical or catheterization techniques.

The myopathic ventricle requires a greater than normal preload to maintain output. If the infant presents with congestive heart failure, pulmonary edema, and a stable systemic blood pressure, diuretics may be useful to reduce LVEDP and relieve pulmonary edema without compromising ventricular output. However, if the infant with a myopathic ventricle presents with hypoperfusion, hypotension, and acidosis, carefully titrated fluid administration may be necessary to optimize preload and increase cardiac output.

Inotropic drugs increase contractility at least in the short term. Unfortunately, inotropic drugs that increase cytosolic Ca^{++} concentration may also impair relaxation of the heart, decrease ventricular compliance, and limit preload (see Chapter 2).[89] In addition, increased inotropy is associated with increased myocardial energy requirements. Therefore, in patients with a pressure overloaded ventricle and risk of myocardial ischemia, inotropic agents with minimal chronotropic activity should be selected. Finally, congestive heart failure may be associated with desensitization of beta-adrenergic receptors and a blunted response to beta-adrenergic agonists.[15] There is an important role for use of inotropes that do not rely on beta-adrenergic stimulation such as milrinone, a phosphodiesterase inhibitor.[7,17]

Treatment of pulmonary edema without pulmonary overcirculation is directed at increasing both oxygen content and delivery. These children benefit from oxygen administration to treat the hypoxia and diuretic therapy to reduce the intravascular volume and left atrial pressure. Positive pressure ventilation with positive end-expiratory pressure (PEEP) can improve end-expiratory lung volume, decrease intrapulmonary shunting by opening collapsed alveoli, improve compliance, increase tidal volume, and decrease the work of breathing.[38] In addition, increased intrathoracic pressure with positive pressure ventilation and PEEP reduces LV afterload, thus improving systemic ventricular function and lowering end-diastolic pressure (LVEDP). Because positive pressure ventilation affects systemic venous return, LV afterload, and pulmonary vascular resistance, the net effect on oxygen delivery depends on intravascular volume status, myocardial function, and lung mechanics. Assisted mechanical ventilation of the child with pulmonary edema may directly increase both CaO_2 and systemic output.

POSTOPERATIVE CARE

Postoperative care requires a thorough understanding of the anatomic defect, the pathophysiology of the preoperative heart as well as any other organ system involvement, the anesthetic regimen used, cardiopulmonary bypass issues, and the details of the operative procedure. Invasive and noninvasive monitoring and laboratory or radiographic monitoring

are tailored to the needs of the individual patient and depend on the lesion, the repair, and expected postoperative issues.

Convalescence after cardiac surgery may be characterized as normal or abnormal. Normal convalescence is recovery that is expected given the preoperative state of the patient, the procedure performed, and the expected effects of cardiopulmonary bypass or other interventions. Abnormal convalescence is recovery that is prolonged or unexpected given what is known about the patient and the interventions that have been performed. It may be due to unknown or underappreciated abnormal preoperative anatomy or physiology, to unexpected complications of bypass, to residual anatomic defects, or to abnormalities in other organ systems such as pneumonia or sepsis. It is crucial to identify abnormal convalescence and to characterize it thoroughly so that appropriate intervention can take place in a timely fashion.

Mechanical Ventilation and Pulmonary Support

Patients who require postoperative mechanical ventilation do so for a variety of reasons: airway control, abnormal lung function, reduction of oxygen delivery needs, significant reactive pulmonary hypertension, assurance of stability during the immediate postoperative period, the beneficial effects of positive pressure ventilation on cardiac loading conditions in certain circumstances, or neurologic concerns or residual anesthesia. Mechanical ventilation, either in the operating room or in the intensive care unit, is usually continued until there is adequate hemostasis, the heart rate and rhythm are stable and close to normal for age, cardiac output is adequate with minimal inotropic support, oxygen saturation is adequate and lung function is close to normal, and the patient is awake enough to have adequate respiratory drive and airway protective reflexes. Depending on a number of factors, these conditions may be met in the operating room or in the intensive care unit much later in the postoperative course (Table 23-4).

Cardiopulmonary interactions can exert important influences on the hemodynamics of the postoperative patient but must be evaluated critically and optimized for the specific patient situation. For example, whereas early extubation and spontaneous ventilation after a Fontan operation is often thought to improve hemodynamics, if atelectasis or hypoventilation occurs, pulmonary vascular resistance will increase and hemodynamics will be adversely affected.

Monitoring of mechanical ventilation and pulmonary adequacy is accomplished via physical examination, noninvasive monitoring of oxygen saturation and end tidal carbon dioxide, and attention to lung mechanics, blood gases, and

Table 23-4 Criteria for Extubation of the Child after Cardiac Surgery

Heart rate close to normal for age
Rhythm normal or stable
Cardiac output adequate with minimal support (<5 mcg/kg/min dopamine, <0.5 mcg/kg/min milrinone)
Oxygen saturation adequate (depending on lesion) with <40% FiO_2
Spontaneously breathing
Airway protective reflexes intact
Hemostasis adequate

chest radiographs. The effects of different modes and strategies of mechanical ventilation on cardiac function should be assessed by monitoring filling pressures, heart rate, blood pressure, and perfusion. The need for tracheal suctioning and the quality and quantity of secretions should be followed as well.

There are minimal data on the optimal strategy for weaning cardiac surgical patients from mechanical ventilation. Weaning must be tailored to the individual patient, taking into consideration the type of repair surgery as well as any difficulties encountered during surgery or the immediate postoperative period. Patients with acyanotic heart disease and good myocardial function can frequently be extubated in the operating room or soon after admission to the intensive care unit. Others who have undergone more extensive repair or who have decreased ventricular function may require several days of support before weaning can occur. Once patients are weaned from mechanical ventilation, care must be taken to avoid atelectasis. Infants and young children will typically move and cry spontaneously, but older children and adolescents frequently will need assistance with sitting and standing and will need encouragement to deep-breathe and to move. Incentive spirometry and a guided program of progressive ambulation are essential and should be initiated as soon as physiologically safe.

Cardiac Evaluation and Support

The routine evaluation of the cardiovascular system after surgery consists of a combination of physical exam, noninvasive monitoring, and invasive monitoring.

Repeated physical examination is an essential part of the evaluation after cardiac surgery. Although a vital part of patient assessment, physical examination remains the least quantifiable and most subjective. Distal extremity temperature, capillary refill, and peripheral pulses suggest the adequacy of tissue perfusion. A prolongation of capillary refill greater than 3 to 4 seconds may indicate poor systemic perfusion but needs to be interpreted in relation to adequacy of the peripheral pulses. Changes in the character of murmur or attenuation of a shunt murmur may reflect significant changes in the child's condition. The child should frequently be examined for changes in cardiorespiratory status.

Noninvasive monitoring includes examination, pulse oximetry, central and peripheral temperatures, and surface electrocardiogram (ECG) monitoring. The surface ECG provides information on heart rate and rhythm. Cool extremities with normal or rising rectal temperature suggest decreasing and inadequate systemic cardiac output.

Before invasive monitoring is planned, the risk to benefit ratio of catheter placement should be considered. Vascular catheters are commonly placed in the operating room and include central venous catheters, right atrial catheters, left atrial catheters, pulmonary artery catheters, and arterial catheters. Central venous and right atrial catheters provide right-sided filling pressures, as well as information about tricuspid valve function. They enable indirect assessment of cardiac output by providing systemic venous oxygen saturation,[43,85] and they provide a site for infusion of pharmacologic agents. Because of their relative safety and extraordinary utility, most cardiac surgery patients will have a central venous/right atrial line. Central venous catheterization can be obtained by percutaneous cannulation of the internal jugular vein/subclavian vein or by placing the catheter directly into the right atrium at the time of surgery.

Left atrial catheterization provides measurement of pressures in the left side of the heart, information about mitral valve function, and measurement of left atrial desaturation due to right-to-left shunting in the lung. The indications for left atrial catheter placement are abnormal mitral valve function, abnormalities of left ventricular diastolic and/or systolic function, and abnormal lung parenchyma. Left atrial catheter placement carries the serious risk of introduction of air into the systemic arterial circulation. This can be kept to a minimum by careful management of these lines, the use of air filters, and appropriate education of the care team. The recent introduction of intraoperative echocardiography has resulted in a more selective use of left atrial lines.[94]

It should be appreciated that a catheter placed into the "right" atrium of a patient with single ventricle is physiologically a "left" atrial line, since it reflects the properties of the single ventricle and it requires the same assiduous management with respect to air as any conventional left atrial catheter. In fact caution must be excercised for any intravenous line in a patient with unrepaired single ventricle, since anything infused (e.g., air) into the line will be carried to the ventricle and subsequently to the systemic circulation. A superior vena cava (SVC) line in a patient with a Glenn shunt (superior cavopulmonary connection) does not carry this risk, since it leads first to the pulmonary arteries. After a Fontan operation (unless it is fenestrated), a venous line once again can be treated as a typical venous line.

Pulmonary artery catheters provide access for measurement of pulmonary pressures, pulmonary arterial saturation, and cardiac output.[32] Indications include the risk of pulmonary hypertension, residual left-to-right shunts, and decreased cardiac output. Pulmonary artery catheters should be used in children whose postoperative pulmonary artery pressure is greater than half systemic arterial pressure and in children who are at a high risk for pulmonary artery hypertension (Table 23-5). Pulmonary artery catheters are placed during surgery through the right ventricular outflow tract and advanced into the main pulmonary artery. Relative contraindications for pulmonary artery catheter placement are a large right ventricular outflow tract patch or any anatomic condition that will not allow placement of the catheter through a muscle bundle.

Arterial catheterization is required in all children who undergo surgery for congenital heart disease and allows for continuous blood pressure monitoring as well as repeated measurements of a variety of laboratory studies.

Table 23-5 Congenital Heart Defects with Increased Risk of Pulmonary Hypertensive Crises in the Postoperative Period

Large ventricular septal defect
Complete atrioventricular canal
Truncus arteriosus
Large patent ductus arteriosus, aortopulmonary window
D-transposition of the great arteries
Total anomalous pulmonary venous return

Support of the cardiovascular system is directed at optimizing cardiac output and oxygen delivery. This is accomplished by optimization of heart rate, preload, afterload, and inotropy and is guided by invasive, noninvasive, and laboratory monitoring. When cardiac output measurement is not available, mixed venous oxygen saturation trends can provide information regarding the adequacy of oxygen delivery. Studies have demonstrated that mixed venous saturations are a reliable and early indicator of cardiovascular dysfunction, and failure to measure this may worsen outcomes in some situations.[5,92] A decreasing mixed venous oxygen saturation, despite escalating support, indicates abnormal convalescence and the need for aggressive intervention.

Another indicator of failing oxygen delivery is the development of lactic acidosis. The sequential evaluation of serum lactate levels provides important assessment of the adequacy of oxygen delivery[18,19] (Fig. 23-2). Lactate levels are usually high immediately after surgery but should decrease to less than 2 mmol/L if oxygen delivery is adequate. Persistent elevation of lactate requires evaluation. The therapeutic strategy implemented should be tailored to the individual patient circumstance but may include volume administration, transfusion, escalation in inotropic or pressor support, alteration of afterload, recognition and management of cardiac rhythm disorders (including pacing), change in ventilator strategy, or mechanical intervention such as opening the sternum or revision of a repair. Occasionally, extracorporeal life support (ECLS) is necessary.[46,98] Metabolic acidosis that is not accompanied by elevated lactate is usually a hyperchloremic metabolic acidosis (non-anion gap metabolic acidosis) and generally resolves without treatment.

Pharmacologic Support of the Heart

Ventricular dysfunction that occurs after cardiac surgery may be due to the preoperative condition of the myocardium, the expected effects of cardiopulmonary bypass or abnormally pronounced response to bypass, suboptimal loading conditions of the heart or abnormal electrolytes, or the presence of residual lesions. Ventricular dysfunction may be systolic or diastolic in nature. The diagnosis of left ventricular dysfuction is suggested by tachycardia, tachypnea, poor perfusion, poor urine output, or elevated serum lactate and acidosis. Left ventricular dysfunction is suggested by elevated left-sided filling pressures. Right ventricular dysfunction may result in similar findings as well as hepatic congestion. Elevation of right-sided filling pressures will be seen if there is diastolic dysfunction. It is important to realize that right and left systolic and diastolic dysfunction often occur simultaneously. Although elevation of filling pressures is apparent in both systolic and diastolic dysfunction, echocardiography can usually distinguish the two by demonstrating the adequacy of ventricular contraction and also the presence of diastolic flow reversal in dysfunction that is primarily diastolic.[60]

Cardiac output is the product of heart rate and stroke volume; hence, optimizing these components results in improved cardiac output (Fig. 23-3). Heart rate can be manipulated by cardiac pacing if the primary problem is a

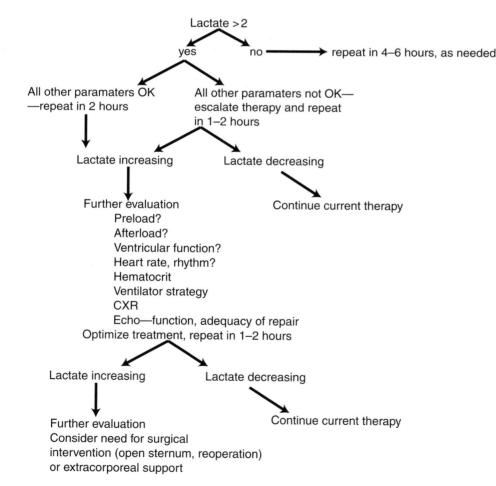

FIGURE 23-2 Suggested treatment algorithm for use when monitoring serum lactate.

Ventricular Dysfunction

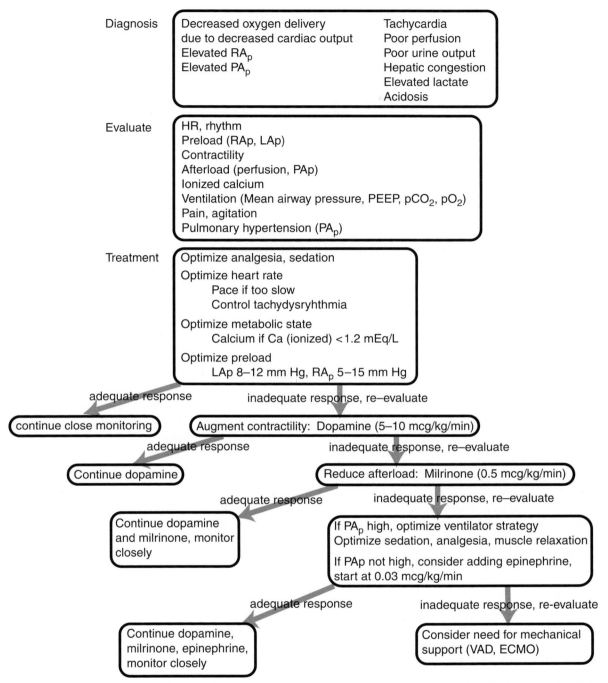

FIGURE 23-3 Evaluation and management of ventricular dysfunction. ECMO, extracorporeal membrane oxygenation; HR, heart rate; LAp, left atrial pressure; PAp, pulmonary artery pressure; pCO₂, partial pressure of carbon dioxide; PEEP, positive end-expiratory pressure; pO₂, partial pressure of oxygen; RAp, right atrial pressure; VAD, ventricular assist device.

slow heart rate compared to what the patient needs. When the primary problem is tachycardia, especially junctional ectopic tachycardia (JET), the heart rate can be manipulated by medications, such as esmolol or amiodarone (see Chapter 8). Patients with low heart rates and neonates with left ventricular dysfunction may increase systemic oxygen delivery by increasing the heart rate, but it should be remembered that coronary blood flow to the left ventricle occurs during diastole.

An increase in heart rate results in a reduction of diastolic filling and can reduce left ventricular myocardial perfusion, especially at heart rates greater than 220 beats per minute.

Stroke volume can be affected by changes in preload, contractility, and afterload. When administering volume to augment preload, one must keep in mind the compliance of the ventricle. If filling pressures are low (<10 mm Hg), small volumes of fluid (5 mL/kg) may increase output.

Noncompliant ventricles with significant diastolic dysfunction likely already have high filling pressures, and one must be cautious with volume administration. Ventricles with poor compliance demonstrate significant increases in filling pressures with very small infusions of volume.

Myocardial contractility can be improved by increasing ionized calcium and by infusing inotropic medications. Calcium supplementation plays an essential role in augmenting left ventricular function in children.[49,71] The underdeveloped sarcoplasmic reticular system in the neonatal myocardium causes the heart to be more dependent on extracellular calcium concentration than is the adult myocardium. Since intracellular calcium plays a central role in myocardial contractility in neonates, normal blood levels of ionized calcium are necessary to augment stroke volume. Although calcium resuscitation in the postoperative period has fallen into some disfavor in adults because of the concerns of reperfusion injury, calcium supplementation remains a central component of the management strategy in infants and children. Wide fluctuations in ionized calcium levels can occur in the perioperative period, and routine monitoring of ionized calcium levels is essential. Infants with chromosome 22q11 deletions (velocardiofacial syndrome, DiGeorge syndrome) are particularly susceptible to low calcium levels.

Positive inotropic medications that are frequently used in the postoperative period include dopamine (1 to 10 mcg/kg/min), milrinone (0.5 to 1 mcg/kg/min), and epinephrine (0.05 to 1 mcg/kg/min). Milrinone may be particularly beneficial, as it improves cardiac output while lowering filling pressures, systemic vascular resistance index (SVRI), and pulmonary vascular resistance index (PVRI) and does not increase myocardial oxygen consumption.[17] There are also data that prophylactic use of milrinone after cardiac surgery in infants and children reduces the risk of developing low cardiac output.[44] Dobutamine is an effective positive inotropic agent but frequently produces unacceptable degrees of tachycardia.[11] Inotropic medications affect both the right and left ventricle and so can be beneficial for both right and left ventricular dysfunction.

Afterload to the left ventricle can be reduced with the use of milrinone or a vasodilator such as nitroprusside. Nitroprusside can have unpredictable effects, however, and should be used with caution. The primary advantage of nitroprusside is that it is an endothelial independent vasodilator and can therefore reliably dilate both the pulmonary and the systemic vasculature, even in the presence of ischemic injury. Nitroprusside also has a very short half-life and can be titrated to the desirable effect and immediately stopped if hypotension occurs. Long-term use of nitroprusside can create cyanide toxicity, so nitroprusside should not be used for long-term management of hypertension or afterload manipulation. Positive pressure ventilation decreases left ventricular afterload and is thus frequently of benefit to patients with left ventricular dysfunction. Afterload to the right ventricle can frequently be reduced by altering the pulmonary vascular resistance through manipulations of the cardiorespiratory interactions, by inducing alkalosis, either pharmacologically with sodium bicarbonate or via hyperventilation, or by increasing inspired oxygen. When these maneuvers are not sufficient and there is pulmonary vascular hypertension that impairs cardiac output, inhaled nitric oxide may be beneficial.

Most pharmacologic approaches to try to reduce pulmonary vascular resistance are problematic because they also reduce systemic vascular resistance and hence produce systemic hypotension. Inhaled nitric oxide is delivered as a gas to the lungs and is rapidly inactivated by binding to hemoglobin,[82] and thus does not produce systemic hypotension.

Vasopressor agents such as norepinephrine and vasopressin are infrequently indicated in the postoperative cardiac surgical patient but sometimes have an important role.[84] Postoperative sepsis is sometimes accompanied by vasodilation and hypotension, which may be reversed with vasopressor agents.

Mechanical Support of the Heart

Application of mechanical circulatory assist is occasionally very beneficial for infants and children after cardiac surgery. Whereas adult patients can benefit from intra-aortic balloon counterpulsation, this modality is fairly ineffective in children. Mechanical assist for children is usually applied as extracorporeal membrane oxygenation (ECMO), which provides support to the entire heart as well as the lungs. Indications range from ventricular dysfunction unresponsive to inotropic support, to severe pulmonary hypertension with resultant right ventricular failure, to circulatory support to meet the increased cardiac output demands after the establishment of single ventricle, shunt-dependent physiology.[2,6,23,24,46,56,81,83,98,102] Most published series suggest that 60% of postcardiac surgery patients who require ECMO survive their hospitalization and 50% are alive at least one year later. Reports vary regarding the risks of ECMO and which patients benefit most from this support. In general, infants who cannot be weaned from CPB represent a high-risk group, although some series suggest that outcomes are better for those who are placed on ECMO in the operating room versus those placed on ECMO in the ICU. Variation in experiences most likely relates to patient selection and to management strategies, especially for shunt management after palliation for complex single ventricle (e.g., hypoplastic left heart syndrome [HLHS]).[46] When it is not possible to wean a patient from CPB, ECMO can be employed with expectation of an increased risk of bleeding due to inability to reverse the heparin used during CPB. This can greatly complicate ICU management, and it is important for the ICU team to work closely with their surgical colleagues in managing anticoagulation, the attendant risk of circuit thrombosis, and the need for mediastinal exploration in the ICU to control tamponade. Usually, these factors can be balanced, but this kind of situation often creates a very eventful evening and good teamwork is essential to a successful outcome.

ECMO can be highly beneficial in the treatment of ventricular dysfunction. With the patient's cardiac output needs supported, excessive inotropes can be removed and afterload can be reduced (either with the use of pharmacologic agents such as milrinone or simply with removal of vasoconstrictive inotropes). The result is usually a well-perfused patient whose heart can recover over a time course that is usually 3 to 5 days. After allowing sufficient time for recovery, infants can usually be weaned from ECMO, occasionally by adding low- to moderate-dose inotropes, and cannulae can be removed. Cardiac support is usually provided with direct atrial and aortic cannulation through an open sternotomy (which is usually covered with a synthetic dressing), and the sternum can usually be closed in the ICU after the cannulae are removed. If chest closure results in significant elevation of the central venous pressure (CVP), it is sometimes important to leave the sternum open (and covered with a synthetic dressing) for a few days while the baby becomes stable off ECMO. Although the literature is conflicted regarding the necessity of venting the left side of the heart when patients are placed on ECMO for cardiac dysfunction (presuming normal, two-ventricle anatomy), it has generally been our experience that this is not only unnecessary but may complicate the ECMO management by introducing a source of thrombus or air to the system.

Some infants with severe pulmonary hypertension are supported by ECMO. A common scenario is pulmonary hypertension after repair of TAPVR (total anomalous pulmonary venous return). It is important to distinguish "primary" pulmonary hypertension from pulmonary hypertension that is "secondary" to LV dysfunction. This differential is possible if the surgeon has placed both a pulmonary artery pressure monitoring catheter and a left atrial line. In primary pulmonary hypertension, the pulmonary artery pressures are elevated and the left atrial pressures may be low to normal. In secondary pulmonary hypertension, which seems to be more common after cardiac repair, the left atrial pressure is elevated (reflecting poor LV function). Echocardiography can help to verify the diagnosis. In either case, ECMO can be very beneficial, but the pre-ECMO therapeutic interventions would include application of nitric oxide and ventilatory management for primary pulmonary hypertension, or inotropic support and afterload reduction if the problem is LV dysfunction. Another option, when confronted with LV dysfunction manifesting as pulmonary hypertension after repair of TAPVR, is to reopen the communicating vein or to reopen the ASD (if it was closed during the repair).

Recently, ECMO has been advocated for the elective management of single ventricle after Norwood procedure to augment cardiac output and enhance neurologic outcomes.[98] An interesting feature of ECMO when applied to infants with shunt-dependent, single ventricle physiology is that it is actually univentricular support; the venous cannula in the atrium decompresses the entire heart and the arterial cannula in the aorta supplies both the systemic and the pulmonary circulation, as long as the shunt is kept open. In this circumstance, the infant's lungs can serve as an oxygenator, and a membrane oxygenator is not necessary in the extracorporeal circuit. This greatly reduces the need for providing anticoagulation until after surgical bleeding has been controlled. However, for these patients, ventilator management is important (in contrast to the full-support ECMO patients for whom ventilation needs are minimal).

ICU management of patients on ECMO requires that the intensivist consider two phases: the acute and the chronic. During the acute phase, the ICU team needs to manage bleeding while balancing the anticoagulation required to protect the extracorporeal circuit from clots. At the same time it is helpful to remove vasoconstrictive inotropes and to enhance the patient's systemic perfusion. It is helpful to follow lactates as a reflection of systemic perfusion.[18,19] After the patient has been stabilized, the ICU team enters into the "chronic" phase. This may be 3 to 7 days in length and

it requires mindfulness toward the goal of removing the patient from ECMO as soon as possible. The stability of patients on ECMO can sometimes lure the ICU team into a sense of complacency. However, it is usually in the patient's best interests to wean from the extracorporeal circuit, since renal function is generally better off ECMO and prolonged exposure to ECMO may increase the risk of mediastinal or systemic infection as well as hematologic complications from prolonged anticoagulation. In general once the patient is well perfused (warm extremities with good capillary refill and normal lactate levels), consideration should be given to weaning from ECMO. If the patient required ECMO for ventricular support, daily echocardiograms can help assess for return of acceptable ventricular function. If ECMO was employed for pulmonary hypertension, pulmonary artery pressures can be monitored as ECMO flow is decreased. Thoughtful collaboration between intensivists, surgeons, and cardiologists can help optimize outcomes for these patients.

Hematology, Thrombosis, and Hemostasis*

Postoperative bleeding is the result of inadequate surgical hemostasis or of coagulopathy due to residual heparin, dilutional effects, or disseminated intravascular coagulation (DIC). If bleeding is not corrected after correction of coagulopathy or if the blood loss is greater than 10 mL/kg/hour, surgical bleeding should be considered and exploration strongly considered. Chest tubes and mediastinal drainage tubes must be kept clear and patent if there is ongoing bleeding to prevent the occurrence of cardiac tamponade. Furthermore, when there is significant bleeding, it is essential to infuse blood and blood products to maintain hemodynamic stability. Typically measured coagulation studies include prothrombin time (PT), activated partial thromboplastin time (aPTT), fibrinogen, and platelet count. These values are frequently abnormal in the immediate postoperative period and require treatment only if there is excessive bleeding. An elevated aPTT usually reflects residual heparin and is treated with protamine. Elevated PT suggests dilutional coagulopathy or DIC and is treated with fresh frozen plasma (10 mL/kg as volume status allows). Low fibrinogen is treated with cryoprecipitate (1 unit per 5 kg body weight). Platelets are usually low due to dilution and should be transfused if the platelet count is less than 100,000 or if there is excessive bleeding. Even if the platelet count is normal, platelet function may be abnormal and platelet transfusion may be helpful. Newly improved methods of thromboelastogram (TEG) evaluation can help delineate the etiology of postoperative bleeding.

Heparin-induced thrombocytopenia and thrombosis (HITT) is increasingly recognized in the pediatric population (Fig. 23-4). HITT is the most common drug-induced thrombocytopenia in adults, complicating 1% to 3% of full-dose exposures to standard heparin.[100] We have reported a similar rate of occurrence of HITT in a pediatric cardiac surgical population.[52] In HITT, the platelet fall is usually 40% to 50% and the thrombocytopenia is moderate (30,000 to 100,000). The onset is 5 to 10 days after first exposure to heparin, and hours to 2 to 3 days with reexposure. Thrombosis may localize to sites of preexisting pathology (central venous lines, shunts, surgical repairs) and be present in unusual locations.

---

*See also Chapter 14

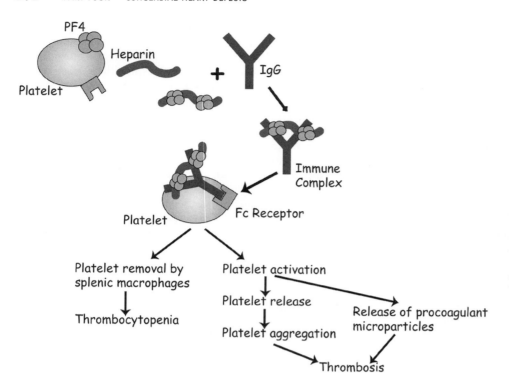

FIGURE 23-4 Heparin-induced thrombocytopenia and thrombosis (HITT) pathophysiology. Heparin forms a complex with platelet factor 4 (PF4), which is released from platelets by platelet activation. Antibody directed against the heparin-PF4 complex binds via its Fab. region. The antibody-heparin-PF4 immune complexes may opsonize platelets, leading to increased clearance. The complexes may also bind to the Fc receptor on the surface of the platelet, leading to platelet activation and generation of procoagulant platelet microparticles. Endothelial cells and monocytes also appear to be targets of the HITT immune complexes.

Less common presentations include delayed thrombocytopenia (two to three weeks), heparin-induced skin necrosis due to subcutaneous injections, adrenal infarction/hemorrhage, heparin resistance, and anaphylactoid reactions.

Antibody (PF4) ELISAs are sensitive but not specific. Positive ELISAs are found in 40% to 60% of asymptomatic adult reoperative cardiac surgery patients.[78] A recent abstract found them in 31 of 64 children (median age 29 months) undergoing reoperative cardiac surgery, only 1 of whom had clinical HITT.[69] Unfortunately, a negative ELISA does not exclude HITT. More specific for clinical HITT are functional assays based on in vitro heparin-dependent platelet activation (^{14}C serotonin release, heparin-dependent platelet aggregation, lumi-aggregometry). Unfortunately, functional assays are less sensitive and often negative or indeterminate in the first 24 to 48 hours of HITT. Both assays usually become negative in about 3 weeks, making it difficult to diagnose previous HITT.[87]

If HITT is diagnosed, all heparin (lines, flushes, heparin-coated catheters, low molecular weight heparins) must be stopped. Platelet transfusion should be avoided (transfusion may precipitate thrombosis) as should warfarin in the acute phase of HITT. Use of alternative anticoagulation is imperative in preexisting or new thrombosis and should be strongly considered for prophylaxis. Argatroban, a hepatically excreted, synthetic antithrombin with a $t_{1/2}$ of approximately 40 to 50 minutes, is presently our choice, with a usual dose of 2 mg/kg/min by continuous infusion. Anticoagulation is monitored by either partial thromboplastin time (PTT) (target 1.5–3.0 × normal) or activated clotting time (ACT) (target on ECMO 180 to 200).[12]

Renal Issues and Fluid Balance

Fluid and electrolyte imbalances after cardiac surgery with cardiopulmonary bypass are the result of the effects of bypass,

reduced cardiac output after surgery, and fluids or diuretics administered in the postoperative period. Cardiopulmonary bypass with hypothermia, nonpulsatile perfusion, and reduced mean arterial pressure causes the release of angiotensin, renin, catecholamines, and antidiuretic hormones.[31,55] These circulating hormones along with reduced cardiac output result in reduced renal blood flow and reduced urine output. Cardiopulmonary bypass and the associated inflammatory process lead to sodium and fluid accumulation during surgery. Ongoing capillary leak and need for preload augmentation in the immediate postoperative period further augment the positive fluid balance.

Most patients who have undergone cardiopulmonary bypass and those who have had non-bypass operations but who have had congestive failure before surgery require diuretic therapy in the postoperative period. Loop diuretics are most commonly used, either intermittently or as a continuous infusion. Continuous infusion of furosemide (0.1mg/kg/hour) produces comparable urinary output for a lower total dose than intermittent furosemide (1 mg/kg/dose), produces less hourly fluctuation in volume status, and consequently lowers the requirement for fluid replacement in hemodynamically unstable patients.[63,88] Traditionally, diuretics have been withheld during the period of ongoing capillary leak after cardiopulmonary bypass (24 to 48 hours), but there are some data to suggest that early diuresis is safe and well tolerated.[63]

During the period of active diuresis, one must pay close attention to potassium, calcium, and magnesium levels, and these electrolytes frequently need supplementation. In addition, loop diuretics such as furosemide and bumetanide usually induce a hypochloremic metabolic alkalosis, though this is usually well tolerated. If the metabolic alkalosis is so severe that it makes weaning from mechanical ventilation difficult, it can often be treated with acetazolamide or arginine chloride.

Severe renal failure is an uncommon occurrence after surgery for congenital heart disease. In those patients, peritoneal dialysis or continuous venovenous or arteriovenous hemofiltration and/or hemodialysis may be used. Patients with significantly elevated filling pressures, as is found in diastolic dysfunction, may have problems mobilizing fluid from their third space; in these patients oliguria is associated with an elevation in blood urea nitrogen (BUN) but not creatinine. This is similar to the type of oliguria found in low cardiac output from poor systolic function. The latter can be treated with inotropic agents, but inotropic support is contraindicated in diastolic dysfunction. It is important to make the distinction between renal failure and diastolic dysfunction leading to inability to mobilize third-spaced fluid. An additional confounding issue might be ongoing capillary leak syndrome from sepsis.

On occasion, when it appears that infants with a noncompliant right ventricle are not mobilizing fluid adequately from their soft tissue, with a rising BUN but a normal creatinine, and sepsis is not an issue, placement of bilateral pleural tubes can be quite beneficial. Even when the infant does not appear to have significant pleural effusions by chest radiograph, pleural tubes can begin to provide substantial drainage, and as the infant begins to mobilize fluid, he or she will diurese. On some occasions, the fluid may appear to be milky, and chylothorax needs to be considered. Pleural fluid can be analyzed for chylomicrons and for triglycerides. If chylothorax is diagnosed, diet should be switched to low and medium chain triglycerides. When oliguria persists, especially when there is electrolyte imbalance, and when the above techniques do not work, dialysis can be helpful. Peritoneal dialysis is generally technically easier to accomplish and does not require large intravascular catheters or anticoagulation, but does not provide as much control over fluid balance as continuous hemodialysis, especially if cardiac output is low or there is ongoing capillary leak (see Chapter 4).

Pain and Sedation

Postoperative pain and agitation or anxiety are expected and must be planned for. The modalities employed to treat pain, agitation, and anxiety depend on the age of the child, the postoperative physiology, and any tolerance or dependence that has developed as a result of long-term pain issues. Effective treatment requires a multidisciplinary approach encompassing physician, nursing, child life specialist, primary caregiver, and family input. Therapies may include regional techniques such as epidural or intrathecal anesthesia, intermittent or continuous infusions of opioids or benzodiazepines, patient-controlled analgesia, or nonsteroidal anti-inflammatory agents. (See Chapter 10 for detailed discussion of analgesic alternatives.)

Infants who undergo cardiopulmonary bypass and cardiac surgery mount a significant stress response including increases in plasma epinephrine, norepinephrine, cortisol, glucagons, and glucose. Anand and colleagues[3] reported that those infants with more profound stress responses had higher mortality, and that the hormonal-metabolic stress response could be attenuated with high-dose synthetic opioid anesthesia that was continued into the initial postoperative period with resultant decreased morbidity and mortality.[4] Although this work was seminal in increasing the awareness of the need for postoperative analgesia in this population, newer data suggest that the use of high-dose opioid anesthesia directed at blunting the endocrine stress response may not be an important factor in determining early outcome after cardiac surgery.[35]

Pulmonary hypertensive crises may occur after repair of congenital heart disease with large left-to-right shunts such as large ventricular septal defect, atrioventricular septal defect, total anomalous pulmonary venous return, large patent ductus arteriosus, truncus arteriosus, and D-transposition of the great arteries. Along with hypoxia and hypercarbia, hypothermia, and hypoglycemia, pain and agitation are potent triggers of pulmonary hypertensive crises (Fig. 23-5). In addition to avoiding triggering conditions, analgesia and sedation in the intensive care unit play a large role in avoiding or treating pulmonary hypertensive crises. High-dose fentanyl boluses do not significantly affect baseline hemodynamics after cardiac surgery[42] but can blunt the response to noxious stimuli such as tracheal suctioning.[41] The use of continuous infusion of opioids such as fentanyl (2 to 4 mcg/kg per hour) alone or in combination with a benzodiazepine (50 to 100 mcg/kg per hour) is generally used in the first 24 to 48 hours postoperatively for infants with pulmonary hypertension. A bolus dose of narcotics or benzodiazepines is used for "breakthrough" episodes. If significant difficulties with pulmonary hypertensive crises continue, the period of deep sedation should be prolonged. Intermittent or continuous neuromuscular blockade is sometimes also used to provide more precise control of ventilation, pH, and systemic carbon dioxide tension ($PaCO_2$) and prevent increases in alveolar pressure and subsequent decrease in pulmonary perfusion caused by coughing or ventilator dyssynchrony. It should be remembered that many of these patients will have elevated pulmonary artery pressures for a prolonged period of time, and if the increased pressures do not compromise cardiac output, they can be tolerated.

Pulmonary Hypertension

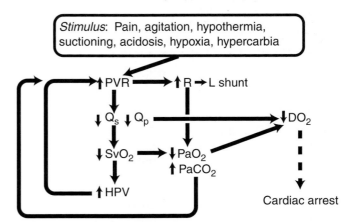

FIGURE 23-5 Pulmonary hypertension. Pulmonary hypertensive crisis leading to decreased oxygen delivery. DO_2, oxygen delivery; HPV, hypoxic vasoconstriction; $PaCO_2$, systemic carbon dioxide tension; PaO_2, systemic arterial oxygen tension; PVR, pulmonary vascular resistance; Q_p, pulmonary blood flow; Q_s, systemic blood flow; SvO_2, systemic venous oxygen saturation.

Nutrition

Nutrition is an essential component of the care of the postoperative patient (see Chapter 15). Early feeding reduces gut translocation of bacteria and the risk of multiorgan system failure and decreases the need for total parenteral nutrition with its attendant risks. Feedings should be withheld in high-risk patients such as those with severe preoperative acidosis and those with poor postoperative hemodynamics. Necrotizing enterocolitis (NEC) can occur in the postoperative period and carries a high incidence of morbidity and mortality.[66,76] It is important to recognize that necrotizing enterocolitis may also occur before surgery and is most common in patients with univentricular hearts with or without arch obstruction.[66]

Patients after cardiac surgery are frequently hyperglycemic in the initial postoperative period. Many infants have received steroids pre- and intraoperatively, and all patients have undergone a physiologically stressful event. There is evidence in the adult literature that administration of insulin to control glucose levels significantly improves outcome in patients in the intensive care unit,[99] although it is unclear if control of hyperglycemia or administration of insulin is responsible for this effect.[28] At the present time there are no data on any beneficial or detrimental effect of control of hyperglycemia in critically ill pediatric patients. If blood glucose is controlled with insulin, care must be taken to avoid hypoglycemia, to which neonates or those with inadequate glycogen stores are particularly vulnerable.

Transpyloric feeding is frequently advocated for mechanically ventilated patients to reduce the incidence of aspiration and to achieve targeted nutritional intake more rapidly, although this has not been demonstrated in the postoperative cardiac surgical population. There is considerable variability in tolerance to the advancement of enteral feedings, and close clinical examination of infants during advancement of nutrition is essential.

Although it has not been well studied, it is not uncommon for neonates, especially those who have had a long or difficult postoperative course, to be poor oral feeders after cardiac surgery. Many such infants require prolonged tube feeding supplementation in addition to trials of oral feeding to ensure adequate caloric intake. There is little understanding of the basis of such poor feeding, but it may include oral aversion, poor pharyngeal coordination, poor cardiac output, or generalized weakness. There is a recent suggestion that the use of transesophageal echocardiography may increase the incidence of postoperative dysphagia and feeding problems.

Infection

Infectious complications and their sequelae after cardiac surgery are among the most common problems encountered in the intensive care unit. Infections can be viral, either community acquired or nosocomial, bacterial, or fungal, and the complications associated with infection in the postoperative period are myriad. The rate of infection after pediatric cardiac surgery varies widely between different reports.

Respiratory syncytial virus (RSV) is a significant pathogen for patients with congenital cardiac disease and is responsible for much more morbidity and mortality in this population than in the population of infants and children without heart disease.[64] Children who undergo cardiac surgery while symptomatic from the RSV infection are at higher risk of postoperative mortality and morbidity, especially pulmonary hypertension. It is not clear what the optimal timing of surgery should be for children who require surgery and who acquire RSV before planned surgery, but it appears that longer waiting periods, if hemodynamically tolerated, to allow optimal recovery from RSV are beneficial. Patients who were infected but asymptomatic before surgery, or who acquire nosocomial RSV, are clearly at risk for a difficult postoperative course. There are also data that suggest that viral upper respiratory infection (URI) in general is predictive of longer length of ICU stay, postoperative bacterial infections, and respiratory complications, though it is not clear if particular pathogens such as RSV or influenza are responsible for the majority of the morbidity.[65] The necessity of performing the operation given the presence of URI must be individualized, but those caring for the patient postoperatively should recognize that those children who undergo surgery with a URI may be at increased risk of postoperative complications.

Bacterial complications after cardiac surgery include line infections and sepsis, mediastinitis, and ventilator associated pneumonia. Risk factors for the acquistion of nosocomial infections after cardiac surgery include younger age, prolonged ICU stay, delayed sternal closure, and more complex cardiac lesion.[59,68,91] Prevention and treatment of infection associated with central lines are particularly important for patients who have a long or difficult postoperative course. Although it is widely accepted that the risk of infection rises with the duration of catheter use, this has been shown not to be true in the pediatric population,[90] although it does appear that the frequency of use of catheters increases their likelihood of being associated with infection.[62] There is good evidence that changing catheters over a wire does not decrease the risk of infection, but placement of new catheters increases the risk of mechanical complications.[20,21] Use of heparin-bonded catheters appears to reduce the risk of infection in a general pediatric ICU population.[77] Although the types of organisms that cause hospital-acquired infections change over time, coagulase-negative *staphylococci*, *enterococci*, and *Staphylococcus aureus* account for the majority of catheter-related infections, although gram-negative organisms and *Candida* (spp.) are increasingly prevalent in pediatric ICUs.[74]

Delayed sternal closure is frequently used in neonates for whom the constrictive effects of immediate sternal closure would prove detrimental in the early postoperative period. The reported incidence of surgical site infection or mediastinitis with delayed sternal closure ranges from 0% to 28%.[27,36,75,91] It is not clear what the optimal antibiotic prophylaxis regimen is to prevent sternal wound infection in the setting of delayed sternal closure, and practice varies widely.

Neurologic Complications

Central nervous system complications after cardiac surgery may include seizures, embolic stroke, intracerebral hemorrhage, choreoathetosis, and long-term cognitive delay (see Chapter 6). Postoperative seizures may occur after simple or complex repairs. The risk of postoperative seizures may be increased in those infants exposed to deep hypothermic circulatory arrest (DHCA), but only when the period of DHCA exceeds 41 minutes.[101] Much attention has been paid to various perfusion techniques utilized during complex operations in infants. Comparison of neurodevelopmental outcomes for patients exposed to CPB as infants with and without the use of DHCA shows no significant differences at 8 years of follow-up,[9] although both groups are developmentally impaired compared to normal. Substantial research has been performed over the past 15 years that has led to significant improvement in the application of CPB to infants, and it appears that neurologic outcomes will continue to improve in the future.[96]

Seizures after cardiopulmonary bypass with or without DHCA are usually transient. The etiology of seizures is unknown and may be related to microemboli during CPB and surgery, especially air emboli. If seizures last more than a few minutes, they should be treated aggressively, recognizing that many anticonvulsants have negative inotropic properties and must be used carefully. Persistent neurologic deficits should be evaluated by computed tomography (CT) or magnetic resonance imaging (MRI) to rule out a more significant embolism or intracerebral hemorrhage that might require more aggressive intervention. The need for and utility of ongoing anticonvulsant therapy for patients who have had a postoperative seizure must be individualized.

Choreoathetosis after cardiac surgery has been reported after cardiopulmonary bypass with or without DHCA.[45] The injury is probably related to hypoxic-ischemic injury to the basal ganglia caused by disturbance to the cerebral blood flow. Some, but not all, patients with postsurgical choreoathetosis have lesions in the basal ganglia that can be seen on CT or MRI (Fig. 23-6). Patients who develop choreoathetosis after cardiac surgery are at high risk of significant long-term developmental and motor delays[26,67] and should receive careful neurologic and cognitive evaluation. Recognition of the groups at higher risk for this complication and application of improved strategies of CPB have virtually eliminated this problem in recent years.[9,47,53,54,95–97,101]

Long-term developmental sequelae of surgery for congenital heart defects are of great concern and the subject of much ongoing research into optimal cerebral protective strategies during cardiopulmonary bypass and DHCA. It has been well documented that mild to moderate cognitive, motor, and behavioral disabilities are prevalent in pediatric patients after cardiac surgery. As one might expect, preoperative risk, postoperative course, as well as operative variables play a role in the development of persistent developmental delays.[29,30,61]

Relatively common peripheral nervous system complications include injury to the phrenic nerve and injury to the recurrent laryngeal nerve. Phrenic nerve injury can be caused by trauma or electrocautery during dissection and will result in a paralyzed hemidiaphragm, which may lead to inability to wean successfully from mechanical ventilation. On routine chest radiographs the paralyzed diaphragm may appear normal when the patient is receiving positive pressure ventilation, but it will appear elevated when the patient is breathing spontaneously. If one cannot successfully wean the patient from mechanical ventilation and a paralyzed diaphragm is suspected, fluoroscopy during spontaneous ventilation while the patient is intubated is frequently diagnostic. Typically, this

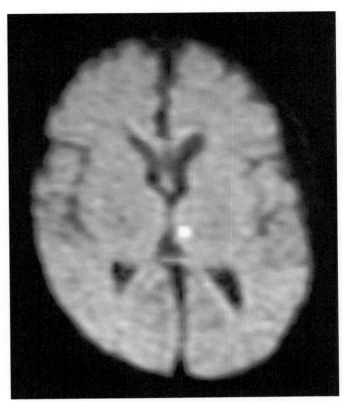

FIGURE 23-6 MRI of infant with choreoathetosis. Diffusion weighted imaging on MRI demonstrates a small area of infarction in the medial thalamus. The infant demonstrated choreoathetosis after repair of total anomalous pulmonary venous return. Subsequently, he had normal cognitive and motor development.

problem can be addressed by plicating the diaphragm to stop paradoxical movement of the diaphragm and place the diaphragm in a more mechanically advantageous position.[1]

Injury to the recurrent laryngeal nerve can result in unilateral vocal cord paralysis, leading to a hoarse voice or weak cry. Damage to the recurrent laryngeal nerve typically results from local trauma during dissection. If the vocal cord paralysis interferes with airway protection, surgical intervention may be necessary, usually with Teflon injection of the affected cord.

Horner's syndrome, consisting of ptosis, anhydrosis, enophthalmus, and miosis, occurs uncommonly after repair of aortic coarctation due to damage to the ophthalmic branch of the cervical sympathetic nerves. It is important to recognize this complication so that the eye can be kept moist and the eyelid closed at night; patients should receive follow-up with an ophthalmologist.[70]

FAMILY-CENTERED CARE

Family-centered care is based on the understanding that the family is the patient's primary source of nurturing and support and that the child and family's desires, perspectives, and observations are important in clinical decision-making. The approach of family-centered care shapes health care policy, facility design, and clinical interactions between patients, families, physicians, nurses, and other health care providers. There is abundant evidence that a family-centered approach to care delivery enhances outcomes and improves patient and family as well as provider satisfaction.[10,40] Such an approach utilizes the abilities and strengths of all team members, including social workers, child life specialists, bedside nurses and nurse educators, physician's assistants, respiratory therapists, surgeons and intensivists, as well as parents and extended family members.

There is relatively little information in the literature to guide the development of a family-centered approach specific to the pediatric cardiac surgical patient. A comprehensive educational approach serves to facilitate the patient's and family members' understanding of surgery, postoperative recovery, the intensive care unit, and longer term recovery and prognosis. Preoperative education of the family and patient, if applicable, regarding the postoperative care is essential. Use of videos demonstrating various types of equipment such as the ventilator or central lines may be useful. Explanations of who the various health care providers are, especially in academic medical settings where there may be physicians and nurses at various levels of training, help to familiarize the family with those they will encounter. If possible to arrange, a tour of the intensive care unit before surgery may make the day of surgery less stressful.

Individual unit policies regarding visitation and family presence during rounds or during procedures vary tremendously. There are some data in the adult literature to support the presence of family members during multidisciplinary rounds.[93] The degree to which parents or patients participate in the discussion obviously varies with different situations, but we have found that the practice does not hinder provider communication or education and greatly enhances the family members' feelings of control and understanding of their child's condition, and often provides the caregivers with important observations or insights into the patient's recovery. It is important that someone, usually the patient's bedside nurse, be available to the parent or patient to answer questions during or after rounds.

There are excellent data in the anesthesia literature that support organized, preplanned parent-present induction as a means of reducing patient anxiety and improving parental satisfaction,[57,58] and there are data that suggest family presence during procedures in the emergency department is beneficial for families and does not detract from care.[14] There has been relatively little work done on the issues surrounding parent presence during invasive procedures in the intensive care unit, though what has been done suggests that parent presence during invasive procedures such as endotracheal intubation, central line placement, and chest tube placement is helpful to parents, patients, and caregivers and does not detract from the quality of care delivered.[79] There are no data to suggest that family presence negatively impacts the successful completion of procedures nor that it increases rates of infection or other complications. As with parent presence during rounds, it is imperative that family members be educated and supported if they choose to remain present during invasive procedures. It is equally important as we embrace an era of family-centered care that health care providers learn effective interpersonal and communication skills when discussing patient care issues in front of the family or with the family.

References

1. Affatato A, Villagra F, De Leon J, et al: Phrenic nerve paralysis following pediatric cardiac surgery: Role of diaphragmatic plication. J Cardiovasc Surg 29:606–609, 1988.
2. Aharon AS, Drinkwater DC, Churchwell KB, et al: Extracorporeal membrane oxygenation in children after repair of congenital cardiac lesions. Ann Thorac Surg 72:2095–2102, 2001.
3. Anand K, Hansen D, Hickey P: Hormonal-metabolic stress responses in neonates undergoing cardiac surgery. Anesthesiology 73:661–670, 1990.
4. Anand K, Hickey P: Halothane-morphine compared with high-dose sufentanil for anesthesia and postoperative analgesia in neonatal cardiac surgery. N Engl J Med 326:1–9, 1992.
5. Bando K, Turrentine MW, Sharp TG, et al: Pulmonary hypertension after operations for congenital heart disease: Analysis of risk factors and management. J Thorac Cardiovasc Surg 112:1600–1609, 1996.
6. Bartlett RH, Andrews AF, Toomasian JM, et al: Extracorporeal membrane oxygenation for newborn respiratory failure: 45 cases. Surgery 92:425–433, 1982.
7. Barton P, Garcia J, Kouatli A, et al: Hemodynamic effects of IV milrinone lactate in pediatric patients with septic shock: A prospective, double-blinded, randomized, placebo-controlled, interventional study. Chest 109:1302–1312, 1996.
8. Beekman R, Rocchini A, Rosenthal A: Hemodynamic effects of nitroprusside in infants with a large ventricular septal defect. Circulation 64:553–558, 1981.
9. Bellinger DC, Wypij D, du Plessis AJ, et al: Neurodevelopmental status at 8 years in children with dextro-transposition of the great arteries: The Boston Circulatory Arrest Trial. J Thorac Cardiovasc Surg 126:1385–1396, 2003.
10. Blesch P, Fisher M: The impact of parental presence on parental anxiety and satisfaction. AORN J 63:761–768, 1996.
11. Bohn D, Poirier C, Edmonds J, Barker G: Hemodynamic effects of dobutamine after cardiopulmonary bypass in children. Crit Care Med 8:367–371, 1980.
12. Boshkov L, Ibsen L, Kirby A, et al: Report of Argatroban infusions for heparin-induced thrombocytopenia (HIT) in a neonate and a 5-month-old congenital cardiac surgery patient. Society for Thrombosis and Hemostasis, 2003 (abstract).
13. Boucek M, Chang R: Effects of captopril on the distribution of left ventricular output with ventricular septal defect. Pediatr Res 24:499–503, 1988.
14. Boudreaux ED, Francis JL, Loyacano T: Family presence during invasive procedures and resuscitations in the emergency department: A critical review and suggestions for future research. Ann Emerg Med 40:193–205, 2002.
15. Bristow M, Ginsburg R, Minobe W, et al: Decreased actecholamine sensitivity and beta-adrenergic-receptor density in failing human hearts. N Engl J Med 307:205–211, 1982.
16. Buchhorn R, Ross R, Bartmus D, et al: Activity of the renin-angiotensin-aldosterone and sympathetic nervous system and their relation to hemodynamic and clinical abnormalities in infants with left-to-right shunts. Int J Cardiol 78:225–230, 2001.
17. Chang AC, Atz AM, Wernovsky G, et al: Milrinone: Systemic and pulmonary hemodynamic effects in neonates after cardiac surgery. Crit Care Med 23:1907–1914, 1995.
18. Charpie JR, Dekeon MK, Goldbert CS, et al: Serial blood lactate measurements predict early outcome after neonatal repair or palliation for complex congenital heart disease. J Thorac Cardiovasc Surg 120:73–80, 2000.
19. Chiefetz I, Kern F, Schulman S, et al: Serum lactates correlate with mortality after operations for complex congenital heart disease. Ann Thorac Surg 64:735–738, 1997.
20. Cobb D, High K, Sawyer R, et al: A controlled trial of scheduled replacement of central venous and pulmonary-artery catheters. N Engl J Med 327:1062–1068, 1992.
21. Cook D, Randolph A, Kernerman P, et al: Central venous catheter replacement strategies: A systematic review of the literature. Crit Care Med 25:1417–1424, 1997.
22. Cordell D, Graham TP Jr, Atwood GF, et al: Left heart volume characteristics following ventricular septal defect closure in infancy. Circulation 54:294–298, 1976.
23. Darling EM, Kaemmer D, Lawson DS, et al: Use of ECMO without the oxygenator to provide ventricular support after Norwood stage I procedures. Ann Thorac Surg 71:735–736, 2001.

24. del Nido P: Extracorporeal membrane oxygenation for cardiac support in children. *Ann Thorac Surg* 61:336–339, 1996.

25. Drummond W, Gregory G, Heymann M, Phibbs R: The independent effects of hyperventilation, tolazoline, and dopamine on infants with persistent pulmonary hypertension. *J Pediatr* 98:603–611, 1981.

26. du Plessis A, Bellinger D, Gauvreau K, et al: Neurologic outcome of choreoathetoid encephalopathy after cardiac surgery. *Pediatr Neurol* 27:9–17, 2002.

27. Fanning W, Vasko J, Kilman J: Delayed sternal closure after cardiac surgery. *Ann Thorac Surg* 44:169–172, 1987.

28. Finney S, Zekveld C, Elia A, Evans T: Glucose control and mortality in critically ill patients. *JAMA* 290:2041–2047, 2003.

29. Galli KK, Zimmerman RA, Jarvik GP, et al: Periventricular leukomalacia is common following neonatal cardiac surgery. *J Thorac Cardiovasc Surg* 127:692–704, 2004.

30. Gaynor JW, Gerdes M, Zackai EH, et al: Apolipoprotein E genotype and neurodevelopmental sequelae of infant cardiac surgery. *J Thorac Cardiovasc Surg* 126:1736–1745, 2003.

31. German J, Chalmers G, Hirai J, et al: Comparison of nonpulsatile and pulsatile extracorporeal circulation on renal tissue perfusion. *Chest* 61:65–69, 1972.

32. Gold J, Jonas R, Lang P, et al: Transthoracic intracardiac monitoring lines in pediatric surgical patients: A 10-year experience. *Ann Thorac Surg* 42:185–191, 1986.

33. Graham T Jr: Ventricular performance in congenital heart disease. *Circulation* 84:2259–2274, 1991.

34. Graham TP: *Ventricular Function in Congenital Heart Disease.* Lancaster, England: MTP Press, 1986.

35. Gruber E, Laussen P, Casta A, et al: Stress response in infants undergoing cardiac surgery: A randomized study of fentanyl bolus, fentanyl infusion, and fentanyl-midazolam infusion. *Anesth Analg* 92:882–890, 2001.

36. Hakimi M, Walters H, Pinsky W, et al: Delayed sternal closure after neonatal cardiac operations. *J Thorac Cardiovasc Surg* 107:925–933, 1994.

37. Hammon J Jr, Lupinetti F, Maples M, et al: Predictors of operative mortality in critical valvular aortic stenosis presenting in infancy. *Ann Thorac Surg* 45:537–540, 1988.

38. Hammon J Jr, Wolfe W, Moran J, et al: The effect of positive end-expiratory pressure on regional ventilation and perfusion in the normal and injured primate lung. *J Thorac Cardiovasc Surg* 72:680–689, 1976.

39. Hansen D, Hickey P: Anesthesia for hypoplastic left heart syndrome: Use of high-dose fentanyl in 30 neonates. *Anesth Analg* 65:127–132, 1986.

40. Hemmelgarn A, Dukes D: Emergency room culture and the emotional support component of family-centered care. *Child Health Care* 30:93–110, 2001.

41. Hickey P, Hansen D, Cramolini G, et al: Pulmonary and systemic hemodynamic responses to ketamine in infants with normal and elevated pulmonary vascular resistance. *Anesthesiology* 62:287–293, 1985.

42. Hickey P, Hansen D, Wessel D, et al: Pulmonary and systemic hemodynamic responses to fentanyl in infants. *Anesth Analg* 64:483–486, 1985.

43. Hijazi Z, Fahey J, Kleinman C, et al: Hemodynamic evaluation before and after closure of fenestrated Fontan: An acute study of changes in oxygen delivery. *Circulation* 86:I196–202, 1992.

44. Hoffman T, Wernovsky G, Atz A, et al: Prophylactic intravenous use of milrinone after cardiac operation in pediatrics (PRIMACORP) study: Prophylactic intravenous use of milrinone after cardiac operation in pediatrics. *Am Heart J* 143:15–21, 2002.

45. Holden K, Sessions J, Cure J, et al: Neurological outcomes in children with post-pump choreoathetosis. *J Pediatr* 132:162–164, 1998.

46. Jaggers JJ, Forbess JM, Shah AS, et al: Extracorporeal membrane oxygenation for infant postcardiotomy support: Significance of shunt management. *Ann Thorac Surg* 69:1476–1483, 2000.

47. Jaggers JJ, Shearer I, Ungerleider RM: Cardiopulmonary bypass in infants and children. In Gravlee GP, Davis RF, Kurusz M, Utley JR (eds): *Cardiopulmonary Bypass: Principles and Practice.* Philadelphia, Lippincott, Williams & Wilkins, 2000, pp. 633–661.

48. Jarmakani J, Graham T Jr, Canent R Jr, Capp M: The effect of corrective surgery on left heart volume and mass in children with ventricular septal defect. *Am J Cardiol* 27:254–258, 1971.

49. Jarmakani J, Nakanishi T, George B, Bers D: Effect of extracellular calcium on myocardial mechanical function in the neonatal rabbit. *Dev Pharmacol Ther* 5:1–13, 1982.

50. Jenkins K, Gauvreau K: Center-specific differences in mortality: Preliminary analyses using the Risk Adjustment in Congenital Heart Surgery (RACHS–1) method. *J Thorac Cardiovasc Surg* 124:97–104, 2002.

51. Katz A: Cardiomyopathy of overload: A major determinant of prognosis in congestive heart failure. *N Engl J Med* 322:100–110, 1990.

52. Kirby A, Ibsen L, Ungerleider R, et al: Heparin induced thrombocytopenia (HIT) in infants. *Pediatr Crit Care Med* 4:A66, 2003.

53. Kirshbom PM, Skaryak LA, DiBerardo LR, et al: Effects of aortopulmonary collaterals on cerebral cooling and cerebral metabolic recovery after circulatory arrest. *Circulation* 92:II490–494, 1995.

54. Kirshbom PM, Skaryak LR, DiBernardo LR, et al: pH-stat cooling improves cerebral metabolic recovery after circulatory arrest in a piglet model of aortopulmonary collaterals. *J Thorac Cardiovasc Surg* 111:147–157, 1996.

55. Kron I, Joob A, Van Meter C: Acute renal failure in the cardiovascular surgical patient. *Ann Thorac Surg* 39:590–598, 1985.

56. Langley SM, Sheppard SV, Tsang VT, et al: When is extracorporeal life support worthwhile following repair of congenital heart disease in children? *Eur J Cardiothorac Surg* 13:520–525, 1998.

57. LaRosa-Nash P, Murphy J: An approach to pediatric perioperative care: Parent-present induction. *Nurs Clin North Am* 32:183–199, 1997.

58. LaRosa-Nash P, Murphy J, Wade L, Clasby L: Implementing a parent-present induction program. *AORN J* 61:526–531, 1995.

59. Levy I, Ovadia B, Erez E, et al: Nosocomial infections after cardiac surgery in infants and children: Incidence and risk factors. *J Hosp Infect* 53:111–116, 2003.

60. Li JS, Bengur AR, Ungerleider RM, et al: Abnormal left ventricular filling after neonatal repair of congenital heart disease: Association with increased mortality and morbidity. *Am Heart J* 136:1075–1080, 1998.

61. Limperopoulos C, Majnemer A, Shevell M, et al: Predictors of developmental disabilities after open heart surgery in young children with heart defects. *J Pediatr* 141:51–58, 2002.

62. Long C, Stashinko E, Byrnes K, et al: Central line associated bacteremia in the pediatric patient. *Pediatr Nurs* 22:247–251, 1996.

63. Luciani G, Nichani S, Chang A, et al: Continuous versus intermittent furosemide infusion in critically ill infants after open heart operations. *Ann Thorac Surg* 64:1133–1139, 1997.

64. MacDonald N, Hall C, Suffin S, et al: Respiratory syncytial viral infection in infants with congenital heart disease. *N Engl J Med* 307:397–400, 1982.

65. Malviya S, Voepel-Lewis T, Siewert M, et al: Risk factors for adverse postoperative outcomes in children presenting for cardiac surgery with upper respiratory tract infections. *Anesthesiology* 98:628–632, 2003.

66. McElhinney D, Hedrick H, Bush D, et al: Necrotizing enterocolitis in neonates with congenital heart disease: Risk factors and outcomes. *Pediatrics* 106:1080–1087, 2000.

67. Medlock M, Cruse R, Winek S, et al: A 10-year experience with post-pump chorea. *Ann Neurol* 34:820–826, 1993.

68. Mrowczynski W, Wojtalik M, Zawadzka D, et al: Infection risk factors in pediatric cardiac surgery. *Asian Cardiovasc Thorac Ann* 10:329–333, 2002.

69. Mullen M, Thomas K, McGowan F, et al: Heparin-induced thrombocytopenia in pediatric patients undergoing cardiopulmonary bypass surgery. *Circulation* 102(Abstract 2276), 2000.

70. Naimer S, Weinstein O, Rosenthal G: Congenital Horner syndrome: A rare though significant complication of subclavian flap aortoplasty. *J Thorac Cardiovasc Surg* 20:419–421, 2000.

71. Nakanishi T, Seguchi M, Takao A: Intracellular calcium concentration in the newborn myocardium. *Dev Pharmacol Ther* 76:455–461, 1987.

72. Nicholson S, Jobes D: Pediatric cardiac anesthesia. In Lake C (ed): *Hypoplastic Left Heart Syndrome.* San Mateo, CA, Appleton and Lange, 1988, pp 243–252.

73. Norwood W: Surgery of the chest. In Sabiston D, Spencer F (eds): *Hypoplastic Left Heart Syndrome.* Philadelphia, WB Saunders, 1995, pp 1659–1666.

74. O'Grady N, Alexander M, Dellinger E, et al: Guidelines for the prevention of intravascular catheter-related infections. *Pediatrics* 110:e51, 2002.

75. Odim J, Tchervenkov C, Dobell A: Delayed sternal closure: A lifesaving maneuver after early operation for complex congenital heart disease in the neonate. *J Thorac Cardiovasc Surg* 98:413–416, 1989.

76. Ostlie DJ, Spilde TL, St. Peter SD, et al: Necrotizing enterocolitis in full-term infants. *J Pediatr Surg* 38:1039–1042, 2003.

77. Pierce C, Wade A, Mok Q: Heparin-bonded central venous lines reduce thrombotic and infective complications in critically ill children. *Intensive Care Med* 26:967–972, 2000.

78. Pouplard C, May MA, Iochmann S, et al: Antibodies to platelet factor 40–heparin after cardiopulmonary bypass in patients anticoagulated with unfractionated heparin or a low-molecular-weight heparin: Clinical implications for heparin-induced thrombocytopenia. *Circulation* 99:2530–2536, 1999.

79. Powers K, Rubenstein J: Family presence during invasive procedures in pediatric intensive care unit: A prospective study. *Arch Pediatr Adolesc Med* 153:955–958, 1999.

80. Rabinovitch M, Haworth SG, Castaneda AR, et al: Lung biopsy in congenital heart disease: A morphometric approach to pulmonary vascular disease. *Circulation* 58:1107–1122, 1978.

81. Raithel SC, Pennington G, Boegner E, et al: Extracorporeal membrane oxygenation in children after cardiac surgery. *Circulation* 86:II305–310, 1992.

82. Rimar S, Gillis C: Selective pulmonary vasodilation by inhaled nitric oxide is due to hemoglobin inactivation. *Circulation* 88:2884–2887, 1993.

83. Rogers AJ, Trento A, Siewers RD, et al: Extracorporeal membrane oxygenation for post-cardiotomy cardiogenic shock in children. *Ann Thorac Surg* 47:903–906, 1989.

84. Rosenzweig E, Starc T, Chen J, et al: Intravenous arginine-vasopressin in children with vasodilatory shock after cardiac surgery. *Circulation* 100:II182–186, 1999.

85. Rossi A, Sommer R, Lotvin A, et al: Usefulness of intermittent monitoring of mixed venous oxygen saturation after state I palliation for hypoplastic left heart syndrome. *Am J Cardiol* 73:1118–1123, 1994.

86. Rudolph A, Yuan S: Response of the pulmonary vasculature to hypoxia and H+ ion concentration changes. *J Clin Invest* 45:399–411, 1966.

87. Severin T, Sutor A: Heparin-induced thrombocytopenia in pediatrics. *Semin Thromb Hemost* 27:293–299, 2001.

88. Singh N, Kissoon N, al Mofada S, et al: Comparison of continuous versus intermittent furosemide administration in postoperative pediatric cardiac patients. *Crit Care Med* 20:17–21, 1992.

89. Slinker B, Wu Y, Green HR, et al: Overall cardiac functional effect of positive inotropic drugs with differing effects on relaxation. *J Cardiovasc Pharmacol* 36:1–13, 2000.

90. Stenzel J, Green T, Fuhrman B, et al: Percutaneous central venous catheterization in a pediatric intensive care unit: A survival analysis of complications. *Crit Care Med* 17:984–988, 1989.

91. Tabbutt S, Duncan B, McLaughlin D, et al: Delayed sternal closure after cardiac operations in a pediatric population. *J Thorac Cardiovasc Surg* 113:886–893, 1997.

92. Tweddell J, Hoffman G, Mussatto K, et al: Improved survival of patients undergoing palliation of hypoplastic left heart syndrome: Lessons learned from 115 consecutive patients. *Circulation* 106:I82–89, 2002.

93. Uhlig P, Brown J, Nason A, et al: Eisenberg patient safety awards. System innovation: Concord Hospital. *Jt Comm J Qual Improv* 28:666–672, 2002.

94. Ungerleider R: *Epicardial Echocardiography during Repair of Congenital Heart Diseases: Advances in Cardiac Surgery.* St. Louis, Mosby–Year Book, 1992.

95. Ungerleider RM: Cerebral protection in infant cardiac surgery. *Ann Surg* 238:S100–103, 2003.

96. Ungerleider RM, Gaynor JW: The Boston Circulatory Arrest Study: An analysis. *J Thorac Cardiovasc Surg,* in press.

97. Ungerleider RM, Shen I: Optimizing response of the neonate and infant to cardiopulmonary bypass. In Mavroudis CM (ed): *Pediatric Cardiac Surgery Annual.* Philadelphia, Elsevier, 2003, pp 140–147.

98. Ungerleider RM, Shen I, Yeh T, et al: Routine mechanical ventricular assist following the Norwood procedure: Improved neurologic outcome and excellent hospital survival. *Ann Thorac Surg* 77:18–22, 2004.

99. van den Berghe G, Wouters P, Verwaest C, et al: Intensive insulin therapy in the critically ill patients. *N Engl J Med* 345:1359–1367, 2001.

100. Warkentin T, Greinacher A: Heparin-induced thrombocytopenia and cardiac surgery. *Ann Thorac Surg* 76:638–648, 2003.

101. Wypij D, Newburger JW, Rappaport LA, et al: The effect of duration of deep hypothermic circulatory arrest in infant heart surgery on late neurodevelopment: The Boston Circulatory Arrest Trial. *J Thorac Cardiovasc Surg* 126:1397–1403, 2003.

102. Ziomek S, Harrell JE, Fasules JW, et al: Extracorporeal membrane oxygenation for cardiac failure after congenital heart operation. *Ann Thorac Surg* 54:861–868, 1992.

Chapter 24

Atrial Septal Defects and Ventricular Septal Defects

J. MARK REDMOND, MD, FRCSI, and ANDREW J. LODGE, MD

ATRIAL SEPTAL DEFECTS

Definition

An atrial septal defect (ASD) is a deficiency of the interatrial septum allowing communication between the right and left atria. It is one of the most common congenital heart anomalies, present in 10% to 15% of patients with congenital heart disease.[21]

Embryology

The atrial septum forms as a result of fusion of several structures. The muscular upper aspect of the atrial septum (septum secundum) is formed by invagination of the roof of the embryologic atrium. Its inferior free margin is marked by the limbus. The lower aspect of the atrial septum is formed by thin septum primum tissue that connects with the fused endocardial cushions. The foramen secundum is an opening in the septum primum where a passage is created between the free edge of the septum primum overlapping the limbus on its left atrial aspect. This anatomic feature creates a one-way valve that allows transit of mainly oxygenated umbilical blood from the right atrium (RA) to the left atrium (LA) during fetal life via the foramen ovale. After birth, increased left atrial pressure causes the mobile septum primum to abut the limbus where ultimate fusion completes atrial septation.[42]

Anatomy

There are multiple types of atrial septal defects. A patent foramen ovale (PFO) occurs in approximately 17% to 35% of the general population.[20,38] A PFO results from inadequate fusion of the septum secundum and the septum primum. This is usually of no consequence clinically as the flap mechanism between these structures prevents shunting from left to right under normal conditions. However, an elevated right atrial pressure with distension widens the foramen, resulting in significant right-to-left shunting and arterial desaturation. This can occur acutely with pulmonary embolism or iatrogenically after procedures on the right side of the heart or after pneumonectomy.

A deficiency of the septum primum results in the *ostium secundum* type atrial septal defect (Fig. 24-1). This is the most

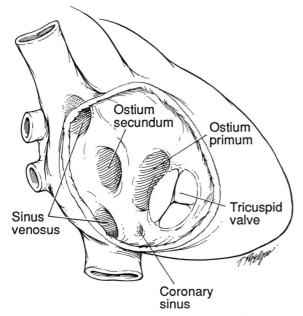

FIGURE 24-1 Various types of atrial septal defects (ASDs) viewed through the right atrium (ostium secundum, ostium primum, sinus venosus). An unroofed coronary sinus may also act as an ASD.

common form of ASD and accounts for two thirds of all ASDs. A secundum ASD is a variably sized opening, usually oval in shape, located in the area of the fossa ovalis. The surrounding septal tissue can be thinned out and fenestrated, resulting in multiple interatrial communications.

About 10% of ASDs are sinus venosus or superior vena cava type in which the interatrial communication occurs just below the junction of the superior vena cava (SVC) and the right atrium (see Fig. 24-1). The inferior margin of the defect is the superior limbic septum. The orifice of the superior vena cava is malpositioned to the left so that it overrides both right and left atria. The defect is almost always associated with partial anomalous connection of the right upper and middle pulmonary veins to the SVC or right atrium.

The inferior vena cava atrial septal defect is a type of secundum ASD and accounts for about 20% of such defects. In this condition there is no rim of septal tissue between the inferior portion of the defect and the orifice of the inferior vena cava. The inferior vena cava may appear to drain partially to the left atrium. These defects are sometimes referred to as inferior sinus venosus type ASDs (see Fig. 24-1). The association with anomalous connection of the right lower lobe pulmonary vein to the right atrium is less common than the anomalous pulmonary drainage occurring in the sinus venosus defect. This defect may be missed with standard transthoracic echocardiography. A transesphogeal study is more accurate for these defects.[45]

In situations where a defect exists in the wall of the coronary sinus as it traverses the left atrium, a communication between the left and right atria results. This defect is termed a coronary sinus ASD or an unroofed coronary sinus. It is often associated with a left superior vena cava.

A primum atrial septal defect, which is a defect in the portion of the atrial septum just cephalad to the atrioventricular

valves, is actually part of an atrioventricular septal (canal) defect and is covered in a separate chapter. Rarely, maldevelopment of the entire atrial septum, including failure of the septum primum to fuse with the endocardial cushions, results in a true common atrium and is therefore classified as part of the spectrum of atrioventricular septal defects as well.

Associated Lesions

ASDs may be an isolated cardiac anomaly and the primary pathophysiologic problem, or they may be associated with a variety of other congenital heart defects including (but by no means limited to) pulmonary stenosis (10%), partial anomalous pulmonary venous return (7%), ventricular septal defects (5%), patent ductus arteriosus (3%), and mitral valve disease (2%).[50] Lutembacher's syndrome consists of rheumatic mitral stenosis and an ASD. Secundum ASDs can be associated, though rarely, with a cleft mitral valve.

There is a high incidence of secundum ASDs in patients with characteristic hand deformities, termed the Holt-Oram syndrome. Patients with Noonan, Marfan, and Turner syndromes also have a higher incidence of ASDs than the general population.[29]

Pathophysiology and Natural History

The direction and volume of blood flow across an ASD depend on the size of the defect and the relative compliance of the downstream chambers (the left and right ventricles)

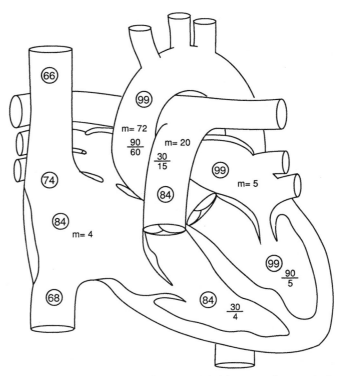

FIGURE 24-2 Pathophysiology of atrial septal defect. Note increase in O_2 saturation from inferior vena cava (68%) to right atrium (84%), indicating a net left-to-right shunt. It is typical for right ventricular (30/4) and pulmonary artery (30/15) pressures to be only minimally elevated despite pulmonary overcirculation. m, mean pressure.

in diastole. Normally the right ventricle is more compliant than the left ventricle, resulting in lower right atrial pressure relative to left atrial pressure. Although respiratory variation in right atrial pressure can cause bidirectional flow, shunting is predominantly left to right. In a patient with an unrestrictive ASD, pulmonary blood flow can be two to four times that of the systemic flow. This produces elevated oxygen saturations in the pulmonary artery (Fig. 24-2).

The highly compliant pulmonary vascular bed can initially accommodate such high flows without significant elevation in pulmonary artery pressure. Pulmonary vascular resistance in children with ASDs is normal or reduced. Although medial hypertrophy and intimal proliferation can develop early in life, advanced and irreversible changes leading to pulmonary hypertension may not occur until the third or fourth decade.[52] The increasing incidence of pulmonary hypertension with age is illustrated by a study that showed a systolic pulmonary arterial pressure greater than 50 mm Hg in 7%, 26%, 32%, and 25% of patients in the third, fourth, fifth, and greater than fifth decades, respectively.[37] Despite the excessive pulmonary blood flow, systemic cardiac output can be maintained at rest and during light exercise. With strenuous activity, however, patients cannot maintain the necessary higher systemic cardiac output, and may become increasingly exercise intolerant.

Spontaneous closure of small secundum ASDs may occur in the first year of life, but is rare thereafter. Although the volume overload of the right ventricle is well tolerated for many years, the incidence of pulmonary vascular disease, right ventricular failure, and atrial dysrhythmias increases in the third and fourth decades of life. As right ventricular compliance falls, the left-to-right shunting decreases and, eventually, with the onset of severe pulmonary vascular disease, the shunt may reverse and cyanosis results (Eisenmenger's syndrome). The average life span of patients with untreated ASDs is 50 years, with most patients succumbing to congestive heart failure (CHF).[12,21]

Diagnosis

Symptoms

Secundum ASDs are often detected in asymptomatic children after evaluation of a murmur during routine physical examination. On questioning, over half of patients admit to easy fatigability and exercise intolerance. Infrequently, infants present with significant congestive heart failure and failure to thrive. Because isolated ASD is an unusual cause of early CHF, such patients should be assessed carefully to rule out a patent ductus arteriosus or left-sided obstructive lesions such as mitral stenosis or aortic coarctation. With failure to thrive and the absence of other signs of heart failure, noncardiac etiologies should be investigated. Adults with ASDs can be asymptomatic or can complain of dyspnea on exertion or palpitations. Adults can also present with atrial flutter or fibrillation.[4,40]

Physical Signs

Patients with large shunts may fall into the lower percentiles for height and weight. A prominent right ventricular impulse can be palpated along the lower left sternal border. A systolic ejection murmur due to increased flow across the pulmonary valve, usually grade 2-3/6, may be heard along the left sternal border. A mid-diastolic murmur heard near the apex is due to the rapid flow of blood across the tricuspid valve. The second heart sound may be split and fixed and is often accentuated. Occasionally, an ASD or PFO will be identified after the patient presents with a transient ischemic attack or stroke.

Electrocardiography

Common electrocardiographic findings include right axis deviation and right ventricular hypertrophy. The P wave morphology may suggest atrial enlargement, and a prolonged PR interval with incomplete right bundle branch block and RSR' pattern in lead V_1 is characteristic.[14]

Chest X-ray

The chest radiograph may be relatively normal or varying degrees of cardiomegaly may be demonstrated due to right atrial and right ventricular dilatation. Pulmonary arterial prominence and increased pulmonary vascularity may also be noted.

Echocardiography

Transthoracic two-dimensional echocardiography and Doppler color flow imaging can demonstrate the size and location of the defect (Fig. 24-3) and the direction of flow across the defect. Right ventricular volume overload and paradoxical ventricular septal motion are characteristic findings. Most associated lesions including anomalous pulmonary venous connection can be detected. Occasionally, the defect may be difficult to image, as with a sinus venosus type. Venous injection of agitated saline with a Valsalva maneuver during the echocardiographic evaluation can often demonstrate an atrial level shunt by revealing left atrial bubble contrast from the right-to-left flow across the defect. In the vast majority of cases echocardiography is the definitive imaging study for an ASD.

Cardiac Catheterization

Diagnosing the presence of an ASD rarely requires cardiac catheterization. This modality can be useful in assessing

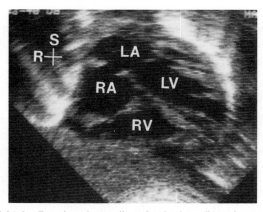

FIGURE 24-3 Transthoracic two-dimensional echocardiography can demonstrate the size and location of most ASDs. In this case a secundum ASD is shown. LA, left atrium; LV, left ventricle; R, right; RA, right atrium; RV, right ventricle; S, superior.

associated anomalies such as those of pulmonary venous connection. In older patients or patients with trisomy 21, catheterization may be indicated to measure pulmonary artery pressures and pulmonary vascular resistance (PVR) to ensure operability. A step-up in oxygen saturation in the right atrium is characteristic of an ASD (see Fig. 24-2), and the degree of left-to-right shunting (Q_p:Q_s) can be determined. In cases of elevated PVR, administration of 100% oxygen or nitric oxide can be performed during catheterization to confirm reversibility. If the PVR falls below 6 Wood units, ASD closure is usually safe.[29]

Indications for Surgical Repair

Generally, repair is recommended for any ASD of appreciable size. In the past, the presence of a measured left-to-right shunt (Q_p:Q_s; see subsequent discussion) of greater than 1.5:1 was used as an indication for surgical closure of an ASD. In asymptomatic patients, the presence of a diastolic murmur at the apex and fixed splitting of the second heart sound, associated with echocardiographic evidence of right ventricular volume overload is a common indication for intervention as this corresponds to a significant left-to-right shunt of greater than 1.5:1. The ideal age for closure is 2 to 5 years, before the child starts school. Infants with an ASD presenting with severe CHF may require intervention in the first year of life.

The potential for paradoxical embolus may also be used as an indication for operative closure. Circumstantial evidence exists for paradoxical systemic embolization through a patent foramen ovale in young patients presenting with stroke.[34] Deep venous thrombosis is the presumed origin of such emboli. The risk of endocarditis is not felt to be elevated in patients with isolated ASD and this is not an indication for repair. If atrial fibrillation is the indication for surgery, an ablative procedure may be necessary concomitantly to control the atrial arrhythmia.[4]

Operative Management

History

An atrial septal defect was the first cardiac lesion successfully corrected using cardiopulmonary bypass (CPB). This was performed in 1953 by Gibbon.[17] Several methods had been used prior to development of the extracorporeal circuit, including the well technique described by Gross,[19] the purse string suture method of Sondergard,[48] and direct suture closure using inflow occlusion and hypothermia described by Lewis.[35]

Surgical Technique

Median sternotomy with a vertical skin incision is the most common approach used. A transverse inframammary incision is occasionally used for cosmetic purposes in female patients. In these cases, median sternotomy is performed after extensive mobilization of subcutaneous flaps. An alternative approach used for cosmetic reasons is the right anterolateral thoracotomy. A skin incision is made in the inframammary crease and the chest is usually entered through the fourth or fifth interspace. This provides limited exposure of the heart and repair of associated lesions is rendered more difficult. If chosen, femoral

arterial cannulation may facilitate this approach. A minimally invasive approach involving a small midline incision (3.5 to 5 cm) over lower sternum, with division of the xiphoid alone or of the lower sternum, is now commonly used for ASD repair and has been shown to be safe and accurate.[5]

After entering the chest, a portion of pericardium is harvested for use as a patch. This may be fixed in gluteraldehyde, depending on surgeon preference. Alternatively, polytetrafluoroethylene (PTFE) patch material can be used to close an ASD. Cardiopulmonary bypass is employed. Ascending aortic and bicaval venous cannulation is performed. The superior vena caval cannula can be positioned through the right atrial appendage or placed directly in the exposed superior vena cava. The cavae are encircled with snares. After initiation of CPB, the core temperature is allowed to drift down but maintained above 34° C. The aorta is cross-clamped and cardioplegia is administered through the aortic root. Alternatively, some surgeons elect to perform isolated ASD closure during a period of induced ventricular fibrillation. Care must be taken to avoid inadvertent defibrillation while the heart is open if this approach is chosen.

The caval snares are secured and an oblique right atrial incision is made. The atrial anatomy is confirmed, including inspection of the pulmonary veins through the defect. Some ASDs can be closed by direct suture closure, though a pericardial (or PTFE) patch is used for larger defects to avoid tension on the margins (Fig. 24-4). Care is taken to avoid the conduction tissue near the coronary sinus. A patch is useful for closing low-lying defects where there is little or no inferior rim near the origin of the inferior vena cava. In this circumstance care must also be used to avoid suturing the inferior margin of the patch to the Eustachian valve and thereby excluding the IVC from the right atrium. A pericardial baffle is required for repair of sinus venosus defects associated with anomalous pulmonary venous drainage of the right upper and middle lobes to direct pulmonary venous flow under the patch, through the defect into the left atrium (Fig. 24-5). With this particular lesion a lateral atriotomy that extends onto the posterolateral aspect of the SVC may be useful. If this incision is chosen or if the ASD patch compromises the lumen of the SVC, a second patch may be used to enlarge the SVC-RA junction. If sufficient pericardium is not available to use as a patch, polytetrafluoroethylene (PTFE) can be used. We prefer to avoid the lateral incision that extends up the SVC, since this incision can create injury to the sinus node and increase the risk of late SVC obstruction (even when the SVC is patched). In most cases, the sinus venosus ASD can be closed with a patch placed over the defect through a standard oblique right atrial incision. The orifices of the pulmonary veins can be identified and directed below this patch. Occasionally, the right upper pulmonary veins drain high (above the level of the right pulmonary artery) and cannot be accessed through an oblique atriotomy. In these cases, if the shunt from these veins is a concern, we recommend the Warden procedure where the SVC is transected at the level of the innominate vein (in these cases the SVC cannulation site needs to be the innominate vein). The cardiac end of the transected SVC is oversewn, transforming the SVC into essentially a receptacle for the pulmonary veins. If an azygous vein is connected to the SVC below the level of transection, it should be ligated. The ASD is then closed by baffling the SVC into the ASD with a patch. In this way, the SVC, which carried the pulmonary

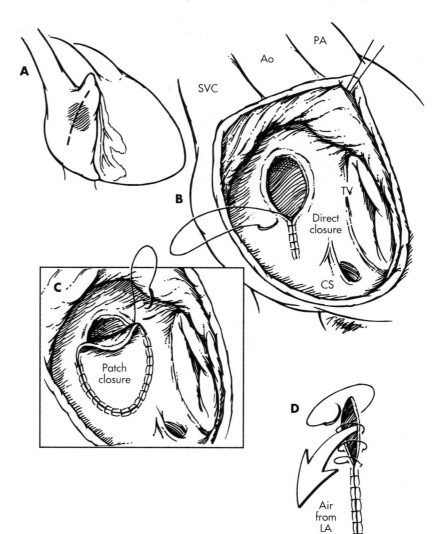

FIGURE 24-4 Surgical procedure for ASD closure. **A,** Orientation of right atriotomy, avoiding area of sinoatrial node. **B,** Direct suture closure of secundum ASD. **C,** Patch closure of secundum ASD. **D,** De-airing of the left atrium. Ao, aorta; CS, coronary sinus; LA, left atrium; PA, pulmonary artery; SVC, superior vena cava; TV, tricuspid valve.

venous flow, is directed into the ASD and no longer connects to the right atrium. The innominate end of the transected SVC is then sutured to the atrial appendage to reconnect venous drainage from the upper body into the right atrium. Although this anastomosis may be somewhat "stretched," it can usually be performed primarily. It is possible to add a "gusset" of pericardium to the top of this connection when necessary.

The left atrium is allowed to fill with blood and the lungs are inflated to facilitate de-airing of the left side of the heart before securing the suture line. The cross-clamp is removed and the heart reperfused with the patient in Trendelenberg position, and further de-airing through the cardioplegia catheter in the ascending aorta is performed. The heart is allowed to fill and eject, and the patient is rewarmed and separated from CPB. Modified ultrafiltration may be instituted at this point, depending on surgeon preference. The heart is decannulated and protamine is administered. A mediastinal drain is placed and once hemostasis is assured, the sternotomy is closed. Temporary epicardial pacing wires may be used but are usually not necessary. They are advisable in older patients following repair of secundum ASDs (since atrial arrhythmias may be common in these patients) and in patients after repair

of sinus venosus (higher incidence of atrial arrhythmia) and often prenum (higher incidence of heart block) defects.

With the burgeoning interest in minimally invasive surgical procedures, alternative methods are being explored. Port access techniques, which are employed in some centers for mitral valve procedures, may be applicable for ASD repair. This approach involves a small right anterolateral thoracotomy, and usually a groin incision for femoral cannulation. Acceptable results have been reported with this technique.[13] Other surgeons favor a limited sternotomy which can yield exceptional cosmetic results if the skin incision is kept no higher than the nipple line. As for limited thoracotomy, a groin incision can be utilized for cannulation. However, in children, where the femoral vessels are too small for safe cannulation, the aorta can be accessed for cannulation through either a right thoracotomy or a limited (partial) sternotomy. Another emerging approach is "totally endoscopic" ASD closure. This procedure has been successfully carried out using the da Vinci robotic system (Intuitive Surgical, Mountain View, Calif.). Four ports in the right hemithorax are required along with a groin incision to establish cardiopulmonary bypass through the femoral vessels. Satisfactory ASD repair, using either primary closure or a patch, and cosmesis have been reported.[2,54] As this is a new technology,

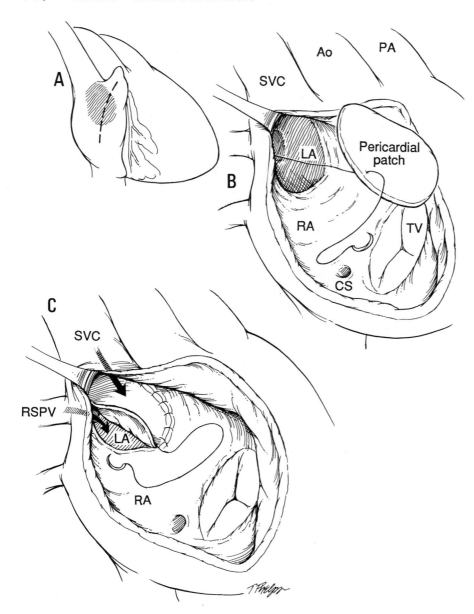

FIGURE 24-5   Surgical correction of sinus venosus defect using a pericardial patch to direct the pulmonary venous blood across the atrial septal defect and into the left atrium. **A,** Right atriotomy *(dashed line)* for repair of sinus venosus defect. **B,** Right atrium (RA) opened to expose subcaval sinus venosus defect through which the left atrium (LA) is viewed. **C,** Anomolous right superior pulmonary vein (RSPV) enters at the superior vena cava (SVC)–right atrium (RA) junction. The defect is closed with a pericardial patch so that blood from the RSPV is baffled into the LA and blood from the SVC enters the RA. Ao, aorta; CS, coronary sinus; PA, pulmonary artery; TV, tricuspid valve.

further study will be needed to document longer term results. ASD repair, however, seems to be a relatively ideal operation for the robotic approach.

Postoperative Care

Most patients are extubated in the operating room or within the first few hours of arrival in intensive care. With transduced radial arterial and central venous lines, hemodynamics are monitored, including heart rate and rhythm, blood pressure, and central venous pressure along with core and peripheral temperature, respiratory rate, and effort. Adequate cardiac output is confirmed by clinical assessment of peripheral perfusion, including peripheral temperature and the strength of peripheral pulses. Low cardiac output is usually secondary to hypovolemia, reflected by a low central venous pressure, and is corrected by judicious volume replacement,

avoiding blood or blood products if possible. Inotropic agents are rarely required in infants and children.

Hematocrit, serum electrolytes, and arterial blood gases are measured on return to the ICU. Serum lactate may also be measured but is usually not necessary. Progressive metabolic acidosis and rising serum lactate may indicate deterioration in cardiac output, and response should be expeditious. A chest radiograph is obtained on arrival in ICU to confirm optimum central line positioning and endotracheal tube placement if applicable, and to rule out air or fluid in the pleural spaces. A postoperative electrocardiogram (ECG) is also usually obtained.

Mediastinal drainage is monitored, and if bleeding of more than 5 mL/kg/hour persists after correction of any abnormality in the coagulation profile, early reexploration may be advisable. Monitoring for 12 to 24 hours in the ICU is usually sufficient. Patients may require diuresis to remove excess interstitial fluid associated with CPB. After the monitoring lines and chest drain are removed, the patient is transferred to the ward. Hospital discharge is usually possible by the third postoperative day.[33] Some patients may be discharged as early as 1 to 2 days after surgery. Some centers have instituted clinical pathways for ASD repair to eliminate unnecessary testing and to streamline the care of these patients.

Outcome

Mortality for isolated ASD repair in infancy and childhood should be close to zero. Elevated PVR and right ventricular dysfunction in older age groups is associated with increased mortality risk. Morbidity includes atrial arrhythmias in older patients, pericarditis, and development of pericardial effusion. The changes associated with right ventricular volume overload should regress as the patient's functional status improves.

Interventional Therapy

Percutaneous ASD closure has been established as a safe and effective alternative to operative repair.[9] The technique involves transcatheter delivery of a device in its retracted state via the femoral vein under fluoroscopic and transesophageal echocardiographic guidance. Most commonly used devices consist of opposing discs made of nickel and titanium (nitinol) with deployment of the first disc on the left atrial aspect of the defect followed by deployment of a second opposing disc on the right atrial side. The expanded discs are tightly approximated, thus closing the defect (Fig. 24-6). The device becomes endothelialized over time. Antiplatelet therapy is usually continued for 6 months. Limitations in the use of this technique include the size of the defect, the absence of adequate margins, proximity to vital cardiac structures and weight of the patient.

The world experience of transcatheter ASD closure using the Amplatzer Septal Occluder has been reported by Omeish.[41] There was a 2.8% minor complication rate and no device-related deaths. In the 3535 patients receiving one or more devices, 97.4% of the procedures were successful. The success rate increased to 99.2% at 3 months and reached 100% at 3 years. It should be noted that "success" was characterized as complete ASD occlusion or the presence of a trivial to small residual shunt. Other studies of mid- and long-term results have revealed residual shunt rates as high as 10% to 40%. Newer devices seem to be more effective, but longer follow-up is needed. More recent studies have demonstrated the efficacy of device closure in the instance of presumed paradoxical embolism.[27]

Comparisons of device occlusion versus surgical closure have been performed prospectively. Hospital stays are shorter, discomfort is less, and time required for convalescence is reduced for patients undergoing successful device closure. Hospital costs are similar. Regression of right ventricular dilatation was similar for both groups of patients.[25,51] There are, however, some specific device-related complications. These may include local complications related to femoral access, as well as device embolization or misplacement. Thrombosis related to septal occluder devices has been reported.[32] The rate of complications is decreased and success is increased with newer devices, and device closure of atrial

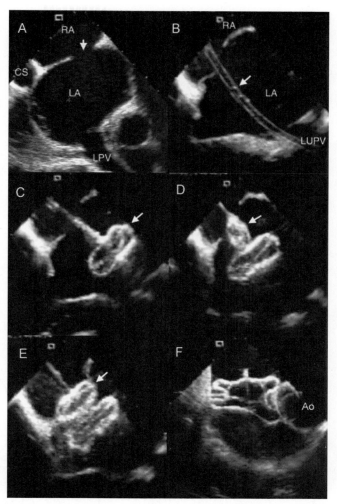

FIGURE 24-6 Catheter-based method of atrial septal defect (ASD) closure using an Amplatzer septal occluder. A series of intracardiac echo images are shown. **A**, A secundum ASD is shown between the right atrium (RA) and left atrium (LA). The coronary sinus (CS) and left upper pulmonary vein (LPV) are also seen. **B**, The device delivery sheath *(arrow)* is shown crossing the defect from the RA to the LA. Its tip is anchored in the left upper pulmonary vein (LUPV). **C**, The left atrial disc *(arrow)* of the device has been deployed. **D**, The connecting waist *(arrow)* of the device has been deployed. **E**, The right atrial disc *(arrow)* has been deployed. **F**, The final position of the ASD closure device. Note the position of the device relative to the aortic root (Ao). (Adapted from Koenig P, Cao Q, Heitschmidt M, Waight DJ, Hijazi ZM: Role of intracardiac echocardiographic guidance in transcatheter closure of atrial septal defects and patent foramen ovale using the Amplatzer device. *J Interv Cardiol* 16:51–62, 2003; with permission.)

septal defects has now become quite standard for uncomplicated ASDs.

VENTRICULAR SEPTAL DEFECTS

Definition

A ventricular septal defect (VSD) is an opening in the interventricular septum resulting in direct communication between the left and right ventricles. VSD can be single or multiple. It is the most commonly diagnosed congenital heart anomaly, present in 20% of patients with congenital heart disease.

Embryology

The interventricular septum is formed by the fusion of three structures. The primary fold at the apex of the heart progresses cephalad, becoming the trabecular portion of the interventricular septum. The inlet septum arises posteroinferiorly and fuses with the trabecular portion, forming the trabecula septomarginalis (septal band). The infundibular or conal septum arises from the downward extension of the conal ridge. The conal ridge fuses with the endocardial cushions to form the membranous portion of the interventricular septum.

Anatomy

There are several schemes for classifying VSDs. Because VSD repair patches are usually placed on the right ventricular aspect of the septum, a commonly used nomenclature relates the defect to the anatomy of the morphologic right ventricle (Fig. 24-7).

Perimembranous (paramembranous) defects comprise up to 80% of all primary VSDs. They are also known as membranous or infracristal defects. They are located between the anterior and posterior divisions of the septal band and between the conal and trabecular interventricular septum. The lateral border is formed by the tricuspid annulus; the superior border is usually the aortic annulus. There may be a variable amount of muscular rim at the superior and lateral borders. The defect can extend into the inlet, trabecular, or outlet portions of the interventricular septum. Extension of the defect to the base of the noncoronary leaflet of the aortic valve may cause aortic regurgitation (AR). The conal septum may be anteriorly malaligned as in tetralogy of Fallot, causing right ventricular outflow tract obstruction, or, less commonly, it may be malaligned posteriorly, causing left ventricular outflow tract obstruction.

Subarterial defects, comprise 5% to 10% of VSDs, are also known as outlet, conal septal, supracristal, or subpulmonary VSDs. They are located beneath the pulmonary valve and

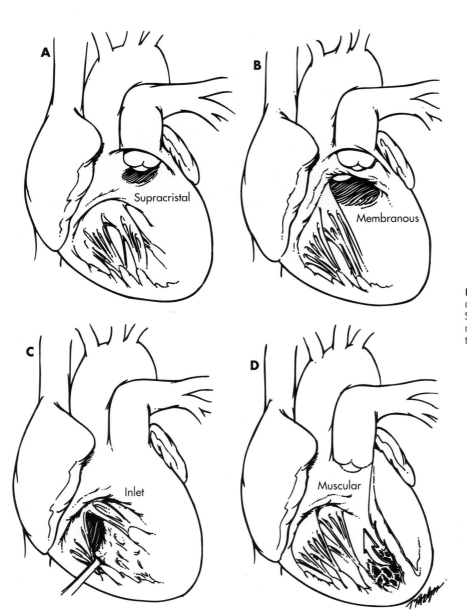

FIGURE 24-7 Various types of ventricular septal defects viewed from within the right ventricle. **A,** Supracristal or subarterial. **B,** Membranous or paramembranous. **C,** Inlet or atrioventricular (AV) canal type. **D,** Muscular or trabecular.

their superior edge is a fibrous ridge between the two semilunar valves. They can be associated with prolapse of the right coronary leaflet of the aortic valve with associated regurgitation. This type of defect is more common in the Asian population.

Inlet defects account for 5% to 10% of VSDs and are also called atrioventricular canal-type defects. The posterior margin of the defect runs along the septal leaflet of the tricuspid valve to the anterior leaflet of the mitral valve, which often has a cleft. The defect extends superiorly to the membranous septum.

Muscular defects represent 5% to 10% of VSDs and are located anywhere in the muscular septum. The margins are characteristically muscular. They are frequently multiple. They may be anterior, mid-muscular, apical, or in the inlet septum. The latter differs from the inlet or atrioventricular canal-type VSD in that it is separated from the tricuspid valve and membranous septum by muscle tissue. Infundibular or outlet muscular VSDs differ from subarterial VSDs because of the presence of a rim of muscle separating the defect from the annuli of the aortic and pulmonary valves.

Associated Anomalies

VSDs can be isolated lesions or part of a variety of major congenital malformations such as tetralogy of Fallot, double outlet right ventricle, transposition of the great vessels, and truncus arteriosus. Fifty percent of patients with VSDs requiring repair have associated cardiovascular anomalies, most commonly patent ductus arteriosus, atrial septal defect, aortic coarctation, aortic stenosis, and pulmonary stenosis.[1]

Pathophysiology and Natural History

The dimension of the defect and pulmonary vascular resistance determine the blood flow across a VSD (shunt).[36] Smaller VSDs are said to be restrictive because there is a pressure gradient across the defect with a greater left ventricular pressure than right ventricular pressure. The left-to-right shunt depends primarily on the pressure differences. Larger defects approximate the size of the aortic annulus and are nonrestrictive with equal right and left ventricular pressures. In these cases the relative resistances in the systemic and pulmonary vasculature determine the left-to-right shunting.

Pulmonary vascular resistance (PVR) is high in the immediate postnatal period and begins to decrease within the first 2 weeks of life.[30] For babies with large nonrestrictive VSDs, the drop in PVR accentuates the left-to-right shunt leading to a large volume load in the pulmonary circulation, increasing left atrial pressure, and causing left ventricular volume overload. CHF develops with decreased peripheral perfusion and increased work of breathing, associated with a drop in stroke volume and tissue oxygen delivery. This results in activation of the renin-angiotensin system, which further increases systemic vasoconstriction and the left-to-right shunting, exacerbating the CHF.[8,18,46]

If infants with nonrestrictive VSDs remain untreated, the pulmonary overcirculation can eventually lead to a fixed elevation of PVR and pulmonary vascular disease. These changes are not reversible after VSD closure. Eisenmenger's complex develops when PVR becomes greater than systemic resistance, reversing the shunt and causing cyanosis.

Infants and children with smaller restrictive VSDs remain asymptomatic. Those with larger nonrestrictive VSDs develop increasingly severe CHF within the first several months of life. This manifests as respiratory symptoms and failure to thrive. These infants have an appreciable mortality within the first year if left untreated.[44] Children with moderate shunting develop a gradual increase in PVR over time, and as the PVR approaches systemic levels, the degree of shunting decreases with improvement in symptoms. If untreated, such patients go on to develop Eisenmenger's complex and die in the third or fourth decade of life. The development of Eisenmenger physiology increases the risk of death 10- to 12-fold and carries a 25-year survival of only 42%.[28]

Spontaneous closure of VSDs is well documented and is more likely to occur within the first several months of life in patients with smaller defects. Muscular defects are the most likely to close by further septal muscular development. This is based mostly on autopsy studies in which most of the postmortem reports of spontaneously closed defects are of the muscular type.[49] Parimembranous VSDs have the next highest rate of spontaneous closure. The mechanism of spontaneous closure of these defects frequently involves the adherence of excess (aneurysmal) tricuspid valve tissue.

Diagnosis

Symptoms

Infants with small defects are usually asymptomatic and the detection of a murmur results in their diagnosis. Moderate defects result in a predisposition to pulmonary infection and varying degrees of growth retardation during the first few years of life but without severe signs of CHF. Larger defects, particularly nonrestrictive VSDs produce signs and symptoms of CHF early in the first year of life, including tachypnea, poor feeding, sweating, irritability, failure to thrive, and poor weight gain. This symptom complex results from the increased work of breathing and energy expenditure associated with pulmonary overcirculation and poor peripheral perfusion.

Physical Signs

Children with smaller defects may present with a harsh holosystolic murmur with no overt signs of CHF. Those patients with larger defects and shunts ($Q_p:Q_s$; see subsequent discussion) in excess of 2:1 may have signs of CHF including poor growth, tachypnea, poor perfusion with reduced peripheral pulses, a palpable thrill along the left sternal border, and a harsh holosystolic murmur loudest over the fourth intercostal space. There may be a diastolic murmur related to increased blood return to the left atrium. There is accentuation of the second heart sound. Hepatomegaly and pulmonary congestion may be present.

Electrocardiography

Typical findings on the electocardiogram include left ventricular hypertrophy and left atrial enlargement reflected in prominent R and T waves in the inferior leads and V_6, particularly with larger defects. Findings of right ventricular hypertrophy with an RSR′ pattern in lead V_1 occurs later in the disease process.

Chest X-ray

Radiographic findings include cardiomegaly and an enlarged main pulmonary artery shadow. Left atrial enlargement and prominence of the pulmonary vasculature are also seen. These radiographic findings are more notable with larger defects and may be absent or more subtle with small VSDs.

Echocardiography

The size, number, and location of medium and large VSDs can be accurately defined by two-dimensional transthoracic echocardiography. Left atrial and ventricular dimensions can be measured and may be important in determining the management of a particular defect. Estimates of pulmonary artery pressure can be made using Doppler imaging of the velocity of a tricuspid regurgitant jet, if present. Other associated cardiac anomalies can also be delineated with this modality. In the majority of cases echocardiography provides sufficient information to proceed with closure of the defect or to follow it expectantly. Transesophageal or epicardial echocardiography is particularly important for providing an intraoperative assessment of VSD closure.

Cardiac Catheterization

For older children with moderate defects and no clinically significant CHF, pulmonary overcirculation, or pulmonary hypertension, echocardiography suffices as the definitive preoperative study. Cardiac catheterization may be indicated where echocardiographic data is unsatisfactory, in patients with large defects and significant pulmonary hypertension, or if there is doubt about the anatomy of associated lesions.

Cardiac catheterization can demonstrate the location, size, and number of defects, along with associated cardiac anomalies. It facilitates direct measurement of left and right heart pressures and oxygen saturations (Fig. 24-8), from which quantification of the intracardiac shunt and PVR may de derived.

The shunt fraction is the ratio of pulmonary blood flow (Q_p) to systemic blood flow (Q_s). It is calculated according to the following formula:

$$Q_p:Q_s = [(AO_2 - MVO_2) / (PVO_2 - PaO_2)]$$

where AO_2 is the aortic oxygen saturation, MVO_2 is the mixed venous oxygen saturation, PaO_2 is the pulmonary arterial saturation, and PVO_2 is the pulmonary venous saturation.[30]

Patients with elevated PVR (5 to 10 U/m²) may be administered 100% oxygen or nitric oxide to test for reversibility. If recalculated PVR falls below 8 U/m², VSD repair can be safely performed. Persistent elevation of PVR suggests irreversible pulmonary hypertension and that VSD closure will likely result in acute right heart failure and death. These recommendations are based primarily on pathologic studies that evaluated lung biopsy findings. Correlations were performed with measured hemodynamics to derive the previous numbers. The most reliable hemodynamic predictor is PVR. In one study, for example, patients with a PVR of less than 8 U/m² had a greater than 90% survival after surgery, whereas patients with a PVR of greater than 8 U/m² had a survival of less than 45%.[55] Heart-lung transplantation or lung transplantation with VSD closure are the only surgical options for this group of patients.[22]

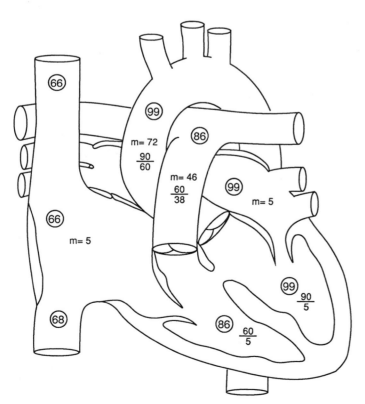

FIGURE 24-8 Pathophysiology of ventricular septal defect (VSD). Note step-up in O_2 saturation from the right atrium (66%) to the right ventricle (86%) indicating left-to-right shunt at the ventricular level. Right ventricular pressure (60/5) is elevated compared with the normal right ventricular pressure, but is less than the left ventricular pressure (90/5), indicating that the VSD is *restrictive*. The pulmonary artery pressure is elevated as well. m, mean pressure.

Indications for Surgical Repair

Infants with a large defect and significant CHF for whom spontaneous closure is unlikely are candidates for early closure, regardless of the patient's size. A trial of diuretic therapy with or without the addition of digoxin may control the symptoms of CHF and allow the infant to grow. The addition of an angiotensin-converting enzyme (ACE) inhibitor to reduce systemic vascular resistance may be helpful in selected cases. In these cases, surgical repair is typically performed between 3 and 6 months of age. If medical therapy fails, surgical repair should be undertaken promptly and can be done safely even in neonates.

Children with moderate-sized defects and shunts greater than 1.5:1 generally have mild to moderate elevations of pulmonary artery pressure and resistance. They can be followed until they are up to 5 years of age to maximize the chance of spontaneous closure. Failing the latter, surgical repair may be performed.

Patients with subarterial or supracristal VSDs can develop progressive aortic regurgitation (AR) due to prolapse of the adjacent aortic valve leaflet caused by Venturi forces associated with left-to-right flow across the defect.[53] The risk of aortic valve prolapse increases with increasing defect size. These defects should be repaired before significant AR develops. Simultaneous aortic valvuloplasty should be considered if the AR has progressed beyond a moderate degree. One study has shown that lesser degrees of AR remained stable after simple defect closure, and more severe AR was associated with a significant need for reintervention despite aortic valvuloplasty at the time of VSD repair.[11]

Children with small VSDs and shunts less than 1.5:1, generally have no symptoms. While they are at risk of bacterial endocarditis, close follow-up and prophylactic antibiotic therapy may be considered as an alternative to surgical repair.[16] The risk of endocarditis is 0.15% to 0.3% per year and, after such a complication, it would seem prudent to repair the VSD after complete resolution of the infectious process. Preemptive surgical closure for such small VSDs is controversial.

A special situation in the neonatal period occurs when an infant is diagnosed with an aortic coarctation and a concomitant VSD. The optimal management strategy for neonates with this combination of lesions is controversial. A two-stage approach, involving coarctation repair and pulmonary artery banding via a left thoracotomy, followed by VSD closure and removal of the band 6 to 12 months later, has been demonstrated to be safe and effective.[26] In the recent era, studies have also shown that the single-stage approach of simultaneous VSD and coarctation repair via a median sternotomy can be performed with comparably low morbidity and mortality, and this is also an acceptable option.[15] It is also a reasonable strategy to repair the coarctation through a left thoracotomy and leave the pulmonary artery unbanded. If the infant remains in severe CHF, even after "unloading" of the systemic output with coarctation repair, the VSD can be closed through a sternotomy with a short period of CPB.

Pulmonary artery banding is rarely indicated for the treatment of VSD except in infants with multiple defects and intractable CHF. Banding in this situation controls the heart failure, allowing the infant to grow, during which time there may be spontaneous closure of some or all of the defects.

Once the infant reaches an appropriate size, the remaining defect(s) can be approached surgically.

Operative Management

With the patient in supine position, a median sternotomy is performed and the thymus subtotally resected to facilitate exposure. The pericardium is opened and suspended. Ascending aortic and bicaval venous cannulation are performed after heparinization. Purse string sutures should all be elongated and narrow. CPB is established and, depending on the anticipated complexity of the procedure, cooling to as low as 28° C is begun. The left heart can be decompressed by placing a vent through the left atrial appendage or, more commonly, the right superior pulmonary vein. Cardioplegia is administered in antegrade fashion after cross-clamping the aorta and redosed at regular intervals if necessary. For infants, another option is to use single venous cannulation through the right atrial appendage and perform the repair under hypothermic circulatory arrest at a rectal temperature of 18° C.

An oblique right atrial incision is made after the caval snares are secured. Placing the incision close to the atrioventricular junction helps with exposure of the defect. Retractors are positioned, after placement of stay sutures. The anatomy is inspected through the tricuspid valve. VSDs are ordinarily closed with a patch (usually PTFE or Dacron), unless they are quite small. Patch material can be sewn into place with either interrupted sutures, or with a continuous technique. Particular care is required with the superior sutures to avoid injury to the aortic valve; inferiorly, sutures are placed away from the margins of the VSD to avoid the conduction tissue. Occasionally, exposure of the defect may be compromised by the tricuspid valve or supporting apparatus. In these cases it may be helpful to partially detach the septal leaflet of the tricuspid valve to facilitate exposure of the lateral and inferior borders. The septal leaflet is then repaired with a running polypropylene suture.

After repair of the VSD is complete, the tricuspid valve is tested for competence and repaired as necessary. An ASD or patent foramen ovale is closed. The right atrium is closed and after de-airing the heart, the cross-clamp is removed. When de-airing and rewarming are complete, the patient is separated from CPB. Modified ultrafiltration can be undertaken before decannulation and protamine administration. Ideally, intraoperative transesophageal or epicardial echocardiography is used to rule out a residual VSD. Information about tricuspid and aortic valve competence and ventricular function is also obtained using this modality. If it is not available or if there is a question about the significance of a residual VSD, direct measurement of pulmonary artery pressure and oxygen saturations can be made, and the Q_p:Q_s can be estimated. For infants with moderate to severe pulmonary hypertension, placement of a pulmonary artery catheter, left atrial line, and even a peritoneal dialysis catheter should be considered to aid in postoperative management. Inhaled nitric oxide can also be helpful in the postoperative management of this subgroup of patients.

The vast majority of membranous and inlet VSDs are closed via the transatrial approach (Fig. 24-9) but can be closed through a ventriculotomy in selected cases. Supracristal defects must be closed through either a ventriculotomy or

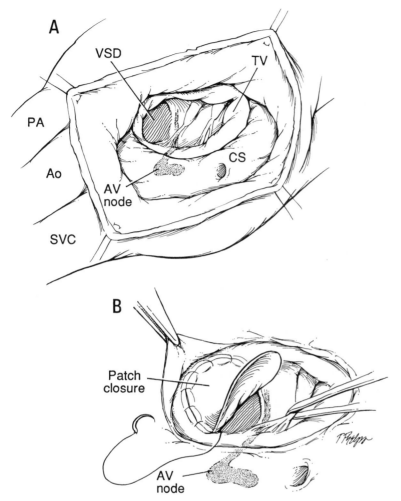

FIGURE 24-9 Ventricular septal defect (VSD) closure via the transatrial approach. **A,** A right atriotomy has been performed and the VSD is seen across the tricuspid valve (TV). Note the position of the atrioventricular node (AV node) and the conduction system that runs along the posterior and inferior border of the VSD. **B,** A Dacron or PTFE patch is used to close the defect. A portion of the TV suspensory apparatus is being retracted. Ao, aorta; CS, conduction system; PA, pulmonary artery; PTFE, polytetrafluoroethylene; SVC, superior vena cava.

through an incision in the pulmonary artery, with sutures anchored to the pulmonary valve annulus.

Muscular VSDs remain a surgical challenge. Whereas inlet and midmuscular defects can be repaired through the tricuspid valve, anterior defects are approached via a right ventriculotomy and apical VSDs through an apical left ventriculotomy. A cardioscope, introduced through the aortic root, can aid in visualization of the muscular defects, permitting direct inspection of the left side of the ventricular septum and illuminating the defects from the right ventricular aspect. Alternatively, a right angle clamp introduced through an aortotomy to probe the septum from the left side can be helpful in identifying the defects. Multiple apical defects can be effectively repaired with the septal obliteration technique in which the defects are excluded from the right ventricular cavity with a pericardial patch.[6] The intraoperative placement of devices designed for transcatheter closure of ASDs or VSDs is another option. This approach has been shown to be safe and effective for muscular VSDs.[39] Creativity in the application of this technology has led to intraoperative placement of catheter delivered devices directly through the right ventricular free-wall, avoiding CPB.[3] Another approach to the multiple VSD patient might involve intraoperative device closure of the muscular VSD(s)

with a device combined with standard patch closure of the paramembranous VSD.

Postoperative Care

Extubation in the operating room for older uncomplicated patients is appropriate. Neonates and infants may require ventilatory support and aggressive diuresis for 24 to 72 hours before safe extubation. If postoperative inotropic support is required, diuresis may not be effective in the initial 24 hours after surgery.

On admission to the ICU a baseline measurement of hemodynamic parameters is performed. The heart rate and rhythm, arterial blood pressure, central venous pressure, and core and peripheral temperatures are monitored. Left atrial or pulmonary artery pressures may also be monitored in complicated cases. Admission hematocrit, serum chemistries, serum lactate, arterial blood gas values, and coagulation parameters are checked. In addition to an electrocardiogram, chest radiography to check support equipment position and the pleural spaces is performed.

Estimates of cardiac output are made on the basis of peripheral perfusion and temperature, strength of pedal pulses, urinary output, serum lactate, and acid-base status. Volume replacement may be required for low filling pressures. For elevated filling pressures (>10 mm Hg) and low output, inotropic support is required. A vasodilating agent is used to treat inadequate cardiac output associated with an elevated mean arterial blood pressure. Milrinone works well in this situation. The majority of patients undergoing straightforward VSD closure require minimal if any inotropic support postoperatively and can be extubated fairly promptly. Most benefit from diuresis instituted within 12 hours of surgery and continued until after the institution of enteral feedings.

Patients that have long-standing pulmonary overcirculation or preoperative evidence of elevated pulmonary vascular resistance are prone to pulmonary hypertensive crises early in their postoperative recovery. A pulmonary artery line may be helpful in these patients. A typical pulmonary hypertension protocol to maintain pulmonary vasodilatation involves full sedation and paralysis, hyperventilation, strict acid-base control, and fastidious pulmonary toilet. For established pulmonary hypertension in the absence of a residual VSD, intravenous vasodilators, such as nitroglycerin, sodium nitroprusside, isoproterenol, or prostaglandin E_1 (PGE_1), can be used. Inhaled nitric oxide (10 to 20 ppm), a potent selective pulmonary vasodilator, has proven very effective for patients unresponsive to these drugs. It has dramatically reduced the need for extracorporeal membrane oxygenation (ECMO) support.

Early postoperative dysrrhythmias occur in up to one third of patients.[43] Supraventricular and junctional ectopic tachycardias are usually accompanied by marked deterioration in cardiac output and must be aggressively treated. Cooling the patient to 33° C or 34° C is effective with simple topical cooling. A peritoneal dialysis catheter, if present, may also be used for this purpose. These interventions require sedation and frequently neuromuscular blockade. An intravenous amiodarone infusion can be used to treat these tachycardias should the response to cooling be insufficient.

Complete heart block is another complication of VSD closure. It is often transient in nature, due to surgical trauma or edema associated with suture placement adjacent to the conduction tissue. Heart block usually resolves in 24 to 48 hours. Disruption of the conduction pathway results in permanent heart block. All patients undergoing VSD repair should have temporary ventricular epicardial pacing wires placed at the time of surgery. Dysrrhythmias in the operating room should prompt the use of temporary atrial wires as well. If there is postoperative heart block, a transvenous or epicardial permanent pacemaker system is required if sinus rhythm is not restored within 7 to 10 days.

Outcome

Mortality rates for isolated VSD closure are less than 1%. For closure of multiple VSDs, the rate may be as high as 5% to 10%.[47] The incidence of residual shunting due to patch dehiscence is very small. On the contrary, it is common to have some degree of residual shunting from small residual defects around the patch. The incidence is reported at 20% to 33%.[28,56] Two thirds of these residual defects are closed by the time of hospital discharge, and the vast majority will eventually close spontaneously.[7,56] Further cardiac surgical intervention for any reason is needed in only 5.5% of patients.[28] Long-term survival is excellent after successful VSD repair,

with only one late (noncardiac) death reported in a recent large series.[7]

Interventional Therapy

Percutaneous transcatheter closure of VSDs with devices is less well established than device closure of ASDs. This technology is most commonly used in the treatment of muscular VSDs and residual postoperative VSDs.[10] The proximity of vital structures such as the aortic valve to the paramembranous VSD makes device closure of this defect more challenging, although newer devices have been developed, and there has been early clinical success with their use. Transcatheter closure of paramembranous VSDs has been reported in six patients with ages ranging from 3.5 to 19 years. The technique appears safe and effective in select patients, though further studies to assess long-term safety and results are required.[23] One important current limitation to the application of percutaneously placed devices is patient size. As most infants with VSDs present with failure to thrive, the requirement of weight greater than 5 kg is unrealistic for many patients who require VSD closure.

A staged approach to treating infants with multiple VSDs involving initial pulmonary artery banding followed by delayed catheter-based closure of the muscular VSDs that have failed to close spontaneously in the intervening period may prove effective in the management of these challenging patients. As above, a combined approach in the operating room could also be effective. As the technology improves, the indications for these procedures will expand. Patient follow-up will be important, as the long-term outcomes of these procedures are currently unknown.

References

1. Arciniegas E: Ventricular septal defect. In Baue AE, Geha AS, Hammond GL, et al (eds): *Glenn's Thoracic and Cardiovascular Surgery.* Norwalk, CT, Appleton & Lange, 1991, pp 1007–1016.
2. Argenziano M, Williams MR: Robotic atrial septal defect repair and endoscopic treatment of atrial fibrillation. *Semin Thorac Cardiovasc Surg* 15:130–140, 2003.
3. Bacha EA, Cao QL, Starr JP, et al: Periventricular device closure of muscular ventricular septal defects on the beating heart: Technique and results. *J Thorac Cardiovasc Surg* 126:1718–1723, 2003.
4. Berger F, Vogel M, Kramer A, et al: Incidence of the atrial flutter/fibrillation in adults with atrial septal defect before and after surgery. *Ann Thorac Surg* 68:75–78, 1999.
5. Bichell DP, Geva T, Bacha EA, et al: Minimal access approach for the repair of atrial septal defect: The initial 135 patients. *Ann Thorac Surg* 70:115–118, 2000.
6. Black MD, Shukla V, Rao V, et al: Repair of isolated multiple muscular ventricular septal defects: The septal obliteration technique. *Ann Thorac Surg* 70:106–110, 2000.
7. Bol-Raap G, Weerheim J, Kappetein AP, et al: Follow-up after surgical closure of congenital ventricular septal defect. *Eur J Cardiothorac Surg* 24:511–515, 2003.
8. Boucek MM, Chang R, Synhorst DP: Renin-angiotensin II response to the hemodynamic pathology of ovines with ventricular septal defect. *Circ Res* 64:524–531, 1989.
9. Brockmeier K, Schmidt KG, Ulmer HE, Gorenflo M: Occlusion of interatrial communications with the Amplatzer device: Experience in 48 consecutive patients. *J Interv Cardiol* 14:325–328, 2001.
10. Chessa M, Carminati M, Cao QL, et al: Transcatheter closure of congenital and acquired muscular ventricular septal defects using the Amplatzer device. *J Invasive Cardiol* 14:322–327, 2002.
11. Cheung YF, Chiu CS, Yung TC, Chau AK: Impact of preoperative aortic cusp prolapse on long-term outcome after surgical closure of subarterial ventricular septal defect. *Ann Thorac Surg* 73:622–627, 2002.

12. Dalen JE, Haynes FW, Dexter L: Life expectancy with atrial septal defect: Influence of complicating pulmonary vascular disease. *JAMA* 200:442–446, 1967.

13. De Mulder W, Vanermen H: Repair of atrial septal defects via limited right anterolateral thoracotomy. *Acta Chir Belg* 102:450–454, 2002.

14. Garson A Jr: *The Electrocardiogram in Infants and Children: A Systemic Approach.* Philadelphia, Lea & Febiger, 1983.

15. Gaynor JW, Wernovsky G, Rychik J, et al: Outcome following single-stage repair of coarctation with ventricular septal defect. *Eur J Cardiothorac Surg* 18:62–67, 2000.

16. Gersony WM, Hayes CJ: Bacterial endocarditis in patients with pulmonary stenosis, aortic stenosis, or ventricular septal defect. *Circulation* 56:I84–I87, 1977.

17. Gibbon JH Jr: Application of a mechanical heart and lung apparatus to cardiac surgery. *Minn Med* 37:171, 1954.

18. Gidding SS, Bessel M: Hemodynamic correlates of clinical severity in isolated ventricular septal defect. *Pediatr Cardiol* 14:135–139, 1993.

19. Gross RE, Watkins E Jr, Pomeranz AA, Goldsmith EI: A method for surgical closure of interauricular septal defects. *Surg Gynecol Obstet* 96:1, 1953.

20. Hagen PT, Scholz DG, Edwards WD: Incidence and size of patent foramen ovale during the first 10 decades of life: An autopsy study of 965 normal hearts. *Mayo Clin Proc* 59:17–20, 1984.

21. Hamilton WT, Haffajee CI, Dalen JE, et al: Atrial septal defect secundum: Clinical profile with physiologic correlates in children and adults. In Roberts WC (ed): *Congenital Heart Disease in Adults.* Philadelphia, Davis, 1979, pp 257–277.

22. Haworth SG: Pulmonary vascular disease in ventricular septal defect: Structural and functional correlations in lung biopsies from 85 patients, with outcome of intracardiac repair. *J Pathol* 152:157–168, 1987.

23. Hijazi ZM, Hakim F, Haweleh AA, et al: Catheter closure of perimembranous ventricular septal defects using the new Amplatzer membranous VSD occluder: Initial clinical experience. *Catheter Cardiovasc Interv* 56:508–515, 2002.

24. Hitchcock JF, Suijker WJ, Ksiezycka E, et al: Management of ventricular septal defect with associated aortic incompetence. *Ann Thorac Surg* 52:70–73, 1991.

25. Hughes ML, Maskell G, Goh TH, Wilkinson JL: Prospective comparison of costs and short-term health outcomes of surgical versus device closure of atrial septal defect in children. *Heart* 88:67–70, 2002.

26. Isomatsu Y, Imai Y, Shin'oka T, et al: Coarctation of the aorta and ventricular septal defect: Should we perform a single-stage repair? *J Thorac Cardiovasc Surg* 122:524–528, 2001.

27. Khositseth A, Cabalka AK, Sweeney JP, et al: Transcatheter Amplatzer device closure of atrial septal defect and patent foramen ovale in patients with presumed paradoxical embolism. *Mayo Clin Proc* 79:35–41, 2004.

28. Kidd L, Driscoll DJ, Gersony WM, et al: Second natural history study of congenital heart defects: Results of treatment of patients with ventricular septal defects. *Circulation* 87:I38–I51, 1993.

29. Kirklin JW, Barratt-Boyce BG: Atrial septal defect and partial anomalous pulmonary venous connection. In Kirklin JW, Barratt-Boyes BG (eds): *Cardiac Surgery.* New York, Churchhill Livingstone, 1993, pp 617.

30. Kirklin JW, Barratt-Boyce BG: Ventricular septal defect. In Kirklin JW, Barratt-Boyes BG (eds): *Cardiac Surgery.* New York, Churchhill Livingstone, 1993, pp 751–764.

31. Koenig P, Cao Q, Heitschmidt M, et al: Role of intracardiac echocardiographic guidance in transcatheter closure of atrial septal defects and patent foramen ovale using the Amplatzer device. *J Interv Cardiol* 16:51–62, 2003.

32. Krumsdorf U, Ostermayer S, Billinger K, et al: Incidence and clinical course of thrombus formation on atrial septal defect and patent foramen ovale closure devices in 1,000 consecutive patients. *J Am Coll Cardiol* 43:302–309, 2004.

33. Laussen PC, Bichell DC, McGowan FX, et al: Postoperative recovery in children after minimum versus full-length sternotomy. *Ann Thorac Surg* 69:591–596, 2000.

34. Lechat P, Mas JL, Lascault G, et al: Prevalence of patent foramen ovale in patients with stroke. *N Engl J Med* 318:1148–1152, 1988.

35. Lewis FJ, Taufic M: Closure of atrial septal defects with the aid of hypothermia: Experimental accomplishments and report of one successful case. *Surgery* 33:52, 1953.

36. Lucas RV, Adams P, Anderson RC, et al: The natural history of isolated ventricular septal defect: A serial physiologic study. *Circulation* 24:1372, 1961.

37. Markman P, Howitt G, Wade EG: Atrial septal defect in the middle-aged and elderly. *Q J Med* 34:409–426, 1965.

38. Meier B, Lock JE: Contemporary management of patent foramen ovale. *Circulation* 107:5–9, 2003.

39. Okubo M, Benson LN, Nykanen D, et al: Outcomes of intraoperative device closure of muscular ventricular septal defects. *Ann Thorac Surg* 72:416–423, 2001.

40. Oliver JM, Gallego P, Gonzalez A, et al: Predisposing conditions for atrial fibrillation in atrial septal defect with and without operative closure. *Am J Cardiol* 89:39–43, 2002.

41. Omeish A, Hijazi ZM: Transcatheter closure of atrial septal defects in children and adults using the Amplatzer Septal Occluder. *J Interv Cardiol* 14:37–44, 2001.

42. O'Rahilly R, Muller F: *Human Embryology and Teratology.* New York, Wiley-Liss, 1992.

43. Pfammatter JP, Wagner B, Berdat P, et al: Procedural factors associated with early postoperative arrhythmias after repair of congenital heart defects. *J Thorac Cardiovasc Surg* 123:258–262, 2002.

44. Rein JG, Freed MD, Norwood WI, Castaneda AR: Early and late results of closure of ventricular septal defect in infancy. *Ann Thorac Surg* 24:19–27, 1977.

45. Ricou FJ, Reynard CA, Lerch R: Transesophageal echocardiography in the diagnosis of inferior caval secundum atrial septal defect. *Am Heart J* 128:196–199, 1994.

46. Scammell AM, Diver MJ: Plasma rennin activity in infants with congenital heart disease. *Arch Dis Child* 62:1136–1138, 1987.

47. Serraf A, Lacour-Gayet F, Bruniaux J, et al: Surgical management of isolated multiple ventricular septal defects: Logical approach in 130 cases. *J Thorac Cardiovasc Surg* 103:437–442, 1992.

48. Sondergaard T: Closure of atrial septal defects: Report of three cases. *Acta Chir Scand* 107:492, 1954.

49. Suzuki H: Spontaneous closure of ventricular septal defects: Anatomic evidence in six adult patients. *Am J Clin Path* 52:391–402, 1969.

50. Tandon R, Edwards JE: Clinicopathologic correlations. Atrial septal defect in infancy: Common association with other anomalies. *Circulation* 49:1005–1010, 1974.

51. Thomson JD, Aburawi EH, Watterson KG, et al: Surgical and transcatheter (Amplatzer) closure of atrial septal defects: A prospective comparison of results and cost. *Heart* 87:466–469, 2002.

52. Thurlbeck WM (ed): *Disorders of the Vascular System in Pathology of the Lung.* Stuttgart, NY, Thieme Medical, 1988.

53. Tohyama K, Satomi G, Momma K: Aortic valve prolapse and aortic regurgitation associated with subpulmonic ventricular septal defect. *Am J Cardiol* 79:1285–1289, 1997.

54. Torracca L, Ismeno G, Quarti A, Alfieri O: Totally endoscopic atrial septal defect closure with a robotic system: Experience with seven cases. *Heart Surg Forum* 5:125–127, 2002.

55. Yamaki S, Mohri H, Haneda K, et al: Indications for surgery based on lung biopsy in cases of ventricular septal defect and/or patent ductus arteriosus with severe pulmonary hypertension. *Chest* 96:31–39, 1989.

56. Yang SG, Novello R, Nicolson SC, et al: Evaluation of ventricular septal defect repair using intraoperative transesophageal echocardiography: Frequency and significance of residual defects in infants and children. *Echocardiography* 17:681–684, 2000.

Chapter 25

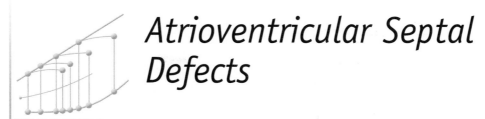

Atrioventricular Septal Defects

SHAUN P. SETTY, MD, and IRVING SHEN, MD

DEFINITION

Atrioventricular septal defects (AVSDs) are characterized by defects in the atrial and ventricular septum immediately above and below the atrioventricular (AV) valves (tricuspid and mitral). Traditionally, this congenital abnormality has also been referred to as AV canal defect, endocardial cushion defect, persistent atrioventricular ostium, and canalis atrioventricularis communis. The defects usually involve the AV valves to some degree, and the pathophysiology of the lesion depends on the extent of shunting at both the atrial and ventricular levels, as well as regurgitation from the involved valves. When limited to the atrial septum, the condition is called an ostium primum atrial septal defect (primum ASD) or partial AVSD. Complete AVSDs combine deficiency of both the atrial and ventricular septum with severe abnormality of the mitral and tricuspid valves, creating what is in essence a common AV valve that serves both ventricles. AVSDs occur in approximately 4% to 5% of people with congenital heart defects.[45] Forty percent of children with Down syndrome have some type of congenital heart disease, and just less than half of these have AVSDs.

EMBRYOLOGY

Partitioning of the AV canal and the atrium begins about the middle of the fourth week of gestation and is essentially complete by the end of the fifth week. The atrial septum is initially partitioned by a thin membrane (septum primum) that appears to grow toward the region of the endocardial cushions from the roof of the atrium. Concurrent with atrial septation, thickenings of subendocardial tissue, called endocardial cushions, develop in the dorsal and ventral walls of the heart in the region of the AV canal. During the fifth week, the AV endocardial cushions grow toward each other and fuse, dividing the AV canal into right and left sides. At the same time, endocardial cushion tissue grows in an upward direction to meet the primum septum and to close the intervening space (referred to as the ostium primum). These cushions give rise to the inferior portion of the atrial septum, ventricular septum (immediately below the tricuspid valve in the inlet to the right ventricle), and septal leaflets of both the

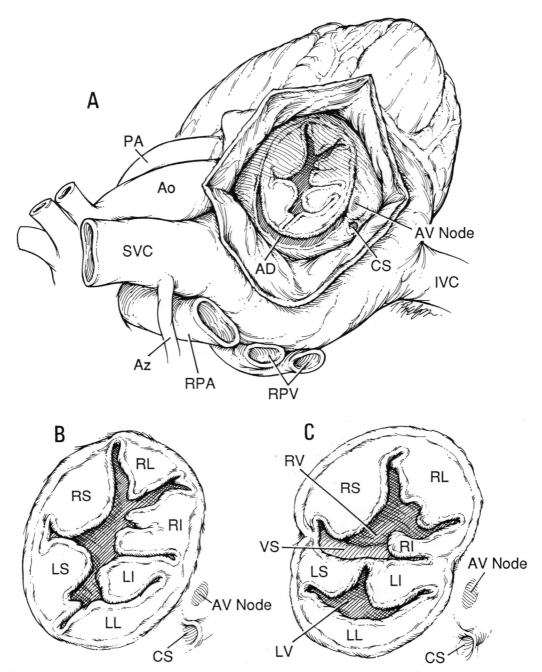

FIGURE 25-1   Native anatomy of the atrioventricular septal defect (AVSD). **A,** Surgeon's view from patient's right side, looking through the right atriotomy of the common AV valve of a complete defect. The left-sided valve can be seen through the atrial defect (AD). Note the location of the AV node and coronary sinus (CS). **B,** Valve anatomy of complete AV septal defect. Note a single orifice and ventricular septum (VS). Right superior (RS), inferior (RI), and lateral (RL) and left inferior (LI), superior (LS), and lateral leaflets (LL) are shown. **C,** Partial AV septal defect, valve anatomy. There are two orifices with separate but complete valve rings. A cleft in the mitral leaflet (between LS and LI) reveals the ventricular septum. Ao, aorta; AVN, AV node; Az, azygous vein; IVC, inferior vena cava; LV, left ventricle; PA, pulmonary artery; RPA, right pulmonary artery; RPV, right pulmonary vein; RV, right ventricle; SVC, superior vena cava.

mitral and tricuspid valves. Therefore, abnormal growth in this region produces a deficiency in the lowermost part of the atrial septum (often with associated abnormalities such as "cleft" of the mitral and tricuspid valves). The most extensive form of this developmental anomaly produces a ventricular septal deficiency as well and what essentially amounts to a hole in the middle of the heart (complete AVSD) with communication at this level between all four cardiac chambers (Fig. 25-1).

CLASSIFICATION AND ANATOMY

The main anatomic feature of the AVSD is a deficiency of the AV septum. This septum between the left ventricle (LV) and the right atrium is created by the attachment of the mitral valve at a slightly higher level (cephalad) than the tricuspid valve. In patients with AVSDs, the mitral and tricuspid valves "attach" to the septum at the same level.

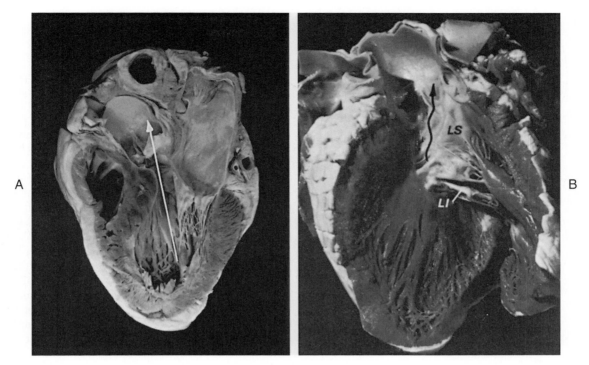

FIGURE 25-2   A, The left ventricular outflow tract (LVOT) viewed from the left ventricular aspect of a normal heart demonstrates how the chordal attachments of the mitral valve are attached to free wall papillary muscles. The attachments of the mitral valve do not encroach on the LVOT (*arrow*). **B,** The LVOT in a heart from a patient with partial AV septal defect, viewed from the same left ventricular orientation, demonstrates that the attachments of the left superior (LS) and left inferior (LI) components of the mitral valve cross the LVOT. In some cases, these attachments can create subaortic obstruction to left ventricular outflow. (From Anderson RH, Baker EJ, Rigby ML, Ebels T: The morphology and diagnosis of atrioventricular septal defects. *Cardiol Young* 1:290–305, 1991; with permission.)

Partial AVSDs consist of an absence of the AV septum without a defect in the ventricular septum.[2] Usually, there is a cleft in the anterior leaflet of the mitral valve, but the heart has two separate orifices for the AV valves. Since the ventricular septum is intact, the only septal defect is atrial, above the AV valves. Nevertheless, the mitral valve should not be considered normal. Its attachments to the ventricular septum are not normal, and the leaflets of the mitral valve are truly part of a common AV valve. The superior bridging leaflet will have attachments into the LV outflow tract (LVOT) instead of attaching to papillary muscles on the LV free wall. These outflow tract attachments can cause LVOT obstruction (Fig. 25-2). Furthermore, the left AV valve may be abnormal, with a spectrum from a relatively pliable valve that opens widely and closes with minimal insufficiency to a thickened, irregular, dysplastic valve with poorly defined commissures that causes poor apposition resulting in mitral valve insufficiency of varying grades. The LVOT is displaced anteriorly and is not trapped between the AV valves, thus giving the LVOT a "gooseneck" appearance on angiogram (elongated and narrow).

Complete AVSDs present as a single-orifice AV valve with deficiency of both the atrial and the ventricular septum. These defects can be extremely complex, depending on the anatomy of the valve tissue and how it relates to the intracardiac anatomy.[2] In 1966, Rastelli and colleagues[50] provided a classification of these valves based on the differing degrees of bridging of the superior bridging leaflet, its chordal attachment pattern, and the degree of associative hypoplasia of the tricuspid anterosuperior leaflet (Fig. 25-3). This classification does not take into consideration the anatomy of the inferior bridging leaflet, because the inferior leaflet has much greater morphologic variation and does not always demonstrate a consistent pattern. The simplest way to distinguish a Rastelli type A defect is that the superior bridging leaflet appears to be clefted over the interventricular septum, and there are numerous chordal attachments between the superior bridging leaflet and the septum. Rastelli type B defect is rare. In this defect, there are chordal attachments from the right side of the interventricular septum to the left side of the common superior bridging leaflet. A Rastelli type C defect has a large superior bridging leaflet that overrides the interventricular septum and has few or no attachments to the septum. This lack of septal attachment can result in a large communication between the ventricles. It is most common in patients with associated cardiac and extracardiac anomalies such as in tetralogy of Fallot and Down syndrome.

The superior bridging leaflet in complete AVSD can encroach on the LVOT and create obstruction to LV outflow after repair. The AV valve tissue itself can also be quite variable, ranging from relatively normal-appearing valvular tissue with minimal incompetence to severely limited, dysplastic tissue with marked valvular incompetence.

ASSOCIATED DEFECTS

Atrioventricular septal defects have no gender predilection and are frequently associated with other cardiac defects

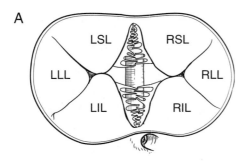

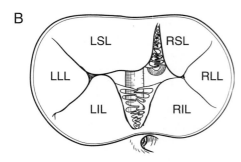

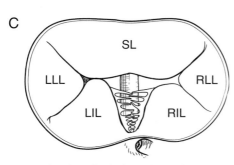

FIGURE 25-3 Superior view of valvular variants of complete atrioventricular septal defects. Based on Rastelli's three classifications. **A,** Rastelli type A defect: The common superior (anterior) bridging leaflet (SL) is completely over its own respective ventricle. The superior leaflet is divided and attached to the ventricular septum. **B,** Rastelli type B defect: A rare defect in which papillary muscles attach from the right side of the septum to the left side of the superior valve. Note that the left superior leaflet has some overlap with the site of the deficient septum. **C,** Rastelli type C defect: The superior leaflet bridges the ventricular septum but is not attached to it. LIL, left interior (posterior) leaflet; LLL, left lateral leaflet; LSL, left superior (anterior) leaflet; RIL, right inferior (posterior) leaflet; RLL, right lateral leaflet; RSL, right superior (anterior) leaflet; SL, superior (anterior) leaflet. (From Jacobs JP, Burke RP, Quintessenza JA, Mavroudis C: Congenital heart surgery nomenclature and database project: Atrioventricular canal defect. *Ann Thorac Surg* 69(4 Suppl):S36–S43, 2000 with permission.)

(ranging between 7% and 25%).[57,66] These other defects include heterotaxy syndromes,[25] tetralogy of Fallot,[8,27] double-outlet right ventricle,[8,25] total anomalous pulmonary venous return,[57] and transposition of the great arteries.[8] It is common for patients with complete AVSD to also have small secundum ASDs.[63] A patent ductus arteriosus is seen in as many as 10% of these patients,[25,57,63] especially when the diagnosis is in infancy. There is clearly an association between Down syndrome and AVSDs, and some form of the defect may be present in as many as 30% of children with this syndrome.[5,24,53]

NATURAL HISTORY

Partial Atrioventricular Septal Defect

The natural history of patients with AVSDs depends on the extent of the lesion (partial or complete), the degree of mitral insufficiency, and the nature of any associated lesion (both cardiac and noncardiac). The clinical course of patients with partial AVSDs and only mild mitral insufficiency parallels those for patients with simple secundum ASDs.[56] There is a tendency for these patients to develop atrial arrhythmias, which may determine the age at which they demonstrate symptoms. This may be due to the location of this defect near (and displacing) the AV node, as well as to the fact that most of these patients have large left-to-right shunts with distention of the right atrium and ventricle. Partial AVSDs associated with moderate to severe mitral insufficiency have a more pronounced natural history. As many as one fifth of these patients have symptoms of congestive heart failure (CHF), dyspnea, and arrhythmias in infancy,[25] and some die during the first decade of life. This reflects the degree of intracardiac shunting as well as the diminished forward cardiac output secondary to mitral insufficiency. It is important to note that the ejection fraction in the setting of substantial mitral regurgitation grossly overestimates cardiac function.

Complete Atrioventricular Septal Defect

The natural history of complete AVSD is not well understood, since it is unusual for patients with this condition to be treated without surgical intervention. Nevertheless, the addition of an intracardiac shunt at the ventricular level, combined with the atrial level shunt and AV valve insufficiency, makes this a particularly morbid lesion with high mortality if left untreated. A few small series have confirmed this suspicion and suggest that 80% of patients who do not undergo surgery will die by 2 years of age.[7,25,45] Even an infant who survives to 1 year of age only has a 15% chance of living to the age of 5 years. These patients die from overwhelming CHF with respiratory distress, arrhythmias, endocarditis, and/or pulmonary infections. Those infants who survive do so by elevation of pulmonary artery resistances, which decreases the intracardiac shunt. They almost invariably go on to develop irreversible pulmonary hypertension at a young age[46]; this is expected in as many as 90% of children who survive until their first birthday. Rapid development of irreversible pulmonary hypertension has been described in infants with Down syndrome within the first 2 months of life.[1,71] Such rapid development of irreversible pulmonary hypertension in these patients may be in part due to their high incidence of laryngotracheomalacia.[44] Although patients who develop severe pulmonary hypertension have less intracardiac shunting and may be clinically improved, their prognosis is dismal because corrective surgery becomes extremely risky, if not impossible. Also, it is of interest that 14% of women with repaired AVSDs who survive to have children risk passing along a congenital heart defect trait (usually tetralogy of Fallot or an AVSD) to their offspring.[18] This is substantially higher than the 2% to 4% risk that mothers with other types of congenital heart defects have of giving birth to children with a heart lesion.[25]

PATHOPHYSIOLOGY

The natural history described in the previous section is created by abnormal blood flow patterns that result in excessive pulmonary blood flow, increased cardiac work, and decreased systemic cardiac output due to mitral regurgitation.

Partial Atrioventricular Septal Defect

Ventricular Compliance and Q_p:Q_s

The physiology of shunt flow in partial AVSDs is similar to that of any ASD and is determined by the compliance of the ventricles[11] and not by the size of the defect (unless the defect is small and restrictive). Thus, quantifying the size of the shunt does not predict the size of the defect.[36] The amount of pulmonary blood flow (Q_p) may be three to four times the amount of systemic blood flow (Q_s) (Q_p:Q_s = 3 or 4:1) in patients who are otherwise asymptomatic. In patients with large shunts, the right ventricular (RV) volume is increased, and this displaces the interventricular septum into the LV. As a result, the LV size may appear to be small, even though the size is often large enough to provide adequate cardiac output after the repair.[10,67] This repeated chronic volume loading and distention, however, may affect RV function.[10,72] The long-term ability of the RV to recover is probably related to the age of the child at the time of repair.[38,48] As the RV compliance begins to approach that of the LV, the intracardiac shunt may decrease, and the patient may have a Q_p:Q_s of 1:1. This shunt ratio actually reflects net pulmonary versus net systemic blood flow and does not mean that there is no shunting across the defect. In reality, patients who develop pulmonary hypertension, which limits the left-to-right shunt flow, begin to develop right-to-left shunting during some phases of the cardiac cycle. This shunt reversal balances out the left-to-right shunting that still continues during the remaining phases so that even though they have no net increase in pulmonary flow versus systemic flow, they do have bidirectional shunting of blood. The right-to-left component results in a significant quantity of desaturated blood crossing to the systemic circulation, which causes these patients to be mildly cyanotic. This is often a sign that the defect is no longer correctable.

Mitral Insufficiency

Without the development of significant RV hypertrophy from RV outflow tract obstruction or pulmonary hypertension, the intracardiac shunt continues to produce excessive pulmonary blood flow with increased blood return to the left atrium. Most of this blood shunts back across the ASD to produce volume loading of the right atrium and ventricle with signs of CHF. In partial AV canal defects, the degree of mitral valve insufficiency plays a large role in determining the severity of the lesion. When there is severe mitral insufficiency, the regurgitant jet is often aimed directly at the atrial septal defect into the right atrium. This not only increases the shunt to the right side but also requires an obligatory increase in LV stroke volume to maintain forward cardiac output. The resultant demands on LV and RV function hasten the onset of biventricular heart failure.

Children with partial AVSDs and moderate to severe mitral insufficiency usually present with symptoms early in life.

Complete Atrioventricular Septal Defect

In children with a complete AVSD, left-to-right shunting occurs at both the atrial and ventricular levels. It is the shunting at the ventricular level that produces the more serious problems. This shunting occurs at systemic pressures and leads to RV and pulmonary artery pressures that equal LV and systemic arterial pressures (Fig. 25-4). To protect against torrential pulmonary blood flow, pulmonary vascular resistance (PVR) quickly rises and may become fixed and permanent during the first month of life.[1,71] Although elevated PVR decreases the net left-to-right shunt at the ventricular level (by decreasing compliance of the pulmonary vascular bed), permanent histologic changes in the pulmonary arterioles prevent PVR from returning to normal when the defect is surgically repaired. This can impose an intolerable impedance to flow that impairs the RV from performing as a pulmonary ventricle when the defect is corrected. Once the PVR has reached this level (greater than 12 Wood's unit/m²),[25] cases are usually considered to be inoperable, because the RV will no longer be capable of supporting pulmonary blood flow once the defect in the interventricular septum is closed.

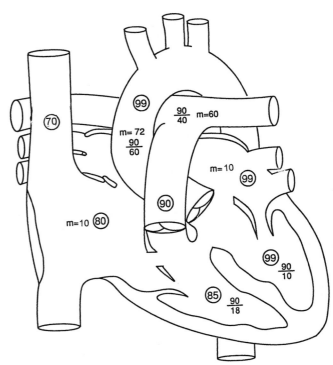

FIGURE 25-4 Pathophysiology of complete septal defect. There is a left-to-right shunt at the atrial level, which is exacerbated by the incompetent atrioventricular valve and elevated left atrial pressure (LAP) (mean LAP = 10 mm Hg) and is reflected in the elevated right atrial oxygen saturation (80%). An additional left-to-right shunt occurs at the ventricular level, which is consistent with systemic right ventricular pressures (90/18) and a further increase in oxygen saturation (85%). In this example:

$$Q_p:Q_s = (Ao - SVC\ sat)/(PV - PA\ sat) = (99 - 70)/(99 - 90) \approx 3/1$$

where Ao = aorta, PV = pulmonary vein, PA = pulmonary artery, SVC = superior vena cava
m, mean.

DIAGNOSTIC ASSESSMENT

Physical Findings

In patients with partial AVSD, abnormal physical findings may not be obvious. The height and weight of these patients may be smaller than normal, as seen on serial growth charts, but they may appear otherwise healthy. There may be a visible left parasternal heave with a palpable RV lift. In some patients, this can produce a localized chest wall deformity with protuberance of the costal cartilage in the left parasternal region. Auscultation will reveal a hyperactive precordium and a prominent first heart sound with fixed splitting of the second heart sound. A short (grade II or III) systolic ejection murmur will be present in the second or third left intercostal space from the increased flow across the pulmonary valve. A mid-diastolic tricuspid flow rumble may also be audible in the fourth or fifth left intercostal space. If the patient is in CHF, there may be jugular venous distention, hepatomegaly, and cardiomegaly. Increased intensity of the RV lift with accentuation of the second heart sound suggests the presence of elevated pulmonary artery pressures and the possibility of increased PVR. In patients with partial AV canal defects and moderate to severe mitral insufficiency, there are usually more pronounced signs of heart failure, and pulmonary edema may be present and detected by the appearance of bibasilar rales. These patients usually have pronounced cardiomegaly, and auscultation discloses a distinct, apical holosystolic murmur of mitral regurgitation.

Patients with complete AVSDs usually present in severe heart failure during the first year of life with tachypnea, poor feeding, failure to grow, and evidence of poor peripheral perfusion. This presentation usually parallels the normal postnatal fall in PVR. Signs of RV overload, interventricular shunting (loud pansystolic murmur), and pulmonary hypertension (loud second heart sound) will be obvious. Occasionally, however, PVR will not fall to the point that the shunt becomes clinically apparent, and as changes of fixed pulmonary vascular disease take over, the patient may seem clinically well.

Patients with partial or complete AVSDs present a risk for subacute bacterial endocarditis because of the turbulence created by the AV valve incompetence and the interventricular shunting. It is possible for these patients to first present with signs of an intracardiac infection.[28,49]

Diagnostic Tests

In children with an AVSD, the chest radiograph usually shows mild to moderate cardiomegaly, prominence of the pulmonary artery shadow, and increased pulmonary vascular markings (Fig. 25-5). The LV and aorta should be normal or slightly smaller than normal. Partial AVSDs with moderate or severe mitral insufficiency may produce prominence of the LV with distinctive biventricular enlargement and signs of pulmonary edema. Patients with complete AVSD usually have a chest x-ray picture consistent with severe heart failure during infancy, with marked cardiomegaly and pulmonary overcirculation. As pulmonary hypertension develops, the lung markings become clearer and the central pulmonary arteries appear larger.

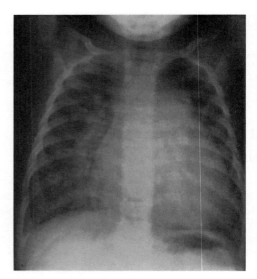

FIGURE 25-5 Chest radiograph of an infant with a complete atrioventricular septal defect (AVSD) shows cardiomegaly, pulmonary overcirculation, and congestive heart failure.

The electrocardiogram can be distinctive. Patients with partial or complete AVSD usually demonstrate marked RV hypertrophy with prolongation of the P-R interval. There may also be LV hypertrophy. Usually, left axis deviation is present and the vector loop in the frontal plane is counterclockwise. Although left-axis deviation and a counterclockwise loop strongly suggest an AVSD, this pattern can occur in approximately 10% of patients with secundum ASDs.[28,49]

Diagnosis can be obtained by using either transthoracic or transesophageal two-dimensional echocardiography with color flow mapping.[29] This will clarify the physiologic alterations created by this defect. Resolution from echocardiography is so good with currently available instruments (especially with the transesophageal approach) that precise details of the nature of the defect can be obtained. Echocardiography with color flow Doppler is now the diagnostic modality of choice to demonstrate partial AVSDs and in most cases obviates the necessity for cardiac catheterization before surgery. In patients with partial AVSDs the degree of mitral insufficiency is nicely demonstrated, and the cleft in the mitral valve can usually be outlined (Fig. 25-6).[4] Patients with complete AVSD can also be evaluated with echocardiography alone. It is easy to disclose the presence of a ventricular level shunt, which distinguishes partial from complete forms of this lesion (Fig. 25-7).[62,69] Doppler techniques can also accurately predict gradients across areas of stenosis. Therefore, patients suspected of having significant RV or LV outflow obstruction or aortic coarctation may not require cardiac catheterization for adequate evaluation of anatomy before repair. This depends on the quality of the echocardiographic images obtained and the experience of the surgical and cardiology team in making these types of assessments on the basis of echocardiography alone. Infants older than 6 months with complete AVSD (especially if they have Down syndrome) may have increased PVR. If physical examination (e.g., loud S2) or Doppler study suggests elevated pulmonary artery pressure and lack of pulmonary reactivity, cardiac catheterization is justified.[1,71]

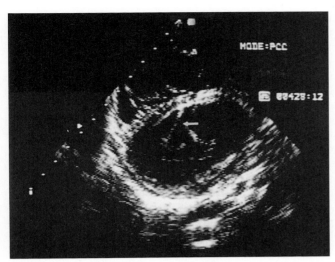

FIGURE 25-6 Echocardiogram (short-axis epicardial view) of the ventricles obtained at the time of surgical repair demonstrates the "cleft" (*arrow*) in the anterior leaflet of the mitral valve found in patients with partial atrioventricular septal defects.

Cineangiography during cardiac catheterization can demonstrate the elongation of the LV outflow tract in relationship to the inflow tract, which produces a characteristic "gooseneck" deformity.[28] Although this finding is characteristic of AVSDs, the anatomic detail provided by the less-invasive echocardiography has replaced the necessity of demonstrating this angiographic feature to establish the diagnosis of AVSD. Catheterization, however, does provide data that enable calculation of pulmonary and systemic blood flow so that the magnitude of the intracardiac shunt can be quantified. Moreover, the degree of pulmonary hypertension, when present, can be measured and, along with pulmonary blood flow calculations, can enable determination of PVR. Patients with PVR greater than 12 Wood's unit/m^2 are considered unable to undergo corrective repair. If the PVR is less than 6 Wood's unit/m^2, the patient's condition usually can be safely corrected, although long-term survival may be shorter in patients with elevated resistance than in those with normal values. Patients with PVR between 6 and 12 Wood's unit/m^2 may benefit from measurement of pulmonary and systemic arterial pressure changes with simultaneous calculation of shunt fractions when breathing high levels of supplemental oxygen or nitric oxide or with intravenous infusion of sodium nitroprusside. Patients who have elevated PVR but are responsive to supplemental oxygen or pulmonary vasodilator challenge may still be able to undergo surgery. Cases in which no significant decrease in PVR occurs or systemic vascular resistance falls with an increase in right-to-left shunting during pulmonary vasodilator challenge may be best left uncorrected. These patients may eventually be candidates for heart-lung transplant or bilateral lung transplant with simultaneous correction of intracardiac defects.

PREOPERATIVE CRITICAL CARE MANAGEMENT

Partial Atrioventricular Septal Defect

Patients with partial AVSD are usually asymptomatic. The indications for repair are the same as for other types of ASDs. Occasionally, an infant presents in moderate to severe CHF from a partial AVSD. These children are usually managed on diuretics and digoxin as outpatients until the time of surgery. Patients with severe AV valve regurgitation may be managed with afterload reduction but only after subaortic obstruction has been ruled out.[56] These defects do not close spontaneously, and surgical correction is recommended for any severely symptomatic patient and for all patients before 5 years of age.

Complete Atrioventricular Septal Defect

The diagnosis of complete AVSD is often established in infancy because most patients with this condition are symptomatic. Although newborn infants may initially be asymptomatic, the substantial left-to-right shunting that accompanies the fall in PVR, along with the potential for marked AV valve insufficiency, usually produces severe CHF

FIGURE 25-7 Echocardiogram demonstrating a complete atrioventricular septal defect in **(A)** diastole and **(B)** systole. The total communication between all chambers of the heart can be appreciated during diastole, as blood entering the atria (*arrow*) can shunt easily toward whichever ventricle has the highest compliance. During systole, there is shunting (*arrow*) across the large ventricular level communication into the pulmonary circulation. CA, common atrium; LV, left ventricle; RV, right ventricle.

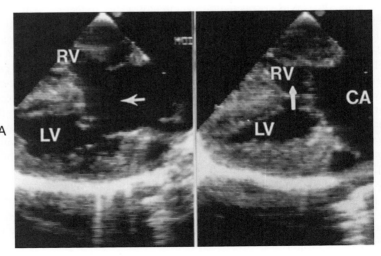

and concomitant failure to thrive. Even after the diagnosis is made, many of these infants can be managed successfully as outpatients on a combination of diuretics and digoxin until elective repair. The ability to manage these patients depends in part on their PVR. Patients with low PVR may be in severe CHF. Furthermore, those patients with severe mitral insufficiency tend to have more significant heart failure. In these patients, there may be a role for afterload reduction. In addition, these patients often have feeding difficulties leading to growth failure. Gavage feeding before surgical repair may be considered, providing the patient can tolerate the increased volume of supplemental feedings. Cases in which a patent ductus arteriosus is present may be even more difficult to manage, and early surgery may be indicated. If there is a contraindication for early repair, ligation of the patent ductus and pulmonary artery banding may be performed to decrease the amount of pulmonary overcirculation followed by complete repair as soon as possible.

The challenge lies in treating those infants who are in severe heart failure and require ventilator support. Hyperventilation with high oxygen concentration may exacerbate the heart failure, and attention to the physiology of pulmonary shunt lesions is important in the management of these patients. It is usually the best policy to operate on infants with complete AVSD immediately if their management becomes complicated, as any medical intervention provided to support these patients does not treat the underlying pathophysiology. Occasionally, however, immediate surgery is contraindicated (e.g., in infants who have severe heart failure secondary to sepsis and who require a few days of antibiotics and stabilization in an intensive care setting before surgery). In these patients, surgery should be performed as soon as their clinical condition allows, since they have a surgically correctable problem that should not invite prolonged attempts at preoperative "fine-tuning," especially if this requires prolonged preoperative mechanical ventilation or placement of centrally located intravenous catheters.

SURGICAL CORRECTION

Surgical correction of AVSDs is performed via a median sternotomy on cardiopulmonary bypass (CPB). The use of pulmonary artery bands to control heart failure in infants with complete AVSD is used only in unusual circumstances. In fact, the use of pulmonary artery bands can be harmful, especially in infants with pulmonary hypertension and/or severe AV valve insufficiency. After exposure of the heart, the anatomy is delineated, especially for the presence of previously unrecognized associated defects, such as a persistent left superior vena cava (SVC) that might affect the surgical approach. The patient is then heparinized and cannulated for CPB. Arterial perfusion is best obtained by direct cannulation of the aorta. In most cases, bicaval venous cannulation should be used so that the patient can be placed on total bypass to allow easy visualization of intracardiac anatomy. These patients usually have excessive intravascular volume and, as a result, it is often safer to place the patient on CPB initially with a single venous cannula in the right atrium. This allows decompression of the heart, which will make direct cannulation of the vena cavae easier with less hemodynamic fluctuation. Before CPB, it is

helpful to perform epicardial or transesophageal echocardiography with Doppler color flow imaging to clearly evaluate the nature of the defect, the degree of mitral insufficiency, and the presence of additional lesions.[60-62] It is possible for the pre-CPB echocardiogram to demonstrate previously unappreciated details of the patient's anatomy or unsuspected associated defects, which may lead to modification of the operative procedure.[62] Once CPB is initiated, the ductus arteriosus should be routinely ligated, even if the echocardiogram does not demonstrate flow.

The repair is usually performed using continuous CPB under mild to moderate hypothermic (25° C to 32° C) conditions. Myocardial protection using aortic cross-clamping and cold antegrade cardioplegic solution to arrest the heart is preferred over induced ventricular fibrillation. Once the heart has been arrested, the right atrium is opened to expose the defect for repair.

Partial Atrioventricular Septal Defect

An oblique right atriotomy is performed, and the intracardiac anatomy can be inspected (Figs. 25-8 and 25-9). The mitral valve leaflets should be visible through the defect in the AV septum, and the cleft in the anterior leaflet should be identified. The annulus between the left- and right-sided AV valves is inspected to make certain it is complete. The inlet portion of the ventricular septum is also carefully examined. If there is no VSD and if the annulus between the two AV valves is complete, the lesion is a partial AVSD. Some authorities believe that the cleft in the anterior leaflet of the mitral valve does not routinely require repair[12,28] if there is no echocardiographic evidence of significant regurgitation, and that the mitral valve will function well as a trileaflet structure. However, the long-term failure rate of this approach is not trivial. Ebels[16] recommends an individualized approach to each defect, determining whether the cleft should be repaired on the basis of the size of the posterior mitral leaflet. He reported excellent results in terms of limiting valvular insufficiency and preventing valvular stenosis by repairing the cleft only in those mitral valves in which the posterior leaflet is large.[16] There are other surgeons who believe that all mitral clefts should be closed routinely in the repair of partial and complete AVSDs (unless there is a parachute mitral valve, in which case closing the cleft is contraindicated). The careful approximation of the cleft anterior leaflet provides excellent long-term results.[34] The cleft in the anterior leaflet of the mitral valve is repaired with nonpledgetted interrupted fine sutures to diminish the risk of late valvular dysfunction from calcification of the pledget material.[58] There are reports of postoperative hemolysis in the presence of prosthetic material and residual mitral insufficiency.[22,54,65] Some surgeons favor the use of pericardial pledgets for the valve repair. The use of the saline injection test can allow tailoring of any AV valve leaking to limit postoperative regurgitation.

The atrial septal communication is closed with either a pericardial or a polytetrafluoroethylene (PTFE) patch. In certain cases where the ostium primum defect is small, the defect can be closed primarily.[14] The surgeon must be cognizant of the location of the AV node to avoid injuring this structure while repairing the ASD.[9,35] The AV node in AVSDs is displaced inferiorly and is located in between the orifice of the

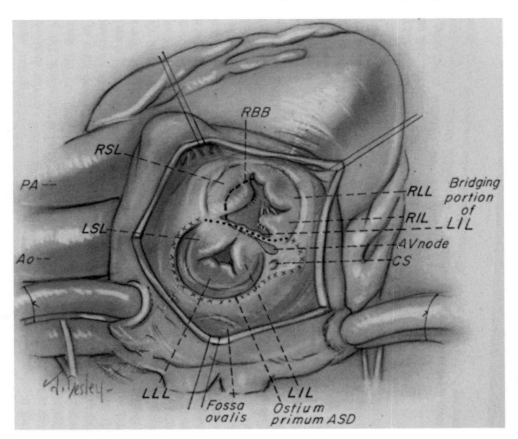

FIGURE 25-8 Note the location of the conduction system in an ostium primum atrial septal defect (ASD) is very close to the coronary sinus (CS) and can be injured by sutures placed in this region. The Xs in this illustration demonstrate one of the locations for placement of sutures to secure the pericardial patch that closes the atrial septal defect but baffles the CS return to the left atrial side. Ao, aorta; CS, coronary sinus; LIL, left inferior leaflet; LSL, left superior leaflet; PA, pulmonary artery; RBB, right bundle branch; RIL, right inferior leaflet; RLL, right lateral leaflet (all these pertain to the portions of the common AV valve); RSL, right superior leaflet.

coronary sinus and the annulus of the AV valve. Multiple techniques have been described to secure the ASD patch near this region to avoid injuring the conduction system. One option is to take care that the sutures placed near the region of the AV node are placed more superficially and travel in the substance of the mitral valve rather than the atrioventricular septum. Alternatively, the ASD patch can be tailored so that it will cover the coronary sinus orifice and baffle the coronary sinus return to the left atrial side. The suture line is carried in between the orifice of the coronary sinus and the orifice of the inferior vena cava onto the right atrial wall before turning in front of the coronary sinus and back toward the edge of the ASD. This technique is contraindicated in patients with a persistent left SVC (LSVC). It is advisable to place temporary atrial and ventricular pacing wires to be used in the postoperative period if necessary.

Complete Atrioventricular Septal Defect

If the defect is a complete AVSD, the anatomy can look quite different from that of a partial AVSD. The single large AV valve bridges the canal defect and can be considered to have a superior and an inferior common leaflet. There is no "annulus" between the left and right AV valves, and the intracardiac defect extends from the atrial to the ventricular septum. Although the surgical technique may vary depending on the precise anatomy of the common AV valve (Rastelli classification),[28,50,51] the principles essentially involve closing the ventricular septal defect (VSD), subdividing the common AV valve into a left-sided and a right-sided AV valve, and

suspending these newly created valves from the top of the VSD patch. Frequently, it has been noted that patients with Down syndrome usually have better and more pliable valves than those without Down syndrome. Exceptional care is necessary in the repair of the left-sided AV valve to prevent insufficiency.[30,31] The ASD is then closed in the same manner as an ostium primum defect.

Surgical repair of complete AVSD can be accomplished by using one of several well-described techniques. A single-patch technique uses one large patch to repair the atrial and the ventricular component of the defect (Fig. 25-10). A double-patch repair uses a patch to close the VSD and another patch to close the primum ASD. A simplified single-patch technique[47,68] involves closing the ventricular septal defect by direct suturing of the common AV valve leaflets to the crest of the ventricular septum using plegetted horizontal mattress sutures. A patch is then used to close the primum ASD. Regardless of the repair technique, placement of temporary pacing wires is advisable. The performance of modified ultrafiltration at the end of the case may be helpful in removing excess fluid, improving the hematocrit, and removing inflammatory mediators, which can worsen pulmonary vascular resistance.

Regardless of the type of defect, it is recommended that the adequacy of the surgical repair be evaluated before the patient leaves the operating room. A residual VSD can be detected by measuring right atrial and pulmonary arterial oxygen saturation to look for an oxygen saturation step-up. Significant left-sided AV valve insufficiency is more difficult to demonstrate by indirect techniques, but many surgical

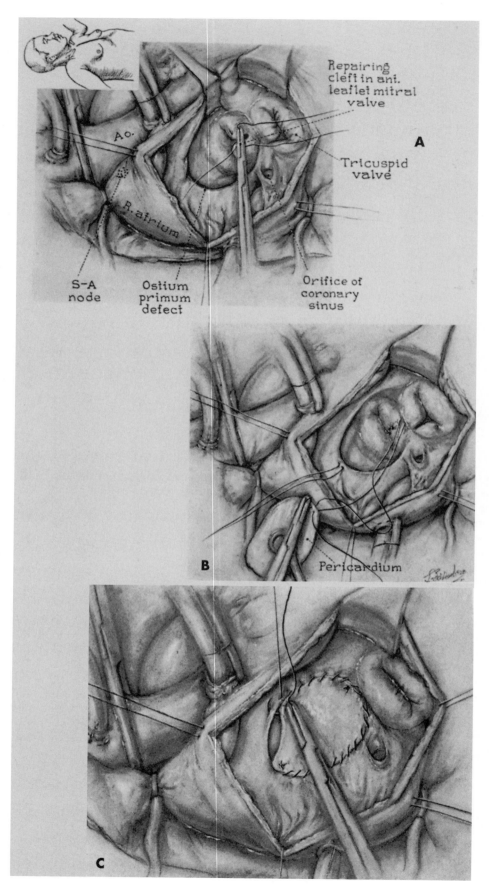

Repairing cleft in ant. leaflet mitral valve

Tricuspid valve

Ao.

R. atrium

S-A node

Ostium primum defect

Orifice of coronary sinus

A

B

Pericardium

C

FIGURE 25-9 **A,** A partial atrioventricular septal defect is exposed so that the "cleft" in the anterior mitral leaflet can be repaired with interrupted sutures. The valve competency can be checked by instilling cold saline into the left ventricle cavity. The aorta has been cross-clamped and the heart arrested with cold cardioplegia solution. **B,** The beginning of the suture line to secure the pericardial patch to the annulus between the tricuspid and repaired mitral valve. **C,** Placement of a pericardial patch to close an ostium primum atrial septal defect can be secured in such a manner as to keep the coronary sinus on the right atrial side. Sutures can be carefully placed to avoid injuring the AV node by keeping them in the tissue of the mitral valve until they are well beyond the coronary sinus. This technique is especially important in patients who have a large coronary sinus from a persistent left superior vena cava. Ao, aorta; S-A, sinoatrial. (From Ebert PA: *Atlas of Congenital ardiac Surgery,* New York, 1989, Churchill Livingstone; with permission.)

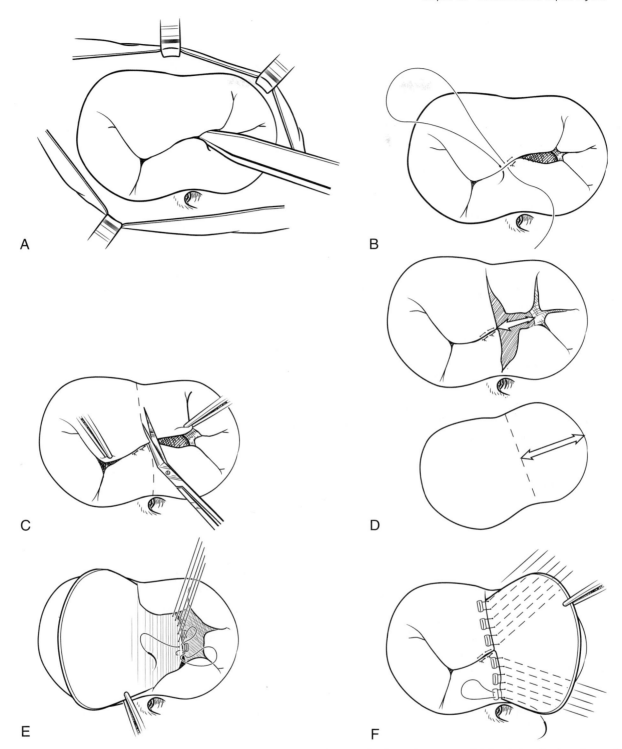

FIGURE 25-10 Single patch repair of complete atrioventricular (AV) septal defect. Repair of complete AV septal defect is usually through a median sternotomy. Cardiopulmonary bypass is achieved through arterial cannulation of the distal ascending aorta and separate venous cannulation of each cava. The defect is exposed through an oblique right atriotomy. **A,** Cold saline is injected into the ventricular cavities to float the AV valve leaflets up. This will help determine the optimal coaptation point of the left superior and inferior bridging leaflets. **B,** The optimal coaptation point of the left superior and inferior bridging leaflets is approximated with either fine mattress or simple sutures. **C,** The superior and inferior bridging leaflets are incised. **D,** A single piece of Gore-tex patch is cut to the appropriate size and shape. **E,** One end of the patch is secured to the right side of the ventricular septum using either pledgetted horizontal mattress sutures or simple running suture. **F,** After repairing the ventricular component of the defect, the leaflets of the left AV valve are attached to the patch using pledgetted horizontal mattress sutures.

(Continued)

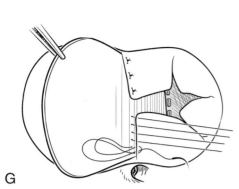

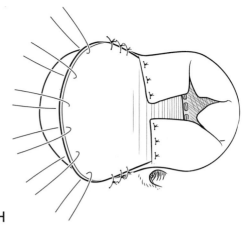

G

H

FIGURE 25-10   Cont'd   **G,** After bringing the sutures from the left side of the patch to the right, they are passed through the leaflets of the right AV valve to secure them to the patch. **H,** The rest of the patch is used to close the atrial component of the defect. This is accomplished using a running suture. (Redrawn from Merill WH, Hammon JW Jr, Bender HW Jr: Technique of repair of atrioventricular septal defect with a comment atrioventricular orifice. *Cardiol Young* 1:379, 1991.)

teams look for V waves on the left atrial line tracing. Intraoperative transesophageal echocardiography with Doppler color flow imaging provides a specific and sensitive method to assess the quality of repair and detect any residual defect. This can direct any necessary revision in the repair before allowing the patient to leave the operating room and provide prognostic information regarding the likelihood of an optimal long-term outcome.

Special Situations

Complete AVSDs are frequently repaired during infancy because of the potential life-threatening complications that can result if surgery is not performed early. Repairing AVSDs in small patients can often be simplified by using techniques of deep hypothermic circulatory arrest with the core body temperature down to 18° C. This enables the surgeon to work in a bloodless field unencumbered by distortion produced from the cannulae necessary to sustain CPB. Although the effects of these techniques on long-term neuropsychiatric development remain obscure, it appears that a period of deep hypothermic circulatory arrest is well tolerated by infants for as long as 60 minutes[28] and perhaps even longer if the period of circulatory arrest is interposed with short periods of low-flow reperfusion (50 mL/kg for 2 minutes).[32] Improvements in technology now make it easier to perform repair of complete AVSD in tiny infants using techniques of continuous CPB and moderate hypothermia as described previously. In tiny (<2.5 kg) infants, especially when there are anomalies in systemic venous return (such as LSVC), the use of brief periods of hypothermic circulatory arrest can greatly simplify cannulation and the technical features of the operation with minimal, if any, added risk.

Two-ventricular repair may not be possible in patients with unbalanced AVSD. Complete AVSD with aortic outflow obstruction resulting in a hypoplastic left ventricle may need to be palliated with a Norwood-type procedure. Other variants of unbalanced AVSDs are eventually staged to a univentricular Fontan circulation.

Persistent Left Superior Vena Cava

Some patients with AVSDs have persistence of the left SVC. This structure usually drains into the coronary sinus. This is not a problem if the intracardiac repair is performed under the conditions of deep hypothermic circulatory arrest. Otherwise, the extra venous drainage from the left SVC can be controlled with a cardiotomy sucker placed into the coronary sinus. In older children, another option is to selectively cannulate the left SVC where it is located near the left pulmonary artery. When a left SVC drains to the coronary sinus, the ASD patch must place the coronary sinus on the right atrial side, since diversion of the coronary sinus into the left atrium will produce a substantial right-to-left shunt.

Complete Atrioventricular Septal Defect with Tetralogy of Fallot

The combination of complete AVSD and tetralogy of Fallot (TOF) is rare, occurring in approximately 8% of patients with complete AVSD. The anterior and superior displacement of the infundibular septum results in the anterior extension of the inlet VSD into the subaortic region, overriding of the aorta, and subpulmonary stenosis. Although the ventricular component of the defect is large, the amount of pulmonary overcirculation and symptoms of heart failure may be limited due to the presence of RV outflow tract obstruction. As a result, corrective surgery can be delayed beyond infancy because surgical mortality was reported to be lower in older patients who undergo complete repair.[64] Occasionally, some patients will be cyanotic during infancy due to inadequate pulmonary blood flow. In these patients, initial palliation with a systemic to pulmonary shunt may be indicated to delay corrective repair until after infancy.

Repair of complete AVSD with TOF can be done using either the single- or the double-patch technique. The double-patch technique may allow better tailoring of the VSD patch near the subaortic region. This area of the VSD patch should be slightly oversized to minimize the potential of creating subaortic obstruction after repair. Although it is possible to close the VSD and perform infundibular resection all through the right atriotomy, this can result in a higher incidence of residual VSD.[21] The anterior portion of the VSD is easily visualized through the infundibular incision, which is made for relieving the RV outflow tract obstruction. In some patients, it is necessary to carry this incision across the pulmonary valve annulus to adequately enlarge the RV outflow tract. In these cases, it may be helpful to create a monocusp pulmonary valve to decrease the risk of substantial pulmonary valve insufficiency. Due to the large defect in the ventricular septum, some patients may have low cardiac output after repair and will need temporary mechanical circulatory support with extracorporeal membrane oxygenation.

POSTOPERATIVE CRITICAL CARE

Partial Atrioventricular Septal Defect

Management of these patients after surgery depends on their age, the type of defect repaired, and the preoperative physiology. Patients with partial AVSD usually have volume-loaded right ventricles from the left-to-right atrial level shunt and the effects of mitral insufficiency that is usually directed into the right atrium. However, closure of the defect and repair of the mitral valve eliminates this volume load and provides substantial improvement over the preoperative physiology. Occasionally, hemodynamically significant LVOT obstruction can result after repair of this defect.[17,58] In older patients who have adapted to the physiologic impact of the defect over years, there may be some RV dysfunction after repair, but patients usually recover quickly with minimal need for specialized postoperative care after partial AVSD repair. Infants may have a reactive pulmonary artery vasculature and may occasionally require mechanical hyperventilation for 12 to 24 hours until they adjust to the diminished RV volume load. It is not common for patients to have conduction abnormalities, but owing to the proximity of the AV nodal tissue to the area of surgical repair, varying degrees of heart block may be present and may require temporary AV sequential pacing. It is rarely indicated to leave permanent pacing wires on the heart, even if the patient is in complete heart block at the completion of the procedure, since this damage is rarely permanent, and normal conduction usually resumes within a few days of surgery. There is also a small incidence of junctional ectopic tachycardia after partial AVSD repairs. Patients who exhibit hemodynamic instability due to junctional ectopic tachycardia may benefit from atrial overdrive pacing and/or mild surface body cooling from 33 to 35° C. Amiodarone (5 to 15 mg/kg loading dose over 30 to 60 minutes follow by 5 to 15 µg/kg/min continuous intraveneous infusion) is becoming the drug of choice for the treatment of junctional ectopic tachycardia, although the Federal Drug Administration does not currently approve it for this purpose. Procainamide has also been demonstrated to be efficacious, although it has a higher incidence of proarrhythmic effects than amiodarone.

Patients who present with low cardiac output after partial AVSD repair may be demonstrating the effect of inadequate

myocardial protection during the repair. Significant ventricular hypertrophy may limit the ability of cardioplegic protection to preserve systolic function. This usually resolves with some inotropic therapy over 24 to 36 hours. Ventricular hypertrophy can also lead to postoperative diastolic dysfunction due to myocardial edema. Both postoperative systolic and diastolic dysfunction can be exacerbated by tachycardia. If low cardiac output persists beyond 48 hours, especially after repair of a partial AVSD, further investigation is warranted. Transthoracic or transesophageal echocardiography can be used to evaluate RV and LV function, as well as the presence of residual defects. It is important to look for LVOT obstruction, especially in patients with partial AVSDs. This can be caused by the attachments of the superior bridging leaflet onto the ventricular septum below the aortic valve and may require surgical intervention ranging from detachment of the valve attachments and repair of the ventricular septum to mitral valve excision and replacement.[16,33,34]

Complete Atrioventricular Septal Defects

Although it is not usually necessary to place pulmonary arterial or left atrial lines in patients who have had repair of partial AVSDs, the use of these lines is often desirable to enhance monitoring after repair of complete AVSDs. Even when these defects are repaired during infancy, pulmonary hypertensive episodes in the postoperative recovery period are not uncommon and can be readily diagnosed and treated if pulmonary artery pressures are monitored. The usual therapy for postoperative pulmonary hypertension is sedation and hyperventilation with 100% inspired oxygen until the patient has adjusted to the diminished RV load. Occasionally, it is helpful to fully paralyze the child to prevent patient-ventilator asynchrony. In extreme cases of pulmonary hypertension, nitric oxide can be added to the ventilator gas mixture to reduce pulmonary hypertension and thereby improve RV function. The left atrial line is useful for monitoring and optimizing LV preload and cardiac output.

Dysrhythmias are more common after repair of complete AVSDs, and placement of temporary atrial and ventricular pacing wires is essential. Varying degrees of heart block or junctional ectopic tachycardia may present in the immediate postoperative period and require treatment. Nevertheless, it is unusual for significant rhythm problems to persist beyond 3 to 5 days unless direct permanent damage has occurred to the conduction tissue.

It is not uncommon to see low cardiac output state following repair of complete AVSDs. Common clinical findings include persistent base deficit, lactic acidosis, cool extremities, and poor peripheral pulses and capillary refill. This is due not necessarily to inadequate myocardial protection during the repair but rather, at least in part, to the sudden change in physiology imparted by the repair. The afterload to the LV is increased after repair because the LV is no longer ejecting against the low resistance provided by mitral insufficiency or by the VSD. Instead, after repair of the defect, the LV is forced to eject exclusively against systemic vascular resistance. These patients need to be supported with inotropic agents during the postoperative period. Nevertheless, they usually recover quickly, especially if they undergo surgery during infancy. Inotropic therapy can usually be withdrawn within 24 to 48 hours. Because of the immense increase in LV afterload created by closure of the defect and repair of the mitral valve, milrinone is an excellent pharmacologic agent to consider for those patients with inadequate cardiac output and elevated systemic vascular resistance. Dopamine and epinephrine in low doses are also excellent inotropic agents when necessary. Because the use of inotropes may exacerbate tachycardia and dysrhythmias, patients with problematic rhythms should be weaned from inotropes as rapidly as possible.

Severe residual mitral insufficiency after repair of complete AVSD is no longer as common with the use of intraoperative echocardiography to assess the repair. Nevertheless, an occasional patient may have significant postoperative heart failure, failure to wean from mechanical ventilation, and severe insufficiency of the repaired mitral valve. The strategy to deal with this problem depends on whether the mitral insufficiency is due to an anatomically inadequate repair or to left ventricular dysfunction, AV valve annular dilatation, and elevated systemic vascular resistance. Options include taking the patient back to the operating room for mitral valve repair or replacement, treating the problem conservatively with inotropic support and afterload reduction, and allowing time for the ventricular function to improve. The results of mitral valve replacement in the immediate postoperative period are discouraging, and the incidence of permanent complete heart block is as high as 25%.[23] Therefore, the decision should be based on careful echocardiographic evaluation of the mitral abnormality, the physiologic response to inotropes and afterload reduction, as well as the patient's condition.

Left ventricular outflow tract obstruction is less of a problem after repair of complete AVSD, but it can cause low cardiac output. Residual intracardiac shunts are becoming less frequent with the use of intraoperative echocardiographic evaluation of the repair and immediate revision of any problems before the patient leaves the operating room. Occasionally, the combination of LV dysfunction, pulmonary hypertension, and mitral insufficiency due to elevated systemic vascular resistance can lead to low cardiac output after repair and require the use of temporary mechanical support with extracorporeal membrane oxygenation. Most patients can be weaned from inotropic therapy and mechanical ventilation within a few days after surgery.

OUTCOME

The risk of AVSD repair depends on the nature and extent of the lesion, as well as the presence of any associated malformations. The mortality rate associated with the repair of uncomplicated partial AVSDs, with minimal or no mitral incompetence, should be less than 2%.[28] The presence of significant preoperative mitral insufficiency increases this risk to 4%.[37,52] Repairing the partial AVSD, including repair of the mitral valve, usually will improve the amount of mitral regurgitation. This repair is quite durable, with excellent long-term results. However the overall long-term prognosis can be affected by late mitral valve functional deterioration and arrhythmias.[15,20,39,42] Long-term development of subaortic stenosis has also been reported and requires follow-up.[17,59]

The operative mortality rate for repair of complete AVSDs is highly inconsistent because of the wide variation in the anatomic patterns of this anomaly. With the refinement of current surgical techniques and preoperative and postoperative care, mortality following repair of complete AVSDs has dramatically improved. In fact, early correction (at younger than 4 months of age) before onset of heart failure can prevent annular dilatation of the common AV valve with a low reoperative rate for residual AV valve regurgitation.[59] The risk of repair is influenced by the nature of the common AV valve, adequacy of the size of the right and left ventricles,[28] presence of pulmonary hypertension, body weight of the patient, and preoperative nutritional status. Patients with Down syndrome have not been consistently shown to have an increased risk of mortality after repair of complete AVSDs, although they tend to have higher postoperative PVR[1,71] and worse hemodynamics when compared with patients without Down syndrome. Pulmonary hypertension with elevation of PVR can affect operative mortality in patients coming to surgical correction after 6 months of age (or even earlier in patients with Down syndrome).[19] Unless repair is undertaken by this age, it may be necessary to place a pulmonary artery band to limit pulmonary blood flow and protect the pulmonary vascular bed from progressing to irreversible damage. Although pulmonary artery banding is still applied with good success by some groups in small or seriously ill infants with complete AVSDs (with repair then deferred for 1 to 2 years),[55,70] current techniques allow safe and effective complete repair of this defect in most small infants as a one-stage procedure.* Long-term results are excellent, even for patients with Down syndrome[53] and especially for those patients with good mitral valve function. Survivors usually have excellent long-term outcome with good results.

References

1. Alt B, Shikes RH: Pulmonary hypertension in congenital heart disease: Irreversible vascular changes in young infants. *Pediatr Pathol* 1:423–434, 1983.
2. Anderson RH, Baker EJ, Rigby ML, Ebels T: The morphology and diagnosis of atrioventricular septal defects. *Cardiol Young* 1:290, 1991.
3. Bender HW Jr, Hammon JW Jr, Hubbard SG, et al: Repair of atrioventricular canal malformation in the first year of life. *J Thorac Cardiovasc Surg* 84:515–522, 1982.
4. Beppu S, Nimura Y, Sakakibara H, et al: Mitral cleft in ostium primum atrial septal defect assessed by cross-sectional echocardiography. *Circulation* 62:1099–1107, 1980.
5. Berg JM, Crome L, France NE: Congenital cardiac malformations in mongolism. *Br Heart J* 22:331, 1960.
6. Berger TJ, Blackstone EH, Kirklin JW, et al: Survival and probability of cure without and with operation in complete atrioventricular canal. *Ann Thorac Surg* 27:104–111, 1979.
7. Berger TJ, Kirklin JW, Blackstone EH, et al: Primary repair of complete atrioventricular canal in patients less than 2 years old. *Am J Cardiol* 41:906–913, 1978.
8. Bharati S, Kirklin JW, McAllister HA Jr, Lev M: The surgical anatomy of common atrioventricular orifice associated with tetralogy of Fallot, double outlet right ventricle and complete regular transposition. *Circulation* 61:1142–1149, 1980.
9. Bharati S, Lev M, Kirklin JW: *Cardiac Surgery and the Conduction System.* New York, Wiley, 1983.

*See references 3, 6, 13, 25, 26, 30, 31, 40, 41, 43, 60, and 63.

10. Bonow RO, Borer JS, Rosing DR, et al: Left ventricular functional reserve in adult patients with atrial septal defect: Pre and postoperative studies. *Circulation* 63:1315–1322, 1981.

11. Brannon ES, Weens HS, Warren JV: Atrial septal defect: Study of hemodynamics by technique of right heart catheterization. *Am J Med Sci* 210:480, 1945.

12. Carpentier A: Surgical anatomy and management of the mitral component of atrioventricular canal defects. In Anderson RH, Shinebourne EA (eds): *Pediatric Cardiology.* London, Churchill Livingstone, 1978, pp 477–490.

13. Castaneda AR, Mayer JE Jr, Jonas RA: Repair of complete atrioventricular canal in infancy. *World J Surg* 9:590–597, 1985.

14. Chikada M, Sekiguchi A, Miyamoto T, et al: Direct closure of ostium primum defect in the repair of atrioventricular septal defect. *Ann Thorac Surg* 72:430–433, 2001.

15. Crawford FA Jr, Stroud MR: Surgical repair of complete atrioventricular septal defect. *Ann Thorac Surg* 72:1621–1628, 2001.

16. Ebels T: Surgery of the left atrioventricular valve and the left ventricular outflow tract in atrioventricular septal defects. *Cardiol Young* 1:344, 1991.

17. Ebels T, Meijboom EJ, Anderson RH, et al: Anatomic and functional "obstruction" of the outflow tract in atrioventricular septal defects with separate valve orifices ("ostium primum atrial septal defect"): An echocardiographic study. *Am J Cardiol* 54:843–847, 1984.

18. Emanuel R, Somerville J, Inns A, Withers R: Evidence of congenital heart disease in the offspring of parents with atrioventricular defects. *Br Heart J* 49:144–147, 1983.

19. Frescura C, Thiene G, Franceschini E, et al: Pulmonary vascular disease in infants with complete atrioventricular septal defect. *Int J Cardiol* 15:91–103, 1987.

20. Goldfaden DM, Jones M, Morrow AG: Long-term results of repair of incomplete persistent atrioventricular canal. *J Thorac Cardiovasc Surg* 82:669–673, 1981.

21. Guo-wei H, Mee RBB: Complete atrioventricular canal associated with tetralogy of Fallot or double-outlet right ventricle and right ventricular outflow tract obstruction: A report of successful surgical treatment. *Ann Thorac Surg* 41:612–615, 1986.

22. Hines GL, Finnerty TT, Doyle E, Isom OW: Near fatal hemolysis following repair of ostium primum atrial septal defect. *J Cardiovasc Surg (Torino)* 19:7–10, 1978.

23. Kadoba K, Jonas RA: Replacement of the left atrioventricular valve after repair of atrioventricular canal. *J Thorac Cardiovasc Surg* 78:32–34, 1979.

24. Keith JD, Rowe RD, Vlad P: *Heart Disease in Infancy and Childhood.* New York, Macmillan, 1978.

25. Kirklin JW, Barratt-Boyes BG: *Cardiac Surgery.* New York, Wiley, 1986.

26. Kirklin JW, Blackstone EH: Management of the infant with complete atrioventricular canal. *J Thorac Cardiovasc Surg* 78:32–34, 1979.

27. Kirklin JW, Blackstone EH, Pacifico AD, et al: Routine primary repair vs two-stage repair of tetralogy of Fallot. *Circulation* 60:373–386, 1979.

28. Kirklin JW, Pacifico EH, Kirklin JK: The surgical treatment of atrioventricular canal defects. In Arciniegas E (ed): *Pediatric Cardiac Surgery.* Chicago, Mosby-Year Book, 1985, pp 155–170.

29. Kisslo JA, Adams DB, Belkin RN: *Doppler Color Flow Imaging.* New York, Churchill Livingstone, 1988.

30. Lacour-Gayet F, Comas J, Bruniaux J, et al: Management of the left atrioventricular valve in 95 patients with atrioventricular septal defects and a common atrioventricular orifice: Ten years' review. *Cardiol Young* 1:367, 1991.

31. Laks H, Capouya ER, Pearl JM, et al: The technique of management of the left atrioventricular valve in the repair of atrioventricular septal defect with a common atrioventricular valve. *Cardiol Young* 1:356, 1991.

32. Langley SM, Chai PJ, Miller SE, et al: Intermittent perfusion protects the brain during deep hypothermic circulatory arrest. *Ann Thorac Surg* 68:4–13, 1999.

33. Lappen RS, Muster AJ, Idriss FS, et al: Masked subaortic stenosis in ostium primum atrial septal defect: Recognition and treatment. *Am J Cardiol* 52:336–340, 1983.

34. LeCompte Y, Crupi G: Atrioventricular septal defect: The need for a flexible surgical approach in a lesion with markedly individual features. *Cardiol Young* 1:261, 1991.

35. Lev M: The architecture of the conduction system in congenital heart disease: I. Common atrioventricular orifice. *AMA Arch Pathol* 65:174, 1958.

36. Levin AR, Spach MS, Boineau JP, et al: Atrial pressure-flow dynamics in atrial septal defects (secundum type). *Circulation* 37:476–488, 1968.

37. Levy S, Blondeau P, Dubost C: Long-term follow-up after surgical correction of the partial form of atrioventricular canal (ostium primum). *J Thorac Cardiovasc Surg* 67:353–363, 1974.

38. Liberthson RR, Boucher CA, Strauss HW, et al: Right ventricular function in adult atrial septal defect: Preoperative and postoperative assessment and clinical implications. *Am J Cardiol* 47:56–60, 1981.

39. Losay J, Rosenthal A, Castaneda AR, et al: Repair of atrial septal defect primum. Results, course, and prognosis. *J Thorac Cardiovasc Surg* 75:248–254, 1978.

40. Mavroudis C, Weinstein G, Turley K, Ebert PA: Surgical management of complete atrioventricular canal. *J Thorac Cardiovasc Surg* 83:670–679, 1982.

41. McGrath LB, Gonzalez-Lavin L: Actuarial survival, freedom from reoperation, and other events after repair of atrioventricular septal defects. *J Thorac Cardiovasc Surg* 94:582–590, 1987.

42. Meijboom EJ, Ebels T, Anderson RH, et al: Left atrioventricular valve after surgical repair of atrioventricular septal defect with separate valve orifices ("ostium primum atrial septal defect"): An echo-Doppler study. *Am J Cardiol* 57:433–436, 1986.

43. Merrill WH, Hammon JW Jr, Bender HW Jr: Technique of repair of complete atrioventricular septal defect. *Cardiol Young* 1:379, 1991.

44. Michielon G, Stelin G, Rizzoli G, Casarotto DC: Repair of complete common atrioventricular canal defects in patients younger than four months of age. *Circulation* 96:II-316–322, 1997.

45. Mitchell SC, Korones SB, Berendes HW: Congenital heart disease in 56,109 births. Incidence and natural history. *Circulation* 43:323–332, 1971.

46. Newfeld EA, Waldman D, Paul MH, et al: Pulmonary vascular disease after systemic-pulmonary arterial shunt operations. *Am J Cardiol* 39:715–720, 1977.

47. Nicholson IA, Nunn GR, Sholler GF, et al: Simplified single patch technique for the repair of atrioventricular septal defect. *J Thorac Cardiovasc Surg* 118:642–647, 1999.

48. Pearlman AS, Borer JS, Clark CE, et al: Abnormal right ventricular size and ventricular septal motion after atrial septal defect closure: Etiology and functional significance. *Am J Cardiol* 41:295–301, 1978.

49. Rahimtoola SH, Kirklin JW, Burchell HB: Atrial septal defect. *Circulation* 38:2–12, 1968.

50. Rastelli G, Kirklin JW, Titus JL: Anatomic observations on complete form of persistent common atrioventricular canal with special reference to atrioventricular valves. *Mayo Clin Proc* 41:296–308, 1966.

51. Rastelli GC: *Atrioventricular Canal Defects.* Philadelphia, WB Saunders, 1976.

52. Rastelli GC, Weidman WH, Kirklin JW: Surgical repair of the partial form of persistent common atrioventricular canal, with special reference to the problem of mitral valve incompetence. *Circulation* 31/32(suppl I): I–31, 1965.

53. Rizzoli G, Mazzucco A, Maizza F, et al: Does Down syndrome affect prognosis of surgically managed atrioventricular canal defects? *J Thorac Cardiovasc Surg* 104:945–953, 1992.

54. Sayd HM, Dacie JV, Handley DA, et al: Hemolytic anemia of mechanical origin after open heart surgery. *Thorax* 16:356, 1961.

55. Silverman N, Levitsky S, Fisher E, et al: Efficacy of pulmonary artery banding in infants with complete atrioventricular canal. *Circulation* 68:148–153, 1983.

56. Somerville J: Ostium primum defects: Factors causing deterioration in the natural history. *Br Heart J* 27:413, 1965.

57. Studer M, Blackstone EH, Kirklin JW, et al: Determinants of early and late results of repair of atrioventricular septal (canal) defects. *J Thorac Cardiovasc Surg* 84:523–542, 1982.

58. Sugimura S, Okies JE, Litchford B, Starr A: Late results of mitral cleft closure for ostium primum atrial septal defect in adolescents and adults. *Am Surg* 45:670–675, 1979.

59. Taylor NC, Somerville J: Fixed subaortic stenosis after repair of ostium primum defects. *Br Heart J* 45:689–697, 1981.

60. Ungerleider RM: The use of intraoperative epicardial echocardiography with color flow imaging during the repair of complete atrioventricular septal defects. *Cardiol Young* 2:56, 1992.

61. Ungerleider RM, Greeley WJ, Sheikh KH, et al: The use of intraoperative echo with Doppler color flow imaging to predict outcome after repair of congenital cardiac defects. *Ann Surg* 210:526–533, 1989.

62. Ungerleider RM, Greeley WJ, Sheikh KH, et al: Routine use of intraoperative epicardial echocardiography and Doppler color flow imaging to guide and evaluate repair of congenital heart lesions: A prospective study. *J Thorac Cardiovasc Surg* 100:297–309, 1990.

63. Ungerleider RM, Kisslo JA, Greeley WJ, et al: Intraoperative prebypass and postbypass epicardial color flow imaging in the repair of atrioventricular septal defects. *J Thorac Cardiovasc Surg* 98:90–99, 1989.

64. Uretzky G, Puga FJ, Danielson GK, et al: Complete atrioventricular canal associated with tetralogy of Fallot: Morphologic and surgical considerations. *J Thorac Cardiovasc Surg* 87:756–766, 1984.

65. Verdon TA Jr, Forrester RH, Crosby WH: Hemolytic anemia after open-heart surgery of ostium primum defects. *N Engl J Med* 269:444, 1963.

66. Waldenhausen JA, Tyers GFO: Atrial septal defects, ostium primum defects, and atrioventricular canals. In Sabiston DC Jr (ed): *Textbook of Surgery*, 13th ed. Philadelphia, WB Saunders, 1986.

67. Wanderman KL, Ovsyshcher I, Gueron M: Left ventricular performance in patients with atrial septal defect: Evaluation with noninvasive methods. *Am J Cardiol* 41:487–493, 1978.

68. Wilcox BR, Jones DR, Frantz EG, et al: Anatomically sound, simplified approach to repair of "complete" atrioventricular septal defect. *Ann Thorac Surg* 64:487–494, 1997.

69. Williams RG, Rudd M: Echocardiographic features of endocardial cushion defects. *Circulation* 49:418–422, 1974.

70. Williams WH, Guyton RA, Michalik RE, et al: Individualized surgical management of complete atrioventricular canal. *J Thorac Cardiovasc Surg* 86:838–844, 1983.

71. Yamaki S, Horiuchi T, Sekino Y: Quantitive analysis of pulmonary vascular disease in simple cardiac anomalies with Down syndrome. *Am J Cardiol* 51:1502–1506, 1983.

72. Young D: Later results of closure of secundum atrial septal defect in children. *Am J Cardiol* 31:14–22, 1973.

Chapter 26

Left Ventricular Outflow Tract Obstruction

JAMES D. ST. LOUIS, MD, and JAMES JAGGERS, MD

Left ventricular (LV) outflow tract (LVOT) obstruction (LVOTO) may be defined as an obstruction to the flow of blood from the systemic ventricle to the ascending aorta that occurs as a result of a defect present at birth. The obstructive process can occur at any level of the systemic ventricular outflow tract, including the aorta. LVOTO often presents with numerous associated anomalies, including coarctation of the aorta, patent ductus arteriosus, ventricular septal defects, pulmonary stenosis, and mitral stenosis.[24] LV chamber size can also be affected. Infants with LVOTO may have relative hypoplasia of the left ventricle and diffuse endothelial scarring that is also termed endocardial fibroelastosis (EFE). The clinical presentation of LVOTO depends on the anatomic site of obstruction, the age at which the child presents, and the associated cardiac abnormalities. The obstructive process can be classified based on the level of the narrowing of the LVOT. These anatomic classifications include valvular, supravalvular, and subvalvular stenosis. A fourth form, caused by hypertrophy of the interventricular septum, presents as a

unique variety of subvalvular obstructions that varies in its physiology and treatment from other forms of stenotic lesions.

Valvular aortic stenosis is the most common anatomic type, with deformities of both number and structure of the valve leaflets. Subvalvular aortic stenosis consists of a discrete membrane or muscular tunnel below the aortic valve. This type of obstruction will usually present in early adulthood with increasing exercise intolerance. Supravalvular aortic stenosis is equivalent to coarctation of the aorta with narrowing of the ascending aorta just distal to the aortic valve. Several inherited syndromes are often seen in association with this defect.

VALVULAR AORTIC STENOSIS

Historical Aspects

Stenosis of the aortic valve was initially described by Riverius in 1646 and then by Morgagni in 1769.[13] However, it was not until 1844 that the congenital etiology of this form of stenosis was detailed by Paget's description of a bicuspid aortic valve.[27] Tuffier first successfully dilated a calcified aortic valve, thus demonstrating that it was possible to restore flow through the normal anatomic pathway. The first open cardiac procedures were performed for this lesion utilizing direct vision valvotomy of stenotic aortic valves during a brief period of vena caval occlusion.[38] Spencer and colleagues[36] initially described open aortic valvotomy utilizing cardiopulmonary bypass in 1958.

Natural History, Clinical Presentation, and Diagnosis

Abnormalities of the aortic valve leaflets account for 70% to 80% of LVOTO. Stenosis of the aortic valve can present at any age, from the neonatal period to late adulthood. Valvular stenosis is three to four times more common in male than in female patients. The natural history is influenced by the age at presentation and morphology of the valve.

Patients who present during the early neonatal period with critical aortic stenosis are usually in cardiogenic shock with severe hypoperfusion and profound acidosis. Critical aortic stenosis in the neonate is a serious, life-threatening lesion that is significantly different than aortic stenosis as it

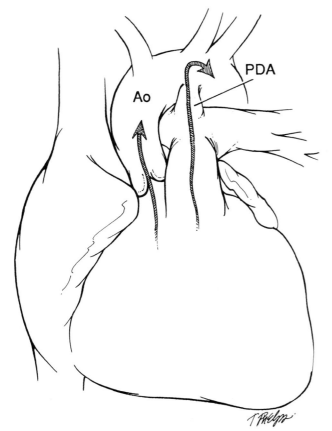

FIGURE 26-1 The physiology of critical aortic stenosis in the neonate is such that the patent ductus arteriosus (PDA) can provide a substantial amount of blood flow to the aorta (Ao) by shunting right ventricular output right to left. This ductal-level shunt is helpful in maintaining systemic perfusion and decompressing pulmonary hypertension (which may exist until the left ventricular outflow obstruction is relieved).

is commonly understood in older patients. This presentation results from the limited antegrade flow of blood across the LVOT and closure of the ductus arteriosus (Fig. 26-1). Severe systemic hypoperfusion results without intervention. Individuals who present during this period often have anomalies of the mitral valve, hypoplasia of the LV cavity, hypoplasia of the subaortic LVOT, and coarctation of the distal aorta.

Children who present after one year of age initially have little in the way of symptoms and generally manifest only mild exercise intolerance. These children do, however, have an increased risk of developing bacterial endocarditis on the abnormal valves and an ongoing risk of sudden death. The degree of stenosis present in children at the time of diagnosis predicts their likelihood of developing severe obstruction; only 20% of mild lesions progress in severity within 10 years, as opposed to 60% of moderate lesions that become severe within that time.

The valve leaflet morphology also dictates the presentation of the individual and the need for early intervention. In patients with stenosis severe enough to require operation in infancy or early childhood, the valve is bicuspid in approximately 70% of cases and consists of thickened leaflets with fusion of the anterior and posterior commissure and a slit-like orifice. In approximately 30% of cases, the valve is tricuspid, with three thickened leaflets of equal size and three recognizable

commissures that are fused peripherally to varying degrees, creating a dome with a central stenotic orifice.[30] Rarely, the valve is unicuspid with only one commissure. This morphology is more common in infants presenting with severe stenosis, but occasionally the stenosis is not severe, and signs and symptoms develop in later life as the valve thickens and calcifies.

Preoperative Critical Care Management

Neonates

As stated, the course of treatment largely depends on the degree of obstruction to forward flow from the left ventricle and the presence of systemic hypoperfusion. Neonates that present in florid heart failure and cardiac collapse require emergent treatment and intervention. If the ductus arteriosus is closed, these infants demonstrate all the signs of severe low cardiac output with cold extremities, diminished pulses, pulmonary edema, acidosis, and tachypnea. When the diagnosis of critical aortic stenosis has been made in the neonate, prostaglandin E_1 should be started to reestablish ductal-dependent systemic flow (see Fig. 26-1).

Reestablishing ductal blood flow not only restores systemic perfusion by shunting blood right to left, but also alleviates the pulmonary hypertension seen with severe LV dysfunction. Intubation and mechanical ventilation may also be required to assist in correction of severe acidosis and to aid in the control of the pulmonary hypertension. Laboratory examination reveals hypoxia with acidosis due to congested pulmonary vasculature and low cardiac output. Hypoxia is caused by the pulmonary congestion associated with LV outflow obstruction as well as the shunting of deoxygenated blood across the ductus. Acidosis is a sign of a compromised circulation and indicates inadequate cardiac output to supply tissue demands.

The use of inotropic drugs such as dopamine and epinephrine increases the inotropic response of the ventricle and aids in resuscitation of the infant. In some cases, when the left ventricle is inadequate or the LVOT is severely stenotic, the infant requires the presence of an atrial-level shunt to decompress the pulmonary venous return over to the right side of the heart. When there is no atrial communication in these patients, pulmonary hypertension may be severe and associated with rapid postnatal deterioration. Resuscitation in these unusual circumstances may require emergent atrial septostomy or even management with extracorporeal life support (e.g., extracorporeal membrane oxygenation). When infants have been adequately resuscitated, a semi-elective procedure for relief of the obstruction can be planned.

In neonates with critical aortic stenosis, it is important to determine whether the left heart and aortic structures are compatible with a two-ventricle repair. In this regard, *neonatal critical aortic stenosis* describes a spectrum or continuum of lesions that range from normal left heart and aorta anatomy, except for a stenotic aortic valve, to a variant of hypoplastic left heart syndrome with diminutive left-sided structures that are not capable of sustaining systemic circulation. The decision of whether to attempt to incorporate the small left ventricle and associated abnormal structures into a biventricular repair versus a single-ventricle palliation can be difficult. The decision has often been based on echocardiographic information regarding the ventricular size and the presence of additional left-sided obstructive lesions such as mitral stenosis and coarctation of the aorta. Infants with an LV volume of less than 20 mL/m^2, LV inflow dimension less than 25 mm, endocardial fibroelastosis, or an aortic valve annulus less than 5 mm in diameter have been shown to have poor outcomes with biventricular repair. In these infants, the ability of the left ventricle to adequately participate in the circulation is marginal. It may be more prudent for the infant to be staged toward a univentricular repair.

Quantification of the severity of aortic stenosis in the neonate is also problematic. Gradients across the aortic valve cannot be accurately assessed in the presence of a patent ductus arteriosus. Furthermore, ventricular function is often severely depressed, with the majority of the systemic flow being provided by the ductus. Consequently, the outflow across the aortic valve is not a true reflection of cardiac output, and, in the most severe cases, the output across the aortic valve may be negligible. Therefore, the gradient across the aortic valve may be lowest when the aortic stenosis is most severe. Mitral insufficiency is often present and can contribute to false estimations of the transvalvular gradient. Doppler velocity cannot provide an accurate index of valve orifice area because of variable transvalvular flow. The aortic valvuvar stenosis often coexists with other left-sided obstructive lesions such as coarctation, which can result in overestimation of the clinical severity of the valvuvar stenosis.

Rhodes and colleagues[29] attempted to resolve this dilemma by evaluating several echocardiographically measured left-sided heart structures and determining which were associated with an adverse outcome. The intent was to determine which patients with critical aortic stenosis and small left-sided structure would be candidates for two-ventricle repair and which would be better served with a single-ventricle palliative approach.[29] Four variables seemed to have predictive value: (1) LV/heart long axis ratio of 0.8 or less, (2) indexed aortic root area of 3.5 cm^2/m^2 or less, (3) indexed mitral valve area of 4.75 cm^2/m^2 or less, and (4) LV mass index of 35 g/m^2 or less. When taken alone, each of these variables did not have any predictive value for biventricular repair. However, when two or more of these variables were present, there was 95% predicted mortality when a biventricular repair was attempted. Other factors that have been identified as possible predictors for increased mortality after a two-ventricle repair in the neonate and infant include mean pulmonary artery pressure, LV peak systolic pressure, LV end-diastolic pressure, peak transvalvular gradient, LV end-diastolic volume, and ejection fraction.[14]

Recently, Lofland and colleagues[21] described a standardized formula for predicting outcome in neonates who present with critical aortic stenosis. In a multi-institutional study of 320 neonates, using predictions from separate multivariable hazard models for survival of either biventricular repair or single-ventricle palliation, the authors determined the predicted optimal pathway and survival benefit for each patient. Independent factors associated with greater survival benefit for the Norwood procedure versus a biventricular repair included younger age at entry, lower aortic valve z-score, LV length, higher grade of endocardial fibroelastosis, absence of important tricuspid regurgitation, and large ascending aorta. A prediction of survival at 5 years could be calculated for all patients. Their final result was a multiple linear regression

equation that predicted the magnitude and the direction of the survival benefit for the optimal pathway. The regression equation can be solved for characteristics of an individual patient to give the predicted 5-year survival benefit of a univentricular palliation versus a biventricular repair.

In neonates with critical aortic valvular stenosis who are selected for biventricular repair, valvotomy has been the mainstay of initial therapy. Historically, open surgical valvotomy and resection of redundant tissue with or without the aid of cardiopulmonary bypass had been considered the standard approach for these critically ill infants. There was concern regarding the published high mortality using this approach. In retrospect, this likely reflected the clinical condition of these infants prior to these procedures and the lack of any substantive resuscitation measures.[8] Percutaneous balloon dilatation has become a dependable alternative to open surgical valvotomy, and, in fact, balloon valvuloplasty is considered by most centers to be the procedure of choice in the neonate with critical aortic stenosis. Although randomized, prospective comparisons of these two treatments have not been performed, multi-institutional comparisons have been reviewed.

McCrindle and coworkers,[22] in association with the Congenital Heart Surgeons Society, reviewed the cases of 320 patients with critical aortic stenosis in a prospective nonrandomized study of 18 institutions. The study compared outcomes of patients who underwent either a surgical or a percutaneous balloon aortic valvotomy. Only those patients (110) whose initial procedure was a valvotomy, indicating an intended biventricular repair, were evaluated. The initial procedure was a surgical valvotomy in 28 patients and a transcatheter balloon aortic valvotomy in 82 patients. Early results revealed that surgical patients had a lower mean percent change in their peak instantaneous systolic gradient and a higher median residual peak instantaneous systolic gradient. Patients who had a balloon valvotomy had a significant trend toward higher grades of aortic regurgitation after the procedure. A similar proportion of patients in each group died before hospital discharge. A higher proportion of patients in the surgical group required reintervention for aortic valve dysfunction. Midterm survival between the two groups was identical. These results indicated that the outcomes of surgical versus percutaneous balloon aortic valvotomy in neonates with critical aortic stenosis have comparable mortality and risk of reintervention, even after adjustment for differences in patient characteristics.

This multi-institutional study does support the sole use of balloon dilatation for neonatal critical aortic stenosis as a primary treatment. Although the use of a catheter-based palliation has certainly been justified by this study, several other well-constructed retrospective reviews have confirmed the efficacy and safety of open valvotomy in properly resuscitated patients. Hawkins and colleagues[15] reviewed the midterm results of 37 infants with critical aortic stenosis who had undergone an open surgical valvotomy. Actuarial survival at 1 and 10 years was 78% + 9% and 73% + 10%, respectively. The actuarial freedom from reintervention postoperatively was demonstrated as 97% at 1 month, 73% at 1 year, and 55% at 11 years. These results are certainly acceptable in terms of both survival and need of reintervention when compared with balloon dilatation. Alexiou and colleagues[1] reviewed the cases of 18 consecutive neonates with critical isolated aortic stenosis who underwent open valvotomy at a mean age of 9 days. There were no operative deaths. At discharge, the mean aortic valve gradient was 37.2 mm Hg, with six patients having mild, and two, moderate aortic regurgitation. Midterm survival was comparable to balloon dilatation. Because of lack of randomized prospective studies evaluating the various treatment options, surgical valvotomy can still be considered an option for relief of valvular aortic stenosis in the neonate, although it is clear that both nonrandomized prospective and retrospective data have not clearly delineated an advantage to one procedure over the other.

Individual patient characteristics, as well as institutional expertise, should dictate which procedure a particular center should consider as first-line therapy. It does seem clear that survivors of neonatal valvotomy, regardless of how it is performed, will most likely come to further surgical intervention within 10 years,[12] and recent, unpublished data reviewing a large cohort of patients from Oregon suggest that infants left with aortic insufficiency may come to surgical intervention (valve replacement) sooner than those left with predominantly aortic stenosis following valvotomy. Considering the palliative nature of valvotomy and the fact that a majority of patients will require surgical intervention for their aortic valve within 10 years, careful balloon valvotomy performed in the cardiac catheterization laboratory (with an attentiveness to limit the creation of aortic insufficiency) offers the advantage of limiting the number of surgical interventions.

Older Infants and Children

Aortic stenosis that presents beyond the neonatal age is a less critical issue. These patients, by virtue of having survived, have essentially demonstrated adequacy of their left heart–aorta complex. Intervention is indicated when the pressure gradient (peak-to-peak) across the valve exceeds 50 mm Hg or when the patient has symptoms such as syncope or chest pain related to the aortic stenosis. Once again, these patients may be treated with either surgical or balloon valvotomy performed in the cardiac catheterization laboratory. In older children or young adults, in whom the annulus has become heavily calcified, valve replacement is certainly a reasonable consideration as a first-line procedure in lieu of valvotomy.

Surgical Treatment: Aortic Valvotomy

Surgical valvotomy is performed via a median sternotomy with cardiopulmonary bypass and cardioplegic cardiac arrest (Fig. 26-2). Cannulation for cardiopulmonary bypass (CPB) is carried out with a standard aortic cannula and single venous cannula in the right atrial appendage. The ductus is ligated with a heavy tie. The aorta is cross-clamped, and cardioplegia is administered. The ascending aorta is opened transversely, approximately 1 cm above the right coronary artery. In infants, the valve leaflets are usually extremely dysplastic. If discrete commissural fusion is detectable (as it often is in older patients), a scalpel blade is used to incise the fused commissures to within 2 mm of the aortic annulus. Overzealous incision of the commissures or division of a nonexistent or rudimentary raphe may result in gross aortic insufficiency. Some authorities recommend more aggressive reconstructive techniques to restore tricommissural function

to abnormal valves in older children, but the long-term outcome for these patients is still in question.[3] One must also pay special attention to the subaortic area and rule out the presence of additional subaortic obstruction. If present, this must also be excised. The results of a precise commissurotomy can be long lasting if there is adequate development of the valve. When severe deformity and maldevelopment of the valve are present, surgical relief is only temporary and should be considered palliative. This latter scenario is most often the case in neonates who present with critical heart failure.

Critical Care Management Following Valvotomy

The requirements for postoperative care depend on the severity of the lesion, the preoperative condition, the associated defects, and the age of the patient. Neonates who require urgent valvotomy may have significant pulmonary hypertension in the postoperative period that can last several days. They may have low cardiac output, manifested by poor peripheral perfusion and mild to moderate acidosis. They are best managed with inotropes to improve cardiac function, sedation, and hyperventilation with high concentrations of inspired oxygen to treat the pulmonary vascular reactivity. Recent published data support the use of inhaled nitric oxide to treat the pulmonary hypertension in patients with extremely poor LV compliance. In patients with significant pulmonary hypertension or questionable ability of the left ventricle to support the systemic circulation, it is occasionally reasonable to leave the ductus arteriosus patent with infusion of prostaglandin for a few postoperative days.[39] In these infants, a patent ductus in the immediate postoperative period helps maintain systemic perfusion and decompress the pulmonary artery hypertension while LV compliance improves.

In selected patients who fail valvotomy because of anatomic limitations at the aortic annulus and who have adequate mitral valves and left ventricles, a neonatal aortic valve replacement, usually as a Ross-Konno, can be life saving and very effective. Because of the difficulties that can be encountered in the postoperative course, neonates who undergo operative valvotomy should have right atrial, pulmonary artery, and left atrial lines placed in the operating room. If ductal patency is still required beyond 3 to 5 days, the adequacy of the LVOT to provide systemic function should be questioned. Failure of the pulmonary hypertension to resolve and continued poor systemic perfusion may be an indication that the child's associated lesions may prohibit adequate left-sided heart function. In this case, alternative therapeutic options should be entertained, such as the use of postoperative extracorporeal membrane oxygenation (if it is thought that the pulmonary hypertension is reversible and the underlying anatomy is acceptable for normal function); staging toward a Fontan procedure (with a Norwood-type repair, if it is thought that the underlying left-sided heart-to-aorta complex is not consistent with normal function); or placement of the patient on a heart transplant list.

Older infants and children are usually much easier to care for in the postoperative period. Their response to valvotomy is usually uncomplicated, and they can be guided through their postoperative recovery quickly. The major risk factors for older children are the occasional neurologic complications,

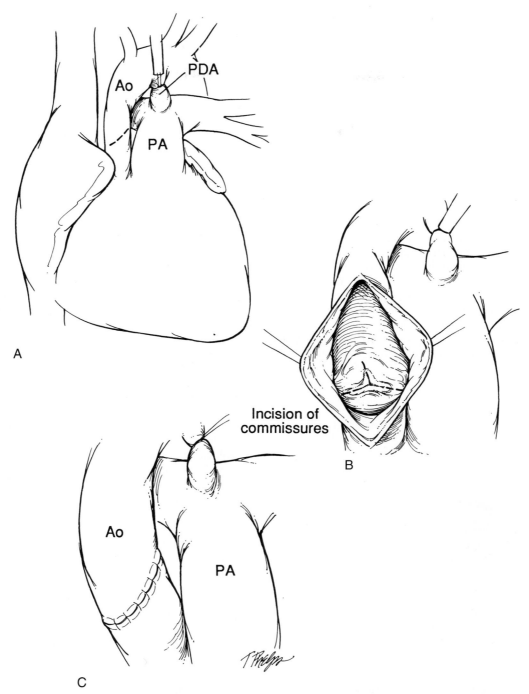

FIGURE 26-2 **A,** In neonates with critical aortic stenosis, the heart is approached through a median sternotomy. The pulmonary artery (PA) often appears to be distended and much larger than the aorta (Ao). In fact, in severe cases the Ao may be only 5 to 7 mm in diameter. Valvotomy is performed on cardiopulmonary bypass by cannulating the ascending Ao and the right atrium (not shown). The patent ductus arteriosus (PDA) (which can be quite large) is controlled with a snare. **B,** An aortotomy is performed, revealing the stenotic aortic valve. The line of commissural fusion is appreciated and opened with a knife blade so that the commissurotomy extends to but not into the annulus. **C,** The aortotomy is closed, and the patient is weaned from cardiopulmonary bypass. The ductus arteriosus can be tied securely at the completion of the procedure unless, in unique circumstances, it is felt prudent to leave the ductus open with the patient on prostaglandin E_1 for a few postoperative days.

which are usually first recognized in the intensive care unit, and the potential for rhythm disturbances (such as third-degree heart block) that necessitate cardiac monitoring.

It is hoped that valvotomy will reduce the aortic valve gradient and enable the child to grow. It has been predicted that as many as 35% of patients who have undergone either a balloon or surgical valvotomy will require some sort of procedure on their LVOT within 10 years. Reasons for repeat operation range from recurrent stenosis to progressive aortic insufficiency. Typical freedom from reintervention following valvotomy is 7 years.[18]

Aortic Valve Replacement

Eventually, many children who undergo neonatal or infant aortic valvotomy will require aortic valve replacement. In a previous era, when mechanical valves were the predominant valve replacement option for children, a typical strategy was to delay valve replacement as long as possible. This enables the child to grow to a size large enough to allow placement of an adult-size prosthesis. With the increased use of nonmechanical valve replacement therapy, early repair has been advocated.

Mechanical Valves

Mechanical valves have numerous disadvantages that discourage their use in children. These include lifestyle limitations due to the need for indefinite anticoagulation, bleeding and thrombotic complications, somatic outgrowth of the valve (when it is placed in young children), hemodynamic limitations imposed by valves that are too small, the need for extensive annular enlargement procedures when the valve is placed in small children (Fig. 26-3), and the continued risk of endocarditis and perivalvular leaks, which necessitate reoperation. As a result, prosthetic mortality and morbidity rates have tended to be higher in children undergoing valve replacement than in adults.[16,32,33] Several centers have reported excellent results with some forms of antiplatelet therapy for children with mechanical aortic prosthesis.[41] Nevertheless, the multiple limitations and risks of mechanical valves make them an unattractive option for children.

Bioprosthetic Valves

After initial early enthusiasm for their use, it is now well demonstrated that bioprosthetic valves may undergo early

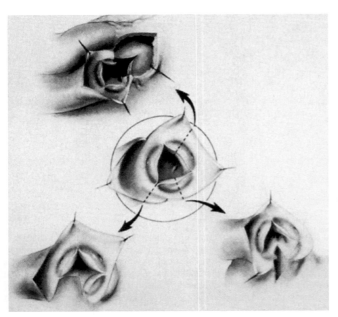

FIGURE 26-3 The locations around the aortic annulus where it is safe to make an incision for annular enlargement. An incision in the commissure between the left and noncoronary cusps (*lower left*) will extend onto the anterior leaflet of the mitral valve. This Manougian annular enlargement can be repaired with a patch and enlarges the annulus by 2 to 3 mm. Likewise, the Nicks enlargement (*lower right*) extends into the roof of the left atrium and, once repaired with a patch, enlarges the annulus by 2 to 3 mm. The Konno Rastan aortoventriculoplasty (*upper left*) is created with an incision across the interventricular septum, between the right and left coronary arteries, and can create annular enlargement of >1 cm when necessary.

degeneration in children and young adults. Allografts had been considered an excellent option for LV reconstruction in children because of superior hemodynamics and freedom from anticoagulation. Recent studies, however, have documented an accelerated rate for tissue calcification and degeneration in young children and infants.[10,43] Because of the lack of growth potential and the inability to oversize the graft in small children and infants, replacement of the allograft is often required. For these reasons and the difficulties associated with mechanical valve replacement, interest in use of autografts for aortic valve replacement has been renewed.

Pulmonary Autograft (Ross Procedure)

The use of pulmonary autografts (Ross procedure) for reconstruction of the LVOT has undergone an evolution over recent years. It was less than 2 decades ago that age younger than 3 years was considered a relative contraindication to the Ross procedure. With several centers providing midterm experience and ever-growing experience with the arterial switch operation, routine use of the pulmonary autograft has become common for LVOT reconstruction. Several distinct advantages exist over other replacement options. Because the pulmonary autograft is the patient's own living tissue, the potential for continued growth of the graft exists. There does exist controversy as to whether this observed growth of the autograft involves a pathologic process of annular dilatation or somatic growth of the graft. Animal studies have shown an increase in both volume and weight of the pulmonary autograft when it is placed in the higher pressured systemic circulation.[34] Histologic specimens from these studies demonstrated an increase in collagen content, which accounted for the weight increase. These studies also indicated that a certain amount of annular dilatation does occur but that it occurs very early and is not of clinical significance. Clinical studies by Solymar and associates[35] have documented two phases of valve enlargement. First, an early period occurs within 6 months of surgery. This period correlates with the initial dilatation of the annulus seen in previous studies. The second phase occurs at a much slower rate, over a period of several years. This phase correlates with the somatic growth of the child and continues at a rate similar to that observed in a control group, which most likely corresponds with normal growth. Further concern exists regarding the potential for significant autograft dysfunction in the face of preoperative aortic valve insufficiency and the existence of a bicuspid aortic valve.[34]

Laudito and colleagues[20] reviewed their experience with 72 patients who had undergone a Ross procedure. The majority of these patients were younger than 15 years. Seven patients required reoperation because of severe neoaortic insufficiency. Moderate insufficiency was identified in five additional patients. Among the seven patients requiring reoperation, six had operative findings consistent with dilatation of the aortic annulus, dilatation of the sinotubular junction, and lack of central leaflet coaptation. All patents who required reoperation had as the primary preoperative diagnosis either aortic insufficiency or the dominant physiologic defect of a combined lesion. Of the possible preoperative risk factors, including preoperative aortic stenosis (AS), gender, aortic valve annulus size, pulmonary valve–to–aortic valve mismatch, aortic cross-clamp time, total bypass time, and previous aortic valve repair, only preoperative aortic insufficiency was statistically significant for postoperative autograft failure. The authors concluded that although the preoperative diagnosis of aortic insufficiency is not an absolute contraindication to the Ross procedure in the pediatric population, it needs to be considered a risk factor for reoperation, and the procedure should be applied on an individual basis.

Several surgical techniques were initially developed for implantation of the pulmonary autograft into the LVOT. Ross's original description for transplantation of the patient's own pulmonary valve complex into the LVOT was in the subcoronary position.[9] This procedure was technically demanding, requiring precise alignment of the commissures to prevent autograft incompetence. The lack of success many experienced

with this technique led to an initial reluctance to use the autograft in infants and young children.

Currently, a modified version of the Ross technique has gained widespread acceptance for complex outflow tract reconstruction. It involves the complete aortic root replacement with the reimplantation of the coronary ostia into the autograft (Fig. 26-4). When subaortic obstruction coexists with valvular pathology, a Konno operation can be used in combination with replacement with the autograft (Fig. 26-5).

The Ross procedure is performed via a median sternotomy, hypothermic cardiopulmonary bypass, and intermittent cold-blood cardioplegia (see Fig. 26-4). The aortic pathology is excised, and root enlargement (or fixation) is undertaken if necessary. The pulmonary artery is opened via a transverse

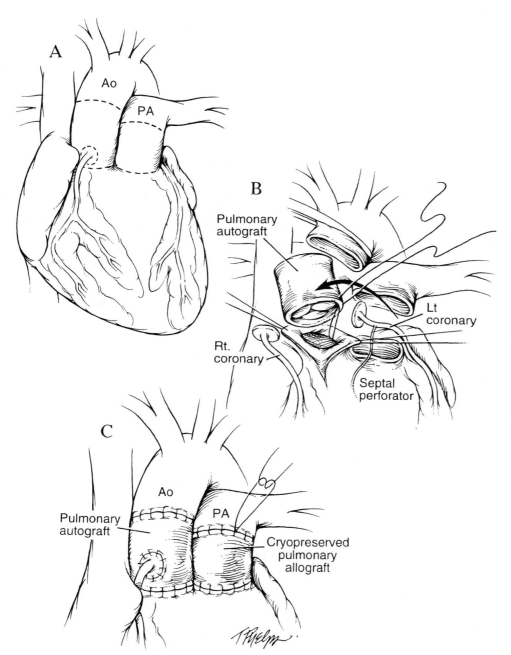

FIGURE 26-4 Ross procedure. **A,** Great arteries are transected above the sinotubular ridge. Aortic sinuses are excised and coronary arteries are mobilized. **B,** Pulmonary autograft is excised from the right ventricular outflow tract to avoid injury to the septal perforator branches of the left coronary artery. The proximal end of the autograft is anastomosed to the annulus with interrupted or continuous sutures. **C,** The coronary arteries are anastomosed to the pulmonary autograft. Autograft-to-aorta (Ao) anastomosis is completed and the right ventricular outflow tract is reconstructed usually with a cryopreserved pulmonary allograft. PA, pulmonary artery.

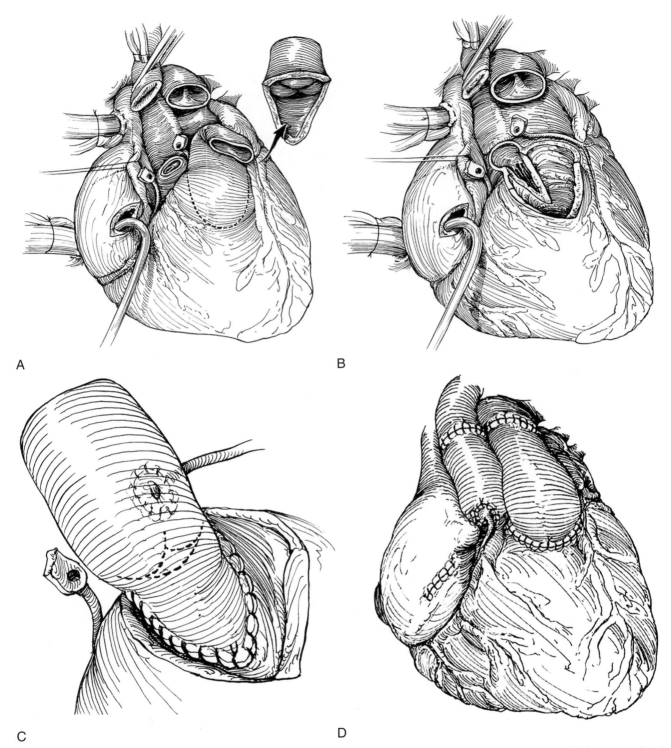

FIGURE 26-5   The Ross-Konno procedure is performed by (**A**) harvesting the pulmonary valve with an extra "tongue" of infundibular muscle after the aorta has been divided and the coronary arteries removed as buttons. **B,** An incision is then made across the infundibular septum by cutting into the septum between the right and left coronary arteries. This is especially easy to visualize after the pulmonary autograft has been removed. **C,** The pulmonary autograft is then anastomosed to the aortic root using the infundibular muscle to repair the interventricular septal defect. The coronary arteries are placed into this neoaorta. **D,** The procedure is completed with a pulmonary homograft to repair the right ventricular outflow tract.

incision just proximal to the bifurcation. The valve is inspected, and if no leaflet pathology is observed, the pulmonary artery is transected and the autograft harvested. The most tedious portion of the procedure is the precise harvesting of the pulmonary valve and its supporting structure. Great care must be taken so as to not injure the left main coronary artery

or its first perforating branch. The dissection is begun on the posterior aspect of the right ventricular outflow tract in a plane between the pulmonary artery and the left main coronary artery. The dissection is carried down into the outflow tract until muscle is reached. The pulmonary artery is then dissected off the aorta, taking care not to injure the right coronary artery. An infundibular incision is then made approximately 0.5 cm below the pulmonary valve annulus (unless a Konno operation is planned, in which case additional infundibular muscle is taken; see Fig. 26-5). This incision is then taken to the left until the prior posterior dissection is encountered. The dissection is then completed to the right. The autograft is removed and the muscle bed is inspected for small coronary artery branches, which need to be coagulated or ligated, as they can be a source of postoperative bleeding. The autograft is then implanted into the LVOT at the annular level, with either a running or an interrupted suture technique.

Some surgeons believe that the proximal suture line should be reinforced with a circumferential Dacron pledget to prevent annular dilatation, especially in patients with an enlarged aortic annulus. The coronary ostia are reimplanted into the autograft, and the distal anastomosis is completed. Next, the right ventricular outflow tract is reconstructed with a homograft in a standard fashion. The heart is then de-aired, and the cross-clamp is removed. In older patients who have annular dilatation and aortic insufficiency, an inclusion technique, which enables implantation of the autograft within the native aorta to prevent dilatation of the autograft, has been gaining in popularity.[28]

Outcome following aortic valve replacement with the Ross procedure is generally excellent. Postoperative convalescence is normally uncomplicated, and patients are often ready for hospital discharge within 3 to 4 days following surgery.[17] The most common complication of pulmonary autograft replacement of the aortic valve is bleeding requiring reexploration in a small percentage of patients. Arrhythmias are uncommon, but heart block and the need for a pacemaker are possible, so patients should not be discharged from the intensive care unit until it is determined that they have normal cardiac rhythm. Patients are usually extubated within hours of surgery, once it is determined that they have adequate hemostasis.

SUBVALVULAR STENOSIS

Overview

Defined as obstruction of the LVOT below the aortic valve, subvalvular stenosis occurs in 8% to 20% of patients with LVOTO. This type of congenital aortic stenosis morphologically consists of four subtypes: (1) a discrete membranous obstruction located anteriorly, immediately below the aortic valve; (2) a diffuse tunnel-like obstruction extending to include the muscular septum; (3) a hypertrophic cardiomyopathy; and (4) other unusual space-occupying lesions (such as duplication of the anterior leaflet of the mitral valve). Other unusual variants include accessory endocardial cushion tissue and anomalous chordal and papillary muscle insertion on the interventricular septum.[42]

Discrete subvalvular stenosis rarely presents in infancy, with most occurring in children and young adults. The obstruction consists of a diaphragm of muscular or fibrous tissue just below the aortic valve. The membrane is circular or crescentic, attaching to the interventricular septum and extending around the outflow tract to involve the anterior leaflet of the mitral valve. Historically considered an acquired form of aortic stenosis, there is evidence that an abnormal angulation of the connection between the left ventricle and the aorta may establish a flow pattern that forms the substrate for this lesion.

A subaortic discrete membrane can be seen in association with a ventricular septal defect or after a ventricular septal defect that has spontaneously closed. The membrane creates abnormal blood flow jets that can lead to valvular insufficiency by preventing normal leaflet motion. Patients generally present with an asymptomatic murmur or increasing exercise intolerance. Indications for surgical intervention include a gradient of greater the 40 mm Hg, progressive aortic insufficiency, and/or symptoms associated with LVOTO.

Surgical Treatment

Resection of the discrete membrane is relatively straightforward, with low morbidity and near-zero mortality (Fig. 26-6). Cardiopulmonary bypass is utilized, with cold-blood cardioplegia to arrest the heart. An LV vent is placed via the right superior pulmonary vein. A transverse aortotomy is placed approximately 2 cm distal to the takeoff of the right coronary artery. The membrane is visualized by gently retracting the leaflets of the aortic valve. The membrane is approximately 5 mm beneath the commissure of the right and left coronary cusp but can extend farther into the heart or, conversely, immediately below and adjacent to the aortic valve leaflets. Beginning at the septum, sharp dissection is used to remove the membrane. The plane of dissection should include a shallow rim of endocardium and be carried in a counterclockwise fashion until the anterior leaflet of the mitral valve is encountered. Any attachment to the mitral valve is removed by gently feathering the membrane off the leaflet, taking care not to perforate the leaflet. Care should be taken to avoid the area of conduction tissue below the right noncoronary commissure. The resection is then continued in a clockwise fashion toward the right. Following removal of the membrane, a 2- to 3-mm wedge of muscular septum is resected beneath the commissure that separates the right and left coronary leaflets. This additional maneuver is believed to decrease the incidence of long-term recurrence, which has been reported to be as high as 15% at 10 years.[40]

Repair of the LVOTO caused by more diffuse fibromuscular lesions may be amenable to resection of enough of the obstructing tissue to relieve the stenosis, although there is a danger of damaging the integrity of the interventricular septum, the mitral valve, or the conduction system. Some obstruction cannot be safely relieved by transaortic resection and requires more complicated procedures, such as a modified Konno operation.[31] A modified Konno can be performed by opening the right ventricular outflow tract below the pulmonary valve. A right angle placed through the aortic valve is used to identify a part on the interventricular septum. A large ventricular septal defect is created in the area of the muscular subaortic stenosis. Sufficient muscle is removed to reduce the subaortic muscular obstruction. The ventricular septal defect is then closed with a prosthetic patch, the right ventricular outflow tract incision is closed primarily, and the aortotomy is also closed (Fig. 26-7). This operation spares the aortic valve and guides safe, extensive resection of the subaortic obstruction. The mid- and long-term results of this procedure are excellent provided the aortic leaflets are of normal structure and the aortic valve annulus is not hypoplastic.

Most patients who present for surgical resection of their subvalvular stenosis are beyond the neonatal age and do not

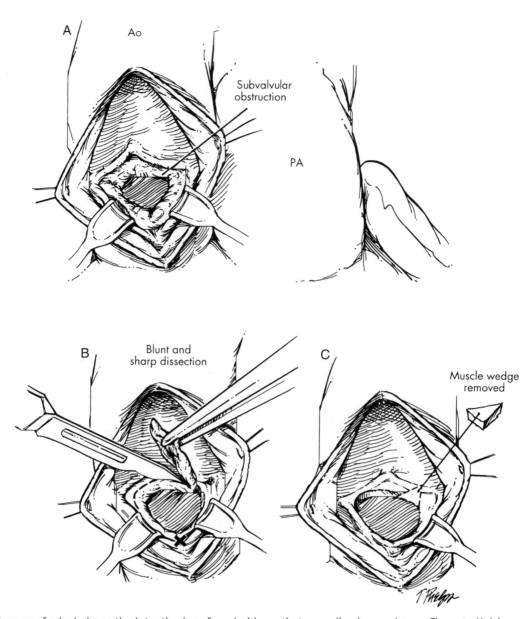

FIGURE 26-6 Exposure of subvalvular aortic obstruction is performed with a patient on cardiopulmonary bypass. The aorta (Ao) is cross-clamped and the heart is protected with cardioplegia solution. After an aortotomy has been performed, the region of subvalvular obstruction can be identified by carefully retracting the aortic valve leaflets **(A)**, This area of obstruction is then removed with a combination of blunt and sharp dissection. **(B)**, taking care to keep the area of dissection superficial between the right and noncoronary cusps (X) so as to limit the risk of injury to the conduction system. **C,** It is helpful to remove a wedge of muscle between the right and left coronary cusps to further the resection of subvalvular stenosis. This may not only limit the likelihood of recurrence but also enlarge the resulting subvalvular outflow tract. PA, pulmonary artery.

have the same postoperative problems demonstrated by infants who have undergone a valvotomy for critical aortic stenosis. In the occasional neonate with severe valvular and subvalvular stenosis, a Ross-Konno can be very effective, and the postoperative convalescence can be relatively uncomplicated, unless the infant has other associated defects that limit the LV functional capability. Older patients who have undergone resection of subaortic membranes usually have a very uncomplicated convalescence. Those patients who have had extensive muscle resection are at risk for third-degree heart block. Patients who have undergone a more extensive cardiac reconstruction by aortoventriculoplasty are at greater risk of complete heart block and may have significant ventricular dysfunction after surgery.

SUPRAVALVULAR STENOSIS

Overview

Left ventricular outflow tract obstruction can occur above the aortic valve at the level of the sinotubular junction or proximal ascending aorta. Supravalvular stenosis is the least common type of LVOTO, presenting in three distinct fashions: as part of Williams syndrome, in a sporadic form, or in a familial form transmitted as an autosomal dominant trait. The underlying defect in the sporadic form is a spontaneous inherited mutation of the elastin gene 5,7. When infants present with symptomatic supravalvular stenosis, it is most often in the familial form. In patients who present with asymptomatic

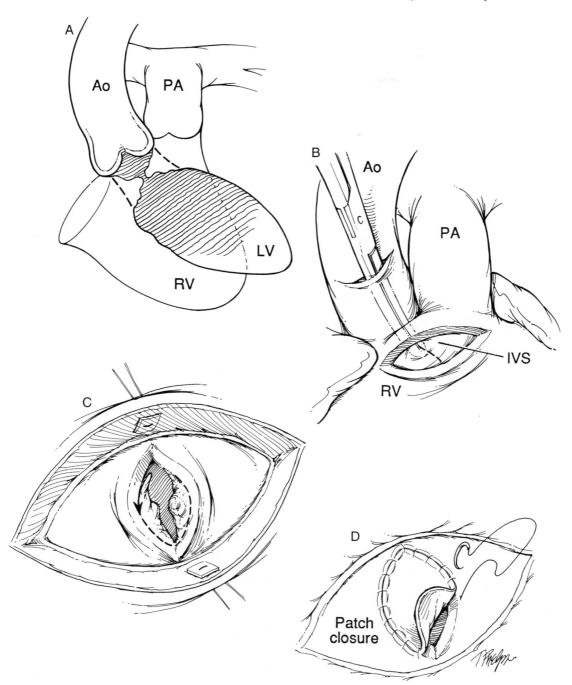

FIGURE 26-7 **A,** In patients with subaortic obstruction who have an otherwise normal aortic valve and annulus, a modified aortoventriculoplasty can be performed after the patient has been placed on cardiopulmonary bypass and the aorta (Ao) has been cross-clamped. The heart is protected with cardioplegia solution. The left ventricular (LV) and right ventricular (RV) outflow tracts overlap at right angles, facilitating exposure of the left ventricular outflow tract through the ventricular septum. **B,** Incisions are made in the Ao as well as on the infundibular surface of the right ventricle. A clamp is placed through the aortic valve and used to identify the interventricular septum (IVS, below the aortic valve) that is accessible through the right ventricular outflow tract. **C,** This area of the IVS is incised (*dashed line*) and the septal muscle causing LV outflow obstruction is removed. **D,** The incision in the IVS is then patched with pericardium or prosthetic material and the incisions in the Ao and right ventricle are closed (not shown). PA, pulmonary artery.

supravalvular stenosis, as many as 50% have the defect as part of Williams syndrome.

In 1961, Williams and associates described the association of supravalvular aortic stenosis, mental retardation, and elfin facies (Fig. 26-8) in a syndrome that now bears the author's name.[4] Subsequently, the presence of severe infantile hypercalcemia and pulmonary stenosis has been added to the syndrome.[11] The first surgical correction was reported in 1961 by McGoon and colleagues,[23] in which the stenotic aortic segment was enlarged by patching along the defect. Other repairs have since been described, most of which entail a more radical augmentation and/or resection of the diseased segment of aorta.

Patients generally present in the early first, or sometimes second, decade of life with progressive obstruction and worsening of LV hypertrophy. The presentation of symptomatic

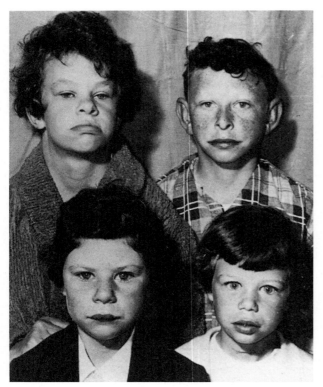

FIGURE 26-8 The elfin facies prominent in patients with supravalvular stenosis. Note the features of the ears, nose, and lips in these patients. (From Williams JCF, Barrett-Boyes BG, Lowe JB: Supravalvular aortic stenosis. *Circulation* 24:1311, 1961; with permission.)

children is similar to other forms of LV obstruction, with the exception of the coronary pathology that occurs. The coronary ostia originate below the level of obstruction; this exposes the coronaries to continued high pressures not normally seen with other levels of stenosis. Degenerative changes of the coronary arteries are likely accelerated secondary to this continued exposure to such pressures. The position of the coronaries below the obstruction also results in their filling during systole instead of diastole, leading to increased tortuosity and aneurysmal dilatation.[26] Because of these changes in the coronary arteries and the LV hypertrophy resulting from the outflow gradient, children with supravalvular stenosis present an increased risk of sudden death. This may account for the fact that presentation in adulthood is uncommon, with the majority of affected individuals succumbing prior to their second decade. The clinical presentation may also be complicated by the associated peripheral pulmonary artery stenosis.

The classic description of the supravalvular anatomy can vary from a discrete ring-like obstruction at the sinotubular junction to a diffusely hypoplastic ascending aorta that may extend to the transverse arch and great vessels (Fig. 26-9). The ring-like membranous obstruction, often having an hourglass appearance, generally occurs just above the commissures of the aortic valve. The initial descriptions of this entity as a discrete supravalvular membrane are probably incorrect, in that these lesions behave more like a coarctation of the ascending aorta with varying degrees of intimal hyperplasia. This intimal thickening and disorganization resides primarily

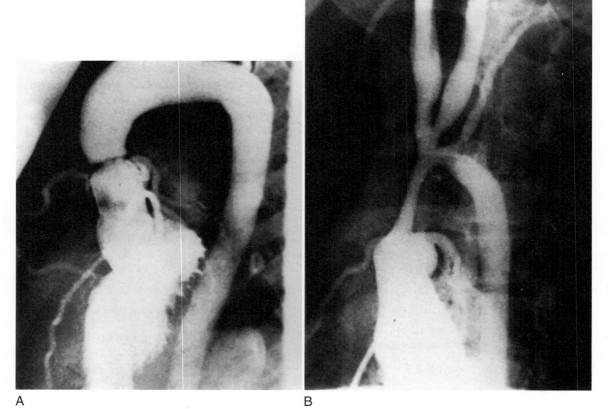

A   B

FIGURE 26-9 The angiographic appearance of supravalvular stenosis can be discrete (**A**), or diffuse (**B**). In (**B**), the stenosis continues to the innominate, carotid, and subclavian arteries. (From Kirklin, JW, Barratt-Boyes, BG: *Cardiac Surgery*. New York, Wiley, 1986, pp 1226–1227, with permission.)

in the medial layer of the aortic wall. The thickening may also extend to and involve the leaflets and commissures of the valve. This intimal proliferation at the sinus of Valsalva also contributes to the resultant coronary insufficiency. The diffuse form is generally seen in individuals who present at an earlier age. This extensive involvement of the aorta is often associated with hypoplasia of the main pulmonary artery as well.

Infants and children who present with the physical stigmata of Williams syndrome (elfin facies, gregarious personality, and mental retardation; see Fig. 26-8) should undergo investigation for possible supravalvular stenosis. Echocardiography delineates the level of obstruction and degree of LV hypertrophy. Cardiac catheterization is indicated to document the supravalvular anatomy, determine gradients, evaluate inflow

to the coronary arteries, and evaluate peripheral arteries, including the visceral and pulmonary vascular beds.

Surgical Treatment

Initial surgical correction addressed the lesion as a discrete membranous obstruction of the ascending aorta by augmenting the diameter of the vessel with a simple diamond-shaped patch placed in the noncoronary sinus.[19] This philosophy did not account for the actual coarctation that existed, resulting in a high incidence of recurrence. It was not long after these initial repairs that Doty and associates[6] reported a more involved technique that addressed two of the sinuses of Valsalva with a bifurcated patch (Fig. 26-10). This operation

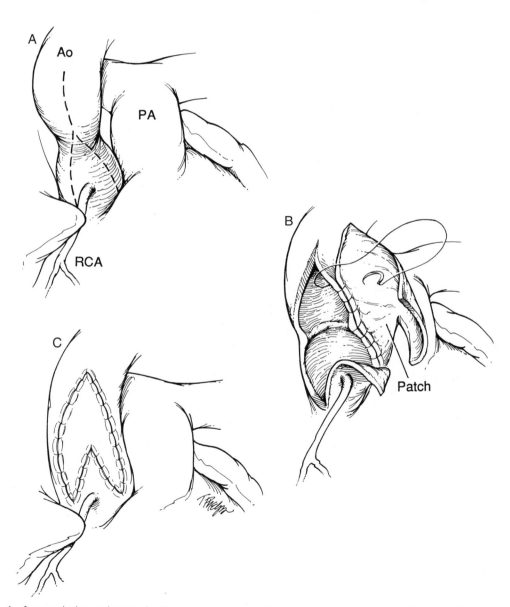

FIGURE 26-10   Repair of supravalvular aortic stenosis. Discrete supravalvar aortic stenosis can be repaired after the patient has been placed on cardiopulmonary bypass, the aorta (Ao) cross-clamped, and the heart protected with cardioplegia solution. **A,** An incision is made through the area of stenosis and extended into the sinuses on either side of the right coronary artery (RCA). This incision results in the ability to enlarge the ascending aorta without distortion of the aortic valve. **B,** The aorta is enlarged with a patch of Gore-Tex fashioned as an inverted Y. **C,** The resulting reconstruction provides enlargement of the supravalvular stenosis. PA, pulmonary artery.

results in improved gradient reduction and better geometry of the aortic root, but, like the previously described procedures, it did not address the underlying pathology of the coarctation and intimal ridge. Some investigators have reported on the dual-sinus repair with a Y graft as described by Doty and colleagues[6] in combination with the resection of the intimal ridge in the sinotubular junction. Reports suggesting that resection of this intimal ridge opposite the patch increases the risk of aneurysm formation probably justify the omission of this technique from the surgical repair.[25]

Brom[2] presented his technique, which involves insertion of patches in all three sinuses after transection of the aorta. With the growing experience with the arterial switch operation and the Ross procedure, approaches have been devised to completely remove and reconstruct the coarcted segment of the aorta. Myers and associates[25] described a technique similar to that of Brom but without the use of synthetic patches. The technique involves creating an incision in each of the three sinuses, with corresponding incisions in the distal segment of the aorta. The transected aorta is then anastomosed together, effectively eliminating the coarctation ring. To date, there is no clear evidence of a survival advantage to any technique over the other, but there is probable improved freedom from reoperation related to stenosis with all techniques compared with the diamond-shaped single patch procedure.[37]

As may be expected, repair of the localized form of congenital aortic stenosis carries a lower hospital mortality rate and good long-term prognosis. Operative mortality in the localized form should approach 0%, whereas it can be as high as 40% in the diffuse form. Similarly, late survival is good, and the reoperation rate should be low. Because this is a form of LVOTO, indications for surgery are similar to those for valvular or subvalvular stenosis.

Postoperative convalescence depends on the nature of the initial defect. Ordinarily, the convalescence is uncomplicated in patients with the discrete form of supravalvular stenosis but can be more complex in those with the more diffuse forms. Pulmonary hypertension can be present, and patients with Williams syndrome can have main pulmonary artery stenosis as well as branch pulmonary artery stenosis. Thoughtful collaboration between cardiologists, surgeons, and intensivists can be helpful in the more complicated forms of supravalvular aortic stenosis.

References

1. Alexiou C, Langley SM, Dalrymple-Hay MJ, et al: Open commissurotomy for critical isolated aortic stenosis in neonates. *Ann Thorac Surg* 71: 489–493, 2001.
2. Brom AG: *Obstruction of the Left Ventricular Outflow Tract*. Rockville, Md, Aspen, 1988.
3. Caspi J, Ilbawi MN, Roberson DA, et al: Extended aortic valvuloplasty for recurrent valvular stenosis and regurgitation in children. *J Thorac Cardiovasc Surg* 107:114–120, 1994.
4. Cornell WP, Elkins RC, Criley JM, Sabiston DC Jr: Supravalvular aortic stenosis. *J Thorac Cardiovasc Surg* 51:484–492, 1996.
5. Dedic J, Weiss AS, Katahira J, et al: A novel elastin gene mutation (1281delC) in a family with supravalvular aortic stenosis: A mutation cluster within exon 20. *Hum Mutat* 17:81, 2001.
6. Doty DB, Polansky DB, Jenson CB: Supravalvular aortic stenosis. Repair by extended aortoplasty. *J Thorac Cardiovasc Surg* 74:362–371, 1977.
7. Duba HC, Doll A, Neyer M, et al: The elastin gene is disrupted in a family with a balanced translocation t(7;16)(q11.23;q13) associated with a variable expression of the Williams-Beuren syndrome. *Eur J Hum Genet* 10:351–361, 2002.
8. Duncan K, Sullivan I, Robinson P, et al: Transventricular aortic valvotomy for critical aortic stenosis in infants. *J Thorac Cardiovasc Surg* 93:546–550, 1987.
9. Elkins RC, Lane MM, McCue C, Ward KE: Pulmonary autograft root replacement: Mid-term results. *J Heart Valve Dis* 8:499–503, 1999.
10. Gallo R, Kumar N, Prabhakar G, et al: Accelerated degeneration of aortic homograft in an infant. *J Thorac Cardiovasc Surg* 107:1161–1162, 1994.
11. Garcia RE, Friedmen WF, Kaback MM, Rowe RD: Idiopathic hypercalcemia and supravalvular aortic stenosis: Documentation of a new syndrome. *N Engl J Med* 271:117–120, 1964.
12. Gaynor JW, Bull C, Sullivan ID, et al: Late outcome of survivors of intervention for neonatal aortic valve stenosis. *Ann Thor Surg* 60:122–126, 1995.
13. Hallman GL, Cooley DA: Congenital aortic stenosis. In Sabiston DC Jr, Spencer FC (eds): *Gibbon's Surgery of the Chest*. Philadelphia, WB Saunders, 1983, pp 1109–1115.
14. Hammon JW Jr, Lupinetti FM, Maples MD, et al: Predictors of operative mortality in critical valvular aortic stenosis presenting in infancy. *Ann Thorac Surg* 45:537–540, 1988.
15. Hawkins JA, Minich LL, Tani LY, et al: Late results and reintervention after aortic valvotomy for critical aortic stenosis in neonates and infants. *Ann Thorac Surg* 65:1758–1763, 1998.
16. Ilbawi MN, Idriss FS, DeLeon SY, et al: Valve replacement in children: Guidelines for selection of prosthesis and timing of surgical intervention. *Ann Thorac Surg* 44:398–403, 1987.
17. Jaggers J, Harrison JK, Bashore TM, et al: The Ross procedure: Shorter hospital stay, decreased morbidity, and cost effective. *Ann Thor Surg* 65:1553–1558, 1998.
18. Johnson RG, Williams GR, Razook JD, et al: Reoperation in congenital aortic stenosis. *Ann Thorac Surg* 40:156–162, 1985.
19. Keane JF, Fellows KE, LaFarge CG, et al: The surgical management of discrete and diffuse supravalvar aortic stenosis. *Circulation* 54:112–117, 1976.
20. Laudito A, Brook MM, Suleman S, et al: The Ross procedure in children and young adults: A word of caution. *J Thorac Cardiovasc Surg* 122:147–153, 2001.
21. Lofland GK, McCrindle BW, Williams WG, et al: Critical aortic stenosis in the neonate: A multi-institutional study of management, outcomes, and risk factors. Congenital Heart Surgeons Society. *J Thorac Cardiovasc Surg* 121:10–27, 2001.
22. McCrindle BW, Blackstone EH, Williams WG, et al: Are outcomes of surgical versus transcatheter balloon valvotomy equivalent in neonatal critical aortic stenosis? *Circulation* 104:1152–1158, 2001.
23. McGoon DC, Mankin HT, Vlad P, Kirkland JW: The surgical treatment of supravalvular aortic stenosis. *J Thorac Cardiovasc Surg* 41:125, 1961.
24. Mulder DG, Katz RD, Moss AJ, Hurwitz RA: The surgical treatment of congenital aortic stenosis. *J Thorac Cardiovasc Surg* 55:786–796, 1968.
25. Myers JL, Waldhausen JA, Cyran SE, et al: Results of surgical repair of congenital supravalvular aortic stenosis. *J Thorac Cardiovasc Surg* 105: 281–287, 1993.
26. Neufeld HN, Wagenvoort CA, Ongley PA, Edwards JE: Hypoplasia of ascending aorta. An unusual form of supravalvular aortic stenosis with special reference to localized coronary arterial hypertension. *Am J Cardiol* 10:746–751, 1962.
27. Paget J: On obstruction of the branches of the pulmonary artery. *Med Chir Trans* 27:162, 1844.
28. Pessotto R, Wells WJ, Baker CJ, et al: Midterm results of the Ross procedure. *Ann Thor Surg* 71:S336–S339, 2001.
29. Rhodes LA, Colan SD, Perry SB, et al: Predictors of survival in neonates with critical aortic stenosis. *Circulation* 84:2325–2335, 1991.
30. Robicsek F, Sanger PW, Daugherty HK, Montgomery CC: Congenital quadricuspid aortic valve with displacement of the left coronary orifice. *Am J Cardiol* 23:288–290, 1969.
31. Roughneen PT, DeLeon SY, Cetta F, et al: Modified Konno-Rastan procedure for subaortic stenosis: Indications, operative techniques, and results. *Ann Thorac Surg* 65:1368–1375, 1998.
32. Sade RM, Crawford FA Jr, Fyfe DA, Stroud MR: Valve prostheses in children: A reassessment of anticoagulation. *J Thorac Cardiovasc Surg* 95:553–561, 1988.
33. Schaffer MS, Clarke DR, Campbell DN, et al: The St. Jude Medical cardiac valve in infants and children: Role of anticoagulant therapy. *J Am Coll Cardiol* 9:235–239, 1987.
34. Schoof PH, Hazekamp MG, van Wermeskerken GK, et al: Disproportionate enlargement of the pulmonary autograft in the aortic position in the growing pig. *J Thorac Cardiovasc Surg* 115:1264–1272, 1998.

35. Solymar L, Sudow G, Holmgren D: Increase in size of the pulmonary autograft after the Ross operation in children: Growth or dilation? *J Thorac Cardiovasc Surg* 119:4–9, 2000.

36. Spencer FC, Neill CA, Sank L, Bahnson HT: Anatomical variations in 46 patients with congenital aortic stenosis. *Am Surg* 26:204–216, 1960.

37. Stamm C, Kreutzer C, Zurakowski D, et al: Forty-one years of surgical experience with congenital supravalvular aortic stenosis. *J Thorac Cardiovasc Surg* 118:874–885, 1999.

38. Ungerleider RM: Direct vision aortic valvotomy: Predecessor to modern aortic surgery. *Ann Thor Surg* 57:1351–1353, 1994.

39. Ungerleider RM: Is there a role for prosthetic patch aortoplasty in the repair of aortic coarctation? *Ann Thorac Surg* 52:601–603, 1991.

40. van Son JA, Schaff HV, Danielson GK, et al: Sugical treatment of discrete and tunnel subaortic stenosis: Late survival and risk of operation. *Circulation* 88:159–169, 1993.

41. Verrier ED, Tranbaugh RF, Soifer SJ, et al: Aspirin anticoagulation in children with mechanical aortic valves. *J Thorac Cardiovasc Surg* 92:1013–1020, 1986.

42. Wright PW, Wittner RS: Obstruction of the left ventricular outflow tract by the mitral valve due to a muscle band. *J Thorac Cardiovasc Surg* 85:938–940, 1983.

43. Yankah AC, Alexi-Meskhishvili V, Weng Y, et al: Accelerated degeneration of allografts in the first two years of life. *Ann Thorac Surg* 60:S71–S76, 1995.

Chapter 27

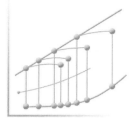

Coarctation of the Aorta and Interrupted Aortic Arch

LAURA A. HASTINGS, MD, and DAVID G. NICHOLS, MD, MBA

DEFINITIONS

Aortic coarctation and interruption are obstructive anomalies of the aortic arch. Coarctation of the aorta is a hemodynamically significant narrowing of the thoracic aorta, directly opposite, proximal, or distal to the ductus arteriosus, resulting in a pressure gradient (Fig. 27-1). True coarctation is a distinct, shelf-like thickening or infolding of the aortic media into the lumen of the aorta.[108] It is distinguished from hypoplasia of the aortic isthmus, previously referred to as "preductal" coarctation. Aortic hypoplasia is defined as a narrowed diameter of an aortic segment with a normal aortic media. An *atretic arch* refers to two patent ends with an interposed ligamentous strand. Aortic interruption consists of complete discontinuity between two parts of the aortic arch. In almost all cases, there is an associated ventricular septal defect (VSD), and the patent ductus arteriosus provides blood flow to the distal aorta.[5]

COARCTATION OF THE AORTA

History

Coarctation of the aorta (CoA) was first described in the 18th century, but it was not until the 1920s that it became recognized as a cause of shortened lifespan, hypertension, endocarditis, and congestive heart failure (CHF). Of the patients with

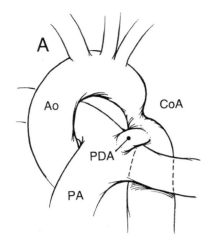

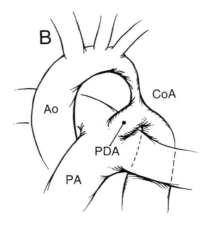

FIGURE 27-1 A, Representation of isolated coarctation of the aorta (CoA). The coarctation is most typically proximal to the patent ductus arteriosus (PDA) or ligamentum arteriosum. **B,** Aortic arch hypoplasia frequently accompanies CoA but can be found independently. Ao, aorta; PA, pulmonary artery.

CoA who survived infancy, mean life expectancy in the presurgical era was only 3 decades; most of these patients died of aortic aneurysm, endocarditis, aortitis, cerebrovascular accident, or CHF.[92] Surgical repair was pioneered by Crafoord and Nylin[19] and Gross[32] in the 1940s. Through their work, it was established that the aorta could be clamped for an extended time without sequelae.

Epidemiology

Aortic coarctation is recognized in 5% to 8% of patients with congenital heart disease excluding mitral valve prolapse or related bicuspid aortic valve. More than 60% of the patients with discrete coarctation of the aorta are male. This male-to-female ratio is less striking in infants with coarctation syndrome, consisting of coarctation plus hypoplasia of the aortic isthmus and intracardiac defects.[77]

Classification and Anatomy

Aortic coarctation lies in close proximity to the ductus arteriosus or ligamentum arteriosum, commonly just distal to the left subclavian artery. Variable presentations occur. An isolated coarctation is more commonly found in older children. In infants, CoA is a syndrome commonly found in association with hypoplasia of the aortic isthmus and other cardiac anomalies.[7,39,94] Sinha and colleagues[108] reviewed the cases of 78 infants with "coarctation" and CHF and found that 71 of 78 had infolding of the media. Seven patients had tubular hypoplasia without medial involvement, and 55 of the 78 had a combination of tubular hypoplasia with distinct juxtaductal coarctation. Some degree of arch hypoplasia is present in most normal neonates;[78,96] isthmus hypoplasia can be defined as less than 40% of the diameter of the ascending aorta. Proximal and distal transverse arch hypoplasia are defined as 60% and 50%, respectively, of the diameter of the ascending aorta.[5]

Historically, coarctations were classified as either adult (postductal) or infantile (preductal). The adult form referred to a discrete narrowing, which was more properly described as juxtaductal in location. The infantile or preductal form was characterized by more diffuse narrowing of an aortic segment in addition to the juxtaductal narrowing. A more modern practical classification, which guides the surgical approach,

recognizes three categories: (1) isolated coarctation, (2) coarctation with ventricular septal defect (VSD), and (3) coarctation with complex intracardiac anomaly.[6] Amato and colleagues[1] introduced a third approach to classification of coarctation that combines coarctation, hypoplasia, and intracardiac defects (Box 27-1). Each of these categories has two subcategories: A, with VSD; and B, with other major cardiac defects.

Associated Defects

Numerous cardiovascular defects may accompany this condition (Box 27-2). Patent ductus arteriosus and patent foramen ovale are so common in neonatal CoA that they are not considered associated defects. A VSD constitutes the most common, hemodynamically significant associated defect in newborns and infants with CoA. Notable also is the association of CoA with bicuspid aortic valve, reported to be 25% to 85% in some series.[22] Aortic insufficiency may develop

---

BOX 27-1   *Classification System of Coarctation, Hypoplasia, and Associated Cardiac Defects Proposed by Amato and Colleagues*

Type I: Coarctation with or without PDA
   IA: With VSD
   IB: With other major cardiac defects
Type II: Coarctation with isthmus hypoplasia, with or without PDA
   IIA: With VSD
   IIB: With other major cardiac defects
Type III: Coarctation with tubular hypoplasia of isthmus and segment between left carotid and subclavian arteries, with or without PDA
   IIIA: With VSD
   IIIB: With other major cardiac defects

From Amato JJ, Galdieri RJ, Cotroneo JV: Role of extended aortoplasty related to the definition of coarctation of the aorta. Ann Thorac Surg 52:615–620, 1991.
PDA, patent ductus arteriosus; VSD, ventricular septal defect.

secondarily in a child with CoA and bicuspid aortic valve. In his study of autopsy specimens, Rosenquist[95] noted that 35 of 44 patients with CoA had abnormal mitral valves. Coarctation of the aorta may be part of a complex of left-sided obstructions identified as Shone's syndrome that consists of coarctation, supravalular mitral stenosis, parachute mitral valve, and subaortic stenosis.[107] Syndromes that have low pulmonary blood flow, such as tetralogy of Fallot, tricuspid atresia, pulmonary stenosis, and atresia, are rarely associated with CoA. Intracranial aneurysms represent a potentially life-threatening associated extracardiac abnormality.[132] Coarctation of the aorta was noted in 9 of 23 patients with a vein of Galen malformation.[70]

Coarctation of the aorta is frequently a component of several chromosomal abnormality syndromes. It is relatively common in trisomy 13 and trisomy 18. Sybert[115] found 136 of 244 Turner syndrome patients to have heart disease. More than 50% of the cardiac malformations were CoA and bicuspid aortic valve, alone or in combination.

Embryology

The embryology and causation of coarctation have focused on ductal tissue migration and fetal hemodynamics as possible explanations of this malformation. Several investigators have suggested the concept of ductal tissue spreading into the aorta and subsequently causing constriction after birth as the origin of coarctation.[96,97] The constriction has been described as a posterior shelf of tissue opposite the ductus that progressively invaginates during ductal closure or on exposure to oxygen. Normally, extension of ductal tissue into the aorta does not exceed one third of the aortic circumference. However, in local

coarctation, the ductal tissue sometimes completely encircles the lumen of the aorta.

Theories of flow as a cause of coarctation are supported by the fact that constellations of intracardiac anomalies with decreased aortic flow patterns have an increased incidence of arch anomalies and that constellations with increased aortic flow (because of decreased pulmonary flow) have no coarctation.[75,79,96,106] Another model for the flow theory may be Turner syndrome. Lymphatic obstruction results in distended thoracic ducts that compress the ascending aorta, alter intracardiac blood flow, and cause neck webbing. Redirection of the intracardiac blood flow is presumed to cause the left-sided heart defects. Coarctation is eight times more common in Turner syndrome patients with webbed neck than those without webbed neck.[13] Other syndromes that can have webbed neck are not usually associated with left-sided heart lesions (e.g., Noonan and fetal hydantoin), but probably are associated with a mechanism different than lymphatic obstruction.

Pathophysiology

Newborns and Infants

Coarctation of the aorta presents a spectrum of severity, in which young age at presentation closely correlates with severity of obstruction and associated defects. Ductal closure in neonates occurs within a predictable time frame and morphologic pattern.[27] The pulmonary end of the ductus closes first. Many infants with CoA will not present until the aortic end of the ductus arteriosus closes. When ductal closure at the aortic end causes aortic constriction, a severe increase in left ventricular (LV) afterload results. Left ventricular ejection fraction decreases acutely in response to the higher afterload, and there is no time for compensatory development of muscle hypertrophy that might improve ejection fraction and hemodynamics. Such increased afterload results in elevated ventricular wall tension, decreased myocardial perfusion pressure, and, in extreme cases, ischemic myocardium (Fig. 27-2).

The increased LV end-diastolic pressure and increased left atrial pressure cause a left-to-right shunt at the foramen ovale and, hence, increased pulmonary blood flow (Q_p). Pulmonary hypertension occurs as a result of (1) increased Q_p and (2) increased pulmonary venous pressures secondary to left atrial hypertension.[31] Right-sided heart enlargement ensues because of volume overload of the right ventricle. All of these pathophysiologic events summate to produce the clinical picture of CHF.

This pattern is exaggerated in the presence of severe coarctation with a large VSD (Fig. 27-3). Left ventricular blood is ejected into the right ventricle and pulmonary circulation at systemic pressures, leading to a substantially increased pulmonary-to-systemic blood flow ratio ($Q_p:Q_s$). As the ductus closes, Q_s decreases further, and $Q_p:Q_s$ is much greater than 1. Systemic hypoperfusion leads to the oliguria and metabolic acidosis observed in many infants on presentation.[31]

Other associated cardiac lesions aggravate the hemodynamic burden. For instance, in some cases, the ductus remains patent, allowing the right ventricle to support systemic perfusion. In all cases of severe coarctation in infancy, adequate systemic cardiac output can be maintained by the right ventricle only across a patent ductus arteriosus. These infants present

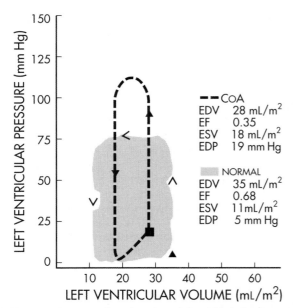

FIGURE 27-2 Pressure-volume loop in an infant with isolated coarctation of the aorta (CoA) compared with normal perinatal values. EDP, end-diastolic pressure; EDV, end-diastolic volume; EF, ejection fraction; ESV, end-systolic volume. (From Graham TP Jr: Ventricular performance in congenital heart disease. *Circulation* 84:2259–2274, 1991; with permission.)

in profound hemodynamic collapse and shock with systemic hypotension, acidosis, and tachypnea (from pulmonary hypertension) when the ductus closes and require intravenous prostaglandin (PGE_1) to open the ductus and restore systemic perfusion. To maintain adequate cardiac output, the right ventricle experiences both hypertrophy and volume overload, especially in the presence of a VSD. Infants with atrioventricular septal defects and coarctation experience more severe heart failure for equivalent degrees of aortic obstruction than infants without atrioventricular septal defects because of the addition of atrioventricular valve regurgitation to the left-to-right shunting described previously.

Older Children

Coarctation in the older child is usually an isolated and asymptomatic lesion, which is discovered following an evaluation for upper extremity hypertension. The coarctation leads to excessive pressure work of the left ventricle. Two major compensatory mechanisms arise in this setting—(1) LV hypertrophy to increase systolic pressure without increasing wall stress and (2) aortic collateralization to decrease LV afterload. Consequently, patients develop varying degrees of LV hypertrophy, depending on the coarctation gradient and the presence of collateral circulation. Collateral circulation may decrease the gradient across the stenotic area, leading to misinterpretation regarding the degree of stenosis.

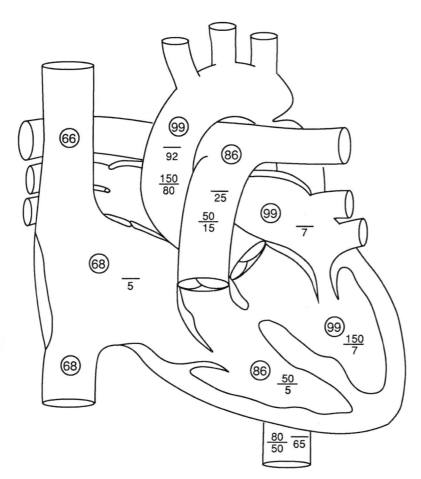

FIGURE 27-3 Pathophysiology of coarctation of the aorta and ventricular septal defect in infancy. There is a step-up in oxygen saturation between the right atrium (68%) and the right ventricle (86%), indicating a left-to-right shunt at the ventricular level, which increases pulmonary blood flow and pressure (50/15). Left ventricular pressure (150/7) and ascending aortic pressure (150/80) are elevated compared to descending aortic pressure (80/65) because of the coarctation.

Diagnostic Assessment

Presentation in Infants

Infants under 3 months of age with CoA have characteristic presenting signs (Box 27-3). CHF is often present. Poor peripheral perfusion, acidosis, tachypnea, and failure to thrive are common.[30,105,130] The physical examination reveals an ejection murmur along the left sternal border and in the left subscapular area. The precordial impulse is prominent and often accompanied by a systolic thrill if the infant has intracardiac defects. Hepatomegaly and a gallop rhythm point to CHF. Femoral pulses are diminished in most, but not all, cases.

Coarctation of the aorta or interrupted aortic arch (IAA) may be difficult conditions to diagnose early in the newborn period. Patients often are not referred until they are in shock or renal failure. Only 10% to 30% of infants with physical findings of CoA are referred with the correct diagnosis.[119,126] Most are thought to have other diagnoses despite decreased femoral pulses in 88% of cases,[126] since decreased femoral pulse can also be a sign of shock from numerous causes (such as neonatal sepsis). Conversely, patients may be erroneously suspected to have a coarctation when they are in shock. Even in patients over 1 year of age, the diagnosis is usually delayed despite classic findings of murmur and upper extremity hypertension.[29] In contrast to older children, infants presenting before 5 days of age rarely have upper extremity hypertension. This is usually related to depressed cardiac output related to the afterload faced by the left ventricle. After 5 days, hypertension becomes more common, and after 15 days the incidence is 86%.[126] Aortic obstruction is the likely diagnosis, when these physical findings are accompanied by a gradient between upper and lower extremity pulses and systolic pressure. However, the absence of such a gradient does not rule out the diagnosis of aortic obstruction, and in fact, when distal (systemic) perfusion is maintained by a patent ductus arteriosus, the pressures in the lower extremities may be equal to or even higher than those in the upper extremities.

The absence of a systolic pressure gradient in patients with CoA usually has one of three anatomic or physiologic explanations: (1) The ductus may be patent such that the right ventricle (RV) provides flow to the lower body. These patients may have differential cyanosis with lower oxygen saturations recorded from the toe than the preductal hand. (2) Left ventricular function may be so poor that systemic hypotension makes it impossible to detect a gradient between upper and lower extremities. (3) Finally, in rare instances, the right subclavian artery (RSCA) has an aberrant origin distal to the coarctation, thus eliminating any gradient. The physician should never exclude the diagnosis of CoA solely because of failure to detect a gradient in pulse volume or systolic pressures between upper and lower extremities.

Presentation in Older Children

Among children over 1 year of age with CoA who are otherwise asymptomatic, 89% to 92% have upper extremity hypertension.[113,119] This is best assessed after obtaining four extremity blood pressures. However, in most cases, it is the gradient between right arm and lower extremity pressures that is most revealing, because the left subclavian artery (and hence the left arm) may be involved in the coarcted segment. Some patients do not have a gradient at rest but develop one upon exercise. Therefore, stress testing is recommended preoperatively and postoperatively to reveal occult gradients.[21]

The minority of older children with CoA who are symptomatic show signs of ischemia or hypertensive organ damage. Lower extremity pain, paresthesia, and muscle weakness may occur from a dilated and tortuous anterior spinal artery compressing the spinal cord or a branch compressing a nerve root.[77] Some children complain of dyspnea on exertion or claudication. Consistent with the presence of upper extremity hypertension in older patients, patients with longstanding CoA have arteriolar tortuosity of the retinal vessels, a finding not seen in patients with early coarctation repair.[46] Subarachnoid hemorrhage and coma from a ruptured intracranial aneurysm represent a devastating presentation of CoA in the older child. Rupture may occur with only moderate elevations of systolic blood pressure.[131]

Murmurs are present in most patients with CoA who are over 1 year of age. The murmurs tend to be systolic and at least grade 3/6 in intensity. Most are heard best in the left upper sternal border, are crescendo-decrescendo in quality, and can be accompanied by an apical diastolic rumble.

Diagnostic Tests

Electrocardiographic (ECG) findings are influenced by the presence of associated intracardiac anomalies and the age at presentation. Infants most commonly show right ventricular hypertrophy (RVH) and later develop biventricular hypertrophy (Fig. 27-4). A minority have LV hypertrophy alone. Some studies report normal electrocardiogram readings in older children with isolated coarctation, but the most common ECG abnormality in older children is LV hypertrophy. ST-segment depression and T-wave inversion can be found in infants as well as older children. ECG abnormalities are present in most patients with associated intracardiac defects.

As with the ECG, the chest radiograph of infants with CoA or interrupted aortic arch may be different from that of older patients with isolated CoA. In infancy,

---

BOX 27-3   *Signs, Symptoms, or Associated Diagnoses: Presenting Signs of Infants Less than 3 Months of Age with Either Coarctation or Interrupted Aortic Arch*

Tachypnea
Cyanosis
Poor perfusion
Difficulty feeding
Failure to thrive
Hepatomegaly
Cardiomegaly
Decreased femoral pulses
Murmur
Metabolic acidosis
Respiratory failure

Data from references 15, 30, 85, 105, and 130.

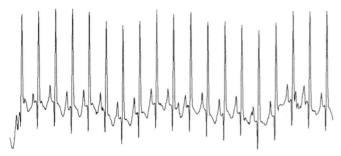

FIGURE 27-4   Lead V_2 of the electrocardiogram of a 10-day-old infant with isolated coarctation of the aorta who presented in shock. There is evidence of right ventricular hypertrophy and ST-segment depression.

cardiomegaly and, frequently, pulmonary congestion are the hallmarks (Fig. 27-5).[72,85] Later in life, classic findings of isolated CoA include LV enlargement, irregularity or notching of the aortic arch, and rib notching (Fig. 27-6).[45] Rib notching, which is created by tortuous collaterals, correlates directly with age and inversely with the diameter of the coarctation.[29]

Two-dimensional echocardiography with Doppler (echo Doppler) has become a sensitive and specific diagnostic method for children with coarctation (Fig. 27-7) and associated intracardiac anomalies.[80,122] In experienced hands, diagnosis of CoA by echo Doppler achieved 95% sensitivity and 99% specificity.[42] Furthermore, echocardiography also demonstrates the presence of associated defects and enables measurements of left ventricular chamber size and aortic valve annulus. Prenatal diagnosis of CoA through the use of normal in utero aortic arch growth curves has been evolving.[40,41,129]

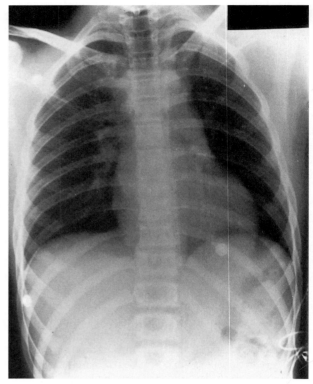

FIGURE 27-6   Chest radiograph of a school-age child with coarctation of the aorta, demonstrating classic findings of left ventricular enlargement and rib notching.

The role of cardiac catheterization in CoA continues to evolve in light of the greater use of noninvasive diagnostic techniques. Cardiac catheterization and angiography are desirable if echocardiography fails to delineate the anatomy completely or where balloon angioplasty or stent placement offers definitive treatment (see later). Data from the mid-1990s suggest that 20% to 25% of neonates with CoA undergo cardiac catheterization before surgery.[33] Fewer patients now require catheterization for diagnosis.

Most recently, magnetic resonance imaging (MRI), which may be combined with angiography, offers a valuable tool to

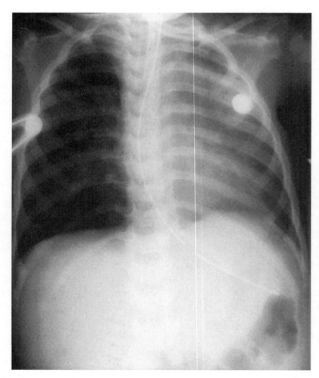

FIGURE 27-5   Chest radiograph of an infant with coarctation of the aorta, showing hallmark signs of cardiomegaly and pulmonary congestion.

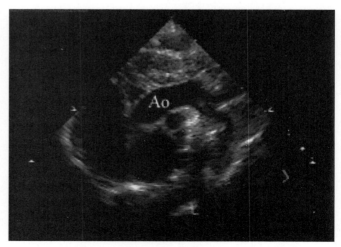

FIGURE 27-7   Echocardiogram of coarctation of the aorta (Ao).

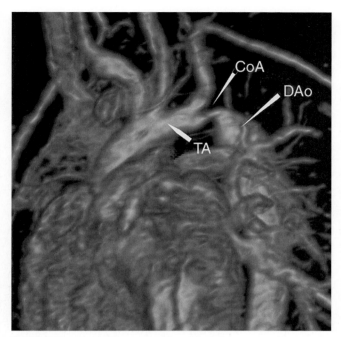

FIGURE 27-8 Magnetic resonance imaging defines coarctation anatomy. CoA, coarctation; DAo, descending aorta; TA, transverse arch.

define coarctation anatomy (Fig. 27-8) (see Chapter 17, Noninvasive Diagnosis of Heart Disease). Mendelsohn and colleagues[73] compared transthoracic echo to MRI and cardiac catheterization and found no significant difference between echo and MRI measurements, except in the diameter of the diaphragmatic aorta and the isthmus length. MRI was superior in identifying aortic collaterals. The echocardiogram was better at assessing myocardial function and intracardiac abnormalities. MRI also can be used to evaluate the aorta after surgery or balloon angioplasty.[109,127] However, it is limited by the time required to perform the test and the need for heavy sedation or general anesthesia in small children.

Preoperative Critical Care Management

Newborns and Infants

A pivotal time in the evolution of the treatment of infants with aortic arch anomalies was the late 1970s, when prostaglandin E_1 became available to maintain patency of the ductus arteriosus. This drug allows preoperative stabilization of critically ill neonates, who often present with heart failure, shock, and renal failure. Coceani and Olley[16] first demonstrated the efficacy of PGE_1 in maintaining ductal patency under both aerobic and anaerobic conditions. Leoni and associates[59] showed the efficacy of PGE_1 therapy in 52 neonates with CoA or IAA. A total of 29% of patients who did not receive PGE_1 died, compared with 0% in the treated group. Renal failure, metabolic acidosis, and survival to the time of surgery were significantly improved in the treatment group. Dopamine and positive-pressure ventilation also contributed to better resuscitation before surgery.[72,104,133]

Prostaglandin E_1 is given initially in doses of 0.05 mcg/kg/min to 0.1 mcg/kg/min, but can be increased gradually to 0.2 mcg/kg/min if it is not effective at the lower dose. Maximal response occurs 15 minutes to 4 hours after the start of the infusion.[24] Initial studies of the drug's effectiveness reported clinical improvement in 80% of patients. Infants 14 days and younger tend to benefit from the drug, but, in general, infants whose ductus closed before infusion showed no benefit.[24,62] Side effects and complications of PGE_1 include cutaneous vasodilation, hypotension, rhythm or conduction disturbances, jitteriness or seizure activity, fever, respiratory depression, increased infection, diarrhea, metabolic derangements, and (rarely) coagulopathy. Many side effects are related to high doses, longer infusion periods, and poorer general medical condition at the start of therapy.[37] McElhinney and coworkers[71] found an elevated risk of necrotizing enterocolitis in neonates whose highest dose of prostaglandin was greater than 0.05 mcg/kg/min. Therefore, the infusion rate should be decreased to 0.01 to 0.02 mcg/kg/min as soon as the desired effect has been achieved.[55] Beat-to-beat blood pressure measurement with an intraarterial catheter may be desirable during PGE_1 infusion, but PGE_1 administration should not be delayed because of lack of arterial access. Reliable venous access is essential for infants who have ductus-dependent lesions. It is our practice to administer PGE_1 to every newborn in shock until critical coarctation, IAA, or other ductus-dependent lesions have been excluded.

Endotracheal intubation and mechanical ventilation are frequently required in the newborn with critical coarctation because of CHF, shock, and the risk of apnea from PGE_1 therapy. If PGE_1 is begun in the absence of shock, ventilatory support is not mandatory, provided that the infant is not apneic and the facilities for intubation are immediately at hand. In newborns with isolated CoA, the expected decrease in the pulmonary vascular resistance from ventilation and PGE_1 does not affect the hemodynamics. Conversely, in those with CoA and VSD, more blood will be shunted left to right as the pulmonary vascular resistance falls. Ventilation must be carefully controlled to restore the pulmonary-to-systemic blood flow ratio ($Q_p:Q_s$) to the range of 1:1 in patients with arch obstruction and left-to-right intracardiac shunt. This requires a ventilation strategy designed to increase pulmonary vascular resistance by lowering the FiO_2 to maintain O_2 saturations of approximately 85% and adjusting minute ventilation to achieve a pCO_2 of 40 to 50 mm Hg. This strategy for balanced $Q_p:Q_s$ is necessary to maintain adequate systemic blood flow. Normal acid-base balance with lactate levels (<2 mmol/L) can provide an indication of adequate oxygen delivery. Mixed venous oxygen saturation is not useful as a measure of systemic oxygen delivery if the measurement is obtained from the right atrium in the presence of a significant atrial shunt, which raises right atrial saturation. Low-dose dopamine may be needed as inotropic support for ventricular failure or to increase renal blood flow by dopaminergic effect when used in doses of less than 5 mcg/kg/min. With a patent ductus, balanced circulation, and necessary inotropic support, the infant should be readily stabilized during the preoperative period.

Fluid and electrolyte balance should be restored as much as possible before operation. Severe metabolic acidosis (pH < 7.2) from systemic hypoperfusion is corrected with bicarbonate administration (0.5 to 1 mEq/kg), given slowly. Bicarbonate doses can be repeated until the metabolic acidosis has resolved; however, inability to correct the acidosis with multiple doses of bicarbonate suggests persistent acid production. This could be associated with poor myocardial function or ischemic tissue, such as ischemic bowel. Severe anemia can also contribute to persistent acidosis.

While it is appropriate to correct dehydration, fluid volume expansion, even in the hypotensive infant with critical coarctation or IAA, may be hazardous. Hypotension is usually not caused by hypovolemia in this setting but rather by aortic obstruction, ductus closure, and ventricular failure. During the initial resuscitation in the emergency department, a small fluid bolus (normal saline, 5 mL/kg) may be useful as a therapeutic trial. An additional bolus is justified only if there is a favorable response to the first bolus. Infants with prolonged shock and acidosis who develop fluid loss from capillary leak syndrome may require repeated fluid boluses. Some infants develop systemic vasodilation after PGE_1 and require titrated isotonic fluid administration (5 mL/kg/dose).

Conversely, the newborn with an established diagnosis of CoA and CHF who is responding to PGE_1 therapy should receive fluid restriction (70% to 80% of maintenance requirements) to limit the salt and water load in the face of heart failure. A second scenario involves the newborn who remains hypotensive despite restoration of ductal patency with PGE_1. Poor ventricular function is the likely cause of persistent hypotension in this setting, and the infant may benefit from inotropic support rather than volume expansion. Table 27-1 summarizes preoperative management strategies for children with CoA and IAA.

Most infants can be adequately stabilized with the measures described here, and surgery should be delayed for 12 to 24 hours until metabolic derangements have been corrected. Symptomatic infants who are unresponsive to PGE_1 have a high mortality. The options for these patients include emergency repair of CoA with or without cardiopulmonary bypass. Additional diagnoses should be sought if the patient is difficult to stabilize.

Older Children with Isolated Coarctation

Older children with isolated coarctation usually present for elective surgical repair, yet preoperative management is also important for this group. Preexisting hypertension occurs in many patients with CoA and may be exacerbated by aortic cross-clamping, which carries the risk of myocardial failure, dysrhythmia, reflex cardiac arrest, or cerebral hemorrhage. All such patients should receive beta-adrenergic–blocking drugs to control hypertension before surgery. Successful control of perioperative hypertension has been reported with the use of propranolol 1.5 mg/kg/day for 2 weeks preoperatively and 1 week postoperatively.[28] Failure to provide preoperative beta blockade may lead to marked hypertensive responses to intubation. Vasodilators are contraindicated before surgery in the hypertensive child with CoA. Left ventricular function may not increase cardiac output sufficiently to compensate for vasodilation because of the relatively fixed obstruction from CoA. Furthermore, tachycardia associated with vasodilation may lead to myocardial ischemia.

Anesthetic Management

Infants

Standard anesthetic management includes careful assessment of the airway before anesthetic induction. Some patients with aortic arch malformations have associated facial anomalies such as those seen in velocardiofacial syndrome/DiGeorge syndrome and the Turner syndrome webbed neck. In addition, induction strategies may be affected by associated intracardiac defects. An intraarterial catheter in the right radial artery is a desirable addition to standard monitors. With its location proximal to the CoA, the response to the aortic cross-clamp can be monitored. The only exception to the use of the right

Table 27-1   Preoperative Management Strategies in Infants and Children

Strategy	Infants with CoA or IAA	Children with Isolated CoA
Drugs	PGE_1 0.05–0.2 mcg/kg/min Dopamine 3–5 mcg/kg/min Calcium supplement $NaHCO_3$ for pH <7.25	Beta blockade for HTN
Ventilation	IAA or CoA with VSD: Controlled ventilation to maintain balance circulation (Q_p:Q_s 1:1) Isolated CoA: Controlled ventilation in patients requiring PGE_1 if apneic	Spontaneous
Fluid management	Hypotensive patient: 5 mL/kg isotonic fluid aliquots; may repeat if improvement observed Normotensive patient: Fluid restriction 70%–80% maintenance requirements	Maintenance fluid
Laboratory studies	Serial electrolytes Calcium Creatinine Type and cross-match CBC Arterial blood gas Liver function tests	Hematocrit Type and cross-match
Intensive Care Department	Yes	No, unless course is complicated by malignant HTN, CHF, CVA, or myocardial ischemia

CBC, complete blood count; CHF, congestive heart failure; CoA, coarctation of aorta; CVA, cerebrovascular accident; HTN, hypertension; IAA, interrupted aortic arch; PGE_1, prostaglandin E_1; VSD, ventricular septal defect.

radial artery would be the case of the anomalous right subclavian artery arising distal to the obstruction. Although one series has reported the use of temporal artery pressure monitoring in CoA with anomalous RSCA,[43] we believe the threat of retrograde propagation of an air or blood clot embolism to the brain during flushing of the catheter makes this technique prohibitively risky. The options in this setting are for the surgeon to place a needle attached to a transducer proximal to the CoA or IAA for monitoring purposes or to perform the repair without direct proximal arterial pressure monitoring.

A postductal (femoral) arterial pressure monitor can be placed to evaluate the adequacy of repair by observing resolution of the systolic pressure gradient between ascending and descending aorta (Fig. 27-9). The arterial line is also utilized to monitor acid-base status, hemoglobin, and calcium levels. Hypotension is a particular threat during release of the aortic cross-clamp, after completion of the repair.

Large-bore venous access is necessary in the event of intraoperative hemorrhage. Central venous access is important for drug administration and pressure monitoring, particularly with more complex intracardiac lesions. A urinary catheter is also placed. All patients require antibiotics for endocarditis prophylaxis; those with DiGeorge syndrome and those receiving PGE$_1$ carry increased infection risks.[37]

Fentanyl is commonly used for pain control, and the anesthetic tends to be narcotic based. Inspired gases can be used to help titrate the blood pressure. Infants and neonates are usually kept intubated at the end of the surgical procedure.

Older Children

In older patients, well-developed collaterals increase the risk of blood loss, which can be minimized by a controlled hypotensive technique. This technique also makes an otherwise tense aorta easier to mobilize. In larger patients, lung isolation with a double-lumen endotracheal tube or bronchial blocker can facilitate exposure when the procedure is done through a thoracotomy. No single anesthetic technique has been universally advocated, as both inhaled and intravenous agents have been used with success. An older technique consists of the combined use of halothane (= 1%) and labetalol (1 mg/kg) to provide titratable hypotension during the aortic cross-clamp time.[49] The children in this series ranged in age from 1 to 14 years; none had heart failure or were receiving treatment for hypertension. More recently, isoflurane has been used for both anesthetic and blood pressure

titration, and fentanyl has been used for pain control. Thoracic epidurals remain controversial due to potential risks associated with heparinization and spinal cord injury. Some opt to place the epidurals after the procedure is completed and the patient has moved the lower extremities.

Vasoactive agents should be available to treat sudden alterations in the blood pressure associated with clamping and unclamping of the aorta. Consideration should also be given to the use of drugs that can be titrated, such as sodium nitroprusside, nitroglycerin, and esmolol. Given the increased ventricular wall tension that occurs during aortic cross-clamping, control of heart rate with esmolol may be desirable to limit myocardial oxygen consumption, since increased wall tension limits myocardial perfusion pressure. The risk of spinal cord ischemia due to hypoperfusion during aortic cross-clamping must be weighed against the level of controlled hypotension.

On release of the cross-clamp, metabolic acidosis and acute hypotension may ensue. In anticipation of this "declamping syndrome," blood loss should have been replaced and normovolemia ensured. Any metabolic acidosis should be corrected. An alpha-adrenergic infusion and bolus doses (e.g., phenylephrine) should be immediately available in the event of hypotension. Calcium administration can treat the hypotension associated with declamping. Finally, and most important, the surgeon must release the aortic cross-clamp slowly.

Surgical Repair of Coarctation

Overview

The objective of surgical treatment is relief of aortic obstruction with minimal risk of repeat stenosis. Over the years, there has been debate about the ideal age for repair of CoA. The discussion has focused on the issues of operative mortality in infancy, the risk of restenosis, and the likelihood of persistent hypertension after repair. There is no disagreement over the need for neonates presenting with CHF to undergo repair as soon as they are metabolically stable. However, debate over the issues of optimal surgical technique and whether single- or two-stage repair of associated defects is appropriate has persisted. There has been a trend of decreasing operative mortality in all age groups, making earlier surgical intervention a more attractive option.[135] Long-term outcome studies suggest that residual hypertension and cardiovascular morbidity and mortality are increased when repairs are made later in life. Recoarctation is the most common late complication among

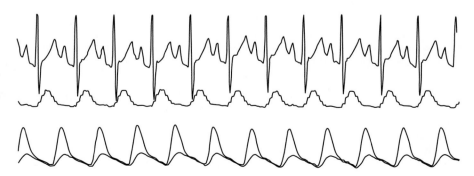

FIGURE 27-9 Pre- and postductal arterial pressure tracings in a patient with coarctation anatomy (CoA) showing the pressure gradient between ascending and descending aorta.

patients repaired in infancy. Operative mortality for repair of CoA is 2% to 3% in patients older than 1 year[74] and 7% in infants.[18] Conte and colleagues[18] reviewed the cases of 307 consecutive neonates at a single institution for coarctation repair and found that mortality is primarily dependent on the complexity of the cardiac associations: 2% mortality in patients with isolated CoA and 17% mortality in patients with complex intracardiac lesions. Operative mortality for repair of restenosis has been decreasing; a recent study reported a 7% mortality.[87] Of note, 26% of the 43 patients required augmentation of the aorta with hypothermic circulatory arrest. A review by the Congenital Heart Surgeons Society of 326 neonates with coarctation noted a 7% mortality rate in those neonates with no VSD and a mortality of 13% in the presence of a VSD. Additional associated defects in the LV outflow tract (such as hypoplastic left ventricle) increased the mortality further.[85a] Improvements in surgical techniques have changed the outcome and favor earlier repair.

Four operative procedures are commonly used to repair CoA: (1) resection of the stenotic segment and end-to-end aortic anastomosis, (2) patch augmentation, (3) subclavian flap aortoplasty, and (4) extended resection with primary anastomosis (Fig. 27-10). The optimal procedure depends on the age of the patient, the need for growth of the repair, the length of the stenosis, and the surgeon's preference.

Newborns

Resection with end-to-end anastomosis is one of the surgical procedures commonly used in the newborn. The left thoracotomy approach is generally used. It has the advantage of removing all ductal tissue from the repair site and of preserving the left subclavian artery. Unfortunately, many neonates have some degree of hypoplasia of the aortic arch as well as extensive ductal tissue in the periductal aorta so that simple end-to-end resection and anastomosis will not always be sufficient to provide adequate relief from the coarctation. A modification of end-to-end resection and anastomosis called extended end-to-end anastomosis, which involves end-to-side anastomosis of the descending aorta to a separate incision extended onto the underside of the aortic arch, proximal to the hypoplastic segment, provides superior relief from the various levels of obstruction found in neonatal coarctation.[86] The incidence of recurrent coarctation may be decreased with this approach because all ductal tissue and tissue with tubular hypoplasia excised. Extended end-to-end repair has become the procedure of choice for neonatal coarctation in most centers even though tension on the anastomosis can lead to restenosis, especially in small neonates, and the technique has a more demanding learning curve. Extended end-to-end repair is usually performed through a left thoracotomy but can be performed via a median sternotomy on cardiopulmonary bypass (CPB) when associated defects are repaired at the same setting (e.g., VSD closure).

The subclavian flap repair uses the ipsilateral subclavian artery as a fold-down flap to enlarge the coarctation site (see Fig. 27-10).[125] It is performed via a left thoracotomy approach. The use of viable autograft potentially allows growth of the repaired segment. Tension is avoided at the anastomosis, and the procedure is technically simpler than end-to-end anastomosis. Criticism of the technique includes the obligatory

sacrifice of the subclavian artery, inability to correct arch hypoplasia in some cases, and the low but constant risk of extremity ischemia.[125] Subtle impairment of arm strength or length may develop, as well as late cerebral ischemic syndromes by a steal mechanism.[123] The late recurrence rate of coarctation following this procedure now appears not to be substantially better than more aggressive surgical treatments such as extended end-to-end anastomosis, and, consequently, the use of subclavian flap repair is used with diminishing frequency. If subclavian flap repair is contemplated, arterial monitoring lines, blood pressure cuffs, and even blood gas sampling are forbidden on the repair side, lest ischemic complications develop.

Prosthetic patch augmentation is a third surgical option that has been used successfully in neonates. A longitudinal incision opens the coarcted segment, which is then covered with a Dacron (polyester) or polytetrafluoroethylene (PTFE, GoreTex) patch. This approach avoids an extensive dissection and the attendant risk of sacrificing intercostal collaterals. Unfortunately, long-term follow-up shows that children with a prosthetic patch aortoplasty are at risk for aneurysm development on the aortic wall opposite the patch. Nevertheless, avoidance of resection of the intimal ridge at the site of coarctation and use of PTFE seem to have eliminated the risk of late aneurysm formation, and this remains a viable option for neonates. Patch aortoplasty has a unique benefit in that it can be performed without ligating the ductus arteriosus and has been reported in cases where the coarctation is associated with relative left ventricular hypoplasia. In these instances, repair of the coarctation with a prosthetic patch can create unloading to the affected ventricle, which still might require several days until it is capable of providing adequate systemic output. During this time, the patient is maintained on PGE_1, and right to left shunting across the ductus augments systemic perfusion and helps to unload the "backed-up" pulmonary circulation. When the ductal shunt reverses to left to right (signaling improvement of LV function, compliance, and output), the prostaglandins can be stopped. If the ductus does not close at this point, it can be safely ligated.

When concomitant cardiac procedures or transverse arch repairs are performed, CoA can be repaired by the anterior midline approach. In neonates in particular, the proximal descending aorta can be mobilized and brought cephalad and anterior to join the undersurface of the arch. Deep hypothermic cardiopulmonary bypass and circulatory arrest are required. The technique used is similar to that described for repair of IAA (see later).

Prematurity and low birth weight have been reported as risk factors for coarctation repair. With advancing techniques, survival in small infants is improving. Bacha and associates[4] reported a series of 18 patients with median weight of 1.33 kg, with one early and two late deaths. Five-year freedom from intervention was 60%.

Older Infants and Children

Children 1 to 10 years of age are usually treated by resection and end-to-end anastomosis. As in neonates, the approach is via a left thoracotomy. Children presenting at this age typically have focal stenoses without tubular hypoplasia of the distal

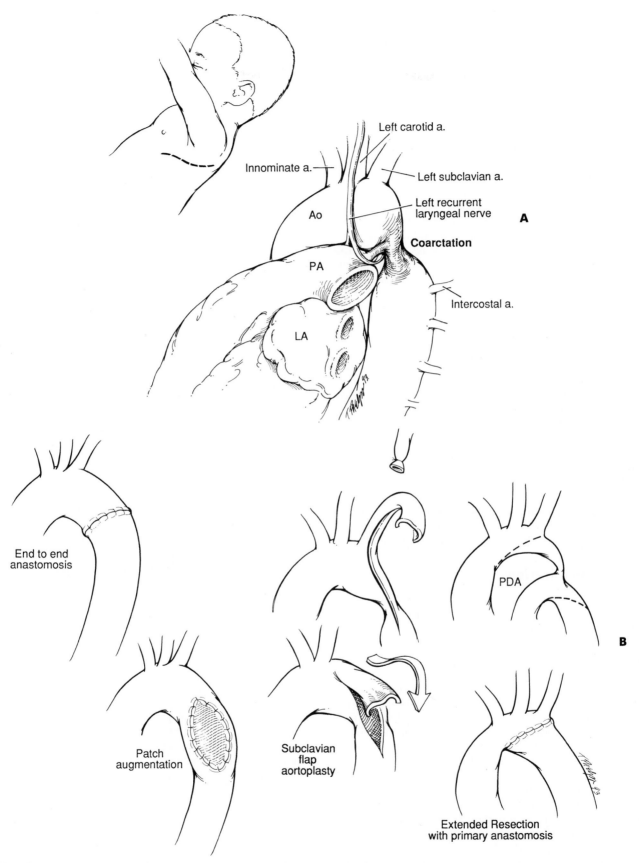

FIGURE 27-10   Surgical approach to coarctation of the aorta. **A,** Placement of a typical surgical incision and surgical anatomy. **B,** Four operative procedures commonly used in repair of coarctation of the aorta: resection of the stenotic segment and end-to-end aortic anastomosis, patch augmentation, subclavian flap aortoplasty, and extended resection with primary anastomosis. a, artery; Ao, aorta; LA, left atrium; PA, pulmonary artery; PDA, patent ductus arteriosus.

transverse arch or isthmus. This anatomic pattern is most conducive to resection followed by a tension-free anastomosis. An enlarged collateral circulation is likely to be the most common anatomic variation in this age group. Hemorrhage can be difficult to control if one of these enlarged vessels is damaged during the dissection.

Adolescents and Young Adults

Repair in the adolescent age group is usually accomplished by prosthetic patch aortoplasty, tubular graft replacement of the stenotic segment (rare), or prosthetic graft bypass of the coarctation. With these patients, growth of the repair is not necessary, and mobilization and clamping of the aorta for end-to-end anastomosis can be dangerous because of the presence of extensive arterial collaterals and the greater risk of paraplegia in the mature central nervous system. Cross-clamping of the aorta in some patients in whom collaterals are not well developed will produce unacceptable hypotension in the distal aorta (< 50 mm Hg), raising the risk of paraplegia.

For patients at greater risk of spinal cord ischemia, several strategies have been suggested for preservation of spinal cord blood flow, including use of temporary vascular heparin-bonded shunts, venoarterial cardiopulmonary bypass, and mild systemic hypothermia. The anterior spinal artery is the sole blood supply to the motor portion of the cord and receives several collateral branches from intercostal arteries. The largest branch is the artery of Adamkiewicz, which arises at the lower thoracic region. During clamping of the aorta, this artery becomes the sole source of collateral circulation to the cord. In general, retrograde flow is much less efficient than caudally directed flow. Some anesthesiologists and surgeons place an arterial catheter in the femoral artery to ensure an adequate distal mean arterial pressure of at least 50 mm Hg. Decreasing the downstream pressure by draining the cerebrospinal fluid can also augment the perfusion pressure.

Surgical Complications

Surgical morbidity after repair of CoA includes anastomotic leak, cardiac arrest, chylothorax, gastrointestinal bleeding, phrenic nerve injury, postcoarctectomy hypertension, recurrent laryngeal nerve injury, seizures, and spinal cord injury (Fig. 27-11). In the landmark review by Brewer and associates,[10] 12,532 coarctectomies were described, and spinal cord ischemic injury occurred in 51 cases (0.41%), but rarely in infants and neonates. There was no association with cross-clamp time. Lack of collaterals and the intrinsic anatomy of the anterior spinal artery may contribute. A higher incidence (1.5%) was reported from a single institutional experience.[60] Aneurysm developing at the site of repair was noted in 5.4%, predominately after patch aortoplasty, using the older techniques of extensive intimal ridge resection and Dacron patch material.[54] Ischemic complications from subclavian artery ligation are rare. The most common abnormal findings after sacrifice of the left subclavian artery are temperature differences between the right and left arm and mild shortening of the left arm.[120] CoA repair before 1 year of age has been associated with a low incidence of late hypertension; relief after 1 year of age results in a sixfold increase in occurrence.[103]

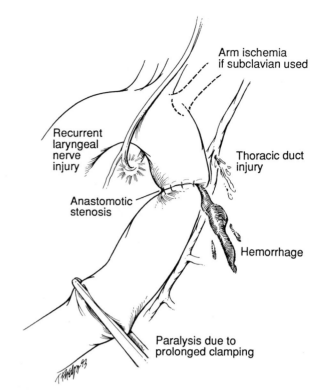

FIGURE 27-11   Complications following repair of coarctation of the aorta.

Postoperative Critical Care Management

Respiratory Function

Older or asymptomatic children are frequently extubated in the operating room or relatively quickly after CoA repair. Newborns and infants with CoA and VSD may have a reactive pulmonary circulation and may experience pulmonary hypertension. Patients at risk should receive intravenous sedation and controlled ventilation during the first 12 to 24 hours after surgery. Documented pulmonary hypertension should be treated with inhaled nitric oxide. Thereafter, these patients can usually be weaned from mechanical ventilation and extubated.

Stridor may become evident at the time of extubation because of recurrent laryngeal nerve injury leading to unilateral vocal cord paralysis. The impact of this partial airway obstruction depends on the age of the patient and the magnitude of other coexisting cardiopulmonary problems. Newborns and infants are at greatest risk because the compliant chest wall retracts during partially obstructed inspiration, and poor lung expansion may result. The markedly negative intrathoracic pressures during obstructive breathing impose an additional afterload on the left ventricle, which may exacerbate heart failure. Those with respiratory distress should be reintubated. If the nerve was traumatized but not severed, function may return after several days. Nutrition should be optimized in preparation for another extubation attempt. If there is evidence of obstruction in a newborn, nasal continuous positive pressure can be evaluated as a means of overcoming the obstruction in a less-invasive manner. Failed extubation for 7 to 10 days secondary to recurrent laryngeal nerve injury warrants airway evaluation by an otolaryngologist and consideration for tracheostomy.

Phrenic nerve injury leading to hemidiaphragmatic paralysis may be diagnosed initially by chest radiograph. Typically, the hemidiaphragm is elevated, although this can be masked by positive-pressure ventilation. Diagnosis is made by fluoroscopy or ultrasound study of the diaphragm, with the patient momentarily removed from positive-pressure ventilation and breathing spontaneously. Older children are usually asymptomatic with hemidiaphragmatic paralysis, and intervention is not necessary. However, a paralyzed hemidiaphragm may prohibit separation of the infant from mechanical ventilation. In that setting, definitive management involves plication of the diaphragm, which some surgeons perform immediately on diagnosis. Others wait 7 to 10 days in the event that the nerve was traumatized and may have better function with time. If the second extubation fails, a diaphragmatic plication is indicated.

Thoracic duct injury may lead to chylothorax, which usually presents as a milky pleural effusion after the initiation of postoperative feeds. If the diagnosis is unclear, triglyceride levels or lipoprotein electrophoresis looking for chylomicrons can be diagnostic. Chylothorax may require repeated aspiration or chest tube drainage, which can improve lung function and enable monitoring of the amount drained. In addition to compromised lung function, persistent chylothorax may lead to hypoproteinemia, hypogammaglobulinemia, and lymphopenia with resultant nutritional debilitation. There is debate over whether chylothorax after CoA repair is best treated by immediate thoracic duct ligation or conservatively with dietary maneuvers alone. Conservative treatment with dietary manipulation alone excludes long-chain fatty acids in favor of medium-chain fatty acids, which can be absorbed directly by the portal system and bypass the thoracic duct. If necessary, flow through the thoracic duct can be further reduced by resting the gastrointestinal tract and providing total intravenous nutrition. Enteral feeds without long-chain fatty acids may resume after 1 to 2 weeks of rest. If the chyle recurs with restarting enteral feeds, the thoracic duct can be surgically ligated, or, sometimes, simply reexploration of the thoracotomy will reveal the area (most often in the region of the superior intercostal vein; just above the area of coarctation repair) that is oozing chyle, and this area can be easily controlled with a few ligatures. Nutrition is an important consideration during this process. If the patient's nutritional status deteriorates during persistent chylothorax, surgical ligation of leaking lymphatics should be undertaken earlier in the course. The postoperative management strategies are summarized in Table 27-2.

Cardiovascular Function after Complex Repairs

Coarctation patients with complex intracardiac defects necessitating cardiopulmonary bypass may have myocardial dysfunction, pulmonary hypertension, or arrhythmias, which are similar to the problems after interrupted aortic arch repair. Therefore, management of this scenario is discussed under "Interrupted Aortic Arch," below.

Postoperative Systemic Hypertension

The cardiac problems for patients with isolated coarctation generally involve hypertension or ischemia. Early postoperative control of hypertension protects the aortic anastomosis, minimizes the risk of aneurysm formation in the dilated poststenotic segment, and alleviates the postcoarctectomy syndrome. Hence, mean arterial pressure is rigidly maintained in the normal range for age. During the immediate postoperative period, this may be achieved by titration of nitroprusside and esmolol[128] infusions, or labetalol alone and adequate pain relief. Some institutions have started to use nicardipine infusions for blood pressure control in this period.[79a] Once the patient is ready for discharge from the intensive care unit, intermittent doses of propranolol, atenolol, labetalol, or captopril may be substituted.

Postoperative hypertension is seen in patients with persistent stenosis or recoarctation but can also be found in the absence of a significant residual postoperative gradient. The hypertension can last for variable lengths of time. Patel and colleagues[85] suggest a higher incidence of postoperative hypertension in patients repaired later in life. Renal function is normal, but plasma renin levels are elevated in these patients. The series by Seirafi and coworkers[103] reported a 4.2% incidence of late hypertension in the group repaired during infancy, compared with 16.8% in the group that underwent later repair.

The study of postcoarctectomy hypertension suggests a biphasic and multifactorial etiology. The incidence of postcoarctectomy hypertension ranges from 37% to 100% in several series. Postrepair hypertension may be explained by surgical stimulation of sympathetic nerve fibers located between the media and adventitia of the aortic isthmus; this stimulation

Table 27-2 Postoperative Management Strategies after Repair of Coarctation in the Infant or Older Child; Management Strategies after IAA Are Similar to Those for Infantile Coarctation

	Infants with CoA or IAA	Older Child with CoA
Drugs	Dopamine, milrinone	Antihypertensives (nitroprusside, esmolol)
Ventilation	Controlled ventilation	Spontaneous
	Monitor for pulmonary hypertension	Monitor for atelectasis or pneumothorax associated with thoracotomy
Fluid management	2/3 maintenance fluids	Maintenance fluids
Laboratory tests	Serial electrolytes	Serial hematocrits
	Serial hematocrits	
	Creatinine	
	Serial ABG	
Intensive Care Department	Yes	Yes

ABG, arterial blood gases; CoA, coarctation of aorta; IAA, interrupted aortic arch.

causes release of norepinephrine with consequential blood pressure elevation. This sympathetic stimulation also causes the juxtaglomerular cells to release renin.[134] Benedict and colleagues[9] demonstrated a 750% increase in norepinephrine concentrations in the first 12 postoperative hours, a finding unique to coarctectomy patients. Lioy and associates[63] showed that aortic stimulation had direct adrenergic effects on blood pressure, and these responses could be avoided by infiltrating the aortic wall with lidocaine. The presence of numerous myelinated and unmyelinated sympathetic fibers in the aortic arch has been confirmed by Khaisman.[53] Postoperative elevation of plasma epinephrine and norepinephrine was demonstrated by Gidding and associates[28] and Leenen and colleagues,[57] who also blocked the postoperative systolic hypertension by pretreatment with propranolol.

A second blood pressure change has been observed 2 to 3 days postoperatively, consisting primarily of increased diastolic blood pressure. This second blood pressure response has been associated with mesenteric arteritis. Rocchinni and colleagues[93] showed an elevation in plasma renin activity in the first postoperative week, compared with a non-CoA control surgical group. Elevated renin activity is important in early postoperative hypertension but not in chronic postrepair hypertension, as renin levels return to normal by the seventh postoperative day. Therefore, it can be postulated that manipulation of the aorta during surgical repair causes sympathetic discharge, resulting in immediate postoperative hypertension. This in turn leads to renin release, which causes secondary hypertension.[23] The hypertensive response to surgical repair is not seen after balloon angioplasty, nor is there a rise in plasma catecholamine levels or plasma renin activity.[12]

Altered baroreceptor function was reported in a group of children with mild arm systolic hypertension despite good surgical repair. Their baroreflex was reset to operate at a higher arterial pressure with reduced sensitivity to changes in arterial pressure compared with control children.[8] Clarkson and associates[14] demonstrated that most patients were normotensive 5 to 10 years after their repair, but blood pressure increased in later years. This observation was independent of age of repair (study population had repair at >1 year of age).

Postcoarctectomy Syndrome

Postcoarctectomy syndrome is a well-described complication after CoA repair. The primary symptom is severe abdominal pain, accompanied by hypertension, fever, abdominal tenderness, vomiting, ileus, melena, and leukocytosis. It occurs 2 to 3 days after surgery. There is a higher incidence in patients with severe aortic constriction and hypertension,[110] and it is rare in neonates. It has been suggested that the sudden increase in blood pressure to vessels below the CoA causes postcoarctectomy syndrome, resulting in necrotizing arteritis of the small arteries of the mesentery and small intestine. Alternatively, the increased postoperative renin levels in some patients might cause abdominal pain by shunting blood from mesenteric vessels.[23] These changes have been demonstrated by angiography, laparotomy, and autopsy. The changes are reversible, and the syndrome is treated and/or prevented by control of postoperative hypertension.[38,52,68] Postcoarctectomy syndrome has not been seen in infants and children after successful treatment of native CoA by balloon angioplasty.[74]

Bleeding and the Collateral Circulation

Postoperative bleeding is a common problem following CoA repairs.[77] The aortic repair itself, by definition, is a high-pressure suture line that is relatively extensive. Loss of integrity of the suture line results in catastrophic bleeding. In older children with longstanding CoA, collaterals may have formed. The collateral system has an anterior and posterior collateral circulation. The anterior connects the internal mammary arteries and the external iliac arteries via the epigastric system. The posterior connects the thyrocervical arteries and the descending aorta via retrograde flow through dilated intercostal arteries. The intercostals can cause significant bleeding after a CoA repair; it takes time for the collaterals to regress. Heparin is frequently given for CoA repair in older children and is not always antagonized with protamine. This can contribute to postoperative bleeding. The intensive care management of bleeding involves careful blood pressure control and correction of a heparin-induced coagulopathy with protamine or fresh frozen plasma.

Pain Control

Postoperative care must include adequate pain management. Cardiac catheterization patients have mild pain, which is treated with acetaminophen. Ibuprofen can be considered after hemostasis is adequate. For surgical repair of CoA, pain management is initiated in the operating room by the anesthesiologist with regional anesthesia or intravenous narcotic. Thoracotomy incisions are more painful than sternotomy incisions. Acceptable regional techniques include epidural or intrathecal narcotics, epidural local anesthetics, or intercostal blocks. With a small risk of paraplegia associated with CoA repair, some opt to place the regional block after the repair is completed and the patient has demonstrated movement in the lower extremities. Regional (thoracic epidural) blockade can then be placed prior to the patient experiencing pain. If lower extremity movement is questionable, any local anesthetic infusion should be stopped to permit assessment. Narcotics by any route—intravenous, epidural, or intrathecal—can cause respiratory depression. Epidural or intrathecal narcotics should be monitored for 24 hours after the dose. An option with intravenous narcotics is patient- or nurse-controlled analgesia. In a monitored setting, this can increase the comfort safely.[76]

Angioplasty
Technique and Complications

In 1983, Lock and associates reported the first series of balloon angioplasties.[64] They described eight patients, three with native CoA who did not benefit from the procedure despite an initial decrease in the gradient, and four patients with re-CoA who were dilated five times with resultant increase in diameter of the CoA site and decrease in the gradient at 24 hours. In three of five successful dilations, the post-dilatation angiography showed evidence of intimal tears.[64] There were no complications reported in the series.

The dilation balloon is positioned via the femoral or umbilical artery. The actual inflation is painful. Immediate results can be evaluated by a change in pressure gradient and angiographic evidence. Potential complications include aortic aneurysm formation, aortic rupture, cerebrovascular accidents, and femoral vessel trauma. Infants are more likely to have femoral artery complications.[131] Aneurysm formation represents a major complication after angioplasty because the mechanism of CoA relief is intimal tearing. The incidence of aneurysms is 1% to 5%.[84,90,131] McCrindle and colleagues[69] reported on 970 procedures in 907 patients from a registry of 25 institutions (Table 27-3). There were complications in 14%, death in 0.7%, neurologic event in 0.6%, intimal tear/flap in 5.2% of cases with native CoA and 1.6% of cases with recurrent CoA, and pulse loss in 3%, with surgery required for 31% of those. Blood products were required in 4.1% of cases with native CoA and in 15% of cases of recurrent CoA.

Angioplasty for Recoarctation

Balloon angioplasty has evolved as the procedure of choice for recoarctation. Recurrent CoA after surgical end-to-end anastomosis, patch angioplasty, and subclavian flap have all been successfully treated with angioplasty. It has been hypothesized that the scar and fibrosis surrounding the anastomotic site may be a protective factor in dilation of patients with recoarctation. Initial success rates for relief of recoarctation are reported to be 75% to 91%.[66,88,131] Yetman and coworkers[131] reported on long-term follow-up of 90 patients for 3 to 144 months (median, 39 months); repeat angioplasty or surgical repair was required for recurrent aortic arch narrowing in 33% of their patients over the 12-year period. They found no relation between time to reintervention and type of initial surgery, age or weight at balloon angioplasty, and percent increase in coarctation diameter. Predictors of time to reintervention included transverse arch diameter less than 2 standard deviations below the mean and higher pre- and postangioplasty pressure gradient.[131] In a study of 22 infants, Maheshwari and colleagues[66] reported that the risk of restenosis with growth in childhood is low and can be successfully treated with repeat angioplasty. Long-term follow-up (median, 56 months) revealed a restenosis rate after initial optimal results of 16%. With reintervention, the success rate

was 95%. Lower infant weight correlated with a suboptimal long-term outcome.

Angioplasty for Native Coarctation

The use of balloon angioplasty in *native* CoA has been evolving and remains controversial. The initial series by Lock and coworkers[64] predicted a higher failure rate with dilation of native CoA and noted that the initial gradient fall was not predictive of long-term outcome. The acute success rates are reported as 79% to 90%,[50,69,84] although the study with 90% success rates did not include infants or neonates.[84] Rao and associates[90] followed the cases of 67 patients and found a recoarctation rate of 25% 14 months after the angioplasty and 2% at 5 to 9 years. They found higher incidence of recoarctation in infants and neonates. In a study by Kaine and colleagues,[50] patients who had early angioplasty failures and those who developed recoarctation during follow-up were younger at angioplasty. However, the high-risk group appears to be concentrated among those infants whose aortic isthmus is hypoplastic for age.

Comparison of angioplasty versus surgical results has been problematic for several reasons: There is no agreement on the optimal surgical approach. Surgical results have steadily improved with decreasing mortality and recoarctation rates.[34] Comparisons with older surgical outcomes data introduce bias. To date, there has not been a randomized controlled trial, which would settle the relative risks and benefits of angioplasty versus surgery for native coarctation.

Stents

Advances in endovascular stent technology have enabled their use in congenital heart disease, including CoA. With the elastic recoil of the aorta negating some of the beneficial balloon dilating effects, the stent has been recently pursued as an alternative. In 1991, O'Laughlin and coworkers[83] reported the first use of a stent to treat CoA. Subsequent reports have focused on the indications and benefits of the stent. Thanopoulos and colleagues[118] reported on 17 patients 0.4 to 15 years of age with isolated CoA to complex long-segment CoA. Their median follow-up was 33 months. All of the patients had good results without complication after stent placement. Fifteen of 17 were normotensive at follow-up. Although the stents can be redilated, the long-term outcome has yet to be determined, particularly in the younger patients who have growth potential. Marshall and associates[67] reported on 33 patients 5 to 60 years of age, 45% with significant structural defects accompanying the CoA who underwent successful stent placement. Notably, they reported an elevated ventricular end-diastolic pressure (17 mm Hg) despite only mild coarctation that decreased to 14 mm Hg after the stent placement. Long-term studies and more patients will help define the role of the stent in CoA, particularly compared with surgery or balloon angioplasty.

Critical Care Management after Angioplasty or Stent Placement

After angioplasty or stent placement, patients are generally observed in the intensive care unit. Their care is similar to

Table 27-3 Complications Associated with Balloon Angioplasty for CoA

	Native CoA (%)	Recurrent CoA (%)
Complication	15	13
Death	0.7	0.7
Neurologic event	0.7	0.6
Intimal tear/flap	5.2	1.6
Pulse loss	4.5	3.7
Blood products required	4.1	15

CoA, coarctation of aorta.
Modified from McCrindle BW, Jones TK, Morrow WR, Hagler DJ, Lloyd TR, Noun S, Latson LA: Acute results of balloon angioplasty of native coarctation versus recurrent aortic obstruction are equivalent. *J Am Coll Cardiol* 28:1810–1817, 1996; with permission.

that of postoperative surgical patients, although their monitoring will likely be less invasive. Commonly, they are breathing spontaneously and not intubated. Fluid balance must be assessed. Difficult access in the catheterization laboratory or multiple laboratory evaluations can result in significant blood loss during the procedure. Pneumothorax is possible if access was obtained from the internal jugular or subclavian vein. Bleeding can occur at the site of the stent or balloon dilation, the puncture site of the access, or any place along the course of the catheter. Retroperitoneal bleeding associated with catheter access is difficult to detect initially, as a large volume of blood may fill the space prior to any obvious signs except for falling hematocrit. Therefore, we recommend routine measurement of the hematocrit 6 hours after the procedure.

Special attention should be paid to evaluation of the groin puncture site and circulation in the corresponding limb. If pulses are lacking in the affected side (assuming that they are present elsewhere), attempts should be made to ensure perfusion to the affected limb. If the leg is cold and poorly perfused, surgical intervention including clot removal and vessel repair should be considered. If the leg is cool, less-invasive measures, including tissue plasminogen activator, heparin, or low-molecular-weight heparin can be considered. The uncomplicated poststent or balloon patient is monitored overnight in the intensive care setting and discharged to home the next day.

Outcome

Early (perioperative), intermediate, and long-term morbidity and mortality define the outcomes of coarctation of the aorta. The operative mortality for coarctation depends primarily on the complexity of coexisting lesions. Newborns and infants with isolated coarctation have less than 1% operative mortality after surgical repair in large multi-institutional series.[33] The operative mortality rate increases to 5% to 7% among infants with CoA and VSD based on results from the Pediatric Cardiac Care Consortium and the University Hospital Consortium.[33,81] More recently, small single-center studies report 2% to 4% hospital mortality rates for repair of CoA with VSD.[26,44] The management of the VSD does not appear to impact the early and intermediate results. This has led to considerable controversy over the best approach to treating infants with CoA and VSD, with advocates for each of the available strategies. Some have argued for coarctation repair only with the expectation for spontaneous VSD closure. Opponents of this approach contend that it will leave some infants with persistent CHF and possible ventilator dependency.

The second option of a two-stage approach involves repair of the coarctation and banding of the pulmonary artery during the first stage. This prevents CHF from pulmonary overcirculation but commits the infant to a second operation for debanding alone (if the VSD has closed spontaneously) or debanding plus VSD closure. The third option entails a single-stage repair via median sternotomy, in which the VSD is closed and the coarctation repaired. This approach also permits reconstruction of a hypoplastic proximal aortic arch or repair of subaortic stenosis, if necessary. Opponents of this approach have worried about neurologic complications if the

single-stage repair is carried out under deep hypothermic circulatory arrest. Because the current data suggest that both single- and two-stage approaches have low early and intermediate mortality rates (< 5%), the approach depends on institutional preference, the size of the VSD (i.e., the likelihood of spontaneous VSD closure), the presence of proximal arch hypoplasia, and the presence of subaortic stenosis.

The infant with complex cardiac anatomy or confounding medical problems has a higher operative mortality rate. The University Hospital Consortium data suggest that coarctation repair as part of surgery for hypoplastic left heart syndrome carries a 50% mortality rate. When hypoplastic left heart syndrome is excluded, the mortality rate for coarctation repair as a component of complex cardiac repairs is 28.6%.[33]

Follow-up now spanning several decades has illuminated the long-term health outlook for the patient after coarctation repair. Toro-Salazar and coworkers[121] analyzed the course over several decades of 252 patients who survived to hospital discharge after repair of isolated CoA from 1948 to 1976. Cumulative long-term survival for isolated coarctation decreased over time from 95% at 10 years to 89% at 20 years, 82% at 30 years, and 79% at 40 years (Fig. 27-12). The major explained causes of late death in this population included coronary artery disease, intraoperative death during a second cardiac operation, and aortic dissection. Ninety-two of the 207 long-term survivors were examined, and 31% were found to have an undiagnosed cardiovascular abnormality, of which systemic hypertension was most common. The etiology of chronic hypertension in the absence of recoarctation may relate to increased stiffness of the repaired aorta. The proximal aortic wall is more rigid than the post-coarctation wall and has more collagen and less smooth muscle.[102]

Recoarctation is one of the most common complications of CoA surgery. It can be due to several mechanisms: (1) incomplete initial repair; (2) residual abnormal aortic tissue that may proliferate; (3) failure of the anastomotic site

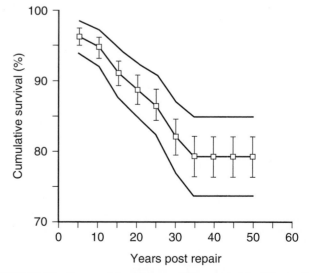

FIGURE 27-12 The overall long-term cumulative survival for 252 operative survivors of coarctation of the aorta at the University of Minnesota. Patients underwent surgery between 1948 and 1976. (From Toro-Salazar OH, Steinberger J, Thomas W, et al: Long-term follow-up of patients after coarctation of the aorta repair. *Am J Cardiol* 89:541–547, 2002, with permission.)

Table 27-4 Complications of Angioplasty
for Aortic Recoarctation

Complication Type	Frequency (%)
Balloon rupture	9.5
Thrombosis (femoral)	5.5
Decreased pulses (femoral)	3
Death	2.5
Postcoarctectomy syndrome	2
Neurologic event	1.5
Intimal dissection	1.5

From Hellenbrand WE, Allen HD, Golinko RJ, Hagler DJ, Lufin W, Kan J: Balloon angioplasty for aortic recoarctation: Results of valvuloplasty and angioplasty of Congenital Anomalies Registry. *Am J Cardiol* 65:793–797, 1990.

to grow; (4) thrombus formation at the suture line; or (5) intimal and medial hyperplasia at the anastomotic site.[74] Recoarctation rates have been highest in patients repaired during infancy. Use of the end-to-end anastomosis has also been implicated. However, there was less reported recoarctation with absorbable sutures with end-to-end anastomosis.[3,135] In his 1991 review of risk factors for recoarctation, Jonas[47] found no conclusive data to support the use of end-to-end anastomosis versus subclavian flap aortoplasty. It is generally felt that with the best techniques available, restenosis occurs in about 20% of neonatal repairs, 10% to 15% of infant repairs, and 5% of childhood repairs. When significant restenosis occurs (resting gradient >20 mm Hg), reoperation or balloon dilation is warranted. Surgical repair of recurrent CoA usually involves prosthetic patch enlargement of the stenotic site or bypass of the segment with a tubular graft.

A multicenter prospective study of 200 patients with recoarctation treated by balloon angioplasty showed that 50% had the gradient reduced to less than 10 mm Hg, 28.4% had the gradient reduced to 11 to 20 mm Hg, and 21.6% had residual gradients greater than 21 mm Hg.[36] Complications among these 200 patients are listed in Table 27-4. Deaths were due to (1) aortic rupture, (2) sudden death in the first 24 hours after angioplasty, (3) cerebral edema, or (4) LV failure. The mortality rate was 2.5%; other series report rates of 0% to 2.5%, while surgical operative mortality for recoarctation ranges from 3% to 33%.[89] Long-term follow-up for balloon angioplasty of recoarctations reported 72% to 82% free of reintervention.[88,131] Results were similar despite various original surgical procedures, which included end-to-end anastomosis, patch aortoplasty, subclavian flap aortoplasty, IAA repair, and palliation of hypoplastic left heart syndrome.[99]

INTERRUPTED AORTIC ARCH

Classification and Anatomy

Interrupted aortic arch is a rare but highly lethal form of congenital heart disease, carrying a mortality rate higher than 90% in the neonatal period if not treated.[100] The incidence of IAA is 1% of all congenital heart defects. Celoria and Patton[11] described the currently used anatomic definitions, in which type A is interrupted distal to the left subclavian artery; type B, between the left subclavian and left carotid

arteries; and type C, proximal to the left carotid artery (Fig. 27-13). Type B IAA is the most common (78%), followed by type A (20%), and type C (2%).[72,101,104] Associated intracardiac anomalies are the rule and are listed in Box 27-4. All have a patent ductus arteriosus, and most have a VSD; also seen are aortic valve anomalies, truncus arteriosus, and double-outlet right ventricle. The VSD is typically conoventricular in origin and is associated with posterior malalignment of the conal septum.[56] The posterior malalignment of the conal septum is associated with left ventricular outflow tract obstruction (LVOTO) at the subvalvuvar and valvuvar levels.

Many patients with IAA have extracardiac anomalies. Unlike those with CoA, the predominant extracardiac abnormality in these patients is DiGeorge syndrome (see Chapter 46,

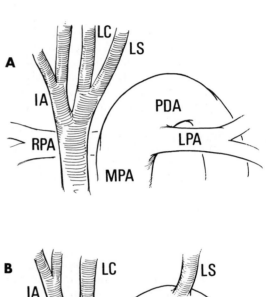
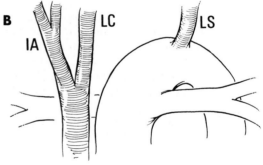
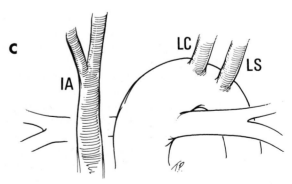

FIGURE 27-13 Celoria and Patton classification of interrupted aortic arch. *Type A* is interrupted distal to the left subclavian artery, *type B* between the left subclavian and left carotid arteries, and *type C* proximal to the left carotid artery. IA, innominate artery; LC, left carotid artery; LPA, left pulmonary artery; LS, left subclavian artery; MPA, main pulmonary artery; PDA, posterior descending artery; RPA, right pulmonary artery.

BOX 27-4   *Defects Associated with Interrupted Aortic Arch*

Ventricular septal defect
Left ventricular outflow tract obstruction
Anomalous right subclavian artery
Aortopulmonary window
Truncus arteriosus
Transposition of the great arteries
Single ventricle

Syndromes and Congenital Heart Defects).[72,104] The association of DiGeorge syndrome with type B IAA suggests that both are part of a causally heterogeneous developmental field defect.[112] Using fluorescence in situ hybridization (FISH) analysis, Lewin and colleagues[61] and Rauch and associates[91] demonstrated that 50% to 80% of patients with IAA type B have 22q11.2 chromosomal deletions. IAA is usually a rare anomaly, but in DiGeorge syndrome, it is a common defect.[17,35] Conley and associates[17] reported that 36% of their patients with DiGeorge syndrome had type B IAA, and all of their autopsied patients had congenital heart disease. Reports of IAA type A with DiGeorge syndrome are rare.[116] The presence of IAA type B with or without the DiGeorge phenotype is an indication for genetic screening for the 22q11 deletion in the patient.

Embryology

The normal embryology of the aortic arch is a complex interaction of tissues arising from the primitive aortic arches, truncus arteriosus, and left dorsal aorta. Schematic drawing of the postnatal aortic arch illustrates the origins of the various portions of the arch complex (Fig. 27-14). The fourth aortic arch is of particular interest in the pathogenesis of IAA type B. As shown in Figure 27-14, aortic arch tissue between the left carotid and left subclavian arteries is derived from the fourth primitive aortic arch. The right subclavian artery (RSCA), also derived in part from the fourth arch, is often malposed in patients with IAA. This anomaly is especially prevalent in patients with IAA type B, but it can also be associated with CoA or can be an independent anomaly. When anomalous, the origin of the RSCA is distal to the left subclavian artery, and the artery courses posteriorly to the esophagus, potentially causing esophageal or tracheal compression.[45] When an aberrant RSCA arises distal to the interruption or coarctation, the patient may have decreased blood pressure in the right arm or right vertebral-subclavian steal.[43,45]

Decreased aortic flow potentially leads to atresia or interruption. However, not all children with obstructive arch lesions have intracardiac lesions that decrease aortic flow. Freedom and associates[25] studied this issue in patients with IAA and VSD and found no definitive mechanism for decreased aortic flow, although 50% had LV outflow tract narrowing that was characterized as conoventricular malalignment.

Left-sided outflow tract and arch anomalies may be due to neural crest migratory problems. Cranial neural crest gives rise to ectomesenchyme, which populates pharyngeal arches III, IV, and VI. These primitive vessels contribute to the carotid arteries, a portion of the aortic arch, the right subclavian artery, and the ductus arteriosus. The tunica media of the aortic arch consists entirely of cranial neural crest cell derivatives.[51,58] Thus, abnormal migration of neural crest cells may have structural consequences and change blood flow patterns. Chromosomal abnormalities may induce abnormalities of the neural crest cells. There is also experimental evidence that fibronectin plays a role in neural crest cell migration and that fibronectin deficiency might result in obliteration of the fourth arch artery in the chick embryo.[114]

Pathophysiology

The pathophysiology of IAA is similar to that of neonatal CoA with VSD. Systemic blood flow is dependent on patency of the ductus. As the ductus closes, the infant develops shock, acidosis, and renal failure. The increasing systemic resistance redirects blood flow to the pulmonary circulation, which ultimately results in volume and pressure overload of the heart, pulmonary edema, and biventricular failure. Any LVOTO further exacerbates pressure overload to the left side of the heart.

Diagnostic Assessment

Interrupted aortic arch presents in a fashion similar to critical coarctation in the newborn. The infant develops tachypnea and poor perfusion as the ductus closes, generally within the first 7 to 10 days of life. Physical examination reveals rales, tachycardia, a loud systolic murmur, hepatomegaly, and decreased femoral pulses. Differential cyanosis between the upper and lower body is usually difficult to appreciate because of significant mixing at the VSD. However, pulse oximetry may show higher oxygen saturation levels in the preductal arm compared with the lower body if the great vessels are normally related. If the great vessels are transposed, the oxygen saturation may be higher in the lower body (reversed differential cyanosis).

Given the common association between IAA type B and DiGeorge syndrome, every infant with suspected IAA should be examined for the DiGeorge stigmata. These include a broad nasal bridge, malar hypoplasia, narrow palpebral fissures, hypertelorism, low-set posteriorly rotated ears, retrognathia, small mouth, and submucosal cleft palate. These stigmata may be difficult to appreciate in the newborn. Therefore, every infant with IAA should be presumed to have DiGeorge syndrome until this can be ruled out by fluorescent in situ hybridization, which probes for submicroscopic deletions in chromosome 22q11.2. Because patients with DiGeorge syndrome have thymic and parathyroid deficiency of variable degree, the physician must anticipate the possibility of T cell deficiency and hypocalcemia. The major risk of T cell deficiency in this patient population is graft-versus-host disease after transfusion with nonirradiated blood.

The ECG and chest x-ray point to heart disease but do not establish a specific diagnosis. The ECG shows right ventricular hypertrophy, and the chest x-ray shows cardiomegaly with pulmonary overcirculation.

Echocardiography establishes the specific diagnosis. The suprasternal long-axis view shows the ductus ending in the

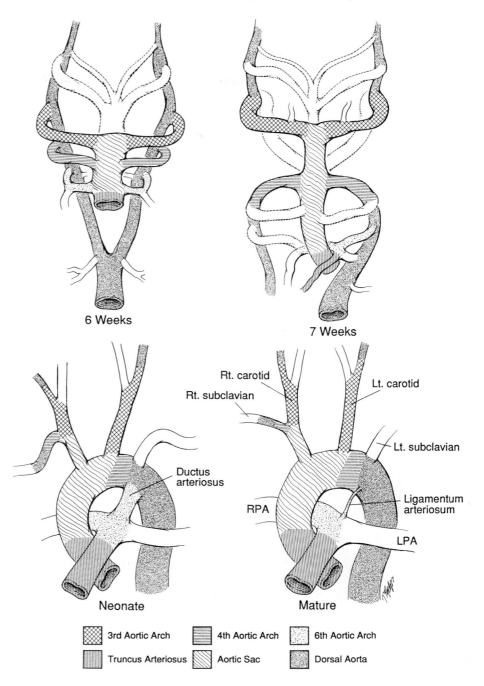

FIGURE 27-14 The postnatal aortic arch, illustrating the embryologic origins at the sixth and seventh gestational weeks of the various portions of the arch complex. LPA, left pulmonary artery; Lt, left; RPA, right pulmonary artery; Rt, Right.

6 Weeks

7 Weeks

Rt. carotid

Rt. subclavian

Lt. carotid

Lt. subclavian

Ductus arteriosus

RPA

Ligamentum arteriosum

LPA

Neonate

Mature

| | 3rd Aortic Arch | | 4th Aortic Arch | | 6th Aortic Arch |
| | Truncus Arteriosus | | Aortic Sac | | Dorsal Aorta |

descending aorta. There is no continuity between the ascending and descending aorta. The presence of coexisting defects should be carefully explored (see Box 27-4). Of particular importance is the diagnosis of LVOTO, which may be under-recognized preoperatively. Several echocardiographic indices may identify LVOTO, including the indexed cross-sectional area of the LV outflow tract, the subaortic diameter index, and the subaortic diameter Z score.[2] Although the measurement of LV outflow tract area is more sensitive, the measurement of subaortic diameter is more reproducible and equally predictive. Salem and associates[98] showed that patients with aortic valve diameter less than 4.5 mm (Z score <−5) subsequently developed LVOTO, whereas those with aortic valve

diameter greater than 4.5 mm (Z > −5) did not. Failure to diagnose and correct LVOTO surgically is likely to result in persistent heart failure in the postoperative period. Cardiac catheterization is rarely indicated unless the arch anatomy or intracardiac defects remain ambiguous after echocardiography.

Preoperative Critical Care Management of Interrupted Aortic Arch

The preoperative critical care management of IAA is similar to that of neonatal CoA. The primary objective is to maintain ductal patency with PGE$_1$. Shock and CHF usually improve after PGE$_1$ administration. However, some infants will require inotropic support and mechanical ventilation in addition to PGE$_1$. Hyperoxia and hypocarbia should be avoided to lessen the chances for pulmonary overcirculation.

Hypocalcemia is a common finding in patients with IAA, even those who do not have DiGeorge syndrome, and these infants require calcium replacement.[17,82] They are at increased risk for symptomatic hypocalcemia during hyperventilation and transfusion of citrated blood products. Irradiated blood products should be used to prevent graft-versus-host disease in all infant CoA and IAA repairs unless DiGeorge syndrome has been specifically excluded. At the Johns Hopkins Hospital, all pediatric blood products are irradiated as an extra safety precaution.

Interrupted Aortic Arch Repair

Surgical treatment of IAA is more complex than that for simple coarctation (Fig. 27-15). For repair, cardiopulmonary bypass with deep hypothermic circulatory arrest is required. An arterial cannula is placed in the ascending aorta, and a venous cannula is placed in the right atrium. When the ductus is still patent, a second arterial cannula is placed in the main pulmonary artery to supply circulation to the descending aorta via the ductus.

The currently favored approach is single-stage repair of the interruption via median sternotomy and total correction of the intracardiac defects, which usually entails closure of the VSD and atrial septal defect. This approach has largely replaced the older two-stage procedure of left thoracotomy and graft interposition between ascending and descending aorta with pulmonary artery banding, followed months to years later by sternotomy and closure of the VSD and pulmonary artery debanding. The single-stage approach avoids prosthetic materials in reconstruction of the arch. However, recurrent arch obstruction complicates more than 50% of the repairs, and late development of subaortic narrowing is common. Subaortic obstruction is frequently implicated in mortality and reoperation.[101] Luciani and associates[65] described a surgical approach utilizing the VSD patch to open the left ventricular outflow tract, with relief of the subaortic stenosis.

When the posterior deviation of the infundibular septum creates unacceptable restriction to LV outflow, the surgical decision-making is more complicated. If the aortic annulus Z score predicts the possibility of two-ventricle repair, then it

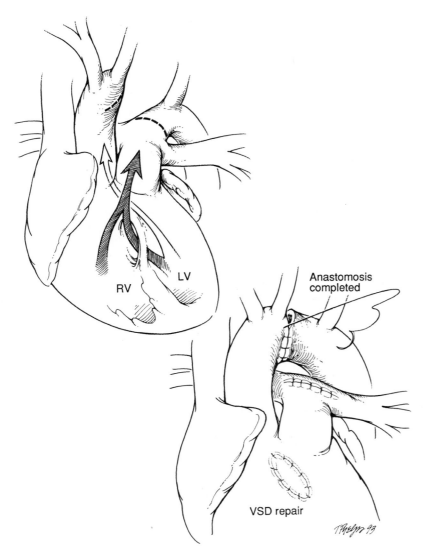

RV
LV
Anastomosis completed
VSD repair
TPhelps 93

FIGURE 27-15 Surgical repair of interrupted aortic arch. RV, right ventricle; LV, left ventricle; VSD, ventricular septal defect.

is possible to resect a large portion of the infundibular septum to enlarge the LV outflow. If the LV outflow obstruction is prohibitive, then the surgeon has two options. One is to perform closure of the VSD (with VSD enlargement if necessary) such that the LV outflow is diverted into the pulmonary valve. A Damus-Kaye-Stansel connection of the aorta and the pulmonary artery then creates a "double outlet" for the left ventricle, and this constructed outflow is anastomosed to the reconstructed ascending aorta and aortic arch. RV to PA continuity is restored with a conduit. Alternatively, an atrial septectomy can be performed and combined with a Damus-Kaye-Stansel. Instead of an RV to PA conduit, pulmonary blood flow is restored with an aortopulmonary shunt. This is a modification of a Norwood operation and predicts that the LV outflow tract will be prohibitive for eventual two-ventricle repair, thus creating the first stage toward Fontan. A final alternative for prohibitive LV outflow tract obstruction is to perform a neonatal Ross/Konno aortic valve replacement in conjunction with the VSD closure and the aortic arch repair. Clearly, these patients require careful surgical judgment that is enhanced by experience.

In addition to the complications following CoA repair, infants with IAA must be evaluated for anastomotic stenosis, aortic and subaortic obstruction, residual atrial or ventricular shunts, pulmonary hypertension, heart block, and left bronchial compression by the reconstructed aortic arch.

Postoperative Critical Care Management

The general principles of critical care management after surgical correction depend on multiple factors including age, preoperative condition, surgical anatomy, intraoperative course, and many others, which are reviewed in Chapter 23, Perioperative Management. The more specific scenarios that usually apply to complex coarctation or IAA repair are outlined in Table 27-2. Specific organ system considerations are discussed in the following sections.

Cardiovascular Function

Cardiovascular events after IAA repair are anticipated with invasive monitoring. Central venous, left atrial (LA), pulmonary artery (PA), and two arterial lines may be useful invasive monitors for IAA repair. The IAA repair involves significant aortic suture lines that are at risk for bleeding. Blood pressure control with vasodilators such as nitroglycerin or nitroprusside reduces this risk and is guided by arterial pressure monitoring. However, vasodilators should be avoided in the face of LVOTO or anastomotic stenosis because of the risk of vasodilation in the face of fixed left ventricular output leading to refractory hypotension. Right radial and femoral arterial pressure monitoring identifies an aortic pressure gradient, which would suggest a stenosis at the site of the repair. Elevations in left atrial pressure may point to residual LVOTO or LV dysfunction following deep hypothermic circulatory arrest. Milrinone is useful as the initial therapy for ventricular dysfunction. An arterial pressure gradient or left atrial pressure elevation should be further investigated with echocardiography. The pulmonary arterial line may signal pulmonary hypertension requiring nitric oxide inhalation.

Respiratory Function

Respiratory management is similar to that in patients undergoing other complex congenital heart surgeries. Left mainstem bronchus compression and malacia from the aortic root and arch represent a rare complication of IAA repair. This complication presents with left lung hyperinflation or atelectasis and may not become evident until several months after the repair. The diagnosis is made with bronchoscopy or computed tomographic scan of the chest. Management is individualized. Various operative approaches have been attempted, including aortopexy, repair of aortic aneurysm, pulmonary artery mobilization and patch augmentation, resection of tracheal stenoses, and bronchial wall suspension.[101] In others cases, the patient requires long-term mechanical ventilation with possible stenting of the airway.[20]

DiGeorge Syndrome

Patients with IAA and DiGeorge syndrome usually require calcium supplementation in the postoperative period. However, there is a wide spectrum, ranging from normal calcium and parathyroid hormone levels to frank hypoparathyroidism and hypocalcemia. Late-onset hypoparathyroidism is also possible. Therefore, calcium levels should be monitored very closely in the postoperative period and periodically after discharge from the hospital.

Immunodeficiency represents the other concern in the DiGeorge syndrome population. In addition to the need for blood product irradiation to prevent graft-versus-host disease, there may be an increased risk for pneumonia and sepsis in this population. Schreiber and associates[101] have shown that nearly 50% of the late deaths after IAA repair result from pneumonia and sepsis.

Outcome

Large series of single-stage IAA repair reveal a 12% early mortality and a 20% late mortality.[101] Both early and late mortality rates increase substantially in the presence of LVOTO.[48,101]

Recurrent arch stenosis represents the primary reason for reoperation or intervention with balloon angioplasty in the IAA population. Freedom from reintervention is estimated at 76% at 1 year, 67% at 5 years, and 53% at 10 years.[101] The etiology of recurrent arch stenosis may relate to incomplete excision of ductal tissue or tension at the primary anastomotic site.

Neurologic disorders including seizures and mental retardation may be present in as many as 20% of survivors.[101] It is unclear whether this results from genetic defects, preoperative shock, or the effects of the CPB strategies necessary for repair.

Some patients will develop late subaortic obstruction which can be treated with Ross/Konno aortic valve replacement. This can provide very effective long-term outcome for these selected patients.

References

1. Amato JJ, Galdieri RJ, Cotroneo JV: Role of extended aortoplasty related to the definition of coarctation of the aorta. *Ann Thorac Surg* 52:615–620, 1991.

2. Apfel HD, Levenbraun J, Quaegebeur JM, Allan LD: Usefulness of preoperative echocardiography in predicting left ventricular outflow obstruction after primary repair of interrupted aortic arch with ventricular septal defect. *Am J Cardiol* 82:470–473, 1998.

3. Arenas JD, Myers JL, Gleason MM, et al: End-to-end repair of aortic coarctation using absorbable polydioxanone suture. *Ann Thorac Surg* 51:413–417, 1991.

4. Bacha EA, Almodovar M, Wessel DL, et al: Surgery for coarctation of the aorta in infants weighing less than 2 kg. *Ann Thorac Surg* 71:1260–1264, 2001.

5. Backer CL, Mavroudis C: Congenital heart surgery nomenclature and database project: Patent ductus arteriosus, coarctation of the aorta, interrupted aortic arch. *Ann Thorac Surg* 69:S298–S307, 2000.

6. Backer CL, Paape K, Zales VR, et al: Coarctation of the aorta: Repair with polytetrafluoroethylene patch aortoplasty. *Circulation* 92:132–136, 1995.

7. Becker AE, Becker MJ, Edwards JE: Anomalies associated with coarctation of aorta: Particular reference to infancy. *Circulation* 41:1067–1075, 1970.

8. Beekman RH, Katz BP, Moorehead-Steffens C, Rocchini AP: Altered baroreceptor function in children with systolic hypertension after coarctation repair. *Am J Cardiol* 52:112–117, 1983.

9. Benedict CR, Grahame-Smith DG, Fisher A: Changes in plasma catecholamines and dopamine beta-hydroxylase after corrective surgery for coarctation of the aorta. *Circulation* 57:598–602, 1978.

10. Brewer LA, Fosburg RG, Mulder GA, Verska JJ: Spinal cord complications following surgery for coarctation of the aorta. A study of 66 cases. *J Thorac Cardiovasc Surg* 64:368–381, 1972.

11. Celoria GC, Patton RB: Congenital absence of the aortic arch. *Am Heart J* 58:407–413, 1959.

12. Choy M, Rocchini AP, Beekman RH, et al: Paradoxical hypertension after repair of coarctation of the aorta in children: Balloon angioplasty versus surgical repair. *Circulation* 75:1186–1191, 1987.

13. Clark EB: Neck web and congenital heart defects: A pathogenic association in 45 X-O Turner syndrome? *Teratology* 29:35–-361, 1984.

14. Clarkson PM, Nicholson MR, Barratt-Boyes BG, et al: Results after repair of coarctation of the aorta beyond infancy: A 10- to 28-year follow-up with particular reference to late systemic hypertension. *Am J Cardiol* 51:1481–1488, 1983.

15. Cobanoglu A, Teply JF, Grunkemeier GL, et al: Coarctation of the aorta in patients younger than three months. A critique of the subclavian flap operation. *J Thorac Cardiovasc Surg* 89:128–135, 1985.

16. Coceani F, Olley PM: The response of the ductus arteriosus to prostaglandins. *Can J Physiol Pharmacol* 51:220–225, 1973.

17. Conley ME, Beckwith JB, Mancer JF, Tenckhoff L: The spectrum of the DiGeorge syndrome. *J Pediatr* 94:883–890, 1979.

18. Conte S, Lacour-Gayet F, Serraf A, et al: Surgical-management of neonatal coarctation. *J Thorac Cardiovasc Surg* 109:663–675, 1995.

19. Crafoord C, Nylin G: Congenital coarctation of the aorta and its surgical treatment. *J Thorac Surg* 14:347–362, 1945.

20. Davis DA, Tucker JA, Russo P: Management of airway obstruction in patients with congenital heart defects. *Ann Otol Rhinol Laryngol* 102:163–166, 1993.

21. Engyall J, Sonnhag C, Nylander E, et al: Arm-ankle systolic blood pressure difference at rest and after exercise in the assessment of aortic coarctation. *Br Heart J* 73:270–276, 1995.

22. Folger GM Jr, Stein PD: Aortic valvular malformation associated with coincident cardiovascular anomalies: Morphologic considerations. *Angiology* 35:779–784, 1984.

23. Fox S, Pierce WS, Waldhausen JA: Pathogenesis of paradoxical hypertension after coarctation repair. *Ann Thorac Surg* 29:135–141, 1980.

24. Freed MD, Heymann MA, Lewis AB, et al: Prostaglandin E$_1$ infants with ductus arteriosus–dependent congenital heart disease. *Circulation* 64:899–905, 1981.

25. Freedom RM, Bain HH, Esplugas E, et al: Ventricular septal defect in interruption of aortic arch. *Am J Cardiol* 39:572–582, 1977.

26. Gaynor JW, Wernovsky G, Rychik J, et al: Outcome following single-stage repair of coarctation with ventricular septal defect. *Eur J Cardiothorac Surg* 18:62–67, 2000.

27. Gentile R, Stevenson G, Dooley T, et al: Pulsed Doppler echocardiographic determination of time of ductal closure in normal newborn infants. *J Pediatr* 98:443–448, 1981.

28. Gidding SS, Rocchini AP, Beekman R, et al: Therapeutic effect of propranolol on paradoxical hypertension after repair of coarctation of the aorta. *N Engl J Med* 312:1224–1228, 1985.

29. Glancy DL, Morrow AG, Simon AL, Roberts WC: Juxtaductal aortic coarctation. Analysis of 84 patients studied hemodynamically, angiographically, and morphologically after age 1 year. *Am J Cardiol* 51:537–551, 1983.

30. Goldman S, Hernandez J, Pappas G: Results of surgical treatment of coarctation of the aorta in the critically ill neonate. Including the influence of pulmonary artery banding. *J Thorac Cardiovasc Surg* 91:732–737, 1986.

31. Graham TP Jr: Ventricular performance in congenital heart disease. *Circulation* 84:2259–2274, 1991.

32. Gross RD: Coarctation of the aorta: Experimental studies regarding its surgical correction. *N Engl J Med* 233:287–293, 1945.

33. Gutgesell HP, Barton DM, Elgin KM: Coarctation of the aorta in the neonate: Associated conditions, management, and early outcome. *Am J Cardiol* 88:457–459, 2001.

34. Hanley FL: The various therapeutic approaches to aortic coarctation: Is it fair to compare? *J Am Coll Cardiol* 27:471–472, 1996.

35. Harvey JC, Dungan WT, Elders MJ, Hughes ER: Third and fourth pharyngeal pouch syndrome, associated vascular anomalies and hypocalcemic seizures. *Clin Pediatr (Phila)* 9:496–499, 1970.

36. Hellenbrand WE, Allen HD, Golinko RJ, et al: Balloon angioplasty for aortic recoarctation: Results of valvuloplasty and angioplasty of Congenital Anomalies Registry. *Am J Cardiol* 65:793–797, 1990.

37. Heymann MA: Pharmacologic use of prostaglandin E$_1$ in infants with congenital heart disease. *Am Heart J* 101:837–843, 1981.

38. Ho EC, Moss AJ: The syndrome of "mesenteric arteritis" following surgical repair of aortic coarctation. Report of nine cases and review of the literature. *Pediatrics* 49:40–45, 1972.

39. Ho SY, Anderson RH: Coarctation, tubular hypoplasia, and the ductus arteriosus. Histological study of 35 specimens. *Br Heart J* 41:268–274, 1979.

40. Hornberger LK, Sahn DJ, Kleinman CS, et al: Antenatal diagnosis of coarctation of the aorta: A multicenter experience. *J Am Coll Cardiol* 23: 417–423, 1994.

41. Hornberger LK, Weintraub RG, Pesonen E, et al: Echocardiographic study of the morphology and growth of the aortic arch in the human fetus. Observations related to the prenatal diagnosis of coarctation. *Circulation* 86:741–747, 1992.

42. Huhta JC, Gutgesell HP, Latson LA, Huffines FD: Two-dimensional echocardiographic assessment of the aorta in infants and children with congenital heart disease. *Circulation* 70:417–424, 1984.

43. Irwin ED, Braunlin EA, Foker JE: Staged repair of interrupted aortic arch and ventricular septal defect in infancy. *Ann Thorac Surg* 52:632–636, 1991.

44. Isomatsu Y, Imai Y, Shin'oka T, et al: Coarctation of the aorta and ventricular septal defect: Should we perform a single stage repair? *J Thorac Cardiovasc Surg* 122:524–528, 2001.

45. Jaffe RB: Radiographic manifestations of congenital anomalies of the aortic arch. *Radiol Clin North Am* 29:319–334, 1991.

46. Johns KJ, Johns JA, Feman SS: Retinal vascular abnormalities in patients with coarctation of the aorta. *Arch Ophthalmol* 109:1266–1268, 1991.

47. Jonas RA: Coarctation: Do we need to resect ductal tissue? *Ann Thorac Surg* 52:604–607, 1991.

48. Jonas RA, Quaegebeur JM, Kirklin JW, et al: Outcomes in patients with interrupted aortic arch and ventricular septal defect. A multiinstitutional study. Congenital Heart Surgeons Society. *J Thorac Cardiovasc Surg* 107:1099–1109, 1994.

49. Jones SE: Coarctation in children. Controlled hypotension using labetalol and halothane. *Anaesthesia* 34:1052–1055, 1979.

50. Kaine SF, Smith EO, Mott AR, et al: Quantitative echocardiographic analysis of the aortic arch predicts outcome of balloon angioplasty of native coarctation of the aorta. *Circulation* 94:1056–1062, 1996.

51. Kappetein AP, Gittenberger-de Groot AC, et al: The neural crest as a possible pathogenetic factor in coarctation of the aorta and bicuspid aortic valve. *J Thorac Cardiovasc Surg* 102:830–836, 1991.

52. Kawauchi M, Tada Y, Asano K, Sudo K: Angiographic demonstration of mesenteric arterial changes in postcoarctectomy syndrome. *Surgery* 98:602–604, 1985.

53. Khaisman EB: An adrenergic component of the nervous apparatus of the aortic reflexogenic zone. *Bull Exp Biol Med* 77:825–828, 1975.

54. Knyshov GV, Sitar LL, Glagola MD, Atamanyuk MY: Aortic aneurysms at the site of the repair of coarctation of the aorta: A review of 48 patients. *Ann Thorac Surg* 61:935–939, 1996.

55. Krammer HH, Sommer M, Rammos S, Krogmann O: Evaluation of low dose prostaglandin E$_1$ treatment for ductus dependent congenital heart disease. *Eur J Pediatr* 154:700–707, 1995.

56. Kreutzer J, Van Praagh R: Comparison of left ventricular outflow tract obstruction in interruption of the aortic arch and in coarctation of the aorta, with diagnostic, developmental, and surgical implications. *Am J Cardiol* 86:856–862, 2000.

57. Leenen FH, Balfe JA, Pelech AN, et al: Postoperative hypertension after repair of coarctation of aorta in children: Protective effect of propranolol? *Am Heart J* 113:1164–1173, 1987.

58. LeLievre CS, LeDouarin NM: Mesenchymal derivatives of the neural crest: Analysis of chimeric quail and chick embryos. *J Embryol Exp Morphol* 34:125–154, 1975.

59. Leoni F, Huhta JC, Douglas J, et al: Effect of prostaglandin on early surgical mortality in obstructive lesions of the systemic circulation. *Br Heart J* 52:654–659, 1984.

60. Lerberg DB, Hardesty RL, Siewers RD, et al: Coarctation of the aorta in infants and children: 25 years of experience. *Ann Thorac Surg* 33:159–170, 1982.

61. Lewin MB, Lindsay EA, Jurecic V, et al: A genetic etiology for interruption of the aortic arch type B. *Am J Cardiol* 80:493–497, 1997.

62. Lewis AB, Takahashi M, Lurie PR: Administration of prostaglandin E$_1$ in neonates with critical congenital cardiac defects. *J Pediatr* 93:481–485, 1978.

63. Lioy F, Malliani A, Pagani M, et al: Reflex hemodynamic responses initiated from the thoracic aorta. *Circ Res* 40:78–84, 1974.

64. Lock JE, Bass JL, Amplatz K, et al: Balloon dilation angioplasty of aortic coarctations in infants and children. *Circulation* 68:109–116, 1983.

65. Luciani GB, Ackerman RJ, Chang AC, et al: One-stage repair of interrupted aortic arch, ventricular septal defect, and subaortic obstruction in the neonate: A novel approach. *J Thorac Cardiovasc Surg* 111: 348–358, 1996.

66. Maheshwari S, Bruckheimer E, Fahey JT, Hellenbrand WE: Balloon angioplasty of postsurgical recoarctation in infants. *J Am Coll Cardiol* 35: 209–213, 2000.

67. Marshall AC, Perry SB, Deane JF, Lock JE: Early results and medium-term follow-up of stent implantation for mild residual or recurrent aortic coarctation. *Am Heart J* 139:1054–1060, 2000.

68. Mays ET, Sergeant GA: Postcoarctectomy syndrome. *Arch Surg* 91: 58–66, 1965.

69. McCrindle BW, Jones TK, Morrow WR, et al: Acute results of balloon angioplasty of native coarctation versus recurrent aortic obstruction are equivalent. *J Am Coll Cardiol* 28:1810–1817, 1996.

70. McElhinney DB, Halbach VV, Silverman NH, et al: Congenital cardiac anomalies with vein of Galen malformations in infants. *Arch Dis Child* 78:548–551, 1998.

71. McElhinney DB, Hedrick HL, Bush DM, et al: Necrotizing enterocolitis in neonates with congenital heart diesase: Risk factors and outcomes. *Pediatrics* 106:1080–1087, 2000.

72. Menahem S, Rahayoe AU, Brawn WJ, Mee RB: Interrupted aortic arch in infancy: A 10-year experience. *Pediatr Cardiol* 13:214–221, 1992.

73. Mendelsohn AM, Banerjee A, Donnelly LF, Schwartz DC: Is echocardiography or magnetic resonance imaging superior for precoarctation angioplasty evaluation? *Cathet Cardiovasc Diagn* 42:26–30, 1997.

74. Mitchell SE, Kan JS, White RI Jr: Interventional techniques in congenital heart disease. *Semin Roentgenol* 20:290–311, 1985.

75. Moene RJ, Oppenheimer-Dekker A, Moulaert AJ, et al: The concurrence of dimensional aortic arch anomalies and abnormal left ventricular muscle bundles. *Pediatr Cardiol* 2:107–114, 1982.

76. Monitto CL, Greenberg RS, Kost-Byerly S, et al: The safety and efficacy of parent-/nurse-controlled analgesia in patients less than six years of age. *Anesth Analg* 91:573–579, 2000.

77. Morriss MJH, McNamara DG: Coarctation of the aorta and interrupted aortic arch. In Garson A, Bricker JT, Fisher DJ, Neish SR (eds): *The Science and Practice of Pediatric Cardiology*, 2nd ed. Baltimore: Williams & Wilkins, 1998, pp 1317–1346.

78. Morrow WR, Huhta JC, Murphy DJ Jr, McNamara DG: Quantitative morphology of the aortic arch in neonatal coarctation. *J Am Coll Cardiol* 8:616–620, 1986.

79. Moulaert AJ, Bruins CC, Oppenheimer-Dekker A: Anomalies of the aortic arch and ventricular septal defects. *Circulation* 53:1011–1015, 1976.

79a. Nakagawa TA, Sartori, SC, Morris A, Schneider DS: Intravenous nicardipine for treatment of postcoarctectomy hypertension in children. *Pediatr Cardiol* 25:26–30, 2004.

80. Nihoyannopoulos P, Karas S, Sapsford RN, et al: Accuracy of two-dimensional echocardiography in the diagnosis of aortic arch obstruction. *J Am Coll Cardiol* 10:1072–1077, 1987.

81. Norton JBJ: Coarctation of the aorta. In Moller JH (ed): *Surgery of Congenital Heart Disease: Pediatric Cardiac Care Consortium 1984–1995.* Armonk, NY: Futura, 1998, pp 143–158.

82. Norwood WI, Lang P, Castaneda AR, Hougen TJ: Reparative operations for interrupted aortic arch with ventricular septal defect. *J Thorac Cardiovasc Surg* 86:832–837, 1983.

83. O'Laughlin MP, Perry SB, Lock JE, Mullins CE: Use of endovascular stents in congenital heart disease. *Circulation* 83:1923–1939, 1991.

84. Ovaert C, McCrindle BW, Nykanen D, et al: Balloon angioplasty of native coarctation: Clinical outcomes and predictors of success. *J Am Coll Cardiol* 35:988–996, 2000.

85. Patel R, Singh SP, Abrams L, Roberts KD: Coarctation of aorta with special reference to infants. Long-term results of operation in 126 cases. *Br Heart J* 39:1246–1253, 1977.

85a. Quaegebeur JM, Jonas RA, Weinberg AD, et al: Outcomes in seriously ill neonates with coarctation of the aorta. A multiinstitutional study. *J Thorac Cardiovasc Surg* 108:841–851, 1994.

86. Rajasinghe HA, Reddy VM, van Son JA, et al: Coarctation repair using end-to-side anastomosis of descending aorta to proximal aortic arch. *Ann Thorac Surg* 61:840–844, 1996.

87. Ralph-Edwards AC, Williams WG, Coles JC, et al: Reoperation for recurrent aortic coarctation. *Ann Thorac Surg* 60:1303–1307, 1995.

88. Rao PS: Long-term follow-up results after balloon dilatation of pulmonic stenosis, aortic stenosis, and coarctation of the aorta: A review. *Prog Cardiovasc Dis* 42:59–74, 1999.

89. Rao PS, Chopra PS: Role of balloon angioplasty in the treatment of aortic coarctation. *Ann Thorac Surg* 52:621–631, 1991.

90. Rao PS, Galal O, Smith PA, Wilson AD: Five- to nine-year follow-up results of balloon angioplasty of native aortic coarctation in infants and children. *J Am Coll Cardiol* 27:462–470, 1996.

91. Rauch A, Hofbeck M, Leipold G, et al: Incidence and significance of 22q11.2 hemizygosity in patients with interrupted aortic arch. *Am J Med Genet* 78:322–331, 1998.

92. Reifenstein GH, Levine SA: Coarctation of the aorta. *Am Heart J* 33: 146, 1947.

93. Rocchini AP, Rosenthal A, Barger AC, et al: Pathogenesis of paradoxical hypertension after coarctation resection. *Circulation* 54:382–387, 1976.

94. Rosenberg HS: Coarctation of the aorta: Morphology and pathogenetic considerations. *Perspect Pediatr Pathol* 1:339–368, 1973.

95. Rosenquist GC: Congenital mitral valve disease associated with coarctation of the aorta: A spectrum that includes parachute deformity of the mitral valve. *Circulation* 49:985–993, 1974.

96. Rudolph AM, Heymann MA, Spitznas U: Hemodynamic considerations in the development of narrowing of the aorta. *Am J Cardiol* 30:514–525, 1972.

97. Russell GA, Berry PJ, Watterson K, et al: Patterns of ductal tissue in coarctation of the aorta in the first three months of life. *J Thorac Cardiovasc Surg* 102:596–601, 1991.

98. Salem MM, Starnes VA, Wells WJ, et al: Predictors of left ventricular outflow obstruction following single-stage repair of interrupted aortic arch and ventricular septal defect. *Am J Cardiol* 86:1044–1047, 2000.

99. Saul JP, Keane JF, Fellows KE, Lock JE: Balloon dilation angioplasty of postoperative aortic obstructions. *Am J Cardiol* 59:943–948, 1987.

100. Schumacher G, Schreiber R, Meisner H, et al: Interrupted aortic arch: Natural history and operative results. *Pediatr Cardiol* 7:89–93, 1986.

101. Schreiber C, Eicken A, Vogt M, et al: Repair of interrupted aortic arch: Results after more than 20 years. *Ann Thorac Surg* 70:1896–1899, 2000.

102. Sehested J, Baandrup U, Mikkelsen E: Different reactivity and structure of the prestenotic and poststenotic aorta in human coarctation. Implications for baroreceptor function. *Circulation* 65:1060–1065, 1982.

103. Seirafi PA, Warner KG, Geggel RL, et al: Repair of coarctation of the aorta during infancy minimizes the risk of late hypertension. *Ann Thorac Surg* 66:1378–1382, 1998.

104. Sell JE, Jonas RA, Mayer JE, et al: The results of a surgical program for interrupted aortic arch. *J Thorac Cardiovasc Surg* 96:864–877, 1988.

105. Serraf A, Lacour-Gayet F, et al: Repair of interrupted aortic arch: A ten-year experience. *J Thorac Cardiovasc Surg* 112:1150–1160, 1996.

106. Shinebourne EA, Elseed AM: Relation between foetal flow patterns, coarctation of the aorta, and pulmonary blood flow. *Br Heart J* 36:492–498, 1974.

107. Shone JD, Sellers RD, Anderson RC, et al: The developmental complex of "parachute mitral valve," supravalvular ring of left atrium, subaortic stenosis, and coarctation of aorta. *Am J Cardiol* 11:714–725, 1963.

108. Sinha SN, Kardatzke ML, Cole RB, et al: Coarctation of the aorta in infancy. *Circulation* 40:385–398, 1969.

109. Soulen RL, Kan J, Mitchell S, White RI Jr: Evaluation of balloon angioplasty of coarctation restenosis by magnetic resonance imaging. *Am J Cardiol* 60:343–345, 1987.

110. Srouji MN, Trusler GA: Paradoxical hypertension and the abdominal pain syndrome following resection of coarctation of the aorta. *Can Med Assoc J* 92:412–416, 1965.

111. Stansel HC, Tabry IF, Poirier RA, et al: One hundred consecutive coarctation resections followed from one to thirteen years. *J Pediatr Surg* 12:279–286, 1977.

112. Stevens CA, Carey JC, Shigeoka AO: DiGeorge anomaly and velo-cardiofacial syndrome. *Pediatrics* 85:526–530, 1990.

113. Strafford MA, Griffiths SP, Gersony WM: Coarctation of the aorta: A study in delayed detection. *Pediatrics* 69:159–163, 1982.

114. Sumida H, Nakamura H, Satow Y: Distribution of vitronectin in the embryonic chick heart during endocardial cell migration. *Arch Histol Cytol* 53:81–88, 1990.

115. Sybert VP: Cardiovascular malformations and complications in Turner syndrome. *Pediatrics* 101:e11, 1998.

116. Takahashi K, Kuwahara T, Nagatsu M: Interruption of the aortic arch at the isthmus with DiGeorge syndrome and 22q11.2 deletion. *Cardiol Young* 9:516–518, 1999.

117. Tawes RL Jr, Aberdeen E, Waterston DJ, Carter RE: Coarctation of the aorta in infants and children. A review of 333 operative cases, including 179 infants. *Circulation* 39:I173–I184, 1969.

118. Thanopoulos BD, Hadjinikolaou L, Konstadopoulou GN, et al: Stent treatment for coarctation of the aorta: Intermediate term follow up and technical considerations. *Heart* 84:65–70, 2000.

119. Thoele DG, Muster AJ, Paul MH: Recognition of coarctation of the aorta. A continuing challenge for the primary care physician. *Am J Dis Child* 141:1201–1204, 1987.

120. Todd PJ, Dangerfield PH, Hamilton DI, Wilkinson JL: Late effects on the left upper limb of subclavian flap aortoplasty. *J Thorac Cardiovasc Surg* 85:678–681, 1983.

121. Toro-Salazar OH, Steinberger J, Thomas W, et al: Long-term follow-up of patients after coarctation of the aorta repair. *Am J Cardiol* 89:541–547, 2002.

122. Tworetzky W, McElhinney DB, Brook MM, et al: Echocardiographic diagnosis alone for the complete repair of major congenital heart defects. *J Am Coll Cardiol* 33:228–233, 1999.

123. Ungerleider RM, Ebert PA: Indications and techniques for midline approach to aortic coarctation in infants and children. *Ann Thorac Surg* 44:517–522, 1987.

124. Van Praagh R, Bernhard WF, Rosenthal A, et al: Interrupted aortic arch: Surgical treatment. *Am J Cardiol* 27:200–211, 1971.

125. Waldhausen JA, Nahrwold DL: Repair of coarctation of the aorta with a subclavian flap. *J Thorac Cardiovasc Surg* 51:532–533, 1966.

126. Ward KE, Pryor RW, Matson JR, et al: Delayed detection of coarctation in infancy: Implications for timing of newborn follow-up. *Pediatrics* 86:972–976, 1990.

127. Weber HS, Mosher T, Mahraj R, Baylen BG: Magnetic resonance imaging demonstration of "remodeling" of the aorta following balloon angioplasty of discrete native coarctation. *Pediatr Cardiol* 17:184–188, 1996.

128. Wiest DB, Garnber SS, Uber WE, Sade RM: Esmolol for the management of pediatric hypertension after cardiac operations. *J Thorac Cardiovasc Surg* 115:890–897, 1998.

129. Yagel S, Weissman A, Rotstein Z, et al: Congenital heart defects: Natural course and in utero development. *Circulation* 96:550–555, 1997.

130. Yee ES, Soifer SJ, Turley K, et al: Infant coarctation: A spectrum in clinical presentation and treatment. *Ann Thorac Surg* 42:488–493, 1986.

131. Yetman AT, Nykanen D, McCrindle BW, et al: Balloon angioplasty of recurrent coarctation: A 12-year review. *J Am Coll Cardiol* 30:811–816, 1997.

132. Young RS, Liberthson RR, Zalneraitis EL: Cerebral hemorrhage in neonates with coarctation of the aorta. *Stroke* 13:491–494, 1982.

133. Zahka KG, Roland JM, Cutilletta AF, et al: Management of aortic arch interruption with prostaglandin E$_1$ infusion and microporous expanded polytetrafluoroethylene grafts. *Am J Cardiol* 46:1001–1005, 1980.

134. Zanchetti A, Stella A: Neural control of renin release. *Clin Sci Mol Med* 48:215, 1975.

135. Zehr KJ, Gillinov AM, Redmond JM, et al: Repair of coarctation of the aorta in neonates and infants: A 30-year experience. *Ann Thorac Surg* 59:33–41, 1995.

Chapter 28

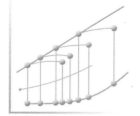

Mitral Valve Diseases

JOHN J. NIGRO, MD, MS, ROBERT D. BART, MD, and
VAUGHN A. STARNES, MD

Isolated congenital abnormalities of the mitral valve are relatively rare, often associated with other congenital heart anomalies, including Shone complex (multiple levels of left heart obstruction including supravalvular mitral ring, parachute mitral valve, subaortic stenosis, and coarctation of the aorta), and metabolic disorders.[22,27,55,57,60,63,67] When there is ventriculoarterial concordance, the left ventricle is systemic and the inlet is the mitral valve. Altered pathophysiology may occur when the inlet valve of the systemic ventricle is not a "mitral" valve but is found to be a tricuspid valve or an Ebstein's type malformation of the atrioventricular valve or developmentally derived from a common atrioventricular orifice. Additionally, systemic atrioventricular valvular abnormalities occur in single-ventricle physiology.

Mitral valve disease may involve congenital stenosis or insufficiency or elements of both. Mitral atresia and severe mitral stenosis occur both in classic hypoplastic left-sided heart syndrome and in other univentricular hearts. The mitral valve is not the central feature in these congenital heart diseases, as diagnosis and treatment are based on strategies of single-ventricle palliation. However, once patients progress to the third stage of single-ventricle palliation (e.g., Fontan), insufficiency of the systemic atrioventricular valve may be a determinant of risk and long-term survival.[41] Insufficiency of the systemic atrioventricular valve can occur after biventricular repair of atrioventricular septal defects.[40,48] Primary management and surgery for hypoplastic left-sided heart syndrome, atrioventricular septal defect, and Ebstein's anomaly are discussed in Chapters 40, 25, and 37, respectively. This chapter focuses on the management of congenital mitral valve stenosis and insufficiency, where the mitral valve is the systemic atrioventricular valve and can be repaired or replaced.

HISTORY

The first report of surgery for mitral valve disease in a child was in 1923, when Cutler operated on an 11-year-old girl with rheumatic mitral stenosis. She survived with mitral insufficiency for more than 4 years.[21] In 1959, the first experience for repair of congenital mitral stenosis and insufficiency was reported; this included both closed and open techniques.[72] In 1964, Young and Robinson reported a successful mitral valve replacement in a 10-month-old child.[83] In 1976, Carpentier and colleagues[14] proposed a systematic and surgically oriented classification of congenital mitral valve disease. Since then, early diagnosis and improved medical management have allowed mitral valve surgery to develop to where mitral valve repair or replacement has relatively low mortality and morbidity.[15,66,82]

EMBRYOLOGY

Mitral valve formation begins during the fourth week of gestation and continues through the sixth month.[23,77,80] Rudimentary atrioventricular valves are defined during the fifth and sixth weeks.[23] Further progression of endomyocardial tissue results in primitive leaflets by the seventh week.[77] During the third month, leaflet endomyocardial tissue is resorbed and replaced by muscle. Primitive trabeculations of the endomyocardial cushion and left ventricular wall develop and fuse, forming the two papillary muscles and chordae by the 24th week. During the sixth month, muscular tissue of the leaflets and chordae is replaced by collagen, completing the development of leaflets and chordae.[79,81]

ANATOMY

Critical to understanding mitral valve function and to successful surgical interventions is an understanding of mitral valve anatomy and surrounding structures (Fig. 28-1).[28] The mitral valve forms the functional union between left atrium and left ventricle. It is situated between the ventricular septum on its anterior aspect and posteriorly of the left ventricle at the sulcus. Surrounding structures include the aortic valve annulus at the junction of the noncoronary and left coronary sinus. The anterior leaflet forms the posterior boundary of the left ventricular outflow tract. The atrioventricular node is adjacent to the atrioventricular valve at the posterior medial commissure of the mitral valve. The posterior aspect of the mitral valve annulus is in continuity with the posterior aspect of the left ventricle and the atrioventricular groove, where the circumflex artery runs. Due to proximity, intricate knowledge of the aortic valve, atrioventricular node, and circumflex artery is required for successful mitral valve surgery.

The valvular portion of the mitral valve is composed of the annulus and leaflets (Fig. 28-2). The annulus is a pliable, functional zone of fibrous and muscular tissue connecting the left atrium and left ventricle. It is normally D shaped and forms the anchor for the base of the mitral leaflets. The atrioventricular groove and the circumflex artery surround it posteriorly, the coronary sinus laterally, and the interventricular septum and tricuspid valve annulus medially. The anterior third of the annulus lies between the right and left fibrous trigones. The rigid fibrous tissue connecting these trigones is a portion of the fibrous skeleton of the heart; it subtends the anterior leaflet supporting it like a curtain rod and is a fixed portion of the annulus. The posterior half defines the posterior annulus; devoid of fibrous tissue, it is not fixed and is the portion that dilates with valvular or ventricular dysfunction. The commissures form the junction between the anterior and posterior annulus and the corresponding leaflets. They are at the corners of the anterior and posterior leaflets denoted by "fan-shaped" chordae tendineae and are designated as the anterolateral and posteromedial commissures by location.

Although the intertrigonal portion of the valve is fixed, the annulus is a dynamic structure that can contract 20% to 40% during systole. The sail-like anterior leaflet is triangular shaped and subtends roughly 150 degrees of the annulus. It emanates from the intertrigonal fixed portion of the annulus and is in direct continuity with the left and noncoronary aortic valve leaflets. It also forms the posterior boundary of the left ventricular outflow tract. Coaption with the posterior leaflet forms a competent valve between the left atrium and left ventricle.[28] The posterior leaflet has an area equal to that of the anterior leaflet but is narrow and long, subtending the remaining 210 degrees of the annulus and forming a crescent shape.

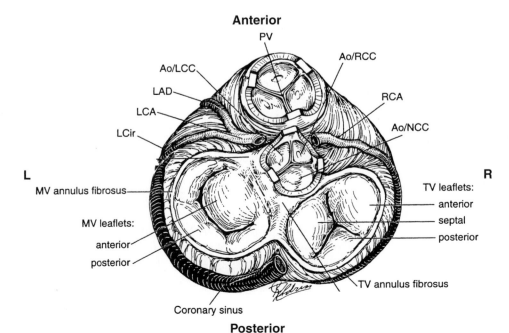

FIGURE 28-1 Cross-sectional anatomy showing the mitral valve (MV) and surrounding structures. Ao/LCC, left coronary cusp aortic valve; Ao/NCC, noncoronary cusp aortic valve; Ao/RCC, right coronary cusp aortic valve; LAD, left anterior descending coronary artery; LCA, left coronary artery; LCir, left circumflex coronary artery; MV, mitral valve; PV, pulmonary valve; RCA, right coronary artery; TV, tricuspid valve. (From Lamberti JJ, Mitruka SN: Congenital anomalies of the mitral valve. In Mavroudis C, Becker CL [eds]: *Pediatric Cardiac Surgery*. Philadelphia: Mosby, 2003; with permission.)

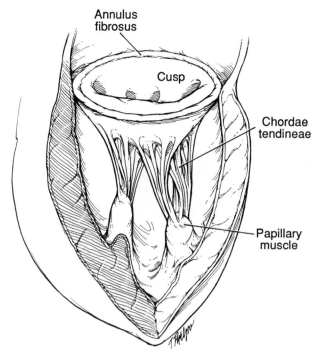

FIGURE 28-2 Four structures of the mitral valve: The valvular portion is composed of the annulus fibrosus and cusp (leaflet) tissue, and the subvalvular portion is composed of the chordae tendineae and papillary muscles.

It is usually scalloped into three separate portions. Taken together, the leaflet areas are twice that of the mitral orifice. Coaption of these two leaflets is critical for proper valve function.[59] Coaption occurs along the leaflet edge in the "rough" zone. A "clear" zone is adjacent to the rough zone and is the portion of the leaflet between the rough-edge zone and the annulus.

The subvalvular apparatus is composed of chordae tendineae and papillary muscles (see Fig. 28-2). The two papillary muscles emanate from left ventricular mid-wall and are located in the anterolateral and posteromedial positions. The anterolateral papillary muscle is usually a single muscle trunk, which is supplied by the left anterior descending artery/diagonal system or the circumflex artery. The posteromedial papillary muscle is usually composed of multiple small trunks and derives 85% of its vascular supply from the right coronary (15% from the posterior circumflex artery). Each papillary muscle anchors chordae from both valve leaflets.[61] The chordae are fibrous thread-like structures connecting papillary muscles to valve leaflets and have been classified into three subtypes based on their origins and insertions.[42]

First-order chordae emanate from the papillary muscle head and attach to the edge of the valve leaflets; they act to prevent valve prolapse during systole. Second-order chordae are thicker and fewer in number, emanating from the papillary muscle to the rough zone of the leaflets a few millimeters from the leaflet edge, strongly anchoring the leaflet. They are more prominent on the anterior leaflet. Third-order chordae arise from the posterior ventricular endocardium (trabeculae carneae) of the adjacent ventricular wall and extend to the posterior leaflet adjacent to the annulus. Commissural chordae emanate from both papillary muscles, with the anterolateral papillary giving rise to chordae, which go to the anterolateral

commissure, and the posterior papillary giving rise to the commissure chordae of the posterior commissure. These commissures arise as a main stem that branches radically like a fan inserting into the free margin of the commissural apparatus. The extent of commissural area is defined by the lateral spread of the attachments of the branches of commissural chordae.

OBSTRUCTIVE (STENOTIC) LESIONS OF THE MITRAL VALVE

Mitral valve pathology can be divided into two major categories: obstructive lesions and incompetent lesions. We first discuss the obstructive lesions.

Congenital obstruction may occur with functional or anatomic alterations of any component of the mitral valve. Classically, a segmental approach to analysis of congenital mitral stenosis has been used, although medical and surgical treatment may be more functionally oriented.[22] Most cases involve abnormalities of several components of the mitral valve.[63]

Supravalvular Mitral Ring

This lesion is caused by the presence of extra left atrial connective tissue, enshrouding the mitral valve and causing an obstruction to transvalvular flow. It is attached at the level of the annulus or just above the annular ring (Fig. 28-3).[74] This tissue can be directly adherent to the leaflets, fixing them in

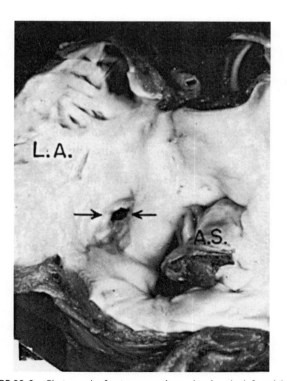

FIGURE 28-3 Photograph of autopsy specimen showing the left atrial view of a supravalvular mitral ring. The arrows indicate the narrowed orifice of the ring. Left atrial endocardium is thickened. AS, atrial septal defect of the fossa ovalis type; LA, superior view of left atrium. (From Davachi F, Moller JH, Edwards E: Diseases of the mitral valve in infancy. An anatomic analysis of 55 cases. *Circulation* 43:565–579, 1971; with permission.)

position, or can be on the adjacent tissues constraining leaflet motion.[19] This lesion is usually associated with other defects, including parachute mitral valve, subaortic stenosis, and aortic coarctation.[4,62,67] The subvalvular apparatus is usually abnormal, resulting in severe obstruction to flow; this lesion should always be considered when a child presents with signs of left-sided heart obstruction.[18] The ring acts to constrain leaflet motion, providing a small orifice for cardiac output to flow through.[74] There is often a single eccentric opening in the membrane. Relief of obstruction at the valvular level usually can be obtained by removal of the ring, which results in increased leaflet motion. Subvalvular anomalies can cause persistent obstruction and be more difficult to alleviate.

Mitral Valve Atresia

With this lesion, all components of the mitral valve apparatus are small. The annulus is small, and diminutive papillary muscles are closely placed. The interchordal distance is reduced, providing for reduced flow area below the valve and for tethering on the leaflets. The majority (80%) are associated with severe left ventricular hypoplasia and left ventricular outflow tract obstruction. Infants with this condition present with symptoms of left-sided heart obstruction in the initial neonatal period and require immediate surgical therapy. Generally, patients with left ventricular size less than 70% during the neonatal period do not survive without surgery.

Mitral valve atresia is often associated with complex ventricular anatomy, double-outlet right ventricle and single left ventricle with transposition of the great vessels. Those patients with mitral valve atresia and normal left ventricle size tend to have a large ventricular septal defect or a straddling tricuspid valve. Presentation and symptoms vary with the associated lesions, diameter of the foramen ovale, left atrial hypertension, size of the ventricular septal defect, and pulmonary blood flow.

Congenital Mitral Stenosis

Stenosis of the mitral valve is the most common form of congenital mitral valve obstruction. All valve components can be involved, including abnormalities of the leaflets, chordae, chordal insertions, and papillary muscles. Although most involve abnormalities of the entire valve complex, the most severely abnormal portion of the valve is used to describe the form of stenosis. Two basic forms involve symmetric and asymmetric chordal-papillary attachments.

In symmetric congenital mitral stenosis, the distribution of chordae from each leaflet is normal, but the leaflets and annular components are hypoplastic. The leaflets are constrained by shortened (but normally spaced) chordae, so that the centrally located valve orifice is smaller than the annular orifice. This narrowed orifice provides significant obstruction.

In asymmetric mitral stenosis or unbalanced chordae distribution, the cords attach predominantly or exclusively to one of the papillary muscles.[22,67,75] Often, the anterior papillary muscle is absent, and the leaflet is attached to a posterior papillary muscle. Some have labeled those cases with only one papillary muscle as "true parachute" mitral valve (Fig. 28-4). Commissures tend to be absent, forming a funnel-like mitral valve. The posterior lateral papillary muscle is most commonly the sole papillary muscle. This causes a "parachute-like" mitral

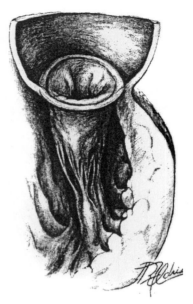

FIGURE 28-4   Stenotic parachute mitral valve. Single/fused papillary muscle arises from posterior left ventricular wall. (From Lamberti JJ, Mitruka SN: Congenital anomalies of the mitral valve. In Mavroudis C, Becker CL [eds]: *Pediatric Cardiac Surgery*. Philadelphia: Mosby, 2003; with permission.)

valve with an eccentric and small orifice. This lesion is associated with aortic coarctation or aortic valve stenosis but usually has a normal-size ventricle.[62]

Fusion of Mitral Valve Commissures

This form of obstruction is usually part of other forms of valvular abnormalities. It is characterized by poorly formed valve commissures and poorly developed chordae.

Excessive Mitral Valve Chordal Tissue

Redundant chordal tissue or extra leaflet tissue can obstruct flow at the subvalvular level and left ventricular outflow tract. This can be due to obstructing or redundant chordal tissue in the subvalvular area and extra leaflet tissue in the left ventricular outflow tract.

Double-Orifice Mitral Valve

A bridge of extraneous tissue or fusion of leaflets can divide the mitral valve inlet into two separate orifices leading into the left ventricle (Fig. 28-5).[7] About 50% of the time, this lesion is associated with valvular dysfunction, both stenosis and insufficiency.[12] In the majority of these valves, the septation is unbalanced, and in those with the smaller orifice toward the posteromedial commissure, there is commonly an associated atrial septal defect. Those with an intact septum tend to be associated with stenosis. The bridging tissue can be normal valve tissue. Resection generally leads to valvular incompetence.

Mitral Arcade

In mitral arcade, subvalvular and leaflet components are severely dysmorphic, such that the leaflets are thickened and almost directly attach to the papillary muscles with

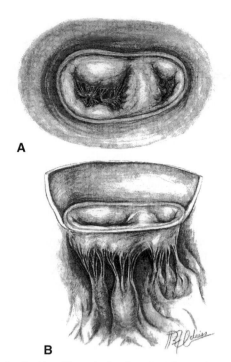

A

B

FIGURE 28-5 Double-orifice mitral valve. **A,** Left atrial view. **B,** Atrioventricular view. (From Lamberti JJ, Mitruka SN: Congenital anomalies of the mitral valve. In Mavroudis C, Becker CL [eds]: *Pediatric Cardiac Surgery.* Philadelphia: Mosby, 2003; with permission.)

dysplastic chordae. This leads to abnormal valvular tethering and excursion, with resultant obstruction to flow into the left ventricle.

Pathophysiology of Mitral Valve Obstruction

Obstructive lesions restrict blood flow from the left atrium into the left ventricle. Mitral stenosis typically results in decreased left ventricular filling. The significant pressure gradient required between the left atrium and left ventricle for blood to cross the mitral valve results in increased pulmonary venous and pulmonary capillary wedge pressures. Left ventricular dysfunction has been shown in patients with pure mitral stenosis, where significantly lower ejection fractions were present with abnormal contractility compared with patients with normal ventricular function.[34] The combination of decreased left ventricular volume and left ventricular dysfunction results in diminished cardiac output.

The increase in left atrial, pulmonary venous, and pulmonary capillary wedge pressures results in increased interstitial and alveolar fluid and congestion of bronchial veins. This causes increased airway resistance due to narrowing of the small airways. This adversely affects pulmonary mechanics and gas exchange, resulting in hypoxemia, hypercapnia, increased work of breathing, and potentially permanent damage to pulmonary parenchyma and vascular architecture. The increase in pulmonary vascular resistance results in pulmonary artery hypertension and right ventricular hypertrophy. If long-standing, this leads to right ventricular dysfunction with tricuspid regurgitation. Poor right ventricular performance results in further reduced cardiac output and oxygen delivery, resulting in end-organ damage and dysfunction.

Left ventricular filling across an obstructed mitral valve occurs during diastole. As heart rate increases, diastolic time decreases, limiting blood flow, further decreasing cardiac output, and worsening pulmonary symptoms. Individuals with mitral stenosis do not tolerate tachycardia well, regardless of cause. As atrial dilation can be a component of long-standing mitral stenosis, there is an increased risk of atrial dysrhythmias. The combined loss of atrial contraction and a rapid ventricular response from atrial fibrillation is tolerated poorly.[54] These individuals develop an acute decrease in cardiac output.

Diagnosis of Mitral Valve Obstruction

Clinical manifestation is dependent on the degree of mitral valve obstruction, pulmonary hypertension, associated lesions, and nutrition and growth of the infant.[63] Given that a fetus tolerates hypoplastic left-sided heart syndrome and develops normally, mitral valve obstruction or complete atresia is of little consequence until birth. Infants and small children with less severe mitral valve obstruction may have no symptoms at rest. However, easy fatigability, irritability, feeding difficulties, poor weight gain, and tachypnea may be signs of progressive mitral valve obstruction. Infants with associated pulmonary hypertension may have failure to thrive or a history of recurrent pulmonary infections. In older children, the inability to increase cardiac output becomes apparent during evaluation, although it is common for the patient or family to minimize exercise limitations when giving the history.

In isolated congenital mitral valve disease, the physical findings may be subtle. As obstruction increases, the concomitant decrease in cardiac output is associated with diminished peripheral perfusion and pulses. With further progression, heart failure and pulmonary hypertension are present, and physical findings become characteristic of mitral valve obstruction in older patients. Mitral stenosis produces an apical mid-diastolic murmur, with the opening mitral snap often absent. The first heart sound is usually soft, and the second varies from narrow to widely split. When marked pulmonary hypertension exists, there is accentuation of the second heart sound, an active precordium, and development of a right ventricular lift (heave).

The diagnosis of mitral valve stenosis is usually established by noninvasive techniques. The electrocardiogram reflects left atrial dilation, right ventricular enlargement, and reduced left ventricular forces. Atrial fibrillation is rare in infants and children, but other atrial arrhythmias may occur. When mitral stenosis is not isolated, the electrocardiogram reflects the associated physiologic abnormality. The chest x-ray reveals left atrial enlargement, prominence of pulmonary vascularity, and enlargement of the right ventricle.

Two-dimensional echocardiography in combination with color-flow studies and Doppler can provide precise information regarding the anatomy and function of the mitral valve. Two-dimensional and Doppler echocardiography are useful for determining mitral valve flow velocities and calculating the orifice area.[24,29] Echocardiography can provide all the information needed for management and correction of stenotic mitral valve pathology.[33,78]

Cardiac catheterization can be employed to measure physiologic pressures and oxygen saturations. Typical findings include elevated left atrial pressure, pulmonary venous pressures, and pulmonary artery pressures. Systemic desaturation may be present in advanced disease due to pulmonary congestion. Most of these determinations can be achieved noninvasively, and cardiac catheterization is unnecessary.

Medical Management

Infants and children exhibiting signs and symptoms of compromise from obstructive mitral valve disease represent both a medical and a surgical management challenge. There is no ideal substitute for the mitral valve in a child of any age, and repair is not always possible. Infants with either isolated mitral valve obstruction or disease where mitral stenosis is the dominant physiology tend to be managed medically as long as possible. Mainstays of therapy are diuretics and dietary supplementation. Digoxin therapy is often instituted, although the utility of digoxin in mitral stenosis is minimal unless there is ventricular dysfunction.[8] Beta-adrenergic antagonists (β-blockers) may benefit patients in sinus rhythm who have exertional symptoms that worsen or occur with higher heart rates.[9,10,46,50]

Patients with mitral stenosis are prone to developing atrial arrhythmias, particularly atrial fibrillation. Treatment of acute episodes of rapid atrial fibrillation consists of anticoagulation with heparin and control of ventricular rate response. Digoxin, β-blockers, or amiodarone should be used to control ventricular response by slowing atrioventricular nodal conduction. If there is hemodynamic instability, cardioversion should be undertaken urgently, with heparin anticoagulation before, during, and after cardioversion. Patients in atrial fibrillation for longer than 1 to 2 days without anticoagulation are at risk for developing atrial thrombi and subsequent embolic events, even after cardioversion.[17,20,64] Cardioversion is usually successful, especially when combined with amiodarone pretreatment and maintenance therapy.[31,39,45] Although amiodarone is rapidly becoming the drug of choice, digoxin and β-blockers are considered mainstays of pharmacologic therapy.[44]

Careful monitoring is needed throughout a course of medical management, as stronger diuretics may allow for prolonged medical therapy as left ventricular function deteriorates or pulmonary hypertension worsens. Prolonged elevation in both left atrial pressures and pulmonary pressures can result in right-sided heart dysfunction. The effects of prolonged pulmonary hypertension resulting from left atrial pressure elevation are not well known.[18]

As symptoms progress, medical management includes routine critical care modalities. Frequently, respiratory decompensation precedes myocardial failure, bringing children with mitral stenosis into the intensive care unit.

Because bronchial venous congestion and interstitial edema occur, wheezing may be a symptom of mitral stenosis. Often beta-adrenergic bronchodilators are prescribed. These worsen the child's condition. Diuretics are preferable. Beta-adrenergics may precipitate tachycardia and arrhythmias; both are detrimental. Additionally, the increased oxygen consumption places a further burden on a child with decreased cardiac output. Finally, beta-adrenergics dilate the submucosal vascular plexus and worsen airway resistance; they also increase dyspnea, wheezing, and the work of breathing.

Beta-adrenergic mimetics should be avoided in the child with wheezing caused by heart disease.

Endotracheal intubation with initiation of mechanical ventilation decreases or eliminates increased work of breathing and cardiac workload. Positive end-expiratory pressure may improve ventilation and perfusion matching in edematous lungs, resulting in improved gas exchange. If tachycardia is a significant problem, β-blockers should be initiated. However, beta-blockade when ventricular dysfunction exists must be initiated with caution. Children requiring intensive care need to be considered candidates for either mitral valve surgery or interventional cardiac catheterization.

Transvenous mitral commissurotomy by a balloon catheter was first performed by Inoue and coworkers[35] in 1984. This transseptal technique requires a guide wire to be introduced across the atrial septum into the left atrium and into the left ventricle. Subsequently, a balloon catheter is positioned across the mitral valve and inflated. There are now several series in children and adults reporting consistent hemodynamic improvement with minimal complications.[1,6,25,26,71] A second technique, found to cause less trauma to the atrial septum and femoral veins, utilizes a double-balloon transseptal valvuloplasty technique (Fig. 28-6).[3,6,30,36,37,68] Comparison of the two catheter techniques shows the single-balloon technique to result in less procedure-induced mitral regurgitation but provide less relief of mitral stenosis. Potential complications of percutaneous balloon mitral valvuloplasty relate to the catheter course and valve manipulation. Most commonly, the transseptal catheter course results in a residual atrial shunt detected in as many as one third of patients.[25,26] As with most interventional catheter procedures, atrial perforation, cardiac tamponade, and cerebrovascular accidents have been reported. In a few cases, mitral valvuloplasty has resulted in severe mitral regurgitation. Attempts to select patients at risk for postprocedure mitral regurgitation have not been successful.[49] Children with preexisting mitral regurgitation are not good candidates for balloon valvuloplasty. Restenosis of the mitral valve occurs after balloon dilation, although the degree and time course of restenosis are unpredictable. Frequently, medical intervention through balloon mitral valvuloplasty is a palliative procedure, allowing a child to grow while awaiting definitive surgery at an older age.

Surgical Management

Mitral stenosis is rarely caused by an isolated abnormality of the valve; surgical repair is challenging, can be complex, and yields variable results. Indications for surgery depend on the anatomy and the child's physiology. Congestive heart failure refractory to medical therapy and pulmonary hypertension secondary to mitral obstruction are traditional indications for surgical intervention. Other indications include obvious changes in atrial dimensions (echocardiographic) and the onset of atrial arrhythmias. Repair with preservation of the native valve is important, because mitral replacement is associated with poor short-term and long-term survival.[32] Because mitral valve preservation is the goal, the threshold for surgery is affected by valvular anatomy and the likelihood of repair. There is a lower intervention threshold for valves with lesions such as isolated mitral ring, while a more conservative

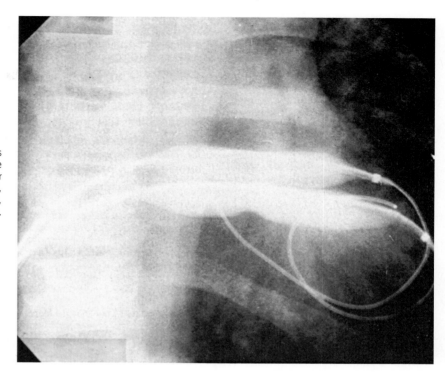

FIGURE 28-6 Angiogram showing two balloon catheters over guidewires through the atrial septum, across the mitral valve, and inflated. There is a "waist" in the lower balloon from the stenotic mitral valve. (From Grifka RG, O'Laughlin MP, Nihill MR, Mullins CE: Double-transseptal, double-balloon valvuloplasty for congenital mitral stenosis. *Circulation* 85:123–129, 1992; with permission.)

approach is used for those that are more complex (parachute and mitral arcade). Factors associated with mortality include young age (<10 months) and replacement of the mitral valve. Actuarial survival for mitral valve repair is between 89% and 97%, and for those who undergo mitral valve replacement, between 52% and 75%.[13,66,73,76] For repaired valves, freedom from reoperation is between 70% and 76%.[13,56]

Open operation of the mitral valve is completed on cardiopulmonary bypass with bicaval venous cannulation and hypothermic cardioplegic arrest. Prior to the initiation of bypass, the valve is carefully analyzed with transesophageal echocardiography, looking at each of the valve components and the valvular function and checking for associated defects or anomalies. The valve can be exposed by a variety of approaches: through the left atrium, through the interatrial septum, or a combination of both. Once exposed, the valve is systematically analyzed, starting with the annular/leaflet components, then the subvalvular apparatus, and, ultimately, the left ventricle.[14,15] Repair for isolated supravalvular mitral ring is generally the most reproducible and provides for the most consistent good result. The ring is carefully incised and removed from the leaflet/annular complex using a combination of sharp and blunt dissection (Fig. 28-7). Most lesions other than mitral ring involve multiple levels of the mitral complex; repair is more complicated, with less predictable results. Repair of these lesions is individualized and involves a combination of techniques. Commissure to papillary muscle fusion requires fenestration of the subvalvular apparatus with splitting of the individual papillary muscles and commissurotomy of the leaflets (Fig. 28-8). Leaflet tissue, which obliterates the interchordal space, is resected to eliminate obstruction to blood flow. Repair of the parachute mitral valve involves all of these techniques.

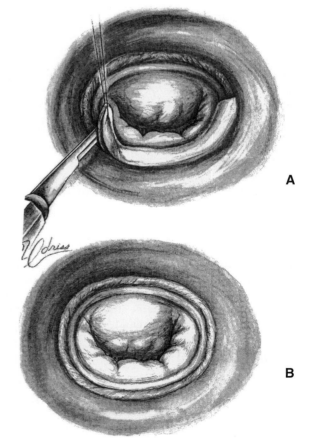

FIGURE 28-7 Resection of supravalvular mitral ring. **A,** Sharp dissection with a suture placed for traction. **B,** Final result. (From Lamberti JJ, Mitruka SN: Congenital anomalies of the mitral valve. In Mavroudis C and Backer CL (eds): Pediatric Cardiac Surgery. Philadelphia: Mosby, 2003; with permission.)

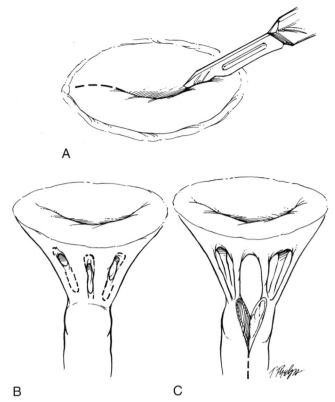

FIGURE 28-8 Surgical correction of mitral stenosis includes the following: **A,** Simple commissurotomy. **B,** Chordal fenestration. **C,** Papillary muscle splitting.

The completed repair is assessed under direct vision and, subsequently, with postbypass transesophageal echocardiography. Degree of acceptable postoperative residual mitral stenosis is proportional to the complexity of the mitral anomaly. Lesions with commissure to papillary muscle fusion are likely to ultimately require replacement, but mitral repair is attempted to allow growth prior to valve replacement. Combined severe mitral regurgitation and residual stenosis is poorly tolerated, difficult to repair, and likely to require valve replacement. Replacement with bioprosthetic valves is avoided because of accelerated tissue degeneration and the need for subsequent valve re-replacement seen in younger children.[5,11] Although mechanical valve replacement with subsequent anticoagulation is the conventional approach, recent experience suggests that the severely diseased mitral valve can be replaced with a pulmonary valve autograft (Ross-Mitral).[38,53,65] This option holds the promise of an effective valve replacement: The patient does not require long-term anticoagulation therapy, and the valve will grow with the child.

Postoperative Critical Care

Postoperative care is dictated by the physiology after repair. Children with residual mitral stenosis and little or no regurgitation should receive medical therapy, as outlined in "Medical Management," to optimize blood flow across a restrictive mitral orifice. Left atrial pressures may need to be higher than normal to optimize left ventricular filling. Due to residual mitral obstruction limiting left ventricular inflow, systemic afterload reduction does not increase cardiac output significantly. It may lead to

tachycardia and hypotension with decreased coronary perfusion. As in preoperative management, avoidance of tachycardia and tachydysrhythmias is important. Maintenance of sinus rhythm is a vital contribution to cardiac output and may require the use of temporary epicardial pacing.

Postoperative low cardiac output syndrome may be related to either 1) limited left ventricular filling from residual mitral stenosis or 2) right ventricular dysfunction related to pulmonary hypertension. Pulmonary hypertension may or may not have been known to exist preoperatively. When in place, a pulmonary artery catheter may be helpful in differentiating these two causes of low cardiac output syndrome. Otherwise, a clinical scenario that may include elevated central venous pressure, decreased peripheral perfusion, low systemic blood pressure, tachycardia, metabolic acidosis, and hypoxemia may lead to a diagnosis of pulmonary hypertension. Echocardiography may provide confirmation of pulmonary hypertension. Therapeutic interventions are aimed at improving right ventricular function and decreasing pulmonary vascular resistance. Inotropic support is usually needed to improve contractility and decrease right ventricle distention. To further reduce the risk of postoperative right ventricular distention and tricuspid regurgitation, pulmonary vasodilator therapy may be added. This includes hyperventilation, pain management, oxygen, and nitric oxide.

In combination with direct cardiorespiratory support, sedation with benzodiazepines and fentanyl analgesia is important for at least 24 hours. The addition of neuromuscular blockade may be needed in individuals with reactive pulmonary circulation. Occasionally, in extreme cases of ventricular dysfunction, leaving the sternum open and closing the skin with a Silastic (silicone) patch improves diastolic function and prevents cardiac compression, which may be significant due to mediastinal and myocardial edema. The open sternum also facilitates ventilation at lower airway pressures and consequently decreases right ventricular afterload. Additionally, because intrathoracic pressure is optimized, the effect on vascular resistance is minimized. The sternum can be closed 3 to 4 days postoperatively when myocardial function has improved and edema has decreased.

REGURGITANT LESIONS OF THE MITRAL VALVE

Isolated insufficiency of the mitral valve is rare and is associated with underlying states such as connective tissue disorders and metabolic or storage diseases. Mitral insufficiency is more commonly present with other cardiac anomalies, such as endocardial cushion defect, ventricular septal defects, patent ductus arteriosus, and anomalous left coronary artery. Acquired valvular incompetence during childhood is due to diverse causes that include trauma, endocarditis, rheumatic fever, and collagen vascular diseases such as Kawasaki's disease. Any process leading to left ventricular dysfunction and altered ventricular geometry, such that the mitral apparatus no longer coapts properly, can result in mitral regurgitation.

Mitral valve prolapse (myxomatous) is the most common cause of significant mitral incompetence for adults in developed countries; however, it is rarely the cause of significant regurgitation in infants and children. The leaflet tissue is

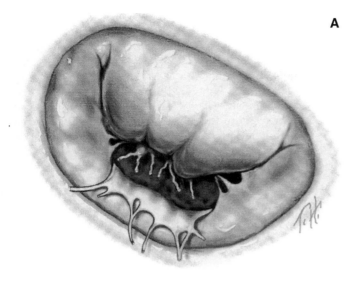

A

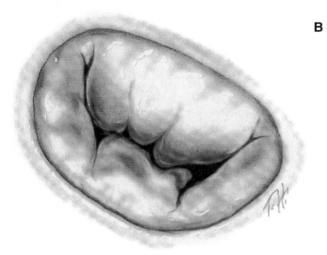

B

FIGURE 28-9 Myxomatous mitral valve. **A**, Redundant nature of myxomatous mitral valve. **B**, Rupture of chordae to the middle scallop of the posterior leaflet, resulting in prolapse and severe regurgitation. (From Nigro JJ, Swartz DS, Bart RD, et al: Neochordal repair of the posterior mitral leaflet. *J Thorac Cardiovasc Surg* 127: 440–447; with permission.)

redundant, and the most common site of prolapse is the middle portion of the posterior leaflet (Fig. 28-9). Valve repair for this lesion has proven to be safe and durable; it consists of resection of prolapsed leaflet segment, leaflet reconstruction, and annuloplasty.

Cleft Mitral Leaflet

Mitral leaflet clefts usually occur in endocardial cushion defect (atrioventricular septal defects), which are described in Chapter 25. Mitral clefts rarely occur as an isolated defect and are usually located in the anterior leaflet; posterior leaflet involvement rarely occurs. Mitral regurgitation due to cleft mitral leaflet is repaired by direct suture closure and posterior (protecting) annuloplasty. The subvalvular apparatus (chordae and papillary muscle) can cross the left ventricular outflow tract and provide for varying degrees of left ventricular outflow tract obstruction and complicate valve repair.

Rarely, these structures cause severe left ventricular outflow tract obstruction, necessitating resection and either complex mitral reconstruction or valve replacement.

Other Lesions

Lesions in which the chordae are thickened and shortened have been variously described as "hammock valve" or anomalous mitral arcade. These lesions produce mitral regurgitation by restriction of leaflet motion and are difficult to repair. Occasionally, arcade fenestration provides for a competent valve. Various other anomalies of valve leaflets and subvalvular apparatus result in regurgitation, and repair for these lesions can be complex. Acquired lesions include infective endocarditis and trauma; in both situations, need for repair is dictated by the degree of regurgitation, cardiac dilation, or the presence of symptoms of congestive heart failure. Emphasis is placed on repair whenever possible. Other congenital anomalies having associated mitral regurgitation are described elsewhere in this text.

Pathophysiology of Mitral Insufficiency

In mitral regurgitation, a portion of the ventricular output flows retrograde into the left atrium, diminishing systemic cardiac output. This results in increased left ventricular fractional shortening and ejection fraction. Compensation for lost cardiac output includes increased stroke volume, ejection fraction, and heart rate. Volume overload leads to gradual dilation of the left atrium and left ventricle. The progressive enlargement in left ventricular dimension leads to progression of mitral regurgitation in a positive feedback manner. The end result is congestive heart failure with pulmonary congestion, pulmonary hypertension, and atrial dilation with the onset of atrial arrhythmias (atrial fibrillation). Acute-onset mitral regurgitation is poorly tolerated with little or no time for cardiac compensation, and the patient experiences severe congestive heart failure.

Diagnosis

Significant mitral regurgitation has characteristic physical findings, which depend on regurgitant fraction and rapidity of regurgitation onset. Classic physical findings include a hyperdynamic precordium. The first heart sound is reduced, P2 is accentuated, and there is a holosystolic high-frequency blowing murmur, which is maximal at the apex. This murmur radiates to the left axilla and back. A third heart sound suggests the presence of poorly tolerated mitral regurgitation with congestive heart failure. Infants tolerate significant mitral regurgitation poorly and manifest signs of congestive heart failure, which consist of failure to thrive, diaphoresis, pallor, tachypnea, and poor feeding. Older children may experience exercise intolerance. Rapid-onset mitral regurgitation, such as that secondary to infective endocarditis or trauma, leads to rapid clinical decompensation with severe congestive heart failure. If cardiac output is significantly decreased and end-organ function is compromised despite aggressive medical therapy (afterload reduction, diuresis, and cardiotonic agents), urgent surgery may be required.

Echocardiography has become the principal modality for diagnosing mitral regurgitation. Two-dimensional and B-mode echocardiography allow for the diagnosis of mitral regurgitation and provide insight into the anatomic basis of regurgitation; these modalities also provide valuable information about ventricular function and the presence of other associated anomalies. Progressive increase in atrial or ventricular dimensions also can be determined and is an important consideration concerning operative timing. Doppler analysis provides information related to regurgitant flow, including the direction of regurgitation and quantification, which depends on the length and width of the regurgitant jet (into the left atrium). Alone, echocardiography can provide sufficient information to proceed to valve surgery. Transesophageal echocardiography provides better resolution of the mitral mechanism and should be utilized prior to operative intervention and perioperatively in the operating room to evaluate repaired valve function. Development of three-dimensional echocardiography holds the promise of improved delineation of anatomy and more accurate determination of regurgitant fraction. Cardiac catheterization can be used as an adjunct to echocardiography when pulmonary arterial pressures or critical anatomic details not evident by echocardiogram are needed prior to operative intervention. Magnetic resonance imaging holds the promise of highly detailed anatomic information, along with accurate assessment of regurgitant fraction and hemodynamics; however, it usually requires sedation and possibly a general anesthetic.

Medical Management

Medical therapy is predicated on the precepts of afterload reduction (to maximize forward flow), diuresis, and inotropic support. Outpatient therapy consists of combining angiotensin-converting enzyme inhibitors (ACE inhibitors), furosemide, and digoxin. When this regimen fails to control symptoms, patients are evaluated for surgical intervention. If hospitalization is required prior to surgery, the child's medical condition can be optimized in the intensive care unit with intravenous inotropes and afterload-reducing agents such as sodium nitroprusside, milrinone, dopamine, and dobutamine. Evidence of continuing or progressive end-organ dysfunction is a sign of inadequate forward flow and an indication for urgent surgery.

Surgical Management

Valve repair is preferred over valve replacement. Repair has been associated with better operative and long-term survival. Repair maintains optimal ventricular function, avoids long-term anticoagulation, and "grows" with the child. Repair generally involves one or a combination of the following valve components: the valve annulus, the leaflets, and the subvalvular apparatus (chordae and papillary muscles). A systematic description of mitral valve incompetence has been developed for acquired adult valvular disease, and application of this system to congenital lesions is useful conceptually and aids in developing a repair strategy. In this description, incompetence with normal leaflet motion is related to annular dilation, such that although the rest of the valve mechanism is normal, a central regurgitant jet is present due to poor

leaflet coaption. Lesions associated with this type of mitral regurgitation include dilated cardiomyopathies, ischemic states (e.g., anomalous coronary artery with ventricular dilation), congenital lesions that provide for left ventricular overload and dilation, and some lesions in which leaflets are deficient (usually the posterior leaflet). This type of valvular dysfunction is usually treated with annular reconstruction/annuloplasty using techniques ranging from placement of a posterior annuloplasty ring to annular plication techniques, depending on the degree of annular dilation and the age of the patient (Fig. 28-10).

Increased leaflet motion or prolapse of the leaflets occurs when leaflet free edge overrides the plane of the annulus, thus resulting in poor leaflet coaptation. The prolapse can be due to a single portion of a single leaflet or generalized bileaflet process, in which both leaflets suffer from excessive leaflet motion. This can be associated with a cleft mitral leaflet and is usually caused by the absence of chordae, redundant leaflets, stretched or elongated chordae, or papillary muscle pathology. This can be caused by myxomatous changes of the mitral valve, trauma, infective endocarditis, collagen-vascular diseases, and infarct/ischemia related chordal rupture or elongation. Classic repair for lesions of this type depends on the site of prolapse; posterior leaflet lesions are generally repaired by leaflet resection and reconstruction with protective leaflet annuloplasty (see Fig. 28-10B and C). Clefts are usually found in the anterior leaflet and are usually repaired by direct suture closure of the cleft (see Fig. 28-10A). Anterior leaflet prolapse is more difficult to repair and is associated with higher recurrence rates; these lesions are usually repaired with chordal shortening techniques or placement of polytetrafluoroethylene (PTFE) neochordae to restore coaptation. Repair utilizing polytetrafluoroethylene has proven to be highly successful. In 2004, we successfully applied this approach to the posterior leaflet, minimizing the requirement for leaflet resection (Fig. 28-11).[51] In regurgitation due to restricted leaflet motion, many portions of the valve apparatus may be pathologic and lead to a state in which the leaflets are "restricted" from completely coapting. This form of mitral regurgitation can be subdivided into two groups: patients with abnormal papillary muscles and those with normal papillary muscles. Abnormal papillary muscles are found in those patients with parachute mitral valves, mitral arcade, and a hammock mitral valve. These lesions are generally difficult to repair completely, with residual regurgitation not uncommonly present, and often require mitral valve replacement. In lesions with normal papillary muscles, chordae can be shortened and thickened, as in rheumatic disease. These are difficult to repair as well. In those patients with narrowed interchordal distance or tethering of the chordae, chordal fenestration and freeing can result in an acceptable repair.

Postoperative Critical Care

Postoperative care is guided by the underlying physiology after repair. Children who have undergone mitral surgery for valvular insufficiency may have residual mitral regurgitation. This may result in low cardiac output due to mitral regurgitation and left ventricular dysfunction. Inotropic support of left ventricular function is important for contractility and to

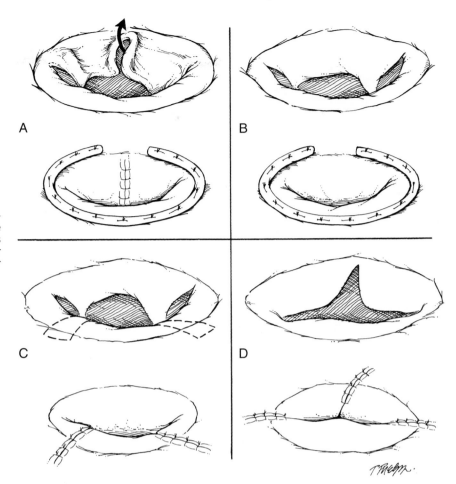

FIGURE 28-10 Surgical correction of mitral insufficiency. Top figure in each quadrant shows preoperative condition. Bottom figure in each quadrant shows surgical correction. **A,** Cleft closure with posterior annuloplasty. **B,** Reduction annuloplasty. **C,** Posterior leaflet quadrangular resection. **D,** Commissuroplasty.

decrease ventricular dilation. Vasodilator therapy with nitroprusside or milrinone decreases systemic vascular resistance and promotes left ventricular output. In addition, decreasing left ventricular afterload aids in "protecting" the integrity of the mitral repair. Diuretic administration with the concomitant decrease in pulmonary interstitial and alveolar edema may facilitate gas exchange and, ultimately, weaning from mechanical ventilation.

In combination with direct cardiorespiratory support, sedation with benzodiazepines and fentanyl analgesia is important for at least the initial 24 hours. Occasionally, in extreme cases of ventricular dysfunction, leaving the sternum open and closing the skin with a Silastic patch improves diastolic function and prevents cardiac compression, which may be significant due to mediastinal and myocardial edema. The open sternum also facilitates ventilation at lower airway pressures and consequently decreases right ventricular afterload. Additionally, because intrathoracic pressure is optimized, the effect on vascular resistance is minimized. The sternum can be closed 3 to 4 days postoperatively when myocardial function has improved and edema has decreased.

RESULTS

With recent improvements in the understanding of mitral pathology and valvuloplasty techniques, the outcome of

mitral valve surgery has steadily improved. Valve repair offers the advantages of low operative mortality, valve growth, and the lack of long-term anticoagulation. Operative risk and long-term results are directly related to the complexity of the underlying valvular pathology and the associated congenital heart defect. Risks appear highest for those with complex heart disease and mitral stenosis, in whom mortality rates as high as 30% have been reported in the past.[47] Most recent series suggest that in well-selected patient populations, valvuloplasty has good short- and long-term results, with an operative mortality risk of 1.5% to 5%, excellent freedom from reoperation, and survival at 10 to 15 years of follow-up.[2,16,43,52,66,84]

MITRAL VALVE REPLACEMENT

A decision for mitral valve replacement is made after assessing the outcome of suboptimal valve repair, factoring in the child's age, weight, clinical condition, and left ventricular function. Mitral valve replacement is associated with higher operative risks and poorer long-term survival than valve repair; however, some valves require replacement. Mitral valve replacement in older infants and children is performed using a technique similar to replacement in adults. When the mitral valve is replaced, functional integrity of the subvalvular apparatus by chordal preservation is considered important in conserving ventricular geometry and function.[69,70] Adjustments in technique

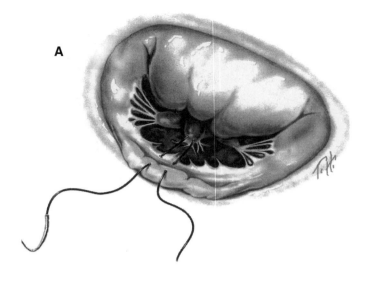

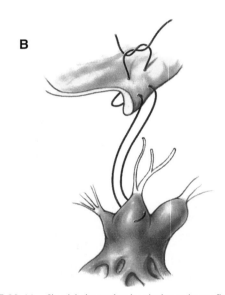

FIGURE 28-11   Chordal shortening by placing polytetrafluoroethylene neochordae to restore coaption. **A,** Placing polytetrafluoroethylene neochordae to posterior leaflet. **B,** Close-up of neochordae from papillary muscle to leaflet edge. (From Nigro JJ, Swartz DS, Bart RD, et al: Neochordal repair of the posterior mitral leaflet. *J Thorac Cardiovasc Surg* 127: 440–447; with permission.)

are needed when a small valve annulus is encountered and unfortunately may require excising portions of the subvalvular apparatus to allow placement of an adequately sized prosthesis.

Operative mortality for replacement in infants has been reported to be as high as 33%.[18,47] At 5 years, survival after mitral replacement has been reported to be 52% to 75%, with a freedom from reoperation of 81%.[13,58,76] Complications after valve replacement include complete heart block, endocarditis, thrombosis, and stroke. For most children younger than 5 years, size and durability dictate placing a mechanical valve requiring long-term anticoagulation. Anticoagulation management is problematic in childhood. Bleeding with the risk of strokes or poor compliance with embolic sequelae occurs. Coagulation monitoring is lifelong and difficult.

CONCLUSIONS

Isolated mitral valve pathology is rare in childhood. Symptomatology and presentation are related to the degree of regurgitation or stenosis and acuity of onset. Medical therapy for stenosis relies on diuretics. Medical therapy for regurgitation consists of afterload reduction, diuretic therapy, and inotropic agents. Operative intervention is indicated when medical therapy fails to control symptoms or, in some cases, based on increasing cardiac dimensions (by echocardiogram). Valve repair is the goal of surgical intervention for mitral disease and is based on the mechanism of valve dysfunction. Mitral replacement is possible and can provide long-term survival but is less desirable than valve repair.

References

1. Abascal VM, Wilkins GT, O'Shea JP, et al: Prediction of successful outcome in 130 patients undergoing percutaneous balloon mitral valvotomy. *Circulation* 82:448–456,1990.
2. Aharon AS, Laks H, Drinkwater DC, et al: Early and late results of mitral valve repair in children. *J Thorac Cardiovasc Surg* 107:1262–1270, 1994.
3. Al Zaibag M, Ribeiro PA, Al Kasab S, Al Fagih MR: Percutaneous double-balloon mitral valvotomy for rheumatic mitral-valve stenosis. *Lancet* 1:757–761, 1986.
4. Anabtawi IN, Ellison RG: Congenital stenosing ring of the left atrioventricular canal (supravalvular mitral stenosis). *J Thorac Cardiovasc Surg* 49:994–1005, 1965.
5. Antunes MJ, Vanderdonck KM, Sussman MJ: Mechanical valve replacement in children and teenagers. *Eur J Cardiothorac Surg* 3:222–228, 1989.
6. Arora R, Nair M, Rajagopal S, et al: Percutaneous balloon mitral valvuloplasty in children and young adults with rheumatic mitral stenosis. *Am Heart J* 118:883–887, 1989.
7. Bano-Rodrigo A, Van Praagh S, Trowitzsch E, Van Praagh R: Double-orifice mitral valve: A study of 27 postmortem cases with developmental, diagnostic and surgical considerations. *Am J Cardiol* 61:152–160, 1988.
8. Beiser GD, Epstein SE, Stampfer M, et al: Studies on digitalis. XVII. Effects of ouabain on the hemodynamic response to exercise in patients with mitral stenosis in normal sinus rhythm. *N Engl J Med* 278:131–137, 1968.
9. Bhatia ML, Shrivastava S, Roy SB: Immediate haemodynamic effects of a beta adrenergic blocking agent—propranolol—in mitral stenosis at fixed heart rates. *Br Heart J* 34:638–644, 1972.
10. Boon NA, Bloomfield P: The medical management of valvular heart disease. *Heart* 87:395–400, 2002.
11. Bottio T, Rizzoli G, Gerosa G, et al: Mid-term follow-up in patients with Biocor porcine bioprostheses. *Cardiovasc Surg* 10:238–244, 2002.
12. Brieger DB, Ward C, Cooper SG, et al: Double-orifice left atrioventricular valve—diagnosis and management of an unexpected lesion. *Cardiol Young* 5:267, 1995.
13. Caldarone CA, Raghuveer G, Hills CB, et al: Long-term survival after mitral valve replacement in children aged <5 years: A multi-institutional study. *Circulation* 104:I143–147, 2001.
14. Carpentier A, Branchini B, Cour JC, et al: Congenital malformations of the mitral valve in children. Pathology and surgical treatment. *J Thorac Cardiovasc Surg* 72:854–866, 1976.
15. Chauvaud S, Fuzellier JF, Houel R, et al: Reconstructive surgery in congenital mitral valve insufficiency (Carpentier's techniques): Long-term results. *J Thorac Cardiovasc Surg* 115:84–92, 1998.
16. Chauvaud SM, Mihaileanu SA, Gaer JAR, et al: Surgical treatment of congenital mitral valvular stenosis: "The Hospital Broussais" experience. *Cardiol Young* 7:15, 1997.
17. Christakis GT, Kormos RL, Weisel RD, et al: Morbidity and mortality in mitral valve surgery. *Circulation* 72:II120–II128, 1985.
18. Collins-Nakai RL, Rosenthal A, Castaneda AR, et al: Congenital mitral stenosis. A review of 20 years' experience. *Circulation* 56:1039–1047, 1977.

19. Coto EO, Judez VM, Juffe A, et al: Supravalvular stenotic mitral ring. A new case with surgical correction. *J Thorac Cardiovasc Surg* 71:537–539, 1976.

20. Coulshed N, Epstein EJ, McKendrick CS, et al: Systemic embolism in mitral valve disease. *Br Heart J* 32:26–34, 1970.

21. Cutler EC, Levin SA: Cardiotomy and valvulotomy for mitral stenosis, experimental observations and clinical notes concerning an operated case with recovery. *Boston Med Surg J* 188:1023, 1923.

22. Davachi F, Moller JH, Edwards JE: Diseases of the mitral valve in infancy. An anatomic analysis of 55 cases. *Circulation* 43:565–579, 1971.

23. De la Cruz MV, Gimenez-Ribotta M, Saravalli O, Cayre R: The contribution of the inferior endocardial cushion of the atrioventricular canal to cardiac septation and to the development of the atrioventricular valves: Study in the chick embryo. *Am J Anat* 166:63–72, 1983.

24. Driscoll DJ, Gutgesell HP, McNamara DG: Echocardiographic features of congenital mitral stenosis. *Am J Cardiol* 42:259–266, 1978.

25. Fawzy ME, Mimish L, Awad M, et al: Mitral balloon valvotomy in children with Inoue balloon technique: Immediate and intermediate-term result. *Am Heart J* 127:1559–1562, 1994.

26. Fawzy ME, Ribeiro PA, Dunn B, et al: Percutaneous mitral valvotomy with the Inoue balloon catheter in children and adults: Immediate results and early follow-up. *Am Heart J* 123:462–465, 1992.

27. Ferencz C, Johnson AL, Wiglesworth FW: Congenital mitral stenosis. *Circulation* 9:161, 1954.

28. Glasson JR, Komeda MK, Daughters GT, et al: Three-dimensional regional dynamics of the normal mitral anulus during left ventricular ejection. *J Thorac Cardiovasc Surg* 111:574–585, 1996.

29. Grenadier E, Sahn DJ, Valdes-Cruz LM, et al: Two-dimensional echo Doppler study of congenital disorders of the mitral valve. *Am Heart J* 107:319–325, 1984.

30. Grifka RG, O'Laughlin MP, Nihill MR, Mullins CE: Double-transseptal, double-balloon valvuloplasty for congenital mitral stenosis. *Circulation* 85:123–129, 1992.

31. Gronefeld GC, Li YG, Bogun F, Hohnloser SH: Efficacy and safety of transvenous atrial cardioversion in patients with mitral valve disease and long-standing atrial fibrillation. *Pacing Clin Electrophysiol* 23:1894–1897, 2000.

32. Gunther T, Mazzitelli D, Schreiber C, et al: Mitral-valve replacement in children under 6 years of age. *Eur J Cardiothorac Surg* 17:426–430, 2000.

33. Hatle L: Noninvasive assessment of valve lesions with Doppler ultrasound. *Herz* 9:213–221, 1984.

34. Heller SJ, Carleton RA: Abnormal left ventricular contraction in patients with mitral stenosis. *Circulation* 42:1099–1110, 1970.

35. Inoue K, Owaki T, Nakamura T, et al: Clinical application of transvenous mitral commissurotomy by a new balloon catheter. *J Thorac Cardiovasc Surg* 87:394–402, 1984.

36. Iung B, Cormier B, Ducimetiere P, et al: Immediate results of percutaneous mitral commissurotomy. A predictive model on a series of 1514 patients. *Circulation* 94:2124–2130, 1996.

37. Jarrar M, Betbout F, Gamra H, et al: Successful percutaneous double balloon valvuloplasty for congenital mitral stenosis. *Int J Cardiol* 56:193–196, 1996.

38. Kabbani SS, Jamil H, Hammoud A, et al: Use of the pulmonary autograft for mitral replacement: Short- and medium-term experience. *Eur J Cardiothorac Surg* 20:257–261, 2001.

39. Kavthale SS, Fulwani MC, Vajifdar BU, et al: Atrial fibrillation: How effectively can sinus rhythm be restored and maintained after balloon mitral valvotomy? *Indian Heart J* 52:568–573, 2000.

40. Kirklin JW, Blackstone EH, Bargeron LM Jr, et al: The repair of atrioventricular septal defects in infancy. *Int J Cardiol* 13:333–360, 1986.

41. Kirklin JK, Blackstone EH, Kirklin JW, et al: The Fontan operation. Ventricular hypertrophy, age, and date of operation as risk factors. *J Thorac Cardiovasc Surg* 92:1049–1064, 1986.

42. Lam JH, Ranganathan N, Wigle ED, Silver MD: Morphology of the human mitral valve. I. Chordae tendineae: A new classification. *Circulation* 41:449–458, 1970.

43. Lamberti JJ, Jensen TS, Grehl TM, et al: Late reoperation for systemic atrioventricular valve regurgitation after repair of congenital heart defects. *Ann Thorac Surg* 47:517–522, 1989.

44. Luedtke SA, Kuhn RJ, McCaffrey FM: Pharmacologic management of supraventricular tachycardias in children. Part 2: Atrial flutter, atrial fibrillation, and junctional and atrial ectopic tachycardia. *Ann Pharmacother* 31:1347–1359, 1997.

45. Maisel WH, Rawn JD, Stevenson WG: Atrial fibrillation after cardiac surgery. *Ann Intern Med* 135:1061–1073, 2001.

46. Meister SG, Engel TR, Feitosa GS, et al: Propranolol in mitral stenosis during sinus rhythm. *Am Heart J* 94:685–688, 1977.

47. Moore P, Adatia I, Spevak PJ, et al: Severe congenital mitral stenosis in infants. *Circulation* 89:2099–2106, 1994.

48. Moran AM, Daebritz S, Keane JF, Mayer JE: Surgical management of mitral regurgitation after repair of endocardial cushion defects: Early and midterm results. *Circulation* 102:III160–III165, 2000.

49. Nair M, Agarwala R, Kalra GS, et al: Can mitral regurgitation after balloon dilation of the mitral valve be predicted? *Br Heart J* 67:442–444, 1992.

50. Nakhjavan FK, Katz MR, Maranhao V, Goldberg H: Analysis of influence of catecholamine and tachycardia during supine exercise in patients with mitral stenosis and sinus rhythm. *Br Heart J* 31:753–761, 1969.

51. Nigro JJ, Schwartz DS, Bart RD, et al: Neochordal repair of the posterior mitral leaflet. *J Thorac Cardiovasc Surg* 127:440–447, 2004.

52. Okita Y, Miki S, Kusuhara K, Ueda Y, et al: Early and late results of reconstructive operation for congenital mitral regurgitation in pediatric age group. *J Thorac Cardiovasc Surg* 96:294–298, 1988.

53. Oswalt JD: Complex valvular procedures: Ross, mitral, redos—time enough? *Semin Thorac Cardiovasc Surg* 13:38–41, 2001.

54. Parris TM, McAllister M, Ross JJ, Mintz GS: Doppler-echocardiographic evaluation of left atrial contribution to left ventricular filling in mitral stenosis at rest and during exercise. *Am J Cardiol* 64:1058–1060, 1989.

55. Phornphutkul C, Rosenthal A, Nadas AS: Cardiac manifestations of Marfan syndrome in infancy and childhood. *Circulation* 47:587–596, 1973.

56. Prifti E, Vanini V, Bonacchi M, et al: Repair of congenital malformations of the mitral valve: Early and midterm results. *Ann Thorac Surg* 73:614–621, 2002.

57. Pyeritz RE, McKusick VA: The Marfan syndrome: Diagnosis and management. *N Engl J Med* 300:772–777, 1979.

58. Raghuveer G, Caldarone CA, Hills CB, et al: Predictors of prosthesis survival, growth, and functional status following mechanical mitral valve replacement in children aged <5 years, a multi-institutional study. *Circulation* 108:II174–179, 2003.

59. Ranganathan N, Lam JH, Wigle ED, Silver MD: Morphology of the human mitral valve. II. The value leaflets. *Circulation* 41:459–467, 1970.

60. Roberts WC: Morphologic features of the normal and abnormal mitral valve. *Am J Cardiol* 51:1005–1028, 1983.

61. Roberts WC, Cohen LS: Left ventricular papillary muscles. Description of the normal and a survey of conditions causing them to be abnormal. *Circulation* 46:138–154, 1972.

62. Rosenquist GC: Congenital mitral valve disease associated with coarctation of the aorta: A spectrum that includes parachute deformity of the mitral valve. *Circulation* 49:985–993, 1974.

63. Ruckman RN, Van Praagh R: Anatomic types of congenital mitral stenosis: Report of 49 autopsy cases with consideration of diagnosis and surgical implications. *Am J Cardiol* 42:592–601, 1978.

64. Scott WC, Miller DC, Haverich A: Operative risk of mitral valve replacement: Discriminant analysis of 1329 procedures. *Circulation* 72:II108–119, 1985.

65. Serraf A, Bruniaux J, Planche C: Ross mitral procedure for massive congenital mitral insufficiency. *Arch Mal Coeur Vaiss* 94:509–512, 2001.

66. Serraf A, Zoghbi J, Belli E: Congenital mitral stenosis with or without associated defects: An evolving surgical strategy. *Circulation* 102:III166–III171, 2000.

67. Shone JD, Sellers RD, Anderson RC: The developmental complex of "parachute mitral valve," supravalvular ring of left atrium, subaortic stenosis, and coarctation of the aorta. *Am J Cardiol* 11:714–725, 1963.

68. Shrivastava S, Mathur A, Dev V, et al: Comparison of immediate hemodynamic response to closed mitral commissurotomy, single-balloon, and double-balloon mitral valvuloplasty in rheumatic mitral stenosis. *J Thorac Cardiovasc Surg* 104:1264–1267, 1992.

69. Sintek CF, Pfeffer TA, Kochamba G, et al: Preservation of normal left ventricular geometry during mitral valve replacement. *J Heart Valve Dis* 4:471–475, 1995.

70. Sintek CF, Pfeffer TA, Kochamba GS, Khonsari S: Mitral valve replacement: Technique to preserve the subvalvular apparatus. *Ann Thorac Surg* 59:1027–1029, 1995.

71. Spevak PJ, Bass JL, Ben-Shachar G, et al: Balloon angioplasty for congenital mitral stenosis. *Am J Cardiol* 66:472–476, 1990.

72. Starkey GWB: Surgical experiences in the treatment of congenital mitral stenosis and mitral insufficiency. *J Thorac Cardiovasc Surg* 38:336, 1959.

73. Stellin G, Padalino M, Milanesi O, et al: Repair of congenital mitral valve dysplasia in infants and children: Is it always possible? *Eur J Cardiothorac Surg* 18:74–82, 2000.

74. Sullivan ID, Robinson PJ, de Leval M, Graham TP Jr: Membranous supravalvular mitral stenosis: A treatable form of congenital heart disease. *J Am Coll Cardiol* 8:159–164, 1986.

75. Tandon R, Moller JH, Edwards JE: Anomalies associated with the parachute mitral valve: A pathologic analysis of 52 cases. *Can J Cardiol* 2:278–281, 1986.

76. van Doorn C, Yates R, Tsang V, et al: Mitral valve replacement in children: Mortality, morbidity, and haemodynamic status up to medium-term follow-up. *Heart* 84:636–642, 2000.

77. Van Mierop LH, Alley RD, Kausel HW, Stranahan A: The anatomy and embryology of endocardial cushion defects. *J Thorac Cardiovasc Surg* 43:71–83, 1962.

78. Vitarelli A, Landolina G, Gentile R, et al: Echocardiographic assessment of congenital mitral stenosis. *Am Heart J* 108:523–531, 1984.

79. Wenink AC: Quantitative morphology of the embryonic heart: An approach to development of the atrioventricular valves. *Anat Rec* 234:129–135, 1992.

80. Wenink AC, Gittenberger-de Groot AC: Embryology of the mitral valve. *Inter J Cardiol* 11:75–84, 1986.

81. Wenink AC, Gittenberger-de Groot AC, Brom AG: Developmental considerations of mitral valve anomalies. *Int J Cardiol* 11:85–101, 1986.

82. Yoshimura N, Yamaguchi M, Oshima Y, et al: Surgery for mitral valve disease in the pediatric age group. *J Thorac Cardiovasc Surg* 118:99–106, 1999.

83. Young D, Robinson G: Successful valve replacement in an infant with congenital mitral stenosis. *N Engl J Med* 270:660–644, 1964.

84. Zias EA, Mavroudis C, Backer CL, et al: Surgical repair of the congenitally malformed mitral valve in infants and children. *Ann Thorac Surg* 66:1551–1559, 1998.

Chapter 29

Aortopulmonary Septal Defects and Patent Ductus Arteriosus

CHARLES D. FRASER, JR., MD

AORTOPULMONARY SEPTAL DEFECTS

Aortopulmonary (AP) septal defect, also known as aortopulmonary window (AP window), represents less than 2% of all congenital heart defects. This condition consists of a communication or fenestration between the ascending aorta and the pulmonary artery in hearts with separate aortic and pulmonary valves (Fig. 29-1). The defect may be round, oval, or spiral and can vary in location. AP window was first described in 1830 by Eliotson.[26] The first reports of correct clinical diagnosis of this condition were made in 1949 and 1951.[24,28] Subsequent reports by Somerville,[68] Morrow and colleagues,[50] and Neufeld and colleagues[53] further characterize the nature of this lesion and its clinical and hemodynamic significance. The first successful surgical closure of aortopulmonary window was reported by Gross in 1952[31] and was accomplished by means of a simple ligature.

Classification

Classification of AP septal defect is based on location, as described by Richardson and colleagues.[60] Classic AP septal defects or type I AP window defects are located on the posteromedial wall of the ascending aorta just above the sinus of Valsalva. Thus, the left main coronary artery orifice is near the defect and must be closely guarded during surgical repair. Defects more cephalad on the ascending aorta are classified as type II; these involve the origin of the right pulmonary artery from the main pulmonary artery trunk (see Fig. 29-1). Type III defects are located more laterally on the aorta, so that the right pulmonary artery arises from the posterior or posterolateral ascending aorta. In type III defects, the right pulmonary artery is completely separate from the main pulmonary artery trunk. A significant proportion of patients with type I and type III AP window defect have some other associated congenital cardiac anomaly, including anomalous origin of a coronary artery, ventricular septal defect (VSD), atrial septal defect, or patent ductus arteriosus (PDA).[38] A syndrome of distal AP window, aortic origin of the right pulmonary artery and intact ventricular septum, PDA, and hypoplasia of the aortic isthmus was recognized and described by Berry and associates in 1982.[9] Without surgical intervention, this particular constellation of anomalies is particularly lethal, usually early in the neonatal period.

Embryology

The embryogenesis of AP window is related to incomplete fusion and/or malalignment of the right and left conotruncal ridges, which normally completely septate the truncus arteriosus between the fifth and eighth weeks of intrauterine life. When the right conotruncal ridge arises more posteriorly than normal, unequal partitioning of the AP trunk may result. The aorta may develop more posteriorly than normal, and a portion of the AP trunk may come into contact with the right sixth aortic arch, which eventually becomes the right pulmonary artery. Thus, the right pulmonary artery may connect to the main pulmonary artery as well as having an orifice into the aorta (type II defect). More dorsal development of the aorta may result in the right sixth arch being completely in contact with the aorta, producing anomalous origin of the right pulmonary artery from the ascending aorta (type III defect).[19]

Natural History

The natural history of AP window is that of early congestive heart failure (CHF), gradual development of irreversible pulmonary hypertension, and ultimately, death. Signs and

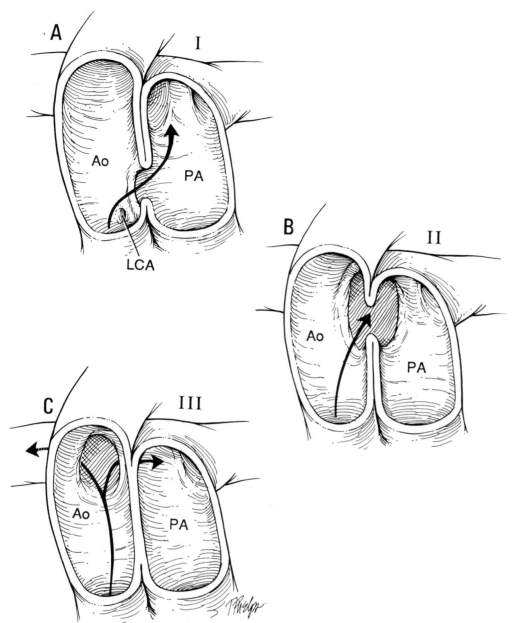

FIGURE 29-1 Native anatomy and classification of aortopulmonary septal defect. **A,** In Type I, the communication is between the ascending aorta and the main pulmonary artery on the posterior medial wall of the ascending aorta. The left main coronary artery (LCA) orifice may be close to the defect. **B,** In Type II, the defect is more cephalad on the ascending aorta. In Type III, the defect is more posterior and lateral in the aorta. **C,** The communication is with the right pulmonary artery, which may be completely separate from the main pulmonary artery.

symptoms of CHF usually appear early in infancy with a presentation that may be similar to that of infants with other large left-to-right shunts, including VSDs and PDA. Thus, these infants tend to be small, underdeveloped, and tachypneic, possibly with a tendency toward recurrent respiratory infections.[71] Acute decompensation may result from intercurrent respiratory infection. In patients with large defects, symptoms may appear very early in life, especially if associated with other cardiac anomalies.

On physical examination, cyanosis is absent, but there is usually the nonspecific history of poor feeding and delayed growth. Peripheral pulses are bounding. Cardiac enlargement is present with a prominent apical impulse and a loud, harsh systolic murmur. There may also be a systolic thrill. Patients who develop elevated pulmonary vascular resistance (PVR)

may display increasing cyanosis, a loud pulmonic ejection sound, and a loud single second heart sound.[25]

The differential diagnosis of this physical spectrum includes large PDA, ruptured sinus of Valsalva aneurysm, coronary arteriovenous fistula, truncus arteriosus, pulmonary arteriovenous fistula, and VSD with aortic insufficiency.

Diagnostic Assessment

Evaluation of the chest x-ray and electrocardiogram (ECG) in children with AP window reveals findings similar to those in children with VSD or large PDA. The chest x-ray film shows cardiomegaly and pulmonary plethora. The electrocardiogram may show left ventricular or biventricular hypertrophy. Evidence of left atrial enlargement also may be present.[11]

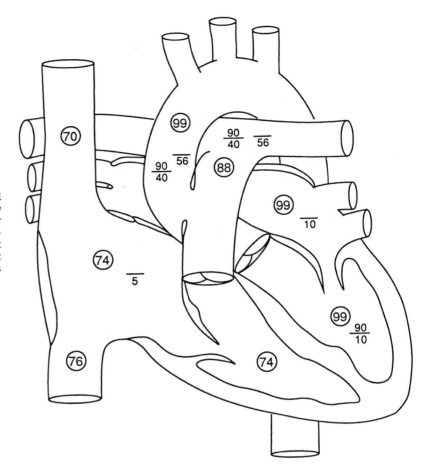

FIGURE 29-2 Pathophysiology of aortopulmonary septal defect. There is communication between the main pulmonary artery and the aorta. Both right and left atrial and ventricular saturations are normal; however, there is an increase in saturation in the main pulmonary artery indicating a left-to-right shunt. This is accompanied by systemic or near-systemic pressure in the main pulmonary artery. In this example pressures are equal, indicating a large defect.

Diagnosis of AP window can usually made with echocardiography. Two-dimensional imaging will reveal the aortopulmonary defect associated with two separate semilunar valves, and color flow imaging will confirm the aortopulmonary shunt. Echocardiography also may identify other associated cardiac defects.[34,47,59] Cardiac catheterization and angiography may be necessary on occasion to provide definitive diagnosis; this study will reveal elevated pulmonary arterial oxygen saturations compared with right ventricular saturations (Fig. 29-2). In patients with late presentation, catheterization may be useful in determining pulmonary vascular resistance. In patients presenting at an older age (>3 months), operability can be ascertained by documenting that the pulmonary vascular bed remains reactive to oxygen or inhaled nitric oxide. Ascending aortic angiography will show rapid filling of a pulmonary artery through the AP window as well as separate aortic and pulmonic valves. Catheterization also may identify the origin of the coronary arteries or confirm aortic origin of the right pulmonary artery in some forms of AP septal defects. In complicated cases, cardiac magnetic resonance imaging may be very helpful in delineating the anatomy, particularly in cases with aortic arch involvement.

Surgical Intervention

Operative repair of AP window is indicated in all infants at the time of diagnosis. Our team prefers to operate before the age of

3 months to prevent irreversible pulmonary vascular changes. Patients presenting later in life should be evaluated for evidence of irreversible pulmonary vascular disease. Decisions regarding operative intervention at this time should be based on the reversibility of pulmonary hypertension.

As mentioned previously, in 1952 Gross performed the first successful surgical closure of AP window by simple ligature.[31] In 1953, interruption by division and direct suture was performed by Scott and Sabiston.[66] Before the availability of cardiopulmonary bypass (CPB), the most common approach for surgical management of AP window was division and oversewing between vascular clamps. This approach is hazardous, with significant risk of rupture and hemorrhage. It has been abandoned since the advent of CPB.

Currently, the procedure of choice for isolated AP septal defect involves transaortic closure of the defect using a prosthetic patch while providing CPB support (Fig. 29-3). Alternatively, the aorta and pulmonary arteries can be separated, and the resultant aortic and pulmonary arterial defects are each closed with pericardium or prosthetic material. In either case, these approaches require optimal visualization of the coronary ostia, which may be in close proximity to the edge of the defect.[15,60,73] The technique of transaortic placement of a patch over the AP window, as described by Deverall and associates,[21] is the preferred method of management because it avoids distortion or narrowing of the great vessels and may be useful in both proximal and distal AP septal defects.

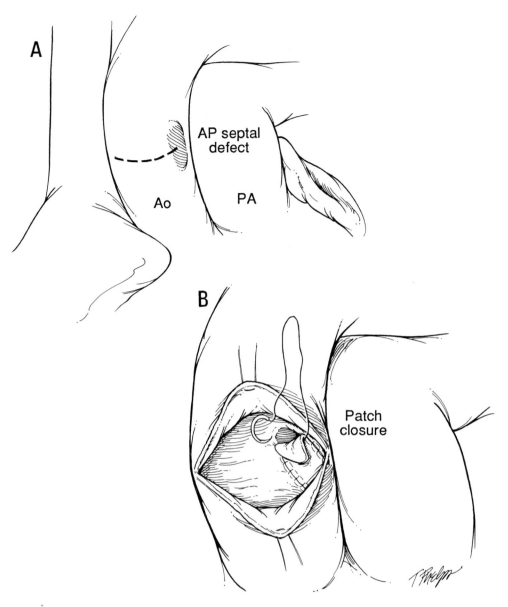

FIGURE 29-3 **A,** Surgical exposure of aortopulmonary septal defect includes transverse incision in ascending aorta. **B,** Aortopulmonary septal defect is closed by suturing a patch over the aortic side of the defect.

The current technique for closure of AP window on CPB includes high aortic cannulation to allow sufficient room for aortic cross-clamping and access to even more distal AP septal defects. Both pulmonary arterial branches are dissected and encircled with Silastic (polymeric silicone) vessel loops to be occluded at the institution of bypass to avoid excessive pulmonary blood flow. It is notable that these patients may have very "irritable" hearts prone to fibrillation (presumably from the diastolic "run-off" into the pulmonary arteries with resultant coronary ischemia), and care should be exercised during sternotomy to avoid undue handling of the heart. Furthermore, the team should be prepared to proceed rapidly toward cannulation and initiation of CPB, because resuscitation of these infants, once the heart fibrillates, is difficult until after the defect is repaired. Venous cannulation can be achieved by either bicaval venous cannulas or direct right atrial cannulation. After aortic cross-clamping, with the pulmonary artery branches occluded, cardioplegia can be instilled in the aorta.

Usually, the repair can be accomplished with moderate hypothermia (28°C to 32°C), but in complex cases involving tiny neonates, some surgeons may prefer to use deep hypothermia with a limited period of circulatory arrest. In type I and II defects, a transverse or longitudinal aortotomy may be used to visualize the defect, which can then be closed with a prosthetic patch consisting of either autologous pericardium or polytetrafluoroethylene. When this incision is made over the anterior portion of the AP window, the patch used to close the defect can be easily placed around the borders of the defect by working through the incision, and the patch can then be incorporated into the suture line as the anterior incision is closed. Alternatively, the aorta and pulmonary artery can be separated. The aortic defect is repaired with pericardium or prosthetic material. The cross-clamp can be released as the pulmonary defect is likewise repaired, often with a piece of pulmonary homograft material. Type III defects may require full mobilization of the right pulmonary artery with creation of pulmonary arterial continuity via direct anastomosis and then direct closure of the aortic defect or patch closure in association with larger defects.[22]

An interesting technique of closure of AP window using a flap of anterior pulmonary arterial wall to reconstruct the posterolateral aortic deficit, followed by closure of the pulmonary arterial deficit with a pericardial patch, was described in 1992 by Matsuki and colleagues.[45] Although theoretically attractive, this technique requires significant pulmonary arterial reconstruction. The theoretical advantage of this is to allow for more normal aortic growth because of its reconstruction with native pulmonary arterial wall. However, this problem has not been significant in patients undergoing standard transaortic approach. Other innovative and creative techniques have been described to address AP septal defects associated with more complex congenital anomalies. These complex anomalies include tricuspid atresia,[29] anomalous coronary arterial origins,[12,14,23] transposition of the great vessels,[4] and the association of cardiac defects described by Berry et al.[9]

To emphasize that AP windows can accompany complex anatomic defects of the aortic arch, we have recently encountered a very interesting and challenging case at Texas Children's Hospital. This premature neonate had caudal regression syndrome with severe CHF. Transthoracic echo imaging documented a distal, type III aortopulmonary window

with type B interrupted aortic arch (interrupted between the left common carotid and subclavian arteries). At surgery, the anatomy was confirmed, but an additional, unexpected defect was encountered. The left main coronary ostium arose completely from the mid-right pulmonary artery. Repair required directed anastomosis to the interrupted arch. The anomalous coronary was mobilized as a button of pulmonary artery and implanted on the posterior ascending aorta in a fashion comparable to an arterial switch procedure. The pulmonary arterial defect and aortopulmonary window were reconstructed with autologous pericardium, and the patient did well after surgery. This unusual association underscores the necessity of careful examination of the coronary ostia at the time of surgical repair (Fig. 29-4).

Critical Care Management

Preoperative and intraoperative care in children presenting with AP window is similar in all respects to other patients presenting with lesions resulting in excessive pulmonary blood flow, such as truncus arteriosus or large VSDs. In infants presenting in severe CHF, significant resuscitation may be required before surgical intervention, including the necessity of endotracheal intubation and mechanical ventilation and correction of metabolic abnormalities in preparation for surgery.

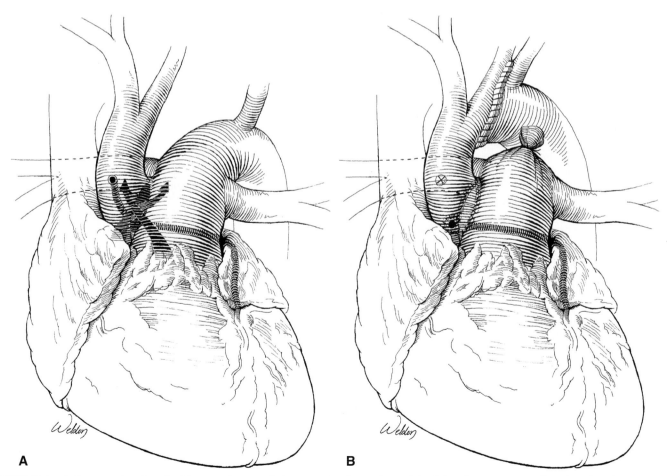

A   **B**

FIGURE 29-4   A, Interrupted aortic arch with aortopulmonary window type III and anomalous origin of the left coronary artery from the right pulmonary artery. **B,** Completed result after repair.

Once this is achieved, however, there is generally no benefit to the patient in trying to temporize with medical therapy. AP window remains a surgical disease not otherwise treatable. We recommend prompt repair, even in the very small neonate, as these patients may have enormous shunt flow. They are at significant risk of ongoing complications, including necrotizing enterocolitis and sepsis.

Detailed consideration concerning anesthetic management for patients with AP window is beyond the scope of the chapter (see Chapter 10 on anesthetic management). One must be alerted, however, to the risks attendant to anesthetic induction in these patients. If the patient becomes hypotensive during induction, significant myocardial ischemia may result from the very low diastolic blood pressure. As a consequence of the enormous "diastolic run-off," coronary blood flow may be jeopardized during periods of hypotension, and ventricular fibrillation may ensue. The anesthesiologist and surgeon should be alerted to this possibility and be prepared to respond appropriately, which might require emergent sternotomy, cannulation, and placement on CPB. For this reason, it is advisable that induction not proceed until the surgical team is available and ready.

At surgery, control of the AP window, either directly or via bilateral pulmonary arterial snares, should be achieved on institution of CPB to prevent excessive pulmonary blood flow and coronary arterial steal. Other aspects of bypass management are as with other forms of congenital heart disease. We prefer to avoid deep hypothermic circulatory arrest for repair, although this may be necessary, particularly where repair of an interrupted aortic arch or some other associated defect warrants its use, such as in very distal defects, in very tiny infants (e.g., <2 kg), or in those patients such as the one described earlier.

The postoperative care of individuals undergoing primary repair of AP window defects is similar to that of other children undergoing corrective open-heart surgery. As in other lesions associated with excessive pulmonary blood flow, the possibility of postoperative pulmonary hypertension exists, and measures aimed at combating this problem should be instituted in the early postoperative period. These include adequate analgesia and sedation, usually in the form of continuous narcotic infusions, as well as complete neuromuscular blockade using either intermittent or continuous infusions. In addition, mild hyperventilation to achieve a $PaCO_2$ near 35 mm Hg and adequate oxygenation are important. Systemic and pulmonary vasodilators, including milrinone, sodium nitroprusside, nitroglycerin, prostaglandin E_1, and phentolamine, also have a role in the early postoperative management of these patients. Our protocol has included the placement of small catheters in the left atrium and pulmonary artery to allow for the accurate assessment of filling pressures and pulmonary vasoreactivity during the various stages of postoperative recovery. Some patients may require inhaled nitric oxide to modulate pulmonary vasoreactivity for some time after surgery. In unusual circumstances, the use of extracorporeal life support such as extracorporeal membrane oxygenation might be required.

Outcomes

The hospital mortality rate for repair of isolated AP window should be low; various series report excellent results in infancy and early childhood.[15,41,71] For repairs made later in life, the outcome is dictated by the presence and severity of pulmonary vascular disease. The possibilities for surgical correction in these patients depend on the degree of pulmonary vascular disease at the time of surgery. Over the past 7 years, the mortality rate at Texas Children's Hospital for surgical repair of AP window (10 patients) has been zero. This series includes several neonates presenting in a very ill state. One patient presented from an outside hospital after attempted device closure of a distal type III defect. Successful surgery was still performed. Long-term complications are unusual. Recurrent aortopulmonary fistula can occur, especially following single-patch repair.

PATENT DUCTUS ARTERIOSUS

Patent ductus arteriosus is a postnatal communication, usually between the main pulmonary trunk and descending thoracic aorta that is due to persistent patency of the fetal ductus arteriosus. This section concentrates on the isolated PDA in infants, children, and adults, with brief mention of issues relating to PDA in preterm newborns. For a more in-depth discussion of the diagnosis of PDA in preterm newborns, the reader is referred to an excellent review by Evans.[27] PDA is also often associated with other congenital cardiac anomalies, but this is not discussed here.

The ductus arteriosus is patent at birth and appears as a muscular artery with an intact internal elastic lamina. The media of the ductus is composed of circularly arranged smooth muscle cells with minimal elastin fibers. Mucoid lakes are present, which are large pools filled with mucoid substance. Postnatal ductal closure occurs in two stages. Initially, medial smooth muscle contraction produces increased wall thickness and shortening and protrusion of the intimal cushions and mucoid lakes. This results in functional closure 10 to 15 hours after birth in full-term infants.[51,63] The next stage of closure is usually completed by 2 to 3 weeks of life and results from infolding of the endothelium, proliferation of subintimal layers, and small subintimal hemorrhages, ultimately resulting in a fibrous band known as the ligamentum arteriosum. The precise mechanism of ductus closure is not fully understood, but it is known to be mediated by the release of vasoactive substances and by variations in pH level, oxygen tension, and circulating prostanoids (prostaglandin E_1, prostaglandin E_2, and prostacyclin).[16,46] Increasing oxygen tension acts to promote ductal constriction, and prostaglandins promote ductal dilatation. This relationship is also known to be affected by gestational age; thus, the ductus is much more sensitive to PaO_2 in the mature full-term infant and to prostaglandin E_1 in the preterm newborn.

As an isolated anomaly, PDA occurs in approximately 1 in 2000 to 2500 live births and is believed to represent approximately 10% of all congenital heart lesions. There is an approximate 2:1 female-to-male preponderance. It has been noted that exposure to rubella during the first trimester of pregnancy is associated with the high frequency of multiple congenital anomalies, and the cardiovascular system is affected in 60% of these infants. PDA is generally present in these patients and is often associated with peripheral pulmonary stenosis and renal artery stenosis.[5,48]

Embryology

Embryologically, the ductus arteriosus develops from the distal portion of the left sixth aortic arch and normally connects the main pulmonary trunk or the proximal left pulmonary trunk with the descending thoracic aorta approximately 5 to 10 mm distal to the origin of the left subclavian artery. A left, right, or bilateral ductus may be present, and the ductus may connect from either the proximal right or left pulmonary artery to any location on the aortic arch or proximal portion of the brachiocephalic vessels. With a right aortic arch, a PDA usually arises from the distal left sixth arch, either an isolated structure off of the right descending aorta or via an anomalous left subclavian artery; thus, the ductus will travel in a retroesophageal position, creating a vascular ring.[6,69] A typical PDA has a conical shape with a large aortic end tapering toward a smaller pulmonary arterial end. This connection may be short and broad or long and narrow; may also have a long, tubular or finger-like shape; and may be very tortuous in its course. The length of the PDA is highly variable regardless of its shape or size and may vary from millimeters to centimeters.

Physiology

The ductus arteriosus is normally functionally closed by about 10 to 15 hours postnatally. In situations of persistent ductal patency, pathophysiology relates to reversal of ductal flow due to the normal decline in PVR that occurs after birth with aeration and ventilation of the lungs. This results in a left-to-right shunt from aorta to pulmonary artery. Fully saturated aortic blood passes from the descending thoracic aorta to the pulmonary artery via the ductus and eventually goes through the lungs into the left atrium, into the left ventricle, and back to the aorta (Fig. 29-5). This results in an increased volume and workload on the left atrium and left ventricle. The increase in left ventricular stroke volume is proportionate to the size of the left-to-right shunt. Ultimately, left atrial dilation occurs along with left ventricular dilation and hypertrophy.

The degree of left-to-right shunting via the ductus is dependent on the relationship between systemic and pulmonary vascular resistance. As systemic vascular resistance remains high after birth, the major determinant of the degree of left-to-right shunting through the PDA is PVR.[62,64]

Pathophysiologic changes caused by left-to-right shunts through the PDA relate to the size of the shunt and the ability of the left ventricle to handle the extra volume load. In situations of a small duct with moderate left-to-right shunting, the left heart may be able to compensate for the extra volume load, and no symptoms may result. However, in situations of a large duct with significant left-to-right shunting, left ventricular and atrial dilatation will ensue, with left heart failure and pulmonary edema. Right ventricular failure may develop later if there is significant pulmonary hypertension.[64]

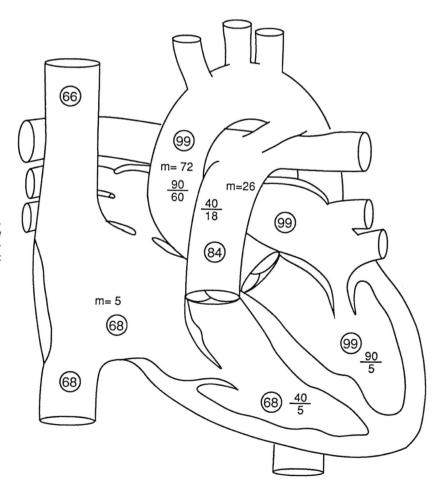

FIGURE 29-5 Pathophysiology of patent ductus arteriosus. There is a step-up in saturation in the main pulmonary artery indicating a left-to-right shunt. Right-sided pressure is elevated, but only approximately half-systemic. End-diastolic pressures are low, indicating the absence of failure.

The net effect of a large left-to-right shunt on the pulmonary circulation may be a delay in the normal postnatal pulmonary vascular changes. Early on, with increased pulmonary blood flow and increased resistance, histologic views may demonstrate increases in medial smooth muscle. Pulmonary vascular disease may develop with intimal damage and cellular proliferation and finally, thrombosis and fibrosis of small pulmonary arteries.[33] In children with a large PDA, aortic and pulmonary artery pressures may be nearly equal, and as mentioned previously, the degree of shunting is affected primarily by PVR. With a normal fall in PVR after birth, there is significant left-to-right shunting, and these infants may develop severe CHF by the before-mentioned mechanisms within the first 4 to 6 weeks of life.[42]

With moderate-sized PDAs, the degree of left-right shunts is regulated by the size of the duct, and pulmonary artery pressure may be only moderately elevated. In these patients, the degree of left ventricular hypertrophy and volume load may be reasonably well tolerated, so that symptoms do not occur. However, these patients may exhibit growth retardation, breathlessness, and poor feeding.[42]

In patients with a small patent ductus, the net left-to-right shunt is small, and pulmonary blood flow is not significantly increased. Left ventricular enlargement and failure do not occur. In this situation, symptoms may be delayed until late in life.

Infants with large PDAs present early in life with signs and symptoms of severe CHF. Other complications are possible with persistent ductus, including bacterial endocarditis. Before the advent of surgical repair and routine use of prophylactic antibiotics, endocarditis was one of the leading causes of death in patients with PDA. This is now an extremely rare complication.[37,40] Nevertheless, on occasion a case of ductus-related endocarditis does occur. In general, the vegetations related to this infection tend to occur on the pulmonic end of the ductus; thus, septic emboli are showered to the lungs, and pulmonary abscesses may occur. The treatment of choice in this situation consists of antibiotics until blood cultures are negative, followed by surgical intervention.

Another complication of PDA occurs when the ductus becomes aneurysmal. This is extremely rare and may occur as an isolated event in a patient after surgery or with endocarditis. In neonates, aneurysmal dilatation of the ductus is very rare but may lead to lethal rupture.[20,35] We recently repaired a giant ductal aneurysm in a newborn diagnosed in utero. This patient was asymptomatic following delivery, but serial postnatal echocardiographic evaluation documented a large ductal aneurysm with no evidence of regression. Surgery was recommended due to the known propensity of these structures to rupture.[67] The infant underwent surgery via left thorocotomy with complete resection of the aneurysm. Recovery was uneventful (Fig. 29-6).[67] Patients with PDA also may present with mediastinal masses and symptoms related to compression of adjacent structures. Treatment of choice for these lesions is surgical correction.[8,18,39,61]

A late complication of long-standing left-to-right shunts and increased pulmonary blood flow is the occurrence of fixed pulmonary vascular resistance and right-sided heart failure. This occurs primarily in patients with long-standing PDAs and ultimately results in right-to-left shunts at the ductal

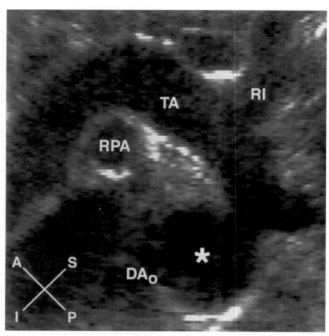

FIGURE 29-6 Suprasternal notch view of the aortic arch demonstrating the dilated ductus arteriosus (*). A, anterior; DA$_o$, descending aorta; I, inferior; P, posterior; RI, right innominate artery; RPA, right pulmonary artery; S, superior; TA, transverse aorta.

level. Patients may also develop severe calcification of the pulmonary artery and ductus. Surgical closure of the duct in patients with irreversible pulmonary vascular disease is contraindicated.

History and Physical Examination

The development of signs and symptoms of CHF in patients with persistent PDA is related to the degree of left-to-right shunt and left ventricular volume overload. In the absence of these findings, patients may be largely asymptomatic, although growth retardation may be evident. The typical patient with PDA usually appears reasonably well with a normal heart rate, but the blood pressure may demonstrate a widened pulse pressure. The classic physical finding of persistent PDA is a continuous machinery murmur,[37] that is, a crescendo, decrescendo murmur, usually of grades III to VI and heard best at the left sternal border. On occasion, a palpable thrill may be present. In patients with significant left ventricular volume overload, a significant left ventricular lift or heave may be present. Electrocardiography may demonstrate evidence of left ventricular hypertrophy or strain. The chest radiographic appearance may range from normal to one demonstrating pulmonary plethora.

Diagnostic Assessment

Most infants with a large PDA exhibit significant symptoms, and the physical examination demonstrates findings consistent with the diagnosis of PDA, including the aforementioned machinery murmur. Confirmation of the diagnosis can be obtained from two-dimensional echocardiography and

Doppler flow studies.[44] The echocardiogram also can be used to determine if other intracardiac anomalies are present.[33]

Cardiac catheterization with cineangiography is generally not indicated in straightforward cases but should be considered when significant pulmonary vascular disease is suspected. As noted, AP window is also in the differential diagnosis, and this lesion should be excluded at catheterization if not already done by echocardiography. Percutaneous device closure of persistent PDA may be performed during the initial catheterization in many cases. This is dealt with in a subsequent section.

An occasional patient presenting in adult life with persistent PDA develops calcification of the duct as well as the pulmonary artery. It is important to be aware of this possibility before surgical intervention, as it affects the surgical approach and management. In these individuals, a computed tomographic scan of the chest may help demonstrate the extent of calcification.

Surgical Intervention

The operative technique of ductal ligation was described in 1907 by Munro.[52] It was not until 1939, however, that Gross and Hubbard[32] reported the first successful ligation of a PDA at Boston Children's Hospital. This landmark operation was a notable event in the development of the field of cardiac surgery. In 1967, Portsmann and colleagues[55] introduced nonsurgical closure of a PDA using an Ivalon plug. Later, in 1979, Rashkind[56] developed a polyurethane foam disc umbrella that could be used in neonates or infants; this technique was further explored by Rashkind and Cuaso[57] and Sato and colleagues.[65].

Surgical ligation or division remains the most common method used for closure of a persistent PDA in newborns, although percutaneous device closure has replaced surgery in older children (Fig. 29-7). The standard approach for surgical closure involves a left posterolateral thoracotomy. This can

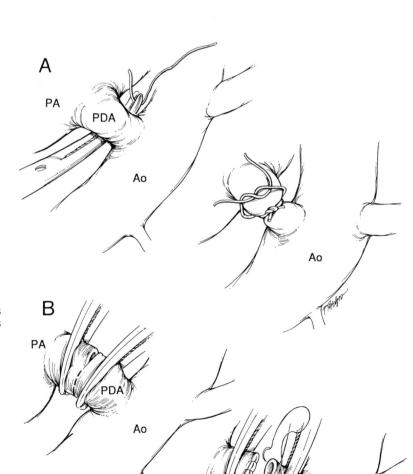

FIGURE 29-7 Surgical correction of patent ductus arteriosus (PDA). **A,** Ligation of ductus arteriosus. **B,** Division of ductus arteriosus. Ao, aorta; PA, pulmonary artery.

be done via the third or fourth intercostal space and generally involves a short incision made in a muscle-sparing fashion. The lung is retracted inferiomedially, and the posterior parietal pleura is incised. The left superior intercostal vein may need to be divided and ligated to provide access. The edges of the pleura are then carefully retracted, avoiding injury to the vagus nerve. Sharp dissection then proceeds on the superior and inferior edge of the ductus. Dissection is best made in the plane closest to the aorta, which is avascular. The left recurrent laryngeal nerve is on the medial reflected pleural flap and is identified and protected. In small patients, especially those with large PDAs, the aortic arch should be carefully identified to avoid confusion. Next, with a blunt, right-angled dissector, circumferential control of the ductus is gained. At this point, the ductus may be either divided and oversewn or ligated, depending on the size and length. Our preference has been to ligate the ductus with multiple large silk ligatures so that it is obliterated in its entire course. In smaller children, this usually amounts to two or three large silk ligatures. Alternatively, in patients with a large PDA, especially older children, adequate mobilization can afford the opportunity to clamp both the pulmonary arterial and aortic ends, followed by ductal division and oversewing of the two stumps. With all techniques, great care must be taken at the time of clamping or ligating because of the occasional extreme friability of the ductal tissue.

On occasion, previous cardiothoracic surgery or calcification of the ductus may require an alternative surgical approach, including the use of CPB. If the PDA is not readily accessible, the patient may be placed on CPB and cooled sufficiently to allow low-flow perfusion and direct closure of the ductus from within the pulmonary artery. If this approach is used, the patient should be cooled on bypass to a nasopharyngeal temperature of 20° C to 25° C, and this is followed by direct suture closure of the duct. In these instances, however, some degree of control on ductal flow must be achieved during the period of bypass cooling to prevent pulmonary overcirculation. This may be provided by a balloon catheter or pulmonary arterial snares.[10] This technique may also be useful in patients with calcified ductus, and sometimes a small prosthetic patch may be needed to achieve ductal closure.

An interesting approach championed by several centers is the use of video-assisted thoracoscopy surgical techniques for interruption of a PDA in small children. This procedure involves the introduction of endoscopic equipment via small counterincisions in the left chest, followed by dissection and application of metallic ligature clips. This has been the source of considerable controversy in terms of its applicability. Although the procedure is theoretically attractive in that it avoids a standard thoracotomy incision, these patients do in fact require multiple chest incisions with some attendant morbidity. The technique is also quite clearly more user dependent than standard open techniques, and this has been demonstrated by an apparent learning curve in the development of this approach. In addition, operating room time and costs are a consideration, not only in terms of length of procedure but also investment in expensive video equipment. A potential and considerable disadvantage lies in the possibility that unexpected surgical bleeding may occur in a video-assisted procedure. One could envision a very difficult situation arising from a transected ductus in which an emergent thoracotomy

has to be performed to gain vascular control.[43] Widespread acceptance of this approach will have to be carefully weighed in comparison with tried and proven direct surgical techniques. One published series of cases of surgical PDA ligation or division involving more than 500 patients revealed no mortality and minimal morbidity relating to the direct surgical approach.[49]

An alternative approach to PDA closure that is now widely accepted is percutaneous catheter introduced device closure. This approach, which involves placement of an intraductal plug or occlusion device, is quite attractive in that it avoids the morbidity of a surgical incision. Initial reports from a variety of centers around the world indicate promise with this technique. Success rates have been reasonable, although at 6-month follow-up, 22% of patients demonstrate small residual shunt, which is higher than in surgical series.[2] As with video-assisted techniques, there are several potential disadvantages to this approach, which must be carefully considered before it can be widely accepted or replace standard surgical procedures. The disadvantages include longer procedure-related times, the necessity to introduce intravascular foreign material with the potential for misplacement and embolization, the small but ever-present risk of device infection, concern over an intravascular rough surface, and obvious differences in procedural experience. In the future, these factors must all be weighed before a firm decision is made as to the applicability of these so-called noninvasive or minimally invasive approaches, especially in the present economic environment in which we may be faced with ever-limited medical resources.[3,7,13,58] A 1993 article by Gray and associates[30] underscores this controversy. These authors examined patients undergoing either standard surgical closure or catheter-introduced device closure over a 5-year period and observed that standard surgical closure was more effective in terms of both success rates and cost.

Between 1995 and 2000, 270 patients underwent percutaneous device PDA occlusions at Texas Children's Hospital. The great majority of those patients (239) had percutaneous coils placed, although others required either sacks or umbrellas. Complete closure was achieved in more than 95% of the patients, although there were several serious complications, including device embolizations (either pulmonary arterial or systemic) and device-related hemolysis. Surgical intervention after unsuccessful device closure may be quite challenging, often involving the necessity of cardiopulmonary bypass.

Results after the classic direct surgical approach have been very good, and the surgical risk in children with isolated PDA is well under 0.5%. Excellent results have been obtained in even the premature age group.[70] Operative morbidity has also been quite small. It is extremely unusual to need to administer blood products.[17]

Critical Care Management

In general, the preoperative and intraoperative care of patients with isolated PDA is simple and straightforward, mainly involving management of pulmonary overcirculation and left ventricular volume overload. Postoperatively, patients generally do quite well and are often extubated in the operating room or in the early postoperative period. Pain management in the form of intercostal nerve blocks with 0.25% bupivacaine may be helpful in postoperative pain management and may allow earlier resumption of normal ventilation.

Complications

Complications related to the procedure have been minimal and include recurrent nerve palsy and chylothorax. In general, the recurrent nerve injury is transient paresis, which responds to expectant management. Chylothorax is unusual and may be treated by pleural tube decompression or pleural sclerosis, plus limiting of fat intake. On rare occasions, reoperation may be required for identification and ligation of the offending lymphatic channel.

Reports of recurrent ductal patency vary widely, but with current surgical methods, the rates should be extremely low, ranging from 0.4% to 3%.[54,72]

One point that merits special attention is the frequent occurrence of gastric distention after PDA ligation. This is likely due in part to traction on the vagus nerve and some degree of gastroparesis; the clinician should watch for this complication carefully in the early postoperative period and manage it with nasogastric intubation and decompression as needed. In general, we have avoided oral intake on the first postoperative day and awaited resumption of normal bowel activity as indicated by the presence of bowel sounds.

As mentioned previously, current operative mortality rates approach zero, and in patients with isolated, uncomplicated PDAs, life expectancy should be near normal. In patients with severe pulmonary vascular disease, however, with a bidirectional or right-to-left shunt, the surgical risk is high, and long-term results are poor because of irreversible pulmonary vascular changes. In patients undergoing surgery late in life who have suffered chronic and long-standing left ventricular volume overload and have developed left ventricular dysfunction, the risk of late death may not be totally alleviated by ductal closure, as a result of irreversible myocardial damage.

The chief controversy today in the management of patients with PDA centers on the most appropriate procedure to use in addressing this lesion. As noted, surgical closure is a tried and proven method, and all other potential options must be measured against this "gold standard" before alternative management schemes are adopted.

References

1. Acherman RJ, Siassi B, Wells W, et al: Aneurysm of the ductus arteriosus: A congenital lesion. *Am J Perinatal* 15:653–659, 1998.
2. Ali Khan MA, al Yousef S, Mullins CE, Sawyer W: Experience with 205 procedures of transcatheter closure of ductus arteriosus in 182 patients, with special reference to residual shunts and long-term follow-up. *J Thorac Cardiovasc Surg* 104:1721–1727, 1992.
3. Ali Khan MA, Mullins CE, Nihill MR, et al: Percutaneous catheter closure of the ductus arteriosus in children and young adults. *Am J Cardiol* 64:218–221, 1989.
4. Amato JJ: Complete transposition of the great arteries with aortopulmonary window. *J Thorac Cardiovasc Surg* 104:1490–1491, 1992.
5. Anderson RC: Causative factors underlying congenital heart malformations. I: Patent ductus arteriosus. *Pediatrics* 14:143–151, 1954.
6. Barger JD, Bregman EH, Edwards JE: Bilateral ductus arteriosus with right aortic arch and right-sided descending aorta. *Am J Roentgenol Radium Ther Nucl Med* 76:758–761, 1956.
7. Bash SE, Mullins CE: Insertion of patent ductus occluder by transvenous approach: A new technique. *Circulation* 70:285, 1984.
8. Berger M, Ferguson C, Hendry J: Paralysis of the left diaphragm, left vocal cord and aneurysm of the ductus arteriosus in a 7-day-old infant. *J Pediatr* 56:800–802, 1960.
9. Berry TE, Bharati S, Muster AJ, et al: Distal aortopulmonary septal defect, aortic origin of the right pulmonary artery, intact ventricular septum, patent ductus arteriosus and hypoplasia of the aortic isthmus: A newly recognized syndrome. *Am J Cardiol* 49:108–116, 1982.
10. Bhati BS, Nandakumaran CP, Shatapathy P, et al: Closure of patent ductus arteriosus during open-heart surgery. Surgical experience with different techniques. *J Thorac Cardiovasc Surg* 63:820–826, 1972.
11. Blieden LC, Moller JH: Aorticopulmonary septal defect. An experience with 17 patients. *Br Heart J* 36:630–635, 1974.
12. Boonstra PW, Talsma M, Ebels T: Interruption of the aortic arch, distal aortopulmonary window, arterial duct and aortic origin of the right pulmonary artery in a neonate: Report of a case successfully repaired in a one-stage operation. *Int J Cardiol* 34:108–110, 1992.
13. Bridges ND, Perry SB, Parness I, et al: Transcatheter closure of a large patent ductus arteriosus with the clamshell septal umbrella. *J Am Coll Cardiol* 18:1297–1302, 1991.
14. Brouwer MH, Beaufort-Krol GC, Talsma MD: Aortopulmonary window associated with an anomalous origin of the right coronary artery. *Int J Cardiol* 28:384–386, 1990.
15. Clarke CP, Richardson JP: The management of aortopulmonary window: Advantages of transaortic closure with a Dacron patch. *J Thorac Cardiovasc Surg* 72:48–51, 1976.
16. Clyman RI, Heymann MA: Pharmacology of the ductus arteriosus. *Pediatr Clin North Am* 28:77–93, 1981.
17. Coster DD, Gorton ME, Grooters RK, et al: Surgical closure of the patent ductus arteriosus in the neonatal intensive care unit. *Ann Thorac Surg* 48:386–389, 1989.
18. Cruickshank B, Marquis RM: Spontaneous aneurysm of the ductus arteriosus. *Am J Med* 25:140–149, 1958.
19. Cucci CE, Doyle EF, Lewis EW Jr: Absence of a primary division of the pulmonary trunk. An ontogenetic theory. *Circulation* 29:124–131, 1964.
20. D'Udekem Y, Rubay JE, Sluysmans T: A case of neonatal ductus arteriosus aneurysm. *Cardiovasc Surg* 5:338–339, 1997.
21. Deverall PB, Lincoln JC, Aberdeen E, et al: Aortopulmonary window. *J Thorac Cardiovasc Surg* 57:479–486, 1969.
22. Di Eusanio G, Mazzola A, Gregorini R, et al: Anomalous origin of right pulmonary artery from the ascending aorta. *J Cardiovasc Surg (Torino)* 30:709–712, 1989.
23. Ding WX, Su ZK, Cao DF, Jonas RA: One-stage repair of absence of the aortopulmonary septum and interrupted aortic arch. *Ann Thorac Surg* 49:664–666, 1990.
24. Dodds JH, Hoyle C: Congenital aortic septal defect. *Br Heart J* 11:390, 1949.
25. Ebert PA, Arciniegas E: Aortopulmonary window. In Arciniegas E (ed): *Pediatric Cardiac Surgery*, Chicago, Mosby-Year Book, 1985, pp 375–379.
26. Eliotson J: Case of malformation of the pulmonary artery and the aorta. *Lancet* 1:247, 1830.
27. Evans N: Diagnosis of patent ductus arteriosus in the preterm newborn. *Arch Dis Child* 68:58–61, 1993.
28. Gasul BM, Fell EH, Casas R: The diagnosis of aortic septal defect by retrograde aortography: Report of a case. *Circulation* 4:251, 1951.
29. Geva T, Ott DA, Ludomirsky A, et al: Tricuspid atresia associated with aortopulmonary window: Controlling pulmonary blood flow with a fenestrated patch. *Am Heart J* 123:260–262, 1992.
30. Gray DT, Fyler DC, Walker AM, et al: Clinical outcomes and costs of transcatheter as compared with surgical closure of patent ductus arteriosus. The Patent Ductus Arteriosus Closure Comparative Study Group. *N Engl J Med* 329:1517–1523, 1993.
31. Gross RE: Surgical closure of an aortic septal defect. *Circulation* 5:858, 1952.
32. Gross RE, Hubbard JP: Ductus arteriosus: Surgical ligation of a patent ductus arteriosus. *JAMA* 8:729, 1939.
33. Hoffman JI, Rudolph AM, Heymann MA: Pulmonary vascular disease with congenital heart lesions: Pathologic features and causes. *Circulation* 64:873–877, 1981.
34. Horimi H, Hasegawa T, Shiraishi H, et al: Detection of aortopulmonary window with ventricular septal defect by Doppler color flow imaging. *Chest* 101:280–281, 1992.
35. Heikkinen ES, Simila S, Laitinen J, Larmi T: Infantile aneurysm of the ductus arteriosus. Diagnosis, incidence, pathogenesis and prognosis. *Acta Paediatr Scand* 63:241–248, 1974.

36. Ingram MT, Ott DA: Concomitant repair of aortopulmonary window and interrupted aortic arch. *Ann Thorac Surg* 53:909–911, 1992.

37. Johnson DH, Rosenthal A, Nadas AS: A forty-year review of bacterial endocarditis in infancy and childhood. *Circulation* 51:581–588, 1975.

38. Keane JF, Maltz D, Bernhard WF, et al: Anomalous origin of one pulmonary artery from the ascending aorta. Diagnostic, physiological and surgical considerations. *Circulation* 50:588–594, 1974.

39. Kerwin AJ, Jaffe FA: Postoperative aneurysm of the ductus arteriosus with fatal rupture of a mycotic aneurysm of a branch of the pulmonary artery. *Am J Cardiol* 3:397–403, 1959.

40. Keys A, Shapiro MJ: Patency of the ductus arteriosus in adults. *Am Heart J* 25:158–186, 1943.

41. Kirklin JW, Barratt-Boyes BG: Aortopulmonary window. In Kirklin JW, Barratt-Boyes BG (eds): *Cardiac Surgery,* New York, Churchill Livingstone, 1992, pp 1153–1156.

42. Krovetz LJ, Warden HE: Patent ductus arteriosus. An analysis of 515 surgically proven cases. *Dis Chest* 42:241, 1962.

43. Laborde F, Noirhomme P, Karam J, et al: A new video-assisted thoracoscopic surgical technique for interruption of patent ductus arteriosus in infants and children. *J Thorac Cardiovasc Surg* 105:278–280, 1993.

44. Lund JT, Hansen D, Brocks V, et al: Aneurysm of the ductus arteriosus in the neonate: Three case reports with a review of the literature. *Pediatr Cardiol* 13:222–226, 1992.

45. Matsuki O, Yagihara T, Yamamoto F, et al: New surgical technique for total-defect aortopulmonary window. *Ann Thorac Surg* 54:991–992, 1992.

46. McMurphy DM, Heymann MA, Rudolph AM, Melmon KL: Developmental changes in constriction of the ductus arteriosus: Responses to oxygen and vasoactive agents in the isolated ductus arteriosus of the fetal lamb. *Pediatr Res* 6:231–238, 1972.

47. Mendoza DA, Ueda T, Nishioka K, et al: Aortopulmonary window, aortic origin of the right pulmonary artery, and interrupted aortic arch: Detection by two-dimensional and color Doppler echocardiography in an infant. *Pediatr Cardiol* 7:49–52, 1986.

48. Mitchell SC, Korones SB, Berendes HW: Congenital heart disease in 56,109 births. Incidence and natural history. *Circulation* 43:323–332, 1971.

49. Morris CD, Menashe VD: 25-year mortality after surgical repair of congenital heart defect in childhood. A population-based cohort study. *JAMA* 266:3447–3452, 1991.

50. Morrow AG, Greenfield LJ, Braunwald E: Congenital aortopulmonary septal defect: Clinical and hemodynamic findings, surgical technique and results of operative correction. *Circulation* 25:463, 1962.

51. Moss AJ, Emmanouilides GC, Duffie ER Jr: Closure of the ductus arteriosus in the newborn infant. *Pediatrics* 32:25–30, 1963.

52. Munro JC: Ligation of the ductus arteriosus. *Ann Surg* 46:335, 1907.

53. Neufeld HN, Lester RG, Adams P, et al: Aortopulmonary septal defect. *Am J Cardiol* 9:12, 1962.

54. Panagopoulos PG, Tatooles CJ, Aberdeen E, et al: Patent ductus arteriosus in infants and children. A review of 936 operations (1946–1969). *Thorax* 26:137–144, 1971.

55. Porstmann W, Wierny L, Warnke H, et al: Catheter closure of patent ductus arteriosus. 62 cases treated without thoracotomy. *Radiol Clin North Am* 9:203–218, 1971.

56. Rashkind WJ: Transcatheter treatment of congenital heart disease. *Circulation* 67:711–716, 1983.

57. Rashkind WJ, Cuaso CC: Transcatheter closure of a patent ductus arteriosus. Successful use in a 3.5 kg infant. *Pediatr Cardiol* 1:3–7, 1979.

58. Rashkind WJ, Mullins CE, Hellenbrand WE, Tait MA: Nonsurgical closure of patent ductus arteriosus: Clinical application of the Rashkind PDA Occluder System. *Circulation* 75:583–592, 1987.

59. Rice MJ, Seward JB, Hagler DJ, et al: Visualization of aortopulmonary window by two-dimensional echocardiography. *Mayo Clin Proc* 57:482–487, 1982.

60. Richardson JV, Doty DB, Rossi NP, Ehrenhaft JL: The spectrum of anomalies of aortopulmonary septation. *J Thorac Cardiovasc Surg* 78:21–27, 1979.

61. Ross RS, Feder FP, Spencer FC: Aneurysm of the previously ligated patent ductus arteriosus. *Circulation* 23:350–357, 1961.

62. Rudolph AM: The changes in the circulation after birth. Their importance in congenital heart disease. *Circulation* 41:343–359, 1970.

63. Rudolph AM, Drorbaugh JE, Auld PAM, et al: Studies on the circulation in the neonatal period: The circulation in the respiratory distress syndrome. *Pediatrics* 27:551–566, 1961.

64. Rudolph AM, Mayer FE, Nadas AS, Gross RE: Patent ductus arteriosus: A clinical and hemodynamic study of patients in the first year of life. *Pediatrics* 22:892–904, 1958.

65. Sato K, Fujino M, Kozuka T, et al: Transfemoral plug closure of patent ductus arteriosus. Experiences in 61 consecutive cases treated without thoracotomy. *Circulation* 51:337–341, 1975.

66. Scott HW, Sabiston DC: Surgical treatment of congenital aorticopulmonary fistula. *J Thorac Surg* 25:26, 1953.

67. Siu BL, Kovalchin JP, Kearney DL, et al: Aneurysmal dilatation of the ductus arteriosus in a neonate. *Pediatr Cardiol* 22:403–405, 2001.

68. Somerville J: Aortopulmonary septal defect: Five cases treated by operation. *Guys Hosp Rep* 108:177, 1959.

69. Steinberg I, Miscall L, Goldberg HP: Congenital absence of left pulmonary artery with patent ductus arteriosi. *JAMA* 190:395, 1964.

70. Taylor RL, Grover FL, Harman PK, et al: Operative closure of patent ductus arteriosus in premature infants in the neonatal intensive care unit. *Am J Surg* 152:704–708, 1986.

71. Tiraboschi R, Salomone G, Crupi G, et al: Aortopulmonary window in the first year of life: Report on 11 surgical cases. *Ann Thorac Surg* 46:438–441, 1988.

72. Trippestad A, Efskind L: Patent ductus arteriosus: Surgical treatment of 686 patients. *Scand J Thorac Cardiovasc Surg* 6:38–42, 1972.

73. van Son JA, Puga FJ, Danielson GK, et al: Aortopulmonary window: Factors associated with early and late success after surgical treatment. *Mayo Clin Proc* 68:128–133, 1993.

Chapter 30

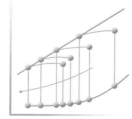

Anomalous Origin of the Coronary Arteries

CHARLES D. FRASER, JR., MD

DEFINITION

An anomalous origin of the coronary artery refers to any pattern that (1) deviates from the normal pattern of the left and right coronary arteries originating from the left and right aortic sinuses, respectively, and that (2) is associated with pathophysiologic disturbances. There are numerous normal variants of coronary anatomy origin that are not associated with pathophysiologic consequences. While occurring infrequently, however, the abnormal patterns of coronary origination associated with pathophysiologic consequences include (1) anomalous origin of one or both coronary arteries *from the pulmonary trunk or one of its branches*; (2) anomalous origin of the coronary artery *from an atypical aortic location*; (3) anomalous origin of the right or left coronary artery (LCA) or the anterior descending or circumflex branches *from the opposite coronary artery or sinus with respect to normal*; (4) ectopic origin of a coronary artery *from an extra cardiac vessel*; or (5) ectopic origin of a coronary artery *from a ventricular cavity*.

For the purpose of this discussion, attention will be turned primarily to anomalous origin of the LCA (ALCA) from the pulmonary artery. This lesion is probably the most frequent important coronary anomaly that must be addressed by pediatric cardiologists, cardiovascular surgeons, and intensivists. Brief attention is also given to anomalous origin of the right coronary artery (RCA) from the pulmonary artery, anomalous origin of both coronary arteries from the pulmonary artery, as well as aberrations in origins of the right and left coronary arteries from the aorta.

EMBRYOLOGY

Most descriptions of the development of the coronary arterial bed mention three separate components. First, the sinusoids are primitive channels representing the sites of metabolic exchange between the blood contained in the cardiac cavities and the cardiac parenchyma, which at this time is composed mainly of cardiac tissue. In humans, the heart starts beating as early as the 22nd day of gestation, and circulation of the blood can be demonstrated a few days later. Second, the in situ vascular endothelial network appears separately in the subepicardium at around 31 days of gestation. Third, the coronary buds arise from the wall of the aortopulmonary trunk as it completes its division into the aorta and pulmonary artery. After completion of aortopulmonary septation, the in situ vascular endothelial network and coronary buds fuse, and the coronary circulation begins to flow normally.

The distribution and size of the major epicardial coronary arteries is strictly related to the extent of their dependent myocardium. A lack of coronary circulation during embryologic development induces hypoplasia of the dependent myocardium. Conversely, a relative reduction in dependent myocardial mass results in relative hypoplasia of its coronary branch.[61]

There are two theories of embryologic development used to explain the occurrence of anomalous coronary origins. The first suggests that coronary arteries originate from two primordial buds on the undivided conotruncus. As the conotruncus septates into the aorta and pulmonary artery, abnormal placement of one of the coronary buds can result in an anomalous coronary origin. Alternatively, abnormal division of the conotruncus can produce an anomalous coronary despite normal placement of the primordial buds.[7,28] The second theory suggests that six coronary buds or anlagen exist on the primitive truncus arteriosus, one from each potential cusp of the aortic and pulmonary sinuses. Normally all but two of these buds regress. However, if some aberration occurs, the wrong sequence of persistence and involution may occur, resulting in anomalous origin of one of the coronaries.

NORMAL VARIATION IN CORONARY ANATOMY

The term *normal coronary anatomy* is somewhat of a misnomer, in that there are frequent variations in the standard coronary anatomic pattern. Usually, however, there are two major coronary arteries that originate from the left and right aortic sinuses of Valsalva (Fig. 30-1). Individual branches of the left and right coronary systems may also have separate orifices from the corresponding sinuses.

It is normal for the coronary ostia to be located at the right and left aortic sinuses. These ostia should be located at the center of each sinus and close to the free edge of the aortic cusp. Ostia located at the other locations on the aortic wall—namely, in the posterior or noncoronary sinus or high in the aortic root—are abnormal. There must be two coronary ostia present for the coronary pattern to be considered normal; however, having three or four separate ostia is clearly considered to be a normal variant. A third ostium is most commonly located in the right coronary sinus as a separate conal branch; this has been noted to be present in 30% to 50% of normal human hearts.[5] Another frequent variant resulting in an accessory coronary ostium is caused by the absence of the left main coronary trunk, such that the left anterior descending and circumflex branches have separate origins from the aorta. The angle of origin of the main coronary stems is usually perpendicular to the aortic wall, but some variation in this angle is commonly noted. An unusual variant occurs when the proximal arterial segment is intramural or embedded in the aortic wall.

Despite the possibility of having three or four separate ostia, an individual normally has only two coronary systems, the left and the right. The term *single coronary artery* or *single coronary system* refers to origin above the right and left coronary arteries from a single ostium. In more than 90% of autopsy cases, the LCA has an initial single stem of variable length and size. For the coronary pattern to be considered normal, both the left anterior descending and the left circumflex coronary arteries must originate from the left coronary cusp, either directly or indirectly through a left main stem.[19,77] The left anterior descending coronary artery (LAD) is characterized by its course all along the anterior interventricular groove. The circumflex branch is characterized by its

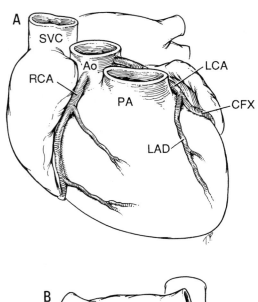

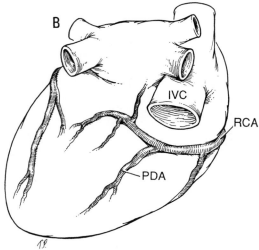

FIGURE 30-1 Normal coronary anatomy. **A,** Anterior aspect. **B,** Posterior aspect. The posterior descending artery originates from the right coronary indicating a dominant right coronary system. Ao, aorta; CFX, circumflex coronary artery; IVC, inferior vena cava; LAD, left anterior descending coronary artery; LCA, left coronary artery; PA, pulmonary artery; RCA, right coronary artery; SVC, superior vena cava.

course all along the left-sided atrioventricular groove. It usually has one or more branches (the circumflex marginal branches) that reach the obtuse margin of the heart, although these branches are not necessary for the pattern to be considered normal. A ramus intermedius branch, or left main diagonal, may be present and is so named because of its location and distribution, intermediate between the LAD and circumflex coronaries.

The RCA normally originates from the right coronary cusp and courses along the right atrioventricular groove. It reaches the acute margin of the heart in all normal cases and then proceeds along the posterior atrioventricular groove to give rise to one or more posterior descending coronary arteries. These posterior descending coronaries are again not necessary for the right coronary system to be considered normal. The term *coronary dominance* is defined by the number of posterior descending arteries and their vessel of origin, either left or right systems.[63,77] With respect to the more distal secondary branches of the major coronary systems, several patterns are consistently observed and are therefore considered to be normal. In 50% of cases, the sinus node artery arises from the left circumflex coronary artery. When it is not a branch of the left circumflex system, it originates from the RCA.

Anterior septal branches originate from the left anterior descending coronary artery. It is abnormal for these branches to arise from other extramural coronary vessels. The LAD does not give rise to large epicardial right ventricular branches. Extramural coronary arteries do not cross each other; therefore, it is considered abnormal for one branch to cross an adjacent branch.[51] The LAD appears to be a continuation of the left main coronary artery rather than a branch of it. The left conus artery is the first branch of the LAD and may anastomose with the conal branch of the RCA, forming the "circle of Vieussens."

As noted previously, right dominance indicates that the preponderance of posterior descending coronary arteries originate from the right coronary system. Ninety percent of individuals have this right-dominant coronary pattern. The artery to the atrioventricular node originates from the posterior descending coronary artery and travels cephalad to reach the atrioventricular node.

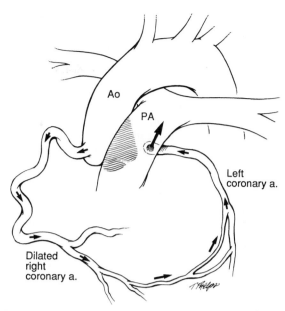

FIGURE 30-2 Schematic representation of a dilated, tortuous right coronary artery (a) associated with anomalous left coronary artery. Arrows indicate coronary "steal," with direction of blood flow from right coronary to left coronary, ultimately draining into the pulmonary artery (PA). Ao, aorta.

ANOMALOUS ORIGIN OF THE LEFT CORONARY ARTERY FROM THE PULMONARY ARTERY

Anomalous origin of the LCA from the pulmonary artery (ALCAPA) occurs in 1 of 300,000 children and constitutes an estimated 0.24% of all congenital cardiac defects.[34] ALCAPA is most commonly an isolated malformation; however, it has been associated with other congenital heart defects, including ventricular septal defect, endocardial cushion defect, tetralogy of Fallot, and truncus arteriosus.[18,54]

Native Anatomy

In anomalous origination of the LCA from the pulmonary artery, the entire left main coronary complex, or only the LAD or circumflex branch may originate from the proximal main pulmonary artery or, more rarely, from the left or right pulmonary arteries (Fig. 30-2). The branching patterns of the anomalously connected LCA remain normal. The RCA arises normally from the aorta and has a normal branching pattern. However, extensive well-developed collaterals from right to left coronary systems may be apparent. The most common site of origin of the anomalous artery was from the posterior main pulmonary artery, followed by a left posterior sinus, the left lateral pulmonary artery, the right posterior sinus, and finally, the right pulmonary artery.[6]

Pathophysiology

Anomalous origin of the LCA from the pulmonary artery was first described in 1886 by Brooks,[10] who postulated that flow in the anomalous coronary artery was retrograde. This report suggested that one of the coronary arteries was not only failing

to supply the myocardium, but was diverting fully oxygenated blood from the heart into the pulmonary artery. This hypothesis was further supported by Case and colleagues in 1958,[15] when they reported a postmortem observation that radiopaque dye injected into the ascending aorta passed out through the normal RCA and, by collaterals, filled the LCA in retrograde fashion.

The current understanding of the pathophysiology of ALCAPA emphasizes the changes in (1) pulmonary artery pressure, (2) intercoronary anastomoses between the right and left coronary systems, and (3) ischemic injury to the myocardium. In utero and in early neonatal life, the right ventricle performs the systemic workload by ejecting blood through the pulmonary artery, ductus arteriosus, and into the aorta. Hence, the perfusion pressure in the anomalous left coronary originating from the pulmonary artery is normal. The left ventricle receives adequate blood supply and functions normally. Later in the postnatal period, pulmonary arterial resistance decreases. This results in decreased pulmonary arterial pressures and, therefore, decreased perfusion of the left coronary system. At this time, perfusion in the left coronary distribution depends on the development of right to left coronary collateral blood flow through intercoronary anastomoses. Once ALCAPA pressure is less than RCA pressure, blood flows from the RCA through intercoronary anastomoses to the ALCAPA and drains into the pulmonary artery (retrograde flow). Because fully oxygenated arterial blood originating from the RCA now drains into the pulmonary artery, a left-to-right shunt is present, although the volume of shunted blood may be insufficient to produce a change in oxygen saturation from the right ventricle to the pulmonary artery.

The absence of antegrade flow in the ALCAPA leads to myocardial ischemia. Ischemia appears to be less severe in patients with a dominant right coronary system who develop extensive collateralization from the right to left coronary systems.[62] With progression of this syndrome in infancy, the left ventricle is generally hypertrophied and dilated. The ischemic injury affects both contraction and relaxation of the left ventricle, and asynchronous motion can be seen in both phases of the cardiac cycle.[14] Diffuse left ventricular fibrosis is present, and patients may have evidence of recent and old myocardial infarction, usually of the anterolateral distribution. The cardiac fibrosis is generally most marked in the subendocardial layer.[55] However, despite the aforementioned pathologic changes, there seems to be significant potential for recovery of myocardial function, as evidenced by cases of individuals with severe left ventricular dysfunction improving after establishment of a two-coronary circulation. This phenomenon is thought to be due to severely ischemic or hibernating myocardium.[42,79]

Mitral insufficiency also may be seen with this lesion. This occurs as the left ventricular myocardium suffers ischemic damage, resulting in changes in and around the mitral valve, including endocardial fibroelastosis, contraction of the chordae tendineae, and papillary muscle ischemia and infarction.[22] Congestive heart failure (CHF) worsens, as mitral insufficiency is superimposed on a hypokinetic, ischemic left ventricle.

Diagnostic Assessment

History and Physical Findings

Patients with ALCAPA may present early in infancy, usually within 1 to 2 weeks of birth, or the lesion may go undetected until adult life. The differences in clinical presentation are due in large part to differences and degrees of collateralization between the right and left coronary systems. Survival into late infancy and beyond also appears to be related to the degree of right coronary dominance.[76] Although the spectrum of presentation represents a continuum, the classic presentations may be conveniently divided into "infantile" and "adult" forms.

The classic description of infants presenting with ALCAPA as described by Bland and colleagues in 1933[8] aptly characterizes the clinical syndrome associated with this lesion. Patients presenting in infancy and early childhood may demonstrate signs and symptoms of severe ischemia or CHF, including tachypnea, pallor, poor feeding, and a history of paroxysms of crying, diaphoresis, severe agitation, and poor weight gain. Infants may exhibit a history of an initial ability to feed followed by sudden cessation of feeding associated with breathlessness, diaphoresis, arching of the back, and crying or screaming. These symptoms are presumed to be due to angina during feeding.[36] Physical examination in infants presenting with ALCAPA may demonstrate circumoral pallor and blueness. Signs and symptoms of CHF may dominate the clinical picture. An apical gallop rhythm and a murmur of mitral insufficiency often may be heard. A precordial lift is common and is associated with the marked cardiomegaly usually found with this lesion. There also may be hepatomegaly and pulmonary rales.[21]

The aforementioned clinical findings associated with ALCAPA may be difficult to distinguish from those of other causes of heart failure in infancy, including myocarditis and cardiomyopathy. In any infant presenting with heart failure,

however, the diagnosis of ALCAPA should be strongly considered. ALCAPA has presented as (near-miss) sudden infant death syndrome.[40] CHF in ALCAPA may lead to wheezing and an erroneous diagnosis of bronchiolitis.[23] Cardiac arrest has occurred during β-agonist administration or induction of anesthesia for bronchoscopy in ALCAPA patients thought to have primary lung disease.[23,65]

In older children and adults with ALCAPA, the clinical spectrum ranges from those who are completely asymptomatic to those with episodic angina and symptoms of CHF. The diagnosis of ALCAPA should be suspected in patients with unexplained cardiomegaly, mitral insufficiency, or continuous cardiac murmur. In particular, in adults there is usually a nonspecific systolic murmur. There may also be an apical pansystolic murmur from the mitral regurgitation. In some instances, mitral regurgitation may dominate the clinical picture, producing CHF.[12,25] The author has treated two adults with ALCA from the main pulmonary artery presenting at 26 and 35 years of life, respectively. In both patients, symptoms of severe mitral insufficiency dominated the clinical picture.

Patients surviving into adulthood usually do so due to extensive collateral circulation from the RCA. This apparently is adequate for the prevention of massive infarction. Although some of these patients remain entirely asymptomatic, many will complain of symptoms consistent with exertional angina. The heart in these patients usually demonstrates a large, thick-walled RCA with large branches evident over the epicardial heart and coursing toward the distal branches of the LCA. The proximal LCA is generally smaller than normal and quite thin walled. The heart size of these individuals is generally normal.

Diagnostic Tests

Electrocardiographic findings in infants who have suffered myocardial infarction resemble those of adults with atherosclerotic coronary artery disease. Most frequently, the infarcts are anterior and anteroseptal, which is related to the fact that it is this aspect of the left ventricle that is supplied exclusively by the LCA. ST elevation and Q wave formation may be present in anterolateral leads, as well as T wave inversions in leads I and AVL and in the left precordial leads (Fig. 30-3).[4] Despite being relatively asymptomatic, adults with ALCAPA may have strikingly abnormal electrocardiographs (ECGs) as well. In these individuals, severe ST segment changes or frank evidence of old anterolateral infarction may be present. ECGs obtained during exercise stress testing usually demonstrate an ischemic response.

Chest radiography will generally demonstrate severe cardiomegaly with or without evidence of interstitial pulmonary edema in infants affected with this syndrome. Adults with ALCAPA, however, may exhibit a normal cardiac silhouette or cardiomegaly, depending on the degree of myocardial damage.

Echocardiography has demonstrated increasing success in identifying anomalous coronary origins. Pulse Doppler echocardiography with color flow mapping may detect the ALCA from the pulmonary trunk, as well as the retrograde direction of flow into the ALCAPA in certain individuals, including small infants.[13,29,31,32] Transesophageal echocardiography may be more effective in identifying the anomalous origin of the

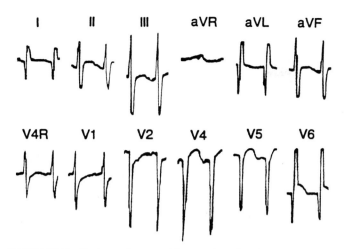

FIGURE 30-3 Electrocardiogram with anterolateral myocardial infarction pattern in a 2-month-old infant with anomalous origin of the left coronary artery. Note deep Q waves in I, aVL, and V6, as well as the QS pattern in V2 through V5. (From Park MK: *Pediatric Cardiology for Practitioners.* Chicago, Mosby–Year Book, 1988, p 280; with permission.)

LCA in adults.[24] Most commonly, the echocardiogram will demonstrate a dilated, poorly contracting ventricle. In addition, Doppler interrogation of the mitral valve may reveal prolapse and/or regurgitation. The papillary muscles also may demonstrate enhanced echogenicity due to fibrosis. Over the past 10 years, echocardiography has become the primary diagnostic modality for patients suspected of having ALCAPA. Characteristic findings include continuous flow in the proximal main pulmonary artery. In our experience, it has become quite unusual for the diagnosis to be missed on transthoracic echo.

For patients with uncertain diagnoses, *selective coronary cineangiography* remains the definitive study in the diagnosis of ALCAPA. Injection of contrast into the pulmonary artery usually does not demonstrate the ALCAPA because of the lack of antegrade flow into the LCA. Aortic root injection always demonstrates only the RCA arising from the aorta. In patients with large, well-developed collaterals, the RCA may be extremely dilated and tortuous. Contrast material can then be followed through the right coronary circulation via collaterals into the left coronary circulation and then, ultimately, into the pulmonary artery. Left ventriculography is performed to assess left ventricular systolic and diastolic function and to document the presence or absence of mitral regurgitation.[36]

Preoperative Critical Care Management

Medical management alone has not been demonstrated to improve outcome for patients with ALCAPA. Although the denominator cannot be known with certainty, it is believed that upwards of 65% of infants born with ALCAPA who do not undergo surgical correction die during the first year of life from protracted left ventricular dysfunction.[74] Only temporary improvement can be achieved in most cases demonstrating CHF. Hence, the goal of medical management is to stabilize the patient awaiting surgery. An aggressive approach should be taken, since ischemic injury in ALCAPA is (at least partially) reversible after surgery, and revascularization can be successfully accomplished in neonates and infants.[3,30,33]

The patient presenting to a critical care unit before surgery is usually an infant with CHF or cardiogenic shock.[6] While preparations for surgery are being made, the critical care management is focused on optimizing myocardial oxygen supply and minimizing myocardial oxygen demand.

For the infant with CHF and stable blood pressure, *diuretic administration* may be beneficial, as long as frank hypovolemia is avoided. Diuresis should decrease myocardial wall tension leading to an improvement in the myocardial oxygen supply-to-demand ratio. Furthermore, the reduction in pulmonary edema may lessen respiratory distress and improve oxygenation. *Supplemental oxygen* should be given as needed to prevent hypoxia. Although cardiac glycosides may be tried, they often do not lead to significant improvement in CHF secondary to myocardial ischemia. Some clinicians have recommended the avoidance of digoxin due to the potential for ventricular dysrhythmias.[72] *Sedation and analgesia* to reduce anginal pain are useful to prevent tachycardia, which increases myocardial oxygen demand and decreases oxygen supply. Patients are at increased risk for life-threatening arrhythmias, including ventricular and supraventricular tachyarrhythmias and sinus or junctional bradycardia. Antiarrhythmic drugs and a defibrillator should be readily available.

Infants with severe CHF and an unstable blood pressure form the highest risk category. Vouhe and colleagues[75] noted 31% perioperative mortality in patients with a left ventricular shortening fraction less than 0.2, whereas there were no deaths when the shortening fraction was greater than 0.2. These infants will invariably require intubation and controlled ventilation. A modest increase in mean airway pressure during positive-pressure ventilation may decrease left ventricular afterload; however, careful monitoring is indicated to prevent excessive rise in mean airway pressure and a reduction in venous return to the heart (see Chapter 9, Pericardial Disease, and Chapter 11, Applied Respiratory Physiology). Vasoactive drugs are needed to support systemic blood pressure, although none of the currently available agents are ideal. Dobutamine and milrinone have the advantage of providing inotropic support without significant tachycardia; however, milrinone in particular may produce vasodilatation. If the diastolic blood pressure is inadequate to maintain coronary perfusion pressure, there may be a role for short-term use of a pure alpha-adrenergic agonist such a phenylephrine, which avoids increased myocardial oxygen demand secondary to tachycardia or increased contractility. The goal of phenylephrine titration is to raise diastolic blood pressure cautiously without producing excessive afterload to the heart. All of these measures are temporary until emergency surgery or extracorporeal membrane oxygenation followed by surgery can be achieved.

Surgical Management

Historical Overview

Attempts at surgical correction were initiated in 1953 when Potts created an aortopulmonary anastomosis in two patients with this anomaly in an attempt to increase the oxygen saturation in the main pulmonary artery.[37] In 1953, Mustard[50] reported an attempted end-to-end anastomosis of the left carotid artery to the ALCAPA. The first successful surgical management of this condition was described in 1960 by

Sabiston and associates from the Johns Hopkins Hospital.[58–60] Their treatment for the ALCAPA was ligation of the anomalous origin. Not only did this result in successful treatment of the patient with resolution of the symptoms, but they were also successful in documenting the right-to-left coronary steal phenomenon by demonstrating an increased LCA pressure after ligation of the anomalous origin.

Later attempts at surgical correction of ALCAPA focused on establishment of a two coronary system. Cooley and associates[17] in 1966 reported revascularization of the ALCAPA with reversed autogenous saphenous vein grafting. In 1968, Meyer and colleagues[46] successfully anastomosed the left subclavian artery to the divided anomalous LCA. More recent techniques of revascularization of the ALCAPA include direct aortic implantation, creation of a coronary tunnel inside the pulmonary artery, and orthotopic cardiac transplantation. These options are discussed in more detail under "Surgical Management."

At one time, it was believed that surgery should be deferred if possible until the age of 1 year because of technical considerations. Successful revascularization in neonates and infants has demonstrated this approach to be unwarranted.[73] Furthermore, postponing surgery until after the age of 1 year exposes these infants to the risk of sudden death at home.[33] Hence, surgical intervention should be carried out as soon as is practical after symptoms have developed and the diagnosis has been made.

Ligation of Anomalous Left Coronary Artery from the Pulmonary Artery

Surgical intervention for ALCAPA has undergone significant evolution since the first successful operative procedure performed by Sabiston in 1959.[58–60] Whereas ligation of the origin of the anomalous left coronary is a technically easy undertaking and therefore a relatively attractive option, a series demonstrated higher mortality rates in patients undergoing this procedure than in those treated by the establishment of a two-coronary system.[6] In addition, it should be noted that while ligation of the anomalous coronary is straightforward, especially when approached via a left thoracotomy (Fig. 30-4), it may be difficult to manage these cases in the event of sudden ventricular fibrillation. Great care must be exercised in manipulating the heart, especially in circumstances where hemodynamic support via cardiopulmonary bypass is not readily available. These patients often have a substrate of enhanced ventricular irritability due to severe ongoing left ventricular ischemia. However, even patients with severe left ventricular dysfunction often show marked improvement after establishment of antegrade LCA perfusion.

Reported mortality rates after ligation of the ALCAPA range from 20% to 50%. Of particular concern is the reported 25% occurrence of late sudden death.[11,47,76] Patients who have undergone previous ALCAPA ligation should undergo follow-up periodically with holter monitoring and stress studies. Consideration should be given to elective coronary revascularization in patients who have survived previous ligation. Modern series of surgical treatment of patients with ALCAPA have clearly documented a survival advantage for those with a surgically created two-coronary system. Ligation of

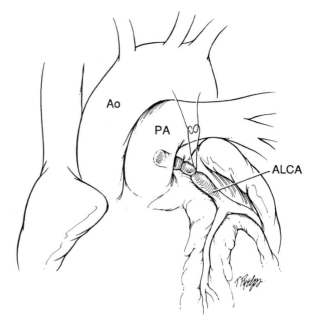

FIGURE 30-4   Ligation of anomalous left coronary artery (ALCA). Ao, aorta; PA, pulmonary artery.

the ALCAPA should be avoided, even in patients with very low ejection fractions.

Left Coronary Artery Transfer

It may be possible to use the operation of coronary artery transfer in many instances of ALCAPA. A sizeable button of pulmonary arterial wall around the coronary ostium of the anomalous left system may be excised and implanted into the aorta (Fig. 30-5). This procedure can be applied regardless of the patient's age or size of the ALCAPA and offers a high rate of patency. When the ALCAPA originates from the right posterior pulmonary sinus or right pulmonary artery, the operation is technically feasible without major mobilization of a left coronary system. Origin of the ALCAPA from the left posterior sinus or left lateral position may make implantation more difficult due to the necessity of significant mobilization of the coronary system and because of the possibility of kinking or torsion of the coronary stem during implantation.[20,27]

The attractive aspect of direct implantation of the ALCAPA into the aorta is that it provides direct aorta-to-coronary perfusion without the necessity of an interposed conduit. This technique can be approached by making a transverse incision into the main pulmonary trunk and demonstrating the LCA ostium from within the pulmonary artery. If the ostium seems to originate from the posterior or right-sided aspect of the pulmonary trunk, the ostium may be excised as button, or the incision may be extended until the pulmonary trunk is completely transected. The button may then be excised and implanted directly onto the aortic wall and then the pulmonary artery reconstructed via primary anastomosis.[26,52] Mortality rates for this procedure have been reported to vary from 0% to 23%.[39,56,74] Long-term patency rates in various series have been excellent.[6,8]

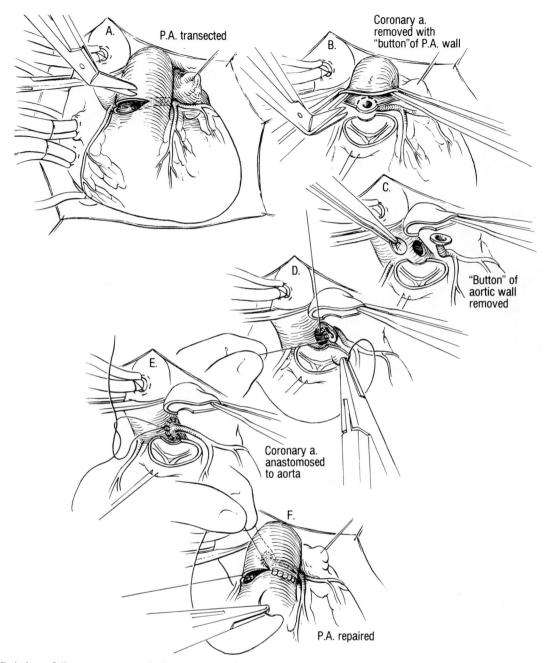

FIGURE 30-5 Technique of direct coronary transfer for anomalous left coronary artery (a.). **A,** Transection of pulmonary artery (PA). **B,** Removal of coronary artery ostial button. **C,** Preparation of aorta. **D,** Coronary anastomosis. **E,** Completion of coronary anastomosis. **F,** Repair of the main PA. (From Hallman GL, Cooley DA, Gutsesell HP: *Surgical Treatment of Congenital Heart Disease,* Philadelphia, Lea & Febiger, 1927; with permission.)

Over the past decade, increasing experience with the arterial switch operation has benefited patients with ALCAPA. As surgeons have become very familiar with coronary ostial transfer, direct aortic implantation has become the procedure of choice for the majority of patients with ALCAPA. Since 1995, the author has treated 13 patients with ALCAPA. In 11 of these patients, direct aortic transfer was possible, with two patients requiring a Takeuchi tunnel (see later). The technique of ostial transfer requires mobilization of the ostium as a generous button of pulmonary artery wall. The anomalous coronary is then mobilized liberally with electrocautery. Next, an appropriate opening is made on the ascending aorta.

Appropriate location for transfer is of critical importance. Determining the site may be facilitated by distending the aorta with cardioplegia. The author favors a "trap-door" type of incision in the aorta, as this functionally extends the ostium and minimizes coronary torsion. The location of the aortic valve pillars should be carefully noted, as aortic valve injury may occur with improper location of the aortotomy. After coronary transfer, the defect in the pulmonary sinus of Valsalva should be reconstructed with a liberal patch of autologous pericardium. This is a critical step to prevent excessive tension in the implanted coronary by the main pulmonary artery.

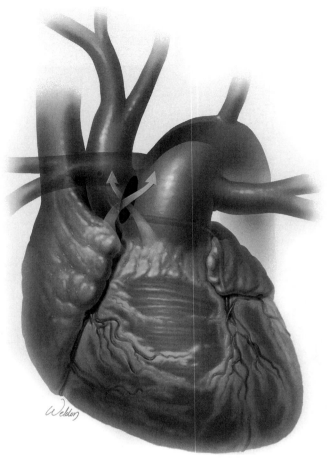

FIGURE 30-6 Interrupted aortic arch with aortopulmonary window type III and anomalous origin of the left coronary artery from the right pulmonary artery. (From McMahon CJ, DiBardino DJ, Undar A, Fraser CD Jr: Anomalous origin of left coronary artery from the right pulmonary artery in association with type III aortopulmonary window and interrupted aortic arch. *Ann Thorac Surg* 74:919–921, 2002; with permission.)

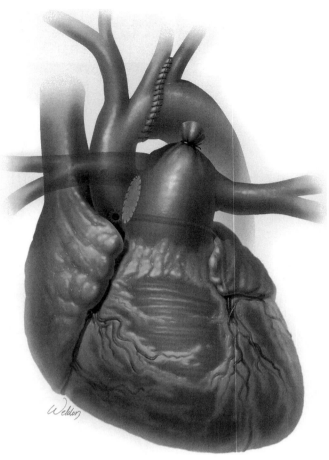

FIGURE 30-7 Completed result after repair of interrupted aortic arch with aortopulmonary window type III and anomalous origin of the left coronary artery. The right pulmonary artery to the main pulmonary artery reanastomosis was not included to avoid further complexity to this figure.[45] (From McMahon CJ, DiBardino DJ, Undar A, Fraser CD Jr: Anomalous origin of left coronary artery from the right pulmonary artery in association with type III aortopulmonary window and interrupted aortic arch. *Ann Thorac Surg* 74:919–921, 2002; with permission.)

We have recently treated a neonate with the unusual constellation of ALCAPA from the right pulmonary artery, Type I aortopulmonary window, and type B interrupted aortic arch. A complete repair was performed, which included direct coronary ostial transfer (Figs. 30-6 and 30-7).[45]

Transpulmonary Tunnel (Takeuchi Repair)

There are some patients in whom it is not technically feasible to directly implant the anomalous coronary button onto the aortic wall. Generally, these cases occur in situations where the anomalous orifice is on the lateral aspect of the main pulmonary artery. In these situations, an intrapulmonary aortocoronary fistula may be created using the method first described by Takeuchi (Fig. 30-8).[68] As with direct implantation of the anomalous coronary, this operation requires cardiopulmonary bypass and elective cardiac arrest. In performing this operation, great care must be taken not to manipulate the heart during the preliminary dissection and cannulation, as even the slightest disturbance of the left ventricle can induce ventricular fibrillation that may prove refractory. It is noteworthy that after the induction of cardiopulmonary bypass in

these patients, the left and right pulmonary arteries should be occluded either by atraumatic vascular clamps or tourniquets to prevent the coronary steal phenomenon, which occurs in the decompressed pulmonary trunk. After the heart is arrested, the main pulmonary artery is incised transversely just distal to the pulmonary valve, and the anomalous orifice is identified. A transverse aortotomy is then made, and a button of aortic wall is excised on the left lateral aspect of the aortic wall at a point in continuity with the pulmonary arterial trunk. Next, an aortopulmonary window is created. Using a flap of either pulmonary arterial wall or pericardium, the tunnel is created, thus diverting blood via the aortopulmonary window into the anomalous coronary orifice. The pulmonary artery is then reconstructed with the pericardial patch.

Preliminary results with the Takeuchi procedure have been encouraging. When appropriately applied, high patency rates can be expected. Several series report minimal operative complications and low mortality rates. Late complications have included moderate aortic regurgitation, supravalvar pulmonary stenosis, and baffle obstruction.[6,11] Autologous tissue should be used in constructing the Takeuchi tunnel.

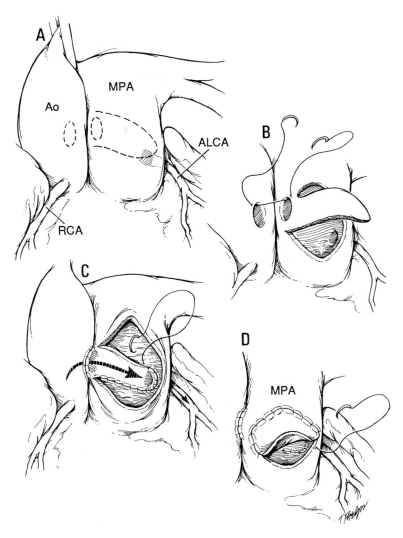

FIGURE 30-8 Technique of intrapulmonary aortocoronary tunnel (Takeuchi repair). **A,** Initial incisions (*dotted lines*) in aorta (Ao) and main pulmonary artery (MPA) in preparation for tunnel to anomalous left coronary artery (ALCA). **B,** Anastomosis of Ao to MPA, creation of flap within MPA. **C,** MPA flap becomes anterior wall of tunnel between the aorta and the ALCA. **D,** Closure of MPA defect with pericardium. RCA, right coronary artery.

This preserves growth potential and minimizes the potential for baffle leak. The author has treated two patients who had significant late baffle leaks after the tunnel had been constructed with a polytetrafluoroethylene tube. Both patients required reoperation.

Bypass Grafting

As noted previously, the first successful creation of a two-coronary system in a patient with ALCAPA was performed by Cooley and associates in 1966[17] using reversed autogenous saphenous vein. Although this technique is technically straightforward, considerable concern exists over the potential for late fibrous changes followed by graft occlusion of the saphenous vein conduits. This is particularly true in infants and small children who must rely on the vein conduit for a lifetime of coronary blood flow. Because of this problem, other procedures have been developed to utilize arterial conduits to revascularize the ALCAPA.

One potential option is the use of divided left subclavian artery (Fig. 30-9). This may be performed either via median sternotomy or left posterolateral thoracotomy, and the divided end of the left subclavian is turned down and anastomosed either end-to-end to the divided ALCAPA or end-to-side to ligated ALCAPA. This may be done either with the heart beating or on cardiopulmonary bypass with cardioplegic arrest. Potential advantages of this approach include the fact that it can be performed in young patients and allows growth of the individuals, and that the arterial conduit has better long-term patency characteristics than saphenous vein conduits. However, technical difficulties may arise due to the fact that in some patients, the anastomosis may not be created without excessive tension on the divided left subclavian artery. In addition, the acute angle resulting from the turning down of the left subclavian can often result in kinking and stenosis of the proximal left subclavian artery. Of course, there are other concerns regarding upper-extremity perfusion, particularly in older children.[35]

Another possible option for an arterial conduit in the creation of a two-vessel coronary system involves the use of the left internal mammary artery as a pedicle of free graft. Although the internal mammary artery may be quite small in infants and young children, it is still technically possible to anastomose this vessel in an end-to-side fashion to the ALCA and thus provide long-term arterial perfusion of the left coronary system.

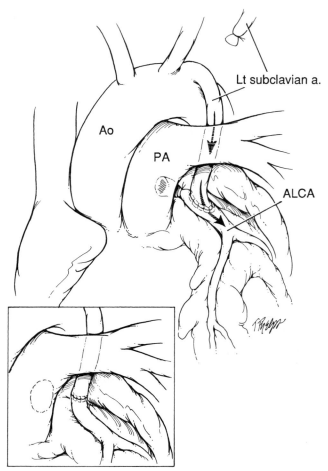

FIGURE 30-9 End-to-side anastomosis of left (Lt) subclavian artery (a.) to the anomalous left coronary artery (ALCA). Inset, Alternatively, the ALCA can be excised from the pulmonary artery (PA) and anastomosed end-to-end to the subclavian artery. Ao, aorta.

Reported mortality rates for the various bypass grafting procedures vary significantly. Reported mortality rates for saphenous vein bypass grafting to the ALCAPA range from 0% to 38%.[16,39,78] Disturbing reports of late conduit fibrosis and occlusion make this choice less desirable, particularly in the younger age group.[1] In any case, ligation of the proximal ALCAPA is an important element of any bypass technique.

Reported mortality rates for left subclavian artery–ALCAPA anastomoses range from 0% to 29%, with graft patency rates ranging from 60% to 80%.[48,67,80] As noted previously, there is significant potential for technical mishap in creation of the left subclavian–to-ALCAPA anastomosis due to kinking of the subclavian artery at the aorta. It also may be technically difficult to perform the subclavian coronary anastomosis on the beating heart, and there is particular risk of inducing ventricular fibrillation in the severely ischemic left ventricle.

Cardiac Transplantation

As noted earlier, many infants presenting with ALCAPA have severely dysfunctional left ventricles and are in profound cardiogenic shock. Fortunately, the majority of these patients may be expected to recover after establishment of antegrade coronary flow, although it may be difficult to predict which ventricle will recover. For the moribund patient with severe impairment of cardiac function, cardiac allograft replacement of the failing heart remains an option. Several series have reported success with this approach to the patient with a failing ventricle due to ALCAPA. In general, however, this procedure should have minimal applications in this lesion due to the significant potential for ventricular recovery and long-term survival.[44,66]

Over the past 18 years, 24 patients have been operated on at the author's institution for ALCAPA. The mean age and weight at operation were 6.8 months (range, 1 to 29 months) and 9.6 kg. Twenty-two of 24 patients underwent direct coronary transfer, with the other two patients undergoing a Takeuchi tunnel. There were two intraoperative deaths, both occurring prior to 1995. There have been no operation deaths since 1995, despite the fact that several patients presented with severe CHF and very depressed ejection fractions (5 of 12 patients with ejection fractions less than 25% since 1995). No patient has required extracorporeal membrane oxygenation or left ventricular assist device support. No patient has required cardiac transplantation.

Postoperative Critical Care Management

Postoperative care is organized as with any other postcardiotomy patient. It must be noted, however, that many individuals have severe impairment of left ventricular function preoperatively and therefore can be expected to need some form of hemodynamic support postoperatively. Progressive improvement in both systolic and diastolic myocardial function, including resolution of mitral insufficiency, can be expected if patients can be supported successfully during the perioperative period.[14] If inotropic drugs are insufficient to maintain adequate hemodynamics, mechanical support devices including extracorporeal membrane oxygenation or left ventricular assist device via a centrifugal pump should be considered in infants.[74] However, the authors have rarely found this to be necessary. Intraaortic balloon counterpulsation may be attempted in older children and adults. Such patients should be considered for cardiac transplantation if they do not exhibit improvement in ventricular function. All patients receive serial ECG and echocardiography. The adequacy of coronary blood flow is assessed using pulsed Doppler and color flow mapping during echocardiography. Serial ECGs reveal gradual resolution of ischemic changes at rest, although T-wave inversion in AVL may persist.[64] Ischemic changes on ECG may become evident during exercise.[53]

ANOMALOUS ORIGIN OF THE RIGHT CORONARY ARTERY FROM THE PULMONARY TRUNK

Anomalous origin of the RCA from the pulmonary artery is a rare anomaly, and its clinical significance is unclear. The anomalous right coronary usually arises from the right pulmonary artery, but it may also originate from the main pulmonary trunk.[9,41] Patients with this lesion are usually entirely asymptomatic, and the anomalous vessel is discovered incidentally at the time of autopsy or during cardiac catheterization for some other reason. There have been some reports, however, that occasionally, this lesion may be associated with sudden death in older children and adults.[41]

Patients with this condition may exhibit a continuous murmur on physical examination. There are usually no associated ECG changes. The anomalous RCA usually courses along the right atrioventricular groove in an otherwise normal location. In this arrangement, coronary blood flow is from an enlarged left coronary system via collaterals into the right coronary circulation. This lesion is usually not associated with myocardial infarction due to the lower intracavitary right ventricular pressure.[2] Surgical correction in these individuals is recommended due to the associated possibility of sudden death.[9] Direct aortic implantation is generally the most technically feasible operation, although coronary artery bypass is another acceptable option.[71]

ANOMALOUS ORIGIN OF A MAIN CORONARY ARTERY FROM THE AORTA

Another condition of anomalous coronary artery origination that may result in significant clinical consequence occurs when either the right or left main coronary artery arises from locations on the aorta other than the appropriate corresponding sinus. It was formerly believed that this situation was only clinically relevant in cases in which the anomalous vessels coursed between the aorta and pulmonary artery.[38] An excellent review by Taylor and colleagues[69] from the Armed Forces Institute of Pathology of the clinicopathologic records of 242 patients with coronary anomalies indicates that other factors of anomalous coronary origin and course result in significant consequences as well. In this study, cardiac death occurred in 59% of patients. Of the 242 patients, 32% experienced sudden cardiac death, and in 45% of this group, death was associated with exercise. In the series, the most common anomaly was origin of the left main from the right coronary sinus or as the first branch of the RCA. The course of the left main was most frequently between the aorta and pulmonary artery, but other conditions included anterior to the pulmonary trunk, posterior to the aorta, posterior to the right ventricular outflow tract, and within the ventricular septum. Anomalous origin of the RCA from the left coronary sinus was the next most frequently observed anomaly. Sudden death occurred most frequently in situations in which the main coronary artery coursed between the aorta and pulmonary artery. Other lesions, however, were also associated with cardiac death, including acute angle takeoff of a single coronary trunk with a valve-like ridge, concomitant coronary atherosclerosis, and intramural and oblique coronary origins.

There are several hypothetical mechanisms responsible for myocardial ischemia and death in patients with coronaries of anomalous aortic origin. As noted previously, the most frequent situation associated with death occurs when the coronary courses between the aorta and pulmonary artery. The presumed mechanism here is intermittent compression of the coronary, especially during exercise. Another possible pathophysiologic mechanism occurs in the arrangement of an acute-angle ostial takeoff of a single coronary artery with a valve-like ridge. In this arrangement, the ostial orifice may be slit-like and become progressively compressed by aortic pulsation, ultimately resulting in coronary insufficiency.

Although most patients with anomalous aortic origin are asymptomatic, some will report symptoms consistent with intermittent or ongoing myocardial ischemia. These symptoms may include angina (particularly exertional), CHF, syncope, and even myocardial infarction.[69] Sudden death from this group of lesions is most frequent in patients younger than 30 years, and anomalous coronary origin should certainly be considered in the differential diagnosis of a young patient presenting with syncope or with complaints consistent with myocardial ischemia.[43,69]

As with other forms of anomalous coronary origin, cineangiography remains the definitive diagnostic modality.[73] In some individuals, however, high-resolution echocardiography, particularly transesophageal, may demonstrate the anomalous vessel.[70] With improving technology and in the hands of an experienced and skilled sonographer, the anatomy of this lesion can be nicely delineated by transthoracic echocardiography.[57]

Management of patients with anomalous aortic origin of a main coronary is somewhat controversial. Most would agree, however, that patients with evidence of intermittent or ongoing myocardial ischemia should undergo surgery.[2,70] The management of individuals without evidence of ischemia is less straightforward, but in general, most believe that patients with an anomalous vessel that courses between the aorta and pulmonary artery should undergo surgery.[36] It may be argued that all patients with major coronary anomalies need some form of revascularization. At the least, patients should be intensively studied for evidence of ischemia, including exercise stress testing. The threshold for surgical intervention should be especially low in those patients with symptoms that can be attributed to coronary insufficiency.

The operative approach to individuals with this problem must be catered to the anatomy and may involve some form of coronary artery bypass conduit. Because many of these patients are quite young, the liberal use of internal mammary artery grafts is preferable.[49] An alternative option in cases in which the anomalous left main courses between the aorta and pulmonary artery is to open the intramural portion of the left main vessel from within the aorta. By unroofing the left main coronary artery, a neo-ostium can be constructed in the left sinus of Valsalva in a normal and unobstructed location.[50,59] A complication of intramural repair is the advent of early or late aortic insufficiency, and great care must be exercised during the procedure to protect the aortic valve commisure (which often must be detached to perform the intramural unroofing) from distortion.

Postoperative Critical Care Management

Management for patients with anomalous origin of a main coronary artery from the aorta is usually less involved than for those patients presenting with severe myocardial ischemia from ALCAPA. Most of these patients are older than those with ALCAPA due to the more insidious presentation of this lesion. Postoperative management should include careful attentiveness to any significant ECG changes with a decision to perform coronary angiography if there is evidence of ongoing myocardial ischemia. In the case of an unroofing procedure, persistent myocardial ischemia could be an indication for adding a bypass graft to the affected area of myocardium. It is debatable whether there is a role for the use of serum troponin levels in the postoperative management of these patients.

References

1. Anthony CL Jr, McAllister HA Jr, Cheitlin MD: Spontaneous graft closure in anomalous origin of the left coronary artery. *Chest* 68:586–588, 1975.
2. Arciniegas E: *Pediatric Cardiac Surgery*. Chicago, Mosby–Year Book, 1985, p 51.
3. Arciniegas E, Farooki ZQ, Hakimi M, Green EW: Management of anomalous left coronary artery from the pulmonary artery. *Circulation* 62:I180–I189, 1980.
4. Askenazi J, Nadas AS: Anomalous left coronary artery originating from the pulmonary artery. Report on 15 cases. *Circulation* 51:976–987, 1975.
5. Austen WG, Edwards JE, Frye RL, et al: A reporting system on patients evaluated for coronary artery disease. Report of the Ad Hoc Committee for Grading of Coronary Artery Disease, Council on Cardiovascular Surgery, American Heart Association. *Circulation* 51(suppl):5–I40, 1975.
6. Backer CL, Stout MJ, Zales VR, et al: Anomalous origin of the left coronary artery. A twenty-year review of surgical management. *J Thorac Cardiovasc Surg* 103:1049–1057, 1992.
7. Blake H, Marion W, Mattingly T, Baroldi G: Coronary artery anomalies. *Circulation* 30:927, 1964.
8. Bland ER, White PD, Garland J: Congenital anomalies of the coronary arteries: Report of an unusual case associated with cardiac hypertrophy. *Am Heart J* 8:787, 1933.
9. Bregman D, Brennan FJ, Singer A, et al: Anomalous origin of the right coronary artery from the pulmonary artery. *J Thorac Cardiovasc Surg* 72:626–630, 1976.
10. Brooks H: Two cases of an abnormal coronary artery arising from the pulmonary artery, with some remarks upon the effect of this anomaly in producing cirsoid dilation of the vessels. *J Anat Physiol* 20:26, 1886.
11. Bunton R, Jonas RA, Lang P, et al: Anomalous origin of left coronary artery from pulmonary artery. Ligation versus establishment of a two coronary artery system. *J Thorac Cardiovasc Surg* 93:103–108, 1987.
12. Burchell HB, Brown AL: Anomalous origin of the coronary artery from pulmonary artery masquerading as mitral insufficiency. *Am Heart J* 63:388, 1962.
13. Caldwell RL, Hurwitz RA, Girod DA, et al: Two-dimensional echocardiographic differentiation of anomalous left coronary artery from congestive cardiomyopathy. *Am Heart J* 106:710–716, 1983.
14. Carvalho JS, Redington AN, Oldershaw PJ, et al: Analysis of left ventricular wall movement before and after reimplantation of anomalous left coronary artery in infancy. *Br Heart J* 65:218–222, 1991.
15. Case RB, Morrow AG, Stainsby W, Nestor JO: Anomalous origin of the left coronary artery: The physiologic defect and suggested surgical treatment. *Circulation* 17:1062, 1958.
16. Chiariello L, Meyer J, Reul GJ Jr, et al: Surgical treatment for anomalous origin of left coronary artery from pulmonary artery. *Ann Thorac Surg* 19:443–450, 1975.
17. Cooley DA, Hallman GL, Bloodwell RD: Definitive surgical treatment of anomalous origin of left coronary artery from pulmonary artery: Indications and results. *J Thorac Cardiovasc Surg* 52:798–808, 1966.
18. Dakalopolous D: Fatal pulmonary artery banding in truncus arteriosus with anomalous origin of circumflex coronary artery from right pulmonary artery. *Am J Cardiol* 52:1363, 1933.
19. Dicicco BS, McManus BM, Waller BF, Roberts WC: Separate aortic ostium of the left anterior descending and left circumflex coronary arteries from the left aortic sinus of Valsalva (absent left main coronary artery). *Am Heart J* 104:153–154, 1982.
20. Doty DB, Chandramouli B, Schieken RE, et al: Anomalous origin of the left coronary artery from the right pulmonary artery. *J Thorac Cardiovasc Surg* 71:787–791, 1976.
21. Driscoll DJ: Congenital coronary artery anomalies. In Garson A, Bricker TJ, McNamara DG (eds): *The Science and Practice of Pediatric Cardiology*. Philadelphia, Lea and Febiger, 1990, pp 1453–1461.
22. Foster HR, Hagstrom JWC, Ehlers KH, Engle MA: Mitral insufficiency due to anomalous origin of the left coronary artery from the pulmonary artery. *Pediatrics* 34:649, 1964.
23. Franklin WH, Dietrich AM, Hickey RW, Brookens MA: Anomalous left coronary artery masquerading as infantile bronchiolitis. *Pediatr Emerg Care* 8:338–341, 1992.
24. Gaither NS, Rogan KM, Stajduhar K, et al: Anomalous origin and course of coronary arteries in adults: Identification and improved imaging utilizing transesophageal echocardiography. *Am Heart J* 122:69–75, 1991.
25. George JM, Knowlan DM: Anomalous origin of the left coronary artery from the pulmonary artery in an adult. *N Engl J Med* 261:993, 1959.
26. Grace RR, Angelini P, Cooley DA: Aortic implantation of anomalous left coronary artery arising from pulmonary artery. *Am J Cardiol* 39:609–613, 1977.
27. Hamilton JR, Mulholland HC, O'Kane HO: Origin of the left coronary artery from the right pulmonary artery: A report of successful surgery in a 3-month-old child. *Ann Thorac Surg* 41:446–448, 1986.
28. Heifetz SA, Robinowitz M, Mueller KH, Virmani R: Total anomalous origin of the coronary arteries from the pulmonary artery. *Pediatr Cardiol* 7:11–18, 1986.
29. Henson KD, Geiser EA, Billett J, et al: Use of transesophageal echocardiography to visualize an anomalous right coronary artery arising from the left main coronary artery (single coronary artery). *Clin Cardiol* 15:462–465, 1992.
30. Househam KC, Human DG, Fraser CB, Joffe HS: Anomalous left coronary artery from the pulmonary artery—a therapeutic dilemma. *S Afr Med J* 63:325–327, 1983.
31. Houston AB, Pollock JC, Doig WB, et al: Anomalous origin of the left coronary artery from the pulmonary trunk: Elucidation with colour Doppler flow mapping. *Br Heart J* 63:50–54, 1990.
32. Jureidini SB, Nouri S, Crawford CJ, et al: Reliability of echocardiography in the diagnosis of anomalous origin of the left coronary artery from the pulmonary trunk. *Am Heart J* 122:61–68, 1991.
33. Kakou Guikahue M, Sidi D, Kachaner J, et al: Anomalous left coronary artery arising from the pulmonary artery in infancy: Is early operation better? *Br Heart J* 60:522–526, 1988.
34. Keith JD, Rowe RD, Vlad P: *Heart Disease in Infancy and Childhood*. New York, Macmillan Company, 1978.
35. Kesler KA, Pennington DG, Nouri S, et al: Left subclavian-left coronary artery anastomosis for anomalous origin of the left coronary artery. Long-term follow-up. *J Thorac Cardiovasc Surg* 98:25–29, 1989.
36. Kirklin JW, Barratt-Boyes BG: Congenital anaomalies of the coronary arteries. In Kirklin JW, Barret-Boyes BG (eds): *Cardiac Surgery*. New York, Churchill Livingstone, 1993, p 1179.
37. Kittle CF, Diehl AM, Heilbrunn A: Anomalous left coronary arising from the pulmonary artery: Report of a case and surgical consideration. *J Pediatr* 47:198, 1955.
38. Kragel AH, Roberts WC: Anomalous origin of either the right or left main coronary artery from the aorta with subsequent coursing between aorta and pulmonary trunk: Analysis of 32 necropsy cases. *Am J Cardiol* 62:771–777, 1988.
39. Laborde F, Marchand M, Leca F, et al: Surgical treatment of anomalous origin of the left coronary artery in infancy and childhood. Early and late results in 20 consecutive cases. *J Thorac Cardiovasc Surg* 82:423–428, 1981.
40. Lalu K, Karhunen PJ, Rautiainen P: Sudden and unexpected death of a 6-month-old baby with silent heart failure due to anomalous origin of the left coronary artery from the pulmonary artery. *Am J Forensic Med Pathol* 13:196–198, 1992.
41. Lerberg DB, Ogden JA, Zuberbuhler JR, Bahnson HT: Anomalous origin of the right coronary artery from the pulmonary artery. *Ann Thorac Surg* 27:87–94, 1979.
42. Levitsky S, van der Horst RL, Hastreiter AR, Fisher EA: Anomalous left coronary artery in the infant: Recovery of ventricular function following early direct aortic implantation. *J Thorac Cardiovasc Surg* 79:598–602, 1980.
43. Lipsett J, Byard RW, Carpenter BF, et al: Anomalous coronary arteries arising from the aorta associated with sudden death in infancy and early childhood. An autopsy series. *Arch Pathol Lab Med* 115:770–773, 1991.
44. Mavroudis C, Harrison H, Klein JB, et al: Infant orthotopic cardiac transplantation. *J Thorac Cardiovasc Surg* 96:912–924, 1988.
45. McMahon CJ, DiBardino DJ, Undar A, Fraser CD Jr: Anomalous origin of left coronary artery from the right pulmonary artery in association with type III aortopulmonary window and interrupted aortic arch. *Ann Thorac Surg* 74:919–921, 2002.
46. Meyer BW, Stefanik G, Stiles QR, et al: A method of definitive surgical treatment of anomalous origin of left coronary artery. A case report. *J Thorac Cardiovasc Surg* 56:104–107, 1968.
47. Montigny M, Stanley P, Chartrand C, et al: Postoperative evaluation after end-to-end subclavian-left coronary artery anastomosis in anomalous left coronary artery. *J Thorac Cardiovasc Surg* 100:270–273, 1990.

48. Moodie DS, Gill C, Loop FD, Sheldon WC: Anomalous left main coronary artery originating from the right sinus of Valsalva: Pathophysiology, angiographic definition, and surgical approaches. *J Thorac Cardiovasc Surg* 80:198–205, 1980.

49. Mustafa I, Gula G, Radley-Smith R, et al: Anomalous origin of the left coronary artery from the anterior aortic sinus: A potential cause of sudden death. Anatomic characterization and surgical treatment. *J Thorac Cardiovasc Surg* 82:297–300, 1981.

50. Mustard WT: Anomalies of the coronary arteries. In *Pediatric Surgery*, vol. I. Chicago, Mosby–Year Book, 1953, p 433.

51. Muyldermans LL, Van den Heuvel PA, Ernst SM: Epicardial crossing of coronary arteries: A variation of coronary arterial anatomy. *Int J Cardiol* 7:416–419, 1985.

52. Neirotti R, Nijveld A, Ithuralde M, et al: Anomalous origin of the left coronary artery from the pulmonary artery: Repair by aortic reimplantation. *Eur J Cardiothorac Surg* 5:368–371, 1991.

53. Paridon SM, Farooki ZQ, Kuhns LR, et al: Exercise performance after repair of anomalous origin of the left coronary artery from the pulmonary artery. *Circulation* 81:1287–1292, 1990.

54. Rao BN, Lucas RV Jr, Edwards JE: Anomalous origin of the left coronary artery from the right pulmonary artery associated with ventricular septal defect. *Chest* 58:616–620, 1970.

55. Rein AJ, Colan SD, Parness IA, Sanders SP: Regional and global left ventricular function in infants with anomalous origin of the left coronary artery from the pulmonary trunk: Preoperative and postoperative assessment. *Circulation* 75:115–123, 1987.

56. Richardson JV, Doty DB: Correction of anomalous origin of the left coronary artery. *J Thorac Cardiovasc Surg* 77:699–703, 1979.

57. Romp RL, Herlong RJ, Landolfo CK, et al: Outcome of unroofing procedure for repair of anomalous aortic origin of left or right coronary artery. *Ann Thoracic Surg* 76:589–596, 2003.

58. Sabiston DC, Neill CA, Taussig HB: The direction of blood flow in anomalous left coronary artery arising from the pulmonary artery. *Circulation* 22:591, 1960.

59. Sabiston DC, Pelagonio S, Taussig HB: Myocardial infarction in infancy: The surgical management of a complication of congenital origin of the left coronary artery from the pulmonary artery. *J Thorac Cardiovasc Surg* 40:321, 1960.

60. Sabiston DC, Ross RS, Criley JM, et al.: Surgical management of congenital lesions of the coronary circulation. *Ann Surg* 157:908, 1963.

61. Saji T, Yamamoto K, Hashiguchi R, et al: Hypoplastic left coronary artery. In association with occlusive intimal thickening of a coronary artery with ectopic ostium and with atresia of the left coronary ostium. *Jpn Heart J* 26:603–612, 1985.

62. Sauer U, Stern H, Meisner H, et al: Risk factors for perioperative mortality in children with anomalous origin of the left coronary artery from the pulmonary artery. *J Thorac Cardiovasc Surg* 104:696–705, 1992.

63. Schlesinger MJ: Relation of anatomic pattern to pathologic conditions at the coronary arteries. *Arch Pathol* 30:403, 1940.

64. Seguchi M, Nakanishi T, Nakazawa M, et al: Myocardial perfusion after aortic implantation for anomalous origin of the left coronary artery from the pulmonary artery. *Eur Heart J* 11:213–218, 1990.

65. Sheinbaum RJ: Cardiac arrest and resuscitation in a child with undetected anomalous left coronary artery. *Anesthesiology* 72:1091–1093, 1990.

66. Starnes VA, Bernstein D, Oyer PE, et al: Heart transplantation in children. *J Heart Transplant* 8:20–26, 1989.

67. Stephenson LW, Edmunds LH Jr, Friedman S, et al: Subclavian–left coronary artery anastomosis (Meyer operation) for anomalous origin of the left coronary artery from the pulmonary artery. *Circulation* 64:II130–II133, 1981.

68. Takeuchi S, Imamura H, Katsumoto K, et al: New surgical method for repair of anomalous left coronary artery from pulmonary artery. *J Thorac Cardiovasc Surg* 78:7–11, 1979.

69. Taylor AJ, Rogan KM, Virmani R: Sudden cardiac death associated with isolated congenital coronary artery anomalies. *J Am Coll Cardiol* 20:640–642, 1992.

70. Thomas D, Salloum J, Montalescot G, et al: Anomalous coronary arteries coursing between the aorta and pulmonary trunk: Clinical indications for coronary artery bypass. *Eur Heart J* 12:832–834, 1991.

71. Tingelstad JB, Lower RR, Eldredge WJ: Anomalous origin of the right coronary artery from the main pulmonary artery. *Am J Cardiol* 30:670–673, 1972.

72. Tokahashi M, Turie P: Abnormalities and diseases of the coronary vessels. In Adams FH, Emmonouilides GC, Reinerschenerder TA (eds): *Moss' Heart Diseases in Infants, Children and Adolescents*. Baltimore, Williams and Wilkens, 1992.

73. Topaz O, DeMarchena EJ, Perin E, et al: Anomalous coronary arteries: Angiographic findings in 80 patients. *Int J Cardiol* 34:129–138, 1992.

74. Vouhe PR, Baillot-Vernant F, Trinquet F, et al: Anomalous left coronary artery from the pulmonary artery in infants. Which operation? When? *J Thorac Cardiovasc Surg* 94:192–199, 1987.

75. Vouhe PR, Tamisier D, Sidi D, et al: Anomalous left coronary artery from the pulmonary artery: Results of isolated aortic reimplantation. *Ann Thorac Surg* 54:621–626, 1992.

76. Wesselhoeft H, Fawcett JS, Johnson AL: Anomalous origin of the left coronary artery from the pulmonary trunk. Its clinical spectrum, pathology, and pathophysiology, based on a review of 140 cases with seven further cases. *Circulation* 38:403–425, 1968.

77. Wilcox BR, Anderson RH: *Surgical Anatomy of the Heart*. New York, Raven Press, 1985, p 31.

78. Wilson CL, Dlabal PW, McGuire SA: Surgical treatment of anomalous left coronary artery from pulmonary artery: Follow-up in teenagers and adults. *Am Heart J* 98:440–446, 1979.

79. Yoshida Y, Emmanouilides GC, Nebon RJ, et al: Anomalous origin of the left coronary artery from the pulmonary artery: A case report with remarkable improvement of myocardial function following subclavian artery–coronary anastomosis. *Cathet Cardiovasc Diagn* 6:293, 1980.

80. Zannini L, Iorio FS, Ghiselli A, et al: Surgical treatment of anomalous origin of the left coronary artery in infancy. *J Cardiovasc Surg* (Torino) 30:706–708, 1989.

Chapter 31

Persistent Truncus Arteriosus

JAMES D. ST. LOUIS, MD

INTRODUCTION AND HISTORY

Persistent truncus arteriosus is a relatively rare cardiac anomaly, occurring in approximately 2.8% of individuals with congenital heart disease.[8] A single arterial vessel arising from the heart, receiving blood from both ventricles, and supplying blood to the aorta, lungs, and coronary arteries characterizes the condition. The pathologic anatomy was first described by Taruffi in 1875,[35] whereas the basic morphology was outlined by Lev and Saphir in 1943.[22] In 1949, Collett and Edwards[7] established a classification system based on the origin of the pulmonary arteries (PAs) from the truncal artery. Van Praagh and Van Praagh[38] reclassified truncus arteriosus based on the morphology of the conotruncal septum and the presence of associated anomalies. In 1968, McGoon[27] and associates reported the first successful repair of truncus arteriosus closing the ventricular septal defect (VSD) and using the work of Rastelli, in which a conduit consisting of a homograft was used to reconstruct the pulmonary outflow tract.[32]

CLASSIFICATION

Two classification systems have been adopted to standardize the reporting of individuals with truncus arteriosus.[17] The system described by Collett and Edwards,[7] based on the origin of the PA from the truncal artery, describes type I as an arterial trunk originating from the common semilunar valve with its immediate bifurcation into a PA and ascending aorta (Fig. 31-1). Type II defects refer to the separate origin of the left and right PAs from the posterior wall of the truncal artery. Type III describes anatomy similar to that of type II but with the right and left PAs originating farther apart. In type IV, often referred to as *pseudotruncus*, the main PA is absent, with the lungs receiving their blood supply through aortopulmonary collaterals. Most would agree that this entity should not be described as a truncus defect, but rather is a form of pulmonary atresia with VSD.

Van Praagh and Van Praagh[38] classified truncus arteriosus based on the presence or absence of the conotruncal septum. When the conal septum fails to form, a conal-type VSD results. The system uses the designation A to represent the presence of a VSD and B for the absence of a VSD. The variable development of the truncal septum defines their specific category (see Fig. 31-1). In Van Praagh type 1, the truncal septum is partially developed, so that a PA and aorta coexist. In type 2, complete absence of the truncal septum is seen, with the main PAs originating from the truncal artery separately. Type 3 is characterized by the absence of one PA originating from the truncal artery. Type 4 describes any type of truncus associated with an interrupted arch defect. The arch anomaly is usually a type B interruption with the descending aorta receiving its blood supply from a large patent ductus arteriosus and the PAs originating from the truncal artery. The Van Praagh system allows a clearer anatomic description of the defect, allowing better preoperative planning for repair. It also eliminates those defects without at least one PA originating from the truncus.

EMBRYOLOGY

Truncal ridges form in the truncus arteriosus during week 5 of gestation and become continuous with the conal septum superiorly. These ridges eventually fuse to separate the

Collett and Edwards

Van Praagh

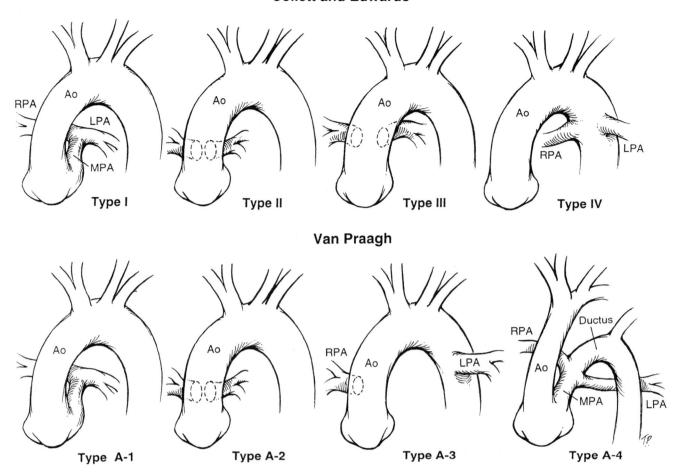

FIGURE 31-1   Collett-Edwards and Van Praagh classifications (see text for details). Collett-Edwards types I, II, and III and Van Praagh types A1 and A2 are similar. Collett-Edwards type IV is now considered a variant of tetralogy of Fallot with pulmonary atresia. Van Praagh type A3 has the right pulmonary artery originating from the truncus and the left pulmonary artery from a ductus off of the descending aorta. In the Van Praagh type A4, the truncus arteriosus occurs with interrupted aortic arch. A patent ductus arteriosus supplies the descending aorta. Pulmonary arteries originate from the posterior aspect of the truncal root. RPA, right pulmonary artery; LPA, left pulmonary artery; MPA, main pulmonary artery; Ao, aorta.

truncus arteriosus into two channels, the aorta and pulmonary trunk. The spiral formation of these ridges results in the normal orientation of the aorta and PA, with the aorta positioned posteriorly and to the right of the PA. The conus cordis gives rise to the left ventricular (LV) and right ventricular (RV) outflow tracts when the conal septum is complete. The truncal and conal septa then fuse, creating RV-to-PA and LV-to-aortic continuity. Persistent truncus arteriosus results from failure of the truncal ridges and aortopulmonary septum to develop and divide into the aorta and pulmonary trunk.[38]

The mechanism for failure of the truncal septation remains unclear. Recent investigation has implicated deficiencies in neural crest development and migration as a possible mechanism for conotruncal anomalies.[19] Several reports have linked truncus arteriosus and other arch anomalies to deletion of chromosome 22q11.[29] Preliminary evidence

suggests that insufficient cranial migration of neural crest cells may be responsible for the associated anomalies in chromosome 22q11 deletion.[12]

ANATOMY AND ASSOCIATED ANOMALIES

The segmental anatomy of truncus arteriosus can be described as situs solitus, a D-looping ventricle, and a single great vessel arising from a common semilunar valve (Fig. 31-2). The truncal artery overrides a large VSD, with frequent malalignment to the right. The truncal valve may have a variable number of cusps, with three cusps reported in 64% of cases, four cusps in 27%, and two cusps in 8%.[1] Truncal valve incompetence has been reported as severe in 6%, moderate in 31%, and absent or minimal in 63% of 167 patients operated on at the

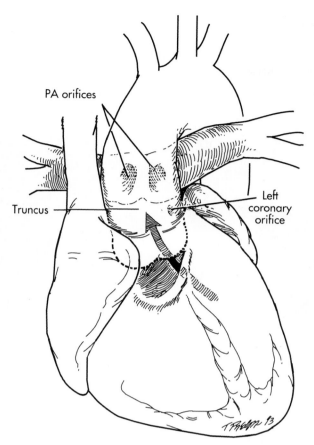

FIGURE 31-2 Relationship of the truncal artery to the truncal valve (*boldface dotted line*), left coronary ostium, and ventricular septal defect (*arrow*).

Mayo Clinic.[9] The position of the valve cusps also has been correlated with the origin and epicardial course of the coronary arteries.[21]

The origin of the coronary ostia and epicardial course of the coronary arteries can be variable in truncus arteriosus. Approximately 15% of patients have some type of coronary anomaly, often with important surgical implications. Coronary ostia can originate in various positions from within the truncal artery or as a single coronary with a variable epicardial course. Anomalous origin of the left coronary artery from the right coronary will cross the RV outflow tract. This is of particular importance when planning the construction of the RV-to-PA conduit. When the left main coronary ostium originates more superiorly in the commissure, care must be taken to avoid injury during separation of the PAs. In 53 hearts studied by Anderson's group, 8 had a single coronary artery, and another 8 had a coronary artery orifice at the upper margin of a commissure.[34]

The VSD in truncus arteriosus, similar to the defect that exists in tetrology of Fallot, results from the failure of the conal septum to develop and rotate. The defect is often large, nonrestrictive, with the superior border being formed by the truncal valve. The inferior and anterior borders are formed by the two limbs of the septomarginalis trabeculation (SMT). In two thirds of cases, the posterior arm of the SMT and the ventriculoinfundibular fold join to separate the VSD from the septal leaflet of the tricuspid valve. This separation places

the conduction system away from the inferior border of the VSD and less likely to be injured during repair. In one third of cases, a deficiency of the ventriculoinfundibular fold and posterior division of the SMT exists, with the defect extending to the annulus of the tricuspid valve. This leaves the conduction system close to the inferior edge of the VSD and vulnerable to injury during closure.[4]

The PA branches are usually of normal caliber; however, stenosis of the origin and diffuse hypoplasia can occur. The pathologic changes that can occur in the pulmonary vasculature are similar to those of other conditions in which a high-pressure, left-to-right shunt is found. This can produce pulmonary vascular obstructive disease, as described by Heath and Edwards.[16]

Other defects of surgical significance occurring with truncus arteriosus include right aortic arch, patent ductus arteriosus, persistent left superior vena cava, atrial septal defect, and an anomalous subclavian artery. Noncardiac anomalies are present in about 20% of cases and may contribute to death. DiGeorge syndrome is associated with truncus arteriosus in 30% of cases.[13] Other less common defects include tethered-cord syndrome, unilateral renal agenesis, and anal atresia.

NATURAL HISTORY

In infants with truncus arteriosus, mortality is the result of low pulmonary vascular resistance and the development of severe congestive heart failure (CHF). As pulmonary vascular resistance decreases during the first few weeks of life, pulmonary blood flow becomes torrential. The left ventricle is subjected to a significant volume overload. The increase in left ventricular end-diastolic volume results in an increase in the pulmonary vascular hydrostatic pressure and severe pulmonary edema. Mortality during the first year of life is more than 80%, with half succumbing during the neonatal period if surgical correction is not undertaken. Pulmonary vascular resistances in infants that survive the neonatal period will increase as the result of increased flows. Irreversible pulmonary vascular disease will eventually develop, usually by the end of the second year, with the infant dying of the effects of chronic, progressive cyanosis. Surgical repair at this age should be approached with caution and may be contraindicated in individuals older than 2 years with pulmonary vascular resistance greater than 8 Woods units.[24] Operative mortality approaches 100% in these children, with the majority of deaths due to acute right heart failure. A small percentage of children will survive past the third year of life with large left-to-right shunts and protected pulmonary circulation. Prenatal death often occurs when truncus is complicated by severe valve regurgitation or interrupted aortic arch.[26]

HEMODYNAMICS

Blood from both the LV and the RV is ejected into the truncal artery. The systemic and pulmonary venous blood mixes and the arterial oxygen saturation depends on the amount of pulmonary blood flow. Pulmonary blood flow may be limited by stenosis of the PAs, but this is uncommon. In most instances, pulmonary blood flow (and thus arterial oxygen saturation) is determined by the resistance to flow in the pulmonary vascular bed. After the second week of life, pulmonary vascular resistance decreases, and the pulmonary-to-systemic flow ratio exceeds 1. Pulmonary blood flow may become torrential, leading to volume overload of the left ventricle, pulmonary edema, and decreased systemic oxygen delivery. The child is seen in florid CHF. Over time, the continued exposure of the pulmonary vascular bed to these flows leads to the development of pulmonary vascular obstructive disease. The pulmonary vascular resistance increases, and the pulmonary-to-systemic ratio approaches 1 or less. The child then has signs of cyanosis. A point is reached at which these changes become irreversible.

DIAGNOSIS

The symptoms associated with truncus arteriosus are related primarily to the amount of pulmonary blood flow. During the first few week of life, when pulmonary vascular resistance is normally increased, symptoms are usually absent unless associated truncal valve incompetence is present. With maturation of the fetal vascular bed, associated with a decrease in pulmonary vascular resistance and an increase in pulmonary blood flow, symptoms of CHF may develop. These include dyspnea, diaphoresis, and failure to thrive. Cyanosis is not usually apparent because the arterial oxygen saturation is generally greater than 85%. With progressive development of pulmonary vascular obstructive disease and the associated decrease in pulmonary blood flow, cyanosis becomes more evident.

Physical examination usually reveals a systolic thrill and murmur over the left third and fourth intercostal spaces parasternally. The infant is typically diaphoretic and in moderate respiratory distress. The patient has a jerky, collapsing arterial pulse due to the rapid run-off from the truncal artery into the pulmonary circulation. The apical impulse is prominent, and signs of cardiomegaly are noted. The second heart sound is single and accentuated. When truncal valve incompetence is present, a diastolic murmur follows the second heart sound.

Chest radiography shows cardiomegaly with biventricular enlargement. The aortic arch is to the right in 20% of patients, and the left PA may be elevated from the normal position. The peripheral pulmonary vasculature is increased, unless advanced pulmonary vascular obstructive disease exists (Fig. 31-3). The electrocardiogram is nonspecific and usually indicates biventricular hypertrophy.

Echocardiography is the diagnostic procedure of choice; in the parasternal long-axis view, a single great vessel is seen overriding the ventricular septum (Fig. 31-4).[37] Echocardiography will also delineate the proximal pulmonary anatomy. Color Doppler evaluation will show the degree of truncal valve incompetence. Echocardiography also may accurately diagnosis truncus arteriosus in the prenatal period.[36]

Cardiac catheterization is reserved for those cases in which the anatomy is unclear, further information is needed concerning the truncal valve, or the status of the pulmonary vasculature is unclear. Systemic pressure is detected in both ventricles. Left atrial pressure (LAP) is frequently elevated because of the increased pulmonary venous return (Fig. 31-5). Pulmonary vascular resistance is usually only mildly elevated (2 to 4 Wood units/m²) in infants younger than 3 months.

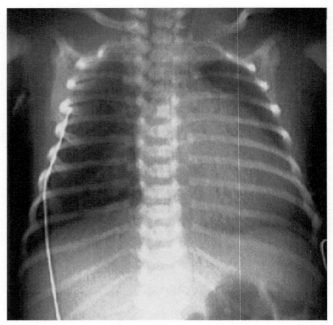

FIGURE 31-3 Chest radiograph of an infant with truncus arteriosus. Note the cardiomegaly, increased pulmonary vascular markings, and right aortic arch.

The elevated pulmonary flow keeps aortic saturation greater than 85%. When arterial oxygen saturation is less than 85%, significant pulmonary vascular disease limiting pulmonary blood flow is usually the cause, and the child may not tolerate correction.

SURGICAL TECHNIQUE

Definitive repair of truncus arteriosus entails separation of the branch PAs from the truncal artery, establishment of RV-to-PA

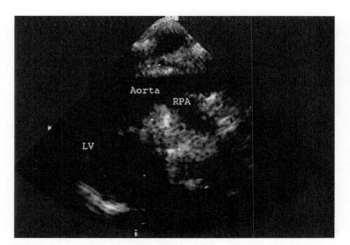

FIGURE 31-4 Echocardiogram (long axis–parasternal view) of truncus arteriosus. Truncal vessel gives rise to the aorta and pulmonary arteries. RPA, Right pulmonary artery; LV, left ventricle.

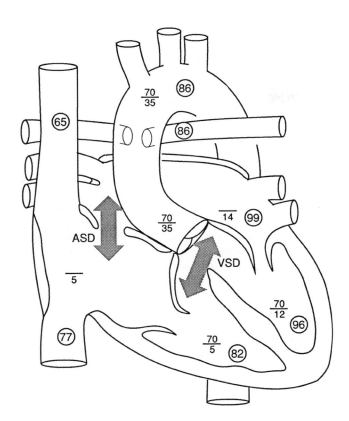

FIGURE 31-5 Pathophysiology of truncus arteriosus. Excessive pulmonary blood flow leads to volume overload of the ventricles. Mixing at the ventricular and arterial level produces similar pulmonary and systemic arterial saturations (*circled values*). Pressure in the right ventricle is at systemic levels to maintain truncal flow. ASD, atrial septal defect; VSD, ventricular septal defect.

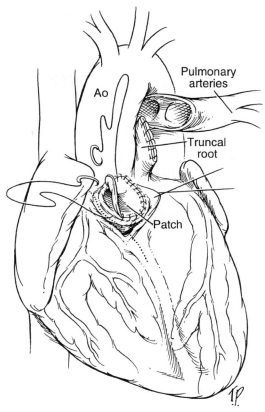

FIGURE 31-6 Repair of truncus arteriosus. The pulmonary arteries are detached from the truncal root. Through the longitudinal infundibulotomy, the malaligned VSD is baffled with a prosthetic patch with base of truncal root directing left ventricular blood to the aorta (Ao).

continuity, closure of the VSD, and repair of associated anomalies. Repair is accomplished through a median sternotomy or cardiopulmonary bypass (CPB). The lower portion of the thymus gland is removed, if present. It is often small, and its absence is suggestive of DiGeorge syndrome. The pericardium is opened, and a rectangular segment is harvested. The pericardial segment is fixed in 0.6% glutaraldehyde for 4 minutes. The aorta is cannulated as distally as possible. We prefer an 8F to 10F DLP (Medtronic, Grand Rapids) aortic cannula for infants weighing less than 5 kg. The right atrium is then cannulated with a 20F metal-tip venous cannula. The mainstem PAs are dissected and encircled with snares. With the establishment of cardiopulmonary bypass, the PAs are occluded to prevent overcirculation. The child is cooled to 25° C. Once cooled, the aorta is cross-clamped, and antegrade cold cardioplegia is administered (30 mL/kg). Subsequent low-K+ cardioplegia (15 mL/kg) is administered at 20-minute intervals.

The PAs are detached from the truncal artery with an elliptical incision (Fig. 31-6). Removal of the PAs from the truncal artery is done with care so as not to injure the coronary arteries. The position of the left main coronary artery ostium, usually just inferior to the PAs, must be identified to prevent injury during separation of the main trunks. A generous cuff of tissue surrounding the orifice of the PAs

should be harvested if possible. If exposure of the PAs is difficult, a longitudinal counterincision in the truncal artery will give excellent exposure. This incision will allow the removal of the PAs from within the truncal artery. In smaller infants, the posterior defect in the truncal artery should be closed with a glutaraldehyde-fixed autologous pericardial patch to avoid distortion of the semilunar valve pillars. The aortic cross-clamp is temporarily released after air has been removed from the aortic root, and the competency of the valve is assessed. If incompetence is severe, valve replacement or repair must be considered.

An anterior right ventriculotomy is made in the RV outflow tract. The orientation of this incision is made slightly to the left, to accommodate construction of the RV-to-PA conduit. The subarterial VSD is closed through the ventriculotomy. If continuous CPB is desired, it may be necessary to create bicaval cannulation before proceeding. In some instances, because of abundant collateral pulmonary blood flow, it may also be helpful to insert a vent into the left side of the heart through the right superior pulmonary vein. The need for all of these cannulae and vents, especially for tiny infants, encourages some to use a simpler system described in the following text. If the septal defect is restrictive, the anterior extension of the SMT can be resected. This will prevent substantial outflow tract obstruction with closure of the VSD. When the inferior border of the VSD is separated from the septal leaflet of the tricuspid valve by the posterior-division SMT, the conduction system is safely behind the margin of the repair. If this muscular rim is absent, the conduction tissue resides close to the inferior border. Complete heart block is avoided by the meticulous placement of sutures in this area. Closure of the VSD is accomplished with a Dacron patch (Fig. 31-7).

An appropriate-sized valved homograft conduit (10 to 13 mm) is cut to the proper length and used to establish continuity between the RV and the PAs. The course of the conduit should be such that kinking and compression with closure of the sternum are avoided. The left pleura can be incised, allowing the heart and conduit to rotate into the left chest. Right ventricular outflow tract reconstruction should always consist of a valved conduit when a high or reactive pulmonary vascular resistance (i.e., neonate) is found. The 12-mm porcine valved conduit has been used successfully for this reconstruction, but the technical ease of insertion and the perhaps greater durability of a cryopreserved-valved homograft support its use when available. The distal anastomosis of the homograft is performed with a running polydioxanone suture (PDS) or monofilament suture. The homograft is positioned as distal as possible so that the valve sits above the shoulder of the heart near the distal anastomosis. The posterior suture line usually can be anchored at the edge of the VSD patch. A Gore-Tex patch or a patch made from the previously harvested pericardium is used to construct a hood over the right venticulotomy. This avoids compression or distortion of the conduit, smoothes the outflow hydraulic profile, and avoids compression of the coronary arteries (Fig. 31-8).

An alternative approach is to systemically cool the infant to 18°C after commencing CPB. During the cooling period, the aorta can be cross-clamped as far distal to the takeoff of the pulmonary arteries as possible. A transverse aortotomy is performed and carried circumferentially to transect the aorta, leaving the orifices of the pulmonary arteries as an "island" around which the posterior aortic incision is carried. While the aorta is transected, the distal pulmonary arteries are dissected and freed from adventitial investments so that they can be "moved" leftward. They are anastomosed to a small homograft (pulmonary or aortic). The aorta is then reconstructed primarily, which is almost always possible in an end-to-end fashion without the need for any material to augment the defect left by removing the pulmonary arteries. The aorta is filled with cardioplegia, and additional cardioplegia is given at this time to test the competency of the truncal valve. An incision is made on the anterior surface of the RV, and the truncal valve can be inspected directly during this infusion of cardioplegia.

At this time, cardiopulmonary bypass is stopped and the VSD can be easily closed with a patch using whatever technique the surgeon prefers. Intermittent cerebral perfusion at 15-minute intervals can be accomplished to improve cerebral

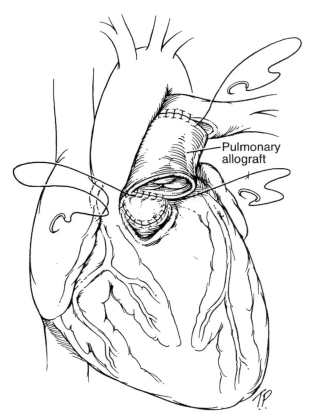

FIGURE 31-7 Repair of truncus arteriosus (*continued*). Right ventricle to pulmonary artery continuity is established by interposition of valved conduit (usually cryopreserved pulmonary allograft).

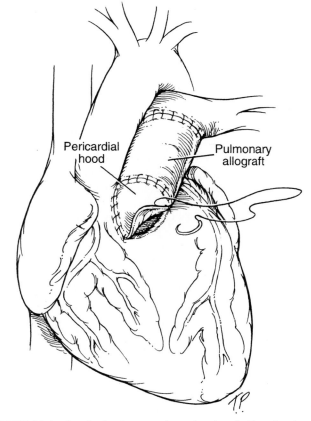

FIGURE 31-8 Repair of truncus arteriosus (*continued*). Use of pericardial patch as proximal hood extension for pulmonary allograft.

protection (see section on cardiopulmonary bypass techniques). If the atrial septal defect (ASD) is large, it can also be partially closed at this time. We prefer to leave foramenal defects open.

Cardiopulmonary bypass is reestablished, and during rewarming, with the cross-clamp still in place (especially if there is some truncal insufficiency), the proximal end of the selected RV-PA conduit is placed to the ventricle, using a hood of previously prepared pericardium or Gore-Tex. As this suture line is completed, the cross-clamp is removed and the heart should begin beating vigorously, further nullifying any effects from mild to moderate truncal insufficiency.

Mild to moderate truncal valve regurgitation is often well tolerated and will improve postoperatively. Severe truncal valve regurgitation is a poor prognostic indicator for long-term survival.[5] Replacement can generally be undertaken with a cryopreserved aortic or pulmonary homograft. The truncal valve is removed, and the homograft is seated in the annulus with interrupted Prolene. The coronary arteries are then reimplanted onto the homograft by using 7.0 Prolene (Fig. 31-9). Distal aortic continuity is then established with running Prolene. Valve repair has been attempted in small numbers of patients with reasonable results in selected patients.[11,25]

When truncus is associated with interrupted arch, repair proceeds differently from the previous description. These infants are generally in extremis and require aggressive preoperative and intraoperative management.[30] Despite the magnitude of the operation, excellent results can be achieved with early repair.[18] The large main pulmonary trunk is used for arterial cannulation. Venous cannulation proceeds as described earlier. The patient is cooled to 18°C. Arch vessels are dissected and encircled with snares. After sufficient cooling, the heart is given a dose of cardioplegia, and the pump is shut off. The arch vessels are snared, and the patient drained of venous blood. The arterial cannula is removed, and the ductus arteriosus is ligated and divided, and the main PA component of the truncal root is transected just above the truncal valve. Ductal tissue is trimmed from the descending aorta, and a pulmonary homograft patch is used as a gusset to establish continuity between separate segments of aorta. Closure of the VSD and reconstruction of the RV outflow tract are accomplished in a fashion similar to that of simple truncus.

POSTOPERATIVE MANAGEMENT

The postoperative course of infants after repair of a persistent truncus arteriosus is generally similar to the postoperative course after repair of other lesions, with a few notable exceptions. Pulmonary hypertensive crisis and low cardiac output are particularly prevalent in infants repaired after the neonatal period. Intraoperative placement of PA and left atrial catheters will assist in the postoperative management of these potentially fatal events. Because of limited space in the mediastinum secondary to placement of an RV-to-PA conduit, adequate drainage is critical to prevent tamponade. It is often useful to leave the sternum open and close the incision with a patch of Silastic or Gore-Tex, until the pulmonary compliance recovers, since premature closure of the chest can create "pulmonary tamponade" with compression of the conduit and decreased filling of the right heart.

Pulmonary hypertension, both sustained and paroxysmal, can be anticipated in infants with preoperative elevation of PA pressures and those that undergo delayed repair. Avoidance of these potentially fatal events has been paramount in the decrease in mortality and morbidity associated with repair.[2] Events that trigger hypertensive crisis, such as hypoxia, hypercapnia, acidosis, pain, airway stimulation, and left ventricular failure, must be avoided. Patients should be kept sedated and paralyzed for the first 24 to 48 hours after repair. The routine use of fentanyl (3 mcg/kg) and pancuronium (0.1 mg/kg) has been shown to prevent the development of hypertensive crisis. Endotracheal suctioning and undue stimulation should be minimized. Keeping the infant well oxygenated and somewhat hypocapnic (pCO_2 30 to 35 mm Hg) is considered ideal.[23] Acidosis must be cautiously corrected with sodium bicarbonate. Correction with sodium bicarbonate with inappropriate minute ventilation will result in an increase in plasma CO_2. Excessive CO_2 will not only increase pulmonary vascular resistance, but also results in depressed myocardial function. An initial dose of 1 mEq/kg can be used, with an additional dose tailored to the arterial blood gas. Use of a high-dose α-agonist must be avoided.

Episodes of pulmonary hypertension are treated in a standard fashion.[3] The infants are hyperventilated and oxygenated. Intravenous calcium is used for short duration of inotropic support. Sedation and paralysis must be maximized.

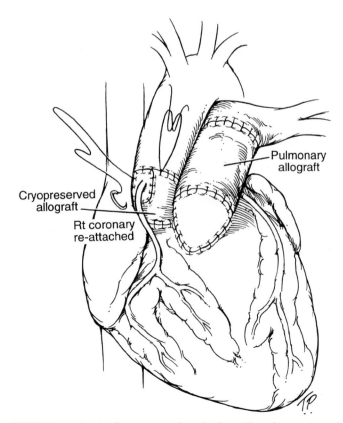

FIGURE 31-9 Repair of truncus arteriosus in the setting of severe truncal insufficiency. Truncal root is replaced with a second cryopreserved allograft, and coronary arteries are reimplanted to the allograft root.

Labels on figure: Pulmonary allograft; Cryopreserved allograft; Rt coronary re-attached

Vasodilator agents such as nitroprusside, isoproterenol, and adenosine may be infused directly into the pulmonary circuit if adequate maintenance of systemic blood pressure is a problem. The liberal use of nitric oxide has been shown to reduce the mortality associated with these episodes, although recent reports question the effectiveness of nitric oxide in reducing the incidence of pulmonary hypertensive episodes.[15] For infants refractory to conventional attempts to reduce pulmonary resistance, extracorporeal membrane oxygenation (ECMO) may be initiated during the immediate postoperative period.[20]

Right ventricular dysfunction may result from elevated pulmonary pressures, insufficient preload relative to a stiff RV, metabolic derangements, volume overload secondary to residual left-to-right shunting, or compression of coronary arteries due to the RV-to-PA conduit. Regardless of the etiology, right heart failure will result in inadequate systemic perfusion, exacerbating the original problem. Low cardiac output will result in persistent acidosis with elevated lactate levels, low mixed venous saturation, elevated arterial-venous gradient, low urine output, and cool extremities. Measures to optimize preload, contractility, and afterload must immediately be initiated. In cases where the cardiac output remains limited, ECMO is justified.

Central venous pressure (CVP) should be maintained at relatively high levels because of the decreased compliance of the RV. CVP of 13 to 18 mm Hg or LAP of 8 to 12 mm Hg should be maintained. The patients must be ventilated at the lowest airway pressure possible. Increased intrathoracic pressure will have a detrimental effect on ventricular filling and output. Because of the stiffness of the ventricle, only moderate increases in stroke volume can be achieved at any given preload. To optimize cardiac output, pacing at heart rates of 140 to 160 beats/minute can be accomplished with epicardial pacing leads placed at the time of repair. Most infants will require some degree of inotropic support for the first 24 to 48 hours. Low-dose dopamine, dobutamine, or epinephrine is commonly used to augment myocardial contractility. Care must be taken to prevent undue effects on the pulmonary vasculature.

Right bundle branch block is nearly always present postoperatively. Other common dysrhythmias include junctional ectopic tachycardia, atrial tachycardias, and atrioventricular block. Complete heart block occurs in 3% to 5% of patients.

CONCLUSIONS

Repair of truncus arteriosus has improved over the past several decades. This improvement is attributed primarily to the emphasis on repair during the neonatal period, before the development of irreversible pulmonary vascular disease. Mortality of children repaired between the ages of 2 and 5 years ranged from 25% to 88%.[33] Ebert[10] was the first to report repair of truncus during the first 6 months of life, with a mortality of 9%. Other reports from Bove,[6] McKay,[28] and Hanley[14] demonstrate improved survival with repair during the neonatal period. Preoperative risk factors that have been described in various reports include older age at time of surgery, severe truncal valve regurgitation, interrupted aortic arch, and coronary artery anomalies.

The major late complication after truncus arteriosus repair is obstruction or stenosis of the conduit. The incidence of obstruction has decreased with the use of homograft conduits.

The reported incidence of homograft obstruction is 14% compared with a 71% incidence of Dacron-porcine graft obstruction over a 6-year period.[18] Although 10- and 20-year survival has dramatically improved with improved conduit material, the need for future conduit replacement adds lifetime risk to these patients.[31]

References

1. Anderson R, Thiene G: Categorization and description of hearts with a common arterial trunk. *Eur J Cardio Thorac Surg* 3:481–487, 1989.
2. Bando K, Turrentine MW, Sharp TG, et al: Pulmonary hypertension after operations for congenital heart disease: Analysis of risk factors and management. *J Thorac Cardiovasc Surg* 112:1600–1609, 1996.
3. Berner M, Beghetti M, Ricou B, et al: Relief of severe pulmonary hypertension after closure of a large ventricular septal defect using low dose inhaled nitric oxide. *Intensive Care Med* 19:75–77, 1993.
4. Bharati S, Karp R, Lev M: The conduction system in truncus arteriosus and its surgical significance: A study of five cases. *J Thorac Cardiovasc Surg* 104:954–960, 1992.
5. Borghi A, Agnoletti G, Valsecchi O, Carminati, M: Aortic balloon dilatation for congenital aortic stenosis: Report of 90 cases (1986–98). *Heart* 82:e10, 1999.
6. Bove EL, Lupinetti FM, Pridjian AK, et al: Results of a policy of primary repair of truncus arteriosus in the neonate. *J Thorac Cardiovasc Surg* 105:1057–1066, 1993.
7. Collett RW, Edwards JE: Persistent truncus arteriosus: A classification according to anatomic types. *Surg Clin North Am* 29:1245, 1949.
8. Crupi G, Macartney FJ, Anderson RH: Persistent truncus arteriosus: A study of 66 autopsy cases with special reference to definition and morphogenesis. *Am J Cardiol* 40:569–578, 1977.
9. DiDonato R, Fyfe D, Puga F, et al: *Fifteen-year Experience with Surgical Repair of Truncus Arteriosus: Annual Meeting of the Western Thoracic Surgical Association*. Maui, Hawaii, June 20–23, 1984.
10. Ebert PA, Turley K, Stanger P, et al: Surgical treatment of truncus arteriosus in the first six months of life. *Ann Thorac Surg* 200:451–456, 1984.
11. Elami A, Laks H, Pearl JM: Truncal valve repair: Initial experience with infants and children. *Ann Thorac Surg* 57:397–401, 1994.
12. Goldmuntz E, Clark B, Mitchell L, et al: Frequency of 22q11 deletions in patients with conotruncal defects. *J Am Coll Cardiol* 32:492–498, 1998.
13. Goldmuntz E, Emanuel B: Genetic disorders of cardiac morphogenesis: The DiGeorge and velocardiofacial syndrome. *Circ Res* 80:437–443, 1997.
14. Hanley FL, Heinemann MK, Jonas RA, et al: Repair of truncus arteriosus in the neonate. *J Thorac Cardiovasc Surg* 105:1047–1056, 1993.
15. Hawkins D, McGough EC, Crezee KL, Orsmond GS: Randomized controlled study of inhaled nitric oxide after operation for congenital heart disease. *Ann Thorac Surg* 69:1907–1912, 2000.
16. Heath D, Edwards J: The pathology of hypertensive pulmonary vascular disease: A description of six grades of structural changes in the pulmonary arteries with special reference to congenital cardiac septal defects. *Circulation* 18:533, 1958.
17. Jacobs M: Congenital heart surgery nomenclature and database project: Truncus arteriosus. *Ann Thorac Surg* 69:S50–S55, 2000.
18. Jahangiri M, Zurakowski D, Mayer J, et al: Repair of the truncal valve and associated interrupted arch in neonates with truncus arteriosus. *J Thorac Cardiovasc Surg* 119:508–514, 2000.
19. Johnson M, Hing A, Wood M, Watson M: Chromosome abnormalities in congenital heart disease. *Am J Med Genet* 70:292–298, 1997.
20. Klein MD, Shaheen KW, Whittlesey GC, et al: Extracorporeal membrane oxygenation for the circulatory support of children after the repair of congenital heart disease. *J Thorac Cardiovasc Surg* 100:498–505, 1990.
21. Lenox C, Debich D, Zuberbuhler J: The role of coronary artery abnormalities in the prognosis of truncus arteriosus. *J Thorac Cardiovasc Surg* 104:1728–1742, 1992.
22. Lev M, Saphir O: Truncus arteriosus communis persistens. *J Pediatr* 20:74, 1943.
23. Lock JE, Einzig S, Bass JL, Moller JH: The pulmonary vascular response to oxygen and its influence on operative results in children with ventricular septal defect. *Pediatr Cardiol* 3:41–46, 1982.
24. Mair DD, Ritter DG, Davis GD: Selection of patients with truncus arteriosus for surgical correction: Anatomic and hemodynamic consideration. *Circulation* 59:144–151, 1974.

25. Mavroudis C, Backer CL: Surgical management of severe truncal insufficiency: Experience with truncal valve remodeling techniques. *Ann Thorac Surg* 72:396–400, 2001.

26. McElhinney D, Reddy M, Rajasinghe H, et al: Trends in the management of truncal valve insufficiency. *Ann Thorac Surg* 65:517–524, 1998.

27. McGoon DC, Rastelli GC, Ongley PA: An operation for the correction of truncus arteriosus. *JAMA* 205:69–73, 1968.

28. McKay R, Miyamoto S, Peart I, et al: Truncus arteriosus with interrupted arch: Successful correction in a neonate. *Ann Thorac Surg* 48:587–589, 1989.

29. Momma K, Ando M, Matsuoka R: Truncus arteriosus communis associated with chromosome 22q11 deletion. *J Am Coll Cardiol* 30:1067–1071, 1997.

30. Pearl JM, Laks H, Drinkwater DC Jr, et al: Repair of conotruncal abnormalities with the use of valved conduit: Improved early and midterm results with the cryopreserved homograft. *J Am Coll Cardiol* 20:191–196, 1992.

31. Rajasinghe H, McElhinney D, Reddy VM, et al: Long-term follow-up of truncus arteriosus repair in infancy: A twenty-year experience. *J Thorac Cardiovasc Surg* 113:869–879, 1997.

32. Rastelli GC, Titus JL, McGoon DC: Homograft of the ascending aorta and aortic valve as a right ventricular outflow: An experimental approach to the repair of truncus arteriosus. *Arch Surg* 95:698–708, 1967.

33. Stark J, Gandhi D, DeLeval M: Surgical treatment of truncus arteriosus in the first year of life. *Br Heart J* 40:1280–1287, 1978.

34. Suzuki A, Ho SY, Anderson RH, Deanfield JE: Coronary arterial and sinusal anatomy in hearts with a common arterial trunk. *Ann Thorac Surg* 48:792–797, 1989.

35. Taruffi C: Sull malattie congenite e sulle anomalie del cuore. *Mem Soc Med Chir Bologna* 8:215, 1875.

36. Tometzki A, Suda K, Kohl T, et al: Accuracy of prenatal echocardiographic diagnosis and prognosis of the fetus with conotruncal anomalies. *J Am Coll Cardiol* 33:1696–1701, 1999.

37. Tworetzky W, McElhinney DB, Brook MM, et al: Echocardiographic diagnosis alone for the complete repair of major congenital heart defects. *J Am Coll Cardiol* 33:228–233, 1999.

38. Van Praagh R, Van Praagh S: The anatomy of common aorticopulmonary trunk (truncus arteriosus communis) and its embryologic implications: A study of 57 necropsy cases. *Am J Cardiol* 16:406–425, 1965.

Chapter 32

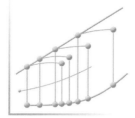

Total Anomalous Pulmonary Venous Return

PETER MARK TRINKAUS, MD, ALLAN J. HORDOF, MD,
ANNE M. MURPHY, MD, and WILLIAM J. GREELEY, MD, MBA

INTRODUCTION

Total anomalous pulmonary venous return (TAPVR) represents a group of congenital heart defects with an array of anatomic and physiologic variants in which the pulmonary veins connect to the remnants of the embryologic venous circulation rather than to the left atrium. This results in an obligatory shunt of the oxygenated pulmonary venous blood to the right side of the heart and is often associated with some degree of pulmonary venous obstruction (PVO).

These anomalies are isolated in approximately two thirds[21] of the cases and in the remainder are associated with complex defects and heterotaxy syndromes that may require univentricular palliation. In this chapter, we address the medical and surgical management of both isolated TAPVR and TAPVR associated with other complex lesions.

EMBRYOLOGY

In very early fetal life, the lungs, larynx, and tracheobronchial tree are derived from the primitive foregut. The splanchnic plexus is the vascular plexus that is shared between the developing lungs and other derivatives of the foregut. This common plexus drains through the paired common cardinal, umbilical, and vitelline veins (Fig. 32-1A).[46] At first, the splanchnic plexus has no direct connection to the heart (see Fig. 32-1A). Later in development, the common pulmonary vein invaginates from the posterior portion of the left atrium and establishes communication with the pulmonary portion of the splanchnic plexus (see Fig. 32-1B). The pulmonary vascular plexus is drained via four individual major pulmonary veins into the common pulmonary vein and into the left atrium. During further differential growth, the common pulmonary vein becomes incorporated into the wall of the left atrium, resulting in the anatomic situation seen normally at birth in which four veins drain into the left atrium (see Fig. 32-1D).[20] Pulmonary blood flow (PBF) may then return directly to the heart via the left atrium. No longer necessary, the primitive pulmonary venous connections attaching to the cardinal and umbilical veins are for the most part lost (see Fig. 32-1D). Disruption of this process of pulmonary venous development during gestation provides the embryologic basis for most of the anatomic abnormalities seen with anomalous pulmonary venous connection.[46] Lack of invagination of the common pulmonary vein directly leads to persistence of the abnormal pulmonary venous connection seen with all types of TAPVR. If failure of common pulmonary vein invagination occurs early during gestation, persistence of the connections for pulmonary venous return to the cardinal or umbilical system veins occurs. The persistence of the primitive connections without any connection of the common pulmonary vein to the left atrium results in TAPVR.

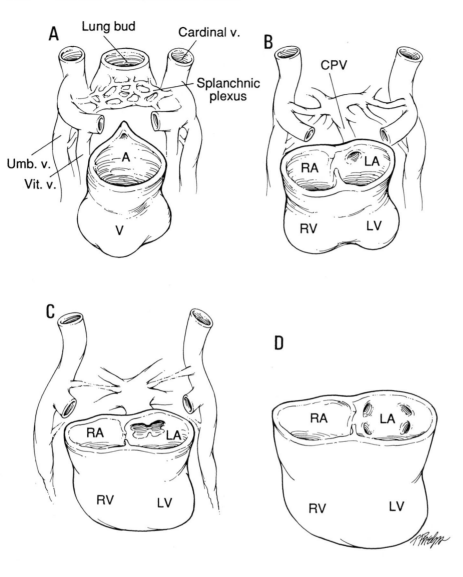

FIGURE 32-1 Normal development of pulmonary veins. **A,** The splanchnic plexus drains the lung buds in early development, with no connection of pulmonary venous drainage to the heart. **B,** The common pulmonary vein (CPV) arises in development from the left atrium (LA) and connects with the developing splanchnic plexus, establishing pulmonary venous return to the heart. **C,** Regression of the cardinal, umbilical (Umb.), and vitelline (Vit.) veins. **D,** Incorporation of the CPV and the individual veins into the LA, establishing normal pulmonary venous drainage. LV, left ventircle; RA, right atrium; RV, right ventricle.

ANATOMY AND CLASSIFICATION

In TAPVR, all the veins drain abnormally outside the left atrium and are connected directly to the right atrium, or indirectly via remnants of the cardinal or umbilical venous system. The classification scheme most commonly used is that of Darling, Rothney, and Craig,[16] based on the anatomic site of the abnormal connection[37]: type 1, supracardiac defect (40% to 50% of cases); type 2, cardiac defect (18% to 31% of cases); type 3, infracardiac defect (13% to 24% of cases); and type 4, mixed defect (5% to 10% of cases). The four most common anatomic defects are illustrated in Figure 32-2. Mixed defects are not shown but involve a combination of the other three variants and are usually further subclassified as either "2+2" or "1+3," depending on how the four main pulmonary veins attach to the heart.[18]

An alternative classification scheme is that of Burroughs and Edwards,[9] in which the anatomy is classified according to the site of embryologic origin of the abnormal connection (Table 32-1). In the typical anatomic configuration, the veins drain to a confluence behind the heart, the common

pulmonary vein.[18] The drainage from the confluence determines further anatomic classification.

In the supracardiac type, the confluence drains to the normal, right-sided, superior vena cava (SVC) via a left SVC or a "vertical vein" (see Fig. 32-2A) that connects to the innominate vein or, less frequently, via a vertical vein that connects directly to the right-sided SVC. Some degree of obstruction to venous drainage has been reported in the majority of these patients[38,57] and usually occurs from compression of the ascending vein between the bronchi and the pulmonary artery or aorta or from stenosis at the orifice of the vertical vein.[53]

In the most common type of intracardiac anomalous connection, the venous confluence drains to the coronary sinus (see Fig. 32-2B). Obstruction once thought to be rare in this form has been reported in one series as occurring in 22% of patients.[33] It usually occurs at the point of connection of the venous channel to the coronary sinus. Rarely, a restrictive atrial communication may also occur. Occasionally the cardiac connection is directly to the posterior wall of the right atrium without a confluence (see Fig. 32-2C).

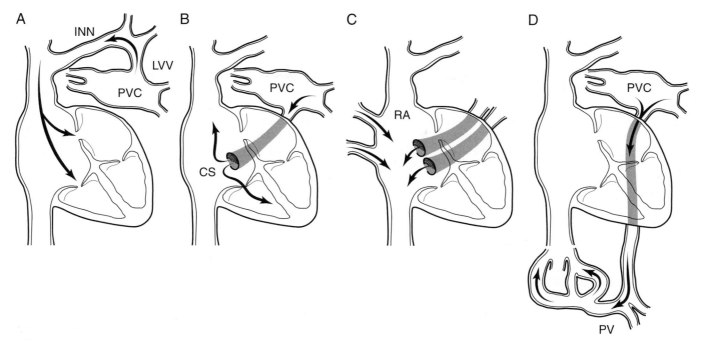

FIGURE 32-2   The four most common anatomic defects in total anomalous pulmonary venous connection (TAPVR). **A,** TAPVR drainage to the innominate vein (INN) via a left vertical vein (LVV). **B,** TAPVR from the common pulmonary venous confluence (PVC) to the coronary sinus (CS). **C,** TAPVR to the right atrium (RA). **D,** Infradiaphragmatic TAPVR from the common pulmonary venous confluence to the portal vein (PV).

With infracardiac TAPVR, a descending vertical vein usually drains the venous confluence, penetrates the diaphragm, and connects with a vessel of the portal system (see Fig. 32-2D). Connections to the ductus venosus, hepatic veins, gastric vein, or inferior vena cava have been reported. Obstruction with infracardiac connection is very common. The point of intersection of the descending vein with the systemic venous system may be stenotic, or some degree of flow limitation may exist in the portal venous system.

The mixed type of TAPVR occurs with two or more sites of anomalous venous connections. The venous confluence is usually diminished in size or absent. Mixed TAPVR can be further classified as "2 + 2" or "3 + 1," depending on whether both veins from each lung segregate together. The most common pattern is a 3 + 1 pattern, in which both the right pulmonary veins and the left lower lobe vein form a confluence that connects directly to the right atrium, usually near the SVC junction. The remaining left upper lobe vein usually connects to the innominate vein via a vertical vein. The second most common form is a 2 + 2 arrangement, in which the right-sided veins join and drain to the right atrium, and the left-sided veins form a confluence that drains to the innominate via a vertical vein. A large number of additional variations have been described, including some in which one or two pulmonary veins appear to drain into a plexus that resembles an embryologic remnant of the splanchnic plexus.[18]

GENETICS

Whereas most cases of TAPVR are sporadic with a recurrence risk of approximately 2.5%,[21] reports have described familial occurrence of TAPVR.[6] Bleyl and colleagues[6] described a large Utah/Idaho kindred with 14 affected individuals over three generations. Anatomic sites of anomalous connection were variable, with five connecting to a vertical vein, two connecting to an infradiaphragmatic vein, and one each with connection to the right atrium, right SVC, and a mixed connection. The gene in this family was localized by using linkage mapping to the centromeric region of the fourth chromosome.[5] Interestingly, this is the same region to which

Table 32-1   Site of Connection in 113 Cases of Uncomplicated Total Anomalous Pulmonary Venous Connection

I. Connection to right atrium	15%
II. Connection to right common cardinal system	
A. (Right) superior vena cava	11%
B. Azygos vein	0%
III. Connection to left common cardinal system	
A. Left innominate vein	36%
B. Coronary sinus	16%
IV. Connection to umbilicovitelline system	
A. Portal vein	6%
B. Ductus venosus	4%
C. Inferior vena cava	2%
D. Hepatic vein	1%
Multiple sites	7%
Unknown	2%

From Burroughs JT, Edwards JE: Total anomalous pulmonary venous connection, *Am Heart J* 59:913, 1960, with permission.

a gene for a vascular endothelial growth factor has been mapped, suggesting that it might be a candidate gene for TAPVR in this kindred.[5]

ASSOCIATED DEFECTS

Approximately one third of patients with TAPVR have other associated major cardiac defects, usually in association with the heterotaxy syndromes, particularly asplenia.[21] Heinemann and colleagues[29] reported their experience with 38 consecutive newborns admitted with heterotaxy syndrome. Twenty-one (55%) had TAPVR, of whom only three had polysplenia and left atrial isomerism. Hashmi and associates[28] reported their 26-year experience with right atrial isomerism. Eighty-seven percent of patients had associated TAPVR, and 63% had single-ventricle physiology. Both atria have right atrial structure in this syndrome, and the pulmonary venous connections are usually via a single orifice to a morphologic right atrium or via a supracardiac connection. In left atrial isomerism, the association with TAPVR is much less pronounced, although partial anomalous pulmonary venous return (PAPVR) is common, with the usual pattern of venous return being for the right-sided pulmonary veins to connect to the right-sided atrium and the left-sided veins to the left-sided atrium.

PATHOPHYSIOLOGY

Patients with TAPVR have an obligatory left-to-right shunt from the pulmonary veins to the right heart and an obligatory right-to-left shunt from the right to the left atrium to maintain systemic output. A pathophysiologic spectrum is determined by the balance of the two main physiologic abnormalities, obstructed pulmonary venous return and increased PBF. In the extreme form of PVO, PBF is decreased, and severe pulmonary edema and pulmonary hypertension (PHT) are present. Significant right-to-left shunting at the atrial and ductal levels occurs. Hypoxemia will be severe because of decreased PBF as well as from pulmonary edema and intrapulmonary shunting. Cardiac output may be critically limited by the anatomic venous obstruction combined with restrictive ductal or foraminal shunting. The result is hemodynamic instability with hypotension, acidosis, and cardiac arrhythmias. These patients have a syndrome similar to severe persistent pulmonary hypertension of the newborn (PPHN), respiratory distress syndrome, or neonatal sepsis. Placement on extracorporeal membrane oxygenation (ECMO) to provide hemodynamic stability and multiple organ system resuscitation by reperfusion may be necessary before the diagnosis is made, although all such symptomatic patients should have a thorough echocardiographic assessment for TAPVR. Emergency surgical therapy to relieve obstruction is necessary. Although a moribund presentation requiring ECMO is unusual and accounts for only 2% to 4% of patients,[38,57] severe PVO requiring mechanical ventilation and inotropic agents for support occurs in approximately one third of infants.[3,7,38,57] Approximately half of these patients will have an infradiaphragmatic connection.[7,57]

The most common pathophysiologic form of TAPVR is a combination of PVO and increased PBF. The most common anatomic variants with this pathophysiology are supracardiac or infracardiac connections. The level of PBF is the most important determinant of the degree of arterial desaturation. As pulmonary vascular resistance decreases and right ventricular compliance increases postnatally, increasing amounts of the pulmonary venous blood entering the right atrium will enter the right ventricle, resulting in increased PBF. This situation results in increasing right ventricular volume overload. PBF may increase to 3 to 5 times normal[21] and may lead to symptoms and signs of congestive failure. An atrial level right-to-left shunt is obligatory to maintain cardiac output and systemic perfusion. Pulmonary artery pressure may range from being mildly elevated to systemic levels, depending on the degree of PVO. These patients require urgent correction in the neonatal or early infant period.

The final pathophysiologic group is those patients without any PVO. This pathophysiology is uncommon, occurring in less than 10% of patients and is often associated with connection to the coronary sinus. This group of patients is usually asymptomatic during infancy. Their mild arterial desaturation and cyanosis may go undetected. The marked increase in PBF will bring most of these patients to attention in later infancy or early childhood with the clinical features of a large secundum atrial septal defect (ASD). Rarely patients may remain undiagnosed until adulthood.[43]

PRESENTATION

History

The clinical presentation depends on the anatomic and pathophysiologic parameters noted earlier, particularly the degree of PVO and PBF and the nature of associated cardiac conditions. As noted, the most common form of TAPVR is the supracardiac variant, with a balance of PVO and increased PBF. Features of congestive heart failure, including tachypnea and failure to thrive, will be present during early infancy. The prominence of cyanosis will be dependent on the degree of PBF. Patients with a high grade of PVO (often with infracardiac connection) are first seen with severe cyanosis, tachypnea, and hemodynamic instability in the newborn period. As noted earlier, this severe form of TAPVR can be mistaken in the neonatal period for persistent fetal circulation, sepsis, or severe respiratory distress syndrome.[14] The severe degree of cyanosis and hemodynamic instability makes these conditions indistinguishable from one another. Rapid progression to profound metabolic acidosis, cardiac failure, and death may occur. Patients with no PVO usually are seen initially in later childhood and may mimic patients with a large secundum ASD.

Physical Examination

The physical manifestations of TAPVR vary with the degree of obstruction and PBF. Tachypnea is frequently present in association with the pulmonary overcirculation. With a high degree of PVO, frank respiratory distress may be present, secondary either to pulmonary edema or to metabolic acidosis associated with a critically diminished cardiac output. Tachycardia, poor peripheral perfusion, and hypotension are present to the extent that systemic cardiac output is compromised. The clinical cardiac examination reflects the degree of pulmonary artery hypertension. A hyperdynamic precordium and increased right ventricular (RV) impulse are frequently present. The pulmonic component of the second heart sound may be increased. Murmurs are not a prominent physical finding, but soft pulmonary outflow murmurs or murmurs of tricuspid insufficiency may be present. Patients without obstruction have physical findings similar to those of an ASD. A parasternal lift, a widely split second heart sound, a pulmonic flow murmur, and a diastolic rumble from tricuspid flow are seen. These patients may have mild tachypnea and arterial desaturation, but this may not be evident clinically.

DIAGNOSTIC ASSESSMENT

The findings on diagnostic assessment once again reflect the pathophysiology that is determined by the degree of PVO, the amount of PBF, and the nature of associated cardiac conditions.

In the presence of severe obstruction, the chest radiograph reveals a heart size that is usually normal, with lung fields that appear diffusely hazy and ground glass in appearance.[23] In patients with lesser degrees of PVO, the chest radiograph shows marked cardiomegaly with right atrial and RV enlargement and pulmonary overcirculation. In older infants and children with a supracardiac connection, the chest radiograph may have the appearance of a "figure eight" or "snowman."

The electrocardiogram shows signs of right atrial and RV pressure and volume overload. These include right-axis deviation, right atrial enlargement, and RV hypertrophy.

The differential diagnoses of these children can be grouped according to the child's age at presentation.[44] Patients with severe obstruction are first seen as neonates and will often be mistaken for having other more common severe illnesses of the newborn associated with acidosis and hypoxemia, including PPHN, sepsis with pneumonia, and hyaline membrane disease, leading to the recommendation that all such critically ill newborns require careful echocardiography to rule out structural heart disease, in particular, TAPVR. Cardiac lesions in the differential diagnosis include severe valvular obstructive lesions, coarctation of the aorta, hypoplastic left heart syndrome (HLHS), and other PVO lesions.[44] Gross cardiomegaly is usually present with aortic valve obstructive lesions and aortic arch obstructions. Pulmonary and tricuspid atresia usually have diminished pulmonary vascular markings on radiograph. HLHS patients also usually have cardiomegaly, as well as increased pulmonary arterial markings, although those with a restrictive ASD may have severe pulmonary edema similar to TAPVR patients. Functional PVO due to heart failure or mitral insufficiency is distinguishable by the presence of left ventricular hypertrophy or biventricular hypertrophy along with cardiomegaly. Mitral stenosis is distinguished by left atrial enlargement on radiograph and electrocardiogram (ECG). *Cor triatriatum* may require echocardiography to distinguish.

Neonates beyond the first few days and infants have varying degrees of hypoxemia as well as signs and symptoms of congestive heart failure. Structural heart disease in the differential diagnosis includes large ventricular septal defects (VSDs), atrioventricular canal defects, truncus arteriosus, single ventricle without pulmonary stenosis, and patent ductus arteriosus (PDA). These lesions are associated with both left atrial and left ventricular (LV) enlargement on radiograph and ECG.

Children and the rare patient first seen as an adult must be distinguished from patients with large ASDs of the primum or secundum type, from patients with common atrium, and from patients with PAPVR. Unlike those with these other lesions, they will usually have some mild degree of arterial desaturation. Primum ASD and common atrium have characteristic ECG findings. A secundum ASD and PAPVR may require echocardiography to distinguish.

The 2-D echocardiogram is the most important diagnostic tool for this lesion. The distinguishing echocardiographic features of TAPVR include RV diastolic volume overload, an absence of pulmonary venous connections to the left atrium, and identification of an alternate drainage site(s) of the pulmonary veins (Fig. 32-3).[59] Multiple reports have confirmed the sensitivity and specificity *in skilled hands* of echocardiography and Doppler techniques for the diagnosis of TAPVR.[13,26]

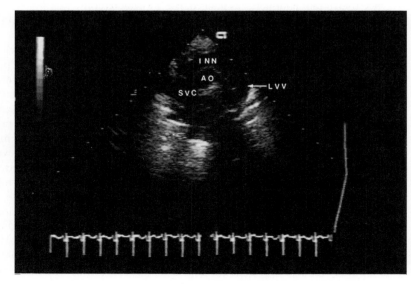

FIGURE 32-3 Echocardiogram of a supracardiac type of total anomalous pulmonary venous connection in a coronal view. Note the left vertical vein (LVV) draining into the innominate vein (INN). AO, aorta; SVC, superior vena cava.

Prenatal diagnosis also has been reported by Printz and Allan[48] and is becoming more common as the sophistication of prenatal ultrasonography has increased. Echo Doppler permits the accurate differentiation of TAPVR from PPHN and the other conditions that mimic it, although a high index of suspicion in this setting is mandatory to avoid a false-negative study.[60] Echo Doppler allows rapid discrimination between normal and abnormal pulmonary venous connections, both above and below the diaphragm, thus facilitating identification of the drainage site. Identification of this lesion is especially important in neonates who are critically ill. The accurate diagnosis of TAPVR usually obviates the need for cardiac catheterization and facilitates direct referral for total surgical correction.

The objectives of the echo Doppler examination in this defect are to (1) identify the pulmonary confluence and all the pulmonary veins; (2) completely trace the anomalous connections; (3) identify the site(s) of obstructed venous flow, by using pulsed and color flow Doppler; (4) identify the presence of other cardiac lesions; and (5) assess the atrial communication.[59] Multiple echocardiographic views are needed to identify the anatomic pathology in TAPVR. In all views, RV dilation may be noted.[50,58]

The position and size of the venous confluence varies with the type of TAPVR. In the supracardiac form, the confluence is superior to the left atrium. This structure is often best visualized from the suprasternal notch view in the short-axis plane, or from the subcostal view. In patients with connection to the coronary sinus, the venous confluence can be viewed from the parasternal long-axis, subxyphoid short-axis, and apical views. In the infracardiac type, the confluence is more inferior and is best viewed in the apical or subcostal views.[13] The confluence may be small in both the mixed and infracardiac types of TAPVR, and for this reason, these types are the most challenging to diagnose. In the single large series of patients with mixed-type TAPVR, Delius and coworkers[18] found that adequate echo Doppler characterization, defined as visualization of at least three pulmonary vein connections, was achieved in only 31% of patients. The current availability of transesophageal probes small enough for the neonate has improved the diagnostic accuracy of echo Doppler in this group.

Once the venous confluence is imaged, the anomalous connection must be traced to its drainage site.[8] The parasternal long- and short-axis views, as well as the apical view, may be used to trace the connection to the coronary sinus. The suprasternal short-axis view is particularly useful for tracing supracardiac drainage. The descending vein in an infracardiac connection can usually be imaged in the subcostal sagittal view anterior to the aorta. Pulsed and color flow Doppler are used to localize the direction and sites of obstruction to flow in the venous channels. In obstructed TAPVR, an abnormal high-velocity, nonphasic pulsed Doppler trace is often seen. Both imaging and Doppler techniques are used to assess the adequacy of the interatrial communication. The availability of transesophageal echo probes of small enough size to use in neonates further enhances the ability to assess the anatomy of TAPVR noninvasively.

With current echocardiographic techniques, it should be possible to define adequately the surgical anatomy in most patients with TAPVR and to avoid cardiac catheterization.[59]

Cardiac catheterization is reserved for patients in whom additional lesions must be further delineated and for those in whom mixed venous return is suspected and the venous-return channels are not satisfactorily defined. In TAPVR, the right atrium is a common mixing chamber. Saturations from the right atrium, left atrium, pulmonary artery, and systemic artery should be similar, although, because of streaming of blood flow along fetal patterns, in infracardiac TAPVR, the systemic arterial saturation may be higher than the pulmonary saturation, and the converse for the supracardiac defects. In infracardiac TAPVR, left atrial saturation may be as much as 15% higher than right atrial, and the finding of an elevated saturation in the portal system during umbilical vein catheterization is virtually diagnostic.[21]

Hemodynamic data will reflect the degree of PBF and PVO. With severe obstruction, systemic or suprasystemic right ventricular and pulmonary arterial pressures are present. Rarely right atrial pressures may be elevated, particularly in the presence of a restrictive atrial defect, and left atrial pressure may be low.

Angiography is used to define the anomalous venous connections. If the anomalous veins can be entered directly, angiography at this site will delineate the anatomy. If this is not possible, selective pulmonary artery angiography is used. Delay in transit of the contrast medium through the pulmonary circuit occurs when severe obstruction exists.

Magnetic resonance imaging (MRI) provides detailed anatomic information in congenital malformations and has particular advantages for imaging posterior structures such as anomalous pulmonary veins.[63] However, this technique is less advantageous than echocardiography for imaging in critically ill, mechanically ventilated infants. In more stable infants, MRI may be used to supplement information obtained by echo Doppler. MRI is particularly useful for delineating the complex systemic and pulmonary venous connections found in the heterotaxy syndromes as well as in mixed lesions when full delineation of anatomy has not been possible by echo Doppler.[62] This technique also has a role in the imaging of residual postoperative pulmonary vein or anastomotic stenosis.

PREOPERATIVE CRITICAL CARE MANAGEMENT

The level of preoperative support required will reflect the spectrum of pathophysiologic states that these patients have and that depend on the degree of PVO and PBF, and the nature of associated defects. Patients who have TAPVR with minimal or no venous obstruction are usually asymptomatic and do not require preoperative critical care management. Those with mild to moderate PVO and increased PBF are seen in early infancy with significant congestive heart failure and require stabilization with anticongestive measures that include diuretics, inotropic agents, and ventilatory support.

Those patients who have TAPVR with a high degree of obstruction are usually severely ill in the newborn period. Unless the child has been diagnosed prenatally, management strategies for severe PPHN will usually be in place before diagnosis. Effective interventions to stabilize these infants include mechanical ventilation with positive end expiratory pressure (PEEP), alkali therapy for metabolic acidosis, and inotropic support with agents such as dopamine, dobutamine, and epinephrine to support cardiac output and systemic perfusion. Induced alkalosis by hyperventilation and alkali therapy, hyperoxygenation with 100% FiO_2, and inhaled nitric oxide also may be in use as pulmonary vasodilators in this setting, which mimics PPHN before diagnosis. Consideration should be given to limiting their use once the diagnosis of severely obstructed TAPVR is made. Preoperative use of inhaled nitric oxide (iNO) has *not* been found to be helpful,[2] and any maneuvers that increase PBF may actually have a deleterious effect in these patients by increasing pulmonary edema. An infusion of prostaglandin E_1 may be initiated in selected patients with low cardiac output to provide systemic perfusion across the ductus arteriosus by providing right-to-left shunting to the systemic circulation. Caution is warranted, however, with prostaglandin E_1, as it improves systemic output at the expense of PBF and oxygenation. Although some reduction of pulmonary edema may be achieved with diuretic therapy, this should be used cautiously when venous obstruction is present, as a noncompliant RV may require a higher preload for optimal function.

When preoperative medical management has failed with progressive acidosis and severe hypoxemia, ECMO may be indicated to provide a period of stability (24 hours or more), in which the residual end-organ effects of metabolic acidosis, ischemia, and hypoxemia can improve.[31] Once stabilized, the patient is taken to the operating room while receiving ECMO[19] and then converted to standard cardiopulmonary bypass (CPB). After the procedure, and depending on the pulmonary artery pressures, the patient can be weaned off CPB and decannulated, and ECMO can be discontinued. In patients with pulmonary hypertension (PHT) and cardiac failure, ECMO may be resumed after CPB for a period of 1 or 2 days to provide additional support.[19] In this setting, iNO may be useful in reducing the need for ongoing ECMO support by controlling PHT.[25]

The timing of surgery for patients with severe obstruction is a matter of judgment. Although in general, emergency repair should be performed to minimize morbidity and mortality,[49] improved preoperative stabilization, including ECMO support, has contributed to the declining perioperative mortality in this group.

SURGICAL INTERVENTION

All patients with TAPVR, except some patients with associated single-ventricle physiology, require surgical correction of the pulmonary venous connection. The urgency with which this is performed is dictated by the anatomy, physiology, and clinical presentation, as discussed earlier. Patients with TAPVR and severe PVO require urgent surgical intervention. Patients with lesser degrees of PVO have pulmonary congestion and congestive heart failure, usually without low cardiac output and systemic acidosis, and can be dealt with in a nonemergent, but still urgent, fashion.

Treatment first requires precise delineation of the pulmonary venous drainage, as discussed earlier. Although echo Doppler usually accurately depicts the anatomy, cardiac catheterization may be necessary if unusual anatomy is found. In addition, it is important for the surgeon to confirm the drainage of all four pulmonary veins at the time of operation.

The surgical principles at the core of correction include (1) CPB for all patients, (2) single-stage repair, (3) establishment of the largest anastomosis between the common venous trunk and the left atrium possible without creating displacement of the heart by using a side-to-side technique, and (4) obliteration of the abnormal pulmonary venous connections to the systemic circulation.[27]

CPB is established by using standard techniques.[7,38,57] Aortic cross-clamping and cardioplegia are universally used. Deep hypothermic circulatory arrest (DHCA) is still commonly used but is no longer universally so.[25,57] Reported average bypass times have ranged from 46 to 85 minutes, cross-clamp times from 32 to 33 minutes, and DHCA times from 26 to 49 minutes.[14,38,57] Bypass and operative times are typically longer in infants with mixed-type lesions and when a low-flow bypass technique is used instead of DHCA.

A number of surgical approaches to these lesions have been described. After median sternotomy, the supracardiac defects are either approached from the right, rotating the heart to gain access to the venous confluence and the posterior wall of the left atrium,[7,30,57] or via a supracardiac[38,39,55] approach, in which aorta and SVC are mobilized and retracted laterally, allowing exposure of the posterior structures for creation of the anastomosis and ligation of the ascending vein (Fig. 32-4). Alternatively, many infracardiac defects can be exposed by dissection of the SVC and the inferior vena cava (IVC) such that the heart can be rolled toward the left chest, thus rotating the posterior left atrium on top of the descending vein. Infracardiac defects require superior rotation of the cardiac apex to expose the venous confluence. The descending vein is ligated and can be divided to reduce traction on the anastomosis (although division of the vein is usually not necessary and may complicate the repair by increasing the likelihood of twisting and distortion), which is created between the posterior left atrial wall and the venous confluence (Fig. 32-5). Intracardiac defects require enlargement of the ASD and baffling of pulmonary venous drainage to the ASD. Finally, for patients with return to the coronary sinus (CS), unroofing of the CS (Fig. 32-6) is usually the preferred procedure. An intra-atrial baffle with pericardium or Gore-Tex is then created that channels the CS flow through the ASD into the left atrium. In cases of anomalous return to the CS with obstruction, the supracardiac approach described earlier is preferred, as the level of obstruction is usually at the point of insertion of the common venous trunk into the CS, and unroofing alone would leave this obstruction uncorrected.[17] Mayer[39] recommended the superior approach for the majority of patients with return to the CS, even if no obstruction is identified. This has the advantage of eliminating the obligatory right-to-left shunt created by channeling the normal CS flow to the left atrium.

The surgical approach to mixed-type TAPVR is determined by the anatomy with which the surgeon is presented. As noted, these lesions in general can be grouped into two categories, depending on the segregation of the pulmonary veins. In patients in whom three of the veins segregate together, usually an adequate common pulmonary vein exists to establish a wide anastomosis between this and the left atrium.[18] Management of the remaining pulmonary vein has generated some controversy. If the vein is obstructed, repair or occasionally lobectomy is undertaken. If the vein

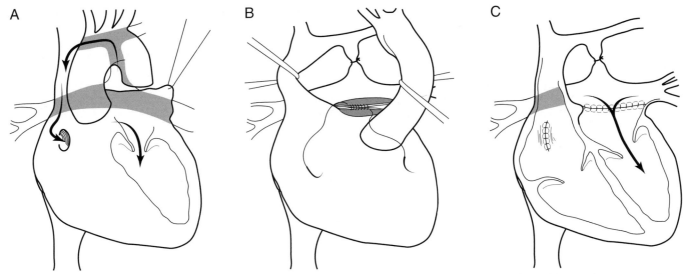

FIGURE 32-4   Technique of repair of supracardiac connection. **A,** Anatomy of supracardiac connection. **B,** Traction of an atrial appendage, aorta, and superior vena cava permit venoatrial repair from a superior, extracardiac approach. **C,** The completed repair. (Reproduced from Lupinetti et al: Correction of total anomalous pulmonary venous connection in infancy. *J Thorac Cardiovasc Surg* 106:880–885, 1993, with permission.)

is unobstructed, the vein is usually left unrepaired, as a single, uncorrected, anomalous pulmonary vein has an excellent prognosis, and achieving a connection between this vein and the left atrium can be difficult. Some caution with this approach may be appropriate, as isolated reports have cited the development of pulmonary vascular disease in patients with a single anomalous pulmonary venous connection.[18]

Patients in whom the pulmonary veins segregate in a 2 + 2 pattern may be more difficult to repair. The right-sided connections are approached by using standard techniques for right-sided partially anomalous venous connection. The left-sided veins are often anastomosed to the left atrial appendage after resection of any potentially obstructing atrial trabeculae.[18] The long-term functional outcome of this approach remains in question, as the possibility exists of stenosis of the relatively muscular orifice.[18]

In patients with functional univentricular anatomy, urgent surgical intervention is needed only to relieve PVO. In patients with an extracardiac connection without PVO, pulmonary vein repair is usually required as part of the staged Fontan palliation.[40] Repair is usually performed at the time that a bidirectional cavopulmonary shunt is performed to lessen the amount of surgery required at the time of Fontan palliation.[41] In patients with an intracardiac connection without obstruction, repair of the venous connection is indicated only if the creation of an intra-atrial conduit will lead to obstruction of the pulmonary venous return.

Postoperative Pulmonary Venous Obstruction

The most significant postoperative complication requiring surgical intervention is the development of postoperative PVO.

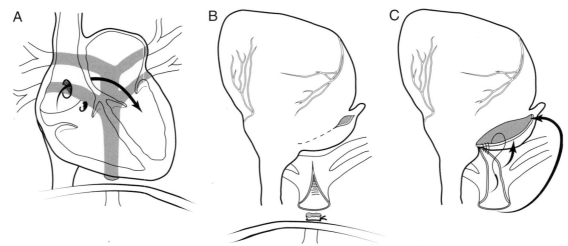

FIGURE 32-5   Technique of repair of infracardiac connection. **A,** Anatomy of infracardiac connection. **B,** Venous confluence is ligated, divided, and longitudinally incised. **C,** Venoatrial anastomosis is performed by aligning the superior end of confluence with the base of left atriotomy. (Reproduced from Lupinetti et al: Correction of total anomalous pulmonary venous connection in infancy. *J Thorac Cardiovasc Surg* 106:880–885, 1993, with permission.)

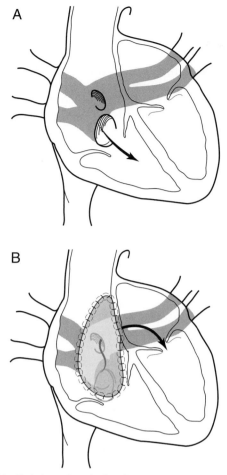

FIGURE 32-6 Technique of repair of cardiac connection to the coronary sinus. **A,** Roof of coronary sinus is incised to allow unrestricted flow between sinus and left atrium. **B,** Redundant patch is used to close interatrial communication and direct all coronary sinus flow into left atrium. (Reproduced from Lupinetti et al: Correction of total anomalous pulmonary venous connection in infancy. *J Thorac Cardiovasc Surg* 106:880–885, 1993, with permission.)

The frequency of this complication ranges from 2.4% to 13.6%.[3,30,33,34] If it occurs in the immediate postoperative period, it usually indicates a technical problem with the original repair, such as torsion or kinking of the anastomosis, and requires immediate repeated repair.

The development of delayed postoperative PVO is the most significant long-term complication. Success rates at reintervention and reoperation are variable and reflect the small numbers of patients being reported on. Moreover, the nature of the pathologic process seems variable, with discrete anastomotic stenosis developing in some patients and diffuse pulmonary vein stenosis with intimal hyperplasia in others. Management of patients with diffuse stenosis has been problematic, as reflected by the relatively low success rates, whereas patients with areas of discrete stenosis are usually amenable to successful repair.

Hyde and associates[30] reported on 12 patients (13.6% of their series on TAPVR) in whom postoperative PVO developed. These patients underwent a total of 18 (1.5 per patient) recatheterizations, including four stents and 23 (1.9 per patient) reoperations to relieve the stenosis. Seven of the patients were alive at the time of the report, but only two

were thriving with no residual obstruction. In a series from Bando and colleagues,[3] 12 (11%) of 105 patients were found to have postoperative PVO. Five patients were early deaths and were found to have small pulmonary venous confluence and diffuse pulmonary vein stenosis at autopsy. Seven patients were reoperated on. Three of these patients died, of whom two had diffuse pulmonary vein stenosis. Those who survived reoperation all had localized stenosis. Lacour-Gayet[34] reported on a larger series of 178 patients operated on for correction of TAPVR, in whom PVO was diagnosed in 16 (8.9%) between 5 weeks and 12 years after operation. All these patients had been shown to have no obstruction after initial repair by echo Doppler. Five (31%) of these patients died, one before reoperation. Only three of the group had isolated anastomotic stenosis, two of whom survived rerepair and were well 41 and 51 months after the report. The only patient with isolated anastomotic obstruction who died had single ventricle and heterotaxy and died of PHT intraoperatively. Nine of the 16 in their series had a mixture of anastomotic stenosis and pulmonary vein intimal hyperplasia. Those whose lesion was unilateral did well. If the lesions were bilateral or involving all four veins, the mortality rates were 57% and 100%, respectively. In general, if a discrete stenotic area at the anastomotic site is identified and accessible to reoperation, the outcome should be excellent. However, in some patients, an obliterative PVO disease develops with increased wall thickness and intimal hyperplasia in the distal pulmonary venous system,[22] and, especially if this is bilateral, they appear to be at higher risk for a poor outcome.

The time of occurrence of reobstruction is usually within the first few postoperative months but can be within the first few days to as late as years after repair and is diagnosed by clinical signs and echo Doppler. Turbulent flow at the anastomotic site as well as abnormal, high-velocity, nonphasic flow on Doppler are often diagnostic. These findings are usually confirmed with angiography.

The etiology of diffuse PVO is not well understood. This complication has been described at autopsy in single-ventricle patients who had no evidence of PVO, suggesting that diffuse PVO with intimal hyperplasia may be an associated primary process in some patients.[22] Evidence also exists that it may be related to the duration of the residual stenosis and has led to the recommendation of aggressive intervention for recurrent venous obstruction.[41] Finally, in some patients with recurrent PVO, a diminutive, abnormal pulmonary venous bed, by estimates from preoperative echo, has been identified, suggesting that overall size of the pulmonary venous bed also is a predictor of poor outcome.[32] The use of continuous, nonabsorbable sutures also has been implicated in the development of recurrent PVO, although Lacour-Gayet[34] challenged this.

In an attempt to address the poor prognosis in patients with progressive pulmonary vein stenosis, Lacour-Gayet,[34] as well as Calderone,[10] described a novel surgical approach termed by Lacour-Gayet *sutureless in situ pericardium repair*. This technique involves incision of the stenotic veins from the orifice to as far distally in the pulmonary vein as is accessible, followed by creation of a neoatrium by using native in situ pericardium. No sutures are placed in the incised pulmonary veins, which are left wide open and draining into the neoatrium. In the few patients described, some long-term success appears to have occurred with this technique.

Catheterization with balloon dilation or stent placement or both has not been found to have a high long-term success rate but may have a role in delaying the need for reoperation.[33]

POSTOPERATIVE CRITICAL CARE MANAGEMENT

The initial patient presentation and the operative indications predict the postoperative hemodynamic issues. Postoperative pulmonary artery hypertension is seen in as many as 45% of patients with isolated TAPVR.[1] Emergency operations performed in the neonatal period are often complicated postoperatively by persistent pulmonary hypertension (Fig. 32-7) and low cardiac output.

In many centers, continuous monitoring of pulmonary arterial and left atrial pressures as well as right atrial pressure has been found to be important in these patients for discerning the primary cause of low cardiac output and for guiding its management. Patients without preoperative PVO are at less risk of postoperative pulmonary hypertensive crisis.

In patients with hemodynamic instability after TAPVR repair, an echo Doppler is an important adjunct. The most important question to answer is whether any significant residual PVO exists at the level of the anastomosis or individual pulmonary veins. It also is an important tool in assessing ventricular function, in looking for any evidence of PHT such as septal flattening or displacement, and in determining the extent and significance of any pericardial fluid accumulation. Transthoracic imaging may be suboptimal in the immediate postoperative period. Transesophageal imaging allows excellent imaging of posterior structures and is thus highly useful for postoperative TAPVR in both the immediate and later postoperative course.

The most serious postoperative hemodynamic problem is a pulmonary hypertensive crisis, manifest as a relatively sudden development of a low-cardiac-output state with hypotension, hypoxemia, and acidosis. Pulmonary artery pressure may be elevated to suprasystemic levels. RV dysfunction ensues, which in turn can contribute to diminished LV function if deformation of the intraventricular septum occurs, leading to a vicious cycle of depressed cardiac function and PHT. Central venous pressure (CVP) increases, and mean arterial pressure decreases. To facilitate the rapid recognition of this condition, placement of a transthoracic pulmonary artery catheter is often recommended.

In anticipation of the risk of PHT, patients who have severe preoperative PVO are treated prophylactically with neuromuscular blocking drugs, high doses of fentanyl, and mild hyperventilation in the early postoperative period (Table 32-2). Stimuli that may trigger a pulmonary hypertensive crisis should be avoided, and even mild degrees of metabolic acidosis should be treated. Because of the possible deleterious impact of aggressive hyperventilation on cerebral perfusion, this should be avoided. The patient is weaned from neuromuscular blockade and analgesia if general hemodynamic and pulmonary artery pressure monitoring indicate stability.

Should evidence of PHT or pulmonary hypertensive crisis develop, the value of iNO has been clearly demonstrated. Atz and Wessel[2] reviewed their experience in 20 infants after repair of TAPVR. In 45%, pulmonary artery hypertension developed. These patients were treated with iNO at a dose of 80 parts per million (ppm) and showed a mean percentage decrease in pulmonary artery pressure of 32% (Fig. 32-8).[1]

Nitric oxide also has been found to be useful in the operating room for infants with severe PHT who cannot be weaned from CPB. Goldman and associates[25] reported their experience with a mixed group of patients, two of whom had TAPVR. Six of ten patients, including both patients with TAPVR who would otherwise have required a period of postoperative extracorporeal life support, received iNO at 20 ppm and were successfully weaned from CPB. In a separate study, this group looked at dose-response in postoperative patients with PHT, including two patients with TAPVR, and showed response with doses as low as 2 ppm (the lowest tested dose).[47]

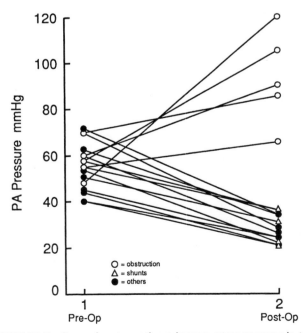

FIGURE 32-7 Pre- and postoperative pulmonary artery pressures in total anomalous pulmonary venous return (TAPVR). Note the persistent elevation of pulmonary artery pressure after repair in patients with an obstructive type of TAPVR. (From Lamb RK, Qureshi SA, Wilkenson JL: Total anomalous venous return. Seventeen-year surgical experience. *J Thorac Cardiovasc Surg* 96:368–375, 1988, with permission.)

Table 32-2   Guidelines for Postoperative Support in the High-Risk Patient

High-dose fentanyl sedation and neuromuscular blockade
Control metabolic acidosis
    Hyperventilation (PaCO$_2$, 30–35 mm Hg)
    Alkali therapy
    High FiO$_2$
Early echocardiography to assess for residual significant PVO
Inhaled nitric oxide (5–20 ppm)
Catecholamines: dobutamine, dopamine, epinephrine
Phosphodiesterase inhibitors: milrinone
Vasopressin (refractory vasodilatory hypotension)
ECMO

ECMO, extracorporeal membrane oxygenation; ppm, parts per million; PVO, pulmonary venous obstruction.

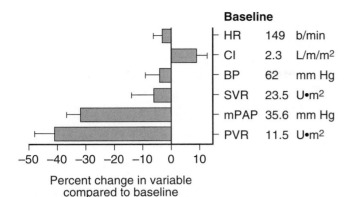

Baseline

HR	149	b/min
CI	2.3	L/m/m²
BP	62	mm Hg
SVR	23.5	U•m²
mPAP	35.6	mm Hg
PVR	11.5	U•m²

Percent change in variable
compared to baseline

FIGURE 32-8   Percentage change in hemodynamic variables from baseline during 15 minutes of nitric oxide at 80 ppm in nine patients with total anomalous pulmonary venous return. Marked specificity is present for the pulmonary circulation. (Reproduced from Atz AM, Wessel DL: Inhaled nitric oxide in the neonate with cardiac disease. *Semin Perinatol* 21:441–445, 1997, with permission.)

Despite a generally favorable response to postoperative iNO, some caution may be warranted, as at least one case report exists of recurrent pulmonary hypertensive crisis shortly after initiation of iNO that responded to discontinuing nitric oxide. The mechanism of deterioration in this case was unclear.[51] When an unfavorable response to iNO occurs, one should strongly suspect residual PVO. Any significant residual venous obstruction after repair contributes to persistent pulmonary artery hypertension and decreased cardiac output.

Although CPB time is usually of moderate length, averaging in one series 63 minutes, occasional cases have been found, especially those with mixed anatomy, that may require bypass times upward of 3 hours.[3] Prolonged bypass time will exacerbate the known deterioration in myocardial function that occurs in the first 12 to 24 hours after CPB. Other intraoperative factors such as the quality of myocardial preservation and the length of any circulatory arrest time also can be significant contributors to postoperative depression of myocardial function. Inotropic support is commonly necessary for the first 24 to 48 hours for recovery of myocardial function, despite evidence of a technically satisfactory repair. With appropriate support, these patients should quickly recover normal function. In our institution, both dobutamine, infused at 3 to 10 mcg/kg/min, and dopamine, infused at 5 to 15 mcg/kg/min, are commonly used. Epinephrine at doses between 0.03 and 0.15 mcg/kg/min also is effective.

Should patients fail to respond to the outlined regimen for control of PHT and for inotropic support, we have found the phosphodiesterase type III inhibitor milrinone to be very useful. Little direct evidence exists of its effectiveness in TAPVR, but it has been shown to improve cardiac output and reduce pulmonary vascular resistance in studies of children with both congenital heart disease[11] and septic shock.[4] Current dosing guidelines follow those developed for the adult of a 50-mcg/kg load followed by a continuous infusion of 0.5 mcg/kg/min. Some evidence indicates that higher doses may be beneficial in children.[36] Its chief limitation is hypotension, and careful monitoring and support of preload is essential when administering milrinone to minimize this.

Vasopressin has been found to be deficient in some adult patients with postoperative shock or post-CPB vasodilatory shock.[12] In these patients, it produces a non–catecholamine-mediated elevation in systemic vascular resistance and mean arterial pressure without depressing cardiac output and with little effect on pulmonary vascular tone. In patients with refractory vasodilatory shock as well as in patients experiencing volume refractory hypotension with milrinone, we have found a vasopressin infusion to be useful starting at a dose of 0.5 mU/kg/min[24,52] and titrating upward to as much as 1.5 mU/kg/min to achieve the desired effect.

In selected cases in which severely depressed cardiac function or severe PHT or both fails to respond adequately to these measures, a period of ECMO support may be required postoperatively for several days to allow recovery. The period of support required may be lengthened by concomitant severe pulmonary edema in these patients.

Supraventricular dysrhythmias occur after repair of TAPVR in approximately 5% to 10% of cases.[54] Atrial flutter or fibrillation may be treated with cardioversion, followed by the use of digoxin. Re-entrant supraventricular tachycardia is treated as an emergency with cardioversion, with atrial overdrive pacing, or with intravenous adenosine. Junctional tachycardias can be treated with overdrive pacing and systemic cooling. If this is unsuccessful, amiodarone has replaced procainamide as the drug of choice to treat junctional ectopic tachycardia, when ventricular pacing wires are in place.

OUTCOME

When left uncorrected, TAPVR carries a high morbidity and mortality rate in the first year of life. Mustard[45] reported the first large surgical series in 1962. He reported a two-stage technique with an overall mortality rate of 51%. Cooley[15] reported shortly thereafter his results by using a one-stage technique with CPB for all patients. Their overall mortality was 39%, and if patients with mixed lesions were excluded, it was 33%. Whereas mortality was high, this report established many of the surgical principles noted earlier that remain at the core of the current approach to surgical correction. Surgical results have continued to improve since the 1960s. In the current era, in the absence of residual or recurrent venous obstruction (postoperative pulmonary venous obstruction) or of complex associated cardiac lesions, the long-term outlook is excellent.

Recent studies reporting outcome are summarized in Table 32-3. Overall mortality ranges from 4.9% to 15.9%, with most of the mortality occurring before mid-1980. Mortality has clearly decreased dramatically in the last 10 to 15 years. Factors implicated in the risk of poor outcome for children with TAPVR after repair in the past have included infracardiac connection, poor preoperative state, persistent acidosis, severe hypoxemia, PVO, delayed operation, small interatrial defect size, pulmonary artery hypertension, and small left heart volume.[35,56] Bando[3] suggested that currently the impact of any preoperative factor other than small pulmonary vein confluence or diffuse pulmonary stenosis has been minimized, although pulmonary arterial and venous hypertension along with postoperative pulmonary hypertensive crisis continue to be significant contributors to early mortality (see Table 32-3). Bando[3] and Sinzobahamvya[57] reported no deaths since the late 1980s in a total of 69 cases. Both of these series excluded

Table 32-3 Surgical Outcome: Isolated TAPVR

Author/ Institution	Series Dates	Total/ Obstructed/ Deaths, (% Deaths)	Supracardiac/ Obstructed/ Deaths	Cardiac/ Obstructed/ Deaths	Infracardiac/ Obstructed/ Deaths	Mixed/ Obstructed/ Deaths	Comments
			TAPVR CHARACTERISTICS				
Lupinetti[38] Mott Children's Hosp, Michigan	1985–1993	41/25/2 (4.9%)	19/10*/1 (*8 severe)	9/4*/0 (*3 severe)	11/11*/1 (*Presumed)	2/1/0	Pulmonary venous obstruction (PVO) postop 1;
Sinzobahamvya[57] Johanniter Kinderkilinik, Sankt-Augustin, Germany	1977–1994	71/45/8 (11.3%)	32/23/NS	17/11/NS	17/11/NS	5/0	Preop: 54 decompensated heart failure, 3 moribund (all died); Postop: Pulmonary hypertensive Crisis (PHC), 27; PVO, 5; 2 reops both died No perioperative deaths last 38 patients (after 1987)
Bando[3] Riley Children's, Indianapolis	1965–1995	105/NS/13 (12.4%)	47/NS/5	27/NS/0	22/NS/3	9/NS/4	Early deaths 10: PHC, 5/10, ventricular failure, 10/10 Autopsy: 8, 5/8 diffuse pulm vein stenosis Late deaths: 2/3 with diffuse PVO No deaths last 31 patients (after 1990)
Hyde[30] Birmingham Children's Hospital, U.K.	1988–1997	88/31/11 (12.5%)	43/12/4	17/0/2	20/17/4	8/2/1	Postop: PVO, 12; deaths, 4; PVO subtypes, intrinsic venous sclerosis, extrinsic anastomotic site obstruction
Bogers[7] Erasmus Medical Center, Rotterdam, The Netherlands	1973–1998	44/15/7 (15.9%)	15/NS/1	10/NS/0	19/NS/6	0	3 deaths last 29 patients (after 1988), postop PVO, 2 patients
Delius[18] Great Ormond St., London, U.K.	1971–1994 Mixed TAPVR only	232 total TAPVR, 20 mixed, 3 obst, 5 deaths (25%)	Cath. 12/20,	Mortality: periop, 3; late, 2	Post op PVO, 1 (died)		3 patients, left upper lobe PVO uncorrected, 3 patients with preop obst died periop

NS, not seen; TAPVR, total anomalous pulmonary venous return.

single-ventricle patients from analysis. The decline in mortality has been attributed to improved pre- and postoperative care, especially with regard to the prevention and management of pulmonary hypertensive crisis and to improved surgical technique. Prophylactic management, as outlined in the section on postoperative critical care (see Table 32-3), has been shown to improve this situation.[49]

Outcome in patients with mixed-type TAPVR has not been well addressed previously, as the lesion frequency is low. Delius[18] reported his results with this lesion in the 232 patients with all types of TAPVR cared for at his institution between 1971 and 1994. He identified 20 (8.6%) patients with mixed-type TAPVR. Three patients had severe preoperative PVO and died after operation. Two additional late deaths occurred, for a mortality rate of 25%. Although it appears that mortality may be higher in this group, the effect of improving surgical and perioperative support techniques over time was not addressed.

Long-term functional status in patients with isolated TAPVR appears to be excellent as well. Most series have reported these patients to be growing normally and to be asymptomatic. Paridon[47] reported the only study of exercise tolerance in this group. He studied nine patients at an average of 10 postoperative years (range, 5 to 18 years), in whom he documented small diminutions in aerobic exercise capacity, chronotropic response, and lung volume, although all patients were asymptomatic.

However, patients with heterotaxy or single ventricle or both associated with TAPVR require specific discussion, as the impact of TAPVR on the outcome of these patients may be significant. When the Fontan procedure was initially described as palliation for single ventricle, anomalies of the pulmonary veins were thought to be a contraindication to repair. Although these anomalies are no longer a contraindication, some series of staged repair of these patients report a very high mortality rate,[22,28] whereas other series suggest that either little specific impact of the venous anomaly is seen on outcome[29,41] or only PVO influences mortality.[40,61] Recent studies reporting experience in this area are summarized in Table 32-4. Gaynor[22] reported on a group of 73 patients with functional single ventricle and TAPVR. The outcome was poor for the group as a whole and particularly poor if repair of TAPVR, usually for PVO, along with aortopulmonary shunt, was required at initial palliation. Overall mortality was 63% at 1 year and 81% at 5 years. Sixteen percent died preoperatively, and 38% died perioperatively. Hashmi[28] reported his experience over a 26-year period with a series of 91 patients with right atrial isomerism. Overall mortality was 69%. Seventy-seven (85%) of the patients had TAPVR. Surgical mortality for pulmonary vein repair was 95%, and, although

Table 32-4 Surgical Outcome in Patients with Heterotaxy and Single Ventricle

Author/Institution	Series Dates	Patient Population Analyzed	Total Patients/ TAPVR Patients/Obstructed	Mortality	Comments
Heinemann,[29] Children's Hospital, Boston, Massachusetts	1981–1991	Patients with visceral heterotaxy and congenital heart disease	38 newborns with heterotaxy/ 21 TAPVR/12 Obst TAPVR	Overall 10/38 died (26%) TAPVR group. 6/21 (29%) TAPVR to systemic vein, 5/18 (27%) Nonobst, 1/6 (17%) Obst, 4/12 (33%)	No statistically significant difference in mortality between group as a whole and group with TAPVR to a systemic vein
McElhinney,[41] Univ of California, San Francisco, California	1990–1995	Bidirectional cavopulmonary shunt (BCPS) and systemic or pulmonary venous anomalies (ven anom)	117 BCPS Ven anom, 36/117; TAPVR, 11/117; Obst TAPVR, 2	Overall, 22/117 died (19%) at 3 years Ven anom, 6/36 (17%) TAPVR, 3/11 (27%)	No significant difference in actuarial survival between groups with or without venous anomalies Statistical analysis of TAPVR subgroup not done
Hashmi,[28] Hospital for Sick Children, Toronto, Ontario, Canada	1970–1996	Outcome of patients with right atrial isomerism (RAI)	91 with RAI/77 with TAPVR/ 25 obst TAPVR	Overall, 63/91 died (69%) TAPVR repair required (14 for PVO), 19/20 (95%)	Association of RAI and TAPVR requiring repair has high mortality with no improvement after 1990
McElhinney,[40] Univ of California, San Francisco, California	1990–1997	Anomalous pulmonary venous return and single-ventricle palliation	32 patients, combined TAPVC and PAPVR	Neonatal palliation, 5/25 died (20%), all had obst TAPVR BCPS, 3/21 (14%), 2 TAPVR, unobst Fontan, 1/7 (14%), TAPVR, obst	TAPVR not separately analyzed from PAPVR, but TAPVR with obstruction thought to be a significant risk factor
Gaynor,[22] Children's Hospital of Philadelphia, Pennsylvania	1984–1997	Single-ventricle patients with TAPVR	73 TAPVR-SV 21 obst TAPVR, heterotaxy, 52	Overall mortality, 61/72 (85%) TAPVR repair required, 24/31 (77%): early, 18; late, 6 with postop PVO; completed Fontan, 10/19 (53%)	Pulmonary pathology: 14 patients, 6 with and 8 without PVO, all had "arterialization" of vein walls

Obst, obstructed; unobst, unobstructed; ven anom, pulmonary venous anomalies; TAPVR, total anomalous pulmonary venous return.

it was not addressed specifically, Hashmi and colleagues concluded that those with TAPVR had "uniformly poor outcomes."

In contrast to these two reports are the series of Heineman[29] and McElhinney.[41] Heineman[29] reported a series of 38 patients with heterotaxy requiring primary palliation for congenital heart disease in the neonatal period. Twenty-one patients had TAPVR, 12 of whom had PVO. The overall mortality rate in the TAPVR group was 29% (6 of 21), and in the obstructed TAPVR group, 33% (4 of 12), little different from the overall mortality in the overall heterotaxy group of 26% (10 of 38). McElhinney[41] reported a series of 117 patients with systemic and pulmonary venous anomalies requiring bidirectional cavopulmonary shunt (BCPS), of whom 11 had TAPVR, 2 with obstruction. Although a TAPVR subgroup was not separately analyzed, early (30-day) mortality in the group of 117 patients was 4.3%, and in the venous anomaly group, it was 5.6%, not significantly different. Moreover, patients were followed up for a mean of 20 months (range, 1 to 47 months), and no significant difference in actuarial survival could be detected between groups with or without systemic or pulmonary venous anomalies.

In both of these reports, statistical analysis comparing TAPVR patients with those without TAPVR was not performed. Nevertheless, whereas the mortality rates may be somewhat higher in the TAPVR groups, outcome appears to be more favorable than that in the reports by Gaynor[22] and Hashmi.[28] The explanation for the differences in outcome in the four series is not clear but may be related to institutional practices, variations in the patient population not presented by the authors, or improvements in management in more recent periods.

McElhinney and Reddy[40] subsequently reported on outcome for a group of 32 patients with functional single ventricle and anomalies of the pulmonary veins (both PAPVR and TAPVR). In the neonatal palliation group, 5 of 25 died, all patients who had obstructed TAPVR. This is similar to our own experience over the last 5-year period with 16 patients with TAPVR and complex intracardiac anatomy requiring single-ventricle palliation.[61] All deaths occurred in the group with PVO, reinforcing this as a major risk factor for death.

In conclusion, accurate, noninvasive diagnosis of TAPVR by means of echo Doppler combined with aggressive preoperative cardiovascular stabilization and an early, expedient one-stage repair can improve the postoperative outcome. Postoperative morbidity in these patients is frequently associated with pulmonary artery and venous hypertension but is manageable with aggressive medical treatment. For most patients with isolated TAPVR, correction in the newborn period is associated with low initial mortality and an excellent long-term outcome. The development of postoperative diffuse pulmonary vein stenosis with intimal hyperplasia is the most serious long-term complication. For patients with heterotaxy syndrome and single ventricle, improvement in the management of single-ventricle physiology has led to improvement in outcome as well, although in this group, the presence of PVO remains a serious threat. Understanding the risk factors for development of recurrent PVO, especially the diffuse form, and the mechanisms responsible for its progression, as well as improving the surgical techniques for its management, remain important challenges for the future.

References

1. Atz AM, Adatia I, Wessel DL: Rebound pulmonary hypertension after inhalation of nitric oxide. *Ann Thorac Surg* 62:1759–1764, 1996.
2. Atz AM, Wessel DL: Inhaled nitric oxide in the neonate with cardiac disease. *Semin Perinatol* 21:441–455, 1997.
3. Bando K, Turrentine MW, Ensing GJ, et al: Surgical management of total anomalous pulmonary venous connection: Thirty-year trends. *Circulation* 94(suppl II):II12–II16, 1996.
4. Barton P, Garcia J, Kouatli A, et al: Hemodynamic effects of I.V. milrinone lactate in pediatric patients with septic shock: A prospective, double-blind, randomized, placebo-controlled, interventional study. *Chest* 109:1302–1312, 1996.
5. Bleyl S, Nelson L, Odelberg SJ, et al: A gene for familial total anomalous pulmonary venous return maps to chromosome 4p13-q12. *Am J Hum Genet* 56:408–415, 1995.
6. Bleyl S, Ruttenberg HD, Carey JC, Ward K: Familial total anomalous pulmonary venous return: A large Utah-Idaho family. *Am J Med Genet* 52:462–466, 1994.
7. Bogers AJJC, Baak R, Lee PC, et al: Early results and long-term follow-up after corrective surgery for total anomalous pulmonary venous return. *Eur J Cardiothorac Surg* 16:296–299, 1999.
8. Brown VE, De Lange M, Dyar DA, et al: Echocardiographic spectrum of supracardiac total anomalous pulmonary venous connection. *J Am Soc Echocardiogr* 11:289–293, 1998.
9. Burroughs JT, Edwards JE: Total anomalous pulmonary venous connection. *Am Heart J* 59:913, 1960.
10. Calderone AC, Najm HK, Kadletz M, et al: Relentless pulmonary vein stenosis after repair of total anomalous pulmonary venous drainage. *Ann Thorac Surg* 66:1514–1520, 1998.
11. Chang AC, Atz AM, Wernovsky G, et al: Milrinone: Systemic and pulmonary hemodynamic effects in neonates after cardiac surgery. *Crit Care Med* 23:1907–1914, 1995.
12. Chen JM, Cullinane S, Spanier TB, et al: Vasopressin deficiency and pressor hypersensitivity in hemodynamically unstable organ donors. *Circulation* 100(suppl II):II244–II246, 1999.
13. Chin AJ, Sanders SP, Sherman F, et al: Accuracy of subcostal two-dimensional echocardiography in prospective diagnosis of total anomalous pulmonary venous connection. *Am Health J* 113:1153–1159, 1987.
14. Cobanoglu A, Menashe VD: Total anomalous pulmonary venous connection in neonates and young infants: Repair in the current era. *Ann Thorac Surg* 55:43–48, 1993.
15. Cooley DA, Hallman GL, Leachman RD: Total anomalous pulmonary venous drainage: Correction with the use of cardiopulmonary bypass in 62 cases. *J Cardiol Vasc Surg* 51:88–101, 1966.
16. Darling RC, Rothney WB, Craig IM: Total pulmonary venous drainage into the right side of the heart. *Lab Invest* 6:44–50, 1957.
17. DeLeon MM, DeLeon SY, Roughneen PT, et al: Recognition and management of obstructed pulmonary veins draining to the coronary sinus. *Ann Thorac Surg* 63:741–745, 1997.
18. Delius RE, de Leval MR, Elliot MJ, Stark J: Mixed total pulmonary venous drainage: Still a surgical challenge. *J Thorac Cardiovasc Surg* 112:1581–1588, 1996.
19. Dudell GG, Evans ML, Krous HF, et al: Common pulmonary vein atresia: The role of extracorporeal membrane oxygenation. *Pediatrics* 91:403–410, 1993.
20. Edwards JE: Pathologic and developmental considerations in anomalous venous connection. *Mayo Clin Proc* 28:441–452, 1953.
21. Fyler DC: Total anomalous pulmonary venous return. In Fyler DC (ed): *Nadas' Pediatric Cardiology*. Philadelphia, Hanley & Belfus, 1992, pp 683–691.
22. Gaynor WJ, Collins MH, Rychik J, et al: Long-term outcome of infants with single ventricle and total anomalous pulmonary venous connection. *J Thorac Cardiovasc Surg* 117:506–514, 1999.
23. Genz T, Locher D, Genz S, et al: Chest x-ray film patterns in children with isolated total anomalous pulmonary vein connection. *Eur J Pediatr* 150:14–18, 1990.
24. Gold JA, Cullinane S, Chen J, et al: Vasopressin as an alternative to norepinephrine in the treatment of milrinone-induced hypotension. *Crit Care Med* 28:249–252, 2000.
25. Goldman AP, Delius RE, Deanfield JE, et al: Nitric oxide might reduce the need for extracorporeal support in children with critical postoperative pulmonary hypertension. *Ann Thorac Surg* 62:750–755, 1996.

26. Goswami KC, Shrivastava S, Saxena A, Dev V: Echocardiographic diagnosis of total anomalous pulmonary venous connection. *Am Heart J* 126:433–440, 1993.
27. Hammon JW: Total anomalous pulmonary venous connection: Then and now. *Ann Thorac Surg* 55:1030–1032, 1993.
28. Hashmi A, Abu-Sulaman R, McCrindle BW, et al: Management and outcomes of right atrial isomerism: A 26-year experience. *J Am Coll Cardiol* 31:1120–1126, 1998.
29. Heinemann MK, Hanley FL, Van Praagh S, et al: Total anomalous pulmonary venous drainage in newborns with visceral heterotaxy. *Ann Thorac Surg* 57:88–91, 1994.
30. Hyde JAJ, Stümper O, Barth MJ, et al: Total anomalous pulmonary venous return: Outcome of surgical correction and management of recurrent venous obstruction. *Eur J Cardiothorac Surg* 15:735–741, 1999.
31. Ishino K, Alexi-Meskishvili V, Hetzer R: Preoperative extracorporeal membrane oxygenation in newborns with total anomalous pulmonary venous connection. *Cardiovasc Surg* 7:473–475, 1999.
32. Jenkins KJ, Sanders SP, Orav EJ, et al: Individual pulmonary vein size and survival in infants with totally anomalous pulmonary venous connection. *J Am Coll Cardiol* 22:201–206, 1993.
33. Jonas RA, Smolinsky A, Mayer JE, Castaneda AR: Obstructed pulmonary venous drainage with total anomalous pulmonary venous connection to the coronary sinus. *Am J Cardiol* 59:431–435, 1987.
34. Lacour-Gayet F, Zoghbi J, Serraf AE, et al: Surgical management of progressive pulmonary venous obstruction after repair of total anomalous pulmonary venous connection. *J Thorac Cardiovasc Surg* 117:679–687, 1999.
35. Lincoln CR, Rigby ML, Mercanti C, et al: Surgical risk factors in total anomalous pulmonary venous connection. *Am J Cardiol* 61:608–611, 1988.
36. Lindsay CA, Barton P, Lawless S, et al: Pharmacokinetics and pharmacodynamics of milrinone lactate in pediatric patients with septic shock. *J Pediatr* 132:329–334, 1998.
37. Lucas RV Jr, Lock JE, Tandon R, Edwards JE: Gross and histologic anatomy of total anomalous pulmonary venous connections. *Am J Cardiol* 62:292–300, 1988.
38. Lupinetti FM, Kulik TJ, Beekman RH III, et al: Correction of total anomalous pulmonary venous connection in infancy. *J Thorac Cardiovasc Surg* 106:880–885, 1993.
39. Mayer JE: Invited commentary. *Ann Thorac Surg* 63:741–745, 1997.
40. McElhinney DB, Reddy VM: Anomalous pulmonary venous return in the staged palliation of functional univentricular heart defects. *Ann Thorac Surg* 66:683–687, 1998.
41. McElhinney DB, Reddy VM, Moore P, Hanley FL: Bi-directional cavopulmonary shunt in patients with anomalies of systemic and pulmonary venous drainage. *Ann Thorac Surg* 63:1676–1684, 1997.
42. Miller OI, Celermajer DS, Deanfield JE, Macrae DJ: Very-low-dose inhaled nitric oxide: A selective pulmonary vasodilator after operations for congenital heart disease. *J Thorac Cardiovasc Surg* 108:487–494, 1994.
43. Misumi K, Berdjis F, Leung C, et al: Adult patient with total anomalous pulmonary venous return undergoing successful pregnancy. *Am Heart J* 128:412–414, 1994.
44. Moss AJ, Adams FH: *Heart Disease in Infants, Children, and Adolescents.* Baltimore, Williams & Wilkins, 1989, pp 595–596.
45. Mustard WT, Keith JD, Trusler GA: Two-stage correction for total anomalous pulmonary venous drainage in childhood. *J Thorac Cardiovasc Surg* 44:477–485, 1962.
46. Neill CA: Development of the pulmonary veins: With reference to the embryology of anomalies of pulmonary venous return. *Pediatrics* 18:880–887, 1956.
47. Paridon SM, Sullivan NM, Schneider J, Pinsky WW: Cardiopulmonary performance at rest and exercise after repair of total anomalous pulmonary venous connection. *Am J Cardiol* 72:1444–1447, 1993.
48. Printz BF, Allan LD: Abnormal pulmonary venous return diagnosed prenatally by pulsed Doppler flow imaging. *Ultrasound Obstet Gynecol* 9:347–349, 1997.
49. Raisher BD, Grant JW, Martin TC, et al: Complete repair of total anomalous pulmonary venous connection in infancy. *J Thorac Cardiovasc Surg* 104:443–448, 1992.
50. Romero-Cardenas A, Vargas-Barron J, Rylaarsdam N, et al: Total anomalous pulmonary venous return: Diagnosis by transesophageal echocardiography. *Am Heart J* 121:1831–1834, 1991.
51. Rosales AM, Bolivar J, Burke RP, Chang AC: Adverse hemodynamic effects observed with inhaled nitric oxide after surgical repair of total anomalous pulmonary venous return. *Pediatr Cardiol* 20:224–226, 1999.
52. Rosenzweig EB, Starc TJ, Chen JM, et al: Intravenous arginine-vasopressin in children with vasodilatory shock after cardiac surgery. *Circulation* 100(suppl II):II182–II186, 1999.
53. Rubino M, Van Praagh S, Kadoba K, et al: Systemic and pulmonary venous connections in visceral heterotaxy with asplenia: Diagnostic and surgical considerations based on seventy-two autopsied cases. *J Thorac Cardiovasc Surg* 110:641–650, 1995.
54. Saxena A, Fong LV, Lamb RK, et al: Cardiac arrhythmias after surgical correction of total anomalous pulmonary venous connection: Late follow-up. *Pediatr Cardiol* 12:89–91, 1991.
55. Serraf A, Belli E, Roux D, et al: Modified superior approach for repair of supracardiac and mixed total anomalous pulmonary venous drainage. *Ann Thorac Surg* 65:1391–1393, 1998.
56. Serraf A, Bruniaux J, Lacour-Gayet F, et al: Obstructed total anomalous pulmonary venous return: Toward neutralization of a major risk factor. *J Thorac Cardiovasc Surg* 101:601–606, 1991.
57. Sinzobahamvya N, Arenz C, Brecher AM, et al: Early and long-term results for correction of total anomalous pulmonary venous drainage (TAPVD) in neonates and infants. *Eur J Cardiothorac Surg* 10:433–438, 1996.
58. Smallhorn JF, Burrows P, Wilson G, et al: Two-dimensional and pulsed Doppler echocardiography in the postoperative evaluation of total anomalous pulmonary venous connection. *Circulation* 76:298–305, 1987.
59. Smallhorn JF, Freedom RM: Pulsed Doppler echocardiography in the preoperative evaluation of total anomalous pulmonary venous connection. *J Am Coll Cardiol* 8:1413–1420, 1986.
60. Trinkaus PM, Biagas KV, Hordof AJ, et al: False negative echocardiography increases morbidity in neonates with isolated total anomalous pulmonary venous connection. *Crit Care Med* 28:A155, 2000.
61. Trinkaus PM, Biagas KV, Hordof AJ, et al: Mortality in total anomalous pulmonary venous connection with associated complex cardiac anatomy is increased by pulmonary venous obstruction. *Crit Care Med* 28:A157, 2000.
62. Wang JK, Li YW, Chiu I, et al: Usefulness of magnetic resonance imaging in the assessment of venoatrial connections, atrial morphology, bronchial situs, and other anomalies of right atrial isomerism. *Am J Cardiol* 74:701–704, 1994.
63. White CS, Baffa JM, Haney PJ, et al: MR imaging of congenital anomalies of thoracic veins. *Radiographics* 17:595–608, 1997.
64. Yee ES, Turley K, Hsieh WR, Ebert PA: Infant total anomalous pulmonary venous connection: Factors influencing timing of presentation and operative outcome. *Circulation* 76:III83–III187, 1987.

Chapter 33

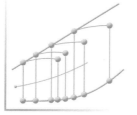

Transposition of the Great Arteries and the Arterial Switch Operation

TOM R. KARL, MD, MS, and PAUL M. KIRSHBOM, MD

INTRODUCTION

The evolution of surgical management of transposition of the great arteries (TGA) parallels that of pediatric cardiac surgery itself. Dating back to the initial attempts at palliation by Blalock and Hanlon in 1950, the treatment of TGA has reflected the evolving capabilities and aspirations of surgeons. As a result, operative success with this entity is the standard by which pediatric cardiac centers are judged. Furthermore, the simpler forms of TGA present the surgeon with the rare opportunity to convert a heart with a lethal abnormality to a nearly normal one within a few weeks of birth.

This chapter focuses on TGA and the role of the arterial switch operation (ASO) in the treatment of newborns and young infants. Although the application of the ASO to more complex problems related to TGA also is addressed, the reader is referred to other publications for details of this experience.[48,50]

EMBRYOLOGY AND ANATOMIC FEATURES

The embryology of TGA is thought to involve abnormal rotation and septation of the arterial truncus. The subject is complex, somewhat speculative, and of limited value for an understanding of the clinical problem, and thus is mainly of academic interest. Therefore this section concentrates on postnatal morphology, which is of paramount importance to the clinical team.

Any heart can be described sequentially by its atrial situs, atrioventricular (AV) connection, and ventriculoarterial (VA) connection. In the broadest sense, TGA refers to any heart in which the aorta is connected primarily to an anatomic right ventricle (RV) and the pulmonary artery (PA) primarily to an anatomic left ventricle (LV), a situation known as discordant VA connection. The term TGA is most frequently used to denote the heart with situs solitus, concordant AV connection, and discordant VA connection, which is the anatomic form most commonly encountered in clinical practice. Included in the TGA "family" are hearts with discordant AV and VA connection (AV and VA discordance or "congenitally corrected" TGA) and hearts with various other anomalies of atrial situs and AV connection (Fig. 33-1). Univentricular hearts such as those with double-inlet left ventricle (DILV) or tricuspid atresia with an outlet chamber of RV morphology giving rise to the aorta also are considered to have TGA.

The spatial orientation of the great arteries varies in TGA. Most patients have an anteroposterior orientation.[54]

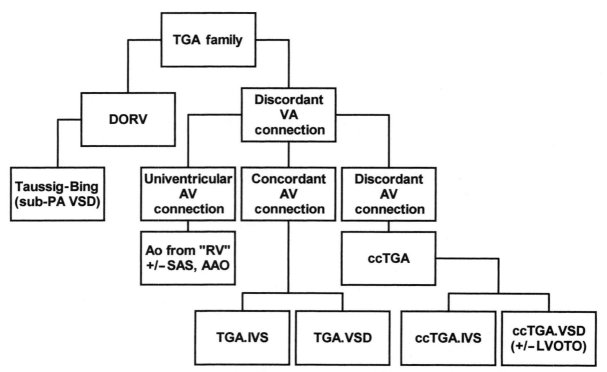

FIGURE 33-1 The family of anatomic lesions considered to be transposition of the great arteries (TGA). The unifying feature is a discordant ventriculoarterial connection. The Taussig-Bing anomaly is technically not TGA, as the VA connection is double outlet; however, from an anatomic, physiologic, and therapeutic point of view, it is so similar as to be included in most TGA and arterial switch operation discussions. AAO, aortic arch obstruction; Ao, aorta; AV, atrioventricular; ccTGA, congenitally corrected transposition of the great arteries; ccTGA.IVS, congenitally corrected transposition of the great arteries with intact ventricular septum; ccTGA.VSD, congenitally corrected transposition of the great arteries with ventricular septal defect; DORV, double-outlet right ventricle; LVOTO, left ventricular outflow tract obstruction; PA, pulmonary artery; RV, right ventricle; SAS, subaortic stenosis; TGA.IVS, transposition of the great arteries with intact ventricular septum; TGA.VSD, transposition of the great arteries with ventricular septal defect; VA, ventriculoatrial; VSD, ventricular septal defect.

The coronary anatomy also is variable.[4,54] A nearly constant feature is that the coronaries arise from the aortic sinuses "facing," or adjacent to, the pulmonary artery.[34] The Leiden classification for describing coronary anatomy in TGA is generally accepted and logical (Fig. 33-2). Although all types of coronary and great vessel anatomy are suitable for ASO, certain types are technically more difficult for the surgeon and carry a higher operative risk in some centers.

Most infants with TGA have a muscular subaortic infundibulum with fibrous continuity between the mitral and pulmonary valves. The exception is the Taussig-Bing (T-B) anomaly.[101,104] Tricuspid and mitral valve anomalies also have been described in TGA, more often in association with complex TGA.[2,41,59,75,86]

Current estimates place the incidence of TGA between 0.02% and 0.05% of live births.[32,35,55] Thus this entity makes up approximately 7% to 8% of all congenital heart defects. About 75% of TGA patients coming for operation have isolated VA discordance with patent foramen ovale (PFO) or patent ductus arteriosus (PDA).[55] A PDA persists until age 2 weeks in 50% of babies with TGA.[108] The PDA improves arterial oxygenation and maintains a favorable LV/RV pressure ratio, albeit at the cost of increased pulmonary blood flow.

Ventricular septal defect (VSD) is present in 20% of TGA cases. As in VA-concordant hearts, the size and location varies. A hemodynamically significant VSD also helps to maintain LV pressure (pLV) at systemic levels. Subpulmonary VSD is found in 30% of cases of double-outlet right ventricle (DORV), the majority being T-B hearts.[56,76] Simplistically, T-B is a DORV with subpulmonary VSD, in this case applying the "50% rule" to the PA rather than to the aorta, which has a uniquely RV origin. The great vessels are parallel and do not spiral. The subpulmonary outlet is unobstructed, although subaortic obstruction may be seen because of hypertrophy of the infundibular septum. The semilunar valves are usually in a side-by-side (or nearly so) position at complementary level. In the T-B anomaly, preferential "streaming" of oxygenated blood from the LV through the VSD to the PA mimics TGA physiology.

Left ventricular outflow obstruction (LVOTO) occurs in 0.7% of cases with intact ventricular septum (IVS) and in 20% of those with a VSD.[55] It may be dynamic obstruction resulting from a shift of the ventricular septum due to the difference in intraventricular pressures (as in TGA/IVS) or anatomic obstruction caused by a subvalvular membrane, tissue tags, or a fibromuscular tunnel (TGA/VSD).[82,88,94,102] LVOTO limits pulmonary blood flow and exacerbates the cyanosis inherent in TGA.

Aortic arch obstruction is rare in TGA/IVS but is present in 7% to 10% of cases of TGA/VSD and the T-B anomaly. Most commonly, the obstruction is a discrete coarctation with hypoplasia of the transverse arch and isthmus.[72,89] Complete aortic interruption is more likely to occur in univentricular hearts with subaortic stenosis.[50] When the distal

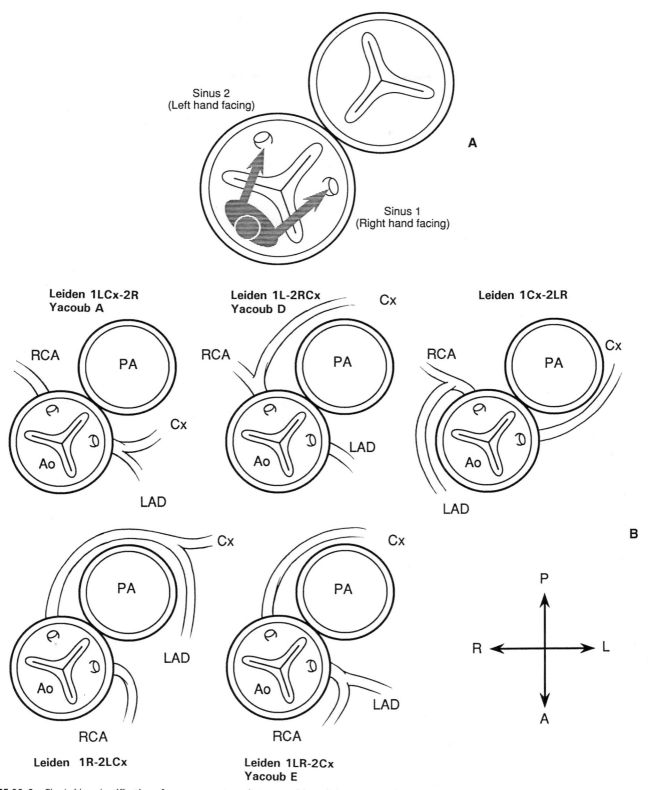

FIGURE 33-2   The Leiden classification of coronary anatomy in transposition of the great arteries. **A,** The coronary arteries are described from the vantage point of a person sitting in the aorta, looking toward the pulmonary artery. The coronary arteries may arise from sinus 1 or sinus 2. Sinus 1 corresponds to the one facing the observer's right hand, whereas sinus 2 faces the left hand. **B,** Coronary artery origins possible in transposition of the great arteries. Yacoub type A is the most common; type D is the second most common. This classification does not account for intramural course of a coronary, which occurs in 5% of cases, but is the most useful classification published to date and is understood by most surgeons. When the great vessels are in a side-by-side configuration, as in the Taussig-Bing heart, a retropulmonary course of the circumflex and single coronary are more common. (From Masuda M, Kado H, Shiokawa Y, et al: Clinical results of arterial switch operation for double-outlet right ventricle with subpulmonary VSD. *Eur J Cardiovasc Surg* 15:283–288, 1999, with permission.)

circulation is ductus dependent, ductal closure can precipitate profound cardiovascular collapse.

PHYSIOLOGY AND NATURAL HISTORY

The pulmonary and systemic circulations in TGA are parallel rather than in series. This may lead to life-threatening arterial desaturation in the systemic circulation (Fig. 33-3). Survival depends on the presence of one or more crossover or mixing points (ASD, VSD, or PDA) between these two circulations to achieve an arterial oxygen saturation that is compatible with life. The amount of mixing of caval and pulmonary venous blood greatly influences the hemoglobin oxygen saturation and the severity of the clinical picture. Newborns with TGA/IVS with a small PFA or ASD have severe cyanosis on the first day of life, sometimes with acidosis and cardiovascular collapse. Those with TGA/VSD or TGA/IVS with a large ASD or PDA have better mixing and hence a higher pO$_2$, but they also have a greater tendency to develop congestive heart failure (CHF).

Without surgical intervention, survival to age 6 months is unlikely, even after balloon atrial septostomy (BAS).[52,53,61,73] The prognosis is worse for patients presenting with severe cyanosis or arch obstruction or both, many of whom do not survive the newborn period without surgical intervention. Those infants who do survive without intervention are prone

to early development of pulmonary vascular disease, even in the presence of IVS.[22,29–31,77,106] Other causes of morbidity and mortality include CHF, stroke, and cerebral abscess secondary to progressive hypoxemia and intracardiac shunts.

At birth, the RV in TGA is abnormally thick walled. This thickness increases with time. In contrast to the heart with VA concordance, the LV mass in TGA remains fairly constant despite somatic growth, resulting in a relatively thin-walled LV by age 2 to 4 months.[8,25,40,63,96] This LV mass involution parallels the normal postnatal decrease in pulmonary vascular resistance. These phenomena significantly influence the timing and nature of surgical correction (see later). LVOTO, a large VSD, or a PDA may maintain high pLV after birth, to some extent preventing LV mass involution in the first year of life.[40,96]

DIAGNOSIS

The diagnosis of TGA should be suspected in any cyanotic infant, especially if a poor response to supplemental oxygen is found. No characteristic features on clinical examination, chest radiography, or electrocardiography (ECG) reliably allow differentiation of TGA from other causes of neonatal cyanosis. Heart murmurs, cardiomegaly, and pulmonary plethora are more likely if a high pulmonary blood flow is present. Absence of femoral pulses suggests aortic arch obstruction.

As is the case for most cardiac lesions in the newborn, the "gold standard" for rapid noninvasive diagnosis is two-dimensional echocardiography, which usually provides excellent detail of the surgically relevant features.[14,58,87] The details of two-dimensional echocardiography diagnosis are beyond the scope of this chapter, but the interested reader is referred to Chapter 17 and to several excellent texts on this subject.[95,97]

Cardiac catheterization is not routinely required for diagnosis of TGA in neonates, although transvenous BAS is usually performed. Older infants with more complex forms of TGA may require catheterization to provide specific hemodynamic data and to define anatomic features such as multiple VSDs. Angiographic delineation of coronary anatomy is usually unnecessary, because almost all coronary patterns can be dealt with surgically by using the ASO strategy. In any case, echocardiography has been refined to the point that coronary anatomy can be demonstrated noninvasively in the majority of cases.

PREOPERATIVE CRITICAL CARE MANAGEMENT

Most infants with TGA are diagnosed shortly after birth. After birth, increasing the FiO$_2$ may improve oxygenation by increasing pulmonary blood flow, but the response is typically poor. Resuscitation with mechanical ventilation, prostaglandin E$_1$ (PGE$_1$), and urgent BAS may be required. BAS may be performed in the intensive care unit (ICU) under echocardiographic guidance.[3,78] Dramatic improvement in oxygenation usually follows, with resolution of metabolic acidosis. Routine BAS converts ASO for TGA from an emergency to a semielective surgical procedure and simplifies management of cardiopulmonary bypass (CPB) by

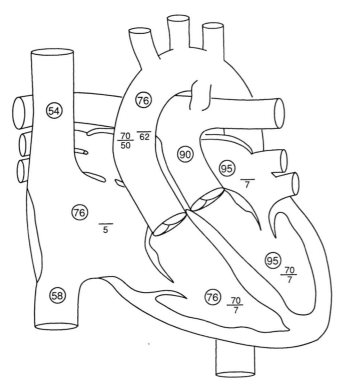

FIGURE 33-3 Circulation in transposition of the great arteries. In its untreated form, the systemic and pulmonary components describe parallel loops. Oxygenation (and therefore survival ex utero) depends on "mixing" of venous and arterial blood at atrial septal defect, ventricular septal defect, or patent ductus arteriosus level. The most efficient mixing occurs at atrial level, as compliance, phasic pressure variation, volume overload, and pulmonary artery pressure are not so critical.

venting the left heart. However, excellent results also have been reported without routine use of BAS.[10] After BAS, most neonates can be extubated and begun on oral feeds on the ward. Patients with arch obstruction or persistent poor oxygenation remain PGE_1 dependent and require operation within 24 to 72 hours. Fever, vasodilation, edema, apnea, and hypertonicity have been observed in infants receiving PGE_1, but these complications occur infrequently at doses of 0.01 to 0.02 mcg/kg/minute. Babies with arch obstruction awaiting operation should be watched carefully for necrotizing enterocolitis (NEC). Enteral feeding should be initiated with care, if at all, in patients receiving PGE_1. Preoperative cranial ultrasonography is recommended as a baseline examination when birth asphyxia or cardiovascular collapse complicates presentation. ASO should be delayed for antibiotic treatment of NEC, and intracranial hemorrhage should be stabilized before the use of CPB. The ideal timing of surgery for other patients is variable and is discussed later. Patients with high pulmonary blood flow may benefit from diuretics, vasodilators, and low-dose inotropic support before operation. In general, the concept of emergency operation for TGA has been replaced by one of resuscitation and stabilization in preparation for semielective ASO.

SURGICAL TREATMENT OF THE INFANT WITH TRANSPOSITION OF THE GREAT ARTERIES

Early surgical procedures for TGA attempted to improve mixing at the atrial level by creating or enlarging an ASD. The Blalock-Hanlon operation created an ASD without the use of CPB, providing dramatic palliation and allowing survival beyond the newborn period.[15] It has been replaced by the Rashkind BAS and is therefore rarely used today.[80,81] BAS achieves a similar result with lower risk and less stress for the critically ill newborn.

Before the mid-1980s, most centers used either the Mustard or Senning operation as definitive surgical treatment of TGA.[71,90,91] These operations, sometimes called "*atrial switch procedures*," direct superior and inferior caval blood to the mitral valve and pulmonary venous blood to the tricuspid valve by use of an intraatrial baffle. The result is serial pulmonary and systemic circuits, but with the RV as the ventricle pumping to the systemic circulation and the LV pumping to the pulmonary circulation (AV/VA discordance). When performed sufficiently early in life, these operations yielded good results.[1,9,66] However, an unacceptably high incidence of late baffle obstruction, arrhythmias, tricuspid insufficiency, dynamic LVOTO, and failure of the systemic RV resulted. Recognition of these long-term complications has led to near-universal acceptance of ASO as preferred treatment for most forms of TGA in the newborn.[6,28,33,38,57,64,103,105,107]

By restoring normal great arterial connections, ASO establishes sequential circulations with concordant AV and VA connections. Concurrent ablation of intracardiac shunts also is performed. Because it is technically impractical to switch the great arteries below the level of the coronary arteries, the latter vessels must be translocated to the PA (neoaorta). Barring other intracardiac or arch anomalies, ASO comes close to complete anatomic correction. The remaining abnormalities are the reversed semilunar valves and sinus segments of the proximal great arteries and the anterior position

of the PA (see later). Despite the technical difficulties of the operation and the problems of postoperative management of the newborn, ASO appeals to most pediatric cardiac surgeons, although excellent early results were not uniformly achievable. Fortunately, since the mid-1980s, steady improvement has occurred in surgical results worldwide. Early mortality is now similar to that of atrial repairs, but late results are superior.[21,24,36,43,62,64,93,105,110]

Indications for and Timing of Operation

Current indications for ASO in newborns and infants are listed in Table 33-1. Although no specific contraindication to ASO exists in infants with TGA and biventricular hearts, the age of the baby must be considered in planning operative strategy. The presence of multiple VSDs or unbalanced ventricles also will influence the decision. Prematurity and low birth weight are relative but not absolute contraindications (the smallest patient at the Royal Children's Hospital in Melbourne [RCH] was a 1.5-kg conjoined twin). Optimal timing of ASO depends on associated anatomic features. The key consideration is LV pressure at the time of presentation.

Because the natural history of TGA/IVS is characterized by progressive postnatal involution of the LV, this ventricle may not function well at systemic pressure and resistance in the older infant. This situation may place some infants with subsystemic pLV at risk for low cardiac output and LV failure after ASO.[55] Initially, success with ASO was limited to older infants with TGA/VSD.[43,111] Indications were later extended to include older infants with TGA/IVS, with preliminary PA banding to induce systemic pLV before ASO.[112] One-stage neonatal switch was a logical but nonetheless bold extension of this concept. Early success was realized in the United Kingdom, the United States, and the Netherlands.[22,82]

Currently, the optimal timing of ASO for TGA/IVS is considered to be around age 5 to 10 days. In our experience, the 15% to 20% of infants who cannot maintain adequate oxygenation after BAS and remain PGE_1 dependent will require earlier operation. Occasionally a baby with TGA/IVS cannot undergo early ASO because of late presentation, late diagnosis or referral or both, or intercurrent medical problems such as NEC or other septic conditions. Our experience and that of others support primary ASO as appropriate therapy for all infants with TGA/IVS up to age 8 weeks.[26] In some centers, a two-stage approach for older babies has been used

Table 33-1 Indications for and Timing of Arterial Switch Operation for Newborns and Infants at the Royal Children's Hospital, Melbourne

Anatomy	Number of Patients	Mean Age	Septostomy	Preoperative Catheter Study
TGA/IVS	152	12 days	88%	52
TGA/VSD	93	82 days	74%	63
Taussig-Bing	25	225 days	48%	13
DILV/SAS	10	4 days	0%	2

TGA/IVS, transposition of the great arteries with intact ventricular septum; TGA/VSD, transposition of the great arteries with ventricular septal defect; DILV/SAS, double-inlet left ventricle with subaortic stenosis.

with good results.[12,44,112] This strategy uses preliminary PA banding combined with a systemic to PA shunt to "retrain" the LV to pump against systemic resistance. The 1- to 2-week interval between PA banding and ASO may be difficult for the infant.[109] A simpler alternative, but one that may be less desirable in the long term, is an atrial-level repair (Senning or Mustard operation), leaving the prepared RV in the systemic circuit. The two-stage PA banding approach has been reserved for older children who had atrial level repairs early in life and in whom late failure of the systemic RV developed.[23,68,69] In such cases, a period of 1 year has sometimes been necessary to achieve adequate LV retraining before arterial switch and atrial reconstruction.

Patients with unrestrictive VSD, T-B anomaly, large PDA, functional (nonanatomic) LVOTO due to septal shift, or a combination of these may maintain systemic pLV well beyond age 2 weeks. In these patients, operation can be deferred until 6 to 8 weeks if they thrive. In practice, however, many infants do not thrive owing to CHF or nutritional problems, and surgical correction may become necessary earlier.

Infants with TGA and severe arch obstruction (usually with univentricular heart or T-B anomaly) typically require urgent operation after adequate resuscitation with PGE₁ and mechanical ventilation. Most of these infants have coarctation with hypoplastic transverse arch or interruption of the aortic arch, in association with complex intracardiac anatomy. A one-stage surgical procedure via median sternotomy is necessary.[48]

Technique of Arterial Switch Operation

ASO was first used in 1975 by Jatene for TGA/VSD and was significantly modified by Lecompte in 1981.[7,51,60] In its current form, it should rightly be known as the Jatene-Lecompte procedure. Our arterial switch technique at RCH and the Children's Hospital of Philadelphia (CHOP) is modified slightly from that of Jatene and Lecompte and has been used in more than 600 patients. It is highly reproducible and applicable to all patients with TGA.[19,23,50] Other variations of the basic Jatene-Lecompte technique are currently in clinical use and have produced good results.

The importance of an anesthetic team with expertise in newborn open-heart surgery cannot be overemphasized.[83] Infants undergoing ASO are anesthetized with fentanyl and paralyzed with pancuronium before insertion of radial artery or umbilical pressure monitoring catheters or both (if not already in place preoperatively). Nasopharyngeal, esophageal, and toe temperature-monitoring probes are attached as well as ECG, capnograph, and oximeter sensors. Hypotension or hypoxemia during the period between induction and CPB is usually due to hypovolemia and is treated with volume expansion (5% albumin solutions, 5 to 10 mL/kg). Aprotinin (30,000 KIU/kg) is administered before CPB, with an initial small test dose.

ASO is performed through a median sternotomy on CPB at 28° C nasopharyngeal temperature. Bicaval and aortic cannulation are used. The CPB priming solution contains fresh blood less than 48 hours old. Alpha-stat pH strategy is used during hypothermia. Full-flow CPB, 150 to 200 mL/kg, is used during most of the operation, and perfusion pressure is maintained at 35 mm Hg. We attempt to avoid both low flow and circulatory arrest during all phases of the ASO.

During cooling, the ductus is divided. The ascending aorta is clamped, and crystalloid cardioplegia solution is administered (30 mL/kg). The ascending aorta is transected just above the commissures, and the left and right coronaries are excised along with a large cuff of aortic sinus tissue (Fig. 33-4). The PA is then transected, and medially based rectangular flaps ("trapdoors") are developed in the pulmonary (neoaortic) sinuses where the coronary arteries are to be implanted. The coronary buttons are then rotated posteriorly and anastomosed to the opened trapdoors by using 8-0 monofilament-running sutures. The distal aorta is moved posteriorly to lie behind the PA bifurcation (the Lecompte maneuver). The neoaortic anastomosis is performed next. Large rectangular patches of autologous pericardium are sutured into the neopulmonary sinuses to fill the defects created by excision of the coronary buttons. The ASD is typically closed by direct suture. The aortic cross-clamp is removed, and the myocardium is inspected for adequacy of perfusion. A reactive hyperemia with distended epicardial coronaries is usually observed. The heart usually begins to beat in slow sinus rhythm. If these events do not occur, a problem with coronary translocation must be suspected, and consideration may be given to revision of the anastomoses. If no problem is encountered, the baby is rewarmed to 37° C. During warming, the neo-PA sinus repair and neo-PA anastomosis are completed.

In infants with TGA/VSD or the T-B anomaly, the VSD is usually closed through the tricuspid valve by using an autologous pericardial patch and pledgeted sutures, during the same period of ischemic arrest. In the case of T-B anomaly, the patch directs blood from the LV through the VSD and into the PA (neoaorta), while the aorta (neo-PA) remains connected to the RV. Enlargement of the VSD in the anterosuperior direction may be required if the VSD is restrictive.

Temporary atrial and ventricular pacing wires are attached in all patients, and both left atrial and PA monitoring catheters are inserted. At the RCH, the aortic cross-clamp and CPB times have averaged 59 and 122 minutes, respectively, for TGA/IVS. For TGA/VSD, these times were 84 minutes and 147 minutes, respectively.

Immediately after discontinuation of CPB, we use modified ultrafiltration to remove the priming and cardioplegia volume. During this 20-minute period, rapid normalization of hemodynamics usually occurs. Ideal hemodynamics (in millimeters of mercury) include arterial systolic pressure of 50 to 60; diastolic pressure, 30 to 40; mean arterial pressure, 40; mean left atrial pressure, 5 to 8; mean PA pressure, 10 to 20; and mean right atrial pressure, 5 to 10. Sinus rhythm should be present with a narrow QRS complex or incomplete right bundle branch block; ST segments should be isoelectric. Most patients receive dopamine (5 mcg/kg/min) and nitroglycerin (1 mcg/kg/min) or a milrinone loading dose (50 mcg/kg) as CPB is discontinued. Protamine administration, decannulation, and chest closure constitute the final steps of the operation.

ANATOMIC FEATURES REQUIRING SPECIAL CONSIDERATION

Left Ventricular Outflow Obstruction

The LVOT may be abnormal in up to 20% of patients with TGA, when all anatomic subsets are considered. LVOTO is a relative contraindication to ASO, although cases with

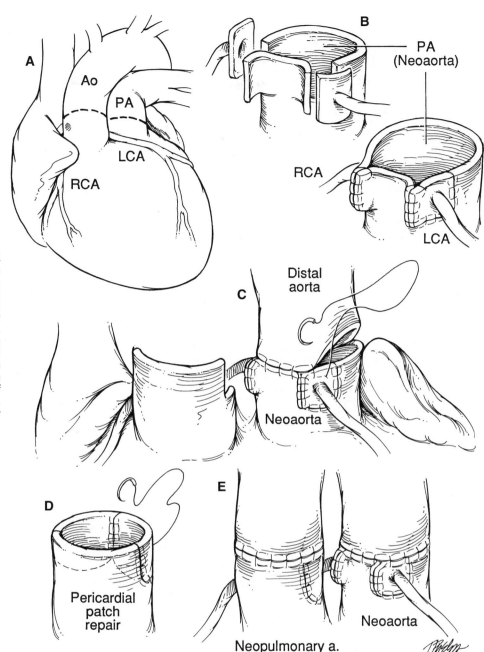

FIGURE 33-4 Technique of the arterial switch operation. **A,** The great arteries are transected above the sinuses of Valsalva. **B,** The coronaries are excised from the aorta (Ao), transposed posteriorly, and anastomosed to the pulmonary artery (PA; neoaorta) by using a "trapdoor technique" (see text). **C,** The distal aorta is brought behind the pulmonary artery (Lecompte maneuver) and anastomosed to the neoaorta. **D,** Separate pericardial patches are sutured to fill in the defects in the aorta created by excision of the coronary arteries. **E,** Completed repair. LCA, left coronary artery. RCA, right coronary artery.

resectable or dynamic obstruction may still be suitable. Resectable forms include minor pulmonary leaflet abnormalities, accessory AV valve tissue, discrete subpulmonary membranes, and anomalous muscle bundles.[98] Dynamic LVOTO may be reversed completely when the normal LV/RV pressure ratio is restored. The technique for dealing with LVOTO is usually a transpulmonary resection, performed just after great vessel transection. Patients with nonresectable forms of LVOTO may be candidates for the Rastelli, REV procedure (*réparation à l'étage ventriculaire*), or Nikaidoh strategies.

Aortic Arch Obstruction

Aortic arch obstruction is more common among patients with complex intracardiac anatomy. Arch obstruction usually consists of either coarctation with hypoplastic transverse arch (arch diameter in millimeters less than the patient's body weight in kilograms plus 1) or type B interruption. In both cases, a one-stage operation is advisable.[48] Cannulation of the ascending aorta is performed with an 8F cervical extracorporeal membrane oxygenation (ECMO) cannula on the rightward aspect (if interrupted aortic arch is present, we use a second arterial cannula in the PA). CPB is used to cool to 18° C, and the PDA is ligated. The aortic cannula is advanced into the innominate artery as flow is reduced to 30%. The head vessels are snared, and the descending aorta is clamped. The aortic arch is ligated just beyond the left subclavian artery and transected distally. A direct anastomosis between descending and ascending aorta is constructed after extensive mobilization and excision of all ductal tissue (Fig. 33-5).

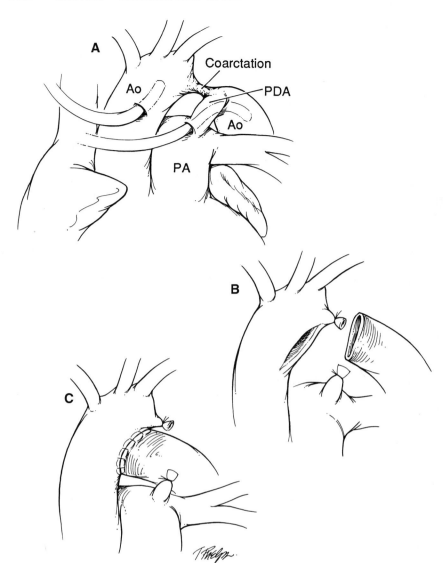

FIGURE 33-5 Technique of aortic arch repair. **A,** Cannulation of the ascending aorta (Ao) is performed with an 8F cervical ECMO cannula on the rightward aspect (if interrupted aortic arch [IAA] is present, a second arterial cannula in the pulmonary artery [PA] is used). **B,** Cardiopulmonary bypass is used to cool to 18° C, and the PDA is ligated proximal to the cannula. The aortic cannula is advanced into the innominate artery (IA) as flow is reduced to 30%. The head vessels are snared, and the descending aorta is clamped. **C,** A direct anastomosis between descending and ascending aorta is constructed after extensive mobilization. Clamps and head vessel snares are removed, and the cannula in the IA is pulled back to the ascending aorta for completion of the arterial switch operation. ECMO, extracorporeal membrane oxygenation; PDA, patent ductus arteriosus.

Clamps and head vessel snares are removed, and the cannula in the innominate artery is pulled back to the ascending aorta for completion of the ASO by using full-flow CPB. If the ascending aorta is less than 6 mm in diameter, enlargement with a patch of allograft pulmonary arterial wall may be advisable.

Variations in Coronary Anatomy

The most challenging pattern of coronary anatomy is the intramural coronary, which may have an eccentrically placed and stenotic ostium (Fig. 33-6).[4] This anomaly has been treated by detaching the posterior commissure of the aortic valve and unroofing the coronary to create a wide ostium. The coronaries are then excised and translocated as described earlier, and the aortic (neo-PA) commissure is resuspended to the pericardial patch used to repair the sinus defect. The single coronary is not problematic unless it branches in both directions between the aorta and PA.[4,54,74] Such cases are treated with a baffle to connect the neoaorta to the single coronary artery without translocation.[5]

The Taussig-Bing Anomaly

The ASO technique in the T-B anomaly requires some modification from the technique used for TGA/VSD. The VSD closure may be performed through the RV or either great artery, but a right atrial approach is generally easier. For coronary translocation, standard principles apply, taking into account the propensity for patterns other than 1 LCx, 2R (see Fig. 33-2).[46] The Lecompte maneuver is used, except in the rare case of anterior PA. The important points in the decision to use or avoid the Lecompte maneuver are avoidance of coronary artery compression and undue tension on the pulmonary anastomosis. The neo-PA anastomosis is constructed on the main pulmonary artery–right pulmonary artery (MPA-RPA) junction, closing a portion of the MPA on its leftward aspect (Fig. 33-7). In selected patients, RVOT obstruction can be treated with a patch enlargement.

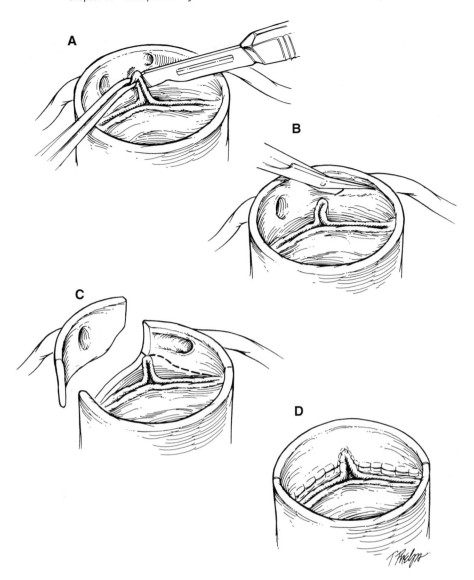

FIGURE 33-6 Surgical technique for management of intramural coronary artery in the arterial switch operation. **A,** Commissure of the aortic valve is detached from the aortic wall. **B,** Intramural portion of the artery can be "unroofed" to create a larger ostium. **C,** Coronaries are detached from the aorta. **D,** Defects in the aorta are repaired by a rectangular pericardial patch. Commissure can be reattached to the pericardial patch.

Previous Atrial-Level Repair

ASO can be performed for late failure of the systemic RV after an atrial (Mustard or Senning) repair.[23,68] Most patients require an interim PA band to "retrain" the LV. At the time of the ASO, the PA band and scarred portion of PA are excised. After the neoaortic anastomosis has been completed, the systemic venous atrium is opened, and the Mustard or Senning baffle is taken down. Atrial reconstruction is performed with autologous pericardium when possible, but a prosthetic patch is usually required after the Mustard operation.

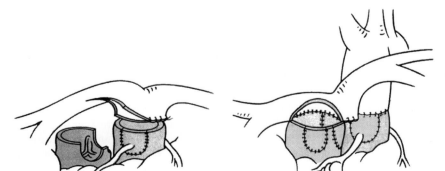

FIGURE 33-7 Pulmonary artery (PA) reconstruction in Taussig-Bing heart, using the Lecompte maneuver. The neo-PA anastomosis is constructed on the MPA-RPA junction, closing a portion of the MPA on its leftward aspect. MPA, main pulmonary artery; RPA, right pulmonary artery.

Arterial Switch Operation for Univentricular Heart with Subaortic Stenosis

Infants with DILV or tricuspid atresia with TGA (aorta arising from the outlet chamber of RV morphology), especially those with aortic arch obstruction, may be candidates for ASO with atrial septectomy.[50] In these patients, systemic cardiac output may be limited by a restrictive bulboventricular foramen. ASO converts this subaortic stenosis to subpulmonic stenosis and establishes a controlled source of pulmonary blood flow without PA banding, which is known to accelerate subaortic stenosis in such hearts. This procedure has generally been abandoned in favor of the modified Norwood operation (arch repair with Damus-Kaye-Stansel connection and modified Blalock-Taussig shunt), but remains in our armamentarium for use in selected cases.

POSTOPERATIVE CRITICAL CARE MANAGEMENT

The aim of postoperative care is to establish a safe homeostatic environment for the infant at minimal metabolic cost. A basic management strategy emphasizes a low-pressure, high-flow circulation to allow gradual hypertrophy of the LV. This requires careful control of temperature, fluid and electrolyte balance, vascular resistance, and other factors. These management issues are important for any newborn undergoing open-heart surgery, but they are critical for the ASO patient. ASO for TGA/IVS is unique in that a ventricle pumping against low pulmonary resistance is placed abruptly in a high-resistance circuit and required to support systemic cardiac output. The ability of the neonatal LV in TGA to adapt to the systemic workload is remarkable, but full adaptation may take days to weeks, depending on the age of the child, preoperative pLV, and other factors.[26] In older infants with unrestrictive VSD and in other patients with high pLV, the LV is already "prepared" and can be expected to function well against systemic vascular resistance.

All infants remain sedated by continuous morphine or fentanyl infusion and are paralyzed with intermittent or continuous pancuronium for 24 postoperative hours. If tachycardia develops, vecuronium is substituted after verifying the adequacy of sedation. After hemodynamic stabilization and cessation of muscle relaxants, gradual weaning from the ventilator takes place over a 12- to 24-hour period.

After ASO for TGA/IVS, the postoperative chest film usually shows a small heart and nonplethoric lungs. In contrast, patients with a preoperative volume load, such as those with TGA/VSD or T-B anomaly, may have persistent cardiomegaly for weeks. Echocardiography typically demonstrates mild global impairment of LV function and paradoxical septal motion. Both improve over the first postoperative week.

ASO patients usually receive milrinone (0.5 mcg/kg/min) for 2 to 3 days. Low-dose dopamine is administered for 2 to 5 days. Progressive improvement of LV function is followed with echocardiography and hemodynamic monitoring.

Interpretation of Hemodynamic Data

The adequacy of the circulation can be assessed by the gradient between core and toe temperature and by acid-base status.

Serum lactate level also is a useful marker.[27] The critical hemodynamic datum in postoperative monitoring of ASO patients is LA pressure, which should remain between 5 and 8 mm Hg. Systolic arterial pressure should be 50 to 60 mm Hg on the first day, with a progressive increase (for a given LA pressure) over the next 72-hour period. Intravenous (IV) fluids are limited to 50% of maintenance. Fluid challenges to increase LA pressure above 8 to 10 mm Hg should be avoided, as the unprepared LV can be forced onto the downslope of the Starling contractility curve, precipitating hemodynamic deterioration. Moderate hypotension (mean arterial pressure, 35 mm Hg) in a well-perfused baby is preferable. If mean arterial pressure decreases to below 35 in the setting of adequate left atrial pressure, norepinephrine, 0.01 to 0.2 mcg/kg/min, may be titrated. Mean PA pressure after newborn ASO is usually one third of systemic mean arterial pressure. Higher PA pressure suggests a residual intracardiac shunt, which should be investigated with Doppler echocardiography and measurement of hemoglobin saturation in the central venous and pulmonary circulations. Inadequate sedation, hypoxia, and hypercapnea are other causes of pulmonary hypertension. Persistence of elevated fetal vascular resistance is rare in newborns after ASO. Similarly, postoperative pulmonary hypertensive crisis per se is unusual in newborns but may occasionally complicate the postoperative course in older infants with complex TGA.

Peritoneal Dialysis

Urinary output is not a reliable guide to cardiac output under postoperative conditions. Some sick infants having open-heart surgery have a peritoneal dialysis catheter inserted at the time of operation. Postoperatively, this catheter drains the abdominal fluid that commonly collects after CPB in newborns. Evidence suggests that proinflammatory cytokines such as interleukin (IL)-6 and IL-8 are concentrated in the peritoneal fluid.[17] If urinary output is less than 1 mL/kg/hr, a single dose of furosemide, 1 mg/kg, is given. Diuretics, however, rarely provide sustained urinary output, and higher doses only complicate the metabolic picture. Transient renal insufficiency is a physiologic response to major surgery and may occur in the presence of satisfactory hemodynamics, adequate hydration, and normal preoperative renal function.

Because even moderate hyperkalemia is a myocardial depressant in newborns, early institution of peritoneal dialysis is advocated, which is greatly facilitated by intraoperative placement of a Tenckhoff catheter. Low-volume peritoneal dialysis provides excellent metabolic support without the diuretic-related complications of metabolic alkalosis, hypokalemia, and nephrotoxicity. Volumes of 10 mL/kg in 30-minute cycles are given to avoid the ventilatory complications of higher-volume dialysis. Isotonic (1.5%) or hypertonic (4.25%) dialysate at 20° C to 40° C is used, according to the patient's fluid status, serum potassium level, and temperature. Cold dialysate provides efficient core cooling for postoperative fever or management of junctional ectopic tachycardia.

Glucose homeostasis is critical in newborns after open-heart surgery. Serum glucose levels should be measured hourly in the immediate postoperative period. Levels less than 7 mmol/L (54 mg/dL) are treated with infusion of 50% glucose, 1 to 2 mL/hr. Similarly, serum ionized calcium levels are maintained at 1.1 to 1.2 mmol/L.

Hemostasis

The extensive anatomic dissection, long suture lines, and long CPB time for ASO predispose to significant bleeding. The use of fresh heparinized blood for the CPB prime, as well as platelets and fresh frozen plasma after CPB, minimize the resultant coagulopathy. Aprotinin also is effective in prevention of coagulopathy bleeding. Most important are patience and perseverance on the part of the surgical team before chest closure. Even mild cardiac tamponade is tolerated poorly by newborns after open-heart surgical procedures. Placement of additional sutures at the coronary anastomoses should be done judiciously. Thrombin-soaked absorbable gelatin sponge (Gelfoam) pledgets and fibrin glue have been useful. Occasionally, several hours are required to obtain hemostasis in the operating room (OR), but the reward is a greatly reduced rate of bleeding in the ICU. The criterion for re-exploration for bleeding is chest drainage exceeding 5 mL/kg/hr in the first hour, 4 mL/kg/hr in the second, and so forth. In practice, the need for re-exploration after ASO has been rare.

Low Cardiac Output

Persistent systemic hypotension, increasing left atrial pressure, poor peripheral perfusion, and signs of LV dysfunction suggest coronary arterial insufficiency or an unprepared LV. Both create an extremely unstable situation. In the case of coronary insufficiency, ST-segment changes may be evident on ECG and regional wall-motion abnormalities seen on echocardiography.[79] Coronary spasm after ASO is probably a real entity, but this has been difficult to prove. Nitroglycerin, 1 mcg/kg/min for 24 to 48 postoperative hours, is believed to be useful if spasm is suspected. Normalization of ST-segment abnormalities has been observed after initiation of this therapy. Technical problems with coronary anastomoses are treatable by exploration and revision if recognized early. If revision is unsuccessful or impossible, an internal thoracic artery–to–coronary artery graft can be applied.[83] Failure of an unprepared LV is more likely to occur in older infants with low preoperative pLV. Additional pharmacologic support is indicated, and delayed closure of the sternum with a synthetic membrane skin closure can be helpful. Institution of mechanical circulatory support with a ventricular assist device may be lifesaving and give added time for ventricular recovery or retraining.[45,49,70,79]

Capillary Leak Syndrome

Occasionally, CPB in newborns and small infants is associated with a profound capillary leak, massive edema, and increased IV fluid requirements. These problems are minimized by the use of aprotinin, avoidance of hypothermic circulatory arrest, and the use of fentanyl rather than morphine anesthesia. Nevertheless, the problem is still encountered and can be life threatening. Abdominal fluid losses via the peritoneal dialysis catheter (if it is used) are replaced with fresh frozen plasma or 5% albumin. Norepinephrine may be required to maintain adequate systemic arterial pressure. The capillary leak usually stabilizes after 24 to 36 hours, and the excess fluid can be removed over the next 2-day period by using hypertonic peritoneal dialysate.

OUTCOME

Hospital mortality for ASO performed at the RCH from 1985 to 1997 was 0.9% (confidence interval [CI], 0 to 3%) for TGA/IVS, 4.1% (CI, 1% to 9%) for TGA/VSD, and 6.6% (CI, 1% to 22%) for T-B anomaly. These results are similar to the results obtained at CHOP between 1995 and July 2001. During this period, 140 ASOs were performed at CHOP, including 90 TGA/IVS and 40 TGA/VSD patients. The operative mortality for this series was 2.2% (CI, 0.6% to 3.8%) for TGA/IVS and 5.0% (CI, 1.3% to 8.7%) for TGA/VSD. The early outcome for TGA/IVS is now comparable to that of tetralogy of Fallot, isolated VSD, and other lesions currently considered to carry a high probability of surgical success. Similar results have been achieved with the ASO in many centers worldwide, documenting the reproducibility of this procedure.[13,19,21,36,55,92,113] The results of ASO for univentricular hearts with subaortic stenosis are comparable to those of the modified Norwood procedure and of VSD enlargement with PA banding. Results for arterial switch conversion after an atrial-level switch must be compared with those of transplantation, which is the only therapeutic alternative.

Several risk factors have been identified for hospital mortality after ASO.[20,67,108,110] Excluding patients with univentricular heart and late RV failure after atrial switch, the presence of a VSD or arch obstruction or both was associated with increased risk of early death in the RCH series ($P < .05$). Age at operation, coronary anatomy (including intramural coronaries and all epicardial patterns), year of operation, and surgeon did not emerge as significant risk factors. Need for LVOTO resection did not increase the operative risk, but did adversely affect the 5-year freedom from reoperation.[98] Wernovsky and colleagues,[110] however, did find that coronary anatomy (Leiden patterns 1R-2LCx and 1LR-2Cx; see Fig. 33-2) increased early risk in their series of 470 ASO procedures performed in Boston between 1983 and 1992. In a follow-up study, Blume and associates[16] reported in 1999 that the risk of operative mortality for 223 babies operated on in Boston was 7%. The risk factors included circulatory arrest time and RV hypoplasia. Inverted and single right coronary artery patterns predicted a longer mechanical ventilation interval and the need for delayed sternal closure, but not mortality.

Tausier and associates[99] reported an 8% early mortality for ASO in 236 infants. Risk factors cited included low birth weight, small RV, arch obstruction, and coronary course between the aorta and pulmonary artery. Fatal and nonfatal coronary events related to these, as well as to intramural coronaries, retropulmonary left main coronary or circumflex arteries, and commissural coronary origin.

After ASO for TGA/IVS, the mean duration of ICU stay at the RCH was 72 hours, which corresponded to the duration of mechanical ventilation. Postoperative feeding problems have been common among newborns undergoing ASO, and prolonged nasogastric tube feeding is sometimes necessary. Long-term follow-up at the RCH has shown that most children are growing and developing normally and that virtually all are in the pediatric equivalent of New York Heart Association functional class I. Exercise testing of 22 randomly chosen TGA patients older than 5 years showed no ST-segment changes or dysrhythmia, although only 6 of 22 performed above the 50th percentile of the Bruce protocol.

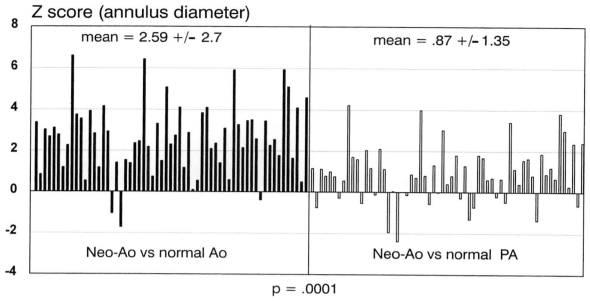

FIGURE 33-8   Neoaortic diameter after the arterial switch operation for 62 patients followed up at 105 (84–180) months postoperatively. At late follow-up, regression of the neo-Ao diameter on native Ao diameter normalized to body surface area suggests that the neo-Ao is abnormally large. This is not the case when regression is performed against a normal pulmonary artery. Median grade of AI was 0 (0–2) and not predicted by age or weight at operation, follow-up interval, or intracardiac anatomy.

Late function of the neoaortic valve has been a concern, based partly on the observation that the neoaortic root appears to be larger than expected. The results of an analysis of this problem performed at the RCH are presented in Figure 33-8. The implication is that the neoaortic valve develops more like a normal pulmonary valve than a normal aortic valve, a not unexpected finding.

Late death after newborn ASO has been rare, with recent reports documenting 10- and 15-year survival probabilities of 92% to 93% and 86%, respectively.[24,36] Given these excellent long-term survival rates, the emphasis for outcomes analysis in ASO patients must now shift from mortality to quality of life. Three lesions that could have an impact on long-term quality of life are late arrhythmias, myocardial ischemia, and neurodevelopmental abnormalities.

Rhodes and colleagues[84] evaluated a series of 390 ASO patients treated at the Boston Children's Hospital between 1983 and 1990. Electrophysiologic studies performed 6 to 12 months postoperatively revealed a low incidence of atrioventricular node dysfunction (4.4% total) with only five (1.7%) of the patients in complete heart block (CHB). All of the CHB patients were in the TGA/VSD group and required permanent pacemaker placement. Supraventricular tachycardia occurred in 5% of patients at late follow-up. Ventricular ectopy, however, was a more frequent finding at follow-up evaluation, with 57% of TGA/IVS and 30% of TGA/VSD patients demonstrating some measure of ventricular dysrhythmia. The vast majority of these patients had isolated premature ventricular beats, with only three patients experiencing ventricular tachycardia.

The topic of late evaluation of myocardial perfusion has been extensively studied with several different modalities, including stress echocardiography, scintigraphy, positron emission tomography (PET), and coronary arteriography.[37,42,85,114]

Although the incidence of late myocardial ischemia after ASO is low, it can be a cause of morbidity and mortality. Hutter and colleagues[42] evaluated all survivors after ASO performed between 1977 and 1999 by using ECG, echocardiography, scintigraphy, and elective coronary arteriography in all patients older than 10 years. Coronary arteriography was performed in 55 patients, 4 of whom were found to have significant ostial lesions, with 2 left ostial occlusions. One of these two children subsequently had an acute cardiac arrest and died, whereas the other required an implantable cardiodefibrillator for documented ventricular fibrillation episodes. Hauser and colleagues[37] evaluated 21 children an average of 11.2 years after ASO with stress echocardiography and PET. All patients were asymptomatic with normal exercise capacity, but two were found to have regional LV dyskinesia on stress echocardiography, whereas five children had perfusion defects on PET. Interestingly, none of these children was found to have coronary abnormalities on coronary arteriography.

Several reports[11,18,100,115] provided further long-term outcome data relating to coronary arteries in TGA. Stenosis or occlusion may occur in 3% to 7% of cases, even in the absence of symptoms, and the problem is more likely with certain coronary patterns (Yacoub D and E). The entire coronary tree may be abnormally small. Low coronary blood flow reserves and regional perfusion defects have been documented by using N-13 PET, adenosine, and Tc-99 sestamibi scans. Late sudden death can occur in patients with coronary abnormalities, but such events have fortunately been rare. Continued surveillance is in order for all TGA patients, at least noninvasively.

Perhaps the most important measure of long-term outcome is the neurodevelopment of children after ASO. Hövels-Gürich and associates[39] recently reported that although evidence of neurologic impairment existed in 21% of the 33 post-ASO patients evaluated, developmental analysis revealed no difference with respect to population norms. Average age at the time of evaluation was 3.6 years, and average deep hypothermic circulatory arrest (DHCA) time was 59 minutes (range, 45 to 99 minutes). In a study performed at the RCH, neurodevelopmental testing was performed on 74 ASO patients and controls.[47] Average age at assessment was 109 months. All patients were repaired by using full-flow CPB with very limited circulatory arrest. As in the prior study, mild neurologic impairment was more frequent in the ASO patients ($P = .002$). Full-scale IQ was higher in the control group; however, both the study and control patients scored higher than the population mean (101.9 and 108.6, respectively). Overall, the data currently available suggest that newborn ASO for TGA results in an extremely low risk of long-term neurodevelopmental impairment.

CONCLUSIONS

ASO has proven to be a reproducible and reliable surgical procedure for most forms of TGA, and this operation may satisfy the goals of every pediatric cardiac surgical intervention (i.e., transformation of a complex anomaly into a near-normal heart very early in life). We must await further long-term results among the large number of survivors to determine whether this goal has been achieved.

References

1. Abe T, Kuribayashi R, Sato M, et al: Successful Jatene operation for transposition of the great arteries with intact ventricular septum: A case report. *J Thorac Cardiovasc Surg* 75:64–67, 1978.
2. Albert HM: Surgical correction of transposition of the great vessels. *Surg Forum* 5:74, 1954.
3. Allan LD, Leanage R, Wainwright R, et al: Balloon atrial septostomy under two dimensional echocardiographic control. *Br Heart J* 47:41–43, 1982.
4. Asou T, Karl TR, Pawade A, Mee RB: Arterial switch operation: Translocation of intramural coronary arteries. *Ann Thorac Surg* 57:461–465, 1994.
5. Aubert J, Pannetier A, Couvelly JP, et al: Transposition of the great arteries: New technique for anatomical correction. *Br Heart J* 40:204–208, 1978.
6. Backer CL, Ilbawi MN, Ohtake S, et al: Transposition of the great arteries: A comparison of results of the Mustard procedure versus the arterial switch. *Ann Thorac Surg* 48:10–14, 1989.
7. Bailey CP, Cookson BA, Downing DF, Neptune WB: Cardiac surgery under hypothermia. *J Thorac Cardiovasc Surg* 28:229, 1954.
8. Bano-Rodrigo A, Quero-Jimenez M, Moreno-Granado F, Gamallo-Amat C: Wall thickness of ventricular chambers in transposition of the great arteries: Surgical implications. *J Thorac Cardiovasc Surg* 79:592–597, 1980.
9. Barratt-Boyes BG, Simpson M, Neutze JM: Intracardiac surgery in neonates and infants using deep hypothermia with surface cooling and limited cardiopulmonary bypass. *Circulation* 43:I25–I30, 1971.
10. Baylen BG, Grzeszczak M, Gleason ME, et al: Role of balloon atrial septostomy before early arterial switch repair of transposition of the great arteries. *J Am Coll Cardiol* 19:1025–1031, 1992.
11. Bengel FM, Hauser M, Duvernoy CS, et al: Myocardial blood flow and coronary flow reserve late after anatomical correction of transposition of the great arteries. *J Am Coll Cardiol* 32:1955–1961, 1998.
12. Bernhard A, Yacoub M, Regensburger D, et al: Further experience with the two-stage anatomic correction of simple transposition of the great arteries. *Thorac Cardiovasc Surg* 29:138–142, 1981.
13. Bertschmann W, Lincoln C: Arterial switch operation in transposition of the great arteries and double outlet right ventricle: Experience at the Brompton Hospital, London. *Helv Chir Acta* 57:545–549, 1991.
14. Bierman FZ, Williams RG: Prospective diagnosis of d-transposition of the great arteries in neonates by subxiphoid, two-dimensional echocardiography. *Circulation* 60:1496–1502, 1979.
15. Blalock A, Hanlon CR: The surgical treatment of complete transposition of the aorta and the pulmonary artery. *Surg Gynecol* 90:1, 1950.
16. Blume ED, Altmann K, Mayer JE, et al: Evolution of risk factors influencing early mortality of the arterial switch operation. *J Am Coll Cardiol* 33:1702–1709, 1999.
17. Bokesch PM, Kapural MB, Mossad EB, et al: Do peritoneal catheters remove proinflammatory cytokines after cardiopulmonary bypass in neonates? *Ann Thorac Surg* 70:639–643, 2000.
18. Bonhoeffer P, Bonnet D, Piechaud JF, et al: Coronary artery obstruction after the arterial switch operation for transposition of the great arteries in newborns. *J Am Coll Cardiol* 29:202–206, 1997.
19. Brawn WJ: Early results for anatomic correction of transposition of the great arteries and for double-outlet right ventricle with subpulmonary ventricular septal defect. *J Thorac Cardiovasc Surg* 95:230–238, 1988.
20. Bridges ND, Perry SB, Keane JF, et al: Preoperative transcatheter closure of congenital muscular ventricular septal defects. *N Engl J Med* 324:1312–1317, 1991.
21. Castaneda AR: Arterial switch operation for simple and complex TGA: Indication criterias and limitations relevant to surgery. *Thorac Cardiovasc Surg* 39:151–154, 1991.
22. Clarkson PM, Neutze JM, Wardill JC, Barratt-Boyes BG: The pulmonary vascular bed in patients with complete transposition of the great arteries. *Circulation* 53:539–543, 1976.
23. Cochrane AD, Karl TR, Mee RB: Staged conversion to arterial switch for late failure of the systemic right ventricle. *Ann Thorac Surg* 56:854–861, 1993.
24. Daebritz SH, Nollert G, Sachweh JS, et al: Anatomical risk factors for mortality and cardiac morbidity after arterial switch operation. *Ann Thorac Surg* 69:1880–1886, 2000.
25. Danford DA, Huhta JC, Gutgesell HP: Left ventricular wall stress and thickness in complete transposition of the great arteries: Implications for surgical intervention. *J Thorac Cardiovasc Surg* 89:610–615, 1985.
26. Davis AM, Wilkinson JL, Karl TR, Mee RB: Transposition of the great arteries with intact ventricular septum: Arterial switch repair in patients 21 days of age or older. *J Thorac Cardiovasc Surg* 106:111–115, 1993.
27. Duke T, Butt W, South M, Karl TR: Early markers of major adverse events in children after cardiac operations. *J Thorac Cardiovasc Surg* 114:1042–1052, 1997.
28. el-Said G, Rosenberg HS, Mullins CE, et al: Dysrhythmias after Mustard's operation for transposition of the great arteries. *Am J Cardiol* 30:526–532, 1972.
29. Ferencz C: Transposition of the great vessels: Pathophysiologic considerations based upon a study of the lungs. *Circulation* 33:232, 1966.
30. Ferguson DJ, Adams P, Watson D: Pulmonary arteriosclerosis in transposition of the great vessels. *Am J Dis Child* 99:653, 1960.
31. Forenz C, Greco JM, Libi-Sylora M: Variability of pulmonary vascular disease in certain malformations of the heart. In Keith JD (ed): *The Natural History and Progressive Treatment of Congenital Heart Defects*. Springfield, Ill, Charles C Thomas, 1971, p 300.
32. Fyler DC, Buckley LP, Hellenbrand WE, Cohn HE: Report of the New England Regional Infant Cardiac Program. *Pediatrics* 65:375–461, 1980.
33. Gewillig M, Cullen S, Mertens B, et al: Risk factors for arrhythmia and death after Mustard operation for simple transposition of the great arteries. *Circulation* 84:III187–III192, 1991.
34. Gittenberger-de Groot AC, Sauer U, Oppenheimer-Dekker A, et al: Coronary artery anatomy in transposition of the great arteries: A morphologic study. *Pediatr Cardiol* 4:15, 1983.
35. Gutgesell HP, Garson A, McNamara DG: Prognosis for the newborn with transposition of the great arteries. *Am J Cardiol* 44:96–100, 1979.
36. Haas F, Wottke M, Poppert H, Meisner H: Long-term survival and functional follow-up in patients after arterial switch operation. *Ann Thorac Surg* 68:1692–1697, 1999.
37. Hauser M, Bengel FM, Kuhn A, et al: Myocardial blood flow and flow reserve after coronary reimplantation in patients after arterial switch and Ross operation. *Circulation* 103:1875–1880, 2001.
38. Hazekamp MG, Ottenkamp J, Quaegebuer JM, et al: Follow-up of arterial switch operation. *J Thorac Cardiovasc Surg* 39:166–169, 1991.
39. Hovels-Gurich HH, Seghaye MC, Sigler M, et al: Neurodevelopmental outcome related to cerebral risk factors in children after neonatal arterial switch operation. *Ann Thorac Surg* 71:881–888, 2001.
40. Huhta JC, Edwards WD, Feldt RH, Puga FJ: Left ventricular wall thickness in complete transposition of the great arteries. *J Thorac Cardiovasc Surg* 84:97–101, 1982.
41. Huhta JC, Hagler DJ, Seward JB, et al: Two-dimensional echocardiographic assessment of dextrocardia: A segmental approach. *Am J Cardiol* 50:1351–1360, 1982.

42. Hutter PA, Bennink GB, Ay L, et al: Influence of coronary anatomy and reimplantation on the long-term outcome of arterial switch. *Eur J Cardiothorac Surg* 18:207–213, 2000.

43. Jatene AD, Fontes VF, Paulista PP, et al: Anatomic correction of transposition of the great vessels. *J Thorac Cardiovasc Surg* 72:364–370, 1976.

44. Jonas RA, Giglia TM, Sanders SP, et al: Rapid, two-stage arterial switch for transposition of the great arteries and intact ventricular septum beyond the neonatal period. *Circulation* 80:I203–I208, 1989.

45. Karl TR, Horton SB, Mee RB: Left heart assist for ischemic postoperative ventricular dysfunction in an infant with anomalous left coronary artery. *J Card Surg* 4:352–354, 1989.

46. Karl TR, Cochrane AD, Brizard CP: Arterial switch operation: Surgical solutions to complex problems. *Tex Heart Inst J* 24:322–333, 1997.

47. Karl TR, Hall S, Ford G, et al: Arterial switch with full-flow cardiopulmonary bypass and limited circulatory arrest: Neurodevelopmental outcome. *J Thorac Cardiovasc Surg* 127:213–222, 2004.

48. Karl TR, Sano S, Brawn W, Mee RB: Repair of hypoplastic or interrupted aortic arch via sternotomy. *J Thorac Cardiovasc Surg* 104:688–695, 1992.

49. Karl TR, Sano S, Horton S, Mee RB: Centrifugal pump left heart assist in pediatric cardiac operations: Indication, technique, and results. *J Thorac Cardiovasc Surg* 102:624–630, 1991.

50. Karl TR, Watterson KG, Sano S, Mee RB: Operations for subaortic stenosis in univentricular hearts. *Ann Thorac Surg* 52:420–427, 1991.

51. Kay EB, Cross FS: Surgical treatment of transposition of the great vessels. *Surgery* 38:712, 1955.

52. Keith JD, Neill CA, Vlad P, et al: Transposition of the great vessels. *Circulation* 7:830, 1953.

53. Kidd BSL: The fate of children with transposition of the great arteries following balloon atrial septostomy. In Kidd BSL, Rowe RD (eds): *The Child with Congenital Heart Disease after Surgery*. New York, Futura, 1953, p 1976.

54. Kirklin JW, Barratt-Boyes BG: Complete transposition of the great arteries. In Kirklin JW, Barratt-Boyes BG (eds): *Cardiac Surgery*. New York, Churchill-Livingstone, 1993, pp 1383–1467.

55. Kirklin JW, Blackstone EH, Tchervenkov CI, Castaneda AR: Clinical outcomes after the arterial switch operation for transposition: Patient, support, procedural, and institutional risk factors: Congenital Heart Surgeons Society. *Circulation* 86:1501–1515, 1992.

56. Kirklin JW, Pacifico AD, Blackstone EH, et al: Current risks and protocols for operations for double-outlet right ventricle. *J Thorac Cardiovasc Surg* 92:913–930, 1986.

57. Kramer HH, Rammos S, Krogmann O, et al: Cardiac rhythm after Mustard repair and after arterial switch operation for complete transposition. *Int J Cardiol* 32:5–12, 1991.

58. LaCorte MA, Fellows KE, Williams RG: Overriding tricuspid valve: Echocardiographic and angiocardiographic features. *Am J Cardiol* 37:911–919, 1976.

59. Layman TE, Edwards JE: Anomalies of the cardiac valves associated with complete transposition of the great vessels. *Am J Cardiol* 37:911–919, 1976.

60. Lecompte Y, Zannini L, Hazan E, et al: Anatomic correction of transposition of the great arteries. *J Thorac Cardiovasc Surg* 82:629–631, 1981.

61. Liebman J, Cullum L, Belloc NB: Natural history of transposition of the great arteries: Anatomy and birth and death characteristics. *Circulation* 40:237–262, 1969.

62. Lupinetti FM, Bove EL, Minich LL, et al: Intermediate-term survival and functional results after arterial repair for transposition of the great arteries. *J Thorac Cardiovasc Surg* 103:421–427, 1992.

63. Maroto E, Fouron JC, Douste-Blazy MY, et al: Influence of age on wall thickness, cavity dimensions and myocardial contractility of the left ventricle in simple transposition of the great arteries. *Circulation* 67:1311–1317, 1983.

64. Martin RP, Qureshi SA, Ettedgui JA, et al: An evaluation of right and left ventricular function after anatomical correction and intra-atrial repair operations for complete transposition of the great arteries. *Circulation* 82:808–816, 1990.

65. Masuda M, Kado H, Shiokawa Y, et al: Clinical results of arterial switch operation for double-outlet right ventricle with subpulmonary VSD. *Eur J Cardiothorac Surg* 15:283–288, 1999.

66. Mauck HP Jr, Robertson LW, Parr EL, Lower RR: Anatomic correction of transposition of the great arteries without significant ventricular septal defect or patent ductus arteriosus. *J Thorac Cardiovasc Surg* 74:631–635, 1977.

67. Mayer JE Jr, Sanders SP, Jonas RA, et al: Coronary artery pattern and outcome of arterial switch operation for transposition of the great arteries. *Circulation* 82:IV139–IV145, 1990.

68. Mee RB: Arterial switch for right ventricular failure following Mustard or Senning operations. In Stark J, Pacifico AD (eds): *Reoperations in Cardiac Surgery*. London, Springer-Verlag, 1989, pp 217–232.

69. Mee RB: Results of the arterial switch procedure for complete transposition with intact ventricular septum. *Cardiol Young* 1:97–98, 1991.

70. Mee RB, Harada Y: Retraining of the left ventricle with a left ventricular assist device (Bio-Medicus) after the arterial switch operation. *J Thorac Cardiovasc Surg* 101:171–173, 1991.

71. Merendino EA, Jesseph JE, Herron PW, et al: Interatrial venous transposition: A one-stage intracardiac operation for the conversion of complete transposition of the aorta and pulmonary artery to corrected transposition. *Surgery* 42:898, 1957.

72. Milanesi O, Thiene G, Bini RM, Pellegrino PA: Complete transposition of great arteries with coarctation of aorta. *Br Heart J* 48:566–571, 1982.

73. Miller RA: Complete transposition of the great arteries. In Morse DP (ed): *Congenital Heart Disease, Pathogenetic Factors, Natural History, Diagnosis, and Surgical Treatment*. Philadelphia, FA Davis, 1962, p 74.

74. Moat NE, Pawade A, Lamb RK: Complex coronary arterial anatomy in transposition of the great arteries: Arterial switch procedure without coronary relocation. *J Thorac Cardiovasc Surg* 103:872–876, 1992.

75. Moene RJ, Oppenheimer-Dekker A: Congenital mitral valve anomalies in transposition of the great arteries. *Am J Cardiol* 49:1972–1978, 1982.

76. Musumeci F, Shumway S, Lincoln C, Anderson RH: Surgical treatment for double-outlet right ventricle at the Brompton Hospital, 1973 to 1986. *J Thorac Cardiovasc Surg* 96:278–287, 1988.

77. Newfeld EA, Paul MM, Muster AJ, Idriss FS: Pulmonary vascular disease in complete transposition of the great arteries: A study of 200 patients. *Am J Cardiol* 34:75–82, 1974.

78. Perry LW, Ruckman RN, Galioto FM Jr, et al: Echocardiographically assisted balloon atrial septostomy. *Pediatrics* 70:403–408, 1982.

79. Quaegebeur J, van Daele M, Stumper O, Sutherland GR: Intraoperative ultrasonographic identification of coronary artery compression after an arterial switch procedure. *J Thorac Cardiovasc Surg* 102:837–840, 1991.

80. Rashkind WJ, Miller WW: Creation of an atrial septal defect without thoracotomy: A palliative approach to complete transposition of the great arteries. *JAMA* 196:991–992, 1966.

81. Rashkind WJ, Miller WW: Transposition of the great arteries: Results of palliation by balloon atrioseptostomy in thirty-one infants. *Circulation* 38:453–462, 1968.

82. Rastelli GC, Wallace RB, Ongley PA: Complete repair of transposition of the great arteries with pulmonary stenosis: A review and report of a case corrected by using a new surgical technique. *Circulation* 39:83–95, 1969.

83. Rheuban KS, Kron IL, Bulatovic A: Internal mammary artery bypass after the arterial switch operation. *Ann Thorac Surg* 50:125–126, 1990.

84. Rhodes LA, Wernovsky G, Keane JF, et al: Arrhythmias and intracardiac conduction after the arterial switch operation. *J Thorac Cardiovasc Surg* 109:303–310, 1995.

85. Rickers C, Sasse K, Buchert R, et al: Myocardial viability assessed by positron emission tomography in infants and children after the arterial switch operation and suspected infarction. *J Am Coll Cardiol* 36:1676–1683, 2000.

86. Rosenquist GC, Stark J, Taylor JF: Congenital mitral valve disease in transposition of the great arteries. *Circulation* 51:731–737, 1975.

87. Sanders SP: Echocardiography and related techniques in the diagnosis of congenital heart defects, III: Conotruncus and great arteries. *Echocardiography* 1:443–493, 1984.

88. Sansa M, Tonkin IL, Bargeron LM Jr, Elliott LP: Left ventricular outflow tract obstruction in transposition of the great arteries: An angiographic study of 74 cases. *Am J Cardiol* 44:88–95, 1979.

89. Schneeweiss A, Motro M, Shem-Tov A, Neufeld HN: Subaortic stenosis: An unrecognized problem in transposition of the great arteries. *Am J Cardiol* 48:336–339, 1981.

90. Senning A: Surgical correction of transposition of the great vessels. *Surgery* 45:966, 1959.

91. Senning A: Surgical correction of transposition of the great vessels. *Surgery* 59:334–336, 1966.

92. Serraf A, Bruniaux J, Lacour-Gayet F, et al: Anatomic correction of transposition of the great arteries with ventricular septal defect: Experience with 118 cases. *J Thorac Cardiovasc Surg* 102:140–147, 1991.

93. Serraf A, Lacour-Gayet F, Bruniaux J, et al: Anatomic correction of Taussig-Bing hearts. *Circulation* 84:III200–III205, 1991.
94. Shrivastava S, Tadavarthy SM, Fukuda T, Edwards JE: Anatomic causes of pulmonary stenosis in complete transposition. *Circulation* 54:154–159, 1976.
95. Silverman NH: *Pediatric Echocardiography*. Baltimore, Williams & Wilkins, 1993.
96. Smith A, Wilkinson JL, Arnold R, et al: Growth and development of ventricular walls in complete transposition of the great arteries with intact septum (simple transposition). *Am J Cardiol* 49:362–368, 1982.
97. Snider RA, Srwer GA: *Echocardiography in Pediatric Heart Disease*. Chicago, Mosby-Year Book, 1990.
98. Sohn YS, Brizard CP, Cochrane AD, et al: Arterial switch in hearts with left ventricular outflow and pulmonary valve abnormalities. *Ann Thorac Surg* 66:842–848, 1998.
99. Tamisier D, Ouaknine R, Pouard P, et al: Neonatal arterial switch operation: coronary artery patterns and coronary events. *Eur J Cardiothorac Surg* 11:810–817, 1997.
100. Tanel RE, Wernovsky G, Landzberg MJ, et al: Coronary artery abnormalities detected at cardiac catheterization following the arterial switch operation for transposition of the great arteries. *Am J Cardiol* 76:153–157, 1995.
101. van Doesburg NH, Bierman FZ, Williams RG: Left ventricular geometry in infants with D-transposition of the great arteries and intact interventricular septum. *Circulation* 68:733–739, 1983.
102. van Gils FA, Moulaert AJ, Oppenheimer-Dekker A, Wenink CG: Transposition of the great arteries with ventricular septal defect and pulmonary stenosis. *Br Heart J* 40:494–499, 1978.
103. Van Praagh R, Jung WK: The arterial switch operation in transposition of the great arteries: Anatomic indications and contraindications. *Thorac Cardiovasc Surg* 39:138–150, 1991.
104. Van Praagh R, Perez-Trevino C, Lopez-Cuellar M, et al: Transposition of the great arteries with posterior aorta, anterior pulmonary artery, subpulmonary conus and fibrous continuity between aortic and atrioventricular valves. *Am J Cardiol* 28:621–631, 1971.
105. Veelken N, Gravinghoff L, Keck EW, Freitag HJ: Improved neurological outcome following early anatomical correction of transposition of the great arteries. *Clin Cardiol* 15:275–279, 1992.
106. Viles PH, Ongley PA, Titus JL: The spectrum of pulmonary vascular disease in transposition of the great arteries. *Circulation* 40:321–341, 1969.
107. Villafane J, White S, Elbl F, et al: An electrocardiographic midterm follow-up study after anatomic repair of transposition of the great arteries. *Am J Cardiol* 66:350–354, 1990.
108. Waldman JD, Paul MH, Newfeld EA, et al: Transposition of the great arteries with intact ventricular septum and patent ductus arteriosus. *Am J Cardiol* 39:232–238, 1977.
109. Wernovsky G, Giglia TM, Jonas RA, et al: Course in the intensive care unit after "preparatory" pulmonary artery banding and aortopulmonary shunt placement for transposition of the great arteries with low left ventricular pressure. *Circulation* 86:II133–II139, 1992.
110. Wernovsky G, Mayer JE Jr, Jonas RA, et al: Factors influencing early and late outcome of the arterial switch operation for transposition of the great arteries. *J Thorac Cardiovasc Surg* 109:289–302, 1995.
111. Yacoub MH, Radley-Smith R, Hilton CJ: Anatomical correction of complete transposition of the great arteries and ventricular septal defect in infancy. *Br Med J* 1:1112–1114, 1976.
112. Yacoub MH, Radley-Smith R, Maclaurin R: Two-stage operation for anatomical correction of transposition of the great arteries with intact interventricular septum. *Lancet* 1:1275–1278, 1977.
113. Yamaguchi M, Hosokawa Y, Imai Y, et al: Early and midterm results of arterial switch operation for transposition of the great arteries in Japan. *J Thorac Cardiovasc Surg* 100:261–269, 1990.
114. Yates RW, Marsden PK, Badawi RD, et al: Evaluation of myocardial perfusion using positron emission tomography in infants following a neonatal arterial switch operation. *Pediatr Cardiol* 21:111–118, 2000.
115. Yatsunami K, Nakazawa M, Kondo C, et al: Small left coronary arteries after arterial switch operation for complete transposition. *Ann Thorac Surg* 64:746–750, 1997.

Chapter 34

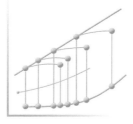

Double-Outlet Right Ventricle and Double-Outlet Left Ventricle

W. REID THOMPSON, MD, DAVID G. NICHOLS, MD, MBA,
PHILIP J. SPEVAK, MD, and ROSS M. UNGERLEIDER, MD

INTRODUCTION

The diagnosis of double-outlet right ventricle (DORV) includes a wide spectrum of pathology and is associated with a variety of other cardiac malformations. An understanding of the common findings in patients with this malformation is an important prerequisite to providing appropriate preoperative and postoperative care.

DEFINITION

The term *double-outlet right ventricle* is most commonly defined as the condition in which both great arteries are related to the morphologic right ventricle (RV). A ventricular septal defect (VSD) is usually (but not always) present, providing the only outlet for the left ventricle (LV). In cases in which either the aorta or the pulmonary artery (PA) appears to be overriding the VSD, deciding which ventricle that artery relates to may be difficult. In those instances, DORV is distinguished from tetralogy of Fallot (TOF) or D-transposition of the great arteries (D-TGA), respectively,

731

if complete lack of fibrous continuity is found between that semilunar valve and the mitral valve, and if more than 50% of both great arteries relates to the RV.

HISTORICAL PERSPECTIVE

Whereas DORV was described pathologically as early as 1703,[94] it was not until relatively recently that it was differentiated from transposition of the great arteries (TGA). TGA has historically been defined as the condition in which ventriculoarterial *discordance* is found (i.e., the pulmonary artery arises above the morphologic LV, and the aorta, above the morphologic RV). Obviously, in DORV, this is only partially true because, although the aorta arises discordantly above the RV, the PA-RV relation is concordant. Consistent with this line of reasoning, DORV was initially called *partial* transposition by Vierordt in 1898, a term that was agreed on by Maude Abbott in 1915.[108] The two other types of TGA, according to Abbott, were *complete* and *corrected* transposition.

In 1949, Taussig and Bing[102] described a heart with "complete transposition of the aorta and levoposition of the pulmonary artery." Although this was not the first report of DORV, it was remarkable for its clarity of pathologic description and because it was the first reported case of a malformation in which not only did both great arteries arise from the RV but the VSD was related to the PA, not to the aorta, as had been the case in all previous reports.

The term *double-outlet RV* was first used by Witham in 1957.[115] McGoon published the first account of a surgical repair for DORV in 1961.[57] Neufeld and colleagues[33,63] published two landmark articles, also in 1961, in which 11 cases with origin of both great vessels from the RV were discussed in an attempt to correlate anatomic findings with clinical and hemodynamic data. These authors divided cases into those with and without pulmonary stenosis (PS) and added a third group for those with "other intracardiac malformations." They found that without significant PS, the clinical features were similar to those of a large VSD with pulmonary hypertension, whereas patients with PS resembled those with the TOF. Their third group contained a single case of DORV with PS and common atrioventricular (AV) canal.

In 1972, Lev[50] emphasized the *position* of the VSD in relation to the two arterial trunks, whether *subaortic, subpulmonary, doubly committed, or noncommitted,* as being of preeminent hemodynamic and surgical importance in DORV. He proposed widening the definition of DORV not necessarily to exclude cases with aortic- or pulmonary-mitral fibrous continuity and required only that two cusps and part of a third of both semilunar valves originate from the RV. He suggested considering as a spectrum hearts that "pass imperceptibly from tetralogy or VSD with overriding aorta into double-outlet right ventricle with subaortic VSD." Likewise, he pointed out that the Taussig-Bing type of DORV also was a spectrum, from hearts in which both great arteries are wholly related to the RV to those with pulmonary-mitral continuity, as in complete transposition. Lev maintained that the acceptance of this continuity from TOF to the common variety of DORV with subaortic VSD to the Taussig-Bing malformation, to D-TGA was consistent with embryologic and anatomic principles and would lead to a better understanding of the clinical features

and the requisite surgical approach associated with each point in the spectrum.[50]

In 1982, after a study of 101 autopsy cases of DORV, Van Praagh and associates[108] published a comprehensive examination of the subject, presenting the summarized anatomic findings of each case individually. They emphasized the distinction between *alignments and connections* between the three main segments of the heart, the visceroatrial situs, the ventricular loop, and the conotruncus. A major segment may be *aligned* with another major segment either *concordantly* (normal) or *discordantly* (abnormal). However, the major segments are physically joined by two *connections*: the AV canal and the infundibulum (or *conus*). This distinction is particularly important for an accurate anatomic understanding of conotruncal malformations. Although the great arteries may be aligned with and arise above a given ventricle, they are actually anatomically connected either to the infundibulum when it is developed or to AV canal tissue when the subarterial infundibulum is absorbed or fails to develop.

EMBRYOLOGY AND GENETICS

In the developing embryonic heart, normal ("D") looping of the ventricles to the right carries the aorta to the right of the PA. Early on, *bilateral* musculature is found beneath *both* semilunar valves. With normal development, the subpulmonary infundibulum grows and expands, resulting in a superior, anterior, and leftward positioning of the pulmonary valve relative to the aortic valve. The subaortic conus, however, normally absorbs, so that the aortic valve descends to an inferior, posterior location, coming into direct fibrous continuity with the left side of the AV canal, the mitral valve. The Taussig-Bing malformation is very similar to the early embryonic arrangement, with the aortic valve directly to the right of and in the same plane as the pulmonary valve and with bilateral subarterial conus.[102] This striking similarity suggests that developmental arrest during formation of the conotruncus may play a role in the etiology of at least some forms of DORV. Recent embryologic studies found that DORV also can result from abnormal development of the AV endocardial cushions,[53] supporting the clinical observation of the frequent coexistence of DORV and complete atrioventricular canal (CAVC) in the heterotaxy syndromes.

Chromosomal abnormalities have been identified in some patients with DORV, although not nearly as frequently as in several other cardiac abnormalities. In the Baltimore-Washington Infant Study, DORV was diagnosed in a few patients with Down syndrome and in trisomies 13 and 18, although the incidence was quite low compared with that of the morphologically similar lesion, TOF.[18,68] Supporting this distinction, the related conotruncal abnormality, complete transposition of the great arteries, was not found in any patient with trisomy in this series, suggesting that DORV and TGA may be etiologically similar and may be fundamentally different from TOF in terms of developmental mechanism. Likewise, DORV and TGA are rarely found in patients with CATCH 22 syndrome (Cardiac defects, Abnormal facies, Thymic hypoplasia, Cleft palate, and Hypocalcemia resulting from 22q11 deletions), although TOF is not uncommon. In a large sample of patients with conotruncal defects prospectively ascertained to evaluate the frequency of 22q11 deletions, only 1 of 20 patients with DORV and none of 45 patients with TGA was found to have a deletion, compared with 50% of patients with interrupted aortic arch, 34.5% with truncus arteriosus, and 15.9% with TOF.[32]

As for most cardiac defects, a single gene defect leading to DORV in humans has not been found. However, increasing evidence suggests that most congenital heart disease may be the result of mutations in one or more of a network of cardiac developmental-control genes.[94] Recent work in avian species has shown that bone morphogenetic proteins 2 and 4 (BMP-2/4), known to be early inducers of the cardiac myocyte lineage, may be required for proper migration of neural crest cells into the developing outflow tract.[3] When BMP-2/4 function was inhibited during development of the conotruncus, a spectrum of abnormalities was seen, including DORV. Targeted gene-knockout experiments in mice have resulted in a variety of cardiac malformations and suggest a role for the protein product of those genes in the normal developmental cascade of signaling and response. Transforming growth factor-β_2 knockout mice have DORV in 87.5%, and associated malformations are those typically seen in humans with this defect.[10] GATA-4 knockout mice exhibit embryonic lethality, and when GATA-4 interaction with a presumptive cardiac cofactor FOG-2 is inhibited, embryos with semilunar valve abnormalities and DORV are produced.[23] Finally, the vitamin A metabolite retinoic acid appears to play a pivotal role in several aspects of normal cardiac morphogenesis, and DORV is among the malformations resulting from mutations in genes encoding various ligand-receptor isoforms.[34,49]

CLASSIFICATION

The many attempts at classification of DORV over the years attest to the complexity of the lesion, which results from three features of DORV: (1) the variable position of the VSD in relation to the great arteries, (2) the variable relation of the great arteries to one another, and (3) the multiplicity of possible segmental connections. Nevertheless, from the surgical- and critical care–management points of view, a useful classification has evolved based on the work of Lev[5,50,63,71,91] and others (Table 34-1).

Table 34-1 Classification of Double-Outlet
Right Ventricle

VSD Location	Outflow Obstruction	Presentation	Differential Diagnosis
Subaortic	None	CHF	Large VSD
Subaortic	PS	Cyanosis	TOF
Subpulmonary	None	CHF with cyanosis	D-TGA with large VSD
	AS	CHF, cyanosis, poor perfusion	D-TGA with VSD and aortic obstruction
Doubly committed	None	CHF	Large VSD
	PS	Cyanosis	TOF
Noncommitted	Rare	CHF	Large VSD

AS, aortic stenosis; CHF, congestive heart failure; PS, pulmonic stenosis; TOF, tetralogy of Fallot; D-TGA and D-transposition of the great arteries; VSD, ventricular septal defect

Elements of Double-Outlet Right Ventricle Classification

The classification scheme of DORV focuses on the predominant morphologic and clinical syndromes, recognizing that many rare variants exist and sometimes defy clear-cut classification (see later under Anatomy). The problem is simplified by the recognition that the vast majority of DORV is in the setting of situs solitus and AV concordance. The relation of the VSD to the great arteries and the presence or absence of outflow-tract obstruction are critically important because they explain (1) the amount and proportion of systemic and pulmonary blood flow and hence the clinical presentation, and (2) the possibilities for surgical repair.

Double-Outlet Right Ventricle Categories

The location of the VSD in relation to the great arteries may be subaortic, subpulmonary, doubly committed, or noncommitted (also referred to as "remote") to a great artery (see Table 34-1).[50] The *subaortic* VSD is most common in DORV (Fig. 34-1A). The great artery relation is most commonly with the aorta to the right of the PA. PS is common in DORV with subaortic VSD. Hence the presentation mimics either a large VSD with congestive heart failure in cases without PS or TOF with cyanosis in cases with PS. When instead subaortic obstruction occurs, cyanosis is less obvious, and the presentation is that of heart failure and poor systemic output. Coarctation is an associated finding.

The *subpulmonary* VSD is the next most common variety of DORV (Fig. 34-1B). PS is rare; however, subaortic stenosis and coarctation of the aorta are frequently associated. The presentation resembles that of TGA with a large VSD, in that the infant is cyanotic with congestive heart failure (CHF). When obstruction to systemic flow is present, poor systemic output and metabolic acidosis may occur.

The *doubly committed* VSD category of DORV resembles the subaortic group, in that PS is relatively frequently associated and governs the presenting signs, as described for the subaortic group (Fig. 34-1C).

In the rare *noncommitted* VSD category of DORV, the VSD is in a remote location from the arterial valve (Fig. 34-1D). PS is usually absent. Patients resemble those with a large VSD and CHF.

DORV rarely occurs with *discordant AV connection*. Battistessa and Soto[11] studied a series of 19 such patients based on angiography and noted that 6 (29%) had subaortic and 11 (52%) had subpulmonic VSD. The VSD was doubly committed in one and noncommitted in two patients. The great artery relationship in DORV with discordant AV connection is usually characterized by the aorta being anterior and to the left of the PA.

ANATOMY

Ventricular Septal Defect

The size and location of the VSD in DORV is of considerable importance in considering the surgical options. Whereas a VSD is almost always present, occasionally none is seen, with

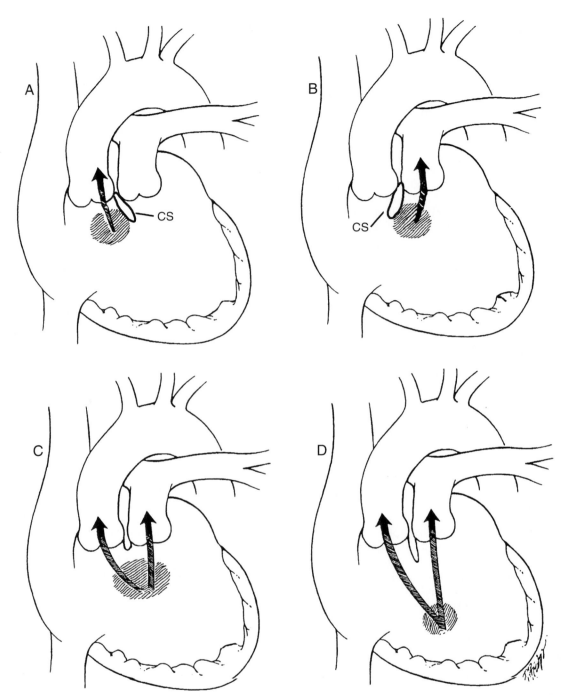

FIGURE 34-1 Four types of ventricular septal defect (VSD) occur in double-outlet right ventricle. The view is of the septal surfaces of the opened right atrium and right ventricle. **A,** Subaortic VSD. Note the anterior and leftward deviation of the conal septum (CS), causing the aorta to be over the VSD and the subpulmonary region to be narrow. **B,** Subpulmonary VSD. Note the posterior and rightward deviation of CS, resulting in the pulmonary artery being over the VSD and subaortic narrowing. **C,** Doubly committed VSD. The CS is deficient and the VSD is large. **D,** Remote VSD, midmuscular. Other remote VSDs not depicted here include apical, anterior and posterior muscular, and some inlet or atrioventicular canal defects.

the only outlet to the LV in these cases being back across an insufficient mitral valve into the left atrium and across an atrial septal defect (ASD) to the right side of the heart.[2,92]

Whether the VSD appears to be subaortic or subpulmonary in location is actually due to the variable position of the conal septum in relation to the VSD. The malformed and malpositioned conus can result in malalignment of the conal septum *superiorly* with the muscular interventricular septum *inferiorly*. Rightward or leftward deviation of the conal septum aligns one or the other semilunar valve more proximal to the defect.[108] The VSD itself, in both cases, is a conoventricular defect (i.e., a defect that lies between the parietal band or conal septum superiorly and the septal band of the muscular ventricular septum inferiorly).

Subaortic Ventricular Septal Defect

Subaortic defects are the most common variety in DORV. The conal septum is usually deviated anteriorly and leftward, aligning the aorta with the VSD and resulting in LV blood streaming preferentially into the aorta. In addition, this conal septal deviation often causes "crowding" of the subpulmonary area, resulting in subpulmonary or pulmonary valvular stenosis or both.

Subpulmonary Ventricular Septal Defect

As mentioned earlier for subaortic VSDs, the subpulmonary VSD in DORV also is a conoventricular defect caused by malalignment of the conal septum, resulting from maldevelopment of the entire infundibulum. This is to be distinguished from the "subpulmonary" VSD found in otherwise normal hearts with a normally aligned but deficient conal septum. The Taussig-Bing malformation is a particular variant of DORV with a subpulmonary VSD, side-by-side great arteries with the aorta to the right, and bilateral subarterial conus.[102] In this case, the conal septum may be deviated anteriorly, aligning the pulmonary artery with the VSD and, not uncommonly, resulting in subaortic stenosis. Subpulmonary stenosis is relatively infrequent.

Doubly Committed Defect

Doubly committed defects are relatively rare, large, conoventricular VSDs that are both subaortic and subpulmonary owing to significant conal septal maldevelopment and malposition. The hemodynamics usually is determined by the presence or absence of subaortic or subpulmonary stenosis.

Noncommitted Defect

Remote VSDs are neither subaortic nor subpulmonary.[96] They can be defects in the anterior, mid, or posterior muscular septum, or can be within the AV canal septum. Because of their lack of proximity to either semilunar valve, surgical options for redirecting LV egress tend to be more limited.

Relation of Great Arteries

From the surgical perspective, the great artery position and interrelation may be grouped into three categories: (1) aorta posterior and rightward to the PA, (2) aorta anterior, pulmonary posterior (with the aorta most commonly to the right of the main PA), and (3) side-by-side orientation (with the aorta most commonly to the right of the PA). The rightward and posterior aorta to the PA is common in DORV with AV concordance, in which the VSD is subaortic, subpulmonary, or doubly committed.[36,44,71] A significant number of cases of DORV with subpulmonary VSD have truly side-by-side great arteries that ascend parallel to each other rather than spiraling around each other, as in normally related great vessels.[5,36] DORV with noncommitted VSD is more likely to have the aorta anterior, either directly or slightly to the right. Despite the utility of these generalizations, it remains true that any type of VSD can occur with any arrangement of the great arteries and any type of subarterial conus.

Associated Anomalies

Many of the associated cardiac lesions in hearts with DORV may be present because of the same dysmorphologic sequence or as a consequence of that sequence. More important, the hemodynamic features are often influenced by the associated malformations.

Outflow-Tract Obstruction

Outflow-tract stenosis in DORV is almost always the result of incomplete growth and expansion of the infundibulum beneath the obstructed artery, usually in association with hypertrophy or deviation of the conal septum, or both. In addition to subarterial stenosis, the structures "downstream" from the narrowed outflow tract are often poorly developed, probably as a result of lower flow states in the artery during development. The semilunar valve itself often has a smaller-than-normal annulus diameter with leaflets that are thickened, bicommissural, and doming in systole.

Pulmonary stenosis is the most common associated lesion in DORV,[92] particularly in cases with a subaortic or doubly committed VSD. The valve leaflets can be malformed or even atretic in rare cases. Often a diminutive subpulmonary conus, a subaortic VSD, and a large aorta are found. Severe malformation of the pulmonary valve can result in pulmonary atresia (technically not meeting some criteria for the diagnosis of DORV, but often referred to as DORV with pulmonary atresia when the atretic valve can be identified and is related to the right ventricle).

Subaortic stenosis occurs frequently in cases with subpulmonary VSD and attenuated subaortic conus.[110] In addition, aortic valvular stenosis, as well as aortic arch anomalies including coarctation and interruption, sometimes is seen. Occasionally the VSD can become restrictive, causing left ventricular outlet obstruction similar to subaortic stenosis.[30,55]

Atrioventricular Valve Malformations

Mitral valve anomalies may occur in DORV, including mitral stenosis and atresia with associated underdevelopment of the LV. Most cases of DORV with intact ventricular septum (IVS) involve severe abnormalities of the mitral valve. In addition, cleft, double orifice, parachute, as well as straddling mitral valve can be associated.[8,29,31,65,77,101,117] When straddling mitral valve is present, it almost always "straddles" the interventricular septum through a large conoventricular defect, attaching into an enlarged infundibular chamber.[108] In addition to mitral valve problems, Ebstein's malformation of the tricuspid valve as well as, rarely, tricuspid atresia can occur in DORV.

Other Associated Intracardiac Malformations

A common AV canal is often seen in association with DORV.[66,67,93,103] When present, it is usually an "unbalanced" canal with the common AV valve opening primarily into the RV, the left-sided structures often being malformed and hypoplastic, although the reverse also can be true, with the great arteries arising from the infundibulum of a hypoplastic RV. Common AV canal is usually associated with a subpulmonary infundibulum and subpulmonary stenosis.[108] The presence of common AV canal in DORV also should raise the possibility of heterotaxy (asplenia/polysplenia syndrome). For many of these patients, if the AV valve is competent, staged reconstruction toward a Fontan may be preferable to attempts at two-ventricle repair.

Ventricular malformations can occur with stenosis or atresia of either the left or right AV valve, leading to hypoplasia of the respective ventricle. When tricuspid atresia and RV sinus hypoplasia are present, both great arteries arise from the infundibular chamber. In severe mitral stenosis or atresia with a VSD, the LV chamber is often hypoplastic, and both great arteries may arise above the RV. In addition, DORV can occur in the setting of double-inlet RV, with a rudimentary hypoplastic LV.

Severe hypertrophy of the septal and parietal bands of the RV can result in a partitioning of the inlet and outlet portions, forming a "double-chambered" RV. Whereas this can occur in the otherwise normal heart with a conoventricular VSD, it also was reported in association with DORV.[22,38]

Occasionally, the atrial appendages can be juxtaposed, either to the left or to the right.[4,6,7] Seventeen percent of cases of juxtaposition of the atrial appendages (JAA) were found to have DORV.[58] In D-looped ventricles, left JAA is more common, whereas in inverted, L-looped ventricles, right JAA is more frequently seen. Left JAA is frequently associated with tricuspid atresia, a hypoplastic inlet portion of the RV, and DORV.

Heterotaxy Syndromes

Both polysplenia and asplenia syndromes frequently have DORV as part of the constellation of heart defects (see Chapter 46 on Syndromes). In *polysplenia* with DORV, usually a subpulmonary infundibulum is noted, and AV canal anomalies with LV hypoplasia are relatively common.[108] Either subaortic or subpulmonary stenosis can occur. The systemic venous connection may be abnormal with azygous continuation of the inferior vena cava.[5]

In *asplenia* syndrome with DORV, subpulmonary stenosis is almost always present, but subaortic stenosis rarely occurs. Almost always, a bilateral infundibulum and common AV canal are present. Common atrium and total anomalous pulmonary venous connection is frequently seen.

Coronary Artery Patterns

The coronary arterial anatomy is "abnormal" in 50% of cases of DORV.[108] If subpulmonary infundibular hypoplasia is seen, occasionally a "conus branch" from the RCA will course across the epicardial surface of the conus to distribute in the territory of (or communicate with, or both) the left anterior descending artery. Alternatively, the left anterior descending itself may arise from this position, as is sometimes seen in TOF. When the aorta is anterior and to the right of the PA, the coronary pattern is similar to that in D-TGA, with the LCA usually coursing *anterior* to the PA. With side-by-side great arteries, as in the Taussig-Bing heart, coronary artery variations in course are frequent.[85] Identification of these coronary artery anomalies is important to avoid coronary injury during the surgical repair.

PATHOPHYSIOLOGY

Once the anatomic variables of DORV are understood, the various physiologic manifestations become both logical and predictable (see Table 34-1; Fig. 34-2). The important variables determining the physiology of a given heart are those mentioned earlier: the position of the VSD in relation to the great arteries, the relation of the great arteries to each other, and the presence or absence of associated defects (in particular, outflow-tract obstruction). The early classification schemes of DORV emphasized the presence or absence of pulmonic stenosis as being the major physiologic determinant in the majority of cases.[33,63] Indeed, with a large, subaortic VSD and side-by-side great arteries (a common situation in DORV), the presence or absence of PS will dictate whether the hemodynamic features suggest TOF or a simple unrestrictive VSD, respectively. However, with a subpulmonary VSD (as in the Taussig-Bing malformation), the physiology is more similar to transposition (D-TGA) with VSD.

Oxygenation

Although both great arteries arise from the RV, often incomplete mixing of oxygenated and unoxygenated blood occurs at the ventricular level because of streaming. The blood in the great artery most closely related to the VSD and therefore most aligned with LV outflow tends to have the highest

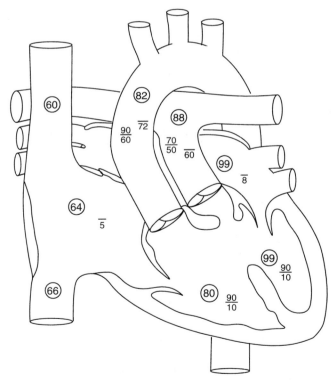

FIGURE 34-2 Schematic diagram of double-outlet right ventricle (DORV) with subaortic ventricular septal defect (VSD) and mild pulmonary stenosis (PS) with O_2 saturations (circled values) and pressures. The position of the VSD allows the left ventricle to be baffled to the aortic valve. The PS is mild and pulmonary flow remains increased, with a calculated Q_p:Q_s ratio of ~3:1. Note that some streaming occurs. Pulmonary saturations may be higher than systemic saturations because of this effect (88% in pulmonary artery vs. 82% in the aorta).

oxygen saturation. Likewise, the great artery that, due to streaming, preferentially receives systemic venous return, tends to have a lower saturation. This can be somewhat different from the situation in true "single-ventricle physiology," in which more complete ventricular-level mixing usually occurs. With complete mixing, as in hypoplastic left heart syndrome with aortic atresia, systemic arterial oxygen saturations can provide an accurate assessment of pulmonary blood flow.

If the VSD is subaortic and no PS is present, pulmonary blood flow will be determined by the relationship of pulmonary (R_p) to systemic (R_s) vascular resistance. When, as is usually the case after the first few weeks of life, R_p is less than R_s, pulmonary blood flow will be greater than systemic flow, with a resulting higher-than-normal pulmonary arterial oxygen saturation and CHF. As R_p inevitably increases in response to this abnormal volume (and pressure) load, pulmonary blood flow correspondingly decreases. Eventually, if left untreated, this usually results in pulmonary vascular obstructive disease with severely and irreversibly elevated R_p, causing progressive cyanosis and early mortality.

With subaortic VSD and PS, either valvular or subvalvular, obstruction to pulmonary blood flow is found, which, depending on the severity of the obstruction, will determine systemic oxygen saturation. As in TOF, a dynamic component to the obstruction may exist, with increased cyanosis occurring during increased inotropic and chronotropic states.

The classic Taussig-Bing anatomy with subpulmonary VSD, side-by-side great arteries, and bilateral conus is characterized by physiology similar to that seen in transposition with VSD. With significant LV-to-PA streaming, essentially two parallel circulations are present, with lower oxygen saturations in the aorta and higher saturations in the PA. If R_p is less than R_s, increased pulmonary blood flow is also found, leading to CHF and early onset of pulmonary vascular obstructive disease if untreated. With associated aortic stenosis or coarctation, the onset of CHF is much sooner, and poor systemic perfusion may be present as the ductus closes.

Pressures

Usually the VSD is unrestrictive, and LV pressure (LV_p) equals RV pressure (RV_p). However, the VSD either can be small from the outset or may become restrictive with time because of increasing septal hypertrophy or occlusive AV valve tissue. If the VSD is restrictive, the LV_p will be greater than RV_p (i.e., suprasystemic LV_p). RV_p will be greater than either aortic or PA pressure if obstruction to flow in either respective artery is present. Occasionally "double-chambered RV" can develop because of muscular hypertrophy of the parietal and septal bands, thereby creating a suprasystemic RV inflow chamber.

DIAGNOSTIC ASSESSMENT

Physical Findings

Most patients with DORV become symptomatic within the first few days to weeks of life, although patients with particularly well-balanced physiology can, although infrequently, go unnoticed for some time. With subaortic VSD and no PS, as in simple, large VSD, increasing signs of pulmonary overcirculation with CHF will often develop as R_p decreases

over the first few weeks of life (see Table 34-1). At presentation, although not necessarily at birth, usually tachypnea, tachycardia, and a loud holosystolic murmur are found. With abnormally high pulmonary blood flow, usually a mid-diastolic murmur of increased flow is heard across the mitral valve. Systemic arterial oxygen saturations may be near normal, depending on the degree of streaming and on the presence of associated pulmonary venous desaturation due to severe CHF and related (or unrelated) lung disease.

In patients with subaortic VSD and PS, moderate to severe cyanosis may be present, depending on the severity of obstruction. As in TOF, the cyanosis may increase over time, and hypercyanotic episodes may occur. The systolic murmur is a harsh ejection-type sound that is due to the outflow-tract obstruction. The intensity of the murmur varies inversely with the degree of obstruction. If pulmonary valve stenosis is present, a pulmonary ejection click may be heard. The second heart sound is often single.

In DORV with subpulmonary VSD, early cyanosis and heart failure are usually the presenting signs. A loud holosystolic murmur as well as an ejection-type systolic murmur often is heard if an associated outflow-tract obstruction exists. As stated earlier, a mid-diastolic rumble may be present with significantly increased pulmonary blood flow.

Diagnostic Tests

Chest Radiograph

The *chest radiograph* appearance varies depending on the type of DORV encountered. In DORV with subaortic VSD and no PS, the pulmonary trunk is prominent, heart size is normal or increased, and pulmonary vasculature appears engorged after the decrease in R_p. In the presence of PS, the pulmonary vasculature is reduced or normal, and the heart size is normal. The chest radiograph in patients with DORV and subpulmonary VSD reveals increased pulmonary vascularity and heart size.

Electrocardiogram

The *electrocardiogram* (ECG) pattern is not diagnostic. Common ECG findings include prolonged PR interval, peaked P waves, and RV or biventricular hypertrophy.

Echocardiography

Echocardiography is now the basis for the diagnosis of DORV with a high degree of accuracy.[82] The key to the diagnosis is visualization of two great arteries committed primarily (each more than 50%) to the RV.[90] This finding can often readily be appreciated by using the subxyphoid short-axis view (Fig. 34-3). The additional demonstration of discontinuity between the posterior semilunar valve annulus and the mitral valve supports this diagnosis and can usually be made by using the parasternal long-axis view. The VSD position relative to the great arteries can be easily investigated from subxyphoid imaging, and the potential pathway from the LV to the aorta examined (Fig. 34-4). Additional VSDs also can be seen from this view.

With a side-by-side great arterial relation, both semilunar valves lie in the same plane, and with bilateral subarterial conus, the valves appear at the same level from subxyphoid

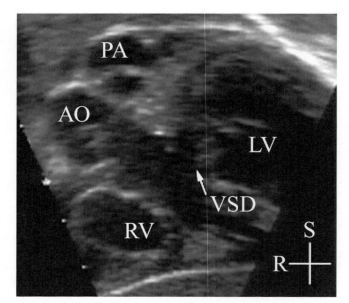

FIGURE 34-3 Echocardiogram, subxyphoid short-axis view, of patient with double-outlet right ventricle. The pulmonary artery (PA) and aorta (AO) both arise above the right ventricle (RV). The conoventricular septal defect is subaortic. LV, left ventricle; R, right; S, superior.

views (Fig. 34-5). This appearance is distinctly different from normally related great arteries, in which the valves are at different heights and lie in nonparallel planes relative to each other. When the aorta is anterior and either rightward or leftward relative to the pulmonary valve, the semilunar valvular relation appears similar on the parasternal short-axis view to D-TGA or corrected transposition (L-TGA), respectively. DORV is differentiated from these latter two diagnoses by tilting the transducer inferiorly so that the muscular interventricular septum is seen and noting that both semilunar valves are on the morphologic RV side of the septum (i.e., *anterior* to the septum with normal, D-looped ventricles).

In addition to making the diagnosis of DORV, the echocardiogram should provide information that can assist in determining the type of surgical repair most suitable for a given heart (Table 34-2). The relative size of both ventricles and their predicted ability to handle their respective, postrepair workloads may influence the decision between a two-versus univentricular repair. The presence of PS or aortic stenosis, either valvular or subvalvular, can usually be imaged in various views and the degree of obstruction estimated by Doppler interrogation. Subaortic stenosis can be caused by a poorly developed subaortic infundibulum, hypertrophied conal septal musculature, or by a narrow, tunnel-like LV outflow

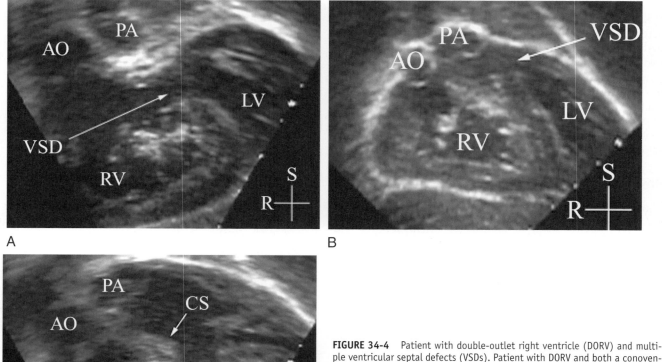

FIGURE 34-4 Patient with double-outlet right ventricle (DORV) and multiple ventricular septal defects (VSDs). Patient with DORV and both a conoventricular septal defect that is primarily subaortic **(A)** as well as a moderate-sized, anterior muscular VSD located under the pulmonary artery **(B)**. **C,** Note conal septum (CS) and the presence of bilateral subarterial conus. AO, aorta; LV, left ventricle; PA, pulmonary artery; R, right; RV, right ventricle; S, superior.

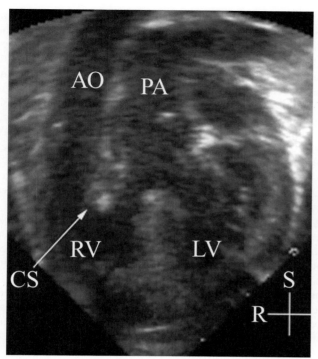

FIGURE 34-5   Double-outlet right ventricle, Taussig-Bing variant. In this view, the side-by-side relation of the great arteries is appreciated. The ventricular septal defect is subpulmonary and results from anterior and rightward displacement of conal septum (CS). The aorta (AO) and pulmonary artery (PA) are simultaneously imaged in the same plane, distinctly different from the normal relation. The AO is directly to the right of the PA, and the bilateral subarterial conus results in the semilunar valves being at approximately the same level. LV, left ventricle; R, right; RV, right ventricle; S, superior.

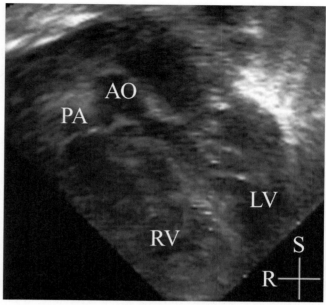

FIGURE 34-6   Double-outlet right ventricle (DORV) with subaortic stenosis. This apical four-chamber view of an infant heart with DORV and mitral stenosis with mild left ventricular hypoplasia demonstrates subaortic stenosis caused by a narrow left ventricular outflow tract and relatively small ventricular septal defect. This patient also had critical coarctation of the aorta. AO, aorta; LV, left ventricle; PA, pulmonary artery; R, right; RV, right ventricle; S, superior.

tract and VSD (Fig. 34-6). The aortic arch should be examined closely in these cases from the suprasternal notch view to rule out coarctation and other arch anomalies.

Associated malformations of the AV canal and the AV valves should be looked for on the apical four-chamber view

Table 34-2   Analysis of the Preoperative Echocardiogram

1. What is the segmental situs?
2. Do both great arteries arise above the morphologic right ventricle?
3. Are there two adequate-sized ventricles?
4. Regarding the VSD (if present)
   a. Size?
   b. Location and position relative to the great arteries?
   c. Additional VSDs?
5. Is there outflow obstruction (pulmonary or aortic)?
6. Are there associated cardiac malformations (CAVC, straddling MV, mitral stenosis, tricuspid atresia, venous anomalies)?
7. Are the coronary arteries normal?
8. Will an interventricular repair be possible?
   a. Can blood from the left ventricle be directed to a great vessel in an unobstructed manner?
   b. Is the tricuspid-to-pulmonary valve distance adequate (at least equal to the aortic diameter)?
   c. Will resection of infundibular septum be required?
   d. Will the VSD have to be enlarged to accommodate the LV-to–great vessel pathway?
   e. Are there tricuspid valve attachments to the infundibular septum or straddling of the AV valves?

VSD, ventricular septal defect; CAVC, common atrioventricular canal; MV, mitral valve; LV, left ventricle.

and from subxyphoid. Additional muscular VSDs should be sought by using plain imaging and color Doppler in parasternal, apical, and subxyphoid views.[99] The coronary artery anatomy should be evaluated, looking in particular for anomalies that would affect a plan to perform an infundibular incision to relieve subpulmonary stenosis (e.g., left anterior descending [LAD] artery or a conal branch from the RCA coursing across the free wall of the conus) or the coronary artery transfer required in the arterial switch operation (ASO).

The preoperative echocardiographic examination also should include specific quantitative information relevant to the respective surgical correction. Measurements of the tricuspid–to–pulmonary valve distance should be made to determine whether an intracardiac repair is feasible (see later).[47] An assessment should be made of whether the infundibular septum will need to be resected to allow for an unobstructed LV-to-aortic tunnel (more commonly a problem when the aorta is *anterior* to the PA and therefore the conal septum is *posterior* to the aortic valve). The VSD also should be assessed not only in terms of its position, but also as to whether it will need to be enlarged to allow unobstructed LV egress. Possible tricuspid valve attachments to the infundibular septum should be looked for and considered when formulating the surgical plan.

Angiography

The classic angiographic features of DORV, as described by Carey and Edwards[20] in 1965, are (1) contrast filling of both great arteries after RV injection, (2) a similar horizontal plane of both the aortic and pulmonary valves, (3) often anterior "malposition" of the aorta, and (4) the impression of a "filling defect," which represents the conal septum dividing the two outflow tracts. Specific issues to address with angiography that may have been incompletely dealt with by echocardiography include (1) position of the VSD in relation to the great arteries, (2) presence of additional (usually mid- and apical-muscular) VSDs, (3) assessment of the size (volume) and function of both ventricles, (4) presence of outflow-tract obstruction including aortic arch defects, (5) coronary artery anatomy, and (6) pulmonary vascular resistance and pressures. Most infants with DORV do not require preoperative cardiac catheterization.

Additional Imaging Techniques

With advances in magnetic resonance imaging (MRI) techniques, including higher spatial resolution, more rapid sequence acquisition, and cine-loop capabilities, this technique is rapidly becoming an essential tool in the evaluation of congenital heart disease, even in the infant. ECG-gated, multislice spin-echo MRI is a useful technique for morphologic assessment of intracardiac and great vessel pathology. For infants and small children referred for evaluation of DORV, the slice thickness can be 3 to 5 mm, resulting in adequate anatomic detail.[64] Multiple-phase gradient-echo MRI allows the evaluation of flow and contractility when displayed in movie or cine format. Gadolinium-enhanced gradient-echo images also are very helpful, particularly in the display of venous and great vessel anatomy.

In addition to MRI, three-dimensional echocardiography, including real-time display techniques, is becoming available for clinical use and should be valuable for the preoperative assessment of DORV, particularly in the setting of unusual anatomic relations and geometry.[9] Transesophageal echocardiography is helpful when transthoracic windows are limited.

PREOPERATIVE CRITICAL CARE MANAGEMENT

Preoperative management of patients with DORV depends primarily on the age of the patient and the presenting signs. Medical management, listed subsequently, represents temporary therapy, and all symptomatic patients require surgical correction or palliation (Table 34-3).

Newborns with severe cyanosis should be initially managed with intravenous prostaglandin E_1 (PGE_1) until the cause of cyanosis is determined and more definitive therapy can be undertaken. If cyanosis is due to severe PS or pulmonary atresia, PGE_1 infusion should be continued to maintain ductal patency and thus provide adequate pulmonary blood flow until the time of surgical intervention. If cyanosis appears to be due to inadequate mixing of pulmonary and systemic venous blood, as in cases of Taussig-Bing DORV with intact atrial septum, consideration of emergency balloon atrial septostomy should be given.

In DORV with increased pulmonary blood flow, signs of CHF may be present. Pulmonary overcirculation is reduced by adjusting the inspired O_2 concentration to maintain a systemic oxygen saturation of 80% to 85%. If mechanical ventilation is required, high FiO_2 and hyperventilation should be strictly avoided, and $PaCO_2$ should be maintained at 40 mm Hg. This may require sedation and paralysis of the patient. The goal of therapy is to maintain a balanced ratio of pulmonary to systemic blood flow (Q_p:$Q_s = 1$). As in other lesions, CHF from increased pulmonary blood flow also may be managed with diuretics, inotropic agents, and systemic afterload-reducing agents.

Shen and coworkers[88] noted that in older patients (10.3 ± 7.8 years), *pre*operative elevation of PA and RA pressures as well as supraventricular tachycardia (perhaps resulting from RA distention) predict late *post*operative sudden death in univariate analysis. Only older age at the time of operation remains an independent predictor of late postoperative death in multivariate analysis. Presumably some form of myocardial damage occurs if repair is delayed. Thus surgical correction should be carried out during infancy in the majority of DORV patients.

In *DORV with decreased pulmonary blood flow* (subaortic or doubly committed VSD and PS) cyanosis may be present. Pulmonary circulation may be ductal dependent (depending on the degree of PS), and these patients may need to be treated like infants with symptomatic TOF, including infusion of PGE_1. In addition to stabilization with prostaglandin, mechanical ventilation may be required. In the situation in which R_p is increased, liberal use of supplemented oxygen, hyperventilation, or administration of nitric oxide may be beneficial.

Table 34-3   Preoperative Problems

DORV Anatomy	Problem	Therapy	Anticipated Result
Subaortic VSD with PS (newborn)	Cyanosis (Q_p:$Q_s < 1$)	PGE_1	Maintain PDA Q_p:$Q_s = 1$
Subaortic VSD with PS (infant/child)	Hypercyanotic ("tet") spell	O_2, morphine, fluid volume, β blockers, neosynephrine	↓ Infundibular spasm ↑ PBF
Subaortic VSD no PS (infant)	CHF (Q_p:$Q_s > 1$)	Respiratory target: SaO_2, 80–85%; $PaCO_2$, 40 mm Hg; diuretics, inotropes	↓ PBF Q_p:$Q_s = 1$ ↓ Heart failure
Subpulmonary VSD (newborn)	Cyanosis (inadequate mixing) and CHF	PGE_1, balloon atrial septostomy SaO_2, 80–85%; $PaCO_2$, 40 mm Hg	↑ Ductal mixing ↑ Atrial mixing ↓ PBF Q_p:$Q_s = 1$
Subpulmonary VSD with AS/CoA (newborn)	Cyanosis, CHF, shock (inadequate mixing, Q_p:$Q_s > 1$)	PGE_1 SaO_2, 80–85%; $PaCO_2$, 40 mm Hg	Maintain PDA for systemic perfusion Q_p:$Q_s = 1$

AS/CoA, Aortic stenosis and/or coarctation of the aorta; CHF, congestive heart failure; $PaCO_2$, arterial CO_2 pressure; PBF, pulmonary blood flow; PDA, patent ductus arteriosus; PGE_1, prostaglandin E_1; PS, pulmonic stenosis; Q_p:Q_s, pulmonary blood flow–to–systemic blood flow ratio; SaO_2, systemic oxygen saturation; VSD, ventricular septal defect.

In *DORV with subpulmonary VSD* (as in the Taussig-Bing malformation), cyanosis is due to incomplete mixing of the (parallel) pulmonary and systemic circulations, as is the case in TGA. Whereas the VSD usually allows adequate mixing, atrial and ductal mixing also may be required, possibly necessitating a balloon atrial septostomy or intravenous PGE_1, respectively, or both. In patients with associated critical aortic obstruction, maintenance of ductal patency with PGE_1 is imperative for adequate systemic perfusion.[95] Once adequate mixing has been assured, maintenance of balanced $Q_p:Q_s = 1$ is achieved with the respiratory management described earlier.

Older patients with DORV and cyanosis due to subpulmonary stenosis may have episodic hypercyanosis ("Tet spells") requiring intervention (see Table 34-3 and Chapter 35). As in TOF, these patients are at increased risk for severe and persistent "spelling" during the preoperative cardiac catheterization and thus should be managed cautiously.

General supportive measures appropriate for all patients include attention to oxygen carrying capacity by maintaining the hematocrit between 40% and 55% for cyanotic patients, avoidance of electrolyte disturbances secondary to diuretic therapy by using appropriate ion-sparing agents or replacement therapy as needed, and the maintenance of adequate nutrition.

SURGICAL PROCEDURE

Surgical management for DORV is determined by the anatomy and physiology of the defect as well as by the age at which the diagnosis is made and at which the need for surgical intervention arises. In most cases, the goal of surgery is to perform a complete two-ventricle repair, which restores normal circulation. Occasionally, such as in patients with heterotaxy and unbalanced ventricles, a two-ventricle repair is not possible, and staging toward a Fontan procedure is warranted. The fact that these lesions can be complex is demonstrated by the study of Wilcox and colleagues.[113] Among 63 hearts with DORV, it was determined that 23 (36.5%) were inoperable as a result of the extent of their anatomic aberrancy. This group of hearts had associated lesions such as straddling valves, multiple septal defects, LV hypoplasia, or other combinations of complex lesions that made the possibility of successful operation unlikely. In most of these patients, the only viable option would be staging toward Fontan, and recognition of this necessity is imperative during the early surgical decision-making process. In an autopsy series of 50 hearts with DORV,[95] 26 were found to be so severely abnormal that surgical correction could not have been performed. Despite these figures, DORV is often a correctable lesion with an increasingly improving surgical outlook.

Goals and Timing of Operation

Since the first reported repair by McGoon[57] in 1961 of the condition now referred to as DORV, many technical advances have been made, but the basic principles of the repair remain the same. The ultimate goals of complete, two-ventricle repair of this defect are to (1) establish unobstructed LV-to-aortic continuity, (2) establish adequate RV-to-PA continuity, and (3) repair associated lesions. When complete repair is not an option, palliative surgery is lesion dependent and has both the short-term goal of providing stable hemodynamics and the longer-term goal of maintaining suitable candidacy of the patient for eventual Fontan procedure.

To plan a suitable surgical repair, the surgeon must know the orientation of the great vessels, the location (and size) of the VSD and its relation to the great arteries, the distribution and location of the coronary arteries, whether PS or aortic stenosis is present, and the nature of any associated intra- or extracardiac anomalies.[113] These data must be combined with information regarding hemodynamics obtained from echocardiographic examination as well as from cardiac catheterization in some cases.[76] The goal of the operation is to separate the systemic and pulmonary circulations. These types of repairs require the use of cardiopulmonary bypass (CPB). In infants, deep hypothermia with total circulatory arrest is sometimes necessary, but increasingly, low-flow bypass techniques are being used to minimize the duration of periods of circulatory arrest. Palliation in infancy (i.e., placement of a systemic-to-pulmonary shunt or PA banding) may be appropriate in some patients, especially in very small infants and those whose anatomy necessitates staging toward Fontan-type operations. The need for initial palliation in those patients whose anatomy is appropriate for a two-ventricle repair is controversial. However, for those patients in whom the location of the VSD would require an extensive intracardiac reconstruction and possibly for those in whom a desire exists to enable growth before placement of an extracardiac conduit, an acceptable role may be found for shunts or PA bands in the neonatal period.

Surgical correction of DORV with increased pulmonary blood flow should be undertaken during the first 3 months of life to minimize the morbidity of heart failure and avoid the risk of development of pulmonary vascular disease. The greatest urgency exists in cases of DORV with subpulmonary VSD and severe aortic obstruction, because these patients do not have a reliable source of systemic blood flow, and surgical correction may be needed in the first few days of life. The timing of repair of subaortic DORV with PS is similar to that for TOF, in that repair is performed electively by 2 to 6 months of life or earlier if the infant becomes symptomatic.

Intraventricular Tunnel Repair of "Classic" Double-Outlet Right Ventricle

The most common form of DORV is that associated with a subaortic VSD with or without PS. The "simple," complete intracardiac repair consists of patching the VSD in such a way that LV blood is baffled to the aorta (Fig. 34-7).[16,52,72,98] In almost all cases, the creation of an unobstructed baffle from the LV to the aorta, which simultaneously serves to patch the interventricular communication, is technically possible. If the VSD is smaller than the orifice of the aortic valve, the VSD may often be safely enlarged by resecting the ventricular septum in an anterior, leftward, and superior direction (Fig. 34-8). Reconstruction of the RV outflow tract is then accomplished to complete the repair. In the best of circumstances, usually when the aortic valve is posterior to the pulmonary valve and no PS is present, the ventricular incision can be closed primarily. Not uncommonly, however, especially in the presence of significant infundibular stenosis,

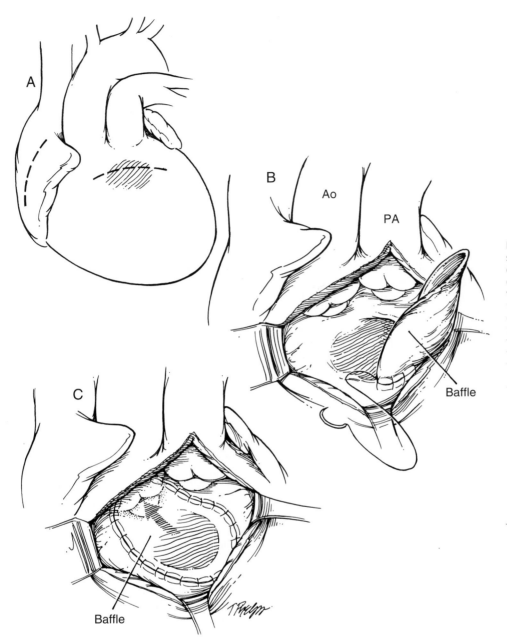

FIGURE 34-7 The intracardiac baffle for a subaortic ventricular septal defect (VSD) in double-outlet right ventricle. A variety of options can be used for closing the ventriculotomy including primary closure, patch closure, transannular patch closure, or a conduit between the right ventricle and pulmonary artery. **A,** Approach can be through either right atriotomy or right ventriculotomy. **B,** Initial placement of baffle for subaortic VSD. **C,** Final closure of defect such that ventricular flow is directed through the VSD toward the aortic valve (*stippled area*).

or to prevent RV outflow obstruction from a large intracardiac baffle, patch closure of the infundibular incision will be required. Occasionally, a transannular patch is necessary, or the use of an extracardiac RV-to-PA conduit may be indicated.

It is crucial that the surgeon be alerted to any additional cardiac defects that might need simultaneous correction. The incidence of associated cardiac anomalies is high,[91,118] especially if ASDs and patent ductus arteriosus (PDA) are included in this definition. Patients with aortic coarctation can have simultaneous repair of the aortic arch at the time of intracardiac repair by use of a median sternotomy approach.[104] The use of routine intraoperative transesophageal or epicardial echocardiography with color-flow imaging has become an invaluable adjunct to the repair of these types of complex lesions because of its ability to accurately and clearly depict intracardiac structures and disclose previously unappreciated details of anatomy at the time of surgical correction (Fig. 34-9).[106,112]

Complications after repair of DORV with subaortic VSD include obstruction to LV outflow from a poorly configured patch or from a restrictive VSD that has not been adequately enlarged or even from progressive obstruction imposed by growth of the infundibular septum.[21,44] Hemolysis across the patch[89] has been less common since the use of Gore-Tex has replaced the use of Dacron in this location. Heart block and other arrhythmias can occur any time a VSD is closed. RV failure also is common for several days after the surgical procedure. The cause is probably multifactorial and may relate to the right ventriculotomy, the ischemia necessary for repair, the suture line on the interventricular septum, and the presence of any pulmonary hypertension that can increase RV afterload in the postoperative period. Because of the potential

When the child has an associated complete AV canal defect, repair of the entire lesion can usually be performed, but once again, careful attention must be given to the intraventricular baffle with anterior-superior enlargement of the inlet-type VSD if necessary. The surgeon must be cautioned that in patients with a noncommitted VSD of the AV canal type, it is likely that the patient may be best staged toward Fontan procedure because often hypoplasia of the RV and straddling of the valvular apparatus exist.

Other Surgical Options

Many patients with DORV and subpulmonary VSD are most reliably repaired by using an arterial switch operation (ASO) after baffling the LV to the PA (through the VSD) (Fig. 34-11).[73,74] Significant PS must not be present; otherwise, aortic stenosis will likely be present postoperatively.

When the aorta is more posterior, it may be possible (although still not necessarily the best option) to construct a baffle to direct LV blood to the aortic valve (referred to by some authors as the "Kawashima procedure," not to be confused with the Kawashima procedure for cavopulmonary anastomosis in the setting of interrupted inferior vena cava with azygous continuation). Although it is sometimes technically possible, the location of the VSD in proximity to the pulmonary orifice and the presence of muscle bands from the infundibular septum can make construction of this baffle technically demanding or even impractical. Nevertheless, careful resection of muscle and placement of the suture line may allow this type of repair in selected patients, particularly those with significant PS or a previous PA band, in whom an ASO may be less appropriate (Fig. 34-12).[116]

The finding of significant subpulmonary stenosis might contraindicate the performance of arterial switch. In these patients, the Damus-Kaye-Stansel procedure can be performed. This requires patching of the VSD into the PA, and diversion of the proximal PA end-to-side into the aorta, with no coronary artery translocation required. RV-to-PA continuity is restored with the use of an external conduit (Fig. 34-13).

If severe subpulmonic stenosis is present and the VSD also can be related to the aortic valve, the arterial switch is contraindicated, and the lesion should be repaired by using the Rastelli procedure. In this operation, the VSD is baffled to the aorta (through a right ventriculotomy), and the PA is divided. The proximal PA is oversewn, and RV-to-PA continuity is established with the use of an external conduit (Fig. 34-14).

Lecompte and associates,[47] on review of 210 patients with abnormal ventriculoarterial connections undergoing 340 operations from 1979 to 1989, reached several conclusions about the requisites for successful intracardiac repair of DORV. They proposed that regardless of the position of the aorta or the VSD, if the pulmonary valve orifice is roughly in its normal location (i.e., the subpulmonary infundibulum is well developed, bringing the pulmonary valve anterior and away from the AV valves), simple intracardiac repair without conduits is usually feasible. The LV-to-aorta tunnel is then able to course posteriorly without impinging on the more anterior pulmonary outflow tract. However, when the subpulmonary infundibulum is less well developed, causing the pulmonary valve to be more posterior and closer to the AV valves, simple intraventricular repair is

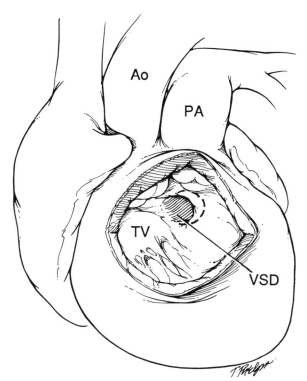

FIGURE 34-8 Double-outlet right ventricle with detailed view of subaortic ventricular septal defect (VSD) anatomy. *Dashed area,* Direction in which a VSD can be enlarged to avoid the risk of complete heart block. Ao, aorta; PA, pulmonary artery; TV, tricuspid valve.

for dysrhythmias, it is recommended that temporary atrial and ventricular wires be left before closure of the chest.

When DORV is associated with a noncommitted VSD, repair follows the same principles but is usually more difficult because the length and configuration of the patch may increase the risk of subaortic baffle obstruction to LV outflow. This problem can be diminished, in part, by generous enlargement of the VSD away from the conduction tissue (Fig. 34-10).

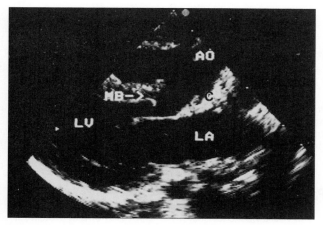

FIGURE 34-9 An intraoperative epicardial echocardiogram of double-outlet right ventricle (DORV) demonstrating the discontinuity between the aortic (AO) and mitral valve leaflets. A large subaortic conus (C) defines the DORV. A fibromuscular membrane (MB) obstructs the left ventricle (LV) outflow tract between the LV and aorta. Intraoperative echocardiography demonstrated this membrane so that it could be resected at the time of surgical repair.

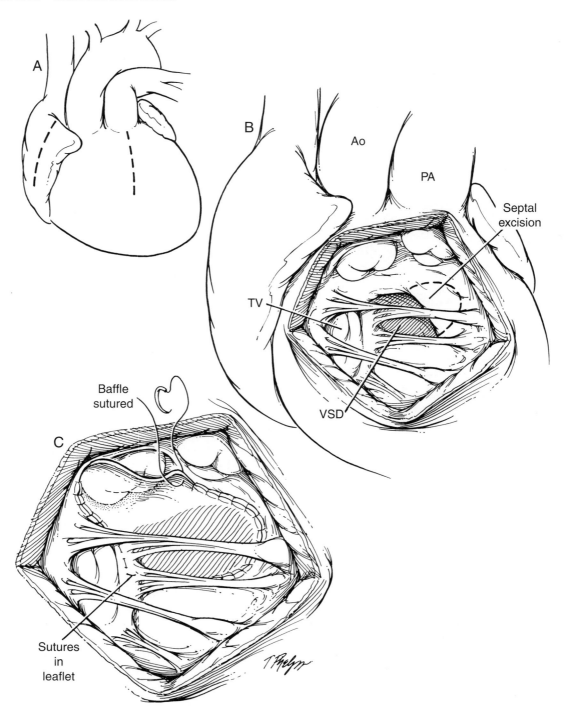

FIGURE 34-10 The anatomy of a patient with an inlet ventricular septal defect (VSD) that is noncommited in double-outlet right ventricle. **A,** Surgical approach may be through a right atriotomy or a right ventriculotomy. **B,** If necessary, the VSD can be enlarged by septal excision. **C,** VSD is patched with a baffle, which directs blood into the aorta (Ao). This is a challenging group of patients; depending on how far the VSD extends into the inlet septum, some are best treated by staging toward a Fontan procedure. PA, pulmonary artery; TV, tricuspid valve.

not usually possible. Options then include the arterial switch operation,[17,19,24,28,39,40,46,51,74,85,114] the Damus-Kaye-Stansel procedure[26] coupled with an RV-to-PA conduit, or baffling when possible the LV to the aorta but with use of either an RV-to-PA conduit (Rastelli procedure[75]) or direct anastomosis of the transected main PA trunk onto the anterior surface of the right ventricle (*REV* procedure, réparation à l'étage ventriculaire).[48]

Palliation

All of these procedures can be performed during infancy, and most forms of DORV lend themselves nicely to early total correction. The advantages of restoring normal circulation early in life are numerous. Even those patients who require external conduits can undergo safe repair in infancy, and the ready availability and excellent performance of homografts

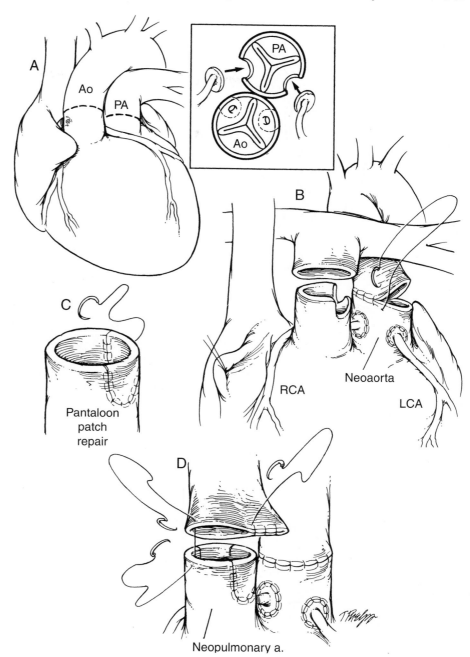

FIGURE 34-11 Arterial switch procedure in double-outlet right ventricle with subpulmonic ventricular septal defect (VSD). **A,** Incision sites in aorta (Ao) and pulmonary artery (PA). **B,** Left and right coronary arteries (LCA, RCA) have been detached from native aorta and reimplanted into neoaorta main PA stump. Aortic arch is pulled leftward and anastomosed to neoaorta. In this diagram, the PA is brought behind the neoaorta, but it is commonly preferred to bring the PA anterior to the neoaorta (Lecompte maneuver) when performing this repair. **C,** Pericardial patch repair of defects in neopulmonary artery. **D,** Partial closure of distal PA is needed to approximate sizes of neopulmonary artery with distal PA.

Pantaloon patch repair

RCA

Neoaorta

LCA

Neopulmonary a.

further favor this approach. Palliation is usually reserved for those patients with complex anatomy (such as severe AV valve abnormalities and unbalanced ventricular dimensions) in whom it may be necessary to stage the patient toward a modified Fontan procedure. In these patients, systemic-to-PA shunts or PA bands should be applied in infancy to palliate the presenting physiology and to provide the necessary growth or protection or both of the pulmonary vasculature that will make it appropriate for Fontan physiology.

If severe cyanosis is present because of PS or atresia, the short-term goal for palliation is, obviously, to provide adequate pulmonary blood flow (i.e., with a systemic-to-PA shunt). Conversely, in the absence of PS, a PA band may be required initially to decrease pulmonary blood flow so that the patient may grow and maintain a "protected" pulmonary

vascular bed until a more definitive repair can be accomplished. In cases of DORV in which either the LV or the inlet portion of the RV is extremely hypoplastic, palliative surgery usually involves a staged application of the Fontan principle: a direct cavopulmonary anastomosis to convey systemic venous return passively to the lungs.[1,35,54,62,80]

POSTOPERATIVE CRITICAL CARE MANAGEMENT

Overview

The postoperative management will depend on the location of the VSD, the presence of associated lesions, the age at

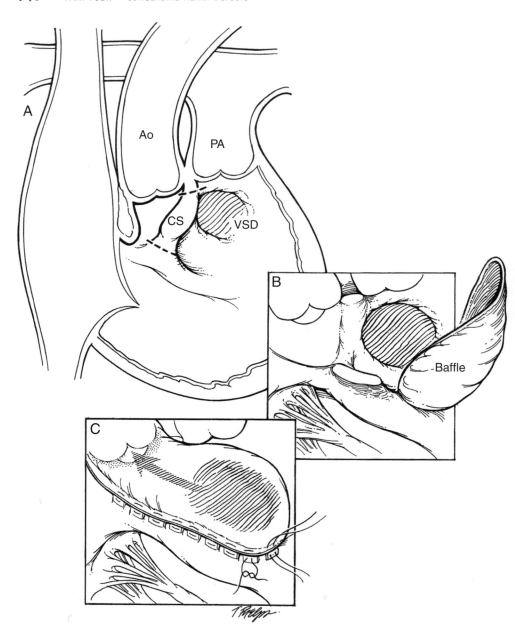

FIGURE 34-12 A subpulmonary ventricular septal defect **(A)** that is effectively blocked from the aorta by the conal septum (CS). The CS can be resected **(B)** so that the VSD can be baffled toward the aorta **(C)**. This is usually possible only if the pulmonary artery annulus is at the same level or slightly anterior to the aortic valve annulus. VSD, ventricular septal defect.

operation, and the surgical reconstruction used. Most infants will return from the operating room with successful separation of the systemic and pulmonary circulations and will be in sinus rhythm. Postoperative care in the first 24 hours is designed to provide afterload reduction and modest inotropic support during recovery of the myocardium from CPB and circulatory arrest and, when necessary, sedation to prevent sudden pulmonary vasospasm in the subgroup without preoperative PS. RV dysfunction can be present after right ventriculotomy and, if so, may transiently compromise cardiac output (Table 34-4).

In some infants, severe hemodynamic problems develop after DORV repair and generally fall into the following categories: LV failure, RV failure, arrhythmias, and residual shunts. Careful monitoring of left and right atrial pressure and PA pressure may help identify the pattern of circulatory failure and the effect of therapy. Intraoperative echocardiography to evaluate the repair before leaving the operating

room has significantly reduced the number of patients discovered in the pediatric intensive care unit (PICU) to have residual defects requiring revision.[105,112]

Left Ventricular Failure

Systemic circulatory failure after DORV repair typically is seen initially with cool extremities, oliguria, and acidosis that may progress to systemic hypotension. If intravascular volume is expanded in the presence of LV failure, LA pressure increases, and pulmonary congestion develops.

A variety of anatomic problems after intracardiac repair of *DORV with subaortic or doubly committed VSD* may occur with signs of systemic circulatory failure. Because LV output is baffled through the VSD to the aorta, obstruction may occur because of insufficient enlargement of VSD size or poor configuration of the patch. Proper configuration of the VSD patch may be especially difficult in *DORV with noncommitted VSD*.

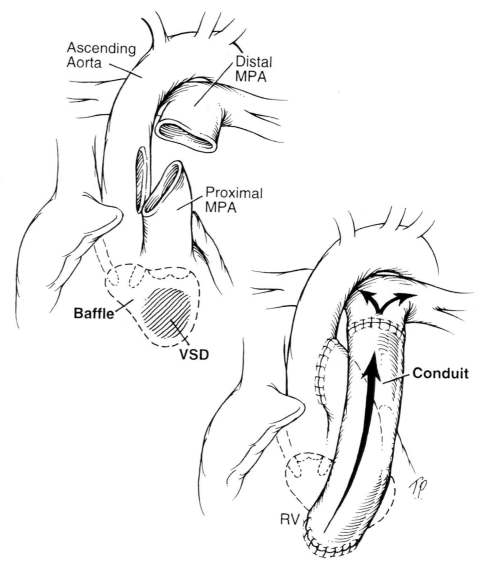

FIGURE 34-13 Damus-Kaye-Stansel procedure for double-outlet right ventricle with subpulmonic ventricular septal defect (VSD). The VSD is baffled into the proximal main pulmonary artery (MPA) and then the pulmonary artery is connected (end-to-side) to the aorta. Alternative technique now preferred for Damus-Kaye-Stansel procedure is as follows: The PA and aorta are transected and attached at their medial borders. This "double-barreled outlet from the heart" is anastomosed to the severed distal aorta by spatulating the end of the distal aorta to enlarge it. The intraventricular patch is placed so that it covers both the aorta and PA, thereby providing a "dual outlet" through the VSD. Right ventricle (RV) reconstruction is provided with a conduit between the RV and severed distal PA.

Table 34-4 Postoperative Problems

Preoperative Anatomy	Type of Repair	Clinical Signs	Potential Problem	Therapeutic Maneuver
DORV, VSD	Any	• Holosystolic murmur	Residual VSD	• Diuretics • Inotropic agents • Reoperate if significant
DORV, VSD	LV to Ao baffle	• Harsh, systolic ejection murmur • Elevated LA$_p$ • Poor systemic perfusion	Subaortic obstruction due to baffle (consider RVOT obstruction too)	• Reoperate if significant
DORV, VSD, no PS	Any	• Elevated PA$_p$ • RV failure	Persistent increase in R$_p$ or residual shunt	• Exclude shunt; if none, use measures to reduce R$_p$
DORV with PS	RVOT patch or RV-to-PA conduit	• Harsh, systolic ejection murmur • RV failure	Residual RVOT obstruction	• Interventional cath or reoperate if significant
DORV with subpulmonary VSD	Arterial switch operation	• Poor systemic perfusion • Elevated LA$_p$	LV dysfunction (may be due to coronary or anastomotic problems)	• Exclude anatomic problem • Avoid rapid volume infusions • Promote afterload reduction

DORV, double-outlet right ventricle; VSD, ventricular septal defect; PA, pulmonary artery; PA$_p$, pulmonary artery pressure; LA$_p$, left atrial pressure; CHF, congestive heart failure; R$_p$, pulmonary resistance; RV, right ventricle; PS, pulmonary stenosis; RVOT, right ventricular outflow tract.

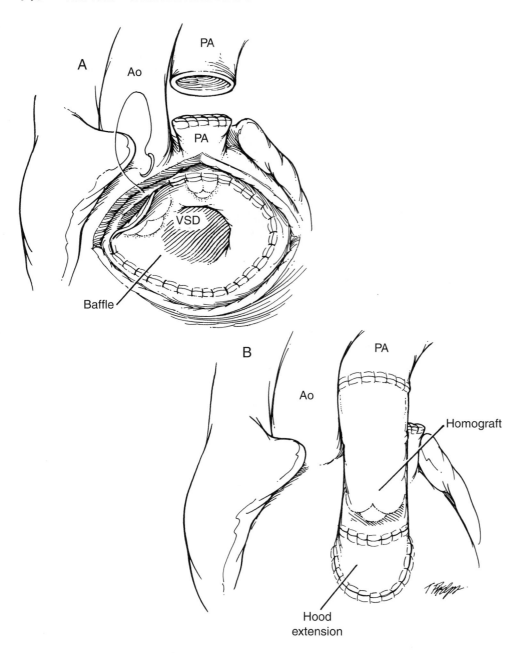

FIGURE 34-14 Rastelli procedure for double-outlet right ventricle with severe subpulmonic stenosis. **A,** An intraventricular baffle directs left ventricular blood to the aorta (Ao) and pulmonary outlet. **B,** Right ventricle to pulmonary artery (PA) continuity is established with a homograft. A piece of pericardium, homograft, or prosthetic material may be used as a hood extension to complete the connection of the homograft with the right ventricle. VSD, ventricular septal defect.

Finally, aortic insufficiency may develop if the aortic valve is injured during resection of the infundibular septum to relieve subpulmonic infundibular stenosis during DORV repair. Although inotropic drugs and mechanical ventilation may provide temporary support, definitive relief of circulatory failure from these anatomic problems will require reoperation.

After repair of *DORV with subpulmonic VSD,* LV failure is most likely related to myocardial ischemia or aortic valve problems. If the ASO was used, patients are at risk for myocardial ischemia due to distortion of the translocated coronary arteries. The postoperative ECG should be compared with the preoperative tracing and scrutinized for ST-T wave abnormalities and regional wall-motion abnormalities identified on echocardiography. If no anatomic problems are present, supportive care includes limiting myocardial O_2 demand. Inotropic support with milrinone also lowers afterload. Aggressive, rapid volume infusion should be avoided because ventricular compliance is often reduced, and volume infusion will increase LV end-diastolic pressure and may decrease coronary perfusion pressure. The mortality rate is high if significant coronary artery distortion occurs, even with optimal supportive care.[84]

The possibility of residual aortic obstruction should be considered if LV failure is encountered after intracardiac baffle repair or after arterial switch of DORV with subpulmonic VSD. The sites of potential residual obstruction are within the baffle, immediately below or at the aortic valve, or within the arch.[79,97] An early gradient in the presence of LV failure likely demands reoperation. In the interim, care is designed to limit further increases in myocardial O_2 demand in the already pressure-overloaded LV. Hence tachycardia and excessive ventricular volume are avoided. Afterload reduction in the face of fixed aortic obstruction is contraindicated because of the risk of sudden hypotension and tachycardia.

Aortic insufficiency may occur in a variety of settings in the infant with DORV and subpulmonic VSD. First, resection of subvalvular aortic stenosis may damage the aortic valve. After the Damus-Kaye-Stansel operation, LV output enters the aorta through a pulmonary-to-aorta (end-to-side) anastomosis. If the aortic valve is incompetent, part of the LV output may regurgitate across the aortic valve into the RV. The increased RV volume may then be ejected through the RV-to-PA conduit, with the result of pulmonary overcirculation. This complication may be managed by oversewing the aortic valve.[25]

After repair of DORV with common AV canal, postoperative AV valve regurgitation may occur. Signs of AV valve regurgitation include a holosystolic murmur at the apex, increased LA pressure, and decreased cardiac output. Definitive diagnosis can be made with echocardiography. Low systemic vascular resistance is maintained when reduced ventricular function is found, and reoperation is considered. Rarely, mitral obstruction may occur after closure of the mitral cleft in DORV with common AV canal and single papillary muscle.[100]

Right Ventricular Failure

Right ventriculotomy combined with the effects of CPB may lead to RV failure after separation of the pulmonary and systemic circulations. RV failure appears with signs of systemic venous congestion, most prominently hepatomegaly in the infant. RA pressure is elevated. Severe RV failure is characterized by worsening systemic venous congestion, such that peripheral edema may become evident in the eyelids, genitalia, and extremities. Decreased systemic (LV) output may occur because of reduced RV output and the negative influence of elevated RV end-diastolic pressure on LV diastolic function.[111]

Pulmonary hypertension is an important cause of life-threatening RV failure in patients with preoperative pulmonary overcirculation; this may occur in any form of DORV without PS. Patients with subpulmonary VSD and aortic obstruction are at greatest risk. A sudden increase in PA pressure can result from a variety of stimuli, such as hypoxia, hypercarbia, and agitation from tracheal suctioning. During the first 24 hours of the postoperative period, sedation, paralysis, hyperventilation, and nitric oxide are used prophylactically in some infants with preoperative pulmonary hypertension. Before concluding that the pulmonary hypertension is due to increased pulmonary resistance, anatomic problems including residual shunt and outflow obstruction must be excluded. Further details of the pathogenesis and management of pulmonary hypertension are given in Chapter 3 on Regulation of Pulmonary Vascular Tone and Chapter 23 on Perioperative Management of Patients with Congenital Heart Disease: A Multidisciplinary Approach.

Residual RV outflow tract obstruction can occur after repair of DORV with subaortic or doubly committed VSD and severe PS, whether the repair required infundibulotomy, outflow tract patch, or some form of RV-to-PA conduit. Obstruction of the valved homograft conduit used in the Rastelli procedure can result from sternal compression, and some groups have advocated delaying sternal closure in this circumstance until myocardial edema resolves.[27] After a few days, compliance of the chest cavity improves sufficiently to accommodate the conduit and permit closure of the sternum. Delayed sternal closure is not required in most patients. Rarely, conduit stenosis may occur months after the original operation. This may necessitate conduit replacement or balloon dilatation or stenting or both.[26]

The various repairs of DORV with subpulmonary VSD may lead to RV failure. Even in the absence of anatomic causes for RV failure, Kawashima and coworkers[41] showed that the intraventricular repair of the Taussig-Bing anomaly is associated with increased RV end-diastolic volume (163% ± 67% of normal) and decreased RV ejection fraction (39% ± 12% of normal), making inotropic support with dopamine or milrinone a rational therapeutic option if clinical signs of RV failure exist in the absence of anatomic causes. A repair with an intraventricular baffle may lead to RV outflow tract obstruction, because the subpulmonary VSD is in proximity to the pulmonary orifice and infundibular septal bands. Tricuspid insufficiency may arise if detachment (and subsequent reattachment) of the tricuspid chordae to the infundibular septum is required to accommodate the baffle.[41]

Certainly after the ASO, obstruction of the neo-PA or branch pulmonary arteries must be excluded.

Other Postoperative Problems

Residual ventricular shunts may be present postoperatively. The source of the shunt may be from VSD patch dehiscence or other unrecognized VSDs. Pulmonary overcirculation and CHF develop. Reoperation is probably required in patients with pulmonary-to-systemic flow ratios in excess of 2:1 and especially those who cannot be weaned from mechanical ventilation.

In the presence of suprasystemic RV pressure secondary to pulmonary hypertension or severe obstruction, those with residual shunts will have hypoxemia from right-to-left shunting. Residual obstruction must be relieved if possible, and elevated pulmonary resistance treated, if present. A residual shunt in such cases may help to preserve systemic output at the expense of some decrease in systemic oxygen saturation.

Postoperative arrhythmias have been related to late postoperative sudden death.[88] Given the proximity of conduction tissue to the rim of the VSD, it is not surprising that third-degree heart block occurs occasionally. All patients should have temporary atrial and ventricular pacing wires present in the early postoperative period. Transient postoperative heart block is an independent predictor of late sudden death, so permanent pacemakers should be placed in those patients still in complete heart block or with high-grade second-degree block 7 to 10 days after operation. Similarly, ventricular tachyarrhythmias (excluding isolated ventricular extrasystoles) may warrant further evaluation and therapy (see Chapter 8 on Pediatric Arrhythmias).

OUTCOME

In general, outcome for patients with DORV is excellent. The results of surgical series from several different institutions have been reported over the last 20-year period.* Kirklin and

---

*See references 13,14,16,17,37,40,43,45,52,56,61,70–72,83,85–87,98

associates[45] summarized results of an 18-year experience (1967 to 1984) involving 127 patients with DORV. Because of inclusion of the early experience and repairs of all forms of DORV in this analysis, the actuarial survival rate at 12 years was only 38%. However, more recent experience in patients with DORV and subaortic VSD repaired by intraventricular tunnel revealed a survival rate of 99% at 2 weeks and 97% at 10 years. Only 1 of 56 patients required reoperation of the tunnel repair. The results were not so good for patients with DORV and subpulmonary VSDs and were relatively bleak for patients with noncommitted or remote VSDs (22% 10-year survival).

Musumeci and colleagues[61] reported the results of operations on 120 patients with DORV from 1973 to 1986. They also found a tremendous improvement in outcome for those patients operated on most recently. In particular, the outcome for the group with DORV and subpulmonary VSD dramatically improved with the introduction of the ASO. In 60 of 68 survivors with intracardiac repair followed up for 2 to 184 (median, 44) months, 5 (8.3%) late deaths and 8 successful reoperations were found, and all but 3 long-term survivors were in New York Heart Association functional class I. Again, patients with noncommitted VSDs did poorly.

At least one more recent study suggests a significant risk of late sudden death after repair of DORV.[88] Shen and coworkers[88] obtained follow-up data on 89 of 95 survivors of corrective operations for DORV performed between 1965 and 1985. Of the 22 late deaths, 16 were sudden. Half of the sudden deaths occurred within 1 year of operation. Risk factors for sudden death included older age at time of repair, perioperative ventricular tachyarrhythmias, and complete heart block. Year at operation did not correlate with risk of sudden death.

Planche and colleauges[13,14,86] have published several important articles regarding their considerable experience at Marie Lannelongue Hospital with the preoperative assessment, surgical management, and outcome of patients with DORV. In most cases in this large series, a biventricular repair, even for complex forms of DORV, both was feasible and resulted in a good outcome. From 1985 through 1996, 154 consecutive patients had a biventricular repair for DORV, with median age at repair of 10 months and median weight of 6.5 kg.[14] An intracardiac baffle approach was used in 75%, and the ASO with VSD-to-PA baffle in 25%. In the 14 hospital deaths and 6 late deaths, the only significant risk factor was the presence of mitral valve anomalies. The presence of PS at the time of presentation appeared to place the patients in a low-risk group for global death. The main reason for reoperation was subaortic obstruction, which was more likely in cases in which the VSD required enlargement at the initial repair or in cases of noncommitted VSD. Residual subaortic obstruction appears to be most often due to protrusion of the inferior rim of the VSD into the LV outflow tract, with progressive septal hypertrophy and membrane development, and can be effectively relieved by an aggressive septoplasty at reoperation.[13] In cases of DORV with straddling of the AV valve(s), 30 of 34 patients underwent biventricular repair with only 4 early and 1 late deaths.[86] Approximately 30% had more than mild residual AV valve regurgitation, and 30% had small residual VSDs.

DOUBLE-OUTLET LEFT VENTRICLE

Double-outlet left ventricle (DOLV) is a rare form of congenital heart disease defined as the condition in which both great arteries arise predominantly above the morphologic LV. The first documented clinical and surgical case was reported in 1967,[81] and the first autopsy-proven case was published in 1970.[69] As in DORV, a variety of different combinations of VSD location, great arterial arrangement, subarterial infundibular anatomy, and associated defects exist for DOLV as well, making an easy but informative classification system difficult.

As a unifying embryologic hypothesis, DOLV often occurs when both the subaortic and subpulmonary infundibula are either absent or poorly developed.[107] The etiology of this lack of subarterial conus is unknown and may be due to either abnormal absorption of early embryonic infundibular musculature or to growth failure of the subpulmonary conus. The subaortic infundibulum, present in early embryonic life, normally absorbs, resulting in aortic-mitral fibrous continuity. When the subpulmonary conus either is absorbed or fails to grow, the result is lack of the normal dextrorotation of the semilunar valves, such that the pulmonary valve fails to move rightward and anterior into the proximity of the RV. Thus in DOLV, either direct or tenuous pulmonary as well as aortic-to-mitral fibrous continuity often is found.

Van Praagh and associates[107] recently summarized the anatomic features of 109 cases of DOLV and found 26 different types. A subaortic location of the VSD was most common, and among these cases, the "tetralogy type" of DOLV, with PS, was most often seen. Subpulmonary defects, most commonly with aortic stenosis, and doubly committed VSDs were somewhat less frequent. No documented cases in this series had two well-developed ventricles, DOLV, and either a remote VSD or an IVS, although a few cases with hypoplastic RV, DOLV, and IVS have been reported.[12,59,69]

As with DORV, a thorough preoperative echocardiographic evaluation can provide not only the diagnosis but also important anatomic details for planning the appropriate surgical solution.[15] On the parasternal long-axis view, both great arteries can be seen arising above the LV. The parasternal short-axis view will demonstrate both semilunar valves to be in the same plane and arising from the LV side of the interventricular septum.

The surgical options will again depend on the anatomy. When possible, a complete intracardiac repair may be appropriate, with the VSD patch serving to direct RV egress into the PA.[60,78] Other approaches include use of a pericardial outflow tract patch to connect the PA to the RV,[42] or an RV-to-PA homograft conduit.[109] Cases with hypoplastic RV will require a Fontan-type approach.

References

1. Abe T, Sugiki K, Komatsu S: Successful repair of double-outlet right ventricle by a modified Fontan operation. *Ann Thorac Surg* 42:554–559, 1986.
2. Ainger LE: Double-outlet right ventricle: Intact ventricular septum, mitral stenosis, and blind left ventricle. *Am Heart J* 70:521–525, 1965.
3. Allen SP, Bogardi JP, Barlow AJ, et al: Misexpression of noggin leads to septal defects in the outflow tract of the chick heart. *Dev Biol* 235:98–109, 2001.

4. Allwork SP, Urban AE, Anderson RH: Left juxtaposition of the auricles with l-position of the aorta: Report of 6 cases. *Br Heart J* 39:299–308, 1977.

5. Anderson RH, Becker AE, Wilcox BR, et al: Surgical anatomy of double-outlet right ventricle: A reappraisal. *Am J Cardiol* 52:555–559, 1983.

6. Anderson RH, Smith A, Wilkinson JL: Right juxtaposition of the auricular appendages. *Eur J Cardiol* 4:495–503, 1976.

7. Anjos RT, Ho SY, Anderson RH: Surgical implications of juxtaposition of the atrial appendages: A review of forty-nine autopsied hearts. *J Thorac Cardiovasc Surg* 99:897–904, 1990.

8. Aziz KU, Paul MH, Muster AJ, Idriss FS: Positional abnormalities of atrioventricular valves in transposition of the great arteries including double outlet right ventricle, atrioventricular valve straddling and malattachment. *Am J Cardiol* 44:1135–1145, 1979.

9. Balestrini L, Fleishman C, Lanzoni L, et al: Real-time 3-dimensional echocardiography evaluation of congenital heart disease. *J Am Soc Echocardiogr* 13:171–176, 2000.

10. Bartram U, Molin DG, Wisse LJ, et al: Double-outlet right ventricle and overriding tricuspid valve reflect disturbances of looping, myocardialization, endocardial cushion differentiation, and apoptosis in TGF-beta(2)-knockout mice. *Circulation* 103:22745–22752, 2001.

11. Battistessa S, Soto B: Double outlet right ventricle with discordant atrioventricular connection: An angiographic analysis of 19 cases. *Int J Cardiol* 27:253–263, 1990.

12. Beitzke A, Suppan C: Double outlet left ventricle with intact ventricular septum. *Int J Cardiol* 5:175–183, 1984.

13. Belli E, Serraf A, Lacour-Gayet F, et al: Surgical treatment of subaortic stenosis after biventricular repair of double-outlet right ventricle. *J Thorac Cardiovasc Surg* 112:1570–1580, 1996.

14. Belli E, Serraf A, Lacour-Gayet F, et al: Biventricular repair for double-outlet right ventricle: Results and long-term follow-up. *Circulation* 98:II360–II367, 1998.

15. Bengur AR, Snider AR, Peters J, Merida-Asmus L: Two-dimensional echocardiographic features of double outlet left ventricle. *J Am Soc Echocardiogr* 3:320–325, 1990.

16. Bjork VO, Henze A, Bergdahl L, et al: Repair of double-outlet right ventricle: Experience of 13 cases. *Scand J Thorac Cardiovasc Surg* 15:229–234, 1981.

17. Borromee L, Lecompte Y, Batisse A, et al: Anatomic repair of anomalies of ventriculoarterial connection associated with ventricular septal defect, II: Clinical results in 50 patients with pulmonary outflow tract obstruction. *J Thorac Cardiovasc Surg* 95:96–102, 1988.

18. Boughman JA, Neill CA, Ferencz C, Loffredo CA: The genetics of congenital heart disease. In Ferencz C, Rubin JD, Loffredo CA, et al (eds): *Perspectives in Pediatric Cardiology*, Vol 4: *Epidemiology of Congenital Heart Disease: The Baltimore-Washington Infant Study 1981–1989.* Mount Kisco, NY, Futura Publishing, 1993, pp 123–167.

19. Brawn WJ: Early results for anatomic correction of transposition of the great arteries and for double-outlet right ventricle with subpulmonary ventricular septal defect. *J Thorac Cardiovasc Surg* 95:230–238, 1988.

20. Carey LS, Edwards JE: Roentgenographic features in cases with origin of both great vessels from the right ventricle without pulmonary stenosis. *AJR Am J Roentgenol* 93:269, 1965.

21. Chaitman BR, Grondin CM, Theroux P, Bourassa MG: Late development of left ventricular outflow tract obstruction after repair of double-outlet right ventricle. *J Thorac Cardiovasc Surg* 72:265–268, 1976.

22. Collan Y, Pesonen E: Double outlet right ventricle with extreme hypertrophy of muscle bundles associated with crista supraventricularis: A heart with three ventricles. *Helv Paediatr Acta* 31:521–526, 1977.

23. Crispino JD, Lodish MB, Thurberg BL, et al: Proper coronary vascular development and heart morphogenesis depend on interaction of GATA-4 with FOG cofactors. *Genes Dev* 15:839–844, 2001.

24. Crupi G, Parenzan L: Arterial repair without coronary relocation for double-outlet right ventricle with subpulmonary ventricular septal defect (Taussig-Bing anomaly). *J Thorac Cardiovasc Surg* 85:800–801, 1983.

25. DeLeon SY, Ilbawi MN, Tubeszewski K, et al: The Damus-Stansel-Kaye procedure: Anatomical determinants and modifications. *Ann Thorac Surg* 52:680–687, 1991.

26. di Carlo DC, Di Donato RM, Carotti A, et al: Evaluation of the Damus-Kaye-Stansel operation in infancy. *Ann Thorac Surg* 52:1148–1153, 1991.

27. Fanning WJ, Vasko JS, Kilman JW: Delayed sternal closure after cardiac surgery. *Ann Thorac Surg* 44:169–172, 1987.

28. Firmin RK, Lima R, Anderson RH, et al: Anatomic problems associated with arterial switch procedures for double outlet right ventricle with subpulmonary ventricular septal defect. *Thorac Cardiovasc Surg* 31:365–368, 1983.

29. Freedom RM, Bini R, Dische R, Rowe RD: The straddling mitral valve: Morphological observations and clinical implications. *Eur J Cardiol* 8:35–50, 1978.

30. Gerlis LM, Dickinson DF, Anderson RH: Disadvantageous closure of the interventricular communication in double outlet right ventricle. *Br Heart J* 51:670–673, 1984.

31. Geva T, Van Praagh S, Sanders SP, et al: Straddling mitral valve with hypoplastic right ventricle, crisscross atrioventricular relations, double outlet right ventricle and dextrocardia: Morphologic, diagnostic and surgical considerations. *J Am Coll Cardiol* 17:1603–1612, 1991.

32. Golmuntz E, Clark BJ, Mitchell LE, et al: Frequency of 22q11 deletions with conotruncal defects. *J Am Coll Cardiol* 32:492–498, 1998.

33. Griffin AJ, Ferrara JD, Lax JO, Cassels DE: Pulmonary compliance: An index of cardiovascular status in infancy. *Am J Dis Child* 123:89–95, 1972.

34. Gruber PJ, Kubalak SW, Pexieder T, et al: RXR alpha deficiency confers genetic susceptibility for aortic sac, conotruncal, atrioventricular cushion, and ventricular muscle defects in mice. *J Clin Invest* 98:1332–1343, 1996.

35. Hagler DJ, Seward JB, Tajik AJ, Ritter DG: Functional assessment of the Fontan operation: Combined M-mode, two-dimensional and Doppler echocardiographic studies. *J Am Coll Cardiol* 4:756–764, 1984.

36. Howell CE, Ho SY, Anderson RH, Elliott MJ: Fibrous skeleton and ventricular outflow tracts in double-outlet right ventricle. *Ann Thorac Surg* 51:394–400, 1991.

37. Judson JP, Danielson GK, Puga FJ, et al: Double-outlet right ventricle: Surgical results, 1970–1980. *J Thorac Cardiovasc Surg* 85:32–40, 1983.

38. Judson JP, Danielson GK, Ritter DG, Hagler DJ: Successful repair of coexisting double-outlet right ventricle and two-chambered right ventricle. *J Thorac Cardiovasc Surg* 84:113–121, 1982.

39. Kanter K, Anderson R, Lincoln C, et al: Anatomic correction of double-outlet right ventricle with subpulmonary ventricular septal defect (the "Taussig-Bing" anomaly). *Ann Thorac Surg* 41:287–292, 1986.

40. Kanter KR, Anderson RH, Lincoln C, et al: Anatomic correction for complete transposition and double outlet right ventricle. *J Thorac Cardiovasc Surg* 90:690–699, 1985.

41. Kawashima Y, Matsuda H, Yagihara T, et al: Intraventricular repair for Taussig-Bing anomaly. *J Thorac Cardiovasc Surg* 105:591–596, 1993.

42. Kerr AR, Barcia A, Bargeron LM Jr, Kirklin JW: Double-outlet left ventricle with ventricular septal defect and pulmonary stenosis: Report of surgical repair. *Am Heart J* 81:688–693, 1971.

43. Kirklin JK, Pacifico AD, Kirklin JW: Intraventricular tunnel repair of double outlet right ventricle. *J Card Surg* 2:231–245, 1987.

44. Kirklin JW, Barratt-Boyes BG (eds): *Double Outlet Right Ventricle, Cardiac Surgery.* New York, Churchill Livingstone, 1993, pp 1469–1500.

45. Kirklin JW, Pacifico AD, Blackstone EH, et al: Current risks and protocols for operations for double-outlet right ventricle: Derivation from an 18 year experience. *J Thorac Cardiovasc Surg* 92:913–930, 1986.

46. Krian A, Kramer HH, Quaegebeur J, et al: The arterial switch-operation: Early and midterm (6 years) results with particular reference to technical problems. *Thorac Cardiovasc Surg* 39(suppl 2):160–165, 1991.

47. Lecompte Y, Batisse A, DiCarlo D: Double-outlet right ventricle: A surgical synthesis. *Adv Card Surg* 4:109–136, 1993.

48. Lecompte Y, Neveux JY, Leca F, et al: Reconstruction of the pulmonary outflow tract without prosthetic conduit. *J Thorac Cardiovasc Surg* 84:727–733, 1982.

49. Lee RY, Luo J, Evans RM, et al: Compartment-selective sensitivity of cardiovascular morphogenesis to combinations of retinoic acid receptor gene mutations. *Circ Res* 80:757–764, 1997.

50. Lev M, Bharati S, Meng CC, et al: A concept of double-outlet right ventricle. *J Thorac Cardiovasc Surg* 64:271–281, 1972.

51. Lincoln C, Redington AN, Li K, et al: Anatomical correction for complete transposition and double outlet right ventricle: Intermediate assessment of functional results. *Br Heart J* 56:259–266, 1986.

52. Luber JM, Castaneda AR, Lang P, Norwood WI: Repair of double-outlet right ventricle: Early and late results. *Circulation* 68:II144–II147, 1983.

53. Manner J, Seidl W, Steding G: Embryological observations on the morphogenesis of double-outlet right ventricle with subaortic ventricular septal defect and normal arrangement of the great arteries. *Thorac Cardiovasc Surg* 43:307–312, 1995.

54. Marcelletti C, Mazzera E, Olthof H, et al: Fontan's operation: An expanded horizon. *J Thorac Cardiovasc Surg* 80:764–769, 1980.

55. Marino B, Loperfido F, Sardi CS: Spontaneous closure of ventricular septal defect in a case of double outlet right ventricle. *Br Heart J* 49:608–611, 1983.

56. Mazzucco A, Faggian G, Stellin G, et al: Surgical management of double-outlet right ventricle. *J Thorac Cardiovasc Surg* 90:29–34, 1985.

57. McGoon DC: Origin of both great vessels from the right ventricle. *Surg Clin North Am* 41:1113, 1961.

58. Melhuish BP, Van Praagh R: Juxtaposition of the atrial appendages: A sign of severe cyanotic congenital heart disease. *Br Heart J* 30:269–284, 1968.

59. Mohan JC, Agarwala R, Arora R: Double outlet left ventricle with intact ventricular septum: A cross-sectional and Doppler echocardiographic diagnosis. *Int J Cardiol* 33:447–449, 1991.

60. Murphy DA, Gillis DA, Sridhara KS: Intraventricular repair of double-outlet left ventricle. *Ann Thorac Surg* 31:364–369, 1981.

61. Musumeci F, Shumway S, Lincoln C, Anderson RH: Surgical treatment for double-outlet right ventricle at the Brompton Hospital, 1973 to 1986. *J Thorac Cardiovasc Surg* 96:278–287, 1988.

62. Myers JL, Waldhausen JA, Weber HS, et al: A reconsideration of risk factors for the Fontan operation. *Ann Surg* 211:738–743, 1990.

63. Neufeld HN, DuShane JW, Edwards JE: Origin of both great vessels from the right ventricle, II: With pulmonary stenosis. *Circulation* 23:603, 1961.

64. Niezen RA, Beekman RP, Helbing WA, et al: Double outlet right ventricle assessed with magnetic resonance imaging. *Int J Card Imaging* 15:323–329, 1999.

65. Ostermeyer J, Korfer R, Frenzel H, Bircks W: Straddling atrioventricular valves in biventricular hearts: Observations made in 5 cases. *Thorac Cardiovasc Surg* 28:233–238, 1980.

66. Pacifico AD, Kirklin JW, Bargeron LM Jr: Repair of complete atrioventricular canal associated with tetralogy of Fallot or double-outlet right ventricle: Report of 10 patients. *Ann Thorac Surg* 29:351–356, 1980.

67. Pacifico AD, Ricchi A, Bargeron LM Jr, et al: Corrective repair of complete atrioventricular canal defects and major associated cardiac anomalies. *Ann Thorac Surg* 46:645–651, 1988.

68. Patel CR, Muise KL, Redline RW: Double-outlet right ventricle with intact ventricular septum in a fetus with trisomy 18. *Cardiol Young* 9:419–422, 1999.

69. Paul MH, Muster AJ, Sinha SN, et al: Double-outlet left ventricle with an intact ventricular septum: Clinical and autopsy diagnosis and developmental implications. *Circulation* 41:129–139, 1970.

70. Pearl JM, Laks H, Drinkwater DC Jr, et al: Repair of conotruncal abnormalities with the use of the valved conduit: Improved early and midterm results with the cryopreserved homograft. *J Am Coll Cardiol* 20:191–196, 1992.

71. Piccoli G, Pacifico AD, Kirklin JW, et al: Changing results and concepts in the surgical treatment of double-outlet right ventricle: Analysis of 137 operations in 126 patients. *Am J Cardiol* 52:549–554, 1983.

72. Pitlick P, French J, Guthaner D, et al: Results of intraventricular baffle procedure for ventricular septal defect and double outlet right ventricle or d-transposition of the great arteries. *Am J Cardiol* 47:307–314, 1981.

73. Quaegebeur JM: The optimal repair for the Taussig-Bing heart. *J Thorac Cardiovasc Surg* 85:276–277, 1983.

74. Quaegebeur JM, Rohmer J, Ottenkamp J, et al: The arterial switch operation: An eight-year experience. *J Thorac Cardiovasc Surg* 92:361–384, 1986.

75. Rastelli GC, Wallace RB, Ongley PA: Complete repair of transposition of the great arteries with pulmonary stenosis: A review and report of a case corrected by using a new surgical technique. *Circulation* 39:83–95, 1969.

76. Replogle RL, Campbell DJ, Campbell CD, Arcilla RA: Double-outlet ventricles. In Arciniegas E (ed): *Pediatric Cardiac Surgery*. Chicago, Year Book Medical Publishers, 1985.

77. Rice MJ, Seward JB, Edwards WD, et al: Straddling atrioventricular valve: Two-dimensional echocardiographic diagnosis, classification and surgical implications. *Am J Cardiol* 55:505–513, 1985.

78. Rivera R, Infantes C, Gil de la Pena M: Double outlet left ventricle (report of a case with intraventricular surgical repair). *J Cardiovasc Surg (Torino)* 21:361–366, 1980.

79. Rocchini AP, Rosenthal A, Castaneda AR, et al: Subaortic obstruction after the use of an intracardiac baffle to tunnel the left ventricle to the aorta. *Circulation* 54:957–960, 1976.

80. Russo P, Danielson GK, Puga FJ, et al: Modified Fontan procedure for biventricular hearts with complex forms of double-outlet right ventricle. *Circulation* 78:III20–III25, 1988.

81. Sakakibara S, Takao A, Arai T, et al: Both great vessels arising from the left ventricle (double outlet left ventricle)(origin of both great vessels from the left ventricle). *Bull Heart Inst Jpn* 66, 1967.

82. Sanders SP, Bierman FZ, Williams RG: Conotruncal malformations: Diagnosis in infancy using subxiphoid 2-dimensional echocardiography. *Am J Cardiol* 50:1361–1367, 1982.

83. Sano S, Karl TR, Mee RB: Extracardiac valved conduits in the pulmonary circuit. *Ann Thorac Surg* 52:285–290, 1991.

84. Serraf A, Bruniaux J, Lacour-Gayet F, et al: Anatomic correction of transposition of the great arteries with ventricular septal defect: Experience with 118 cases. *J Thorac Cardiovasc Surg* 102:140–147, 1991.

85. Serraf A, Lacour-Gayet F, Bruniaux J, et al: Anatomic repair of Taussig-Bing hearts. *Circulation* 84:III200–III205, 1991.

86. Serraf A, Nakamura T, Lacour-Gayet F, et al: Surgical approaches for double-outlet right ventricle or transposition of the great arteries associated with straddling atrioventricular valves. *J Thorac Cardiovasc Surg* 111:527–535, 1996.

87. Sharma S, Cobanoglu A, Dobbs J, Rice M: Clinical results of cryopreserved valved conduits in the pulmonary ventricle–to–pulmonary artery position. *Am J Surg* 165:587–591, 1993.

88. Shen WK, Holmes DR, Porter CJ, et al: Sudden death after repair of double-outlet right ventricle. *Circulation* 81:128–136, 1990.

89. Singh A, Letsky EA, Stark J: Hemolysis following correction of double-outlet right ventricle. *J Thorac Cardiovasc Surg* 71:226–229, 1976.

90. Snider AR, Serwer GA: Abnormalities of ventriculoarterial connection. In Lampert RH (ed): *Echocardiography in Pediatric Heart Disease*. St. Louis, Mosby-Year Book, 1990, pp 190–194.

91. Sondheimer HM, Freedom RM, Olley PM: Double outlet right ventricle: Clinical spectrum and prognosis. *Am J Cardiol* 39:709–714, 1977.

92. Sridaromont S, Feldt RH, Ritter DG, et al: Double outlet right ventricle: Hemodynamic and anatomic correlations. *Am J Cardiol* 38:85–94, 1976.

93. Sridaromont S, Feldt RH, Ritter DG, et al: Double-outlet right ventricle associated with persistent common atrioventricular canal. *Circulation* 52:933–942, 1975.

94. Srivastava D, Olson EN: A genetic blueprint for cardiac development. *Nature* 407:221–226, 2000.

95. Stark J, deLeval M: *Surgery for Congenital Heart Defects*. Philadelphia, WB Saunders, 1994.

96. Stellin G, Ho SY, Anderson RH, et al: The surgical anatomy of double-outlet right ventricle with concordant atrioventricular connection and noncommitted ventricular septal defect. *J Thorac Cardiovasc Surg* 102:849–855, 1991.

97. Stewart JR, Merrill WH, Hammon JW Jr, et al: Reappraisal of localized resection for subvalvar aortic stenosis. *Ann Thorac Surg* 50:197–202, 1990.

98. Stewart RW, Kirklin JW, Pacifico AD, et al: Repair of double-outlet right ventricle: An analysis of 62 cases. *J Thorac Cardiovasc Surg* 78:502–514, 1979.

99. Sutherland GR, Smyllie JH, Ogilvie BC, Keeton BR: Colour flow imaging in the diagnosis of multiple ventricular septal defects. *Br Heart J* 62:43–49, 1989.

100. Tandon R, Moller JH, Edwards JE: Single papillary muscle of the left ventricle associated with persistent common atrioventricular canal: Variant of parachute mitral valve. *Pediatr Cardiol* 7:111–114, 1986.

101. Tandon R, Moller JH, Edwards JE: Anomalies associated with the parachute mitral valve: A pathologic analysis of 52 cases. *Can J Cardiol* 2:278–281, 1986.

102. Taussig HB, Bing RJ: Complete transposition of aorta and levoposition of pulmonary artery. *Am Heart J* 37:551, 1949.

103. Toussaint M, Planche C, Graff WC, et al: Double outlet right ventricle associated with common atrioventricular canal: Report of nine anatomic specimens. *J Am Coll Cardiol* 8:396–401, 1986.

104. Ungerleider RM, Ebert PA: Indications and techniques for midline approach to aortic coarctation in infants and children. *Ann Thorac Surg* 44:517–522, 1987.

105. Ungerleider RM, Greeley WJ, Kanter RJ, Kisslo JA: The learning curve for intraoperative echocardiography during congenital heart surgery. *Ann Thorac Surg* 54:691–696, 1992.

106. Ungerleider RM, Greeley WJ, Sheikh KH, et al: Routine use of intraoperative epicardial echocardiography and Doppler color flow imaging

to guide and evaluate repair of congenital heart lesions: A prospective study. *J Thorac Cardiovasc Surg* 100:297–309, 1990.

107. Van Praagh R, Weinberg PM, Srebro JP: Double-outlet left ventricle. In Adams FH, Emmanouilides GC, Riemenschneider TA (eds): *Moss' Heart Disease in Infants, Children, and Adolescents.* Baltimore, Williams & Wilkins, 1989, pp 461–485.

108. Van Praagh S, Davidoff A, Chin A, et al: Double outlet right ventricle: Anatomic types and developmental implications based on a study of 100 autopsied cases. *Coeur* 13:389–439, 1982.

109. Villani M, Lipscombe S, Ross DN: Double outlet left ventricle: How should we repair it? *J Cardiovasc Surg (Torino)* 20:413–418, 1979.

110. Westerman GR, Norton JB, Kiel EA, Van Devanter SH: Double-outlet right ventricle and severe systemic outflow tract hypoplasia. *Ann Thorac Surg* 44:154–158, 1987.

111. Weyman AE, Wann S, Feigenbaum H, Dillon JC: Mechanism of abnormal septal motion in patients with right ventricular volume overload: A cross-sectional echocardiographic study. *Circulation* 54:179–186, 1976.

112. Wienecke M, Fyfe DA, Kline CH, et al: Comparison of intraoperative transesophageal echocardiography to epicardial imaging in children undergoing ventricular septal defect repair. *J Am Soc Echocardiogr* 4:607–614, 1991.

113. Wilcox BR, Ho SY, Macartney FJ, et al: Surgical anatomy of double-outlet right ventricle with situs solitus and atrioventricular concordance. *J Thorac Cardiovasc Surg* 82:405–417, 1981.

114. Williams WG, Freedom RM, Culham G, et al: Early experience with arterial repair of transposition. *Ann Thorac Surg* 32:8–15, 1981.

115. Witham AC: Double outlet right ventricle: A partial transposition complex. *Am Heart J* 53:928, 1957.

116. Yacoub MH, Radley-Smith R: Anatomic correction of the Taussig-Bing anomaly. *J Thorac Cardiovasc Surg* 88:380–388, 1984.

117. Yoshida Y, Fukuda M, Sasaki T, et al: Echocardiographic features of straddling mitral valve. *Tohoku J Exp Med* 122:387–392, 1977.

118. Zamora R, Moller JH, Edwards JE: Double-outlet right ventricle: Anatomic types and associated anomalies. *Chest* 68:672, 1975.

Chapter 35

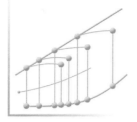

Tetralogy of Fallot with and without Pulmonary Atresia

STEVE DAVIS, MD

INTRODUCTION

Tetralogy of Fallot (TOF) is one of the most common congenital cardiac malformations. It occurs in three to six infants for every 10,000 live births.[58] Fallot originally described the malformation as consisting of (1) stenosis of the pulmonary artery; (2) interventricular communication; (3) deviation of the origin of the aorta to the right; and (4) hypertrophy, almost always concentric, of the right ventricle.[22] Pulmonary atresia

represents extreme right ventricular outflow tract obstruction (RVOTO) within the spectrum of TOF.

ANATOMY

A wide spectrum of anatomic variability exists in TOF with and without pulmonary atresia (TOF/PA). The primary features are generally considered to be (1) RVOTO, and (2) a ventricular septal defect (VSD), which is almost always nonrestrictive, subaortic, and associated with anterior malalignment of the infundibular septum with the muscular septum.[5,46,51] The level of RVOTO may be subvalvular, valvular, or in the pulmonary artery or its branches. The VSD is usually as large as the aortic valve orifice, but variants with a restrictive VSD have been described (Fig. 35-1).[23]

The overriding aorta is associated with dextroposition and abnormal rotation. A right aortic arch is found in 25% of cases, and branching of the arch vessels may be abnormal in these. The subclavian artery may arise from a retroesophageal location in up to 10% of cases, and persistence of the left superior vena cava occurs with about the same frequency,[60] along with the possibility of mitral valve hypoplasia.

Other abnormalities are frequently seen in TOF. Coronary artery abnormalities include an origin of the left anterior descending coronary artery (LAD) from the proximal right coronary. This causes the LAD to cross the right ventricular outflow tract (RVOT) at variable distances from the pulmonary valve annulus.[15,24,25] Less common variations include origin of all coronaries from a single main coronary ostium, in which case, the right coronary artery crosses the RVOT, and origin of the left coronary from the pulmonary artery.[3] Atrial septal defects are routinely encountered. Less commonly seen associated defects include atrioventricular canal defects, muscular VSDs, aortic incompetence, and anomalous pulmonary venous return.[45,55,86,91]

In TOF/PA, the intracardiac anatomy is similar to that of TOF. The VSD is generally a large nonrestrictive malalignment defect, but can occasionally be restrictive, due primarily to the presence of accessory abnormal tricuspid valve tissue. Additional VSDs occur in 5% to 15% of cases.[38] The site of PA is variable and may occur in the infundibulum, at the pulmonary valve, or extend to include the entire main pulmonary artery and intrapericardial branches. The main pulmonary artery may be patent up to the atretic valve, hypoplastic, or

755

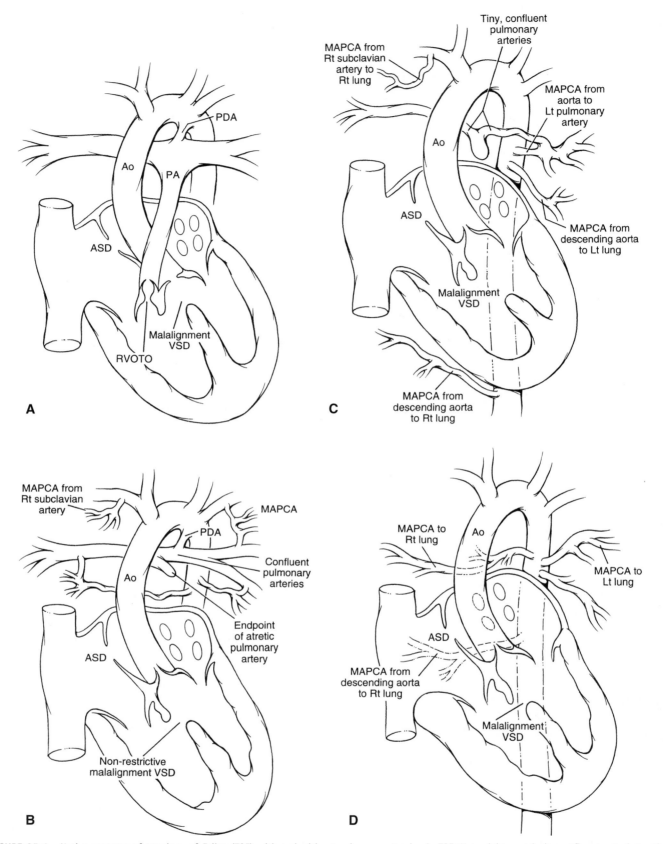

FIGURE 35-1 Native anatomy of tetralogy of Fallot (TOF) with and without pulmonary atresia. **A,** TOF. Note right ventricular outflow tract obstruction (RVOTO) at the infundibular level. The main pulmonary artery (PA) is small in comparison to the size of the aorta (Ao). RVOTO and the anterior malalignment ventricular septal defect allow desaturated blood to enter the systemic circulation. **B,** TOF with long-segment pulmonary atresia and confluent pulmonary arteries. The right and left PAs are confluent, but the main PA is atretic and discontinuous from the RVOT. Pulmonary blood flow is supplied in part via a patent ductus arteriosus (PDA). Major aortopulmonary collateral arteries (MAPCA) arising from the descending AO as well as right and left subclavian arteries also supply pulmonary blood flow. **C,** TOF with long-segment pulmonary atresia and tiny central pulmonary arteries with MAPCAs showing extensive arborization abnormalities. Note the absence of the PDA. **D,** TOF with pulmonary atresia, absent central PA and extensive MAPCAs as the sole source of pulmonary blood flow. ASD, atrial septal defect; VSD, ventricular septal defect.

absent, persisting only as a fibrous cord between the RVOT and the central pulmonary arteries. The aorta is dilated and overrides the VSD, and aortic valve stenosis is rarely encountered. The aortic arch is right-sided in 25% to 50% of cases. An aberrant right or left retroesophageal subclavian artery is present in 18% of cases.[38]

The pulmonary blood supply in PA is responsible for the variable clinical presentation and the challenges of surgical management. Blood supply to the lungs is derived from the systemic arterial circulation, most commonly from a patent ductus arteriosus (PDA) or major aortopulmonary collateral arteries (MAPCAs) or both. A wide spectrum of pulmonary blood supply is seen in this group of patients. In the simplest form, pulmonary blood flow (PBF) is supplied by a PDA, and the central pulmonary arteries are well formed and confluent. The distribution of the pulmonary arteries is typically normal, with occasional arborization abnormalities. This arrangement accounts for one third of the cases with PA.[38] The most complex and technically challenging subset of patients has diminutive or atretic pulmonary arteries. PBF is supplied by MAPCAs with or without connections to the native pulmonary arteries. Native pulmonary artery arborization abnormalities occur frequently.

Central pulmonary arteries are confluent in approximately 75% of cases; however, they may supply only a portion of each lung because of the presence of MAPCAs and arborization abnormalities. Arborization abnormalities are more common and more severe with nonconfluent pulmonary arteries, but occur in up to 50% of patients with confluent pulmonary arteries.[76]

MAPCAs are highly variable in number, size, site of origin, and connections to the central pulmonary arteries. They usually arise from the anterior surface of the descending thoracic aorta, but also can arise from the abdominal aorta, subclavian arteries, intercostal arteries, and the internal mammary arteries. The number of MAPCAs is generally directly related to the incompleteness of arborization of the left and right pulmonary arteries.[17,35,76] Patients with nonconfluent pulmonary arteries have at least one MAPCA, half have at least four MAPCAs, and 4% have five or more.[17] Only 40% of MAPCAs anastomose to the native pulmonary arteries. In the other 60%, blood flow to those lung segments is dependent on the MAPCAs.

GENETICS

In recent years, advances in genetic techniques have allowed earlier detection of chromosomal microdeletions. Microdeletion of chromosome 22q11 is the most common deletion, affecting approximately 1 in 4000 live births and has a significant relation to cardiac, craniofacial, and developmental abnormalities.[11,37] Presentation is variable and depends on the age of the patient. Common findings in the neonatal period include palatal anomalies, hypocalcemia, and dysmorphic facies (microstomia, micrognathia, unusually shaped ears, long nose). In older children, velopharyngeal insufficiency, myopathic facies, short stature, and mild learning difficulties are common.[81] Microdeletions in the region of 22q11 occur in 83% of individuals with velocardiofacial syndrome, 94% of those with DiGeorge syndrome, 20% of

patients with TOF, and 40% with TOF/PA.[45] Fluorescent in situ hybridization techniques allow for rapid detection of this microdeletion. This is important because of the potential for complications in the perioperative period (hypocalcemia and graft-vs.-host reaction with use of nonirradiated blood), associated learning difficulties, and possible hereditary implications for close relatives. In a series of 40 children with 22q11 deletions, 9 were found to have inherited the deleted chromosome, with 8 of 9 from the mother.[81]

PHYSIOLOGY

The variability in anatomy leads to a wide range of physiologic presentations. The primary determinant of preoperative physiology is the degree of RVOTO present. At one end of the spectrum are the patients with mild RVOTO. They have signs and symptoms of pulmonary overcirculation due to a left-to-right shunt at the VSD. Oxygen saturations are normal (leading to the term "pink tetralogy"), and congestive heart failure (CHF) occurs with the normal decrease in pulmonary artery pressures during the first few weeks of life. Those with moderate RVOTO have a near-normal pulmonary-to-systemic blood flow ratio (Q_p:Q_s) and oxygen saturations in the low 90s. Growth and development are normal, and they are usually asymptomatic. If the obstruction is severe, significant right-to-left shunting occurs at the VSD, and oxygen saturations are typically in the 70s (Fig. 35-2).

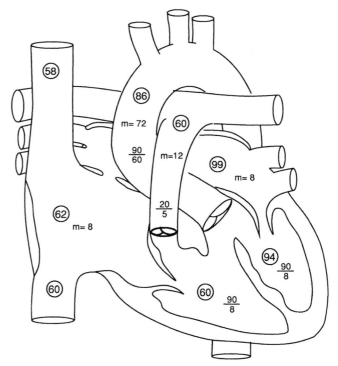

FIGURE 35-2 Schematic diagram of oxygen saturations (*circled values*) and pressures in native anatomy of tetralogy of Fallot. Note systemic pressure in the right ventricle (90/8), with a pressure gradient across the stenotic right ventricle outflow tract resulting in a relatively low pulmonary artery pressure (20/5). A right-to-left shunt into the left ventricle is noted by the decrease in oxygen saturation from the left atrium (99%) to the left ventricle (94%). The overriding aorta receives mixed right ventricular and left ventricular blood and has a saturation of 86%, lower than that of the left ventricle.

Hypercyanotic episodes occur because of a change in the pulmonary-to-systemic blood flow ratio (Q_p:Q_s). A severe hypercyanotic episode is characterized by irritability, hyperpnea, marked cyanosis, pallor, and lethargy or unconsciousness and is known as a "tet spell." A decrease in systemic vascular resistance or an increase in pulmonary vascular resistance leads to increased right-to-left shunting and marked desaturation. The desaturation and resulting metabolic acidosis can increase the pulmonary resistance, thereby worsening the right-to-left shunting. It is imperative to reverse this physiology, or the cycle may continue and lead to irreversible brain damage or death.

Physiology in TOF/PA depends on the amount of PBF. Because all PBF is derived from the systemic circulation, pulmonary and systemic oxygen saturations will be equal. The greater the PBF, the higher the systemic saturation. Saturation levels greater than 85% indicate a Q_p:Q_s of 2:1 or greater, whereas saturations in the 70s indicate a Q_p:Q_s of 1 or less. As in TOF, patients may have evidence of not enough, adequate, or too much PBF. Decreasing arterial oxygen saturations in the neonate may indicate that the ductus arteriosus is closing. High oxygen saturations indicate excessive PBF and will lead to CHF. This high flow through nonrestrictive MAPCAs may lead to pulmonary vascular obstructive disease in the affected lung segments.

In both cyanotic TOF and TOF/PA patients, the presence of a VSD and RVOTO leads to intracardiac right-to-left shunting. Until the patients have undergone closure of the VSD, they are at increased risk of embolic stroke, brain abscess, and the effects of long-term hypoxemia.

DIAGNOSIS

Clinical Manifestations

Because of the variable anatomy, the clinical manifestations of TOF and TOF/PA are diverse. The natural history of these defects is dependent on the severity of the anatomic defect.[46,56] Mortality rates are 30% at 6 months and 50% by 2 years. Fewer than 10% can be expected to reach age 21 years.[8,46] Patients with TOF/PA have a much worse prognosis, with a mortality rate of 50% by 1 year and 85% by age 5 years. Fortunately, it is now rare for children to go unrepaired beyond infancy.

Clinical presentation depends on the severity of the anatomic defects. As noted in the previous section, if the RVOTO is mild, presentation is similar to that of children with VSD. If RVOTO is more significant, right-to-left shunting will result in cyanosis. TOF/PA presentation also is highly variable and dependent on PBF. Development of cyanosis in the neonatal period as the ductus arteriosus closes indicates inadequate collateral circulation. Prompt recognition and institution of prostaglandin E_1 (PGE_1) therapy to maintain ductal patency until surgical palliation or repair is critical to limiting morbidity and mortality. More than half of all infants with TOF/PA will have cyanosis in the neonatal period.

The presence of MAPCAs alleviates cyanosis to a variable degree. As the infant grows, PBF will eventually become inadequate, and cyanosis will develop. This may occur because MAPCAs tend to develop stenoses, and pulmonary vascular obstructive disease can develop in unobstructed MAPCAs.

If PBF is excessive, CHF may develop, and signs and symptoms of CHF, such as tachypnea, failure to thrive, and hepatomegaly, will occur. This occurs as pulmonary vascular resistance decreases during the first few weeks of life. CHF in an infant with TOF/PA is an indication for surgical intervention, either complete repair or palliation, to prevent the development of pulmonary vascular obstructive disease. Approximately 10% of children will go undiagnosed because of adequate but not excessive PBF.[10]

Physical Examination

Infants with TOF and TOF/PA are generally full sized and normal in appearance unless they also have a microdeletion in chromosome 22 (22q11; see section on genetics). Growth failure may develop over time, and cyanosis becomes more easily apparent. Hypertrophic pulmonary osteoarthropathy may develop later in the unrepaired toddler. Signs and symptoms of CHF are related to pulmonary overcirculation and do not differ from those of other cardiac defects. Palpation of the chest will frequently reveal a thrill, indicative of a grade IV/VI systolic murmur. Auscultation of the chest typically reveals a harsh systolic murmur along the left upper sternal border. The murmur reflects flow across the stenotic outflow tract. The second heart sound is usually single and not increased in intensity, and may be accompanied by an ejection click. Absence of a systolic ejection murmur should raise suspicion of pulmonary atresia. A continuous murmur may be present in TOF/PA over the site of a large MAPCA or PDA. As pulmonary vascular resistance decreases, the continuous murmur may become more prominent.

A systolic ejection murmur that decreases in intensity over time is indicative of decreased PBF. In this situation, the child will have progressive cyanosis as the right-to-left shunt increases. During hypercyanotic spells, the murmur may disappear completely. As the spell is treated or resolves, the intensity of the murmur should return to baseline.

Laboratory Studies

The laboratory evaluation is usually nonspecific. Blood gas values and oxygen saturations reflect the level of cyanosis. Hemoglobin increases in proportion to the level and duration of desaturation. A mild bleeding tendency is evident in some patients, particularly those with severe cyanosis and polycythemia. Clotting factors are slightly reduced, as are platelet count and fibrinogen levels. This is not specific for TOF and was first reported in cyanotic heart defects in 1952.[33]

Diagnostic Evaluation

Chest radiographic findings are variable. Pulmonary vascular markings may be decreased, normal, or increased, depending on the degree of RVOT in TOF and collateral circulation in TOF/PA. The great vessel shadow is diminished in the superior mediastinum because of the diminished caliber of the pulmonary artery. The classic finding of a boot-shaped heart with a prominent upturned cardiac apex and concavity in the region of the main pulmonary artery (Fig. 35-3) is a hallmark of TOF and TOF/PA. A right-sided aortic arch occurs in 25% of TOF and 50% of TOF/PA.

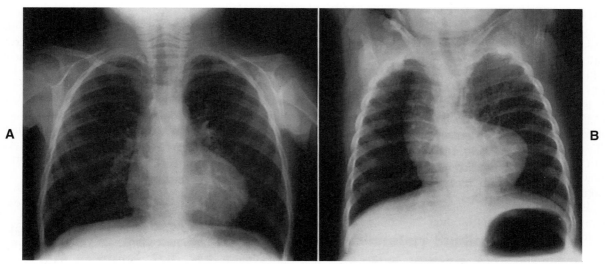

FIGURE 35-3   A, Chest radiograph of a patient with tetralogy of flow and left aortic arch. The absence of the pulmonary artery shadow gives the heart a characteristic "boot-shaped" appearance. **B,** In this patient, the boot-shaped appearance of the heart is even more prominent because the right aortic arch accentuates the absence of the pulmonary arterial shadow.

The electrocardiogram should reflect the degree of RV hypertrophy and includes right axis deviation, upright and peaked T waves in the right precordial leads, and reversal of the R/S ratio. Absence of RV hypertrophy may be seen in TOF/PA in the unusual instance of a hypoplastic RV.

Echocardiography is the mainstay of diagnosis for intracardiac anatomy. Improvements in 2D-echocardiography and color flow Doppler have significantly reduced the need for cardiac catheterization for the majority of patients with TOF.[54,85] The intracardiac anatomy, presence of a patent ductus, and coronary anatomy can accurately be determined with echocardiography.

For patients with TOF/PA, echo can be used to demonstrate the lack of continuity between the RV and the pulmonary arteries. Color flow imaging is used to show lack of prograde flow into the pulmonary arteries. The proximal pulmonary arteries can be visualized, but one must be careful not to confuse the pulmonary arteries with MAPCAs from the descending thoracic aorta. Occasionally the ductus may arise from the innominate or subclavian artery. When this occurs, it can be difficult to distinguish from a MAPCA.[2] Because of the inability to accurately delineate all sources of pulmonary blood supply, cardiac catheterization is necessary in the majority of cases to plan surgical treatment.

Cardiac catheterization is not typically required for patients with TOF. Most centers reserve catheterization for situations in which echo has been unable to identify coronary anatomy clearly (for those centers that perform transventricular repair) or if alternate sources of PBF are suspected. Some added risk occurs during catheterization because intracardiac manipulation may exacerbate RVOTO and precipitate a hypercyanotic episode. Infants who have undergone surgical palliation may require catheterization to assess the degree of distortion of the pulmonary arteries caused by the shunt, if the shunted pulmonary artery cannot be visualized by echocardiogram on both sides of the shunt anastomosis (Fig. 35-4).

Catheterization is necessary to provide a thorough anatomic description of the central pulmonary arteries, ductus arteriosus, branch pulmonary arteries, MAPCAs, and stenosis of MAPCAs. Angiographic assessment of the central pulmonary artery size has been used as a predictor for postoperative RV pressures and mortality.[61,67] A McGoon ratio of 0.8 predicts severely hypoplastic central pulmonary arteries. The Nakata index is determined by measuring the cross-sectional area of the right and left pulmonary artery relative to body surface area. However, both the Nakata index and McGoon ratios were initially developed to look at children whose lesions were repaired at an older age. It is not clear that they are useful tools in younger children.

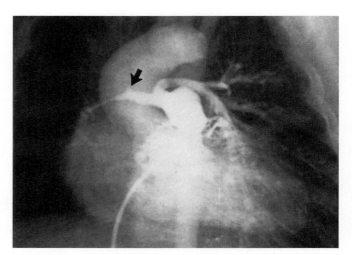

FIGURE 35-4   An angiogram obtained from a patient with tetralogy of Fallot who has severe stenosis of the right pulmonary artery at the site of the previously placed Blalock-Taussig shunt. This patient initially had extreme cyanosis from thrombosis of the shunt (*arrow*). The right pulmonary artery distal to the shunt is virtually obliterated.

INITIAL MEDICAL MANAGEMENT

Initial medical management is dependent on the clinical presentation. The asymptomatic patient with good PBF often requires little in the way of specific medical therapy. Surgical repair can be undertaken electively. If the anatomic defect in TOF is more severe, perioperative stabilization maybe necessary. When obstruction to PBF is severe, neonates will have cyanosis, hypoxemia, and metabolic acidosis. Before the availability of PGE₁, these patients required emergency palliation with creation of a systemic-to–pulmonary artery shunt. PGE₁ allows maintenance of ductal patency to ensure adequate PBF.[19] Correction of acidosis and hypoxemia allows the surgical team to take a hemodynamically stable patient to the operating room. The cardiologist and surgeon then have time to evaluate more thoroughly the anatomy and determine whether palliation or correction is most appropriate. Despite remarkable improvements in neonatal perioperative care, neonatal surgery for TOF and TOF/PA remains a controversial issue.

Management of infants with TOF/PA depends on the degree of PBF. For infants with confluent pulmonary arteries and a PDA, management consists of maintenance of ductal patency with PGE₁ and surgical palliation or repair after stabilization. Occasionally infants will have signs and symptoms of excessive PBF. Medical management of CHF with diuretics and digoxin is appropriate. Provision of adequate calories and attention to growth and symptoms of persistent CHF are important in determining the timing of surgery.

SURGICAL MANAGEMENT

Surgical Management of Tetralogy of Fallot

All patients with TOF and TOF/PA require surgical intervention. Significant advances in perioperative care, anesthesia, and cardiopulmonary bypass (CPB) techniques have spurred earlier correction of congenital heart disease. Early repair may minimize secondary insults to the heart and other organ systems.[9,13,29,63,70,77,82,88] Historically, infants with TOF underwent elective repair at age 2 to 5 years and were palliated by systemic-to–pulmonary artery shunts if symptomatic in the first year of life. With improvements in perioperative care and operative techniques, earlier repair has become standard practice in many centers.[18,28,29,47,82,88] Repair of all children by age 1 year is a reasonable practice. Primary repair of symptomatic neonates is advocated by some centers, but may have a higher mortality rate and increased use of valved conduits and reoperation.[5,6,30,68,73,87]

The argument for repair after the first month of life has centered on the possibility of lower mortality.[5,6,30,73,87] Despite advances in neonatal surgery, most procedures are more easily accomplished in a larger child. Repair at a younger age may lead to a greater use of a transannular patch.[68] The timing of surgical repair should take into account operative and late mortality, attrition rate while waiting for operation, preservation of anatomy and ventricular function, good early and late hemodynamic status, and the need for reoperation. A potential risk to the heart, lungs, and brain may be incurred if surgery is delayed.[14,34,52,93]

Neonatal repair of TOF may be distinctly different from repair of other forms of congenital heart disease. Unlike most corrective procedures, repair of cyanotic TOF actually volume loads the heart with closure of the VSD. The neonatal myocardium does not respond as well to volume loading as does that of the older child because of the inability to significantly increase stroke volume. This may be exacerbated by use of a ventriculotomy, leading to the possibility of low cardiac output and prolonged right heart failure. Additional volume loading of the RV occurs secondary to pulmonary regurgitation and tricuspid regurgitation in a heart that has also been insulted by surgery, CPB, and ischemia.

Neurobehavioral abnormalities in children with congenital heart disease have often been attributed to the effects of prolonged abnormal physiology and intraoperative factors including the risk of CPB. A recent prospective study of newborns with congenital heart disease suggests that other factors are involved.[53] Limperopoulos et al.[53] performed a standardized neonatal behavioral assessment and neurologic examination before surgery on a cohort of neonates referred for evaluation of congenital heart disease. Neurobehavioral and neurologic abnormalities were documented in more than half of the cohort. Additionally, 5% had seizures, 35% were microcephalic, and 12% were macrocephalic.

Other concerns with neonatal repair are the possibility that RVOTO may recur as the child grows,[47] and neonatal repair is most commonly done through a transventricular approach. Non-neonatal transatrial, transpulmonary repair of TOF differs from the transventricular approach in that if an incision in the RV is needed, it is extended from the main pulmonary artery through the pulmonary valve just long enough to relieve the RVOTO. Kawashima et al.[43] showed that this approach results in a lower RV end-diastolic index and higher RV ejection fraction during isoproterenol infusion, and a lower incidence of ventricular dysrhythmias. The postoperative course can be expected to be shorter, with a potential for decreased need for inotropic support and a shorter time on mechanical ventilation. Late RV dilation or dysfunction and an increased risk of ventricular ectopic activity may be related to the presence of a large ventriculotomy scar.[7,31,39,43] Although controversial, dysrhythmias appear to be more problematic after a larger ventriculotomy.[1,7,42,44]

The risk of postoperative dysrhythmias may be due to factors other than the size of the ventriculotomy. Repair outside the infant period may lead to pathologic accumulation of fibrous tissue.[36,78] These changes may increase the incidence of ventricular dysrhythmias.[16,20,36,78] Complicating the issue is that early postoperative dysrhythmias do not necessarily correlate with long-term problems. With neonatal repair, perioperative dysrhythmias occur much more frequently than do those in non-neonatal repair and may be even higher in some centers than the 29% of patients reported by Pigula et al.[68]

Two large series of non-neonatal repair were published in the 1990s.[41,87] Vobecky et al.[87] reviewed their experience with 270 consecutive infants with TOF. Thirty-three were excluded from analysis because of severe noncardiac lesions, major associated cardiac defects, or absent pulmonary valve syndrome. Ninety-six of these patients were asymptomatic until repair after age 18 months. Three (3.1%) of these 96 died awaiting repair. One hundred forty-one underwent initial palliation, with two hospital deaths. In 36 (27.5%), the initial palliation failed, and a second shunt was necessary; 2 of these patients died. An additional 8 died while awaiting complete repair. Total mortality at age 10 years was 11%, with 65% of all deaths occurring while awaiting operation. Karl et al.[41] describe their results in 366 patients, from 1981 to 1991, who underwent non-neonatal transatrial, transpulmonary repair. Only 2 (0.5%) hospital deaths occurred. Mortality rate at a mean follow-up of 42 months was only 2.5%. This compares favorably with results from the most recent series of single-stage repair from the Boston Children's Hospital[68] a decade later, in which mortality at 5 years was 8.4%. Freedom from reoperation in the Karl series was 95% at 5 years versus 88% in the Boston series.

Although most centers now favor the single-stage repair in early infancy, the use of palliative procedures may still have some advantages. It appears that acceptable short- and medium-range results can be achieved with either approach, but at the most experienced centers, mortality appears lower with the non-neonatal approach compared with neonatal repair.[41,68] It may depend on the experience and preference of the surgeon. It is difficult to compare results from one decade to another because of the improvements that have occurred in all aspects of perioperative care. It also is difficult to compare results from one surgeon to another because they may not be generalized to other surgeons less skilled in a particular approach. Long-range results including rates of dysrhythmias, ventricular dysfunction, and need for reoperation may favor one or the other approach.

Surgical Management of TOF/PA

The surgical management of TOF/PA is more controversial. Infants with ductal-dependent PBF and confluent pulmonary arteries can be managed with primary repair or initial shunting followed by secondary repair. Prognosis should be similar to that for patients with TOF. Management of infants with MAPCAs with or without confluent pulmonary arteries is much more complex. Complete repair without unifocalization and ligation of collaterals was the standard until the early 1980s. Prognosis in this era was poor, with survival to age 1 year of 65% and only 50% to 2 years in those patients who appeared operable.[10]

The theoretical feasibility of unifocalization, incorporation of alternative sources of PBF into the central pulmonary arteries, was first suggested by Haworth and McCartney in 1980.[35] Many techniques have been developed to achieve unifocalization, including use of a modified Blalock-Taussig shunt, central aortopulmonary shunts, and transplantation or ligation of MAPCAs.[40,75,79,89,92] The repair is completed by using a valved conduit between the RV and the pulmonary artery. Because of the need for multiple procedures and the difficulty in determining suitability for complete repair, it is difficult to compare results across centers.

Several centers have reported their short and mid-term experience with TOF/PA and MAPCAs by using a staged approach.[35,40,69,75] Iyer and Mee[40] reported on 58 patients of all ages over a 10-year period. Operative mortality was 10.3%. Complete repair was possible in 52% of patients.

Twenty-two (38%) of 58 were deemed unsuitable for complete repair. Sawatari et al.[75] were able to perform a complete repair in 47%, with only 30% deemed to have good results at the end of the 6-year study period. Puga et al.[69] managed 38 patients over a 5-year period with a staged approach. Complete repair was performed in 23 (60%) patients with 2 deaths.

These reports were a considerable improvement over previous results. However, the staged approach is a long, arduous process requiring multiple operations with some attrition along the way. Patients may be unsuitable for complete repair or have unfavorable hemodynamics after this approach. Because of the difficulties in a staged approach, several centers have begun using a strategy of early one-stage unifocalization and complete repair.[49,57,71,80] Possible advantages of early one-stage repair include early reversal of cyanosis, decreased number of operations, probable reduction in pulmonary vascular obstructive disease, reduced need for nonviable tissue, and possibly increased number of patients suitable for complete repair. Disadvantages of the single-stage approach include an extremely long, complex operation with prolonged CPB times, poorer access for some of the small anastomoses, and the likelihood of stenoses of small anastomoses when done at a young age. McElhinney et al.[57] reported their experience over a 6-year period with 67 patients by using a one-stage approach. Forty-six of 67 patients had complete one-stage repair performed; in 23 patients, they were unable to close the VSD. Fourteen of the 23 subsequently underwent VSD closure. Eight early deaths and 6 late deaths occurred, for a combined 20% mortality over the period of the study. Taken as a whole, 21 (31%) of the 67 were unable to undergo complete successful repair. Over the same period, 32 patients underwent a staged approach at the Cleveland Clinic Children's Hospital (unpublished data, Dr. Mee) with no early or late deaths. Sixty percent had already undergone complete repair.

Results continue to improve for both the staged and one-stage repair of TOF/PA. Long-term follow-up is currently lacking. Meticulously planned surgical and interventional catheterization has led to promising short-term results.

The goal of surgical management of these patients is to normalize cardiopulmonary physiology. The pulmonary artery pressure achieved is related to the number of lung segments supplied by the arterial system and the resistance in each segment.[92] Peak RV pressure is the best predictor of outcome after repair, and it is directly related to pulmonary vascular resistance.[62,65] Because of this, it is important to incorporate as many lung segments as possible in the unifocalized pulmonary vascular bed and ensure that the resistance in the individual segments is as low as possible. The natural history of MAPCAs frequently leads to progressive stenosis. Even after unifocalization, progressive stenosis may develop at the site of the MAPCA-to–pulmonary artery connection, at the surgical anastomosis, at the end of an augmentation patch, or in remote intrapulmonary branches. Differential flow may lead to inhibition of growth in some segments and vascular disease in others. Early unifocalization of unobstructed MAPCAs may reduce the incidence of both stenosis and localized vascular disease, thereby increasing the likelihood of successful complete repair.

SURGICAL TECHNIQUES

Palliative Procedures

As previously discussed, the timing and type of intervention for TOF varies from center to center. Among the many options for surgical palliation are the classic Blalock-Taussig shunt, modified B-T shunt, central aortopulmonary shunt, and RV outflow tract patch without closure of the VSD (Fig. 35-5). The choice of palliative procedure depends on the experience and preference of the surgeon and specific anatomic concerns. The goal of palliation is to temporize until total correction is performed, except in rare cases in which other cardiac and extracardiac defects preclude complete repair. Therefore the palliative procedure should aim not only to relieve symptoms and provide for a stable source of PBF but also to provide optimal preparation for complete repair.

Total Correction

Total correction is the goal for TOF patients, except in rare instances in which other issues prevent complete repair. Repair is done on full CPB, deep hypothermic circulatory arrest (DHCA), or deep hypothermia with low-flow CPB. In recent years, the use of DHCA has significantly decreased, as has the use of low-flow CPB. As previously discussed, complete repair can be accomplished either through a transatrial, transpulmonary approach or through a ventriculotomy. The advantages and disadvantages of both approaches were discussed in an earlier section.

POSTOPERATIVE CARE

Postoperative care begins in the operating room after separation from CPB. The VSD closure can be assessed with echocardiography.[83,84] A residual VSD is occasionally seen; however, a residual defect large enough to require further repair occurs rarely (<2%).[26,50] Standard postoperative monitoring includes ECG, arterial line, central venous line, left atrial (LA) line, temporary pacing wires, and a pulmonary artery line if pulmonary resistance is high. A pulmonary artery line maybe useful if a residual VSD, RVOTO, or pulmonary hypertension is a concern.[50] Use of invasive monitoring lines allows more rapid identification of changes in volume status, elevation in pulmonary vascular resistance, early tamponade, and other possible changes. Although evidence is now lacking, they may contribute to shorter intensive care stays, more judicious use of volume, and more timely treatment of pulmonary hypertension. Although not risk free, their use is associated with a low complication rate.[26,32]

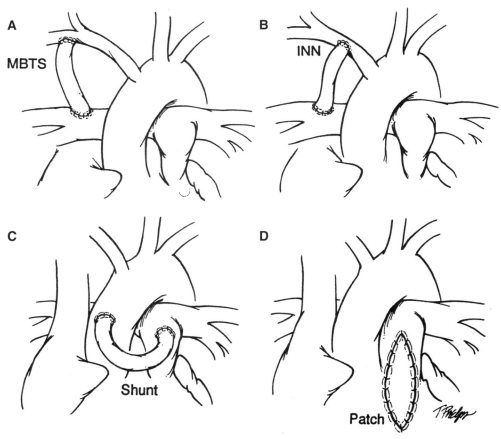

FIGURE 35-5 The most common types of palliative procedures for tetralogy of Fallot. The modified Blalock-Taussig shunt (MBTS) using a Gore-Tex graft either from the right subclavian artery **(A)** or the right innominate (INN) artery **(B)**. **C,** A central aortopulmonary shunt using Gore-Tex. **D,** A right ventricular outflow patch without ventricular septal defect closure.

A significant residual VSD is not well tolerated after TOF repair. Several factors may account for this. After release of the RVOT, the increase in RV volume loading may lead to RV dysfunction. The RV is typically less compliant in patients with TOF, and this is worsened if repair is performed via a ventriculotomy or very early in life because of lower compliance of neonatal myocardium. Other factors may include pulmonary regurgitation after relief of the outflow tract obstruction and LV dysfunction secondary to acute volume loading. These patients may have an LA pressure that is higher than right atrial pressure, and this is easily observed if an LA line is available. Repeated echocardiography may demonstrate a VSD patch leak. Moderate RVOTO is usually fairly well tolerated in the immediate postoperative period but may lead to late problems. Cardiac catheterization is rarely necessary but may be helpful in those patients with an unusual postoperative course. More commonly, right atrial pressure may actually be higher than LA pressure after repair of TOF in infants, reflecting the worse compliance of the RV compared with the LV. In these cases, a patent foramen ovale may allow a small right-to-left shunt, which augments systemic blood flow at the expense of mild systemic oxygen desaturation. More recently, some groups believe that creation of the synthetic monocusp pulmonary valve limits postoperative pulmonary insufficiency and improves initial convalescence after complete repair.

Low cardiac output is not unusual after CPB. This may be related to the size of the ventricular incision, but more likely is produced by the poor compliance of the RV and its inability to fill adequately after repair. Sinus tachycardia (heart rates of 180 to 200 beats/min) is a hallmark of limited cardiac output in this setting. Although advances in technology have made it easier to assess cardiac output, it is still not conveniently measurable in small infants. Clinical assessment of cardiac output includes assessment of peripheral perfusion, central venous and LA pressure, urine output, and acid-base status. Continuous monitoring of core and toe temperatures provides a readily accessible tool to assess adequacy of perfusion. An increasing difference between core and toe temperature is an indicator of decreased cardiac output. Because RV dysfunction and RV failure are the most likely cause of low cardiac output, serial examination of the patient to assess for development of hepatomegaly and peripheral edema must be performed. Some surgeons choose to leave the foramen ovale open to allow right-to-left shunting at the atrial level in situations of anticipated RV failure or dysfunction.[66] This allows greater cardiac output at the expense of oxygen saturation. This is analogous to using a fenestration in the Fontan operation. After the initial few postoperative days, RV compliance should improve, and the right-to-left shunt diminishes.

Dysrhythmias are a common occurrence in the immediate postoperative period. Complete heart block may be seen in the operating room, and temporary pacing may be required. Permanent pacemakers are rarely needed.[48] Right bundle branch block is seen in nearly all patients with a ventriculotomy and in a significant percentage of patients without a ventriculotomy. The most worrisome postoperative dysrhythmia is junctional ectopic tachycardia (JET) (see Chapter 8). JET typically has a warm-up phase with gradual increase in heart rate, occurs on the first postoperative night, and is characterized by atrial-ventricular (AV) dissociation. The degree of hemodynamic impairment during JET is probably related to the degree of RV dysfunction before the onset of JET. Performance of an ECG by using the temporary atrial pacing wires allows rapid identification of dysrhythmias. Adenosine may be useful in differentiating supraventricular tachycardia from JET. Ventricular rates are usually in the range of 200 to 230 beats/min. Cooling to a core temperature less than 36°C may be all that is needed, but antiarrhythmic treatment with amiodarone should not be delayed in those with hemodynamic instability.

Postoperative care for patients with TOF/PA is similar, but may require more thorough assessment of postoperative anatomy and physiology. Serial echocardiography to assess for residual VSDs, RV pressure, RVOTO, or tricuspid or aortic regurgitation may be indicated. If echocardiography reveals elevated RV pressure, cardiac catheterization may be necessary to assess distal pulmonary artery anatomy. If RV pressure is elevated, distal stenoses should be dilated.[74] At this time, residual MAPCAs can be embolized.

OUTCOME

Perioperative outcomes after TOF and TOF/PA have improved significantly over the last few decades. Advances in all areas of care have reduced the mortality rates in some centers to less than 5% with either early complete repair[68] or non-neonatal repair.[41] Improvements in these areas also have reduced morbidity. Thorough preoperative assessment has revealed that a significant percentage of children have preexisting neurobehavioral abnormalities.[53]

Improvements in CPB and operative techniques have reduced but not eliminated early postoperative ventricular dysfunction. Long-term follow-up reveals that ventricular dysfunction, particularly RV dysfunction, in those repaired in the earlier era is common. LV function appears to be well preserved, even in adult TOF patients with chronic pulmonary regurgitation.[21,64,72]

Abnormal RV physiology is a significant long-term problem for TOF patients. Chronic pulmonary regurgitation has been associated with RV dysfunction,[4,12] exercise intolerance,[90] and ventricular dysrhythmias.[94] In a study of ventricular function using Doppler echocardiography by Gatzoulis et al.,[27] restrictive RV dysfunction was evident in 20 (58%) of 38 patients. Antegrade diastolic flow detectable by Doppler was seen in the pulmonary artery. This reflects decreased RV compliance. Similar Doppler phenomena were described previously in adults with restrictive myocardial processes involving the RV.[72] Although prograde pulmonary artery flow during atrial systole represents abnormal physiology, it shortens the duration of pulmonary regurgitation. In the Gatzoulis study, this led to less cardiomegaly and improved exercise performance.

Pulmonary regurgitation and subsequent RV dilation has been shown to be negatively correlated with exercise performance.[90] Eyeskens et al.[21] showed that pulmonary valve replacement in those with severe pulmonary regurgitation substantially improves exercise capacity. However, most of the patients in these studies may not be comparable to current patients. In the current era, age at repair, even in those undergoing palliation before total repair, is significantly younger.

Ventriculotomy, when done, is much smaller. Placement of a transannular patch may be more common in patients undergoing neonatal repair, although Kirklin et al.[48] showed that anatomic considerations, and not age at operation, determined the need for transannular patching.

SUMMARY

In summary, improvements in all aspects of perioperative management of congenital heart disease have led to dramatic improvements in morbidity and mortality. Although a significant push for neonatal repair of TOF has been noted, it is not clear that this approach provides the lowest overall morbidity and mortality. In the best hands, a staged approach yields a lower medium-range mortality than does neonatal repair.[41,47] Currently, both neonatal repair and non-neonatal transatrial, transpulmonary repair can be recommended based on the experience and preference of the surgeon. Although major improvement also has occurred in the outcome for patients with PA/VSD, morbidity and mortality remain higher than those of most other congenital heart defects. One-stage and multistaged approaches are currently being used without the clear superiority of either approach.

References

1. Abe T, Komatsu S: Long term follow-up studies in 211 patients with tetralogy of Fallot after corrective surgery over ten years. *Kyobu Geka* 43:598–604, 1990.
2. Acherman RJ, Smallhorn JF, Freedom RM: Echocardiographic assessment of pulmonary blood supply in patients with pulmonary atresia and ventricular septal defect. *J Am Coll Cardiol* 28:1308–1313, 1996.
3. Akasaka T, Itoh K, Ohkawa Y, et al: Surgical treatment of anomalous origin of the left coronary artery from the pulmonary artery associated with tetralogy of Fallot. *Ann Thorac Surg* 31:469–474, 1981.
4. Appleton CP, Hatle LK, Popp RL: Demonstration of restrictive ventricular physiology by Doppler echocardiography. *J Am Coll Cardiol* 4:757–768, 1988.
5. Arciniegas E, Farooki ZQ, Hakimi M, Green EW: Results of two-stage surgical treatment of tetralogy of Fallot. *J Thorac Cardiovasc Surg* 79:876–883, 1980.
6. Arciniegas E, Farooki ZQ, Hakimi M, et al: Early and late results of total correction of tetralogy of Fallot. *J Thorac Cardiovasc Surg* 80:770–778, 1980.
7. Basagoitia AM, Iturralde P, Galvan O, et al: Disorders of the rhythm and conduction in patients operated on for a total correction of tetralogy of Fallot. *Arch Inst Cardiol Mex* 61:27–32, 1991.
8. Bertranou EG, Blackstone EH, Hazelrig JB, et al: Life expectancy without surgery in tetralogy of Fallot. *Am J Cardiol* 42:458–466, 1978.
9. Borow KM, Green LH, Castaneda AR, Keane JF: Left ventricular function after repair of tetralogy of Fallot and its relationship to age at surgery. *Circulation* 61:1150–1158, 1980.
10. Bull K, Somerville J, Ty E, Spiegelhalter D: Presentation and attrition in complex pulmonary atresia. *J Am Coll Cardiol* 25:491–499, 1995.
11. Burn J, Goodship J: Congenital heart disease. In Rimoin D, Connor J, Pyeritz R (eds): *Emery and Rimoin's Principles and Practice of Medical Genetics.* 3rd ed. New York, Churchill Livingstone, 1996, pp 767–828.
12. Carvalho JS, Shinebourne EA, Busst C, et al: Exercise capacity after complete repair of tetralogy of Fallot: Deleterious effects of residual pulmonary regurgitation. *Br Heart J* 67:470–473, 1992.
13. Castaneda AR, Mayer JE, Jonas RA, et al: The neonate with critical congenital heart disease: repair: A surgical challenge. *J Thorac Cardiovasc Surg* 98:861–875, 1989.
14. Chandar JS, Wolff GS, Garson A Jr, et al: Ventricular arrhythmias in postoperative tetralogy of Fallot. *Am J Cardiol* 65:55–61, 1990.
15. Dabizzi RP, Caprioli G, Aiazzi L, et al: Distribution and anomalies of coronary arteries in tetralogy of Fallot. *Circulation* 61:95–102, 1980.
16. Deanfield JE, McKenna WJ, Presbitero P, et al: Ventricular arrhythmias in unrepaired and repaired tetralogy of Fallot: Relation of age, timing of repair, and haemodynamic status. *Br Heart J* 52:77–81, 1984.
17. DeRuiter MC, Gittenberger-de Groot AC, Bogers AJJC, Elzenga NJ: The restricted surgical relevance of morphologic criteria to classify systemic-pulmonary collateral arteries in pulmonary atresia with ventricular septal defect. *J Thorac Cardiovasc Surg* 108:692–699, 1994.
18. DiDonato RM, Jonas RA, Lang P, et al: Neonatal repair of tetralogy of Fallot with and without pulmonary atresia. *J Thorac Cardiovasc Surg* 101:126–137, 1991.
19. Donahoo JS, Roland JM, Kan J, et al: Prostaglandin E₁ as an adjunct to emergency cardiac operation in neonates. *J Thorac Cardiovasc Surg* 81:227–231, 1981.
20. Ewing LL, Gillette PC, Zeigler V, et al: Only 8% of postoperative tetralogy patients have inducible ventricular dysrhythmias. *J Am Coll Cardiol* 9:36A, 1987.
21. Eyskens B, Reybrouck T, Bogaert J, et al: Homograft insertion for pulmonary regurgitation after repair of tetralogy of Fallot improves cardiorespiratory exercise performance. *Am J Cardiol* 85:221–225, 2000.
22. Fallot ELA: Contribution a l'anatomic pathologique de la maladie bleue (cyanose cardiaque). *Marseille Med* 25:77, 138, 207, 270, 341, 1888.
23. Farre JR: *Pathological Researches: SA I: Malformations of the Human Head: Illustrated by Numerous Cases, and Preceded by Some Observations on the Method of Improving the Diagnostic Span of Medicine.* London, Longmans, Green, 1814.
24. Fellows KE, Freed MD, Keane JF, et al: Results of routine preoperative coronary angiography in tetralogy of Fallot. *Circulation* 51:561–566, 1975.
25. Fellows KE, Smith J, Keane JF: Preoperative angiocardiography in infants with tetrad of Fallot: Review of 36 cases. *Am J Cardiol* 47:1279–1285, 1981.
26. Flori HR, Johnson LD, Hanley FL, Fineman JR: Transthoracic intracardiac catheters in pediatric patients recovering from congenital heart defect surgery: Associated complications and outcomes. *Crit Care Med* 28:2997–3001, 2000.
27. Gatzoulis MA, Clark AL, Cullen S, et al: Right ventricular diastolic function 15 to 35 years after repair of tetralogy of Fallot. *Circulation* 91:1775–1781, 1995.
28. Groh MA, Meliones JN, Bove EL, et al: Repair of tetralogy of Fallot in infancy: Effect of pulmonary artery size on outcome. *Circulation* 84:206–212, 1991.
29. Gustafson RA, Murray GF, Warden HE, et al: Early primary repair of tetralogy of Fallot. *Ann Thorac Surg* 45:235–241, 1988.
30. Hammon JW Jr, Henry CL Jr, Merrill WH, et al: Tetralogy of Fallot: Selective surgical management can minimize operative mortality. *Ann Thorac Surg* 40:280–284, 1985.
31. Harkin AH, Horowitz LN, Josephson ME: Surgical correction of recurrent sustained ventricular tachycardia following complete repair of tetralogy of Fallot. *J Thorac Cardiovasc Surg* 80:779–781, 1980.
32. Harrison AM, Davis SJ, Graney JA, et al: Removal of epicardial pacing wires and intracardiac transthoracic monitoring lines after congenital heart surgery. Abstract 2000. Presented at AAP meeting 55056.
33. Hartmann RC: A hemorrhagic disorder occurring in patients with cyanotic congenital heart disease. *Bull Johns Hopkins Hosp* 91:49–67, 1952.
34. Hausdorf G, Hinrichs C, Nienaber CA, Keck EW: Left ventricular contractile state after surgical correction of tetralogy of Fallot: Risk factors for late left ventricular dysfunction. *Pediatr Cardiol* 11:61–68, 1990.
35. Haworth SG, Macartney FJ: Growth and development of pulmonary circulation in pulmonary atresia with ventricular septal defect and major aortopulmonary collateral arteries. *Br Heart J* 44:14–24, 1980.
36. Hegarty A, Anderson RH, Deanfield JE: Myocardial fibrosis in tetralogy of Fallot: Effect of surgery or part of the natural history? *Br Heart J* 59:123, 1988.
37. Hofbeck M, Rauch A, Buheitel G, et al: Monosomy 22q11 in patients with pulmonary atresia, ventricular septal defect and major aortopulmonary collateral arteries. *Heart* 79:180–185, 1998.
38. Hofbeck M, Sunnegardh JT, Burrows PE, et al: Analysis of survival in patients with pulmonic valve atresia and ventricular septal defect. *Am J Cardiol* 67:737–743, 1991.
39. Horowitz LN, Vetter VL, Harken AH, Josephson ME: Electrophysiologic characteristics of sustained ventricular tachycardia occurring after repair of tetralogy of Fallot. *Am J Cardiol* 46:446–452, 1980.

40. Iyer KS, Mee RBB: Staged repair of pulmonary atresia with ventricular septal defect and major systemic to pulmonary artery collaterals. *Ann Thorac Surg* 51:65–72, 1991.
41. Karl TR, Sano S, Pornviliwan S, Mee RBB. Tetralogy of Fallot: Favorable outcome of nonneonatal transatrial, transpulmonary repair. *Ann Thorac Surg* 54:903–907, 1992.
42. Kato H, Nakano S, Matsuda H, et al: The influence of pulmonary regurgitation on left ventricular function after repair of tetralogy of Fallot. *Nippon Kyobu Geka Gakkai Zasshi* 38:2257–2263, 1990.
43. Kawashima Y, Kitamura S, Nakano S, Hagihara T: Corrective surgery for tetralogy of Fallot without or with minimal right ventriculotomy and with repair of the pulmonary valve. *Circulation* 64:147–153, 1981.
44. Kawashima Y, Kobayashi J, Matsuda A: Long term evaluation after correction of tetralogy of Fallot. *Kyobu Geka* 43:660–665, 1990.
45. Kirklin JW, Barratt-Boyes BG: Ventricular septal defect and pulmonary stenosis or atresia. In Kirklin JW, Barratt-Boyes BG (eds): *Cardiac Surgery*. New York, Churchill Livingstone, 1993, p 861.
46. Kirklin JW, Barratt-Boyes BG: Ventricular septal defect and pulmonary stenosis or atresia. In Kirklin JW, Barratt-Boyes BG (eds): *Cardiac Surgery*. New York, Churchill Livingstone, 1993, p 861.
47. Kirklin JW, Blackstone EH, Covin EV, McConnell ME: Early primary correction of tetralogy of Fallot. *Ann Thorac Surg* 45:231–233, 1988.
48. Kirklin JW, Blackstone EH, Jonas RA, et al: Morphologic and surgical determinants of outcome events after repair of tetralogy of Fallot and pulmonary stenosis: A two-institution study. *J Thorac Cardiovasc Surg* 103:706–723, 1992.
49. Kirklin JW, Blackstone EH, Shimazaki Y, et al: Survival, functional status, and reoperations after repair of tetralogy of Fallot with pulmonary atresia. *J Thorac Cardiovasc Surg* 96:102–116, 1988.
50. Lang P, Chipman CW, Siden H, et al: Early assessment of hemodynamic status after repair of tetralogy of Fallot: A comparison of 24 hour (ICU) and 1 year postoperative data in 98 patients. *Am J Cardiol* 50:795–799, 1982.
51. Lev M, Eckner FAQ: The pathologic anatomy of tetralogy of Fallot and its variations. *Dis Chest* 45:251, 1964.
52. Li RK, Mickle DA, Weisel RD, et al: Effect of oxygen tension on the antioxidant enzyme activities of tetralogy of Fallot ventricular myocytes. *J Mol Cell Cardiol* 21:567–575, 1989.
53. Limeropoulos C, Majnemer A, Shevell MI, et al: Neurologic status of newborns with congenital heart defects before open heart surgery. *Pediatrics* 103:402–408, 1999.
54. Marino B, Corno A, Pasquini L, et al: Indication for systemic-pulmonary artery shunts guided by two-dimensional and Doppler echocardiography: Criteria for patient selection. *Ann Thorac Surg* 44:495–498, 1987.
55. Matsuda H, Ihara K, Mori T, et al: Tetralogy of Fallot associated with aortic insufficiency. *Ann Thorac Surg* 29:529–533, 1980.
56. McCord M, van Elk J, Blount G Jr: Tetralogy of Fallot: Clinical and hemodynamic spectrum of combined pulmonary stenosis and ventricular septal defects. *Circulation* 16:736, 1957.
57. McElhinney DB, Reddy VM, Hanley FL: Tetralogy of Fallot with major aortopulmonary collaterals: Early total repair. *Pediatr Cardiol* 19:289–296, 1998.
58. Mitchell SC, Korones SB, Berendes HW: Congenital heart disease in 56,109 births: Incidence and natural history. *Circulation* 43:323–332, 1971.
59. Moritz A, Marx M, Wollenek G, et al: Complete repair of PA/VSD with diminutive or discontinuous pulmonary arteries by transverse thoracotomy. *Ann Thorac Surg* 61:646–650, 1996.
60. Nagao GI, Daoud GI, McAdams AJ, et al: Cardiovascular anomalies associated with tetralogy of Fallot. *Am J Cardiol* 20:206–215, 1967.
61. Nakata S, Imai Y, Takanashi Y, et al: A new method for the quantitative standardization of cross-sectional areas of the pulmonary arteries in congenital heart diseases with decreased pulmonary blood flow. *J Thorac Cardiovasc Surg* 88:610–620, 1984.
62. Newburger JW, Jonas RA, Wernovsky G, et al: A comparision of the perioperative neurologic effects of hypothermic circulatory arrest versus low flow cardiopulmonary bypass in infant heart surgery. *N Engl J Med* 329:1057–1064, 1993.
63. Newburger JW, Silbert AR, Buckley LP, Fyler DC: Cognitive function and age at repair of transposition of the great arteries in children. *N Engl J Med* 310:1495–1499, 1984.
64. Niezen RA, Helbing WA, van Der Wall EE, et al: Left ventricular function in adult Fallot patients with residual pulmonary regurgitation. *Heart* 82:697–703, 1999.
65. Papagiannis J, Kanter RJ, Armstrong BE, et al: Intraoperative epicardial echocardiography during repair of tetralogy of Fallot. *J Am Soc Echocardiogr* 6:366–373, 1993.
66. Pass RH, Mayer JE Jr, Jonas RA, et al: Course in the intensive care unit after right ventriculotomy and neonatal repair of congenital heart disease. *J Am Coll Cardiol* 29:107a, 1997.
67. Piehler JM, Danielson GK, McGoon DC, et al: Management of pulmonary atresia with ventricular septal defect and hypoplastic pulmonary arteries by right ventricular outflow construction. *J Thorac Cardiovasc Surg* 80:552–567, 1980.
68. Pigula FA, Khalil PN, Mayer JE, et al: Repair of tetralogy of Fallot in neonates and young infants. *Circulation* 100:II157–II161, 1999.
69. Puga FJ, Leoni FE, Julsrud PR, Mair DD: Complete repair of pulmonary atresia, ventricular septal defect, and severe peripheral arborization abnormalities of the central pulmonary arteries. *J Thorac Cardiovasc Surg* 98:1018–1029, 1989.
70. Rabinovitch M, Herrera-deLeon V, Castaneda AR, Reid L: Growth and development of the pulmonary vascular bed in patients with tetralogy of Fallot with or without pulmonary atresia. *Circulation* 64:1234–1249, 1981.
71. Reddy VM, Petrossian E, McElhnnney DB, et al: Surgery for congenital heart disease. *J Thorac Cardiovasc Surg* 113:858–868, 1997.
72. Redington AN, Oldershaw PJ, Shinebourne EA, Rigby ML: A new technique for the assessment of pulmonary regurgitation and its application to the assessment of right ventricular function before and after repair of tetralogy of Fallot. *Br Heart J* 60:57–65, 1988.
73. Rittenhouse EA, Mansfield PB, Hall DG, et al: Tetralogy of Fallot: Selective staged management. *J Thorac Cardiovasc Surg* 89:772–779, 1985.
74. Rome JJ, Mayer JE, Castaneda AR, Lock JE: Tetralogy of Fallot with pulmonary atresia: Rehabilitation of diminutive pulmonary arteries. *Circulation* 88:1691–1698, 1993.
75. Sawatari K, Imai Y, Kurosawa H, et al: Staged operation for pulmonary atresia and ventricular septal defect with major aortopulmonary collateral arteries. *J Thorac Cardiovasc Surg* 98:738–750, 1989.
76. Shimazaki Y, Maehara T, Blackstone EH, et al: The structure of the pulmonary circulation in tetralogy of Fallot with pulmonary atresia. *J Thorac Cardiovasc Surg* 95:1048–1058, 1988.
77. Shimazaki Y, Tokuan Y, Lio M, et al: Pulmonary artery pressure and resistance late after repair of tetralogy of Fallot with pulmonary atresia. *J Thorac Cardiovasc Surg* 100:425–440, 1990.
78. Sullivan ID, Presbitero P, Gooch VM, et al: Is ventricular arrhythmia in repaired tetralogy of Fallot an effect of operation or a consequence of the course of the disease? A prospective study. *Br Heart J* 58:40–44, 1987.
79. Sullivan ID, Wren C, Stark J, et al: Surgical unifocalization in pulmonary atresia and ventricular septal defect: A realistic goal? *Circulation* 78:III5–III13, 1988.
80. Tchervenkov CI, Salasidis G, Cecere R, et al: One-stage midline unifocalization and complete repair in infancy versus multiple-stage unifocalization followed by repair for complex heart disease with major aortopulmonary collaterals. *J Thorac Cardiovasc Surg* 114:727–737, 1997.
81. Tobias ES, Morrison N, Whiteford ML, Tolmie JL: Towards earlier diagnosis of 22q11 deletions. *Arch Dis Child* 81:513–514, 1999.
82. Touati GD, Vouhe PR, Amodeo A, et al: Primary repair of tetralogy of Fallot in infancy. *J Thorac Cardiovasc Surg* 99:396–403, 1990.
83. Ungerleider RM, Greeley WJ, Kanter RJ, Kisslo JA: The learning curve for intraoperative echocardiography during congenital heart surgery. *Ann Thorac Surg* 54:691–696, 1992.
84. Ungerleider RM, Greeley WJ, Sheikh KH, et al: Routine use of intraoperative epicardial echocardiography and Doppler color flow imaging to guide and evaluate repair of congenital heart lesions: A prospective study. *J Thorac Cardiovasc Surg* 100:297–309, 1990.
85. Ungerleider RM, Greeley WI, Sheikh KH, et al: The use of intraoperative echo with Doppler color flow imaging to predict outcome after repair of congenital cardiac defects. *Ann Surg* 210:526–533, 1989.
86. Vargas FI, Coto EO, Mayer JE Jr, et al: Complete atrioventricular canal and tetralogy of Fallot: Surgical considerations. *Ann Thorac Surg* 42:258–263, 1986.
87. Vobecky SI, Williams WG, Trusler GA, et al: Survival analysis of infants under age 18 months presenting with tetralogy of Fallot. *Ann Thorac Surg* 56:944–949, 1993.
88. Walsh EP, Rockenmacher S, Keane JF, et al: Late results in patients with tetralogy of Fallot repaired during infancy. *Circulation* 77:1062–1067, 1988.

89. Watterson KG, Wilkinson JL, Karl TR, Mee RBB: Very small pulmonary arteries: Central end-to-side shunts. *Ann Thorac Surg* 52:1132–1137, 1991.

90. Wessel HU, Cunningham WJ, Paul MH, et al: Exercise performance in tetralogy of Fallot after intracardiac repair. *J Thorac Cardiovasc Surg* 80:582–593, 1980.

91. Westerman GR, Norton IB, Van Devanter SH: Double-outlet right atrium associated with tetralogy of Fallot and common atrioventricular valve. *J Thorac Cardiovasc Surg* 91:205–207, 1986.

92. Yagihara T, Yamamoto F, Nishigaki K, et al: Unifocalization for pulmonary atresia with ventricular septal defect and major aortopulmonary collateral arteries: Surgery for congenital heart disease. *J Thorac Cardiovasc Surg* 112:392–402, 1996.

93. Yamaki S: Pulmonary vascular disease in shunted and non-shunted patients with tetralogy of Fallot. *Tohoku J Exp Med* 162:109–119, 1990.

94. Zakha KG, Horneffer PJ, Rose SA, et al: Long-term valvular function after total repair of tetralogy of Fallot: Relation to ventricular arrhythmias. *Circulation* 78:14–19, 1988.

Chapter 36

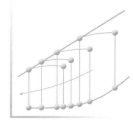

Pulmonary Atresia with Intact Ventricular Septum

DAVID P. BICHELL, MD

INTRODUCTION/DEFINITIONS

Congenital heart defects occur in an estimated 8 of 1000 live births. Pulmonary atresia with intact ventricular septum (PA/IVS) accounts for fewer than 3% of congenital heart defects, making its general incidence less than 3 per 10,000 live births.[19,45] Although an autosomal dominant inheritance pattern has been described in certain families, a majority of cases appear to be sporadic.[11,16,29]

Pulmonary atresia with intact ventricular septum includes a spectrum of disease ranging from simple membranous valvular atresia with a well-developed right ventricle (RV), treated with an anatomic biventricular repair, to a severely hypoplastic RV with RV-coronary fistulae and absent infundibulum, requiring a staged univentricular palliation.

In general, PA/IVS is characterized by abnormalities proximal to the RV-pulmonary artery (PA) junction, whereas PA with ventricular septal defect (VSD) includes a normal RV and tricuspid valve, with a majority of abnormalities distal to the pulmonary valve. These distinctions suggest different pathogenic origins for the two entities.[40,67]

ANATOMY/MORPHOLOGIC CONSIDERATIONS

General

John Hunter's description[34] (1783) endures as an accurate point of departure and overview of the physiology of PA/IVS: The pulmonary artery, which, at its beginning from the right ventricle, was contracted into a solid substance or cord, and absolutely and completely impervious; so that the lungs had not received one drop of blood from the heart by the trunk of the pulmonary artery. The right ventricle, therefore, had been of no use in transmitting the blood, and had scarcely any cavity left ... The blood, which was brought to the right auricle, by the two cavae and the coronary veins, had passed through the foramen ovale, which was very large, into the left side of the heart, and so into the aorta, without passing through the lungs, and of course without receiving the benefit of respiration. The pulmonary artery, except just at its beginning, was everywhere previous; and the canalis arteriosus had supplied it with a scanty share of blood, which was derived,

767

in a retrograde way, from the aorta.... The right auriculoven-tricular aperture was especially small ... The left ventricle (LV) was large and powerful.

Hunter described a severe and typical form of PA/IVS, with significant hypoplasia of the RV, diminutive tricuspid valve orifice, and ductus-dependent pulmonary blood flow. The spectrum of anatomic abnormality associated with PA/IVS ranges from Hunter's description at the severe end of the spectrum to considerably milder forms. The following anatomic descriptions characterize the spectrum of disease as it affects each segment of the heart, starting with the atretic valve and working upstream to associated abnormalities.

Pulmonary Valve

The pulmonary root typically is 75% of normal diameter, and the valve tricommissural, with well-formed sinuses but fused leaflets. A variety of more dysmorphic valves also are described with unicuspid or quadricuspid configurations, as well as the complete absence of any valvular architecture, with a fibrous ventriculoarterial junction.[40]

Right Ventricle

The RV is hypertrophic with a small cavity in 90% of cases of PA/IVS and severely hypoplastic in more than 50% (Fig. 36-1). Ventriculocoronary fistulae are present in 45% of cases, and 9% have RV-dependent coronary circulation. The tripartite classification of the RV, proposed by Goor and Lillehei,[28] describes ventricular morphology according to the presence or absence of inlet, trabecular, and infundibular components. The presence or absence of a tripartite RV was proposed as a gauge of whether a biventricular repair is feasible. More commonly, RV volume, measured or inferred by associated tricuspid valve diameter, is the gauge of the adequacy of a ventricle. The diminutive, hypertrophic RV usually exhibits diffuse fibro-elastic changes from chronic ischemia and hypertension.[7,8,17,67]

Although a majority of cases are characterized by a diminutive RV cavity, rarer variants occur with a dilated RV, presumed secondary to outflow obstruction and tricuspid regurgitation. The Ebstein-like variant of PA/IVS, occurring in 5% to 10% of cases, is characterized by severe tricuspid regurgitation and a dilated RV.[30] Uhl's anomaly, with a dilated parchment-like RV, is a rare accompaniment to PA/IVS.

Tricuspid Valve

The 1993 Congenital Heart Surgeons' Society (CHSS) multi-institutional study of PA/IVS confirmed a strong correlation between the echocardiographically determined tricuspid valve z value and the RV cavity size, as well as with the presence of coronary fistulae and RV-dependent coronary circulation, and the likelihood of success in biventricular versus univentricular repairs.[14,20,30,67] The tricuspid valve is typically small, with a z value less than −2, but is enlarged in the uncommon Ebstein-like variant.[2,3,30] The tricuspid valve is commonly dysplastic and variably regurgitant, severely so in 27% of cases. A parachute tricuspid valve has been described.[4,12,20]

Right Atrium

The right atrium is invariably dilated. A patent foramen ovale (PFO) or atrial septal defect (ASD) is always present, through which all systemic venous return is conducted to the left-sided circulation. A restrictive PFO is indication to perform a balloon atrial septostomy as the initial palliative intervention.

Pulmonary Arteries

Distal to the atretic pulmonary valve, the pulmonary arteries are confluent, and the arterial tree is typically normal in caliber and distribution. Hypoplastic branch pulmonary arteries are found in only 6% of cases.[30] Aortopulmonary collaterals, typically associated with PA with VSD, are rare in PA/IVS, but may be present when a ductus arteriosus is not present.[41]

Coronary Arteries

Ventriculocoronary sinusoids are present in 45% of cases, and probably represent precoronary nutrient connections that persist because of RV hypertension, as evidenced by their

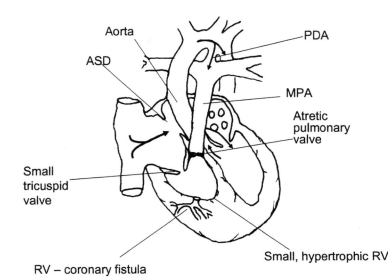

FIGURE 36-1 Native anatomy of pulmonary atresia with intact ventricular septum. The atretic pulmonary valve prevents exit of blood from the small, hypertrophic right ventricle (RV). As a result, the elevated right heart pressures drive systemic venous blood through the atrial septal defect (ASD) to mix with pulmonary venous blood in the left heart. This desaturated blood is ejected into the aorta to supply both the systemic circulation and the pulmonary circulation via the patent ductus arteriosus (PDA). Coronary blood supply to the RV is maintained in part by an RV- coronary fistula. Note also the small tricuspid valve and the normal caliber of the main pulmonary artery (MPA).

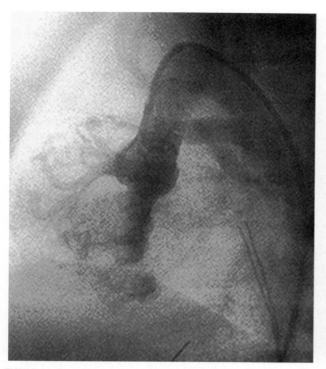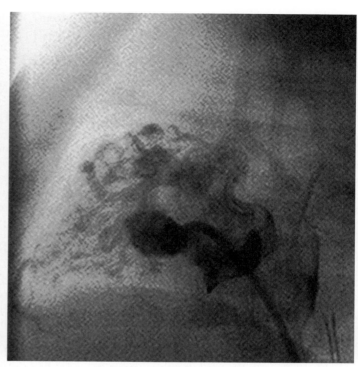

FIGURE 36-2 Angiogram of a newborn with pulmonary atresia with intact ventricular septum. The aortic root injection shows the course of the right coronary artery (*left*). An injection of the diminutive RV shows the retrograde filling of the right coronary artery through extensive ventriculocoronary fistulae (*right*).

prevalence relating to RV pressure and size (Fig. 36-2). A small tricuspid valve predicts the presence of ventriculocoronary fistulae. Two thirds of patients with tricuspid z values of −3, and virtually all of those with z values less than −5, will have ventriculocoronary artery fistulae (Fig. 36-3). Ventriculocoronary fistulae are not present in cases of important tricuspid regurgitation, presumably because RV hypertension does not develop. Coronary artery stenoses form in severe cases because

of myointimal hyperplasia in the true coronary artery proximal to the ventriculocoronary connection, thereby rendering the coronary blood flow dependent on the RV. The etiology of proximal stenoses is presumably related to competitive ventricular versus coronary flow. Coronary stenoses generally progress after birth.[27,30,47,49] With ductal runoff after birth, diastolic blood pressure is relatively low, and in competition with the suprasystemic RV for perfusion of the coronary arteries.

FIGURE 36-3 The relationship between tricuspid diameter (*z* value) and the likelihood of having ventriculocoronary artery fistulae. (Reproduced from Hanley FL, Sade RM, Blackstone EH, et al: Outcomes in neonatal pulmonary atresia with intact ventricular septum. A multi-institutional study. *J Thorac Cardiovasc Surg* 105:406–427, 1993; with permission.)

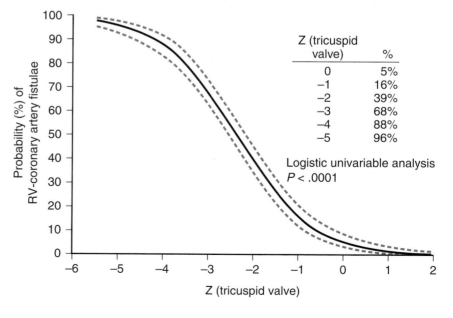

Z (tricuspid valve)	%
0	5%
−1	16%
−2	39%
−3	68%
−4	88%
−5	96%

Logistic univariable analysis
$P < .0001$

The physiology of ventriculocoronary artery fistulae presents important risks and must be understood in planning a strategy for palliation of PA/IVS. A truly RV-dependent coronary artery system, with RV-coronary sinusoids and proximal coronary artery stenoses, cannot undergo procedures to open the obstructed RV, as resultant diastolic coronary steal into the decompressed ventricle will cause myocardial hypoperfusion.

Left Ventricle

Volume overload from the patent ductus arteriosus (PDA), the atrial level right-to-left shunt, and palliative shunts results in left atrial and ventricular enlargement and endocardial fibroelastosis.[30] Septal distortion and hypertrophy from the hypertensive RV can produce LV outflow obstruction and impaired LV function.[22,31,60] In a setting of coronary sinusoids and RV-dependent coronary circulation, desaturated coronary perfusion may promote myocardial changes as a result of chronic hypoxia, further insulting LV performance.

EMBRYOLOGY

Based on prenatal echocardiographic data, it appears that PA/IVS occurs as an RV outflow tract obstruction in the late embryonic period. Forward flow has been observed by fetal echo before the formation of PA/IVS, supporting the hypothesis that PA forms as a late fetal event, rather than being an abnormality of primary morphogenesis. It has been suggested that inflammatory or infectious processes may play a role in the development of embryonic pulmonary artery obstruction.[50]

Associated abnormalities upstream from the atretic valve may occur in response to aberrant flow patterns set up by the atretic valve, disrupting a cascade of signals that direct the normal development of the heart. Mechanical determinants may drive local changes in genes that direct the modeling of the developing heart.[66] It is known that arteries grow and remodel according to shear stresses.[62] Endocardial cells have been shown to align with the direction of flow, supporting evidence for a similar phenomenon affecting the cardiac tube and heart formation.[35] Various animal models of flow disruption resulting in upstream abnormalities of the left and right heart have been described. For example, LV inflow obstruction by atrial clipping in a chick embryo model results in LV hypoplasia with accelerated trabecular compaction, RV trabecular proliferation, and thickening of the compact myocardium. Conotruncal banding results in ventricular dilation and a thickening of compact myocardium and trabeculae.[32,57]

Abnormal flow through the obstructed embryonic right heart logically leads to the associated anatomic findings in PA/IVS. An obstruction of flow at the level of the pulmonary valve in the embryonic heart results in a diversion of right-sided blood flow across the foramen ovale, depriving the RV of a putative shear-stress induction of normal growth and development. Ventriculocoronary artery fistulae presumably persist when the tricuspid valve is competent and the RV hypertensive. Corroborating this hypothesis is the observation

that the Ebstein-like variant of PA/IVS, with a regurgitant tricuspid valve, is not associated with ventriculocoronary artery fistulae.

NATURAL HISTORY

Untreated, 50% of patients die within 2 weeks of birth. Eighty-five percent die by age 6 months. Death follows ductal closure and a resultant cyanosis, acidosis, and cardiovascular collapse. Rarely, survival to adulthood is possible if a PDA persists.[44,52] Hydrops fetalis and embryonic death as a result of tricuspid regurgitation probably accounts for the relative rarity of the Ebstein-like variant of PA/IVS.[2,3]

DIAGNOSTICS

The 1993 CHSS multi-institutional study of PA/IVS observed that more than 90% of patients are initially seen in the first 3 days of life. Presenting physical findings typically include cyanosis, a continuous murmur of a PDA, and a single S2 on auscultation. The PDA murmur is often not present or remains unappreciated. The electrocardiogram (ECG) demonstrates an absence of the usual dominant right forces seen in the newborn and a large P wave consistent with right atrial enlargement. Sinus rhythm is the rule. The cardiac silhouette is normal in size, enlarged in the presence of important tricuspid regurgitation, and pulmonary vascular markings are variable, dependent on ductal flow. The cardiac silhouette progressively enlarges as right atrial enlargement progresses. An echocardiogram confirms the diagnosis and is the most accurate determinant of anatomic detail. Ductal patency and size of PFO are determined, and balloon atrial septostomy is performed when necessary. Although the echocardiogram can often map ventriculocoronary sinusoids, cardiac catheterization more precisely assesses coronary anatomy, the presence or absence of coronary artery stenoses, and the uncommon presence or not of aortopulmonary collaterals.[56] Right ventricular pressure is typically suprasystemic. Systemic arterial desaturation is relative to the atrial level right-to-left shunt and the degree of restriction to ductal left-to-right shunting, on which pulmonary blood flow is dependent.

PREOPERATIVE MANAGEMENT

The newborn with PA/IVS is first seen with hypoxia, progressing to acidosis and cardiovascular collapse as the ductus closes, causing pulmonary blood flow to be progressively compromised. Prostaglandin E_1 (PGE$_1$) infusion at 0.02 to 0.1 mcg/kg/min is initiated promptly to maintain ductus-dependent pulmonary blood flow, and any acidosis is aggressively corrected. A complete characterization of anatomy by echocardiogram is imperative, and a cardiac catheterization is performed in every patient to determine coronary anatomy and ventriculocoronary dependence. Persistent hypoperfusion after the reestablishment of ductal patency suggests the presence of a restrictive inter-atrial communication.

Catheter-based atrial septostomy, performed in the catheterization laboratory or at the bedside under echocardiographic guidance, improves the right-to-left shunting necessary to support the cardiac output and decompresses the systemic venous return to the heart. A 15% to 20% incidence of apnea in newborns receiving PGE$_1$ warrants careful observation and possible elective intubation. Arterial oxygen saturations in the range of 80% are desirable, and a failure to achieve this target with a PDA should prompt an investigation into pulmonary causes of hypoxia such as atelectasis, right main-stem bronchial intubation, mucus plugging, or effusion.

PRINCIPLES OF TREATMENT

The neonate with PA/IVS has ductus-dependent pulmonary blood flow and atrial-level shunting to divert all systemic venous return to the left atrium for complete mixing. This precarious and temporary balance must be replaced by a durable solution, by biventricular, univentricular, or hybrid palliations, depending on anatomic indices that predict the success of one approach over others (Fig. 36-4). The principal goals of treatment consist of

1. An appropriate assignment of patients to univentricular or biventricular pathways at presentation
2. A complete separation of systemic and pulmonary circulations to eliminate cyanosis
3. An optimized contribution of the RV to the pulmonary circulation, optimized opportunity for RV growth, where possible
4. Avoidance of systemic venous hypertension
5. Avoidance of compromised cardiac output

The improved results of univentricular palliations in recent years, and a rational triage of patients to the approach most likely to succeed based on anatomy, has resulted in a marked improvement in outcomes for PA/IVS as compared with those in past decades. Careful patient selection for univentricular versus biventricular approaches for PA/IVS have yielded recent short- and mid-term survival approaching 100%.[36]

CATHETER-BASED INTERVENTIONS

Techniques first reported in 1991 to traverse the atretic valve plate by laser perforation permit catheter-based balloon dilation techniques to be applied to milder forms of PA.[51] Subsequent modifications include straight guide wires, radiofrequency catheters, and other means of perforating the valve.[1,13,25,37,48,65] Controversy remains as to the efficacy of catheter-based interventions, when compared with surgical RV outflow tract procedures, in sufficiently relieving obstruction to optimize the opportunity for a marginal RV to "grow." Although success in crossing and dilating the atretic valve is reported as 80%, procedure-related complications occur in 18%, and mortality of catheter-based approaches is 6%. Furthermore, 50% of catheter-treated patients require an aortopulmonary shunt or a procedure both to relieve RV outflow obstruction and to augment pulmonary blood flow.[55] Recent outcome data for a surgical approach by comparison demonstrated 2% early mortality and are inclusive of all forms of PA/IVS, mild and severe.[36] Surgical valvotomy produces adequate results in only 36% of patients, and, as balloon valvotomy can only approach the efficacy of a surgical valvotomy, it is logical to conclude that balloon dilation alone is largely a suboptimal approach.[9,53] Certainly a subpopulation of PA/IVS patients with membranous valvular atresia and mild right-sided hypoplasia can benefit equivalently from catheter-based or surgical valvotomy, and standards for patient selection are in evolution. Fedderly and associates[18] determined that a

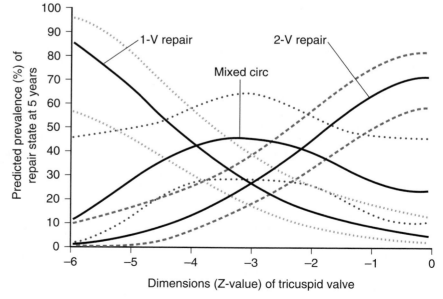

FIGURE 36-4 Predicted prevalence of biventricular, univentricular, and 1.5 ventricle repairs at age 5 years, according to tricuspid diameter (z value). (Reproduced from Hanley FL, Sade RM, Blackstone EH, et al: Outcomes in neonatal pulmonary atresia with intact ventricular septum. A multiinstitutional study. *J Thorac Cardiovasc Surg* 105:406–427, 1993; with permission.)

tricuspid z value greater than -0.5 or a pulmonary valve z value greater than -1.5 predicted a durable result without subsequent need for surgery in a population of neonates with critical pulmonary stenosis and PA/IVS. Additional guidelines included a tricuspid annulus larger than 11 mm, pulmonary valve annulus larger than 7 mm, and RV end-diastolic volume greater than 30 mL/m². Other investigators report RV growth after balloon dilation alone in patients with tricuspid z values less than -2.[48] An additional concern in attempting a purely catheter-based strategy is the experience of a protracted hospitalization for prostaglandin dependence after a successful balloon valvotomy in PA/IVS. In many instances, the non-compliant RV cannot provide adequate pulmonary blood flow, even across a successfully opened right ventricular outflow tract (RVOT), and the patient will require another source of pulmonary blood flow (e.g., aortopulmonary shunt or PDA) for several *weeks* as the RV remodels.

In an effort to further the scope of nonsurgical interventions for PA, and recognizing the additional burden of prolonged prostaglandin dependence even after a successful balloon valvotomy, techniques have been devised to place stents across the ductus arteriosus.[24,26,54] This may create significant future problems for these patients. The world experience with this approach is small, and this is not a feasible approach at a majority of centers today.

Transumbilical fetal cardiac catheterization under fetal transesophageal echocardiographic guidance has been used to perform balloon pulmonary valvuloplasty in a fetal sheep model of PA/IVS.[38] Such advances contribute to our under-standing of embryonic flow patterns as determinants of cardiac dysmorphogenesis and, together with improving pre-natal diagnosis, may point to nearly preventive fetal cardiac interventions in the future.

SURGICAL INTERVENTIONS

Survival for infants with PA/IVS has improved significantly in the last decade, with 50% 5-year survival reported at the outset of the 1990s, as compared with 98% 5-year survival in 2000.[9,36] A large part of improved survival results from a better understanding of anatomy and early, anatomy-based selection of patients for univentricular, biventricular, or hybrid 1.5-ventricle repairs. Improved outcomes for Fontan patients in recent years underscore the principle that the functional result of a good univentricular palliation may exceed that of a marginal biventricular candidate. The subpopulation of Fontan patients consisting of PA/IVS patients enjoys the advantages of having a morphologic left systemic ventricle, and quality of life for these Fontan patients well exceeds that of the marginal biventricular repair with RV hypertrophy, multiple valve and conduit replacements, venous hyperten-sion, and arrhythmias. The 1993 Congenital Heart Surgeons Society multi-institutional prospective study of PA/IVS defined some of the commonly used measures that facilitate the current selection criteria and predict success as a univen-tricular versus biventricular repair.[30]

Predicting the trajectory of growth for the diminutive RV is a challenge. Surely, although unproven, ventricular devel-opment is partially flow dependent. That is to say, a ventricle denied the burden of conducting its capacity would likely remain underdeveloped. Eliminating RVOT obstruction (RVOTO) and encouraging forward flow through the RV permits optimal flow-responsive growth to occur. Supporting evidence for flow-responsive ventricular growth in PA/IVS is the observation that, independent of the initial tricuspid size, z values are preserved or enlarged subsequent to an initial pro-cedure that relieves RVOTO, whereas in shunted patients, the tricuspid z value diminished with patient growth. Multivariate analysis confirmed that these observations were related to the initial procedure and not to the initial anatomic condition.[30] Overestimating the capacity of a small RV and creating overburden, however, promotes ventricular failure, systemic venous hypertension, and unacceptable morbidity.

Flow-responsive myocardial remodeling is likely limited by a finite window of time in the neonatal period when the genetic milieu permits myocyte proliferation in response to flow. Timing flow-corrective surgery beyond this window may produce a response limited to hypertrophy. In the human heart, the total number of cardiomyocytes doubles in the first few months and remains constant thereafter. At birth, cardiomy-ocytes may still be capable of flow-responsive proliferation. By several weeks after birth, apoptosis begins, proliferative growth slows, and remodeling may be limited largely to hyper-trophy. Hypertrophic growth of the heart is accompanied by proportional capillary growth, but not by larger vessel ingrowth; therefore hypertrophy results in a higher coronary vascular resistance, and the delivery of less efficient blood supply to hypertrophic tissue.[33]

Biventricular Pathway

The mildly hypoplastic RV and tricuspid valve with valvular PA can be effectively treated with a procedure to relieve RVOTO, either catheter based or surgical, with a high rate of success. A tricuspid z value greater than -2 suggests a nearly normal-sized RV, assuredly amenable to a biventricular repair.

The 1993 CHSS multi-institutional study observed a greater than 50% incidence of systemic-to-pulmonary shunt required within 1 month of an isolated RVOT procedure, predicted by tricuspid z value at presentation (Fig. 36-5). Forty percent of patients undergoing initial valvotomy alone had an additional transannular patch RVOT procedure by 24 months.[30]

Biventricular repairs, with documented ventricular and tricuspid valve growth, have been routinely achieved with tricuspid z values significantly smaller than -2. Shaddy and colleagues[58] reported 91% success in treating 22 consecutive patients with PA/IVS and a patent RV infundibulum, regard-less of tricuspid z value, by surgical pulmonary valvotomy and aortopulmonary shunt construction as an initial procedure, followed by staged ASD closure and shunt takedown. Test occlusion of the ASD at preoperative cardiac catheterization aids in predicting the readiness for ASD closure and the com-pletion of a biventricular pathway. Steinberger and col-leagues[61] reported an 80% success rate at biventricular repair regardless of the presenting tricuspid or right ventricular size, with a strategy of early and complete surgical relief of RVOTO and protracted maintenance of a PDA with PGE_1 infusion.

Considerable controversy remains as to how much RV and tricuspid valve growth can be induced, and therefore which

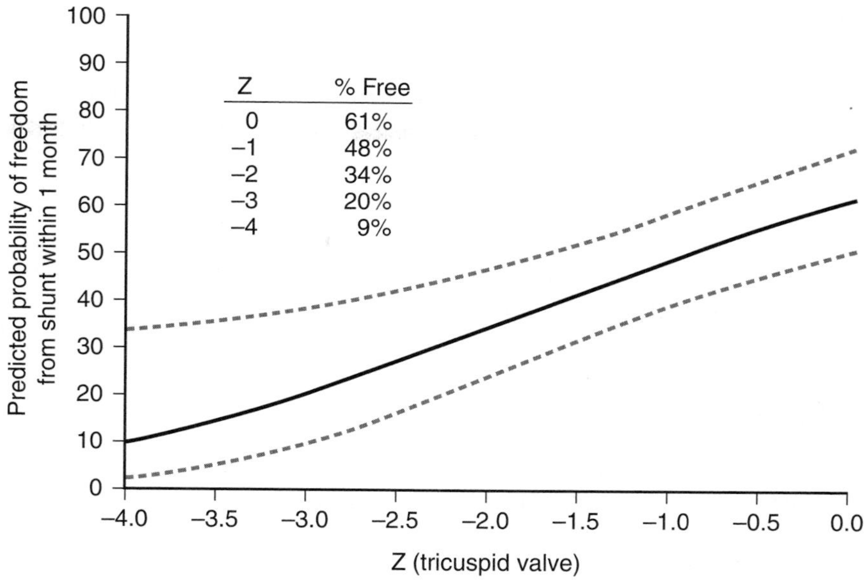

FIGURE 36-5 The relation between tricuspid valve diameter (expressed as z value) and the probability of needing a systemic-to-pulmonary shunt within 1 month of an initial procedure to decompress the RV. (Reproduced from Hanley FL, Sade RM, Blackstone EH, et al: Outcomes in neonatal pulmonary atresia with intact ventricular septum. A multiinstitutional study. *J Thorac Cardiovasc Surg* 105:406–427, 1993; with permission.)

extremes of initial right-sided hypoplasia should proceed as biventricular repairs. General theoretical and practical agreement exists on the principle that RV growth can be optimized by an early and complete relief of RV obstruction, allowing the conduct of blood flow through the ventricle during a finite window of time during which flow-responsive remodeling is possible.

Univentricular Pathway

For patients with diminutive RVs, a palliative univentricular approach is clearly indicated. The CHSS multi-institutional study found that the tricuspid z value less than −4 predicts a univentricular approach.[30] The abandonment of the atriopulmonary Fontan in favor of the lateral baffle or extracardiac conduit, the interim construction of a bidirectional cavopulmonary anastomosis (bidirectional Glenn shunt), and adherence to the principle of early relief of ventricular volume overloading has contributed to significant improvement in Fontan outcomes since the middle 1980s. The low-risk Fontan can clearly produce more favorable long-term results than can the marginal biventricular repair.[14]

For patients with diminutive RVs and RV-dependent coronary circulation with multiple proximal pulmonary stenosis, conversion to Fontan may have long-term disadvantages, as LV function may deteriorate. It is appropriate to consider neonatal heart transplantation for these infants.

One-and-One-Half-Ventricle Repair

De Leval and associates[15] reported 80% mortality for PA/IVS patients undergoing an attempted biventricular repair when the tricuspid z value is less than −3, and 84% survival for a z value greater than −3. Whereas agreement exists at the extremes of RV hypoplasia about univentricular versus biventricular approaches and their respective probabilities of success, controversy remains in the treatment of a broad range of mild and moderate right-sided hypoplasia. A partial biventricular repair, or 1.5-ventricle repair, entails a strategy of encouraging forward flow through the challenged RV and performing a partial right-heart bypass to complement the partial antegrade pulmonary flow and prevent systemic venous hypertension. The construction of a bidirectional cavopulmonary anastomosis diverts one third to one half of an infant's systemic venous return directly to the pulmonary circulation, obligating the RV to conduct only inferior vena caval return. In this manner, a complete separation of systemic and pulmonary circulations is achieved. When the RV is sufficiently hypoplastic not to permit the conduct of inferior vena caval flow, an additional atrial septal fenestration can be used to divert some blood flow to the left circulation, at the cost of some systemic desaturation. A fenestrated atrial septum or postoperative blade septostomy, in conjunction with a bidirectional cavopulmonary anastomosis, can be successful with tricuspid z values less than −6.[64]

Competitive sources of pulmonary blood flow create the potential for pulsatile systemic venous hypertension, and maneuvers are described to alleviate this phenomenon by partially ligating the proximal right pulmonary artery, so as to segregate the pulmonary vascular beds supplied by ventricle-driven antegrade flow and passive cavopulmonary flow.[23] Mainwaring and colleagues[42] and Frommelt and associates[21] found an increased incidence of chylothorax, pleural effusion, and mortality when a competitive source of pulmonary blood flow accompanies a cavopulmonary anastomosis.

POSTOPERATIVE MANAGEMENT

RVOT Procedure

An isolated RVOT procedure obliges the diminutive RV to conduct an entire cardiac output. A fenestration in the atrial septum is advisable in all but the mildest forms of RV hypoplasia to permit adequate left-heart filling, albeit desaturated, until RV recovery and growth is complete. An excessive inotropic requirement and cyanosis in the early postoperative period should prompt an aggressive investigation of the adequacy of RV volume and function, with a low threshold for returning to the operating room to add a systemic-to-pulmonary shunt to augment pulmonary blood flow. The CHSS multi-institutional study of PA/IVS predicts the need for an additional systemic-to-pulmonary shunt in the initial month after an RVOT procedure for 50% of patients undergoing an initial RVOT procedure alone, with an increasing incidence related to small tricuspid z values (Fig. 36-6).

Systemic-to-Pulmonary Shunt

The addition of a systemic-to-pulmonary shunt augments pulmonary blood flow at the expense of volume load to the LV. Antegrade pulmonary blood flow plus pulmonary blood flow derived from a systemic-to-pulmonary shunt risks the phenomenon of pulmonary overcirculation, with resultant systemic hypoperfusion and acidosis. Postoperative pharmacologic interventions to decrease systemic resistance, such as phosphodiesterase inhibitors and angiotensin-converting enzyme (ACE) inhibitors, can improve the balance of pulmonary and systemic circulations. Pulmonary undercirculation and cyanosis can be ameliorated by inotropic support to drive the shunt flow. Excessive cyanosis should prompt an investigation of the adequacy of the shunt, with a low threshold for surgical revision. The incidence of shunt thrombosis may be reduced by the empirical infusion of 10 to 20 mcg/kg/hr of heparin in the perioperative period. As RV function improves with time, saturations improve, indicative of pulmonary blood flow increasing above that supplied by the shunt. Excessive pulmonary blood flow with congestive signs should be an indication to ligate or coil-occlude the systemic-to-pulmonary shunt and close the ASD, completing a biventricular repair. Failure of adequate RV growth results in advancing cyanosis as the patient outgrows the shunt, perhaps indicating the need for a bidirectional cavopulmonary anastomosis to unload the inadequate RV and provide improved pulmonary blood flow.

Bidirectional Cavopulmonary Anastomosis

The basis of perioperative management for patients after bidirectional cavopulmonary anastomosis is the effort to promote the transit of blood through the pulmonary circuit. Positive-pressure ventilation may itself impede pulmonary blood flow. This effect is minimized by strategies of low inspiratory/expiratory (I:E) ratio and early extubation. Hyperventilation impairs oxygenation even as it reduces pulmonary vascular resistance, possibly as a result of an increased cerebrovascular resistance in response to a decreasing PCO_2.[6] An elevation of the patient's head promotes forward flow through the pulmonary circuit and minimizes upper body edema.

Pharmacologic maneuvers to optimize pulmonary blood flow include the routine use of phosphodiesterase inhibitors such as milrinone, which effects pulmonary as well as systemic vasodilatation. Nitric oxide may augment pulmonary blood flow but is seldom necessary in the postoperative period.

Postoperative hypoxia despite these maneuvers prompts an aggressive investigation of possible etiologies. A high level of suspicion is maintained for pulmonary artery or prepulmonary stenosis that could require surgical revision. Decompressing venovenous collaterals from the upper to lower body compartment should be ruled out, presenting the apparent paradox of insufficient pulmonary blood flow with a low transpulmonary gradient. Atrioventricular valve regurgitation or poor ventricular function result in elevated atrial and ventricular end-diastolic pressures and are addressed with appropriate inotropic support or surgical intervention. In rare instances of unrelenting severe hypoxia, it may be necessary to construct a second source of pulmonary blood flow in the form of a systemic-to-pulmonary shunt, although this strategy returns to a volume-loaded ventricle and can exacerbate systemic venous hypertension when left in continuity with the side receiving the cavopulmonary shunt.

Airway and pulmonary abnormalities leading to ineffective ventilation and high ventilatory pressures can create dramatic

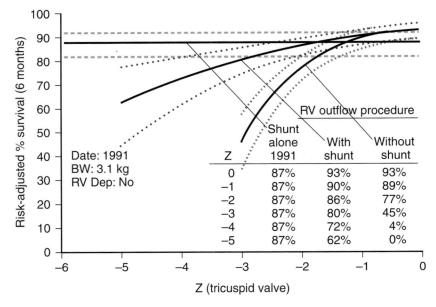

FIGURE 36-6 The effect of tricuspid valve diameter (z value) and 6-month survival for neonates treated by systemic-to-pulmonary shunt alone versus right ventricular outflow procedure (pulmonary valvotomy or transannular patch), with or without the addition of a systemic-to-pulmonary shunt. (Reproduced from Hanley FL, Sade RM, Blackstone EH, et al: Outcomes in neonatal pulmonary atresia with intact ventricular septum. A multiinstitutional study. *J Thorac Cardiovasc Surg* 105:406–427, 1993; with permission.)

Date: 1991
BW: 3.1 kg
RV Dep: No

| | | RV outflow procedure | |
Z	Shunt alone 1991	With shunt	Without shunt
0	87%	93%	93%
−1	87%	90%	89%
−2	87%	86%	77%
−3	87%	80%	45%
−4	87%	72%	4%
−5	87%	62%	0%

hypoxia when pulmonary blood flow is converted to passive, at the creation of the cavopulmonary anastomosis.

Perioperative and late mortality from the construction of a bidirectional cavopulmonary anastomosis in the present era is less than 2%.[39] Fontan morbidity may be reduced when the interim cavopulmonary anastomosis is used. Late sequelae include progressive cyanosis secondary to growth, venovenous collateral formation, or the development of pulmonary arteriovenous malformations. The late development of pulmonary arteriovenous malformations has been reported to occur in 25% to 50% of patients with bidirectional cavopulmonary shunts.[5] These may occur within the first 18 months of life. Fontan completion to include hepatic venous effluent in the pulmonary vascular circuit contributes to their resolution.[59] Aortopulmonary collateral formation may occur in two thirds of patients, requiring coil embolization where possible.[63]

OUTCOME

Mair and colleagues[43] reported operative and late results of the Fontan procedure as palliation for PA/IVS at the Mayo Clinic from 1979 to 1995. Operative mortality among the 40 patients was 8%. Eighty-five percent were alive at a median 6-year follow-up. Ninety-seven percent of survivors were New York Heart Association (NYHA) Class I to II, and 56% were taking no cardiovascular medications. Najm and associates[46] reported the Toronto experience for pulmonary atresia with intact ventricular septum patients undergoing Fontan between 1980 and 1994. Actuarial survival at 10 years after Fontan was 80%. Jahangiri and colleagues[36] reported 98% survival at 1, 5, and 7 years for 47 consecutive PA/IVS patients treated surgically at Children's Hospital, Boston. Fewer than 25% of patients received a biventricular repair, underscoring the principle that, as presently carried out, a favorable univentricular repair with a morphologic left systemic ventricle produces better early and late results than does a marginal biventricular repair.

From 1985 to 2000, 36 patients with PA/IVS were seen in the division of Cardiovascular Surgery at Children's Hospital, San Diego. Twenty-six (72%) had a systemic-to-pulmonary shunt alone in the newborn period, and 8 (22%) had an RVOT procedure and a systemic-to-pulmonary shunt. One (3%) patient had an RVOT procedure alone, and 1 (3%) had no surgical intervention as a newborn. Eventual biventricular repairs were achieved for 5 (13.8%) patients. Overall survival for all PA/IVS patients over the 5-year period was 86%.

Significant improvements in survival and quality of life for patients with PA/IVS have occurred over the last decade. Accurate diagnostic techniques identify patients earlier and characterize anatomic subclasses that predict which palliative pathways will give optimal results. Outcomes have improved largely owing to an early anatomy-based triage of patients to univentricular or biventricular pathways. Adhering to principles of treatment directed toward an early and complete relief of RVOTO for biventricular candidates potentiates optimal RV growth. For the univentricular population, improved outcomes reflect improvements in the Fontan procedure, including early volume unloading with the interim bidirectional cavopulmonary anastomosis, Fontan fenestration, and prophylactic antiarrhythmic maneuvers.

References

1. Akagi T, Hashino K, Maeno Y, et al: Balloon dilation of the pulmonary valve in a patient with pulmonary atresia and intact ventricular septum using a commercially available radiofrequency catheter. *Pediatr Cardiol* 18:61–63, 1997.
2. Allan LD: Development of congenital heart lesions in mid to late gestation. *Int J Cardiol* 19:36, 1988.
3. Allan LD, Crawford DC, Tynan MJ: Pulmonary atresia in prenatal life. *Am J Coll Cardiol* 8:1131–1136, 1986.
4. Becker AE, Becker MJ, Edwards JE: Pathologic spectrum of dysplasia of the tricuspid valve. *Arch Pathol* 91:167, 1971.
5. Bernstein HS, Brook MM, Silverman NH, Bristow J: Development of pulmonary arteriovenous fistulae in children after cavopulmonary shunt. *Circulation* 92(suppl II):II309–II314, 1995.
6. Bradley SM, Simsic JM, Mulvihill DM. Hyperventilation impairs oxygenation after bidirectional superior cavopulmonary connection. *Circulation* 98:II372–II377, 1998.
7. Bryan CS, Oppenheimer EH: Ventricular endocardial fibroelastosis: Basis for its presence or absence in cases of pulmonic or aortic atresia. *Arch Pathol* 87:82, 1969.
8. Bulkey BH, D'Amico B, Taylor AL: Extensive myocardial fiber disarray in aortic and pulmonary atresia: Relevance to hypertrophic cardiomyopathy. *Circulation* 67:191–198, 1983.
9. Bull C, Kostelka M, Sorensen K, de Leval M: Outcome measures for the neonatal management of pulmonary atresia with intact ventricular septum. *J Thorac Cardiovasc Surg* 107:359–366, 1994.
10. Bull C, de Leval MR, Mercanti C, et al: Pulmonary atresia and intact ventricular septum: A revised classification. *Circulation* 66:266–272, 1982.
11. Chitayat D, McIntosh N, Fouron JC: Pulmonary atresia with intact ventricular septum: A single gene disorder. *Am J Med Genet* 72:304–306, 1992.
12. Cole RB, Muster AJ, Leu M, Paul MH: Pulmonary atresia with intact ventricular septum: *Am J Cardiol* 21:23, 1968.
13. Colli AM, Perry SB, Lock JE, Keane JF: Balloon dilation of critical pulmonary stenosis in the first month of life. *Cathet Cardiovasc Diagn* 34:23–28, 1995.
14. Delius RE, Rademecker MA, de Leval MR, et al: Is a high-risk biventricular repair always preferable to conversion to a single-ventricle repair? *J Thorac Cardiovasc Surg* 112:1561–1569, 1996.
15. de Leval M, Bull C, Hopkins R, et al: Decision making in the definitive repair of the heart with a small right ventricle. *Circulation* 72(suppl II):52–60, 1985.
16. Eriksen NL, Buttino LJ, Juberg RC: Congenital pulmonary atresia and patent ductus arteriosus in two sibs. *Am J Med Genet* 32:187–188, 1989.
17. Essed CE, Klein HW, Kredict P: Coronary and endocardial fibroelastosis of the ventricles in the hypoplastic left and right heart syndromes. *Virchows Arch [A]* 368:87–97, 1975.
18. Fedderly RT, Lloyd TR, Mendelsohn AM, Beekman RH: Determinants of successful balloon valvotomy in infants with critical pulmonary stenosis or membranous pulmonary atresia with intact ventricular septum. *Am J Coll Cardiol* 25:460–465, 1995.
19. Freedom RM: *Pulmonary Atresia with Intact Ventricular Septum*. Mount Kisco, NY, Futura Publishing, 1989.
20. Freedom RM, Dische MR, Rowe RD: The tricuspid valve in pulmonary atresia and intact ventricular septum. *Arch Pathol Lab Med* 102:28–31, 1978.
21. Frommelt MA, Frommelt PC, Berger S, et al: Does an additional source of pulmonary blood flow alter outcome after a bidirectional cavopulmonary shunt? *Circulation* 92(suppl II):240–244, 1995.
22. Fyfe DA, Edwards WD, Driscoll DJ: Myocardial ischemia in patients with pulmonary atresia and intact ventricular septum. *J Am Coll Cardiol* 8:402–406, 1986.
23. Gentles TL, Keane JF, Jonas RA, et al: Surgical alternatives to the Fontan procedure incorporating a hypoplastic right ventricle. *Circulation* 90(suppl II):2–6, 1994.
24. Gibbs JL: Stenting the arterial duct. *Arch Dis Child* 72:196–197, 1995.
25. Gibbs JL, Blackburn ME, Uzun O, et al: Laser valvotomy with balloon valvuloplasty for pulmonary atresia with intact ventricular septum: Five years' experience. *Heart* 77:225–228, 1997.
26. Gibbs JL, Rothman MT, Rees MR, et al: Stenting of the arterial duct: A new approach for palliation of pulmonary atresia. *Br Heart J* 67:240–245, 1992.

27. Gittenberger-de Groot AC, Sauer U, Bindl L, et al: Competition of coronary arteries and ventriculocoronary arterial communications in pulmonary atresia with intact ventricular septum. *Int J Cardiol* 18:243–258, 1988.

28. Goor DA, Lillehei CW: *Congenital Malformations of the Heart*. New York, Grune & Stratton, 1975.

29. Grossfeld PD, Lucas VW, Sklansky MS, et al: Familial occurrence of pulmonary atresia with intact ventricular septum. *Am J Med Genet* 72:294–296, 1997.

30. Hanley FL, Sade RM, Blackstone EH, et al: Outcomes in neonatal pulmonary atresia with intact ventricular septum: A multiinstitutional study. *J Thorac Cardiovasc Surg* 105:406–423, 1993.

31. Hausdorf G, Gravinghoff L, Keck EW: Effects of persisting myocardial sinusoids on LV performance in pulmonary atresia with intact ventricular septum. *Eur Heart J* 8:291, 1987.

32. Hogers B, DeRuiter MC, Gittenberger-de Groot AC, Poelmann RE: Unilateral vitelline vein ligation alters intracardiac flow patterns and morphogenesis in the chick embryo. *Circ Res* 80:473–481, 1997.

33. Hudlicka O, Brown MD: Postnatal growth of the heart and its blood vessels. *J Vasc Res* 33:266–287, 1996.

34. Hunter W: Three cases of mal-conformation of the heart. *Med Obs Inquiries* 6:291–299, 1783.

35. Icardo JM: Endocardial cell arrangement: Role of hemodynamics. *Anat Rec* 225:150–155, 1989.

36. Jahangiri M, Zurakowski D, Bichell D, et al: Improved results with selective management in pulmonary atresia with intact ventricular septum. *J Thorac Cardiovasc Surg* 118:1046–1055, 1999.

37. Justo RN, Nykanen DG, Williams WG, et al: Transcatheter perforation of the right ventricular outflow tract as initial therapy for pulmonary valve atresia and intact ventricular septum in the newborn. *Cathet Cardiovasc Diagn* 40:408–413, 1997.

38. Kohl T, Szabo Z, Suda K, et al: Fetoscopic and open transumbilical fetal cardiac catheterization in sheep: Potential approaches for human fetal cardiac intervention. *Circulation* 95:1048–1053, 1997.

39. Kopf GS, Laks H, Stansel HC, et al: Thirty year follow-up of superior vena cava-pulmonary artery (Glenn) shunts. *J Thorac Cardiovasc Surg* 100:662–671, 1990.

40. Kutsche LM, Van Mierop LHS: Pulmonary atresia with and without ventricular septal defect: A different etiology and pathogenesis for the atresia in the 2 types? *Am J Cardiol* 51:932–935, 1983.

41. Luciani GB, Swilley S, Starnes VA: Pulmonary atresia, intact ventricular septum, and major aortopulmonary collateral: Morphogenic and surgical implications. *J Thorac Cardiovasc Surg* 110:853–854, 1995.

42. Mainwaring RD, Lamberti JJ, Uzark K, Spicer RL: Bidirectional Glenn: Is accessory pulmonary blood flow good or bad? *Circulation* 92(suppl II): 294–297, 1995.

43. Mair DD, Julsrud PR, Puga FJ, Danielson GK: The Fontan procedure for pulmonary atresia with intact ventricular septum: Operative and late results. *J Am Coll Cardiol* 29:1359–1364, 1997.

44. McArthur JD, Munsi SC, Sukumar IP, Cherian G: Pulmonary valve atresia with intact ventricular septum. *Circulation* 44:740, 1971.

45. Mitchell SC, Korones SB, Berends HW: Congenital heart disease in 56,109 births. *Circulation* 43:323, 1971.

46. Najm HK, Williams WG, Coles JG, et al: Pulmonary atresia with intact ventricular septum: Results of the Fontan procedure. *Ann Thorac Surg* 63:669–675, 1997.

47. O'Connor WN, Stahr BJ, Cottrill CM, et al: Ventriculocoronary connections in hypoplastic right heart syndrome: Autopsy serial section study of six cases. *J Am Coll Cardiol* 11:1061–1072, 1988.

48. Ovaert C, Qureshi SA, Rosenthal E, et al: Growth of the right ventricle after successful transcatheter valvotomy in neonates and infants with pulmonary atresia and intact ventricular septum. *J Thorac Cardiovasc Surg* 115:1055–1062, 1998.

49. Patel RG, Freedom RM, Moes CAF, et al: Right ventricular volume determinations in 18 patients with pulmonary atresia and intact ventricular septum: Analysis of factors influencing right ventricular growth. *Circulation* 61:428–440, 1980.

50. Perloff J: *Pulmonary Atresia with Intact Ventricular Septum*. Philadelphia, WB Saunders, 1987.

51. Qureshi SA, Rosenthal E, Tynan M, et al: Transcatheter laser-assisted balloon pulmonary valve dilation in pulmonary valve atresia. *Am J Cardiol* 67:428–431, 1991.

52. Robicsek F, Bostoen H, Sander PW: Atresia of pulmonary valve with normal pulmonary artery and intact ventricular septum in a 21-year-old woman. *Angiology* 17:896, 1966.

53. Rome JJ: Balloon pulmonary valvuloplasty. *Pediatr Cardiol* 19:18–24, 1998.

54. Rosenthal E, Qureschi SA, Tynan M: Percutaneous pulmonary valvotomy and arterial duct stenting in neonates with right ventricular hypoplasia. *Am J Cardiol* 74:304–306, 1994.

55. Ruiz CE, Zhang HP: Is balloon a challenge to scalpel in membranous pulmonary atresia or just a partner? *Cathet Cardiovasc Diagn* 40:414–415, 1997.

56. Satou GM, Perry SB, Gauvreau K, Geva T: Echocardiographic predictors of coronary artery pathology in pulmonary atresia with intact ventricular septum. *Am J Cardiol* 85:1319–1324, 2000.

57. Sedmera D, Pexieder T, Rychterova V, et al: Remodeling of chick embryonic myoarchitecture under experimentally changed loading conditions. *Anat Rec* 254:238–252, 1999.

58. Shaddy RE, Sturtevant JE, Judd VE, McGough EC: Right ventricular growth after transventricular pulmonary valvotomy and central aortopulmonary shunt for pulmonary atresia and intact ventricular septum. *Circulation* 82(suppl IV):IV157–IV163, 1990.

59. Shah MJ, Rychik J, Fogel MA, et al: Pulmonary AV malformations after superior cavopulmonary connection: Resolution after inclusion of hepatic veins in the pulmonary circulation. *Ann Thorac Surg* 63:960–963, 1997.

60. Sholler GF, Colan SD, Sanders SP: Effect of isolated right ventricular outflow obstruction on left ventricular function in infants. *Am J Cardiol* 62:778–784, 1988.

61. Steinberger J, Berry JM, Bass JL, et al: Results of a right ventricular outflow patch for pulmonary atresia with intact ventricular septum. *Circulation* 86(suppl II):II167–II175, 1992.

62. Taber LA: Mechanical aspects of cardiac development. *Prog Biophys Mol Biol* 69:237–255, 1998.

63. Triedman JK, Bridges ND, Mayer JE, Lock JE: Prevalence and risk factors for aortopulmonary collateral vessels after Fontan and bidirectional Glenn procedures. *J Am Coll Cardiol* 22:207–215, 1993.

64. Van Arsdell GS, Williams WG, Maser CM, et al: Superior vena cava to pulmonary artery anastomosis: An adjunct to biventricular repair. *J Thorac Cardiovasc Surg* 112:1143–1149, 1996.

65. Wright SB, Radtke WA, Gillette PC: Percutaneous radiofrequency valvotomy using a standard 5 Fr electrode catheter for pulmonary atresia in neonates. *Am J Cardiol* 77:1370–1372, 1996.

66. Yasui H, Nakazawa M, Morishima M, et al: Cardiac outflow tract septation process in the mouse model of transposition of the great arteries. *Teratology* 55:353–363, 1997.

67. Zuberbuhler JR, Anderson RH: Morphologic variations in pulmonary atresia with intact ventricular septum. *Br Heart J* 41:281–288, 1979.

Chapter 37

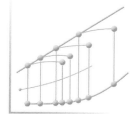

Ebstein's Malformation

ROBERT D. BART, MD, ROSS MACRAE BREMNER, MD, PhD,
and VAUGHN A. STARNES, MD

HISTORY

In 1866, Wilhelm Ebstein described a severe malformation of the tricuspid valve. He concluded this malformation probably occurred during formation of the atrioventricular (AV) valves in the third month of gestation.[15] The eponym "Ebsteinsche Krankheit" (Ebstein's disease) was given by Arnstein in 1927.[4] In 1949, the first in vivo diagnosis of Ebstein's anomaly was made by using cardiac catheterization.[45] Barnard and Schrire[6] reported the first total correction with prosthetic valve replacement in 1963. It was only after Schiebler and associates[39] translated the original article from German into English that this congenital cardiac anomaly received significant attention in the United States.

DEFINITION

Ebstein's anomaly is characterized by abnormal attachment of the posterior and septal tricuspid leaflets in the right ventricular (RV) cavity away from a normally positioned tricuspid valve annulus (Fig. 37-1).[2,7] The degree of leaflet displacement is variable. The leaflets are often hypoplastic, with varying degrees of adherence to the RV wall.[38] The anterior leaflet is normally attached at the annulus; however, it is enlarged, "sail-like," and often abnormally tethered to the RV wall. This anterior leaflet may functionally obstruct the RV outlet. The tricuspid valve orifice is displaced downward into the RV cavity at the junction of the inlet and trabecular components of the right ventricle.[49] The inlet portion of the RV is usually functionally integrated into the right atrium ("atrialization" of the RV), whereas the trabecular and outlet portions of the RV constitute the functional small RV cavity.[19] The proximal, atrialized RV often has a thinner wall than the distal functional RV because of partial thinning of the "atrialized" RV myocardium. The severity of hemodynamic compromise is related to the extent of downward displacement of the leaflets, the degree of functional outlet obstruction, the degree of myocardial dysfunction, and the presence of other associated cardiac abnormalities.

EMBRYOLOGY

The leaflets and tensor apparatus of the tricuspid valve are formed from the interior of the RV myocardium by delamination of the inner layers of the inlet portion of the ventricle.[30,49] Simply, the leaflets of the tricuspid valve develop equally from endocardial cushion tissue and myocardium. In Ebstein's anomaly, the insertions of septal and posterior leaflets are displaced to the junction between inlet and apicotrabecular RV, which suggests that delamination from the inlet portion failed to occur. With the leaflets adherent to the RV myocardium, the fibrous transformation of the leaflets from muscular precursors remains incomplete. Causation is poorly understood.

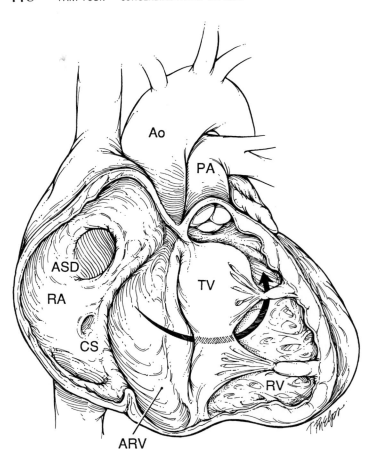

FIGURE 37-1 Native anatomy of Ebstein's anomaly. The tricuspid valve is displaced into the right ventricle (RV), leaving an atrialized portion of the RV (ARV) above the level of the tricuspid valve (TV) leaflets. The anterior leaflet of the TV is large and sail-like and may obstruct the RV outflow tract. The posterior and septal leaflets are small, and a large ostium secundum defect (ASD) is seen. Ao, aorta; PA, pulmonary artery; RA, right atrium; CS, coronary sinus.

Alteration in blood flow (pressures) at a relatively late developmental stage, when delamination of the valve leaflets occurs, is a leading possibility.

Despite the poorly understood etiology, the timing of developmental events is precisely known. The anterior leaflet of the tricuspid valve is completely formed by 44 to 48 days of gestation. At this time, the septal and posterior leaflets are just beginning to develop. A singular event or process initiated at this developmental stage could give rise to Ebstein's anomaly. A continuum of pathologic changes associated with the anomaly is due to variations in the degree of displacement of the proximal leaflet attachments and the topography of the functional orifice between atrium and RV.[49] Some consistent features are atrial dilation, short chordae tendinae, deformed papillary muscles, and thinning of the atrialized RV. Despite the anatomic constant of tricuspid valve leaflet displacement, the pathologic and physiologic effects are unique in each case.

ASSOCIATED DEFECTS

The most common associated defect, found in approximately half of all children diagnosed with Ebstein's anomaly, is a secundum-type atrial septal defect or persistent foramen ovale, which may be a consequence of hemodynamic forces from the abnormal tricuspid valve.[47] Another frequent association is congenitally corrected transposition of the great arteries.

Here the affected tricuspid valve is positioned on the left side of the heart.[1,42] An important association is severe pulmonary artery stenosis or atresia.[18,44] In infants with cyanosis, functional pulmonary atresia was found in 54%.[48] Anatomic pulmonary atresia was noted in a further 24% and was associated with significant mortality.[48] Other associations include ventricular septal defect, tetralogy of Fallot, and mitral valve abnormalities. A Wolff-Parkinson-White (WPW) type of accessory atrioventricular conduction pathway is noted in some of the Ebstein's anomaly patients.

PATHOPHYSIOLOGY

The spectrum of hemodynamic consequences caused by Ebstein's anomaly is related to the severity of tricuspid regurgitation, the degree of right-outflow-tract obstruction, and the reduced chamber capacity of the functional RV. RV output is decreased by decreased RV volume combined with RV obstruction. Poor filling of the RV is a consequence of the distention of the atrialized RV that occurs with atrial systole. Importantly, these alterations in right heart structure and function contribute to altered left ventricular (LV) geometry, resulting in decreased LV systolic function.

In Ebstein's anomaly, a right-to-left shunt occurs at the atrial level, either through the frequently associated atrial septal defects or through a patent foramen ovale induced by elevated right atrial pressures.[33] The elevated right atrial

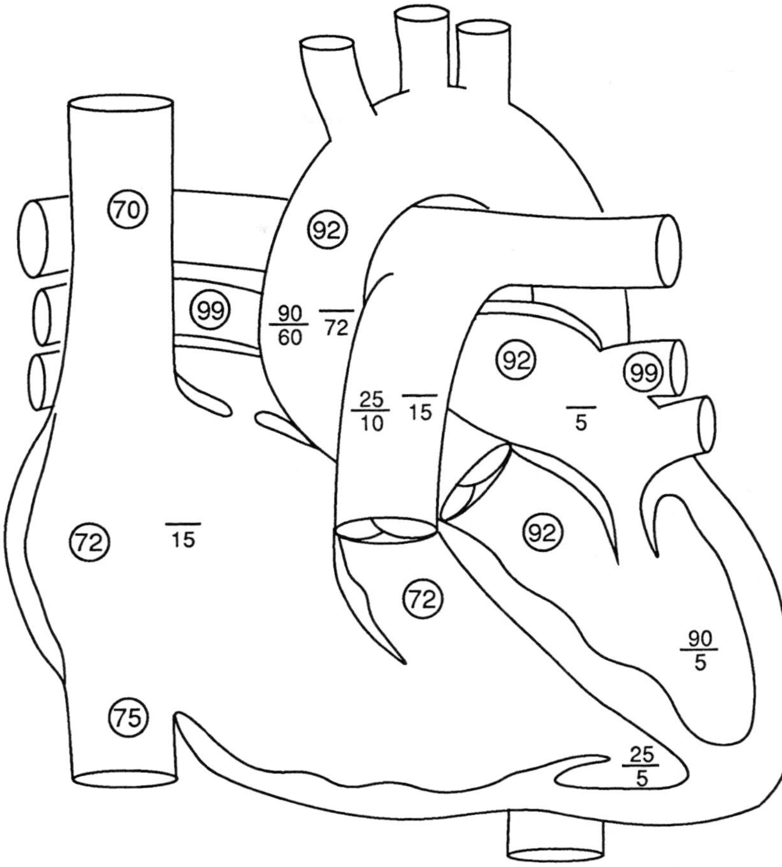

FIGURE 37-2 Schematic diagram of O_2 saturations (*circled values*) and pressures in native anatomy of Ebstein's malformation. Tricuspid regurgitation results in elevated right atrial pressure (15 mm Hg) in the face of normal pulmonary artery pressure (25/5 mm Hg). Right atrial pressure exceeds left atrial pressure (5 mm Hg) and a right-to-left shunt through a patent foramen ovale is reflected in the stepdown of O_2 saturation from the pulmonary vein (99%) to the left atrium (92%).

pressure is a result of stenosis or atresia of the anomalous tricuspid valve orifice, valvular incompetence, or myocardial mechanics of atrialized RV. Right atrial pressure is moderately elevated in most patients; however, if the atrium is severely dilated, the atrial pressure pulse may be normal despite severe tricuspid regurgitation. This physiology is relatively unique to Ebstein's anomaly, creating a circumstance in which tricuspid regurgitation is present with normal pulmonary vascular pressures (Fig. 37-2).

PRESENTATION AND DIAGNOSIS

Ebstein's anomaly has an extremely varied presentation, ranging from normal tricuspid valve function found incidentally at autopsy to severe cyanosis, compromised cardiac function, and neonatal death. Ebstein's hemodynamic abnormality is dependent on the degree of displacement of proximal leaflet attachments and the connection between the right atrium and ventricle. The prevalence among patients with congenital heart disease is approximately 0.5% and about 1 in 20,000 to 50,000 live births.[41] No gender dominance is reported.

The spectrum of abnormalities that occur with Ebstein's anomaly is reflected by the age at clinical presentation. Carpentier and colleagues[8] described four types of abnormality, types A through D, reflecting the severity of the lesion. In type A, a large, freely mobile anterior leaflet is found with minimally displaced posterior and septal leaflets of the

tricuspid valve, and a small atrialized segment of RV. In type A, the RV volume is adequate. In type B, the displacement of the posterior and septal leaflets is more marked, but the anterior leaflet is large and moves freely. The atrialized chamber is thinner than that in type A, and the RV is small. In type C, the anterior leaflet is restricted, with fibrous strands attaching the ventricular aspect of the valve to the infundibulum. The posterior and septal leaflets are markedly displaced and usually hypoplastic. The RV is very small with a thin, noncontractile wall. Type D represents the extreme of the spectrum of Ebstein's anomaly and is sometimes referred to as the "tricuspid sac." In this type, the anterior leaflet partially adheres to the infundibulum and trabecular portion of the RV, with the ventricular edge of the valve adherent to the ventricle in continuity with the abnormal septal and posterior leaflets. A small restrictive ostium at the site of the atrial septal commissure is the site of communication between atrium and ventricle. The ventricular wall is thin and poorly contractile.

The clinical presentation depends on the type and severity of Ebstein's malformation. At birth, pulmonary vascular resistance is high, and the degree of cyanosis will depend on the amount of right-to-left shunting at the atrial level. Two large studies found nearly half of the neonates with Ebstein's anomaly were first seen with cyanosis and cardiac murmur within the first week of life.[22,36] In neonates, with relatively mild tricuspid valve displacement and no RV outflow tract obstruction, shunting will decrease as pulmonary vascular resistance decreases over the ensuing 1 to 2 weeks, and cyanosis will improve. If a significant portion of RV is atrialized, or the anterior leaflet obstructs the outflow tract, cyanosis persists, and the severity of congestive heart failure increases. Classically, these individuals have massive cardiomegaly with a cardiac-to–thoracic cavity ratio greater than 0.65. They usually do not tolerate medical management alone. Indeed, congestive heart failure, dependence on mechanical ventilation, dependence on prostaglandin E$_1$, and massive cardiomegaly in the immediate neonatal period are associated with the failure of medical management and are an indication for surgery.

For infants who improve, a variable interval passes before surgical treatment is necessary. Some remain asymptomatic into childhood, although all individuals ultimately experience congestive heart failure. The initial presentation of young children is often due to cardiac murmur or abnormal cardiac rhythm. In adolescents and teenagers, fatigability, palpitations, dyspnea, and chest pain are often presenting symptoms. In the Carpentier[8] series, the natural history is such that 50% of patients died by age 35 years without surgical intervention. Recent studies have shown a significant incidence of sudden death, which supports earlier surgical intervention as opposed to expectant medical management.[5,20] Growth and development of children with Ebstein's anomaly are generally normal. When cyanosis is present, it does not necessarily correlate with disease severity.

A palpable thrill is often found on initial examination of the chest, between the second and fourth intercostal spaces, left of the sternal border in the midclavicular line. This is the result of turbulence in the dilated right atrium. A second systolic thrill may be present at the left lower sternal border. Ebstein's anomaly is one of the few disorders that may cause a thrill in a neonate.[36] Cardiac impulse is usually normal but may be weaker and diffuse in cyanotic patients. This may reflect greater right heart dilatation in the more cyanotic individuals.

A cardiac murmur may not be auscultated in some individuals. When present, the murmur may vary in intensity, tone, and location, but with sounds all originating from the right heart. Characteristically the tonal quality of the heart sounds is often unusual. A widely split second heart sound is frequently found, and additional third and fourth heart sounds may be present in 50% of patients.[46] Because the sounds originate in the right heart, they become louder during respiratory inspiration.

Arrhythmias occur in more than 50% of patients with Ebstein's anomaly. Most arrhythmias are tachydysrhythmias, including paroxysmal supraventricular tachydysrhythmias, atrial fibrillation, and atrial flutter. Paroxysmal supraventricular tachydysrhythmias are the most common rhythm abnormality, occurring in approximately 15% of patients, and often an accessory conduction pathway can be defined (WPW). However, ventricular tachycardia does occur and may be one cause of early death in Ebstein's anomaly patients.[32] Sudden death occurs in 3% of patients, most likely related to the high arrhythmogenic potential of this lesion. Right heart thromboembolism and paradoxical embolism also have been implicated and may be an additional factor contributing to sudden death.[17] Tachydysrhythmias should be medically controlled by using standard therapy; if they are refractory, ablation of accessory conduction pathways should be considered, even when no hemodynamic impact occurs.[3,32]

Diagnostic tests may help in evaluating the patient suspected of having Ebstein's anomaly. A chest radiograph will frequently reveal an enlarged cardiac silhouette with decreased pulmonary vascular markings. The cardiac size may be closer to normal, the older the age at presentation. Radford and associates[36] found that neonates had an average cardiothoracic ratio of 0.73, children and adolescents averaged 0.57, and adults had an average ratio of 0.55. Right atrial dilatation produces significant enlargement of the cardiac silhouette to the right of the sternum, while concomitantly shifting the pulmonary artery leftward. The right-to-left shunt results in the lack of pulmonary vascularity, providing darkened lung fields. If increased pulmonary vascular markings are seen, the diagnosis of Ebstein's anomaly should be questioned.

The electrocardiogram (ECG) is always abnormal in patients with Ebstein's anomaly. Right bundle branch block accounts for the ECG abnormality in 70% to 80% of patients with Ebstein's anomaly. Prolongation of the terminal QRS depolarization is found, with frequent notching, slurring, or splintering of the QRS complex (Fig. 37-3). Right atrial enlargement is often indicated by a prolonged PR interval and increased height of the P wave. The right bundle branch pattern occurs because of pressure on the upper right septum produced by right atrial enlargement.[21,22] As a patient ages, the ECG demonstrates increasing prolongation of the QRS complex, decreasing QRS voltage, and increasing P-wave height, which correlate with worsening prognosis.

WPW, usually type B, is reported in 5% to 20% of patients with Ebstein's malformation. Atypical WPW morphology can be seen, and in one series, the presentation of ventricular preexcitation with a normal PR interval and delta waves was seen in two patients with paroxysmal tachycardia.[16] Ebstein's anomaly is the most common cardiac defect in children with the WPW pattern on ECG. As previously mentioned, a variety of dysrhythmias can be seen, including supraventricular tachycardias, atrial flutter, atrial fibrillation, junctional rhythms, and ventricular ectopy.

Two-dimensional echocardiography is the standard for confirming diagnosis and delineating the anatomy of patients with Ebstein's anomaly. Echocardiographic features found to correlate with intraoperative findings include the size and presence of tricuspid leaflets, valve tethering and mobility, relative size of the functional RV chamber and dimensions, associated defects, and RV outflow tract anatomy. Echocardiography had less utility in defining features of the cleft, perforation or fenestration of the anterior leaflet, features of the posterior leaflet, and the tricuspid orifice.[40] The displacement index (apical displacement of the septal cusp of the tricuspid valve in millimeters indexed to body surface area) is an important echocardiographic determination. In normal hearts, the septal insertion of the tricuspid valve is at a lower level than the septal insertion of the mitral valve. Measuring the distance between mitral and tricuspid valves provides a displacement; a displacement greater than 8 mm/m^2 of body surface area is a sensitive predictor of Ebstein's anomaly.[23] The apical four-chamber view provides additional information regarding the tethering of the septal leaflet of the tricuspid valve, billowing motion of the anterior leaflet, and relative sizes of the atrialized and functional RV.[36]

Recently, Celermajer and colleagues[9] developed a score for neonates with Ebstein's anomaly based on echocardiographic

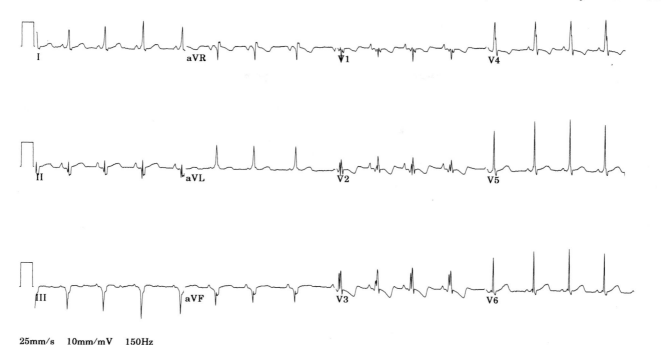

25mm/s   10mm/mV   150Hz

FIGURE 37-3   Electrocardiogram of a patient with Ebstein's malformation. Note rSR pattern in right precordial leads, indicating right bundle-branch block.

findings that identify patients at high risk of neonatal death. The score is based on a ratio of the right atrium and atrialized RV area compared with the area of the functional RV and left heart chambers. When this ratio was greater than 1.5, the observed mortality was 100%, whereas observed mortality is 15% for those with a ratio less than 1.5. Others have validated these findings, with a ratio of 1.1 to 1.4 associated with an early mortality of approximately 10%, and a late mortality of 45% in early childhood.

M-mode echocardiography is of minimal utility in the diagnosis of Ebstein's anomaly. Some features suggestive of Ebstein's anomaly are a tricuspid closure more than 50 milliseconds after mitral valve closure, recording the anterior tricuspid leaflet to the left of the sternum, wide excursion of the tricuspid valve, decreased E-F slope of the tricuspid valve, increased RV dimensions, and paradoxical septal motion.[22]

Fetal echocardiography demonstrates features that correlate well with postnatal echocardiograms. Fetal echocardiography of tricuspid valve disease is associated with mortality; one study found a total neonatal mortality rate of 83%.[27] Interestingly, pulmonary hypoplasia was found at autopsy in just over 50% of the fetuses and infants who died.

The utility of cardiac catheterization in defining the anatomy of Ebstein's anomaly has diminished as echocardiographic quality has improved. Because Ebstein's anomaly patients are predisposed to cardiac dysrhythmias, minimizing the number of cardiac catheterizations is preferred. Watson[47] reported a cooperative study of 505 patients with Ebstein's anomaly, in which 363 underwent cardiac catheterization. All patients were in sinus rhythm at the start of the procedure; paroxysmal tachycardia occurred in 90 patients; 13 deaths and 6 cardiac arrests occurred. Two had ventricular preexcitation, and five had a history of paroxysmal dysrhythmia.[47]

Magnetic resonance imaging (MRI) is a diagnostic tool that may add to the information obtained with transthoracic echocardiography. On occasion, the images provided by two-dimensional echocardiography may be inconclusive or technically difficult. As early as 1988, Link and associates[31] performed ECG-gated MRI in four patients known to have Ebstein's anomaly. MRI provided detailed anatomic information and compared favorably with the cineangiography or two-dimensional echocardiography or both on each patient. More recently, in 2000, Gutberlet and colleagues[24] were able to use preoperative and postoperative MRI on 12 patients who underwent surgery for Ebstein's anomaly. The MRI provided end-systolic and end-diastolic volumes; ejection fraction, stroke volume, and muscle mass was calculated for both ventricles; and a qualitative assessment of tricuspid insufficiency was possible.

MEDICAL MANAGEMENT

In the newborn period, the primary problems facing the child with Ebstein's anomaly are hypoxemia and congestive heart failure. Maintaining patency of the ductus arteriosus and decreasing pulmonary vascular resistance are essential for management. Mild hyperventilation, alkalosis, supplemental oxygen, and, if necessary, nitric oxide may be helpful. Prostaglandin E1 may be necessary for ductal patency. Inotropic agents such as dopamine, dobutamine, milrinone and epinephrine may be necessary to manage congestive heart failure. If symptoms resolve, support can be slowly decreased, but if symptoms persist, further treatment is required. After age 6 months, prognosis improves, and medical management may be continued through childhood or adolescence. However, the recent report by Attie and associates[5] of 148 patients with Ebstein's anomaly suggests that sudden death may occur more frequently than previously recognized in children managed conservatively. The group noted that the risk factors for sudden death included younger age at diagnosis, male gender, anatomic severity on echocardiography, and an increased cardiothoracic ratio. If a child has significant risk factors, early surgery may be warranted.

Complications of Ebstein's anomaly that may occur during medical management include significant dysrhythmias, cerebral abscesses, and paradoxical emboli. Endocarditis is a relatively infrequent complication. The occurrence of any of these complications or a decreasing functional class of congestive heart failure should prompt surgical correction.

A significant percentage of children with Ebstein's will initially be seen with arrhythmias. These children should undergo electrophysiologic study with a view to ablation of accessory pathways. Ablation should be done before surgery, as it will aid in operative and postoperative management. The operative procedure also may render the inciting arrhythmogenic area inaccessible.

SURGICAL TECHNIQUES

Selection of the appropriate surgical procedure depends on the age at presentation and the associated anomalies. Although case reports exist of success with total correction in the newborn period, most have found that a surgical attempt at this stage results in dismal survival rates that make no improvement on medical management alone.[28] An alternative for these patients is a creation of single-ventricle physiology that excludes the RV from the right atrium, thereby alleviating the problems of poor RV function, tricuspid regurgitation, and RV outflow tract obstruction.[43] These patients ultimately go on to a Fontan procedure.

In children, the option of repairing the tricuspid valve mechanism is preferable to valve replacement because the child will outgrow the valve prosthesis. Valve repair is generally not possible in patients with extensively atrialized ventricles, with anterior leaflets adherent to the ventricular wall, or with absent chordae and papillary muscles. In these patients, tricuspid valve replacement is a better option.

The subset of patients with severe pulmonary stenosis, pulmonary atresia, or absent pulmonary valve should have neither an attempt at tricuspid valve repair or replacement nor an attempt at single-ventricle physiology. The results of surgical attempts at RV outflow tract reconstruction combined with either single- or two-ventricle repairs have been uniformly unsuccessful, and the only option for these individuals may be heart-lung transplantation.

Single-Ventricle Repair

This procedure is performed through standard median sternotomy, harvesting pericardium on entry and treating this with glutaraldehyde. After bicaval venous cannulation and institution of cardiopulmonary bypass, the patient is cooled to 20°C. An LV vent is placed through the right superior pulmonary vein. The ascending aorta is clamped, and cold blood cardioplegia administered. Caval tourniquets are applied. The right atrium is opened obliquely, and the atrial septal and tricuspid valve anatomy carefully examined. If the atrial septal defect is small or not present, the septum is excised to ensure complete right-to-left shunting. A preserved pericardial patch is used to close the tricuspid valve orifice with continuous nonabsorbable polypropylene suture. The patch is positioned on the valve annulus, and the suture line travels superior to the coronary sinus to avoid the risk of heart block (Fig. 37-4). The atriotomy is then closed. A systemic-to-pulmonary PTFE (polytetrafluoroethylene, Gore-Tex) shunt

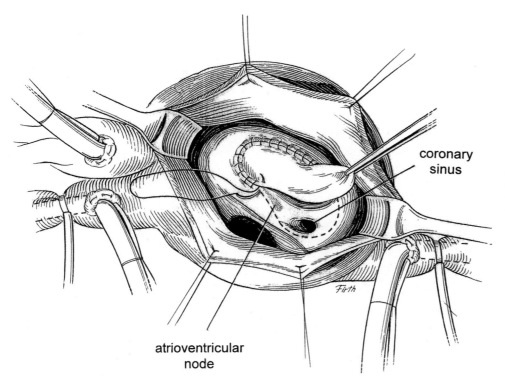

coronary
sinus

FIGURE 37-4 Patch closure of tricuspid valve. Suture injury of the atrioventricular node is avoided by placing stitches outside of the coronary sinus.

atrioventricular
node

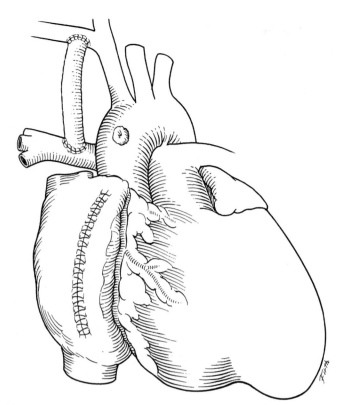

FIGURE 37-5 Atrial closure and systemic-to-pulmonary shunt. The right atriotomy is closed, and a 3.5-mm or 4.0-mm shunt of polytetrafluoroethylene is placed between the innominate artery and the right pulmonary artery.

of 3.5 to 4 mm is constructed either centrally or from innominate artery to right pulmonary artery (Fig. 37-5). Subsequently, the patient is rewarmed and weaned from cardiopulmonary bypass.

One-and-a-Half–Ventricle Repair

Patient selection for a one-and-a-half–ventricle repair comes under consideration in two clinical circumstances. The child is a marginal candidate for two-ventricle repair, and a decision opting for a one-and-a-half–ventricle repair is made to decrease the risk of postoperative RV failure or undue volume stress on a marginal tricuspid valve.[37] The second clinical circumstance is a child who was never considered a candidate for two-ventricle repair, has been staged along single-ventricle palliation, and now it is thought the intracardiac anatomy will tolerate surgical septation. For Ebstein's anomaly, predominant consideration of a one-and-a-half–ventricle repair will be the initial clinical scenario, in which the child does not need a neonatal palliative procedure. This allows time for growth and development and a decrease in the pulmonary vascular resistance. Once the child is out of the neonatal period, selection for a one-and-a-half–ventricle repair comes under consideration for Ebstein's anomaly when either the tricuspid valve apparatus or RV cavity demonstrates concerning morphologic or physiologic characteristics, eliminating consideration for a two-ventricle repair. Generally, children with RV diastolic volumes less than

45% of predicted are treated as single-ventricle hearts, and greater than 90% of predicted normal are treated as biventricular repairs.[29] Those falling in between can be considered for a one-and-a-half–ventricle repair. Additional considerations include RV function and severity of tricuspid valve disease. In either instance, a one-and-a-half–ventricle repair results in a smaller volume load on an RV with compromised function or a tricuspid valve with suboptimal competence, even after repair.[29]

Similar to the two-ventricle repair, the one-and-a-half–ventricle repair aims to transpose the tricuspid leaflets to the tricuspid annulus and thereby obliterate the atrialized ventricle. It also minimizes tricuspid regurgitation and relieves RV outflow obstruction. As in a second-stage palliative surgery, a connection is made between the superior vena cava and proximal right pulmonary artery, resulting in a bidirectional Glenn shunt (Fig. 37-6). Unlike single-ventricle palliation, the RV and RV outflow tract have continuity maintained, allowing pulsatile blood flow into the pulmonary artery.[34] With the exception of the bidirectional Glenn, the surgery is similar to the two-ventricle repair described in detail later. Results from two groups, Chowdhury and associates and

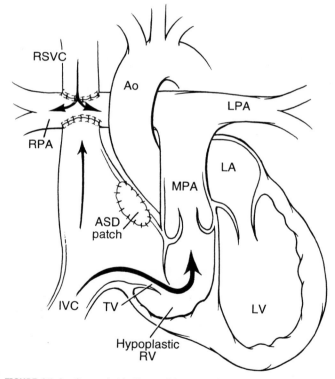

FIGURE 37-6 One-and-a-half–ventricle repair for Ebstein's anomaly with hypoplastic right ventricle (RV). In this patient with significant RV hypoplasia, the right heart is too small to carry a full cardiac output and a one-and-a-half–ventricle repair is performed. In this modification, the right superior vena cava (RSVC) is transected and both segments anastomosed to the right pulmonary artery (RPA). Patch closure of the atrial septal defect (ASD) is performed. This then allows the superior caval circulation to drain directly to the lungs via the caval connection and the hypoplastic right heart to carry only the inferior caval circulation. By preserving the connection of the right atrium (RA) with the RPA, a portion of the flow from the inferior caval circulation can, if necessary, drain to the RPA. Ao, aorta; IVC, inferior vena cava; LA, left atrium; LPA, left pulmonary artery; LV, left ventricle; MPA, main pulmonary artery; RV, right ventricle; TV, tricuspid valve.

Kreutzer and colleagues,[11,29] indicate that the one-and-a-half–ventricle repair compares favorably with the Fontan procedure in both perioperative risk and early outcome. Long-term follow-up is needed, as well as further study providing evidence of either improved function or improved survival with the one-and-a-half–ventricle repair over standard palliative surgeries.

Two-Ventricle Repair

The two-ventricle repair aims to transpose the tricuspid leaflets to the tricuspid annulus and thereby obliterate the atrialized ventricle. It also minimizes tricuspid regurgitation and relieves RV outflow obstruction. The surgery is performed through standard median sternotomy with bicaval venous cannulation and aortic arterial perfusion. A right superior pulmonary vein vent is placed in the LV, and the patient is cooled to 25°C. The aorta is cross-clamped, and cold blood cardioplegia administered antegrade. Caval tourniquets are applied, and the right atrium is opened obliquely, allowing close inspection of the tricuspid valve leaflets and annulus. Multiple techniques have been described to decrease the atrialized portion of the RV and to bring the anterior leaflet into a competent position. Most of these repairs are based on the contributions of Danielson and Carpentier.[8,12,13]

Our preference is a technique using vertically placed mattress sutures, which are passed from the septal and posterior leaflets through the dilated atrialized ventricular wall to the tricuspid annulus. Care must be taken not to injure the posterior descending coronary artery. The spacing between each suture is wider at the annulus than at the leaflet (Fig. 37-7),

effectively narrowing the annulus. No attempt is made to plicate leaflet tissue overlying the septum. Further narrowing of the annulus is performed by plicating the free-wall portion of the annulus to the septal portion by using pledgeted mattress sutures (Fig. 37-8). While performing this aspect of the repair, care must be directed at avoiding distortion of the coronary sinus or the right coronary artery. The posterior annuloplasty is then performed further to decrease the size of the dilated annulus (Fig. 37-9). The annuloplasty sutures should remain lateral to the coronary sinus to avoid heart block. Further clefts or perforations are closed with fine interrupted sutures. The tricuspid valve subsequently functions as either a monocusp valve when a large anterior leaflet is present or as a partial bicuspid or tricuspid valve, depending on individual anatomy. Valvar competency is then tested by saline injection into the RV. The atrial septal defect is closed with a patch (Fig. 37-10); a portion of the right atrial wall is resected to reduce the incidence of atrial arrhythmias, and the atriotomy is closed. The patient is rewarmed and weaned from cardiopulmonary bypass. Inotropic agents are usually needed to enhance ventricular performance. Pulmonary vascular resistance must be maintained low with analgesia, muscle relaxation, increased oxygen, hyperventilation, and nitric oxide. These strategies may be used to reduce RV afterload.

Intraoperative management of these patients is complicated by the frequent occurrence of dysrhythmias, most frequently supraventricular tachycardia. Intravenous amiodarone is useful for intraoperative management of these problems. Intraoperative transesophageal echocardiography provides valuable information both before and after repair.

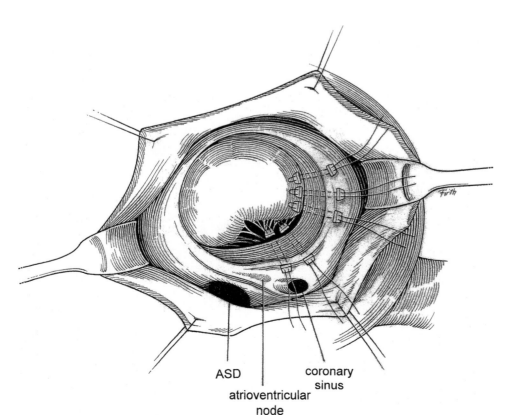

FIGURE 37-7 Plication of the atrialized ventricle. Mattress pledgetted sutures are placed from the free wall of the right ventricle around to the coronary sinus, avoiding the atrioventricular node.

ASD

atrioventricular node

coronary sinus

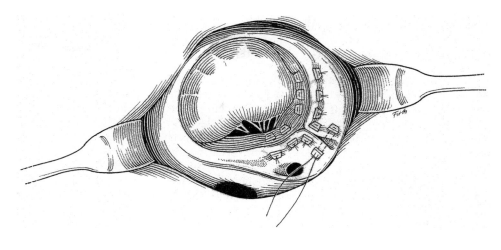

FIGURE 37-8 Lateral tricuspid annuloplasty. One or two sutures plicate the dilated annulus laterally.

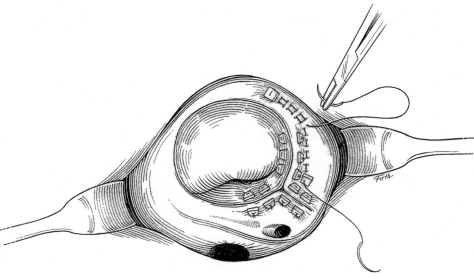

FIGURE 37-9 Semicircular annuloplasty. Further reduction in the tricuspid annuloplasty can be achieved by a circular annuloplasty of the lateral free wall.

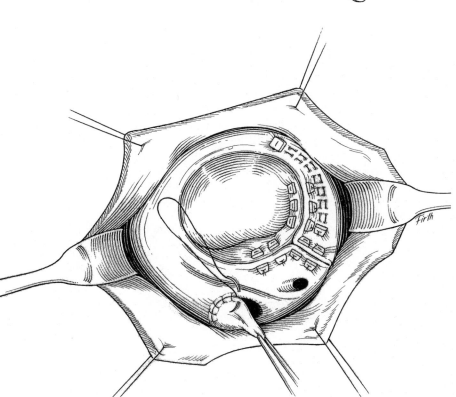

FIGURE 37-10 Atrial septal defect closure.

POSTOPERATIVE CRITICAL CARE

Hemodynamic Management

The neonate, after single-ventricle palliation for Ebstein's anomaly, experiences low cardiac output. Postoperatively, the coronary sinus and thebesian veins continue to empty into the RV. Inotropic support for the RV is necessary, and LV support is needed if significant congestive heart failure existed preoperatively. Similarly, in the two-ventricle repair, postoperative RV failure is common. Inotropic support is usually needed to decrease RV distention and to augment LV performance. LV function may be more compromised in children with preoperative congestive failure. To reduce the risk of postoperative RV distention and tricuspid regurgitation, manipulation of pulmonary vascular resistance may be necessary. This includes pain management, oxygen, nitric oxide, and hyperventilation with appropriate ventilation to support pulmonary perfusion. Maintenance of sinus rhythm is a critical contribution to cardiac output and may require the use of temporary epicardial pacing.

In combination with direct cardiorespiratory support, sedation with benzodiazepines and fentanyl analgesia is important for at least the initial 24 hours. The addition of neuromuscular blockade may be necessary in children with a reactive pulmonary circulation. Occasionally, in extreme cases of ventricular dysfunction, leaving the sternum open and closing the skin with an inert silicone rubber Silastic patch improves diastolic function and prevents cardiac compression, which may be significant because of mediastinal and myocardial edema. The open sternum also facilitates ventilation at lower airway pressures and consequently decreases RV afterload. In addition, because intrathoracic pressure is atmospheric, its effect on vascular resistance is minimized. The sternum can be closed 3 to 4 days postoperatively when myocardial function has improved, and edema has decreased.

After hemodynamic improvement or after the sternum is closed, the patient is allowed to awaken. Monitoring the pulmonary artery pressures is useful as an end point for these medications and assists with the weaning of inotropes and pulmonary vasodilators. Neonates with single-ventricle physiology are begun on digoxin and angiotensin-converting enzyme inhibitors as the intravenous agents are weaned. Continued shunt patency is improved by administration of aspirin on a daily basis. Neonates with single-ventricle repair require construction of a superior cavopulmonary anastomosis (Glenn) at approximately age 6 months, and a complete cavopulmonary anastomosis (Fontan) is constructed at approximately age 2 to 3 years. For the latter procedure, our preference is an external cardiac conduit with PTFE from the inferior vena cava to the pulmonary artery.

Arrhythmias

Postoperative arrhythmias include supraventricular tachycardia, intermittent atrioventricular block, ventricular arrhythmias, and junctional ectopic tachycardia.[10,25,26] These arrhythmias may significantly complicate the postoperative course. In a series of 52 patients from Mayo Clinic, perioperative and postoperative arrhythmias occurred in 42% of the patients, with 36% of the dysrhythmias being ventricular in origin.[35] Five sudden death events occurred, in which four of these patients exhibited perioperative ventricular tachycardia or fibrillation. This suggests that intraoperative ventricular irritability predisposes to postoperative dysrhythmias and probably to sudden death. In this situation, consider intraoperative administration of amiodarone with continuation of this drug through the postoperative period. Slowing of atrioventricular conduction can be overcome by temporary epicardial pacing, should the effect of amiodarone result in bradycardia. Antiarrhythmic agents are usually continued for a period of 6 months, and if arrhythmias do not recur, the medication is tapered. Arrhythmias not responsive to pharmacologic agents may require ablation.

RESULTS

In our series of single-ventricle palliation for cyanotic neonates with severe Ebstein's anomaly, survival is in excess of 60% versus certain mortality associated with medical management in patients with severe congestive heart failure and RV outflow tract obstruction.[14] When possible, tricuspid valve repair has less than 10% early and late mortality, with favorable long-term outcome. Valve replacement with porcine valves is usually durable and may require replacement if the child outgrows the valve. Recent reports indicate a preference toward earlier surgical intervention, as opposed to expectant medical management.

References

1. Anderson KR, Danielson GK, McGoon DC, Lie JT: Ebstein's anomaly of the left-sided tricuspid valve: Pathological anatomy of the valvular malformation. *Circulation* 58:87–91, 1978.
2. Anderson KR, Zuberbuhler JR, Anderson RH, et al: Morphologic spectrum of Ebstein's anomaly of the heart: A review. *Mayo Clin Proc* 54:174–180, 1979.
3. Andress JD, Vander Salm TJ, Huang SK: Bidirectional bundle branch reentry tachycardia associated with Ebstein's anomaly: Cured by extensive cryoablation of the right bundle branch. *Pacing Clin Electrophysiol* 14:1639–1647, 1991.
4. Arnstein A: Eine seltene Missbilding der Trikuspidalklappe ("Ebsteinsche Krankheit"). *Virchows Arch (Pathol Anat)* 266:247–254, 1927.
5. Attie F, Casanova JM, Zabal C, et al: Clinical profile in 174 patients. *Arch Inst Cardiol Mex* 69:17–25, 1999.
6. Barnard CN, Schrire V: Surgical correction of Ebstein's malformation with prosthetic tricuspid valve. *Surgery* 54:302–308, 1963
7. Becker AE, Becker MJ, Edwards JE: Pathological spectrum of dysplasia of the tricuspid valve: Features in common with Ebstein's malformation. *J Pathol* 103:Pxix–Pxx, 1971.
8. Carpentier A, Chauvaud S, Mace L, et al: A new reconstructive operation for Ebstein's anomaly of the tricuspid valve. *J Thorac Cardiovasc Surg* 96:92–101, 1988.
9. Celermajer DS, Cullen S, Sullivan ID, et al: Outcome in neonates with Ebstein's anomaly. *J Am Coll Cardiol* 19:1041–1046, 1992.
10. Chauvaud SM, Brancaccio G, Carpentier AF: Cardiac arrhythmia in patients undergoing surgical repair of Ebstein's anomaly. *Ann Thorac Surg* 71:1547–1552, 2001.
11. Chowdhury UK, Airan B, Sharma R, et al: One and a half ventricle repair with pulsatile bidirectional Glenn: Results and guidelines for patient selection. *Ann Thorac Surg* 71:1995–2002, 2001.
12. Danielson GK, Driscoll DJ, Mair DD, et al: Operative treatment of Ebstein's anomaly. *J Thorac Cardiovasc Surg* 104:1195–1202, 1992.
13. Danielson GK, Fuster V: Surgical repair of Ebstein's anomaly. *Ann Surg* 196:499–504, 1982.
14. Davis JE, Starnes VA: Ebstein's malformation of the tricuspid valve in children. In: Kaiser LR, Kron IL, Spray TL (eds): *Mastery of Cardiothoracic Surgery*. Philadelphia, Lippincott-Raven, 1998, pp 930–937.

15. Ebstein W: Ueber einen sehr seltenen Fall von Insufficienz der Valvula tricuspidalis, bedingt durch eine angeborene hochgradige Missbildung derselben. *Arch Anat Physiol Wissenschafliche Med* 33:238–254, 1866.

16. Follath F, Hallidie-Smith KA: Unusual electrocardiographic changes in Ebstein's anomaly. *Br Heart J* 34:513–519, 1972.

17. Fornace J, Rozanski LT, Berger BC: Right heart thromboembolism and suspected paradoxical embolism in Ebstein's anomaly. *Am Heart J* 114:1520–1522, 1987.

18. Freedom RM, Dische MR, Rowe RD: The tricuspid valve in pulmonary atresia and intact ventricular septum: A morphological study of 60 cases. *Arch Pathol Lab Med* 102:28–31, 1978.

19. Frescura C, Angelini A, Daliento L, Thiene G: Morphological aspects of Ebstein's anomaly in adults. *Thorac Cardiovasc Surg* 48:203–208, 2000.

20. Gentles TL, Calder AL, Clarkson PM, Neutze JM: Predictors of long-term survival with Ebstein's anomaly of the tricuspid valve. *Am J Cardiol* 69:377–381, 1992.

21. Genton E, Blount SG Jr: The spectrum of Ebstein's anomaly. *Am Heart J* 73:395–425, 1967.

22. Giuliani ER, Fuster V, Brandenburg RO, Mair DD: Ebstein's anomaly: The clinical features and natural history of Ebstein's anomaly of the tricuspid valve. *Mayo Clin Proc* 54:163–173, 1979.

23. Gussenhoven EJ, Essed CE, Bos E, de Villeneuve VH: Echocardiographic diagnosis of overriding tricuspid valve in a child with Ebstein's anomaly. *Pediatr Cardiol* 5:209–211, 1984.

24. Gutberlet M, Oellinger H, Ewert P, et al: [Pre- and postoperative evaluation of ventricular function, muscle mass and valve morphology by magnetic resonance tomography in Ebstein's anomaly]. *Rofo Fortschr Geb Rontgenstr Neuen Bildgeb Verfahr* 172:436–442, 2000.

25. Hebe J: Ebstein's anomaly in adults: Arrhythmias: Diagnosis and therapeutic approach. *Thorac Cardiovasc Surg* 48:214–219, 2000.

26. Ho SY, Goltz D, McCarthy K, et al: The atrioventricular junctions in Ebstein malformation. *Heart* 83:444–449, 2000.

27. Hornberger LK, Sahn DJ, Kleinman CS, et al: Tricuspid valve disease with significant tricuspid insufficiency in the fetus: Diagnosis and outcome. *J Am Coll Card* 17:167–173, 1991.

28. Knott-Craig CJ, Overholt ED, Ward KE, Razook JD: Neonatal repair of Ebstein's anomaly: Indications, surgical technique, and medium-term follow-up. *Ann Thorac Surg* 69:1505–1510, 2000.

29. Kreutzer C, Mayorquim RC, Kreutzer GO, et al: Experience with one and a half ventricle repair. *J Thorac Cardiovasc Surg* 117:662–668, 1999.

30. Lamers WH, Viragh S, Wessels A, et al: Formation of the tricuspid valve in the human heart. *Circulation* 91:111–121, 1995.

31. Link KM, Herrera MA, D'Souza VJ, Formanek AG: MR imaging of Ebstein anomaly: Results in four cases. *AJR Am J Roentgenol* 150:363–367, 1988.

32. Lo HM, Lin FY, Jong YS, et al: Ebstein's anomaly with ventricular tachycardia: Evidence for the arrhythmogenic role of the atrialized ventricle. *Am Heart J* 117:959–962, 1989.

33. Mair DD: Ebstein's anomaly: Natural history and management. *J Am Coll Cardiol* 19:1047–1048, 1992.

34. Muster AJ, Zales VR, Ilbawi MN, et al: Biventricular repair of hypoplastic right ventricle assisted by pulsatile bidirectional cavopulmonary anastomosis. *J Thorac Cardiovasc Surg* 105:112–119, 1993.

35. Oh JK, Holmes DR Jr, Hayes DL, et al: Cardiac arrhythmias in patients with surgical repair of Ebstein's anomaly. *J Am Coll Cardiol* 6:1351–1357, 1985.

36. Radford DJ, Graff RF, Neilson GH: Diagnosis and natural history of Ebstein's anomaly. *Br Heart J* 54:517–522, 1985.

37. Reddy VM, McElhinney DB, Silverman NH, et al: Partial biventricular repair for complex congenital heart defects: An intermediate option for complicated anatomy or functionally borderline right complex heart. *J Thorac Cardiovasc Surg* 116:21–27, 1998.

38. Schiebler GL, Gravenstein JS, Van Mierop LH: Ebstein's anomaly of the tricuspid valve: Translation of original description with comments. *Am J Cardiol* 22:867–873, 1968.

39. Schreiber C, Cook A, Ho SY, et al: Morphologic spectrum of Ebstein's malformation: Revisitation relative to surgical repair. *J Thorac Cardiovasc Surg* 117:148–155, 1999.

40. Shiina A, Seward JB, Tajik AJ, et al: Two-dimensional echocardiographic-surgical correlation in Ebstein's anomaly: Preoperative determination of patients requiring tricuspid valve plication vs. replacement. *Circulation* 68:534–544, 1983.

41. Siebert JR, Barr M Jr, Jackson JC, Benjamin DR: Ebstein's anomaly and extracardiac defects. *Am J Dis Child* 143:570–572, 1989.

42. Silverman NH, Gerlis LM, Horowitz ES, et al: Pathologic elucidation of the echocardiographic features of Ebstein's malformation of the morphologically tricuspid valve in discordant atrioventricular connections. *Am J Cardiol* 76:1277–1283, 1995.

43. Starnes VA, Pitlick PT, Bernstein D, et al: Ebstein anomaly appearing in the neonate: A new surgical approach. *J Thorac Cardiovasc Surg* 101:1082–1087, 1991.

44. Stellin G, Santini F, Thiene G, et al: Pulmonary atresia, intact ventricular septum, and Ebstein anomaly of the tricuspid valve: Anatomic and surgical considerations. *J Thorac Cardiovasc Surg* 106:255–261, 1993.

45. Tourniaire A, Deyerieux F, Tortulier H: Maladie d'Ebstein: Essai de diagnostie clinique. *Arch Mal Coeur* 42:1211–1216, 1949.

46. Tuzcu EM, Moodie DS, Ghazi F, et al: Ebstein's anomaly: Natural and unnatural history. *Cleve Clin J Med* 56:614–618, 1989.

47. Watson H: Natural history of Ebstein's anomaly of tricuspid valve in childhood and adolescence: An international co-operative study of 505 cases. *Br Heart J* 36:417–427, 1974.

48. Yetman AT, Freedom RM, McCrindle BW: Outcome in cyanotic neonates with Ebstein's anomaly. *Am J Cardiol* 81:749–754, 1998.

49. Zuberbuhler JR, Allwork SP, Anderson RH: The spectrum of Ebstein's anomaly of the tricuspid valve. *J Thorac Cardiovasc Surg* 77:202–211, 1979.

Chapter 38

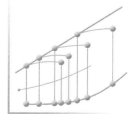

Single-Ventricle Lesions

BRADLEY S. MARINO, MD, MPP, MSCE, GIL WERNOVSKY, MD,
and WILLIAM J. GREELEY, MD, MBA

ANATOMY OF SINGLE-VENTRICLE COMPLEXES

General Anatomic Considerations

Atresia of an atrioventricular or semilunar valve results in single-ventricle physiologic complexes that have complete mixing of the systemic and pulmonary venous circulations. A wide variety of anatomic lesions, usually associated with atresia of an atrioventricular or semilunar valve, have the common physiology of complete mixing of the systemic and pulmonary venous return. Table 38-1 delineates the anatomic lesions that result in variations of single left ventricle, variations of single right ventricle, and two-ventricle hearts with the potential for single-ventricle physiology. In some children, borderline hypoplasia of an atrioventricular valve, outflow tract, or ventricle is found, where a separated two-ventricle circulation is possible. An example of this type of lesion includes Shone's syndrome, in which multiple left-sided obstructive lesions are seen.[54] Controversy exists whether patients with mild to moderate forms of Shone's syndrome or similar left-sided inflow or outflow lesions or both should be converted to a single-ventricle repair, or staged toward a separated two-ventricular circulation.[4,10,11,13,58]

Alternately, some infants are born with two ventricles of normal size, who have malpositioned or straddling atrioventricular valve, or a ventricular septal defect that is remote from either great vessel, that preclude a two-ventricular repair. Although these infants have ventricular chambers and atrioventricular valves suitable in size for a two-ventricle repair, the anatomy is such that single-ventricular management must be undertaken. Examples include patients with double outlet right ventricle with a "remote" ventricular septal defect or patients with a d-transposition of the great arteries, ventricular septal defect and pulmonary stenosis with tricuspid valve chordae that prohibit a Rastelli repair.

Single-Ventricle Physiology

In each of the lesions delineated, essentially complete mixing of the systemic and pulmonary venous return occurs. Mixing typically occurs at the atrial or ventricular level or both. One consequence of the mixing is that the ventricular output must be divided between the pulmonary and systemic arterial circuits, the two competing parallel circuits. In this situation, the pulmonary artery and the aortic oxygen saturations are equal, and the ventricular output is the sum of the pulmonary blood flow (PBF) (Q_p) and the systemic blood flow (Q_s). The proportion of the ventricular output that goes to the pulmonary or systemic vascular bed is determined by the relative resistance to flow into the two circuits. The physiology is in contrast to

Table 38-1 Anatomic Variations in Single-Ventricle Physiology in the Preoperative and Postoperative States

	Preoperative	Postoperative
Variations of Single Left Ventricle		
1. Tricuspid valve atresia		
a. Normally related great arteries	Yes	Yes
b. Transposed great arteries*	Yes	Yes
2. Double-inlet left ventricle		
a. Normally related great arteries*	Yes	Yes
b. Transposed great arteries*	Yes†	Yes
3. Malaligned complete atrioventricular canal with hypoplastic right ventricle	Yes	Yes
4. Pulmonary atresia with intact ventricular septum	Yes	Variable†
Variations of Single Right Ventricle		
1. Mitral valve atresia		
a. Hypoplastic left heart syndrome	Yes	Yes
b. Double-outlet right ventricle	Yes	Yes
2. Aortic valve atresia		
a. Hypoplastic left heart syndrome	Yes	Yes
b. Large ventricular septal defect and normal left ventricular size	Yes	Variable†
3. Malaligned complete atrioventricular canal with hypoplastic left ventricle	Yes	Yes
4. Heterotaxy syndromes: most forms have pulmonary stenosis or atresia	Yes	Yes
Two-Ventricle Hearts with Potential Single-Ventricle Physiology		
1. Tetralogy of Fallot with pulmonary atresia	Yes	Variable†
2. Truncus arteriosus	Yes‡	No
3. Total anomalous pulmonary venous connection	Yes‡	No

*In tricuspid atresia or double-inlet left ventricle with transposed great arteries ([S,D,D] or [S,L,L]), right ventricular hypoplasia, subaortic obstruction, arch hypoplasia, and coarctation frequently exist.

†Single-ventricle physiology will result if a systemic-to-pulmonary artery shunt or pulmonary artery band is placed. Two ventricle repairs with normal series circulation or partial repairs with incomplete mixing are possible in certain anatomic types.

‡Streaming may result in incomplete mixing.

Adapted from Marino BS, Wernovsky G. Preoperative care. In Chang AC, Hanley FL, Wernovsky G, Wessel DL (eds). *Pediatric Cardiac Intensive Care.* Baltimore, Williams & Wilkins, 1998, p 272, with permission.

a "series" circulation, in which the aortic saturation is higher than the pulmonary artery saturation, and "transposition physiology," in which the pulmonary artery saturation is higher than the aortic saturation.

In almost all hearts with single-ventricle physiology, one of the two outflows is obstructed. It is extremely rare to have no outflow obstruction or to have obstruction to *both* the pulmonary and systemic circuits. As a result, patients generally fall into two distinct categories, those with obstructed pulmonary outflow and those with obstructed systemic outflow.

Resistance to pulmonary flow is determined by:
1. The degree of subvalvar, valvar, or supravalvar pulmonary stenosis
2. The pulmonary vascular (arteriolar) resistance
3. The pulmonary venous and left atrial pressure
4. The size of the ductus arteriosus.

The left atrial pressure is determined by the volume of the PBF entering the left atrium and the degree of obstruction to outflow through the left atrioventricular valve and atrial septum.

Resistance to systemic flow is determined by:
1. The degree of subaortic or aortic valvar stenosis, aortic arch hypoplasia, or coarctation of the aorta
2. The systemic vascular resistance
3. The size of the ductus arteriosus.

BALANCING THE PARALLEL CIRCULATIONS

The goal of preoperative management of the neonate with single-ventricle physiology is to have the infant arrive in the operating room with good cardiac output, normal end-organ function, and normal systemic oxygen delivery and blood flow. By achieving balanced blood flow between the systemic and pulmonary vascular beds, usually adequate oxygen delivery will be present to prevent acidosis and a minimization of the volume load to the single ventricle. Inadequate PBF (low Q_p:Q_s) results in unacceptable hypoxemia. Excessive PBF (high Q_p:Q_s) may result in congestive heart failure and inadequate systemic blood flow.

Based on the Fick principle:

$$Q_p:Q_s = \frac{(SaO_2 - SvO_2)}{(SpvO_2 - SpaO_2)}$$

Assuming a pulmonary venous saturation ($SpvO_2$) of 100% and a mixed venous oxygen saturation (SvO_2) of 50%, an arterial oxygen saturation (SaO_2) of 75%, and a pulmonary artery saturation ($SpaO_2$) of 75%, the Q_p/Q_s ratio is approximately 1:1. In single-ventricle physiology, the SaO_2 is equal to the $SpaO_2$ because of complete interatrial or interventricular mixing. A Q_p:Q_s of 1:1 typically results in mild ventricular volume overload (the Q_p *plus* the Q_s), minimal atrioventricular valve regurgitation, and adequate systemic blood flow (SBF) and oxygen delivery (DO_2).

Using only the systemic arterial saturation to estimate the Q_p:Q_s may be misleading. If the practitioner assumes an $SpvO_2$ of 100%, which may not always be the case, a varying SvO_2 from ventricular dysfunction may dramatically alter the Q_p:Q_s. For example, the neonate described earlier with normal ventricular function has a Q_p:Q_s of 1:1 with an SaO_2 of 75%. The same neonate may have significant ventricular dysfunction and have an SvO_2 of 25%, which, assuming an $SpvO_2$ of 100% and the same SaO_2 of 75%, results in a Q_p:Q_s of 2:1. This second infant has a wide arterial-to-venous oxygen difference (AVO$_2$ difference, 75% − 25% = 50%) and has clinically significant "overcirculation." To assist in the management of the clinically unstable single-ventricle patient in the preoperative or postoperative period or both, some institutions have advocated monitoring the systemic venous saturation. This is typically done in the superior vena cava (SVC), as it provides an estimation of the SvO_2.[19,43,47,60] The pulmonary artery saturation cannot be used as the mixed venous saturation because, by definition, intracardiac shunting occurs at the atrial or ventricular level or both in the neonate with single-ventricle anatomy. In the neonate, the umbilical venous catheter (UVC) may be advanced, placing its tip into the SVC. Although the SVC may be the most advantageous position for SvO_2 measurement and assessment of Q_p:Q_s, using the SVC may increase the risk of SVC thrombosis, which will have dramatic implications on subsequent palliation (hemi-Fontan or bidirectional Glenn procedures).

Although SvO_2 measurement is a good indirect measure of DO_2 (when it is low, it represents low DO_2, and when it is within 25% of the SaO_2, it represents adequate DO_2), it does not directly reflect the amount of excess oxygen that is available in the hemodynamic system in question at the time the SvO_2 is obtained. The measure of oxygen excess is Ω.

$$\text{Omega } (\Omega) = \frac{\text{oxygen delivery}}{\text{oxygen consumption}}$$

$$= \frac{(Q_s)(CaO_2)}{(Q_s)(CaO_2 - CvO_2)}$$

$$= \frac{SaO_2}{SaO_2 - SvO_2}$$

where CaO_2 is the systemic arterial oxygen content, and the CvO_2 is the systemic venous oxygen content. Ω is the reciprocal of the oxygen-extraction ratio. In the single-ventricle neonate with excellent ventricular function, with a SaO_2 of 90% and an SvO_2 of 65%, the omega or oxygen-excess factor is 3.6 (90/90 – 65). In the single-ventricle neonate with poor ventricular function, with an SaO_2 of 90% and an SvO_2 of 20%, the Ω or oxygen-excess factor is 1.3 (90/90 – 20), indicating that little if any oxygen excess is available and that oxygen delivery is inadequate. Barnea and associates[2] in an elegant computer simulation, showed that (1) small increases in SaO_2 can be associated with large decreases in overall DO_2, (2) estimation of $Q_p:Q_s$ from SaO_2 results in errors when pulmonary venous desaturation is present, (3) low values of SvO_2 indicate low values of DO_2, and (4) the linear relation between DO_2 and Ω is not altered by changes in cardiac output and $SpvO_2$.[2]

Taeed and colleagues[56] recently showed that a significant variation occurred in pulmonary venous saturation during the early postoperative period after Stage I Norwood palliation, with 32% of the cohort they examined having a pulmonary venous saturation less than 95%. This finding, along with the variability in SvO_2 noted before in this discussion, makes the SaO_2 in isolation a poor estimator of $Q_p:Q_s$, Q_s, and DO_2.

The Transitional Circulation

After birth, over the first few hours to days of life, a decrease occurs in pulmonary vascular resistance (PVR), and in the absence of a significant obstruction to PBF, a relative increase is found in the proportion of PBF from the combined ventricular output. As the $Q_p:Q_s$ ratio approaches 2.0, the single ventricle becomes progressively more volume overloaded, with mildly elevated ventricular end-diastolic and atrial pressures. As the single ventricle dilates, atrioventricular valve insufficiency may be seen. The neonate may show signs of respiratory distress. The normal homeostatic mechanisms to improve systemic output result in an increased stroke volume and an increased heart rate. The greater proportion of pulmonary venous return in the mixed ventricular blood results in elevated SaO_2 (approximately 85% to 90%). Visible cyanosis may be mild or absent.

Some neonates tolerate pulmonary "overcirculation" in the preoperative period without end-organ damage and without

significant intervention, whereas others do not. When the diagnosis of single ventricle is made early and prostaglandin E_1 (PGE_1) is started expeditiously, acidosis may be avoided. At low doses of PGE_1 (0.01 mcg/kg/min), intubation and other side effects of PGE_1 may be avoided. These infants may have a mild degree of restriction at the atrial septum, providing some balance to their $Q_p:Q_s$, and although tachypneic (respiratory rate, 60 to 80) and well saturated ($SaO_2 > 90\%$; PaO_2, 40 to 50 mm Hg), they remain clinically stable with minimal intervention. This group of patients maintains adequate SBF and DO_2 to the tissues despite increased PBF.

Patients with "unbalanced" single-ventricle physiology that require intervention may be grouped into three physiologic extremes:

1. Progressively increasing PBF, resulting in congestive heart failure and inadequate SBF
2. Late diagnosis presenting in shock
3. Inadequate PBF, resulting in hypoxemia.

Before surgical intervention, a number of ventilatory and pharmacologic maneuvers may be used to "balance" the circulation ($Q_p:Q_s \sim 1.0$), resulting in adequate SBF and DO_2. However, in many of these patients, ventilatory and pharmacologic management only temporizes the need for surgical intervention.

Early Diagnosis with Excessive Pulmonary Blood Flow and Inadequate Systemic Blood Flow

Infants with single-ventricle physiology, an open ductus arteriosus, and "high" arterial oxygen saturations (>90%), may develop "steal" of the combined ventricular output into the pulmonary vascular circuit (high $Q_p:Q_s$). Although this phenomenon is rare, the "steal" may result in increased oxygen content in the systemic blood at the expense of reduced systemic blood flow and *decreased* oxygen delivery to the tissues. Inadequate tissue perfusion coupled with a low diastolic blood pressure and retrograde aortic flow may result in hypotension, metabolic acidosis, acute renal failure, necrotizing enterocolitis (NEC), cerebral ischemia, and liver dysfunction. "Overcirculated" infants generally have an unrestrictive atrial communication, low PVR, and high systemic vascular resistance (SVR). In addition, ventricular wall tension and oxygen consumption are increased in the dilated, volume-overloaded single ventricle, potentially contributing to myocardial dysfunction and atrioventricular valve regurgitation. A progressive metabolic acidosis, even if mild, is a worrisome sign in these patients and requires urgent evaluation.

In these patients, once establishment of a patent ductus arteriosus is confirmed, maneuvers to reduce SVR and maximize the PVR should be used. Intubation and mechanical ventilation with sedation, paralysis, and permissive hypoventilation may be used to elevate the pCO_2 to the 40 to 50 mm Hg range, and thereby increase the PVR.[8] Maintaining the hematocrit greater than 45% may increase viscosity and serve to elevate the PVR.

Supplemental inspired gases may be used to increase the PVR and reduce excessive PBF. Several case reports and small case series support the use of inspired carbon dioxide and hypercarbia to stabilize preoperative infants with hypoplastic left heart syndrome.[24,41] Similarly, small case series reported clinical improvement in systemic output with alveolar hypoxia by increasing inspired nitrogen (14% to 19% FiO_2).[12,53] Until recently, prospective controlled studies comparing hypoxia with hypercarbia were limited to studies in shunt-dependent single-ventricle animal models.[36,41,45] Reddy and associates[41] surgically created single-ventricle physiology in fetal sheep and showed that at 3 days of life, both hypercarbia (5% $FiCO_2$) and hypoxia (10% FiO_2) decreased PBF and increased SBF.

In a prospective, crossover study, Tabbutt and colleagues[55] compared the effects of hypoxia, achieved by adding increased inspired nitrogen (FiO_2 17%), with hypercarbia, achieved by adding increased inspired carbon dioxide ($FiCO_2$ 2.7%) in pre-operative infants with hypoplastic left heart syndrome (HLHS) under conditions of anesthesia, paralysis, and fixed minute ventilation. Outcome variables included SvO_2, SaO_2, and mixed cerebral oxygen saturation, with each condition compared with the room air baseline. Both hypoxia and hypercarbia decreased the Q_p:Q_s, -0.8 ± 0.48 and -0.9 ± 0.54, respectively, although the decrease was not statistically significant for hypoxia. Only hypercarbia increased cardiac output (AVO_2 difference decreased by 8.5% $\pm$ 2.3%) and increased mixed cerebral oxygen saturation (9.6% $\pm$ 1.8%).

If inadequate oxygen is delivered to the tissues, decreasing SVR and minimizing oxygen consumption will help improve the neonate's balance of oxygen supply and consumption. Intubation, mechanical ventilation, and sedation will work to decrease oxygen consumption, as most infants who are "overcirculated" have some degree of respiratory distress and increased catecholamine levels. In these "overcirculated" infants, excessive inotropic support (particularly at α-doses) should be minimized, and in extremely rare circumstances, afterload reduction may be helpful in patients with elevated SVR and an adequate blood pressure.[44] Patients with marked "overcirculation" and systemic hypoperfusion should not undergo a lengthy period of "medical management" of their unstable physiology. *If a patient requires intubation, sedation, or inotropic support, or a combination of these, to maintain adequate systemic blood flow, the patient should undergo relatively urgent surgical management to achieve a more favorable physiology, unless concurrent contraindications to surgery exist.*

Necrotizing Enterocolitis before Cardiac Surgery

In general, neonates with single-ventricle physiology with inadequate systemic blood flow, whether it results from excessive PBF and congestive heart failure or from late diagnosis with a restrictive patent ductus arteriosus and shock, are at risk for NEC. A case-control study by McElhinney and associates[35] revealed an incidence of NEC of 3.3% during a 4-year study period of 643 neonates with congenital heart disease. This was substantially higher than that in the control population. Risk factors for developing NEC included a diagnosis of HLHS, truncus arteriosus, and aortopulmonary window. Earlier gestational age and episodes of low cardiac output were the only factors other than the anatomic diagnoses associated with the development of NEC. Episodes of low cardiac output were defined as arterial pH less than 7.2, serum creatinine more than 1.2 mg/dL, and serum aspartate aminotransferase and serum alanine aminotransferase more than 300 U/L.

In patients with significant diastolic runoff through the ductus arteriosus, mesenteric ischemia may predispose the neonate to develop NEC.

Infants with unexplained lactic acidosis, abdominal distention, dilated loops of bowel, persistently heme-positive stools, hypoglycemia, thrombocytopenia, or a combination of these should be carefully evaluated for pneumatosis, free air, or portal air by serial abdominal radiograph examination. If possible, neonates with "medical" NEC should be given a 7- to 10-day course of antibiotics before subjecting the bowel to the ischemia and reperfusion injury associated with cardiopulmonary bypass. It is not clear whether patients with "surgical" NEC need a shorter or longer recovery time before surgical palliation relative to the neonate with "medical" NEC.

Late Diagnosis with Shock

Neonates with single-ventricle anatomy initially seen after the first week of life may appear in shock with inadequate systemic perfusion from either ductal constriction or pulmonary "overcirculation." These infants are typically discharged to home and are seen at age 1 to 2 weeks with tachypnea, decreased feeding, weak peripheral pulses, and poor perfusion. These infants have depressed myocardial function and atrioventricular valve regurgitation, profound metabolic acidosis, usually some degree of hepatic dysfunction and renal failure, occasionally bowel ischemia or disseminated intravascular coagulopathy or both, and in rare cases, severe hypoxic-ischemic encephalopathy or seizures or both.

These infants may require rapid and aggressive resuscitation with PGE_1 (0.1 mcg/kg/min) to open their ductus arteriosus and inotropic support to improve ventricular performance. Sedation, paralysis, and intubation will decrease oxygen consumption and will control ventilation (targeted PCO_2 40 to 45 mm Hg) to increase PVR and decrease Q_p:Q_s. If pulmonary "overcirculation" exists with normoventilation with room air, then inspired CO_2 ($FiCO_2$, 2% to 3%) may be used to improve systemic oxygen delivery.[55] Neonates with a single ventricle, in shock, with end-organ dysfunction, should have their initial palliation delayed if possible to allow recovery of secondary organ function.

Inadequate Pulmonary Blood Flow

Neonates with single-ventricle anatomies that are ductal dependent for PBF may have severe hypoxemia with inadequate PBF due to ductal constriction.

Management strategies to improve PBF in this setting should be tailored to the underlying anatomy or pathophysiology resulting in the decreased PBF. For example, patients who are hypoxemic due to an obstructive left-sided atrioventricular valve and restrictive foramen ovale may have transcatheter dilation of the atrial septum performed.[18,39] If the child is born with intact atrial septum, the neonate should be taken to the operating room or the cardiac catheterization laboratory as an emergency for creation of an atrial communication. Patients with intracardiac obstruction to PBF may have maneuvers performed to increase blood pressure and SVR (e.g., increasing inotropic infusions), thereby "forcing" more blood through the obstructed intracardiac pulmonary outflow. Interventional procedures such as pulmonary valve dilation also may be considered in this group of patients. Patients with ductal-dependent

PBF with a restrictive ductus arteriosus, hypoxemia, and inadequate oxygen delivery to the tissues may need to go to the operating room as an emergency if PGE₁ is unsuccessful in opening the ductus arteriosus. Neonates thought to be hypoxemic because of elevated PVR should have maneuvers performed to decrease PVR (e.g., increased FiO₂, hyperventilation/alkalosis, nitric oxide). Most intravenous pulmonary vasodilators are nonspecific and result in unpredictable relative changes in the PVR and SVR. Possible causes of increased PVR include restrictive or intact atrial communication at birth, primary lung disease, sepsis, and persistent pulmonary hypertension of the newborn with or without meconium aspiration.

GENERAL PRINCIPLES OF NEWBORN SURGICAL MANAGEMENT

Children with single-ventricle complexes will, in most cases, undergo a variation of the Fontan operation as their ultimate surgical palliation. Risk factors for poor outcome after the modified Fontan operation include, among others: (1) ventricular hypertrophy,[9] (2) elevated PVR or pulmonary artery pressure,[17,26,27] (3) pulmonary artery distortion,[33,52] (4) atrioventricular valve regurgitation,[3,21] and (5) ventricular dysfunction.[34] The management strategies for surgical and medical management of newborns with single-ventricle anatomy must minimize these potential risk factors over the long term, even if it means that a more "complex" neonatal palliation must be performed. All newborn procedures for surgical palliation of the single ventricle are performed to achieve the following:

1. Unobstructed systemic blood flow (to minimize ventricular hypertrophy)
2. Limited PBF (to minimize ventricular volume overload and the risk of ventricular dysfunction, atrioventricular valve regurgitation, and pulmonary artery hypertension and secondary damage to the pulmonary vasculature)
3. Minimal atrioventricular valve regurgitation
4. Nondistorted pulmonary arteries
5. Unrestrictive pulmonary venous return (to minimize the risk of left atrial hypertension, pulmonary venous hypertension, and secondary pulmonary artery hypertension).

Surgical palliation in the newborn for the single ventricle may include placement of a systemic-to-pulmonary artery shunt, pulmonary artery banding, pulmonary artery-to-aortic anastomosis (Damus–Kaye–Stansel), Stage I Norwood procedure, or a combination procedure. Typically, surgical palliation occurs early in life. Mahle and associates[31] found age older than 14 days at the time of Stage I palliation to be a risk factor for death in the perioperative period. Similarly, Ianettoni and colleagues[20] reported a 29% survival rate for infants older than 30 days, and a 91% survival rate for infants younger than 30 days after Stage I palliation for HLHS. The risk of palliation is higher in the older single-ventricle neonate for multiple reasons, including labile postoperative PVR and ventricular hypertrophy. Although palliation is clearly a higher risk, it may be performed in some cases with placement of a larger modified Blalock-Taussig (B-T) shunt to augment PBF and decrease hypoxemia.[14]

Palliative Procedures

Systemic-to-Pulmonary Artery Shunt

The modified B-T shunt is the palliative procedure most commonly used to secure PBF in the neonate with single-ventricle physiology with restrictive PBF. Depending on the size of the neonate and the preexisting PVR, a 3.0- to 4.0-mm Gore-Tex tube is placed from the brachiocephalic vessels, usually the subclavian or innominate artery, to the pulmonary artery. Similarly, placement of a central shunt involves inserting a Gore-Tex tube between the ascending aorta and the pulmonary artery. The central shunt is generally used when an aberrant subclavian artery is found, and therefore no innominate artery from which to place the modified B-T shunt. In the past, the Waterston and Potts shunts were used to provide PBF, but fell out of favor because they were associated with a high risk of pulmonary artery hypertension or distortion of the pulmonary arteries or both. Figure 38-1 illustrates the classic B-T, modified B-T, central, Waterston, and Potts shunts.

Experimentation has been done with adjustable systemic-to-pulmonary artery shunts with a hemostatic clip or an adjustable

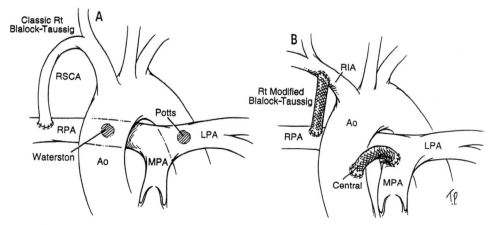

FIGURE 38-1 Systemic-to-pulmonary artery shunts. **A,** Anatomic location of previously used systemic-to-pulmonary artery shunts. These three shunts (classic Blalock-Taussig, Waterston, and Potts) are, for the most part, no longer performed because of the difficulty in takedown and/or the increased potential for branch pulmonary artery (PA) distortion. **B,** Anatomic location of currently used systemic-to-pulmonary artery shunts. Right modified Blalock-Taussig shunt: 3.5-mm prosthetic graft (Gore-Tex) from right innominate artery (RIA) to right pulmonary artery (RPA). Central shunt: Prosthetic 3.5-mm (Gore-Tex) graft from the ascending aorta (Ao) to central branch pulmonary arteries. In the presence of a right aortic arch, a modified Blalock-Taussig shunt is typically performed on the opposite (left) side. LPA, left pulmonary artery; MPA, main pulmonary artery; RSCA, right subclavian artery.

snare to allow further restriction of PBF if the neonate has an elevated Q_p:Q_s in the postoperative period.[28,51] Experimentation also was done with saphenous vein homograft utilization instead or Gore-Tex tube graft in systemic–pulmonary artery shunts because of the smaller size of the saphenous vein homograft.[57] The smaller saphenous vein homograft would result in even more restriction to Q_p than the standard 3.0-mm Gore-Tex tube graft.

Pulmonary Artery Banding

In children with no restriction to systemic blood flow and little to no restriction to PBF, a pulmonary artery band may be placed to limit PBF and pulmonary artery pressure (Fig. 38-2). The pulmonary artery band is placed without cardiopulmonary bypass. Surgical staff must minimize distortion of the branch pulmonary arteries, which, as described earlier, increases the risk for eventual Fontan completion.[22,32] By decreasing the PBF, acute reduction in the volume load on the ventricle occurs, with an immediate decrease in cavity dimension and an increase in wall thickness.[48] These changes may result in acute development of subaortic stenosis, especially if systemic output is dependent on a relatively small ventricular septal defect.

Pulmonary Artery-to-Aortic Anastomosis (Damus-Kaye-Stansel)

The Damus-Kaye-Stansel (D-K-S) palliation is used for children with a single ventricle with subaortic stenosis with or without distal arch obstruction to allow both great arteries and semilunar valves to provide unobstructed systemic blood flow (Fig. 38-3).[7,16,25,29,49] The most common lesions for which the D-K-S operation is used are double-inlet left ventricle with transposition of the great arteries and subaortic obstruction, tricuspid atresia with transposition of the great

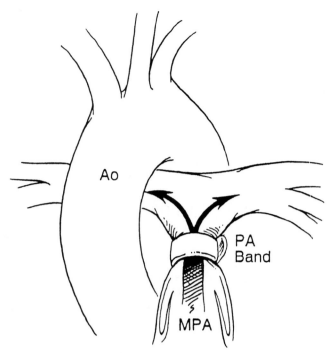

FIGURE 38-2 Pulmonary artery (PA) band. A band is placed on the main PA (MPA) so as to not distort the branch PAs or compromise pulmonary valve function. Ao, *aorta*.

arteries and subaortic obstruction, or double-outlet RV with subaortic obstruction. In each case, subaortic stenosis is present, and the pulmonary artery is relied on to provide unimpeded systemic flow. The palliation involves anastomosis of the main pulmonary artery to the aorta to provide unobstructed SBF. A B-T shunt is placed to provide for PBF. Distal aortic arch augmentation is necessary if distal arch hypoplasia is present,

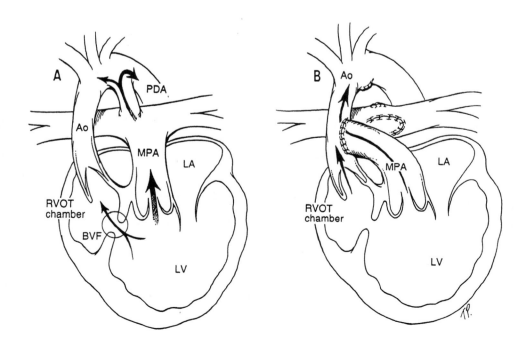

FIGURE 38-3 Damus-Kaye-Stansel procedure in a patient with double-inlet left ventricle with subaortic stenosis. **A,** Preoperative. The aorta (Ao) arises from a hypoplastic right ventricular outflow tract (RVOT) chamber producing subaortic stenosis. The main pulmonary artery (MPA) connects with the left ventricle. **B,** Postoperative. Palliation involves transection of the MPA with end-to-side anastomosis of the proximal PA with the ascending Ao, providing unobstructed systemic blood flow. A systemic shunt, such as a Blalock-Taussig shunt, is placed to provide pulmonary blood flow (*not shown*). BVF, bulboventricular foramen; LA, left atrium; LV, left ventricle; PDA, patent ductus arteriosus.

and an atrial septectomy is usually performed as well. The neoaortic (native pulmonary) valve frequently has trivial to mild insufficiency after the pulmonary-to-aortic anastomosis, but this is rarely hemodynamically significant.[49,61]

Stage I Norwood Procedure

The Stage I palliation, first successfully described by Norwood for HLHS,[37] is used for children with functional single ventricle and aortic atresia or severe aortic arch hypoplasia with subaortic obstruction.[5,15,23] The procedure involves amalgamation of the pulmonary artery and aorta to provide unobstructed SBF, patch augmentation of the aortic arch beyond the ductal insertion site, an atrial septectomy, and placement of a modified B-T shunt to provide restrictive PBF.

In some centers, the Sano modification, which uses a 5.0-mm RV-to-main pulmonary artery shunt, is being performed instead of the modified B-T shunt. Advantages may exist in using the Sano in the case of aortic atresia where the native ascending aorta tends to be smaller and "diastolic steal" into the modified B-T shunt may theoretically decrease coronary perfusion.[50]

A homograft patch is usually used to augment the transverse and distal aortic arch, and the distal main pulmonary artery is typically closed with homograft patch. Technical aspects of the Stage I procedure and risk factors for Stage I mortality are noted in Chapter 40 on hypoplastic left heart syndrome.

Combination Strategies

Combination surgical and interventional catheterization strategies have been used to palliate the neonate with HLHS. Akintuerk and associates[1] reported stenting of the ductus arteriosus to provide unobstructed SBF and, if necessary, balloon atrial septostomy to provide an unobstructed atrial communication, coupled with surgical pulmonary artery banding. Eight of nine patients in the series survived single-stage aortic arch reconstruction and bidirectional cavopulmonary connection at 3.5 to 6 months. Two of three patients listed for heart transplantation survived to transplantation.

IMMEDIATE POSTOPERATIVE MANAGEMENT OF PALLIATIVE PROCEDURES

The physiology of the single ventricle with parallel circulation was described previously. Although the postoperative management is similar, management strategies also must take into account the effects of cardiopulmonary bypass and aortic cross-clamping on myocardial function and the PVR. After the D-K-S and Stage I procedures, PVR may be transiently elevated or even labile. In addition, the effects of myocardial ischemia from aortic cross-clamping may lead to globally depressed myocardial function in the first 24 to 36 hours after surgery.[62]

The postoperative evaluation should assess all aspects of the specific procedure that has been used. The patient with either *low systemic cardiac output*, *excessive cyanosis* (oxygen saturation <65%), or relatively *high oxygen saturations* (>90%) must have the repair and postoperative physiology carefully evaluated.

POSTOPERATIVE SURGICAL COMPLICATIONS

Postoperative complications after single-ventricle palliation may include seizures, vocal cord paralysis, diaphragmatic paresis or paralysis, bleeding, mediastinitis, and sepsis. Chylothorax is generally treated with bowel rest, total parenteral nutrition, and effective chest tube drainage. Portagen via oral or nasogastric route may be used to minimize chylous effusions. If chylous effusions persist after bowel rest and Portagen therapy, thoracic duct ligation may be performed, with or without pleuradesis. Case reports and small case series investigated the use of somatostatin to decrease chylothorax drainage.[40] Chapter 40 discusses the surgical complications after Stage I in greater detail.

Low Cardiac Output

Low cardiac output syndrome may occur in the first 24 to 36 hours after the Stage I Norwood or D-K-S palliations. Signs include tachycardia, hypotension, oliguria, and metabolic acidosis. Assessment of the arterial-venous saturation difference (AVO_2 difference) by intermittent measurement of SvO_2 has been shown to be a sensitive predictor of low systemic blood flow and inadequate oxygen delivery.[19,46,47,60] An AVO_2 difference greater than 40% to 50% suggests low cardiac output and inadequate tissue delivery of oxygen. Hoffman and associates[19] showed that an SVC saturation of less than 30% predicted a 29% risk of anaerobic metabolism after the Stage I procedure for hypoplastic left heart syndrome. Low systemic cardiac output may be due to (1) decreased total cardiac output due to poor ventricular performance or tamponade or both, (2) adequate pump performance with maldistribution of flow (increased $Q_p:Q_s$), and (3) adequate pump performance with atrioventricular valve regurgitation, which may result in maldistribution of flow from a large regurgitant fraction. A combination of these factors is typically present.

The combination of echocardiography, to evaluate ventricular and atrioventricular valve function, and measurement of the AVO_2 difference, to estimate systemic blood flow and $Q_p:Q_s$ ratio, is important in establishing the cause of the low cardiac output and rationally directing therapy.

Globally depressed ventricular function is generally treated by increasing inotropic support, whereas low SBF with adequate pump function and a high $Q_p:Q_s$ ratio may improve by increasing PVR and reducing SVR. The infant with atrioventricular valve regurgitation and low cardiac output may benefit from afterload reduction, which will minimize the regurgitant fraction and improve the maldistribution of flow from the single ventricle. Afterload reduction may be accomplished with milrinone, a phosphodiesterase inhibitor, or phenoxybenzamine, an α_1-receptor blocker.[42,59] Phenoxybenzamine has a very long half-life, and if hypotension is present, it may be necessary to use additional support to maintain adequate blood pressure.[38] Some centers have reported the use of supplemental inspired CO_2 to increase PVR and thereby decrease Q_p, increase Q_s, and maximize DO_2 in those patients in whom hypoventilation (low tidal volume and low ventilatory rate) has not been an effective modulator of Q_p:Q_s.[6,8] A strategy of hypoventilation may be detrimental to DO_2 if the neonate has pulmonary venous desaturation at baseline, which is not uncommon.[56] The reduction in oxygen delivery based on decreased oxygen content in the systemic arterial blood (decreased PvO_2 and SaO_2) may not be offset by increased SBF.

Hypoxemia

The differential diagnosis of hypoxemia (SaO_2 <70%) after surgical palliation includes pulmonary venous desaturation, systemic venous desaturation, and decreased PBF. Pulmonary venous desaturation may result from ventilation/perfusion mismatch in the lung (e.g., pneumothorax, chylothorax, hemothorax, pleural effusion, pulmonary edema, pneumonia, pneumonitis, atelectasis). Systemic venous desaturation is seen with low systemic output, anemia, and high oxygen consumption states. Decreased PBF may occur with elevated PVR, pulmonary venous hypertension, a restrictive atrial septal defect,[30] pulmonary artery distortion resulting in pulmonary artery obstruction, and an inadequate systemic-to-pulmonary artery shunt.

Elevated Oxygen Saturations

The child with single-ventricle physiology who has systemic oxygen saturation greater than or equal to 90% generally has low PVR and PBF far in excess of SBF. This hemodynamic situation may, in time, result in inadequate systemic perfusion, renal hypoperfusion, and an inability to wean the child from mechanical ventilation. In patients with left-sided obstructive lesions, which were palliated with either the Stage I Norwood procedure or the D-K-S procedure, arch obstruction must be ruled out, as distal obstruction may force more blood through the shunt and increase Q_p at the expense of Q_s.

Necrotizing Enterocolitis after Cardiac Surgery

A case-control study by McElhinney and associates[35] showed no difference in hospital mortality between neonates in whom NEC developed and controls. However, all four of the deaths in patients with NEC were directly attributable to NEC or to associated complications such as multisystem organ failure or *Escherichia coli* sepsis. No correlation was found between hospital mortality and the time of onset of NEC, before or after cardiac intervention. In neonates with congenital heart disease, hospital stay was significantly longer in neonates that developed NEC compared with controls (36 ± 22 days vs. 19 ± 14 days). Postoperative NEC is treated with bowel rest, broad-spectrum antibiotics, and hyperalimentation, usually for a minimum of 10 to 14 days. After the period of hyperalimentation and bowel rest, continuous nasogastric feeds may be slowly increased over time. At the first sign of obstruction or significant "residuals" during nasogastric feeds, feeding rate should be reduced and evaluation of the small and large bowel with or without surgical consultation should occur.

CONCLUSIONS

Single-ventricle patients share many management strategies and perioperative risks regardless of the anatomic subtype involved. A careful understanding of the single-ventricle physiology outlined earlier allows the care team to support these patients through a staged palliation to the completion of the Fontan operation.

References

1. Akintuerk H, Michel-Behnke I, Valeske K, et al: Stenting of the arterial duct and banding of the pulmonary arteries: Basis for combined Norwood stage I and II repair in hypoplastic left heart. *Circulation* 105:1099–1103, 2002.
2. Barnea O, Santamore WP, Rossi A, et al: Estimation of oxygen delivery in newborns with a univentricular circulation. *Circulation* 98:1407–1413, 1998.
3. Bartmus DA, Driscoll DJ, Offord KP, et al: The modified Fontan operation for children less than 4 years old. *J Am Coll Cardiol* 15:429–435, 1990.
4. Bolling SF, Iannettoni MD, Dick M 2nd, et al: Shone's anomaly: Operative results and late outcome. *Ann Thorac Surg* 49:887–893, 1990.
5. Bove E, Lloyd T: Staged reconstruction for hypoplastic left heart syndrome: Contemporary results. *Ann Surg* 224:387–394, 1996.
6. Bradley SM, Simsic JM, Atz AM: Hemodynamic effects of inspired carbon dioxide after the Norwood procedure. *Ann Thorac Surg* 72:2088–2094, 2001.
7. Brawn WJ, Sethia B, Jagtap R, et al: Univentricular heart with systemic outflow obstruction: Palliation by primary Damus procedure. *Ann Thorac Surg* 59:1441–1447, 1995.
8. Chang AC, Zucker HA, Hickey PR, Wessel DL: Pulmonary vascular resistance in infants after cardiac surgery: Role of carbon dioxide and hydrogen ion. *Crit Care Med* 23:568–574, 1995.
9. Cohen AJ, Cleveland DC, Dyck J, et al: Results of the Fontan procedure for patients with univentricular heart. *Ann Thorac Surg* 52:1266–1271, 1991.
10. Cohen MS, Jacobs ML, Weinberg PM, Rychik J: Morphometric analysis of unbalanced common atrioventricular canal using two-dimensional echocardiography. *J Am Coll Cardiol* 28:1017–1023, 1996.
11. Cohen MS, Rychik J: The small left ventricle: How small is too small for biventricular repair? *Semin Thorac Cardiovasc Surg Pediatr Card Surg Annu* 2:189–202, 1999.
12. Day RW, Tani LY, Minich LL, et al: Congenital heart disease with ductal-dependent systemic perfusion: Doppler ultra-sonography flow velocities are altered by changes in the fraction of inspired oxygen. *J Heart Lung Transplant* 14:718–725, 1995.
13. Delius RE, Rademecker MA, de Leval MR, et al: Is a high-risk biventricular repair always preferable to conversion to a single ventricle repair? *J Thorac Cardiovasc Surg* 112:1561–1568, 1996.
14. Duncan BW, Rosenthal GL, Jones TK, Lupinetti FM: First-stage palliation of complex univentricular cardiac anomalies in older infants. *Ann Thorac Surg* 72:2077–2080, 2001.
15. Forbess J, Cook N, Roth S, et al: Ten-year institutional experience with palliative surgery for hypoplastic left heart syndrome: Risk factors related to stage I mortality. *Circulation* 92:II262–II266, 1995.
16. Gates R, Laks H, Elami A, et al: Damus-Stansel-Kaye procedure: Current indications and results. *Ann Thorac Surg* 56:111–119, 1993.
17. Gentles TL, Mayer JE Jr, Gauvreau K, et al: Fontan operation in 500 consecutive patients: Factors influencing early and late outcome. *J Thorac Cardiovasc Surg* 114:376–391, 1997.
18. Grady RM, Canter CE, Bridges ND: Transcatheter ASD creation in infants with left heart obstruction. *J Am Coll Cardiol* 484A, 1994.
19. Hoffman GM, Ghanayem NS, Kampine JM, et al: Venous saturation and the anaerobic threshold in neonates after the Norwood procedure for hypoplastic left heart syndrome. *Ann Thorac Surg* 70:1515–1521, 2000.
20. Iannettoni MD, Bove EL, Mosca RS, et al: Improving results with first stage palliation for hypoplastic left heart syndrome. *J Thorac Cardiovasc Surg* 107:934–940, 1994.
21. Imai Y, Takanashi Y, Hoshino S, et al: Modified Fontan procedure in ninety-nine cases of atrioventricular valve regurgitation. *J Thorac Cardiovasc Surg* 113:262–269, 1997.

22. Jenkins KJ, Hanley FL, Colan SD, et al: Function of the anatomic pulmonary valve in the systemic circulation. *Circulation* 84:173–179, 1991.
23. Jacobs M, Rychik J, Murphy J, et al: Results of Norwood's operation of lesions other than hypoplastic heart syndrome. *J Thorac Cardiovasc Surg* 110:1555–1562, 1995.
24. Jobes DR, Nicolson SC, Steven JM, et al: Carbon dioxide prevents pulmonary overcirculation in hypoplastic heart syndrome. *Ann Thorac Surg* 54:150–151, 1992.
25. Karl TR, Watterson KG, Sano S, Mee RBB: Operations for subaortic stenosis in the univentricular heart. *Ann Thorac Surg* 52:420–428, 1991.
26. Kaulitz R, Ziemer G, Luhmer I, Kallfelz H: Modified Fontan operation in functionally univentricular hearts: Preoperative risk factors and intermediate results. *J Thorac Cardiovasc Surg* 112:658–664, 1996.
27. Knott-Craig C, Danielson G, Schaff H, et al. The modified Fontan operation: An analysis of risk factors for early postoperative death or takedown in 702 consecutive patients from one institution. *J Thorac Cardiovasc Surg* 109:1237–1243, 1995.
28. Kuduvalli M, McLaughlin KE, Trivedi DB, Pozzi M: Norwood type operation with adjustable systemic-pulmonary shunt using hemostatic clip. *Ann Thorac Surg* 72:634–635, 2001.
29. Lui RC, Williams WG, Trusler GA, et al: Experience with the Damus-Kaye-Stansel procedure for children with Taussig-Bing hearts or univentricular hearts with subaortic stenosis. *Circulation* 88:II170–III176, 1993.
30. Mahle WT, Rychik J, Gaynor JW, et al: Restrictive atrial communication after reconstructive surgery for hypoplastic left heart syndrome. *Am J Cardiol* 88:1454–1457, 2001.
31. Mahle WT, Spray TL, Wernovsky G, et al: Survival after reconstructive surgery for hypoplastic left heart syndrome: A 15-year experience from a single institution. *Circulation* 102:III136–III141, 2000.
32. Malcic I, Sauer U, Stern H, et al: The influence of pulmonary artery banding on outcome after the Fontan operation. *J Thorac Cardiovasc Surg* 104:743–747, 1992.
33. Mayer JE Jr, Bridges ND, Lock JE, et al: Factors associated with marked reduction in mortality for Fontan operations in patients with single ventricle. *J Thorac Cardiovasc Surg* 103:444–452, 1992.
34. Mayer JE Jr: Risk factors for modified Fontan operations. In Jacobs ML, Norwood WI (eds): *Pediatric Cardiac Surgery.* Boston, Butterworth-Heinemann, 1992, pp 70–82.
35. McElhinney DB, Hedrick HL, Bush DM, et al: Necrotizing enterocolitis in neonates with congenital heart disease: Risk factors and outcomes. *Pediatrics* 106:1080–1087, 2000.
36. Mora GA, Pizarro C, Jacobs ML, Norwood WI: Experimental model of single ventricle: Influence of carbon dioxide on pulmonary vascular dynamics. *Circulation* 90:II43–II46, 1994.
37. Norwood WI, Lang P, Hansen DD: Physiologic repair of aortic atresia with hypoplastic left heart syndrome. *N Engl J Med* 308:23–26, 1983.
38. O'Blenes SB, Roy N, Konstantinov I, et al: Vasopressin reversal of phenoxybenzamine-induced hypotension after the Norwood procedure. *J Thorac Cardiovasc Surg* 123:1012–1013, 2002.
39. Perry SB, Lang P, Keane JF, et al: Creation and maintenance of adequate interatrial communication in left atrioventricular valve atresia or stenosis. *Am J Cardiol* 58:622–626, 1986.
40. Pettit TW, Caspi J, Borne A: Treatment of persistent chylothorax after Norwood procedure with somatostatin. *Ann Thorac Surg* 73:977–979, 2002.
41. Reddy VM, Liddicoat JR, Fineman JR, et al: Fetal model of single ventricle physiology: Hemodynamic effects of oxygen, nitric oxide, carbon dioxide, and hypoxia in the early postnatal period. *J Thorac Cardiovasc Surg* 112:437–449, 1996.
42. Reinoso-Barbero F, Garcia-Fernandez FJ, Diez-Labajo A, et al: Postoperative use of milrinone for Norwood procedure. *Paediatr Anaesth* 6:342–343, 1996.
43. Riordan CJ, Locher JP, Santamore WP, et al: Monitoring systemic venous oxygen saturations in the hypoplastic left heart syndrome. *Ann Thorac Surg* 63:835–837, 1997.
44. Riordan CJ, Randsbaek F, Storey JH, et al: Inotropes in the hypoplastic left heart syndrome: Effects in an animal model. *Ann Thorac Surg* 62:83–90, 1996.
45. Riordan CJ, Randsbaek F, Storey JH, et al: Effects of oxygen, positive end-expiratory pressure, and carbon dioxide on oxygen delivery in an animal model of the univentricular heart. *J Thorac Cardiovasc Surg* 112:644–654, 1996.
46. Riordan CJ, Randsbaek F, Storey JH, et al: Balancing pulmonary and systemic arterial flows in parallel circulations: The value of monitoring systemic venous oxygen saturations. *Cardiol Young* 7:74–79, 1997.
47. Rossi AF, Sommer RJ, Lotvin A, et al: Usefulness of intermittent monitoring of mixed venous oxygen saturation after stage I palliation for hypoplastic left heart syndrome. *Am J Cardiol* 73:1118–1123, 1994.
48. Rychik J, Jacobs ML, Norwood WI: Acute changes in left ventricular geometry after volume reduction operation. *Ann Thorac Surg* 60:1267–1274, 1995.
49. Rychik J, Murdison KA, Chin AJ, Norwood WI: Surgical management of severe aortic outflow obstruction in lesions other than the hypoplastic left heart syndrome: Use of a pulmonary artery to aorta anastomosis. *J Am Coll Cardiol* 18:809–816, 1991.
50. Sano S, Kawada M, Yoshida H, et al: Norwood procedure to hypoplastic left heart syndrome. *Jpn J Thorac Cardiovasc Surg* 46:1311–1316, 1998.
51. Schmid FX, Kampmann C, Kuroczynski W, et al: Adjustable tourniquet to manipulate pulmonary blood flow after Norwood operations. *Ann Thorac Surg* 68:2306–2309, 1999.
52. Senzaki H, Isoda T, Ishizawa A, Hishi T: Reconsideration of criteria for the Fontan operation: Influence of pulmonary artery size on postoperative hemodynamics of the Fontan operation. *Circulation* 89:1196–1202, 1994.
53. Shime N, Hashimoto S, Hiramatsu N, et al: Hypoxic gas therapy using nitrogen in the preoperative management of neonates with hypoplastic left heart syndrome. *Pediatr Crit Care Med* 1:38–41, 2000.
54. Shone JD, Sellars RD, Anderson RC, et al: The developmental complex of parachute mitral valve, supravalvar ring of the left atrium, subaortic stenosis, and coarctation of the aorta. *Am J Cardiol* 11:714–725, 1963.
55. Tabbutt S, Ramamoorthy C, Montenegro LM, et al: Impact of inspired gas mixtures on preoperative infants with hypoplastic left heart syndrome during controlled ventilation. *Circulation* 104:I159–I164, 2001.
56. Taeed R, Schwartz SM, Pearl JM, et al: Unrecognized pulmonary venous desaturation early after Norwood palliation confounds Q_p:Q_s assessment and compromises oxygen delivery. *Circulation* 103:2699–2704, 2001.
57. Tam VK, Murphy K, Parks WJ, et al: Saphenous vein homograft: A superior conduit for the systemic arterial shunt in the Norwood operation. *Ann Thorac Surg* 71:1537–1540, 2001.
58. Tchervenkov CI: Two-ventricle repair for hypoplastic left heart syndrome. *Semin Thorac Cardiovasc Surg Pediatr Card Surg Annu* 4:83–93, 2001.
59. Tweddell JS, Hoffman GM, Fedderly RT, et al: Phenoxybenzamine improves systemic oxygen delivery after the Norwood procedure. *Ann Thorac Surg* 67:161–168, 1999.
60. Tweddell JS, Hoffman GM, Fedderly RT, et al: Patients at risk for low systemic oxygen delivery after the Norwood procedure. *Ann Thorac Surg* 69:1893–1899, 2000.
61. van Son JA, Reddy VM, Haas GS, Hanley FL: Modified surgical techniques for relief of aortic obstruction in [S,L,L] hearts with rudimentary right ventricle and restrictive bulboventricular foramen. *J Thorac Cardiovasc Surg* 110:909–915, 1995.
62. Wernovsky G, Wypij D, Jonas RA, et al: Postoperative course and hemodynamic profile after the arterial switch operation in neonates and infants: A comparison of low-flow cardiopulmonary bypass and circulatory arrest. *Circulation* 92:2226–2235, 1995.

Chapter 39

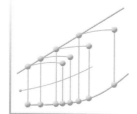

Tricuspid Atresia

JOSEPHINE M. LOK, MD, PHILIP J. SPEVAK, MD, and
DAVID G. NICHOLS, MD, MBA

DEFINITION

Tricuspid atresia (TA) is defined as complete obstruction of the atrioventricular valve of the morphologic right ventricle (RV) and is a type of single ventricle lesion (see Chapter 38). The RV is typically hypoplastic. In some cases of TA, a rudimentary tricuspid valve is present but with membranous atresia, and in other cases, no tricuspid valve is apparent.

EPIDEMIOLOGY

The true prevalence of TA is not known; however, in clinical series of patients with congenital heart disease, prevalence ranges from 0.3% to 3.7%,[112] whereas the prevalence in autopsy series ranges from 2% to 3%.[95,112] TA occurs in approximately 1 in 15,000 live births,[5,112] with 6% of these infants delivered prematurely.[41]

EMBRYOLOGY

The cause of TA is unknown but has been postulated by Van Praagh[137] as the result of malalignment of the ventricular septum in relation to the atria and atrioventricular (AV) canal. Absence of the RV sinus during development results in a shift to the right of the ventricular septum and obliteration of the right AV orifice. The ultimate size of the RV also is determined by the extent to which the septum is shifted to the right and the size of the associated ventricular septal defect. The series of abnormalities during embryologic development of the heart resulting in TA and associated defects occurs between the postconceptional days 25 and 55.[49] The odds of TA appear to increase with maternal febrile illness during pregnancy.[10] Most cases of TA are sporadic, but occurrences in siblings have been reported.[79]

ANATOMY AND CLASSIFICATION

A variety of anatomic characteristics are manifested in TA; however, all forms share (1) lack of communication between the atrium (most commonly the right) and RV, (2) the presence of an interatrial communication, (3) an enlarged mitral valve, and (4) a hypoplastic RV usually in communication with the left ventricle (LV) via a ventricular septal defect (VSD).[139]

TA was first classified by Kuhne[114] in 1906, according to the interrelation of the great arteries. This classification was later expanded by Edwards and Burchell[31] and has been modified by Rao and others since then to include a wider spectrum of associated cardiac malformations.[108,139]

From the clinical standpoint, TA is seen in three major types based on the ventriculoarterial relations. Each type is

Table 39-1   Tricuspid Atresia

Type	Relation	Frequency
I	*Normal Great Arteries*	*70%*
I-A	Pulmonary atresia	9%
I-B	Restrictive VSD, pulmonary stenosis	51%
I-C	Nonrestrictive VSD, no pulmonary stenosis	9%
II	*D-Transposition of Great Arteries*	*28%*
II-A	VSD, pulmonary atresia	2%
II-B	VSD, pulmonary stenosis	8%
II-C	VSD, no pulmonary stenosis	18%
III	*L-Transposition of Great Arteries*	*3%*

VSD, ventricular septal defect.

subdivided further based on the severity of pulmonic stenosis or pulmonary atresia (Table 39-1). The most common form (approximately 70%) of TA is type I, which has *normally related great vessels* (Fig. 39-1). Because the majority of these infants experience some form of obstruction to pulmonary blood flow, the site of obstruction at either the pulmonary valve, infundibulum, or VSD characterizes this category further. Obstruction to pulmonary blood flow may occur at more than one level simultaneously (e.g., restrictive VSD and infundibular stenosis). These anatomic features account for the usual appearance of cyanosis in infants with TA and normally related great vessels. A small number of infants with TA and normally related great vessels have a *non*restrictive VSD and increased pulmonary blood flow. These infants are seen initially with congestive heart failure. However, the VSD may close during later infancy, leading to cyanosis.

Persistent left superior vena cava (LSVC) represents an associated cardiovascular anomaly in patients with TA and normally related great vessels. The LSVC most typically

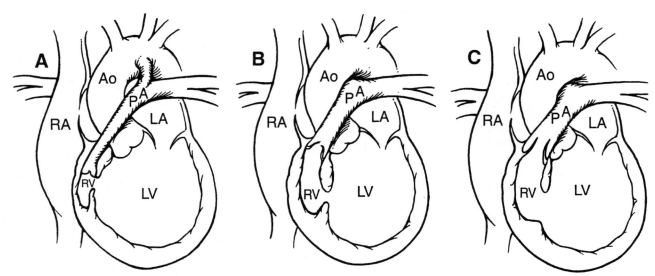

FIGURE 39-1   Native anatomy of tricuspid atresia (TA) with normally related great vessels. **A,** Type Ia: TA with normally related great vessels and pulmonary atresia. **B,** Type Ib: TA with normally related great vessels, restrictive ventricular septal defect (VSD), and pulmonic stenosis. **C,** Type Ic: TA with normally related great vessels and a large VSD. Ao, aorta; LA, left atrium; LV, left ventricle; PA, pulmonary artery; RA, right atrium; RV, right ventricle.

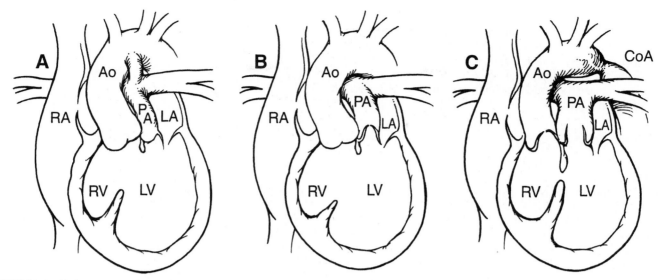

FIGURE 39-2   Native anatomy of tricuspid atresia (TA) with *D*-transposition of the great vessels (D-TGA). **A**, TA with D-TGA, ventricular septal defect (VSD), and pulmonary atresia. **B**, TA with D-TGA, VSD, and pulmonic stenosis. **C**, TA with D-TGA, restrictive VSD, and coarctation of the aorta (CoA). Note the large pulmonary artery (PA) as left ventricle (LV) ejects preferentially into the PA because of restrictive VSD (subaortic stenosis) and coarctation. The patent ductus arteriosus is omitted for clarity, but may be required to supply systemic blood flow in this lesion. LA, left atrium; RA, right atrium; RV, right ventricle.

drains via the coronary sinus to the right atrium (RA). Failure to identify anomalous systemic venous return patterns will lead to persistent hypoxia after any form of cavopulmonary anastomosis.

TA with D-transposed great vessels represents the other major category (type II) of TA (approximately 30%) (Fig. 39-2). The VSD is usually conoventricular or muscular in position. LV blood passes through the VSD into the RV and into the transposed aorta. (Sub)pulmonic stenosis or pulmonary atresia also may produce obstruction to pulmonary blood flow in TA with transposed great vessels. However, the major clinical problem arises when *systemic* blood flow is obstructed by closure of the VSD or by the presence of associated coarctation of the aorta or both.[8,52] Other anomalies in this group include juxtaposition of the atrial appendages and a coronary artery pattern seen in D-transposition of the great arteries (TGA).[8,13,23–25,54]

Rarely, TA (type III) may arise with forms of great artery malposition other than D-TGA. Several anatomic variations exist, but L-TGA is the most common (approximately 3% of all TA). When TA with L-TGA occurs, the malformed morphologic tricuspid valve obstructs flow between the left atrium and the hypoplastic left-sided RV (the systemic ventricle), which ejects into the aorta. Associated anomalies in this group usually include a VSD and LV outflow tract (pulmonary) obstruction.

Tricuspid Valve

Five variants of tricuspid valve morphology are found in TA.[141] The most common (76% to 84%) is a *muscular* atresia, in which no tricuspid valvular tissue is found, but a dimpling in the muscular floor of the anatomic RA is present. This dimple is presumed to be the location of the atretic tricuspid valve.[31]

In the *membranous* form (4% to 12%), the membranous portion of the atrioventricular septum (between the RA and LV) forms part of the floor of the RA in the expected location of the tricuspid valve.[137,140,141]

A *valvular* form (6%) is identified by a thin, imperforate, membrane of tissue consisting of minute fused valve leaflets.[2,33,136] Rudimentary chordae are sometimes attached to the solid membrane.

In the *Ebstein* form (4% to 6%), valvular tissue also is found, with fusion and Ebstein deformity of the tricuspid valve leaflets[2,137] further reducing the size of the RV cavity.

A rare form (2%) occurs with *complete AV canal defect*. Here the orifice of the RV is sealed by the RV aspect of the common AV valve.

Interatrial Communication

An interatrial communication providing an exit for systemic venous return is necessary for survival in types I and II TA. A patent foramen ovale is present in two thirds of patients with TA.[139] The foramen may be widely patent or restrictive to systemic venous outflow. Aneurysmal dilation of the foramen ovale and RA occasionally occurs and may cause obstruction to left atrial blood flow.[39,115] A true atrial septal defect (ASD) is present in about one third of patients and is usually of the ostium secundum type. Less commonly, a primum ASD or complete absence of the atrial septum may occur. Rarely, interatrial communication occurs through a defect between the coronary sinus and the left atrium.[119] This may be an additional source of right-to-left shunt flow in the presence of elevated RA pressure.

Mitral Valve

In TA, both systemic and pulmonary venous return pass through a morphologic mitral valve into the LV. The mitral valve usually has two leaflets and an enlarged orifice.

Although the mitral valve is usually competent, 10% of patients will have mitral insufficiency, and 45% of patients will have some sort of mitral abnormality.[121] It is important to assess the function and morphology of the mitral valve because mitral valve abnormalities can be common in TA, and this can place the patient at higher risk for complications after a Fontan repair.

Left Ventricle

The morphologic LV is enlarged and hypertrophied at least in part because of increased volume load. The overall architecture of the muscle fibers in TA hearts not only is hypertrophied but also is abnormally aligned and irregular.[125] Similarly, the collagen content of the TA hearts is increased compared with that of normal hearts. These findings have been observed in the newborn with TA, suggesting that the myoarchitectural changes may be inherent in the malformation. The remodeled architecture and increased collagen matrix may contribute to abnormal contractility or diastolic function or both, which, in turn, affect the long-term outlook for a successful Fontan repair.

Right Ventricle

The RV is almost always hypoplastic in TA. In general, the size of the RV cavity is determined by the anatomic type of TA and correlates with the size of the VSD.[110] However, even with TGAs and large VSDs, the RV is usually smaller than normal. In rare cases, the RV may be identifiable only on microscopic examination.[31]

The maldevelopment in TA affects the portions of the RV cavity in different ways. The cavity usually contains an infundibulum. The sinus portion is absent or rudimentary with trabeculae and communicates with the LV via the VSD.[7,8,141] The RV inlet is absent in all cases.

PATHOPHYSIOLOGY

TA is an example of single-ventricle physiology. By definition in types I and II TA, no communication exists between the RA and the RV. Systemic and coronary venous return to the RA is shunted across the foramen ovale or an ASD into the left atrium, where it mixes freely with pulmonary venous blood. Thus all venous return flows into the LV, from where it may pass in several ways depending on the ventricular anatomy, the positions of the great arteries, and the presence or absence of pulmonary or systemic arterial obstruction.

Pulmonary Blood Flow

Clinical features and survival of patients with TA are determined largely by the absolute and relative amounts of pulmonary and systemic blood flow, the magnitude of which depends on the degree of outflow tract obstruction, pulmonary vascular resistance (PVR), and patency of the ductus arteriosus.

In the common form of tricuspid atresia (type IB, TA with normally related great arteries, small VSD, and pulmonic stenosis), shunting of LV blood occurs across a VSD, into the

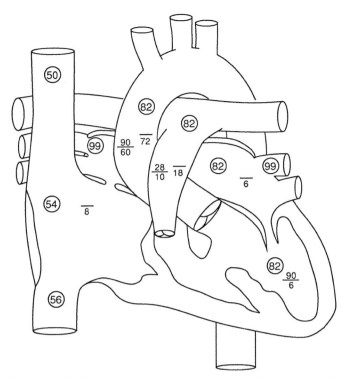

FIGURE 39-3 Pathophysiology of tricuspid atresia (TA) with normally related great vessels, small ventricular septal defect (VSD), and pulmonic stenosis. Note pressure gradient between the right atrium (RA) and left atrium (LA), suggesting restrictive patent foramen ovale. Oxygen saturation rises from RA to LA as systemic venous blood mixes with pulmonary venous blood in the LA and left ventricle (LV). LA O_2 saturation is <85%, reflecting right-to-left intra-atrial shunt. The right ventricle (RV) is not entered because of the small size of the VSD.

hypoplastic right ventricle, providing pulmonary arterial blood flow.[108] These infants typically are cyanotic, because effective pulmonary blood flow is reduced either by a restrictive VSD or by valvar pulmonic stenosis (Fig. 39-3). Systemic blood flow is derived directly from the LV. Because pulmonary blood flow is limited, the LV is more protected against volume overload. During the first year of life, the VSD may close spontaneously, leaving pulmonary blood flow supplied exclusively by a patent ductus arteriosus (PDA) or by aortopulmonary collaterals. Worsening cyanosis heralds these events. TA patients with pulmonary atresia are deeply cyanotic at birth, as pulmonary blood flow is entirely dependent on a PDA or, less commonly, aortopulmonary or bronchopulmonary collateral vessels.

The pathophysiology of the second most common form (type IIC, TA with D-TGA and a large VSD) is characterized by excessive pulmonary blood flow and congestive heart failure (Fig. 39-4).[109,139] Pulmonary blood flow is derived directly from the LV. Systemic blood is routed via the VSD and the RV into the transposed aorta. Hence the RV functions as a subaortic outlet chamber for the main (left) ventricle. In the presence of a nonrestrictive VSD, any associated pulmonic stenosis and the magnitude of the PVR determine pulmonary blood flow. $Q_p:Q_s$ greater than 1.5:1 usually exists, and the infant appears only mildly cyanotic because of the presence of some degree of right-to-left shunting. As PVR decreases during the first few days to weeks, pulmonary overcirculation

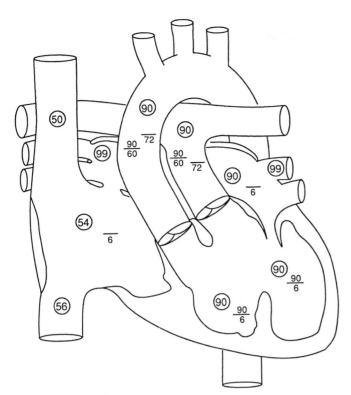

FIGURE 39-4 Pathophysiology of tricuspid atresia (TA) with d-transposition of great arteries and a large ventricular septal defect (VSD). Note significant increase in O_2 saturation from right atrium (RA) to left atrium (LA) as systemic venous blood mixes with large volumes of pulmonary venous blood, reflecting increased pulmonary blood flow. The higher saturations in the aorta (Ao) and pulmonary artery (PA), compared with those in Figure 39-3, reflect greater pulmonary blood flow. Left ventricular (LV) and right ventricular (RV) pressures are equal because of an unrestrictive VSD.

worsens, leading to LV volume overload. In patients without pulmonic stenosis, pulmonary vascular disease may ultimately develop within the first year of life.[24] Similar pathophysiologic events may occur in TA with normally related great arteries, a large VSD, and unrestricted pulmonary blood flow.

In TA with L-TGA,[139] the morphologic RV and its atretic AV valve are on the left side of the heart, resulting in obstruction of left atrial blood flow. Left-to-right shunting occurs at the atrial level, and the blood traverses the morphologic mitral valve, into the morphologic LV (both of which are right-sided). LV blood is pumped directly into the pulmonary artery (PA) and also across the VSD into the morphologic RV, through which it passes to the aorta. Pulmonary or aortic flow may be impeded by subpulmonic or subaortic stenosis in TA with L-TGA.

Left Ventricular Function

The extent of LV dysfunction is an important factor in the short-term and long-term survival of patients with TA.[51,61,116,129] The morphologic LV in TA receives all systemic, coronary, and pulmonary venous return and serves as the pump for both the systemic and pulmonary circulations. The resultant volume overload may be exacerbated by excessive

pulmonary blood flow, often leading to congestive heart failure. Left ventricular end-diastolic volume (LVEDV) is increased in most patients with TA but is increased even further in those with high Q_p:Q_s.[70] Left ventricular ejection fraction is usually decreased in TA and is inversely related to age and LVEDV.[70,92] Chronic hypoxemia may depress LV function further. Various studies have reported that LV ejection fraction may increase, decrease, or remain unchanged after the Fontan procedure, but these changes cannot be predicted reliably. As a result of the volume load of the LV in TA, LV mass is increased.

Acute Hemodynamic Changes

Certain anatomic and physiologic changes may occur with growth and development in the patient with TA. In the neonatal period, closure of the ductus arteriosus in TA patients with pulmonary atresia may result in severe hypoxemia and acidosis as pulmonary blood flow is reduced. Interatrial obstruction leads to systemic venous congestion and may necessitate atrial septostomy. A restrictive ASD is reflected by a giant "a" wave (>5 mm Hg) in the RA pressure tracing or by a gradient between RA and LA pressures of more than 3 mm Hg. Progressive diminution and spontaneous closure of the VSD may occur[44,107,109]; this leads to decreased pulmonary blood flow (Q_p:Q_s <1) in patients with normally related great vessels and to subaortic stenosis and decreased systemic blood flow (Q_p:Q_s >>1) in patients with transposed great vessels.

DIAGNOSTIC ASSESSMENT

Tricuspid Atresia with Normally Related Great Arteries

Most infants with *TA and normally related great vessels* have central cyanosis during the first month of life. In the subset of infants born with a nonrestrictive VSD, cyanosis appears more gradually as the VSD decreases in size and subpulmonic obstruction develops. Hypercyanotic spells similar to those found in patients with tetralogy of Fallot have been reported in 16% to 45% of TA infants.[105] These are characterized by sudden episodes of increased cyanosis, paroxysmal dyspnea, hyperpnea, lethargy, and occasionally, loss of consciousness. These ominous spells may be due to rapidly progressive pulmonic stenosis (infundibular or valvular), closure of the ductus arteriosus,[28,44,107] or spontaneous closure of the VSD[44,111] and are indicative of critically low pulmonary blood flow. Death occurs in 4% of infants; spells are considered an absolute indication for a surgical shunt.

Other findings include tachypnea or hyperpnea, a quiet precordium without thrills, and normal arterial pulses. Prominent jugular venous pulsations may be appreciated in some infants with restrictive interatrial communication. Auscultation reveals a single second heart sound and either an ejection type or a holosystolic murmur at the left lower sternal border. Closure of the VSD or increasing pulmonic stenosis is accompanied by a reduction in the intensity of the murmur. Hepatomegaly is absent, unless the interatrial communication is restrictive.

Tricuspid Atresia with D-Transposition of the Great Arteries

Most infants with TA and D-TGA exhibit signs of congestive heart failure within the first few months of life. The onset of heart failure occurs even earlier in those infants with systemic outflow obstruction in the form of a restrictive VSD or coarctation of the aorta or both. Other symptoms include poor feeding, dyspnea, excessive perspiration, frequent respiratory infections, and growth retardation. Squatting is reported in a few children.[95] Significant findings on examination include mild cyanosis, tachypnea, tachycardia, prominent jugular venous pulsations, and hepatomegaly. Femoral pulses may be diminished in the presence of coarctation of the aorta and a small PDA. Hyperdynamic precordial impulses are noted. A holosystolic murmur, loudest at the left lower sternal border, may be heard and is suggestive of VSD. An apical mid-diastolic rumble reflects increased mitral flow. When significant obstruction to systemic blood flow exists, the infant is in shock with metabolic acidosis.

Diagnostic Tests

The *electrocardiogram* (ECG) may be diagnostic in TA. It demonstrates RA enlargement, LV hypertrophy, and an abnormal superior QRS vector, often described as "left axis deviation" (Fig. 39-5).[109] Tall, peaked P waves with amplitudes greater than 2.5 mm are seen in 70% to 80% of patients with TA.[24,45,106,109] The P waves may be double-peaked, known as "P tricuspidale,"[45] and are usually seen in leads I, II, or V$_{3R}$.[19,24] The two peaks represent RA and LA

depolarization, respectively. Electrophysiologic evidence supports the hypothesis that both the double-peaked nature and increased duration of the P wave in TA are due to RA enlargement, causing prolongation of atrial myocardial pathways and consequently delayed onset of LA activation.[130] As a result of the increased P-wave duration, the PR segment may be short. ST-segment depression may be seen in the lateral chest leads, especially in patients with TGA.

The *chest radiograph* appearance depends largely on the amount of pulmonary blood flow, which separates TA into the two functional categories of increased or decreased pulmonary blood flow. It also provides information regarding cardiac position and the presence of associated anomalies of the lungs, diaphragm, or vertebrae.

In TA with decreased pulmonary blood flow, the radiographic heart size is either normal or slightly enlarged.[32,83] The RA shadow may appear prominent. Absence of the PA segment suggests significant obstruction to pulmonary blood flow. In patients with increased pulmonary blood flow, the heart is moderately to severely enlarged.[32,83] Although more commonly associated with tetralogy of Fallot and truncus arteriosus, a right aortic arch is present in about 8% of TA cases.[139]

Echocardiography is the most important diagnostic tool to define anatomy of the heart and great vessels in patients with TA.[118,131] In TA, two-dimensional (2-D) echocardiography demonstrates the typical enlargement of the RA, LA, and LV, with a hypoplastic RV. The size of the left atrium reflects the volume of systemic and pulmonary blood flow. The hallmark is the atresia of the tricuspid valve with apical, parasternal, and subxiphoid views of the heart revealing a dense echogenic band in the location normally occupied by the tricuspid

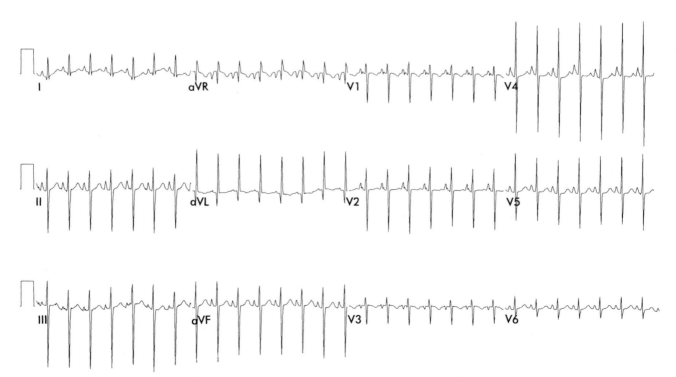

FIGURE 39-5   Characteristic electrocardiogram in tricuspid atresia (TA). Note the tall, peaked P waves in II (right atrial enlargement), tall R wave and inverted T wave in aVL, as well as deep S waves in the right precordial leads (left ventricular hypertrophy). The abnormal superior QRS vector (ASV) is often described as "left axis deviation."

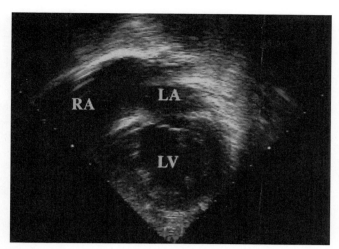

FIGURE 39-6 Echocardiogram of tricuspid atresia (TA), revealing a dense echogenic band in the location normally occupied by the tricuspid valve, indicating the diagnosis of TA. LA, left atrium; LV, left ventricle; RA, right atrium.

valve (Fig. 39-6).[6,68] This finding is pathognomonic for the common muscular type of TA. Two-dimensional echocardiography permits identification of the relative positions of the atrioventricular and semilunar valves, as well as the relation of the atrioventricular valves to the atrioventricular septae. The interatrial communication, the anatomy of the ventricular septum, great vessel relations, and the presence of associated anomalies such as coarctation of the aorta also can be determined with two-dimensional echocardiography. Doppler techniques demonstrate shunt direction across septal defects and measure pressure gradients across stenotic orifices such as restrictive ASDs or VSDs (see Chapter 17 on Noninvasive Diagnosis of Heart Disease).[18,40] This may be useful in determining the need for interventions such as atrial septostomy or septectomy.[122] Although echocardiography is useful in quantitating central PA size, it is limited in determining peripheral PA stenosis, although peripheral stenoses are not common in TA.[40] In addition to its diagnostic value, Doppler echocardiography provides a noninvasive means to evaluate myocardial function and hemodynamics after surgical treatment.[46,53]

Cardiac catheterization is not needed to diagnose TA and is usually unnecessary until the patient is referred for the Glenn or Fontan procedures. Only very rarely, catheterization may provide additional data to guide the surgical repair in newborns.[25] In neonates with profound hypoxemia, angiography may determine the sources of pulmonary blood flow and detect associated cardiovascular anomalies that might complicate management. Because the ductus arteriosus may be the only source of pulmonary blood flow in neonates, preparation of these patients before catheterization should include intravenous administration of prostaglandin E$_1$ (PGE$_1$) to maintain the patency of the ductus arteriosus.[17,37]

Rare infants with a restrictive interatrial communication require balloon atrial septostomy during cardiac catheterization. Because an obligatory shunting of all systemic venous return across the interatrial communication exists in TA, obstruction of the patent foramen ovale or a restrictive ASD results in systemic venous congestion, with peripheral edema, hepatomegaly, and presystolic hepatic and jugular venous pulsations. These clinical signs, a mean interatrial pressure

difference of 3 mm Hg or more, and prominent "a" waves (>5 mm Hg) in the RA constitute evidence of significant interatrial obstruction.[120] Balloon atrial septostomy[113] successfully relieves the obstruction.[77,132] Blade atrial septostomy[104] has been used after failed balloon septostomy and in older infants. In rare cases, surgical atrial septectomy may be required for successful relief of interatrial obstruction.

Typical findings at cardiac catheterization in TA include an inability to pass the catheter directly into the RV from the RA. This is highly suggestive, but not diagnostic of TA. Systemic venous oxygen saturation is typically low in proportion to the degree of systemic arterial desaturation. Right-to-left shunting across the atrial septum is present, yet some left-to-right shunting is reported to occur frequently in TA.[109] This results in an increase of 6% or more in O$_2$ saturations from superior vena cava to RA.[109] Because of mixing of systemic and pulmonary venous return, O$_2$ saturation in LV, RV, PA, and aorta are often similar, although incomplete mixing is common. In general, TA patients with normally related great vessels (type I) have lower oxygen saturation in all cardiac chambers, the vena cava, and the aorta than do patients with TA and D-transposition (type II). Pulmonary oligemia in type I patients accounts for this difference.

LVED pressure is usually normal or increased and may increase further with increasing Q$_p$:Q$_s$ or worsening LV function. LV systolic pressure may be elevated in patients with coarctation of the aorta or subaortic obstruction.[107] RV pressure depends on size of the VSD.

In patients in whom palliative cavopulmonary shunts are planned, cardiac catheterization can provide important hemodynamic and anatomic details. These include measurement of the PVR, the presence of PA distortion, and the location and size of single or bilateral superior venae cavae. Before the modified Fontan procedure, cardiac catheterization and cineangiography are recommended (1) to obtain precise hemodynamic information such as mean PA pressure, pulmonary arteriolar resistance, and LVED pressure; (2) to determine PA size, distribution, and identify distortions or arteriovenous fistulae from previous palliative procedures[30]; and (3) to assess ventricular function and atrioventricular valve competence.

MANAGEMENT OF TRICUSPID ATRESIA

Overview

The treatment of TA is mainly surgical. TA belongs to a family of lesions with single-ventricle anatomy, all of which are managed with a series of staged operations including modified Blalock-Taussig shunt, bidirectional cavopulmonary anastomosis, and completion of the Fontan. In most cases, the ultimate goal is to achieve physiologic "correction" of the anomaly with the Fontan operation or one of its modifications.[9,34,42]

Management of the Newborn with Decreased Pulmonary Blood Flow

Preoperative Critical Care

The neonatal management depends on the anatomic subtype of TA and particularly on whether pulmonary blood flow is decreased or increased. The surgical objective for newborns with TA and *decreased pulmonary blood flow* is to increase pulmonary blood flow with a systemic-to-PA shunt. Before surgical correction, the ductus arteriosus is the main source of pulmonary blood flow in these infants. Ductal closure may lead to severe hypoxemia, metabolic acidosis, and death. Therefore PGE₁ (0.05 mcg/kg/min) should be administered by continuous intravenous infusion to maintain patency of the ductus arteriosus and pulmonary blood flow.[100] Additional supportive therapy to prevent pulmonary vasoconstriction includes correction of acidosis, maintenance of normal blood glucose and calcium levels, and preservation of a neutral thermal environment.

Tracheal intubation or induction of anesthesia requires techniques that maintain normal PVR. The principal goal is to avoid worsening hypoxia and hypercapnia, which may increase PVR at the time of intubation.[71] Because tracheal stimulation may trigger pulmonary vasoconstriction,[55] some form of anesthesia is indicated to blunt pulmonary vasoconstriction at the time of intubation. Ketamine[57] or fentanyl[55] may accomplish this goal.

The Modified Blalock-Taussig Shunt in the Newborn

At present, a modified Blalock-Taussig shunt is the palliative procedure of choice for newborns with TA and decreased pulmonary blood flow.[30,122] The modified Blalock-Taussig shunt, which uses a polytetrafluoroethylene (Gore-Tex) graft interposed between the innominate or subclavian artery and the ipsilateral PA,[21] augments pulmonary blood flow, ideally resulting in a balanced circulation and a systemic arterial oxygen saturation (SaO₂) of approximately 75% to 80%.[30] This results in a Qp:Qs ratio between ~1 and 1.8. The Gore-Tex interposition prevents kinking of the systemic artery at its junction with the aortic arch.[89] The increased pulmonary blood flow provided by the systemic-to-PA shunt appears to enhance growth of the PAs,[43] providing favorable anatomic conditions for future cavopulmonary anastomosis.

Postoperative Critical Care Management after Blalock-Taussig Shunt

The postoperative management after Blalock-Taussig shunt placement is generally uncomplicated. The SaO₂ should be 75% to 80%, assuming absence of lung disease, adequate left ventricular function, and adequate flow through the shunt. Extubation is deferred until pulmonary blood flow is adequate and arterial oxygen saturations are stable. The differential diagnosis for SaO₂ below the desired range includes hypotension, shunt narrowing or occlusion, lung disease, and less commonly, inadequate shunt size. Measurement of a low system versus O₂ saturation (SvO₂) suggests inadequate systemic blood. Thus if lung disease and shunt obstruction can be excluded, supplemental fluid volume administration or inotropic drugs may be needed occasionally to optimize the perfusion-pressure gradient and maintain SaO₂ in the desired range. Anticoagulation by using low-dose heparin in the immediate postoperative period or aspirin in the long term to reduce the risk of shunt thrombosis remains controversial.

Pulmonary overcirculation arises if the shunt is too large and is manifested by pulmonary edema, SaO₂ greater than 85%, and difficulty in weaning from mechanical ventilation. Ipsilateral hemorrhagic pulmonary edema reflects unilateral

pulmonary overcirculation. Significant pulmonary overcirculation is generally an indication for return to the operating room to narrow the shunt size.

Obstruction of the shunt produces severe hypoxemia and represents an emergency. Auscultation for a "shunt murmur" with the bell of the stethoscope is an effective method of promptly assessing shunt flow at the bedside. The absence of the shunt murmur confirms the diagnosis, which may be confirmed by the absence of shunt flow on Doppler color flow imaging.[144] Shunt obstruction immediately after surgery probably requires reoperation, but in some cases, narrowing at the proximal anastomotic site may be treated with percutaneous balloon angioplasty. Local infusion of recombinant tissue plasminogen activator has been described for shunt thrombolysis.[102,117] Unexplained hypoxemia and difficulty with weaning from mechanical ventilation may arise from a variety of pulmonary problems. In addition to the obvious physical and radiographic findings, an increase in SaO₂ saturation with increasing inspired O₂ concentration indicates the presence of lung disease as the major factor in unexplained hypoxemia. Lung disease may take the form of chylothorax from thoracic duct injury, hemothorax from intercostal vessel injury, or atelectasis from phrenic nerve injury.

Management of the Newborn with Increased Pulmonary Blood Flow

Preoperative Critical Care

TA infants with *increased pulmonary blood flow* present with varying degrees of heart failure, depending on their precise anatomy, and may or may not need PGE₁, depending on the presence of obstruction to *systemic* blood flow. The major clinical decisions required in this patient population are whether systemic blood flow is obstructed and whether PA banding alone will limit pulmonary blood flow.

Infants with TA, normally related great vessels, and *increased pulmonary blood flow* (type IC) can initially be managed with medical anticongestive measures without the need for PA banding. However, if sufficient pulmonic stenosis does not develop by a few weeks of life, a PA band is likely needed to control pulmonary blood flow and protect the pulmonary vasculature. If the VSD begins to close, leading to a transition from congestive symptoms to cyanosis, meticulous follow-up will determine whether a modified Blalock-Taussig shunt (for infants younger than 3 months) or a bidirectional Glenn (BDG) shunt (for infants older than 3 months) should be offered as a stable source of pulmonary blood flow. If hypercyanotic spells occur before a surgical shunt is established, the infant receives the same management as for the classic tetrology spell ("tet spell") including 100% oxygen, analgesia (morphine, 0.1 mg/kg), beta blockade (esmolol infusion), or systemic vasoconstrictors (phenylephrine infusion, 1 to 10 mcg/kg/min to increase systemic pressure by 20% to 25%). A hypercyanotic episode represents an urgent indication for surgical palliation to provide stable pulmonary blood flow. Young infants with elevated PVR should receive a modified Blalock-Taussig shunt. Older infants with low pulmonary resistance may go directly to BDG shunt.

TA patients with a large VSD and *transposed* great arteries (type IIC) usually are initially seen with severe congestive heart failure. When these infants become critically ill, the management strategy is designed to achieve a balanced circulation (Q_p:$Q_s \approx 1$). To this end, the inspired O_2 concentration is reduced until SaO_2 equals 75% to 80%. Minute ventilation in mechanically ventilated infants is adjusted to maintain $PaCO_2$ of 40 to 50 mm Hg.

PGE_1 infusion also may be administered to the infant first seen with type IIC TA and aortic obstruction (coarctation of the aorta or aortic arch hypoplasia). Systemic blood flow and relief of heart failure in these patients depends on PGE_1 maintaining a PDA. Prostaglandin administration may be complicated by hypotension, apnea, hyperthermia, and seizures; accordingly, all infants must be closely monitored during this therapy.[78]

Pulmonary Artery Banding in the Newborn

Infants with TA, D-TGA, and nonrestrictive VSD are likely to have torrential pulmonary blood flow and heart failure, which cannot be managed by medical therapy alone, particularly if systemic vascular resistance (SVR) is increased by the presence of aortic obstruction. Furthermore, excessive pulmonary blood flow will lead to pulmonary vascular disease, which will make later Fontan operation impossible. Hence these patients require control of the pulmonary circulation, but the medical team must make this decision with great care, because PA banding entails the risk of accelerated narrowing of the VSD and resultant subaortic obstruction (19%).[38,122] PA distortion and ventricular hypertrophy represent two additional risks that should be considered before submitting the newborn to PA banding. The higher mortality rate for infants with TA and D-TGA compared with other forms of TA reflects these increased risks.[94]

PA banding can be performed through a left anterolateral thoracotomy but increasingly is approached through a median sternotomy because of superior access and the ability to institute bypass if needed. Banding involves passing a tape of synthetic material, such as Teflon, around the main PA and tightening the band until the PA pressure distal to the band is about one third to one half of the aortic pressure. Significant coarctation of the aorta must be corrected at the time of PA banding. Meticulous follow-up is required for optimal timing of the debanding and cavopulmonary anastomosis before significant subaortic obstruction develops.

The Damus–Kaye–Stansel Operation

The Damus–Kaye–Stansel operation (main PA-to-aorta anastomosis) may be useful in eliminating the need for PA banding in type IIC TA. When combined with a systemic-to-PA shunt to supply controlled pulmonary blood flow, the Damus–Kaye–Stansel operation addresses subaortic obstruction (Fig. 39-7).[94] When the VSD is inadequate

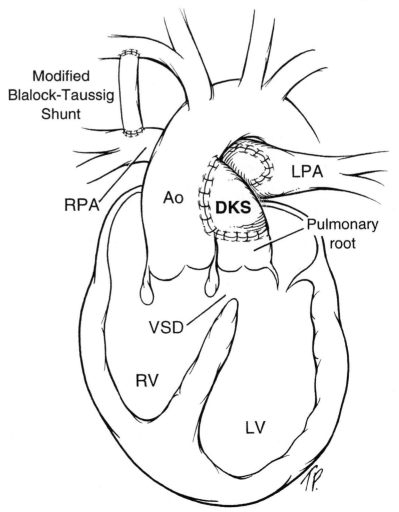

FIGURE 39-7 The Damus–Kaye–Stansel procedure for tricuspid atresia with transposition of the great arteries with subaortic obstruction. The main pulmonary artery (PA) and the proximal stump are anastomosed end-to-side to the ascending aorta. This provides a dependable source of systemic blood flow. A modified right Blalock–Taussig shunt is placed between the right innominate (or subclavian) artery and the right PA to provide pulmonary blood flow.

(less than ~2 cm²/m²), the Damus–Kaye–Stansel procedure combined with a Blalock-Taussig shunt appears superior to a PA band as a means of assuring adequate systemic flow and controlled pulmonary flow.[84] The Damus–Kaye–Stansel operation also has been combined with the BDG shunt to treat older infants with established subaortic obstruction.[26]

Management of the Older Infant

The goals of palliative treatment include alleviation of severe hypoxemia and cyanosis or congestive heart failure, as well as preservation of ventricular function and pulmonary vasculature until such time as the Fontan procedure can be performed safely.[72] The next step in the sequence of palliative operations becomes necessary around age 6 months to avoid ventricular hypertrophy and decreased ventricular function from excess ventricular volume (Blalock-Taussig shunt) or pressure (PA band).

The physiologic burden of volume overload of the LV becomes evident when one considers that an arterial O_2 saturation of 75% to 80% combined with adequate systemic perfusion (mixed venous O_2 saturation of 50% to 60%) implies a Qp:Qs ratio of 1:1 or greater. Even with a Qp:Qs ratio of 1:1, the systemic ventricle must eject a total of 5 L/min/m² to guarantee adequate flow (2.5 L/min/m² each) to the systemic and pulmonary circuits, respectively. Hence an obligatory volume load is associated with a Blalock-Taussig shunt.

The Bidirectional Glenn (Cavopulmonary) Anastomosis

In most cases of TA, the BDG represents the second operation and follows one of the operations performed during infancy and described earlier. For infants with marked pulmonary oligemia (e.g., type IA or IB), the BGD most commonly follows a Blalock-Taussig shunt. In those with pulmonary plethora (for example, type IC), the BDG most commonly follows a PA band. The BDG is performed after the PVR has reached its nadir and pulmonary musculature has regressed. When the BDG has been attempted in patients younger than 2 months, the results have been very unfavorable.

For a subset of infants with TA and pulmonic stenosis, either type IB or less commonly type IIB, the degree of pulmonic stenosis may be perfectly balanced to prevent pulmonary overcirculation (obviating the need for a PA band) without the risk of inadequate pulmonary blood flow (which would necessitate a systemic shunt). In this subset, it is sometimes possible for the BDG or even a fenestrated Fontan procedure to become the first surgical intervention.

Although practices vary somewhat from center to center, our preference is to submit all infants for a BDG anastomosis or the hemi-Fontan at age 6 months, followed by the completion Fontan procedure with an external conduit at about age 4 years and more than ~15 kg body weight. When the Fontan procedure is performed at a younger age, it is typically completed by using a "fenestrated" baffle (see later).

The BDG is usually performed via median sternotomy to allow the use of cardiopulmonary bypass (CPB) and visualization of the branch pulmonary arteries in the event that PA reconstruction is needed. Cardioplegic arrest of the heart is not necessary. The SVC or innominate vein as well as the inferior vena cava (IVC) and aorta are cannulated for CPB.

The SVC is transected, and the cephalad end anastomosed to the right PA with absorbable suture (Fig. 39-8). The cardiac end of the SVC is oversewn. Previous systemic-to-PA shunts are taken down, and other sources of pulmonary blood flow, such as PDA, are interrupted. Some surgeons leave a small amount of RV-to-PA antegrade flow if present, in the hope of reducing the incidence of hepatic arteriovenous malformations and promoting PA growth with pulsatile flow. After the BDG, IVC blood flows through the ASD into the left heart.

Hemi-Fontan Procedure

The hemi-Fontan procedure is physiologically identical to the BDG and carries the same indications. In the hemi-Fontan, a large confluence of the SVC, upper RA, and right PA is created (Fig. 39-9).[29,62] IVC and coronary sinus blood are partitioned from the PA by a homograft or polytetrafluoroethylene (PTFE) baffle. Thus only SVC flow is directed to the PA, whereas IVC blood crosses the ASD, making this a BDG in physiologic terms. At the subsequent Fontan operation, the partition between right PA and RA is excised, and a lateral tunnel or baffle is created from the IVC to the SVC–right PA anastomosis.

Postoperative Critical Care Management after Bidirectional Glenn Anastomosis or Hemi-Fontan Procedure

SaO_2 saturation of 80% to 85% is usually well tolerated after BDG or hemi-Fontan. Ventricular preload and cardiac output are maintained by the contribution of IVC blood flow into the left heart via the ASD. This is in marked contrast to the Fontan operation, in which left heart preload is entirely dependent on pulmonary venous return. The most common postoperative abnormality includes excessive hypoxemia (SaO_2 <70%). Excessive hypoxemia may be due to pulmonary disease, pulmonary hypertension, ventricular dysfunction, or stenosis at the Glenn anastomosis (Fig. 39-10).

Decreased pulmonary blood flow secondary to mechanical obstruction of the SVC-RPA anastomosis should be ruled out intraoperatively by using echocardiography. Elevated systemic venous pressure with normal PA pressure suggests obstruction at the caval-PA anastomotic site or the proximal PA, which may be due to thrombosis or PA distortion after previous PA surgery (e.g., systemic-to-PA shunt or PA band). Even a small SVC-PA pressure gradient (2 to 3 mm Hg) may reflect significant obstruction. If transthoracic echocardiography does not allow adequate visualization of the minor pressure gradients within the atrial baffle or the SVC-PA anastomosis, cardiac catheterization may be required for diagnosis. Management in this setting may consist of thrombolytic therapy, interventional cardiac catheterization, or reoperation.

Elevation of PVR is suggested by a high transpulmonary pressure gradient (SVC pressure – atrial pressure) in the absence of residual anatomic gradient between SVC and PA. Therapy should be directed toward lowering PVR to promote pulmonary blood flow. Mechanical ventilatory parameters are set to maintain mean airway pressure at a minimum consistent with adequate lung inflation (see Chapter 12 on Respiratory Support). Evacuation of pleural effusions and chylothorax may decrease intrathoracic pressure and increase

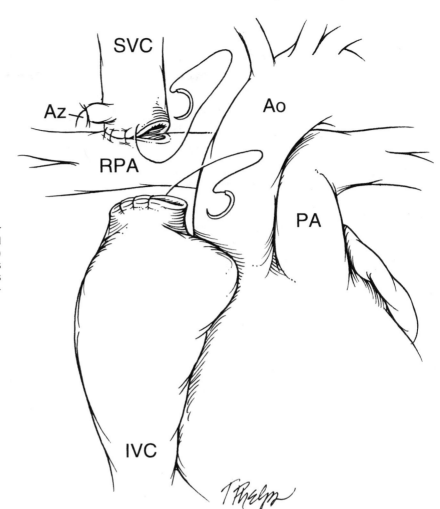

FIGURE 39-8 The bidirectional Glenn operation. After transection of the superior vena cava (SVC), the cephalad end is anastomosed to the right pulmonary artery (RPA) and the cardiac end of the SVC is oversewn. The azygous (Az) vein is ligated. Inferior vena cava (IVC) blood flows through the atrial septal defect (ASD) and thus contributes to left ventricular preload. Ao, aorta.

pulmonary blood flow (see later).[73] Early extubation is attempted when feasible to return intrathoracic pressures to atmospheric levels.[127] If ventilatory failure prevents extubation, phrenic nerve injury must be ruled out. Nitric oxide inhalation (5 to 50 ppm) has become the standard therapy to dilate the pulmonary vascular bed.

Worsening ventricular function after BDG is rare, because removal of a portion of the preoperative volume loading usually results in improved ventricular function. When ventricular dysfunction does occur, it is usually related to preoperative ventricular dysfunction, abnormal loading conditions, or other effects of CPB on myocardial performance. Ventricular dysfunction is diagnosed by the signs of decreased systemic perfusion and oxygen delivery, increased atrial pressures, and abnormal shortening fraction on echocardiography. Administration of milrinone will increase the force of ventricular contraction, decrease SVR and PVR, and may increase cardiac output.

Coronary air embolism represents a preventable cause of postoperative myocardial dysfunction in *any* patient with an intracardiac right-to-left shunt. With the infant in the supine position, air bubbles lodge preferentially in the right coronary artery because of its anterior location. Myocardial dysfunction is due to regional myocardial ischemia from intracoronary air block. The depression in myocardial function is proportional to the size of the air bubble.[135] Prevention of coronary air embolism relies on intraoperative de-airing procedures and postoperative avoidance of air within intravenous lines. Air filters and air detectors within intravenous lines may provide some protection but do not eliminate the need for repetitive, meticulous inspection of intravenous lines so that air can be removed in a timely fashion, particularly from stopcock connections.

Potential Long-Term Complications after Bidirectional Glenn or Hemi-Fontan

"Venous shunts," such as the BDG or hemi-Fontan, do not produce volume overload but have other limitations. Whereas an SaO_2 of 80% to 85% is usually achievable, which allows growth of the young child, this degree of desaturation does not provide good palliation in the older child and adult. As the child grows, the IVC blood assumes a greater proportion of ventricular preload, and pulmonary

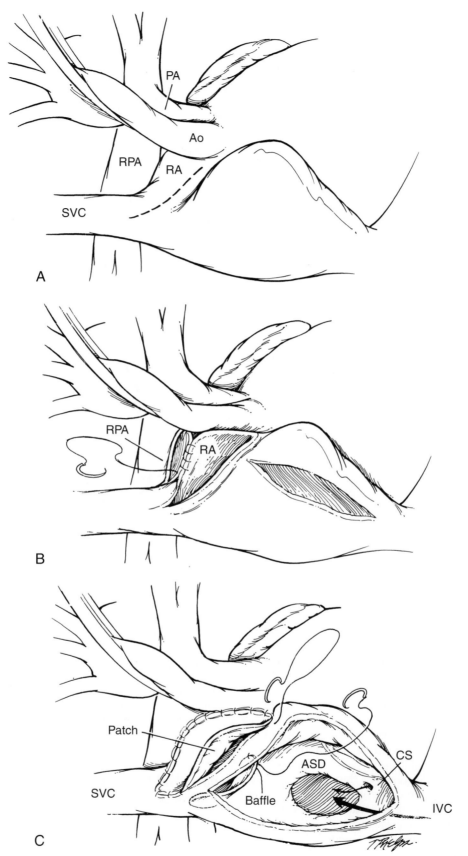

FIGURE 39-9 The hemi-Fontan operation. **A,** The hemi-Fontan operation from the surgical view showing spiral incision extending from the superior vena cava (SVC) onto the surface of the right atrium (RA). **B,** After incision of the right pulmonary artery (RPA), a vascular confluence is created incorporating the cardiac end of the SVC, cephalad portion of the RA, and RPA. **C,** This confluence is roofed with a patch of polytetrafluoroethylene (PTFE). A second PTFE baffle forms the floor of this confluence and separates the inferior vena cava (IVC) and coronary sinus (CS) blood from the SVC blood, thus allowing IVC and coronary blood to enter the left atrium via the atrial septal defect (ASD). Ao, aorta.

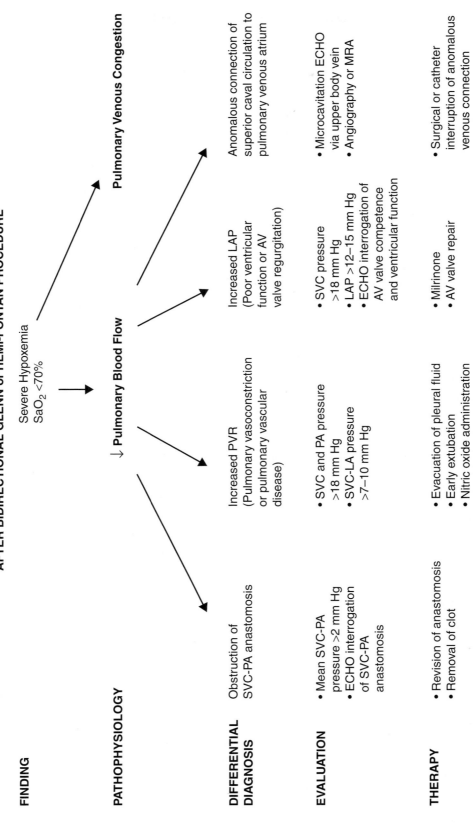

FIGURE 39-10 Management algorithm for hypoxemia after the bidirectional Glenn or hemi-Fontan procedure. AV, atrioventricular; CVP, central venous pressure; ECHO, echocardiogram; IVC, inferior vena cava; LA, left atrium; PA, pulmonary artery; SaO₂, oxygen saturation; SVC, superior vena cava.

venous return from the BDG assumes a lesser proportion. Hence arterial desaturation tends to increase over time.

The development of veno-venous collaterals also may contribute to worsening cyanosis. The elevated central venous pressure (CVP) associated with BDG may recannalize vestigial venous channels (pericardial, azygous, or diaphragmatic veins), which then drain into the pulmonary veins, left atrium, or IVC.[88] Interventional or surgical closure of these collaterals can improve arterial oxygen saturation.

All shunts, whether prosthetic or of native tissue, carry a small risk of endocarditis, probably less than 1% per year. Because of this and the fact that surgical shunts are usually placed in patients with significant intracardiac defects, all shunt patients should receive prophylactic antibiotics according to the recommendations of the American Heart Association for high-risk patients (see Chapter 45 on Endocarditis).

The Fontan Operation

The Fontan operation is not a specific operation but rather a class of operations that separate the pulmonary and systemic circulations in patients with single-ventricle physiology. This separation is accomplished by directing all systemic venous return to the pulmonary vascular bed. The physiologic benefits of the Fontan include better systemic oxygenation, reduced volume loading of the systemic ventricle, and reduced risk of paradoxical embolism through right-to-left shunts. The cost of this physiologic change is elevated systemic venous pressure.

Fontan[34] achieved the first clinical success treating TA by closing the ASD and establishing a connection between the RA and PA. Initially, it was thought that the atrium was needed to pump systemic venous return into the lungs, and that valves were essential to the circuit. However, subsequent studies disproved both assumptions.[27] More recently, establishment of direct connections of the vena cavae to the PAs has been shown to provide superior hemodynamics. Fontan's original operation is no longer performed, and all subsequent modifications of the original procedure have been termed "modified Fontan," although this term is probably unnecessary.

Surgical Options for the Fontan Operation

Total Cavopulmonary Connection Recognition of the excellent hemodynamic results of the BDG shunt and the elegant in vitro experiments by deLeval[20] have made the total cavopulmonary connection an attractive method of connection of the systemic veins to the PA in the Fontan circulation. Now general consensus exists that the goal of this connection should be to preserve laminar, nonpulsatile flow through a straight, nonvalved passageway and to make minimal use of prosthetic material. These goals can be met by use of the BDG shunt in combination with a lateral tunnel within the RA, resulting in a "total" cavopulmonary connection (Fig. 39-11). The latter modification involves septating the RA with a tube of prosthetic material (Gore-Tex) to create a tunnel along the lateral aspect of the atrium through which blood from the IVC is directed to the SVC and then to the undersurface of the right PA.[20]

An alternative approach to the total cavopulmonary connection involves the placement of an extracardiac circumferential prosthetic tube or aortic homograft outside the RA (extracardiac Fontan).[74,82] This conduit or homograft connects the IVC, which has been divided at the RA-IVC junction, to the PA (Fig. 39-12). The extracardiac approach avoids several potential hazards of intracardiac Fontan approaches. It can be performed without CPB. The surgeon does not manipulate the area of the sinus node or place suture lines in the atrium. Finally, the absence of atrial distention and atrial suture lines may decrease the risk of postoperative dysrhythmias.[103] Although the overall operative mortality rate does not differ between extracardiac and lateral-tunnel Fontan patients, comparative data from a single institution suggest that the postoperative course for the lateral-tunnel group may be more complicated with longer duration of ventilatory support, chest tube drainage, and intensive care unit (ICU) stay.[3]

Fenestrated Fontan The sudden diversion of the entire systemic venous return to the pulmonary circuit may result in low systemic blood flow and high systemic venous pressures, particularly in the high-risk Fontan patient (Table 39-2). Fenestration of the lateral-tunnel or extracardiac conduit addresses these problems by shunting systemic venous blood through the fenestration to the left atrium (Fig. 39-13). This decompresses the Fontan circuit and augments systemic blood flow, albeit at the expense of O_2 desaturation. The resultant physiologic state is similar to the BDG shunt (see Fig. 39-8). The fenestration is created with 3- to 6-mm punch hole in the wall of the tunnel or conduit.

Twenty-nine percent of fenestrations close spontaneously within 3 months.[133] For those patients in whom spontaneous closure does not occur, the fenestration can be closed by using a ductal or septal occlusion device in the catheterization laboratory.

The long-term risk/benefit ratio of fenestration remains controversial. Whereas it is clear that many high-risk patients will not tolerate a Fontan operation at all, unless it is accompanied by a fenestration, the situation in the low-risk patient is less clear. Some data suggest that routine fenestration of all Fontan patients (not just high-risk candidates) may decrease pleural drainage and hospital length of stay.[75] However, these immediate benefits must be weighed against the risks of paradoxical embolism, lower O_2 saturation, as well as the risks of interventional catheterization to close the fenestration.

Risk factors for the Fontan operation have been outlined in several large series.[35,86] *Elevated PVR* is an important risk factor for perioperative death.[87,94] In addition to pulmonary vascular disease, pulmonary microthrombi should be considered a possible cause, especially in the polycythemic patient (hemoglobin concentration, 16 to 22 g/dL). Management is further complicated because polycythemia and decreased pulmonary blood flow falsely elevate the calculated PVR.[97] Some groups have found lung biopsy helpful in distinguishing irreversible pulmonary vascular disease from pulmonary microthrombi.[101] Others have found no clear relation between biopsy results and pulmonary arterial lesions or PVR.[48,65,143] Impaired ventricular function, especially diastolic ventricular function, is an important risk factor for the Fontan operation. Decreased compliance of the LV leads to

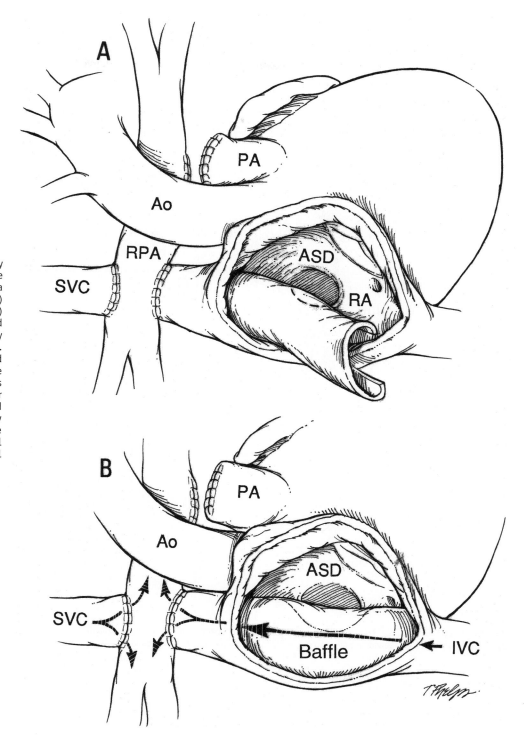

FIGURE 39-11 Total cavopulmonary anastomosis using intracaval baffle technique. Previous superior vena cava (SVC)–right pulmonary artery (RPA) anastomosis (bidirectional Glenn shunt) is in place. SVC cannula was removed during deep hypothermia and circulatory arrest. **A,** Right atrium (RA) is opened. Caudal segment end of the transected SVC is anastomosed to the surface of the RPA. Atrial septal defect (ASD) is enlarged but sparing the atrioventricular node. **B,** Intra-atrial baffle is fashioned from Gore-Tex and positioned to convey inferior vena cava (IVC) blood to the SVC-RPA anastomosis. The posterolateral wall of the pathway is the right atrial wall. Ao, aorta.

increased LVED pressure (LVEDP) and LA pressure, which reduces the perfusion pressure gradient (SVC – LA pressure) for inflow into the LV.

AV valve incompetence also must be considered in the differential diagnosis of elevated LA pressure. If valve incompetence is sufficiently advanced to produce a marginal transpulmonary pressure, valve replacement will have to be considered before or at the time of the Fontan repair.

A small PA size increases the risk of death or take-down after the Fontan operation. The clinical problem has been to define the lower limit of PA size that would permit the Fontan operation. Cineangiographic measures of PA diameter (McGoon ratio) or area (Nakata index) may supplement the clinical impression of small PAs.[96] Even small PAs do not necessarily contraindicate the Fontan operation as long as PA size can be augmented at operation.[11]

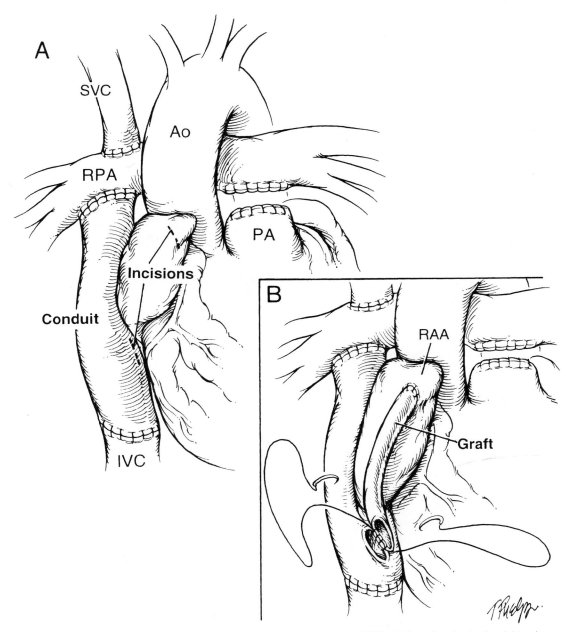

FIGURE 39-12   Extracardiac Fontan. **A,** An external conduit connects the inferior vena cava (IVC) and hepatic veins to the right pulmonary artery (RPA). **B,** If a "fenestration" is needed, a graft can be interposed between the external conduit and the right atrial appendage (RAA), allowing egress of systemic venous blood into the right atrium. Ao, aorta; PA, pulmonary artery.

Subaortic obstruction is a major risk factor for death in candidates for the Fontan operation. Echo-Doppler or cardiac catheterization is used to define the presence of subaortic obstruction. A resting gradient greater than 10 mm Hg between the dominant ventricle and the aorta is a specific (but not sensitive) test for the presence of subaortic obstruction.[36] Morphologic criteria of obstruction such as a VSD diameter less than 0.5 times the aortic ring diameter provide a more sensitive test than pressure gradients; however, the search for obstruction must include all levels of the systemic outflow tract.

The impact of age on operative risk remains controversial. Although large retrospective analyses have found no significant effect of age at operation on outcome,[81] delaying the Fontan operation exposes the child to risks of paradoxical embolism, chronic hypoxia, and subaortic obstruction. Franklin et al.[36] noted that whereas 86% of their patients were considered candidates for later Fontan operation when evaluated as infants, 40% had either died or developed adverse features precluding the Fontan operation by the time they reached age 4 years. The extracardiac Fontan, which has the advantage of not requiring CPB in some patients, must be delayed until the child is large enough to accommodate an 18- to 20-mm diameter conduit. Conversely, the lateral-tunnel Fontan incorporates atrial tissue with growth potential as part of the tunnel wall. This permits an earlier age at operation, albeit at the

Table 39-2 Preoperative Risk Assessment
in Candidates for the Fontan Operation

Variable	Low Risk	Medium Risk	High Risk
PVR (Wood units)	<2	2–4	>4
Mean PAP (mm Hg)	<15	15–20	>20
LVEDP (mm Hg)	<8	8–12	>12
EF (%)	>60	45–60	<45
Systemic outflow obstruction	<10 mm Hg LV-Ao gradient	For TA with TGA: • >10 mm Hg gradient from main ventricle to Ao • Diameter of VSD <0.5× diameter of aortic ring on echocardiography or angiography	

PVR, pulmonary vascular resistance; PAP, pulmonary artery pressure; LVEDP, left ventricular end diastolic pressure; LV, left ventricle; Ao, aorta; TA, tricuspid atresia; VSD, ventricular septal defect; EF, ejection fraction.

cost of requiring bypass and incurring an increased risk of pleural effusions and arrhythmias. To date, no randomized, controlled trial of earlier lateral tunnel versus later extracardiac Fontan has been conducted.

Anesthetic Management for the Fontan Operation

The anesthetic management of Fontan candidates is dictated by the physiology of the Fontan circulation. Some patients may be polycythemic, which is aggravated by preoperative dehydration from a long fasting period. Thus polycythemic patients should have intravenous access established once oral intake is prohibited. Special care is taken to prevent air embolism once the intravenous line is started, as all infants

after BDG or hemi-Fontan have large right-to-left shunts at the atrial level.

Either intravenous or inhalational techniques can be used for induction and maintenance of anesthesia as long as significant increases in PVR and depression of ventricular function are avoided. Neither nitrous oxide nor ketamine produces pulmonary vasoconstriction in infants.[57,58] Thus these agents may be suitable for induction. Fentanyl blunts the increase in PVR and PA pressure associated with laryngoscopy and incision, and thus most groups use high-dose fentanyl and 100% O_2.[59,60]

Standard monitoring is used, as in any pediatric heart operation. The decision on the use of invasive monitoring lines must balance the risk of clot formation in the Fontan circuit against the risk of insufficient information to manage low cardiac output postoperatively. The high-risk Fontan patient undergoing CPB is a candidate for full invasive monitoring. The length of the central venous line in the internal jugular vein must be carefully estimated not to encroach on the surgical field in the SVC. The surgeon can insert additional monitoring lines into the PA and LA after the repair has been completed. Intraoperative transesophageal echocardiography constitutes another valuable monitoring tool to assess patency of the anastomosis, ventricular function, and atrioventricular valve competency.

POSTOPERATIVE PROBLEMS AFTER THE FONTAN OPERATION

Low Cardiac Output Syndrome: Overview

Recent innovations, including the fenestration, the possibility of performing the (extracardiac) Fontan without CPB,

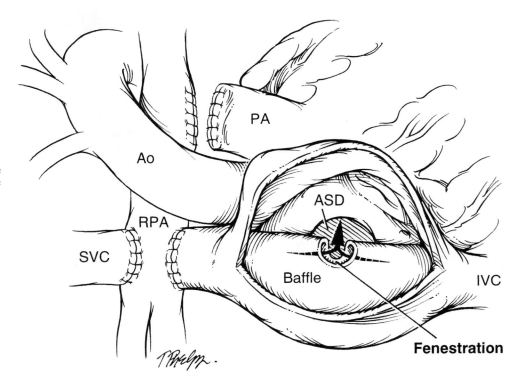

FIGURE 39-13 The fenestrated Fontan. A fenestration is created in the wall of the intra-atrial baffle, allowing egress of systemic venous blood into the atria. Ao, aorta; ASD, atrial septal defect; IVC, inferior vena cava; PA, pulmonary artery; SVC, superior vena cava.

and modified ultrafiltration for Fontan cases done with bypass, have made low cardiac output syndrome much less common than in prior years. However, the consequences can be life-threatening when low cardiac output syndrome does occur, usually in a high-risk patient.

After the Fontan operation, cardiac output is dependent on pulmonary blood flow. Because the single ventricle fills passively, blood return to the left atrium is dependent on the transpulmonary pressure gradient between systemic venous pressure and (left) atrial pressure. In general, adequate pulmonary blood flow requires a transpulmonary pressure gradient of about 7 mm Hg.[22,67]

Any reduction of pulmonary blood flow will reduce systemic oxygen delivery. The major manifestations include poorly perfused extremities, hypotension, metabolic acidosis, and oliguria.[22] Some conditions which limit pulmonary blood flow include hypovolemia, increased PVR or SVR, distortion of the PAs, obstruction of the Fontan circuit, pulmonary venous obstruction, AV valve regurgitation, and systolic or diastolic ventricular dysfunction.[51,64,126] Analysis of systemic venous, PA, and left atrial pressures can provide important insight into the causes of abnormal convalescence, which are manifested clinically by low cardiac output syndrome (Fig. 39-14).

Hypovolemia

The most readily reversible cause of low cardiac output syndrome after the Fontan operation is hypovolemia. Fluid volume administration is frequently required because systemic ventricular output is dependent on adequate preload represented by pulmonary venous return, which, in turn, depends on recruitment of the pulmonary vascular bed. Systemic venous hypertension after the Fontan operation also leads to transudation of fluid from systemic veins into the interstitial space. This loss of intravascular fluid must be replaced to maintain cardiac output. Supplemental fluid volume is typically needed when LA pressure (LAP), cardiac output, and mixed venous O_2 saturation are low (see Fig. 39-14). Additional fluid administration is terminated once LA pressure reaches 8 to 10 mm Hg or the CVP-LAP gradient is less than 5 to 7 mm Hg.

Obstruction of Superior Vena Cava–Pulmonary Artery Anastomosis

Although obstruction of the caval-PA anastomosis is a larger concern at the time of the BDG (see earlier), it remains a threat to the Fontan patient. The causes and management of

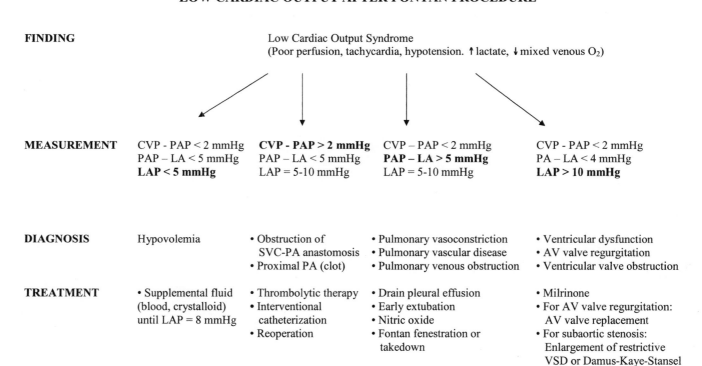

MANAGEMENT ALGORITHM for
LOW CARDIAC OUTPUT AFTER FONTAN PROCEDURE

FINDING	Low Cardiac Output Syndrome (Poor perfusion, tachycardia, hypotension. ↑lactate, ↓mixed venous O_2)			
MEASUREMENT	CVP - PAP < 2 mmHg PAP – LA < 5 mmHg **LAP < 5 mmHg**	**CVP - PAP > 2 mmHg** PAP – LA < 5 mmHg LAP = 5-10 mmHg	CVP – PAP < 2 mmHg **PAP – LA > 5 mmHg** LAP = 5-10 mmHg	CVP - PAP < 2 mmHg PA – LA < 4 mmHg **LAP > 10 mmHg**
DIAGNOSIS	Hypovolemia	• Obstruction of SVC-PA anastomosis • Proximal PA (clot)	• Pulmonary vasoconstriction • Pulmonary vascular disease • Pulmonary venous obstruction	• Ventricular dysfunction • AV valve regurgitation • Ventricular valve obstruction
TREATMENT	• Supplemental fluid (blood, crystalloid) until LAP = 8 mmHg	• Thrombolytic therapy • Interventional catheterization • Reoperation	• Drain pleural effusion • Early extubation • Nitric oxide • Fontan fenestration or takedown	• Milrinone • For AV valve regurgitation: AV valve replacement • For subaortic stenosis: Enlargement of restrictive VSD or Damus-Kaye-Stansel procedure

FIGURE 39-14 Algorithm for management of low-cardiac-output syndrome after Fontan procedure. AV, atrioventricular; CVP, central venous pressure; LAP, left atrial pressure; PA, pulmonary artery; PAP, pulmonary artery pressure; SVC, superior vena cava; VSD, ventricular septal defect.

the obstruction are the same as those after BDG, but the initial manifestation is low cardiac output in the Fontan patient rather than the worsening hypoxemia in the BDG patient.

Pulmonary Vasoconstriction Versus Vascular Disease versus Pulmonary Venous Obstruction

Elevation of both CVP and PA pressures with normal LA pressure suggests (reactive) pulmonary vasoconstriction, (fixed) pulmonary vascular disease, or pulmonary venous obstruction. Several therapeutic and diagnostic steps are indicated. Normoglycemia, normocalcemia, euthermia, and adequate sedation are verified or restored if necessary. Nitric oxide is administered as a pulmonary vasodilator. Ventilator settings are rechecked to ensure normal blood gas values. Positive end-expiratory pressure (PEEP) maintains functional residual capacity and increases PaO_2 after the Fontan procedure.[142] However, PVR is increased at all levels of PEEP (3 to 12 cm H_2O), and cardiac index is decreased at high levels of PEEP (9 to 12 cm H_2O) (Fig. 39-15).[142]

Doppler echocardiography is performed to confirm unobstructed drainage of all four pulmonary veins into the (left) atrium. Stenotic pulmonary veins are very difficult to treat. Although balloon dilation and placement of stents have been used, the results have been poor. Pulmonary venous obstruction should be diagnosed preoperatively and treated, if possible, before the Fontan procedure or at the time of operation, because pulmonary venous obstruction is poorly tolerated.

If these correctable causes of pulmonary hypertension are excluded, then previously unrecognized pulmonary vascular disease is the likely cause. The physician team must urgently consider fenestration of the Fontan pathway or even takedown of the Fontan repair, if pulmonary hypertension is accompanied by low cardiac output and hemodynamic instability.[22] Fontan takedown converts the patient back to BDG physiology such that IVC blood passes through the interatrial communication and supports ventricular output.

Ventricular Dysfunction Versus Atrioventricular Valve Regurgitation Versus Ventricular Outflow Tract Obstruction

Low cardiac output syndrome in the presence of elevated CVP, PA, and LA pressures indicates ventricular dysfunction, AV valvar regurgitation, or ventricular outflow tract obstruction or pericardial effusion or constriction.[98,126] Doppler echocardiography is used to make the definitive diagnosis. The major cause of postoperative ventricular dysfunction is preoperative ventricular dysfunction caused by chronic volume overload and hypoxia. A hypertrophied ventricle with marginal compliance preoperatively may become less compliant postoperatively because of prolonged aortic cross-clamp time and the potential myocardial ischemia.

Chin et al.[16] suggested that immediate relief of ventricular volume overload by the Fontan operation leads to changes in ventricular geometry. The net result is an increase in ventricular wall thickness and a decrease in chamber volume, which may affect diastolic and systolic function unfavorably.

Ventricular dysfunction also may result from failure to incorporate the coronary sinus into the LA. If the coronary

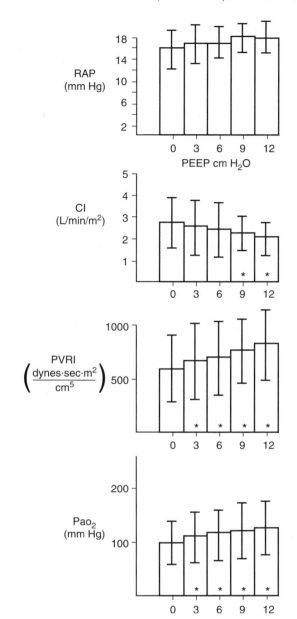

FIGURE 39-15 Effect of positive end-expiratory pressure (PEEP) on right atrial pressure (RAP), cardiac index (CI), pulmonary vascular resistance index (PVRI), and partial arterial oxygen pressure (PaO_2). PEEP has detrimental hemodynamic effects in the Fontan circulation as PVRI is increased and CI decreased. (From Williams DB, Kiernan PD, Metke MP, et al: Hemodynamic response to positive end-expiratory pressure following right atrium–pulmonary artery bypass [Fontan procedure]. *J Thorac Cardiovasc Surg* 87:856–861, 1984, with permission.)

sinus remains in the RA after the Fontan operation, coronary sinus drainage may be impeded by high RA pressures.

Catecholamine inotropic agents, which improve systolic function, may actually worsen diastolic function by impairing ventricular relaxation, in part because of their chronotropic effects. Vasodilators are often helpful when ventricular dysfunction is present. However, cardiac output is preload limited in the postoperative Fontan patient. Therefore vasodilators must be used cautiously in these patients, who are sensitive to reductions in filling pressure.

Phosphodiesterase inhibitors (milrinone) are probably the best agents to treat ventricular dysfunction in the Fontan patient, because they improve both diastolic and systolic function. Extracorporeal membrane oxygenation (ECMO) has been used infrequently to support the circulation after the Fontan procedure.[124]

AV valve regurgitation may be due to either a preexisting abnormal valve or a chronic volume load on the single ventricle in the preoperative period.[126] In either case, AV valve regurgitation is poorly tolerated in the postoperative period, because of the critical dependence of this physiology on ventricular filling. The mortality rate increases when valve replacement is necessary with a Fontan operation.[66] Afterload reduction coupled with preload augmentation and mild increases in inotropy with milrinone, low-dose dopamine, or dobutamine may be helpful in these patients. Valve repair is encouraged to reduce AV valve regurgitation at the time of Fontan.

Ventricular outflow tract obstruction results in a pressure load on a previously volume-loaded heart. This worsens ventricular systolic and diastolic function, increasing the risk of a poor outcome after Fontan.[36] The diagnosis should be made before Fontan surgery is contemplated, and the patency of the systemic outflow tract should be assessed by intraoperative echocardiography. If subaortic obstruction is identified, therapeutic options include enlargement of the restrictive VSD or anastomosis of the proximal PA to the side of the aorta (Damus-Kaye-Stansel) to bypass the obstruction.[15,94]

Unexplained Hypoxemia

Postoperative assessment of oxygenation requires clear understanding of the type of Fontan operation performed. If the tunnel or conduit is intentionally fenestrated, some degree of arterial desaturation is anticipated as systemic venous blood bypasses the lung and contributes to systemic cardiac output. If no fenestration is present, then persistent hypoxemia reflects lung disease, unrecognized right-to-left shunts, or low cardiac output syndrome (Table 39-3). Lung disease is assessed by auscultation, chest radiography, and measurement of lung compliance. Minor pulmonary infiltrates are common after thoracic surgery and CPB; however, arterial O_2 saturation of 100% should be readily achievable with mechanical ventilation and FiO_2 less than 0.6 within the first 12 to 24 hours. This goal may not be achievable in the face of significant lung disease because of atelectasis or increased interstitial fluid after prolonged CPB.

If the hypoxemia is disproportionate to the extent of lung disease on chest radiograph, right-to-left intracardiac shunts should be ruled out with echocardiography by using Doppler or contrast techniques or cardiac catheterization if necessary. Assuming the absence of a fenestration, abnormal systemic venous connections represent the most likely cause, as discussed earlier under BDG. If hypoxemia from abnormal systemic venous connections is sufficiently severe to prevent extubation, reoperation or interventional catheterization will be required.

Low cardiac output may cause hypoxemia by leading to an increase in systemic O_2 extraction, which in turn results in a lowered systemic venous O_2 saturation (SvO_2). In the presence of some degree of ventilation-perfusion mismatch in the

Table 39-3 Differential Diagnosis of Unexpected Hypoxemia after Fontan Procedure

Cause	Diagnosis	Therapy
Lung disease (atelectasis, pneumonia, pulmonary edema)	• Significant infiltrates on chest radiograph • Poor lung compliance (peak airway pressure, >30–35 cm H_2O) • Positive culture from tracheal secretions	• Suctioning, chest physiotherapy • Long exhalation time (I:E = 1:5) • Antibiotics
Unrecognized abnormal systemic venous connections	• Echocardiography (Doppler or micro-cavitation contrast) • Cardiac catheterization	• Observation if patient can be weaned from mechanical ventilation • Coil occlusion (interventional catherization) • Reoperation
Low cardiac output	• SvO_2 <50% • Echocardiography for ventricular function, AV valve competence, patency of cavopulmonary anastomosis, etc.	• Depends on the etiology of low cardiac output (see Fig. 39-14)

CHF, congestive heart failure; AV, atrioventricular.

lung, systemic venous blood with low SvO_2 may not achieve 100% O_2 saturation after passing through the pulmonary circuit. The diagnosis is made by measuring mixed venous SvO_2. Blood samples from the SVC are adequate for this purpose, because SVC O_2 saturation correlates with PA O_2 saturation, with a correlation coefficient of 0.86.[91] The therapy is to improve cardiac output.

Complications of Systemic Venous Hypertension

All patients undergoing Fontan operations have elevated systemic venous pressure. Systemic venous hypertension leads to a hydrostatic pressure gradient favoring transudation of fluid into the interstitium and particularly into serosal cavities. Therefore Fontan patients may exhibit pleural effusions, edema, ascites, and protein-losing enteropathy.[66]

Pleural effusions are the most common postoperative abnormality after a Fontan operation.[47] Fenestration of the Fontan decreases the duration of chest-tube drainage significantly.[75] Some effusions represent true chylothorax or have a composition suggestive of chyle. The etiology may represent injury to peritracheal lymphatics. More commonly, a diffuse oozing of lymphatic fluid is seen within the chest, probably resulting from transmission of elevated systemic venous pressure to the lymphatic system through the thoracic duct.[80,134] Activation of the renin-angiotensin-aldosterone system also may contribute to fluid retention.[80]

The primary management goal for the Fontan patient with a pleural-effusion is to prevent cardiorespiratory embarrassment. Relatively small effusions in any patient after Fontan may exert detectable deleterious effects on hemodynamics in the first few postoperative days. The presence of the effusion leads to a reduction in intrathoracic

Table 39-4 Composition of Pleural Fluid in Different Conditions

Condition	Appearance	Cells/µL	Protein (g/dL)	LDH (IU/L)	Glucose (mg/dL)	Other
CHF	Serous	<1000 lymphs	PF/S, <0.5	PF/S, <0.6	= S	—
Bacterial infection	Variable	>10,000 PMNs	1.4–6.1	<700	= S	—
Viral infection	Serous	<6000 mononuclears	3.2–4.9	PF/S, >0.6	= S	—
Chylothorax	Milky, bloody, turbid, or serous	2000–20,000 lymphs	>3.0	PF/S, >0.6	= S	Triglyceride, >110 mg/dL

CHF, congestive heart failure; PF/S, pleural fluid/serum ratio; lymphs, lymphocytes; PMN, polymorphonuclear leukocyte; S, serum.
From Sahn SA: State of the art: The pleura. *Am Rev Respir Dis* 138:184–234, 1988, with permission.

compliance and an increase in mean airway pressure during mechanical ventilation. This process is further aggravated if ascites is present, which elevates the diaphragm and reduces intrathoracic compliance to an even greater extent. The increase in mean airway pressure limits venous return, pulmonary blood flow, and cardiac output. In these circumstances, a catheter is placed in the affected site to drain the effusion completely.

If the characteristics of the pleural fluid are most consistent with chyle (Table 39-4), the child's nutrition also may require modification. The fat source in the diet should consist of medium-chain triglycerides rather than long-chain triglycerides. It may be necessary to discontinue all enteral feedings and rely exclusively on parenteral nutrition (see Chapter 15 on Nutrition). Serum protein and albumin levels should be monitored closely, as hypoalbuminemia is a frequent complication of persistent chylothorax. The low oncotic pressure resulting from hypoalbuminemia exacerbates the tendency for fluid retention in Fontan patients, and albumin replacement therapy may become necessary.

When a child, who exhibits evidence of a good hemodynamic result, develops an effusion several days after operation, enough reserve usually exists to permit a period of observation. In some cases, diuretic therapy may be tried. Thoracentesis is indicated when early signs of hemodynamic compromise are present (i.e., decreased appetite, irritability, respiratory distress, or evidence of diminished systemic perfusion). Chest roentgenograms, although quantitatively imprecise, constitute the most convenient means to judge pleural effusions. An ultrasound of the chest offers more precise information on the size and location of the effusion.

As the child progresses further into the postoperative course, the volume of effusion necessary to produce symptoms typically increases. When the effusions are voluminous or protracted, a hemodynamic evaluation should be conducted to determine the presence of anatomic pathology amenable to further surgery. Similarly, the late development of effusions in a child who did not have them in the immediate postoperative period, or rapid resurgence of previously quiescent effusions, usually signals a hemodynamically important problem.

Passive congestion of the liver is a common finding after the Fontan operation. Although some elevation of hepatic enzymes often accompanies this congestion, impaired hepatosynthetic function or cholestasis rarely occurs. Liver dysfunction presumably reflects hepatic ischemia, because it correlates with decreased cardiac index, urine output, and hepatic venous O_2 saturation and with increased systemic venous pressure.[63,76,85] Hence the therapy for hepatic dysfunction is to prevent or treat the causes of low cardiac output syndrome after the Fontan operation. The ultimate therapy for systemic venous hypertension and low cardiac output is to take down the Fontan circuit and revert to the BDG.

Chronic systemic venous hypertension may contribute to *protein-losing enteropathy*.[56] This condition reflects the combined effects of gastrointestinal congestion, impaired absorption, and reduced lymphatic drainage. (See Chapter 5 on Splanchnic Function).

Dysrhythmias

Rhythm disturbances may occur after the Fontan operation.[14,69] It was originally thought that the absence of sinus rhythm was a risk factor for Fontan operation; however, more recent evidence suggests that sinus rhythm is not an absolute requirement for successful outcome after the Fontan procedure.[4] However, atrial pacing can improve cardiac output and systemic blood pressure, especially when junctional rhythm is present in the early postoperative period. Atrial pacing reduces left atrial pressure and provides an atrial contribution to systemic stroke volume.[1]

More significant rhythm disturbances such as atrial flutter or junctional ectopic tachycardia increase the risk of hemodynamic instability in the early postoperative period.[69] By using a total cavopulmonary connection rather than an atriopulmonary connection, atrial tachydysrhythmias are less common and more easily controlled with antiarrhythmic therapy, overdrive pacing, or DC cardioversion.[4] Exposure of native atrial tissue to high pressure may contribute significantly to postoperative dysrhythmias in the Fontan patient. This may explain the higher incidence of junctional dysrhythmias in the lateral-tunnel Fontan than in the extracardiac Fontan. The presence of AV valve regurgitation also has been suggested as a risk factor for postoperative dysrhythmias, which also suggest high atrial pressure as a principal factor.[4] It is likely that other mechanisms contribute to arrhythmias, including trauma to the sinoatrial or atrioventricular node, elevated catecholamine levels after CPB, or autonomic imbalance after atrial incision.[106]

Although most junctional and supraventricular rhythm disturbances are transient and well tolerated, rapid junctional ectopic tachycardia (rapid accelerated junctional tachycardia) with heart rate greater than 190 beats/min represents a serious rhythm disturbance after the Fontan operation.[69] It is associated with myocardial dysfunction and low cardiac output.

Medical therapy should be attempted, including amiodarone,[138] discontinuation of catecholamine infusions, atrial pacing,[12] and finally surface cooling (33° C) if other measures are unsuccessful.

Other significant arrhythmias after the Fontan procedure include complete heart block, atrial flutter, and sustained supraventricular tachycardia.[50,69] Complete heart block is treated with epicardial ventricular demand pacing during the immediate postoperative period. Transvenous pacing is not an option in the Fontan patient, because no systemic venous connection to ventricular mass exists.

Thrombosis

Thrombosis in the systemic venous circulation may limit cardiac output and prove life threatening. Patients are first seen with signs of localized systemic venous congestion such as facial plethora (SVC syndrome) or lower-body edema and ascites (IVC obstruction). Although decreased systemic venous flow rates undoubtedly play a major role, fibrinolytic abnormalities also may contribute to the mechanism of venous thrombosis. Children awaiting the Fontan operation have decreased levels of protein C, plasminogen, and antithrombin III.[99] Management of symptomatic venous thrombosis generally requires heparin infusion to achieve a partial thromboplastin time of 2 times control. Twice-daily administration of low-molecular-weight heparin (Lovenox, 1.0 mg/kg SC or IV q12 h) instead of heparin infusion simplifies therapy and may be equally effective.[93] Seipelt et al.[128] suggested that prophylactic anticoagulation of the Fontan patient, preferably with coumadin or with aspirin, prevents thromboembolic complications without significant bleeding events.

CONCLUSION

Improvements in the understanding of the physiology of the Fontan circulation and consequently in surgical technique have lead to steady improvements in outcome. Operative mortality for the Fontan operation in TA patients has declined to 2%.[81] Nevertheless, the multitude of potential perioperative complications highlights the need for careful planning and vigilance in the management of these children.

References

1. Alboliras ET, Porter CB, Danielson GK, et al: Results of the modified Fontan operation for congenital heart lesions in patients without preoperative sinus rhythm. J Am Coll Cardiol 6:228–233, 1985.
2. Anderson RH, Wilkinson JL, Gerlis LM, et al: Atresia of the right atrioventricular orifice. Br Heart J 39:414–428, 1977.
3. Azakie A, McCrindle BW, Van Arsdell G, et al: Extracardiac conduit versus lateral tunnel cavopulmonary connections at a single institution: Impact on outcomes. J Thorac Cardiovasc Surg 122:1219–1228, 2001.
4. Balaji S, Gewillig M, Bull C, et al: Arrhythmias after the Fontan procedure: Comparison of total cavopulmonary connection and atriopulmonary connection. Circulation 84:III162–III167, 1991.
5. Behrendt DM, Rosenthal A: Cardiovascular status after repair by Fontan procedure. Ann Thorac Surg 29:322–330, 1980.
6. Beppu S, Nimura Y, Tamai M, et al: Two-dimensional echocardiography in diagnosing tricuspid atresia: Differentiation from other hypoplastic right heart syndromes and common atrioventricular canal. Br Heart J 40:1174–1183, 1978.
7. Bharati S, Lev M: The concept of tricuspid atresia complex as distinct from that of the single ventricle complex. Pediatr Cardiol 1:57–62, 1979.
8. Bharati S, McAllister HA Jr, Tatooles CJ, et al: Anatomic variations in underdeveloped right ventricle related to tricuspid atresia and stenosis. J Thorac Cardiovasc Surg 72:383–400, 1976.
9. Bjork VO, Olin CL, Bjarke BB, Thoren CA: Right atrial-right ventricular anastomosis for correction of tricuspid atresia. J Thorac Cardiovasc Surg 77:452–458, 1979.
10. Botto LD, Lynberg MC, Erickson JD: Congenital heart defects, maternal febrile illness, and multivitamin use: A population-based study. Epidemiology 12:485–490, 2001.
11. Bridges ND, Farrell PE Jr, Pigott JD, et al: Pulmonary artery index: A nonpredictor of operative survival in patients undergoing modified Fontan repair. Circulation 80:I216–I221, 1989.
12. Case CL, Gillette PC: Automatic atrial and junctional tachycardias in the pediatric patient: Strategies for diagnosis and management. PACE Pacing Clin Electrophysiol 16:1323–1335, 1993.
13. Charuzi Y, Spanos PK, Amplatz K, Edwards JE: Juxtaposition of the atrial appendages. Circulation 47:620–627, 1973.
14. Chen SC, Nouri S, Pennington DG: Dysrhythmias after the modified Fontan procedure. Pediatr Cardiol 9:215–219, 1988.
15. Cheung HC, Lincoln C, Anderson RH, et al: Options for surgical repair in hearts with univentricular atrioventricular connection and subaortic stenosis. J Thorac Cardiovasc Surg 100:672–681, 1990.
16. Chin AJ, Franklin WH, Andrews BA, Norwood WI Jr: Changes in ventricular geometry early after Fontan operation. Ann Thorac Surg 56:1359–1365, 1993.
17. Coceani F, Olley PM: The response of the ductus arteriosus to prostaglandins. Can J Physiol Pharmacol 51:220–225, 1973.
18. Currie PJ, Hagler DJ, Seward JB, et al: Instantaneous pressure gradient: A simultaneous Doppler and dual catheter correlative study. J Am Coll Cardiol 7:800–806, 1986.
19. Davachi F, Lucas RV Jr, Moller JH: The electrocardiogram and vectorcardiogram in tricuspid atresia: Correlation with pathologic anatomy. Am J Cardiol 25:18–27, 1970.
20. de Leval MR, Kilner P, Gewillig M, Bull C: Total cavopulmonary connection: A logical alternative to atriopulmonary connection for complex Fontan operations: Experimental studies and early clinical experience. J Thorac Cardiovasc Surg 96:682–695, 1988.
21. de Leval MR, McKay R, Jones M, et al: Modified Blalock-Taussig shunt: Use of subclavian artery orifice as flow regulator in prosthetic systemic-pulmonary artery shunts. J Thorac Cardiovasc Surg 81:112–119, 1981.
22. DeLeon SY, Ilbawi MN, Idriss FS, et al: Persistent low cardiac output after the Fontan operation: Should takedown be considered? J Thorac Cardiovasc Surg 92:402–405, 1986.
23. Deutsch V, Shem-Tov A, Yahini JH, Neufeld HN: Juxtaposition of atrial appendages: Angiocardiographic observations. Am J Cardiol 34:240–244, 1974.
24. Dick M, Fyler DC, Nadas AS: Tricuspid atresia: Clinical course in 101 patients. Am J Cardiol 36:327–337, 1975.
25. Dick M, Rosenthal A, Bove EL: The clinical profile of tricuspid atresia. In Rao PS (ed): Tricuspid Atresia. Mt. Kisco, Futura Publishing, 1992, pp 117–140.
26. Di Donato RM, Amodeo A, di Carlo DD, et al: Staged Fontan operation for complex cardiac anomalies with subaortic obstruction. J Thorac Cardiovasc Surg 105:398–404, 1993.
27. DiSessa TG, Child JS, Perloff JK, et al: Systemic venous and pulmonary arterial flow patterns after Fontan's procedure for tricuspid atresia or single ventricle. Circulation 70:898–902, 1984.
28. Dolara A, Fazzini PF, Marchi F, Tordini B: Changing clinical features in tricuspid atresia without transposition of great vessels: Report of two cases. Acta Cardiol 24:275–284, 1969.
29. Douville EC, Sade RM, Fyfe DA: Hemi-Fontan operation in surgery for single ventricle: A preliminary report. Ann Thorac Surg 51:893–899, 1991.
30. Driscoll DJ: Tricuspid atresia. In Garson AJ, Bricker TJ, McNamera DG (eds): The Science and Practice of Pediatric Cardiology. Philadelphia, Lea & Febiger, 1990, pp 1118–1126.
31. Edwards JE, Burchell HB: Congenital tricuspid atresia: A classification. Med Clin North Am 33:1117–1196, 1949.
32. Elliott L: The roentgenology of tricuspid atresia. Semin Roentgenol 3:399, 1968.
33. Elster SK: Congenital atresia of pulmonary and tricuspid valves. Am J Dis Child 79:692–697, 1950.
34. Fontan F, Baudet E: Surgical repair of tricuspid atresia. Thorax 26:240–248, 1971.
35. Fontan F, Kirklin JW, Fernandez G, et al: Outcome after a "perfect" Fontan operation. Circulation 81:1520–1536, 1990.

36. Franklin RC, Spiegelhalter DJ, Sullivan ID, et al: Tricuspid atresia presenting in infancy: Survival and suitability for the Fontan operation. *Circulation* 87:427–439, 1993.

37. Freed MD, Heymann MA, Lewis AB, et al: Prostaglandin E₁ infants with ductus arteriosus-dependent congenital heart disease. *Circulation* 64:899–905, 1981.

38. Freedom RM, Benson LN, Smallhorn JF, et al: Subaortic stenosis, the univentricular heart, and banding of the pulmonary artery: An analysis of the courses of 43 patients with univentricular heart palliated by pulmonary artery banding. *Circulation* 73:758–764, 1986.

39. Freedom RM, Rowe RD: Aneurysm of the atrial septum in tricuspid atresia: Diagnosis during life and therapy. *Am J Cardiol* 38:265–267, 1976.

40. Fyfe DA, Taylor AB, Gillette PC, et al: Doppler echocardiographic confirmation of recurrent atrial septal defect stenosis in infants with mitral valve atresia. *Am J Cardiol* 60:410–411, 1987.

41. Fyler DC, Buckley LP, Hellenbrand WE, Cohn HE: Report of the New England Regional Infant Cardiac Program. *Pediatrics* 65:375–461, 1980.

42. Gago O, Salles CA, Stern AM, et al: A different approach for the total correction of tricuspid atresia. *J Thorac Cardiovasc Surg* 72:209–214, 1976.

43. Gale AW, Arciniegas E, Green EW, et al: Growth of the pulmonary annulus and pulmonary arteries after the Blalock-Taussig shunt. *J Thorac Cardiovasc Surg* 77:459–465, 1979.

44. Gallaher ME, Fyler DC: Observations on changing hemodynamics in tricuspid atresia without associated transposition of the great vessels. *Circulation* 35:381–388, 1967.

45. Gamboa R, Gersony WM, Nadas AS: The electrocardiogram in tricuspid atresia and pulmonary atresia with intact ventricular septum. *Circulation* 34:24–37, 1966.

46. Garcia EJ, Riggs T, Hirschfeld S, Liebman J: Echocardiographic assessment of the adequacy of pulmonary arterial banding. *Am J Cardiol* 44:487–492, 1979.

47. Gaynor JW, Bridges ND, Cohen MI, et al: Predictors of outcome after the Fontan operation: Is hypoplastic left heart syndrome still a risk factor? *J Thorac Cardiovasc Surg* 123:237–245, 2002.

48. Geggel RL, Mayer JE Jr, Fried R, et al: Role of lung biopsy in patients undergoing a modified Fontan procedure. *J Thorac Cardiovasc Surg* 99:451–459, 1990.

49. Gessner IH: Embryology of atrioventricular valve formation and embryogenesis of tricuspid atresia. In Rao PS (ed): *Tricuspid Atresia.* Mt. Kisco, Futura Publishing, 1992, pp 39–57.

50. Gewillig M, Wyse RK, de Leval MR, Deanfield JE: Early and late arrhythmias after the Fontan operation: Predisposing factors and clinical consequences. *Br Heart J* 67:72–79, 1992.

51. Gewillig MH, Lundstrom UR, Deanfield JE, et al: Impact of Fontan operation on left ventricular size and contractility in tricuspid atresia. *Circulation* 81:118–127, 1990.

52. Gyepes MT, Marcano BA, Desilets DT: Tricuspid atresia, transposition, and coarctation of the aorta. *Radiology* 97:633–636, 1970.

53. Hagler DJ, Seward JB, Tajik AJ, Ritter DG: Functional assessment of the Fontan operation: combined M-mode, two-dimensional and Doppler echocardiographic studies. *J Am Coll Cardiol* 4:756–764, 1984.

54. Hanes TE, Page DL, Graham TB, et al: Regional myocardial infarction of low-flow type in a neonate with tricuspid atresia. *Arch Pathol Lab Med* 101:86–88, 1977.

55. Hansen DD, Hickey PR: Anesthesia for hypoplastic left heart syndrome: Use of high-dose fentanyl in 30 neonates. *Anesth Analg* 65:127–132, 1986.

56. Hess J, Kruizinga K, Bijleveld CM, et al: Protein-losing enteropathy after Fontan operation. *J Thorac Cardiovasc Surg* 88:606–609, 1984.

57. Hickey PR, Hansen DD, Cramolini GM, et al: Pulmonary and systemic hemodynamic responses to ketamine in infants with normal and elevated pulmonary vascular resistance. *Anesthesiology* 62:287–293, 1985.

58. Hickey PR, Hansen DD, Strafford M, et al: Pulmonary and systemic hemodynamic effects of nitrous oxide in infants with normal and elevated pulmonary vascular resistance. *Anesthesiology* 65:374–378, 1986.

59. Hickey PR, Hansen DD, Wessel DL, et al: Pulmonary and systemic hemodynamic responses to fentanyl in infants. *Anesth Analg* 64:483–486, 1985.

60. Hickey PR, Hansen DD, Wessel DL, et al: Blunting of stress responses in the pulmonary circulation of infants by fentanyl. *Anesth Analg* 64:1137–1142, 1985.

61. Hurwitz RA, Caldwell RL, Girod DA, Wellman H: Left ventricular function in tricuspid atresia: A radionuclide study. *J Am Coll Cardiol* 8:916–921, 1986.

62. Jacobs ML, Norwood WI: Hypoplastic left heart syndrome. In Jacobs ML, Norwood WI (eds): *Pediatric Cardiac Surgery.* Boston, Butterworth-Heinemann, 1992, pp 182–192.

63. Jenkins JG, Lynn AM, Wood AE, et al: Acute hepatic failure following cardiac operation in children. *J Thorac Cardiovasc Surg* 84:865–871, 1982.

64. Jonas RA, Castaneda AR: Modified Fontan procedure: Atrial baffle and systemic venous to pulmonary artery anastomotic techniques. *J Card Surg* 3:91–96, 1988.

65. Juaneda E, Haworth SG: Pulmonary vascular structure in patients dying after a Fontan procedure: The lung as a risk factor. *Br Heart J* 52:575–580, 1984.

66. Kirklin JW, Barratt-Boyes BG: *Cardiac Surgery.* New York, Wiley Medical Publication, 1986.

67. Kirklin JK, Blackstone EH, Kirklin JW, et al: The Fontan operation: Ventricular hypertrophy, age, and date of operation as risk factors. *J Thorac Cardiovasc Surg* 92:1049–1064, 1986.

68. Koiwaya Y, Watanabe K, Orita Y, et al: Contrast two-dimensional echocardiography in diagnosis of tricuspid atresia. *Am Heart J* 101:507–510, 1981.

69. Kurer CC, Tanner CS, Norwood WI, Vetter VL: Perioperative arrhythmias after Fontan repair. *Circulation* 82:IV190–IV194, 1990.

70. La Corte MA, Dick M, Scheer G, et al: Left ventricular function in tricuspid atresia: Angiographic analysis in 28 patients. *Circulation* 52:996–1000, 1975.

71. Laishley RS, Burrows FA, Lerman J, Roy WL: Effect of anesthetic induction regimens on oxygen saturation in cyanotic congenital heart disease. *Anesthesiology* 65:673–677, 1986.

72. Laks H, Pearl JM, Haas GS, et al: Partial Fontan: Advantages of an adjustable interatrial communication. *Ann Thorac Surg* 52:1084–1094, 1991.

73. Lamberti JJ, Spicer RL, Waldman JD, et al: The bidirectional cavopulmonary shunt. *J Thorac Cardiovasc Surg* 100:22–29, 1990.

74. Laschinger JC, Ringel RE, Brenner JI, McLaughlin JS: The extracardiac total cavopulmonary connection for definitive conversion to the Fontan circulation: Summary of early experience and results. *J Card Surg* 8:524–533, 1993.

75. Lemler MS, Scott WA, Leonard SR, et al: Fenestration improves clinical outcome of the Fontan procedure: A prospective, randomized study. *Circulation* 105:207–212, 2002.

76. Lemmer JH, Coran AG, Behrendt DM, et al: Liver fibrosis (cardiac cirrhosis) five years after modified Fontan operation for tricuspid atresia. *J Thorac Cardiovasc Surg* 86:757–760, 1983.

77. Lenox CC, Zuberbuhler JR: Balloon septostomy in tricuspid atresia after infancy. *Am J Cardiol* 25:723–726, 1970.

78. Lewis AB, Freed MD, Heymann MA, et al: Side effects of therapy with prostaglandin E₁ in infants with critical congenital heart disease. *Circulation* 64:893–898, 1981.

79. Lin AE, Rosti L: Tricuspid atresia in sibs. *J Med Genet* 35:1055–1056, 1998.

80. Mainwaring RD, Lamberti JJ, Moore JW, et al: Comparison of the hormonal response after bidirectional Glenn and Fontan procedures. *Ann Thorac Surg* 57:59–63, 1994.

81. Mair DD, Puga FJ, Danielson GK: The Fontan procedure for tricuspid atresia: Early and late results of a 25-year experience with 216 patients. *J Am Coll Cardiol* 37:933–939, 2001.

82. Marcelletti C, Corno A, Giannico S, Marino B: Inferior vena cava-pulmonary artery extracardiac conduit: A new form of right heart bypass. *J Thorac Cardiovasc Surg* 100:228–232, 1990.

83. Marder SH, Seaman WB, Scott WG: Roentgenologic consideration in the diagnosis of congenital tricuspid atresia. *Radiology* 61:174, 1958.

84. Matitiau A, Geva T, Colan SD, et al: Bulboventricular foramen size in infants with double-inlet left ventricle or tricuspid atresia with transposed great arteries: influence on initial palliative operation and rate of growth. *J Am Coll Cardiol* 19:142–148, 1992.

85. Matsuda H, Covino E, Hirose H, et al: Acute liver dysfunction after modified Fontan operation for complex cardiac lesions: Analysis of the contributing factors and its relation to the early prognosis. *J Thorac Cardiovasc Surg* 96:219–226, 1988.

86. Mayer JE Jr, Bridges ND, Lock JE, et al: Factors associated with marked reduction in mortality for Fontan operations in patients with single ventricle. *J Thorac Cardiovasc Surg* 103:444–451, 1992.

87. Mayer JE Jr, Helgason H, Jonas RA, et al: Extending the limits for modified Fontan procedures. *J Thorac Cardiovasc Surg* 92:1021–1028, 1986.

88. McElhinney DB, Reddy VM, Hanley FL, Moore P: Systemic venous collateral channels causing desaturation after bi-directional cavopulmonary anastomosis: Evaluation and management. *J Am Coll Cardiol* 30:817–824, 1997.

89. McKay R, de Leval MR, Rees P, et al: Postoperative angiographic assessment of modified Blalock-Taussig shunts using expanded polytetrafluoroethylene (Gore-Tex). *Ann Thorac Surg* 30:137–145, 1980.

90. Mietus-Snyder M, Lang P, Mayer JE, et al: Childhood systemic-pulmonary shunts: Subsequent suitability for Fontan operation. *Circulation* 76:III39–III44, 1987.

91. Miller HC, Brown DJ, Miller GA: Comparison of formulae used to estimate oxygen saturation of mixed venous blood from caval samples. *Br Heart J* 36:446–451, 1974.

92. Mocellin R, Sauer U: Haemodynamics studies in patients with univentricular hearts. *Herz* 4:242–247, 1979.

93. Monagle P, Michelson AD, Bovill E, Andrew M: Antithrombotic therapy in children. *Chest* 119:344S–370S, 2001.

94. Myers JL, Waldhausen JA, Weber HS, et al: A reconsideration of risk factors for the Fontan operation. *Ann Surg* 211:738–743, 1990.

95. Nadas AS, Fyler DC: *Pediatric Cardiology*. Philadelphia, WB Saunders, 1972.

96. Nakata S, Imai Y, Takanashi Y, et al: A new method for the quantitative standardization of cross-sectional areas of the pulmonary arteries in congenital heart diseases with decreased pulmonary blood flow. *J Thorac Cardiovasc Surg* 88:610–619, 1984.

97. Nihill MR, McNamara DG, Vick RL: The effects of increased blood viscosity on pulmonary vascular resistance. *Am Heart J* 92:65–72, 1976.

98. Nishioka K, Kamiya T, Ueda T, et al: Left ventricle volume characteristics in children with tricuspid atresia before and after surgery. *Am J Cardiol* 47:1105–1110, 1981.

99. Odegard KC, McGowan FX Jr, Zurakowski D, et al: Coagulation factor abnormalities in patients with single ventricle physiology immediately prior to the Fontan procedure. *Ann Thorac Surg* 73:1770–1777, 2002.

100. Olley PM, Coceani F, Bodach E: E-type prostaglandins: A new emergency therapy for certain cyanotic congenital heart malformations. *Circulation* 53:728–731, 1976.

101. Olson TM, Driscoll DJ, Edwards WD, et al: Pulmonary microthrombi: Caveat for successful modified Fontan operation. *J Thorac Cardiovasc Surg* 106:739–744, 1993.

102. Ormiston JA, Neutze JM, Calder AL, Hak NS: Percutaneous balloon angioplasty for early postoperative modified Blalock-Taussig shunt failure. *Cathet Cardiovasc Diagn* 29:31–34, 1993.

103. Ovroutski S, Dahnert I, Alexi-Meskishvili V, et al: Preliminary analysis of arrhythmias after Fontan with extracardiac conduit compared with intra-atrial lateral tunnel. *Thorac Cardiovasc Surg* 49:334–337, 2001.

104. Park SC, Neches WH, Zuberbuhler JR, et al: Clinical use of blade atrial septostomy. *Circulation* 58:600–606, 1978.

105. Patel R, Fox K, Taylor JF, Graham GR: Tricuspid atresia: Clinical course in 62 cases (1967–1974). *Br Heart J* 40:1408–1414, 1978.

106. Randall WC, Wurster RD, Duff M, et al: Surgical interruption of postganglionic innervation of the sinoatrial nodal region. *J Thorac Cardiovasc Surg* 101:66–74, 1991.

107. Rao PS: Natural history of the ventricular septal defect in tricuspid atresia and its surgical implications. *Br Heart J* 39:276–288, 1977.

108. Rao PS: A unified classification for tricuspid atresia. *Am Heart J* 99:799–804, 1980.

109. Rao PS: Left to right atrial shunting in tricuspid atresia. *Br Heart J* 49:345–349, 1983.

110. Rao PS: Is the term "tricuspid atresia" appropriate? *Am J Cardiol* 66:1251–1254, 1990.

111. Rao PS, Linde LM, Liebman J, Perrin E: Functional closure of physiologically advantageous ventricular septal defects: Observations in three cases with tricuspid atresia. *Am J Dis Child* 127:36–40, 1974.

112. Rao PS: Demographic features of tricuspid atresia. In Rao PS (ed): *Tricuspid Atresia*. Mount Kisco, Futura Publishing, 1992, pp 23–37.

113. Rashkind W, Waldhausen J, Miller W, Friedman S: Palliative treatment in tricuspid atresia: Combined balloon atrioseptostomy and surgical alteration of pulmonary blood flow. *J Thorac Cardiovasc Surg* 57:812–818, 1969.

114. Rashkind WJ: Tricuspid atresia: A historical review. *Pediatr Cardiol* 2:85–88, 1982.

115. Reder RF, Yeh HC, Steinfeld L: Aneurysm of the interatrial septum causing pulmonary venous obstruction in an infant with tricuspid atresia. *Am Heart J* 102:786–789, 1981.

116. Redington AN, Knight B, Oldershaw PJ, et al: Left ventricular function in double inlet left ventricle before the Fontan operation: Comparison with tricuspid atresia. *Br Heart J* 60:324–331, 1988.

117. Ries M, Singer H, Hofbeck M: Thrombolysis of a modified Blalock-Taussig shunt with recombinant tissue plasminogen activator in a newborn infant with pulmonary atresia and ventricular septal defect. *Br Heart J* 72:201–202, 1994.

118. Rigby ML, Anderson RH, Gibson D, et al: Two dimensional echocardiographic categorization of the univentricular heart: Ventricular morphology, type, and mode of atrioventricular connection. *Br Heart J* 46:603–612, 1981.

119. Rose AG, Beckman CB, Edwards JE: Communication between coronary sinus and left atrium. *Br Heart J* 36:182–185, 1974.

120. Rudolph AM: *Congenital Diseases of the Heart*. Chicago, Year Book Medical Publishers, 1974.

121. Rydberg A, BarAm S, Teien DE, et al: The abnormal contralateral atrioventricular valve abnormality in mitral and tricuspid atresia in neonates: An echocardiographic study. *Pediatr Cardiol* 20:200–202, 1999.

122. Sade RM, Fyfe DA: Tricuspid atresia: current concepts in diagnosis and treatment. *Pediatr Clin North Am* 37:151–169, 1990.

123. Sahn SA: State of the art: The pleura. *Am Rev Respir Dis* 138:184–234, 1988.

124. Saito A, Miyamura H, Kanazawa H, et al: Extracorporeal membrane oxygenation for severe heart failure after Fontan operation. *Ann Thorac Surg* 55:153–155, 1993.

125. Sanchez-Quintana D, Climent V, Ho SY, et al: Myoarchitecture and connective tissue in hearts with tricuspid atresia. *Heart* 81:182–191, 1999.

126. Sanders SP, Wright GB, Keane JF, et al: Clinical and hemodynamic results of the Fontan operation for tricuspid atresia. *Am J Cardiol* 49:1733–1740, 1982.

127. Schuller JL, Sebel PS, Bovill JG, Marcelletti C: Early extubation after Fontan operation: A clinical report. *Br J Anaesth* 52:999–1004, 1980.

128. Seipelt RG, Franke A, Vazquez-Jimenez JF, et al: Thromboembolic complications after Fontan procedures: Comparison of different therapeutic approaches. *Ann Thorac Surg* 74:556–562, 2002.

129. Seliem M, Muster AJ, Paul MH, Benson DW Jr: Relation between preoperative left ventricular muscle mass and outcome of the Fontan procedure in patients with tricuspid atresia. *J Am Coll Cardiol* 14:750–755, 1989.

130. Serratto M, Pahlajani DB: Electrophysiologic studies in tricuspid atresia. *Am J Cardiol* 42:983–986, 1978.

131. Seward JB, Tajik AJ, Hagler DJ, Ritter DG: Echocardiographic spectrum of tricuspid atresia. *Mayo Clin Proc* 53:100–112, 1978.

132. Singh SP, Astley R, Parsons CG: Haemodynamic effects of balloon septostomy in tricuspid atresia. *Br Med J* 1:225–226, 1968.

133. Sommer RJ: Transcatheter coil occlusion of surgical fenestration after Fontan operation. *Circulation* 94:249–252, 1996.

134. Szabo G, Magyar Z: Effect of increased systemic venous pressure on lymph pressure and flow. *Am J Physiol* 212:1469–1474, 1967.

135. Van Blankenstein JH, Slager CJ, Schuurbiers JC, et al: Heart function after injection of small air bubbles in coronary artery of pigs. *J Appl Physiol* 75:1201–1207, 1993.

136. Van Praagh R: The segmental approach to diagnosis in congenital heart disease. *Birth Defects: Original Article Series* 8:4–23, 1972.

137. Van Praagh R, Ando M, Dungan WT: Anatomic types of tricuspid atresia: Clinical and developmental implications. *Circulation* 44(suppl II):115, 1971.

138. Villain E, Vetter VL, Garcia JM, et al: Evolving concepts in the management of congenital junctional ectopic tachycardia: A multicenter study. *Circulation* 81:1544–1549, 1990.

139. Vlad P: Tricuspid atresia: In Keith JD, Rowe RD, Vlad P (eds): *Heart Disease in Infancy and Childhood*. New York, Macmillan, 1978, p 518.

140. Weinberg PM: Anatomy of tricuspid atresia and its relevance to current forms of surgical therapy. *Ann Thorac Surg* 29:306–311, 1980.

141. Weinberg PM: Pathological anatomy of tricuspid atresia. In Rao PS (ed): *Tricuspid Atresia*. Mount Kisco, Futura Publishing, 1992, pp 81–100.

142. Williams DB, Kiernan PD, Metke MP, et al: Hemodynamic response to positive end-expiratory pressure following right atrium-pulmonary artery bypass (Fontan procedure). *J Thorac Cardiovasc Surg* 87:856–861, 1984.

143. Wilson NJ, Seear MD, Taylor GP, et al: The clinical value and risks of lung biopsy in children with congenital heart disease. *J Thorac Cardiovasc Surg* 99:460–468, 1990.

144. Yoxall CW, Walsh K, Sreeram N: Patency of Blalock-Taussig shunt assessed by Doppler colour flow imaging. *Int J Cardiol* 36:230–231, 1992.

Chapter 40

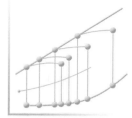

Hypoplastic Left Heart Syndrome

JAMES M. STEVEN, MD, MS, BRADLEY S. MARINO, MD, MPP, MSCE, and DAVID R. JOBES, MD

INTRODUCTION

Definition

Hypoplastic left heart syndrome (HLHS) is the term used to describe a spectrum of congenital cardiac malformations that exhibit varying degrees of underdevelopment of the left-sided heart structures. The central anatomic feature in the most common form of HLHS is aortic valve atresia with resultant hypoplasia of the ascending aorta and aortic arch. The left ventricle is hypoplastic or absent (Fig. 40-1). Nearly all patients with aortic valve atresia have coexisting atresia or stenosis of the mitral valve. Systemic blood flow is maintained by the right ventricle via the pulmonary artery (PA) and a patent ductus arteriosus.

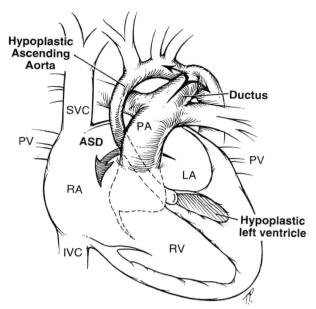

FIGURE 40-1 Native anatomy in hypoplastic left heart syndrome. Note hypoplastic left ventricle, aortic valve atresia, and hypoplastic ascending aorta. Systemic blood flow is propelled by the right ventricle (RV) via the pulmonary artery (PA) and ductus arteriosus. Pulmonary venous return enters the left atrium (LA) and crosses the atrial septal defect (ASD) into the right atrium (RA). Systemic venous flow returns normally from the inferior vena cava (IVC) and superior vena cava (SVC) to the RA.

Approximately one fourth of the children with HLHS have left ventricular hypoplasia and aortic valve atresia in association with either double-outlet right ventricle with mitral atresia or complete common atrioventricular canal defect malaligned over the right ventricle. The anatomic defects that are categorized as HLHS are varied; however, their physiologic similarity has resulted in the persistence of the term. This chapter focuses on the initial stage of reconstructive surgery as a treatment modality for children born with HLHS. Beyond initial reconstruction, these infants are managed in a manner analogous to the management of other univentricular heart malformations destined for a modified Fontan operation. Thus considerations relevant to subsequent stages of the reconstructive sequence culminating in Fontan circulation are discussed in Chapter 41. The other surgical option, cardiac allotransplantation, is discussed in detail in Chapter 16.

Epidemiology and Embryology

HLHS is the most common congenital cardiac malformation where only one developed ventricle is found. It represents the fourth most common defect first appreciated in the neonatal period. The syndrome was described in 1952 by Lev[58] and later termed HLHS by Noonan and Nadas.[79] It accounts for 7.5% of the newborns with congenital heart disease (CHD) and is sufficiently significant to require early therapeutic interventions, as well as 25% and 15% of the cardiac deaths within the first week and month of life, respectively.[33] Longitudinal data from the Atlanta metropolitan region suggest that the incidence of HLHS, at 2.1/10,000 live births, has changed little over the past 30 years.[13] The embryologic cause of HLHS is not fully understood. Because HLHS is

a collection of lesions, multiple developmental anomalies likely are related to a limitation of left ventricular inflow or outflow that results in the syndrome.

PATHOPHYSIOLOGY

Overview

The left ventricle is a nonfunctional structure in the child with HLHS (Fig. 40-2). Pulmonary venous return must be routed to the right atrium through a stretched foramen ovale, an atrial septal defect, or rarely by total anomalous pulmonary venous connection. Systemic and pulmonary venous returns mix in the right atrium. The right ventricle supplies both the systemic and pulmonary circulations in a parallel fashion, because the main PA gives rise to the branch pulmonary arteries, as well as the systemic circulation via the ductus arteriosus. Blood flows retrograde from the ductus arteriosus through the transverse aortic arch to its branches, and through the ascending aorta to the coronary arteries. Flow to the lower body is antegrade from the ductus arteriosus via the descending aorta. Ductal closure results in inadequate

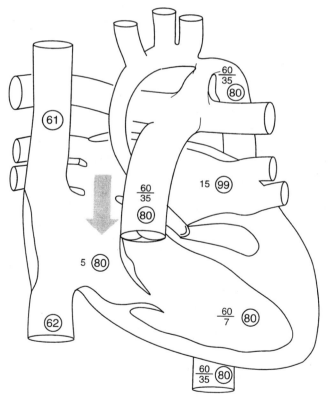

FIGURE 40-2 Schematic diagram of O_2 saturations (circled values) and pressures in native anatomy of hypoplastic left heart syndrome. Note increase in O_2 saturation due to mixing of systemic and pulmonary venous blood in the right atrium. The resultant systemic O_2 saturation of 80% represents balanced pulmonary and systemic blood flow ($Q_p:Q_s = 1$). Left atrial pressure (15 mm Hg) exceeds right atrial pressure (5 mm Hg), indicating restriction to left to right flow through the atrial communication.

$$Q_p:Q_s = \frac{SaO_2\ Ao - SaO_2\ SVC}{SaO_2\ PV - SaO_2\ PA}$$

systemic and coronary perfusion, leading to progressive metabolic acidemia, ischemia, and death.

With the pulmonary and systemic arteries connected in parallel, the $Q_p:Q_s$ depends on a delicate balance between the pulmonary and the systemic vascular resistance (SVR). In addition, two important anatomic elements must be present: (1) a patent, unrestrictive ductus arteriosus, and (2) the presence of an appropriately restrictive interatrial communication. Accordingly, the clinical presenting signs of HLHS are (1) shock related to closure of the ductus arteriosus, or (2) imbalance of $Q_p:Q_s$, resulting in signs of congestive heart failure or hypoxemia (see Chapter 41).

Changes in Pulmonary Vascular Resistance

At birth the pulmonary vascular resistance (PVR) is elevated but eventually decreases in the child with HLHS, as it does in any normal newborn. Because both circulations are supplied in parallel, the unabated decrease in PVR results in ever-increasing pulmonary blood flow, thereby increasing the volume work the right ventricle must perform to preserve adequate systemic output. The growing proportion of saturated blood entering the right atrium as $Q_p:Q_s$ increases may engender a misguided reassurance as the systemic saturation approaches normal values despite progressive clinical signs of congestive heart failure. By this mechanism, HLHS represents the most common cause of congestive heart failure in the first weeks of life. Unless other anatomic features act to limit pulmonary blood flow, the progressive imbalance in $Q_p:Q_s$ will result in high-output failure, acidemia reflecting inadequate systemic perfusion, and potentially death.

Degree of Interatrial Communication

The character of the interatrial communication serves as the most common anatomic determinant of pulmonary blood flow. Because the left ventricle accepts minimal or no flow, the interatrial communication provides the only route for egress of pulmonary venous blood entering the left atrium. In neonates with HLHS and a foramen ovale as the only interatrial communication, left atrial pressure typically exceeds right atrial pressure by 10 to 15 mm Hg so blood will flow left to right at the foramen ovale (see Fig. 40-2). The resultant elevation in pulmonary venous pressure increases PVR and limits pulmonary blood flow. When the foramen ovale or an additional atrial septal defect permits unobstructed interatrial flow of blood from left to right, pulmonary blood flow increases dramatically as PVR decreases. Alternatively, excessive narrowing or obliteration of the foramen ovale imposes severe restriction on pulmonary blood flow. Therefore the systemic saturation reflects the mixture of systemic venous return with variable pulmonary venous return permitted by the interatrial communication (see Fig. 40-2).

DIAGNOSTIC ASSESSMENT

Physical Findings

Fortunately, most neonates exhibit a $Q_p:Q_s$ close to unity. These infants will have adequate systemic perfusion, as evidenced by a normal systemic arterial blood pressure, warm extremities with good peripheral pulses, and the absence of a metabolic acidemia. The skin color is usually dusky. Auscultation reveals a systolic ejection murmur and a single second heart sound. Analysis of their arterial blood while breathing room air will exhibit "ideal" results (pH, 7.40; PaO_2, 40 ± 5 mm Hg; $PaCO_2$, 40 ± 5 mm Hg).

Patients exhibiting marked imbalance in $Q_p:Q_s$ often appear in extremis. Those with widely patent atrial septal defects have a $Q_p:Q_s$ well in excess of 1. Once the ability of the right ventricle to effect a compensatory increase in volume output is exceeded, systemic hypoperfusion develops. The physical findings in this cohort are dominated by evidence of shock and congestive heart failure. These infants appear listless and tachypneic with diminished pulses in all extremities. The liver is enlarged. Acidosis, hyperkalemia, and hypoglycemia signify metabolic decompensation.

Conversely, patients with little or no interatrial communication are deeply cyanotic because of inadequate pulmonary blood flow. Although this cohort may appear vigorous immediately after delivery, the deleterious cardiovascular and metabolic effects of profound hypoxemia, characterized by PaO_2 values of 20 mm Hg or lower in the most severe cases, ultimately become apparent. Myocardial performance deteriorates, and many of the same findings develop as seen in those with excessive pulmonary blood flow; listlessness, diminished peripheral pulses, acidosis, and hypoglycemia.

Diagnostic Tests

The electrocardiogram (ECG) shows right atrial enlargement with peaked P waves in leads II, III, and AVF and right ventricular enlargement with a qR pattern in the right precordial leads. The chest radiograph reveals cardiomegaly because of right atrial, right ventricular, and proximal PA enlargement. The lung fields exhibit pulmonary congestion in the majority. In patients with severely obstructed interatrial communication, the cardiomegaly is less prominent, and the pulmonary vascular markings vary from diminished to congested in a more reticular pattern, which reflects the pulmonary venous hypertension.

Two-dimensional echocardiography is sufficient to diagnose this lesion (Fig. 40-3). Echocardiographic imaging determines the anatomic details. Pulse and continuous-wave Doppler in conjunction with color-flow analysis are then used to evaluate several aspects of the physiology. For example, the relative pulmonary and systemic resistances can be inferred from the direction of flow in the ductus arteriosus during diastole. Assessment of the tricuspid or common atrioventricular valve for regurgitation is particularly important[6] as well as identification of the insertion and drainage of the pulmonary veins (PVs).

Routine cardiac catheterization is not necessary in the evaluation of neonates with HLHS.

Associated Anomalies

Most neonates with HLHS are born at term, and few have noncardiac anomalies in comparison with other infants with structural heart disease (12% to 15% vs. 28%). Although a small series of HLHS diagnosed in utero described an incidence of genetic or extracardiac malformations in eight

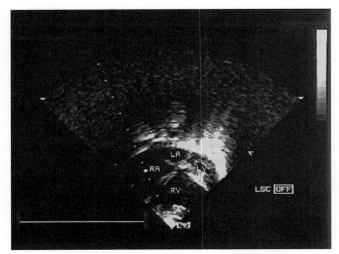

FIGURE 40-3 Echocardiogram (long axis–parasternal view) of hypoplastic left heart. Left ventricle is hypoplastic.

of 20 (40%), such series are notoriously biased by insensitivity of fetal ultrasound diagnosis and the inclusion of fetuses that do not survive to term.[12] Similarly, autopsy series conducted in an era when surgical therapy was offered are vulnerable to sampling bias. Natowicz[75] described genetic or major extracardiac anomalies or both in 28% of a series of 83 autopsies conducted over an 11-year time span. Turner's syndrome[76] and two rare chromosomal abnormalities, duplication of the short arm of chromosome 12[86] and trisomy 18,[44] are reported to have a higher incidence of HLHS. A karyotype should be included in the preoperative evaluation of any female neonate with HLHS as well as in boys who have somatic abnormalities.

Structural brain malformations occur in HLHS. The prevalence of structural brain malformation varies with the method of data collection. The New England infant cardiac data bank reported central nervous system (CNS) abnormalities in fewer than 5% of infants with HLHS.[33] Glauser and associates[37] conducted a retrospective evaluation of 41 autopsies and concluded that 29% of infants with HLHS exhibited some brain anomaly, although only 10% were characterized as overt. These include such lesions as holoprosencephaly (2%) and absence of the corpus callosum (7%). Although this study provides a very comprehensive catalogue of minor and major brain malformations, it may not depict a representative sample of neonates with HLHS. The autopsy series represents a selected population among whom 50% had died after surgical palliation and 41% of whom were characterized as dysmorphic. Our recent series including 102 newborns with HLHS indicates that approximately 15% have some genetic syndrome or significant noncardiac malformation.[35]

The magnitude and distribution of acquired vital organ dysfunction usually relates to circulatory instability at the time of diagnosis. Infants that have had a profound or protracted shock state at the time of diagnosis can demonstrate a wide spectrum of injury to renal, central nervous, cardiac, gastrointestinal, or hepatic systems. These derangements may necessitate a delay in operative intervention to permit recovery.

PREOPERATIVE CRITICAL CARE MANAGEMENT

All interventions in the preoperative period are directed toward two goals: (1) preserving ductal patency and (2) establishing or maintaining the $Q_p:Q_s$ ratio at unity.

Prostaglandin E₁ Infusion

Prenatal ultrasound diagnosis and the growing awareness of potential survival after surgical intervention have increased the number of patients with HLHS presenting for surgery within the first week of life. A continuous infusion of prostaglandin E₁ (PGE₁), 0.01 to 0.1 mcg/kg/min should be instituted once the diagnosis has been made because all infants with HLHS have a ductal-dependent systemic circulation. Oral PGE₂[32] has been substituted in the rare circumstance in which PGE₁ is unavailable or its administration impractical. Patients who were not diagnosed prenatally should receive PGE₁ infusion as soon as the diagnosis is suspected. Hence any newborn with unexplained shock is a candidate for PGE₁ infusion until HLHS or other forms of ductal-dependent systemic circulation have been specifically excluded.

Physiologic Assessment and Manipulation of the Ratio of Pulmonary Blood Flow to Systemic Output

Much of the preoperative management of neonates with HLHS entails optimizing the condition of the cardiovascular and other organ systems. Because the right ventricle must perfuse the pulmonary and systemic circulations in parallel, emphasis is placed on strategies that promote optimal systemic oxygen delivery with minimal overall volume work imposed on the ventricle. This goal is usually attained when pulmonary blood flow approximates systemic output (i.e., $Q_p:Q_s = 1$). Although HLHS is not unique in posing the need to balance $Q_p:Q_s$, the subtle difference exhibited by this cardiac malformation is a tendency for high pulmonary blood flow and marginal systemic output. Perhaps the anatomic relation whereby the systemic flow must traverse the main PA on its way to the aorta contributes to this phenomenon. In addition, speculation persists as to whether the right ventricle is intrinsically less well suited to the excess volume work imposed by a high $Q_p:Q_s$ state.

The key to management of HLHS perioperatively rests with the ability to assess systemic perfusion and $Q_p:Q_s$. Unfortunately, these variables often cannot be quantified precisely under typical clinical circumstances. In the past decade, however, significant progress has been made in our ability to predict, measure, and manipulate this complex physiology. At the core of many of these assessments is the calculation of $Q_p:Q_s$ according to the Fick equation:

$$Q_p:Q_s = (Ao - SVC)/(PV - PA)$$

where Ao, SVC, PV, and PA all represent oxygen-content values at the aorta (Ao), superior vena cava (SVC), pulmonary vein (PV), and pulmonary artery (PA), respectively.

In patients with cardiac lesions that result in complete mixing and parallel systemic and pulmonary circulations, one can assume that content in the Ao and PA are equal, and the former is usually conveniently measured. When significant pulmonary disease does not complicate the clinical situation, clinicians typically assume that the PV is fully saturated with oxygen, or nearly so. That leaves the SVC content to be either measured or assumed. In the clinical environment, measurement of oxygen saturation usually replaces calculation of content because accurate measurement instruments of the former are readily available, and the relation of the two values is reasonably constant.

Until recently, the clinical estimate of $Q_p:Q_s$ was made on the basis of a single value, determined in the systemic arterial circulation. From that, estimates were made as to the pulmonary venous and systemic venous saturation, and a $Q_p:Q_s$ value calculated. For example, if the systemic oxygen saturation were 80%, the following assumptions for SVC and PV saturation would result in a calculation such as

$$Q_p:Q_s = (80 - 60)/(100 - 80) = 1$$

The assumed values imply normal systemic AV extraction (and thus systemic cardiac output) and full oxygen saturation of the pulmonary venous blood. By using similar assumptions and a systemic oxygen saturation of 60%, one might calculate $Q_p:Q_s$ as

$$Q_p:Q_s = (60 - 40)/(100 - 60) = 0.5$$

A systemic oxygen saturation of 90% might yield the following:

$$Q_p:Q_s = (90 - 70)/(100 - 90) = 2$$

Although such determinations often provide a reasonable estimate, values can be significantly altered by changing the underlying assumptions, even within normal boundaries. For example, with a systemic oxygen saturation of 80%:

$$Q_p:Q_s = (80 - 50)/(95 - 80) = 2$$

On occasion, these estimates can lead to serious misinterpretation and inappropriate therapy. For example, the conclusion that low systemic arterial saturation represents low $Q_p:Q_s$ may lead to measures directed at reducing PVR. If, however, the systemic oxygen saturation reflected low cardiac output, as illustrated later, such measures would be counterproductive.

$$Q_p:Q_s = (70 - 35)/(95 - 70) = 1.4$$

Data from Rychik and colleagues[95] comparing the accuracy of various methods used to estimate $Q_p:Q_s$ reveal a weak correlation between aortic oxygen saturation and measured $Q_p:Q_s$ (Fig. 40-4A). Although cumbersome for routine evaluations, aortic Doppler flow patterns are substantially more accurate and precise in evaluation of $Q_p:Q_s$ (Fig. 40-4B and C).

When available, the addition of data to quantify systemic output and $Q_p:Q_s$ accurately, such as mixed venous oxygen saturation or Doppler aortic flow patterns, substantially improves the assessment and appropriate intervention in patients with HLHS. This information assumes even greater importance in the context of volatile physiologic changes characteristic during the early postoperative period.

Limiting Excessive Pulmonary Blood Flow

In the preoperative period, neonates with HLHS who have been resuscitated and stabilized and who are not impaired by other vital organ system dysfunction are initially assumed to be able to maintain satisfactory balance in $Q_p:Q_s$. The goal for such patients is to allow spontaneous ventilation via a natural airway. The majority of neonates meet this objective. The most common imbalance of $Q_p:Q_s$ typically manifests itself with signs of inadequate systemic output and relative excess in pulmonary blood flow. These signs might include hypotension, lactic acidosis, and diminished urine flow in the context of relatively high systemic oxygen saturation. Once assured of an adequate circulating intravascular volume and oxygen-carrying capacity, we often direct therapeutic measures at increasing PVR. To obtain selective constriction of the pulmonary vasculature, clinicians have used gas mixtures that either reduced alveolar PO_2 (P_AO_2), promoting hypoxic pulmonary vasoconstriction, or increased alveolar PCO_2 (P_ACO_2) to achieve constriction via local effects on pH or tissue CO_2. Either of these ambient gas manipulations can be accomplished by placing the infant in a hood, supplemented with nitrogen or carbon dioxide, respectively. Caution must be used when altering the inspired gas mixtures in neonates breathing spontaneously while receiving PGE_1 by infusion. Mild hypoventilation can result in significant hypoxemia in neonates breathing an FiO_2 less than 0.21. This is illustrated by using a modification of the alveolar gas equation listed:

$$P_AO_2 = 713 \text{ mm Hg} \times FiO_2 - \frac{P_ACO_2}{0.8}$$

Under conditions of hypoxia (FiO_2 of 0.17), if the neonate hypoventilates or is apneic to the point that the P_ACO_2 reaches 70 mm Hg or both, this will result in a P_AO_2 of only 34 mm Hg. The systemic arterial PO_2 will be significantly lower, as it represents a combination of the mixed venous and alveolar PO_2. Although increased inspired carbon dioxide has been shown to improve oxygen delivery in the anesthetized neonate under conditions of controlled ventilation,[102] the increased oxygen consumption associated with carbon dioxide–induced tachypnea in the spontaneously breathing patient might negate the benefits observed in the anesthetized patient.

The only alteration anticipated in a selected proportion of this group is tracheal intubation and ventilatory support necessitated by apnea, an adverse effect of PGE_1 administration (Table 40-1). After measures that establish the $Q_p:Q_s = 1$, a neonate with HLHS awaiting surgery will rarely require inotropic support for low cardiac output. Dopamine in a dose of 3 to 5 mcg/kg/min can be efficacious by improving ventricular function in those rare circumstances. High doses of inotropic agents are likely to be counterproductive by further increasing an already elevated SVR.

The ability to adjust alveolar P_ACO_2 rapidly is the most important variable governing the approach to mechanical ventilation. An increase in P_ACO_2 will result in an increase in PVR and a reduction in pulmonary blood flow.[71] In cases

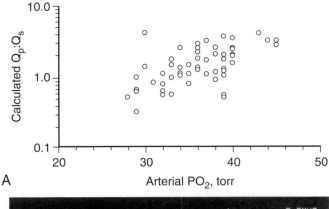

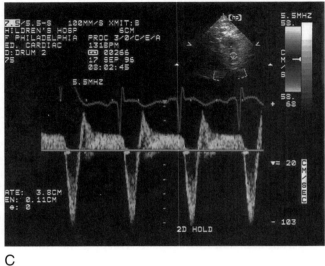

FIGURE 40-4   Comparison of methods used to estimate $Q_p:Q_s$. **A,** While arterial PO_2 exhibited trend correlation with Fick determinations of $Q_p:Q_s$, at any one value, a low correlation coefficient translates into a wide variation in $Q_p:Q_s$ for any given arterial PO_2 (p = .84, $R^2 = 0.78$). **B,** Conversely, estimates of $Q_p:Q_s$ made using Doppler diastolic flow reversal exhibit a much higher coefficient of determination (P<.001, $R^2 = 0.94$). **C,** Illustrates Doppler flow pattern in the distal aortic arch. (Data and graphic from Rychik J, Bush DM, Spray TL, et al: Assessment of pulmonary/systemic blood flow ratio after first-stage palliation for hypoplastic left heart syndrome: Development of a new index with the use of Doppler echocardiography. *J Thorac Cardiovasc Surg* 102:81–87, 2000.)

of increased $Q_p:Q_s$, we have tried adjusting ventilatory parameters (frequency, tidal volume, FiO₂, airway pressures including positive end-expiratory pressure [PEEP]) to prevent hypocarbia and increase P_ACO_2, while ensuring oxygenation. This approach demonstrates how changes in mechanical ventilatory parameters may have multiple interdependent effects. For example, reduction of minute ventilation to prevent hypocarbia often leads to atelectasis and alveolar

Table 40-1   Physiologic Spectrum of Neonates with HLHS

Anatomic Features	$Q_p:Q_s$	Sequelae	Management
Restrictive IAC	1:1	Apnea (PGE₁)	• Ventilate if apneic
Unrestrictive IAC	>>1:1	Systemic hypoperfusion	• Correct acidosis
			• Volume resuscitation
			• Inotropic agents
			• Inspired CO₂
			• Paralysis with judicious ventilation
Severely restrictive IAC	<<1:1	Profound hypoxemia	• Hyperventilation
			• Increase FiO₂
			• Increase SVR
			• Hypothermia
			• Immediate surgery (atrial septectomy ± stage I palliation)

IAC, interatrial communication; PGE₁, prostaglandin E₁; CO₂, carbon dioxide; FiO₂, fraction of inspired oxygen; SVR, systemic vascular resistance.

hypoxemia, thus reducing pulmonary venous oxygen saturation independent of pulmonary blood flow. Increasing PVR from hypoxemia, atelectasis, and perhaps hypercarbia and acidosis may progressively result in unacceptable hypoxemia. Attempts to correct the situation lack precision and accuracy and result in yet more changes in ventilatory mechanics, most often resulting in excessive pulmonary blood flow. The inherent number of variables in this approach introduces sufficient uncertainty about pulmonary venous oxygen saturation as to impair the estimates of $Q_p:Q_s$ that direct management, even when the patient and environment are stable. Assessment of $Q_p:Q_s$ becomes virtually impossible in an unstable patient or during anesthesia, cooling, and surgery in an operating room.

In our opinion, the simplest and most successful strategy directed at increasing PVR has been the addition of carbon dioxide to the inspired gas mixture.[53] During mechanical ventilation, the frequency, tidal volume, airway pressures, and FiO₂ can be kept constant while altering only the FiCO₂. This approach adds the capability of increasing the P_ACO_2 virtually within seconds and changing FiO₂ to meet oxygen requirements that are unrelated to pulmonary blood flow.

Hypoplastic Left Heart Syndrome with Severe Pulmonary Venous Obstruction

In contrast, those who have severely obstructed pulmonary venous return, such as the few who are first seen with an intact atrial septum and no alternative decompressing vein, have an extremely low Q_p:Q_s. Despite transient hemodynamic and metabolic stability that might ensue with aggressive therapeutic maneuvers designed to reduce PVR and promote pulmonary blood flow (see Table 40-1), these infants exhibit marked hypoxemia that requires urgent intervention to decompress pulmonary venous return to have any hope of survival.[2,96] Tracheal intubation facilitated by neuromuscular blocking agents and anesthetic agents, as tolerated, is accompanied by hyperventilation with an FiO_2 of 1.0. In addition, measures should be undertaken to augment the right ventricular pressure to promote pulmonary blood flow, including ensuring adequate intravascular volume and metabolic status, and in some infants, inotropic agents. If, despite these maneuvers, the PaO_2 remains less than 20 mm Hg with evidence of metabolic decompensation, deliberate hypothermia should be considered to minimize oxygen consumption until cardiopulmonary bypass (CPB) can be instituted. This can be accomplished by removing the overhead warmer, placing ice bags around the head and body, and using a cooling blanket until transport to the operating room, where these measures are continued.

The use of sodium bicarbonate to address a metabolic acidemia in the face of extremely limited pulmonary blood flow offers limited benefit and may even be hazardous. The elimination of carbon dioxide after bicarbonate hydrolysis is severely impaired. Hence, bicarbonate administration will often result in a shift from metabolic to respiratory acidemia, with little change in pH, and the attendant prospect of a highly undesirable increase in PVR. Tromethamine may be an appropriate alternative to sodium bicarbonate in this clinical situation to treat acidosis secondary to hypoxemia, as it does not create carbon dioxide as it buffers the metabolic acidosis.

SURGICAL INTERVENTION

Historical Overview

Historically, HLHS was considered fatal with or without surgery. With only sporadic exceptions, no intervention was undertaken once that diagnosis was made. Approaches to surgical palliation based on autopsy findings were proposed as early as 1968,[99] and isolated case reports or small series began to appear in 1970.[18,31] However, these infants did not have HLHS, but rather aortic stenosis with mild left ventricular hypoplasia or aortic atresia with ventricular septal defect and a developed left ventricle. Short-term survival after surgical palliation for classic aortic valve atresia was reported in the late 1970s.[26,59,70] Short-term survival also occurs if continued patency of the ductus arteriosus is ensured and a balanced Q_p:Q_s is maintained. However, prolonged parallel connection of the pulmonary and systemic circulations will ultimately result in either intractable congestive heart failure or development of pulmonary vascular obstructive disease. Thus additional steps were necessary for long-term survival.

Development of the Staged Repair of Hypoplastic Left Heart Syndrome

In the early 1970s, Fontan[29] and Kreutzer[57a] independently introduced operative treatment of tricuspid atresia that resulted in nearly normal systemic arterial oxygen saturation and normal volume work for the single ventricle (see also Chapter 39 on Tricuspid Atresia). Fontan created a series circulation, which requires the single ventricle to pump fully saturated blood only to the systemic circulation. The systemic venous drainage passes directly through the pulmonary vascular bed without benefit of a ventricular pump. The child's PVR must be low to maintain the pulmonary circulation. Since that time, the principle of Fontan's operation has been applied to a variety of cardiac lesions with one functional ventricle. It was recognized that long-term survival with HLHS, a more common univentricular lesion, would depend on the creation of this same physiology.

The first report of an attempt to provide surgical therapy to a patient with HLHS was reported by Redo and colleagues[90] in 1961. A 2.5-month-old infant with mitral atresia underwent atrial septectomy under inflow occlusion through a right thoracotomy. The next major advance in surgical treatment was provided by Sinha and coworkers[99] who analyzed 30 autopsy cases of infants with HLHS and established the primary principles for successful first-stage reconstruction. The authors suggested that provision of an unobstructed interatrial communication for free left-to-right shunting of pulmonary venous blood was a primary objective in addition to providing a continuing right-to-left shunt at the ductal level and banding of the pulmonary arteries to limit pulmonary blood flow. The first successful attempts to use these principles of reconstruction were performed by Cayler and associates,[18] who banded the right and left pulmonary arteries, created an atrial septal defect, and maintained aortic flow with anastomosis of the right PA to the ascending aorta.

A different procedure, described by Litwin, van Praagh, and Bernard[60] in 1972, provided the basis for a surgical approach for patients with HLHS. The original description of the operative interventions by Litwin and colleagues were for patients with interrupted aortic arch and combined placement of a graft from the main PA to the descending aorta with distal PA banding. This approach was subsequently used in early operations by Mohri and coworkers[70] in 1979 and Levitsky and associates[59] in 1980.

Despite early unsuccessful attempts at palliative reconstruction, other more aggressive attempts were undertaken to provide a one-stage Fontan-type circulation in patients with HLHS. In 1977 Doty and Knott[25] described five unsuccessful cases of primary reconstruction for HLHS, including Fontan connection of the right atrium directly to the pulmonary arteries. In these patients, under deep hypothermic circulatory arrest, the patent ductus was ligated, the atrial septum excised, and the atrium repartitioned with a pericardial baffle so that the pulmonary venous return was directed to the tricuspid valve and right ventricle. The PA was then connected to the aortic arch with a tubular Dacron prosthesis, and the pulmonary arteries directly connected to the right atrium. All of these infants died of inadequate right ventricular performance or compromised coronary blood flow. This experience established the principle that one-stage complete reconstruction to the Fontan circulation would not likely be successful in newborns because of elevated PVR and the complexity of the operation, and therefore established the principle of *staged* reconstructive surgery, culminating in a Fontan circulation at a later age.

Development of the staged reconstructive approach for HLHS is appropriately accredited to William I. Norwood, who provided much of the development of the early staged operations for this condition. The initial report by Norwood[81] in 1980 described three cases of newborns with HLHS who underwent first-stage reconstruction. In the first patient, an attempt was made to perform a Glenn anastomosis to the right PA artery; however, this patient died with progressive acidosis 7 hours after operation. Two additional infants underwent a modification of Litwin's procedure, with anastomosis of a valved conduit from the right ventricle to the descending aorta and distal pulmonary arterial banding. Both patients survived and were released from the hospital in satisfactory condition. Norwood described a proposed second-stage operation to separate the systemic and pulmonary circulations with utilization of as much autologous tissue as possible. In his proposed physiologic repair of aortic atresia at the second stage, the proximal PA and origin of the right PA were to be anastomosed to the diminutive ascending aorta to create an all-autologous reconstruction from the right ventricle to the arch of the aorta, with excision of the previously placed conduit from right ventricle to descending aorta. The divided right PA would then be anastomosed to the SVC in a Glenn anastomosis, and the left PA reconstructed with a valved conduit. These descriptions made the first note of the fact that autologous reconstruction of the aortic arch would be a necessary and desirable component to ultimate repair of HLHS when severe aortic stenosis or atresia was present. A variation on this technique was described by Behrendt and Rocchini,[8] who suggested a simplified technique for creating a fixed pulmonary band by use of a punch in the PA anterior wall, which was then used to occlude the pulmonary bifurcation. Arch reconstruction was to be undertaken at the first neonatal procedure, with patch augmentation of the main PA connecting to the ascending aorta to beyond the aortic arch. This innovative technique was described in a single successful infant in their original report, and the principle for second-stage repair also was described.[8]

With the evolution of multiple approaches to first-stage reconstruction, it was inevitable that success would eventually be achieved with staged reconstruction to serial completion of the Fontan circulation. The first successful physiologic repair of aortic atresia with HLHS was described by Norwood, Lange, and Hansen in 1983.[83] This success was accomplished with two separate operations, confirming the principle of staged reconstruction. The patient described in this report was recently seen at The Children's Hospital of Philadelphia (CHOP) and is now older than 20 years with signs of chronic stable protein-losing enteropathy and atrial arrhythmias. Evolution of the initial surgical therapies, however, continued, and much of the development of the successful first-stage reconstruction is credited to William I. Norwood, who gradually refined and developed the surgical principles, which have led to successful outcomes in infants with HLHS.[80] The first successful palliation operation with staged reconstruction, as described by Norwood, has changed little over the past 20-year period; however, recently several technical modifications have been proposed, which aim to limit the use of prosthetic material in the reconstruction and to decrease the use and duration of deep hypothermic circulatory arrest.[50,57] The approach to staged reconstructive surgical correction of

HLHS is based on the principle that carefully planned and appropriately timed palliative operations will result in suitable physiology for the modified Fontan procedure.[80] Norwood[83] described an initial palliative reconstruction allowing survival and growth until the PVR decreases. The initial palliation (stage I) results in construction of a "neo-aorta" and connection of the systemic and pulmonary circulations at the arterial level via a modified Blalock-Taussig shunt (Fig. 40-5). The volume work of the single ventricle is equal to the sum of the systemic and pulmonary blood flows. After a period of maturation of the pulmonary vasculature, systemic venous return may be directed to the PAs, thus placing the two circulations in series (stages II and III). This goal of the Fontan operation is undertaken in stages in an effort to reduce the volume load of the ventricle as early as possible and to minimize the impact of rapid changes in ventricular geometry and diastolic function that accompany primary Fontan.[80]

Because our experience has demonstrated that infants with HLHS achieve early outcomes from Fontan operation comparable to other univentricular heart malformations,[34] we limit the detailed discussion in this chapter to perioperative management of stage I reconstruction (i.e., the Norwood operation). The Fontan operation is discussed in Chapters 39 and 41.

Heart Transplantation for Hypoplastic Left Heart Syndrome

In 1986, Bailey described successful allotransplantation methods for HLHS.[4] Despite intermediate-term reports indicating 70% 7-year survival of recipients,[89] two major limitations arise when contemplating adopting this strategy widely: donor organ availability and long-term transplant outcome. At present, fewer than 70 infants receive heart transplants annually for all indications,[48] whereas population demographics suggest that as many as 1000 children are born with HLHS.[13] Even in the minority of infants with HLHS who are listed for transplant, the waiting period can extend as long as 6 months with the mortality as high as 30% during that interval.[51] Multicenter efforts to submit this conundrum to rigorous decision analysis result in varying recommendations depending on a given center's success with reconstructive surgery and the regional waiting time for infant donor hearts.[51,101] This model also fails to incorporate differences in long-term outcome. The consequences of chronic immunosuppression and rejection limit 12-year survival to 50% in all pediatric heart recipients.[14] Infants with congenital heart malformations fare significantly less well. Once beyond the initial year, mortality in pediatric transplant recipients decreases to approximately 3% per year, whereas the comparable mortality after Fontan operation is less than 1% per year.[14,51]

INITIAL PALLIATIVE RECONSTRUCTION (STAGE I)

Anesthetic Considerations

The anesthetic considerations before CPB are identical, regardless of whether the child has stage I reconstruction or heart replacement. Anesthesia should be induced and maintained while preserving the delicate balance between

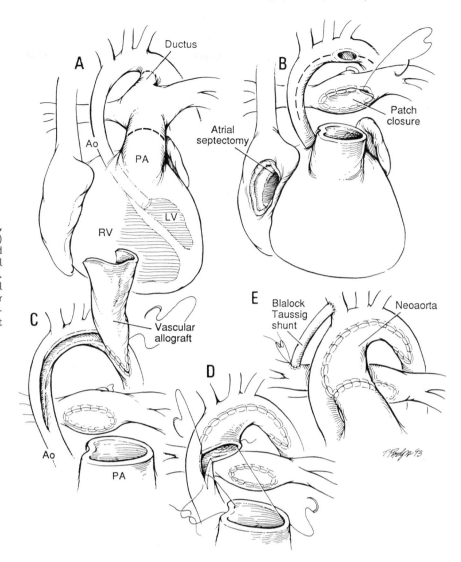

FIGURE 40-5 Stage I Norwood Procedure. **A,** Transection points of the main pulmonary artery (PA) and ductus arteriosus. **B,** Atrial septectomy to avoid pulmonary venous hypertension. Patch closure of distal main PA. Division and ligation of the ductus arteriosus. **C–D,** Construction of a "neoaorta" using the proximal main PA, diminutive ascending aorta, and vascular allograft. **E,** Pulmonary blood flow supplied by a modified right Blalock–Taussig shunt connecting the right innominate artery to the right PA.

SVR and PVR and minimizing myocardial depression. An undesirable increase in $Q_p:Q_s$ will be reflected in an increase in the child's PaO_2 and a decrease in systemic arterial blood pressure. Because the arterial oxygen saturation is ideally between 75% and 85% in these infants, oximetry will provide some indication of alterations in pulmonary blood flow, assuming alveolar oxygen availability is maintained. The anesthetic goals can be met by using either a narcotic or an inhalational agent or both in conjunction with neuromuscular blockade. Anesthetic agents appear to have comparable direct vascular effects in these patients as in others. Narcotic anesthesia with a synthetic opioid, such as fentanyl, is most frequently chosen because of minimal apparent effects on the heart and vasculature.

In our experience, 10 mcg/kg is the lowest dose of fentanyl that reliably results in minimal or no change in heart rate or blood pressure with laryngoscopy, intubation, and surgical procedures before bypass. Others have recommended high-dose fentanyl[40,45] or sufentanil.[1] Although earlier reports suggested that massive doses of opioid exert a beneficial impact on outcome after neonatal cardiac surgical correction by ablating

endogenous stress responses, recent investigations have concluded that outcome measures are not adversely affected by traditional high-dose opioid techniques that do not completely inhibit stress hormone release.[39] Pancuronium offers vagolytic properties that offset the bradycardia associated with narcotic induction; however, we have observed that optimal relaxation requires larger (0.2 mg/kg) than usual (0.1 mg/kg) doses in patients receiving PGE_1.

When managing infants who demonstrate the typical physiologic proclivity to increased pulmonary blood flow on induction of anesthesia and transition from spontaneous to positive pressure ventilation, the anesthesiologist must take care not to use ventilatory maneuvers that further reduce PVR, such as hyperventilation with a high FiO_2. Some means of increasing PVR should be immediately available in the operating room. Until recently, no data existed to compare the efficacy of nitrogen (i.e., hypoxic gas mixtures) with carbon dioxide in this setting. Tabbutt and colleagues[102] recently compared the effects of hypoxia (FiO_2, 0.17) with those of hypercarbia, achieved by adding supplemental carbon dioxide (2.7% or 20 torr CO_2), in a uniform group of 10 neonates with HLHS immediately before stage I reconstruction under identical conditions of anesthesia, paralysis, and fixed minute ventilation (Fig. 40-6). With a prospective, randomized, crossover design, the investigators measured SvO_2 and SaO_2 from catheters placed in the SVC and systemic artery, respectively, and mixed cerebral oxygen saturation (ScO_2) via near-infrared spectroscopy (NIRS) with each condition compared with the baseline in room air. Both hypoxia and hypercarbia resulted in small, but significant, changes in arterial blood gas data. Both conditions decreased $Q_p:Q_s$ (see Fig. 40-6), although the decrease achieved statistical significance only with hypercarbia. Only hypercarbia improved oxygen delivery. Unlike patients without intracardiac shunting, it is not possible to measure a true mixed venous oxygen saturation accurately in neonates with HLHS. This method cannot differentiate between cerebral and systemic oxygen delivery. Hypercarbia significantly increased ScO_2, whereas hypoxia had no effect.[88,102]

Assuming no difference in cerebral oxygen extraction between the two conditions, the increase in ScO_2 with hypercarbia may reflect an increase in global cardiac output or a selective effect on cerebral blood flow.

Other advantages of inspired carbon dioxide over nitrogen include the following: it does not require neutralization of all safety systems designed to avoid delivery of a hypoxic gas mixture, and it is available with flow meters in appropriate clinical ranges. In addition, inspired carbon dioxide serves to augment systemic arterial pressure, whereas hypoxic gas mixtures will not (see Fig. 40-6).[102]

We therefore elect to balance $Q_p:Q_s$ in the prebypass period by sustaining the $PaCO_2$ at or above 40 mm Hg by the addition of sufficient carbon dioxide to the fresh gas flow while maintaining the functional residual capacity with an appropriate tidal volume and respiratory rate. Surface cooling instituted before bypass results in decreased carbon dioxide production. $FiCO_2$ requirements can reach 4% to 5% as the core temperature decreases to 30°C to 32°C.

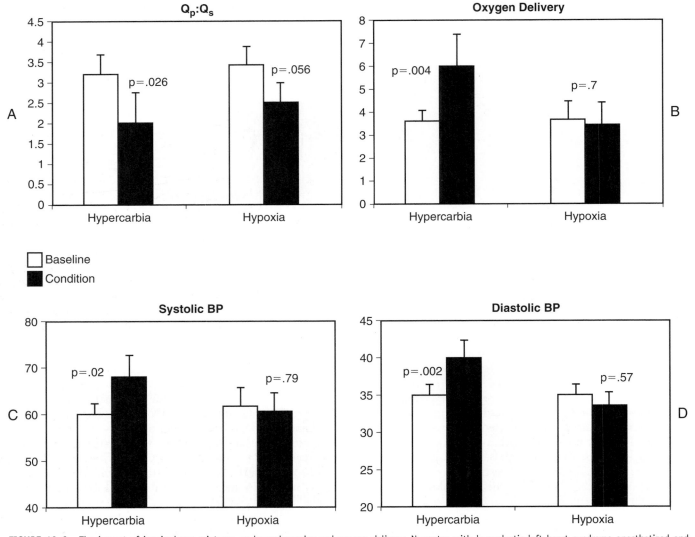

FIGURE 40-6   The impact of inspired gas mixtures on hemodynamics and oxygen delivery. Neonates with hypoplastic left heart syndrome anesthetized and intubated in a crossover study comparing hypercarbia ($FiCO_2$ 2.7%) versus hypoxia (FiO_2 17%). Although both gas mixtures reduced $Q_p:Q_s$ **(A)**, only hypercarbia increased oxygen delivery **(B)**, systolic blood pressure **(C)**, or diastolic blood pressure **(D)**. (Data from Tabbutt S, Ramamoorthy C, Montenegro LM, et al: Impact of inspired gas mixtures on preoperative infants with hypoplastic left heart syndrome during controlled ventilation. *Circulation* 104:I159–164, 2001.)

Temporary occlusion of the right PA during prebypass dissection represents an option that is rarely necessary to reduce pulmonary blood flow, thus preserving systemic perfusion.

Surgical Procedure (Stage I Reconstruction)

The three goals of stage I reconstruction are (1) to provide systemic perfusion independent of the ductus arteriosus, (2) to preserve function of the single ventricle by minimizing excess pressure and volume work, and (3) to allow normal maturation of the pulmonary vasculature (see Fig. 40-5). The creation of an unobstructed communication from the right ventricle to the systemic circulation satisfies the first goal completely and the second partially. This is achieved by transection of the main PA and constructing a "neoaorta" by using the proximal main PA, diminutive ascending aorta, and vascular allograft (see Fig. 40-5). The incorporation of a longitudinal strip of native aorta, albeit narrow, confers growth potential to this neoaorta, obviating further aortic operation. Pulmonary blood flow arises from a right modified Blalock-Taussig shunt or, less frequently, a central systemic-to-PA shunt connecting the neoaorta to the confluence of the branch PAs. In the absence of confounding anatomic or physiologic variables, a 3.5- to 4-mm modified Blalock-Taussig shunt reliably limits pulmonary blood flow to approximate a balanced $Q_p:Q_s$. An atrial septectomy is necessary to avoid obstruction of pulmonary venous return. Regulation of pulmonary blood flow with a shunt of fixed diameter and length coupled with creation of a nonrestrictive interatrial communication enables normal development of the pulmonary vasculature while avoiding excessive ventricular volume overload (i.e., $Q_p:Q_s>1$).

Right Ventricle–Pulmonary Artery Shunt Placement (Sano Modification)

Maldistribution of cardiac output associated with the systemic-to-pulmonary shunt has been implicated as a major cause of death after stage I palliation.[50,72] A review of 122 postmortem cases after the Norwood procedure at the Children's Hospital Boston indicated that the most important causes of death were impairment of coronary perfusion, excessive pulmonary blood flow, and obstruction of pulmonary blood flow.[7] Coronary hypoperfusion secondary to the systemic-to-PA shunt has been proposed to be a cause of late mortality after the Norwood palliation.[65,66,85]

The advantage to using a right ventricle–to-PA shunt instead of a systemic-to-PA shunt is that coronary hypoperfusion secondary to diastolic runoff through the systemic-to-PA shunt may be eliminated in both the perioperative period and interstage period before the superior cavopulmonary anastomosis, and that coronary perfusion is independent of the pulmonary-to-systemic flow ratio.

The first attempts to use a right ventricle–to-PA shunt to reestablish a stable source of PA blood flow after stage I palliation were by Norwood and associates in 1981.[82] These early attempts at utilization of the right ventricle–to-PA shunt failed because the shunts used were too large for the neonate (8–12 mm). All four patients died soon after surgery of excessive pulmonary blood flow and right ventricular failure. Kishimoto and coworkers[57] revived use of the right ventricle–to-PA shunt by using a xenopericardial valved

conduit and reported stable postoperative hemodynamics with a high diastolic blood pressure. Similar to those after Norwood's early right ventricle–to-PA shunt, Kishimoto's patients ultimately died of excessive PA blood flow and right ventricular dysfunction.

Sano and colleagues used a small (5 mm) nonvalved polytetrafluoroethylene (Gore-Tex) right ventricle–to-PA shunt to provide stable pulmonary blood flow to avoid the effects of diastolic run-off into the pulmonary circulation that occurs with the systemic-to-PA shunt (Fig. 40-7B).[98] Between February 1998 and November 2003, 33 consecutive neonates with HLHS or a variant underwent modified Norwood palliation with placement of a right ventricle–to-PA shunt at Okoyama University Hospital in Japan. Comparison between the right ventricle–to-PA shunt and systemic-to-pulmonary shunt revealed a lower $Q_p:Q_s$, smaller right ventricular end-diastolic diameter, and tricuspid valve annulus in the right ventricle–to-PA shunt group. The small right ventriculotomy for shunt placement in the right ventricle–to-PA group did not negatively affect right ventricular function significantly. Stenosis at the distal anastomosis site was common, and despite pulsatile blood flow into the PAs, PA growth was limited after right ventricle–to-PA shunt.[97]

Although theoretical advantages exist to using a right ventricle–to-PA shunt in patients with HLHS, a multicenter trial is needed to evaluate outcomes prospectively after the stage I palliation, comparing the standard systemic-to-PA shunt and the right ventricle–to-PA shunt.

Preparation for Termination of Bypass

During the terminal phases of warming on CPB, preparations for separation and early postbypass management include resumption of pulmonary function, monitoring of the cardiovascular system, hemodynamic support, and anticipatory evaluation of PVR. Accumulated secretions are removed from the airway, and the lungs are carefully expanded to eliminate atelectasis and assure normal pulmonary venous oxygen saturation. To provide the most consistent alveolar ventilation, we use volume-preset mode of ventilation. The precise ventilatory targets vary according to physiologic expectations, as delineated subsequently. In addition to the routine cardiopulmonary monitoring established in the prebypass period, the surgical team positions transthoracic catheters in the atrium and SVC to monitor intravascular volume, diastolic function, and permit determination of mixed venous oxygen saturation.

Despite a technically perfect operation, this procedure does not result in any reduction of the volume or pressure burden placed on the single ventricle, as the physiology of parallel systemic and pulmonary circulations in which $Q_p:Q_s = 1$ remains the objective throughout the postoperative period. Yet the myocardium has incurred the physiologic insult inflicted by CPB and a period of hypothermic ischemia. In the absence of major deficiencies in myocardial protection or persistent anatomic residua, such as arch obstruction, coronary compromise, or valvar insufficiency, these sequelae are usually ameliorated with relatively modest doses of dopamine (3 to 5 mcg/kg/min).

Although the fundamental circulatory principles do not change after surgery, the underlying tendencies have (Fig. 40-8). The proclivity to excessive pulmonary blood flow is virtually

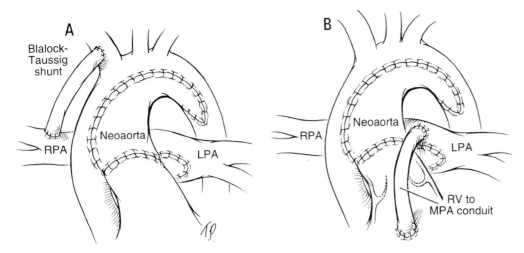

FIGURE 40-7 A, Stage I Norwood procedure with pulmonary blood flow provided by a modified right Blalock-Taussig shunt. **B,** In the Sano modification, a 5-mm right ventricle (RV)-to-main pulmonary artery (MPA) conduit is placed to provide pulmonary blood flow. LPA, left pulmonary artery; RPA, right pulmonary artery.

eliminated by the interposition of a restrictive prosthetic shunt. To promote maximal systemic perfusion and warming, this shunt is temporarily occluded during the warming period on bypass. Transiently opening the systemic-to-PA shunt during the terminal phase of bypass provides an estimate of PVR by the magnitude of the decrease in mean systemic arterial pressure. When coupled with the assessment of SVR made with the shunt occluded (i.e., mean systemic arterial pressure), one can anticipate the immediate postbypass $Q_p:Q_s$, thereby guiding initial ventilator targets. For example, assuming a constant pump flow rate of 150 mL/kg/min and SVR in the normal range, one would expect to see a mean systemic pressure between 50 and 70 mm Hg with the shunt occluded during the terminal phases of warming. Opening the shunt most commonly results in a decrease of 20 to 30 mm Hg in the mean systemic pressure. If the decrease is less than 10 mm Hg, the differential diagnosis includes high PVR or obstruction to pulmonary blood flow related to the shunt. A decrease greater than 30 mm Hg implies an extremely low PVR. Patients demonstrating a low pulmonary-to-SVR ratio (i.e., either a high mean systemic pressure with the shunt occluded or a large decrease when opened) are likely to have luxuriant pulmonary blood flow on separation from bypass, requiring normocapnic ventilation with a lower FiO_2. Those with a high pulmonary-to-SVR ratio exhibit a low $Q_p:Q_s$ on termination of bypass that necessitates more aggressive ventilation with higher FiO_2.

Early Postbypass Management

Much of the comprehensive perioperative management plan is initiated in the early postbypass period. Although a variety of reasonable strategies exist for neonates after the Norwood operation, optimal quality of care can be achieved only if surgeons, anesthesiologists, cardiologists, intensivists, and nurses arrive at a shared set of common goals that will carry across the continuum from operating room (OR) to intensive care unit (ICU). Although individual adjustments are necessary in virtually every patient, comprehensive goals help guide the choice of intervention within the bounds of shared objectives.

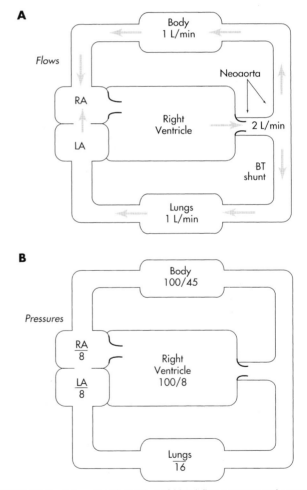

FIGURE 40-8 Schematic illustration of blood flow patterns and pressures in an infant after palliation for hypoplastic left heart syndrome. **A,** In a parallel circulation at the arterial level, the right ventricle must provide enough flow to adequately perfuse both the systemic and pulmonary circulations. In this example, pulmonary and systemic flow are equal ($Q_p:Q_s = 1$), but a variety of anatomic and physiologic issues can alter this relation, as described in the text. **B,** Pressures in the body and lung compartments represent systemic arterial and pulmonary arterial data. Body, systemic circulation; LA, left atrium; lungs, pulmonary circulation; RA, right atrium.

On termination of CPB, the shunt is opened and the heart filled to achieve satisfactory systemic arterial pressure without excessive distension. Ideally, this goal can be attained at an atrial pressure of 10 mm Hg or less. When cardiac performance fails to meet these objectives, prompt evaluation of potential issues with ventilation, oxygenation, metabolic variables, and technical aspects of the reconstruction is conducted. In the absence of remediable findings, adjustments to inotropic support may be necessary.

Modified Ultrafiltration

Whenever possible, we perform modified ultrafiltration (MUF) at the termination of CPB after stage 1 reconstruction. Once satisfactory hemodynamics have been established, MUF is instituted. When conducted immediately after CPB, MUF has been demonstrated to exert beneficial effects on hematocrit, hemodynamics, hemostasis, pulmonary function, and CNS recovery.[5,22,28,74,100] Perioperative weight gain is reduced significantly, as are certain inflammatory mediator levels. Occasionally, the position of the bypass cannulae or the continuous flux of blood through the MUF circuit results in unfavorable hemodynamic changes, precluding completion of the filtration. In our experience, the perturbations of MUF have contributed to unsatisfactory hemodynamics in 3 of the last 100 stage 1 reconstruction procedures.

Restoration of Hemostasis

Stage 1 reconstruction entails substantial suture lines in creation of the neoaorta. Thus rapid restoration of normal hemostasis represents an important early postoperative objective. Once satisfied with the technical and physiologic result of the repair after MUF, heparin effect is immediately reversed with protamine. Although patients with HLHS are not known to be associated with a specific bleeding etiology, they are included with groups exhibiting the most blood loss and the highest transfusion rates (i.e., youngest having complex surgery).[5,17,19,24,56,67,69,84,109,110] The goal for control of bleeding after CPB is to reduce transfusion requirement and the associated morbidity including surgical re-exploration and cardiac tamponade. After stage I reconstruction, initial blood loss can be attributed largely to the combination of extensive suture lines, most in high-pressure vessels, and coagulopathy. The relative contributions of dilution, fibrinolysis, or platelet dysfunction to coagulopathy are not clearly defined in HLHS or in neonates as a specific population. However, abnormalities of all three are documented as a result of CPB.[24,49,56,91,108] The performance of routine tests of coagulation has not been shown to be beneficial in attenuating bleeding in these patients. The most effective management (defined as the fewest donor exposures per patient) is associated with programs in which "fresh" whole blood is routinely used. Whole blood 24 to 48 hours old administered in the pump prime and to replace postbypass losses can result in a median donor exposure rate of two in the perioperative period.[24,67] Programs in which blood components are preferentially used report six to eight donor exposures in similar patient populations. Reports of antifibrinolytic therapy in the very young are limited largely to aprotinin.[17,24] The volume of blood loss can be reduced by high-dose aprotinin, but it may not be clinically important because donor exposures are not necessarily affected.

Prompt control of hemostasis, resulting in reduced transfusion requirements, can be associated with a diminished need for reexploration for bleeding. Reexploration in children younger than 2 years undergoing complex repairs at our institution, which includes all patients with HLHS, was reduced (from 3% to 0.8%) after the adoption of the routine use of fresh whole blood.

Cardiac tamponade can easily occur from a small quantity of mediastinal blood accumulated in the early postoperative period before bleeding has completely ceased. Continuous removal is essential because blockage easily occurs in the relatively small mediastinal drainage tubes of these neonates. A technique of active, continuous aspiration of accumulating blood from the mediastinum has virtually eliminated this complication.[52]

Optimize Systemic Perfusion

Maximizing the ratio of oxygen delivery to extraction represents the underlying physiologic goal that dominates early postbypass management.[106] However, in a manner characteristic of many major cardiac interventions in neonates and young infants, myocardial performance may deteriorate appreciably in the first 6 to 12 postoperative hours before starting to improve.[107] As a result, we routinely take measures to reduce metabolic demands by infusing continuous muscle relaxant (e.g., pancuronium, 0.05 to 0.1 mg/kg/hr) and opioid (e.g., fentanyl, 2 to 5 mcg/kg/hr). In addition, we usually add an inotrope/vasodilator infusion of the phosphodiesterase III-inhibitor class (e.g., milrinone: load, 50 to 100 mcg/kg; infusion, 0.5 to 1 mcg/kg/min) in the early postbypass period. Infants demonstrating increased SVR during rewarming on CPB often receive the milrinone loading dose at that time. In the event that milrinone is administered while the patient is connected to an extracorporeal circuit, the loading dose is increased by 300 mcg/L of pump prime to compensate for the increased volume of distribution.[87]

Fluid Administration

In the immediate postoperative period, intravascular volume supplementation serves to replace blood and urine losses, as well as the changes in capacitance that occur with warming. Volume requirements are guided by heart rate, systemic arterial pressure, and physical examination of peripheral perfusion, including temperature and capillary refill in the distal extremities. Although a transthoracic catheter placed in the common atrium at the time of surgery provides some information with respect to the intravascular volume status, it also reflects the compliance of the ventricle. In the face of satisfactory hemodynamics, ventricular compliance usually improves in the early postoperative period; hence the atrial pressure at a given intravascular volume should decrease concomitantly. To avoid excessive transfusion, the least amount of fluid necessary to produce satisfactory systemic hemodynamics and perfusion is administered, rather than rigidly adhering to a specific atrial pressure target. If the hemodynamic goals cannot be achieved despite a common atrial pressure consistently in excess of 10 mm Hg and no evidence of tamponade is found, consideration should be given to augmenting inotropic support. Fresh whole blood reliably supplements intravascular volume and promotes hemostasis while limiting multiple donor exposure. In the vast majority of neonates after stage I reconstruction, it satisfies all fluid requirements above maintenance glucose and electrolyte solutions. Once mediastinal hemorrhage has subsided, and hemoglobin concentration exceeds 16 g/dL, any additional volume requirements are met with colloid solutions.

Digoxin and furosemide are reinstituted expectantly in the postoperative period to ameliorate the impact of the obligatory increased volume load under which the single ventricle must operate. Because the systemic and pulmonary circulations remain connected in parallel at the arterial level, the volume work of the right ventricle continues to be equal to the sum of the systemic and pulmonary blood flow ($Q_p + Q_s$).

Common Problems in the Early Postbypass Period

Hypoxemia

Excessive hypoxemia represents one of the more commonly encountered problems in the early postbypass period. Although inadequate Q_p:Q_s was usually the assumed cause, factors that impair systemic oxygen delivery, thereby reducing mixed venous oxygen saturation, are now known to be significantly more common than previously appreciated (see Fig. 40-8).[47,92,93,95] One typically observes a progressive increase in systemic oxygen saturation during MUF, for example, probably because of the impact that hemoconcentration and the resulting increased oxygen delivery have on mixed venous oxygen saturation. Thereafter, measures directed at maintaining hematocrit above 40% may alleviate excessive demands placed on the recovering heart to increase systemic output. The distinction between systemic hypoxemia due to low Q_p:Q_s, low pulmonary venous oxygen saturation, or low mixed venous saturation is a critical one, as the therapies are diametrically different. Measures designed to reduce PVR will impose a further volume load on a heart already struggling to provide marginal systemic perfusion. Patients demonstrating low SvO_2 would be better served with therapies that promote systemic output, such as inotropic agents or vasodilators.

Those with low pulmonary venous oxygen saturation require a strategy of ventilatory support designed to reduce atelectasis and promote gas exchange in impaired alveoli. Unfortunately, the latter diagnosis is rarely made definitively in the OR or postoperative ICU, as blood sampling from the PVs presents logistic challenges. Intraoperatively, expectant measures directed at complete expansion of the lungs and maintenance of normal functional residual capacity usually suffice to avoid PV desaturation. Among the three etiologies of persistent systemic hypoxemia, this was believed to be the least common, but a recent series found PV desaturation in as many as 30%.[103]

When systemic hypoxemia occurs because of low Q_p:Q_s, other manifestations provide supporting evidence. Trial opening of the shunt during the latter phases of rewarming on CPB typically fails to produce a significant decrease in systemic arterial pressure. The early postbypass hemodynamics reveal a relatively narrow systemic pulse pressure or diastolic pressure that exceeds expectations (i.e., normal). A substantial discrepancy often exists between arterial and end-tidal CO_2 measurements. These suggestive pieces of inferential evidence can be confirmed by aortic Doppler flow analysis or calculation of a Fick ratio by using oxygen saturation determinations. Most commonly, diminished pulmonary blood flow reflects a subtle technical aspect of the arch reconstruction, innominate artery dimension, or the Blalock-Taussig shunt. Physiologic derangements may exacerbate PVR (e.g., hypoventilation, hypoxemia, acidosis, or hypothermia). However, certain patient subsets exhibit profound abnormalities in the pulmonary vasculature that cause excessive PVR elevations. Neonates with HLHS routinely demonstrate extremely high and volatile PVR when born with extreme pulmonary venous obstruction due to intact atrial septum without alternative decompressing veins. Even the typical HLHS anatomic constellation is associated with marked abnormalities in the number and muscularization of the pulmonary vasculature by pathologic examination.[41] Hypotheses attribute these changes to chronic fetal pulmonary venous obstruction.[42] Pathology studies confirm that these developmental abnormalities become more extreme in the context of the marked obstruction caused by HLHS with intact atrial septum.[96] Fetal echocardiography has demonstrated that alteration in pulmonary venous flow pattern correlates with the magnitude of restriction at the atrial septum.[10]

In the context of hypoxemia due to low Q_p:Q_s, interventions fall into three categories: technical, pulmonary vasodilators, and systemic vasoconstriction. For patients expected to have unusually elevated PVR, modifications in the surgical technique might entail placement of a larger shunt or interposition between a larger systemic vessel (e.g., aorta) and PA. Pulmonary vasodilator therapy includes the strategies one might use in any patient demonstrating elevated PVR, such as high FiO_2, moderate hyperventilation, normothermia, alkali, and nitric oxide.[3,71,94] Should those measures prove insufficient to result in adequate pulmonary blood flow, the focus might be expanded to include measures designed to increase the driving pressure across the shunt, by using increased inotropic stimulant infusions or even vasoconstrictors. The latter necessitates careful monitoring to avoid jeopardizing perfusion of other vital organs and should be used only as a temporizing measure until more definitive diagnostic and therapeutic interventions can occur.

Myocardial Dysfunction

Depressed myocardial performance represents another potential problem in the early postbypass period. As mentioned previously, some degree of myocardial dysfunction typically occurs after this operation, as no hemodynamic benefit is achieved to offset the cost of CPB and an ischemic interval. When this dysfunction becomes more significant than usual, specific causes should be sought. Even in the context of the typical conduct of stage 1 reconstruction, the consequences of aortic atresia make routine myocardial protection measures challenging, such as the infusion of cardioplegia solutions. Thus inadequate myocardial preservation represents one potential cause for persisting or excessive myocardial depression.

Technical considerations represent the predominant cause of myocardial dysfunction after this extraordinarily complex operative intervention. One of the most intricate aspects of this procedure is the reconstruction of an aortic arch in such a way that the small ascending aorta, which serves principally to provide coronary flow, is not compromised. This subtle finding may not become evident until the cardiac volume is restored in anticipation of terminating CPB. Residual hemodynamic derangement represents another potential cause of myocardial dysfunction. Because one emerges from the Norwood operation with no appreciable hemodynamic benefit, one would expect a heart facing a newly imposed volume or pressure load to tolerate it poorly. Examples of such findings include residual aortic arch obstruction, atrioventricular valve dysfunction, and semilunar valve obstruction or regurgitation.

Metabolic disturbances also result in significant myocardial dysfunction. This fragile right ventricle struggling to cope with significantly increased volume output demands at systemic pressure is perhaps more susceptible to what might otherwise be modest metabolic disturbances. As such, one should meticulously track and address those variables that have some impact on myocardial performance, such as ionized calcium and lactic acidosis. The rapid administration of blood products, for example, which contain calcium-binding drugs, high levels of potassium and lactic acid, as well as other vasoactive mediators, can result in an acute, profound deterioration in cardiac performance in the early postoperative period. In our experience, myocardial performance will deteriorate during the early postoperative period in neonates with HLHS when the arterial pH falls below 7.3 and may contribute to further reduction in systemic perfusion. The administration of intravenous sodium bicarbonate, calculated to eliminate the base deficit completely, often exerts a beneficial effect on both myocardial performance and systemic perfusion. In addition to the inherent cardiac sensitivity, inescapable anatomic peculiarities accentuate this vulnerability. Blood carrying the transfused products from the systemic venous circulation enters the right ventricle and is directed immediately to the reconstructed aorta, whereby the first branch is the coronary circulation. Thus any constituent of the transfused blood (e.g., citrate, potassium, lactate) infused into the venous circulation arrives at the coronary arteries with greater speed and concentration than might have occurred had it followed a normal circulatory pattern and been dissipated over the course of the pulmonary vasculature before entering the aorta. This effect is further accentuated if central venous catheters are used to infuse the blood product. As such, we abide by a protocol whereby blood transfused via central catheters or rapidly through peripheral catheters is either fresh whole blood or washed packed cells.

Arrhythmias

Arrhythmias most commonly occur as manifestations of the problems described previously. When they become manifest early in the process of rewarming on CPB, coronary insufficiency represents the most common cause, particularly if the arrhythmia is ventricular in origin. Metabolic disturbances produce the same qualitative rhythm changes seen in normal hearts, although the manifestations might be more extreme. Given the predominantly extracardiac nature of the Norwood procedure, acquired heart block rarely follows this operation,

unless it existed preoperatively. On very rare occasions, a patient has HLHS and a primary arrhythmia, such as Wolf-Parkinson-White syndrome.

Excessive Pulmonary Blood Flow

Excessive pulmonary blood flow may complicate the early postoperative period; however, this diagnosis should be entertained cautiously. In many instances, the apparent excess pulmonary blood flow really reflects a relative imbalance with respect to significantly diminished systemic cardiac output. The latter should be specifically excluded and addressed before invoking extreme measures to restrict pulmonary blood flow. Of course, subtle technical differences in the conduct of the operation can result in an anatomic propensity to an excessive $Q_p:Q_s$, and this can, in turn, jeopardize systemic perfusion. Such patients typically exhibit an extremely wide pulse pressure or low diastolic pressure reflecting pulmonary "runoff." If myocardial performance otherwise appears robust, the specific measures used to increase PVR preoperatively are appropriate in this circumstance. However, no data exist comparing inspired carbon dioxide versus nitrogen in this setting. In most patients, this condition dissipates as the infant recovers from surgery. Should the problem persist beyond the first postoperative day, a cardiac catheterization might be warranted to evaluate the need for further surgical intervention aimed at diminishing pulmonary blood flow.

Transition to the Intensive Care Unit

After transport from the OR, infants are returned to a volume-cycled mechanical ventilator at settings designed to mimic closely those that have proven satisfactory in the OR. The inotropic drug infusions initiated in the OR are maintained throughout transport. Given the marginal cardiac performance that typifies the early postoperative course after the Norwood operation, we initiate opioid and muscle relaxant infusions to diminish systemic metabolic demands and blunt the volatile PVR changes for which these patients are renowned. Before routine use of opioid-relaxant infusions in the ICU, Murdison and associates[72] examined the clinical course and outcome after stage I reconstruction and before modified Fontan in 200 neonates born with HLHS treated at The Children's Hospital of Philadelphia. Seventy percent of the mortality of these patients occurred during their initial hospitalization, the majority of which was associated with an acute or unrelenting mismatch between pulmonary and systemic flow on the first postoperative night. Cardiovascular collapse appeared to be related to events associated with sudden increases in PVR, often temporally associated with early spontaneous motor activity or interventions such as endotracheal suctioning. Endotracheal suctioning might precipitate acute elevations in PVR, either by reduction in alveolar ventilation and oxygenation or by a reflex mechanism.[46]

To anticipate further deterioration in cardiac performance over the first few postoperative hours, an infusion of milrinone is routinely initiated. If the systemic arterial pressure exceeds desired goals, further vasodilator therapy (e.g., nitroprusside) is added rather than reduction of inotropic support. This tactic emerges from the systematic observation of SvO_2

values that regularly indicate marginal or low systemic cardiac output during this period of recovery.

Armed with knowledge of these early postoperative objectives, the anesthesiologist may elect to begin any or all of these interventions in the early postbypass period, should they be indicated. Transition is further smoothed by ongoing communication with the ICU team to discuss which measures have been instituted in the OR and which will be initiated in the ICU. In addition, the other unique aspects of any given infant's care with respect to the conduct of surgery or anesthetic management should be transmitted to the ICU staff (e.g., hemorrhage/hemostasis, hemodynamics, airway issues, or arrhythmia).

Recovery Issues in the Intensive Care Unit

The harbinger of recovering cardiac function is often spontaneous diuresis. In uncomplicated cases, this typically occurs 24 to 36 hours postoperatively. This phase of care includes withdrawal of respiratory and cardiovascular support measures, removal of monitoring catheters, and the initiation of enteral nutrition.

Pulmonary Mechanics and Weaning from Mechanical Ventilation

Pulmonary mechanics are most commonly abnormal in these infants because of changes in airway resistance, lung compliance, or bellows function. Increased airway resistance usually results from luminal narrowing related either to intrinsic accumulation of secretions or to extrinsic compression from interstitial edema or dilated neighboring vessels or both in the bronchovascular pedicle associated with pulmonary venous hypertension. Although many pathologic processes culminate in reduced lung compliance, the most common mechanism in these neonates is the perioperative accumulation of interstitial lung water.[105] DiCarlo[23] demonstrated reduced mean lung compliance in all of 28 neonates (17 with HLHS) after cardiac surgical procedures. The subgroup in whom respiratory failure developed after initial withdrawal of mechanical ventilatory support also exhibited increased airway resistance. The routine use of MUF has dramatically reduced the frequency and magnitude of these intrinsic problems with pulmonary mechanics. In patients who have had the benefit of MUF, abnormalities of pulmonary mechanics of sufficient magnitude to cause respiratory failure are limited almost entirely to the subset of patients with significant hemodynamic issues or infection. Apart from the residual effects of neuromuscular blockade, the most common cause of bellows dysfunction in these neonates is diaphragmatic paresis, presumably resulting from phrenic nerve injury.

Because confirmation of sufficient cardiac reserve and manageable abnormalities in pulmonary mechanics is difficult to quantify in neonates, we empirically taper mechanical ventilatory support on the first or second postoperative day once hemodynamics are satisfactory. Minimal support is maintained to offset the resistance to breathing imposed by the endotracheal tube. The infant is evaluated at each step, with particular attention to the effort expended in spontaneous breaths and cardiovascular evidence of excessive sympathetic response to the increased metabolic demand (i.e., increased heart rate, systemic arterial pressure, atrial pressure).

Tracheal extubation is performed if the neonate exhibits minimal effort with spontaneous respiration and no evidence is noted of sympathetic response to the metabolic demand posed by the threshold level of support. When either of these criteria is not met, an attempt is made to identify and treat the underlying cause while continuing an appropriate level of ventilatory support. A decision to proceed with a trial of extubation may be made in the absence of a clearly identified cardiopulmonary etiology (e.g., inadequate cardiac reserve, abnormal pulmonary mechanics, increased work imposed by spontaneous respiration through a tracheal tube), recognizing the potential for immediate respiratory failure.

Reintubation is as frequently based on cardiovascular signs as on blood gas–tension abnormalities. In a 1988 series of 56 neonates extubated after stage I, the 30% who were ultimately reintubated manifested significant increases in heart rate, systemic arterial pressure, and atrial pressure during the period of spontaneous ventilation.[30] These changes probably reflected sympathetic discharge and diminished ventricular compliance. Analysis of arterial blood in these infants before and after extubation demonstrated reduced arterial pH (diminished metabolic alkalemia), but gas tensions were no different compared with those in patients successfully weaned. Recent experience indicates that the median duration of mechanical ventilation after stage I is 2 to 3 days, with 85% to 90% of patients successfully weaned from mechanical ventilatory support by the fifth postoperative day.

Central Nervous System

Systematically determined neurologic status before and after reconstruction (I and II) or transplantation is not often reported in the literature and is usually limited to clinically evident seizures, focal abnormality, or coma. The knowledge of the relative contribution of developmental and acquired abnormalities is limited, but some evidence is found from postmortem examinations of infants with HLHS. In an autopsy series, subject to the limitations of such cohorts described previously, 29% had major or minor developmental anomalies of the brain, whereas acquired hypoxic-ischemic lesions or intracranial hemorrhage were present in 45%.[36,37] The acquired lesions could have been present before surgery or subsequently. Genetic abnormalities and other syndromes are found with HLHS and may be associated with brain dysfunction. The prevalence of these findings in HLHS is variously reported between 5% and 40%; however, figures at the higher end represent potentially biased samples, such as autopsy series and fetal diagnoses.[12,33,75] Evaluation of a large, inclusive cohort of viable neonates presenting for treatment of HLHS demonstrated 3% with chromosomal abnormalities and a further 4% with syndromes or major extracardiac anomalies that might be associated with diminished brain function.[35]

After stage I, the incidence of clinically evident neurologic abnormalities (seizure, coma, stroke, developmental delay) is reported to be between 6% (n = 120) and 22% (n = 216).[16,20,61] Both congenital and acquired etiologies were included. Magnetic resonance imaging of the brain in neonates with CHD demonstrates structural abnormalities, predominantly periventricular leukomalacia, in 25% of patients before neonatal heart surgery and new lesions or worsening of pre-existing lesions in 66% postoperatively.[64] The postoperative changes were not different for patients with HLHS (half the group) compared with patients with other CHD. The functional significance of these findings is as yet unknown.

Several opportunities occur throughout the perioperative course during which an acquired brain injury may occur in infants with HLHS. Shock occurring as the ductus arteriosus closes, or as a result of inappropriate early management of an infant who exhibits severely imbalanced $Q_p:Q_s$ before diagnosis, may produce ischemic injury of all vital organs, including the brain. Even after diagnosis, certain subsets of infants with HLHS, notably those at the extremes of $Q_p:Q_s$, may have ongoing injury from inadequate oxygen delivery. HLHS is increasingly being diagnosed in utero, allowing planned management at delivery, suggesting greater stability through more controlled circumstances. A study of patients with critical left heart obstructive lesions (including HLHS) showed greater hemodynamic stability and a lower incidence of preoperative neurologic events in those patients with prenatal diagnosis.[27] A lower incidence of postoperative seizures was found in the prenatal group when neurologic outcome after stage I was compared.

Little attention has been given to the potential contribution of postoperative states to neurologic issues. Hyperthermia after CPB in adults is associated with neurologic impairment.[38] The recent observation of cerebral hyperthermia occurring in a pediatric population during the immediate postoperative period is particularly worrisome, but its etiology and impact have yet to be determined.[11] Patients frequently have low diastolic blood pressure and low arterial oxygen saturation after stage I reconstruction. The combination of these elements suggests the potential for adversely affecting brain function.

Gastrointestinal System

Between January 1995 and December 1998, 7.6% of the 131 neonates with HLHS treated at CHOP manifest signs resulting in the clinical diagnosis of necrotizing enterocolitis.[68] When compared with the cardiac ICU population as a whole, infants with HLHS demonstrated an odds ratio of 3.8 for the development of necrotizing enterocolitis. Although the incidence of necrotizing enterocolitis among infants with HLHS was similar to that in a previous study in our institution,[43] the mortality was dramatically lower (19% vs. 93%). This may

represent a consequence of using the more sensitive Bell criteria to establish the diagnosis of necrotizing enterocolitis in the recent study or a lower incidence of unrecognized inadequate systemic perfusion (Q_s).

Late Postoperative Issues

After discharge, regular cardiovascular evaluations enable prompt detection of hemodynamically significant complications that would impose further pressure or volume loads on the right ventricle or impede pulmonary blood flow (Table 40-2). Aortic arch obstruction occurs most commonly at the distal arch, although it can develop more proximally at the anastomoses joining the main PA, ascending aorta, and homograft gusset. Whereas some infants may show signs of congestive heart failure, many with arch obstruction are without symptoms. Immediate relief via balloon dilation or patch aortoplasty should be performed to prevent progressive right ventricular hypertrophy.[73] If obstruction occurs distal to the systemic-to-PA shunt, a maldistribution of $Q_p:Q_s$ may impose an added volume burden on the right ventricle.

Impediments to pulmonary blood flow causing progressive cyanosis usually occur as a result of either obstruction at the systemic-to-PA shunt or progressive restriction to flow at the interatrial communication. Timing of these complications dictates treatment. If the shunt becomes inadequate before the child reaches age 3 to 4 months, when the PVR is likely to still be elevated, it is surgically revised. Likewise a restrictive interatrial communication is addressed by balloon dilation or repeated atrial septectomy early in life. Similar problems occurring when the child is older than 4 months are most commonly handled by performing an SVC-PA anastomosis earlier than planned, presuming favorable maturation of PVR and other hemodynamic variables.

ANESTHESIA FOR NONCARDIAC SURGERY IN CHILDREN WITH HLHS

A number of patients with HLHS require noncardiac surgical interventions, both before and between the reconstructive stages.[54] These procedures encompass a wide spectrum of complexity and urgency. It is our impression that a carefully administered anesthetic, appropriate for age and surgical procedure, is tolerated, provided that the unique ventilatory

Table 40-2 Late Complications after Stage I Reconstruction

Presenting Sign	Pathophysiology	Therapy
Congestive heart failure (CHF)	• AV valve regurgitation • Distal arch obstruction	• AV valve repair • Balloon dilation or surgical aortoplasty
Right ventricular hypertrophy	• Arch obstruction	• Balloon dilation or surgical aortoplasty
Hypoxemia	• Shunt stenosis • Pulmonary artery distortion • Restrictive IAC • Pulmonary vein stenosis • Congestive heart failure • Anemia	• Shunt revision ± pulmonary arterioplasty • Early bidirectional Glenn or hemi-Fontan • Balloon atrial septostomy or surgical atrial septectomy • Sutureless pulmonary vein repair or orthotopic heart transplantation • See above for CHF therapy • Packed red cell transfusion

IAC, interatrial communication; AV, atrioventricular; CHF, congestive heart failure.

and circulatory requirements of these patients are consistently met. For example, one must clearly appreciate the expected range of arterial oxygenation and the physiologic significance of both increased and decreased saturation to avoid potentially disastrous manipulations in PVR.

Preoperative Assessment and Planning

When possible, one might defer elective major noncardiac surgery until the infant with HLHS has recovered from an SVC-PA anastomosis (i.e., hemi-Fontan or bidirectional Glenn procedure).[78] At this stage of the reconstructive sequence, hemodynamic performance tends to be most resilient, as the right ventricle is no longer encumbered with extra volume output demands, and the Q_p:Q_s is not subject to wide variation in relation to manipulation of PVR. Nor is the cardiac output entirely dependent on the subtle factors that influence "passive" pulmonary blood flow, as occurs after Fontan operation. However, any potential impact that moderate elevation in SVC pressure has on the surgery should be weighed against the benefits of hemodynamic stability.

Unfortunately, many interventions will not wait for optimal hemodynamic stability. Urgent and emergency surgery often transpires when hemodynamics are least favorable. Under these circumstances, the principles of perioperative management and critical care for HLHS pertain, as described previously.

Whatever the timing, a clear understanding of each patient's anatomy and physiology constitutes the essential foundation of any perioperative plan. These details can usually be obtained most succinctly from the child's cardiologist. When a considerable time interval has elapsed since the cardiologist has evaluated the patient, the cardiologist should be included in preoperative assessment plans. From this information, a set of physiologic goals develops. In consultation with the surgeon involved, the anesthesiologist must anticipate the magnitude of the planned intervention.

Between July 1998 and June 2001, 247 infants and children with HLHS and comparable single-ventricle lesions underwent noncardiac surgery at the CHOP. Although noncardiac surgery was performed at every stage of the reconstructive sequence, including nine patients with native anatomy before stage 1, the majority of interventions occurred between SVC-PA anastomosis and Fontan procedure. Emergency surgery accounted for 27 (11%). Procedures ranged in complexity from simple, superficial operations (n = 190; 77%) to highly complex interventions (e.g., major intracavitary, CNS, craniofacial, or orthopedic) (n = 57; 23%).

Intraoperative Management

The conduct of anesthesia varies according to the physiologic state of the infant and the magnitude of the planned intervention. The important conditions necessary for the procedure should be reviewed with the surgeon and modified as necessary to accommodate the condition of the patient. For superficial surgery in a patient with HLHS who has good hemodynamics, short-acting anesthetics that allow prompt recovery and routine noninvasive monitoring are perfectly satisfactory. Conversely, those with significant hemodynamic impairment or volatile physiology who are undergoing major surgical interventions (e.g., preoperative neonate with HLHS

and a perforated bowel) would benefit from invasive monitoring. This strategy enables clinicians to track hemodynamic and ventilatory changes as well as therapies designed to optimize cardiac performance and systemic perfusion.

Postoperative Management

Postoperative surveillance ranges from discharge according to protocols established for healthy children of similar age through admission to an ICU. Although some extra caution is warranted, patients with HLHS are eligible for outpatient surgery when permitted by their cardiac function and surgical procedure. Should any aspect of the infant's condition render them vulnerable to the routine consequences of anesthesia and surgery; however, overnight admission to the hospital might represent the most prudent course. These consequences include such things as nausea, vomiting, pain, and limited ability to ingest fluids or medication orally. If one could envision a dramatic or life-threatening physiologic change (e.g., infant with profound baseline hypoxemia or after major surgery), surveillance in the ICU is advisable. In our series, the majority of children had day surgery (n = 127; 51%) or "same-day" surgery, in which they were admitted from home on the day of surgery (n = 42; 17%).

OUTCOME

General

The outcome after stage I reconstruction for HLHS has improved substantially since its introduction. In a large retrospective survey of 840 patients who underwent the Norwood procedure between 1984 and 1999, the overall 1-year survival was 51%.[63] In the cohort treated in the last 4 years of that study, the survival had increased to 71%. In a more recent review of 158 patients who underwent stage I reconstruction at the CHOP between January 1998 and June 2001, the operative survival was 77%.[35] In the cohort that had no associated risk factors, operative survival was 88%, compared with 63% with one or more risk factors. The risk factors for adverse outcome included low birth weight (<2.5 kg), associated cardiac and noncardiac malformations, and prolonged extracorporeal support (e.g., ventricular assist device [VAD] or extracorporeal membrane oxygenation [ECMO]). In this population, 23% had low birth weight, and nearly half (46%) had either low birth weight, an associated anomaly, or both. Either VAD or ECMO was used in 18 (11%) patients. Although prolonged extracorporeal support can permit extended favorable outcomes, the odds ratio for mortality in this very high-risk cohort is more than 17 (95% CI, 4.4–71).

Other centers with significant experience in treating HLHS have recently reported similar results. Bove[15] reported 76% operative survival in a series of 253 patients treated between 1990 and 1997. He also described significantly better outcome in patients with no associated risk factors (86% vs. 42%), such as noncardiac congenital conditions and severe preoperative pulmonary venous obstruction. Daebritz[21] reported a series of 194 patients undergoing stage I between 1990 and 1998. Those treated in the latter half of the period demonstrated a 79% operative survival. In this series, patients with HLHS, strictly defined as aortic and mitral atresia or severe stenosis, intact ventricular septum, and hypoplasia of the left ventricle, fared less well than other variants treated with stage I. The latter included double-outlet right ventricle with mitral atresia, malaligned atrioventricular canal defect, and tricuspid atresia with transposition of the great arteries. The operative survival was 63% with HLHS versus 81% with the other variants. This discrepancy has not been found in the other large series. Finally, Tworetzky[104] reported a series of 52 patients with HLHS who underwent stage I reconstruction with a 75% operative survival. In this series, a significant difference was noted between the outcome of those diagnosed prenatally (n = 14; survival, 100%) versus those diagnosed postnatally (n = 38; survival, 66%).

Despite remarkable improvements in operative outcome, most large series report additional mortality in the first year of life.[16,62] Gaynor[35] reported 15 deaths among the 122 survivors of stage I reconstruction. Most (n = 11; 73%) occurred before SVC-PA anastomosis. The most common cause of death in the first year was sudden unexplained cardiac death (n = 10; 67%). Documented perioperative arrhythmia has been identified as an independent risk factor in those who subsequently died suddenly, but accounts for only a minority of deaths.[62] The operative mortality from hemi-Fontan was extremely low (1.1%). Many hypotheses exist to explain this finding, including coronary insufficiency, arrhythmia, and acute shunt occlusion. The only risk factor identified in the Gaynor series was presence of associated anomalies (either cardiac or noncardiac). Patients with an anatomic diagnosis of aortic atresia, which may contribute to coronary insufficiency, demonstrated a trend toward unfavorable 1-year survival, but it did not achieve statistical significance. However, this factor may contribute to the discrepancy reported by Daebritz.[21]

Neurologic Outcome

Abnormal neurologic states exist to a notable degree in HLHS but may not be different from those in patients with major congenital heart malformations requiring similar treatment. Brain dysfunction results from congenital anomalies and the insults occurring in the immediate perioperative and interval periods between surgical procedures. The discovery of coexisting anomalies early in pregnancy influences treatment choices and thus the profiles of survivors. Assessment of neurologic function early in life is limited, but as patients grow older, testing methods become applicable and are being reported with increasing frequency. A high degree of selection bias is present in every study population that has been reported, and the application of findings to local populations should be undertaken with caution.

Virtually all reports of stage I reconstruction describe the use of circulatory arrest with deep hypothermia for neuroprotection. The relative merits of the components of hypothermic management (e.g., acid-base, cooling time, rate, and degree) remain controversial because they are based on surrogate outcome measures or retrospective observations in small numbers of patients. Some have even postulated that neonates with HLHS are particularly vulnerable because of the necessary modifications in cannulation procedures and perfusion of the aortic arch vessels.[55] However, current strategies offer limited protection because virtually all reports find an association between neurologic deficit and prolonged circulatory arrest time, although the definition of *prolonged* varies. It is appealing to apply methods of continuous perfusion instead of circulatory arrest. However, in a comparative analysis of arrest and low flow in neonates with transposition of the great arteries, the incidence of neurologic abnormality at hospital discharge was not statistically different (23% vs. 17% for arrest vs. low flow).[77] Long-term developmental follow-up of this population has not revealed clinically important differences.[9]

The neurologic outcome of a population of patients who essentially did not exist until the last decade is in the process of being defined. Although initially the focus was on operative interventions as the most likely cause of adverse neurologic outcomes, it is increasingly apparent that preoperative issues, and perhaps postoperative states as well, must be scrutinized as major contributors. The impact of genetic factors, management techniques, and chronically abnormal perfusion and oxygenation are likely to be additive and synergistic and are just beginning to be understood.

CONCLUSIONS

Over the past two decades, incredible progress has been forged in the treatment of HLHS. Infants are now delivered to the threshold of a cavopulmonary connection sequence in a condition virtually indistinguishable from that with other forms of single ventricle.[34] Early and intermediate-term outcomes rival those of other serious congenital heart malformations. The success of both surgical options in selected centers raises the question as to whether one can ethically continue to offer the option of no therapy selectively to families of infants with HLHS in contradistinction to other congenital malformations whose outcome is far less favorable.

Opportunities remain to improve outcome further still. The factors that contribute to sudden death in the late postoperative period after stage I reconstruction demand more attention, although they will be difficult to study. Further refinements in surgical technique offer the prospect of adequate pulmonary blood flow without necessitating the low diastolic pressure that potentially jeopardizes coronary and systemic perfusion after stage I. Although not limited to HLHS, methods that enhance organ protection, especially the heart and brain, during CPB and circulatory arrest offer the promise of better outcome.

Although myriad challenges confront clinicians caring for these patients that are remarkably complex, both technically and physiologically, unique rewards also ensue.

References

1. Anand KJ, Hickey PR: Halothane-morphine compared with high-dose sufentanil for anesthesia and postoperative analgesia in neonatal cardiac surgery. *N Engl J Med* 326:1–9, 1992.
2. Atz AM, Feinstein JA, Jonas RA, et al: Preoperative management of pulmonary venous hypertension in hypoplastic left heart syndrome with restrictive atrial septal defect. *Am J Cardiol* 83:1224–1228, 1999.
3. Atz AM, Wessel DL: Inhaled nitric oxide in the neonate with cardiac disease. *Semin Perinatol* 21:441–455, 1997.
4. Bailey LL, Nehlsen-Cannarella SL, Doroshow RW, et al: Cardiac allotransplantation in newborns as therapy for hypoplastic left heart syndrome. *N Engl J Med* 315:949–951, 1986.

5. Bando K, Turrentine MW, Vijay P, et al: Effect of modified ultrafiltration in high-risk patients undergoing operations for congenital heart disease. *Ann Thorac Surg* 66:821–827, 1998.

6. Barber G, Helton JG, Aglira BA, et al: The significance of tricuspid regurgitation in hypoplastic left-heart syndrome. *Am Heart J* 116:1563–1567, 1988.

7. Bartram U, Grunenfelder J, Van Praagh R: Causes of death after the modified Norwood Procedure: A study of 122 postmortem cases. *Ann Thorac Surg* 64:1795–1802, 1997.

8. Behrendt DM, Rocchini A: An operation for the hypoplastic left heart syndrome: Preliminary report. *Ann Thorac Surg* 32:284–288, 1981.

9. Bellinger DC, Wypij D, Kuban KC, et al: Developmental and neurological status of children at 4 years of age after heart surgery with hypothermic circulatory arrest or low-flow cardiopulmonary bypass. *Circulation* 100:526–532, 1999.

10. Better DJ, Apfel HD, Zidere V, Allan LD: Pattern of pulmonary venous blood flow in the hypoplastic left heart syndrome in the fetus. *Heart* 81:646–649, 1999.

11. Bissonnette B, Holtby MH, Davis AJ, et al: Cerebral hyperthermia in children after cardiopulmonary bypass. *Anesthesiology* 93:611–618, 2000.

12. Blake DM, Copel JA, Kleinman CS: Hypoplastic left heart syndrome: Prenatal diagnosis, clinical profile, and management. *Am J Obstet Gynecol* 165:529–534, 1991.

13. Botto L, Correa A, Erikson JD: Racial and temporal variations in the prevalence of heart defects. *Pediatrics* 107:e32, 2001.

14. Boucek MM, Faro A, Novick RJ, et al: The registry of the International Society for Heart and Lung Transplantation: Fourth official pediatric report-2000. *J Heart Lung Transplant* 20:39–52, 2001.

15. Bove EL: Current status of staged reconstruction for hypoplastic left heart syndrome. *Pediatr Cardiol* 19:308–315, 1998.

16. Bove EL, Lloyd TR: Staged reconstruction for hypoplastic left heart syndrome: Contemporary results. *Ann Surg* 224:387–394, 1996.

17. Carrel TP, Schwanda M, Vogt PR, Turina MI: Aprotinin in pediatric cardiac operations: A benefit in complex malformations and with high-dose regimen only. *Ann Thorac Surg* 66:153–158, 1998.

18. Cayler GG, Smeloff EA, Miller GE Jr: Surgical palliation of hypoplastic left side of the heart. *N Engl J Med* 282:780–783, 1970.

19. Chambers LA, Cohen DM, Davis JT: Transfusion patterns in pediatric open heart surgery. *Transfusion* 36:150–154, 1996.

20. Clancy RR, McGaurn SA, Goin JE, et al: Allopurinol neurocardiac protection trial in infants undergoing heart surgery using deep hypothermic circulatory arrest. *Pediatrics* 108:61–70, 2001.

21. Daebritz SH, Nollert GD, Zurakowski D, et al: Results of Norwood stage I operation: Comparison of hypoplastic left heart syndrome with other malformations. *J Thorac Cardiovasc Surg* 119:358–367, 2000.

22. Davies MJ, Nguyen K, Gaynor JW, Elliott MJ: Modified ultrafiltration improves left ventricular systolic function in infants after cardiopulmonary bypass. *J Thorac Cardiovasc Surg* 115:361–369, 1998.

23. DiCarlo JV, Raphaely RC, Steven JM, et al: Pulmonary mechanics in infants after cardiac surgery. *Crit Care Med* 20:22–27, 1992.

24. Dietrich W, Mossinger H, Spannagl M, et al: Hemostatic activation during cardiopulmonary bypass with different aprotinin dosages in pediatric patient having cardiac operations. *J Thorac Cardiovasc Surg* 105:712–720, 1993.

25. Doty DB, Knott HW: Hypoplastic left heart syndrome: Experience with an operation to establish functionally normal circulation. *J Thorac Cardiovasc Surg* 74:624–630, 1977.

26. Doty DB, Marvin WJ Jr, Schieken RM, Lauer RM: Hypoplastic left heart syndrome: Successful palliation with a new operation. *J Thorac Cardiovasc Surg* 80:148–152, 1980.

27. Eapen RS, Rowland DG, Franklin WH: Effect of prenatal diagnosis of critical left heart obstruction on perinatal morbidity and mortality. *Am J Perinatol* 15:237–242, 1998.

28. Elliott MJ: Ultrafiltration and modified ultrafiltration in pediatric open-heart operations. *Ann Thorac Surg* 56:1518–1522, 1993.

29. Fontan F, Baudet E: Surgical repair of tricuspid atresia. *Thorax* 26:240–248, 1971.

30. Frankville D, Steven JM, Raphaely RC, Norwood WI: Ventilatory support after palliative surgery (the Norwood operation) for hypoplastic left heart syndrome. *Proc Pediatr Crit Care Colloquium* 1989.

31. Freedom RM, Williams WG, Dische MR, Rowe RD: Anatomical variants in aortic atresia: Potential candidates for ventriculoaortic reconstitution. *Br Heart J* 38:821–826, 1976.

32. Fujiseki Y, Yamamoto H, Hattori M, et al: Oral administration of prostaglandin E$_2$ in the hypoplastic left heart syndrome. *Jpn Heart J* 24:481–487, 1983.

33. Fyler DC, Buckley LP, Hellenbrand WE, Cohn HE: Report of the New England Regional Infant Cardiac Program. *Pediatrics* 65:375–461, 1980.

34. Gaynor JW, Bridges ND, Cohen MI, et al: Predictors of outcome after the Fontan operation: Is hypoplastic left heart syndrome still a risk factor? *J Thorac Cardiovasc Surg* 123:237–245, 2002.

35. Gaynor JW, Mahle WT, Cohen MI, et al: Risk factors for mortality after the Norwood procedure. *Eur J Cardiothorac Surg* 22:82–89, 2002.

36. Glauser TA, Rorke LB, Weinberg PM, Clancy RR: Acquired neuropathologic lesions associated with the hypoplastic left heart syndrome. *Pediatrics* 85:991–1000, 1990.

37. Glauser TA, Rorke LB, Weinberg PM, Clancy RR: Congenital brain anomalies associated with the hypoplastic left heart syndrome. *Pediatrics* 85:984–990, 1990.

38. Grocott HP, Mackensen GB, Grigore AM, et al: Postoperative hyperthermia is associated with cognitive dysfunction after coronary artery bypass graft surgery. *Stroke* 33:537–541, 2002.

39. Gruber EM, Laussen PC, Casta A, et al: Stress response in infants undergoing cardiac surgery: A randomized study of fentanyl bolus, fentanyl infusion, and fentanyl-midazolam infusion. *Anesth Analg* 92:882–890, 2001.

40. Hansen DD, Hickey PR: Anesthesia for hypoplastic left heart syndrome: Use of high-dose fentanyl in 30 neonates. *Anesth Analg* 65:127–132, 1986.

41. Haworth SG: Pulmonary vascular disease in different types of congenital heart disease: Implications for interpretation of lung biopsy findings in early childhood. *Br Heart J* 52:557–571, 1984.

42. Haworth SG, Reid L: Structural study of pulmonary circulation and of heart in total anomalous pulmonary venous return in early infancy. *Br Heart J* 39:80–92, 1977.

43. Hebra A, Brown MF, Hirschl RB, et al: Mesenteric ischemia in hypoplastic left heart syndrome. *J Pediatr Surg* 28:606–611, 1993.

44. Helton JG, Aglira BA, Chin AJ, et al: Analysis of potential anatomic or physiologic determinants of outcome of palliative surgery for hypoplastic left heart syndrome. *Circulation* 74:I70–I76, 1986.

45. Hickey PR, Hansen DD: High-dose fentanyl reduces intraoperative ventricular fibrillation in neonates with hypoplastic left heart syndrome. *J Clin Anesth* 3:295–300, 1991.

46. Hickey PR, Hansen DD, Wessel DL, et al: Blunting of stress responses in the pulmonary circulation of infants by fentanyl. *Anesth Analg* 64:1137–1142, 1985.

47. Hoffman GM, Ghanayem NS, Kampine JM, et al: Venous saturation and the anaerobic threshold in neonates after the Norwood procedure for hypoplastic left heart syndrome. *Ann Thorac Surg* 70:1515–1520, 2000.

48. Hosenpud JD, Bennett LE, Keck BM, et al: The registry of the International Society for Heart and Lung Transplantation: Eighteenth official report-2001. *J Heart Lung Transplant* 20:805–815, 2001.

49. Ichinose F, Uezono S, Muto R, et al: Platelet hyporeactivity in young infants during cardiopulmonary bypass. *Anesth Analg* 88:258–262, 1999.

50. Ishino K, Stumper O, De Giovanni JJ, et al: The modified Norwood procedure for hypoplastic left heart syndrome: Early to intermediate results of 120 patients with particular reference to aortic arch repair. *J Thorac Cardiovasc Surg* 117:920–930, 1999.

51. Jenkins PC, Flanagan MF, Sargent JD, et al: A comparison of treatment strategies for hypoplastic left heart syndrome using decision analysis. *J Am Coll Cardiol* 38:1181–1187, 2001.

52. Jobes DR, Nicolson SC, Pigott JD, Norwood WI: An enclosed system for continuous postoperative mediastinal aspiration. *Ann Thorac Surg* 45:101–102, 1988.

53. Jobes DR, Nicolson SC, Steven JM, et al: Carbon dioxide prevents pulmonary overcirculation in hypoplastic left heart syndrome. *Ann Thorac Surg* 54:150–151, 1992.

54. Karl HW, Hensley FA Jr, Cyran SE, et al: Hypoplastic left heart syndrome: Anesthesia for elective noncardiac surgery. *Anesthesiology* 72:753–757, 1990.

55. Kern FH, Jonas RA, Mayer JE Jr, et al: Temperature monitoring during CPB in infants: Does it predict efficient brain cooling? *Ann Thorac Surg* 54:749–754, 1992.

56. Kern FH, Morana NJ, Sears JJ, Hickey PR: Coagulation defects in neonates during cardiopulmonary bypass. *Ann Thorac Surg* 54:541–546, 1992.

57. Kishimoto H, Kawahira Y, Kawata H, et al: The modified Norwood palliation on a beating heart. *J Thorac Cardiovasc Surg* 118:1130–1132, 1999.

57a. Kreutzer G, Galindez E, Bono H, et al: An operation for the correction of tricuspid atresia. *J Thorac Cardiovasc Surg* 66: 613–621, 1973.

58. Lev M: Pathologic anatomy and interrelationship of hypoplasia of the aortic complexes. *Lab Invest* 1:61–70, 1952.

59. Levitsky S, van der Horst RL, Hasteiter AR, et al: Surgical palliation in aortic atresia. *J Thorac Cardiovasc Surg* 79:456–461, 1980.

60. Litwin SB, Van Praagh R, Bernhard WF: A palliative operation for certain infants with aortic arch interruption. *Ann Thorac Surg* 14:369–375, 1972.

61. Mahle WT, Clancy RR, McGaurn SP, et al: Impact of prenatal diagnosis on survival and early neurologic morbidity in neonates with the hypoplastic left heart syndrome. *Pediatrics* 107:1277–1282, 2001.

62. Mahle WT, Spray TL, Gaynor JW, Clark BJ: Unexpected death after reconstructive surgery for hypoplastic left heart syndrome. *Ann Thorac Surg* 71:61–65, 2001.

63. Mahle WT, Spray TL, Wernovsky G, et al: Survival after reconstructive surgery for hypoplastic left heart syndrome: A 15-year experience from a single institution. *Circulation* 102:III136–III141, 2000.

64. Mahle WT, Tavani F, Zimmerman RA, et al: An MRI study of neurologic injury before and after congenital heart surgery. *Circulation* 106:I109–I114, 2002.

65. Mair R, Tulzer G, Sames E, et al: Right ventricle to pulmonary artery conduit instead of modified Blalock-Taussig shunt improves post-operative hemodynamics in newborns after the Norwood procedure. *J Thorac Cardiovasc Surg* 126:1378–1384, 2003.

66. Malec E, Januszewska K, Kolcz J, et al: Right ventricle to pulmonary artery shunt versus modified Blalock-Taussig shunt in the Norwood procedure for hypoplastic left heart syndrome: Influence on early and late hemodynamic status. *Eur J Cardiothorac Surg* 23:728–734, 2003.

67. Manno CS, Hedberg KW, Kim HC, et al: Comparison of the hemostatic effects of fresh whole blood, stored whole blood and components after open heart surgery in children. *Blood* 77:930–936, 1991.

68. McElhinney DB, Hedrick HL, Bush DM, et al: Necrotizing enterocolitis in neonates with congenital heart disease: Risk factors and outcomes. *Pediatrics* 106:1080–1087, 2000.

69. Miller BE, Mochizuki T, Levy JH, et al: Predicting and treating coagulopathies after cardiopulmonary bypass in children. *Anesth Analg* 85:1196–1202, 1997.

70. Mohri H, Horiuchi T, Haneda K, et al: Surgical treatment for hypoplastic left heart syndrome: Case reports. *J Thorac Cardiovasc Surg* 78:223–228, 1979.

71. Morray JP, Lynn AM, Mansfield PB: Effect of pH and PCO$_2$ on pulmonary and systemic hemodynamics after surgery in children with congenital heart disease and pulmonary hypertension. *J Pediatr* 113:474–479, 1988.

72. Murdison KA, Baffa JM, Farrell PE Jr, et al: Hypoplastic left heart syndrome: Outcome after initial reconstruction and before modified Fontan procedure. *Circulation* 82:IV199–IV207, 1990.

73. Murphy JD, Sands BL, Norwood WI: Intraoperative balloon angioplasty of aortic coarctation in infants with hypoplastic left heart syndrome. *Am J Cardiol* 59:949–951, 1987.

74. Naik SK, Knight A, Elliott MJ: A successful modification of ultrafiltration for cardiopulmonary bypass in children. *Perfusion* 6:41–50, 1991.

75. Natowicz M, Chatten J, Clancy R, et al: Genetic disorders and major extracardiac anomalies associated with the hypoplastic left heart syndrome. *Pediatrics* 82:698–706, 1988.

76. Natowicz M, Kelley RI: Association of Turner syndrome with hypoplastic left-heart syndrome. *Am J Dis Child* 141:218–220, 1987.

77. Newburger JW, Jonas RA, Wernovsky G, et al: A comparison of the perioperative neurologic effects of hypothermic circulatory arrest versus low-flow cardiopulmonary bypass in infant heart surgery. *N Engl J Med* 329:1057–1064, 1993.

78. Nicolson SC, Steven JM, Kurth CD, et al: Anesthesia for noncardiac surgery infants with hypoplastic left heart syndrome following hemi-Fontan operation. *J Cardiothorac Vasc Anesth* 8:334–336, 1994.

79. Noonan JA, Nadas AS: The hypoplastic left heart syndrome: An analysis of 101 cases. *Pediatr Clin North Am* 5:1029–1056, 1958.

80. Norwood WI, Jacobs ML, Murphy JD: Fontan procedure for hypoplastic left heart syndrome. *Ann Thorac Surg* 54:1025–1029, 1992.

81. Norwood WI, Kirklin JK, Sanders SP: Hypoplastic left heart syndrome: Experience with palliative surgery. *Am J Cardiol* 45:87–91, 1980.

82. Norwood WI, Lang P, Castaneda AR, Campbell DN: Experience with operation for hypoplastic left heart syndrome. *J Thorac Cardiovasc Surg* 82:511–519, 1981.

83. Norwood WI, Lang P, Hansen DD: Physiologic repair of aortic atresia-hypoplastic left heart syndrome. *N Engl J Med* 308:23–26, 1983.

84. Petaja J, Lundstrom U, Leijala M, et al: Bleeding and use of blood products after heart operations in infants. *J Thorac Cardiovasc Surg* 109:524–529, 1995.

85. Pizarro C, Malec E, Maher KO, et al: Right ventricle to pulmonary artery conduit improves outcome after stage I Norwood for hypoplastic left heart syndrome. *Circulation* 108:II155–II160, 2003.

86. Qazi QH, Kanchanapoomi R, Cooper R, et al: Dup(12p) and hypoplastic left heart. *Am J Med Genet* 9:195–199, 1981.

87. Ramamoorthy C, Anderson GD, Williams GD, Lynn AM: Pharmacokinetics and side effects of milrinone in infants and children after open heart surgery. *Anesth Analg* 86:283–289, 1998.

88. Ramamoorthy C, Tabbutt S, Kurth CD, et al: Effects of inspired hypoxic and hypercapnic gas mixtures on cerebral oxygen saturation in neonates with univentricular heart defects. *Anesthesiology* 96:283–288, 2002.

89. Razzouk AJ, Chinnock RE, Gundry SR, et al: Transplantation as a primary treatment for hypoplastic left heart syndrome: Intermediate-term results. *Ann Thorac Surg* 62:1–8, 1996.

90. Redo SF, Farber S, Gross RE: Atresia of the mitral valve. *Arch Surg* 82:678–694, 1961.

91. Rinder CS, Gaal D, Student LA, Smith BR: Platelet-leukocyte activation and modulation of adhesion receptors in pediatric patients with congenital heart disease undergoing cardiopulmonary bypass. *J Thorac Cardiovasc Surg* 107:280–288, 1994.

92. Riordan CJ, Locher JP Jr, Santamore WP, et al: Monitoring systemic venous oxygen saturations in hypoplastic left heart syndrome. *Ann Thorac Surg* 63:835, 1997.

93. Rossi AF, Sommer RJ, Lotvin A, et al: Usefulness of intermittent monitoring of mixed venous oxygen saturation after stage I palliation for hypoplastic left heart syndrome. *Am J Cardiology* 73:1118–1123, 1994.

94. Russell IA, Zwass MS, Fineman JR, et al: The effects of inhaled nitric oxide on postoperative pulmonary hypertension in infants and children undergoing surgical repair of congenital heart disease. *Anesth Analg* 87:46–51, 1998.

95. Rychik J, Bush DM, Spray TL, et al: Assessment of pulmonary/systemic blood flow ratio after first-stage palliation for hypoplastic left heart syndrome: Development of a new index with the use of Doppler echocardiography. *J Thorac Cardiovasc Surg* 102:81–87, 2000.

96. Rychik J, Rome JJ, Collins MH, et al: The hypoplastic left heart syndrome with intact atrial septum: Atrial morphology, pulmonary vascular histopathology and outcome. *J Am Coll Cardiol* 34:554–560, 1999.

97. Sano S, Ishino K, Kawada M, Honjo O: Right ventricle-pulmonary artery shunt in first-stage palliation of hypoplastic left heart syndrome. *Semin Thorac Cardiovasc Surg* 7:22–31, 2004.

98. Sano S, Kawada M, Yoshida H, et al: Norwood procedure to hypoplastic left heart syndrome. *Jpn J Thorac Cardiovasc Surg* 46:1311–1316, 1998.

99. Sinha SN, Rusnak SL, Sommers HM, et al: Hypoplastic left ventricle syndrome: Analysis of thirty autopsy cases in infants with surgical considerations. *Am J Cardiol* 21:166–173, 1968.

100. Skaryak LA, Kirshbom PM, DiBernardo LR, et al: Modified ultrafiltration improves cerebral metabolic recovery after circulatory arrest. *J Thorac Cardiovasc Surg* 109:744–751, 1995.

101. Starnes VA, Griffin ML, Pitlick PT, et al: Current approach to hypoplastic left heart syndrome: Palliation, transplantation, or both? *J Thorac Cardiovasc Surg* 104:189–194, 1992.

102. Tabbutt S, Ramamoorthy C, Montenegro LM, et al: Impact of inspired gas mixtures on preoperative infants with hypoplastic left heart syndrome during controlled ventilation. *Circulation* 104:I159–164, 2001.

103. Taeed R, Schwartz SM, Pearl JM, et al: Unrecognized pulmonary venous desaturation early after Norwood palliation confounds Qp:Qs assessment and compromises oxygen delivery. *Circulation* 103:2699–2704, 2001.

104. Tworetzky W, McElhinney DB, Reddy VM, et al: Improved surgical outcome after fetal diagnosis of hypoplastic left heart syndrome. *Circulation* 103:1269–1273, 2001.

105. Vincent RN, Lang P, Elixson EM, et al: Measurement of extravascular lung water in infants and children after cardiac surgery. *Am J Cardiol* 54:161–165, 1984.

106. Wernovsky G, McElhinney DB, Tabbutt S: Postoperative management after first-stage palliation. In Rychik J, Wernovsky G (eds): *The Hypoplastic Left Heart Syndrome*. Boston, Kluwer Academic Publishing, 2002.

107. Wernovsky G, Wypij D, Jonas RA, et al: Postoperative course and hemodynamic profile after the arterial switch operation in neonates and infants: A comparison of low-flow cardiopulmonary bypass and circulatory arrest. *Circulation* 92:2226–2235, 1995.

108. Williams GD, Bratton SL, Nielsen NJ, Ramamoorthy C: Fibrinolysis in pediatric patients undergoing cardiopulmonary bypass. *J Cardiothorac Vasc Anesth* 12:633–638, 1998.

109. Williams GD, Bratton SL, Riley EC, Ramamoorthy C: Association between age and blood loss in children undergoing open heart operations. *Ann Thorac Surg* 66:870–875, 1998.

110. Williams GD, Bratton SL, Riley EC, Ramamoorthy C: Coagulation tests during cardiopulmonary bypass correlate with blood loss in children undergoing cardiac surgery. *J Cardiothor Vasc Anesth* 13:398–404, 1999.

Chapter 41

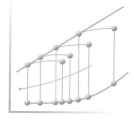

Separating the Circulations: Cavopulmonary Connections (Bidirectional Glenn, Hemi-Fontan) and the Modified Fontan Operation

BRADLEY S. MARINO, MD, MPP, MSCE, THOMAS L. SPRAY, MD, and WILLIAM J. GREELEY, MD, MBA

Atresia of an atrioventricular or semilunar valve results in single-ventricle anatomies that have complete mixing of the systemic and pulmonary venous circulations. Structural defects that are generally managed with a staged palliation include variations of single left ventricle (e.g., tricuspid atresia with normally related great arteries or transposition of the great arteries, double-inlet left ventricle with normally related great arteries or transposition of the great arteries, malaligned atrioventricular canal with hypoplastic right ventricle, and pulmonary atresia with intact ventricular septum) and variations of single right ventricle (e.g., hypoplastic left heart syndrome [HLHS], double-outlet right ventricle with mitral atresia, malaligned atrioventricular canal with hypoplastic left ventricle, and heterotaxy syndromes). Children with single-ventricle anatomy generally undergo palliative surgery in the neonatal period that will result in unobstructed systemic blood flow, limited pulmonary blood flow, undistorted pulmonary arteries, unobstructed pulmonary venous

845

return, and minimal atrioventricular valve regurgitation. Newborn surgical palliation allows the neonate to survive into infancy but is not a stable anatomic or physiologic long-term solution. Children with single-ventricle anatomy will ultimately undergo some variation of the Fontan operation as their final surgical palliation.[17,79,94]

Risk factors for poor outcome after the modified Fontan operation include ventricular hypertrophy, elevated pulmonary vascular resistance (PVR) or pulmonary artery (PA) pressure, PA distortion, atrioventricular valve regurgitation, and ventricular dysfunction. Newborn surgical palliation for single-ventricle anatomy is performed to minimize these potential risk factors for poor outcome at the time of the superior cavopulmonary anastomosis and total cavopulmonary anastomosis.

This chapter discusses the history, surgical indications, surgical technique, postoperative physiology, and postoperative issues for the superior cavopulmonary anastomoses (hemi-Fontan and bidirectional Glenn [BDG]) and the modified Fontan procedures.

GENERAL PRINCIPLES OF SUPERIOR AND TOTAL CAVOPULMONARY CONNECTIONS

The goal of surgical palliation for the various single-ventricle lesions is to separate the systemic and pulmonary circuits, resulting in normal or near-normal oxygen saturation. Cavopulmonary connections are used to divert systemic venous return directly into the pulmonary vascular bed, providing more "effective" pulmonary blood flow and reducing the volume load on the single ventricle. After these procedures, the single ventricle ejects blood only to the systemic circuit, with pulmonary blood flow derived by "passive flow" into the pulmonary vascular bed at the expense of higher central venous pressure. Although cavopulmonary connections improve cyanosis and minimize ventricular work, the elevated PVR in the neonate precludes their use until approximately 3 months of age.

The cavopulmonary connections used to stage the single-ventricle patient to the modified Fontan include the BDG and the hemi-Fontan. Staging to Fontan is presently performed because of the high incidence of pleural effusions and low-output myocardial failure that occurred when patients were taken directly from a neonatal single-ventricle palliation to the Fontan.[46] Creation of the superior cavopulmonary anastomosis with ligation of the systemic-PA or right ventricle-to-PA shunt or removal of the PA band with ligation of the PA provides a single stable source of pulmonary blood flow.

BIDIRECTIONAL GLENN/HEMI-FONTAN

History

In the 1950s and 1960s in Italy, the United States, and Russia, many surgeons were concurrently discovering and harnessing the utility of the cavopulmonary connection. An experimental model of the cavopulmonary anastomosis was used in dogs by Carlon in the 1950s.[16] This model identified many of the hemodynamic and surgical advantages of the cavopulmonary anastomosis relative to the Blalock-Taussig shunt. Carlon ligated the proximal right pulmonary artery (RPA)

and superior vena cava (SVC) and used the azygos vein to anastomose the SVC to the RPA. Azzolina[5] promulgated the concept of bidirectionality, using his technique in nine patients with tricuspid atresia. Many other surgeons, including Glenn, Haller, Norwood, Jacobs, and Kawashima, made further modifications and adjustments to the cavopulmonary shunt that allowed it ultimately to be used extensively in single-ventricle palliation.[67]

The first significant clinical use of the cavopulmonary anastomosis in the United States was performed by Glenn.[48] He used unidirectional (classic) and bidirectional superior cavopulmonary anastomoses and inferior cavopulmonary anastomosis (inferior vena cava [IVC]-to-PA connection). Interim palliation with a BDG shunt has now become the standard of care over the past decade, typically in infancy (4 to 9 months of age).[1,11,19,38,39,54,92,103,108]

Indications for Surgery

The timing of superior cavopulmonary connection is variable. With a decrease in PVR, infants with single ventricle who have had a neonatal palliation become candidates for the superior cavopulmonary anastomoses by 3 to 6 months of age. Mahle and associates[80] showed that early ventricular unloading after neonatal single-ventricle palliation improved aerobic exercise performance in preadolescents with the Fontan palliation. An additional advantage of an early superior cavopulmonary anastomosis is the opportunity to address distorted pulmonary arteries from previous bands or shunts and to create a better distribution of PA blood flow and growth of the pulmonary vascular bed. A number of specific scenarios should prompt expedited consideration of a cavopulmonary anastomosis. These scenarios include cyanosis secondary to inadequate pulmonary blood flow after neonatal palliation or congestive heart failure from an excessive volume load caused either by severe atrioventricular valve regurgitation or by an elevated $Q_p:Q_s$.[109] Atrioventricular valve regurgitation and ventricular dysfunction increase the risk of performing the superior cavopulmonary anastomosis.

The benefits of early cavopulmonary anastomosis must be weighed against the risks of elevated SVC pressure and cyanosis. Bradley and colleagues[11] found that cavopulmonary anastomosis at younger than 3 months was associated with lower oxygen saturation in the early postoperative period and a risk of PA thrombosis. Some infants with severe ventricular dysfunction or atrioventricular valve regurgitation may not be suitable for further staged palliation and may require heart transplantation.

Before cavopulmonary anastomosis, the child should have an echocardiogram and cardiac catheterization for anatomic and hemodynamic assessment of the pulmonary arteries, aortic arch, ventricular and atrioventricular valve function, caval anatomy, and the presence of decompressing veins that may result in cyanosis after superior cavopulmonary anastomosis.

Surgical Technique: Bidirectional Glenn Procedure

The BDG and hemi-Fontan are used to create the superior cavopulmonary anastomosis.[56,61] Although the BDG and hemi-Fontan are comparable physiologically, differences occur in bypass technique, utilization of patch material,

Table 41-1 Summary of Advantages and Disadvantages of the Bidirectional Glenn and Hemi-Fontan Procedures

Consideration	Bidirectional Glenn	Hemi-Fontan
Bypass technique	Normothermic, beating heart CPB, totally extracardiac repair. Can be done without CPB in some cases.	Cardioplegic arrest or total circulatory arrest for intracardiac work
Added material	Can be performed with no added prosthetic material	Requires patch material (usually allograft)
Cannulation	Usually SVC, RA, and Ao	RA and Ao only, if done with circulatory arrest
Prospects for PA enlargement	Requires additional PA plasty if enlargement is required	Excellent central PA enlargement is part of the operation
Fontan completion options	Extracardiac Fontan completion can be performed with normothermic beating heart CPB	Lateral tunnel TCPC is obligatory (barring takedown of the hemi-Fontan connection), with need for ischemia and/or circulatory arrest
Technique ease	Straightforward to learn and perform	More demanding technically, but works well in experienced hands
SA node blood supply	Untouched	Compromised, but may not be important for outcome[23]
Risk of operation	Low	Low
Postoperative physiology	Equivalent	Equivalent
Eventual Fontan outcome	Very good in current era	Better than those achieved with BDG in some institutions (see text)

Ao, aorta; BDG, bidirectional Glenn; CPB, cardiopulmonary bypass; PA, pulmonary artery; RA, right atrium; SA, sinoatrial; SVC, superior vena cava; TCPC, total cavopulmonary connection.

From Karl TR: Staged reconstruction for hypoplastic left heart syndrome: The bi-directional cavopulmonary shunt. In Rychik J, Wernovsky G (eds): *Hypoplastic Left Heart Syndrome.* Boston, Kluwer Academic Publishers, 2003, p 135; with permission.

cannulation, methods of PA augmentation, Fontan completion options, and ease of technique that should be considered. Table 41-1 summarizes the advantages and disadvantages of the two strategies.

Cardiopulmonary Bypass Technique

The BDG operation is performed via median sternotomy (Fig. 41-1). At the initiation of cardiopulmonary bypass (CPB), the shunt is ligated with a vascular clip or ligature. Preservation of the proper spatial orientation of the SVC relative to the PA is essential. Therefore the azygos vein is ligated but not divided. The SVC is then divided, and the cardiac end is oversewn. The cephalic end is anastomosed end to side to the ipsilateral PA, as indicated in Figure 41-1. The distal end of the shunt is completely excised from the RPA. Modified ultrafiltration (MUF) may be used to remove the priming volume of the CPB circuit, resulting in hemoconcentration, usually with a concurrent improvement in hemodynamics. The use of MUF reduces blood use, chest-tube losses, pleuropericardial effusion incidence, and hospital stay for both hemi-Fontan and BDG patients.[69]

Technique Without Cardiopulmonary Bypass

Unlike the hemi-Fontan, the BDG may be performed without the utilization of CPB. Patients with sources of pulmonary blood flow that do not need interruption as part of the cavopulmonary anastomosis (e.g., antegrade flow through a stenotic pulmonary valve or banded PA) and have no specific intracardiac pathology requiring revision may be candidates for cavopulmonary anastomosis without CPB. Patients with bilateral superior vena cavae also may be candidates for

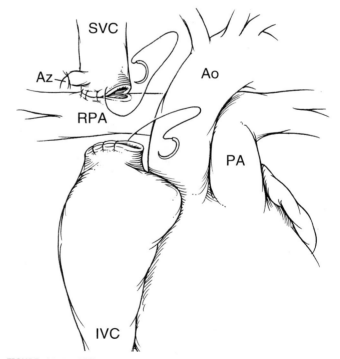

FIGURE 41-1 Bidirectional superior cavopulmonary anastomosis (bidirectional Glenn). The superior vena cava (SVC) is transected at the level of the right pulmonary artery (RPA), the cardiac end is oversewn, and the cephalad portion of the superior vena cava is anastomosed end-to-side into the proximal right pulmonary artery. Ao, aorta; IVC, inferior vena cava; PA, pulmonary artery.

superior cavopulmonary anastomosis without CPB, because a single-branch PA is occluded at a time to accomplish the bicaval connections. In some cases, an SVC to RA or PA shunt may be needed to decompress upper systemic venous blood flow. HLHS patients are generally not candidates for superior cavopulmonary anastomosis without CPB because their pulmonary blood flow is shunt dependent, and because they may require PA reconstruction and other intracardiac procedures at the time of their superior cavopulmonary anastomosis.

Surgical Technique: The Hemi-Fontan Procedure

Alternatively, a hemi-Fontan may be performed, in which a temporary "dam" is placed in the orifice of the SVC separating the SVC from the atrium, and an anastomosis is created superior to the dam between the SVC and the ipsilateral PA.[60,61,95] Norwood and Jacobs[95] initially described this technical modification of the BDG to be used in HLHS patients after the stage I reconstruction. Although the hemi-Fontan enlarges the central PAs at the time of the cavopulmonary anastomosis with a triangular-shaped patch and makes the Fontan completion simpler (lateral tunnel Fontan completion), it is technically more difficult and requires aortic cross-clamping with cardioplegic arrest with or without circulatory arrest. The use of the hemi-Fontan (rather than BDG) facilitates the lateral tunnel Fontan completion, which requires only an atriotomy and fenestrated baffle placement. In contrast, after the BDG, the extracardiac Fontan completion is more complicated. The technical steps of the hemi-Fontan operation are outlined in Figure 41-2A through C.

Concurrent Procedures in Hypoplastic Left Heart Syndrome Patients Undergoing Superior Cavopulmonary Anastomosis Completion

Obstruction of the Aortic Arch

It is not uncommon after neo–aortic arch reconstruction as part of the stage I HLHS procedure to encounter re-coarctation at the distal aspect of the homograft patch arch augmentation. In some centers, the re-coarctation is balloon dilated in the cardiac catheterization laboratory before cavopulmonary anastomosis. Reduction of the re-coarctation gradient may result in hypoxemia secondary to decreased flow through an aortopulmonary shunt. If the hypoxemia is severe, the child may require an early cavopulmonary anastomosis or shunt revision. Distal neo–aortic arch re-coarctation that is not deemed suitable for balloon dilation angioplasty or proximal neo–aortic arch obstruction may require patch augmentation at the time of the cavopulmonary anastomosis.

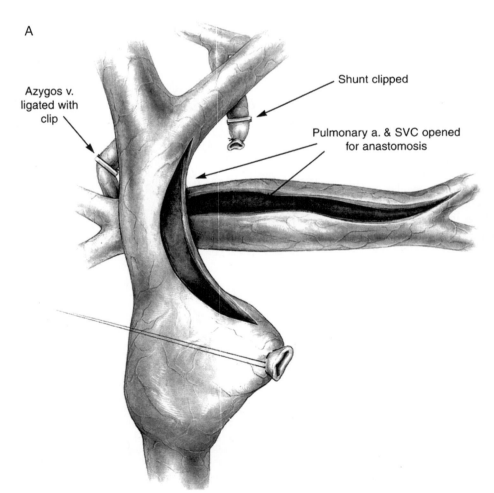

A

Azygos v. ligated with clip

Shunt clipped

Pulmonary a. & SVC opened for anastomosis

FIGURE 41-2 Steps of hemi-Fontan procedure. **A,** An incision is made in the pulmonary artery (a.) from hilum to hilum to allow the widest possible opening of the pulmonary bifurcation. An incision also is made in the medial aspect of the superior vena cava (SVC) across the cavoatrial junction onto the right atrial appendage, as delineated in this figure. The azygos vein (v.) is ligated with a clip if it is readily accessible; however, this is not necessary in all patients.

(Continued)

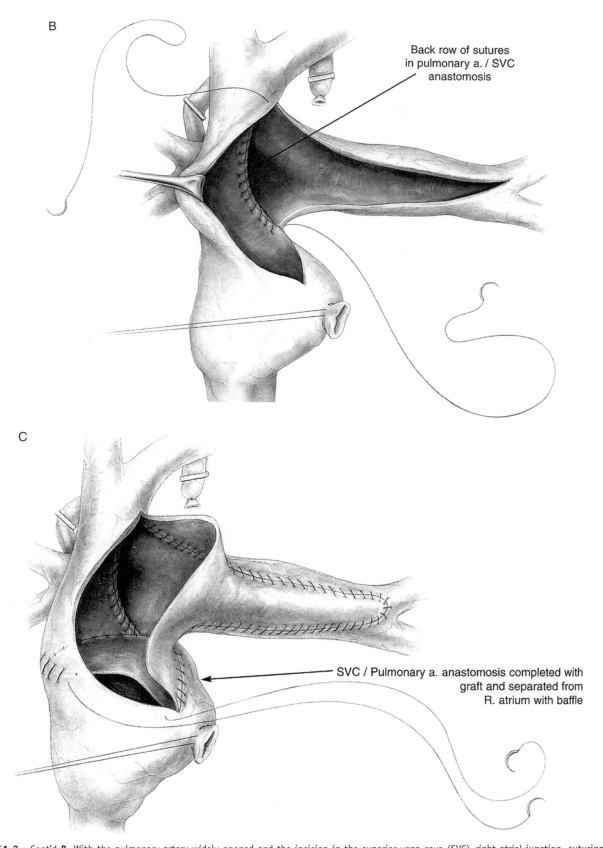

FIGURE 41-2 Cont'd **B,** With the pulmonary artery widely opened and the incision in the superior vena cava (SVC)–right atrial junction, suturing is initiated connecting the posterior aspect of the superior vena cava and right (R.) atrium to the right pulmonary artery by using a running 6-0 polypropylene suture. In this fashion, a wide connection between the superior vena cava and pulmonary artery can be ensured. **C,** After the posterior suture line is created, a large triangular patch of pulmonary homograft is used to augment the pulmonary artery bifurcation. As the suture line along the inferior aspect of the pulmonary bifurcation is created, the suture line is carried into the cavoatrial junction, using the pulmonary homograft to create a dam between the superior vena cava and right atrium. The suture line is brought completely across the cavoatrial junction to the anterior incision across the cavoatrial junction. Next, the homograft is folded down to create the dam at the level of the atrium and secured with a 5-0 polypropylene suture. Care must be taken with this suture line to incorporate the doubled flap of pulmonary homograft completely along the right lateral aspect of the suture line to prevent any baffle leaks entering the right atrium after the repair. (From Cox L, Sundt TM III, eds: *Operative Techniques in Cardiac and Thoracic Surgery: A Comparative Atlas*. Philadelphia: WB Saunders, 1997, pp. 242–244, with permission.)

Atrioventricular Valve Regurgitation

The tricuspid valve has a different papillary muscle structure than the mitral valve and lacks a well-formed annulus. As a result, it may become regurgitant under a systemic pressure load and the volume load placed on the right ventricle by an aortopulmonary shunt. Common causes of atrioventricular valve insufficiency include prolapse of the septal leaflet and leaflet deficiency or displacement or both. The superior cavopulmonary anastomosis decreases the volume load to the right ventricle and may reduce atrioventricular valve regurgitation. Tricuspid valvuloplasty performed concurrent with the superior cavopulmonary anastomosis may improve outcome in patients after single-ventricle palliation who are left with severe atrioventricular valve regurgitation.[109] Commisuroplasty, annuloplasty, chordal shortening, and leaflet extension may all be used to minimize regurgitation. These valvuloplasty techniques all require aortic cross-clamping with cardioplegic arrest with or without circulatory arrest.

Anesthetic Considerations

Anesthetic management is detailed in Chapter 10 on cardiovascular anesthesia.

Postoperative Physiology

After completion of the superior cavopulmonary anastomosis, the circulation to the lungs is from the upper body systemic venous return. The pulmonary blood flow results from upper body blood flow; all SVC return must pass through the lungs to reach the heart (in the absence of decompressing venous collaterals; see later). The principal physiologic advantage of conversion to a superior cavopulmonary anastomosis (drainage of the SVC to the PA and the IVC to the systemic ventricle) at an early age is the reduction of the volume work of the single ventricle and a predictable Q_p:Q_s of approximately 0.6 to 0.7. This ratio may be higher in young infants because of the relative size of the head and the upper extremities in young infants as opposed to those in older children,[51] but in general, systemic arterial oxygen saturations (SaO_2) are 75% to 85%.[1,19,54,103]

The immediate reduction in the volume load of the single ventricle by removing the aortopulmonary shunt decreases the work of the single ventricle and may improve long-term atrioventricular valve and myocardial function.[80] Atrioventricular valve regurgitation resulting from physiologic rather than structural abnormalities may decrease as the ventricular geometry normalizes.[109]

After superior cavopulmonary anastomosis, oxygen is delivered more efficiently to the body because only deoxygenated blood (from the SVC) rather than admixed blood (from the ventricle) is presented to the lungs for oxygen uptake. The net result of the more efficient oxygen uptake in the lungs is a reduction in cardiac output needed to achieve a given tissue O_2 delivery.[116]

After superior cavopulmonary anastomosis, there is an acute decrease occurs in single-ventricle end-systolic and end-diastolic volume, resulting in a decrease in stroke volume index with no change in myocardial mass. This results in an increase in mass/volume ratio and ventricular wall thickness (Fig. 41-3).[34,100,114] These changes result in

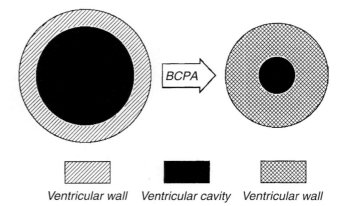

Ventricular wall   Ventricular cavity   Ventricular wall

FIGURE 41-3   Physiology of volume unloading in the univentricular heart: changes that occur immediately include a volume reduction without a change of mass, increased wall thickness-to-cavitary volume ratio, decreased rate of pressure decay, incoordinate relaxation, and increased filling pressure. These effects may be generically termed *diastolic dysfunction*. BCPA, bilateral cardiopulmonary anastomosis. (From Rychik J, Wernovsky G, eds: *Hypoplastic Left Heart Syndrome*. Boston: Kluwer Academic Publishers, 2003, p 133, with permission.)

short-term diminished ventricular compliance and impaired diastolic function.[34] After the BDG or hemi-Fontan, ventricular filling is not absolutely dependent on pulmonary venous return, because IVC flow is still diverted directly to the single ventricle and maintains preload. As a result, the acute volume reduction noted after superior cavopulmonary anastomosis is better tolerated than in the case of transitioning a child from a neonatal palliation directly to the Fontan completion without an intervening superior cavopulmonary anastomosis.

In children with single left ventricle with transposition of the great arteries that have a bulboventricular foramen and are dependent on an unrestricted ventricular septal defect (VSD) for systemic ventricular outflow, ventricular unloading may result in restrictive VSD physiology.[29,87] Careful assessment of the subaortic area in patients with these anatomic subtypes should be performed.

SaO_2 after creation of a BDG shunt tends to be lower in very young (younger than 3 months) patients. Although some patients as young as 4 weeks have had satisfactory BDG shunt creation,[11,108] patients younger than 3 months have a higher incidence of early cyanosis, PA thrombosis, and vascular congestion.[11,108] Therefore a delay of the procedure until the child is older than 3 months is generally recommended. By age 6 months, the mortality risk approaches 0 in many centers.[19,54,69,103]

Although the BDG is associated with good palliation, and midterm growth and development are satisfactory, the late development of progressive cyanosis is common. The development of cyanosis can occur from the development of pulmonary arteriovenous malformations,[81,121] the development of collateral venous drainage (see later), or the redistribution of flow between the upper and lower body as the child ages. The use of an intermediate superior cavopulmonary connection allows relative ease of completion of the Fontan operation[60,61] and a lower incidence of effusions and morbidity after the completion operation.[46]

Additional physiologic changes that occur after the superior cavopulmonary anastomosis include the elimination of first-pass hepatic venous blood from the PA circulation (see later), elevation of serum levels of angiotensin II, aldosterone, arginine vasopressin, atrial natriuretic factor (ANF), and brain natriuretic peptide.[55] Despite the bidirectional nature of the connection, a dominance of right lung perfusion is common and can be demonstrated by 99mTc microsphere injection and other techniques.[104,115]

The physiologic differences between the Norwood reconstruction, superior cavopulmonary connection, and the Fontan circulations are presented in Figure 41-4.

Postoperative Issues

Mechanical Ventilation

Positive pressure ventilation with increased mean airway pressures may adversely affect PVR and ventricular filling; early institution of spontaneous ventilation may improve hemodynamics in the awake patient. Intraoperative anesthetic management should be designed with a planned early extubation. Spontaneous breathing may also increase PCO_2, which will promote increased cerebral blood flow and, thereby, increase pulmonary blood flow.

"Physiologic" (3 to 5 cm H_2O) positive end-expiratory pressure (PEEP) is generally well tolerated, does not significantly affect PVR or cardiac output, and may improve oxygenation by reducing areas of microatelectasis, reestablishing functional residual capacity, and improving ventilation/perfusion matching.

Elevated Cavopulmonary Pressures

The goal of postoperative cavopulmonary anastomosis management is to *minimize the transpulmonary gradient* (PA mean pressure – common atrium mean pressure) to allow passive pulmonary blood flow through the lungs and back to the single ventricle. An elevated transpulmonary gradient may result from pulmonary venous obstruction, elevated PVR, or pleural effusion, hemothorax, or pneumothorax. Extubating the patient expeditiously will reduce the common atrial pressure and promote flow through the lungs by creating a greater transthoracic gradient from the extrathoracic space to the intrathoracic space. If the patient requires reintubation or persistent intubation, normocapnea or slight hypercapnea is recommended. Low PCO_2 will dilate the pulmonary vasculature, but will more importantly decrease cerebral blood flow and thereby decrease SVC return into the cavopulmonary circulation.[12,33] Diminished cavopulmonary blood flow will reduce systemic SaO_2. Elevation of PVR from the inflammatory effects of CPB may be minimized with pulmonary vasodilators such as nitric oxide at 5 to 20 parts per million in inspired gas.[41,131] Mild facial edema after superior cavopulmonary anastomosis may persist for up to 72 hours. Improved patient selection and increased utilization of modified ultrafiltration after CPB have reduced the incidence of significant postoperative pleural effusions after cavopulmonary anastomosis.[69] The majority of pleural effusions after superior cavopulmonary anastomosis will diminish over time with judicious diuretic use and fluid restriction. Diuretics are used for several months after cavopulmonary anastomosis. If chylothorax is present, a diet of medium-chain triglycerides (e.g., Portagen) may reduce lymphatic drainage. Cessation of enteral feeds and the use of parenteral nutrition are set aside for those

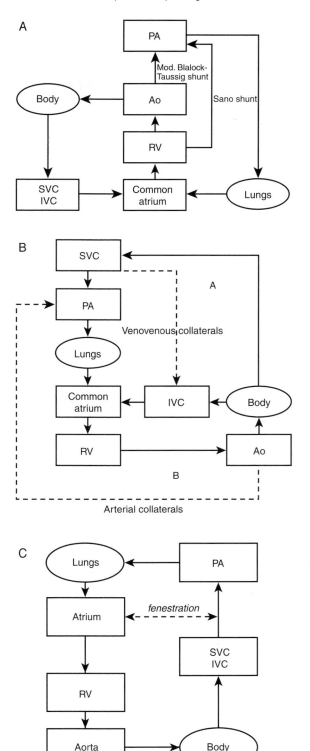

FIGURE 41-4 The physiologic differences between the stage I Norwood reconstruction (**A**), superior cavopulmonary connection (**B**), and the Fontan completion (**C**). In A, note that pulmonary blood flow may be provided either by an aorta-to-pulmonary artery (modified Blalock-Taussig shunt) or a right ventricle-to-pulmonary artery (Sano modification) shunt. In B, note the presence of venovenous collaterals, which will decrease pulmonary blood flow and result in systemic venous desaturation, as well as arteriopulmonary collaterals, which will increase pulmonary blood flow and superior cavopulmonary pressures. (Adapted from Rychik J, Wernovsky G, eds: *Hypoplastic Left Heart Syndrome*. Boston: Kluwer Academic Publishers, 2003, p 135, with permission.)

patients with intractable effusions. Patients are typically given aspirin (5 mg/kg/day) after superior cavopulmonary anastomosis to reduce the risk of thrombosis of the superior cavopulmonary circuit.

Patients with clinical signs of significantly *elevated SVC pressure* (upper extremity plethora and edema) may have obstruction at the cavopulmonary anastomosis, distal PA distortion, or marked elevations in PVR. In these patients, it is not uncommon to see immediately after surgery a visible line of demarcation of venous congestion across the chest, in the distribution of the upper body venous return. Significant elevations of pressure in the SVC may limit cerebral blood flow, which may be further decreased by hyperventilation and alkalosis used to decrease PVR. If the SVC pressure is more than 18 mm Hg, the etiology should be promptly investigated, including early catheterization, if necessary.

Hypertension and Bradycardia

Transient postoperative hypertension and bradycardia have been frequently observed in the first 24 to 72 hours after the cavopulmonary shunt.[19] Hypertension may be due to pain, catecholamine secretion, intracranial hypertension, or a combination of these. We speculate that acute elevation of the central venous pressure may result in a reflex similar to that seen in head trauma, such that systemic hypertension is necessary to preserve adequate cerebral perfusion. Therefore aggressive lowering of the blood pressure may adversely affect the cerebral perfusion pressure, and vasodilators should be used cautiously. Transient bradycardia also is typically seen after a cavopulmonary

connection and may be due to the acute reduction of the volume load of the single ventricle, or may be due to injury to the sinus node or its arterial supply.[23,84]

Low Cardiac Output

Low cardiac output is relatively uncommon after the cavopulmonary anastomosis because the ventricle has been volume unloaded, and, as noted earlier, oxygen delivery tends to be more efficient. The exception to that general rule is when the child has preexisting ventricular dysfunction or severe atrioventricular valve regurgitation. In these volume-loaded ventricles, which need high filling pressures to generate adequate output, volume reduction and the effects from CPB may significantly reduce cardiac output and oxygen delivery to the tissues.

Cyanosis

Excessive *hypoxemia* (SpO_2 <75%) should be investigated promptly, especially in infants, where a greater proportion of systemic output is dedicated to the upper half of the body and should result in oxygen saturations closer to 85%. The differential diagnosis of excessive or unexplained cyanosis can be grouped into three broad categories: *pulmonary venous desaturation, systemic venous desaturation,* or *decreased pulmonary blood flow* (Table 41-2).

Decreased pulmonary blood flow may be due to decompressing venovenous collaterals, an undiagnosed contralateral (usually left) SVC, or a baffle leak (only for "hemi-Fontan").[30,61,125] Factors related to the development of decompressing venous

Table 41-2   Differential Diagnosis of Cyanosis after the Superior Cavopulmonary Anastomosis and the Fontan Completion

	Bidirectional Glenn/Hemi-Fontan	Fontan Completion
Pulmonary venous desaturation	Ventilation/perfusion mismatch Pleural effusion Pneumothorax Hemothorax Chylothorax Pulmonary edema Atelectasis Bacterial pneumonia/viral pneumonitis Arteriovenous malformation	Ventilation/perfusion mismatch Pleural effusion Pneumothorax Hemothorax Chylothorax Pulmonary edema Atelectasis Bacterial pneumonia/viral pneumonitis Arteriovenous malformation
Systemic venous desaturation	Decreased oxygen delivery Anemia Low cardiac output Decreased ventricular function Severe atrioventricular valve regurgitation Pericardial tamponade Increased oxygen consumption Sepsis Decompressing vein Venovenous collateral from superior cavopulmonary circuit via the systemic venous circuit to the systemic ventricle Baffle leak (only for hemi-Fontan)	Decreased oxygen delivery Anemia Low cardiac output Decreased ventricular function Severe atrioventricular valve regurgitation Pericardial tamponade Increased oxygen consumption Sepsis Decompressing vein Venovenous collateral from superior cavopulmonary circuit to the systemic ventricle Baffle leak (only for lateral tunnel fontan completion) Fenestration that is too large
Decreased pulmonary blood flow	Increased pulmonary vascular resistance Pulmonary venous hypertension Restrictive atrial communication Decompressing vein Baffle leak	Increased pulmonary vascular resistance Pulmonary venous hypertension Restrictive atrial communication Decompressing vein Baffle leak Pulmonary artery obstruction

collaterals include bilateral superior vena cava,[77] a higher early postoperative transpulmonary gradient, and elevated pressure in the SVC.[43,77,93,111] A left SVC to coronary sinus, which appeared closed on the cardiac catheterization before the superior cavopulmonary anastomosis, may re-canalize, resulting in significant desaturation after superior cavopulmonary anastomosis.[31] Successful transcatheter coil embolization of these vessels can be accomplished with good results.[93]

An additional cause of pulmonary venous desaturation after a BDG is the development of pulmonary arteriovenous malformations, particularly in patients with heterotaxy syndrome.[3,8,119,121] It has been postulated that the diversion of normal hepatic venous flow from the pulmonary circulation may be related to development of these abnormal pathways,[121] and some have been noted to regress after incorporation of hepatic venous flow into the lungs.[119] Pulmonary arteriovenous malformations have been associated with young age at the time of the superior cavopulmonary anastomosis, polysplenia (interrupted IVC with azygos continuation to the SVC), and the time elapsed since the cavopulmonary connection was completed. These pulmonary arteriovenous malformations typically cause gradual hypoxemia *months to years* after the surgical procedure, rather than in the immediate postoperative period. Studies have shown that a pulsatile second source of pulmonary blood flow may minimize the development of pulmonary arteriovenous malformations.[66,128] In most cases, the malformations diminish or disappear completely after Fontan completion.[64,81] Although theoretic advantages exist to an IVC-PA cavopulmonary anastomosis relative to the formation of pulmonary arteriovenous malformations, the elevation in hepatic venous pressure and the detrimental effects on liver function may be prohibitive.[52]

The Superior Cavopulmonary Anastomosis as "Definitive Palliation"

The strategy for the treatment of neonates with single-ventricle anatomy has been to palliate to a Fontan circulation at most large centers. Although this strategy works for many of the children with single-ventricle complexes, the Fontan is palliative, not curative. Complications may occur after the Fontan completion, some severe enough to require cardiac transplantation to prevent death. Most of these complications rarely occur after superior cavopulmonary anastomosis. Some patients may be palliated equally well (from a hemodynamic point of view) with a superior cavopulmonary connection, especially if there is a second source of antegrade pulmonary blood flow.[9]

Patients with HLHS cannot be well palliated in the long term with a superior cavopulmonary anastomosis as their only source of pulmonary blood flow, because of diminishing oxygen saturations over time. Older age is associated with progressive cyanosis, as a relatively lower proportion of the cardiac output is directed to the head and the upper extremities in older patients.[51]

THE MODIFIED FONTAN OPERATION

The goal of staged reconstructive surgery for children with HLHS and other single-ventricle defects is ultimately to achieve a modified Fontan circulation. The modified Fontan circuit allows systemic venous blood from both the SVC and IVC to return to the PAs directly, thereby separating the systemic and pulmonary circulations. The Fontan circuit relieves cyanosis and volume load of the single ventricle, while permitting an adequate cardiac output at acceptable systemic venous pressures. The multiple technical modifications of the Fontan completion[37] in the past two decades, combined with improved patient selection and postoperative management, have reduced the operative mortality to less than 2.5% in many centers, with acceptable perioperative and midterm morbidity.[46,47,60,65] Despite improvements in mortality and perioperative morbidity, the long-term outcome in this high-risk population remains uncertain.[36,130]

History

Many investigators, including Glenn and others, experimented with a variety of right heart bypass procedures prior to 1971 when Fontan and Baudet reported the first "physiologic" correction of tricuspid atresia with a "Fontan" procedure.[35] In 1973, Kreutzer and colleagues[70] reported the first Fontan procedure with a direct connection of the right atrium to the PA. Norwood and colleagues[96] reported the first successful Fontan operation in a patient with HLHS in 1983. Subsequent investigators described further technical modifications including the total cavopulmonary connection (lateral tunnel),[27,120,127] extracardiac conduits,[27,74,85,105] and the recent use of adjustable atrial defects[73] or fixed fenestrations in the intraatrial baffle.[13]

The intraatrial lateral tunnel supplanted the direct atrial-pulmonary anastomosis because of salient hydrodynamics of blood flow in more constricted atrial pathways,[28,120,127] which do not allow stasis of blood and loss of hydraulic energy as blood flows passively into the pulmonary vascular bed. The lateral tunnel also may result in a decreased incidence of late tachyarrhythmias relative to the atriopulmonary Fontan completion.[32,45]

The most recent modification of the Fontan operation is the use of an extracardiac conduit from the IVC to the PA. One advantage of this approach is the elimination of atrial suture lines, which in other Fontan connections—such as the atriopulmonary connections and intracardiac lateral tunnel—may isolate the sinus node from the atrioventricular node and disrupt intraatrial conduction, in addition to contributing to sinus node dysfunction. These suture lines have been shown to participate in reentrant circuits and atrial flutter and fibrillation late after the Fontan operation.[6,32,42,45]

Despite the multiple modifications to the Fontan completion over the past two decades, the early mortality and morbidity (e.g., prolonged effusions and Fontan takedown for inadequate hemodynamics) associated with the Fontan completion operation remained high until the last decade.[18,46] The presence of a systemic right ventricle was noted to be a risk factor for poor outcome. The incidence of prolonged effusions was higher in patients who did not have an intervening superior cavopulmonary anastomosis.[102,132] The single-stage Fontan also was found to result in an acute decrease in single-ventricle end-systolic and end-diastolic volume, and a decrease in stroke volume index with no change in myocardial mass. These geometric changes caused an increase in the mass/volume ratio, ventricular wall thickness, and filling pressures with impaired diastolic function (compliance) and low cardiac output.[49,61] As a result of these findings, several centers began intervening with a superior cavopulmonary connection at approximately 6 months of age between the neonatal palliation and the Fontan completion.[14,38,72,95]

The presence of a persistent aortopulmonary shunt from the neonatal palliation to the single-stage Fontan completion resulted in ventricular hypertrophy and dilation. The intervening superior cavopulmonary anastomosis reduced the volume load caused by the aortopulmonary shunt at a younger age, which allowed regression of the ventricular hypertrophy and dilation. This regression made the child a better candidate for modified Fontan completion.

A major advance in the completion of the Fontan operation has been the use of a temporary communication or fenestration between the systemic venous and pulmonary venous pathways, which allows a right-to-left shunt in the immediate postoperative period, and improves cardiac output and system oxygen delivery at the cost of mild systemic desaturation. The fenestration has been shown to reduce mortality,[46] decrease the incidence of early effusions after the procedure, and maintain left ventricular preload in times of hemodynamic stress.[13,14,68] Hemodynamic studies have shown that with temporary occlusion of such fenestrations or adjustable atrial septal defects (ASDs),[14,15,53,68,71,72] the cardiac output decreases, although the increase in oxygen saturation maintains oxygen delivery to the tissues. Rychik and colleagues[113] showed that late surgical fenestration for high cavopulmonary pressures after the Fontan may be beneficial.

Several techniques have been used for fenestration, including creation of an adjustable interatrial communication,[53,72] creation of a fixed fenestration by punching a hole in the Fontan baffle,[4] or exclusion of a single hepatic vein, allowing drainage into the pulmonary venous atrium. Progressive right-to-left shunting via intrahepatic collaterals resulted from hepatic vein exclusion, which has been abandoned as a means to provide a fenestration in the Fontan baffle.[117]

Utilization of an intervening superior cavopulmonary connection and fenestration creation at the time of Fontan completion has dramatically reduced the early mortality and morbidity associated with the single-stage Fontan completion. Outcomes after single-ventricle staged palliation are equivalent for patients with systemic right ventricle (e.g., HLHS) and other forms of the univentricular heart.[10,44,91,126]

Indications for Surgery

Criteria for Fontan completion have included normal ventricular function, absence of atrioventricular valve regurgitation, normal systemic and pulmonary venous drainage, absence of PA distortion, and low PVR. The multiple modifications to the Fontan completion have decreased the occurrence and potential impact of these risk factors.

PA stenosis and hemodynamically significant atrioventricular valve regurgitation can be addressed at the time of the superior cavopulmonary anastomosis or Fontan completion. Patients with discrete pulmonary vein stenosis may undergo Fontan completion and sutureless pulmonary vein repair simultaneously. Severe ventricular dysfunction and fixed elevated PVR (>4 Wood units) remain the most

significant contraindications to Fontan completion. Until recently, patients who were evaluated for Fontan completion typically underwent an echocardiogram and cardiac catheterization to assess anatomic and hemodynamic fitness for the Fontan operation. Additional significant hemodynamic lesions noted were addressed either during the preoperative cardiac catheterization or at the time of the Fontan completion. A study by Ro and associates[110] retrospectively assessed the utility of the pre-Fontan cardiac catheterization. Patients had a low incidence of unexpected additional lesions identified at cardiac catheterization if they had an SaO_2 greater than 76% and a hemoglobin concentration less than 18 g/dL, and had an echocardiogram that demonstrated an unobstructed left pulmonary artery (LPA), absence of significant atrioventricular valve regurgitation, normal ventricular function, no neo–aortic arch obstruction, an unrestricted atrial communication, and no evidence of a decompressing vessel. The negative predictive value for the criteria was 93%, meaning that 93% of the time, no additional hemodynamically significant lesion would have been identified if the patient had had a preoperative cardiac catheterization.[110] If a cardiac catheterization before Fontan completion is not performed based on the Ro criteria noted, cardiac magnetic resonance imaging (MRI) may be helpful to delineate further abnormalities of the PAs, systemic veins, and pulmonary veins that may not be fully appreciated on echocardiogram.

The present standard sequence of single-ventricle palliation for HLHS includes the stage I reconstruction during the neonatal period, an intervening superior cavopulmonary anastomosis at age 4 to 8 months, and performance of the modified Fontan completion at age 18 to 24 months. The modified Fontan completion is performed at 18 to 24 months to provide improved systemic arterial oxygen saturation and to increase blood flow through the pulmonary vasculature during a period of significant lung growth. Depending on the superior cavopulmonary anastomosis chosen, the modified Fontan completion may be either an extracardiac (previous BDG) or a lateral tunnel completion (previous hemi-Fontan). In patients with heterotaxy syndrome, anomalies of pulmonary and systemic venous return are common. These venous anomalies may increase the risk of systemic or pulmonary venous pathway obstruction if a lateral tunnel completion is performed. As a result, a BDG shunt with an extracardiac Fontan completion is recommended for these patients.

Some institutions perform the Fontan completion with excellent results without intervening cavopulmonary anastomosis, fenestration, or the use of CPB.[59,123,124] These case series include few patients with HLHS.

Surgical Technique

Lateral Tunnel Fontan Completion after the Hemi-Fontan Procedure

Children with HLHS who have undergone previous hemi-Fontan may have lateral tunnel Fontan completion at age 18 months to 5 years, depending on center-specific preference. The lateral tunnel modified Fontan completion requires limited mobilization of the neo-aorta and lateral aspect of the right atrium.

The lateral aspect of the right atrium is opened up to the base of the hemi-Fontan baffle (Fig. 41-5A). This permits access to the homograft dam that divides the right atrium and the SVC. The dam is then removed under direct vision. The resultant opening allows creation of a baffle to shunt IVC blood into the pulmonary arteries (Fig. 41-5B). A 10-mm polytetrafluoroethylene (PTFE) graft is used to create the intra-atrial baffle. The graft is opened longitudinally so that a larger-diameter tunnel can be created than the diameter of the graft. Before placement, a 4-mm punch-hole (fenestration) is made in the lower portion of the graft (Fig. 41-6). A suture line along the posterior aspect of the right atrium secures the baffle so the right pulmonary veins are excluded from the systemic venous side of the baffle. The suture line is continued between the graft and between the two walls of the right atrium to complete the lateral tunnel and close the atriotomy (Fig. 41-7). Transthoracic monitoring lines are placed in each side of the newly placed baffle in the PA and pulmonary venous atrium, respectively (Fig. 41-8).

This procedure is usually performed under a short period of circulatory arrest by using hypothermic CPB. The CPB causes a significant inflammatory response that increases total body water and causes tissue edema and multisystem organ dysfunction. The myocardium and lung parenchyma are especially affected. Myocardial edema causes decreased single-ventricle compliance, elevated filling pressures, and decreased cardiac output. These myocardial changes are particularly problematic in the Fontan circuit, where the goal is to have the highest cardiac output at the lowest filling pressure possible. Edema of the lung parenchyma and pulmonary endothelium results in decreased lung compliance and increased PVR, respectively. These pulmonary effects worsen with an increasing duration of exposure to CPB. The lateral tunnel completion after intervening hemi-Fontan reduces the time required on CPB, as well as the duration of aortic cross-clamping.

Extracardiac Fontan Completion after the Bidirectional Glenn

Children who have had an intervening BDG for their superior cavopulmonary anastomosis will generally undergo an extracardiac Fontan completion. Similar to the lateral tunnel Fontan completion, the extracardiac Fontan completion may be performed at age 18 to 24 months, depending on center preference. An 18- to 20-mm PTFE extracardiac conduit is

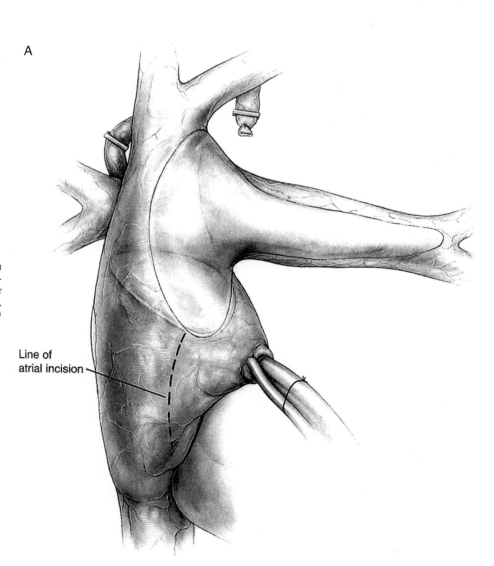

A

Line of atrial incision

FIGURE 41-5 Lateral tunnel completion Fontan. **A,** Working through the right atrial incision, the homograft dam between the superior vena cava and right atrium is readily identified.
(Continued)

B   Removal of baffle between
inferior and superior venous
systems

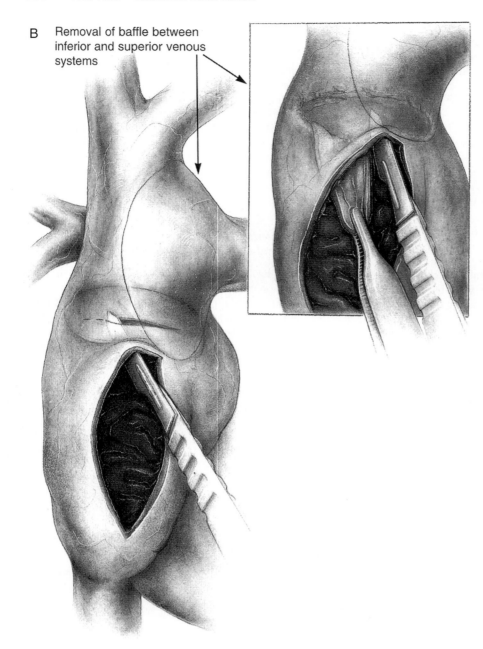

FIGURE 41-5   Cont'd **B,** This dam of tissue is excised under direct vision, creating an opening that is adequate in size for baffling of the inferior vena cava flow into the pulmonary arteries. This opening is created in such a way that a rim of tissue can be used for the suture line of the intracardiac lateral tunnel (inset). (From Cox L, Sundt TM III, eds: *Operative Techniques in Cardiac & Thoracic Surgery: A Comparative Atlas.* Philadelphia: WB Saunders, 1997, p 247, with permission.)

inserted between the IVC and the superior cavopulmonary anastomosis to complete the Fontan circuit.

Some institutions complete the extracardiac Fontan procedure without the use of CPB or cardioplegic arrest, whereas others use CPB either with circulatory arrest or with bicaval cannulation and continuous CPB. After mobilization of the IVC at the level of the hepatic veins, the IVC is divided at its entrance site into the right atrium, and the right atrium is closed by using a running suture. An end-to-end anastomosis between the conduit and IVC is created (Fig. 41-9). The graft is cut to an appropriate length. The extracardiac conduit is fenestrated by creating a punch-hole (4 mm) in the graft, and the IVC opening in the right atrium is sewn to the exterior of the graft, exposing the fenestration to the atrium with a side-to-side anastomosis. At some institutions, a 5- to

8-mm PTFE shunt is placed between the conduit and the right atrium to provide a physiologic fenestration.

To complete the anastomosis of the conduit to the superior cavopulmonary anastomosis, the underside of the right PA is incised and sutured to the superior aspect of the conduit (Fig. 41-10). A pulmonary arterioplasty for pulmonary stenosis may be performed with homograft patch material or a PTFE graft that may be beveled to cross any stenotic areas at the PA end of the anastomosis. If the BDG has been directed slightly leftward toward the midline, this will allow offsetting of the superior and inferior cavopulmonary connections to minimize energy losses.

After the lateral tunnel or extracardiac Fontan completion, we avoid placing lines directly in the internal jugular vein, innominate vein, or SVC to reduce the risk of

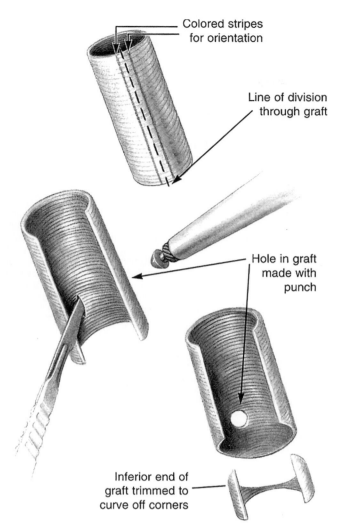

Colored stripes
for orientation

Line of division
through graft

Hole in graft
made with
punch

Inferior end of
graft trimmed to
curve off corners

FIGURE 41-6   Lateral tunnel completion Fontan. A polytetrafluoroethylene graft 10 mm in diameter is opened longitudinally, so that a larger lateral tunnel can be created than the diameter of the graft used. Before implantation, an incision is made in the left lower portion of the graft, and a 4-mm punch hole is made in the graft, which can be easily performed before implantation and avoids manipulating the graft after it is sewn in place. The inferior rim of the graft is then trimmed to a gentle curve and sewn into the lateral aspect of the right atrium. (From Cox L, Sundt TM III, eds: *Operative Techniques in Cardiac & Thoracic Surgery: A Comparative Atlas*. Philadelphia: WB Saunders, 1997, p 248, with permission.)

postoperative thrombosis. Given the incidence of postoperative arrhythmias after Fontan completion, temporary atrial and ventricular pacing wires are placed on the myocardium. After separation from CPB, MUF is performed to minimize the effects of CPB. A mediastinal chest tube is placed for bleeding.

Modified Ultrafiltration

MUF minimizes the inflammatory effects of CPB in neonates. After separation from CPB, the patient's blood is ultrafiltered, and red cells are salvaged from the CPB circuit. MUF after Fontan completion decreases the transfusion requirement and significantly decreases the incidence and duration of pleural effusions.[69] The lower incidence and duration of pleural effusions decrease the total hospital length of stay. MUF is thought to remove inflammatory mediators, which may result in less capillary leak and tissue edema, and improved ventricular function and decreased PVR.

Management of Associated Lesions

Left Pulmonary Artery Stenosis

Compression from the large neo-aorta or involution of the ductus arteriosus or both may lead to left pulmonary artery stenosis after stage I reconstruction for HLHS. The triangular baffle that is placed as part of the hemi-Fontan procedure generally augments the LPA and addresses LPA stenosis that may be present. A separate homograft augmentation of the LPA is necessary in patients who undergo BDG as the cavopulmonary anastomosis. In certain patients, the LPA remains diffusely small despite augmentation at the intervening cavopulmonary anastomosis. Balloon dilation angioplasty with or without stent placement can be performed at the time of pre-Fontan cardiac catheterization, or a repeated pulmonary arterioplasty can be performed at the time of the Fontan completion.

Tricuspid Regurgitation

Atrioventricular valve regurgitation is common in patients with HLHS, occurring in 16% to 33% of patients.[109,122] Tricuspid regurgitation causes an additional volume load on the single right ventricle and may contribute to ventricular dysfunction. Either an abnormality of the valve (e.g., dysplasia and Ebsteinoid malformation) or annular dilation with poor leaflet coaptation produces tricuspid regurgitation. A concurrent valvuloplasty may be performed at the time of the Fontan completion for moderate to severe atrioventricular valve regurgitation. Tricuspid valvuloplasty improves the severity of regurgitation in patients after hemi-Fontan or Fontan completion at a median follow-up of 24 months.[109]

Neo–aortic Arch Obstruction

Neo–aortic arch obstruction may occur at either the proximal or distal end of the arch reconstruction, but distal obstruction at the end of the homograft patch augmentation near the ductal insertion site is more common. Re-coarctation is generally addressed by balloon dilation angioplasty at the time of the pre-Fontan cardiac catheterization. Cases of significant proximal arch obstruction and rare cases of distal arch obstruction are fixed by patch augmentation at the time of the Fontan completion.

Anesthetic Considerations

Anesthetic management is detailed in Chapter 10 on cardiovascular anesthesia.

Postoperative Physiology

After the Fontan operation, patients may have systolic and diastolic myocardial dysfunction, abnormal arterial hemodynamics, abnormal venous hemodynamics, or a combination of these.

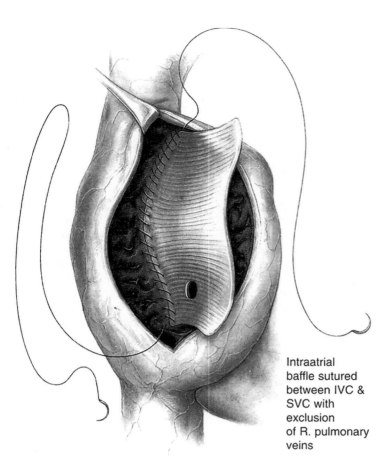

Intraatrial
baffle sutured
between IVC &
SVC with
exclusion
of R. pulmonary
veins

FIGURE 41-7 Lateral tunnel completion Fontan. The opened polytetrafluoroethylene graft with the previously created fenestration is secured in the right atrium, excluding the right pulmonary veins behind the baffle. The suture line along the posterior aspect of the right atrium, which is then carried down inferiorly to the eustachian valve, where the graft is sutured along the eustachian valve up to the margin of the incision in the right atrium. Superiorly, the graft is sutured along the wall of the atrial septum up to the level of the excised dam in the cavoatrial junction. Then the graft is brought to the right and sewn to the margins of the previous excision of the homograft dam up to the level of the incision in the right atrium. The graft at this point can be trimmed if it is excessively wide and then the suture line continued, sandwiching the graft free margin between the two walls of the right atrium to complete the lateral tunnel suture line. After completion of this suture line, the atrium can be filled with the saline solution and the venous cannula reinserted. IVC, inferior vena cava; SVC, superior vena cava. (From Cox L, Sundt TM III, eds: *Operative Techniques in Cardiac & Thoracic Surgery: A Comparative Atlas*. Philadelphia: WB Saunders, 1997, p 249, with permission.)

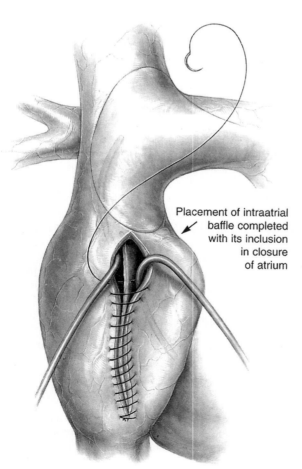

Placement of intraatrial
baffle completed
with its inclusion
in closure
of atrium

FIGURE 41-8 Lateral tunnel completion Fontan. An advantage of incorporating the wall of the lateral tunnel in the suture line is the ability to place lines easily for postoperative monitoring. Transthoracic atrial lines are positioned on either side of the polytetrafluoroethylene baffle, which places one line on the left atrial side of the baffle and the other on the pulmonary arterial side for measurement of pressures postoperatively. In this fashion, no lines must be placed directly in the internal jugular vein, innominate vein, or superior vena cava, reducing the risk of postoperative caval thrombosis. (From Cox L, Sundt TM III, eds: *Operative Techniques in Cardiac & Thoracic Surgery: A Comparative Atlas*. Philadelphia: WB Saunders, 1997, p 250, with permission.)

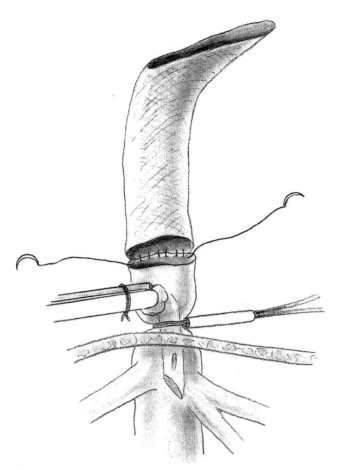

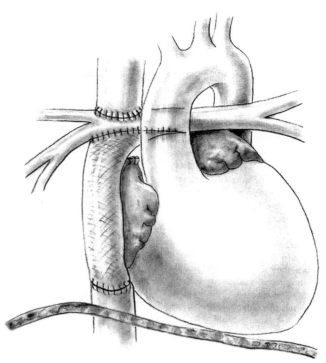

FIGURE 41-10 Extracardiac Fontan completion. The completed extracardiac conduit Fontan is as shown. A fenestration is placed by performing a 4- to 5-mm side-to-side anastomosis between the conduit and the right atrial free wall. Another option for fenestration is to place a synthetic tube graft (5 to 8 mm) from the conduit to the free wall. (From Cox L, Sundt TM III, eds: *Operative Techniques in Cardiac & Thoracic Surgery: A Comparative Atlas.* Philadelphia: WB Saunders, 1997, p 227, with permission.)

FIGURE 41-9 Extracardiac Fontan completion. After the institution of bypass, the inferior vena cava (IVC) is clamped just inferior to the cavoatrial junction and transected between the clamp and the snared IVC cannula. The cardiac end of the transected IVC is doubly oversewn with running 4-0 or 5-0 nonabsorbable monofilament suture. The extracardiac conduit of polytetrafluoroethylene vascular tube graft is then tailored. The size of the conduit usually ranges from 20 to 25 mm in diameter. The cross-sectional diameter of the conduit is usually slightly oversized with respect to the diameter of the IVC. An end-to-end anastomosis between the conduit and the IVC is performed with 4-0 or 5-0 monofilament suture. After completion of the inferior anastomosis, the conduit is clamped at midlevel, and the IVC cannula snare is released, allowing the inferior half of the conduit to fill with blood. Any anastomotic suture-line bleeding can be repaired at this time. Cardiopulmonary bypass is continued with the cannula unsnared to allow more accurate approximation of conduit position in the mediastinum. The length of the conduit is then tailored to the undersurface of the right pulmonary artery. The superior orifice of the conduit is beveled at an angle less than or equal to 45 degrees relative to the long axis of the conduit. This allows an oblique conduit-to-pulmonary artery anastomosis with a substantially greater anastomotic surface area rather than with direct end-to-side connection. In addition, this allows greater offsetting of the superior and inferior cavopulmonary connections, which has been shown by computational fluid dynamics to minimize energy losses at the cavopulmonary junction. Furthermore, this oblique anastomosis effectively serves as a central pulmonary arterioplasty, and the angle of the bevel can be adjusted to maximize this effect. At this point, the superior vena cava is cannulated and snared, and full cardiopulmonary bypass is instituted. (From Cox L, Sundt TM III, eds: *Operative Techniques in Cardiac & Thoracic Surgery: A Comparative Atlas.* Philadelphia: WB Saunders, 1997, p 225, with permission.)

Systolic dysfunction has been reported in many studies. Mahle and colleagues[78] demonstrated this finding by using two new methods to assess right ventricular function: automatic detection of borders and the myocardial performance index. In the study, they compared 35 asymptomatic Fontan patients with single right ventricles with 32 age-matched normal controls. They found that the Fontan patients, based on automatic detection of borders, had diminished systolic function based on a lower fractional change in area and diminished diastolic function based on a greater reliance on atrial contraction to achieve ventricular filling. The mean myocardial performance index in the single-right-ventricle patients also was significantly higher than that in controls, and the indexed ejection time was shorter, suggesting less efficient ventricular mechanics.

Cheung and associates[21] demonstrated that significant diastolic dysfunction exists in the Fontan patient. The study was a case series evaluating 13 Fontan patients who had serial assessment of diastolic function of the systemic single ventricle, (median) 2.8 years and 11.4 years after Fontan.[21] The isovolumic relaxation time, E-wave deceleration time, E- and A-wave velocities, and E:A velocity ratio were reduced compared with normal, both early and late after Fontan. Diastolic function remained highly abnormal, with reduction in ventricular compliance and persistent "incoordinate relaxation."

In an elegant evaluation of ventricular afterload and ventricular work in the Fontan patient, Sensaki and colleagues[118] described inefficient ventricular vascular coupling. They compared the normal two-ventricle circulation, the single ventricle with a modified Blalock-Taussig shunt, and the Fontan circulation in the cardiac catheterization laboratory. They measured aortic impedance and ventricular hydraulic power at rest and under dobutamine stress. They noted that in the Fontan circulation, an elevated systemic vascular resistance was present that they believed to be reflective of the nonpulsatile properties of vascular load. The pulsatile component of vascular afterload, low-frequency impedance, is markedly elevated at rest and under β-adrenergic stimulation. Not only diminished cardiac output, but also higher power expenditure per unit cardiac output, was found in the Fontan group. The limited β-adrenergic response was thought to be due in part to limited preload reserve.

Fontan patients also have abnormal venous hemodynamics. They have an elevated central venous pressure and a limited venous capacitance. Increased venous tone limits the ability to mobilize blood from the capacitance vessels, thereby impairing cardiac output. Hsia and associates[57] described the effects of respiration and gravity on infradiaphragmatic venous flow in patients with normal biventricular hearts (n = 20) and in patients with a Fontan completion (n = 48). They noted that gravity exerts a detrimental effect on lower body venous return and that inspiration is an important factor in hepatic venous return. After the Fontan completion, loss of the normal augmentation in portal venous flow takes place with expiration. Elevated hepatic venous wedge pressures reflect elevated splanchnic venous pressures. Hsia and her colleagues[58] then showed that the fenestration moderates these findings. They found that although the fenestration reduces venous pressures and partially restores the transhepatic venous pressure gradient, its beneficial effects on flow in the total cavopulmonary connection are mediated primarily by an inspiration-derived hepatic venous forward flow and reduced flow reversal. This augmentation of hepatic venous forward flow may decompress the splanchnic circulation, which may theoretically modulate the development of protein-losing enteropathy.

Postoperative Issues

Postoperative care after the Fontan completion is goal-directed to provide for the highest cardiac output at the lowest atrial filling pressure. Most children after Fontan completion are hemodynamically stable without excessive bleeding, require minimal inotropic support, and are extubated as soon as possible after arrival in the intensive care unit. Extubation reduces atrial filling pressures and improves blood flow across the pulmonary vascular bed. Anesthetic management should be optimized such that an early extubation, within 4 to 6 hours of surgery completion, is possible. These improvements in postoperative care reflect the use of the staged superior cavopulmonary anastomosis, baffle fenestration, and MUF.

Mechanical Ventilation

Mechanical positive pressure ventilation with increased mean airway pressures may adversely affect PVR and ventricular filling; early institution of spontaneous ventilation may improve hemodynamics in the awake patient.[101] "Physiologic" (3 to 5 cm H_2O) PEEP is generally well tolerated, does not significantly affect PVR or cardiac output, and may improve oxygenation by reducing areas of microatelectasis, reestablishing functional residual capacity, and improving ventilation/perfusion matching.

Low Cardiac Output

The patient with low cardiac output after surgery should have prompt investigation of the repair and physiology. In addition to postoperative echocardiography, "physiologic" right atrial (RA) and left atrial (LA) catheters are invaluable in the diagnosis and management of these patients (Table 41-3). Low cardiac output may be due to
1. Inadequate preload; typically due to hypovolemia (low RA and LA pressures),
2. Elevated PVR (high RA and low LA pressures),
3. Anatomic obstruction in the systemic venous pathway (high RA and low LA pressures), or
4. Pump failure (high RA and high LA pressures).

Low cardiac output in the face of *high* LA pressure is an ominous sign and may be due to ventricular dysfunction, loss of atrioventricular synchrony, atrioventricular valve regurgitation, or ventricular outflow obstruction (e.g., subaortic stenosis). Prompt investigation of the surgical repair, including catheterization and angiography, is indicated in the patient with persistent low cardiac output, if the combination of ECG monitoring, echocardiography, and intracardiac pressure monitoring does not readily identify the cause.

Twenty to thirty years ago, a single-stage non-fenestrated Fontan procedure often led to severe low cardiac output with elevation of central venous pressures in the early postoperative period because of the changes in ventricular geometry noted previously.[46,83] This low-output state often resulted in death or necessitated takedown of the Fontan circuit to an aortopulmonary shunt. In the current era, the utilization of the intervening superior cavopulmonary anastomosis has removed the long-standing volume load on the ventricle. The net effect is a reduction of ventricular hypertrophy, dilation, secondary diastolic dysfunction, and elevated filling pressures. Fenestration of the baffle also has improved cardiac output by providing a right-to-left shunt to maintain adequate single-ventricle

Table 41-3 Differential Diagnosis of Low Cardiac Output after Fontan

RA_p	LA_p	Cause(s)	
Low	Low	Hypovolemia	
High	Low	PVR, baffle obstruction, pulmonary artery hypoplasia or branch stenoses	
High	High	Ventricular dysfunction, A-V valve stenosis or regurgitation, arrhythmia, outflow obstruction, tamponade	

preload and cardiac output. Despite the relative systemic desaturation from the fenestration, the overall oxygen delivery is improved based on increased cardiac output. In addition, systemic venous pressures are reduced with baffle fenestration, which in turn decreases the incidence and duration of pleural effusions.

Although the dramatic improvements in early mortality and morbidity after the Fontan completion may be largely attributed to the intervening superior cavopulmonary anastomosis and fenestration creation, advances also have been made in CPB management, surgical technique, and postoperative care.

Milrinone, a potent phosphodiesterase-3 inhibitor, is an effective inotrope-vasodilator in infants and children after superior cava-pulmonary anastomosis or modified Fontan procedures in the treatment of low cardiac output. Studies of milrinone in neonates after open-heart surgery reveal significant reductions in SVR and PVR and increases in cardiac index, primarily due to larger stroke volume.[20] Infants and children demonstrate a larger volume of distribution and clearance of milrinone compared with adults.[106] In infants, the loading dose of milrinone during CPB is 100 mcg/kg, followed by a continuous infusion to be started within 90 minutes of the load dose at a rate of 0.2 mcg/kg/min to maintain a therapeutic level. In older infants and children, the rate of continuous infusion is higher, usually 0.5 to 1.0 mcg/kg/min.

Arrhythmias

Significant arrhythmias, especially those with *loss of atrioventricular synchrony* (e.g., junctional ectopic tachycardia), are tolerated particularly poorly in this patient population. With progressive tachycardia, usually continued hemodynamic deterioration occurs. Frequently, it is difficult to decide whether the arrhythmia is a result of poor hemodynamics or is its cause. Given the predilection toward perioperative sinus node dysfunction, atrial pacing may be necessary in the immediate postoperative period. Transthoracic atrial and ventricular pacing wires are therefore placed in all patients undergoing a Fontan operation.

The temporary pacing atrial wires may be used to obtain an atrial electrogram, which may be helpful to differentiate among various arrhythmias. No difference is found in the frequency of sinus node dysfunction with junctional rhythm with lateral tunnel completion after an intervening hemi-Fontan versus extracardiac conduit completion after an intervening BDG.[22] The sinus node dysfunction probably reflects dissection in the area of the sinoatrial node. Most of these patients will have recovery of sinus function before hospital discharge. The long-term incidence of junctional rhythm and its importance as a risk factor for late atrial arrhythmias are not known. Significant tachyarrhythmias are rare in the early postoperative period; however, if these are present, they should be treated as indicated. Treatment with amiodarone has been particularly effective for atrial flutter and junctional ectopic tachycardia.

One of the theoretical advantages of the extracardiac Fontan completion is the minimization of suture lines and the avoidance of right atrial hypertension that may predispose the Fontan patient to atrial arrhythmias and sinus

node dysfunction. However, Cohen and colleagues[24] reported that no difference was noted in the incidence of early postoperative sinus node dysfunction between those patients who underwent lateral tunnel Fontan procedure and extracardiac Fontan completion. In contrast, Ovroutski and associates[99] found that their extracardiac Fontan cohort (n = 23) had a decreased incidence of atrial tachyarrhythmias and bradyarrhythmias relative to their lateral tunnel cohort (n = 24). The extracardiac patients maintained sinus rhythm to a greater degree compared with lateral tunnel patients (91% vs. 51%), and whereas 33% of lateral tunnel patients required a pacemaker for sinus node dysfunction, no patients who had the extracardiac completion required a pacemaker at 3 years of follow-up. Similarly, Azakie and colleagues[4] showed that a lateral tunnel cohort (n = 47) had a significantly higher rate of early postoperative sinus node dysfunction (45% vs. 15%), supraventricular tachycardia (33% vs. 8%), and need for temporary postoperative pacing (32% vs. 12%), relative to an extracardiac Fontan cohort (n = 60). Furthermore, Holter analysis at 3 years revealed a higher incidence of atrial arrhythmias in the lateral tunnel group (23% vs. 7%). Multivariate analysis showed lateral tunnel Fontan as the only risk factor for early postoperative and intermediate arrhythmias.

Cyanosis

The evaluation of excessive *cyanosis* after the Fontan completion is similar to that outlined earlier for the patient after superior cavo-pulmonary anastomosis. *Systemic venous desaturation* may be due to low systemic cardiac output, anemia, a decompressing vein, baffle leak, a fenestration that is too large, or increased oxygen-consumption states. In patients with fenestrated baffles, low cardiac output or anemia causes a very low mixed venous saturation and will result in excessive systemic arterial desaturation, as the blood crossing the fenestration is lower in oxygen content than usual. Causes of *pulmonary venous desaturation* after the Fontan procedure include pneumothorax, pleural effusions, pneumonia, atelectasis, and importantly, preexisting pulmonary arteriovenous malformations, such as those that may occur after a Kawashima procedure or after a long-standing cavopulmonary shunt. *Decreased pulmonary blood flow* also may be due to high PVR (in patients with the potential for right-to-left shunting), additional baffle leaks, "too large" an ASD or fenestration, decompressing venous collaterals to the systemic ventricle or pulmonary venous hypertension or PA obstruction resulting in increased shunting at the fenestration (see Table 41-2).

Pleural and Pericardial Effusions

The duration and frequency of pleural and pericardial effusions, typically the most frequent postoperative problem requiring prolonged hospitalization, have been recently reduced with the use of baffle fenestrations, the adjustable ASD, and modified ultrafiltration. Drainage of the effusion, with appropriate replacement of intravascular volume, electrolytes, protein, clotting factors and immunoglobulins, are necessary in cases of prolonged drainage. Patients with prolonged drainage (e.g., >2 to 3 weeks) should undergo cardiac catheterization to rule out potentially correctable causes, such as baffle obstruction, innominate vein thrombosis, and PA distortion. Diuretic therapy is usually sufficient to manage small pleural effusions. Larger effusions may require pleural catheter (5 to 8 French) placement. Patients usually have serous instead of chylous effusions. An enteral diet of medium-chain fatty acids or a period of parenteral nutrition usually results in diminution of the chylous drainage. Thoracic duct ligation and pleurodesis are rarely used.

Thrombosis

After the Fontan operation, patients (especially those with low cardiac output) may be at increased risk for venous thrombosis[40,63,112] and central nervous system complications. Anticoagulation with heparin or warfarin, or antiplatelet medications, may be useful in this subgroup of patients. Coagulation abnormalities[26,62] and acute liver dysfunction[88] have been described in patients after the Fontan operation. The reported incidence of adverse neurologic sequelae after the Fontan operation is approximately 2% to 3%.[86,89,90,129]

Causes of thrombotic complications after the Fontan include the low-flow state through the cavopulmonary circuit, a hypercoagulable state, atrial arrhythmias, and suture lines and scarring. Coagulopathy may result from clotting factor loss in pleural effusion fluid in the early postoperative period or from protein-losing enteropathy later in time or from both. In the past, Fontan patients have been shown to have normal liver function but a hypercoagulable state due to deficiency of protein C, protein S, and antithrombin III.

A pair of studies by Odegard and colleagues[97,98] showed actual abnormalities to the coagulation system before both the superior cavopulmonary anastomosis and the Fontan completion. Before the superior cavopulmonary anastomosis and the Fontan completion, procoagulant factors (factors II, V, VII, IX, and X, plasminogen, fibrinogen) as well as anticoagulant factors (protein C and antithrombin III) were lower than those in normal controls. Before the Fontan completion, Ravn and co-workers showed increased platelet reactivity.[107]

Thrombosis after Fontan completion has been reported to be as high as 20% to 30%. Coon and associates[25] reviewed transthoracic echocardiograms in 592 Fontan patients retrospectively after Fontan (median, 22 months; range, 1 day to 20 years). Thrombus was identified in 9% of patients. Freedom from thrombus was 92% at 1 year, 90% at 3 years, 84% at 8 years, and 82% at 10 years. No difference in freedom from thrombus was found between atriopulmonary and lateral tunnel Fontans, and no difference was found between fenestrated and nonfenestrated Fontans. Thrombus was just as likely on the pulmonary venous side (44%) as on the systemic venous side (48%). Balling and colleagues[7] also sought to determine the incidence of intracardiac thrombus and to define predisposing risk factors including type of Fontan modification. They found an incidence of 33% in a cohort of 52 asymptomatic Fontan patients by using transesophageal echocardiography. No predisposing factors could be identified. The study of Ballings et al.[7] would suggest that the resolution of transesophageal echocardiography is better than transthoracic echocardiography for identifying thrombus in the heart after Fontan, and that transthoracic echocardiography may be missing a large number of clots in the heart or Fontan circuit.

How to screen for thrombus formation is uncertain (transthoracic echocardiogram vs. transesophageal echocardiogram). It also is not clear whether prevention of thromboembolic phenomena should occur through platelet function inhibition (acetylsalicylic acid; ASA), inhibition of the coagulation cascade (warfarin; Coumadin), or replacement of insufficient anticoagulant factors. Multicenter randomized clinical trials are needed.

EARLY OUTCOME AFTER THE FONTAN PROCEDURE

To appreciate the dramatic improvement in the outcome after Fontan completion, it is useful to review results from earlier eras. The initial patients in the cohort of 500 patients undergoing the Fontan completion at Boston Children's Hospital had nonstaged, nonfenestrated atriopulmonary Fontan completions.[46] The most recent patients in the cohort had intervening superior cavopulmonary anastomosis and fenestrated lateral tunnel Fontan completion. The incidence of death or Fontan takedown decreased from 27.1% to 7.5% over the study period. HLHS was a risk factor for early failure in study of Gentles and colleagues.[46] Several studies have documented improved outcomes after intervening superior cavopulmonary anastomosis.[38,60,95]

Improving early mortality over time is not exclusive to those patients with HLHS. Mair and associates[83] from the Mayo Clinic reported on their 25-year experience with 216 patients with tricuspid atresia who underwent a nonfenestrated Fontan completion. Patients were arbitrarily grouped into early (1973 to 1980), middle (1981 to 1987), and late (1988 to 1997) surgical eras. Overall survival was 79% for the entire cohort. Similar to the study by Gentles and colleagues,[46] early mortality decreased dramatically over the three eras; the most recent era had a 2% mortality rate. Late survival also increased significantly from the earliest era to the most recent. The only risk factor for late mortality was nonfenestrated Fontan completion after age 18 years.

Baffle fenestration also has clearly improved outcomes. Bridges and associates[14] showed that baffle fenestration significantly decreased the incidence of "Fontan failure" from 11% to 7%, prolonged pleural effusions from 38% to 13%, and prolonged hospitalization from 20% to 12%.

Gaynor and colleagues[44] described a cohort using intervening superior cavopulmonary anastomosis and fenestrated Fontan completion. One hundred eighteen patients underwent Fontan completion between January 1996 and June 1999 at The Children's Hospital of Philadelphia. Sixty-eight patients had HLHS (n = 44) or HLHS variant (n = 24). Lateral tunnel fenestrated Fontan completion was performed in 34 of 44 patients with HLHS and 21 of 24 patients with HLHS variants. Eighty of the 118 patients in the cohort underwent lateral tunnel Fontan completion, and 38 underwent extracardiac Fontan completion. An intervening superior cavopulmonary connection was performed in 112 of 118 patients. All the patients with HLHS or HLHS variant had an intervening superior cavopulmonary anastomosis.

An intervening BDG was done in 91% of the patients who later underwent extracardiac Fontan completion, and the hemi-Fontan was done in 97% of the patients who later underwent lateral tunnel Fontan completion. The median age at Fontan completion was 24 months (range, 12 to 218 months), and the median weight was 11.3 kg (range, 6.7 to 52 kg). No difference in age or weight was found between the patients who underwent lateral tunnel and extracardiac Fontan completion. Of the patients who underwent a lateral tunnel completion, 98% had fenestration creation. The only patients who did not have fenestration creation in the lateral tunnel group were those with existing significant venous collaterals or pulmonary arteriovenous malformations. Of the patients who underwent the extracardiac Fontan completion, 84% had fenestration creation. A brief period of circulatory arrest was used in the lateral tunnel Fontan completion group. The median duration of circulatory arrest was 18 minutes (range, 12 to 59 minutes). Circulatory arrest also was used in 26 of 38 patients who underwent extracardiac Fontan completion.

Illustrating the significant improvement in outcomes after Fontan completion, no hospital or 30-day mortality was noted. One non-HLHS patient did not tolerate the Fontan and required transplantation. The rate of early mortality or "Fontan failure" was 0.8%. The median period of mechanical ventilation was 6 hours (range, 1 hour to 56 days). Only 6.8% of the patients were ventilated for more than 24 hours. The median intensive care unit (ICU) length of stay was 1 day (range, 1 to 56 days), and only 6.8% of the patients had an ICU length of stay longer than 7 days. The median hospital length of stay was 6 days, and only 6.8% were hospitalized for more than 14 days. The duration of mechanical ventilation, ICU, or hospital length of stay did not differ between those patients who had lateral tunnel or the extracardiac Fontan completion. The diagnosis of HLHS was not a risk factor for prolonged ventilation or ICU or hospital length of stay.

The median duration of mediastinal chest tube drainage was 1 day (range, 1 to 10 days). Pleural effusions needing either thoracentesis or placement of a chest tube occurred in 21% of the cohort; 32% after extracardiac and 16% after lateral tunnel. Readmission within 30 days for pleural effusion occurred in seven patients. The incidence of prolonged pleural effusions was very low. Including patients who were readmitted for pleural effusions, the median duration of pleural effusions requiring drainage was 1 day (range, 1 to 24 days). Only 4.2% of the cohort required pleural drainage for longer than 14 days. The mean period of drainage was greater for the extracardiac Fontan group relative to the lateral tunnel group—5 ± 6.5 days compared with 2.5 ± 3.5 days (P = 0.02). The diagnosis of HLHS was not a risk factor for prolonged pleural effusions.

Mosca and colleagues[91] at C.S. Mott Children's Hospital also illustrated the utility of intervening superior cavopulmonary anastomosis and MUF in a study. Outcomes were analyzed after Fontan completion in 100 consecutive patients with HLHS. A lateral tunnel Fontan completion was done in 48 patients by using bicaval cannulation and continuous CPB, whereas 52 patients underwent a lateral tunnel Fontan completion with circulatory arrest and MUF after an intervening hemi-Fontan cavopulmonary anastomosis. Mortality and morbidity (greater duration of mechanical ventilation, ICU, and total hospital length of stay) were significantly greater in the first group that did not have an intervening hemi-Fontan cavopulmonary anastomosis or the utilization of circulatory arrest and MUF during Fontan completion.

Three studies focused on mortality and morbidity in the early postoperative period after Fontan. The first was reported from by Gaynor and associates,[44] in which the Fontan completion experience from 1992 to 1999 was reviewed to assess for predictors of mortality and morbidity (duration of pleural effusions and hospital length of stay). During the 7-year period, 332 Fontan completions were performed on children with HLHS and other single-ventricle variants at a median age of 22 months. Overall mortality was 6.6% (22 of 332). Between 1992 and 1999, the surgical mortality after a modified Fontan operation decreased significantly; only two deaths occurred after 1994. Decreased morbidity with a decreased duration of pleural effusions and decreased hospital length of stay also were found. The diagnosis of HLHS was not a risk factor for death. The presence of a common atrioventricular valve and the presence of an increased preoperative PA pressure were associated with an increased risk of early death, whereas the use of single-punch fenestration in a lateral tunnel Fontan and the use of MUF decreased the risk of death. The risk of prolonged pleural effusions (longer than 3 days) was increased in patients with HLHS and was decreased by the use of a single-punch fenestration in a lateral tunnel Fontan and with the use of MUF. The risk of prolonged effusions lasting longer than 14 days was less in patients with extracardiac conduit with side-by-side fenestration and in patients who underwent lateral tunnel Fontan with single-punch fenestration. Prolonged hospital stay was defined as a length of stay longer than 14 days. A risk for prolonged length of stay existed in those diagnosed with HLHS, and a decreased risk of prolonged length of stay occurred in those patients with single-punch fenestration or the use of MUF.

The second study was a randomized clinical trial evaluating the effects of baffle fenestration on standard-risk single-ventricle patients undergoing the Fontan procedure. Lemler and associates[75] enrolled 49 consecutive patients randomized to either fenestrated (n = 25) or nonfenestrated (n = 24) Fontan procedure. Patients in the fenestrated group had 55% less total chest-tube drainage, a length of stay that was 41% shorter, and 67% fewer additional procedures in the postoperative period than did those in the nonfenestrated group. Fenestration at the time of modified Fontan surgery improves short-term outcome in standard-risk patients by decreasing pleural drainage, hospital length of stay, and the need for additional postoperative procedures. No difference in mortality was noted between the fenestrated and nonfenestrated Fontan groups.

The third study was a case-control study comparing early postoperative morbidity after the modified Fontan operation in patients with and without hemidiaphragmatic paralysis. Amin and colleagues[2] compared 10 patients with documented hemidiaphragmatic paralysis and 30 patients with normal diaphragmatic function, who were matched for diagnosis, fenestration, and age. Patients with hemidiaphragmatic paralysis had a longer hospital length of stay and had an increased risk of ascites, prolonged pleural effusions, and readmission. After the Fontan completion, pulmonary blood flow is augmented during inspiration through negative intrathoracic pressure. With hemidiaphragmatic paralysis, the inspiratory augmentation of pulmonary blood flow is diminished or lost.

Modifications in the procedure and improvements in perioperative care have dramatically reduced the mortality and morbidity associated with the Fontan procedure. The results for Fontan completion demonstrated that even for patients with HLHS, a protocol of routine staging, routine baffle fenestration, and use of MUF results in very low mortality and morbidity for completion of the Fontan procedure. Interinstitutional and intrainstitutional differences in technique, timing, and staging, and variations in perioperative management, make comparing studies on survival after Fontan completion problematic. Despite these confounding variables, analyses on the evolution of Fontan completion over the past decade, from the original valveless atriopulmonary connection to the staged total pulmonary cavopulmonary connection (lateral tunnel vs. extracardiac) with fenestration, have shown a progressive and dramatic improvement in operative survival.

Neurodevelopmental Outcome

One of the most active and important areas of outcomes research after the modified Fontan completion is neurodevelopmental outcome. The category of complex congenital heart disease in which neurodevelopmental outcome is of the greatest concern is the univentricular heart. Patients with single ventricles today undergo a three-staged palliation during which their brains may experience inadequate blood flow. In most cases, the initial palliative procedure requires low-flow or deep hypothermic circulatory arrest. Subsequent palliations are often performed on CPB. In addition, patients with single ventricles may experience inadequate cerebral blood flow because of hypotension during the perioperative period of one of their palliative procedures. Furthermore, many Fontan patients have survived with chronic hypoxemia. Limperopolous and associates[76] documented brain abnormalities in more than 50% of neonates with congenital heart disease before surgery. How these potential operative and perioperative insults, chronic hypoxemia, and preexisting brain anomalies come together to affect the neurodevelopmental outcome is not known.

Three important studies have assessed neurodevelopmental outcome after the Fontan completion. The first study is by Wernovsky and colleagues,[129] in which cognitive development after the Fontan was assessed. In a study of 133 patients palliated with a Fontan operation at Boston Children's Hospital for various subtypes of single ventricle, Wernovsky and associates found that these patients had a mean full-scale IQ significantly lower than that of the normal population (95.7 ± 17.4); 7.8% of patients scored below the threshold for mental retardation. Among several independent variables associated with lower IQ in this cohort was a diagnosis of HLHS. In a separate study at The Children's Hospital of Philadelphia looking at neurodevelopmental outcome in school-aged children and adolescents with HLHS after Fontan completion, the median IQ was 86, and 18% of the patients met criteria for mental retardation.[82] Goldberg and colleagues[50] at the C.S. Mott Children's Hospital did not find the same significant depression in IQ in Fontan patients that the Boston and Philadelphia groups found. Goldberg and co-workers[50] found that neurodevelopmental and behavioral outcome in patients who have undergone the Fontan procedure, including patients with HLHS, is good in the preschool and early school years, with Wechsler Intelligence scores generally in the normal range. Although the HLHS group had significantly lower scores (93.8 ± 7.3) than the non-HLHS univentricular group (107.0 ± 7.0), neither subgroup scored significantly different from the standard population on the Wechsler Scales.

The first attempt to quantify the quality of life of Fontan patients was made by the cardiovascular group at Babies Hospital in New York. Williams and colleagues[130] assessed the quality of life of 106 children and adolescents with HLHS who had undergone the staged palliation from 1990 through 1999. They used the Children's Health Questionnaire Parent Form 28 to assess quality of life. They used parent proxy reporting only; the children were not assessed. The Mean Physical Health summary score was slightly lower than that for normal subjects, and the Mean Psychosocial summary score was significantly lower than that for normal subjects. One of the difficulties in translating these studies into clinical practice is that the data reflect outcomes of perioperative management, surgical technique, and technology of 10 to 15 years ago.

References

1. Albanese SB, Carotti A, Di Donato RM, et al: Bi-directional cavopulmonary anastomosis in patients under two years of age. *J Thorac Cardiovasc Surg* 104:904–909, 1992.
2. Amin Z, McElhinney DB, Strawn JK, et al: Hemidiaphragmatic paralysis increases postoperative morbidity after a modified Fontan operation. *J Thorac Cardiovasc Surg* 122:856–862, 2001.
3. Amodeo A, Di Donato R, Carotti A, et al: Pulmonary arteriovenous fistulas and polysplenia syndrome. *J Thorac Cardiovasc Surg* 107:1378–1379, 1994.
4. Azakie A, McCrindle BW, Van Arsdell G, et al: Extracardiac conduit versus lateral tunnel cavopulmonary connections at a single institution: Impact on outcomes. *J Thorac Cardiovasc Surg* 122:1219–1228, 2001.
5. Azzolina G, Eufrate S, Pensa P: Tricuspid atresia: Experience in surgical management with a modified cavopulmonary anastomosis. *Thorax* 27:111–115, 1972.
6. Balaji S, Gewellig M, Bull C, et al: Arrhythmias after the Fontan procedure. *Circulation* 84:III162–III167, 1991.
7. Balling G, Vogt M, Kaemmerer H, et al: Intracardiac thrombus formation after the Fontan. *J Thorac Cardiovasc Surg* 119:745–752, 2000.
8. Bernstein HS, Brook MM, Silverman NH, et al: Development of pulmonary arteriovenous fistulae in children after cavopulmonary shunt. *Circulation* 92:II309–II314, 1995.
9. Bonnet D, Acar P, Aggoun Y, et al: Can partial cavo-pulmonary connection be considered as an alternative to the Fontan procedure? *Arch Mal Coeur Vaiss* 91:569–573, 1998.
10. Bove EL: Current status of staged reconstruction for hypoplastic left heart syndrome. *Pediatr Cardiol* 19:308–315, 1998.
11. Bradley SM, Mosca RS, Hennein HA, et al: Bidirectional superior cavopulmonary connection in young infants. *Circulation* 94:II5–II111, 1996.
12. Bradley SM, Simsic JM, Mulvihill DM: Hyperventilation impairs oxygenation after bidirectional superior cavopulmonary connection. *Circulation* 98:II372–II376, 1998.
13. Bridges ND, Lock JE, Castaneda AR: Baffle fenestration with subsequent transcatheter closure: Modification of the Fontan operation for patients at increased risk. *Circulation* 82:1681–1689, 1990.
14. Bridges ND, Mayer JE Jr, Lock JE, et al: Effect of baffle fenestration on outcome of the modified Fontan operation. *Circulation* 86:1762–1769, 1992.
15. Bridges ND, Lock JE, Mayer JE Jr, et al: Cardiac catheterization and test occlusion of the interatrial communication after the fenestrated Fontan operation. *J Am Coll Cardiol* 25:1712–1717, 1995.
16. Carlon CA, Mondini PG, de Marchi R: Su una nuova anastomosi vasale per la terapia chirurgica di alcuni visi cardiovasculari. [A new vascular anastomosis for surgical treatment of some cardiovascular anomalies]. *Ital Chir* 6:760–765, 1950.

17. Castaneda AR: Congenital heart disease from Glenn to Fontan: A continuing evolution. *Circulation* 86:II80–II84, 1992.

18. Cetta F, Feldt RH, O'Leary PW, et al: Improved early morbidity and mortality after Fontan operation: The Mayo Clinic experience, 1987 to 1992. *J Am Coll Cardiol* 28:480–486, 1996.

19. Chang AC, Hanley FL, Wernovsky G, et al: Early bidirectional cavopulmonary shunt in young infants: Postoperative course and early results. *Circulation* 88:149–158, 1993.

20. Chang AC, Atz AM, Wernovsky G, et al: Milrinone: Systemic and pulmonary hemodynamic effects in neonates after cardiac surgery. *Crit Care Med* 23:1907–1914, 1995.

21. Cheung YF, Penny DJ, Redington AN: Serial assessment of left ventricular diastolic function after Fontan procedure. *Heart* 83:420–424, 2000.

22. Cohen MI, Wernovsky G, Vetter VL, et al: Sinus node function after a systemically staged Fontan procedure. *Circulation* 98:II352–II358, 1998.

23. Cohen MI, Bridges ND, Gaynor JW, et al: Modifications to the cavopulmonary anastomosis do not eliminate early sinus node dysfunction. *J Thorac Cardiovasc Surg* 120:891–900, 2000.

24. Cohen MI, Bridges ND, Gaynor JW, et al: Modifications to the cavopulmonary anastomosis do not eliminate early sinus node dysfunction. *J Thorac Cardiovasc Surg* 120:891–900, 2000.

25. Coon PD, Rychik J, Novello RT, et al: Thrombus formation after the Fontan. *Ann Thorac Surg* 71:1990–1994, 2001.

26. Cromme-Dijkhuis AH, Hess J, Hahlen K, et al: Specific sequelae after Fontan operation at mid- and long-term follow-up. *J Thorac Cardiovasc Surg* 106:1126–1132, 1993.

27. de Leval MR, Kilner P, Gewillig M, et al: Total cavopulmonary connection: A logical alternative to atriopulmonary connection for complex Fontan operations: Experimental studies and early clinical experience. *J Thorac Cardiovasc Surg* 96:682–695, 1988.

28. de Leval MR, Dubini G, Migliavacca F, et al: Use of computational fluid dynamics in the design of surgical procedures: Application to the study of competitive flows in cavopulmonary connections. *J Thorac Cardiovasc Surg* 111:502–513, 1996.

29. Donofrio MT, Jacobs ML, Norwood WI, et al: Early changes in ventricular septal defect size and ventricular geometry in the single left ventricle after volume-unloading surgery. *J Am Coll Cardiol* 26:1008–1015, 1995.

30. Elizari A, Somerville J: Experience with the Glenn anastomosis in the adult with cyanotic congenital heart disease. *Cardiol Young* 9:257–265, 1999.

31. Filippini LH, Ovaert C, Nykanen DG, et al: Reopening of persistent left superior caval vein after bidirectional cavopulmonary connections. *Heart* 79:509–512, 1998.

32. Fishberger SB, Wernovsky G, Gentles TL, et al: Factors that influence the development of atrial flutter after the Fontan operation. *J Thorac Cardiovasc Surg* 113:80–86, 1997.

33. Fogel MA, Weinberg PM, Fychik J, et al: Caval contribution to flow in the branch pulmonary arteries of Fontan patients using a novel application of magnetic resonance presaturation pulse. *Circulation* 94:I181, 1996.

34. Fogel MA, Weinberg PM, Chin AJ, et al: Late ventricular geometry and performance changes of single ventricle throughout staged fontan reconstruction assessed by magnetic resonance imaging. *J Am Coll Cardiol* 28:212–221, 1996.

35. Fontan F, Baudet E: Surgical repair of tricuspid atresia. *Thorax* 26:240–248, 1971.

36. Fontan F, Kirklin JW, Fernandez G, et al: Outcome after a "perfect" Fontan operation. *Circulation* 81:1520–1536, 1990.

37. Fontan F, Baudet E: Surgical repair of tricuspid atresia. *Thorax* 26:240–248, 1971.

38. Forbess JM, Cook N, Serraf A, et al: An institutional experience with second- and third-stage palliative procedures for hypoplastic left heart syndrome: The impact of the bidirectional cavopulmonary shunt. *J Am Coll Cardiol* 29:665–670, 1997.

39. Freedom RM, Nykanen D, Benson LN: The physiology of the bidirectional cavopulmonary connection. *Ann Thorac Surg* 66:664–667, 1998.

40. Fyfe DA, Kline CH, Sade RM, et al: Transesophageal echocardiography detects thrombus formation not identified by transthoracic echocardiography after the Fontan operation. *J Am Coll Cardiol* 18:1733–1737, 1991.

41. Gamillscheg A, Zobel G, Urlesberger B, et al: Inhaled nitric oxide in patients with critical pulmonary perfusion after Fontan-type procedures and bidirectional Glenn anastomosis. *J Thorac Cardiovasc Surg* 113:435–442, 1997.

42. Gandhi SK, Bromberg BI, Rodefeld MD, et al: Lateral tunnel suture line variation reduces atrial flutter after the modified Fontan operation. *Ann Thorac Surg* 61:1299–1309, 1996.

43. Gatzoulis MA, Shinebourne EA, Redington AN, et al: Increasing cyanosis early after cavopulmonary connection caused by abnormal systemic venous channels. *Br Heart J* 73:182–186, 1995.

44. Gaynor JW, Bridges ND, Cohen MI, et al: Predictors of outcome after the Fontan operation: Is HLHS still a risk factor? *J Thorac Cardiovasc Surg* 123:237–245, 2002.

45. Gelatt M, Hamilton RM, McCrindle BW, et al: Risk factors for atrial tachyarrhythmias after the Fontan operation. *J Am Coll Cardiol* 24:1735–1741, 1994.

46. Gentles TL, Mayer JE Jr, Gauvreau K, et al: Fontan operation in five hundred consecutive patients: Factors influencing early and late outcome. *J Thorac Cardiovasc Surg* 114:376–391, 1997.

47. Gentles TL, Gauvreau K, Mayer JE Jr, et al: Functional outcome after the Fontan operation: Factors influencing late morbidity. *J Thorac Cardiovasc Surg* 114:392–403, 1997.

48. Glenn WWL: Circulatory bypass of the right side of the heart: IV shunt between the superior vena cava and distal right pulmonary artery: Report of clinical application. *N Engl J Med* 259:117–120, 1958.

49. Gewillig M, Daenen W, Aubert A, et al: Abolishment of chronic volume overload: Implications for diastolic function of the systemic ventricle immediately after Fontan repair. *Circulation* 86:II93–II99, 1992.

50. Goldberg CS, Schwartz EM, Brunberg JA, et al: Neurodevelopmental outcome of patients after the Fontan operation: A comparison between children with hypoplastic left heart syndrome and other functional single ventricle lesions. *J Pediatr* 137:646–652, 2000.

51. Gross GJ, Jonas RA, Castaneda AR, et al: Maturational and hemodynamic factors predictive of increased cyanosis after bidirectional cavopulmonary anastomosis. *Am J Cardiol* 74:705–709, 1994.

52. Haller JA Jr: Bidirectional inferior vena cava–pulmonary artery shunt. *J Thorac Cardiovasc Surg* 114:1123, 1997.

53. Harake B, Kuhn MA, Jarmakani JM, et al: Acute hemodynamic effects of adjustable atrial septal defect closure in the lateral tunnel Fontan procedure. *J Am Coll Cardiol* 23:1671–1676, 1994.

54. Hawkins JA, Shaddy RE, Day RW, et al: Mid-term results after bidirectional cavopulmonary shunts. *Ann Thorac Surg* 56:833–837, 1993.

55. Hjortdal VE, Stenbog EV, Ravn HB, et al: Neurohormonal activation late after cavopulmonary connection. *Heart* 83:439–443, 2000.

56. Hopkins RA, Armstrong BE, Serwer GA, et al: Physiological rationale for a bidirectional cavopulmonary shunt: A versatile complement to the Fontan principle. *J Thorac Cardiovasc Surg* 90:391–398, 1985.

57. Hsia TY, Khambadkone S, Redington AN, et al: Effects of respiration and gravity on infradiaphragmatic venous flow in normal and Fontan patients. *Circulation* 102:III148–III153, 2000.

58. Hsia TY, Khambadkone S, Redington AN, et al: Effect of fenestration on the subdiaphragmatic venous hemodynamics in the total-cavopulmonary connection. *Eur J Cardiothorac Surg* 19:785–792, 2001.

59. Hsu DT, Quaegebeur JM, Ing FF, et al: Outcome after the single-stage, nonfenestrated Fontan procedure. *Circulation* 96:II335–II340, 1997.

60. Jacobs ML, Norwood WI: Fontan operation: Influence of modifications on morbidity and mortality. *Ann Thorac Surg* 58:945–952, 1994.

61. Jacobs ML, Rychik J, Rome JJ, et al: Early reduction of the volume work of the single ventricle: The hemi-Fontan operation. *Ann Thorac Surg* 62:456–461, 1996.

62. Jahangiri M, Shore D, Kakkar V, et al: Coagulation factor abnormalities after the Fontan procedure and its modifications. *J Thorac Cardiovasc Surg* 113:989–993, 1997.

63. Kaulitz R, Ziemer G, Bergmann F, et al: Atrial thrombus after the Fontan operation: Predisposing factors, treatment and prophylaxis. *Cardiol Young* 7:37–43, 1997.

64. Knight WB, Mee RB: A cure for pulmonary arteriovenous fistulas? *Ann Thorac Surg* 59:999–1001, 1995.

65. Knott-Craig CJ, Danielson GK, Schaff HV, et al: The modified Fontan operation: An analysis of risk factors for early postoperative death or takedown in 702 consecutive patients from one institution. *J Thorac Cardiovasc Surg* 109:1237–1243, 1995.

66. Kobayashi J, Matsuda H, Nakano S, et al: Hemodynamic effects of bidirectional cavopulmonary shunt with pulsatile pulmonary flow. *Circulation* 84:III219–III225, 1991.

67. Konstantinov IE, Alexi-Meskishvit VV: Cavo-pulmonary shunt: From the first experiments to clinical practice. *Ann Thorac Surg* 68:1100–1106, 1999.

68. Kopf GS, Kleinman CS, Hijazi ZM, et al: Fenestrated Fontan operation with delayed transcatheter closure of atrial septal defect. *J Thorac Cardiovasc Surg* 103:1039–1048, 1992.

69. Koutlas TC, Gaynor JW, Nicolson SC, et al: Modified ultrafiltration reduces postoperative morbidity after cavopulmonary connection. *Ann Thorac Surg* 64:37–43, 1997.

70. Kreutzer G, Galindez E, Bono H, et al: An operation for the correction of tricuspid atresia. *J Thorac Cardiovasc Surg* 66:613–621, 1973.

71. Kuhn MA, Jarmakani JM, Laks H, et al: Effect of late post-operative atrial septal defect closure on hemodynamic function in patients with a lateral tunnel Fontan procedure. *J Am Coll Cardiol* 26:259–265, 1995.

72. Laks H, Pearl JM, Haas GS, et al: Partial Fontan: Advantages of an adjustable interatrial communication. *Ann Thorac Surg* 52:1084–1095, 1991.

73. Laks H, Ardehali A, Grant PW, et al: Modifications of the Fontan procedure: Superior vena cava to left pulmonary artery connection and inferior vena cava to right pulmonary artery connection with adjustable atrial septal defect. *Circulation* 91:2943–2947, 1995.

74. Laschinger JC, Redmond JM, Cameron DE, et al: Intermediate results of the extracardiac Fontan procedure. *Ann Thorac Surg* 62:1261–1267, 1996.

75. Lemler MS, Scott WA, Leonard SR, et al: Fenestration improves clinical outcome of the Fontan procedure: A prospective, randomized study. *Circulation* 105:207–212, 2002.

76. Limperopoulos C, Majnemer A, Shevell MI, et al: Neurologic status of newborns with congenital heart defects before open heart surgery. *Pediatrics* 103:402–408, 1999.

77. Magee AG, McCrindle BW, Mawson J, et al: Systemic venous collateral development after the bidirectional cavopulmonary anastomosis: Prevalence and predictors. *J Am Coll Cardiol* 32:502–508, 1998.

78. Mahle WT, Coon PD, Wernovsky G, et al: Quantitative echocardiographic assessment of the performance of the functionally single right ventricle after the Fontan operation. *Cardiol Young* 11:399–406, 2001.

79. Mahle WT, Spray TL, Wernovsky G, et al: Survival after reconstructive surgery for hypoplastic left heart syndrome: A 15-year experience from a single institution. *Circulation* 102:II36–II41, 2000.

80. Mahle WT, Wernovsky G, Bridges ND, et al: Impact of early ventricular unloading on exercise performance in preadolescents with single ventricle Fontan physiology. *J Am Coll Cardiol* 34:1637–1643, 1999.

81. Mahle WT, Rychik J, Rome JJ: Clinical significance of pulmonary arteriovenous malformations after staging bidirectional cavopulmonary anastomosis. *Am J Cardiol* 86:239–241, 2000.

82. Mahle WT, Clancy RR, Moss EM, et al: Neurodevelopmental outcome and lifestyle assessment in school-aged and adolescent children with hypoplastic left heart syndrome. *Pediatrics* 105:1082–1089, 2000.

83. Mair DD, Puga FJ, Danielson GK: The Fontan procedure for tricuspid atresia: Early and late results of a 25 year experience with 216 patients. *J Am Coll Cardiol* 37:933–939, 2001.

84. Manning PB, Mayer JE Jr, Wernovsky G, et al: Staged operation to Fontan increases the incidence of sinoatrial node dysfunction. *J Thorac Cardiovasc Surg* 111:833–840, 1996.

85. Marcelletti C, Como A, Giannico S, et al: Inferior vena cava–pulmonary artery extracardiac conduit: A new form of right heart bypass. *J Thorac Cardiovasc Surg* 100:228–232, 1990.

86. Mathews K, Bale JF Jr, Clark EB, et al: Cerebral infarction complicating Fontan surgery for cyanotic congenital heart disease. *Pediatr Cardiol* 7:161–166, 1986.

87. Matitiau A, Geva T, Colan SD, et al: Bulboventricular foramen size in infants with double-inlet left ventricle or tricuspid atresia with transposed great arteries: Influence on initial palliative operation and rate of growth. *J Am Coll Cardiol* 9:142–148, 1992.

88. Matsuda H, Covino E, Hirose H, et al: Acute liver dysfunction after modified Fontan operation for complex cardiac lesions. *J Thorac Cardiovasc Surg* 96:219–226, 1988.

89. Miller G, Eggli KD, Contant C, et al: Postoperative neurologic complications after open heart surgery on young infants. *Arch Pediatr Adolesc Med* 149:764–768, 1995.

90. Miller G, Mamourian AC, Tesman JR, et al: Long-term MRI changes in brain after pediatric open heart surgery. *J Child Neurol* 9:390–397, 1994.

91. Mosca RS, Kulik TJ, Goldberg CS, et al: Early results of the Fontan procedure in one hundred consecutive patients with hypoplastic left heart syndrome. *J Thorac Cardiovasc Surg* 119:1110–1118, 2000.

92. McElhinney DB, Reddy VM, Moore P, et al: Bidirectional cavopulmonary shunt in patients with anomalies of systemic and pulmonary venous drainage. *Ann Thorac Surg* 63:1676–1684, 1997.

93. McElhinney DB, Reddy VM, Hanley FL, et al: Systemic venous collateral channels causing desaturation after bidirectional cavopulmonary anastomosis: Evaluation and management. *J Am Coll Cardiol* 30:817–824, 1997.

94. Norwood WI, Kirklin JK, Sanders JP: Hypoplastic left heart syndrome: Experience with palliative surgery. *Am J Cardiol* 45:87–91, 1980.

95. Norwood WI, Jacobs ML: Fontan's procedure in two stages. *Am J Surg* 166:548–551, 1993.

96. Norwood WI, Lang P, Hansen DD: Physiologic repair of aortic atresia–hypoplastic left heart syndrome. *N Engl J Med* 308:23–26, 1983.

97. Odegard KC, McGowan FX Jr, DiNardo JA, et al: Coagulation abnormalities in patients with single ventricle physiology precede the Fontan procedure. *J Thorac Cardiovasc Surg* 123:459–465, 2002.

98. Odegard KC, McGowan FX Jr, Zurakowski D, et al: Coagulation factor abnormalities in patients with single-ventricle physiology immediately prior to the Fontan procedure. *Ann Thorac Surg* 73:1770–1777, 2002.

99. Ovroutski S, Dahnert I, Alexi-Meskishvili V, et al: Preliminary analysis of arrhythmias after Fontan operation with extracardiac conduit compared with intra-atrial lateral tunnel. *Thorac Cardiovasc Surg* 49:334–337, 2001.

100. Penny DJ, Redington AN: Diastolic ventricular function after the Fontan operation. *Am J Cardiol* 69:974–975, 1992.

101. Penny DJ, Redington AN: Doppler echocardiographic evaluation of pulmonary blood flow after the Fontan operation: The role of the lungs. *Br Heart J* 66:372–374, 1991.

102. Pennington DG, Nouri S, Ho J, et al: Glenn shunt: Long-term results and current role in congenital heart operations. *Ann Thorac Surg* 31:532–539, 1980.

103. Pridjian AK, Mendelsohn AM, Lupinetti FM, et al: Usefulness of the bidirectional Glenn procedure as staged reconstruction for the functional single ventricle. *Am J Cardiol* 71:959–962, 1993.

104. Pruckmayer M, Zacherl S, Salzer-Muhar U, et al: Scintigraphic assessment of pulmonary and whole-body blood flow patterns after surgical intervention in congenital heart disease. *J Nucl Med* 40:1477–1483, 1999.

105. Puga FJ, Chiavarelli M, Hagler DJ: Modifications of the Fontan operation applicable to patients with left atrioventricular valve atresia or single atrioventricular valve. *Circulation* 76:III53–III60, 1987.

106. Ramamoorthy C, Anderson GD, Williams GD, et al: Pharmacokinetics and side effects of milrinone in infants and children after open-heart surgery. *Anesth Analg* 86:283–289, 1998.

107. Ravn HB, Hjortdal VE, Stenbog EV, et al: Increased platelet reactivity and significant changes in coagulation markers after cavopulmonary connection. *Heart* 85:61–65, 2001.

108. Reddy VM, Liddicoat J, Hanley F: Primary bidirectional superior cavopulmonary shunt in infants between 1 and 4 months of age. *Ann Thorac Surg* 59:1120–1126, 1995.

109. Reyes A 2nd, Bove EL, Mosca RS, et al: Tricuspid valve repair in children with hypoplastic left heart syndrome during staged surgical reconstruction. *Circulation* 96:II341–II343, 1997.

110. Ro PS, Rome JJ, Cohen MS, et al: Diagnostic assessment before Fontan operation in patients with bidirectional cavopulmonary anastomosis: Are noninvasive methods sufficient? *J Am Soc Echocardiogr* 13:452, 2000.

111. Ro PS, Weinberg PM, Delrosario J, et al: Predicting the identity of decompressing veins after cavopulmonary anastomoses. *Am J Cardiol* 88:1317–1320, 2001.

112. Rosenthal DN, Friedman AH, Kleinman CS: Thromboembolic complications after Fontan operations. *Circulation* 92:II287–II293, 1995.

113. Rychik J, Rome JJ, Jacobs ML: Late surgical fenestration for complications after the Fontan operation. *Circulation* 96:33–36, 1997.

114. Rychik J, Jacobs ML, Norwood WI Jr: Acute changes in left ventricular geometry after volume reduction operation. *Ann Thorac Surg* 60:1267–1273, 1995.

115. Salzer-Muhar U, Marx M, Ties M, et al: Doppler flow profiles in the right and left pulmonary artery in children with congenital heart disease and a bidirectional cavopulmonary shunt. *Pediatr Cardiol* 15:302–307, 1994.

116. Santamore WP, Barnea O, Riordan CJ, et al: Theoretical optimization of pulmonary-to-systemic flow ratio after a bidirectional cavopulmonary anastomosis. *Am J Physiol* 274:H694–H700, 1998.

117. Schneider DJ, Banerjee A, Mendelsohn AM, et al: Hepatic venous malformation after modified Fontan procedure with partial hepatic vein exclusion. *Ann Thorac Surg* 63:1177–1179, 1997.

118. Senzaki H, Masutani S, Kobayashi J, et al: Ventricular afterload and ventricular work in Fontan circulation: Comparison with normal

two-ventricle circulation and single-ventricle circulation with Blalock-Taussig shunts. *Circulation* 105:2885–2892, 2002.

119. Shah MJ, Rychik J, Fogel MA, et al: Pulmonary AV malformations after superior cavopulmonary connection: Resolution after inclusion of hepatic veins in the pulmonary circulation. *Ann Thorac Surg* 63:960–963, 1997.

120. Sharma S, Goudy S, Walker P, et al: In vitro flow experiments for determination of optimal geometry of total cavopulmonary connection for surgical repair of children with functional single ventricle. *J Am Coll Cardiol* 27:1264–1269, 1996.

121. Srivastava D, Preminger T, Lock JE, et al: Hepatic venous blood and the development of pulmonary arteriovenous malformations in congenital heart disease. *Circulation* 92:1217–1222, 1995.

122. Stamm C, Anderson RH, Ho SY: The morphologically tricuspid valve in hypoplastic left heart syndrome. *Eur J Cardiothorac Surg* 12:587–592, 1997.

123. Tam VKH, Miller BE, Murphy K: Modified Fontan without use of cardiopulmonary bypass. *Ann Thorac Surg* 68:1698–1704, 1999.

124. Thompson LD, Petrossian E, McElhinney DB, et al: Is it necessary to routinely fenestrate an extracardiac Fontan? *J Am Coll Cardiol* 34:539–544, 1999.

125. Triedman JK, Bridges ND, Mayer JE Jr, et al: Prevalence and risk factors for aortopulmonary collateral vessels after Fontan and bidirectional Glenn procedures. *J Am Coll Cardiol* 22:207–215, 1993.

126. Tweddell JS, Litwin B, Thomas JP, et al: Recent advances in the surgical management of the single ventricle pediatric patient. *Pediatr Clin North Am* 46:465–480, 1999.

127. Van Haesdonck JM, Mertens L, Sizaire R, et al: Comparison by computerized numeric modeling of energy losses in different Fontan connections. *Circulation* 92:II322–II326, 1995.

128. Vettukattil JJ, Slavik Z, Lamb RK, et al: Intrapulmonary arteriovenous shunting may be a universal phenomenon in patients with the superior cavopulmonary anastomosis: A radionuclide study. *Heart* 83:425–428, 2000.

129. Wernovsky G, Stiles KM, Gauvreau K, et al: Cognitive development after the Fontan operation. *Circulation* 102:883–889, 2000.

130. Williams DL, Gelijns AC, Moskowitz AJ, et al: Hypoplastic left heart syndrome: Valuing the survival. *J Thorac Cardiovasc Surg* 119:720–731, 2000.

131. Yahagi N, Kumon K, Tanigami H, et al: Cardiac surgery and inhaled nitric oxide: Indication and follow-up (2–4 years). *Artif Organs* 22:886–891, 1998.

132. Zellars TM, Driscoll DJ, Humes RA, et al: Glenn shunt: Effect on pleural drainage after modified Fontan operation. *J Thorac Cardiovasc Surg* 98:725–729, 1989.

PART FIVE

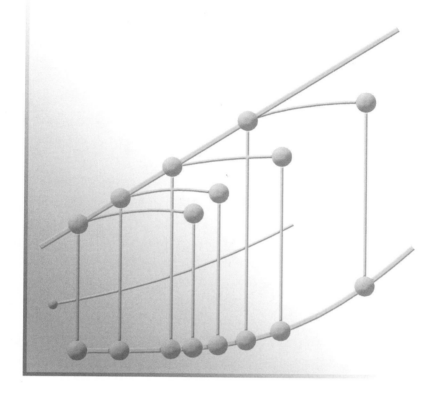

Medical Conditions

Chapter 42

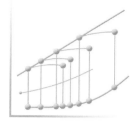

The Critical Appraisal and Use of Evidence about Therapy

BRIAN W. MCCRINDLE, MD, MPH, FRCPC

TRYING TO SORT OUT WHAT WORKED: A CASE STUDY

Van Arsdell and colleagues[17] performed a retrospective* case review of consecutive patients who had undergone the Fontan procedure at a single institution. The impetus for the study was the observation of a period of 50 consecutive procedures having been performed from November, 1993 to November 1995, with no operative (<30 days) mortality. The characteristics, management, and outcomes for these patients were compared with those of the previous 50 consecutive procedures performed from January 1992 to October 1993, during which four operative deaths occurred. The investigators wished to define what changes in management could have caused the decrease in mortality. No significant differences were noted between the two periods in patient demographics, underlying anatomy, previous procedures, and preoperative risk factors, including data obtained at preoperative cardiac catheterization. The only exception was a greater likelihood of staging with a bidirectional cavopulmonary anastomosis in the second period. However, several significant differences were found regarding operative and perioperative interventions. Procedures performed in the second period were more likely to include extracardiac conduits

---

*This chapter uses the terms *retrospective* to mean data that were collected from the past and *prospective* to mean data collected from the present into the future. Although this is the common usage, it is inaccurate. The actual terms for this would be nonconcomitant and concomitant data collection and reflect when the measurements were made. The terms *retrospective* and *prospective* refer to which information was collected first, the predictor or risk factor or exposure, or the outcome. If the outcomes for the subjects are known at the start of the study and data regarding risk factors are then obtained from previously collected or data collected in the present, then the study is retrospective, the most common type of design being the case-control study. If the risk factors are assessed in the past and the patients monitored forward in time to determine in whom the outcomes develop, then the study is prospective, the most common designs being the cohort study and the clinical trial. More commonly, studies can have an element of both, in that a medical record review simultaneously collects nonconcomitant data regarding both risk factors and outcomes, and a cross-sectional study may collect data regarding both risk factors and outcomes from a single period in the present. Further, some studies may begin with assembly of a cohort of patients from the past, nonconcomitantly review their past records, and then obtain more up-to-date data in the present with concomitant follow-up into the future.

(8% vs. 38%), baffle fenestration (58% vs. 76%), non–Gore-Tex patch material (52% vs. 72%), no or single-dose cardioplegia (6% vs. 42%), magnesium-rich cardioplegia (39% vs. 100%), modified ultrafiltration (4% vs. 62%), and greater use of inotropes and vasodilators in the operating room. The mean duration of cardiopulmonary bypass was significantly shorter in the second period (141 vs. 121 minutes). In addition to operative mortality, a number of other outcomes were better in the second period, including shorter duration of stay in the intensive care unit, shorter total hospital stay, less baffle leak, less low cardiac output syndrome, and less need for early postoperative cardiac catheterizations. No significant differences were found in postoperative physiologic measurements. However, when the patients from the two periods were pooled together, the only independent factor significantly associated with decreased odds of mortality was a shorter duration of cardiopulmonary bypass, and none of the many interventions was significantly associated.

This study illustrates what happens when evidence of therapeutic effect is sought from clinical practice and not from systematic study. Many changes in practice were made over the period of review. A literature search for evidence from clinical trials to support any of the therapies adopted found only two studies (both published after the period of review for this study), one by Lemler and associates[11] published in 2002, showing the benefit of fenestration, and one by Bando and coworkers,[2] published in 1998, showing the benefit of modified ultrafiltration. Thus it is not known on what evidence the changes in practice were based at the time of their adoption. The study also highlights several methodologic issues. The division of the study period into two halves was arbitrary. With only four deaths or outcome events, very little statistical power existed to detect any associated factors. The many changes in therapy occurring over the same period make it very difficult to dissect out the independent contribution of each. The study can conclude that mortality improved and that many therapies were adopted but cannot make any assertions as to a causal relation. Unfortunately, this is the predominant form in which evidence currently is found in clinical pediatric cardiology, and decisions to reject or adopt certain therapies are often based on the results of studies such as this.

THE ERA OF EVIDENCE-BASED MEDICINE

Evidence-based medicine (EBM) is not a new concept, but it has taken on a new imperative quality and importance. The greatest reason is that an acceleration in the development and application of new technologies and therapies has occurred, which has caused health care costs to escalate. These advances are likely to benefit fewer patients and to have a smaller incremental effect on outcomes, making it harder to detect a benefit and to exclude random error as an explanation. Yet a shift in the management and financing of health care has ensued, and an increasing demand to adopt only innovations of proven benefit that can be applied in a cost-effective manner.

Whereas an explosion has occurred in the medical literature and wide access via the Internet, health care providers are left to search, appraise, and filter the literature on their own, but often lack the necessary resources and skills.

An assumption is found that just because someone is qualified to practice clinical medicine, he or she is automatically qualified to perform and appraise clinical research, an assumption that impairs the effectiveness of the peer-review process. Although it may appear that a glut of information exists, the overall quality of the evidence is poor, with important gaps in which no evidence is available.

A focus on use and critical appraisal of the literature has emerged as one potential solution to this situation. This has gradually led to both support and debate for a field of study now known as EBM or evidence-based clinical decision-making.[5,15,16] Detractors claim that this focus on the literature will lead to a "cookbook" approach to clinical practice, yet EBM has been defined as the integration of the best research evidence with clinical expertise and patient values. EBM must, therefore, include an awareness of the role of the patient and his or her beliefs, milieu, and preferences, and the clinician should consider this context when weighing the balance of potential benefits versus risks for the individual patient. EBM recognizes an art as well as a science in clinical practice, but that sound decision making must be first based on the best science. The artful application of therapies that have no or unknown scientific merit is unlikely to be in the best interest of anyone other than financial investors.

STEPS IN THE PRACTICE OF EVIDENCE-BASED MEDICINE

The practice of EBM is defined by a series of steps as noted in Table 42-1, by which critically appraised evidence is brought to a clinical question and incorporated into the decision-making process. The process begins with the recognition of the need for information. This is often not as simple as it sounds. In a busy clinical practice, particularly in a critical care setting, we may not have the time to contemplate our gaps in knowledge or anxieties about uncertainty while trying to deal with the situation at hand. We then rely on the foundations of our knowledge, usually derived from didactic teaching, tempered with experience, either our own or that imparted to us as "wisdom" by others. Often we suppress rather than address our knowledge gaps and areas of uncertainty. Our time for improving and updating our knowledge and skills is scarce, and we often rely on others through didactic

Table 42-1 Steps in the Practice of Evidence-Based Medicine

1. To give the process the most immediate relevance, begin with a clinical scenario, and phrase the need for information to resolve the scenario in terms of an answerable question.
2. Develop and implement a strategy to obtain the best available evidence.
3. Critically appraise the evidence in terms of its validity, the magnitude and reliability of the reported effect, and its applicability and relevance to the clinical scenario at hand.
4. In addition to the appraised evidence, take into account the uniqueness of the clinical scenario in terms of the individual patient's pathophysiology, social and cultural milieu, and preferences and values. From this integration, make the best-informed clinical decision.
5. Record, track, and update the results of the preceding process. Assess the process itself, and strive for greater efficiency and benefit in future clinical scenarios.

teaching methods, such as continuing educational events, textbooks, and review articles, to help fill in the gaps. The anxiety we feel by "not knowing" is ignored rather than acted on. The practice of EBM is an effective and efficient method to help deal with that knowledge-deficit anxiety.

Formulating the Question

Learners, colleagues, and patients may pose questions to us directly, or questions may arise when we delve into those areas of uncertainty we might feel about specific aspects of a clinical scenario. Many questions may arise simultaneously, and we may have to assign priorities to which ones should be pursued. Regardless, the first step is to phrase the question as an answerable question. "What about milrinone?" is not an answerable question. "What are the pharmacologic mechanisms of action of milrinone?" may be too broad, but it is better, and is an example of a question that arises from gaps in foundation knowledge; these are often the questions raised by persons early in their clinical training. "Does prophylactic use of milrinone decrease the prevalence of low cardiac output syndrome in neonates after cardiopulmonary bypass?" is a specific, focused, and answerable question that likely has immediate relevance to a clinical scenario. Indeed, this question was addressed by a recent multicenter clinical trial.[6] An answerable question thus has several characteristics. First, it is phrased in the format of a question. Second, it is specific and focused, rather than broad and vague. Third, the answer to the question should have immediate relevance to the clinical scenario at hand. These questions tend to focus on aspects of diagnosis, therapy, and prognosis.

Searching for Evidence

In the search for medical evidence, the clinician may consult specialists, read textbooks, search evidence-based review journals and databases, or attend continuing education courses. Although each has its place, they all have limitations, and the clinician is left with sifting through the peer-reviewed scientific medical literature through databases such as MEDLINE through PubMed (http://www.ncbi.nlm.nih.gov/entrez/ query.fcgi).

The search involves specification of particular terms of key relevance to the question. One can then progressively focus the results of an initial search by providing further specification, particularly of research design. The PubMed website offers a service called "clinical queries," which automatically filters articles based on research design. For identified initial articles of interest, using a "related articles" search feature can identify both more specific and more recent articles. The search process thus involves some contraction and expansion, until one is satisfied that the most rigorous and most relevant article has been identified. One usually first screens titles, and then abstracts, and then study purposes and methods, before settling on one article.

Critical Appraisal

Critiquing and appraising evidence usually focuses on two main activities. The first is evaluating the extent to which the design and execution of a study have been performed with a sufficient degree of scientific rigor and freedom from bias and error so that the results will be an accurate and reliable reflection of the truth. The second is an evaluation of the magnitude, reliability, and generalizability of the reported results. These concepts are specified later in the chapter.

Application of Results

On critical appraisal of the actual findings of the study, one must then weigh the risks versus the benefits for the individual patient, which requires taking into consideration unique aspects of the setting and the patient. If the study has reported the results with sufficient detail and clarity, it may be possible to apply prediction formulas, likelihood ratios, and calculate estimates of numbers needed to treat for benefit and harm that take into account some important patient characteristics. However, this information is often not analyzed or reported in many important clinical trials, and it is left to the reader to attempt to apply the formulas with that information that is reported. Many of these formulas are available in the *JAMA User's Guides to the Medical Literature* or textbooks of EBM. The incorporation of patient's preferences and values is best approached by performing a clinical decision analysis, but this is rarely available in the medical literature and not easily performed in the clinical scenario. A more feasible approach might be to communicate the patient-specific risks and benefits to the patient, ensuring comprehension, and then to elicit not only the patient's preferences but also the magnitude of those preferences. These magnitudes can then be used to adjust some of the specific estimates of benefit and risk derived from the literature and communicated to the patient again for feedback and further adjustment, until an appropriate decision has been reached. Critical care providers often go through this process informally when working with families through decisions regarding high-risk interventions versus withdrawal of support.

Tuning the Process

Going through the steps of EBM is inherently a learning activity. Recording the results is an additional way to ensure that the process has ongoing benefits and gives the potential for the critical appraisal to be disseminated and available to other providers. However, the use of the critical appraisal reported by others must be considered with caution. The users must assure themselves that the appraisal was performed in a correct manner. The date of all reported appraisals must be recorded. Because the process is designed to bring the most current as well as the best evidence to the clinical scenario, one must be careful not to bypass the process by relying on appraisals beyond their expiration date. If appraisals are recorded and stored for retrieval, then mechanisms should be in place by which they can be revised, updated, and accumulated. In addition, the process of EBM itself is not a stagnant process, and practitioners should strive to evaluate their efforts to achieve greater efficiency, overcome barriers, and provide the best benefit to future clinical scenarios.

BUILDING A BODY OF EVIDENCE

In appraising a study about a therapy or intervention, the type of study design used and the degree of rigor and care with which it is executed directly affect the confidence we might

Table 42-2 Seven Questions to Consider Before Widespread Adoption of a New Therapy as the Standard of Care

1. Is there a sound rationale for the therapy based on current knowledge of physiology and pathophysiology (in the specific patient population)?
2. Can the therapy be applied in the clinical setting?
3. Does the therapy have a beneficial effect on the primary outcome of interest, particularly an outcome associated with improved prognosis or enhanced health status or quality of life?
4. What is the full spectrum of beneficial and adverse effects of the therapy?
5. What factors influence the effects of the therapy in the clinical setting?
6. How does the therapy compare with currently applied therapies?
7. What are patients' preferences for the therapy? Is the therapy cost-effective? What are the practical limitations for widespread delivery of the therapy?

have in accepting the conclusions. The study design is often the most important element defining the validity of the evidence provided. Validity determines the degree to which the results represent the truth. Study designs can be ranked regarding the quality of evidence they provide, which also correspond with the ease with which they are performed and appraised, and the degree to which biases might be evident and detectable. No individual study answers all questions about a therapy or intervention, and each study design has its place in the development of a chain of evidence. Table 42-2 gives seven questions regarding a new therapy that should be answered in sequence, although often overlapping, to provide the complete body of evidence in support of widespread adoption of the therapy as the standard of care.

When investigating a new therapy, one does not immediately begin with a large-scale clinical trial. The first question that must be addressed is whether the therapy is based on a sound rationale and that it makes sense in terms of our knowledge of physiology and pathophysiology. This knowledge often comes from basic science studies. In addition, the rationale for many therapies currently in widespread use in children rests solely on the basis of studies performed in adults, often with different underlying pathophysiologic processes. The current widespread use of angiotensin-converting enzyme inhibitors aimed at the long-term preservation of ventricular function in patients who have had the Fontan procedure is largely based on extrapolation from studies of adults with structurally normal failing hearts. The only randomized clinical trial in this setting failed to show any benefit,[10] yet in many institutions, the practice is widespread.

The next question is whether the therapy can be applied. This early evidence is usually provided from case reports and short-term case series, that may be either prospective or, more commonly, retrospective. Some therapies, particularly surgical and interventional cardiac catheterization procedures, can require special resources and expertise and experience before they can be applied. When this is the case, early results may not be as impressive, and some rationale may exist for persisting. Early experience with the arterial switch operation for transposition of the great arteries showed a high early mortality, but important multi-institutional studies demonstrated a learning curve before more optimal results

could be achieved.[9] A similar experience has evolved regarding the Norwood procedure.

Usually at the same time one is considering aspects of the application of a therapy, information is gathered to support whether the therapy has the intended beneficial effect on the primary outcomes of interest. This evidence usually comes from case series, predominantly retrospective and descriptive in design. At this stage, the priority of outcomes under consideration starts with mortality, reinterventions, and then medical morbidity. These studies could be more correctly classified as studies of prognosis, albeit after a specific intervention. One often uses these studies as a comparison with other previously published studies of alternative and often more established therapies. The comparison with other studies of outcomes is fraught with a multitude of biases. The studies may involve different institutions with different patient populations having therapies applied in a different era in which many other aspects of patient selection and management may differ, as well as differences in the definition and assessment of those outcomes. To provide the greatest chance for minimizing both detectable and unknown biases, a randomized, double-blinded clinical trial should be performed. Unfortunately, this is a rare occurrence.

If a given therapy shows some promise of beneficial effect, then the next priority is to define the full spectrum of both beneficial and adverse outcomes that are attributable to the therapy. This ideally involves a large-scale cohort study, with the cohort being defined and followed up prospectively, preferably in a standardized manner. More often, these studies are retrospective, and the data collection is not well standardized and spans a long era, reflecting an evolving practice in a single institution. Nonetheless, some multi-institutional groups have adopted the prospective cohort approach to tracking outcomes. The Congenital Heart Surgeons Society has performed several studies of prospectively enrolled patients with particular congenital heart lesions. Likewise, the Pediatric Heart Transplantation Study Group has tracked outcomes of prospectively enrolled patients both after listing and transplantation. These groups have used advanced statistical methods to define outcomes and associated factors, and to even provide prediction models to guide selection of optimal therapy.

Concomitant with the definition of the spectrum of outcomes, an analysis often is aimed at defining patient selection and management factors that affect the risk of those outcomes. The identification of these factors allows more specific prognostication for an individual patient after a given therapy. It also may identify factors that might be amenable to additional interventions to improve outcomes. The failure to identify explanatory factors is one of the greatest limitations of studies with only descriptive analyses.

A critical question for any new therapy is whether it will be more or less beneficial or risky than doing nothing or in comparison to the currently available standard therapy. The criterion standard for this comparison is the randomized, double-blind clinical trial. The key value of a clinical trial in minimizing bias and confounding rests with the randomization, in which study subjects are randomly assigned to either the study intervention or a placebo or alternative therapy. This allows random (and we hope equal) distribution of baseline characteristics and gives the best chance that the final study groups will have been very similar at baseline before any study maneuver. If the subsequent assessment of outcomes is done in a blinded manner with no knowledge of the study assignment of the subject, then this also minimizes further bias. However, comparisons regarding therapy are more commonly made from data obtained as part of individualized routine clinical care, usually abstracted from retrospective medical record review. Thus the assignment of interventions is not random, and it is well known that certain patients will be preferentially selected for certain therapies based on certain patient and clinical milieu characteristics. This has the potential to introduce a great deal of bias and confounding into any comparison, and this can be further compounded if the clinical data are obtained from a long period in which many important changes in patient and management characteristics may have occurred. Studies of therapy without a concomitant comparison are really studies of the prognosis after a given therapy. Nonetheless, many investigators will not be content with only this descriptive aspect and will attempt comparison with other published studies (which may differ to a variable degree in their subjects, design, intervention, and analysis) or with "historical controls" (those patients who were treated with an alternative therapy in the period preceding the adoption of the therapy of the current cohort). These studies are the least valid and provide the weakest evidence that the therapy is causally related to the outcomes demonstrated.

Most often in critical heart disease in children, therapies become widely entrenched based on a variable body of evidence that never includes investigation with randomized clinical trials. This situation has arisen for several reasons. Many clinicians do not have the skills to appraise the literature critically, and thus are not aware of the absence or quality of the data on which their decisions are based. A great tendency exists to rely on authorities for direction, and these authorities are more often the innovators and not the evaluators. Pediatric cardiology involves diseases that are rare, and increasingly studies must be collaborative within and between institutions, yet a limited history exists of collaborative efforts in a technical field in which innovation is more highly valued. Many therapies have a technical performance aspect and often a degree of operator dependence on the applications and outcomes of the therapy, reflected in learning curves and disparities between institutions. Clinical trials are relatively easy to critique but difficult to organize, design, and perform. They require considerably more advanced training in research methods than many pediatric clinicians currently possess. The ethical concerns regarding clinical research are magnified when the subject is a child, and restrictions regarding tolerance for potential harms are more stringent. For many drug evaluations, specific pediatric pharmacologic information is often missing. With some therapies, the effect of the intervention may not become apparent for many years, spanning periods that are not feasible for prospective study. Finally, great difficulties are found in obtaining funding for pediatric clinical trials, as the medical industry does not readily sponsor pediatric studies because of increased perceived risks and lack of a substantial product market.

The bridge from the "cookbook" or clinical investigation to individualization and widespread adoption of a new therapy requires some higher-level studies that are rarely performed but are increasingly relevant. Patients' preferences or aversion for the nature of a therapy, such as its degree of invasiveness, as well as the level of risk they will tolerate to achieve or avoid certain outcomes, should be factored into evaluation and clinical decision making. This often takes the form of a clinical decision-analysis type of study, in which patients' values are assessed and multiplied by the probabilities of different outcomes. Alternatively, a cost-effectiveness or cost-benefit analysis uses costs to assign values to therapies and outcomes. Finally, many therapies may work well in the scenario of a clinical study but fail in their application in clinical practice when issues of health care provider and patient compliance, availability and costs, and use in more diverse clinical scenarios come to bear. Thus ongoing study in clinical practice should be performed.

PITFALLS IN DATA INTERPRETATION

When reviewing the literature regarding a given therapy, the main emphasis of the study is usually to determine if the observed outcomes occurred as a direct result of that therapy. From a clinical study, four main types of relations exist between the therapy and the outcome that may be evident. An assumption exists on the part of the unaware reader that any reported relation is a causal one, especially if the P value is less than .05. However, this error usually reflects a lack of knowledge on the part of the reader or a lack of specification of the details of the study on the part of the authors.

Bias

Associations are said to be biased when some known or unknown factor influences the patient selection, application of the therapy, and ascertainment of the outcomes in a systematic rather than a random way. Regarding patient selection, decisions to apply one therapy versus another are often based on specific patient and system characteristics that also are factors that influence the outcome. The key feature of randomization of patient assignment is to distribute these characteristics randomly. Some studies have shown that patients who choose to participate in clinical studies may differ in potentially important ways from those who do not. The therapy also should be applied in a uniform manner, which can be a key source of bias when comparing therapies that have a high degree of operator dependence in their successful application. A specific therapy may induce the application of other therapies, or co-interventions, which also may influence the outcomes. Outcomes may be sought more aggressively for one therapy versus another, particularly when comparing new experimental treatments that are greatly scrutinized versus those that have been long established. The potential sources of bias are infinite, and every step should be made to address as many as possible. Bias tends to refer to factors that are errors in the experimental process.

Confounding

When assessing the effect of a therapy on an outcome, many factors other than the therapy under study also can affect the outcome, and if any of those factors also is associated with the therapy assignment or application, then the factors can distort or confound our ability to detect the true effect. Confounding factors can include the characteristics of the patients and the management of their condition, differences in the way in which the therapy under study was applied, such as compliance, and concomitant therapies or interventions. Confounding tends to refer to factors outside of the experimental process, over which we have no control, and often are the biggest challenge in accepting results from observational studies, in which much of the potential confounding is unknown.

Chance

Chance relations are random occurrences. We often have little control over them in the complex clinical scenario. However, we can use the science of probability both to quantitate and to minimize the occurrence of random errors. In general, a random error is less likely to occur in a study of a large versus a small number of patients. The calculated P value is the predicted probability that a study result may have occurred by chance alone. We generally accept a smaller than 5% chance, or $P < .05$, of concluding that the results are true when in fact they are due to a random error.

Causality

When considering a therapy, we would like to be confident that the outcome we observe occurs as a direct result of that therapy. Whereas it is important that the observation be free of bias, confounding, and chance errors, other criteria give further information that the relation is causal. These are usually satisfied in well-designed and -executed clinical trials, but may not be evident in other types of observational study designs, as bias, confounding, and chance may predominate. The time relation must be correct, in that the therapy must be applied before the patient develops the outcome or change in the outcome. Strong relations or powerful effects are more likely to be causal, as are dose-response relations. Treatment effects that are consistent within the study and specific to the study imply causation. The effect of the therapy should be consistent in other relevant populations and should be consistent with other evidence. The action of the treatment in causing the effect should be biologically plausible. All of these characteristics improve one's confidence that the treatment caused the effect observed in the study.

CRITICAL APPRAISAL OF THE CLINICAL TRIAL

The properly designed and executed clinical trial gives the best evidence that a specific intervention exerts a causal effect on an outcome or adverse effect. It also gives the best likelihood that the relation is free of bias, confounding, and chance errors, if confidence limits are appropriately provided. Because the criteria and flaws are more obvious, clinical trials are, in spite of being more difficult to perform, easier to appraise critically (Table 42-3). However, because more of the flaws are evident, this also increases the risk of their not reaching the level for publication, although a suboptimal

Table 42-3   Critical Appraisal of the Clinical Trial

1. Is the study well designed and executed such that the results are likely to be free of bias and therefore representative of the truth?
   a. Was treatment assignment randomized? If so,
      i. Is the ramdomization strategy specified?
      ii. Was it tamper proof?
      iii. Was it successful, in that baseline characteristics are comparable between comparison groups?
   b. Are all of the study subjects accounted for throughout the study and analyzed according to their initial assignment?
   c. Were the groups treated equally in all other respects besides the study maneuver?
   d. Are the primary and secondary outcomes relevant and sufficient?
   e. Was the study period sufficiently long for the outcomes to occur?
   f. Was the study maneuver, assessments, and data analysis blinded to the initial assignment?
   g. Is there a stated hypothesis, and are sample-size calculations provided?
2. What are the results, and is the analysis and presentation in a format that allows assessment of the magnitude and reliability of treatment effects?
   a. What are the magnitudes of the treatment effects?
      i. Absolute effects
      ii. Relative effects
   b. How reliable are the estimates of the treatment effects?
      i. Are standard errors or confidence intervals provided?
      ii. Are power calculations provided for nonsignificant differences?
3. Are the results relevant and applicable to the clinical scenario at hand?
   a. Are inclusion and exclusion criteria described in sufficient detail?
   b. Is the treatment described in sufficient detail to enable implementation?
      i. Is the treatment feasible in the clinical scenario?
   c. Is any information provided that would allow further specification of the treatment effects to the characteristics of an individual patient?
      i. What are the benefits and harms for the specific patient?
   d. What are the values and preferences for the specific patient?

clinical trial gives better evidence than a suboptimal, but harder to evaluate, observational study. In addition, clinical trials that do not show a significant effect of the studied intervention on the primary outcomes of interest often fail to be published, even though the negative results may be very important. Given that no one study definitively resolves all issues related to the evaluation of a therapy, and that the cumulative body of evidence is important, this publication bias in favor of positive studies imparts an unfair bias in favor of rejection of what might be an effective therapy.

Several aspects of the clinical trial should be appraised before acceptance of the results and application to a clinical population.

Specification of the Study Population

The first paragraph of the paper's section on study methods should give the *source population* that was evaluated for possible enrollment. The source population is a subset of the target population, which is a specified population of present and future patients to which the results of the trial might be applicable. The source population consists of those patients who are accessible for this particular trial to these particular investigators. This source population may be a group of identified patients already known to have a given condition.

In this scenario, we have the patients and simply must recontact them. Alternatively, we may wish to enroll only newly identified patients as they present for medical care and are diagnosed or undergo a specific intervention. Either way, not everyone in the source population may be eligible for the trial. The determination of eligibility is based on the presence of predefined *inclusion criteria* and the absence of *exclusion criteria*. These criteria should be stated explicitly and definitions provided for each criterion. Sometimes, additional measurements may be used to assess some criteria. Inclusion criteria tend to define the unifying characteristics of our eligible population, as well as a few logistic criteria that may make the study more feasible. Exclusion criteria tend to define characteristics that would confound the effects or create contraindications for the study intervention, such as the presence of other medical complications. Critical appraisal of these criteria and definitions, together with an assessment of the characteristics of the actual study participants, is necessary to determine the applicability of the study and its results to our own individual clinical scenarios to which we are trying to bring evidence to bear.

Sometimes the investigators may have more potential study subjects than they need, and they are faced with the problem of how to take just some of the subjects. This can occur at the level of the source or eligible population and is solved by *sampling*. The sampling strategy should be clearly specified and tamper-proof and should produce a sample that has the same characteristics as the population from which it was taken. The best chance for this to occur is if the subjects are chosen randomly after enumeration of the population. Particularly when the sample to be drawn is small, a chance exists that the randomly chosen sample is not similar to the population from which it was drawn. To minimize this happening, at least for the important characteristics, the investigators may divide or *stratify* the population according to the characteristic of interest into smaller sets, and then randomly take a number of subjects from that set that is proportionate to the size of the set relative to the size of the population, which is known as *proportionate stratified sampling*. More commonly, the investigators specifically wish to see how the study intervention might work in these individual sets and thus may take equal or even greater numbers from each set, which is known as *disproportionate stratified sampling*. If sampling is used, the investigators should report their specific strategy.

From the eligible population or sample, the investigators will then recruit their study participants. Not all patients will agree to participate and give informed consent, and those that do might be different in important ways from those that do not participate. The study should report their numbers at each stage of specification toward the study participants, and explore and report any deviations from the source population.

Baseline Assessment and Randomization

The key to the success of a randomized clinical trial is the rigor and success of the randomization. Assurances should be given that patient assignment was truly random, and that randomization did not occur until after the patient had been deemed eligible and had consented for participation, with the commitment on the part of the patient and investigator to comply with the treatment assignment. The goal of randomization is to distribute evenly both known and unknown factors equally between the comparison groups. However, for some studies, particularly those with relatively small sample sizes, it may be important to make sure that key confounding factors are perfectly distributed between comparison groups. In this situation, the randomization may be stratified, in that the study participants are randomized within a classification group. An example might be to randomize male separately from female subjects, and thus ensure that the gender distribution in the comparison groups is identical. In multi-institutional studies, it is common to stratify randomization by study center. An additional goal of randomization is to ensure that equal or proportional numbers of subjects are assigned to each group. Again, if the sample size is small, the risk of unequal proportions increases. This can be controlled by doing a block randomization, in that patients are randomized in subsets or blocks to achieve perfect proportions. For example, if the block size is four, and randomization assigned patient 1 to placebo, patient 2 to treatment, and patient 3 to treatment, then patient 4 is arbitrarily assigned to placebo to maintain the perfect proportion. Clearly, block randomization must be completely blinded, and it is often necessary to vary the size of the blocks randomly. Randomization is best done either by computer or by using a random-number generator by a person not directly involved in the study maneuver and who makes it impossible for the study personnel to predict the assignment of the next patient.

Appropriate baseline assessment is very important. First, it allows assurance that inclusion and exclusion criteria are satisfied. Second, it allows characterization of the study subjects, which is very important when describing the study population. If information is collected on all potential subjects, then one has the opportunity to compare participants versus nonparticipants to exclude bias. Third, it allows the characterization of study subjects in terms of important confounders that may influence the impact of the treatment on outcomes. This leads to the first task in data analysis of a clinical trial, the comparison of the groups' baseline characteristics. This is a test of the success of randomization, in that no clinically or statistically important differences should be present. This is often the first table in the report of a clinical trial. Although *P* values are important, they are highly dependent on sample size. In a small study, large differences between groups may be present, yet *P* values will be nonsignificant. The converse is true in very large studies. Thus attention should first be paid to the magnitude of differences in characteristics between groups. If a certain characteristic seems to have an important difference, then one must decide the degree and the direction in which that characteristic might influence or bias the outcome.

Bias in the Execution

Blinding

The more subjective the treatment effects, the more important it is to ensure that everyone involved in the implementation of the study is unaware as to the treatment assignments. It is amazing the number of study subjects that report hallucinations (and miraculous cures) while taking placebo, or the number of investigators that unwittingly bias their results by looking harder for outcomes in those patients they know are receiving the treatment (for which the manufacturer is generously sponsoring the study). Every attempt should be made to blind the treatment assignment at as many levels as possible. Important people to blind are the personnel applying the treatment, the study subject, the personnel making study assessments and interpretations, and the personnel analyzing and reporting the data. Blinding should be tamper-proof at each level. Sometimes the inherent nature of the treatment and comparison precludes certain levels of blinding, such as the comparison of medical versus surgical interventions. This should not preclude best efforts to blind the study assessments and the data analysis.

Accounting for All Patients in the Study

Many things can happen to study subjects during the course of a clinical trial that cause them to deviate from the assigned group. Patients may choose to withdraw their participation before study completion. Investigators also may choose to withdraw a patient from the trial if they perceive complications or adverse effects. Crossovers also may occur, whereby a patient or their provider decides to implement the alterative therapy. Patients also may become lost to follow-up before study completion. Co-interventions can influence the outcome. All of these problems can introduce bias into the study, and every attempt should be made to minimize their occurrence. In published studies, the investigators must give a complete accounting of all study subjects enrolled in the study. If withdrawals, crossovers, loss-to-follow-ups, or co-interventions seem to be occurring more frequently in one group than another, then something about the intervention may be causing this to occur, which may bias the study results. It is important that in the analysis, patients be analyzed according to their initial study assignment, also known as an intention-to-treat analysis.

Choosing the End Points of Relevance

Investigators often labor over the selection of primary and secondary end points or outcomes. The primary end point must be relevant, in that it should have a direct impact or be a direct measure of the well-being of the patients. It is the end point from which a hypothesis is made, and this hypothesis is a major determinant of the sample size for the study, which should be specified in the report. Secondary end points also are important, but tend to be proxy measures or mechanistic in nature. The investigators should ensure that the end points are relevant and sufficiently complete to assess the important benefits and risks of the therapy. Once the end points are specified, the investigators should ensure that the duration of the study is sufficiently long that these relevant outcomes have a chance to occur. In addition, the assessments should be made with the utmost accuracy and reliability, and objective definitions should be used wherever possible.

Assessment of Safety and Adverse Outcomes

In addition to benefit, the study also must consider all relevant aspects of safety and adverse effects. This allows the reader to weigh the relative benefits of a therapy versus its associated risks. The methods for monitoring for adverse outcomes should be clearly specified in the report. Certain therapies may be known to be associated with certain specific adverse effects, and monitoring of such things as laboratory tests and physiologic measurements is often an integral part of the clinical trial protocol. For example, anticoagulation with warfarin has the benefit of preventing thrombosis and thrombosis-related events, but safety monitoring of coagulation tests such as INR, as well as specific adverse events such as bleeding episodes, is essential. In addition, adverse-effect monitoring should include more generic measures, such as study subject reporting of all symptoms or signs, regardless of any presumption of whether they may or may not be related to the study intervention. Reporting can be investigator initiated, with telephone or questionnaire follow-ups, or patient initiated, by maintaining ready access to study personnel throughout the trial. Independent data- and safety-monitoring committees are becoming an established part of clinical trials, often mandated by institutional research ethics boards. These committees should review adverse-effect reports throughout the trial and may perform interim analyses at prespecified intervals. They may make judgments regarding the attribution of usually major adverse effects to the study interventions and may elect to terminate a clinical trial prematurely in the face of serious adverse effects or overwhelming evidence of benefit. Only if the methods and results of safety and adverse effects are reported and adequate can one then evaluate the relative risks versus benefits.

Reporting and Relevance of the Results

It is not enough to give numbers concerning what happened in one group and what happened in the other, and then some P values (Table 42-4). The difference in an outcome between the treatment and the comparison group is the most relevant piece of information, both in absolute and in relative terms. If a study shows a prevalence of an outcome of 1% in the treatment group and 2% in the comparison group, the relative treatment effect is to reduce the prevalence by 50%, but the absolute difference is only 1%. It is important to note both numbers, as they will affect the decision to adopt or not to adopt the therapy. An additional indicator of the magnitude of the treatment effect that is more clinically interpretable is calculation of the number of patients you might need to treat with the therapy versus its alternative to achieve or prevent an outcome occurring in one patient. The greater the number needed to treat, the less relevant or important the therapy, although many other factors, such as costs, harms, and patient preferences may modify this interpretation. Although the P value is important to tell us the degree to which chance may explain the difference, it is not sufficient. The confidence intervals around the difference should be provided and specified. This interval will tell us the range of possible differences over which we might conclude that a true difference exists. The intervals widen with diminishing sample size, and we become less confident that we have defined the possible treatment effect. If the confidence interval includes clinically unimportant differences, we might be more reluctant to adopt the therapy based on the evidence provided. Alternatively, if the confidence interval is wide and includes no difference but ranges to clinically important treatment effects, we might be reluctant to accept the conclusion that no treatment effect exists and might be

Table 42-4 Assessing the Relevance of the Results of a Valid Clinical Trial

1. How large is the effect of the therapy relative to the alternative?
   a. Absolute effect = outcome incidence in the treatment group minus outcome incidence in the alternative group
   b. Relative effect = absolute effect divided by outcome incidence in the alternative group
   c. Number needed to treat to achieve or prevent one outcome = 1/absolute effect (e.g., A [hypothetical] 2-year clinical trial of anticoagulation after Fontan procedure showed a 10% incidence of thrombosis in those treated with warfarin versus 25% in those treated with aspirin).
      Absolute effect = 10% − 25% = −15% (15% absolute reduction)
      Relative effect = −15%/25% = −60% (60% relative reduction)
      Number needed to treat with warfarin versus aspirin for 2 years to prevent one thrombosis = 1/0.15 = 6.7 patients
2. How precise is the effect of the therapy relative to the alternative?
   a. Confidence intervals around measures of the magnitude of effect (see Table 42-5)
3. Can the study results be applied to my individual patient?
   a. Does my patient meet important inclusion and exclusion criteria for the study?
   b. Is the care setting for my patient similar to that of the study?
   c. Can the therapy be feasibly applied to my patient?
   d. Does my patient have specific characteristics that may modify the risk for outcomes or harms of the therapy?
   e. What are my patient's specific preferences and expectations regarding the therapy?

reluctant to stop using the therapy (Table 42-5). Results relevant to risks or harms of the treatment should be reported in the same manner.

Given the validity and importance of the results, one must then ask if the results are relevant and applicable to a particular patient. In general, careful review of the study's inclusion and exclusion criteria should be performed to determine whether the patient meets the majority or important

Table 42-5 Issues to Consider Regarding Confidence Intervals

1. Are they provided? If not, is the information required to calculate them (measures of variation such as standard error or standard deviation) reported?
2. Is the level of confidence enclosing the interval around the observed difference specified? (e.g., 70% vs. 95% confidence intervals)
3. What and how wide is the confidence interval? (affected by sample size, measure of variation, and level of confidence)
   a. Does the interval include no difference (a difference of 0)?
   b. Does the interval exceed a clinically meaningful threshold value such that we would conclude that the therapy is of benefit? (e.g., Consider the [hypothetical] example from Table 42-4. The absolute effect was −15%, or a 15% reduction in the incidence of thrombosis in favor of warfarin. The investigators made a case that a reduction of ≥10% would be the minimal clinically important benefit to justify use of warfarin.
      i. The 95% confidence interval was −18% to −12%. Interpretation: Conclude with sufficient confidence that warfarin has a clinically important benefit.
      ii. The 95% confidence interval was −35% to +5%. Interpretation: Cannot exclude with sufficient confidence that no benefit was found, yet the interval does include a potentially important clinical benefit. The results are suggestive but inconclusive, and likely the sample size was too small.
      iii. The 95% confidence interval was −25% to −5%. Interpretation: Conclude with sufficient confidence that a benefit does exist but do not have sufficient confidence that it is a clinically important benefit).

criteria, and the care setting is similar. The study intervention should be described in sufficient detail that it can be determined whether the intervention is feasible and can be replicated with sufficient accuracy in the clinical scenario and setting at hand. Given that clinical care is necessarily individualized, details of the study should be reviewed to determine whether any factors may modify the benefits, harms, or application of the study therapy, and whether these factors are present in the clinical scenario or setting. Because the practice of EBM involves the incorporation of patients' values and preferences for therapies and outcomes, these should be elicited and consolidated, together with the critically appraised evidence and the clinical expertise of the care providers in the clinical decision-making process.

CAUTIONS REGARDING OBSERVATIONAL STUDIES OF THERAPY

Almost all observational studies of therapy will be based largely on data abstracted either prospectively or retrospectively from the medical record. As a result, they are all subject to the limitations of the use of secondary data, or data collected for purposes other than the research study at hand. The medical record is a documentation of clinical care, which is individualized and not standardized. For research purposes, important information may be missing or recorded unreliably. Recording is from the perspectives of multiple levels of providers and multiple individuals, using different definitions and interpretations. Because clinical care is largely individualized, the use of pooled clinical data in an observational study of therapy is fraught with many potential sources of bias that are difficult to detect. Often important discrepancies exist between the results from randomized clinical trials and observational studies that may affect clinical care.[8]

Many observational studies report the outcomes of a group of patients who are uniformly given the same therapy. These studies are often only descriptive and provide little information other than the prognosis of patients who receive that therapy. However, many of them report improved outcomes compared with their previous (often unstudied) cohort of patients who were treated in a different manner, and attempt to conclude that the improved outcomes were as a direct result of the more recently applied therapy. This is erroneous, as noted in the introduction of this chapter, as the use of historical reports or a previous cohort for comparison introduces many confounding factors, biasing the comparison. As a result, studies of a completely descriptive nature with no comparison group provide almost no useful information and may be misleading. Some of these studies may provide useful information if they attempt to determine factors associated with outcomes within the uniformly treated study population.

However, in clinical care, changes in therapy are often not introduced suddenly or uniformly, and for variable periods, a transition may occur, during which both therapies may be used. Some observational studies will therefore look at this cohort of patients and attempt to make comparisons regarding outcomes between the therapies. Although these studies may lack some of the bias related to comparison with historical cohorts, the patients have not been randomized and thus may differ in important ways that may affect outcomes other than the therapy received. Because care is individualized, patients with certain characteristics may be more likely to receive one therapy versus the alternative. For the comparison to be valid, the patients must be similar. The most common way to equalize the comparison is to use statistics, usually in the form of multiple regression techniques, to adjust for important differences in characteristics. Usually the important factors associated with the outcomes can be recognized if the study population is sufficiently large to give adequate statistical power. These techniques tend to adjust only for those independent factors that achieve statistical significance. Another method is to make some arbitrary judgment about the severity or complexity of illness of the patient. These judgments are often based on a limited number of factors that are then debated by a group of experts who, based on their training, experience, and sometimes an interpretation of the published literature, assign an empirical score to the individual patient, a score that reflects their predisposition to the outcome. These scores are to be viewed with great caution, as they are not based on actual data.

A more recent method of adjustment is to calculate an adjustment factor called the propensity score. The propensity score uses multiple logistic regression analysis and all available information about the patients to derive a probability (or propensity) that a given patient will have received one therapy versus the alternative. This probability, or the propensity score, can then be used as an adjustment factor in a multiple regression before testing whether an impact is attributable to the therapy. McCrindle and colleagues[13] reported a multi-institutional observational study from the Congenital Heart Surgeons Society comparing transcatheter balloon valvotomy with surgical valvotomy for neonatal critical aortic stenosis deemed suitable for biventricular repair. Both therapies were used over the period of observation, but the surgical patients tended to have more factors indicating more severe and complex disease. In an unadjusted comparison of time-related mortality, the surgical patients indeed fared worse. However, when the comparison was adjusted with the propensity score, the therapies were nearly identical in terms of mortality. An alternative use of the propensity score would be to do a matched comparison between pairs of patients with the therapy and its alternative, matching for propensity score. Although the propensity score makes use of the maximal amount of information available, it must be recognized that it is not a perfect adjustment and does not take into account potentially important factors for which information was not available. No amount of statistical adjustment can perfectly or confidently make up for the lack of randomization, and thus the properly designed and executed clinical trial remains the best evidence to appraise therapies.

IMPORTANT ANALYSIS ISSUES RELATED TO APPRAISAL OF OUTCOMES OF THERAPY

One of the more difficult aspects of the critical appraisal of a published study is whether the statistical analyses are appropriate. This often requires some advanced expertise on the part of readers and reviewers. In general, when the data analysis of a study is flawed, it is often more as a result of failure of the plan for the analysis rather than as a result of the actual statistical tests used. This most commonly results from a failure to recognize the particular aspects by which the outcomes occur. Rarely in clinical studies can outcomes be meaningfully evaluated immediately after an intervention (however, more exceptions to this may exist in the intensive care unit [ICU] than elsewhere). An example might be the response of a tachyarrhythmia to a bolus of adenosine. Much more commonly, outcomes occur either as discrete events or evolve in a graded manner over a period of time. For example, death can almost always be defined in a given patient as a discrete event. These types of outcomes are simpler and tend to be easier to measure and analyze. In contrast, the grade of valvar regurgitation, the change in dimension of a cardiovascular structure, or the degree of quality of life occurs not as a discrete event but in a continuous and changing manner over a period of time. These types of outcomes require continuous or, more feasibly, periodic measurements to detect and document changes and are more difficult to measure and analyze. Sometimes a discrete event may mark the development of a given level in a continuous and evolving outcome, such as when valvar regurgitation progresses to a threshold level (often together with other criteria) at which point an intervention or reintervention occurs. This is an example of how one type of outcome may either be reflected as or evolve into another type of outcome. Adding a further level of complexity, a patient is often simultaneously at risk for a variety of outcomes, some of which may be mutually exclusive (such as death and reoperation) or interrelated. Fortunately, approaches are available for data analysis in each of these situations.

Time-Related Events

Many of the outcomes in pediatric cardiology occur after a given period, and failure to recognize when this is so results in one of the more common errors in data analysis. This time period may be very short or very long, but the event occurs unambiguously at a discrete time. Sometimes we know the exact date and time the event occurred, or the time that the subject was last known to be free of the event (censored observation). Sometimes we may know only a time when the subject was free of the event and a subsequent time when the event was known to have occurred, with the actual event having occurred sometime between the two times (interval event). Any analysis of an event must take into account the time to the event or the duration of follow-up. Reports of the incidence of an outcome after a given therapy are rather useless unless the time period of observation also is known. For example, the report of 50% mortality after Fontan procedure is a meaningless number. However, a mortality of 50% after 1 year is much different from a mortality of 50% after 30 years. Clearly, the proportion of patients who have experienced a given event after a given period is a reflection of the cumulative effect of variations in the number of patients at risk for the event and the instantaneous risk of that event. If the risk of an event is constant and does not change over time, then the proportion of patients who have had the event after given period is a reflection of a multiple of the risk by duration of the period. More often the risk is changing over time. In addition, the number of patients at risk also changes over time. We generally do not follow up all patients until they have experienced the event. More commonly, the members of a cohort are followed up for a variable period, during which some patients who have yet to experience the event either will be lost to follow-up or have reached the end of the period of observation. Usually we know the date or time when this occurred. This is commonly referred to as a censored observation. Up until that time, these patients are at risk for the outcome and contribute to the denominator for any estimate of cumulative risk. Statistical methods that give estimates of this time-related cumulative risk in the setting of changing risk and changing denominator are available, with the most common being the *Kaplan–Meier curve*. In appraising a Kaplan–Meier curve, four specific aspects should be present: The Kaplan–Meier should step and not be smoothed, confidence intervals or bars should be provided, the number of patients at risk should be present along the time axis, and it should be documented which event or outcome was being studied and how other competing outcomes were handled. For example, when presenting a Kaplan–Meier curve of freedom from reoperation, it should be stated how patients who died without having reoperation were handled. Most authors will just handle the deaths as censored observations, which is inaccurate, unless the number of deaths is extremely small. Sometimes authors will combine several somewhat related events in an outcome event analysis, such as combining death, reoperation, and cardiac transplantation, but often the risk and associated factors for these events are completely different, and rarely is there adequate justification for their combination, even when trying to maximize the number of events for analysis.

Phases of Risk, Modeling, and Prediction

As previously mentioned, the instantaneous risk of an event is rarely constant over the complete period of follow-up. Particularly for major outcomes, the risk can be divided into three phases: an early phase, a constant phase, and a late phase. This can often be seen when noting the shape of a Kaplan–Meier curve, especially if the follow-up is very long. For example, when examining the risk of mortality after the Mustard procedure for transposition of the great arteries, clearly a great risk of mortality exists before and immediately after the procedure, related to complications of cyanosis and operative mortality. After this, a constant risk or hazard phase is seen, with a low but ongoing risk of mortality, presumably related to evolving problems with brady- and tachyarrhythmias. If follow-up is long enough, a late hazard phase is noted with a more precipitate decrease in survival, related to the late onset of ventricular failure and its associated complications. With short periods of follow-up, only the early-risk phase is evident and a few events indicative of a constant phase. Both the Kaplan–Meier analysis and its multivariable counterpart, Cox's proportionate hazard analysis, do not distinguish these different phases of time-related outcomes, which differ not only in the instantaneous risk of an event but in the associated and predictive factors as well. Blackstone and coworkers[3] recognized these three phases of risk and developed methods to model each of them based on the instantaneous risk at a given time. These models, like any model, are not the real thing but are the best simulation of the truth based on the data. But unlike the real thing, a model can be manipulated and tested and used for prediction. This is the strength of this

technique over the "nonparametric" techniques of the Kaplan–Meier and Cox's methods commonly used.

These "parametric" methods have been most commonly used in the analysis of large multicenter outcomes data from both the Congenital Heart Surgeons Society and the Pediatric Heart Transplantation Study Group. The best example of this type of analysis and its use in prediction is from Lofland and associates [12] in the analysis of risk of mortality after interventions for neonatal critical aortic stenosis. A cohort of patients with critical aortic stenosis was prospectively enrolled in a multi-institutional outcomes study, in which patients underwent therapy as selected by their participating teams of clinicians. Often with critical aortic stenosis, variable degrees of hypoplasia or stenosis of the aortic valve and other left heart structures may be present. Some patients may have minimal disease and have adequate left heart structures whereby the left heart is fully capable of sustaining the systemic circulation in the long term. However, some patients, with severe stenosis or hypoplasia of the aortic valve or other left heart structures, may be unable to sustain systemic circulation and are therefore on a single-ventricle palliation pathway, usually starting with a Norwood procedure and culminating in the Fontan procedure. However, because the degree of disease severity occupies a continuum, the decision for a biventricular pathway versus a single-ventricle pathway may be ambiguous. In the study by Lofland and associates, the survival function of those patients who underwent a biventricular pathway was modeled separately from that of those who underwent a single-ventricle pathway, with multivariable models of predictive factors being determined separately for both. The models were then solved separately for every patient in the dataset. The first model assumed the biventricular route, and the second, the single-ventricle route. This then gave the prediction for every patient, based on the individual characteristics, of the survival "curves" if the patient had had either a biventricular repair or a single-ventricle repair. For the biventricular pathway, those characteristics that increased time-related mortality were the presence and severity of endocardial fibroelastosis, size of the left ventricular outflow tract at the level of the aortic valve sinuses, and earlier age at presentation. For the single-ventricle pathway, those characteristics were a smaller aortic root size and the presence and severity of tricuspid valve regurgitation. An arbitrary end point of survival at 5 years after enrollment was chosen, and the difference for every patient in the predicted survival was calculated from the models. This difference, or survival benefit, was then modeled in multivariable linear regression, entering patient characteristics as potential associated factors, and a regression equation was derived that, when solved for an individual patient's characteristics, predicted the survival benefit, and therefore the optimal pathway that predicted the best 5-year survival, for every patient. The factors that were included in the final predictive survival-benefit model included those in the separate pathway models, together with the length of the left ventricle. When the survival benefit was calculated, it was noted that a large proportion of patients who went down the biventricular pathway would have had better survival if they had gone down a single-ventricle pathway, and to a lesser extent, vice versa. The published formula, with a calculator available on the Society's website (www.chssdc.org), can therefore be used to predict for subsequent patients. However, it must be stated that any predictive formula always performs best in the patient population from which the formula is derived, and less so in subsequent populations. Thus any predictive formula must be submitted for external validation. Many predictive formulas also are completely applicable to subsequent periods in which changes in patient selection and management may have further improved outcomes subsequent to the period of the initial study. Most predictive formulas should therefore be used only as a guideline for informing which factors must be evaluated when guiding clinical decisions for individual patients and should not be viewed as binding. This study, however, demonstrates the use of parametric modeling of phases of risk and their subsequent use for prediction, particularly in an area in which clinical decision making remains somewhat problematic.

Competing Outcomes and Markov Modeling

Often in pediatric cardiology, a given patient is simultaneously at risk for a multitude of outcomes, each with its own time course of risk and associated factors. As mentioned previously, many authors ignore this concept. However, the use of parametric modeling of time-related events allows the analysis of competing outcomes or risks, and therefore the prediction of the proportion of patients who have achieved each outcome at any given time point after the start point. One also could calculate the Kaplan–Meier function for each type of outcome, censoring at the occurrence of other outcomes, but when combined, they tend to account for a greater proportion of patients than actually exists. This was best illustrated in the analysis of outcomes after listing for heart transplantation in pediatric patients from the Pediatric Heart Transplantation Study Group published by McGiffin and colleagues.[14] If a patient is listed for heart transplantation, a number of things might happen. The patients may die without a transplant, have a transplant, be removed from listing because they are too well or because they become too sick (and ineligible), or they may remain on the list without having reached any of these mutually exclusive outcomes. The risk or hazard for each of these outcomes can be modeled separately, and associated factors for each time-related event determined in multivariable models. These models can then be combined to predict more accurately the overall proportion of patients having achieved each outcome at a given time or, more important, be used to predict the same for an individual patient's characteristics. However, patients may have further time-related outcomes after having achieved an initial time-related outcome. An example might be a patient who is given a transplant after listing (the initial outcome) who subsequently dies of coronary vascular disease (the subsequent outcome). These series of outcomes can be modeled and predicted by using techniques known as Markov modeling, but have not yet been applied in pediatric cardiology. A similar analysis has recently looked at outcomes after the Norwood procedure in patients with critical aortic stenosis or aortic atresia.[1]

Serial Measurements

When an outcome is not associated with a discrete occurrence, it usually is something that changes continuously or evolves in a graduated manner over time. The collected data are usually serial or repeated measurements that are made in an individual patient usually over varying time intervals. In reality, a lot of the measurements we make are serial measurements, whether they are repeated vital signs or hemodynamic parameters assessed in the ICU, or repeated echocardiographic measurements made in outpatient follow-up. The most common way authors handle this type of data is to take the first and the last measurement while ignoring all intervening measurements, and to look at the change, often ignoring the time interval over which that change occurred, or dividing the change by the time interval to get a linear or constant rate of change. This is simple but erroneous and does not take advantage of intervening data or allow detection of nonlinear or variable rates of change. Rarely are the newer methods of longitudinal data analysis used. For outcomes that have a continuous value, such as cardiac dimensions or hemodynamic parameters, mixed linear regression analysis can be used to determined relations with the time of observation, and multivariable relations among associated factors that may influence both the outcome measurements and their relation with time. This technique has recently been used by Humpl and coworkers[7] to show a lack of catch-up growth of right heart structures after percutaneous transcatheter valve perforation and dilation for patients with pulmonary atresia and intact ventricular septum. For outcomes that have a discrete or ordinal value, such as grade of valvar regurgitation, general estimating equations can serve the same purpose. This technique was recently used by Chiu and associates[4] to determine factors related to success of repeated overdrive conversions of atrial reentrant tachycardia episodes in children using their permanent atrial-based pacemakers.

SUMMARY

Decisions regarding therapy are often the most important decisions that a health care provider must make on behalf of individual patients under their care. They should be based on the best available evidence in support of their benefit, relative to their risks. This can occur only when evidence is appropriately sought, available, and critically appraised. This must be incorporated into the clinician's expertise based on local experience as well as the patient's values and preferences for therapies and outcomes. For the field of pediatric cardiology to advance, health care providers must become greater and more knowledgeable consumers of the best available evidence. In addition, the academic milieu must respond to this call for better and more complete evidence.

Suggested Readings

Altman DG: *Practical Statistics for Medical Research*. Boca Raton, FL, CRC Press, 1990. (An excellent statistics textbook that does not get bogged down in probability theory and mathematics.)

Altman DG, Machin D, Bryant TN, Gardner MJ (eds): *Statistics with Confidence*, 2nd ed. London, British Medical Journal, 2000. (Excellent reference regarding confidence intervals and includes software for their calculation.)

Campbell MJ, Machin D: *Medical Statistics: A Commonsense Approach*, 3rd ed. Philadelphia, John Wiley & Sons, 1999. (Another readable and practical book with real examples from the current literature.)

Elwood JE: *Critical Appraisal of Epidemiological Studies and Clinical Trials*, 2nd ed. Oxford, UK, Oxford University Press, 1998. (An excellent, thorough, and readable book discussing all aspects of critical appraisal of common clinical study designs.)

Guyatt G, Rennie D (eds): *Users' Guides to the Medical Literature: A Manual for Evidence-Based Clinical Practice.* Chicago, AMA Press, 2002. (A compilation of the Users' Guides article series published in *JAMA*, together with a CD. A pocket-sized version is available as well, and both allow access to a website. The Users' Guides articles also can be accessed through www.cche.net/usersguides/main.asp. The original series remains one of the best resources.)

Hulley SB, Cummings SR, Browner WS, et al: *Designing Clinical Research: An Epidemiologic Approach*, 2nd ed. Philadelphia, Lippincott Williams & Wilkins, 2000. (A readable and practical textbook for those setting out for the first or subsequent time to design a clinical research study.)

Hunick M, Glasziou P, Siegel J, et al: *Decision Making in Health and Medicine: Integrating Evidence and Values.* Cambridge University Press, 2001. (A readable and practical book that emphasizes the keys integrations to EBM from a tutorial approach. With CD.)

Norman GR, Streiner DL: *Biostatistics: The Bare Essentials*, 2nd ed. Lewiston, NY, BC Decker, 2000. (An expansion of the PDQ statistics book, with the same sense of humor but more detail.)

Riegelman RM: *Studying a Study and Testing a Test: How to Read the Medical Evidence*, 4th ed. Philadelphia, Lippincott Williams & Wilkins, 1999. (An excellent book that also comes with a CD.)

Sackett DL, Haynes RB, Guyatt GH, Tugwell P: *Clinical Epidemiology: A Basic Science for Clinical Medicine*, 2nd ed. Boston, Little, Brown, 1991. (An earlier classic.)

Sackett DL, Straus SE, Richardson WS, et al: *Evidence-Based Medicine. How to Practice and Teach EBM*, 2nd ed. London, Churchill Livingstone, 2000. (The standard reference, inexpensive and fits in a pocket. Comes with a CD, and links to a website: www.cebm.utoronto.ca for updates and resources for handheld devices. Very practical and highly recommended.)

Silverman WA: *Where's the Evidence? Debates in Modern Medicine.* New York, Oxford University Press, 1998. (A collection of excellent and thought-provoking essays on the subject of evidence-based medicine.)

Streiner DL, Norman GR: *PDQ Statistics*, 3rd ed. Lewiston, NY, BC Decker, 2003. (Small pocketbook, big on practical information with a sense of humor. A truly readable introduction to statistics for busy clinicians.)

References

1. Ashburn DA, McCrindle BW, Tchervenkov CI, et al: Outcomes after the Norwood operation in neonates with critical aortic stenosis or aortic valve atresia. *J Thorac Cardiovasc Surg* 125:1070–1082, 2003.
2. Bando K, Vijay P, Turrentine MW, et al: Dilutional and modified ultrafiltration reduces pulmonary hypertension after operations for congenital heart disease: A prospective randomized study. *J Thorac Cardiovasc Surg* 115:517–525, 1998.
3. Blackstone EH, Naftel DC, Turner ME Jr: The decomposition of time-varying hazard into phases, each incorporating a separate stream of concomitant information. *J Am Stat Assoc* 81:615–624, 1986.
4. Chiu CC, McCrindle BW, Hamilton RM, et al: Clinical use of permanent pacemaker for conversion of intraatrial reentry tachycardia in children. *Pacing Clin Electrophysiol* 24:950–956, 2001.
5. Cook DJ, Levy MM: Evidence-based medicine: A tool for enhancing critical care practice. *Crit Care Clin* 14:353–358, 1998.
6. Hoffman TM, Wernovsky G, Atz AM, et al: Efficacy and safety of milrinone in preventing low cardiac output syndrome in infants and children after corrective surgery for congenital heart disease. *Circulation* 107:996–1002, 2003.
7. Humpl T, Soderberg B, McCrindle BW, et al: Percutaneous balloon valvotomy in pulmonary atresia with intact ventricular septum: Impact on patient care. *Circulation* 108:826–832, 2003.
8. Ioannidis JP, Haidich AB, Pappa M, et al: Comparison of evidence of treatment effects in randomized and nonrandomized studies. *JAMA* 286:821–830, 2001.
9. Kirklin JW, Blackstone EH, Tchervenkov CI, Castaneda AR: Clinical outcomes after the arterial switch operation for transposition: Patient, support, procedural, and institutional risk factors: Congenital Heart Surgeons Society. *Circulation* 86:1501–1515, 1992.
10. Kouatli AA, Garcia JA, Zellers TM, et al: Enalapril does not enhance exercise capacity in patients after Fontan procedure. *Circulation* 96:1507–1512, 1997.
11. Lemler MS, Scott WA, Leonard SR, et al: Fenestration improves clinical outcome of the Fontan procedure: A prospective, randomized study. *Circulation* 105:207–212, 2002.
12. Lofland GK, McCrindle BW, Williams WG, et al: Critical aortic stenosis in the neonate: A multi-institutional study of management, outcomes, and risk factors: Congenital Heart Surgeons Society. *J Thorac Cardiovasc Surg* 121:10–27, 2001.
13. McCrindle BW, Blackstone EH, Williams WG, et al: Are outcomes of surgical versus transcatheter balloon valvotomy equivalent in neonatal critical aortic stenosis? *Circulation* 104:I152–I158, 2001.
14. McGiffin DC, Naftel DC, Kirklin JK, et al: Predicting outcome after listing for heart transplantation in children: Comparison of Kaplan-Meier and parametric competing risk analysis: Pediatric Heart Transplant Study Group. *J Heart Lung Transplant* 16:713–722, 1997.
15. Norman GR: Examining the assumptions of evidence-based medicine. *J Eval Clin Pract* 5:139–147, 1999.
16. Straus SE, McAlister FA: Evidence-based medicine: A commentary on common criticisms. *CMAJ* 163:837–841, 2000.
17. Van Arsdell GS, McCrindle BW, Einarson KD, et al: Interventions associated with minimal Fontan mortality. *Ann Thorac Surg* 70:568–574, 2000.

Chapter 43

Pulmonary Hypertension

ARTHUR J. SMERLING, MD, CHARLES L. SCHLEIEN, MD, and ROBYN J. BARST, MD

pulmonary capillary wedge pressure (PCWP) ≤15 mm Hg and a pulmonary vascular resistance (PVR) >3 Wood units. Pulmonary arterial hypertension unassociated with any identifiable disease was termed *primary* or *idiopathic*. Pulmonary hypertension associated with an underlying disease was termed *secondary*. Researchers now understand that patients with pulmonary hypertension due to many of the associated etiologies share many of the same genetic, histologic, cellular, and mechanical characteristics. Pathologists, for example, cannot distinguish by histopathologic analyses between patients with pulmonary arterial hypertension associated with human immunodeficiency virus (HIV) disease, medications such as diet pills, familial causes, or portal hypertension.[17,18] In addition, patients with various etiologies for pulmonary hypertension may have abnormalities in the endothelial production of locally active mediators, and thus they may respond to vasodilator therapy.[16,72] Finally, in all patients with pulmonary hypertension, right-sided heart failure may develop. A more useful way of defining patients with pulmonary hypertension is by describing the mechanism of the development of pulmonary hypertension by the associated disease.

Three basic mechanisms cause pulmonary hypertension. These include (1) increased pulmonary blood flow into a normal vascular bed, (2) increased resistance in the precapillary pulmonary vessels, and (3) abnormal resistance in the postcapillary vascular bed (Table 43-2).[87] Precapillary resistance is further defined as vascular constriction, obstruction, or

DEFINITION/NOMENCLATURE

Recent advances in the understanding of the pathophysiology and pathobiology of pulmonary hypertension have enabled clinicians to prevent acute exacerbations and to treat patients with acute and chronic disease more effectively. Pulmonary hypertension is defined as a mean pulmonary artery pressure (PAP) of greater than 25 mm Hg at rest or more than 30 mm Hg during exercise (Table 43-1).[3] Traditionally, several ways of classifying patients with pulmonary hypertension have been used. The term *cor pulmonale* was reserved for right ventricular enlargement associated with elevated PAP secondary to neuromuscular, skeletal, parenchymal, or vascular lung disease.[29] Pulmonary *arterial* hypertension is defined as pulmonary hypertension (see previous) combined with a

Table 43-1 Values for Normal Pulmonary Hemodynamics at Sea Level (Rest and Mild Exercise) and at Elevated Altitude (Rest)*

	Sea Level Rest	Sea Level Mild Exercise	Altitude (~15,000 ft) Rest
Pulmonary arterial pressure†	20/10, 15	30/13, 20	38/14, 26
Cardiac output (L/min)	6.0	12.0	6.0
Left atrial pressure (mm Hg)	5.0	9.0	5.0
Pulmonary vascular resistance (units)	1.7	0.9	3.3

*For a 70-kg adult male
†Systolic/diastolic, mean mm Hg

Table 43-2 Basic Mechanisms That Cause Pulmonary Hypertension

Increased pulmonary blood flow	Increased cardiac output
	Left-to-right shunts
Increased precapillary resistance	Constriction
	Obliteration
	Obstruction
Increased postcapillary resistance	Pulmonary vein obstruction
	Left atrial obstruction
	(e.g., cor triatriatum, myxoma)
	Mitral or aortic valve disease
	Left ventricular dysfunction

Table 43-3 The 2003 Venice Classification of Pulmonary Hypertension

1. Pulmonary aterial hypertension (PAH)
   1.1. Idiopathic (IPAH)
   1.2. Familial (FPAH)
   1.3. Associated with (APAH):
       1.3.1 Collagen vascular disease
       1.3.2 Congenital systemic-to-pulmonary shunts
       1.3.3 Portal hypertension
       1.3.4 HIV infection
       1.3.5 Drugs and toxins
       1.3.6 Other (thyroid disorders, glycogen storage disease, Gaucher's disease, hereditary hemorrhagic telangiectasia, hemoglobinopathies, myeloproliferative disorders, splenectomy)
   1.4. Associated with significant venous or capillary involvement
       1.4.1 Pulmonary veno-occlusive disease (PVOD)
       1.4.2 Pulmonary capillary hemangiomatosis (PCH)
   1.5. Persistent pulmonary hypertension of the newborn
2. Pulmonary hypertension with left heart disease
   2.1. Left-sided atrial or ventricular heart disease
   2.2. Left-sided valvular heart disease
3. Pulmonary hypertension associated with lung diseases and/or hypoxemia
   3.1. Chronic obstructive pulmonary disease
   3.2. Interstitial lung disease
   3.3. Sleep-disordered breathing
   3.4. Alveolar hypoventilation disorders
   3.5. Chronic exposure to high altitude
   3.6. Developmental abnormalities
4. Pulmonary hypertension due to chronic thrombotic and/or embolic disease
   4.1. Thromboembolic obstruction of proximal pulmonary arteries
   4.2. Thromboembolic obstruction of distal pulmonary arteries
   4.3. Nonthrombotic pulmonary embolism (tumor, parasites, foreign material)
5. Miscellaneous
   Sarcoidosis, histocytosis X, lymphangiomatosis, compression of pulmonary vessels (adenopathy, tumor, fibrosing mediastinitis)

From: Simonneau G, Galie N, Rubin LJ, et al: Clinical classification of pulmonary hypertension. *J Am Coll Cardiol* 43:55–125, 2004.

obliteration. The specific mechanism of the development of pulmonary hypertension in a given patient dictates treatment. Specific therapies are then directed at either decreasing pulmonary blood flow, dilating precapillary pulmonary vessels, or relieving postcapillary resistance. Furthermore, therapy may be directed at the patient's underlying disease. We discuss the specific etiologies causing pulmonary hypertension, the biophysical descriptors, the clinical presentation of patients acquiring this disease, specific pathophysiologic principles, and present-day management of the patient with pulmonary hypertension due to its various causes.

ETIOLOGY

Pulmonary arterial hypertension is observed in different patterns in the population: in epidemics, at constant rates in certain societies, and in isolated cases. Epidemics of pulmonary arterial hypertension have been associated with toxins, pollutants, and medications such as mercury, vinyl chloride, ergotamine, tryptophan, rapeseed oil, alkaloids, and most recently, diet pills (e.g., fenfluramine or dexfenfluramine).[23] In the industrialized world, smoking-induced chronic lung disease is the most common cause of mild pulmonary hypertension. In the developing world, infestation usually due to *Schistosomiasis mansoni* is the most common cause of pulmonary hypertension.[60] Finally, sporadic cases occur throughout the world and are associated with underlying familial, endocrine, cardiac, pulmonary, or rheumatologic disease.

The associated underlying disease often determines the mechanism of pulmonary hypertension (Table 43-3). Hyperthyroidism, pheochromocytoma, systemic-to-pulmonary shunts result in increased pulmonary blood flow. Eventually these shear forces on the pulmonary vascular wall cause hypertrophy in the wall itself, resulting in obstruction of forward flow. Precapillary vasoconstriction occurs with hypoxia, chemical exposure, and familial pulmonary arterial hypertension. Thromboembolic disease results in obstruction of precapillary vessels. Connective tissue disease, parenchymal lung disease, and surgically induced loss of the pulmonary vascular tree lead to an obliteration of the pulmonary vessels. Finally, patients with pulmonary hypertension associated with systemic hypertension, a noncompliant left ventricle, an abnormal mitral or aortic valve, or pulmonary venous obstruction are associated with postcapillary pulmonary hypertension.

Patients with congenital heart disease and pulmonary hypertension may have increased pulmonary blood flow, precapillary or postcapillary pulmonary hypertension.[92]

Treatment with pulmonary vasodilators is indicated only in patients with reversible precapillary pulmonary vasoconstriction. Aggressive pulmonary vasodilation in patients with systemic-to-pulmonary may worsen the amount of shunt flow, resulting in an increased volume load on the heart. Aggressive pulmonary vasodilation in patients with postcapillary obstruction may result in an increase in the intrapulmonary vascular pressure, resulting in pulmonary edema.[91]

BIOPHYSICS/MEASUREMENT

At the most fundamental level, pressure in a fluid-filled system is dependent on flow and resistance. Patients with congenital heart disease and pulmonary hypertension may have reversible vasoconstriction and/or irreversible obstruction of the pulmonary vasculature or both. The degree of vasoconstriction and reactivity of the pulmonary vascular bed is particularly important in these patients because it may influence the type of surgical repair, predict perioperative morbidity, and determine the viability of heart transplantation for a given patient.[3]

Pulmonary hypertension is characterized physiologically by the Poiseuille-Hagen equation that relates flow to resistance factors:

$$Q = \Delta Pap \; \pi \; r^4 / \, l\eta$$

where Q is the flow or cardiac output, ΔPap is the pressure decrease across the pulmonary bed (i.e., the difference between the mean PAP and mean left atrial pressure), r is the radius of the vessel, l is the length, and η is the viscosity of the blood.

For example, an increase in blood viscosity secondary to an increased hematocrit in a cyanotic patient results in either an increase in the transpulmonary pressure gradient (ΔPap) or a decrease in flow. Even a small decrease in vessel radius, as in vasoconstriction of the pulmonary arterioles, will have a profound effect by decreasing flow or increasing PAP.

The equation can be simplified to a modification of Ohm's law:

$$PVR = \Delta Pap/CO$$

where PVR is the pulmonary vascular resistance, ΔPap is the pressure decrease across the pulmonary bed, and CO is the cardiac output.

The pressure across the pulmonary bed and the cardiac output both change dramatically during the respiratory and cardiac cycles. Because it is impractical to measure pressure and flow continuously in a pulsatile circulation, we customarily use mean pressures to calculate resistance. The ΔPap, therefore, is calculated as the difference between the mean PAP and the mean pulmonary capillary wedge pressure (PCWP). By using mean pressures, the equation becomes

$$PVR = \text{Mean pulmonary artery pressure} - \text{Mean pulmonary capillary wedge pressure}/\text{Cardiac output}$$

where PVR is the pulmonary vascular resistance, measured in mm, Hg/L/min (Wood). If the PVR in Wood units is multiplied by 80, the units become dynes/sec/cm^{-5}. Pulmonary artery pressure and PCWP are measured in mm Hg. Cardiac output (CO) is measured in L/min.

Pulmonary vascular resistance is used to evaluate medical therapy and to predict the ability to tolerate cardiac surgery in a patient with pulmonary hypertension. Normal PVR is generally considered to be less than 3 Wood units · m^2. A PVR greater than 6 Wood units · m^2 is considered to be significant pulmonary hypertension, with an increased risk of postoperative pulmonary hypertension. Having a PVR greater than 10 Wood units · m^2 is considered a grave operative risk. These patients may not be candidates for corrective cardiac surgery.[55] For example, with the earlier equation, a patient with a ventricular septal defect (VSD) and a mean PAP of 25 mm Hg, PCWP of 5 mm Hg, and a cardiac output of 5 L/min has a PVR of 4 Wood units. This patient would be considered a good candidate for surgical closure of the VSD. Conversely, a patient with congestive heart failure and a mean PAP of 55 mm Hg, PCWP of 30 mm Hg, and a cardiac output of 1.5 L/min has a PVR of 15 Wood units. This patient has a high likelihood of pulmonary hypertension and right ventricular failure developing after a heart transplant. This patient would be tested preoperatively with a vasodilator (e.g., nitroprusside) in an attempt to decrease the PVR. In our example, the mean PAP subsequently decreases to 49 mm Hg, the PCWP decreases to 25 mm Hg, and the cardiac output increases to 4 L/min. The PVR is now 6 Wood units, and so the patient would be considered a candidate for heart transplantation, albeit with the expected perioperative administration of vasodilators. A medical therapy should decrease PAP without decreasing

the cardiac output. If the medication decreases both the mean PAP and the cardiac output equally, PVR does not change. This type of therapy is rarely helpful. Unfortunately, the equation is not useful for predicting the effect of changing only one of the three variables. A medication that increases cardiac output, for instance, may increase PAP, decrease PVR, or affect both depending on the reserve capacity of the pulmonary vasculature. It may not become apparent that a patient with low cardiac output has pulmonary hypertension until the cardiac output is improved.

Not all maneuvers that reduce PVR will benefit the patient. Any physiologic maneuver that increases the wedge pressure more than the mean PAP will decrease PVR, decrease the cardiac output, or decrease both. Increasing the wedge pressure, for example, by administering fluid to a patient with poor cardiac function, may decrease the PVR by elevating downstream pressure and passively distending the pulmonary vessels. This elevated pulmonary venous pressure may not cause active vasodilation of the pulmonary arteries and often results in pulmonary edema.

The PVR calculation, although clinically useful, does not fully describe the frequency-dependent, elastic components of the pulmonary vasculature. The impedance to flow from the right ventricle is dependent on the patient's heart rate, a factor not considered by the PVR equation. Furthermore, this calculation assumes that the pulmonary pressure–flow relation is linear, an inaccurate assumption. As PAP increases, the increase in pulmonary blood flow becomes incrementally greater. This pulmonary pressure–flow relation is dependent on the magnitude of the pulmonary blood flow, vascular pressures, alveolar pressures, and patient position.[38] For example, at the same PAP, decreasing the alveolar pressure will decrease the PVR. In addition, although a patient with a PAP of 110/70 mm Hg may have the same mean (PAP$_m$) as another patient with a PAP of 130/45 mm Hg (i.e., PAP$_m$ of 80 mm Hg for both patients), they behave differently. Remember that Poiseuille developed his equation in a system in which a newtonian fluid passed continuously with laminar flow through rigid glass tubes. The pulmonary circulation has non-newtonian fluid (e.g., hematocrit matters), pulsating through elastic conduits (systolic pressures and absolute magnitude of the pressures also matter) without laminar flow. When attempting to reduce a patient's PAP, it is important, therefore, to consider the effects on cardiac output, wedge pressure, pulmonary systolic pressure, blood viscosity, and heart rate.

The pulmonary diastolic pressure (PAP$_d$) may assist in determining the mechanism of pulmonary hypertension. During diastole when the pulmonic valve is closed, the PAP and left atrial pressure equilibrate. The pulmonary artery diastolic pressure, then, should approximate the wedge pressure (PAP$_d$ is usually 1 to 3 mm greater than the PCWP). When the pulmonary arterial diastolic pressure is much greater than the wedge pressure, an obstruction between the pulmonary artery and left atrium is likely; its causes include pulmonary vascular constriction, obstruction, obliteration, or a combination of these.

Indexing PVR to body surface area further improves the ability to identify those patients at risk for right heart failure after cardiac transplantation.[1]

$$PVRI = \text{Mean pulmonary artery pressure} - \text{Mean pulmonary capillary wedge pressure}/\text{Cardiac index}$$

where PVRI, the pulmonary vascular resistance index, is measured in mm $Hg/L/min/m^2$ = Wood units · m^2; Cardiac index is the cardiac output/m^2). Having a PVRI greater than 6 Wood units · m^2 increases the risk of developing right ventricular failure and death after cardiac transplantation.[1]

Some common pitfalls exist when measuring PAP and cardiac output in patients with pulmonary hypertension. PCWP is accurate only when a patent fluid channel exists between the catheter tip lying in the pulmonary artery and the pulmonary veins into the left atrium. Thus the balloon tip should be in West zone 3, where the PAP is greater than the pulmonary vein pressure, which in turn is greater than the alveolar pressure. With the patient in a supine position, the catheter should be posterior to the left atrium, have the standard central venous pressure waveform with "A" – "C" – "V" waves, minimal respiratory variation, and a pulmonary arterial diastolic pressure greater than the PCWP. In addition, cardiac output may not be accurately measured by thermodilution techniques in patients with pulmonary hypertension and tricuspid regurgitation or pulmonary insufficiency or both. Thermodilution also is inaccurate in patients with shunts. In these patients, use of the Fick equation may be a more accurate method to calculate cardiac output. The Fick equation is:

$$\text{Cardiac output} = O_2 \text{ consumption/Arterial } O_2 \text{ content} - \text{Venous } O_2 \text{ content}$$

Oxygen consumption varies widely because of changes in heart rate or level of sedation and so must be measured directly and not assumed from published tables.

CLINICAL PRESENTATION

Children with pulmonary arterial hypertension often initially have nonspecific and subtle findings. Symptoms include dyspnea with exertion, fatigue, chest pain, syncope, and hypoxic seizures. It is not uncommon for these patients to be treated for another disease such as epilepsy or reactive airway disease before the diagnosis of pulmonary hypertension is made. The physical examination also is often unrevealing. The second heart sound may be accentuated, but a gallop and hepatomegaly are found only in severe cases. Digital clubbing occurs in patients with pulmonary hypertension associated with cardiac, parenchymal lung, or hepatic disease, although it rarely occurs in familial or primary pulmonary hypertension.

Patients with pulmonary artery hypertension related to increased pulmonary blood flow either have a left-to-right cardiac shunt or endocrine disease (see Table 43-3). Clinically, these patients are first seen with tachypnea, poor growth, congestive heart failure, and hazy lung fields on chest radiographs. Initially, the pulmonary circulation will accommodate the increased volume by recruiting and distending previously collapsed pulmonary vessels. Eventually, however, sustained high flow (especially at high pressure) leads to medial hypertrophy and intimal thickening of the pulmonary arterioles that is grossly indistinguishable from other forms of pulmonary hypertension. In extreme cases, the pulmonary resistance increases to suprasystemic levels, and the systemic-to-pulmonary shunt reverses direction, becoming right-to-left. These patients with Eisenmenger syndrome are seen with cyanosis and clubbing. Furthermore, all patients with systemic-to-pulmonary shunting can develop reversal of shunt flow, decreased pulmonary blood flow, and hypoxemia in the face of other causes of pulmonary hypertension. Once the pulmonary pressures increase to suprasystemic levels and the pulmonary vascular endothelial and smooth muscle cells have hypertrophied, correction of the anatomic abnormality resulting in the left-to-right shunt will not immediately relieve the pulmonary arterial hypertension and may be contraindicated. Months may be required for the vessels to remodel.

Patients with pulmonary hypertension related to increased precapillary resistance have symptoms of their underlying disease, dyspnea, chest pain, signs of decreased cardiac output, and chest radiographs with prominent central pulmonary arteries and clear lung fields (see Table 43-3).

Patients with postcapillary pulmonary hypertension typically have elevated downstream vascular pressure that is transmitted via the pulmonary microcirculation to the pulmonary arteries (see Table 43-3). Clinically, dyspnea, pulmonary hemorrhage, pulmonary edema, and hazy chest radiographs develop in these patients. The combination of a hazy chest radiograph with an underfilled left ventricle on echocardiogram points to an abnormality of pulmonary venous drainage. Sustained increased downstream pressure eventually leads to the development of medial hypertrophy and intimal thickening of the precapillary pulmonary arteries. Again, once this pathologic stage occurs and the vessels remodel, relieving the downstream pressure (i.e., by replacing the mitral valve) may not immediately relieve the pulmonary artery hypertension. The pulmonary hypertension may take months to resolve.[4]

PATHOPHYSIOLOGY

Right Ventricle

The right ventricle is designed to accommodate an increase in blood volume in response to physiologic changes, including exercise, peripheral vasoconstriction, and orthostatic changes. The thin-walled, crescentic right ventricle easily accepts more fluid by assuming a globular shape, with only a modest increase in transmural pressure (much the way a collapsed beach ball accepts more air). Unfortunately, the thin, compliant walls that allow the right ventricle to hold an increased fluid volume are the cause of its failure in the face of an increased afterload. A chronic, moderate increase in PAP causes the right ventricle first to hypertrophy, then to dilate, and finally to encroach on left ventricular filling, resulting in decreased cardiac output.[54] Coronary perfusion pressure also decreases in this situation because of the increase in intraventricular pressure with no increase and often a decrease in systemic arterial pressure. The decreased coronary blood flow in the setting of increased right ventricular mass and elevated right ventricular systolic and diastolic pressures results in right ventricular ischemia and chest pain. Oxygen demand of any muscle is proportional to the tension generated by that muscle. According to Laplace, the tension developed in the ventricle is proportional to the pressure (now elevated) times the radius (now dilated) divided by twice the wall thickness.

$$\text{Laplace's law: } T = Pr/2h$$

where T is total wall tension, P is transmural pressure, h is ventricular muscle thickness, and r is the radius of the sphere.[50]

The right ventricular oxygen demand in patients with chronic pulmonary hypertension, then, increases in the face of decreasing oxygen supply, resulting in failure of the right ventricle and further decrease in cardiac output. Dyspnea with exertion, the most frequent presenting complaint in patients with pulmonary hypertension, is due to impaired oxygen delivery during physical activity as a result of an inability to increase cardiac output in the presence of increased oxygen demands. Syncope, which is often exertional or postexertional, implies a severely restricted cardiac output, leading to diminished cerebral blood flow.[4]

An acute pulmonary hypertension crisis causes an even more dramatic failure of the right ventricle. This crisis may be triggered by an increase in serum catecholamines, hypoxemia, metabolic or respiratory acidosis, pulmonary embolism, or a normal right ventricle transplanted into an organ recipient with pulmonary vascular obstructive disease. The pulmonary and intraventricular pressures increase, and the right ventricular radius increases without the necessary time for the right ventricular wall to hypertrophy. The oxygen demand, again, is proportional to the now elevated intraventricular pressure times the now dilated right ventricular radius divided by twice the wall thickness, which is actually thinner. The oxygen demand, then, increases immediately while the coronary perfusion pressure, cardiac output, and oxygen supply all decrease, leading to dilation of the right ventricle and eventual right ventricular failure. Bradycardia may develop as a result of conduction system disturbance due to subendocardial ischemia in the right ventricle and atrium. Ultimately, the rhythm may deteriorate into ventricular fibrillation as the ischemia worsens.

At the molecular level, the chronically hypertensive right ventricle expresses a fetal genetic pattern. In the fetus, nearly all of the ventricular contractile protein is β-myosin heavy chain. After birth, 30% of the contractile protein is α-myosin heavy chain, which is threefold to fourfold more enzymatically active than the β-myosin heavy chain. The chronically hypertensive right ventricle downregulates the gene for the α-myosin heavy chain and upregulates the gene for the β-myosin heavy chain. This conversion to the enzymatically slower contractile protein could account for a 24% decrease in shortening velocity.[11,15,54] The gene for atrial natriuretic peptide, associated with both the fetal genetic pattern and ventricular hypertrophy, also is upregulated in the hypertensive right ventricle.[15,54] Plasma levels of both atrial and brain natriuretic peptide are elevated in patients with hypertensive right ventricles.[2] In animal models of chronic pulmonary hypertension, the messenger RNA (mRNA) for phosphodiesterase-3 is downregulated. In humans with pulmonary hypertension, the β1 receptor is downregulated and considered to be related to the systolic dysfunction.[54] It is, therefore, not surprising that β agonists and phosphodiesterase inhibitors may be relatively ineffective in treating patients with right ventricular failure because of the decreased numbers of β receptors and the decreased formation of phosphodiesterase.[80]

Pulmonary Vasculature

The pulmonary circulation is designed for maximal compliance. In normal patients, it must accept the entire

cardiac output at less than 20% of the systemic pressure. The normal pulmonary circulation can accept two and a half times the usual cardiac output without an increase in PAP. To maximize compliance, pulmonary arteries have more elastic tissue and less muscle tissue than similar-sized systemic arteries. The pulmonary veins also are more compliant because they lack valves that can obstruct flow. Finally, the lungs have reserve vascular capacity that can be recruited to handle extra blood volume without an increase in PAP.[92]

When pulmonary hypertension is present, the pulmonary circulation is less compliant with less elastic tissue and more endothelial and smooth muscle tissue. This decreased compliance is associated with distinct histologic changes (Fig. 43-1). Nearly all patients with severe pulmonary hypertension, for example, demonstrate medial hypertrophy of the muscular arterioles and the development of muscle layers in previously nonmuscularized arterioles. Early studies associate this proliferation with abnormal vasoconstriction.[65,89] More recent studies implicate the endothelial cell in the vasoconstriction, vascular wall remodeling, and thrombosis that is seen in pulmonary hypertension. Endothelial cells in normal arteries form orderly ridges. Those in hypertensive arteries are twisted, intertwined, and contain an increased amount of rough endoplasmic reticulum and microfilaments.[68] The elastic layer that separates the endothelial cell from the smooth muscle cell also is injured in pulmonary hypertension. In most forms of pulmonary hypertension, the abnormal endothelial cells proliferate to form plexiform lesions and eventually form concentric-obliterative lesions that obstruct the pulmonary vessels.[18] The endothelial cell proliferation appears to be monoclonal in patients with sporadic, familial, and anorexigen-induced pulmonary hypertension and polyclonal in patients with congenital systemic-to-pulmonary shunts and connective tissue disease.[51] Interestingly, in patients with either hypoxemia-associated pulmonary hypertension or veno-occlusive disease, medial hypertrophy develops without prominent endothelial cell proliferation.[84,87] Finally, in situ thrombosis is often seen in patients with pulmonary arterial hypertension.[88]

The abnormal pulmonary endothelial cells are thought to produce increased amounts of vasoconstrictors and prothrombotic mediators while producing decreased amounts of vasodilators and antithrombotics (Table 43-4).[3] Christman and colleagues[16] showed that patients with pulmonary arterial hypertension excrete an increased amount of a metabolite of thromboxane, a vasoconstrictor and promoter of platelet aggregation produced in the endothelium. At the same time, these patients excrete a decreased amount of a metabolite of prostacyclin, an endothelium-derived vasodilator and antiplatelet mediator. Production of nitric oxide, another important endothelium-derived vasodilator, also is decreased in patients with pulmonary arterial hypertension.[35] Endothelin, one of the most potent endothelium-derived vasoconstrictors identified to date, is increased in patients with congenital systemic-to-pulmonary shunts with pulmonary hypertension.[36,81,85] Endothelin and thromboxane are also vascular smooth muscle cell and fibroblast mitogens; in contrast, prostacyclin and nitric oxide have antiproliferative effects.[22,67] Plasma levels of the procoagulants, plasminogen-activator inhibitor, von Willebrand factor (vWF), and P-selectin, are also increased in patients with pulmonary hypertension.[45,69,75] Plasminogen-activator inhibitor is synthesized in endothelial

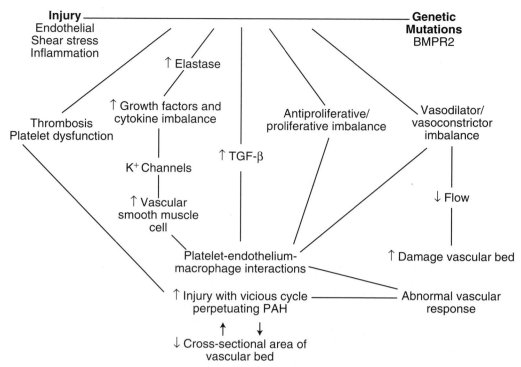

FIGURE 43-1   Pathobiology of pulmonary arterial hypertension (PAH). Various types of injury and genetic mutations lead to a decrease in cross-sectional area of the pulmonary vascular bed. BMPR2, bone morphogenetic protein receptor II; TGF-β, transforming growth factor beta.

cells, platelets, and hepatocytes. It impairs fibrinolysis and is produced in high concentration in the lungs of patients with primary pulmonary hypertension.[45] vWF and P-selectin are both glycoproteins that are stored in the Weibel-Palade bodies of endothelial cells and activate platelets upon release. Plasma vWF, a carrier protein for factor VIII, is increased but dysfunctional in pulmonary hypertension patients because of the absence of the high-molecular-weight multimers. High plasma concentration of vWF in pulmonary hypertension patients is associated with poor prognosis. In one study, a plasma vWF antigenic activity greater than 240%

Table 43-4   Mediators in Pulmonary Hypertension

Mediators That Are Elevated in Pulmonary Hypertension	Mediators That Are Decreased in Pulmonary Hypertension
Platelet-derived growth factor A	Prostacyclin
Basic fibroblast growth factor	Matrix metalloproteinases
Transforming growth factor B	Nitric oxide
Insulin-like growth factor 1	Thrombomodulin
Epinephrine	
Angiotensin II	
Endothelin 1	
TPA	
Fibrinopeptide A	
Thromboxane A$_2$	
Serotonin	
Plasminogen activating inhibitor	
P-selectin	
Von Willebrand factor	

TPA, tissue plasminogen activator.

was 54% sensitive and 93% specific for identifying patients who would not survive one year.[52,53] Plasma concentration of thrombomodulin, an endothelial cell protein that acts as an anticoagulant, is decreased in primary pulmonary hypertension patients.[75] Interestingly, treatment with continuous intravenous epoprostenol may reverse the abnormalities in P-selectin, thrombomodulin, and vWF.[31,75] Although it is unclear whether the imbalance in the levels of these vasoactive and coagulant mediators is a cause, a result, or a marker of pulmonary hypertension, treatment directed at these abnormalities appears to improve patient outcome.[3]

Serotonin, or 5-hydroxytryptamine, also is considered a potential cause of pulmonary hypertension. It is a smooth muscle cell mitogen, a pulmonary vasoconstrictor, a systemic vasodilator, and causes local thrombosis.[23,25] Normally serotonin is produced in the enterochromaffin cells in the intestine. It is usually filtered by the liver, taken up by the platelets, and not seen in high concentrations in the lung. In some forms of pulmonary hypertension, however, pulmonary neuroendocrine cells produce large amounts of serotonin. In other patients with liver disease or abnormal platelet uptake and release, serotonin is not cleared from the blood. Many of the diet pills that are linked to pulmonary hypertension are serotonergic drugs. Other drugs with serotonergic effects may be related to pulmonary arterial hypertension (Table 43-5). Limited cutaneous systemic sclerosis (previously termed the CREST variant of scleroderma) also is associated with both a high plasma serotonin level and an increased incidence of pulmonary arterial hypertension.[24] Similarly, the antiphospholipid syndrome is associated with both a high plasma

Table 43-5 Drugs with Serotonergic Effects That May Be Related to Pulmonary Arterial Hypertension

Cocaine
Dopamine
Doxapram
Fluoxetine
Lithium
Methamphetamine
Methysergide
Pentazocine
Phenmetrazine
Protamine
Sertaline
Tryptophan (Egermayer)

Table 43-6 Risk Factors and Associated Conditions for Pulmonary Hypertension

A. Drugs and toxins
1. Definite
   - Aminorex
   - Fenfluramine
   - Dexfenfluramine
   - Toxic rapeseed oil
2. Very likely
   - Amphetamines
   - L-tryptophan
3. Possible
   - Meta-amphetamines
   - Cocaine
   - Chemotherapeutic agents
4. Unlikely
   - Antidepressants
   - Oral contraceptives
   - Estrogen therapy
   - Cigarette smoking
B. Demographic and medical conditions
1. Definite
   - Gender (females)
2. Possible
   - Pregnancy
   - Systemic hypertension
3. Unlikely
   - Obesity
C. Diseases
1. Definite
   - HIV infection
2. Very likely
   - Portal hypertension/liver disease
   - Collagen vascular diseases
   - Congenital systemic-pulmonary cardiac shunts
3. Possible
   - Thyroid disorders

HIV, human immunodeficiency virus.
From Proceedings of the 3rd World Symposium on pulmonary arterial hypertension. Venice, Italy, June 23–25. 2003. *J Am Coll Cardiol* 43:1S–90S, 2003.

serotonin level and an elevated incidence of pulmonary arterial hypertension.[23] Experimentally, the fawn-hooded rat, which has a defect in platelet serotonin uptake, develops severe pulmonary hypertension when exposed to hypoxia.[77]

RISK FACTORS

Genetic risk factors exist for developing pulmonary arterial hypertension (Table 43-6). It has long been known that young adult women have a 1.7-to-1 greater incidence of primary pulmonary hypertension than do men. In addition, familial primary pulmonary hypertension occurs in at least 6% of all cases of primary pulmonary hypertension. Patients with both sporadic and familial primary pulmonary hypertension have a decreased expression of genes encoding several kinases and phosphatases, while having increased expression of several oncogenes and genes for ion channel proteins.[34] Recent studies have identified a gene mutation for familial primary pulmonary hypertension in the bone morphogenetic protein receptor 2 gene on chromosome 2q31-32. Approximately 50% of familial cases and 10% to 25% of patients with sporadic primary pulmonary hypertension have mutations in that gene.[46] Patients with sporadic but not familial primary pulmonary arterial hypertension have increased expression of several other genes, including the gene encoding the 5-hydroxytryptamine (serotonin) receptor 1B.[34]

Because most of the intra-acinar arteries are formed during the first 18 months of life, a physiologic insult during this period may increase the risk of developing pulmonary arterial hypertension later in life. Sartori and colleagues,[76] who studied 10 adults with previous persistent fetal circulation at birth, showed a significantly greater pulmonary vasoconstrictor response to high altitude than did control subjects. Similarly, rats exposed to hypoxia during the first few days of life have an increased vasoconstrictor response when exposed to hypoxia as adults.[39,83]

Living at high altitude with long-term exposure to hypobaric hypoxia also increases the risk of pulmonary hypertension. Five percent of the population living at an altitude between 3000 and 5000 feet show evidence of right ventricular hypertrophy. Approximately 25% of those living between 4500 and 5000 feet demonstrate evidence of pulmonary hypertension.[37] Evidence also exists of a genetic susceptibility to high-altitude pulmonary hypertension.[59]

Asplenia due to any cause may be a risk factor for developing pulmonary hypertension.[82] It is thought that the lack of a vascular filter allows abnormal cells and activated platelets to reach the lung. In a recent series, the prevalence of asplenia in patients with pulmonary hypertension was 11.5% compared with none in the patients without pulmonary hypertension.[43]

Pulmonary hypertension after cardiopulmonary bypass has been ascribed to increased production of thromboxane, microemboli, pulmonary sequestration of leukocytes, atelectasis, adrenergic hyperactivity, and the decreased release of nitric oxide.[91] Patients undergoing cardiopulmonary bypass with an active respiratory syncytial virus infection are even more likely to develop pulmonary hypertension postoperatively than are those who undergo bypass when they are fully recovered from this infection.[48]

Prior to the 1970s, researchers concentrated on the effects of hypoxia on the pulmonary vasculature. With the discovery of clinically effective vasodilators, attention shifted to dilating constricted vessels. Now, by using the tools of molecular biology, researchers are focusing on improving endothelial cell function, limiting the growth of smooth muscle cells, increasing the elastic tissue, and correcting coagulopathies. Recent work has identified a host of mediators that are abnormal in patients with pulmonary hypertension. Researchers must still determine which mediators are clinically important and which mediators can be tampered with. For example, the orally active ET_A-ET_B-receptor antagonist, bosentan, reduces PAP in some patients otherwise resistant to vasodilators[14]; dose-related liver toxicity is a side effect of endothelin-receptor antagonists.[26]

PRINCIPLES OF MANAGEMENT

Avoid Harm

Although patients with "fixed" or "permanent" pulmonary hypertension may not have pulmonary vessels that can dilate immediately, these vessels often retain the ability to constrict further and worsen the right ventricular failure. The first principle of management, then, is to avoid an acute increase in PAP while maintaining coronary perfusion pressure. Common triggers for pulmonary hypertension include hypoxia, acidosis, elevated intrathoracic pressure, and increased blood concentrations of vasoconstrictors or procoagulants.

Hypoxia, like serotonin, causes pulmonary vasoconstriction and systemic peripheral vasodilation. In areas of regional pulmonary hypoxia (e.g., atelectasis), this mechanism is beneficial because it diverts blood away from areas of low oxygenation and matches ventilation to perfusion. Unfortunately, global pulmonary hypoxia causes pulmonary hypertension, while the peripheral vasodilation further worsens coronary perfusion pressure by decreasing aortic diastolic pressure. Patients with pulmonary hypertension, therefore, should avoid exposure to even moderate degrees of hypoxia. Commercial airplanes, for example, are pressurized only to 8000 feet, and so a given passenger's PaO_2 may decrease by 35%.[20] These patients are therefore advised to fly with supplemental oxygen and not to visit high-altitude locations. Patients who desaturate during sleep or activity are, likewise, advised to use supplemental oxygen.[3] When children with pulmonary hypertension develop pneumonia, they too should receive oxygen to maintain systemic arterial oxygen saturation greater than 95%. In addition to supplemental oxygen, some patients may require bronchodilators, antibiotics, corticosteroids, or a combination of these to maintain normal oxygen saturation. Antipyretics should be administered for fever greater than 101°F (38°C) to minimize the consequences of increased metabolic demands.

Similarly, acidosis causes pulmonary vasoconstriction and systemic peripheral vasodilation. It acts synergistically with hypoxia to increase PAP. Most studies show that acidosis, not the level of $PaCO_2$, causes vasoconstriction, so metabolic acidosis should be promptly corrected with bicarbonate, fluid, and vasopressors, or a combination of these.[12] Patients with uncompensated respiratory acidosis also should receive immediate ventilatory support to correct hypercarbia, even though tracheal intubation and positive pressure ventilation pose a risk in these patients. Prolonged hyperventilation, however, is not recommended in these children. The respiratory alkalosis that reduces the PAP immediately does not protect the pulmonary circulation from subsequent vasoconstrictive stimuli.[58] In addition, overdistention of the lung parenchyma that often accompanies hyperventilation will, like atelectasis, increase the PVR. The goals of ventilatory support for patients with

pulmonary hypertension, therefore, should be maintenance of arterial oxygen saturation greater than 95%, $PaCO_2$ in the range of 35 to 40 mm Hg, and pH in the range of 7.35 to 7.40 at the lowest possible alveolar distending pressure.

Respiratory maneuvers that increase intrathoracic pressure also increase PAP. More important, these maneuvers decrease venous return to a preload-dependent right ventricle. Straining on an endotracheal tube or violent coughing has triggered pulmonary hemorrhage in patients with pulmonary hypertension. Therefore the intubated pulmonary hypertensive patient should be treated with opioids and sedatives to suppress cough and agitation.[47] The Valsalva maneuver also can cause a decrease in cardiac output, resulting in syncope, as well as fatalities; therefore stool softeners are recommended as needed.

Some systemic medications as well as blood product transfusions may affect the pulmonary vasculature. Drugs that cause vasoconstriction or hypercoagulability (e.g., α agonists or oral contraceptives) should be avoided. Platelet transfusions contain serotonin, thromboxane A_2, and other vasoactive substances, which can trigger a pulmonary hypertensive crisis. These transfusions should be given slowly, carefully monitored, after pretreatment with steroids, acetaminophen and diphenhydramine (Benadryl) to decrease the likelihood of an idiosyncratic reaction. Blood transfusions increase oxygen-carrying capacity, but, as noted earlier, a higher hematocrit increases viscosity and PVR. Clinicians must weigh the benefits of increased oxygen-carrying capacity versus the risk of increased PVR. In the face of an elevated PAP, the right ventricle is dependent on preload for cardiac output. Dehydration associated with diuretics or diarrhea causes a decrease in right ventricular filling and cardiac output.

Endogenous increases of stress hormones also may cause an increase in PVR in patients with pulmonary hypertension.[61] Invasive medical procedures should be avoided, if possible, because they will increase sympathetic nervous system activation. If necessary, anesthetic agents can be used to blunt this increase in PVR, but these drugs may cause hypoventilation and a decrease in systemic blood pressure. Conventional treatment of pulmonary hypertensive crises includes deep sedation to blunt a catecholamine surge, but care must be taken to avoid decreasing coronary perfusion pressure.[47] Intubated patients, for example, should be gently sedated before suctioning. Fentanyl blunts pulmonary artery response to noxious stimuli and is usually well tolerated by children with pulmonary hypertension.[42]

Nitrous oxide (50% inspired concentration) does not cause or exacerbate pulmonary hypertension in children and may, therefore, be considered safe as an adjunct to general anesthesia in these patients.[41] Mild reductions in mean systemic arterial pressure and cardiac output accompany the use of nitrous oxide, making it an unwise choice in patients with severely limited cardiovascular reserve. In contrast, nitrous oxide may exacerbate pulmonary hypertension in adults with mitral valve disease.[49,78]

Ketamine did not increase PAP among postoperative patients in one study.[40] However, two subsequent studies showed a dramatic increase in PAP in patients with pulmonary hypertension undergoing cardiac catheterization with the use of ketamine sedation.[9,93] Ketamine, therefore, probably should be avoided in these patients. Narcotics, benzodiazepines, propofol, volatile agents, barbiturates, and etomidate all have been given safely without an immediate increase in PAP, taking care that systemic blood pressure, respiratory drive, and a patent airway are all maintained.

GENERAL PHARMACOLOGIC MEASURES

Pharmacologic management of the patient with pulmonary hypertension includes decreasing PAP, supporting right ventricular contractility, improving cardiac output, and maintaining coronary perfusion pressure. Administering intravenous fluids to a patient with a pulmonary hypertensive crisis, for example, increases coronary perfusion pressure but does not directly alter PAP or cardiac contractility. Medications often given to patients with pulmonary hypertension include oxygen, diuretics, inodilators, anticoagulants, and vasodilators. As mentioned earlier, supplemental oxygen is used to achieve normal oxygen saturation, and diuretics may be useful in reducing the increased intravascular volume and hepatic congestion that can occur in patients with right heart failure. There is, however, no reason to make the patient hyperoxic. Diuretics must be used judiciously to avoid decreased preload. Rich and colleagues[71] demonstrated that digoxin increases cardiac output in patients with pulmonary hypertension and right heart failure. Studies in adults suggest that the concomitant use of digoxin and a calcium channel blocker may counteract the potentially negative inotropic effects of the calcium channel blocker alone.[70] Concomitant use of digoxin and calcium channel blockers may increase digoxin levels. Therefore digitalis toxicity, which also may be enhanced by hypoxemia or diuretic-induced hypokalemia, should be avoided.

Some patients with severe right ventricular dysfunction associated with pulmonary hypertension improve with intravenous inotropes. Dobutamine may be used to improve systemic blood pressure to restore right ventricular coronary perfusion pressure.[61] It is not clear whether dobutamine decreases PVR or only improves right coronary perfusion pressure.[10,21] In animal studies of right ventricular failure, dobutamine as well as dopamine improved right ventricular function, but only epinephrine decreased PVR.[56] Interestingly, in other animal models of right ventricular failure, even treatment with the vasoconstrictor phenylephrine improved right ventricular function by improving coronary blood flow.[86] Milrinone, a phosphodiesterase III inhibitor, decreases the breakdown of cyclic adenosine monophosphate (cAMP) and effectively increases the intracellular concentration of calcium. Milrinone increases cardiac contractility, decreases systemic vascular resistance (SVR), and, in some reports, decreases PVR.[27] Caution is advised when administering the loading dose of milrinone because the sudden decrease of SVR can lower coronary perfusion and cause ischemia.

Survival rates of adults with primary pulmonary arterial hypertension are increased when these patients are treated with prolonged anticoagulation.[30,32] Although the efficacy of anticoagulation has not been studied in children, warfarin is often used. The role of anticoagulation in patients with pulmonary hypertension associated with systemic-to-pulmonary shunts is unclear because of the risk of hemoptysis.[61] Further work must be done to evaluate the efficacy of anticoagulation in children with pulmonary hypertension and to compare the efficacy of heparin versus warfarin versus antiplatelet agents (e.g., aspirin, clopidogrel).

Pulmonary Vasodilators

Clinicians attempt to dilate the pulmonary vasculature by replacing the missing endothelium-derived vasodilators (e.g., nitric oxide, prostacyclin, and heparin-like mediators). Another approach is to inhibit the action and/or secretion of pulmonary vasoconstrictors (e.g., endothelin, thromboxane, and serotonin). The "ideal" drug would selectively dilate the pulmonary vasculature and remodel the pulmonary arteries without causing peripheral systemic vasodilation. Titration of the drug dose is often used to maximize pulmonary vasodilation while minimizing systemic vasodilation (e.g., calcium channel blockade, prostacyclin). In addition, delivery of vasodilators directly into the pulmonary vasculature is used to dilate the pulmonary vasculature selectively (e.g., inhaled nitric oxide, aersolized iloprost).

The rationale for the use of vasodilator agents to treat patients with pulmonary hypertension is based on the premise that there may be an element of reversible pulmonary vasoconstriction. The goal of vasodilator therapy, then, is to reduce PAP and increase cardiac output without causing systemic hypotension. The mechanisms of action of commonly used vasodilators include increasing cAMP, increasing cyclic guanosine monophosphate (cGMP), or blocking calcium channels. Unfortunately, none of these medications is absolutely selective for the pulmonary vasculature.

Acute pulmonary vasodilation occurs in 40% of children with idiopathic pulmonary arterial hypertension, also referred to as primary pulmonary hypertension, in response to a short-term dose of an oral calcium channel blocker. The youngest children have the greatest likelihood of a positive response (Fig. 43-2).[3] Long-term oral calcium channel blocker treatment in these patients increases survival, improves hemodynamics, and relieves symptoms.[6,94] When these children have respiratory infections, however, the nonspecific vasodilating effect of calcium channel blockers may cause a mismatch of ventilation to perfusion, resulting in hypoxemia. Children who do not respond to short-term drug testing with calcium channel blockers have not benefited from prolonged calcium channel blockade therapy.[6] Pulmonary arterial hypertension patients must undergo brief drug testing before starting therapy with calcium channel blockade.

Various drugs have been used for brief vasodilator testing in patients with pulmonary hypertension (Fig. 43-3).[90] The criteria to indicate acute active pulmonary vasodilation with vasodilator testing is at least a 20% decrease in mean PAP, no change or an increase in cardiac index, and a decrease in PVR/SVR.[6] Most of the drugs used for short-term vasodilator testing carry a risk for systemic hypotension, which can result in decreased right coronary perfusion and right ventricular failure. The present consensus is to use short-acting drugs that are as specific as possible for the pulmonary circulation.[61] Commonly used drugs include intravenous (IV) adenosine, IV epoprostenol, and inhaled nitric oxide.[61] The short-term administration of inhaled nitric oxide should identify virtually all the vasoreactive primary pulmonary hypertension patients without causing systemic hypotension.[79] Patients with pulmonary hypertension associated with

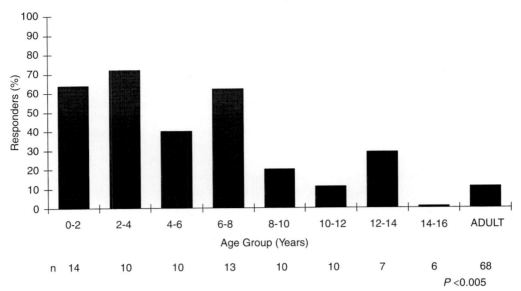

FIGURE 43-2 Response to acute vasodilator drug testing by age. The younger the child at the time of testing, the greater the likelihood of eliciting acute pulmonary vasodilation ($P < .005$).[6]

congenital heart disease also should be tested. The response to the short-acting agents IV epoprostenol and inhaled nitric oxide has been used to determine which children should be tested with longer-acting agents such as oral calcium channel blockers. Children who respond to a brief dose of oral calcium channel blocker will likely have a favorable response to prolonged calcium channel blockade. Those who do not respond to a dose of oral calcium channel blocker and have significant symptoms may be treated with continuous IV epoprostenol (prostacyclin).

Prostacyclin, produced by the endothelial cell, acts via a cAMP mechanism to inhibit platelet aggregation, dilate vessels, repair endothelial cell injury, inhibit vascular cell proliferation, and improve the pulmonary clearance of endothelin. Continuous IV epoprostenol has been used to treat patients with pulmonary arterial hypertension. Long-term IV epoprostenol administration to pulmonary arterial hypertension patients improves hemodynamics, relieves symptoms, and increases survival in idiopathic pulmonary arterial hypertension, even in patients who do not respond to acute vasodilator drug testing with IV epoprostenol.

Epoprostenol, the most commonly used form of prostacyclin, causes dose-dependent vasorelaxation, as well as flushing, headache, jaw pain, foot pain, and diarrhea. It is effective in treating patients with pulmonary arterial hypertension associated with scleroderma, lupus, congenital heart disease, portal hypertension, human immunodeficiency virus, Gaucher's disease, and primary pulmonary hypertension. When it is used for patients with pulmonary veno-occlusive disease or pulmonary capillary hemangiomatosis, however, a significant incidence exists of pulmonary edema.[66] Presumably, this is due to the increased pulmonary blood flow into an area of "fixed" downstream obstruction. Because the half-life of IV epoprostenol is only 2 to 3 minutes, it must be administered continuously by pump via an intravenous catheter. Adverse events include pump malfunction, sepsis, thromboembolic events, catheter obstruction, and resultant rebound pulmonary

hypertension. To avoid these complications, investigations are under way with more stable analogues of prostacyclin that can be administered sub-cutaneously, orally, or by inhalation.

Treprostinil sodium is an analogue of prostacyclin that is more stable with longer half-life. It can be administered continuously via a subcutaneous catheter as well as IV with a reduction in PVR and relief of symptoms. The most common side effect with the subcutaneous administration is pain and redness at the infusion site.[5,8,33] Iloprost is a stable prostacyclin analogue that can be administered by IV infusion as well as by inhalation. It reduces PVR, relieves symptoms, and lasts several hours.[44,63] Finally, beraprost is a stable prostacyclin analogue that can be administered orally. Early results suggest a decrease in PVR and an improvement of symptoms.[62,74]

Endothelin-receptor antagonists also have been studied in patients with pulmonary arterial hypertension. At least two different receptor subtypes are known: ET_A receptors are localized on vascular smooth muscle cells and cardiac myocytes, whereas ET_B receptors are found on vascular endothelial cells, vascular smooth muscle cells, and cardiac fibroblasts. Both ET_A and ET_B receptors on vascular smooth muscle cells mediate pulmonary vasoconstriction, inflammation, proliferation of smooth muscle cells, cell hypertrophy, fibrosis, and bronchoconstriction. ET_B receptors on endothelial cells are associated with endothelium-dependent vasorelaxation through the release of prostacyclin and nitric oxide.[57] ET-1 is cleared by the ET_B receptor. Bosentan, an ET_A/ET_B-receptor antagonist, improved hemodynamics and relieved symptoms in two randomized, placebo-controlled trials.[14,73] Sitaxsentan, a selective ET_A-receptor antagonist, improved hemodynamics and relieved symptoms in a pilot study with pulmonary arterial hypertension patients; a follow-up randomized trial demonstrated increased exercise capacity, improved hemodynamics, and improved symptoms.[7] Adverse events associated with endothelin-receptor antagonists include increase in hepatic transaminases teratogenicity, and possible irreversible male infertility.

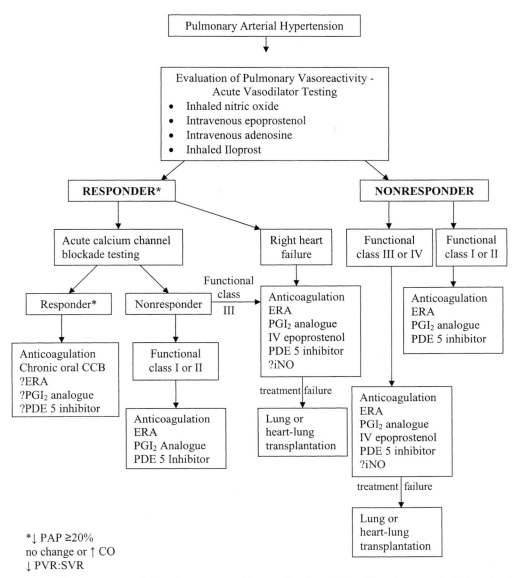

FIGURE 43-3 Evaluation of pulmonary vasoreactivity using acute vasodilator testing in patients with pulmonary arterial hypertension.[6] Clinically-based treatment algorithm in children with pulmonary arterial hypertension. *CCB*, calcium channel blockade. *CO*, cardiac output; *ERA*, endothelin receptor antagonist; *iNO*, inhaled nitric oxide; *PAP*, pulmonary artery hypertension; *PDE 5*, phosphodiesterase type 5; *PGI₂*, prostacyclin *PVR:SVR*, pulmonary vascular resistance–to–systemic vascular resistance ratio.

Nitric oxide, produced by endothelial cells, acts via a cGMP mechanism to inhibit platelet aggregation, dilate vessels, and inhibit vascular cell proliferation. It is vital to maintaining normal pulmonary vascular tone. Delivered in gaseous form, it vasodilates pulmonary arterial vessels, is absorbed and inactivated by hemoglobin, and has little effect on the systemic vasculature. Because it is relatively specific for the pulmonary circulation, it is useful for acute drug testing, management of acute postoperative pulmonary hypertensive crises, and treatment of persistent pulmonary hypertension of the newborn and acute sickle cell chest syndrome. It has been delivered over the long term to pulmonary hypertension patients with improvement in hemodynamics.[13]

Because the active moiety in nitroglycerin is nitric oxide, nebulized nitroglycerin also has been used to decrease PAP selectively in children with congenital heart disease.[64]

Phosphodiesterase inhibitors may be particularly useful when combined with inhaled nitric oxide. Type 5 phosphodiesterase inhibitors (e.g., sildenafil) increase the concentration of cGMP, whereas type 3/4 inhibitors (e.g., milrinone) increase the concentration of cAMP. In trials, sildenafil and dipyridamole increase the concentration of cGMP and have effects comparable to those of inhaled nitric oxide.[64,95] Carefully designed studies of the therapeutic efficacy of phosphodiesterase inhibitors alone and in combination with nitric oxide appear warranted. Sildenafil improved hemodynamics and symptoms in a randomized placebo-controlled trial.*

---

* Galie N, Ghofrani HA, Torbicki A, et al, for the Sildenafil Use in Pulmonary Arterial Hypertension (SUPER) studies groups: Sildenafil citrate therapy for pulmonary arterial hypertension. *N Engl J Med* 2005 (in press).

CONCLUSIONS

Critically ill children have pulmonary hypertensive crises associated with systemic diseases, cardiac surgery, or an acute exacerbation of chronic pulmonary hypertension. Understanding the pathobiology and pathophysiology of pulmonary hypertension is important for preventing, palliating, and treating pulmonary hypertensive crises. Although a number of promising new drugs are on the horizon, the basic goal remains to vasodilate and remodel the pulmonary vasculature. Any new drug should decrease PAP, maintain coronary perfusion pressure, and improve cardiac output. Combination therapy may further improve the efficacy of pulmonary arterial hypertension treatment (e.g., combining endothelin-receptor antagonists with IV epoprostenol may be more effective than either drug alone). In the near future, we may be able to tailor the treatment to the individual child's pathophysiology and apply the new pharmacologic discoveries to critically ill patients. Discoveries in vascular biology will improve our understanding of the etiologies and pathobiology of pulmonary hypertension and lead to specific and novel medical therapies.

References

1. Addonizio LJ, Gersony WM, Robbins RC, et al: Elevated pulmonary vascular resistance and cardiac transplantation. *Circulation* 76:V52–V55, 1987.
2. Bando M, Ishii Y, Sugiyama Y, Kitamura S: Elevated plasma brain natriuretic peptide levels in chronic respiratory failure with cor pulmonale. *Resp Med* 93:507–514, 1999.
3. Barst RJ: Recent advances in the treatment of pediatric pulmonary artery hypertension. *Pediatr Clin North Am* 46:331–345, 1999.
4. Barst, RJ: Pulmonary hypertension. In Goldman L (ed): *Cecil Textbook of Medicine*, 22nd ed. Philadelphia, WB Saunders, 2003, pp 363–370.
5. Barst RJ, Horn EM, Widlitz AC, et al: Efficacy of long-term subcutaneous infusion of UT-15 in primary pulmonary hypertension. *Eur Heart J* 21:315, 2000.
6. Barst RJ, Maislin G, Fishman AP: Vasodilator therapy for primary pulmonary hypertension in children. *Circulation* 99:1197–1208, 1999.
7. Barst RJ, Langleben D, Frost A, et al: Sitaxsentan therapy for pulmonary arterial hypertension. *Am J Respir Crit Care Med* 169:441–447, 2004.
8. Barst RJ, Simonneau G, Rich S, et al: Efficacy and safety of chronic subcutaneous infusion of UT-15 (Uniprost) in pulmonary arterial hypertension (PAH). *Circulation* 102:II100–II101, 2000.
9. Berman W, Fripp RR, Rutter M, Aldrete L: Hemodynamic effects of ketamine in children undergoing cardiac catheterization. *Pediatr Cardiol* 11:72–76, 1990.
10. Berner M, Rouge JC, Friedli B: The hemodynamic effect of phentolamine and dobutamine after open-heart operations in children: Influence of the underlying heart defect. *Ann Thorac Surg* 35:643–650, 1983.
11. Bouvagnet P, Neveu S, Montoya M, Leger JJ: Development changes in the human cardiac isomyosin distribution: An immunohistochemical study using monoclonal antibodies. *Circ Res* 61:329–336, 1987.
12. Chang AC, Zucker HA, Hickey PR, Wessel DL: Pulmonary vascular resistance in infants after cardiac surgery: Role of carbon dioxide and hydrogen ion. *Crit Care Med* 23:568–574, 1995.
13. Channick RN, Newhart JW, Johnson FW, et al: Pulsed delivery of inhaled nitric oxide to patients with primary pulmonary hypertension: An ambulatory delivery system and initial clinical tests. *Chest* 109:1545–1549, 1996.
14. Channick RN, Simonneau G, Sitbon O, et al: Effects of the dual endothelin-receptor antagonist bosentan in patients with pulmonary hypertension: A randomised placebo-controlled study. *Lancet* 58:1119–1123, 2001.
15. Chien KR, Zhu H, Knowlton KU, et al: Transcriptional regulation during cardiac growth and development. *Annu Rev Physiol* 55:77–95, 1993.
16. Christman BW, McPherson CD, Newman JH, et al: An imbalance between the excretion of thromboxane and prostacyclin metabolites in pulmonary hypertension. *N Engl J Med* 327:70–75, 1992.
17. Cool CD, Kennedy D, Voelkel NF, Tuder RM: Pathogenesis and evolution of plexiform lesions in pulmonary hypertension associated with scleroderma and human immunodeficiency virus infection. *Hum Pathol* 28:434–442, 1997.
18. Cool CD, Voelkel NF, Wheeler LJ, Tuder RM: Analysis of vascular lesions in familial primary pulmonary hypertension: Insights into the endothelial cell as the common denominator of a morphologically heterogeneous disorder. *Am J Resp Crit Care Med* 155:A628, 1997.
19. Deb B, Bradford K, Pearl RG: Additive effects of inhaled nitric oxide and intravenous milrinone in experimental pulmonary hypertension. *Crit Care Med* 28:795–799, 2000.
20. Dillard TA, Berg BW, Rajagopal KR, et al: Hypoxemia during air travel in patients with chronic obstructive pulmonary disease. *Ann Intern Med* 111:362–367, 1989.
21. Driscoll D, Gillette P, Duff D, et al: Hemodynamic effects of dobutamine in children. *Am J Cardiol* 43:581–585, 1979.
22. Dubin D, Pratt RE, Dzau VJ: Endothelin, a potent vasoconstrictor, is a smooth muscle mitogen. *J Vasc Biol Med* 1:150–154, 1989.
23. Egermayer P: Epidemics of vascular toxicity and pulmonary hypertension: What can be learned? *J Intern Med* 247:11–17, 2000.
24. Egermayer P, Town GI, Peacock AJ: Role of serotonin in the pathogenesis of acute and chronic pulmonary hypertension. *Thorax* 54:161–168, 1999.
25. Fanburg BL, Lee SL: A new role of an old molecule: Serotonin as a mitogen. *Am J Physiol* 272:L795–L806, 1997.
26. Fattinger K, Funk C, Pantze M, et al: The endothelin antagonist bosentan inhibits the canalicular bile salt export pump: A potential mechanism for hepatic adverse reactions. *Clin Pharmacol Ther* 69:223–231, 2001.
27. Feneck RO: Milrinone and postoperative pulmonary hypertension. *J Cardiothorac Vasc Anesth* 7:21–23, 1993.
28. Fishman AP: Clinical classification of pulmonary hypertension. *Clin Chest Med* 22:385–391, 2001.
29. Fishman AP: State of the art: Chronic cor pulmonale. *Am Rev Respir Dis* 114:775–794, 1976.
30. Frank H, Mlczoch J, Huber K, et al: The effect of anticoagulant therapy in primary and anorectic drug-induced pulmonary hypertension. *Chest* 112:714–721, 1997.
31. Friedman R, Mears JG, Barst RJ: Continuous infusion of prostacyclin normalizes plasma markers of endothelial cell injury and platelet aggregation in primary pulmonary hypertension. *Circulation* 96:2782–2784, 1997.
32. Fuster V, Steele PM, Edwards WD, et al: Primary pulmonary hypertension: Natural history and the importance of thrombosis. *Circulation* 70:580–587, 1984.
33. Gaine SP, Barst RJ, Rich S, et al: Acute hemodynamic effects of subcutaneous UT-15 in primary pulmonary hypertension. *Am J Resp Crit Care Med* 159:A161, 1999.
34. Geraci MW, Moore M, Gesell T, et al: Gene expression patterns in the lungs of patients with primary pulmonary hypertension: A gene microarray analysis. *Circ Res* 88:555–562, 2001.
35. Giaid A, Saleh D: Reduced expression of endothelial nitric oxide synthase in the lungs of patients with pulmonary hypertension. *N Engl J Med* 333:214–221, 1995.
36. Giaid A, Yanagisawa M, Langleben D, et al: Expression of endothelin-1 in the lungs of patients with pulmonary hypertension. *N Engl J Med* 328:1732–1739, 1993.
37. Groves BM, Droma T, Sutton JR, et al: Minimal hypoxic pulmonary hypertension in normal Tibetans at 3,658 m. *J Appl Physiol* 74:312–318, 1993.
38. Hakim TS, Chang HK, Michel RP: The rectilinear pressure-flow relationship in the pulmonary vasculature: Zones 2 and 3. *Respir Physiol* 61:115–123, 1985.
39. Hampl V, Herget J: Perinatal hypoxia increases hypoxic pulmonary vasoconstriction in adult rats recovering from chronic exposure to hypoxia. *Am Rev Respir Dis* 142:619–624, 1990.
40. Hickey PR, Hansen DD, Cramolini GM, et al: Pulmonary and systemic hemodynamic responses to ketamine in infants with normal and elevated pulmonary vascular resistance. *Anesthesiology* 62:287–293, 1985.
41. Hickey PR, Hansen DD, Strafford M, et al: Pulmonary and systemic hemodynamic effects of nitrous oxide in infants with normal and elevated pulmonary vascular resistance. *Anesthesiology* 65:374–378, 1986.
42. Hickey PR, Hansen DD, Wessel DL, et al: Blunting of stress responses in the pulmonary circulation of infants by fentanyl. *Anesth Analg* 64:1137–1142, 1985.
43. Hoeper MM, Niedermeyer J, Hoffmeyer F, et al: Pulmonary hypertension after splenectomy? *Ann Intern Med* 130:506–509, 1999.
44. Hoeper MM, Schwarze M, Ehlerding S, et al: Long-term treatment of primary pulmonary hypertension with aerosolized iloprost: A prostacyclin analogue. *N Engl J Med* 342:1866–1870, 2000.

45. Hoeper MM, Sosada M, Fabel H: Plasma coagulation profiles in patients with severe primary pulmonary hypertension. *Eur Respir J* 12:1446–1449, 1998.

46. Humbert M, Nunes H, Sitbon O, et al: Risk factors for pulmonary arterial hypertension. *Clin Chest Med* 22:459–475, 2001.

47. Journois D, Pouard P, Mauriat P, et al: Inhaled nitric oxide as a therapy for pulmonary hypertension after operations for congenital heart defects. *J Thorac Cardiovasc Surg* 107:1129–1135, 1994.

48. Khongphatthanayothin A, Wong PC, Samara Y, et al: Impact of respiratory syncytial virus infection on surgery for congenital heart disease: Postoperative course and outcome. *Crit Care Med* 27:1974–1981, 1999.

49. Konstadt SN, Reich DL, Thys DM: Nitrous oxide does not exacerbate pulmonary or ventricular dysfunction in patients with mitral valve disease. *Can J Anaesth* 37:603–607, 1990.

50. Lake CL: Cardiovascular anatomy and physiology. In Barash PG, Cullen BF, Stoelting RK (eds): *Clinical Anesthesia*, 2nd ed. Philadelphia, JB Lippincott, 1992, p 1010.

51. Lee SD, Shroyer KR, Markham NE, et al: Monoclonal endothelial cell proliferation is present in primary but not secondary pulmonary hypertension. *J Clin Invest* 101:927–934, 1998.

52. Lopes AA, Maeda NY: Circulating von Willebrand factor antigen as a predictor of short-term prognosis in pulmonary hypertension. *Chest* 114:1276–1282, 1998.

53. Lopes AA, Maeda NY, Bydlowski SP: Abnormalities in circulating von Willebrand factor and survival in pulmonary hypertension. *Am J Med* 105:21–26, 1998.

54. Lowes BD, Minobe W, Abraham WT, et al: Changes in gene expression in the intact human heart: Downregulation of alpha-myosin heavy chain in hypertrophied, failing ventricular myocardium. *J Clin Invest* 100:2315–2324, 1997.

55. Mair DD, Ritter DG, Ongley PA, Helmholz HF Jr: Hemodynamics and evaluation for surgery of patients with complete transposition of the great arteries and ventricular septal defect. *Am J Cardiol* 28:632–640, 1971.

56. McGovern JJ, Cheifitz IM, Craig DM, et al: Right ventricular injury in young swine: Effects of catecholamines on right ventricular function and pulmonary vascular mechanics. *Pediatr Res* 48:763–769, 2000.

57. Miyauchi T, Masaki T: Pathophysiology of endothelin in the cardiovascular system. *Annu Rev Physiol* 61:391–415, 1999.

58. Moreira GA, O'Donnell DC, Tod ML, et al: Discordant effects of alkalosis on elevated pulmonary vascular resistance and vascular reactivity in lamb lungs. *Crit Care Med* 27:1838–1842, 1999.

59. Morrell NW, Sarybaev AS, Alikhan A, et al: ACE genotype and risk of high altitude pulmonary hypertension in Kyrghyz highlanders. *Lancet* 353:814, 1999.

60. Morris W, Knauer CM: Cardiopulmonary manifestations of schistosomiasis. *Semin Respir Infect* 12:159–170, 1997.

61. Naeije R, Vachiery JL: Medical therapy of pulmonary hypertension: Conventional therapies. *Clin Chest Med* 22:517–527, 2001.

62. Nagaya N, Uematsu M, Okano Y, et al: Effect of orally active prostacyclin analogue on survival of outpatients with primary pulmonary hypertension. *J Am Coll Cardiol* 4:1188–1192, 1999.

63. Nikkho S, Seeger W, Baumgartner R, et al: One-year observation of iloprost inhalation therapy in patients with pulmonary hypertension. *Eur Respir J* 16:324, 2001.

64. Omar HA, Gong F, Sun MY, Einzig S: Nebulized nitroglycerin in children with pulmonary hypertension secondary to congenital heart disease. *W V Med J* 95:74–75, 1999.

65. Palevsky HI, Schloo BL, Pietra GG, et al: Primary pulmonary hypertension: Vascular structure, morphometry, and responsiveness to vasodilator agents. *Circulation* 80:1207–1221, 1989.

66. Palmer SM, Robinson LJ, Wang A, et al: Massive pulmonary edema and death after prostacyclin infusion in a patient with pulmonary venoocclusive disease. *Chest* 113:237–240, 1998.

67. Peacock AJ, Dawes KE, Shock A, et al: Endothelin-1 and endothelin-3 induce chemotaxis and replication of pulmonary artery fibroblasts. *Am J Respir Cell Mol Biol* 7:492–499, 1992.

68. Rabinovitch M: Pathobiology of pulmonary hypertension, extracellular matrix. *Clin Chest Med* 22:433–449, 2001.

69. Rabinovitch M, Andrew M, Thom H, et al: Abnormal endothelial factor VIII associated with pulmonary hypertension and congenital heart defects. *Circulation* 76:1043–1052, 1987.

70. Rich S, Kaufmann E, Levy PS: The effect of high doses of calcium-channel blockers on survival in primary pulmonary hypertension. *N Engl J Med* 327:76–81, 1992.

71. Rich S, Seidlitz M, Dodin E, et al: The short-term effects of digoxin in patients with right ventricular dysfunction from pulmonary hypertension. *Chest* 114:787–792, 1998.

72. Rosenzweig EB, Kerstein D, Barst RJ: Long-term prostacyclin for pulmonary hypertension with associated congenital heart defects. *Circulation* 99:1858–1865, 1999.

73. Rubin LJ, Badesch DB, Barst RJ, et al: Bosentan therapy for pulmonary arterial hypertension. *N Engl J Med* 346:896–903, 2002.

74. Saji T, Ozawa Y, Ishikita T, et al: Short-term hemodynamic effect of a new oral PGI_2 analogue, beraprost, in primary and secondary pulmonary hypertension. *Am J Cardiol* 78:244–247, 1996.

75. Sakamaki F, Kyotani S, Nagaya N, et al: Increased plasma P-selectin and decreased thrombomodulin in pulmonary arterial hypertension were improved by continuous prostacyclin therapy. *Circulation* 102:2720–2725, 2000.

76. Sartori C, Allemann Y, Trueb L, et al: Augmented vasoreactivity in adult life associated with perinatal vascular insult. *Lancet* 353:2205–2207, 1999.

77. Sato K, Webb S, Tucker A, et al: Factors influencing the idiopathic development of pulmonary hypertension in the fawn hooded rat. *Am Rev Respir Dis* 145:793–797, 1992.

78. Schulte-Sasse U, Hess W, Tarnow J: Pulmonary vascular responses to nitrous oxide in patients with normal and high pulmonary vascular resistance. *Anesthesiology* 57:9–13, 1982.

79. Smerling AJ, Kerstein D, Rosenzweig EB, et al: Acute drug testing in pulmonary hypertension: Congenital versus primary pulmonary hypertension. *Anesth Analg* 92:S63, 2001.

80. Smith CJ, He J, Ricketts SG, et al: Downregulation of right ventricular phosphodiesterase PDE-3A mRNA and protein before the development of canine heart failure. *Cell Biochem Biophys* 29:67–88, 1998.

81. Stewart DJ, Levy RD, Cernacek P, Langleben D: Increased plasma endothelin-1 in pulmonary hypertension: Marker or mediator of disease? *Ann Intern Med* 114:464–469, 1991.

82. Stewart GW, Amess JA, Eber SW, et al: Thrombo-embolic disease after splenectomy for hereditary stomatocytosis. *Br J Haematol* 93:303–310, 1996.

83. Tang JR, Le Cras TD, Morris KG Jr, Abman SH: Brief perinatal hypoxia increases severity of pulmonary hypertension after reexposure to hypoxia in infant rats. *Am J Physiol Lung Cell Mol Physiol* 278: L356–L364, 2000.

84. Tuder RM, Groves B, Badesch DB, Voelkel NF: Exuberant endothelial cell growth and elements of inflammation are present in plexiform lesions of pulmonary hypertension. *Am J Pathol* 144:275–285, 1994.

85. Tutar HE, Imamoglu A, Atalay S, et al: Plasma endothelin-1 levels in patients with left-to-right shunt with or without pulmonary hypertension. *Int J Cardiol* 70:57–62, 1999.

86. Vlahakes GJ, Turley K, Hoffman JI: The pathophysiology of failure in acute right ventricular hypertension: Hemodynamic and biochemical correlations. *Circulation* 63:87–95, 1981.

87. Voelkel NF, Tuder RM: Severe pulmonary hypertensive diseases: A perspective. *Eur Respir J* 14:1246–1250, 1999.

88. Wagenvoort CA, Mulder PG: Thrombotic lesions in primary plexogenic arteriopathy: Similar pathogenesis or complication? *Chest* 103:844–849, 1993.

89. Wagenvoort CA, Wagenvoort N: Primary pulmonary hypertension: A pathologic study of the lung vessels in 156 clinically diagnosed cases. *Circulation* 42:1163–1184, 1970.

90. Weir EK, Rubin LJ, Ayres SM, et al: The acute administration of vasodilators in primary pulmonary hypertension: Experience from the National Institutes of Health Registry on Primary Pulmonary Hypertension. *Am Rev Respir Dis* 140:1623–1630, 1989.

91. Wessel DL: Managing low cardiac output after congenital heart surgery. *Crit Care Med* 29:S220–S230, 2001.

92. West JB: *Pulmonary Pathophysiology, the Essentials*. 5th ed. Baltimore, Williams & Wilkins, 1998, p 111.

93. Wolfe RR, Loehr JP, Schaffer MS, Wiggins JW Jr: Hemodynamic effects of ketamine, hypoxia and hyperoxia in children with surgically treated congenital heart disease residing greater than or equal to 1,200 meters above sea level. *Am J Cardiol* 67:84–87, 1991.

94. Yung D, Widlitz AC, Rosenzweig EB, et al: Outcomes in children with idiopathic pulmonary arterial hypertension. *Circulation* 110:660–665, 2004.

95. Ziegler JW, Ivy DD, Wiggins JW, et al: Effects of dipyridamole and inhaled nitric oxide in pediatric patients with pulmonary hypertension. *Am J Respir Crit Care Med* 158:1388–1395, 1998.

Chapter 44

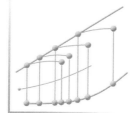

Inflammatory Heart Disease

JOSEPH D. TOBIAS, MD, JAYANT K. DESHPANDE, MD, MPH,
JAMES A. JOHNS, MD, and DAVID G. NICHOLS, MD, MBA

INTRODUCTION

Inflammatory heart disease encompasses a wide array of entities including idiopathic, infectious, rheumatic, autoimmune, toxic, and allergic diseases, among others. Although isolated pericarditis or myocarditis is the most common presentation, in some cases all three layers of the myocardium are involved, resulting in a pancarditis. Myocardial or pericardial involvement may be the primary, isolated component of the disease process or just one manifestation of a systemic, multiorgan disease. The cardiac involvement may be the first manifestation of a systemic disease or may occur years after the primary disease process has been identified. The cardiologist, intensivist, and surgeon must often collaborate in the management of these patients, as they may be initially seen with life-threatening cardiac dysfunction, require invasive procedures to drain fluid, or progress to chronic heart failure, for which transplantation is the only option.

PERICARDITIS

The pericardium is a dual-layered structure consisting of the visceral pericardium (epicardium) that adheres closely to the myocardium and the outer parietal pericardium. Between the two layers of the pericardium is a potential space, containing 10 to 30 mL of fluid in the adult. The fluid provides protection to the heart and limits intrapericardial pressure changes that occur with changes in posture and during respiration. With inflammatory or infectious processes affecting the pericardium, the amount of fluid may increase dramatically, resulting in an effusion that can significantly compromise myocardial filling and function. The pathophysiology of the pericardium is reviewed in detail in Chapter 9.

Acute pericarditis has a long list of potential causes, but the presentation and management tend to be generic. We review the common features of the various causes of acute pericarditis before considering the distinguishing features of the differential diagnosis.

Etiology

By definition, pericarditis is an inflammatory process. It may be infectious (including bacterial, viral, mycobacterial, or fungal) or noninfectious. Noninfectious pericarditis may result from various etiologies including autoimmune, uremic, neoplastic, postpericardiotomy, and hypersensitivity. Idiopathic pericarditis may represent infectious pericarditis in which the infectious agent is not identified. Causes of pericarditis in infants and children are summarized in Table 44-1.

Idiopathic and Viral Pericarditis

The spectrum of viruses associated with pericarditis is similar to that for myocarditis, with enteroviruses (especially coxsackievirus and enteric cytopathic human orphan [ECHO] virus) being isolated most frequently (Table 44-2). Other childhood viruses, including adenovirus, influenza, measles, mumps, varicella, hepatitis B, and Epstein-Barr viruses, have been implicated in the pathogenesis of pericarditis. Cytomegalovirus (CMV) can cause pericarditis in immunocompetent individuals but is more common in immunosuppressed patients. Patients with the acquired immunodeficiency syndrome (AIDS) also may develop pericarditis, but it is not always clear whether the pericarditis is the result of the human immunodeficiency virus (HIV) infection itself or other opportunistic infectious agents (see later).[30,97,98,108]

Table 44-1   Etiology of Pericarditis in Infants and Children

Infectious
Viral (coxsackie, echovirus, adenovirus, mumps, measles, varicella, HBV, HIV, EBV, cytomegalovirus)
Bacterial (*Streptococcus pneumoniae, Staphylococcus aureus, Haemophilus influenzae, Neisseria meningitidis, Klebsiella pneumonia,* anaerobic species)
Fungal (histoplasmosis, coccidioidomycosis, *Candida*)
Other (*Mycobacterium, Mycoplasma,* Lyme disease, rickettsia, *Toxocara canis*)
Noninfectious
Idiopathic
Cardiac injury (trauma, postsurgical, postpericardiotomy syndrome, post–myocardial infarction, radiation)
Rheumatic fever
Chylous effusions
Autoimmune diseases (systemic lupus erythematosus, juvenile rheumatoid arthritis, inflammatory bowel disease)
Kawasaki syndrome
Hypothyroidism
Uremia
Hypersensitivity to drugs/toxins
Neoplasia
Amyloidosis

HBV, hepatitis B virus; HIV, human immunodeficiency virus; EBV, Epstein-Barr virus.

Table 44-2   Viruses Implicated in Myocarditis/Pericarditis

RNA Viruses	DNA Viruses	Retroviruses
Coxsackie A, B	Adenovirus	Human immunodeficiency virus
Echovirus	Cytomegalovirus	
Hepatitis A	Epstein-Barr	
Influenza A, B	Hepatitis B	
Lymphocytic choriomeningitis virus	Varicella	
	Variola	
Mumps	Rubeola	
Poliovirus	Togavirus	
Rhabdovirus	Rubella	
Rhinovirus		

The true incidence of viral pericarditis is difficult to determine, because rigorous attempts at direct viral isolation or detection of an increase in viral antibody titers are not performed in all patients. Many cases of idiopathic pericarditis may be viral. In several pediatric and adult series, idiopathic pericarditis accounts for up to 40% to 90% of all cases of pericarditis.[44,119,134,150] These numbers may change with refined techniques of viral isolation/culture and the recent advances in molecular biology, thereby allowing effective identification of viral genomes in body-fluid samples.

Bacterial Pericarditis

Bacterial pericarditis may be the result of direct spread from an adjacent pneumonia/empyema or mediastinal infection or hematogenous spread from either a primary bacteremia or a distant site of infection. In postoperative patients, the pericardial space may be infected directly from the surgical procedure or along the track of pacing wires and mediastinal drainage tubes. The most common pathogens in bacterial pericarditis have been *Staphylococcus aureus, Streptococcus pneumoniae, Neisseria meningitidis,* and *Haemophilus influenzae.*[17,46,57,126,164] The latter three organisms may be associated with concurrent meningitis and pericarditis. With the routine vaccination of children against *Haemophilus influenzae* type B, invasive disease from this organism has markedly decreased.[147] The same may soon be said for *Streptococcus pneumoniae,* with the recommendations for the use of the polyvalent pneumococcal vaccine as part of routine childhood immunization. Bacterial pericarditis remains a major cause of pericarditis in developing countries.[81] Most of these cases involve disseminated sepsis with *S. aureus.*

Tuberculous, Fungal, and Other Infectious Causes of Pericarditis

Although *Mycobacterium tuberculosis* is often considered a potential cause of pericarditis,[49] Fyler[53] reported in 1992 that in the previous 30 years, there had not been a case of tuberculosis (TB) pericarditis at Boston Children's Hospital. However, TB pericarditis, as an early manifestation of disseminated TB, is spreading rapidly in the developing world, particularly in Africa, where it may appear with or without coexistent AIDS.[64] Diagnostic features of TB pericarditis include a lymphocytic infiltrate in the pericardial fluid and an echocardiographic appearance of a layer of shaggy fibrin around the heart. Cultures may be negative, as the isolation rate from culture of pericardial fluid ranges from 40% to 70%.

Fungal agents including histoplasmosis can cause pericarditis, especially in the southern and midwestern regions of the United States, where they are endemic. The pericarditis associated with histoplasmosis most likely results from inflammation adjacent to mediastinal lymph nodes. *Aspergillus* pericarditis occurs largely in the severely immunocompromised host after direct invasion from the lung or myocardium.[94] Only approximately one third of cases are diagnosed premortem. Any immunocompromised patient with diagnosed or suspected pulmonary aspergillosis, in whom pericardial disease develops, should be presumed to have aspergillus pericarditis until proven otherwise.

Candida pericarditis is rare. It has a similar demographic profile in the immunocompromised patient population, but also is seen after cardiac surgery.[136] The disease progresses more slowly than that from *Aspergillus*, with unexplained fever and gradual accumulation of pericardial fluid. Pericardiocentesis and culture of *Candida* from the fluid provide the diagnosis. Hence, *Candida* pericarditis can usually be diagnosed prior to the patient's demise.

Other less common infectious causes of pericarditis include *Mycoplasma*, Lyme disease, and parasitic infections such as *Toxocara canis*.

Constrictive Pericarditis

In some patients, pericarditis may result in excessive fibrosis and constriction of the pericardium. Granulomatous disease (TB and histoplasmosis) is thought of as a common cause of constrictive pericarditis. However, most other forms of acute pericarditis can evolve into constrictive pericarditis.[16] In children, bacterial pericarditis may be the most common cause of constrictive pericarditis.[159]

Constrictive pericarditis impairs filling of the ventricles during diastole. The fibrotic pericardium forms a tight sac around the heart, which impairs ventricular filling as soon as the elastic limits of the pericardium have been reached. Most of the filling occurs during an early diastolic dip of ventricular pressure, with little additional filling later in diastole. This results in a plateau of the diastolic pressure, producing what is known as the "square root sign" because of similarity of the right or left ventricular pressure tracing to the square root symbol ($\sqrt{}$).

Constrictive pericarditis may be difficult to distinguish clinically from restrictive cardiomyopathy or pericardial tamponade. The most prominent features of the physical examination reflect evidence of marked systemic venous hypertension with hepatomegaly, ascites, and even splenomegaly. A protein-losing enteropathy may occur. The heart sounds are distant, and the apical pulse is diminished. In contrast to tamponade or restrictive cardiomyopathy, the heart size is normal or only minimally enlarged, and pulmonary edema is rare in constrictive pericarditis.

The combination of echocardiography and computed tomography (CT) scan or magnetic resonance imaging (MRI) may help establish the diagnosis of constrictive pericarditis. Pericardial biopsy is sometimes needed. Pericardiectomy is the only effective therapy and should be undertaken early before the fibrotic process also has affected the myocardium. The patient's rate of recovery will depend on the extent of comorbid disease and especially the degree of coexistent myocardial fibrosis.

Noninfectious Pericarditis

Noninfectious pericarditis can result from a number of systemic diseases, reactions to drugs/toxins, or hypersensitivity responses. When pericarditis is the by-product of another disease process, the timing and severity of presentation will be highly variable. For example, the pericarditis seen in systemic lupus erythematosus (SLE) is often a manifestation of a generalized serositis associated with a flare-up of the lupus, although pericarditis also may be the primary complaint identified at the time of the initial presentation of the disease.[102,152] Other autoimmune diseases or those presumed to have autoimmune components, such as juvenile rheumatoid arthritis and inflammatory bowel disease, also may have pericarditis as part of the systemic disease process.[59,115,117,152]

Procainamide and hydralazine are commonly implicated drugs in the pericarditis associated with drug-induced hypersensitivity reactions. Both can be associated with a drug-induced lupus-like disease process resulting in serositis. Other drugs implicated as possible etiologic agents of pericarditis include methyldopa, heparin, warfarin, dantrolene, and cromolyn sodium. Pericarditis also has been reported as a complication of stellate ganglion block,[143] presumably as a result of an inflammatory response to the local anesthetic agent that can spread along fascial planes from the prevertebral space into the mediastinum.

The postpericardiotomy syndrome may occur after any open-heart procedure that involves opening of the pericardium. It has been potentially linked to viruses, irritation of the pericardial space by blood, or immunologic mechanisms.[39] The frequency of this syndrome seems to have decreased over the past decade.

Clinical Manifestations

Chest pain and fever are the most common presenting symptoms of pericarditis. The pain may be substernal or may radiate to the middle of the back or the trapezius muscle. The pain is generally sharp, increasing with inspiration. Patients with pericarditis often find that the pain is reduced by leaning forward. Patients with large pericardial effusions may have dyspnea, shortness of breath, or even shock or respiratory failure or both. On auscultation of the precordium, a pericardial friction rub may be heard, most commonly with three components. A large effusion may not produce a rub because the visceral and parietal pericardial surfaces are not in apposition, and the heart sounds may be muffled. Arrhythmias are rarely a sign of pericarditis without concomitant myocarditis.[153]

In the presence of cardiac tamponade, peripheral perfusion may be decreased, the jugular veins distended, and hepatomegaly present because of venous congestion from an increase in right-sided filling pressures. With this degree of cardiac compromise, pulsus paradoxus is generally present. To detect pulsus paradoxus, one takes a blood pressure in the usual manner but allows the cuff pressure to decrease very slowly as the patient breathes normally. The pressure at which Korotkoff sounds are first heard is the systolic pressure during expiration. At this pressure, no sounds will be heard during inspiration, because the cuff pressure exceeds the inspiratory systolic blood pressure. The cuff pressure is slowly released, and when the cuff pressure is equal to the systolic blood pressure in inspiration, the Korotkoff sounds will be heard throughout the respiratory cycle. The difference between the point at which Korotkoff sounds are first heard in expiration and when they are heard throughout the respiratory cycle reflects the difference between the expiratory and inspiratory systolic blood pressures. This difference is the pulsus paradoxus. A pulsus paradoxus of up to 10 mm Hg may be normal. Patients with increased respiratory effort may have pulsus paradoxus even without pericardial disease.

Laboratory Data

Laboratory findings are nonspecific, with leukocytosis, an elevation of the erythrocyte sedimentation rate (ESR), and occasionally a modest elevation of cardiac enzymes (CPK-MB). Chest radiograph reveals enlargement of the cardiothymic silhouette in the presence of a pericardial effusion. The cardiac size may be normal in patients with pericarditis without a significant effusion. In the presence of tamponade, pulmonary edema may occur with Kerley B lines. Pneumonias may be associated with pleural effusion. Figure 44-1 shows chest radiographs of a patient with purulent pericarditis before and after pericardiocentesis. Various electrocardiogram (ECG) patterns are possible in pericarditis/myocarditis, including ST- and T-wave changes with ST-segment elevation (concave upward ST-segment elevation), T-wave inversion, and PR-segment depression.[25,103] The ECG also may reveal decreased QRS amplitude if an associated pericardial effusion is present.

Echocardiography will demonstrate the presence and location of the pericardial effusion. With a subcostal approach, the echocardiogram can be used to guide pericardiocentesis (see later). In patients with pericarditis with no significant effusion, echocardiography may be normal. If cardiac tamponade is seen, it is often possible to see diastolic collapse of the right atrium. Figure 44-2 shows an echocardiogram of a patient with a large pericardial effusion and tamponade. Pulsed Doppler flow mapping of mitral valve inflow can demonstrate decreased mitral inflow during inspiration in patients with tamponade. Doppler flow analysis of the superior vena caval flow pattern can be helpful in diagnosing constrictive pericarditis.[22]

Management

The management of patients with pericarditis depends in large part on its etiology and on whether a significant pericardial effusion appears. Cardiac tamponade is a medical emergency, and relief of the tamponade must be carried out as quickly as possible. Despite the presence of an already high central venous pressure, fluid administration and volume resuscitation may be helpful in improving ventricular filling while preparations are made for pericardiocentesis. Use of diuretics may further impair cardiac filling and may have catastrophic results. In the presence of a significant pericardial effusion, stroke volume is fixed, and any change in systemic vascular resistance or myocardial contractility can result in cardiovascular collapse. Similarly, the switch from spontaneous to positive-pressure ventilation can significantly decrease ventricular filling, resulting in cardiovascular collapse.

Pericardiocentesis

Pericardiocentesis may be performed in the intensive care unit or in the catheterization laboratory, with or without echocardiographic/fluoroscopic guidance. We prefer to perform emergency pericardiocentesis in the intensive care unit, because it avoids the need to transport a critically ill patient

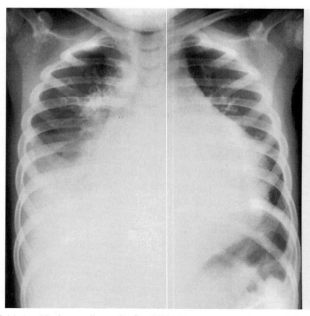 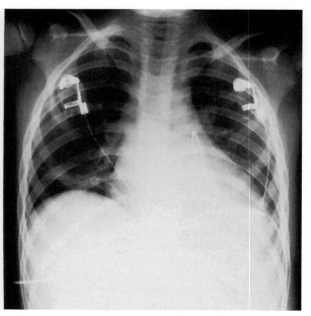

FIGURE 44-1   AP chest radiograph of a child with purulent pericarditis before (*left*) and after (*right*) drainage of the effusion with a percutaneous catheter. Note the decrease in the cardiac silhouette after drainage. The catheter is seen on the x-ray on the right.

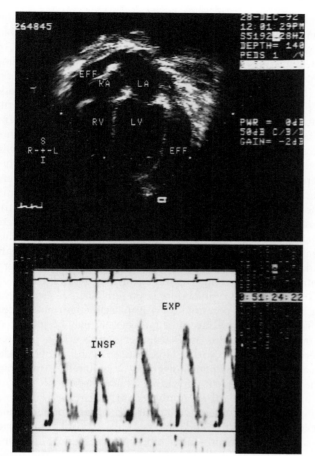

FIGURE 44-2 Echocardiogram of a child with a large pericardial effusion and cardiac tamponade. *Top,* An apical four-chamber view shows the atria (RA and LA), the ventricles (RV and LV), and the effusion (EFF). Note the collapse of the right atrium. *Bottom,* The mitral inflow velocity is measured by pulsed Doppler flow measurement. With inspiration (INSP), the flow is markedly decreased as compared with expiration (EXP).

should establish the position of the needle relative to the pericardial sac before advancing the needle farther. If echocardiography is not available for the procedure, the physician can monitor the ECG signal for the presence of an "injury current." One of the chest (V) leads of the ECG is attached to the needle with an alligator clip. When the needle comes in contact with the heart, an injury current produces elevation of the ST segment (Fig. 44-3). However, disagreement exists in the literature as to the value of ECG monitoring.[101,179] If an injury current is observed on ECG monitoring, the needle is withdrawn slightly.

Sedation before the procedure with a combination of a benzodiazepine, an opioid, or other agent is desirable unless the patient is unconscious or extremely unstable. When sedative/analgesic agents are administered, the previously mentioned issues concerning spontaneous ventilation and changes in systemic vascular resistance and cardiac contractility should be considered. As pericardiocentesis is a superficial procedure, it can be performed with infiltration of a local anesthetic agent in the older cooperative patient. Pericardiocentesis in a struggling child can be dangerous and should be avoided until adequate sedation has been achieved. The patient's ECG should be monitored continuously, and blood pressure and respiratory rate should be checked frequently throughout the procedure. It is helpful to elevate the head of the bed slightly for the procedure. We use a technique similar to that previously described by Lock[101] and Zahn.[179] The subxiphoid approach is generally used, with the entry site just below and to the left of the xiphoid process. The area is cleansed with an iodine solution, and the skin and subcutaneous tissues are anesthetized with 1% lidocaine. The needle is directed toward the left shoulder and is angled inferior to the anterior chest wall (~30 degrees posteriorly). We prefer to use either a thin-walled vascular-access needle or an over-the-needle intravenous catheter (18 or 20 gauge, depending on the patient's age) to perform the pericardiocentesis, although in larger patients, it may be necessary to use a spinal needle (3 or 3.5 inches) to reach the effusion. Prepackaged kits containing needles, guide wires, and pigtail catheters are available from several manufacturers. Often, a "pop" is felt as the needle punctures the parietal pericardium. As soon as fluid returns, the needle is held in place. The return of bloody fluid is disconcerting, but it may indicate that the pericardial fluid is bloody, rather than puncture of the ventricular cavity. If echocardiography is not immediately available, several techniques can exclude ventricular puncture. A lower hematocrit of the effusion compared with the

to the cardiac catheterization laboratory. An echocardiogram from the subcostal approach is helpful before the procedure, because it shows the size of the effusion anterior and inferior to the heart, which is where the pericardiocentesis needle is directed. The echocardiogram also provides an estimate of the distance from the skin to the effusion. We generally perform the echocardiogram before, but not during, the actual pericardiocentesis. However, if pericardial fluid is not encountered at the expected depth, an echocardiographic examination

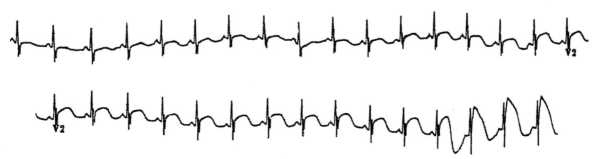

FIGURE 44-3 Electrocardiogram obtained from a needle during pericardiocentesis. As the needle contacts the epicardial surface of the heart, an injury current is produced, resulting in ST-segment elevation. With withdrawal of the needle, the ST segment returns to normal (not shown).

peripheral blood hematocrit or failure of the pericardial blood to clot (or both) suggests that pericardial fluid and not intraventricular blood is being aspirated. It is often not possible to determine the difference between blood and pericardial fluid simply by visual inspection.

Once the physician is confident that the tip of the needle is in the pericardial space, if an over-the-needle catheter is used, the catheter is then advanced off the needle. Whether an introducer needle or an over-the-needle catheter is used, we prefer to use a flexible guide wire (usually a 0.035-inch diameter, 150-cm wire) to replace the initial needle or catheter with a pigtail angiographic catheter by using the Seldinger technique before withdrawal of the fluid. By using a pigtail catheter, the risk of accidental dislodgment of the needle or perforation of the heart is reduced, and it is easier to drain the fluid completely. Additionally, the pigtail catheters have multiple lumens, not just one at the tip of the catheter, so that fluid can be drained even if the end hole is against a structure or becomes occluded with debris. The pigtail catheter may be removed at the end of the procedure, or it may be left in place with a bio-occlusive dressing covering the entry site. If the catheter is left in place, strict aseptic technique must be used whenever the catheter is entered. Flushing the catheter with 1 to 2 mL of heparin (10 units/mL), several times daily, may help keep the catheter patent. The catheter may be either connected to a closed drainage system or manually aspirated as needed. Echocardiography can determine whether a loculated area of effusion is not adequately drained. The catheter also may be used for intermittent injection of a thrombolytic agent such as streptokinase to promote lysis of fibrin and other adhesive processes that may occur with purulent pericarditis.[86]

Laboratory Examination of Pericardial Fluid

The pericardial fluid that is removed should be sent to the laboratory for cell count, Gram stain, and culture (bacterial, fungal, acid-fast bacteria, and viral), as well as cytology if malignant effusion or SLE is suspected. Polymerase chain reactions (PCRs) allows the amplification and identification of viral and *Mycoplasma* genomes, thereby eliminating the need to wait for cultures. As these techniques become more widely applicable, their use may increase the likelihood of identifying a host of infectious agents.

The effusion of bacterial pericarditis typically has a high white blood cell count, predominantly with polymorphonuclear cells, frequently with a positive Gram stain. Viral pericarditis often produces lymphocyte predominance, although significant overlap is present, suggesting that a definite conclusion of the etiology cannot be based on the cell count. Uremic, tuberculous, and histoplasmosis pericarditis often cause bloody effusions. Protein and lactate dehydrogenase (LDH) of the pericardial fluid are generally elevated in most types of pericarditis. Although these measurements are not very specific, they are generally performed.

Specific Management Approaches

Once the effusion is drained and tamponade is relieved, attention is turned toward identification and treatment of the underlying cause of the pericarditis. Patient history

may reveal exposure to a drug or toxin responsible for the inflammatory reaction, a history of trauma, previous exposure to ionizing radiation, a recent surgical procedure, or chronic symptoms suggestive of a malignancy or autoimmune process.

Management approaches beyond the relief of tamponade depend on the specific etiology of the pericarditis. In patients without tamponade who do not have evidence of bacterial infection (fever and leukocytosis), pericardiocentesis may not be necessary. Nonsteroidal anti-inflammatory agents remain the mainstay of therapy for viral, idiopathic, and noninfectious pericarditis. Bed rest may be helpful. Patients with purulent pericarditis require broad-spectrum antibiotic coverage until the organism and its sensitivities are identified. With the possibility of resistant staphylococcal species and the recent increase in the incidence of penicillin-resistant *Pneumococcus*, gram-positive coverage should include vancomycin. Additional gram-negative coverage with a broad-spectrum, third-generation cephalosporin also is suggested. If the possibility of anaerobic infection is present (i.e., if esophageal disease or other potential for a primary mediastinal process is suspected), clindamycin or meropenem may be indicated. Controversy remains as to whether drainage of a purulent pericardial effusion with a large-bore pericardial tube is adequate, or whether pericardiectomy is required to minimize the risk of subsequent pericardial constriction.[116]

Therapy for other nonbacterial infectious causes is directed at the causative organisms. If cultures of pericardial fluid remain negative and the potential for fungal or mycobacterial disease remains high, biopsy of the pericardium may be indicated to allow histologic examination of the tissue. A course of corticosteroids as an adjunct to antituberculous therapy may help prevent constrictive pericarditis and reduce mortality.[64,158]

Management of fungal pericarditis requires aggressive antifungal medications combined with surgical drainage. In histoplasmosis pericarditis, the organism is not present in the pericardial space, and antimicrobial drugs may not be required. Pericardiocentesis may be life-saving in the event of tamponade, but rapid reaccumulation of pericardial fluid is possible.

Some forms of pericarditis, including uremic, viral, and idiopathic pericarditis, may recur. Local instillation of corticosteroids such as triamcinolone has been used with some success in recurrent uremic pericarditis.[112] In patients who have recurrent pericardial effusions despite medical therapy, a pericardial window may be required. Similarly, in patients in whom constrictive pericarditis develops, removal of the pericardium is generally the treatment of choice.[168]

MYOCARDITIS

Overview

Like the pericardium, inflammatory processes of the myocardium have a wide spectrum of clinical presentations and multiple possible etiologic agents. As these disease processes progress, progressive myocyte necrosis can lead to the development of a congestive, dilated cardiomyopathy (DCM). It is estimated that roughly 10% to 15% of cases of DCM are due to biopsy-proven myocarditis.[174] The following discussion considers inflammatory processes of the myocardium.

Although frequently diagnosed as myocarditis, many of the processes involve all three layers of the heart, including the pericardium, myocardium, and endocardium. As such, *pancarditis* may be a more accurate term. Presentations vary from an absence of clinical findings to isolated chest pain, congestive heart failure with a DCM, or dysrhythmias. This wide range of symptoms makes the determination of the exact incidence of myocarditis difficult. Furthermore, a significant discrepancy may exist between myocarditis diagnosed in autopsy studies and that noted clinically, because many cases are subclinical and never manifest symptoms severe enough to warrant medical care, whereas others may present as sudden death due to arrhythmias. Although all ages may be affected, a bimodal pattern is seen, with a higher incidence in infants and teenagers, whereas toddlers and younger children are relatively spared. The reasons for the disparity in the clinical presentation, age at onset, and course of patients are poorly understood.

Etiology

The spectrum of possible infectious and noninfectious etiologies for myocarditis is similar to that of pericarditis (Table 44-3). Infectious agents may produce cardiac damage by direct invasion of myocardial cells, an abnormal immunologic response of the host, or in rare cases, toxin production by the invading organism (e.g., *Corynebacterium diphtheriae*). Despite refinements in identification and viral-isolation techniques and the increased use of PCR, many cases of myocarditis remain idiopathic with no identifiable infectious agent isolated.

Viral Myocarditis

In cases in which the cause can be established, the majority of cases of myocarditis in North America are of a viral etiology. Given its prevalence and the major advances in understanding the molecular biology of viral myocarditis, we discuss it as a prototype. The peculiarities in the presentation and management of other forms of myocarditis are reviewed in separate sections later.

Although several viral agents have been implicated as possible causes of myocarditis (see Table 44-3), enteroviruses (members of the picornavirus family) have been the most frequently identified.[176] Of these agents, coxsackie B is the culprit in more than half of the cases.[60] Other enteroviruses associated with myocarditis include ECHO E6, 9, 11, 22 serotypes. More recently, with the advent of PCR technology, adenovirus has been implicated in a significant percentage of cases.[104,131] A subsequent section of this chapter reviews acquired immunodeficiency virus as a specific cause of myocarditis.

Pathogenesis

The pathogenesis of myocarditis may result from a combination of direct viral infection and immunologic reaction.[100] Viral particles and nucleic acid sequences have been

Table 44-3   Etiology of Myocarditis

Infectious Agents	Noninfectious Etiologies
RNA viruses	Toxins
Adenovirus	Cocaine
Coxsackie A, B	Toluene
Hepatitis A	Chemotherapy
Influenza A, B	Interleukin-2
Lymphocytic	Ethanol
choriomeningitis virus	Cobalt
Mumps	Drug hypersensitivity
Poliovirus	(see Table 44-5)
Echovirus	Autoimmune diseases
Rhabdovirus	SLE
Rhinovirus	JRA
DNA viruses	Giant cell arteritis
Adenovirus	Takayasu arteritis
CMV	Sarcoidosis
Epstein-Barr	Kawasaki syndrome
Hepatitis B	Transplant rejection
Herpes	Peripartum
Varicella	
Variola	
Rubeola	
Togavirus	
Rubella	
Retroviruses	
HIV	
Bacteria	
Streptococcus	
Corynebacterium diphtheriae	
Neisseria meningitidis	
Mycoplasma pneumoniae	
Chlamydia psittaci	
Staphylococcus aureus	
Shigella sonnei	
Enterococcus	
Borrelia burgdorferi	
Parasitic diseases	
Toxoplasmosis	
Trypanosoma cruzi	
Trichinella spiralis	
Echinococcosis	

CMV, cytomegalovirus; SLE, systemic lupus erythematosus; JRA, juvenile rheumatoid arthritis; HIV, human immunodeficiency virus.

identified in myocardial cells after coxsackie infection.[14,20,82,180] Endomyocardial biopsies have yielded a highly variable recovery rate of viral genome in the myocardium of patients with suspected myocarditis, presumably because of the patchy nature of the disease and the variability of sampling techniques.

Virus enters the myocyte via receptor-mediated endocytosis (Fig. 44-4). The details of the cellular events after virus entry have been elucidated in the mouse model. The first step in this process is the attachment of the virus to a myocyte cell-surface adhesion molecule. The prototype adhesion molecule in myocarditis is the coxsackie-adenoviral receptor (CAR). The predominance of coxsackievirus B group and adenovirus as etiologic agents for myocarditis probably results from the fact that they share a common myocardial cell-surface receptor.[12] CAR belongs to the immunoglobulin superfamily. Although its normal cellular function is unknown, the structural features of CAR suggest that it may act as a homophilic cell-adhesion molecule.[170] With the help of certain cofactors that increase the binding efficiency, adeno- or coxsackievirus may attach to CAR on the myocyte surface, after which the CAR

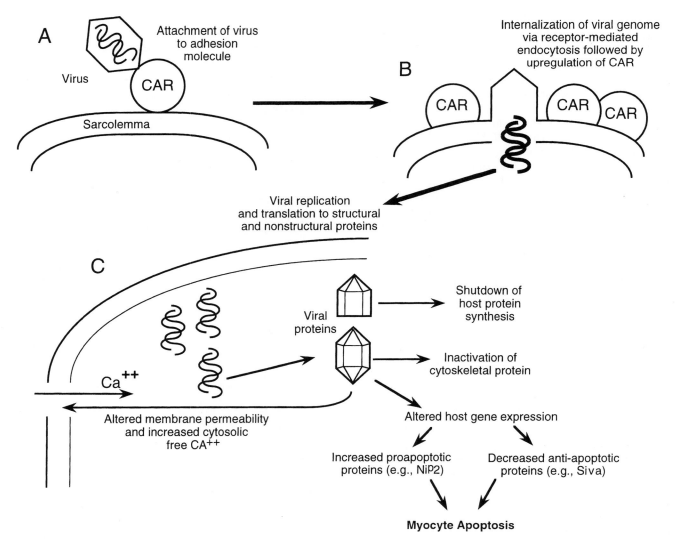

FIGURE 44-4   Sequence of events leading to myocyte apoptosis. **A,** Viral attachment to coxsackie-adenoviral receptor (CAR). **B,** Internalization of viral genome via endocytosis, and **C,** viral replication and translation, which results in cell death.

complex facilitates internalization of the virus.[106,145] In experimental animals, the newborn heart expresses CAR to a far greater extent than does the adult heart, which may partially explain the prevalence of coxsackievirus infection and the acute life-threatening nature of myocarditis in the infant.[79]

After the virus gains entry into the myocyte, it is translated into a single polyprotein, which is then cleaved into structural and nonstructural proteins by virus-specific proteases. Viral genome replication occurs as the viral RNA polymerase transcribes viral negative-strand RNA. As viral replication proceeds, viral products may damage several host cellular processes. Host cellular protein synthesis may be shut down.[43] Cytoskeletal proteins are inactivated.[10] Cytosolic free calcium concentration increases as the coxsackievirus alters plasma membrane and endoplasmic reticulum permeability.[34,169]

Viral infection may promote programmed cell death (apoptosis) in the host myocardium. The mechanism involves up- or downregulation of several host genes by viral products. In particular, mRNA levels of murine *Nip21*, which is equivalent to human *Nip2*, are decreased. Under normal circumstances, *Nip2* binds to Bcl 2 to promote cell survival.[177]

Presumably, reduced levels of *Nip2* would lead to apoptosis. Similarly, infection with coxsackievirus B3 increases transcription of the proapoptotic protein Siva.[70] Apoptosis appears to follow the binding of Siva to the viral capsid protein VP2 and then to the CD27 surface receptor. The Siva-VP2-CD27 complex may lead to caspase 3 production, which in turn initiates apoptosis. These findings may explain the fact that susceptible mice die within 4 days of coxsackievirus infection, even though no histologic evidence of myocarditis is seen.[69]

The immune response to viral infection is crucial in the pathogenesis of myocarditis. Several observations support this theory, including the demonstration of immune complexes in the myocardium,[127] the occurrence of myocarditis in autoimmune diseases such as SLE, and the clinical response of some patients to immunosuppressive and other immune-modulating therapies.

The details of the immune response to myocardial infection have emerged from numerous experiments using murine models of enterovirus infection (Fig. 44-5).[45,89] The initial phase of acute myocarditis occurs within the first 4 days

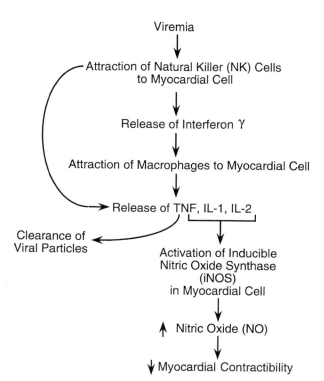

Viremia

↓

Attraction of Natural Killer (NK) Cells to Myocardial Cell

↓

Release of Interferon γ

↓

Attraction of Macrophages to Myocardial Cell

↓

Release of TNF, IL-1, IL-2

Clearance of Viral Particles

Activation of Inducible Nitric Oxide Synthase (iNOS) in Myocardial Cell

↓

↑ Nitric Oxide (NO)

↓

↓ Myocardial Contractibility

FIGURE 44-5 Acute (day 1–4) white blood cell and cytokine response in the myocardium after viremia. TNF, tumor necrosis factor; IL, interleukin.

of viral infection and is characterized by viremia. Natural killer (NK) cells are the first white blood cells to invade the myocardium. NK cells release interferon γ, which attracts macrophages. Subsequently, NK cells and macrophages express a number of cytokines, which amplify the inflammatory response, including interleukins 1 and 2 and tumor necrosis factor.

The inflammatory and cytokine responses have both beneficial and detrimental effects. NK cells appear to target only virus-infected myocytes and thus retard viral replication.[58] The rapid clearance of viral particles appears dependent on tumor necrosis factor. Interferon inhibits viral proliferation. Conversely, interleukins 1 and 2 and tumor necrosis factor have profound negative inotropic effects.[173] Nitric oxide may be responsible for mediating the cytokine-induced myocardial depression.[47] However, complex effects also apply to nitric oxide, as suggested by the fact that inducible nitric oxide synthase–deficient mice exhibit delayed clearance of virus and more severe myocarditis.[181]

Cell-mediated immunity affects the host response during the subacute phase of myocarditis (days 4 to 14) (Fig. 44-6). Cytotoxic T-lymphocytes, which express the CD4 or CD8 co-receptor molecule, invade the myocardium. The major histocompatibility complex class I antigens on the myocyte surface present viral particles to the cytotoxic T lymphocytes. Tumor necrosis factor α and interferon γ facilitate cell-to-cell adhesion necessary for lysis of the infected cardiomyocyte by the cytotoxic T lymphocyte. Lysis proceeds after a second, co-stimulatory signal from the antigen-bearing cardiomyocyte fully activates the lymphocyte.[118] Whereas cell-mediated immunity is necessary for viral clearance, persistent T-cell activation may aggravate myocardial damage and lead to

chronic myocarditis or DCM.[128] Chronic autoimmune myocarditis may involve T cells targeted against cardiac myosin epitopes, which mimic those of the infecting agent.[32] Humoral immunity with the production of neutralizing antibody by B lymphocytes also aids in viral clearance. High-dose immunoglobulin therapy is clearly beneficial in myocarditis secondary to Kawasaki disease and also may benefit patients with viral myocarditis.[36]

Clinical Manifestations

Manifestations of myocarditis range from an asymptomatic patient to obvious signs of congestive heart failure. Most older children are somewhere in between these two extremes, with an acute febrile illness and a minor degree of cardiovascular involvement, such as tachycardia or isolated ECG changes. The most common cardiovascular symptom is chest pain, which may be the sole complaint in some patients.[65,68] Other presentations include isolated ventricular ectopy without obvious signs of cardiac failure. Syncope may result from ventricular tachycardia or less frequently from high-grade atrioventricular (AV) block. The ECG may be normal in between spells, making it more difficult to establish the diagnosis. Sudden death is the most severe presentation, and in such cases, the diagnosis of myocarditis is made only at autopsy.[124] Myocarditis and cardiomyopathy also can be causes of sudden death during general anesthesia and surgery among patients not previously suspected of having heart disease.[160]

In most cases, the multisystem effects and symptoms of the underlying viral illness outweigh the symptoms related to the cardiovascular system. However, signs and symptoms related to cardiac involvement may be seen. A tachycardia out of proportion to the fever may be present. Signs of cardiac failure such as cardiomegaly, pulsus alternans, hepatomegaly, and third or fourth heart sounds may be present. Decreased exercise tolerance, dyspnea, and easy fatiguability may be the only complaints in some children. In infants, poor feeding may be the presenting sign. Associated symptoms such as myalgias, pneumonitis, exanthems, or lymphadenopathy may be suggestive of a viral etiology.

The presentation in infants stands out because it is often very acute and life-threatening. Irritability and poor feeding give way after a few hours to signs of overwhelming shock and heart failure. Respiratory distress, cyanosis, thready pulses, and gallop rhythm all suggest an infant in extremis. Because of the similarity of this presentation to ductal-dependent left-sided obstructive lesions such as coarctation, prostaglandin E_1 is sometimes given before the recognition of the myocarditis in very young infants.

Laboratory and Electrocardiographic Findings

The majority of laboratory and ECG findings of myocarditis are nonspecific. Elevations of CPK and LDH are present in 50% to 75% of cases with ST-segment abnormalities.[67] However, cardiac troponin I (cTnI) levels now are the most sensitive diagnostic test for biopsy-proven myocarditis.[149] In addition, cTnI levels may be of prognostic value, because they correlate with ejection fraction and clinical heart failure.[15] The complete blood count reveals a leukocytosis in 50% of patients.[55] The presence of eosinophilia should prompt

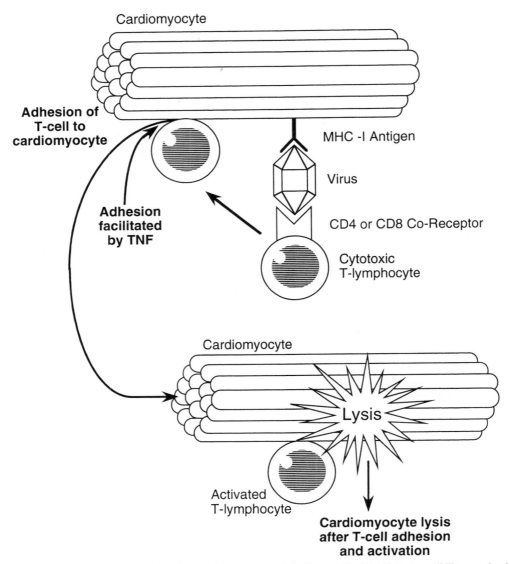

FIGURE 44-6   Effects of cell-mediated immunity during subacute phase of myocarditis (day 4–14). Major histocompatibility complex (MHC) class I antigen on myocyte presents virus to CD4 or CD8 receptor on T lymphocyte. Tumor necrosis factor (TNF) facilitates T-cell adhesion to cardiomyocyte. Cardiomyocyte lysis occurs after T-cell activation.

the search for a parasitic etiology of the myocarditis. Another nonspecific indicator of an inflammatory process is an elevated ESR.[76]

ECG changes in myocarditis also are nonspecific and only support the diagnosis. The ECG most commonly reveals nonspecific, ST-T–wave abnormalities. Other abnormalities include ventricular and atrial ectopy, conduction defects, sinus tachycardia, and T-wave inversion. The presence of ventricular ectopy in a febrile, irritable infant represents myocarditis until proven otherwise and should prompt immediate admission to an intensive care unit. Occasionally the ECG may point toward an alternate diagnosis. For example, Pompe disease has a characteristic ECG pattern of a short PR interval with very large precordial voltages. Similarly, the presence of ventricular pre-excitation (Wolff-Parkinson-White syndrome) may raise the question of unrecognized sustained tachyarrhythmias as a cause of ventricular dysfunction.

Diagnostic Approach

Because of the wide clinical spectrum in presentation and the diversity of etiologic agents, the diagnostic approach to the patient with myocarditis must include a strategy that attempts to include several etiologic possibilities. A thorough history is imperative and should focus on the possibility of toxic ingestion, drug ingestion (including illicit and over-the-counter medications), trauma, and possible exposure to infectious agents (including a complete travel history). Past history should include immunization status, because several infectious diseases of childhood (diphtheria, polio virus) are included in the differential diagnosis. Additionally, the history may reveal signs or symptoms of previously undiagnosed collagen vascular disorder or inflammatory bowel disease. Although echocardiography will not establish the diagnosis, it will rule out complicating features such as pericardial effusion and structural cardiac lesions, which may be confused with myocarditis. Additionally, echocardiography can provide an estimate of myocardial function. In infants with an ECG pattern consistent with acute myocardial infarction, anomalous origin of the left coronary artery from the pulmonary artery should be considered and excluded, either by echocardiography or by cardiac catheterization. Cardiac catheterization and endomyocardial biopsy may be indicated to rule out other disorders associated with congestive failure such as glycogen storage disease type II (Pompe disease), endocardial fibroelastosis, and structural cardiac defects. Also included in the list are metabolic abnormalities that may affect cardiac function, including hypoglycemia, hypocalcemia, and disorders of carnitine metabolism.

The diagnosis of viral myocarditis is generally based on circumstantial evidence such as a recent viral infection and the sudden onset of cardiac dysfunction while ruling out other diagnostic possibilities. Although viral cultures (pharyngeal, rectal) should be obtained, the "window of opportunity" for viral isolation is narrow, and therefore isolation of the virus is often not possible. Use of PCR may allow identification of the viral genome even when cultures are negative. Supportive evidence for a viral etiology can be obtained by a fourfold or greater increase in antibody titer between acute and convalescent sera. In addition to these titers, the presence of Epstein-Barr virus infection should be investigated with serology. Routine bacterial and fungal cultures of blood should be obtained in addition to serology to rule out treponemal infection (VDRL or RPR).

Because of the varied etiologic and clinical spectrum of myocarditis, the diagnosis of infectious myocarditis may require endomyocardial biopsy. Edwards and associates[38] suggested a criterion for myocarditis that includes five or more lymphocytes per 20 high-power fields during histologic examination of the endomyocardial specimen. Several biopsy specimens (5 to 10) may be needed because the inflammatory process is focal. These criteria were subsequently refined with the introduction of the so-called Dallas criteria, which state that *active* myocarditis is present when routine light-microscopy examination of the biopsy specimen reveals lymphocytic infiltration and myocytolysis.[6] Borderline or ongoing myocarditis exists in the presence of lymphocytic infiltration alone without myocytolysis. The specimen is considered negative if both lymphocytic infiltration and myocytolysis are absent. Although the Dallas criteria remain in widespread use, most clinicians believe that they underestimate the true incidence of myocarditis, probably because of the patchy nature of myocardial inflammation and the high degree of interobserver variability.[146]

Endomyocardial biopsy also may be valuable in ruling out other disorders in the differential diagnosis such as endocardial fibroelastosis and Pompe disease. In addition to histologic examination, new techniques of RNA/DNA hybridization allow virus identification in the biopsy specimen.[181] Martin and colleagues[104] used PCR to analyze 38 myocardial samples of patients with myocarditis obtained during endomyocardial biopsy. In 26 of the 38 samples, viral genome was isolated by using PCR. The viral genomes isolated included adenovirus (15), enterovirus (8), herpesvirus (2), and CMV (1). Four patients had positive viral cultures that matched the PCR findings. The authors concluded that PCR offered a rapid and accurate means of diagnosing viral infection in patients with myocarditis. They also noted that the most prevalent virus they isolated was adenovirus, as opposed to the enteroviruses that are generally thought to be the most common viral pathogens in myocarditis.

In addition to endomyocardial biopsy, nuclear medicine imaging techniques may provide a means of identifying myocardial inflammation. Indium-111 monoclonal antimyosin antibody imaging has been shown to diagnose myocarditis accurately.[178] In patients with tracer uptake in the left ventricular myocardium, active myocarditis also was present on biopsy. Further studies are needed to define the role of these methods in the diagnosis of myocarditis.

Management

Pharmacologic and General Supportive Care The cornerstones of treatment for myocarditis, regardless of the etiology, include removal of any offending agent/toxin and supportive care. Once the diagnosis is established, continuous monitoring in an intensive care unit is recommended because of the risks of ventricular ectopy. Offending factors such as toxins, pharmacologic agents, or excessive catecholamines should be eliminated. Limitation of activity or bed rest is recommended, because clinical experience suggests that early ambulation and activity may favor viral replication and ongoing myocardial damage. Supportive care is directed at maintaining adequate cardiac output and systemic oxygen delivery. The use of invasive hemodynamic monitoring is based on the patient's clinical status. Although routine use of a pulmonary artery catheter is not recommended, invasive hemodynamic monitoring may be required for the appropriate monitoring of intravascular status and response to inotropic medications. However, the benefits of such monitoring should be weighed against the risks of ventricular ectopy during insertion. Additionally, proper placement may be difficult, requiring fluoroscopic guidance, in the child with a dilated, poorly contractile heart.

The use of inotropic agents may be indicated in patients with signs of poor cardiac output. Because of the irritable state of the myocardium, arrhythmias may be seen with catecholamine administration. In our experience, such patients may respond to the phosphodiesterase (PDE) inhibitor milrinone with less arrhythmogenicity. This agent, which inhibits PDE and thereby increases the intracellular concentration of cyclic adenosine monophosphate (cAMP), possesses cardiovascular properties similar to those of dobutamine (see Chapter 7). As such, a positive inotropic effect with peripheral vasodilation is seen. In addition, milrinone improves the diastolic function of the myocardium, which may result in improved ventricular relaxation and increased filling volumes during diastole. For patients with no signs of ectopy, empiric administration of dobutamine at low doses (5 to 10 mcg/kg/min) may be tried without invasive monitoring. More aggressive inotropic intervention, such as the combination of inotropic agents and vasodilators, may require direct measurements of cardiac output and systemic vascular resistance.

Although cardiac failure responds to inotropic agents in the majority of patients, ongoing cardiac dysfunction may require mechanical support. Because of the reversible nature of many of the etiologies of myocarditis, mechanical support with ventricular assist devices (VADs), intra aortic balloon counterpulsation, or extracorporeal membrane oxygenation (ECMO) may be indicated in some patients. The indication for VAD or ECMO usually involves the patient with shock who is either unresponsive to inotropes or in whom ventricular or supraventricular arrhythmias are increasing while receiving inotropes. The choice between ECMO and VAD depends on the size of the patient and the anticipated duration of mechanical support (see Chapter 21). ECMO can be used in the smallest patients, but the duration of support is usually limited to approximately 3 weeks, during which continuous anticoagulation is required. Separate left atrial drainage or decompression via a patent foramen ovale may be required to prevent overdistention of the left heart. Other disadvantages include platelet and red cell destruction by the pump, necessitating frequent transfusions. Despite these limitations, ECMO has been a very useful tool to support the myocarditis patient, because a significant portion will recover sufficient myocardial function to allow weaning from ECMO in 2 to 3 weeks. In the adult-sized patient, the paracorporeal VAD allows support for months, even years, without the need for continuous anticoagulation, so that bridge to transplantation is a viable option. The large blood chamber volume (>50 mL) has limited the pediatric application until recently. Hetzer and coworkers[72] reported a miniaturized, pneumatically driven, pediatric biventricular assist device (the "Berlin Heart") with a chamber volume as low as 12 mL, which has allowed support for up to 98 days in patients as small as the newborn. Bleeding may occur as patients using this system receive continuous heparin administration.

Arrhythmias constitute the second life-threatening complication of myocarditis. High-degree AV block may occur in viral myocarditis, but it is especially characteristic of lupus carditis and Lyme carditis. Although patients may respond to isoproterenol administration, such chronotropic drugs entail the risk of inducing ventricular tachycardia, particularly in viral myocarditis. (The risk of developing ventricular tachyarrhythmias after chronotropic therapy is perhaps less pronounced in other, nonviral forms of myocarditis.) Therefore cardiac pacing is the preferred therapy for life-threatening bradyarrhythmias. Transcutaneous pacing can be placed rapidly and is effective during the resuscitation phase. A temporary transvenous pacemaker can be substituted after the resuscitation is complete. If heart block persists for more than 2 to 3 weeks, the physician should consider replacing the temporary pacemaker with an implanted permanent pacemaker.

Aside from AV block, ventricular ectopy and even sudden death from ventricular fibrillation may occur in myocarditis.[124] Whereas lidocaine has been considered standard therapy for ventricular ectopy, no controlled studies support its efficacy in myocarditis. Both clinical experience and studies in other populations, such as cardiac arrest or myocardial infarction, have failed to support its efficacy in ventricular tachyarrhythmias.[142] Conversely, amiodarone may improve survival after cardiac arrest due to ventricular tachyarrhythmias.[92] The American Heart Association now recommends amiodarone, 5 mg/kg IV, as the first-line antiarrhythmic therapy in pulseless ventricular tachycardia or ventricular fibrillation after defibrillation has been attempted.[3] Lidocaine has become a second-tier choice. Antiarrhythmic agents other than lidocaine and amiodarone have a high likelihood of worsening

ventricular function and thus are problematic in patients with myocarditis. Aside from pharmacologic therapy, correction of electrolyte imbalances such as hypokalemia and hypomagnesemia may be particularly effective in the treatment of ventricular ectopy. The occurrence of such electrolyte disturbances should be evaluated both initially and periodically during therapy, because diuretic therapy can cause excessive urinary losses of both of these cations.

Supraventricular tachyarrhythmias (SVTs) based on a re-entrant mechanism (AV nodal re-entrant tachycardia or AV re-entrant tachycardia) are treated initially with adenosine, 50 to 200 mcg/kg IV, if the patient is hemodynamically stable. Intra-atrial re-entry tachycardia (atrial flutter) often is not responsive to adenosine. In such cases, and in patients with frequent reinitiation of SVTs, amiodarone is usually the drug of choice. Electrical cardioversion is the treatment of choice in the unstable patient but is of no value in patients with termination and immediate reinitiation of their tachycardia. In the past, digoxin has been used to treat SVT in myocarditis. However, experimental and clinical evidence suggests caution with this approach during the acute phase of myocarditis, because digoxin was found to increase myocardial cytokine production.[109] The intracellular calcium loading caused by digoxin may induce or worsen ventricular arrhythmias.

Once the patient's cardiovascular status is stabilized, a gradual switch to more prolonged, oral therapy is indicated. This therapy may include diuretics and peripheral vasodilators. These agents also may be the first-line therapy in patients with minimal to moderate degrees of myocardial dysfunction. The role of digoxin in chronic congestive failure remains controversial for several reasons. If the heart is still inflamed, digoxin use will increase the risk of arrhythmias. Patients with myocarditis also usually have poor diastolic function, which is not improved with digoxin. If the choice is made to administer digitalis, digitalization should be accomplished over a 24- to 36-hour period, with 75% of the usual dose, because of an increased risk of ventricular arrhythmias with active myocarditis and the administration of digoxin.

Diuretics are used in the initial and long-term treatment of congestive failure after myocarditis. Several appropriate choices for intravenous diuretic therapy are available, including furosemide and bumetanide. The addition of the oral agent metolazone may improve diuresis in resistant patients. With the use of diuretic therapy, careful monitoring of serum potassium and magnesium is recommended, so as not to increase the risk of ventricular ectopy. Additionally, low doses of diuretics should be administered initially (furosemide, 0.1 to 0.25 mg/kg), as excess diuresis may lead to an excessive reduction of preload and cardiac output. Once the acute episode of congestive failure has been controlled, thiazide diuretics may be adequate, while avoiding the risk of hypercalciuria and nephrocalcinosis seen with furosemide. The addition of spironolactone to this long-term regimen may limit the need for potassium supplementation. Recent data in adults with congestive heart failure suggest that spironolactone also may improve survival,[134a] although these data may or may not apply to children or to patients with myocarditis.

Vasodilators, in particular, the angiotensin-converting enzyme (ACE) inhibitors, may improve symptoms in the chronic setting. Although several new options for ACE inhibitors exist that make once-a-day dosing possible, little clinical experience is available with their use in children. Therefore we prefer to use either captopril (3 to 4 times a day) or twice-a-day dosing with enalapril. During the acute phase, the ACE inhibitor enalaprilat may be administered intravenously, when oral drug administration is not possible.

Immunosuppressive Therapy Although direct viral damage to myocardial cells may be responsible for the cardiac dysfunction in myocarditis, clinical and laboratory evidence also points to immune dysfunction and altered cellular immunity as playing the primary role in many cases.[90] Based on these findings, it is speculated that immunosuppressive therapy may alter the course of viral myocarditis.[24] However, the possible beneficial effects must be weighed against the risks of progressive viral replication during the administration of immunosuppressive agents. Both dramatic improvement and fatal progression of myocarditis have been described after immunosuppressive therapy.[2,36,144] Once myocarditis is confirmed by biopsy, the decision to administer such therapy must take into account the morbidity and mortality associated with the use of such agents versus that associated with myocarditis. It also has been recommended that the decision to administer immunosuppressive therapy be based on the histologic findings. Patients with significant lymphocyte infiltration on the biopsy are the primary group in whom immunosuppressive therapy is indicated. Myocardial uptake of gallium-67 also has been suggested to be helpful in predicting those patients that will have a beneficial response to immunosuppressive agents.[125]

Drucker and colleagues[36] noted improved ventricular function and a trend toward improved survival at 12 months for children who received intravenous immunoglobulin, 2 g/kg, as a single dose to treat biopsy-proven myocarditis. To date no randomized controlled trial of immunoglobulin therapy has been conducted in pediatric viral myocarditis. Randomized controlled trials of either prednisone alone or prednisone plus cyclosporine in adults with viral myocarditis have shown either small or no treatment effect.[107,130] At this point, the efficacy and optimal combination of agents (corticosteroids, cyclosporine, azathioprine, immunoglobulin, anti-thymocyte monoclonal antibodies) as well as their impact on the natural history of myocarditis remain to be demonstrated. This uncertainty about the benefits of immunomodulation in viral myocarditis stands in marked contrast to the proven benefits of such therapy in autoimmune myocarditis from lupus erythematosus, Kawasaki syndrome, polymyositis, and others (see later).

Antiviral Therapy Effective antiviral therapy against the common causes of viral myocarditis is under development. Pleconaril represents a new class of drugs targeted specifically against picornaviruses, including the enteroviruses.[140] This agent integrates into the capsid of the picornavirus and thereby prevents viral attachment to myocyte receptors. Isolated reports have been made of benefit from pleconaril among children with life-threatening viral infections. However, the drug is still considered experimental, and special waivers from an Institutional Review Board and the Food and Drug Administration are required for its use.

Outcome and Natural History

Various factors affect the eventual outcome and natural history of myocarditis, including the etiology, the patient's general state of health before the onset of the illness, and the extent of myocardial inflammation. Although mortality early in the course is rare, death may occur related to ventricular arrhythmias, progressive cardiac failure, or conduction disturbances. Early mortality is especially high in infants and young children, approaching 10% to 15%.[111,178] McCarthy and colleagues[111] recently suggested that adolescent and adult patients may have a better long-term prognosis after fulminant myocarditis, with up to 93% transplant-free survival after 11 years. "Fulminant" was defined by the need for inotropes or VAD. Patients with acute (nonfulminant) myocarditis had worse outcomes, with only 45% long-term, transplant-free survival.

Dilated Cardiomyopathies

After the acute phase, the long-term outcome of patients with myocarditis follows one of three courses: complete recovery, mild residual cardiac dysfunction, or chronic congestive failure that requires long-term medication. The latter patients may have frequent relapses of congestive failure that require hospital admission and inotropic administration. It is this group that may have progressive cardiovascular dysfunction and eventually require cardiac transplantation. This group bears striking similarities to patients with dilated hearts and congestive heart failure of unknown etiology. The use of PCR to detect viral genome in patients with DCM has established a causal link between myocarditis and DCM.[14,50] Approximately one third of children with DCM may exhibit gradual improvement, to the point of normal cardiac function, after a mean duration of 4.5 years.[96] See Chapters 47 and 48 for further discussion of DCM.

Other Causes of Dilated Cardiomyopathies

An unusual cause of DCM is chronic catecholamine excess related to a pheochromocytoma. Although other signs and symptoms, including hypertension, palpitations, or headaches, are the usual presenting symptoms of pheochromocytoma, at least three reports in the literature describe the occurrence of congestive heart failure with a DCM eventually linked to a pheochromocytoma.[31,56,175] We previously reported a 14-year-old boy with left-sided weakness after a cerebrovascular accident.[31] Workup revealed a DCM and a mural thrombus. Persistent hypertension prompted further investigation that resulted in the diagnosis of a pheochromocytoma.

Cardiomyopathy is a well-recognized and potentially reversible consequence of catecholamine excess. Degenerative and fibrotic myocardial changes have been described in autopsy specimens of patients dying with pheochromocytoma since the early 1900s. In some cases, lymphocytic infiltration and cell necrosis may mimic those changes seen with postviral myocarditis. The majority of patients with pheochromocytoma have changes in the myocardium on autopsy; however, evidence of myocardial dysfunction may not be observed clinically. The pathogenesis of catecholamine-induced cardiomyopathy is multifactorial. Excessive catecholamine levels lead to (1) downregulation of β-adrenergic receptors and a reduction of myofibers; (2) increased sarcolemmal permeability to calcium and increased calcium concentration in the cytosol with a direct toxic effect on the myocardium; (3) the potential for coronary vasospasm and ischemia; (4) reperfusion injury and free radical formation after vasospasm; and (5) direct toxic myocardial effects of the intermediates of catecholamine metabolism.

The treatment of DCM secondary to pheochromocytoma consists primarily of adrenergic blockade. Effective adrenergic blockade can result in a dramatic and relatively rapid reversal, even with severe left ventricular systolic dysfunction. After stabilization and control of blood pressure with medical therapy, removal of the pheochromocytoma is indicated.

Acquired Immunodeficiency Syndrome

Cardiac manifestations of AIDS include pericardial effusion, myocarditis, DCM, endocarditis, pulmonary hypertension, malignant neoplasms, coronary artery disease, and drug-induced cardiotoxicity. Cardiomyopathy associated with AIDS and HIV infection is being recognized more frequently as experience with AIDS accumulates. Cardiomyopathy and congestive heart failure associated with HIV were first reported in 1986 by Cohen and colleagues.[26] The authors reported three adults with AIDS who died of DCM. None of these patients had clinical or pathologic evidence of Kaposi's sarcoma in the myocardium, suggesting that the cardiomyopathy was a result of the HIV infection. Subsequently, DCM and myocarditis with HIV infection have been reported numerous times.[1,26,61,74,84,85,95] Himelman and coworkers[74] presented a prospective study of cardiac abnormalities in HIV-positive patients (51 with AIDS, 13 with AIDS-related complex, and 6 without symptoms). Echocardiography revealed DCM in 11% with a DCM, pericardial effusions in 10%, and pleural effusions in 6%. The inpatient population in this study had a higher incidence of echocardiographic abnormalities.

More recently, the potential for cardiac involvement in infants and children with AIDS has been increasingly recognized. In a prospective cohort study in infants with vertical transmission of HIV, the incidence of cardiomyopathy was 3.8 per 100 person-years during the first 6 months of life and 9 per 100 person-years after the second 6 months of life.[33] In the same cohort of patients, the incidence of cardiomyopathy was 30% in infants in whom encephalopathy developed.[28] The exact process responsible for cardiomyopathy in HIV-infected infants remains unknown. Postulated etiologies include direct viral invasion/destruction of cardiac myocytes,[95] immune-mediated disease, drug-related complications, and opportunistic infections. Among the opportunistic infections, *Toxoplasma gondii*, *Mycobacterium tuberculosis*, and *Cryptococcus neoformans* are the organisms most commonly associated with AIDS myocarditis. Less frequently, *Mycobacterium avium-intracellulare* complex, *Aspergillus fumigatus*, *Candida albicans*, *Histoplasma capsulatum*, *Coccidioides immitis*, CMV, adenovirus, and herpes simplex have been associated with AIDS myocarditis.

Grody and associates[61] found evidence suggesting that HIV may be a direct cardiac pathogen. The authors studied myocardial tissue from 23 patients who had died of AIDS. With in situ DNA hybridization techniques, the investigators detected HIV sequences in 6 of 22 patients examined. The principal site appeared to be the cardiac myocyte. However, the authors found no correlation with location of the cells showing a positive hybridization signal or their number and the patient's clinical course.

DCM is a clinically significant form of cardiac involvement among children with AIDS. Patients with a history of myocarditis, a low CD4 cell count, and elevated antiheart antibodies may be at increased risk for DCM.[71] The DCM in children with AIDS appears with signs similar to those of DCM from other causes: shortness of breath, easy fatiguability, tachypnea, sinus tachycardia, rales, hepatosplenomegaly, and cardiomegaly. ECG changes include ST-T–wave abnormalities, reduced voltage, and left ventricular hypertrophy. The echocardiogram shows dilation of the left atrium and left ventricle, ventricular hypokinesis, and decreased shortening fraction. Progressive right atrial and right ventricular enlargement also may occur, along with thickening of the tricuspid valve. Because of repeated pulmonary infections, pulmonary hypertension may ensue, which subsequently produces right ventricular enlargement and hypertrophy and right atrial enlargement.[84,85]

Infants and children receiving immune globulin for prophylaxis against bacterial infection have demonstrated a decreased incidence of cardiomyopathy compared with controls.[99] The latter effect has been attributed to the immune-modulating effects of IV immune globulin. Although left ventricular function has been correlated with the initial extent of immune suppression, the degree of cardiac dysfunction does not necessarily follow the overall disease progression, so that worsening cardiac function appears to be independent of worsening immune function.

Poor nutritional status has been shown to affect the progression of HIV-associated cardiomyopathy, as has co-infection with the Epstein-Barr virus. Case reports have suggested that AIDS cardiomyopathy may be associated with selenium deficiency, as selenium supplementation appeared to improve cardiac function.[88] Drug toxicity may lead to cardiac manifestations in the AIDS patient. Amphotericin B, foscarnet, zidovudine, and interferon have all been associated with cardiomyopathy in this population.[8,18,35,151]

The treatment of myocarditis or DCM is aimed at both symptomatic improvement and treating the underlying cause. Children with AIDS and cardiac involvement due to viral or nonviral opportunistic infections will benefit from appropriate antimicrobial therapy. In addition, the child should receive anticongestive therapy with cardiotonic agents such as dobutamine or milrinone, afterload reduction, and diuretics. Patients also should be treated for the primary disease with the evolving armamentarium of anti-HIV agents. However, the drugs used to treat various infections in AIDS patients or to treat the disease itself may have a direct cardiotoxic effect that can exacerbate the compromised myocardial function.

Other Infectious Etiologies

Although viruses lead the list of etiologies of myocarditis, several nonviral infectious agents have been implicated in the pathogenesis of myocarditis, including bacterial, rickettsial, protozoal, fungal, mycobacterial, and parasitic agents. Primary bacterial invasion of the myocardium is rare; however, myocardial invasion and abscess formation may occur with any overwhelming bacterial infection.[13] Additionally, a hypersensitivity reaction resulting in myocarditis has been reported with meningococcemia. This hypersensitivity myocarditis occurs 4 to 7 days after the initial presentation of the illness and may lead to serious dysrhythmias and conduction block.[66]

Diphtheria and Shigella

Other organisms such as *Corynebacterium diphtheriae* and *Shigella sonnei* can produce myocardial damage through exotoxin production without direct myocardial involvement. Although the incidence of diphtheria continues to decline because of widespread immunization, sporadic cases continue to occur. Diphtheria is caused by infection with a strain of *C. diphtheriae* that is infected with a bacteriophage carrying the gene for the production of an exotoxin. This exotoxin interferes with the function of nicotinamide adenine dinucleotide (NAD), thereby inhibiting protein synthesis. The toxin, produced at the site of infection (usually the respiratory tract), is carried via the bloodstream to the heart. Myocarditis generally occurs 7 to 14 days after the onset of infection. The presence of AV block in a child with presumed infectious myocarditis should raise the possibility of diphtheria.[132]

A similar toxemia with myocarditis also has been described in association with gastrointestinal infection with *S. sonnei*.[141] As with diphtheria, the cardiac dysfunction is thought to be the result of an exotoxin produced by the bacteria and occurs in the absence of bacteremia or direct myocardial invasion or both.

Lyme Disease

Lyme disease is a tick-borne illness caused by the spirochete *Borrelia burgdorferi*. The clinical manifestations of the illness consist of a pathognomonic skin rash (erythema chronicum migrans), carditis, meningitis, and arthritis. The disease has been found worldwide and is transmitted by species of the deer tick, *Ixodes*. The three different clinical stages of Lyme disease consist of cutaneous manifestations, disseminated infection, and persistent infection. Table 44-4 lists the features of these stages.

Carditis occurs during the disseminated phase of the illness (stage II) in a minority of patients with Lyme disease (4% to 10%). Thus cardiac manifestations appear 1 to 2 months after the onset of infection or approximately 3 weeks after identification of erythema chronicum migrans. Patients may complain of shortness of breath, palpitations, chest pain, or lightheadedness. Although it is possible for the patient to have cardiac manifestations as the sole evidence of Lyme disease, most patients will have coexisting musculoskeletal or central nervous system (CNS) symptoms. The most common cardiac manifestation involves varying degrees of AV conduction defects. Bundle branch block and fascicular block also have been described. A smaller number of patients will exhibit atrial or ventricular tachyarrhythmias or mild contractile dysfunction with cardiomegaly. Isolated, nonspecific ST-T–wave abnormalities may be the only ECG abnormality.

Histologic examination of biopsy material shows an interstitial infiltration with lymphocytes accompanied by varying amounts of myocyte necrosis, edema, or fibrosis. In contrast to viral myocarditis, Lyme carditis also demonstrates a plaque-like endocardial infiltrate of lymphocytes and plasma cells. *B. burgdorferi* has been grown from cardiac biopsy material,

Table 44-4 Clinical Stages of Lyme Disease (Lyme Borreliosis)

Stage I	Cutaneous Manifestations
	Easy fatiguability
	Erythema chronicum migrans
	Malar rash
	Conjunctivitis
	Lymphadenopathy (occasional)
	Elevated erythrocyte sedimentation rate
	Elevated liver enzymes
Stage II	Disseminated Infection
	Myalgias
	Headaches
	Cranial neuropathies (e.g., facial palsies)
	Peripheral neuropathies
	Cardiac involvement (conduction abnormalities, pericarditis, myocarditis)
Stage III	Persistent Infection
	Chronic (sometimes progressive) arthritis
	Chronic CNS involvement

CNS, central nervous system.

suggesting that live organism in the heart causes Lyme carditis.[154]

Both the diagnosis and treatment rely on a high index of suspicion and recognition of the signs and symptoms of Lyme disease. In addition to the history of a tick bite or potential exposure, the findings of erythema chronicum migrans and an elevated ESR may be helpful in determining the diagnosis. The definite diagnosis relies on serology testing with the demonstration of elevated antibody titers against the infecting organism, *B. burgdorferi*. However, these tests are not yet standardized, and false positives and false negatives are common. Erythema chronicum migrans and other symptoms may resolve with antibiotic therapy with erythromycin, penicillin, or tetracycline. The primary treatment for the disease should be prevention by reducing tick exposure or removing ticks on children as soon as possible.[155] Early medical treatment should prevent subsequent progression to carditis and other late manifestations of the disease. Amoxicillin may be used in younger children (30 mg/kg/day) for 10 to 30 days. In the penicillin-allergic patient, doxycycline, 2 to 4 mg/kg/day PO, divided BID for 14 to 28 days, offers an alternative. Disseminated infection to the heart or the CNS is usually treated with ceftriaxone, 50 to 80 mg/kg IV daily for 14 to 28 days. Up to one third of patients with heart block may require temporary cardiac pacing, but most recover completely. Heart block usually resolves within a few days.

Parasitic and Protozoal Myocarditis

A final group of infectious diseases that may involve the myocardium are parasitic or protozoal organisms. Although myocardial involvement is rare, it can occur with trichinosis, American trypanosomiasis, toxoplasmosis, malaria, and amebic meningoencephalitis. Myocardial damage is related to direct myocardial invasion by the parasite or to the subsequent immune response. Both the primary invasion and a secondary inflammatory response can result in alterations in contractility and the conduction system.

Chagas disease, caused by *Trypanosoma cruzi,* is the most common cause of myocarditis in Central and South America, affecting 16 to 18 million people. This protozoal disease is carried by an insect vector. The acute infection usually affects children or young adults in areas in which it is endemic. A small percentage of patients will die shortly after infection because of myocarditis or meningoencephalitis. However, most patients are not diagnosed during the acute phase because of the nonspecific nature of the complaints and poor access to medical care. When the disease is diagnosed, treatment with the antiparasitic drug benznidazole is effective. In 20% to 40% of infected individuals, chronic myocarditis develops with myocardial thinning and fibrosis, and aneurysms may form 10 to 30 years after the acute infection. In addition to the symptoms of chronic heart failure, these patients may have ventricular tachyarrhythmias, heart block, thromboembolism, or sudden death. Physicians in nonedemic countries should be aware of Chagas disease because of the immigration patterns from countries in which it is endemic to North America and because *T. cruzi* may be transmitted through blood transfusion or organ donation.

Drug-Induced (Toxic) Myocarditis

Several noninfectious etiologies may lead to the development of myocarditis, including hypersensitivity reactions to drugs, autoimmune diseases, and toxin exposure. Of paramount importance is drug-related myocarditis, because early identification and discontinuation of the offending drug may allow recovery. Drug-associated myocarditis may be the result of a hypersensitivity reaction or a direct toxic effect of the drug. A hypersensitivity reaction with myocarditis has been reported with several drugs (Table 44-5). After documentation of myocardial dysfunction, a thorough history of possible exposure to any of a number of toxins or medications (including over-the-counter and herbal medications) should be elicited.

In addition to hypersensitivity reactions, certain drugs, particularly the chemotherapeutic agents, may directly damage the myocardium. Although the majority of information has centered on the cardiac effects of the anthracyclines (doxorubicin and daunorubicin), several other chemotherapeutic agents may cause myocardial damage (Table 44-6). Chemotherapy-related effects may appear early during the infusion of the drug or become manifest several months to years after cessation of therapy.

Table 44-5   Drugs Associated with Hypersensitivity Myocarditis

Acetazolamide	Methyldopa
Amitriptyline	Neomercazole
Carbamazepine	*Para*-aminosalicylic acid
Cephalosporins	Penicillin
Chloramphenicol	Phenylbutazone
Cyclophosphamide	Phenytoin
Emetine	Spironolactone
Hydrochlorothiazide	Streptomycin
Indomethacin	Sulfonamide
Isoniazid	Tetracycline
Lithium	

Table 44-6   Chemotherapy Associated with Cardiac Toxicity

Anthracyclines: doxorubicin, daunorubicin
Cyclophosphamide
5-Fluorouracil
Amsacrine
Cis-Platinum
Mithramycin
Mitomycin C
Vincristine
Actinomycin D

Doxorubicin (Adriamycin) and daunorubicin are the most commonly used anthracyclines and are integral components of the chemotherapeutic regimens for acute myelogenous leukemia, Hodgkin's lymphoma, and various solid tumors of childhood. Severe cardiovascular manifestations can occur with other agents, including cyclophosphamide, *cis*-platinum, amsacrine (AMSA), and 5-fluorouracil (5-FU). These agents may be associated with acute cardiac disturbances by themselves, in addition to potentiating the cardiotoxicity of the anthracyclines. Cyclophosphamide-induced toxicity is manifested by acute congestive failure, which is not dose related.[113] ECG findings include loss of R-wave progression and ST-T–wave changes. Histologic examination reveals hemorrhagic necrosis of cardiac cells. Although much of the evidence concerning the cardiotoxicity is anecdotal, the clinical significance of these findings cannot be ignored.

5-FU inhibits DNA and RNA synthesis. Although most commonly used in solid tumors in the adult population, it has found some clinical utility in relatively uncommon malignancies of childhood, such as carcinoma of the colon. The toxicity of 5-FU is an acute effect, occurring during administration, manifested by myocardial ischemia with chest pain and ECG changes.[80,93] The toxicity is not dose related, occurs in 1% to 2% of patients, and has a mortality of 10% to 15%. Postulated mechanisms for the ischemia include coronary vasospasm, inhibition of myocardial cell DNA synthesis, and depletion of high-energy phosphate compounds. 5-FU is metabolized to fluorocitrate, which inhibits aconitase, an enzyme of the Krebs cycle, leading to citrate accumulation and depletion of high-energy phosphate compounds. In addition to the acute ischemic changes associated with 5-FU administration, acute cardiac failure also has been described.[114] Clinical manifestations include hypotension and cardiac failure occurring during 5-FU administration. These changes may occur without ECG evidence of ischemia or alterations in cardiac enzymes.

Anecdotal evidence also supports the potential cardiac toxicity of *cis*-platinum.[80,172] Reported cardiac effects have included congestive failure with ECG evidence of myocardial ischemia, myocarditis, and alterations in cardiac conduction (left bundle branch block). The exact cardiotoxicity of *cis*-platinum is difficult to define, as the majority of the anecdotal reports have included patients receiving several different chemotherapeutic agents.

AMSA is the most recently introduced agent that also has been associated with cardiotoxic effects. AMSA is an acridine derivative that inhibits DNA synthesis, with activity in various hematologic and solid malignancies. The toxicity of this new agent is acute with both arrhythmias and congestive failure.[156] Arrhythmias, both atrial and ventricular, have been reported during the infusion. Ventricular premature beats, ventricular tachycardia, and ventricular fibrillation can occur. Additionally, acute congestive failure may occur, especially in patients who have received previous doses of anthracyclines. In particular, patients who have received more than 400 mg/m² of anthracycline, those receiving more than 200 mg/m² of AMSA, and those receiving a total dose of the two agents of more than 600 mg/m² are at risk for cardiotoxicity (Table 44-7).[156]

The sedative drug propofol has been associated with fatal myocardial failure when given at high doses for prolonged periods to children in intensive care. Parke and associates[129] originally reported five children in whom progressive metabolic acidosis, lipemic serum, bradyarrhythmias, and ultimately, myocardial failure developed, unresponsive to resuscitative measures. A detailed case report by Cray and colleagues[29] found severe lactic acidosis, liver and muscle necrosis, and bradyarrhythmias in a child who had received propofol, 10 mg/kg/hr for 50 hours. Analysis of muscle biopsy material demonstrated a reduction in cytochrome C oxidase activity. Furthermore, the patient improved after receiving continuous venovenous hemofiltration. Some investigators argue that prolonged low-dose propofol infusions (≤4 mg/kg/hr) may be safe in children.[105,138] The safest approach is to obey the manufacturer's warning against the use of propofol for prolonged sedation in the pediatric ICU.

Aside from pharmacologic agents, a toxic myocarditis may be seen with certain exogenous toxins including phosphorus, ethanol, heavy metals, radiation therapy, and envenomation (scorpions, spiders). Although relatively uncommon in children, diffuse myocardial inflammation and progressive myocardial failure may occur in association with these toxicities.

Radiation therapy can have significant adverse effects on the cardiac system. Adverse effects have included congestive failure, conduction block, pericarditis, and sick sinus syndrome.[5,135] Although such effects are generally transient, permanent alterations in conduction as well as magnification of the toxic effects of various chemotherapeutic agents may occur with mediastinal irradiation.

Autoimmune and Inflammatory Diseases

Myocardial involvement also may occur with several of the autoimmune diseases, including SLE, rheumatoid arthritis, and ulcerative colitis.[19,117] Although myocardial involvement may be a prominent feature of these disorders, it generally does not occur as an isolated finding or as the initial symptom of the disease process. Associated symptoms or organ system involvement is usually present.[42,59,102] Cardiac involvement manifested as either a pericarditis or primary carditis occurs most commonly in patients with SLE.[133] Although these autoimmune disorders rarely are seen initially with myocardial involvement, this possibility must always be kept in mind. A history of vague symptoms of arthritis or intermittent skin rashes or both may be a clue to the diagnosis. Myocardial involvement also may be seen in other inflammatory disease entities of undetermined etiology including Kawasaki syndrome, Takayasu's disease, sarcoidosis, and Reye syndrome.

Kawasaki Syndrome

Kawasaki syndrome was first described in Japan by Dr. Kawasaki in 1967. Since then, the syndrome has been recognized around the world and has now become the most common cause of acquired heart disease among children in the United States.[163] The syndrome consists of a constellation of specific diagnostic signs and symptoms that are outlined in Table 44-8.[166] Fever plus four of the remaining five diagnostic criteria are required to confirm the diagnosis. Children with Kawasaki disease usually are initially seen with sudden high fever, a polymorphous skin rash, nonpurulent conjunctivitis, cracked and fissured red lips, erythematous buccal mucosa, cervical lymphadenitis, and swelling and erythema of the hands and feet. Often the skin lesions appear in the diaper area and spread centrifugally. In the early stages, erythema and induration of the hands and feet, accompanied by swelling of the distal extremities, are common. In the third to fourth week of illness, the palms and soles and the subungual areas may desquamate. Early in the illness, arthralgia or arthritis may develop and can persist for months.[73] If the patient remains untreated, the febrile illness may persist for up to 3 weeks. During this time, the child also may manifest anemia, leukocytosis, and thrombocytosis. The acute-phase reactants (C-reactive protein, ESR, and α_1-antitrypsin) are elevated for up to 8 weeks of illness.

The presentation of Kawasaki syndrome may be highly variable and may not conform to the classic syndrome

Table 44-7 Factors Increasing Anthracycline Cardiotoxicity

Doses in excess of 550 mg/m²
Preexisting myocardial dysfunction
Uncontrolled hypertension
Extremes of age (younger than 1 year or older than 70 years)
Mediastinal irradiation
Concurrent use of other chemotherapeutic agents
Cyclophosphamide
Actinomycin D
Cis-platinum
Mithramycin
5-Fluorouracil
Mitomycin C
Vincristine
Amsacrine
Other drugs
Propranolol
Calcium channel blockers

Table 44-8 Diagnostic Criteria of Kawasaki Syndrome

Fever (≥5 days)
Polymorphous exanthem of the trunk
Lymphadenopathy
Nonvesicular, oral mucosal changes
Swelling of the hands and feet
Bilateral, nonpurulent conjunctival injection

described earlier. In addition to the primary diagnostic signs and symptoms, associated findings are common. Tizard and coworkers[166] noted the following associated findings among 81 children with Kawasaki syndrome: irritability ($n = 41$; 51%), diarrhea ($n = 27$; 33%), vomiting ($n = 18$; 22%), joint pain and tenderness ($n = 18$; 22%), preceding upper respiratory infection ($n = 10$; 12%), hydrops of the gallbladder ($n = 9$; 11%), pneumonia ($n = 2$; 2%), and abnormality on electroencephalogram, elevated serum creatinine, and hypertension, each in 1 (1%) patient. Some patients will be labeled "atypical Kawasaki syndrome" because of a presentation with coronary abnormalities on echocardiogram but fewer than the classically required number of other diagnostic criteria.

The majority (>80%) of the children affected are younger than 5 years, with a slight preponderance (1.5:1) of boys to girls. The disease is first seen most frequently in the winter and spring months. The specific etiology is still unidentified, although an autoimmune mechanism is suspected. None of the proposed etiologies (including rickettsiae, propionibacteria, streptococcal toxins, dust-mite antigens, mercury, and others) has been proven to be a causative factor. In up to 20% of untreated patients, coronary artery aneurysms may develop, which accounts for the mortality and long-term morbidity of Kawasaki syndrome. Aneurysms develop most commonly during the subacute phase of the disease, 10 to 30 days after the onset of fever. The risk of aneurysmal dilation is greatest in children younger than 6 months or older than 8 years.[21,157] Persistent fever or laboratory evidence of ongoing inflammation signifies an increased risk of aneurysm formation.[78]

Histologically, the disease is characterized by a microvasculitis followed by myocarditis.[51] The vasculitic involvement particularly affects coronary arteries and is characterized by mononuclear cell infiltration, intimal necrosis, and necrosis of the various layers of the vascular wall. Up to 50% of children exhibit diffuse, mild dilation of the coronary arteries during the acute phase. In up to 20% of untreated patients, this may progress to aneurysmal dilation (Fig. 44-7). Typically, the aneurysms are found in the left main coronary artery and the left anterior descending branch. The aneurysms rarely rupture. However, the vasculitis may cause occlusion and thrombosis of the lumen. The etiology of the thrombosis is a combination of vascular inflammation, stagnation of flow, and activation of platelets. Furthermore, decreased production of thromboxane A_2 by the inflamed endothelium also contributes to thrombus formation. More than 50% of the patients with coronary artery aneurysms show regression of the aneurysm over a 2-year period. This development most commonly occurs in younger patients who have fusiform dilation and small aneurysms. The long-term prognosis and effect on coronary artery function of these lesions are unclear. In some patients, coronary artery stenosis may develop, which can lead to angina or myocardial infarction. Additional late findings (2 months after the onset of the disease) include fibrosis of the myocardium, coagulation necrosis, lesions of the conduction system, and endocardial fibroelastosis.

Signs of acute myocarditis are present early and manifested as tachycardia, gallop rhythm, and muffled heart sounds.[75] Congestive failure is rarely noted early in the disease, and cardiogenic shock requiring therapy is extremely rare. Although pericarditis may be diagnosed on echocardiography in up to a third of all the cases, pericardial effusion and tamponade rarely occur. A systolic ejection murmur may be related to increased cardiac output and decreased hematocrit. Rarely, mitral or aortic insufficiency may be present early in

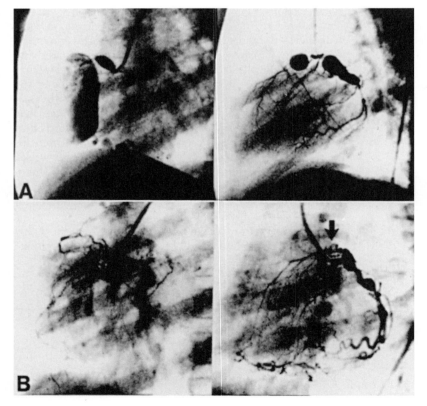

FIGURE 44-7 Coronary angiogram showing aneurysmal dilation of the coronary arteries in Kawasaki syndrome. **A,** Giant aneurysms at the right coronary artery, left anterior descending artery, and circumflex artery. **B,** Recanalization at the right coronary artery and left anterior descending artery *(arrow)* in the recuperative phase. (From Tatara K, Kusakawa S: Long-term prognosis of giant coronary aneurysm in Kawasaki disease. An angiographic study. *J Pediatr* 111:705–710, 1987, Fig. 1; with permission.)

the course. Patients with severe aneurysmal dilation of the coronary vessels may be at risk for acute myocardial infarction, even during the early stages of the disease.[51] According to one survey of 195 patients with Kawasaki syndrome in Japan, 73% of myocardial infarctions occurred within 12 months of the onset of the disease.[87] Clinical symptoms of myocardial infarction are similar to those found in adults, with the exception of chest pain. Hemodynamic compromise, vomiting, irritability, crying, and abdominal pain are frequently seen. Up to one third of the patients may be asymptomatic. These infarctions seem unrelated to physical exertion and occur most commonly during sleep or at rest. Repeated myocardial infarction increases the chance of mortality.

Characteristic ECG findings of Kawasaki syndrome include sinus tachycardia, slightly prolonged PR and QT intervals, and decreased QRS voltages (Fig. 44-8). Frequently, ST-T–wave changes, including flattened T waves, are seen. The presence of acute myocardial infarction is suggested by the presence of significant ST elevation and inversion of T waves. Q waves also may be seen in the distribution of the involved area. Radiologic studies are occasionally helpful. Although the routine chest radiograph is rarely helpful, it may reveal "eggshell-like calcifications," which outline aneurysms that have been present for longer than 1 year. Gallium scans (gallium 67 scintiphotographs) may show myocardial involvement. In one study, positive uptake was noted in 19 of 46 patients, indicating acute myocarditis.[110] Perfusion scans with a thallium 201 may be useful to delineate ischemic areas of the myocardium, although the study has no pathognomonic signs for Kawasaki syndrome.

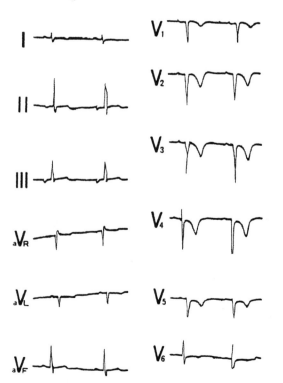

FIGURE 44-8 Electrocardiographic changes of myocardial infarction in Kawasaki disease. Note the inverted T waves across the precordial leads and Q waves in V 1–3. (From Hayashi H, Kisamori K, Kaneko M, et al: Unstable angina in a patient with mucocutaneous lymph node syndrome. *Japanese Heart J* 25:661–668, 1984, Fig. 1; with permission.)

Echocardiography is useful for diagnosing and monitoring the cardiac involvement, including aneurysmal dilation of the coronary vasculature. Pericardial effusions, dilation of the ventricles, decreased systolic function, and valvular involvement can be detected with this technique. Although selective coronary arteriography may be used to delineate further the abnormal anatomy, it is best postponed until recovery from the acute inflammatory disease occurs, as evidenced by a normal ESR and platelet count, to minimize the risk of aneurysmal rupture or myocardial infarction.

Acute therapy consists of IV gamma globulin and enteral salicylates, which have been shown to decrease morbidity and mortality. Aspirin in high, anti-inflammatory doses (80 to 100 mg/kg/day) has been used in addition to IV immunoglobulin during the acute inflammatory phase of the illness. Because of impaired gastrointestinal absorption during the acute stages of the illness, high doses of salicylates are needed to achieve therapeutic levels. During this time, salicylate levels may be monitored to ensure a therapeutic level and avoid toxicity. After the acute phase of the illness (first 2 weeks), the salicylate dose is generally decreased to a low-dose regimen of 4 to 5 mg/kg once a day. Some clinicians prefer to start the aspirin at low dose, because it is difficult to achieve the higher anti-inflammatory levels during the acute phase. Salicylates are often discontinued at 6 to 8 weeks, if echocardiography shows no coronary abnormalities.

Intravenous gamma globulin (IVIG) also has been shown to improve significantly the outcome and reduce coronary artery involvement, especially when administered during the acute phase of the illness.[52,123] Immediate administration of IVIG decreases the prevalence of coronary dilation to less than 5% and that of giant coronary aneurysms to less than 1%.[37] Initial studies used regimens of IVIG of 400 mg/kg every day for 5 days. This regimen has now been replaced by a single dose of 2 g/kg administered over a 12-hour period. The combination of IVIG and aspirin results in decreased duration of symptoms, including fever and improvement in laboratory studies such as the ESR.[122] Adequate therapy given early (before day 10) in the course reduces the mortality from 1% to 0.1%.[120]

Children who have dilated coronary aneurysm (>8 mm in diameter) are at significant risk for myocardial ischemia despite therapy. These children should be monitored closely. The role of prolonged anticoagulation with warfarin in patients with giant coronary aneurysms is controversial. In the event of acute myocardial infarction, thrombolytic therapy may be considered. Children in whom coronary artery stenosis or occlusion develops because of thrombosis or stricture of the vessels may require coronary artery bypass grafts. However, the success of bypass grafting in this setting depends on technique. Kitamura[91] found only a 38% incidence of patency with saphenous vein grafts compared with 82% with internal mammary artery grafts in children younger than 8 years. In addition, the internal mammary grafts may actually grow with the patient, providing ongoing myocardial blood flow to the susceptible area.

Systemic Lupus Erythematosus

SLE is a diffuse autoimmune vasculitis with CNS, cardiac, renal, and skin manifestations (Table 44-9). The etiology

Table 44-9　Clinical Signs and Symptoms of SLE in Children

Malaise
Weight loss
Growth retardation
Cutaneous abnormalities
Hematologic abnormalities (anemia, thrombocytopenia, leukopenia)
Fever
Nephritis
Hematuria, proteinuria
Musculocutaneous complaints
Pleural and pulmonary disease
Hepatosplenomegaly
Lymphadenopathy
Neurologic disease (seizures, cerebritis, psychosis)
Cardiac abnormalities
Hypertension
Ocular abnormalities
Gastrointestinal symptoms
Raynaud's phenomenon

SLE, Systemic lupus erythematosus.

of the disease is unknown. Drugs such as hydralazine, procainamide, practolol, and phenytoin are associated with a systemic lupus-like syndrome. It is hypothesized that SLE is a disease of the immune system with altered immune regulation. Patients with SLE have elevated serum immunoglobulins and antibodies that react against nuclear constituents, ribonucleic acid, gamma globulin, red cells, and other blood products. Circulating immune complexes also are found in patients with SLE. These complexes may be deposited in the kidneys, heart, and other tissue beds.

The clinical manifestations may begin as an acute illness or evolve more gradually. Patients may have symptoms for months or years before the diagnosis of SLE is made. Table 44-9 lists some of the clinical signs and symptoms of SLE in children. SLE is a great masquerader and can appear as a variety of illnesses. The pathognomonic presentation includes a "butterfly rash" in the malar distribution. The scaly erythematous patches are usually photosensitive and may involve the face, scalp, neck, chest, and extremities. Children also may have other skin manifestations including a macular rash on the palms, soles, and phalanges or erythema nodosum and erythema multiforme. Arthralgias or arthritis may appear in the early stages and may progress to recurrent arthritis in later stages. Polyserositis (including pleuritis, pericarditis, and peritonitis) is common and may produce pain in the affected areas. Hepatosplenomegaly and lymphadenopathy also may occur. Children also may have pulmonary disease and gastrointestinal problems with diffuse SLE. Ocular involvement includes scleritis, iritis, or retinitis.

Cardiovascular manifestations of SLE, most commonly pericarditis or pericardial effusion, occur at some point in the disease process in up to 40% of patients.[19,42] The pericarditis may be focal or diffuse and is commonly of the fibrinous type. In addition to pericarditis, patients also may have myocarditis manifested as cardiomegaly, friction rubs, or heart murmurs. Myocardial infarction can occur because of coronary vasculitis and myocardial ischemia. Rarely, children may die suddenly because of acute myocardial infarction. Verrucous endocarditis has been seen on echocardiography or on autopsy.

However, hemodynamically significant AV valve regurgitation is uncommon. Valvular involvement is associated with the presence of antiphospholipid antibodies.

The newborn may experience a distinct lupus syndrome characterized by the transplacental passage from the mother to the fetus of autoantibodies, in particular anti-Ro (SS-A), anti-La (SS-B), or both. The majority of infants with neonatal lupus exhibit isolated congenital heart block or cutaneous lesions analogous to subacute cutaneous lupus erythematosus in the adult. Fetal heart block may be sufficiently severe to produce hydrops fetalis. Despite the presence of these maternal antibodies, many of these mothers are not yet clinically affected by lupus at the time the fetus or infant is affected. In some mothers, clinical lupus may develop years later.

Congenital complete heart block (CHB) carries a mortality rate up to 16%, with the majority of deaths occurring during the first 12 months of life even if early cardiac pacing is instituted.[40] It has recently been recognized that the cardiac manifestations of neonatal lupus may not be limited to the conduction system, as approximately one fourth of newborns with congenital CHB later develop DCM, which carries a poor prognosis.[40] The risk of DCM makes close follow-up mandatory in this population. Until recently, the general approach to infants and children with high-grade heart block from neonatal lupus was to implant a permanent pacemaker only if symptoms or profound bradycardia were found. Michaelsson and associates[112a] found a 5% mortality between the ages of 15 and 30 years in patients with congenital heart block, and that 75% of those who died or had a cardiac arrest had had no prior symptoms. This finding has prompted many physicians caring for patients with congenital heart block to recommend a permanent pacemaker sometime in the second decade of life, even in asymptomatic patients. It is important to recognize that infants with neonatal lupus do not generally develop other symptoms of lupus, as their disease is related to passive transfer of maternal antibodies from their mothers with lupus, rather than lupus in the fetus or infant.

Because SLE can easily mimic other diseases, making the correct diagnosis is important. The diagnosis is based on the presence of the previously mentioned clinical signs/symptoms plus confirmatory laboratory tests documenting the presence of autoantibodies: a positive lupus erythematous cell preparation, antibodies against double-stranded DNA, antibodies against the Sm nuclear antigen, or false-positive tests for syphilis. The diagnostic criteria for SLE are outlined in reference 161.

A pericardial friction rub often is the first sign of cardiovascular involvement in children with SLE. On occasion, this may progress to pericardial tamponade or constrictive disease. The systolic murmur is commonly that of mitral insufficiency. Overt congestive failure is rare and may result from valvular involvement. A variety of ECG changes range from nonspecific ST-T–wave changes to frank conduction block.

The primary therapy for SLE remains immunosuppressive medications including corticosteroids. Salicylates or other nonsteroidal anti-inflammatory drugs (NSAIDs) may be effective in improving and relieving arthralgias or the pain of arthritis. Other agents such as chloroquine and hydroxychloroquine or anti-inflammatory agents such as cyclophosphamide or azathioprine also may prove useful. However, because of the potential toxicity, these drugs should be used with great caution.

CNS manifestations may require anticonvulsant therapy as well as more aggressive anti-inflammatory treatment with steroids and adjunct medications. Renal dialysis may be required for end-stage renal disease. The prognosis for children with SLE has improved remarkably because of supportive therapy with antibiotics, corticosteroids, and cytotoxic drugs. The 5-year survival rate for children is greater than 90%. However, children may have significant morbidity during these 5 years and beyond.

Rheumatic Fever

Rheumatic fever was first identified as a separate entity during the 17th century; however, its association with cardiac disease and group A streptococcus was not recognized for more than 100 years. Although rheumatic fever involves several different organ systems including the skin, musculoskeletal, and CNS, the major morbidity and mortality relate to its effects on the cardiovascular system and the development of rheumatic heart disease.

Rheumatic fever requires prior infection with group A, β-hemolytic streptococci. Patients may have had an antecedent asymptomatic upper respiratory infection and subsequently have negative cultures at the time of presentation. In these patients, evidence of recent infection (elevated antibody titers) must be present to make the diagnosis of rheumatic fever.

The factors predisposing patients to rheumatic fever remain poorly defined, as many patients have streptococcal pharyngitis, whereas in very few does rheumatic fever develop. Acute rheumatic fever occurs most commonly in children from ages 5 to 15 years with no gender predilection. The exact incidence after streptococcal infection varies from 0.3% in the general population to rates as high as 2% during epidemics of streptococcal pharyngitis. The incidence is higher with more severe infections, inadequate treatment of the primary infection, and factors that predispose to the spread of contagious diseases, including patients of lower socioeconomic background and those living in crowded environments.[77] The highest incidence has been reported in developing countries in tropical and subtropical regions of the world, where the disease also may appear in a particularly virulent form.[7,9] Even before the antibiotic era, a decrease in the incidence of rheumatic fever was noted in the United States, with speculation that rheumatic fever would cease to be a clinical problem. However, in the 1980s and 1990s, a resurgence of rheumatic fever occurred, with several outbreaks being reported.[170a,173a] Interestingly, these outbreaks did not follow the demographic patterns of previous outbreaks, and several occurred in middle-class suburban populations. It is possible that changes in the streptococcus organism have contributed to the return of rheumatic fever. To paraphrase Mark Twain, the report of the death of rheumatic fever was an exaggeration.

Although rheumatic fever is known to be a direct sequel of infection with group A, β-hemolytic streptococci, the exact pathogenesis has not been determined. The initial theory of direct invasion of tissue by the offending organism was disproved by the inability to isolate the organism from affected tissue. Other theories have involved an autoimmune process related to a state of immune hyperreactivity initiated by exposure to streptococcal antigens or the production of toxins by the invading organisms. Although various streptococcal toxins may damage myocardial tissue in cell cultures,[165] this theory does not explain the latency period that is present between the initial infection and the onset of cardiac involvement. The currently accepted theory is that an aberrant immunologic mechanism, either humoral or cellular, which is triggered by the streptococcal infection, is responsible for the tissue damage. It is postulated that cross-reactivity exists between the antigens of the streptococcal organism and the host tissue, such that induction of host immunity is directed at the streptococcal organisms and the host tissue with antigenic similarity. Such antigen similarity is present between streptococci and the proteins of the sarcolemma of the heart, valvular tissue, neuronal tissue, and cartilage. This immunologic similarity of the streptococci and proteins in several different organ systems explains the specific organ involvement seen in acute rheumatic fever. Several recent studies support this view. Evidence of a humoral immunologic mechanism emerged from the demonstration of cytotoxic cross-reactivity between the antistreptococcal antibody N-acetyl-β-D-glucosamine and the extracellular matrix protein laminin.[54] The cellular immunologic component may arise after activation of the surface of the valvular endothelium with antivascular cell adhesion molecule-1.[139] Subsequently, CD4(+) and CD8(+) T lymphocytes adhere to valve endothelium and ultimately penetrate the subendothelial layer.

The clinical manifestations follow the symptoms of upper respiratory infection by a latency period of 2 to 5 weeks. The initial manifestations may include the skin, musculoskeletal, central nervous, or cardiovascular systems or a combination of these. Musculoskeletal complaints with joint symptoms (arthralgias or arthritis) are the most common presenting symptoms. These symptoms occur in up to 80% of patients during the initial presentation. Isolated polyarthritis involving the large joints without other manifestations can be confused with other diseases. Joint involvement varies from arthralgia to arthritis with effusion. The arthritis tends to be migratory, with involvement of the large joints (wrists, knees, ankles, and elbows). The joint symptoms are self-limiting even without medical intervention and do not lead to permanent damage or residual arthritic changes.

Myocardial involvement or carditis is the most serious manifestation of acute rheumatic fever, occurring in 40% to 50% of cases. Primary myocarditis leading to decreased contractility and ventricular arrhythmias accounts for the mortality seen during the acute stage, whereas cardiac sequelae such as valvular damage account for the majority of the long-term complications. Although the overall incidence of rheumatic fever may be declining,[4] the incidence of carditis may be increasing, with reports of cardiac involvement in up to 90% of cases.[167,171] One explanation for this increased incidence of cardiac involvement is the variation in the techniques used to determine whether cardiac involvement is present. Older studies used auscultation alone, whereas more recent investigators have relied on more sensitive measures such as echocardiography. It may be that the incidence of cardiac involvement has not changed, but our ability to detect it has.

Although carditis may be the sole manifestation or the presenting symptom, it also may occur with other organ system involvement, most commonly arthritis. The usual clinical scenario is a patient with the acute onset of fever and joint involvement, followed by the demonstration of clinical or echocardiographic signs of cardiac involvement. Primary symptoms referable to the heart are generally absent, except in patients with either pericarditis or myocarditis. The presentation of pericarditis is similar to that with other etiologies and includes chest pain, effusion, friction rub, ECG findings, or a combination of these. Isolated pericarditis is rare without other features of carditis.

The manifestations of carditis are variable, ranging from asymptomatic involvement with the development of valvular disease (silent carditis) to acute involvement with congestive heart failure and arrhythmias. More commonly, relatively subtle clinical signs of cardiac involvement are present including tachycardia or ECG changes. During the acute phase, although uncommon, valvular involvement may be present, with evidence of mitral or aortic insufficiency. In the absence of a murmur or other evidence of carditis, mild mitral or aortic regurgitation may be evident on echocardiographic examination.[48]

Mitral valve involvement is most common with a holosystolic murmur and a low-pitched mid-diastolic rumble (Carey-Coombs) murmur. The diastolic component of the murmur results from increased blood flow during diastole as a result of the large regurgitant volume. Aortic involvement with insufficiency occurs in up to 20% of patients with cardiac involvement. Overt congestive failure occurs in 5% of patients. Debate continues about the extent to which valvular dysfunction or primary myocardial dysfunction contributes to congestive heart failure in rheumatic carditis. However, isolated mitral or combined mitral and aortic insufficiency appear to be major factors in the development of congestive heart failure in the rheumatic fever patient. These left-heart regurgitant lesions lead to left-heart volume overload with increased left ventricular end-diastolic diameter, which improves significantly after valve replacement.[41] It has also been suggested that the increased cardiac work from left ventricular volume overload exacerbates the direct effects of rheumatic fever on the heart.[11] Later on in the course of acute rheumatic fever or years afterward, pulmonary edema and congestive heart failure can develop from pulmonary venous hypertension as a result of mitral stenosis. Pulmonary hypertension also can occur, and its severity correlates with the severity of mitral stenosis.[148]

The duration of rheumatic carditis varies from 4 weeks to 6 months. Although most patients recover from the acute process, residual involvement of cardiac valves may lead to chronic insufficiency or more commonly to stenosis. Symptoms of such involvement may not appear for years after the initial bout of rheumatic fever. Additionally, subsequent subclinical episodes of rheumatic fever may lead to cardiac symptoms years later, with decompensation from valvular insufficiency or stenosis. Even in the absence of overt valvular involvement, residual scarring may predispose these patients to endocarditis, necessitating antibiotic prophylaxis for specific surgical/dental procedures.

Other less common manifestations of rheumatic fever include Sydenham's chorea, erythema marginatum, and

Table 44-10   Jones Criteria for Diagnosis of Acute Rheumatic Fever

Major Manifestations
Carditis
Polyarthritis
Chorea
Erythema marginatum
Subcutaneous nodules
Minor Manifestations
Clinical findings
Arthralgia
Fever
Previous rheumatic fever
Laboratory findings
Elevated acute phase reactants
Erythrocyte sedimentation rate
C-reactive protein
White blood cell count
Prolonged PR interval
Supporting Evidence of Antecedent Group A Streptococcal Infections
Positive throat culture
Positive rapid streptococcal antigen test
Elevated or increasing streptococcal antibody titer

If supported by evidence of preceding group A streptococcal infection, the presence of two major manifestations or one major and two minor manifestations indicates a high probability of acute rheumatic fever.

subcutaneous nodules. These latter three clinical findings, in addition to arthritis and carditis, form the five major manifestations according to the revised Jones criteria (Table 44-10).[83] Sydenham's chorea (St. Vitus dance) reflects the inflammatory involvement of the basal ganglia. It occurs in 10% to 15% of patients. The characteristic movements are involuntary, nonpurposeful, and rapid, usually involving the face and upper extremities. Paresis of the affected muscle groups also is common. Other more subtle neurologic findings include emotional lability, changes in personality, moodiness, or a change in school performance. Although the other manifestations generally occur early on (<4 weeks), the neurologic manifestations of rheumatic fever may have a long latency period after the initial streptococcal infection by up to 6 months.[162] The chorea is generally self-limited and resolves in 1 to 2 weeks, although isolated cases have lasted up to 2 years.

Erythema marginatum may be found in 3% to 5% of patients with acute rheumatic fever. The characteristic rash is described as macular, nonpruritic, with a serpiginous border. These lesions are found most commonly on the thighs and trunk and may become more evident after exposure to heat. Because of their evanescent nature, these lesions may be impossible to detect in patients with dark skin.

Subcutaneous nodules are the least common of the major manifestations, occurring in 1% of patients. They are located on the extensor surface of joints, most commonly the elbows, knees, hands, and ankles. They are freely moveable, nonpainful, and vary in size from 0.5 to 2 cm.

The diagnosis of acute rheumatic fever relies on recognition of both the major and minor manifestations. In many cases, a clear history of preceding streptococcal infection is not present, as many infections are subclinical. The diagnosis rests on the identification of two of the major criteria or one major and two minor criteria. The minor criteria include both clinical and laboratory findings (see Table 44-10). The clinical findings of the minor criteria include fever, arthralgia, and previous rheumatic fever. The laboratory findings include a prolonged PR interval and elevation of acute-phase reactants (ESR, C-reactive protein, white blood cell count). Aside from helping in the diagnostic process, the ESR may be used to monitor the response to therapy, because it decreases as the rheumatic fever subsides or in response to effective anti-inflammatory treatment with either salicylates or corticosteroids.

In addition, evidence of a recent streptococcal infection is required. Serologic testing is often needed to document a recent streptococcal infection, as the history may be negative in many cases, and pharyngeal cultures may fail to isolate the organism (60% to 70% of cases) because of the latency period between the primary infection and the development of acute rheumatic fever. Several serologic tests are available to document preceding streptococcal infection and rely on the identification of serum antibodies to various streptococcal antigens or extracellular enzymes: anti-streptolysin O (ASO) or anti-deoxyribonuclease B (anti-DNAse B). Antibody levels to one of these antigens will be present in 80% to 85% of patients.[9] The use of both tests increases the probability of a positive finding to 92% in patients with acute rheumatic fever.[9]

No specific tests for rheumatic carditis improve on the clinical diagnosis with the revised Jones criteria. Endomyocardial biopsy rarely provides specific diagnostic information in children with clinically diagnosed rheumatic carditis.[121] Biopsy may be a means of excluding other possibilities, such as a postviral DCM. Similarly, echocardiography should be viewed as a tool to supplement clinical diagnosis of rheumatic carditis and valvulitis[62] and is used primarily to evaluate myocardial/valvular function and demonstrate the presence or absence of pericardial effusion.

The treatment of acute rheumatic fever is aimed primarily at eradication of the offending organism, administration of anti-inflammatory agents (either salicylates or corticosteroids), and support of the cardiovascular system. Several appropriate choices are available to eradicate pharyngeal colonization with streptococci, including penicillin and erythromycin. In addition to initial therapy, ongoing prophylaxis is required, because recurrences of acute rheumatic fever are common after the initial attack. Monthly injection of benzathine penicillin (1.2 million units) is the most commonly used form of prophylaxis, although daily oral administration of penicillin also is possible.

After the initial diagnosis, strict bed rest is recommended, with evaluation at 2-week intervals to determine the presence of carditis. The exact duration of bed rest will vary depending on the extent of cardiac involvement. In the absence of carditis, bed rest is recommended for 2 weeks, whereas bed rest for 4 weeks is recommended for patients with carditis without cardiac enlargement. The presence of cardiomegaly increases the recommendations for bed rest to 6 weeks.

The treatment of carditis remains somewhat controversial concerning the use of salicylates or corticosteroids. Current recommendations include the use of salicylates for patients with mild carditis and the restriction of corticosteroid administration to patients with severe cardiac involvement and overt congestive failure or pancarditis.[27] Salicylates are administered in doses of 80 to 100 mg/kg/day in four divided doses

and adjusted as needed to maintain therapeutic serum levels. Salicylate therapy is continued for 4 to 8 weeks and then slowly tapered over a 4- to 8-week period, provided a continued decline is seen in the acute-phase reactants (ESR). Corticosteroids, prednisone or methylprednisolone, 2 mg/kg/day, are administered for 2 weeks and then tapered over a 2-week period. Before tapering the corticosteroid dose, therapeutic doses of salicylates should be administered as outlined earlier.

Supportive care, such as that provided for congestive failure of other etiologies, may be required by some patients. Although digitalis and diuretics are commonly recommended, caution is required with digitalis because of the risks of increasing ventricular ectopy, especially in the presence of inflammatory diseases of the heart. Additionally, the role of digoxin preparations in the treatment of congestive failure remains controversial. Patients with mild degrees of myocardial dysfunction may respond to anticongestive therapy with diuretics and afterload reduction with ACE inhibitors. These agents also may provide improvement in children with left heart volume overload secondary to mitral or aortic regurgitation. Severe cases may require intravenous inotropic agents (dobutamine, milrinone). With these supportive measures, mortality is rare in children with mild to moderate rheumatic carditis.

Severe heart failure secondary to valvular regurgitation may require valve replacement, which should not be delayed.[11] Rheumatic mitral stenosis can be treated with percutaneous mitral balloon valvotomy.[23] Heart transplantation has been attempted for end-stage rheumatic cardiomyopathy but may result in severe allograft rejection and death.[63] Graft rejection may be related to the streptococcal antigen–induced induction of host immunity against heart tissue.

SUMMARY

Myocarditis is a descriptive term based on histologic findings showing an inflammatory process of the heart with isolated areas of myocardial cell necrosis. In many cases, the process may involve all three layers of the heart, resulting in what may more appropriately be considered a pancarditis. The primary consequences of the inflammatory process are alterations in myocardial function or the potential for arrhythmias or both. Various etiologies include infectious agents, autoimmune diseases, and drugs/toxins. Autoimmune phenomena may be part of the primary disease process, as with cardiac involvement in SLE or an aberrant immunologic reaction directed at the myocardium such as a postviral myocarditis or the carditis associated with rheumatic fever. With improvements in viral isolation techniques such as PCR, fewer cases are now considered idiopathic. Treatment includes treatment of primary infectious etiologies, removal of the offending toxin/drug, control of the underlying autoimmune process, and provision of pharmacologic support of the failing myocardium. Additional/future therapies may involve better control of the aberrant immune response with immunosuppressive agents or the use of gamma globulin.

References

1. Acierno LJ: Cardiac complications in acquired immunodeficiency syndrome (AIDS): A review. *J Am Coll Cardiol* 13:1144–1154, 1989.

2. Ainger LE: Acute aseptic myocarditis: Corticosteroid therapy. *J Pediatr* 64:716–720, 1964.

3. American Heart Association: Guidelines 2000 for cardiopulmonary resuscitation and emergency cardiovascular care. *Circulation* 102(8 suppl): I140–I141, 2000.

4. Annegers JF, Pillman NL, Weidman WH, Kurland LT: Rheumatic fever in Rochester, Minnesota, 1935–1978. *Mayo Clin Proc* 57:753–757, 1982.

5. Applefeld MM, Wiernik PH: Cardiac disease after radiation therapy for Hodgkin's disease: Analysis of 48 patients. *Am J Cardiol* 51:1679–1681, 1983.

6. Aretz HT, Billingham ME, Edwards WD, et al: Myocarditis: A histopathologic definition and classification. *Am J Cardiovasc Pathol* 1:3–14, 1987.

7. Arora R, Nair M, Kalra GS, et al: Non-surgical mitral valvuloplasty for rheumatic mitral stenosis. *Indian Heart J* 42:329–334, 1990.

8. Arsura EL, Ismail Y, Freeman S, et al: Amphotericin B–induced dilated cardiomyopathy. *Am J Med* 97:560–562, 1994.

9. Ayoub EM, Wannamaker LW: Evaluation of the streptococcal deoxyribonuclease B and diphosphopyridine nucleotidase antibody tests in acute rheumatic fever and acute glomerulonephritis. *Pediatrics* 29:527–538, 1962.

10. Badorff C, Lee GH, Lamphear BJ, et al: Enteroviral protease 2A cleaves dystrophin: Evidence of cytoskeletal disruption in an acquired cardiomyopathy. *Nat Med* 5:320–326, 1999.

11. Barlow JB, Marcus RH, Pocock WA, et al: Mechanisms and management of heart failure in active rheumatic carditis. *S Afr Med J* 78:181–186, 1990.

12. Bergelson JM, Cunningham JA, Droguett G, et al: Isolation of a common receptor for coxsackie B viruses and adenoviruses 2 and 5. *Science* 275:1320–1323, 1997.

13. Bohm N: Adrenal, cutaneous and myocardial lesions in fulminating endotoxinemia (Waterhouse-Friderichsen syndrome). *Pathol Res Pract* 174:92–105, 1982.

14. Bowles NE, Richardson PJ, Olsen EGJ, Archard LC: Detection of coxsackie-B-virus-specific RNA sequences in myocardial biopsy samples from patients with myocarditis and dilated cardiomyopathy. *Lancet* 1:1120–1123, 1986.

15. Briassoulis G, Papadopoulos G, Zavras N, et al: Cardiac troponin I in fulminant adenovirus myocarditis treated with a 24-hour infusion of high-dose intravenous immunoglobulin. *Pediatr Cardiol* 21:391–394, 2000.

16. Brockington GM, Zebede J, Pandian NG: Constrictive pericarditis. *Cardiol Clin* 8:645–661, 1990.

17. Brook I, Frazier EH: Microbiology of acute purulent pericarditis: A 12 year experience in a military hospital. *Arch Intern Med* 156:1857–1860, 1996.

18. Brown DL, Sather S, Cheitlin MD: Reversible cardiac dysfunction associated with foscarnet therapy for cytomegalovirus esophagitis in an AIDS patient. *Am Heart J* 125:1439–1441, 1993.

19. Bulkley BH, Roberts WC: The heart in systemic lupus erythematosus and the changes induced in it by corticosteroid therapy: A study of 36 necropsy patients. *Am J Med* 58:243–264, 1975.

20. Burch GE, Sun SC, Colcolough HL, et al: Coxsackie B viral myocarditis and valvulitis identified in routine autopsy specimens by immunofluorescent techniques. *Am Heart J* 74:13–23, 1967.

21. Burns JC, Wiggins JW Jr, Toews WH, et al: Clinical spectrum of Kawasaki disease in infants younger than 6 months of age. *J Pediatr* 109:759–763, 1986.

22. Byrd BF, Linden RW: Superior vena cava Doppler flow velocity patterns in pericardial disease. *Am J Cardiol* 65:1464–1470, 1990.

23. Carroll JD, Feldman T: Percutaneous mitral balloon valvotomy and the new demographics of mitral stenosis. *JAMA* 270:1731–1736, 1993.

24. Chan KY, Iwahara M, Benson LN, et al: Immunosuppressive therapy in the management of acute myocarditis in children: A clinical trial. *J Am Coll Cardiol* 17:458–460, 1991.

25. Chan TC, Brady WJ, Pollack M: Electrocardiographic manifestations: Acute myopericarditis. *J Emerg Med* 17:865–872, 1999.

26. Cohen IS, Anderson DW, Virmani R, et al: Congestive cardiomyopathy in association with the acquired immunodeficiency syndrome. *N Engl J Med* 315:628–630, 1986.

27. Combined Rheumatic Fever Study Group: A comparison of the effect of prednisone and acetylsalicylic acid on the incidence of residual rheumatic heart disease. *N Engl J Med* 262:895–902, 1960.

28. Cooper ER, Hanson C, Diaz C, et al: Encephalopathy and progression of human immune deficiency virus disease in a cohort of children with perinatally acquired human immunodeficiency virus infection: Women and Infants Transmission Study Group. *J Pediatr* 132:808–812, 1998.

29. Cray SH, Robinson BH, Cox PN: Lactic acidemia and bradyarrhythmia in a child sedated with propofol. *Crit Care Med* 26:2087–2092, 1998.

30. Dacso CC: Pericarditis in AIDS. *Cardiol Clin* 8:697–699, 1990.

31. Dagartzikas MI, Sprague K, Tobias JD: Cerebrovascular event, dilated cardiomyopathy, and pheochromocytoma. *Pediatr Emerg Care* 18:33–35, 2002.

32. Davies JM: Molecular mimicry: Can epitope mimicry induce autoimmune disease? *Immunol Cell Biol* 75:113–126, 1997.

33. Diaz C, Hanson C, Cooper ER, et al: Disease progression in a cohort of infants with vertically acquired HIV infection observed from birth: The Women and Infants Transmission Study. *J Acquired Immune Defic Syndr Hum Retrovirol* 18:221–228, 1998.

34. Doedens JR, Kirkegaard, K: Inhibition of cellular protein secretion by poliovirus proteins 2B and 3A. *EMBO J* 14:894–907, 1995.

35. Domanski MJ, Sloas MM, Follmann DA, et al: Effect of zidovudine and didanosine treatment on heart function in children infected with human immunodeficiency virus. *J Pediatr* 127:137–146, 1995.

36. Drucker NA, Colan SD, Lewis AB, et al: Gamma-globulin treatment of acute myocarditis in the pediatric population. *Circulation* 89:252–257, 1994.

37. Durongpisitkul K, Gururaj VJ, Park JM, Martin CF: The prevention of coronary artery aneurysm in Kawasaki disease: A meta-analysis on the efficacy of aspirin and immunoglobulin treatment. *Pediatrics* 96: 1057–1061, 1995.

38. Edwards WD, Holmes DR Jr, Reeder GS: Diagnosis of active lymphocytic myocarditis by endomyocardial biopsy: Quantitative criteria for light microscopy. *Mayo Clin Proc* 57:419–425, 1982.

39. Engle MA, Ehlers KH, O'Loughlin JE Jr, et al: The postpericardiotomy syndrome: Iatrogenic illness with immunologic and virologic components. *Cardiovasc Clin* 11:381–391, 1981.

40. Eronen M, Siren MK, Ekblad H, et al: Short- and long-term outcome of children with congenital complete heart block diagnosed in utero or as a newborn. *Pediatrics* 106:86–91, 2000.

41. Essop MR, Wisenbaugh T, Sareli P: Evidence against a myocardial factor as the cause of left ventricular dilation in active rheumatic carditis. *J Am Coll Cardiol* 22:826–829, 1993.

42. Estes D, Christian CL: The natural history of systemic lupus erythematosus by prospective analysis. *Medicine (Baltimore)* 50:85–95, 1971.

43. Etchison D, Milburn SC, Edery I, et al: Inhibition of HeLa cell protein synthesis following poliovirus infection correlates with the proteolysis of a 220,000-dalton polypeptide associated with eukaryotic initiation factor 3 and a cap binding protein complex. *J Biol Chem* 257: 14806–14810, 1982.

44. Farinha NJ, Bartolo A, Trindale L, et al: Acute pericarditis in childhood: The 9 year experience of a tertiary referral center. *Acta Med Portuguesa* 10:157–160, 1997.

45. Feldman AM, McNamara D: Medical progress: Myocarditis. *N Engl J Med* 343:1388–1398, 2000.

46. Feldman WE: Bacterial etiology and mortality of purulent pericarditis in pediatric patients: Review of 162 cases. *Am J Dis Child* 133:641–644, 1979.

47. Finkel MS, Oddis CV, Jacob TD, et al: Negative inotropic effects of cytokines on the heart mediated by nitric oxide. *Science* 257:387–389, 1992.

48. Folger GM Jr, Hajar R, Robida A, Hajar HA: Occurrence of valvular heart disease in acute rheumatic fever without evident carditis: Colourflow Doppler identification. *Br Heart J* 67:434–438, 1992.

49. Fowler NO: Tuberculous pericarditis. *JAMA* 266:99–103, 1991.

50. Fujioka S, Koide H, Kitaura Y, et al: Molecular detection and differentiation of enteroviruses in endomyocardial biopsies and pericardial effusions from dilated cardiomyopathy and myocarditis. *Am Heart J* 131:760–765, 1996.

51. Fujiwara H, Hamashima Y: Pathology of the heart in Kawasaki disease. *Pediatrics* 61:100–107, 1978.

52. Furusho K, Kamiya T, Nakano H, et al: High-dose intravenous gammaglobulin for Kawasaki disease. *Lancet* 2:1055–1058, 1984.

53. Fyler DC: Pericardial disease. In Fyler DC (ed): *Nadas' Pediatric Cardiology.* Philadelphia, Hanley and Belfus, 1992.

54. Galvin JE, Hemric ME, Ward K, Cunningham MW: Cytotoxic mAb from rheumatic carditis recognizes heart valves and laminin. *J Clin Invest* 106:217–224, 2000.

55. Gardiner AJ, Short D: Four faces of acute myopericarditis. *Br Heart J* 35:433–442, 1973.

56. Gatzoulis K, Tolis G, Theopistou A, et al: Cardiomyopathy due to a pheochromocytoma: A reversible entity. *Acta Cardiol* 53:227–229, 1998.

57. Gersony WM, McCracken GH Jr: Purulent pericarditis in infancy. *Pediatrics* 40:224–232, 1967.

58. Godeny EK, Gauntt CJ: Murine natural killer cells limit coxsackievirus B3 replication. *J Immunol* 139:913–918, 1987.

59. Goldenberg J, Ferraz MB, Pessoa AP, et al: Symptomatic cardiac involvement in juvenile rheumatoid arthritis. *Int J Cardiol* 34:57–62, 1992.

60. Grist NR, Bell EJ: A six-year study of Coxsackie virus B infections in heart disease. *J Hyg (Lond)* 73:165–172, 1974.

61. Grody WW, Cheng L, Lewis W: Infection of the heart by the human immunodeficiency virus. *Am J Cardiol* 66:203–206, 1990.

62. Guidelines for the diagnosis of rheumatic fever. Jones Criteria, 1992 update. Special Writing Group of the Committee on Rheumatic Fever, Endocarditis, and Kawasaki Disease of the Council on Cardiovascular Disease in the Young of the American Heart Association. *JAMA* 268:2069–2073, 1992.

63. Gulizia JM, Engel PJ, McManus BM: Acute rheumatic carditis: Diagnostic and therapeutic challenges in the era of heart transplantation. *J Heart Lung Transplant* 12:372–380, 1993.

64. Hakim JG, Ternouth I, Mushangi E, et al: Double blind randomised placebo controlled trial of adjunctive prednisolone in the treatment of effusive tuberculous pericarditis in HIV seropositive patients. *Heart* 84:183–188, 2000.

65. Hallagan LF, Dawson PA, Eljaiek LF Jr: Pediatric chest pain: Case report of a malignant cause. *Am J Emerg Med* 10:43–45, 1992.

66. Hardman JM, Earle KM: Myocarditis in 200 fatal meningococcal infections. *Arch Pathol Lab Med* 87:318–325, 1969.

67. Heikkila J, Karjalainen J: Evaluation of mild acute infectious myocarditis. *Br Heart J* 47:381–391, 1982.

68. Helin M, Savola J, Lapinleimu K: Cardiac manifestations during a coxsackie B5 epidemic. *Br Med J* 3:97–99, 1968.

69. Henke A, Huber S, Stelzner A, Whitton JL: The role of CD8+ T lymphocytes in coxsackievirus B3-induced myocarditis. *J Virol* 69:6720–6728, 1995.

70. Henke A, Launhardt H, Klement K, et al: Apoptosis in coxsackievirus B3–caused diseases: Interaction between the capsid protein VP2 and the proapoptotic protein siva. *J Virol* 74:4284–4290, 2000.

71. Herskowitz A, Willoughby SB, Vlahov K, et al: Dilated heart muscle disease associated with HIV infection. *Eur Heart J* 16(suppl O):50–55, 1995.

72. Hetzer R, Loebe M, Potapov EV, et al: Circulatory support with pneumatic paracorporeal ventricular assist device in infants and children. *Ann Thorac Surg* 66:1498–1506, 1998.

73. Hicks RV, Melish ME: Kawasaki syndrome. *Pediatr Clin North Am* 33:1151–1175, 1986.

74. Himelman RB, Chung WS, Chernoff DN, et al: Cardiac manifestations of human immunodeficiency virus infection: A two-dimensional echocardiographic study. *J Am Coll Cardiol* 13:1030–1036, 1989.

75. Hiraishi S, Yashiro K, et al: Clinical course of cardiovascular involvement in the mucocutaneous lymph node syndrome: Relation between clinical signs of carditis and development of coronary arterial aneurysm. *Am J Cardiol* 47:323–330, 1981.

76. Hohn AR, Stanton RE: Myocarditis in children. *Pediatr Rev* 9:83–88, 1987.

77. Holmberg SD, Faich GA: Streptococcal pharyngitis and acute rheumatic fever in Rhode Island. *JAMA* 250:2307–2312, 1983.

78. Ichida F, Fatica NS, Engle MA, et al: Coronary artery involvement in Kawasaki syndrome in Manhattan, New York: Risk factors and role of aspirin. *Pediatrics* 80:828–835, 1987.

79. Ito M, Kodama M, Masuko M, et al: Expression of coxsackievirus and adenovirus receptor in hearts of rats with experimental autoimmune myocarditis. *Circ Res* 86:275–280, 2000.

80. Jakubowski AA, Kemeny N: Hypotension as a manifestation of cardiotoxicity in three patients receiving cisplatin and 5-fluorouracil. *Cancer* 62:266–269, 1988.

81. Jayashree M, Singhi SC, Singh RS, Singh M: Purulent pericarditis: Clinical profile and outcome following surgical drainage and intensive care in children in Chandigarh. *Ann Trop Paediatr* 19:377–381, 1999.

82. Jin O, Sole MJ, Butany JW, et al: Detection of enterovirus RNA in myocardial biopsies from patients with myocarditis and cardiomyopathy using gene amplification by polymerase chain reaction. *Circulation* 82:8–16, 1990.

83. Jones Criteria (revised) for guidance in the diagnosis of rheumatic fever. *Circulation* 69:204A–208A, 1984.

84. Joshi VV, Gadol C, Connor E, et al: Dilated cardiomyopathy in children with acquired immunodeficiency syndrome: A pathologic study of five cases. *Hum Pathol* 19:69–73, 1988.

85. Joshi VV, Pawel B, Connor E, et al: Arteriopathy in children with acquired immune deficiency syndrome. *Pediatr Pathol* 7:261–275, 1987.

86. Juneja R, Kothari SS, Saxena A, et al: Intrapericardial streptokinase in purulent pericarditis. *Arch Dis Child* 80:275–277, 1999.

87. Kato H, Ichinose E, Kawasaki T: Myocardial infarction in Kawasaki disease: Clinical analyses in 195 cases. *J Pediatr* 108:923–927, 1986.

88. Kavanaugh-McHugh AL, Ruff AL, Perlman E, et al: Selenium deficiency and cardiomyopathy in acquired immunodeficiency syndrome. *JPEN J Parenter Enteral Nutr* 15:347–349, 1991.

89. Kawai C: From myocarditis to cardiomyopathy: Mechanisms of inflammation and cell death: Learning from the past for the future. *Circulation* 99:1091–1100, 1999.

90. Kereiakes DJ, Parmley WW: Myocarditis and cardiomyopathy. *Am Heart J* 108:1318–1326, 1984.

91. Kitamura S, Kawachi K, Seki T, et al: Bilateral internal mammary artery grafts for coronary artery bypass operations in children. *J Thorac Cardiovasc Surg* 99:708–715, 1990.

92. Kudenchuk PJ, Cobb LA, Copass MK, et al: Amiodarone for resuscitation after out-of-hospital cardiac arrest due to ventricular fibrillation. *N Engl J Med* 341:871–878, 1999.

93. Labianca R, Beretta G, Clerici M, et al: Cardiac toxicity of 5-fluorouracil: A study on 1083 patients. *Tumori* 68:505–510, 1982.

94. Le Moing V, Lortholary O, Timsit JF, et al: Aspergillus pericarditis with tamponade: Report of a successfully treated case and review. *Clin Infect Dis* 26:451–460, 1998.

95. Levy WS, Simon GL, Rios JC, Ross AM: Prevalence of cardiac abnormalities in human immunodeficiency virus infection. *Am J Cardiol* 63:86–89, 1989.

96. Lewis AB: Late recovery of ventricular function in children with idiopathic dilated cardiomyopathy. *Am Heart J* 138:334–338, 1999.

97. Lipshultz SE, Chanock S, Sanders SP, et al: Cardiovascular manifestations of human immunodeficiency virus infection in infants and children. *Am J Cardiol* 63:1489–1497, 1989.

98. Lipshultz SE, Fox CH, Perez-Atayde AR, et al: Identification of human immunodeficiency virus-1 RNA and DNA in the heart of a child with cardiovascular abnormalities and congenital acquired immune deficiency syndrome. *Am J Cardiol* 66:246–250, 1990.

99. Lipshultz SE, Orav EJ, Sanders SP, Colan SD: Immunoglobulins and left ventricular structure and function in pediatric HIV infection. *Circulation* 92:2220–2225, 1995.

100. Liu PP, Opavsky MA: Viral myocarditis: Receptors that bridge the cardiovascular with the immune system? *Circ Res* 86:253–254, 2000.

101. Lock JE, Bass JL, Kulik TJ, Fuhrman BP: Chronic percutaneous pericardial drainage with modified pigtail catheters in children. *Am J Cardiol* 53:1179–1182, 1984.

102. Mandell BF: Cardiovascular involvement in systemic lupus erythematosus. *Semin Arthritis Rheum* 17:126–141, 1987.

103. Marinella MA: Electrocardiographic manifestations and differential diagnosis of acute pericarditis. *Am Fam Phys* 57:699–704, 1998.

104. Martin AB, Webber S, Fricker FJ, et al: Acute myocarditis: Rapid diagnosis by PCR in children. *Circulation* 90:330–339, 1994.

105. Martin PH, Murthy BV, Petros AJ: Metabolic, biochemical and haemodynamic effects of infusion of propofol for long-term sedation of children undergoing intensive care. *Br J Anaesth* 79:276–279, 1997.

106. Martino TA, Petric M, Brown M, et al: Cardiovirulent coxsackieviruses and the decay-accelerating factor (CD55) receptor. *Virology* 244:302–314, 1998.

107. Mason JW, O'Connell JB, Herskowitz A, et al: A clinical trial of immunosuppressive therapy for myocarditis. *N Engl J Med* 333:269–275, 1995.

108. Mast HL, Haller JO, Schiller MS, Anderson VM: Pericardial effusion and its relationship to cardiac disease in children with acquired immunodeficiency syndrome. *Pediatr Radiol* 22:548–551, 1992.

109. Matsumori A, Igata H, Ono K, et al: High doses of digitalis increase the myocardial production of proinflammatory cytokines and worsen myocardial injury in viral myocarditis: A possible mechanism of digitalis toxicity. *Jpn Circ J* 63:934–940, 1999.

110. Matsuura H, Ishikita T, Yamamoto S, et al: Gallium-67 myocardial imaging for the detection of myocarditis in the acute phase of Kawasaki disease (mucocutaneous lymph node syndrome): The usefulness of single photon emission computed tomography. Br Heart J 58:385–392, 1987.

111. McCarthy RE III, Boehmer JP, Hruban RH, et al: Long-term outcome of fulminant myocarditis as compared with acute (non-fulminant) myocarditis. N Engl J Med 342:690–695, 2000.

112. Medani CR, Ringel RE: Intrapericardial triamcinolone hexacetonide in the treatment of intractable uremic pericarditis in a child. Pediatr Nephrol 2:32–33, 1988.

112a. Michaelsson M, Riesenfeld T, Jonzon A: Isolated congenital complete atrioventricular block in adult life: A prospective study. Circulation 92:442–449, 1995.

113. Mills BA, Roberts RW: Cyclophosphamide-induced cardiomyopathy: A report of two cases and review of the English literature. Cancer 43:2223–2226, 1979.

114. Misset B, Escudier B, Leclercq B, et al: Acute myocardiotoxicity during 5-fluorouracil therapy. Intens Care Med 16:210–211, 1990.

115. Molnar T, Hogye M, Nagy F, Lonovics J: Pericarditis associated with inflammatory bowel disease. Am J Gastroenterol 94:1099–1100, 1999.

116. Morgan RJ, Stephenson LW, Woolf PK, et al: Surgical treatment of purulent pericarditis in children. J Thorac Cardiovasc Surg 85:527–531, 1983.

117. Mowat NA, Bennett PN, Finlayson JK, et al: Myopericarditis complicating ulcerative colitis. Br Heart J 36:724–727, 1974.

118. Mueller DL, Jenkins MK, Schwartz RH: Clonal expansion versus functional clonal inactivation: A costimulatory signalling pathway determines the outcome of T cell antigen receptor occupancy. Annu Rev Immunol 7:445–480, 1989.

119. Mueller XM, Tevaearai HT, Hurni M, et al: Etiologic diagnosis of pericardial disease: The value of routine tests during surgical procedures. J Am Coll Surg 184:645–649, 1997.

120. Nakamura Y, Yanagawa H, Kato H, et al: Mortality among patients with a history of Kawasaki disease: The third look: The Kawasaki Disease Follow-up Group. Acta Paediatr Jpn 40:419–423, 1998.

121. Narula J, Chopra P, Talwar KK, et al: Does endomyocardial biopsy aid in the diagnosis of active rheumatic carditis? Circulation 88:2198–2205, 1993.

122. Newburger JW, Takahashi M, Beiser AS, et al: A single intravenous infusion of gamma globulin as compared with four infusions in the treatment of acute Kawasaki syndrome. N Engl J Med 324:1633–1639, 1991.

123. Newburger JW, Takahashi M, Burns JC, et al: The treatment of Kawasaki syndrome with intravenous gamma globulin. N Engl J Med 315:341–347, 1986.

124. Noren GR, Staley NA, Bandt CM, Kaplan EL: Occurrence of myocarditis in sudden death in children. J Forens Sci 22:188–196, 1977.

125. O'Connell JB, Robinson JA, Henkin RE, Gunnar RM: Immunosuppressive therapy in patients with congestive cardiomyopathy and myocardial uptake of gallium-67. Circulation 64:780–786, 1981.

126. Okoroma EO, Perry LW, Scott LP: Acute bacterial pericarditis in children: Report of 25 cases. Am Heart J 90:709–713, 1975.

127. Okuni M, Yamada T, Mochizuki S, Sakurai I: Studies on myocarditis in childhood, with special reference to the possible role of immunological process and the thymus in the chronicity of the disease. Jpn Circ J 39:463–470, 1975.

128. Opavsky MA, Penninger J, Aitken K, et al: Susceptibility to myocarditis is dependent on the response of alpha beta T lymphocytes to coxsackieviral infection. Circ Res 85:551–558, 1999.

129. Parke TJ, Stevens JE, Rice AS, et al: Metabolic acidosis and fatal myocardial failure after propofol infusion in children: Five case reports. BMJ 305:613–616, 1992.

130. Parrillo JE, Cunnion RE, Epstein SE, et al: A prospective, randomized, controlled trial of prednisone for dilated cardiomyopathy. N Engl J Med 321:1061–1068, 1989.

131. Pauschinger M, Bowles NE, Fuentes-Garcia FJ, et al: Detection of adenoviral genome in the myocardium of adult patients with idiopathic left ventricular dysfunction. Circulation 99:1348–1354, 1999.

132. Perles Z, Nir A, Cohen E, et al: Atrioventricular block in a toxic child: Do not forget diphtheria. Pediatr Cardiol 21:282–283, 2000.

133. Perlroth MG: Connective tissue diseases and the heart. JAMA 231:410–412, 1975.

134. Permanyer-Miralda G, Sagrista-Sauleda J, Soler-Soler J: Primary acute pericardial disease: A prospective series of 231 consecutive patients. Am J Cardiol 56:623–630, 1985.

134a. Pitt B, Zannad F, Remme WJ, et al: The effect of spironolactone on morbidity and mortality in patients with severe heart failure. N Engl J Med. 341:709–717, 1999.

135. Pohjola-Sintonen S, Totterman KJ, Kupari M: Sick sinus syndrome as a complication of mediastinal radiation therapy. Cancer 65:2494–2496, 1990.

136. Rabinovici R, Szewczyk D, Ovadia P, et al: Candida pericarditis: Clinical profile and treatment. Ann Thorac Surg 63:1200–1204, 1997.

137. Reddy PS, Curtiss EI: Cardiac tamponade. Cardiol Clin 8:627–637, 1990.

138. Reed MD, Yamashita TS, Marx CM, et al: A pharmacokinetically based propofol dosing strategy for sedation of the critically ill, mechanically ventilated pediatric patient. Crit Care Med 24:1473–1481, 1996.

139. Roberts S, Kosanke S, Terrence Dunn S, et al: Pathogenic mechanisms in rheumatic carditis: Focus on valvular endothelium. J Infect Dis 183:507–511, 2001.

140. Rotbart HA, Webster AD, Pleconaril Treatment Registry Group: Treatment of potentially life-threatening enterovirus infections with pleconaril. Clin Infect Dis 32:228–235, 2001.

141. Rubenstein JS, Noah ZL, Zales VR, Shulman ST: Acute myocarditis associated with Shigella sonnei gastroenteritis. J Pediatr 122:82–84, 1993.

142. Sadowski ZP, Alexander JH, Skrabucha B, et al: Multicenter randomized trial and a systematic overview of lidocaine in acute myocardial infarction. Am Heart J 137:792–798, 1999.

143. Sayed IM, Elias M: Acute chemical pericarditis following celiac plexus block: A case report. Middle East J Anesth 14:201–206, 1997.

144. Segal JP, Harvey WP, Gurel T: Diagnosis and treatment of primary myocardial disease. Circulation 32:837–844, 1965.

145. Shafren DR, Bates RC, Agrez MV, et al: Coxsackieviruses B1, B3, and B5 use decay accelerating factor as a receptor for cell attachment. J Virol 69:3873–3877, 1995.

146. Shanes JG, Ghali J, Billingham ME, et al: Interobserver variability in the pathologic interpretation of endomyocardial biopsy results. Circulation 75:401–405, 1987.

147. Shapiro ED, Berg AT: Protective efficacy of Haemophilus influenza type b polysaccharide vaccine. Pediatrics 85:643–647, 1990.

148. Shrivastava S, Tandon R: Severity of rheumatic mitral stenosis in children. Int J Cardiol 30:163–167, 1991.

149. Smith SC, Ladenson JH, Mason JW, Jaffe AS: Elevations of cardiac troponin I associated with myocarditis: Experimental and clinical correlates. Circulation 95:163–168, 1997.

150. Soler-Soler J, Permanyer-Miralda G, Sagrista-Sauleda J: A systematic diagnostic approach to primary acute pericardial disease: The Barcelona experience. Cardiol Clin 8:609–620, 1990.

151. Sonnenblick M, Rosin A: Cardiotoxicity of interferon: A review of 44 cases. Chest 99:557–561, 1991.

152. Spodick DH: Pericarditis in systemic diseases. Cardiol Clin 8:709–716, 1990.

153. Spodick DH: Frequency of arrhythmias in acute pericarditis determined by Holter monitoring. Am J Cardiol 53:842–845, 1984.

154. Stanek G, Klein J, Bittner R, Glogar D: Isolation of Borrelia burgdorferi from the myocardium of a patient with longstanding cardiomyopathy. N Engl J Med 322:249–252, 1990.

155. Steere AC: Lyme disease. N Engl J Med 321:586–596, 1989.

156. Steinherz LJ, Steinherz PG, Mangiacasale D, et al: Cardiac abnormalities after AMSA administration. Cancer Treat Rep 66:483–488, 1982.

157. Stockheim JA, Innocentini N, Shulman ST: Kawasaki disease in older children and adolescents. J Pediatr 137:250–252, 2000.

158. Strang JIG: Rapid resolution of tuberculous pericardial effusions with high dose prednisone and anti-tuberculous drugs. J Infect 28:251–254, 1994.

159. Strauss AW, Santa-Maria M, Goldring D: Constrictive pericarditis in children. Am J Dis Child 129:822–826, 1975.

160. Tabib A, Loire R, Miras A, et al: Unsuspected cardiac lesions associated with sudden unexpected perioperative death. Eur J Anaesthesiol 17:230–235, 2000.

161. Tan EM, Cohen AS, Fries JF, et al: The 1982 revised criteria for the classification of systemic lupus erythematosus. Arthritis Rheum 25:1271–1277, 1982.

162. Taranta A, Stollerman GH: Relation of isolate recurrences of Sydenham's chorea to preceding streptococcal infections. N Engl J Med 260:1204–1210, 1959.

163. Taubert KA, Rowley AH, Shulman ST: Seven-year national survey of Kawasaki disease and acute rheumatic fever. *Pediatr Infect Dis J* 13:704–708, 1994.

164. Thebaud B, Sidi D, Kachaner J: Purulent pericarditis in children: A 15 year experience. 3:1084–1090, 1996.

165. Thompson A, Halbert SP, Smith U: The toxicity of streptolysin O for beating mammalian heart cells in tissue culture. *J Exp Med* 131:745–763, 1970.

166. Tizard EJ, Suzuki A, Levin M, Dillon MJ: Clinical aspects of 100 patients with Kawasaki disease. *Arch Dis Child* 66:185–188, 1991.

167. Tolaymat A, Goudarzi T, Soler GP, et al: Acute rheumatic fever in north Florida. *South Med J* 77:819–823, 1984.

168. Tuna IC, Danielson GK: Surgical management of pericardial diseases. *Cardiol Clin* 8:683–696, 1990.

169. van Kuppeveld, FJ, Hoenderop JG, Smeets RL, et al: Coxsackievirus protein 2B modifies endoplasmic reticulum membrane and plasma membrane permeability and facilitates virus release. *EMBO J* 16:3519–3532, 1997.

170. van Raaij MJ, Chouin E, van der Zandt H, et al: Dimeric structure of the coxsackievirus and adenovirus receptor D1 domain at 1.7 A resolution. *Structure Fold Des* 8:1147–1155, 2000.

170a. Veasy LG, Tani LY, Hill HR: Persistence of acute rheumatic fever in the intermountain area of the United States. *J Pediatr* 124:9–16, 1994.

171. Veasy LG, Wiedmeier SE, Orsmond GS, et al: Resurgence of acute rheumatic fever in the intermountain area of the United States. *N Engl J Med* 316:421–427, 1987.

172. Von Hoff DD, Schilsky R, Reichert CM, et al: Toxic effects of cis-dichlorodiammineplatinum (II) in man. *Cancer Treat Rep* 63:1527–1531, 1979.

173. Weisensee D, Bereiter-Hahn J, Schoeppe W, Low-Friedrich I: Effects of cytokines on the contractility of cultured cardiac myocytes. *Int J Immunopharmacol* 15:581–587, 1993.

173a. Westlake RM, Graham TP, Edwards KM: An outbreak of acute rheumatic fever in Tennessee. *Pediatr Infect Dis J* 9:97–100, 1990.

174. Wiles HB, McArthur PD, Taylor AB: Prognostic features of children with idiopathic dilated cardiomyopathy. *Am J Cardiol* 68:1372–1376, 1991.

175. Wilkenfeld C, Cohen M, Lansman SL, et al: Heart transplantation for end-stage cardiomyopathy caused by an occult pheochromocytoma. *J Heart Lung Transplant* 11:363–366, 1992.

176. Woodruff JF: Viral myocarditis: A review. *Am J Pathol* 101:425–484, 1980.

177. Yang, D, Yu J, Luo Z, et al: Viral myocarditis: Identification of five differentially expressed genes in coxsackie-virus B3-infected mouse heart. *Circ Res* 84:704–712, 1999.

178. Yasuda T, Palacios IF, Dec GW, et al: Indium 111-monoclonal antimyosin antibody imaging in the diagnosis of acute myocarditis. *Circulation* 76:306–311, 1987.

179. Zahn EM, Houde C, Benson L, Freedom RM: Percutaneous pericardial catheter drainage in childhood. *Am J Cardiol* 70:678–680, 1992.

180. Zahringer J, Stangl E, Aschauer W, Van der Walt M: Virus myocarditis: Molecular hybridization allows the detection of virus-RNA in heart muscle after virus infection. *J Mol Cell Cardiol* 17:83–85, 1985.

181. Zaragoza C, Ocampo C, Saura M, et al: The role of inducible nitric oxide synthase in the host response to coxsackievirus myocarditis. *Proc Natl Acad Sci USA* 95:2469–2474, 1998.

Chapter 45

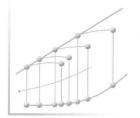

Infective Endocarditis

FRANK E. BERKOWITZ, MBBCh, MPH

INTRODUCTION

Since the first edition of this textbook was published, the main advances in infective endocarditis have concerned criteria for diagnosis and new recommendations for treatment and prophylaxis.

927

Infective endocarditis (IE), often referred to as bacterial endocarditis, is an infection of the endothelium of the heart; *infective endocarditis* is a better term because it recognizes that nonbacterial infections, such as fungal and viral, can occur. Although it affects mainly the heart valves, it may also affect other endothelium-lined cardiac structures and vascular protheses. This discussion includes infections of the great vessels, patent ductus arteriosus, artificial conduits, and systemic-to-pulmonary shunts.

Because IE is more commonly encountered in adults than in children, much of the information about this disease is derived from studies on adults and has been extrapolated to children.

Infective endocarditis has relevance to pediatric critical care for three main reasons: (1) patients with IE may develop complications, especially affecting the heart, for which they may require cardiac surgery or critical care management; (2) cardiac surgery is an important precedent of IE; and (3) patients in the critical care unit, even those without underlying heart disease, are subjected to various invasive procedures that place them at risk for developing IE.

INCIDENCE

Most data on the frequency of IE are based on the number of cases per 1000 hospital admissions, which is inevitably influenced by referral patterns to the respective hospitals. Frequencies in children vary from 0.149 to 1.35 per 1000 admissions.[68,98,143,181,202] In adults, IE accounts for 0.16 to 5.4 per 1000 hospital admissions.[72]

A study at a single institution in Boston showed an increase in frequency of IE in children from 0.22 per 1000 admissions in the period of 1943 to 1952, to 0.55 per 1000 admissions in 1963 to 1972.[87] A study in Tel Aviv, however, showed a decrease in frequency from 0.55 per 1000 admissions in the period of 1965 to 1974 to 0.149 per 1000 admissions in 1975 to 1984.[68] The only population-based study of the incidence of IE in children is that by Schollin and colleagues in Sweden, who showed an incidence in children younger than 15 years of 0.34 cases per 100,000 per year.[175] In adults, the incidence is about 2 cases per 100,000 population per year.[72,185]

If there is indeed an increase in the frequency of IE in children, there are several possible explanations for it: (1) survival of children with congenital heart disease, particularly cyanotic heart disease, as a result of advances in cardiac surgery; (2) cardiac surgery itself, an important precursor of IE; (3) increasing use of invasive intravascular devices (e.g., central venous lines); and (4) increasing recognition of IE, especially in the neonate. The changing pattern of IE, as described in the section on patterns of IE in children, suggests that the first three of these reasons are indeed operating.

PATHOGENESIS OF INFECTIVE ENDOCARDITIS

There are two essential requirements for the development of IE; namely, damaged or abnormal endothelium and presence of infectious organisms (usually bacteria) in the bloodstream.[16,107,173,182] Damaged endothelium occurs as the result of either mechanical stress on it from turbulent blood flow or from direct trauma. For example, turbulent flow is created by a stenotic or regurgitant valve. Most endothelial damage occurs on the low-pressure side of a pressure gradient (e.g., the ventricular side of a regurgitant aortic valve, the atrial side of a regurgitant mitral valve, or the right ventricular wall opposite the jet created by a ventricular septal defect).[160] Direct trauma to the endothelium is usually caused by intracardiac catheters (e.g., central venous lines and Swan-Ganz catheters), pacemaker leads, and cardiac surgery.

Damaged endothelium causes local activation of the coagulation system, resulting in a noninfected thrombotic lesion called nonbacterial thrombotic endocarditis (NBTE). This sterile lesion consists of platelets, red cells, and fibrin. NBTE also may develop in the absence of direct endothelial damage in individuals with malignancies, burns, systemic lupus erythematosus, and uremia and in the neonate.

Nonbacterial thrombotic endocarditis forms a nidus for infection by bacteria that may be present in the bloodstream. Any condition causing bacteremia can result in IE if endothelial abnormalities are present. However, certain bacteria (e.g., staphylococci and streptococci), when present in the blood, are much more likely to cause IE than are others (e.g., enteric bacilli). The following factors explain the predilection of certain bacteria for causing IE: First, the adherence of certain bacteria to endothelial cells is facilitated by several factors; namely, (1) dextran, produced by certain streptococci; (2) fibronectin, a glycoprotein produced by endothelial cells, which facilitates adherence to endothelial cells of *Staphylococcus aureus*, streptococci, and *Candida* spp. but not gram-negative bacilli; (3) lipoteichoic acid in streptococci; and (4) slime layer in coagulase-negative staphylococci. Second, the endothelium ingests certain organisms (e.g., staphylococci and *Candida* spp). Finally, many enteric bacilli, despite their ability to cause bacteremia, are susceptible to the bactericidal activity of serum, exerted by the activation of complement and the lytic effect of the terminal complement complex. This impedes their ability to cause IE.

The bacteremia leading to IE may be mild and asymptomatic or associated with severe clinical illness. It may arise from an infection, such as pneumonia, furuncle, or dental abscess, or from a procedure, such as dental or genitourinary, in which case it is often transient.

Once bacteria adhere to the endothelium or NBTE, the adherence of platelets and fibrin progresses to form a vegetation. The bacteria become enmeshed and buried within the growing vegetation, where they are protected from the host's phagocytes. Deep within the vegetation, they become relatively inactive metabolically. This protection from phagocytes and metabolic inactivity has important implications for antimicrobial therapy of IE, namely, that bactericidal rather than bacteriostatic agents are necessary and that therapy must be prolonged.

PATHOLOGY

The hallmark of IE is the vegetation. This consists of platelets, fibrin, some red cells, a few leukocytes (mainly neutrophils), and microorganisms.[116,182] Vegetations vary in appearance and texture from grey, pink, soft, and friable to grey, yellow, brown, and firm. They may be smooth or rough and single or multiple. They are usually located at two sites: (1) on the low-pressure side of a pressure gradient (e.g., the atrial side of a regurgitant mitral valve, the ventricular side of a regurgitant aortic valve, the pulmonary side of a patent ductus arteriosus, the right ventricular side of a ventricular septal defect, or the distal end of a coarctation of the aorta) or (2) at the site of impingement of a jet (e.g., the left atrial wall in mitral regurgitation, the ventricular surface of the anterior mitral leaflet in aortic regurgitation, or the right ventricular wall or tricuspid valve in a ventricular septal defect).[158,159,182] The vegetations on heart valves develop close to lines of closure but may extend to involve the cusps themselves, the chordae tendineae, or the sinuses of Valsalva.

The complications of IE may be considered as cardiac or systemic. Cardiac complications include (1) the mass of the vegetation that may interfere with valvular function by causing obstruction or regurgitation; (2) destruction of valve tissue that may cause perforation of the cusp, with resultant insufficiency or aneurysm formation in the cusp; and (3) extension of the infection into contiguous structures, which accounts for many of the severe complications of IE. The infection may spread into the valve ring, causing a valve ring abscess, and thence into the myocardium. Extension in this fashion, especially from the aortic valve, may result in damage to the conduction system of the heart. The infection may spread further into other heart chambers and the pericardium.[182] Valve damage may create an abnormal jet of blood flow, which can impinge on and cause infection of a noncontiguous part of the heart. For example, IE on a regurgitant aortic valve can lead to infection on the septal leaflet of the mitral valve.

Systemic complications of IE result from (1) the presence of microorganisms in the bloodstream (bacteremia, fungemia) with metastatic infection; (2) emboli of vegetations; and (3) immune stimulation and antigen-antibody complex formation, which occurs where IE develops over a period of weeks to months.

Bacteremia or septic emboli may result in metastatic infection in any organ, including the brain, lung, kidney, spleen, bone, joint, skin, or eye. These secondary foci may undergo suppuration. Emboli resulting in ischemia affect mainly the brain, lung, intestine, skin, kidneys, and peripheral blood vessels. In children, emboli to the brain and lungs are the most common.* Cerebral emboli may result in major infarcts, especially in the distribution of the middle cerebral artery; multiple petechial hemorrhages; multiple microabscesses or macroscopic abscesses; meningitis; or major intracerebral or subarachnoid hemorrhage. Hemorrhage may result from rupture of a mycotic aneurysm, from septic arteritis without mycotic aneurysm formation, or as a complication of infarction.[18,73,149,166] Pulmonary emboli can lead to pneumonia, lung abscess and empyema, and infarction.[93] (See "Intravenous Drug Abusers.")

Immune stimulation results in two important clinical features; namely, splenomegaly, thought to be caused by chronic reticuloendothelial hyperplasia, and glomerulonephritis due to circulating immune complexes. The glomerulonephritis, recognized primarily by the presence of hematuria, may be either focal, segmental, or diffuse.[95,116,132]

---

*See references 9, 21, 68, 82, 86, 87, 91, 96, 98, 123, 127, 129, 143, 175, 181, 190, 202, and 220.

THE PATTERN OF INFECTIVE ENDOCARDITIS IN CHILDREN

Underlying Heart Disease

The underlying cardiac diseases and microbiological causes of IE in children are described in this section. The data on underlying disease (Table 45-1) are derived from 884 patients from 20 published series spanning 1933 to 1989 from the following countries: Australia, Canada, Germany, India, Israel, Japan, South Africa, Spain, Sweden, United Kingdom, and the United States. Although these series include cases of neonatal IE, nosocomial IE, and IE on prosthetic valves, these specific forms of disease, as well as IE in intravenous drug abusers, are discussed separately in more detail.

The most common underlying heart diseases are congenital heart defects, of which ventricular septal defect, tetralogy of Fallot, and aortic stenosis prevail.* Fifty-seven percent of children with congenital heart disease who also have IE have undergone previous cardiac surgery (Table 45-2). In the presence of cyanotic heart disease, 88% of children with IE had previous surgery.[9,82,127,190,202]

Rheumatic heart disease precedes IE in 20% to 70% of cases in India and South Africa,[21,22,82,96,123] while in the United States, there was a decline in the proportion of rheumatic-related IE from 22% during 1933 to 1942[87] to 3% to 6% in the 1960s and 1970s.[87,190,202] In Western Europe, Japan, and Australia, rheumatic heart disease is associated with 0% to 3% of cases of childhood IE.[98,127,129,143,175,220]

Table 45-1 Underlying Heart Disease in Children with Infective Endocarditis

Congenital Heart Disease	Cases (n)	% of Total
Acyanotic Heart Lesions		
Ventricular septal defect	194	21.8
Ventricular septal defect and other	18	2.0
Patent ductus arteriosus	25	2.8
Aortic stenosis	89	10.0
Subvalvar aortic stenosis	9	1.0
Coarctation of aorta	25	2.8
Pulmonary stenosis	21	2.4
Atrioventricular defect	16	1.8
Atrial septal defect	11	1.2
Mitral valve abnormality	16	1.8
Mitral valve prolapse	8	0.9
Cyanotic Heart Lesions		
Tetralogy of Fallot	143	16.0
Transposition of great vessels	35	3.9
Truncus arteriosus	8	0.9
Tricuspid atresia	9	1.0
Pulmonary atresia	8	0.9
Single ventricle	9	1.0
Other	79	8.9
Rheumatic heart disease	86	9.7
No Heart Disease	75	8.4
Total	884	100

Data from references 9, 21, 68, 82, 86, 87, 91, 96, 98, 123, 127, 129, 143, 175, 181, 190, 202, and 220.

Table 45-2 Underlying Congenital Heart Disease in Children with Infective Endocarditis, Who Had or Had Not Undergone Cardiac Surgery

Congenital Heart Disease	Total	No Surgery	Surgery	% Surgery
Acyanotic Heart Lesions				
Ventricular septal defect	36	29	7	19
Ventricular septal defect and other	7	1	6	86
Patent ductus arteriosus	7	5	2	29
Aortic valve abnormality	30	15	15	50
Subaortic valvar stenosis	2	2	0	0
Coarctation of aorta	1	1	0	0
Pulmonary stenosis	3	3	0	0
Atrioventricular defect	9	1	8	89
Atrial septal defect	3	1	2	67
Mitral valve abnormality	8	3	5	63
Mitral valve prolapse	7	7	0	0
Subtotal	113	68	45	40
Cyanotic Heart Lesions				
Tetralogy of Fallot	19	1	18	95
Transposition of great vessels	13	3	10	77
Truncus arteriosus	5	1	4	80
Pulmonary/tricuspid atresia	8	2	6	75
Single ventricle	7	0	7	100
Other	12	1	11	92
Subtotal	64	8	56	88
Total	177	76	101	57

Data from references 9, 91, 127, 190, and 202.

The proportion of IE cases with no identifiable underlying heart disease is approximately 9%, ranging from 0% to 32%. Of importance is the fact that many of these children have other iatrogenic factors that predispose to IE, particularly the presence of central venous catheters, which constitute an increasingly important predisposing factor to IE, accounting for as many as 18% of cases.[164] This is discussed further in the section on nosocomial IE.

More recently published series are not included in Table 45-1. In the series by Stockhein and colleagues,[193] in which 111 cases of IE seen between 1978 and 1996 were reviewed, the most common underlying congenital defects were ventricular septal defect (VSD) with other abnormalities (25 cases), pulmonary atresia (14 cases), tetralogy of Fallot (11 cases), atrial septal defect (ASD) with other abnormalities (12 cases), coarctation of the aorta (11 cases), transposition of the great vessels (12 cases), and pulmonary stenosis (10 cases). In this series, 8 children had prosthetic valves, 18 had systemic-to-pulmonary shunts, 9 had corrective conduits, and 7 had had IE previously. In the series by Martin and associates[113] of 76 cases of IE from 1958 to 1992, 23 had systemic-to-pulmonary shunts. In the series of 62 IE cases reported by Saiman and coworkers,[164] 22 patients had complex cyanotic heart disease. These cases included children with palliative shunts, conduits, or prosthetic valves.

In an excellent prospective study, Morris and colleagues[125] determined the incidence rates (number of cases per 1000 person-years of follow-up) for the development of IE following surgery for 12 different congenital heart diseases. These were as follows: pulmonary atresia with VSD, 11.5; tetralogy of Fallot with palliative systemic-to-pulmonary shunt, 8.2; aortic stenosis, 7.2; pulmonary atresia, 6.4; unoperated VSD, 3.8; primum ASD with cleft mitral valve, 1.8; coarctation of the aorta, 1.2; complete atrioventricular septal defect, 1.0; tetralogy of Fallot, 0.7; dextrotransposition of the great arteries, 0.7; and VSD, 0.6. All the cases with a VSD had a residual defect or an associated abnormality. There were no cases of IE in patients who had had surgery for ASD, PDA, or pulmonary stenosis.

Microorganisms

Although many different bacterial and nonbacterial microorganisms have been reported to cause IE, the vast majority of cases are caused by a limited number of organisms. The causes of IE in 24 pediatric series are summarized in Table 45-3. Clinical reports of IE cases caused by specific organisms, especially unusual ones, abound and are important but are likely to present a distorted view of their *relative* importance. Approximately two thirds of cases of IE in children are caused by viridans streptococci (a group consisting of several species, including *Streptococcus mitior*, *Streptococcus sanguis*, *Streptococcus milleri*, *Streptococcus salivarius*, and *Streptococcus mutans*,[27,158] and by *Staphylococcus aureus* (see Table 45-3). In a recently published series, the proportions of cases caused by viridans streptococci (33%) and *Staphylococcus aureus* (27.9%) are very similar to those of the overall series shown in the table.

Of the organisms included as "gram-negative bacilli," the most common were enteric bacilli and *Pseudomonas aeruginosa*. Considering the frequency with which these bacteria cause bacteremia, especially nosocomial bacteremia, they are relatively unusual causes of IE. This is due, at least in part, to their poor ability to adhere to endothelium and their susceptibility to the bactericidal effects of serum.[80,107]

A wide variety of gram-negative bacteria have been reported to cause IE. These include *Neisseria* spp., *Acinetobacter* spp., *Brucella* spp., *Bartonella* spp., *Legionella* spp., and anaerobes, in addition to enteric bacilli and *Pseudomonas* spp.[19,37,200]

Table 45-3 Microorganisms Causing Infective Endocarditis in Children*

Microorganism	Number	Percentage
viridans streptococci	362	31.7
Other streptococci and enterococci	75	6.4
Streptococcus pneumoniae	31	2.6
Staphylococcus aureus	295	25.1
Coagulase-negative staphylococcus	69	5.9
HACEK[†] + diphtheroids	60	5.1
Gram-negative bacilli[‡]	50	4.3
Fungi	25	2.1
Others	32	2.7
Negative cultures	164	14
Total	1173	100

*Several cases had more than one isolate.
†*Haemophilus* spp., *Actinobacillus*, *Cardiobacterium*, *Eikenella*, *Kingella*.
‡Enteric bacilli and *Pseudomonas* spp.
Data from references 6, 9, 21, 47, 68, 82, 86, 87, 91, 96, 98, 113, 123, 127, 129, 143, 175, 181, 190, 193, 202, and 220.

A group of gram-negative bacilli of particular importance is the so-called HACEK group, which consists of *Haemophilus* spp., *Actinobacillus actinomycetemcomitans*, *Cardiobacterium hominis*, *Eikenella corrodens*, and *Kingella* spp. These are constituents of normal human oropharyngeal flora and are susceptible to β-lactam agents. They may be fastidious in growth requirements and therefore must be specifically sought in suspected IE if initial blood cultures are negative. The *Haemophilus* spp. most commonly associated with IE are *Haemophilus aphrophilus*, *Haemophilus paraphrophilus*, and *Haemophilus parainfluenzae*.[37] *Haemophilus influenzae* type b, a common cause of childhood bacteremia prior to widespread vaccination against this organism, and nontypeable *H. influenzae* strains are uncommon causes of IE.[41]

Of the gram-positive bacilli causing IE, various species of the genus *Corynebacterium* (diphtheroids) are the most frequently reported. Although they cause infection mainly on prosthetic heart valves, they may also infect native valves.[21,52,75,210,214]

Because most organisms causing IE are constituents of normal oropharyngeal or skin flora and are often considered blood culture contaminants, several blood cultures should be drawn for confirmation of the diagnosis of IE (see "Diagnosis of Infective Endocarditis") before antimicrobial therapy is initiated in suspected cases of IE. About 14% of patients with IE have negative blood cultures (see Table 45-3).

The most important reason for failure to isolate a microorganism from blood in a patient with IE is that the patient has received antimicrobial therapy.[202] A few antibiotic doses, even orally administered, may render blood cultures negative for up to 2 weeks.[146,148] Therefore, if a patient suspected of having IE is not severely ill and has received antimicrobial therapy, the antimicrobial therapy should not be continued until definitive blood culture results are available. If cultures are negative, additional cultures should be performed.[146] (See "Diagnosis of Infective Endocarditis" and "Management.")

There are other reasons for negative blood cultures. The causative organism may not grow readily in the usual blood culture systems because it is (1) a fastidious bacterium requiring special media for growth (e.g., *Abiotrophia defectiva*, formerly called nutrient-deficient streptococcus, which requires pyridoxine or cysteine) or longer incubation periods (e.g., *Brucella* spp.); (2) a fungus; (3) *Coxiella burnetii*, the rickettsia-like organism causing Q fever, which is diagnosed serologically; (4) *Chlamydia* spp.; (5) *Mycobacterium* spp.; or (6) *Bartonella* spp.[14,151] Negative blood cultures are also seen in right-sided endocarditis and noninfective endocarditis.[203] The fastidious microorganisms causing IE are discussed in an excellent review by Berbari and colleagues.[19]

Clinical Features of Infective Endocarditis*

Infective endocarditis is usually a subacute infection but may be acute. Its clinical manifestations can be considered in terms of nonspecific features of infection, cardiac manifestations, manifestations of emboli and metastatic infections, and evidence

---

*See references 31, 78, 173, and 195.

Table 45-4 Clinical Features of Infective Endocarditis in Children

Clinical Feature	Cases(n)*	Those with Abnormality (n)	Those with Abnormality (%)
Fever	419	368	88
Anemia	152	122	80
Heart murmur	152	99	65
New/changing murmur	242	68	28
Heart failure	317	114	36
Peripheral manifestations	175	29	17
Cerebral manifestations	175	39	22
Pulmonary emboli	133	22	17
Other emboli	37	137	27
Splenomegaly	397	211	53
Hematuria	318	62	19

*Number of cases for which abnormality was evaluated.
Data from references 9, 21, 68, 82, 86, 87, 91, 96, 98, 123, 127, 129, 143, 175, 181, 190, 202, and 220.

of immune stimulation or immune complex disease. The main manifestations seen in children are shown in Table 45-4.

Nonspecific Features

Fever is the most common clinical manifestation of IE and is present in almost all cases. Fever is usually low grade, but in acute endocarditis in which the nonspecific features of infection dominate the clinical picture, fever may be high and associated with clinical toxicity and the hemodynamic effects of septicemia. In the series depicted in Table 45-4, fever was present for 1 to 210 days before a diagnosis was made. On average, fever preceded diagnosis by 27 to 43 days. Other nonspecific features include malaise, anorexia, weight loss, night sweats, myalgias, and arthralgias.

Anemia is the second most common abnormality in children with IE. It has the features of anemia of chronic disease, which is due to depression of the bone marrow and its failure to utilize iron. The anemia is usually not hemodynamically significant.[59] Occasionally, if anemia is severe, hemolysis due to intravascular damage to red cells should be suspected; this occurs mainly in individuals with prosthetic valves.[20,63,130,133]

Cardiac Manifestations

Because most patients with IE have underlying structural heart abnormalities, most cases of IE are associated with heart murmurs. However, in acute endocarditis, especially of the tricuspid valve or mural endocardium, murmurs may not be present. Appearance of a new murmur or a change in an old murmur is of particular significance, as it implies distortion of the valve aperture with or without stenosis or incompetence.

Development of heart failure is the most important and common complication of IE. It is also the most common cause of death from IE and develops in approximately one third of children with IE.* It is caused primarily by valvular incompetence or, much less frequently, by obstruction but may be due to other cardiac complications, including myocardial infection and conduction defects.[182] In the series of Johnson and colleagues,[87] heart failure was present in 51 of the 58 patients on admission.

Embolic Manifestations

Embolic manifestations occur in the minority of children but, when present, provide important clues to the diagnosis of IE. Clinically apparent major emboli lodge most commonly in the cerebral or pulmonary circulations.

Cerebral manifestations occur in 30% to 40% of adults with IE.[144,149,166] They include focal neurologic deficits, meningeal symptoms and signs, seizures, encephalopathy, visual disturbances, psychiatric disturbances, and evidence of intracranial hemorrhage. In several pediatric IE series, about 22% of cases overall had evidence of cerebral complications.* These were not described in detail.

It is important to examine all the peripheral pulses of patients suspected of having IE, as absence or loss of such a pulse suggests the possibility of an embolus. Such an embolus should be viewed as an important source of material for making a histologic and microbiologic diagnosis of the cause of IE.

Several peripheral manifestations of IE, seen in the minority of childhood cases, are thought to be caused by emboli. Petechiae may occur in the skin and buccal and conjunctival mucosae. Roth spots are oval-shaped retinal hemorrhages with a white center. In cases of suspected IE, the pupils should be dilated with a mydriatic so that the retinae can be adequately examined for Roth spots. Subungual splinter hemorrhages may be present. Janeway lesions are hemorrhagic macules on the palms and soles, most commonly seen in cases of IE caused by S. aureus. Acute endocarditis caused by this organism may be associated with areas of skin infarction, resembling those seen in cases of meningococcemia. Aspirates of these lesions should be examined with Gram's stain and cultured to provide immediate information as to the cause of the infection. Osler's nodes are small (2 to 15 mm in diameter), tender, purple nodules on the pulp of the digits. Digital clubbing may occur. However, its pathogenesis is unclear.

Immune Manifestations

Immune manifestations are most common in subacute or chronic cases. Splenomegaly occurs in about one half of cases, and hematuria, a manifestation of glomerulonephritis, in about one fifth of cases.*

Source of Bacteremia Leading to Infective Endocarditis

The sources of bacteremia resulting in IE, derived from 11 pediatric series, are shown in Table 45-5. A source was identified in the minority of cases. The infection was hospital acquired in 15.8% of cases. Cardiac surgery and dental procedures were the most common identified factors leading to the development of IE. (See "Nosocomial Endocarditis" and "Prevention of Infective Carditis.")

Table 45-5 Source of Bacteremia, Where Known, in Children with Infective Endocarditis

Source of Bacteremia	Number	Percentage of All Cases of Infective Endocarditis
Nosocomial	91	15.8
Intravascular catheters	17	3.0
Cardiac surgery	47	8.2
Cardiac catheterization	8	1.4
Noncardiac surgery	13	2.3
Other sources	6	1.0
Dental Procedures	29	5.0
No Procedure	82	14.3
Dental infection	13	2.3
Ear, nose, throat infection	20	3.5
Skin infection	17	3.0
Pulmonary infection	5	0.8
Other infections*	27	4.7
Total with Identified Source	202	35.1
Total Number of Cases	575	100

*Not specified, 15; urinary tract infection, 2; meningitis, 3; burns, 2; bone infection, 2; gastrointestinal infection, 2; ventriculoperitoneal shunt infection, 1.

Data from references 9, 21, 68, 82, 86, 87, 91, 96, 98, 123, 127, 129, 143, 175, 181, 190, 202, and 220.

NEONATAL ENDOCARDITIS

Infective endocarditis in the neonate has been recognized with increasing frequency during the past decade.* This is probably due to a true increase in its frequency as a result of the management of babies, especially premature babies, in intensive care units, and to an increase in awareness of the disease. In this section, features of IE peculiar to the neonate are discussed.

Predisposing Factors

The great majority of neonates with IE have no underlying heart disease. The pathogenetic factors leading to IE in neonates (see "Pathogenesis of Infective Endocarditis") are somewhat different from those in older children. NBTE in the neonate occurs mostly on the right side of the heart and follows hypoxia resulting from conditions such as persistent fetal circulation and hyaline membrane disease, as well as disseminated intravascular coagulation. This has been found in 8% to 10% of all neonatal autopsies.[196] Persistent fetal circulation and hyaline membrane disease might result in IE by causing the release of vasoactive substances (e.g., thromboxane A_2 or other eicosanoids), which cause platelet aggregation.[126] Endothelial damage is caused by intravascular catheters, either percutaneous central venous catheters or catheters passed through the umbilical vein. In a report by Mecrow and colleagues,[119] all 12 patients with neonatal endocarditis with normal hearts had central venous catheters. In the series by Daher and Berkowitz,[42] there were two groups of neonates with different patterns of endocarditis, one consisting of premature infants with medical problems related to prematurity, including patent ductus arteriosus, but

---

*See references 9, 21, 68, 82, 86, 87, 91, 96, 98, 123, 127, 129, 143, 175, 181, 190, 202, and 220.

*See references 81, 112, 121, 134, 138, 139, 147, 180, 196, and 221.

no other underlying heart disease and another consisting of term infants who developed IE following surgery for congenital heart disease.

Causative Organisms

Almost all cases of neonatal IE are nosocomial. The most common causative organisms are *S. aureus* (which accounts for about half of all cases), coagulase-negative staphylococcus, streptococci (including group B streptococcus) and *Candida* spp.[42,81,112,120,134,138,139,180,196]

Clinical Features

Clinical features are nonspecific and the same as those of other infections, such as septicemia, in this age group (e.g., temperature instability and poor feeding). The more specific features are the same as those occurring in older children. Thrombocytopenia is common.[81,112,120,134,138,139,180,196]

PROSTHETIC VALVE ENDOCARDITIS

Infection of prosthetic valves is a major complication of valve replacement.[52,75,172,214] It occurs at some time in 1% to 4% of all patients with prosthetic valves with a risk of 0.32% to 1.20% per patient year.[5,52,55] The period of highest risk for developing prosthetic valve endocarditis (PVE) is the first 2 months after surgery. Nevertheless, because of high patient survival rates, most cases of PVE occur after this period.[75] PVE differs from native valve endocarditis in several ways.

Causative Organisms

In the early postoperative period (<2 months) staphylococci, both *S. aureus* and coagulase-negative staphylococci, account for about 50% of cases, and gram-negative bacilli, diphtheroids, and fungi (particularly *Candida* spp.) account for a significant proportion of cases. After 1 year, the most common causative organisms are essentially the same as those in native valve endocarditis, with the exception that coagulase-negative staphylococci remain important.[52,75,214] Although the tags attached to prosthetic valves may grow microorganisms when cultured, in one study, these cultures did not predict the development of endocarditis.[69]

Complications

The initial focus of infection may be at the site of suture of the valve into the valve ring. Therefore, complications such as valve dehiscence and valve ring abscesses with extension into deeper cardiac tissue are common.

Diagnosis

Making the diagnosis of PVE may be difficult in certain circumstances. In the early postoperative period, PVE may be difficult to differentiate from other causes of postoperative fever (see "Diagnosis of Infective Endocarditis"). In the case of valve ring abscesses, bacteremia may not be continuous.[73] Transthoracic two-dimensional (2-D) echocardiography is far less sensitive in detecting vegetations associated with endocarditis of mechanical prosthetic valves than those associated with native valve endocarditis, due to the echodensity of the mechanical prosthesis itself. Transesophageal echocardiography is more sensitive in this situation.[45,188] This has been used in infants as small as 2.2 kg.[176]

Prognosis and Management

The case fatality rate of PVE is higher than in native valve infection, and surgery, in addition to medical therapy, is often necessary in PVE. The data on prosthetic valve endocarditis are derived largely from studies in adults. However, many cardiac procedures in children involve patches, conduits, and shunts. Infections on these types of protheses are not well addressed in the literature. Furthermore, diagnosis of infection localized to these structures is difficult because specific physical signs may be absent, and the lesions may not be readily detected by echocardiography.

NOSOCOMIAL ENDOCARDITIS

A significant proportion of cases of IE are hospital acquired.[209] Although IE complicating cardiac surgery is well recognized, that complicating nosocomial bacteremia in individuals with or without underlying heart disease is less well appreciated.[21,65,187,198,209,211] The combined data from three series of IE in adults show that 66 of 436 (14%) cases were nosocomial and that only 7 of these were related to cardiac surgery. Thirty (45%) of these 66 cases were caused by intravascular procedures or devices. Forty-three cases (65%) were caused by staphylococci, the other major pathogen being enterococcus.[34,65,198] In a study of 76 cases of *S. aureus* bacteremia, 35 were nosocomial, of which 6 were associated with endocarditis,[122] and in a study of 119 cases of *S. aureus* endocarditis, 38% were nosocomial.[60] The intravascular devices and procedures leading to nosocomial endocarditis include not only central venous lines but also peripheral intravenous catheters, diagnostic cardiac catheterizations, pacemakers, and Swan-Ganz catheters.[211] In an autopsy study of patients who had had Swan-Ganz catheters placed, 4 of 55 (7.3%) had IE.[162] Infection of long-term indwelling catheters used for outpatient intravenous access (e.g., Broviac catheters) also may lead to IE.[17,35,104,114]

Intravascular devices predispose to bloodstream infections by forming a bridge between the external environment and the bloodstream. Most device-related infections are caused by cutaneous organisms infecting the catheter tip at the time of its insertion or growing down along the insertion track.[111] Once the catheter tip is infected, it becomes a nidus of infection within the bloodstream. The infection may spread hematogenously to any focus in the body, including the endocardium, and to other intravascular devices. The organisms that are the most important causes of catheter-related bacteremia, namely coagulase-negative staphylococci, *S. aureus* and *Candida* spp.,[111] have the propensity to attach to endothelium (see "Pathogenesis of Infective Endocarditis"). This renders them important causes of catheter-associated endocarditis. Intravascular devices may lead to endocarditis not only by causing bacteremia but also, in the case of catheters entering the heart, by causing endocardial damage and NBTE.

Several variables influence the risks of particular types of catheters becoming infected (e.g., their duration of usage and site of insertion). Overall, in adults, septicemia is associated with about 0.2% of peripheral venous catheters, 1% of arterial catheters, and 3% of percutaneous central venous catheters inserted.[111] For cuffed central venous catheters (e.g., Broviac, Hickman), these rates are about 0.2 per 100 device days, and for subcutaneous central venous ports, about 0.04 per 100 device days.[111] In a study of 91 newborns, Cronin and colleagues[39] showed that microbial colonization occurred in 13% of peripheral venous and umbilical venous catheters, 27% of central venous catheters, 15% of umbilical arterial catheters, and 36% of peripheral arterial catheters. There were seven device-related bacteremias in this series.

Diagnosis of Catheter-Related Bacteremia and Endocarditis

In any febrile patient who has or who has had an intravascular device in situ, the device or its track should be considered a possible focus of infection. Bacteremia caused by staphylococci, *Candida* spp., *Bacillus* spp., or *Corynebacterium* spp. is likely to be caused by an intravascular device, while that caused by gram-negative bacilli is not.[111,150] A positive culture of blood drawn through the catheter does not allow differentiation between bacteremia arising from the catheter and that arising from a distant focus. This problem can sometimes be resolved by quantitative blood cultures, in which the bacterial counts of blood drawn through the catheter are compared with those of blood drawn percutaneously. A ratio of greater than 10:1 (catheter-to-percutaneous) suggests a catheter-related bacteremia.[84,111,150] Unfortunately, quantitative blood cultures are usually not readily available. Examination of a gram-stained smear of the buffy coat of blood drawn through the catheter has been useful in the diagnosis of catheter-related fungemia caused by *Malassezia furfur* in neonates.[139] Once the catheter has been removed, semi-quantitative culture of its tip, by the roll-plate method, can suggest whether it had been infected.[111]

Management

Ideally, in a patient with catheter related bacteremia, the catheter should be removed. This is not always possible. When catheter removal is not considered to be in the patient's best interest, antimicrobial therapy should be attempted.[150] This is often successful. The absolute need to remove the catheter in cases caused by specific organisms (e.g., *Candida* spp. or gram-positive bacilli) is controversial.[150] The antimicrobial therapy must be infused through the infected catheter and, in alternate doses, through each port of the catheter. If bacteremia persists despite appropriate antimicrobial therapy, the catheter should be removed. If bacteremia persists for more than 48 hours after catheter removal, a diagnosis of septic phlebitis, infected thrombus, or infective endocarditis should be considered likely. These entities may be impossible to differentiate from one another unless an anatomic study (e.g., echocardiogram) indicates a vegetation or thrombus.

Prevention

Factors that can reduce the risk of catheters becoming infected include meticulous aseptic technique and cleansing of the site at the time of catheter insertion, adequate immobilization of the catheter, and regular inspection of the insertion site for evidence of inflammation. Occlusive dressings increase the risk of catheter infections.[111,150] Peripheral venous catheters, which are the catheters most readily replaced, should be removed after 48 to 72 hours.[184] The upper limits of duration for which other temporary catheters should be allowed to remain in situ are unclear, because the risks of infection in different studies are so variable.[33,44,66,136] As seen in Table 45-5, 15.8% of pediatric IE cases were nosocomial, and only half of these followed cardiac surgery.

INFECTIVE ENDOCARDITIS IN INTRAVENOUS DRUG ABUSERS

Although IE in intravenous drug abusers (IVDAs) is a disease primarily of young adults, it also affects older teenagers. IE is a very important infective complication of intravenous drug abuse.[152,157,168] IVDAs, including those with no underlying heart disease, are at a very high risk of developing IE, estimated to be 1.5 to 2 per 1000 per year.[183] Predisposing factors include (1) damage to the heart valves, especially the tricuspid valve, by injected foreign material; (2) phlebitis and other foci of infection resulting in bacteremia; (3) injection of skin flora; (4) contamination of the injecting paraphernalia; and (5) contamination of the diluent. Although contamination of the drug would be expected to be a factor, this has not been demonstrated.[152,157,168]

The clinical features are generally the same as those of IE in other individuals, but certain peculiar features deserve comment. Most affected individuals have no underlying heart disease. The infection is caused by *S. aureus* in about 50% of cases and is often acute in onset. Other predominant causative organisms vary with time and geographic area. Epidemics caused by specific organisms (e.g., *Serratia marcescens* and *P. aeruginosa*) have been described.[133] Most cases of polymicrobial endocarditis occur in IVDAs.[10]

About half of cases affect the right side of the heart, primarily the tricuspid valve. The main complications are therefore pulmonary—namely, pulmonary emboli—and hematogenous pneumonia, sometimes followed by the development of cavities and extension to the pleura. Management of these patients is complicated by their risky behavior, which makes them susceptible to repeated infections.

Although IE is the most important diagnosis to consider in an IVDA with fever, such individuals are at risk for developing numerous other infections, the bacterial causes of which may themselves lead to endocarditis. These infections include bacterial infection of the skin, soft tissue, and skeleton; pneumonia; hepatitis B and C; HIV infection and its complications; and malaria.[74,167,179]

FUNGAL ENDOCARDITIS

Although fungi cause a small proportion of cases of IE in children overall (see Table 45-3; approximately 2%) and adults[200] (approximately 1%), fungal endocarditis is an important disease in the critical care unit for the following reasons: (1) many critical care patients, whether cardiac or noncardiac, are at risk for developing this infection; (2) it is difficult to diagnose; (3) the treatment usually entails cardiac surgery; and (4) the case fatality rate is extremely high.[117,128,163] Fungi account for a high proportion of IE cases in the neonate.[42] In the series by Aspesberro and colleagues, 5 of 16 cases of IE were caused by fungi.[7]

Microbiology

A large number of different fungi, including yeasts, molds, and dimorphic fungi, have been reported to cause IE.[117,128] However, about 85% of cases are caused by *Candida albicans*, other species of *Candida* (*Candida tropicalis*, *Candida parapsilosis*, *Candida krusei*, *Candida stellatoidea*, *Candida guillermondii*, and *Candida glabrata*) and species of *Aspergillus* (*Aspergillus fumigatus*, *Aspergillus flavus*, *Aspergillus niger*, *Aspergillus glaucus*, *Aspergillus ustus*, *Aspergillus terreus*, *Aspergillus sydowi*, and *Aspergillus nidulans*).[16,117,128,163,219] *Histoplasma capsulatum* causes about 7% of cases,[94] the majority of which occur in patients without underlying heart disease.[25]

Predisposing Factors and Pathogenesis

Three main categories of patients are at risk for developing fungal endocarditis, namely, those who have undergone cardiac surgery, those with various derangements of their host defenses, and IVDAs.

Cardiac Surgery Patients

Fungi account for about 10% of cases of IE in the first year after prosthetic valve surgery.[52] These cases are caused mainly by *C. albicans*, other *Candida* spp., and *Aspergillus* spp.[52] The infections caused by *Aspergillus* spp. are thought to occur as a result of inoculation of the heart or bloodstream during surgery by fungal spores present in the environment.[89] This was shown to have been very likely in a specific cluster of cases.[120]

Candida spp. have a predilection for causing endocarditis because of their ability to attach to fibrin-platelet thrombi. Platelets stimulate the germination of the yeast cells, and yeast cell wall fragments cause complement fixation, which, in turn, causes platelet aggregation.[161] Individuals undergoing cardiac surgery are at risk for developing *Candida* endocarditis because of their structural abnormalities and disrupted endothelium, as well as their host defense derangements.

Host Defense Derangements

Several derangements of host defenses affecting the skin and mucous membranes, the immune system, and the normal microbial flora predispose to fungemia, which can lead to fungal endocarditis. These include immunosuppressive therapy (e.g., corticosteroids, cancer chemotherapy, and transplant immunosuppression), intravascular catheters, and prolonged broad-spectrum antimicrobial therapy. These factors predispose particularly to *Candida* endocarditis, but also to *Aspergillus* endocarditis.[3,89,117,161,219] Several cases of fungal endocarditis have developed in individuals being treated for bacterial endocarditis.[3,161]

Intravenous Drug Abusers

The main causative fungi in this group of individuals, who are discussed in greater detail in a previous section, are non-*albicans* species of *Candida*.[3,117,163] Fungal endocarditis affects both valvular and mural endocardium. Myocardial involvement is frequent and is thought, in some cases, to precede the endocardial involvement.[3,89,117,161]

Clinical Features

These are essentially the same as those of other forms of endocarditis. However, embolism is frequent and often the presenting feature of the illness. The emboli often impact in large vessels, especially in the extremities, brain, and lung, but all viscera may be affected.[117,128,161]

Diagnosis

Whereas blood cultures are usually positive in *Candida* endocarditis, this is rarely so in cases of endocarditis caused by other fungi.[117,128,161] Most cases of *Aspergillus* endocarditis have been diagnosed at autopsy.[15,161,219] The most useful material for diagnosing non-*candida* endocarditis is the embolus. When removed, this should be processed immediately for diagnosing the cause of the endocarditis (see "Diagnosis of Infective Endocarditis"). Serologic tests may be helpful in diagnosing systemic histoplasma and cryptococcal infections.[128] Such tests for the diagnosis of systemic *Candida* and *Aspergillus* infections are currently being developed but are not in general use at present.

Therapy and Outcome

The outcome is influenced by the type of the causative fungus and whether the infection occurs on a native or prosthetic valve. Because fungal endocarditis may progress very slowly and recurrences may manifest after long delays, patients should not be considered cured without a follow-up period of at least 2 years.[88,103] This criterion is not necessarily met in all reported cases.

Therapy consists of antifungal therapy and, in most cases, surgery. The mainstay of medical therapy is amphotericin B, used together with 5-flucytosine in cases of yeast endocarditis (*Candida* and *Cryptococcus*; Tables 45-6 and 45-7). In cases in which there is significant impairment of renal function, consideration should be given to the use of one of the lipid complex preparations of amphotericin B. In the cases treated successfully with medical therapy alone, therapy was given for 6 to 12 weeks.[61,128,161,221] The role of triazoles

Table 45-6 Antimicrobial Therapy of Infective Endocarditis Caused by Gram-Negative Bacteria and by Fungi

Organism	Antimicrobial Agent	Duration (wk)
HACEK organisms	Third-generation cephalosporin or	4
	ampicillin + gentamicin (if susceptibility demonstrated)	4
Enteric bacilli†	Third-generation cephalosporin	6
	+ aminoglycoside	6
Pseudomonas aeruginosa*	Antipseudomonal penicillin	6
	+ aminoglycoside	6
	or	
	ceftazidime	6
	+ aminoglycoside	6
Fungi	Amphotericin B	At least 6
	+	
	flucytosine (for infection with yeast)	At least 6

*Depending on susceptibilities.
Data from references 13, 117, 128, 173, 217, and 221.

(e.g., fluconazole and itraconazole) in the treatment of fungal endocarditis is unclear. In experimental animals, fluconazole was inferior to amphotericin B in treating or preventing Candida endocarditis.[218] However, this drug might have a role in chronic suppression of an infection.[7,88] Surgery usually entails valve replacement,[128,161] but surgical débridement has been successful in a case of Candida endocarditis.[197]

In an analysis of 319 cases of fungal endocarditis, McLeod and colleagues[117] found that in patients with non-Aspergillus infections of native valves, medical treatment alone was associated with a survival rate of 73% (8 of 11 cases), compared with 58% (15 of 26 cases) for combined medical and surgical therapy. However, in patients who had had previous cardiac surgery, 19% (4 of 21) treated only medically versus 50% (11 of 22) treated with combined therapy survived.

Of the few reported survivors of Aspergillus endocarditis, all had undergone valve replacement.[128,161]

DIAGNOSIS OF INFECTIVE ENDOCARDITIS

Infective endocarditis should be considered a diagnostic possibility in any individual with a fever and a risk factor for IE (e.g., structural heart disease or intravenous drug abuse) or in any individual with prolonged unexplained fever (Table 45-8). Making a microbiologic diagnosis of IE is of the utmost importance for optimal management of the patient. Because the hallmark of the disease is persistent bacteremia, the diagnosis is confirmed by the demonstration of repeatedly positive blood cultures.[94]

Blood Cultures

The levels of bacteremia in IE are often low (less than 100 organisms per milliliter of blood[8,94]); therefore, adequate volumes of blood should be drawn and diluted 1:5 to 1:10 in the blood culture medium. In adults, at least 10 mL of blood should be drawn for each bottle.[94,206,207,208] This cannot be done in infants and young children. Nevertheless, as large a volume as is reasonable should be drawn for each culture, preferably 3 to 5 mL. The organisms causing endocarditis include those that may be considered skin contaminants of blood cultures, especially coagulase-negative staphylococci and diphtheroids. Therefore, the blood should be drawn with a meticulously aseptic technique and percutaneously, not through indwelling intravascular catheters.

At least three sets of blood cultures should be drawn over a period of 24 hours to (1) demonstrate persistent bacteremia, (2) increase the probability of a positive culture (which is accomplished to only a small degree), and (3) increase the likelihood that the isolate is significant and not a contaminant.[94,206-208]

Table 45-7 Dosages, Routes, and Dosing Schedules for Antimicrobial Agents Used in the Treatment of Infective Endocarditis

Drug	Pediatric Dosage and Route	Adult Dosage and Route	Schedule
Amphotericin B	1 mg/kg/24 hr IV	1 mg/kg/24 hr IV	Daily
Ampicillin	300 mg/kg/24 hr IV	12 g/24 hr IV	Continuously or q4 hr
Cefazolin	80–100 mg/kg/24 hr IV	2 g/dose IV	q8 hr
Cefotaxime	100–200 mg/kg/24 hr IV	2 g/dose IV	q6 hr
Ceftazidime	100–150 mg/kg/24 hr IV	2 g/dose IV	q8 hr
Ceftriaxone	50–100 mg/kg/24 hr IV or IM	2 g/24 hr IV or IM	q12–24 hr
Cephalothin*	100–150 mg/kg/24 hr IV	2 g/dose IV	q6 hr
Ciprofloxacin	20–30 mg/kg/24 hr IV	800 mg/24 hr IV	q12 hr
	30–40 mg/kg/24 hr PO	1500 mg/24 hr PO	
Flucytosine	100–150 mg/kg/24 hr PO	100–150 mg/kg/24 hr PO	q6 hr
Gentamicin	2.0–2.5/kg/dose IV or IM	1 mg/kg/dose IV or IM	q8 hr
Imipenem/cilastatin	60–100 mg/kg/24 hr IV	2 g/24 hr IV	q6 hr
Meropenem	60 mg/kg/24 hr IV	3 g/24 hr IV	q8 hr
Nafcillin	150–200 mg/kg/24 hr IV	12 g/24 hr IV	q4–6 hr
Oxacillin	150–200 mg/kg/24 hr IV	12 g/24 hr IV	q4–6 hr
Penicillin G	150,000–200,000 U/kg/24 hr IV	10–20 million U/24 hr IV	Continuously or q4 hr
Penicillin G high dosage	200,000–300,000 U/kg/24 hr IV	20–30 million U/24 hr IV	Continuously or q4 hr
Rifampin	10 mg/kg/dose PO	300 mg/dose PO	q12 hr
Streptomycin	7.5–10 mg/kg/dose IM	7.5 mg/kg/dose IM	q12 hr
Vancomycin	40 mg/kg/24 hr IV	30 mg/kg/24 hr IV	q6–12 hr

*No longer available in the USA.
Data from references 24, 131, 171, and 217.

Table 45-8 Conditions Other than Infective Endocarditis Associated with Fever and Occurring in Individuals at Risk for Infective Endocarditis or in Individuals with Heart Disease

Risk Factor	Other Diagnosis
Rheumatic heart disease	Acute rheumatic fever
Congenital heart disease	Common childhood infections: viral exanthems, upper respiratory tract infections; otitis media; bacteremia due to *Streptococcus pneumoniae* or *Haemophilus influenzae* type b
Cyanotic heart disease	Brain abscess
Intravenous drug abusers*	Phlebitis; hepatitis B; HIV infection with opportunistic infection; tuberculosis
After cardiac surgery*	Infections: lung, urinary tract, vascular catheters, wound; postcardiotomy syndrome; postperfusion syndrome
New onset of cardiac disease and fever	Acute rheumatic fever; systemic lupus erythematosus; rheumatoid disease; acute myocarditis
Afebrile cardiac disease, emboli	Atrial myxoma
Murmur, anemia	Functional murmur from anemia

*See "Differential Diagnosis" in text.

In a severely ill patient in whom the diagnosis of IE is very likely and the pace of the illness is acute, three sets of blood cultures should be drawn over a period of 1 to 2 hr, and appropriate antimicrobial therapy should be instituted. However, in patients with a more indolent course of illness or in whom the diagnosis is not as clear—and especially if prior antimicrobial therapy has been given—one should not initiate antimicrobial therapy for IE until the results of blood cultures become available. If the blood cultures are negative at 48 hr and the diagnosis of IE is still considered likely, additional cultures should be performed and the various causes of culture-negative endocarditis should be considered (see "Microorganisms"). The optimal methods for identifying these causes should be discussed with the microbiology laboratory staff.[203]

If antimicrobial therapy has been initiated and the blood cultures are negative, it may become impossible to confirm the diagnosis of IE. If the patient improves because of—or in spite of—this therapy, the most reasonable approach is to complete therapy as for culture-negative endocarditis, unless an alternative diagnosis becomes apparent.

Several criteria have been used for categorizing the likelihood of a diagnosis of IE. Those proposed by von Reyn and colleagues[204] have been widely used as inclusion criteria for studies of IE. Of note is the fact that echocardiographic findings are not included in these criteria. More recently, a set of diagnostic criteria often referred as the "Duke criteria" have been proposed by Durack and associates.[53] These have been evaluated in children and considered to be superior to the von Reyn criteria.[192] They are noteworthy for including echocardiographic findings. These criteria are shown in Table 45-9A, and the definitions used for this criteria are shown in Table 45-9B.

In addition to blood cultures, culture and Gram's stain of any potentially infected fluid should be performed. Gram's stain of the urine may give a rapid microbiologic diagnosis, especially in the case of *S. aureus* infection.[102,135] In cases of bacteremia, this organism is commonly present in the urine in the absence of urinary tract infection. Emboli or vegetations

removed surgically should be examined by the following methods: (1) histologic analysis should be performed with appropriate tissue Gram's stains and fungal stains (e.g., periodic acid–Schiff and silver impregnation stains) and mycobacterial stains; (2) smears should be stained for the same organisms; and (3) cultures should be performed on media appropriate for aerobic, anaerobic, and fastidious bacteria, *Legionella* spp., mycobacteria, and fungi.

Echocardiography

Echocardiography is useful in the diagnosis and management of some cases of IE.[188] Initially M-mode echocardiography was used, but this has been superseded by 2-D echocardiography, which is more sensitive for the detection of valvular vegetations. When compared with clinicopathologic criteria for the diagnosis of IE, transthoracic 2-D echocardiography has been shown to detect as many as 80% of cases of IE in adults. The findings in various adult studies have been summarized by Sokil.[188] In children, Bricker and coworkers[28] found M-mode echocardiography to detect cardiac vegetations in only 7 of 35 (20%) cases and 2-D echocardiography to detect them in 16 of 28 (57%), whereas Kavey and colleagues[92] found 2-D echocardiography to detect vegetations in 9 of 11 (82%) pediatric cases. Of importance is the fact that these pediatric studies do not report detection of abnormalities of prosthetic conduits, patent ductus arteriosus, or coarctation of the aorta, and most of the abnormalities detected were left sided.

Although transthoracic echocardiography is useful in both detecting vegetations and evaluating cardiac function, its limitations should be appreciated. These include the inability to detect vegetations smaller than about 2 mm in diameter and vegetations on mechanical prosthetic valves, differentiate between vegetations and some other valvular abnormalities (e.g., myxomatous degeneration), and determine whether a vegetation is infected or healed.[11,188]

In some studies, the presence of echocardiographic vegetations has been correlated with a higher risk of adverse outcomes, including the development of congestive heart failure, significant embolism, requirement for surgery, or death.[30,109,137,192] This is controversial and certainly does not indicate that all patients with echocardiographic vegetations should undergo surgery.

A recent advance in echocardiography is transesophageal echocardiography. With the probe placed within the esophagus and close to the heart, a higher sound frequency can be used, resulting in a greater degree of resolution of the image. This technique has been shown to have a higher sensitivity for detecting vegetations in adults than does transthoracic echocardiography and is particularly useful for detecting valve ring abscesses[45] and prosthetic mitral valve infections.[23] In a study of transesopohageal echocardiography in children, Scott and colleagues[176] showed that a 13-mm adult probe could be used in children weighing as little as 7 kg and that a 7-mm probe could be used in a 2.2-kg infant. They demonstrated in two children vegetations that were not detected by transthoracic echocardiography.

Radionucleide Imaging

Various radionucleide scans, including gallium 67 citrate and indium 111–labeled leukocytes and platelets, have been used for diagnosing IE but with very little success.[188]

Table 45-9A Criteria for Diagnosis of Infective Endocarditis

Definite Infective Endocarditis

Pathologic criteria
  Microorganisms: demonstrated by culture or
  Histology in a vegetation or
  In a vegetation that has embolized or
  In an intracardiac abscess or
  Pathologic lesions: Vegetation or intracardiac abscess present confirmed by histology showing active endocarditis
Clinical criteria, using specific definitions listed in Table 45-9B
  Two major criteria or
  One major and three minor criteria or
  Five minor criteria

Possible Infective Endocarditis

  Findings consistent with infective endocarditis that fall short of "definite" but not "rejected"

Rejected

  Firm alternate diagnosis for manifestations of endocarditis or
  Resolution of manifestations of endocarditis, with antibiotic therapy for ≤4 days or
  No pathologic evidence of infective endocarditis at surgery or autopsy, after antibiotic therapy for ≤4 days

From Durack DT, Lukes AS, Bright DK, Duke Endocarditis Service: New criteria for diagnosis of infective endocarditis: Utilization of specific echocardiographic findings. *Am J Med* 96:200–209, 1994; with permission from Excerpta Medica, Inc.

Indium 111–labeled nonspecific immunoglobulin G may be of some value in detecting IE on vascular prostheses, as may gallium 67.[93,141] Technetium 99–labelled anti–NCA-95 antigranulocyte antibodies may help in the diagnosis in some cases.[124]

Various hematologic parameters, including leukocyte count, erythrocyte sedimentation rate, C-reactive protein and serum gamma globulin concentrations are often abnormal in IE, and abnormal proteins, such as rheumatoid factor and circulating immune complexes, are often present in the blood. However, these abnormalities are neither sensitive nor specific for diagnosing IE. Of particular note is the fact that the leukocyte count is often normal in IE.[94,213]

DIFFERENTIAL DIAGNOSIS

Various conditions associated with fever and occurring in individuals with heart disease or in those at risk of developing IE are listed in Table 45-8. A situation in which a diagnosis is particularly difficult to make is in the patient after cardiac surgery who has fever, with or without positive blood cultures. Such patients are at risk for developing IE, but they also have numerous other possible foci of infection, including the lungs, the chest wound, intravenous and intra-arterial catheter sites, and the urinary tract. This problem was studied by Sande and associates,[169] who showed that early onset of persistent bacteremia (less than 25 days postoperatively) in the presence of a potentially infected focus was unlikely to be

Table 45-9B Definitions of Terminology Used in the Criteria

Major Criteria	
Positive blood culture for infective endocarditis	Typical microorganism for infective endocarditis from two separate blood cultures *viridans streptococci* ,* *Streptococcus bovis*, HACEK group or Community-acquired *Staphylococcus aureus* or enterococci in the absence of a primary focus or
Persistently positive blood culture	Defined as recovery of a microorganism consistent with infective endocarditis from Blood cultures drawn more than 12 hr apart or All of three or a majority of four or more separate blood cultures, with first and last drawn at least 1 hr apart
Evidence of endocardial involvement	Positive echocardiogram for infective endocarditis Oscillating intracardiac mass, on valve or supporting structures, or in the path of regurgant jets or on implanted material, in the absence of an alternative anatomic explanation or Abscess or New partial dehiscence of prosthetic valve or New valvular regurgitation (increase or change in preexisting murmur not sufficient)
Minor Criteria	
Predisposition	Predisposing heart condition or IV drug use
Fever	≥38.0°C (100.4°F)
Vascular phenomena	Major arterial emboli, septic pulmonary infarcts, mycotic aneurysm, intracranial hemorrhage, conjunctival hemorrhages, Janeway lesions
Immunologic phenomena	Glomerulonephritis, Osler's nodes, Roth spots, rheumatoid factor
Microbiologic evidence	Positive blood culture but not meeting major criterion as noted previously† or serologic evidence of active infection with organism consistent with infective endocarditis
Echocardiogram	Consistent with infective endocarditis but not meeting major criterion as noted previously

*Including nutritional variant strains.
†Excluding single positive cultures for coagulase-negative staphylococci and organisms that do not cause endocarditis.
HACEK, *Haemophilus* spp., *Actinobacillus actinomycetemcomitans*, *Cardiobacterium hominis*, *Eikenella* spp., and *Kingella kingae*.
From Durack DT, Lukes AS, Bright DK, Duke Endocarditis Service: New criteria for diagnosis of infective endocarditis: utilization of specific echocardiographic findings. *Am J Med* 96:200–209, 1994; with permission of Excerpta Medica, Inc.

caused by IE, especially if the organism was a gram-negative bacillus. Parker and colleagues showed similar findings.[142]

Two important syndromes following cardiac surgery may suggest the possibility of IE; namely, the postpericardiotomy syndrome and the postperfusion syndrome of lymphocytosis and hepatosplenomegaly.[57] The postpericardiotomy syndrome, which develops 1 to 3 weeks after pericardiotomy, is characterized by fever, pericarditis, and pleuritis. It occurs in 25% to 30% of patients undergoing pericardiotomy but is uncommon in children younger than 2 years.[57] An acute or reactivated viral infection is thought to play a role in its pathogenesis.[58] The postperfusion syndrome, which is usually caused by infection with cytomegalovirus or occasionally by Epstein-Barr virus in the transfused blood, develops 4 to 6 weeks after extracorporeal circulation and is characterized by fever, splenomegaly, and lymphocytosis, with or without hepatomegaly, lymphadenopathy, and a transient rash.[57,71,118] Other blood transfusion–transmitted infections should also be considered in patients with fever in the postoperative period.[26,71,177]

MANAGEMENT

Management consists of four elements: (1) supportive care, primarily treatment of heart failure, which is not discussed here; (2) antimicrobial therapy; (3) surgical therapy; and (4) management of complications.

General Principles of Antimicrobial Therapy

Because the infectious agent in IE is buried within a fibrin-platelet vegetation, where its metabolic rate is reduced and where the host's phagocytes cannot act, antimicrobial therapy must be microbicidal and administered at high dosage for a prolonged period.

Optimal management requires close collaboration between the clinician and the personnel in the microbiology laboratory.[12] Once a causative organism has been isolated and identified, a subculture should be stored for possible future use in additional tests. Appropriate antimicrobial susceptibilities should be determined as rapidly as possible.[13] In addition, the minimal inhibitory concentration (MIC) and minimal bactericidal concentration should be determined. Peak and trough serum levels of antibiotics with a narrow therapeutic index, primarily vancomycin and aminoglycosides, should be measured once steady state has been attained and then weekly. Often serum levels of these antibiotics are inadequate rather than excessive during the early stages of therapy.

In vitro testing of the bactericidal activity of the patient's serum (presumably containing antibiotic) can be performed. This assay, called the serum bactericidal test, serum activity test, or Schlichter test, essentially entails testing serial twofold dilutions of the patient's serum for their ability to inhibit and kill the patient's own bacterial isolate. The test is widely used, but its value is controversial. Peak bactericidal titers (i.e., when the antibiotic concentration should be at a peak) of dilutions equal to or greater than 1:64 or trough titers equal to or greater than 1:32 generally predict a good outcome from a bacteriological viewpoint.[153] However, activities at lower dilutions do not necessarily predict bacteriologic failure,[105,153] and many authors consider peak bactericidal titers of 1:8 or

greater as desirable.[24,201] Blood cultures should be repeated daily until they have become negative. They should also be repeated 1 and 2 months after cessation of therapy to detect a relapse, which usually occurs within this period.[170]

Antimicrobial Therapy Against Specific Microorganisms

Recommended antimicrobial agents for the treatment of IE caused by different microorganisms are summarized in Tables 45-6 and 45-10.[13,24,117,128,173,217,221] The dosages, routes of administration, and dosing schedules of these antimicrobial agents are shown in Table 45-7.[131,171,189,217]

Streptococci

Most streptococci causing IE belong to the *viridans* group. Although generally susceptible to penicillin, their degree of susceptibility varies. Whereas those streptococci that are inhibited by low concentrations of penicillin (MIC ≤ 0.1 mcg/mL) are readily killed by this drug, those with a higher MIC (>0.5 mcg/mL) might not be killed. In cases of IE caused by the latter, bactericidal activity is best achieved by the addition of an aminoglycoside (gentamicin or streptomycin). Streptococci are resistant to aminoglycosides alone, but penicillin damages the organism's cell wall, allowing the aminoglycoside to enter more readily and exert its bactericidal effect. For accomplishing this synergistic effect, the necessary peak serum concentrations of aminoglycoside are lower than those necessary for the treatment of gram-negative bacillary infections (e.g., for gentamicin, 3 mcg/mL rather than 8 mcg/mL).[13,158]

The recommended therapy of streptococcal endocarditis is shown in Table 45-10.[24,217] The duration of therapy and aminoglycoside requirement are based on the following penicillin susceptibility categories: MIC ≤ 0.1 mcg/mL, MIC >0.1 to <0.5 mcg/mL, and MIC ≥0.5 mcg/mL. Treatment of cases with the most resistant streptococci is the same as for those with enterococci.

Enterococci

Enterococci were formerly classified among group D streptococci (see Table 45-10).[24] They comprise *Enterococcus faecalis*, *Enterococcus faecium*, and several other species. They are resistant to all cephalosporins. Other cell-wall–active agents (namely, penicillin or ampicillin and vancomycin) exert only a bacteriostatic effect against them. Penicillin and vancomycin can achieve bactericidal activity only by the addition of an aminoglycoside, either gentamicin or streptomycin. Unfortunately, high-level resistance to these aminoglycosides, which can be demonstrated in the laboratory, has become fairly widespread. Cross-resistance between gentamicin and streptomycin is not always present. Bactericidal activity against aminoglycoside-resistant strains is impossible to achieve.[51]

Because antimicrobial resistance among enterococci has increased, the therapy of cases of enterococcal endocarditis must be individualized. There are several patterns of resistance in enterococci[100]:

1. Resistance to the synergistic effect of aminoglycosides, namely gentamicin (MIC > 500 mg/mL) or streptomycin (MIC > 2000 mg/mL). Resistance to one does not

Table 45-10 Antimicrobial Therapy of Infective Endocarditis Caused by Gram-Positive Cocci

Organism	Antimicrobial Agent	Duration
Streptococcus viridans **or** *Streptococcus bovis* MIC ≤ 0.1 mcg/mL	Penicillin G* **or** Penicillin G + streptomycin or gentamicin† **or** ceftriaxone Penicillin-allergy, type 1 Vancomycin	4 wk 2–4 wk 2 wk 4 wk 4 wk
Streptococcus viridans **or** *Streptococcus bovis* MIC > 0.1 and < 0.5 mcg/mL	Penicillin G + streptomycin or gentamicin† Penicillin-allergic, not type 1 cephalothin or cefazolin + streptomycin or gentamicin† Penicillin-allergic, type 1 vancomycin	4 wk 2 wk 4 wk 2 wk 4 wk
Streptococci viridans **or** enterococci MIC ≥ 0.5 mcg/mL **or** nutritionally deficient streptococci **or** if symptoms >3 mo **or** prosthetic material	Penicillin G (high dosage)‡ + streptomycin or gentamicin† **or** ampicillin + streptomycin or gentamicin† Penicillin-allergic, all types Vancomycin + streptomycin or gentamicin†	4–6 wk 4–6 wk 4–6 wk 4–6 wk 4–6 wk 4–6 wk
Staphylococci Methicillin-susceptible no prosthetic material	Nafcillin or oxacillin ± gentamicin Penicillin-allergic, not type 1 Cephalothin§ or cefazolin ± gentamicin Penicillin-allergic, type 1 vancomycin	4–6 wk 3–5 days 4–6 wk 3–5 days 4–6 wk
Staphylococci Methicillin-resistant no prosthetic material	Vancomycin	4–6 wk
Staphylococci Methicillin-susceptible prosthesis present	Nafcillin or oxacillin + rifampin + gentamicin	6–8 wk 6–8 wk 2 wk
Staphylococci Methicillin-resistant Prosthesis present	Vancomycin + rifampin + gentamicin	6–8 wk 6–8 wk 2 wk

*Aqueous crystalline penicillin G.
†To achieve peak serum concentrations of approximately 3 mcg/mL and trough <1 mcg/mL for gentamicin or peak of 20 mcg/mL for streptomycin.
‡Higher dosage.
§No longer available in the USA.
From Wilson WR, Karchmer AW, Dajani AS, et al: Antibiotic treatment of adults with infective endocarditis due to Streptococci, enterococci, staphylococci, and HACEK microorganisms. *JAMA* 274:1706–1713, 1995.

necessarily imply resistance to the other. If there is resistance to gentamicin, susceptibility to streptomycin should be tested. If there is resistance to both aminoglycosides, then therapy should consist of penicillin or ampicillin for 8 to 12 weeks.[217]

2. Resistance to penicillin and ampicillin. With *E. faecium*, this is due to resistance at the level of the penicillin-binding protein, in which case, vancomycin together with an aminoglycoside should be used. With *E. faecalis*, penicillin resistance may be due to the production of a β-lactamase. In such cases, treatment should consist of an ampicillin–β-lactamase inhibitor, such as ampicillin sulbactam, in addition to an aminoglycoside.[56,76,77]

3. Resistance to vancomycin. Vancomycin-resistant enterococci have become a very troubling microbiologic problem, especially within hospitals. There are several different types of vancomycin resistance in enterococci. In one form, the organism remains susceptible to teicoplanin, another glycopeptide, not licensed in the United States. In the other types, glycopeptides are ineffective. If this occurs together with penicillin resistance, there may be no effective antimicrobial therapy, and surgery may be the only possible therapy. Nevertheless, attempts should be made by the microbiology laboratory to determine effective antimicrobial combinations that might be effective, despite the individual drugs being ineffective. Drugs that should be tested include ampicillin, ceftriaxone, rifampin, doxycycline, chloramphenicol, fluoroquinolones, imipenem, and quinupristin/dalfopristine.[40] Quinupristin/dalfopristin, a combination of two streptogramins, is an antimicrobial agent that has activity against vancomycin-resistant *E. faecium* but not *E. faecalis*.[70,85] This has been used successfully in combination with rifampin and doxycycline to treat a case of *E. faecium* endocarditis.[115]

Pneumococci

As antibiotic resistance in *Streptococcus pneumoniae* has emerged to penicillin and other drugs, treatment recommendations for severe infections, particularly meningitis, have changed.[38,90] There is little experience with endocarditis caused by multiresistant strains of this organism. Aronin and colleagues[4] have recommended the same treatment regimens for pneumococcal endocarditis as are used for pneumococcal meningitis. These are as follows: If the isolate is susceptible to penicillin (MIC < 0.1 mcg/mL), use penicillin; if resistant to penicillin (MIC ≥ 0.1 mcg/mL) but susceptible to cefotaxime and ceftriaxone (MIC ≤ 0.5 μg/mL), use one of these third-generation cephalosporins (but not ceftazidime); if intermediately resistant to the third-generation cephalosporin (MIC = 1 mcg/mL), use the cephalosporin plus vancomycin; and if resistant to the third-generation cephalosporins (MIC ≥ 2 mcg/mL), use the third-generation cephalosporin plus vancomycin plus rifampin.[90] Whitby and associates[212] successfully treated a patient with endocarditis caused by a strain of pneumococcus with high-level resistance to penicillin and to third-generation cephalosporins with vancomycin plus rifampin.

Staphylococci

Presently, *S. aureus* and the various species of coagulase-negative staphylococci (mainly *Staphylococcus epidermidis*) are almost always resistant to penicillin and ampicillin due to their production of a β-lactamase (see Table 45-10).[24] Various semi-synthetic penicillins (e.g., methicillin, nafcillin, oxacillin, and cloxacillin) are active against most strains of *S. aureus* and some strains of coagulase-negative staphylococci. However, some strains of *S. aureus* and many strains of coagulase-negative staphylococci are also resistant to these semi-synthetic penicillins due to alterations in their penicillin-binding proteins, the molecular target of the penicillins. These strains, known as methicillin-resistant *S. aureus* (MRSA) and methicillin-resistant *S. epidermidis*, are also resistant to cephalosporins.[29] In the past, MRSA infections have been primarily a nosocomial problem, but the number of community-acquired MRSA infections is increasing.[79] In the study by Herold and colleagues,[79] most MRSA isolates from patients with risk factors for MRSA infections (e.g., prior hospitalizations) were more likely to be multiply resistant than those from patients without such risk factors. Vancomycin is the mainstay of therapy of patients infected with such strains.[24,145,217] However, strains of staphylococci with reduced susceptibility to vancomycin have now been reported. These have been called glycopeptide-intermediate *S. aureus*.[186,205] Cases of IE caused by such strains would be very difficult to treat. There is experimental evidence that a combination of vancomycin plus oxacillin or other β-lactam agents with antistaphylococcal activity may be valuable in this situation.[36]

Vancomycin, compared with the penicillins, has the disadvantages of being very expensive and, at high serum levels, being ototoxic and nephrotoxic. Therefore, serum concentrations should be monitored. Peak concentrations, drawn 1 hour after the end of a 1-hour infusion, should be 20 to 35 mcg/mL if four daily doses are given, as is generally the case in children, or 30 to 45 mcg/mL if two daily doses are given.[13,24,217]

In the treatment of *S. aureus* endocarditis, the addition of gentamicin has been shown to shorten the duration of bacteremia but not to influence the ultimate outcome of the infection.[97] Its use may be considered for the first 3 to 5 days of therapy.

Rifampin is an extremely active antistaphylococcal agent to which resistance develops very rapidly if it is used alone. It should be added to the therapeutic regimen in prosthetic valve endocarditis.[24,217]

In suspected staphylococcal IE acquired in a hospital or community in which methicillin-resistant staphylococci are prevalent, vancomycin should be used instead of—or in addition to—a semi-synthetic penicillin until antimicrobial susceptibilities of the isolate are known. In cases of endocarditis caused by staphylococci susceptible to methicillin, one should be wary of using vancomycin for the convenience of twice-daily infusions, because it might not be as effective as a semi-synthetic penicillin.[217]

HACEK Organisms (see "Microorganisms")

These organisms tend to grow relatively slowly, and their antimicrobial susceptibilities may not be readily determined. Although in the past they have been susceptible to ampicillin, this is now not always the case, as they may produce a β-lactamase. Therefore, a third-generation cephalosporin should be used unless susceptibility to ampicillin is demonstrated (see Table 45-6).[217]

Gram-Negative Bacteria

Because of the wide variety of possible causative gram-negative bacteria in IE and their wide spectra of antimicrobial susceptibilities, optimal treatment must be based on their identification and antimicrobial susceptibilities. Generally, treatment of enteric bacillary endocarditis should consist of a third-generation cephalosporin and an aminoglycoside, and that of *P. aeruginosa* endocarditis should consist of ceftazidime plus an aminoglycoside or an antipseudomonal penicillin (e.g., piperacillin) in addition to an aminoglycoside.[13,173] In cases of *Pseudomonas* or other gram-negative endocarditis in which a β-lactam antibiotic together with an aminoglycoside is ineffective, addition of a fluoroquinolone should be considered. Depending on antimicrobial susceptibilities and response to therapy, carbapenem drugs (e.g., imipenem/cilastatin or meropenem) may be preferable to β-lactam drugs.

Empiric Treatment of Infective Endocarditis

I would categorize patients in whom treatment for IE is being considered and before microbiologic information is available into three groups. In the first group are those with acute endocarditis, which is usually caused by *S. aureus* and is usually associated with severe illness. After drawing three separate blood cultures over a few minutes, I would initiate therapy with vancomycin plus oxacillin or nafcillin plus gentamicin. Rifampin should be added in the case of prosthetic valve endocarditis.

The second group consists of those who have many features of endocarditis and about whom a decision has been made that a full course of therapy for endocarditis will be given even if the blood cultures are negative. In such cases, I would initiate therapy with oxacillin or nafcillin plus penicillin plus gentamicin. The reasons for using penicillin in addition to oxacillin are that it is much more active than oxacillin against viridans streptococci, and oxacillin is inactive against enterococci.[99] If methicillin-resistant staphylococcal infection is likely, vancomycin should be used rather than oxacillin or nafcillin, and penicillin would not be necessary.

The third group is made up of those who might have endocarditis but in whom the evidence is not very strong. I would not initiate antimicrobial therapy for endocarditis until results of blood cultures were available.

Route of Administration and Duration of Therapy

Treatment should be administered intravenously with few exceptions. In cases of native valve endocarditis, therapy should be given for 4 to 6 weeks, while in prosthetic valve infection, it should be continued for 6 to 8 weeks.[13,24,217]

Outpatient Therapy

The high cost of hospitalization has led to the outpatient treatment of patients whose conditions are stable and who require prolonged parenteral antimicrobial therapy.[83] There are few published reports of outpatient treatment of IE. Recent studies in adults showed that a once-daily injection of ceftriaxone (2 g) for 4 weeks was very effective treatment for patients with IE caused by highly susceptible streptococci.[64,178,189] It seems prudent at present to reserve outpatient treatment of patients with IE for those in whom the infection is caused by highly susceptible streptococci and affects a native valve with no significant complications. In addition, the necessary social environment, home care services, and follow-up medical care must be available.

Surgery for Active Endocarditis

Valve surgery during active infection can be life saving. It usually entails valve replacement, but valve débridement and repair have also been performed. Fear of spreading infection in the surgical field or of infecting the new valve should not be a deterrent to submitting the patient with appropriate indications to surgery.[4,49,51]

The indications for surgery can be classified as hemodynamic or infective. The most common indications for surgery for IE in the current era are hemodynamic factors. These are congestive heart failure that is moderate to severe and refractory to medical therapy, valvular obstruction, and an unstable prosthesis. The infective indications are persistent bacteremia, despite adequate doses of appropriate antimicrobial therapy, which usually means beyond 7 days of therapy; fungal endocarditis, for which antimicrobial therapy alone is predictably ineffective; and extension of suppuration into deeper structures, such as the valve annulus, myocardium, or pericardial space.[2,49,51]

Several other factors have been identified that predict failure of medical therapy and are thus relative indications for surgery. These include infection by staphylococci or gram-negative bacilli, presence of large vegetations on echocardiogram (which occurs in up to 80% of cases), history of major emboli, recurrent infection in an adequately treated patient, and prosthetic valve infection. However, while the failure rate of medical therapy for prosthetic valve endocarditis is higher than for native valve endocarditis, not all cases of prosthetic valve infection require surgery.[51]

The type of operation performed for IE depends on the organism, the valve affected, the extent of its destruction, and patient-related factors such as age, size, and suitability for long-term therapeutic anticoagulation. Generally, aortic and mitral endocarditis require valve replacement, though small leaflet perforations of these valves can occasionally be débrided and patched with pericardium. Indeed, early aggressive surgical treatment has been advocated in children to maximize the chance that valve repair rather than replacement can be performed. Pulmonary and tricuspid valves can be débrided ("vegetectomy") or even excised with acceptable hemodynamic consequences in an otherwise normal heart, but in the presence of congenital heart disease or pulmonary hypertension, repair or replacement may be necessary.

When valve replacement with prosthesis is necessary, either mechanical prostheses or bioprosthetic valves (glutaraldehyde-treated porcine aortic valves or bovine pericardial valves) can be used; there is no significant difference between bioprosthetic and mechanical valves with respect to risk of reinfection of the prosthesis (approximately 5% each). However, there are several considerations important to selection of the appropriate prosthesis for a particular patient. First, mechanical valves require long-term (lifetime) anticoagulation with sodium warfarin. The hemorrhagic complication rate and management challenge of therapeutic anticoagulation in infants and small children are legion. Second, although bioprostheses do not require anticoagulation, they undergo accelerated degeneration in young children, possibly related to the calcium metabolism peculiar to the growing patient. Bioprostheses with durability of 10 to 15 years in older adults may last only 2 to 5 years in small children. Third, neither mechanical nor bioprosthetic valves have growth potential, so re-replacement may become necessary as growth proceeds.

Another option for replacement of aortic or pulmonary valves is the cryopreserved human allograft, more commonly called the homograft. These valves are human pulmonary or aortic valves taken from organ donors. They contain viable fibroblasts, but whether viability is important to graft durability and resistance to infection remains controversial. As with other tissues for transplantation, they are in short supply. Homografts do not necessitate immunosuppression and indeed offer significant advantages over bioprostheses and mechanical valves in resistance to infection when implanted in contaminated surgical sites. Disadvantages include limited availability, durability only somewhat better than heterograft bioprostheses, and suitability for use only in the aortic and pulmonary positions. Perhaps their greatest usefulness is for severe infections of the aortic root, in which replacement of the aortic valve and the lowermost cylinder of the ascending aorta must be replaced, and for treatment of aortic and pulmonary prosthetic valve infections.

Infections of prosthetic patches (VSD, coarctation, or right ventricular outflow tract patches) and prosthetic shunts (such as Gore-Tex [polytetrafluoroethylene] systemic-to-pulmonary artery shunts) deserve a trial of antibiotic therapy if the organisms are identifiable and reasonably susceptible to antimicrobials, such as viridans streptococci. However, prosthetic infections by staphylococcal species, gram-negative, or fungal organisms or associated with pseudoaneurysm, dehiscence, or excessive local turbulence are unlikely to become sterilized with antibiotics and are better treated by early surgery.

A recent report reviewed surgery for active endocarditis in 192 children younger than 19 years, from 1940 to 1989.[199] The most common sites of infection were the aortic valve (40%), mitral valve (18%), tricuspid valve (14%), pulmonic valve (5%), patent ductus arteriosus (13%), and prosthetic or suture material at previous operative sites (15%; Fig. 45-1). The most common indication for surgery was persistent bacteremia or infection (not defined; 23%), repeated embolic events (23%), and worsening congestive heart failure (21%). Overall survival was 77%; of note, survival among neonates was 65% (11 of 17).[199] Alsip and coworkers[1] have suggested a point scoring system as a guideline for recommending surgical intervention in IE (Table 45-11); a score of 5 or greater suggests the need for valve replacement.

Fleming and associates[62] recently reported a case of a premature infant (weight, 815 g) with tricuspid valve endocarditis, persistently positive blood cultures, and a vegetation enlarging from 5 mm by 5 mm to 10 mm by 6 mm in diameter who was successfully treated with tissue plaminogen activator. This was given through a left subclavian venous catheter in a dosage of 0.5 mg/kg over 10 minutes, followed by a continuous infusion of 0.2 mg/kg for 3 days. This was used because surgery was indicated but was considered not to be an option.

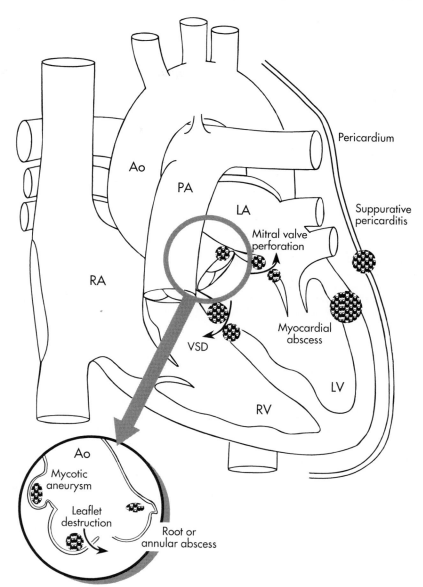

FIGURE 45-1 Common sites of infection in patients requiring surgery for active endocarditis. (Reprinted with permission from Berkowitz FE: Infective endocarditis. In Nichols DG, Cameron DE, Greeley WJ, et al [eds]: *Critical Heart Disease in Infants and Children*. St Louis, Mosby, 1995, p 978.)

MANAGEMENT OF COMPLICATIONS

The most important complication of IE is heart failure. Its management is not discussed in this chapter. Patients with IE and deteriorating cardiac function refractory to medical therapy should undergo cardiac surgery.

The other important complications are related to emboli, especially those to the brain. It is important to note that not all episodes of cerebral dysfunction in patients with IE are necessarily caused by emboli. Encephalopathy or seizures in individuals being treated for IE also may be caused by electrolyte or metabolic disturbances, shock, hypoxia, or drug toxicity (e.g., excessive doses of penicillin or imipenem in the presence of renal dysfunction).[174] Similarly, renal dysfunction may be caused not only by renal emboli or immune complex glomerulonephritis, characteristic of IE, but also by shock or drug therapy (e.g., aminoglycosides, vancomycin, or amphotericin B).

The optimal forms of management of cerebral emboli and mycotic aneurysms are unclear with respect to anticoagulation and surgery, respectively. Although cerebral emboli may occur after institution of antimicrobial therapy, their frequency decreases with increasing duration of therapy.[144,191] In considering the role of anticoagulation, patients with prosthetic valves should be differentiated from those without. In a study by Wilson and colleagues[215] of patients with prosthetic valve endocarditis, anticoagulation appeared to reduce the risk of cerebral embolism, whereas in that of Delahaye and associates,[48] in patients with native valve endocarditis, anticoagulation was associated with a higher risk of cerebrovascular accidents (hemorrhage or emboli) and of death. In the series of cases of PVE reported by Carpenter and McAllister,[32] 5 of 14 anticoagulated patients developed cerebral hemorrhage, of whom 4 died. Therefore, anticoagulation should not be used unless there are other specific indications, as in patients with certain types of prostheses.[46] If such a patient has a cerebral embolus, anticoagulation should probably be discontinued, if possible, for a few days. If the patient remains stable, anticoagulation should then be restarted.[191,216]

Table 45-11 Point System for Cardiac Surgery during Active Infective Endocarditis*

Disorder	Native Valve Endocarditis	Prosthetic Valve Endocarditis
Heart failure		
Severe	5	5
Moderate	3	5
Mild	1	2
Fungal etiology	5	5
Persistent bacteremia	5	5
Organism other than "susceptible" *Streptococcus*	1	2
Relapse	2	3
One major embolus	2	2
Two or more systemic emboli	4	4
Vegetations by echocardiography	1	1
Early mitral valve closure by echocardiography	2	N/A
Ruptured chordae tendineae or papillary muscle	3	N/A
Heart block	3	3
Ruptured sinus of Valsalva or ventricular septum	4	4
Unstable prosthesis	N/A	5
Early prosthetic valve endocarditis (<60 days)	N/A	2
Periprosthetic leak	N/A	2

*Accumulation of five or more points suggests the need for valve replacement.
From Alsip SG, Blackstone EH, Kirklin JW, Cobbs CG: Indications for cardiac surgery in patients with active infective endocarditis. *Am J Med* 78:138–148, 1985; with permission.

Whether mycotic aneurysms are frequently or rarely associated with clinical symptoms prior to their rupture is controversial.[165,191] Most heal with antimicrobial therapy. Nevertheless, if they bleed, the fatality rate is very high. In patients developing a focal neurologic deficit, imaging of the brain should be performed as soon as possible, and, depending on the findings, a cerebral angiogram should be performed between 48 hr and 2 weeks after the episode. This should be done by magnetic resonance imaging if possible. If the angiogram is negative, it should be repeated at the end of antimicrobial therapy if anticoagulation therapy is planned.[165,216] If an aneurysm is present, depending on its size and location, the patient should undergo cerebrovascular surgery or undergo follow-up with periodic angiograms.[50,216]

OUTCOME

The prognosis of IE is influenced by many factors, including age, causative organism, site of infection, and whether the infection is postoperative and affects a native or prosthetic valve. In various pediatric series, the case fatality has varied from 8% to 60%. Children younger than 2 years have a higher fatality rate than older children.*

RESPONSE TO THERAPY

Fever, the most common clinical feature of IE and that most readily monitored, usually declines within the 1st week of antimicrobial therapy. In a study of 150 adults, Lederman and colleagues[101] showed that after institution of therapy, 50% of cases were afebrile by 72 hr, 72% by 7 days, and 84% by 14 days. The clinical abnormalities independently associated with prolonged fever were microvascular phenomena and large-vessel emboli.

When fever persists for longer than 7 days or recurs after initially subsiding, the following possible reasons should be considered: (1) inadequate antimicrobial therapy, either due to an inappropriate agent or inadequate dosage; (2) the presence of a primary focus of infection leading to IE or a metastatic focus requiring surgical drainage; (3) thrombophlebitis caused by an intravenous catheter; (4) other nosocomial infections; or (5) drug fever.[106,110] It is very important that primary sources of infection and metastatic foci be sought and appropriately treated to reduce the chances of reinfection.

RELAPSE

When relapse occurs, it usually does so within 2 months of completion of antimicrobial therapy. It is more likely to occur when the initial infection had been caused by an organism relatively resistant to antimicrobial agents or when it had been present for more than 3 months before institution of therapy. When relapse occurs, the identification and antimicrobial susceptibilities of the isolate from the original infection and the therapy of that infection should be reviewed. Therefore, in all cases of IE, the blood culture isolates should be stored. Although relapses can be treated medically, the fact that the infection is a relapse, together with other factors, should be taken into account in the consideration of surgical therapy.[135]

PREVENTION OF INFECTIVE ENDOCARDITIS

Infective endocarditis lends itself to chemoprophylaxis under certain circumstances for several reasons: (1) it carries a significant morbidity and mortality; (2) many individuals at risk are readily identified; (3) most cases are caused by a limited number of organisms; and (4) the medical and surgical procedures causing transient bacteremia with important IE pathogens are recognized. Although prophylaxis is not of

---

*See references 9, 21, 68, 82, 86, 87, 91, 96, 98, 123, 127, 129, 143, 175, 181, 190, 202, and 220.

Table 45-12 Cardiac Conditions Associated with Endocarditis

Endocarditis Prophylaxis Recommended

High-risk category
  Prosthetic cardiac valves, including bioprosthetic and homograft valves
  Previous bacterial endocarditis
  Complex cyanotic congenital heart disease (e.g., single ventricle states, transposition of the great arteries, tetralogy of Fallot)
  Surgically constructed systemic pulmonary shunts or conduits
Moderate-risk category
  Most other congenital cardiac malformations (other than those cited here)
  Acquired valvar dysfunction (e.g., rheumatic heart disease)
  Hypertrophic cardiomyopathy
  Mitral valve prolapse with valvar regurgitation and/or thickened leaflets*

Endocarditis Prophylaxis Not Recommended

Negligible-risk category (no greater risk than the general population)
  Isolated secundum atrial septal defect
  Surgical repair of atrial septal defect, ventricular septal defect, or patent ductus arteriosus (without residua beyond 6 mo)
  Previous coronary artery bypass graft surgery
  Mitral valve prolapse without valvar regurgitation*
  Physiologic, functional, or innocent heart murmurs*
  Previous Kawasaki disease without valvar dysfunction
  Previous rheumatic fever without valvar dysfunction
  Cardiac pacemakers (intravascular and epicardial) and implanted defibrillators

*From Dajani AS, Taubert KA, Wilson W, et al: Prevention of bacterial endocarditis. Recommendations by the American Heart Association. *JAMA* 277:1794–1801, 1997; with permission.

Table 45-13 Dental Procedures and Endocarditis Prophylaxis

Endocarditis Prophylaxis Recommended*

Dental extractions
  Dental procedures including surgery, scaling and root planing, probing, and recall maintenance
  Dental implant placement and reimplantation of avulsed teeth
  Endodontic (root canal) instrumentation or surgery only beyond the apex
  Subgingival placement of antibiotic fibers or strips
  Initial placement of orthodontic bands but not brackets
  Intraligamentary local anesthetic injections
  Prophylactic cleaning of teeth or implants where bleeding is anticipated

Endocarditis Prophylaxis Not Recommended

Restorative dentistry† (operative and prosthodontic) with or without retraction cord‡
Local anesthetic injections (nonintraligamentary)
Intracanal endodontic treatment; after placement and buildup
Placement of rubber dams
Postoperative suture removal
Placement of removable prosthodontic or orthodontic appliances
Taking of oral impressions
Fluoride treatments
Taking of oral radiographs
Orthodontic appliance adjustment
Shedding of primary teeth

*Prophylaxis is recommended for patients with high- and moderate-risk cardiac conditions.
†This includes restoration of decayed teeth (filling cavities) and replacement of missing teeth.
‡Clinical judgment may indicate antibiotic use in selected circumstances that may create significant bleeding.
From Dajani AS, Taubert KA, Wilson W, et al: Prevention of bacterial endocarditis. Recommendations by the American Heart Association. *JAMA* 277:1794–1801, 1997; with permission.

proven value,[54,201] its potential benefits are thought to outweigh its risks. Important principles in chemoprophylaxis during procedures are that there should be a high concentration of the antibiotic in the blood at the time the procedure is performed and that the prophylaxis should be of short duration.[43] Bacteria of dental origin, especially viridans streptococci, constitute a very important group of causes of IE. Therefore, situations that result in bacteremia from these bacteria are considered opportunities for prophylaxis, as recommended by the American Heart Association.[43] Nevertheless, there is controversy as to whether dental procedures are really the cause of IE due to dental bacteria.[108,193,194] Roberts and colleagues[155,156] quote data showing that the intensity of bacteremia associated with dental procedures is low compared with that necessary to cause IE in experimental models. They also showed that the cumulative exposure to bacteremia from normal activities (e.g., brushing teeth and chewing) is orders of magnitude greater than that from dental procedures. Dental and

Table 45-14 Other Procedures and Endocarditis Prophylaxis

Endocarditis Prophylaxis Recommended

Respiratory tract
  Tonsillectomy and/or adenoidectomy
  Surgical operations that involve respiratory mucosa
  Bronchoscopy with a rigid bronchoscope
Gastrointestinal tract*
  Sclerotherapy for esophageal varices
  Esophageal stricture dilatation
  Endoscopic retrograde cholangiography with biliary obstruction
  Biliary tract surgery
  Surgical operations that involve intestinal mucosa
Genitourinary tract
  Prostatic surgery
  Cystoscopy
  Urethral dilatation

Endocarditis Prophylaxis Not Recommended

Respiratory tract
  Endotracheal intubation
  Bronchoscopy with a flexible bronchoscope, with or without biopsy†
  Typanostomy tube insertion
Gastrointestinal tract
  Transesophageal echocardiography†
  Endoscopy with or without gastrointestinal biopsy†
Genitourinary tract
  Vaginal hysterectomy†
  Vaginal delivery†
  Cesarean section
In uninfected tissue
  Urethral catheterization
  Uterine dilatation and curettage
  Therapeutic abortion
  Sterilization procedures
  Insertion or removal of intrauterine devices
Other
  Cardiac catheterization, including balloon angioplasty
  Implanted cardiac pacemakers, implanted defibrillators, and coronary stents
  Incision or biopsy of surgically scrubbed skin
  Circumcision

*Prophylaxis is recommended for high-risk patients; optional for medium-risk patients.
†Prophylaxis is optional for high-risk patients.
From Dajani AS, Taubert KA, Wilson W, et al: Prevention of bacterial endocarditis. Recommendations by the American Heart Association. *JAMA* 277:1794–1801, 1997; with permission.

Table 45-15 Prophylactic Regimens for Dental, Oral, Respiratory Tract, or Esophageal Procedures

Situation	Agent	Regimen*
Standard general prophylaxis	Amoxicillin	Children: 50 mg/kg PO 1 hr before procedure Adults: 2.0 g
Unable to take oral medications	Ampicillin	Children: 50 mg/kg IM or IV within 30 min before procedure Adults: 2.0 g IM or IV
Allergic to penicillin	Clindamycin or	Children: 20 mg/kg PO 1 hr before procedure Adults: 600 mg
	Cephalexin or cefadroxil or	Children: 50 mg/kg PO 1 hr before procedure Adults: 2.0 g
	Azithromycin or clarithromycin	Children: 15 mg/kg PO 1 hr before procedure Adults: 500 mg
Allergic to penicillin and unable to take oral medications	Clindamycin or	Children: 20 mg/kg IV within 30 min before procedure Adults: 600 mg
	Cefazolin	Children: 25 mg/kg IM or IV within 30 min before procedure Adults: 1.0 g

*Total children's dose should not exceed adult dose. Cephalosporins should not be used in individuals with immediate-type hypersensitivity reaction (urticaria, angioedema, or anaphylaxis) to penicillins.
From Dajani AS, Taubert KA, Wilson W, et al: Prevention of bacterial endocarditis. Recommendations by the American Heart Association. *JAMA* 277:1794–1801, 1997; with permission.

periodontal health would seem to be important in preventing IE and should be actively promoted in cardiology clinics. Unfortunately, this is not widely practiced.[140]

The recommendations of the American Heart Association for chemoprophylaxis against IE are shown in Tables 45-12 to 45-16.[43] Similar recommendations have been made by the British Society for Antimicrobial Chemotherapy.[3] The European Society of Gastrointestinal Endoscopy has recently published guidelines for antibiotic prophylaxis for gastrointestinal endoscopy.[154] This group considers esophageal dilatation, laser therapy of the upper gastrointestinal tract, and variceal sclerotherapy to be procedures with a particularly high risk of causing bacteremia with organisms that cause IE. It is important to note that these are guidelines that cannot address prophylaxis in all circumstances. Prophylaxis should be influenced by clinical circumstances, by prevalent antimicrobial susceptibility patterns, and whether the patient has recently received antimicrobial therapy (e.g., hospitalized patients who have received antibiotics might require regimens different from those recommended here).

Although IE is a relatively uncommon complication of cardiac surgery, a significant proportion of IE cases result from cardiac surgery. Because staphylococci are the most important causes of these infections, prophylaxis should be directed against these organisms. Cephalosporins are widely used for this purpose. Although it has been suggested that in centers in which methicillin-resistant *S. aureus* is prevalent, prophylaxis with vancomycin should be considered,[43] this is fraught with the hazard of encouraging the growth and spread of vancomycin-resistant bacteria and therefore generally should be discouraged.

References

1. Alsip SG, Blackstone EH, Kirklin JW, Cobbs CG: Indications for cardiac surgery in patients with active infective endocarditis. *Am J Med* 78: 138–148, 1985.
2. Andriole VT, Kravetz HM, Roberts WC, Utz JP: Candida endocarditis: Clinical and pathologic studies. *Am J Med* 32:251–285, 1962.
3. Antibiotic prophylaxis of infective endocarditis. Recommendations from the Endocarditis Working Party of the British Society for Antimicrobial Chemotherapy. *Lancet* 335:88–89, 1990.
4. Aronin SI, Mukherjee SK, West JC, Cooney EL: Review of pneumococcal endocarditis in adults in the penicillin era. *Clin Infect Dis* 26:165–171, 1998.
5. Arvay A, Lengyel M: Incidence and risk factors of prosthetic valve endocarditis. *Eur J Cardiothorac Surg* 2:340–346, 1988.
6. Ashkenazi S, Levy O, Blieden L: Trends of childhood infective endocarditis in Israel with emphasis on children under 2 years of age. *Pediatr Cardiol* 18:419–424, 1997.
7. Aspesberro F, Beghetti M, Oberhansli I, Friedli B: Fungal endocarditis in critically ill children. *Eur J Pediatr* 158:275–280, 1999.
8. Auckenthaler RW: Laboratory diagnosis of infective endocarditis. *Eur Heart J* 5(suppl C):49–51, 1984.
9. Awadallah SM, Kavey RE, Byrum CJ, et al: The changing pattern of infective endocarditis in childhood. *Am J Cardiol* 68:90–94, 1991.
10. Baddour LM, Meyer J, Henry B: Polymicrobial infective endocarditis in the 1980s. *Rev Infect Dis* 13:963–970, 1991.

Table 45-16 Prophylactic Regimens for Genitourinary and Gastrointestinal (Excluding Esophageal) Procedures

Situation	Agents*	Regimen
High-risk patients	Ampicillin + gentamicin	Adults: Ampicillin 2.0 g IM or IV + gentamicin 1.5 mg/kg (not to exceed 120 mg) within 30 min of starting the procedure; 6 hr later, ampicillin 1 g IM/IV or amoxicillin 1 g PO Children: Ampicillin 50 mg/kg IM or IV (not to exceed 2.0 g) + gentamicin 1.5 mg/kg within 30 min of starting the procedure; 6 hr later, ampicillin 25 mg/kg IM/IV or amoxicillin 25 mg/kg PO
High-risk patients allergic to ampicillin/amoxicillin	Vancomycin + gentamicin	Adults: Vancomycin 1.0 g IV over 1–2 hr + gentamicin 1.5 mg/kg IV/IM (not to exceed 120 mg); complete injection/infusion within 30 min of starting the procedure Children: Vancomycin 20 mg/kg IV over 1–2 hr + gentamicin 1.5 mg/kg within 30 min
Moderate-risk patients	Amoxicillin or ampicillin	Adults: Amoxcillin 2.0 g orally 1 hr before procedure, or ampicillin 2.0 g IM/IV within 30 min of starting the procedure Children: Amoxicillin 50 mg/kg PO 1 hr before procedure, or ampicillin 50 mg/kg IM/IV within 30 min of starting the procedure
Moderate-risk patients allergic to ampicillin/amoxicillin	Vancomycin	Adults: Vancomycin 1.0 g IV over 1–2 hr; complete infusion within 30 min of starting the procedure Children: Vancomycin 20 mg/kg IV over 1–2 hr; complete infusion within 30 min of starting the procedure

*Total children's dose should not exceed adult dose. No second dose of vancomycin or gentamicin is recommended.
From Dajani AS, Taubert KA, Wilson W, et al: Prevention of bacterial endocarditis. Recommendations by the American Heart Association. *JAMA* 277:1794–1801, 1997; with permission.

11. Bain RJ, Geddes AM, Littler WA, McKinlay AW: The clinical and echocardiographic diagnosis of infective endocarditis. *J Antimicrob Chemother* 20(suppl A):17–27, 1987.

12. Bain RJ, Glover D, Littler WA, Geddes AM: The impact of a policy of collaborative management on mortality and morbidity from infective endocarditis. *Int J Cardiol* 19:47–57, 1988.

13. Baldassarre JS, Kaye D: Principles and overview of antibiotic therapy. In Kaye D (ed): *Infective Endocarditis.* New York, Raven Press, 1992, pp 169–190.

14. Baorto E, Payne RM, Slater LN, et al: Culture-negative endocarditis caused by *Bartonella henselae. J Pediatr* 132:1051–1054, 1998.

15. Barst RJ, Prince AS, Neu HC: Aspergillus endocarditis in children: Case report and review of the literature. *Pediatrics* 68:73–78, 1981.

16. Bayer AS: New concepts in the pathogenesis and modalities of the chemoprophylaxis of native valve endocarditis. *Chest* 96:893–899, 1989.

17. Becton DL, Friedman HS, Armstrong BE, et al: Bacterial endocarditis in a child with a Broviac catheter. *Pediatr Hematol Oncol* 4:131–136, 1987.

18. Bell WE, McCormick WF: Neurologic infection in children. In Markowitz M (ed): *Major Problems in Clinical Pediatrics.* Philadelphia, WB Saunders, 1981, pp 227–233.

19. Berbari EF, Cockerill FR, Steckelberg JM: Infective endocarditis due to unusual or fastidious microorganisms. *Mayo Clin Proc* 72:532–542, 1997.

20. Berkowitz FE: Hemolysis and infection: Categories and mechanisms of their interrelationship. *Rev Infect Dis* 13:1151–1162, 1991.

21. Berkowitz FE, Dansky R: Infective endocarditis in black South African children: Report of 10 cases with some unusual features. *Pediatr Infect Dis J* 8:787–791, 1989.

22. Bhandari S, Kaul U, Shrivastava S, et al: Infective endocarditis in children. *Indian J Pediatr* 51:529–532, 1984.

23. Birmingham GD, Rahko PS, Ballantyne F: Improved detection of infective endocarditis with transesophageal echocardiography. *Am Heart J* 123:774–781, 1992.

24. Bisno AL, Dismukes WE, Durack DT, et al: Antimicrobial treatment of infective endocarditis due to viridans streptococci, enterococci, and staphylococci. *JAMA* 261:1471–1477, 1989.

25. Blair TP, Waugh RA, Pollack M, et al: Histoplasma capsulatum endocarditis. *Am Heart J* 99:783–788, 1980.

26. Bove JR: Transfusion-transmitted diseases: Current problems and challenges. *Prog Hematol* 14:123–147, 1986.

27. Brennan RG, Durack DT: The viridans streptococci in perspective. In Schwartz MN, Remington JS (eds): *Current Clinical Topics in Infectious Diseases.* New York, McGraw-Hill, 1985, pp 253–289.

28. Bricker JT, Latson LA, Huhta JC, Gutgesell HP: Echocardiographic evaluation of infective endocarditis in children. *Clin Pediatr (Phila)* 24:312–317, 1985.

29. Brumfitt W, Hamilton-Miller J: Methicillin-resistant *Staphylococcus aureus. N Engl J Med* 320:1188–1196, 1989.

30. Buda AJ, Zotz RJ, LeMire MS, Bach DS: Prognostic significance of vegetations detected by two-dimensional echocardiography in infective endocarditis. *Am Heart J* 112:1291–1296, 1986.

31. Bush LM, Johnson JJ: Clinical syndrome and diagnosis. In Kaye D (ed): *Infective Endocarditis.* New York, Raven Press, 1992, pp 99–115.

32. Carpenter JL, McAllister CK: Anticoagulation in prosthetic valve endocarditis. *South Med J* 76:1372–1375, 1983.

33. Casado-Flores J, Valdivielso-Serna A, Perez-Jurado L, et al: Subclavian vein catheterization in critically ill children: Analysis of 322 cannulations. *Intensive Care Med* 17:350–354, 1991.

34. Chen SC, Dwyer DE, Sorrell TC: A comparison of hospital and community-acquired infective endocarditis. *Am J Cardiol* 70:1449–1452, 1992.

35. Citak M, Rees A, Mavroudis C: Surgical management of infective endocarditis in children. *Ann Thorac Surg* 54:755–760, 1992.

36. Climo MW, Patron RL, Archer GL: Combinations of vancomycin and β-lactams against staphylococci with reduced susceptibilities to vancomycin. *Antimicrob Agents Chemother* 43:1747–1753, 1999.

37. Cohen PS, Maguire JH, Weinstein L: Infective endocarditis caused by gram-negative bacteria: A review of the literature, 1945–1977. *Prog Cardiovasc Dis* 22:205–242, 1980.

38. Committee of Infectious Diseases, American Academy of Pediatrics: Therapy for children with invasive pneumococcal infections. *Pediatrics* 99:289–299, 1997.

39. Cronin WA, Germanson TP, Donowitz LG: Intravascular catheter colonization and related bloodstream infection in critically ill neonates. *Infect Control Hosp Epidemiol* 11:301–308, 1990.

40. Cross JT Jr, Jacobs RF: Vancomycin-resistant enterococcal infections. *Semin Pediatr Infect Dis* 7:162–169, 1996.

41. Csukas SR, Elbl F, Marshall GS: Type b and non-type b *Haemophilus influenzae* endocarditis. *Pediatr Infect Dis J* 11:1053–1056, 1992.

42. Daher AH, Berkowitz FE: Infective endocarditis in neonates. *Clin Pediatr* 34:198–206, 1995.

43. Dajani AS, Taubert KA, Wilson W, et al: Prevention of bacterial endocarditis. Recommendations by the American Heart Association. *JAMA* 277:1794–1801, 1997.

44. Damen J, Van der Tweel I: Positive tip cultures and related risk factors associated with intravascular catheterization in pediatric cardiac patients. *Crit Care Med* 16:221–228, 1988.

45. Daniel WG, Mugge A, Martin RP, et al: Improvement in the diagnosis of abscesses associated with endocarditis by transesophageal echocardiography. *N Engl J Med* 324:795–800, 1991.

46. Davenport J, Hart RG: Prosthetic valve endocarditis 1976–1987. Antibiotics, anticoagulation, and stroke. *Stroke* 21:993–999, 1990.

47. del Pont JM, de Cicco LT, Vartlitis C, et al: Infective endocarditis in children: Clinical analyses and evaluation of two diagnostic criteria. *Pediatr Infect Dis J* 14:1079–1086, 1995.

48. Delahaye JP, Poncet P, Malquarti V, et al: Cerebrovascular accidents in infective endocarditis: Role of anticoagulation. *Eur Heart J* 11:1074–1078, 1990.

49. DiNubile MJ: Surgery in active endocarditis. *Ann Intern Med* 96:650–659, 1982.

50. DiNubile MJ, Calderwood SB, Steinhaus DM, Karchmer AW: Cardiac conduction abnormalities complicating native valve active infective endocarditis. *Am J Cardiol* 58:1213–1217, 1986.

51. Douglas DL, Dismukes WE: Surgical therapy of infective endocarditis on natural valves. In Kaye D (ed): *Infective Endocarditis.* New York, Raven Press, 1992, pp 397–411.

52. Douglas JL, Cobb CG: Prosthetic valve endocarditis. In Kaye D (ed): *Infective Endocarditis.* New York, Raven Press, 1992, pp 375–396.

53. Durack DT, Lukes AS, Bright DK, Duke Endocarditis Service: New criteria for diagnosis of infective endocarditis: Utilization of specific echocardiographic findings: *Am J Med* 96:200–209, 1994.

54. Durack DT: Prevention of infective endocarditis. *N Engl J Med* 332:38–44, 1995.

55. el Makhlouf A, Friedli B, Oberhansli I, et al: Prosthetic heart valve replacement in children: Results and follow-up of 273 patients. *J Thorac Cardiovasc Surg* 93:80–85, 1987.

56. Eliopoulus GM: Enterococcal endocarditis. In Kaye D (ed): *Infective Endocarditis.* New York, Raven Press, 1992, pp 209–223.

57. Engle MA: Postoperative problems. In Adams FH, Emmanouilides GC, Riemenschneider TA (eds): *Moss' Heart Disease in Infants, Children and Adolescents.* Baltimore, Williams and Wilkins, 1989, pp 964–972.

58. Engle MA, Zabriskie JB, Senterfit LB, et al: Viral illness and the postpericardiotomy syndrome: A prospective study in children. *Circulation* 62:1151–1158, 1980.

59. Erslev AJ: Anemia of chronic disorders. In Williams WJ, Beutler E, Erslev AJ, Lichtman MA (eds): *Hematology.* New York, McGraw-Hill, 1990, pp 540–546.

60. Espersen F, Frimodt-Moller N: *Staphylococcus aureus* endocarditis. A review of 119 cases. *Arch Intern Med* 146:1118–1121, 1986.

61. Faix RG, Feick HJ, Frommelt P, Snider AR: Successful medical treatment of *Candida parapsilosis* endocarditis in a premature infant. *Am J Perinatol* 7:272–275, 1990.

62. Fleming RE, Barenkamp J, Jureidini SB: Successful treatment of a staphylococcal endocarditis vegetation with tissue plasminogen activator. *J Pediatr* 132:535–537, 1998.

63. Forshaw J, Harwood L: Red blood cell abnormalities in cardiac valvular disease. *J Clin Pathol* 20:848–853, 1967.

64. Francioli P, Etienne J, Hoigne R, et al: Treatment of streptococcal endocarditis with a single daily dose of ceftriaxone sodium for 4 weeks: Efficacy and outpatient treatment feasibility. *JAMA* 267:264–267, 1992.

65. Friedland G, Von Reyn CF, Levy B, et al: Nosocomial endocarditis. *Infect Control* 5:284–288, 1984.

66. Furfaro S, Gauthier M, Lacroix J, et al: Arterial catheter-related infections in children. A 1-year cohort analysis. *Am J Dis Child* 145:1037–1043, 1991.

67. Gavalda J, Torres C, Tenorio C, Lopez P, et al: Efficacy of ampicillin plus ceftriaxone in treatment of experimental endocarditis due to *Enterococcus faecalis* strains highly resistant to aminoglycosides. *Antimicrob Agents Chemother* 43:639–646, 1999.

68. Geva T, Frand M: Infective endocarditis in children with congenital heart disease: The changing spectrum, 1965–85. *Eur Heart J* 9:1244–1249, 1988.

69. Giladi M, Szold O, Elami A, et al: Microbiological cultures of heart valves and valve tags are not valuable for patients without infective endocarditis who are undergoing valve replacement. *Clin Infect Dis* 24:884–888, 1997.

70. Gray JW, Darbyshire PJ, Beath SV, et al: Experience with quinupristin/dalfopristin in treating infections with vancomycin-resistant *Enterococcus faecium* in children. *Pediatr Infect Dis J* 19:234–238, 2000.

71. Gurevich I: Infectious complications after open heart surgery. *Heart Lung* 13:472–481, 1984.

72. Harris SL: Definitions and demographic characteristics. In Kaye D (ed): *Infective Endocarditis*. New York, Raven Press, 1992, pp 1–18.

73. Hart RG, Kagan-Hallet K, Joerns SE: Mechanisms of intracranial hemorrhage in infective endocarditis. *Stroke* 18:1048–1056, 1987.

74. Haverkos HW, Lange WR: From the Alcohol, Drug Abuse, and Mental Health Administration: Serious infections other than human immunodeficiency virus among intravenous drug abusers. *J Infect Dis* 161:894–902, 1990. [Published erratum appears in *J Infect Dis* 162(6):1421, 1990.]

75. Heimberger TS, Duma RJ: Infections of prosthetic heart valves and cardiac pacemakers. *Infect Dis Clin North Am* 3:221–245, 1989.

76. Herman DJ, Gerding DN: Antimicrobial resistance among enterococci. *Antimicrob Agents Chemother* 35:1–4, 1991.

77. Herman DJ, Gerding DN: Screening and treatment of infections caused by resistant enterococci. *Antimicrob Agents Chemother* 35:215–219, 1991.

78. Hermans PE: The clinical manifestations of infective endocarditis. *Mayo Clin Proc* 57:15–21, 1982.

79. Herold BC, Immergluck LC, Maranan M, et al: Community-acquired methicillin-resistant *Staphylococcus aureus* in children with no identified predisposing risk. *JAMA* 279:593–598, 1998.

80. Hessen MT, Abrutyn E: Gram-negative bacterial endocarditis. In Kaye D (ed): *Infective Endocarditis*. New York, Raven Press, 1992, pp 57–83.

81. Heydarian M, Werthammer JW, Kelly PJ: Echocardiographic diagnosis of *Candida* mass of the right atrium in a premature infant. *Am Heart J* 113:402–404, 1987.

82. Hugo-Hamman CT, de Moor MM, Human DG: Infective endocarditis in South African children. *J Trop Pediatr* 35:154–158, 1989.

83. Huminer D, Bishara J, Pitlik S: Home intravenous antibiotic therapy for patients with infective endocarditis. *Eur J Clin Microbiol Infect Dis* 18:330–334, 1999.

84. Johnson A, Oppenheim BA: Vascular catheter-related sepsis: Diagnosis and prevention. *J Hosp Infect* 20:67–78, 1992.

85. Johnson A, Livermore DM: Quinupristin/dalfopristin, a new addition to the antimicrobial arsenal. *Lancet* 354:2012–2013, 1999.

86. Johnson CM, Rhodes KH: Pediatric endocarditis. *Mayo Clin Proc* 57:86–94, 1982.

87. Johnson DH, Rosenthal A, Nadas AS: A forty-year review of bacterial endocarditis in infancy and childhood. *Circulation* 51:581–588, 1975.

88. Johnston PG, Lee J, Domanski M, et al: Late recurrent *Candida* endocarditis. *Chest* 99:1531–1533, 1991.

89. Kammer RB, Utz JP: *Aspergillus* species endocarditis: The new face of a not so rare disease. *Am J Med* 56:506–521, 1974.

90. Kaplan SL, Mason EO: Management of infections due to antibiotic-resistant *Streptococcus pneumoniae*. *Clin Microbiol Rev* 11:628–644, 1998.

91. Karl T, Wensley D, Stark J, de Leval M, et al: Infective endocarditis in children with congenital heart disease: Comparison of selected features in patients with surgical correction or palliation and those without. *Br Heart J* 58:57–65, 1987.

92. Kavey RE, Frank DM, Byrum CJ, et al: Two-dimensional echocardiographic assessment of infective endocarditis in children. *Am J Dis Child* 137:851–856, 1983.

93. Kawamura S, Ono Y, Kamiya T, et al: Diagnosing infection of extracardiac conduit in children. *Heart and Vessels* 10:214–217, 1995.

94. Kaye KM, Kaye D: Laboratory findings including blood cultures. In Kaye D (ed): *Infective Endocarditis*. New York, Raven Press, 1992, pp 117–124.

95. Kim Y, Michael AF, Tarshish P: Infection and nephritis. In Edelman CM Jr (ed): *Pediatric Kidney Disease*. Boston, Little Brown Company, 1992, pp 1569–1584.

96. Kohli RS, Anand IS, Nagrani B, et al: Infective endocarditis in children. *Indian J Pediatr* 20:439–443, 1983.

97. Korzeniowski O, Sande MA: Combination antimicrobial therapy for *Staphylococcus aureus* endocarditis in patients addicted to parenteral drugs and in nonaddicts: A prospective study. *Ann Intern Med* 97:496–503, 1982.

98. Kramer HH, Bourgeois M, Liersch R, et al: Current clinical aspects of bacterial endocarditis in infancy, childhood, and adolescence. *Eur J Pediatr* 140:253–259, 1983.

99. Kucers A, Bennett N McK: *The Use of Antibiotics. A Comprehensive Review with Clinical Emphasis*, 3rd ed. Philadelphia, Lippincott, 1988, pp 67–68.

100. Landman D, Quale JM: Management of infections due to resistant enterococci: A review of therapeutic options. *J Antimicrobial Chemother* 40:161–170, 1997.

101. Lederman MM, Sprague L, Wallis RS, Ellner JJ: Duration of fever during treatment of infective endocarditis. *Medicine (Baltimore)* 71:52–57, 1992.

102. Lee BK, Crossley K, Gerding DN: The association between *Staphylococcus aureus* bacteremia and bacteriuria. *Am J Med* 65:303–306, 1978.

103. Leisen JC, Lang DM, Quinn EL: Fungal organisms. In Magilligan DJ Jr, Quinn EL (eds): *Endocarditis: Medical and Surgical Management*. New York, Marcel Dekker, 1986.

104. Leung WH, Lau CP, Tai YT, et al: *Candida* right ventricular mural endocarditis complicating indwelling right atrial catheter. *Chest* 97:1492–1493, 1990.

105. Levison ME: In vitro assays. In Kaye D (ed): *Infective Endocarditis*. New York, Raven Press, 1992, pp 151–167.

106. Lipsky BA, Hirschmann JV: Drug fever. *JAMA* 245:851–854, 1981.

107. Livornese LL Jr, Korzeniowski OM: Pathogenesis of infective endocarditis. In Kaye D (ed): *Infective Endocarditis*. New York, Raven Press, 1992, pp 19–35.

108. Lockhart PB, Durack DT: Oral microflora as a cause of endocarditis and other distant site infections. *Infect Dis Clin N Am* 13:833–850, 1999.

109. Lutas EM, Roberts RB, Devereux RB, Prieto LM: Relation between the presence of echocardiographic vegetations and the complication rate in infective endocarditis. *Am Heart J* 112:107–113, 1986.

110. Mackowiak PA, LeMaistre CF: Drug fever: A critical appraisal of conventional concepts: An analysis of 51 episodes in two Dallas hospitals and 97 episodes reported in the English literature. *Ann Intern Med* 106:728–733, 1987.

111. Maki DG: Infections due to infusion therapy. In Bennett JV, Brachman PS, Sanford JP (eds): *Hospital Infections*. Boston, Little, Brown and Co, 1992, pp 849–898.

112. Marcy M, Klein JO: Focal bacterial infections. In Remington JS, Klein JO (eds): *Infectious Diseases of the Fetus and Newborn Infant*. Philadelphia, WB Saunders, 1990, pp 700–741.

113. Martin JM, Neches WH, Wald ER: Infective endocarditis: 35 years of experience at a children's hospital. *Clin Infect Dis* 24:669–675, 1997.

114. Martino P, Micozzi A, Venditti M, et al: Catheter-related right-sided endocarditis in bone marrow transplant recipients. *Rev Infect Dis* 12:250–257, 1990.

115. Matsumura S, Simor AE: Treatment of endocarditis due to vancomycin-resistant *Enterococcus faecium* with quinupristin/dalfopristin, doxycycline, and rifampin: A synergistic drug combination. *Clin Infect Dis* 27:1554–1556, 1998.

116. McFarland MM: Pathology of infective endocarditis. In Kaye D (ed): *Infective Endocarditis*. New York, Raven Press, 1992, pp 57–83.

117. McLeod R, Remington JS: Fungal endocarditis. In Rahimtoola SH (ed): *Infective Endocarditis*. New York, Grune and Stratton, 1978, pp 211–290.

118. McMonigal K, Horwitz CA, Henle W, et al: Post-perfusion syndrome due to Epstein-Barr virus: Report of two cases and review of the literature. *Transfusion* 23:331–335, 1983.

119. Mecrow IK, Ladusans EJ: Infective endocarditis in newborn infants with structurally normal hearts. *Acta Paediatrica* 83:35–39, 1994.

120. Mehta G: *Aspergillus* endocarditis after open heart surgery: An epidemiological investigation. *J Hosp Infect* 15:245–253, 1990.

121. Millard DD, Shulman ST: The changing spectrum of neonatal endocarditis. *Clin Perinatol* 15:587–608, 1988.

122. Mirimanoff RO, Glauser MP: Endocarditis during *Staphylococcus aureus* septicemia in a population of non-drug addicts. *Arch Intern Med* 142:1311–1313, 1982.

123. Moethilalh R, Coovadia HM: Infective endocarditis in thirteen children: A retrospective study (1974–1981). *Ann Trop Paediatr* 2:57–62, 1982.

124. Morguet AJ, Muntz DL, Ivancevic V, et al: Immunoscintigraphy using technetium-99m–labeled anti–NCA-95 antigranulocyte antibodies as an adjunct to echocardiography in subacute infective endocarditis. *J Am Coll Cardiol* 23:1171–1178, 1994.

125. Morris CD, Reller M, Menashe VD: Thirty-year incidence of infective endocarditis after surgery for congenital heart defect. *JAMA* 279:599–603, 1998.

126. Morrow WR, Haas JE, Benjamin DR: Nonbacterial endocardial thrombosis in neonates: Relationship to persistent fetal circulation. *J Pediatr* 100:117–122, 1982.

127. Moy RJ, George RH, de Giovanni JV, Silove ED: Improving survival in bacterial endocarditis. *Arch Dis Child* 61:394–399, 1986.

128. Moyer DV, Edwards JE Jr: Fungal endocarditis. In Kaye D (ed): *Infective Endocarditis.* New York, Raven Press, 1992, pp 299–312.

129. Naganuma M: Infective endocarditis in children. *Jpn Circ J* 49:545–552, 1985.

130. Naidoo DP, Seedat MA, Vythilingum S: Isolated endocarditis of the pulmonary valve with fragmentation haemolysis. *Br Heart J* 60:527–529, 1988.

131. Nelson JD: *1998–1999 Pocket Book of Pediatric Antimicrobial Therapy,* 13th ed. Baltimore, Williams and Wilkins, 1998, pp 68–88.

132. Neugarten J, Baldwin DS: Glomerulonephritis in bacterial endocarditis. *Am J Med* 77:297–304, 1984.

133. Nishiura T, Miyazaki Y, Oritani K, et al: *Aspergillus* vegetative endocarditis complicated with schizocytic hemolytic anemia in a patient with acute lymphocytic leukemia. *Acta Haematol* 76:60–62, 1986.

134. Noel GJ, O'Loughlin JE, Edelson PJ: Neonatal *Staphylococcus epidermidis* right-sided endocarditis: Description of five catheterized infants. *Pediatrics* 82:234–239, 1988.

135. Nolan CM, Beaty HN: *Staphylococcus aureus* bacteremia. Current clinical patterns. *Am J Med* 60:495–500, 1976.

136. Norwood SH, Cormier B, McMahon NG, et al: Prospective study of catheter-related infection during prolonged arterial catheterization. *Crit Care Med* 16:836–839, 1988.

137. O'Brien JT, Geiser EA: Infective endocarditis and echocardiography. *Am Heart J* 108:386–394, 1984.

138. O'Callaghan C, McDougall P: Infective endocarditis in neonates. *Arch Dis Child* 63:53–57, 1988.

139. Oelberg DG, Fisher DJ, Gross DM, et al: Endocarditis in high-risk neonates. *Pediatrics* 71:392–397, 1983.

140. Olderog-Hermiston EJ, Nowak A, Kanellis MJ: Practices and attitudes concerning oral health in pediatric cardiology clinics to prevent infective endocarditis. *Am J Cardiol* 81:1500–1502, 1998.

141. Oyen WJ, Claessens RA, van der Meer JW, et al: Indium-111–labeled human nonspecific immunoglobulin G: A new radiopharmaceutical for imaging infectious and inflammatory foci. *Clin Infect Dis* 14:1110–1118, 1992.

142. Parker FB Jr, Greiner-Hayes C, Tomar RH, et al: Bacteremia following prosthetic valve replacement. *Ann Surg* 197:147–151, 1983.

143. Parras F, Bouza E, Romero J, Buzon L, et al: Infectious endocarditis in children. *Pediatr Cardiol* 11:77–81, 1990.

144. Paschalis C, Pugsley W, John R, Harrison MJ: Rate of cerebral embolic events in relation to antibiotic and anticoagulant therapy in patients with bacterial endocarditis. *Eur Neurol* 30:87–89, 1990.

145. Patrick CC: Coagulase-negative staphylococci: Pathogens with increasing clinical significance. *J Pediatr* 116:497–507, 1990.

146. Pazin GJ, Saul S, Thompson ME: Blood culture positivity: Suppression by outpatient antibiotic therapy in patients with bacterial endocarditis. *Arch Intern Med* 142:263–268, 1982.

147. Pearlman SA, Higgins S, Eppes S, et al: Infective endocarditis in the premature neonate. *Clin Pediatr* 37:741–746, 1998.

148. Pesanti EL, Smith IM: Infective endocarditis with negative blood cultures. An analysis of 52 cases. *Am J Med* 66:43–50, 1979.

149. Pruitt AA, Rubin RH, Karchmer AW, Duncan GW: Neurologic complications of bacterial endocarditis. *Medicine (Baltimore)* 57:329–343, 1978.

150. Raad II, Bodey GP: Infectious complications of indwelling vascular catheters. *Clin Infect Dis* 15:197–208, 1992.

151. Raoult D, Fournier PE, Drancourt M, et al: Diagnosis of 22 new cases of *Bartonella* endocarditis. *Ann Intern Med* 125:646–652, 1996.

152. Reisberg BE: Infective endocarditis in the narcotic addict. *Prog Cardiovasc Dis* 22:193–204, 1979.

153. Reller LB: The serum bactericidal test. *Rev Infect Dis* 8:803–808, 1986.

154. Rey JR, Axon A, Budzynska A, Kruse A, Nowak A (working group): Guidelines of the European Society of gastrointestinal endoscopy (E.S.G.E.). Antibiotic prophylaxis for gastrointestinal endoscopy. *Endoscopy* 30:318–324, 1998.

155. Roberts GJ, Holzel HS, Sury MRJ, et al: Dental bacteremia in children. *Pediatr Cardiol* 18:24–27, 1997.

156. Roberts GJ: Dentists are innocent! "Everyday" bacteremia is the real culprit: A review and assessment of the evidence that dental surgical procedures are a principal cause of bacterial endocarditis in children. *Pediatr Cardiol* 20:317–325, 1999.

157. Roberts R, Slovis CM: Endocarditis in intravenous drug abusers. *Emerg Med Clin North Am* 8:665–681, 1990.

158. Roberts RB: Streptococcal endocarditis: The viridans and beta hemolytic streptococci. In Kaye D (ed): *Infective Endocarditis.* New York, Raven Press, 1992, pp 191–208.

159. Roberts WC: Characteristics and consequences of infective endocarditis (active or healed or both) learned from morphologic studies. In Rahimtoola SH (ed): *Infective Endocarditis.* New York, Grune and Stratton, 1978, pp 55–123.

160. Rodbard S: Blood velocity and endocarditis. *Circulation* 27:18–28, 1963.

161. Rotrosen D, Calderone RA, Edwards JE Jr: Adherence of *Candida* species to host tissues and plastic surfaces. *Rev Infect Dis* 8:73–85, 1986.

162. Rowley KM, Clubb KS, Smith GJ, Cabin HS: Right-sided infective endocarditis as a consequence of flow-directed pulmonary-artery catheterization: A clinicopathological study of 55 autopsied patients. *N Engl J Med* 311:1152–1156, 1984.

163. Rubinstein E, Noriega ER, Simberkoff MS, et al: Fungal endocarditis: Analysis of 24 cases and review of the literature. *Medicine (Baltimore)* 54:331–334, 1975.

164. Saiman L, Prince A, Gersony WM: Pediatric infective endocarditis in the modern era. *J Pediatr* 122:847–853, 1993.

165. Salgado AV, Furlan AJ, Keys TF: Mycotic aneurysm, subarachnoid hemorrhage, and indications for cerebral angiography in infective endocarditis. *Stroke* 18:1057–1060, 1987.

166. Salgado AV, Furlan AJ, Keys TF, et al: Neurologic complications of endocarditis. A 12-year experience. *Neurology* 39:173–178, 1989.

167. Samet JH, Shevitz A, Fowle J, Singer DE: Hospitalization decision in febrile intravenous drug users. *Am J Med* 89:53–57, 1990.

168. Sande MA: Endocarditis in intravenous drug abusers. In Kaye D (ed): *Infective Endocarditis.* New York, Raven Press, 1992, pp 345–359.

169. Sande MA, Johnson WD Jr, Hook EW, Kaye D: Sustained bacteremia in patients with prosthetic cardiac valves. *N Engl J Med* 286:1067–1070, 1972.

170. Santoro J, Ingerman M: Response to therapy: Relapses and reinfections. In Kaye D (ed): *Infective Endocarditis.* New York, Raven Press, 1992, pp 423–433.

171. Schaad UB: Pediatric use of quinolones. *Pediatr Infect Dis J* 18:469–470, 1999.

172. Schachner A, Salomon J, Levinsky L, Blieden LC, Levy MJ: Prosthetic valve replacement in infants and children. *J Cardiovasc Surg (Torino)* 25:537–544, 1984.

173. Scheld WM, Sande MA: Endocarditis and intravascular infections. In Mandell GL, Douglas RG Jr, Bennett JE (eds): *Principles and Practice of Infectious Diseases.* New York, Churchill Livingstone, 1990, pp 670–706.

174. Schliamser SE, Cars O, Norrby SR: Neurotoxicity of beta-lactam antibiotics: Predisposing factors and pathogenesis. *J Antimicrob Chemother* 27:405–425, 1991.

175. Schollin J, Bjarke B, Wesstrom G: Infective endocarditis in Swedish children: I. Incidence, etiology, underlying factors and port of entry of infection. *Acta Paediatr Scand* 75:993–998, 1986.

176. Scott PJ, Blackburn ME, Wharton GA, et al: Transoesophageal echocardiography in neonates, infants, and children: Applicability and diagnostic value in everyday practice of a cardiothoracic unit. *Br Heart J* 68:488–492, 1992.

177. Seidl S, Kuhnl P: Transmission of diseases by blood transfusion. *World J Surg* 11:30–35, 1987.

178. Sexton DJ, Tenenbaum MJ, Wilson WR, et al: Ceftriaxone once daily for four weeks compared with ceftriaxone plus gentamicin once daily for two weeks for treatment of endocarditis due to penicillin-susceptibile streptococci. *Clin Infect Dis* 27:1470–1474, 1998.

179. Shepherd SM, Druckenbrod GG, Haywood YC: Other infectious complications in intravenous drug users: The compromised host. *Emerg Med Clin North Am* 8:683–692, 1990.

180. Shinefield HR: Staphylococcal infections. In Remington JS, Klein JO (eds): *Infectious Diseases of the Fetus and Newborn Infant.* Philadelphia, WB Saunders, 1990, pp 866–900.

181. Sholler GF, Hawker RE, Celermajer JM: Infective endocarditis in childhood. *Pediatr Cardiol* 6:183–186, 1986.

182. Silver MD: Infective endocarditis. In Silver MD (ed): *Cardiovascular Pathology.* New York, Churchill Livingstone, 1991, pp 895–931.

183. Simberkoff MS: Narcotic associated infective endocarditis. In Kaplan EL, Taranta AV (eds): *Infective Endocarditis.* Dallas, The American Heart Association, 1977, pp 46–50.

184. Simmons BP, Wong ES: Guideline for prevention of nosocomial pneumonia. *Infect Control* 3:327–333, 1982.

185. Skehan JD, Murray M, Mills PG: Infective endocarditis: Incidence and mortality in the North East Thames Region. *Br Heart J* 59:62–68, 1988.

186. Smith TL, Pearson ML, Wilcox KR, et al for the glycopeptide-intermediate *Staphylococcus aureus* working group: Emergence of vancomycin resistance in *staphylococcus aureus*. *N Engl J Med* 340:493–501, 1999.

187. Sobel JD: Nosocomial infective endocarditis. In Kaye D (ed): *Infective Endocarditis*. New York, Raven Press, 1992, pp 361–373.

188. Sokil AB: Cardiac imaging in infective endocarditis. In Kaye D (ed): *Infective Endocarditis*. New York, Raven Press, 1992, pp 125–150.

189. Stamboulian D, Bonvehi P, Arevalo C, et al: Antibiotic management of outpatients with endocarditis due to penicillin-susceptible streptococci. *Rev Infect Dis* 13(suppl 2):S160–S163, 1991.

190. Stanton BF, Baltimore RS, Clemens JD: Changing spectrum of infective endocarditis in children. Analysis of 26 cases, 1970–1979. *Am J Dis Child* 138:720–725, 1984.

191. Steckelberg JM, Murphy JG, Wilson WR: Management of complications of infective endocarditis. In Kaye D (ed): *Infective Endocarditis*. New York, Raven Press, 1992, pp 435–453.

192. Steckelberg JM, Murphy JG, Ballard D, et al: Emboli in infective endocarditis: The prognostic value of echocardiography. *Ann Intern Med* 114:635–640, 1991.

193. Stockheim JA, Chadwick EG, Kessler S, et al: Are the Duke criteria superior to the Beth Israel criteria for the diagnosis of infective endocarditis in children? *Clin Infect Dis* 27:1451–1456, 1998.

194. Strom BL, Abrutyn E, Berlin JA, et al: Dental and cardiac risk factors for infective endocarditis: A population-based, case-control study. *Ann Intern Med* 129:761–769, 1998.

195. Stull TL, LiPuma JJ: Endocarditis in children. In Kaye D (ed): *Infective Endocarditis*. New York, Raven Press, 1992, pp 313–327.

196. Symchych PS, Krauss AN, Winchester P: Endocarditis following intracardiac placement of umbilical venous catheters in neonates. *J Pediatr* 90:287–289, 1977.

197. Tanaka M, Abe T, Hosokawa S, et al: Tricuspid valve *Candida* endocarditis cured by valve-sparing debridement. *Ann Thorac Surg* 48:857–858, 1989.

198. Terpenning MS, Buggy BP, Kauffman CA: Hospital-acquired infective endocarditis. *Arch Intern Med* 148:1601–1603, 1988.

199. Tolan RW Jr, Kleiman MB, Frank M, et al: Operative intervention in active endocarditis in children: Report of a series of cases and review. *Clin Infect Dis* 14:852–862, 1992.

200. Tunkel AR, Mandell GL: Infecting microorganisms. In Kaye D (ed): *Infective Endocarditis*. New York, Raven Press, 1992, pp 85–97.

201. Van der Meer JT, Van Wijk W, et al: Efficacy of antibiotic prophylaxis for prevention of native-valve endocarditis. *Lancet* 339:135–139, 1992.

202. Van Hare GF, Ben-Shachar G, Liebman J, et al: Infective endocarditis in infants and children during the past 10 years: A decade of change. *Am Heart J* 107:1235–1240, 1984.

203. Van Scoy RE: Culture-negative endocarditis. *Mayo Clin Proc* 57:149–154, 1982.

204. Von Reyn CF, Levy BS, Arbeit RD, Friedland G, Crumpacker CS: Infective endocarditis: An analysis based on strict case definitions. *Ann Intern Med* 94:505–518, 1981.

205. Waldvogel FA: New resistance in *Staphylococcus aureus*. *N Engl J Med* 340:556–557, 1999.

206. Washington JA: The role of the microbiology laboratory in the diagnosis and antimicrobial treatment of infective endocarditis. *Mayo Clin Proc* 57:22–32, 1982.

207. Washington JA: The microbiological diagnosis of infective endocarditis. *J Antimicrob Chemother* 20(suppl A):29–39, 1987.

208. Washington JA, Ilstrup DM: Blood cultures: Issues and controversies. *Rev Infect Dis* 8:792–802, 1986.

209. Watanakunakorn C: Infective endocarditis as a result of medical progress. *Am J Med* 64:917–919, 1978.

210. Watanakunakorn C: Prosthetic valve infective endocarditis. *Prog Cardiovasc Dis* 22:181–192, 1979.

211. Watanakunakorn C, Baird IM: *Staphylococcus aureus* bacteremia and endocarditis associated with a removable infected intravenous device. *Am J Med* 63:253–256, 1977.

212. Whitby S, Pallera A, Schaberg DR, Bronze MS: Infective endocarditis caused by *Streptococcus pneumoniae* with high-level resistance to penicillin and cephalosporin. *Clin Infect Dis* 23:1176–1177, 1996.

213. Williams RC: Rheumatoid factors in subacute bacterial endocarditis and other infectious diseases. *Scand J Rheumatol* (suppl 75):300–308, 1988.

214. Wilson WR, Danielson GK, Giuliani ER, Geraci JE: Prosthetic valve endocarditis. *Mayo Clin Proc* 57:155–161, 1982.

215. Wilson WR, Geraci JE, Danielson GK, et al: Anticoagulant therapy and central nervous system complications in patients with prosthetic valve endocarditis. *Circulation* 57:1004–1007, 1978.

216. Wilson WR, Giuliani ER, Danielson GK, Geraci JE: Management of complications of infective endocarditis. *Mayo Clin Proc* 57:162–170, 1982.

217. Wilson WR, Karchmer AW, Dajani AS, et al: Antibiotic treatment of adults with infective endocarditis due to streptococci, enterococci, staphylococci, and HACEK microorganisms. *JAMA* 274:1706–1713, 1995.

218. Witt MD, Bayer AS: Comparison of fluconazole and amphotericin B for prevention and treatment of experimental *Candida* endocarditis. *Antimicrob Agents Chemother* 35:2481–2485, 1991.

219. Woods GL, Wood RP, Shaw BW Jr: *Aspergillus* endocarditis in patients without prior cardiovascular surgery: Report of a case in a liver transplant recipient and review. *Rev Infect Dis* 11:263–272, 1989.

220. Yokochi K, Sakamoto H, Mikajima T, et al: Infective endocarditis in children: A current diagnostic trend and the embolic complications. *Jpn Circ J* 50:1294–1297, 1986.

221. Zenker PN, Rosenberg EM, Van Dyke RB, et al: Successful medical treatment of presumed *Candida* endocarditis in critically ill infants. *J Pediatr* 119:472–477, 1991

Chapter 46

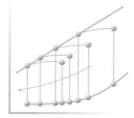

Syndromes and Congenital Heart Defects

ANNE M. MURPHY, MD, CATHERINE A. NEILL, MD,
and AARON L. ZUCKERBERG, MD

INTRODUCTION

Since the first edition of this textbook, continuing advances have been made in syndrome recognition and understanding. It is not feasible to describe here the burgeoning literature concerning genetics and molecular biology. The availability on the Internet of the McKusick catalogue of inherited disorders in humans[128,129] is a great resource to those seeking to keep abreast of new developments. In this chapter, we summarize some of the major new findings, particularly in the 22q11.2 deletion syndromes, while maintaining primary emphasis on the clinical aspects of syndromes confronted by the pediatric cardiac intensive care team.

The frequent coexistence of cardiac and extracardiac malformations has long been recognized.[142] Interest in cardiac syndromes has been stimulated by genetic,[107,154] cellular,[110] and epidemiologic studies.[59,60] Such studies have led to recognition that "isolated" cardiac malformations, although accounting for almost three fourths of all cardiac defects, are often less severe and accompanied by less long-term morbidity than are those associated with extracardiac defects or syndromes. Indeed, the extraordinary advances in cardiac surgical treatment have been accompanied by decreases in mortality and morbidity, such that syndromic associations now play an increasing role in determining overall prognosis and utilization of resources.[99] Thus both scientific and clinical reasons exist for considering syndromes in a textbook such as this.

Despite their importance, syndromes have been somewhat underemphasized in the pediatric cardiac literature, which has tended to focus on diagnostic techniques and surgical approaches. This is in part because of the rapidly increasing number of syndromes; in part because some associations (as for example, that of Down syndrome with atrioventricular [AV] septal defect) are too well established to cause clinical comment; and in part and perhaps most important, natural resistance to the idea that successful cardiac surgery and postoperative care are inadequate to ensure a normal life for some children.

Terminology can be a problem, because some authors prefer to confine the term *syndrome* to conditions of known etiology, such as trisomies and other chromosomal syndromes, or to known mendelian disorders such as Marfan syndrome. They use an alternative term such as DiGeorge *anomaly*, when the etiology is heterogeneous, and Vacterl *association* when the disorder is sporadic and the phenotype variable. No complete consensus exists on the use of these alternatives.

The relevance of different syndromes in the intensive care setting varies widely. Some, such as Down syndrome, are of great importance to the intensivist, because of the frequency and association with multiple defects that may complicate care. Others, for example, trisomy 18, have such a poor prognosis that serious ethical issues are raised regarding the appropriate use of intensive care. Still others, such as Holt-Oram syndrome, are of diagnostic importance and certainly require recognition and genetic counseling[141] but do not have any significant impact on perioperative management.

This chapter emphasizes four major cardiac syndromes of significance to the pediatric cardiac intensivist: Down syndrome, a frequently encountered chromosomal anomaly; Noonan syndrome, a cardiac syndrome with an autosomal dominant mode of inheritance; DiGeorge and other syndromes representing the spectrum of anomalies caused by chromosome 22q11.2 deletions; and heterotaxy syndrome, also known as Ivemark, cardiosplenic, or isomerism syndrome, involving extremely complex cardiac and noncardiac anomalies. Following this discussion is a brief tabulation of some other syndromes likely to be encountered in intensive care settings and a discussion of some ethical issues encountered in critical cardiac care.

DOWN SYNDROME OMIM 1906851

Definition, Prevalence, and General Concepts

Down syndrome, or trisomy 21, is the most frequent syndrome causing congenital heart disease. It is estimated to affect more than 300,000 individuals in the United States,[108]

and congenital cardiac malformations are present in between 40% and 50% of affected children. The association of trisomy 21 with defects in AV septation (also called endocardial cushion or AV canal defect) is well established.[58] Abnormalities are found in almost all organ systems (Fig. 46-1),[36,163] but the most important are mental retardation, delayed growth,[36] facial dysmorphism,[100] and congenital cardiac[66] and gastrointestinal anomalies.[114] Other problems, which are increasingly recognized, are upper airway obstruction,[94,193] atlantoaxial instability,[202] frequent hypothyroidism,[36] thymic hypoplasia, and immune deficiency.[205] Transient leukemia of the newborn usually resolves spontaneously; however, leukemia of childhood occurs at about 15 times the normal rate, and other hematologic disorders can occur.[222] A risk of early-onset Alzheimer's disease has been demonstrated.[91]

The cytogenetic abnormality in Down syndrome is trisomy 21 (47, +21) in 93% to 96% of cases and translocation in 2% to 5% of cases.[53] About 2% to 4% of all cases are associated with mosaicism, in which case the clinical findings are usually milder. Although advanced maternal age is a risk factor, approximately 80% of Down syndrome mothers are between ages 18 and 35 years.

The precise pathogenetic mechanism for the Down syndrome phenotype in relation to trisomy of chromosome 21 is not yet understood. Studies of patients with partial duplications of chromosome 21 have revealed regions of 21q that may contribute to abnormalities in various organ systems, including a region that may be critical to congenital cardiac defects on distal 21q.[106] Mouse models, which duplicate some features of Down syndrome, also are under investigation. These models are problematic, in that the Ts16 mouse, which mimics the cardiac defects in Down syndrome, results in fetal lethality (as summarized[53]), whereas a more recently developed model does not feature cardiac defects, at least in live-born mice.[167] The recent completion of the sequence of human chromosome 21 may hasten the understanding of the contribution of increased gene dosage of specific genes or gene sets to the Down syndrome phenotype.[81]

The prevalence of Down syndrome is estimated at 1/700 live births. In the Baltimore Washington Infant Study (BWIS), a 10-year regional study of all live-born infants younger than 1 year diagnosed with congenital heart defects,[58] the importance of this syndrome as a cause of severe heart defects was made clear. Among 4390 live-born infants diagnosed with heart defects in the region during the study period, 385 had Down syndrome.[59] Of the Down syndrome infants in the study, 60% had AV septal defects, whereas almost 70% of all study infants with this form of cardiac defect had Down syndrome.

Changing concepts about the appropriateness of care have occurred among our society and the healthcare community.[82] The overwhelming majority of these children now live at home, and the emphasis is on allowing them to reach their maximal potential. Early cardiac surgery has transformed the clinical course of infants with heart defects and Down syndrome. Early detection and treatment of severe defects is now the rule.[177] Children with and without heart defects have benefited from enrollment in infant-stimulation programs, the growth of the Special Olympics, and other participatory activities. The mean life expectancy is now more than 50 years, a dramatic change from even 20 years ago.

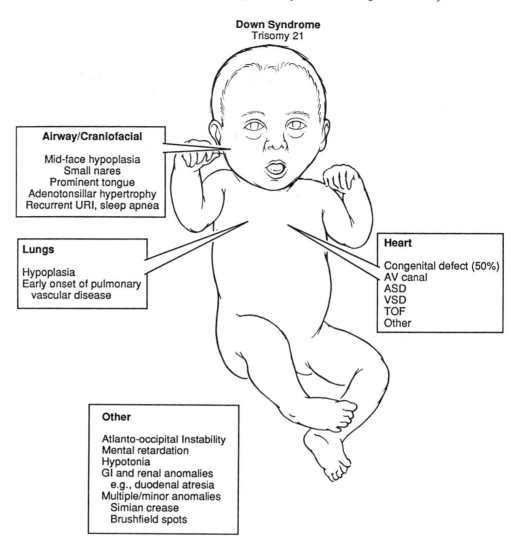

Down Syndrome
Trisomy 21

Airway/Craniofacial

Mid-face hypoplasia
Small nares
Prominent tongue
Adenotonsillar hypertrophy
Recurrent URI, sleep apnea

Lungs

Hypoplasia
Early onset of pulmonary
    vascular disease

Heart

Congenital defect (50%)
AV canal
ASD
VSD
TOF
Other

Other

Atlanto-occipital Instability
Mental retardation
Hypotonia
GI and renal anomalies
    e.g., duodenal atresia
Multiple/minor anomalies
    Simian crease
    Brushfield spots

Evaluation

Echocardiogram
Karyotyping

FIGURE 46-1 Associated defects of Down syndrome. AV, atrioventricular, ASD, atrial septal defect; VSD, ventricular septal defect, ToF, tetralogy of Fallot,

Nevertheless, the syndrome remains an important problem with significant morbidity.

Relevance of Down Syndrome in the Intensive Care Setting

Cardiac Findings

Congenital heart defects are present in between 40% and 50% of live-born infants with Down syndrome and show a distribution pattern significantly different from that in the euploid population. In the Baltimore Washington Infant Study,[58,59] AV septal defects were the most frequent (60%), followed by ventricular septal defect (VSD; 19%), atrial septal defects (ASDs; 9%), and tetralogy of Fallot (7%). Dextrocardia and complete transposition did not occur,

confirming findings of earlier investigators. Korenberg and colleagues[107] recently demonstrated differences in chromosomal abnormalities in infants with trisomy 21 with and without cardiac defects. Other studies of animal models[133] and of the molecular biology of the endocardial cushions[110] are helping to clarify the strong association of Down syndrome with defects in AV septation.

Pulmonary vascular obstructive disease can occur early in the course of infants with large left-to-right shunts and Down syndrome.[30] This finding has several implications of clinical importance: (1) *early repair* of AV canal (or other large left-to-right shunt) is indicated, usually by age 6 months; (2) *postoperative protocols* may be necessary to address the management of pulmonary hypertension (Chapter 46); (3) infants with marked midfacial hypoplasia and other upper airway problems may present particular perioperative difficulties and may contribute to the reported increased surgical risk in Down syndrome infants undergoing repair of AV canal defects.[136,168]

Because of the high incidence of severe cardiac defects[120,203] and the difficulty in auscultation of cardiac murmurs, any infant with Down syndrome should have a cardiac consultation and echocardiography by age 4 weeks, or earlier if admitted for care of an acute respiratory illness or if any other operations are required.

Upper Airway and Pulmonary Problems

Multiple anomalies contribute to the increased incidence of sleep apnea and upper airway obstruction seen in infants with Down syndrome (see Fig. 46-1).[103,193] In addition to excessive secretions and narrow upper airway passages, some pathologic evidence exists of pulmonary alveolar hypoplasia.[53] The generalized hypotonia (which is constantly present but variable in severity) could contribute to reducing the effectiveness of coughing and other responses to viral or bacterial respiratory infection. In some children, obesity is a complicating factor. Whatever the mechanism, recurrent upper respiratory infections and repeated otitis media may lead to adenotonsillar hyperplasia, with exacerbation of upper airway obstruction and alveolar hypoventilation. Respiratory syncytial viral (RSV) infections are particularly poorly tolerated, especially in those infants who also have a cardiac defect with pulmonary overcirculation, thus prophylaxis against RSV should be considered. This interaction of cardiac and respiratory disorders undoubtedly contributed to the high infant mortality seen in past studies.[123] In addition, recurrent otitis and abnormally narrow auditory passages may contribute to hearing loss.[18]

Intubation and ventilatory support are required for operative procedures and occasionally for other pulmonary problems. Because of potential cervical spine instability,[202] preoperative cervical spine films are recommended in some institutions. Screening children with Down syndrome with cervical spine films, however, remains controversial.[34,162]

Extracardiac Problems

Gastrointestinal anomalies are present in 2% to 3% of Down syndrome infants, the most usual being duodenal stenosis or atresia, and occasionally, Hirschsprung disease or tracheoesophageal fistula.[53,114] In the Baltimore Washington Infant Study,[58,59] among 218 live-born infants with Down syndrome and heart defects, 15 (6.9%) had a gastrointestinal anomaly, and 4 (1.8%) had an abnormality of the genitourinary tract. Thus an infant with Down syndrome may need urgent neonatal surgery, usually even while a severe cardiac malformation is unrepaired. In recent years, most such infants have done well, although a planned approach to timing and coordination of the healthcare team members involved is crucial for the infant and family. Even infants with structurally normal gastrointestinal systems may experience feeding difficulties due to oral motor difficulties or reflux disease.

A few medical problems encountered with more than usual frequency include petechial rashes, giving rise to concern as to infective endocarditis or possibly leukemia[7,97]; increased susceptibility to infections, including hepatitis B; and hypothyroidism. In most instances, widespread petechial rashes are due to transient thrombocytopenia and platelet dysfunction.[222]

The Whole Child: Additional Special Problems

The whole child and the family are always of great concern in the intensive care setting. Effective communications in children with Down syndrome are made more difficult than usual by the child's mental retardation, which complicates the participation of the child in treatment decisions. Occasionally, the family has already become frustrated by the number of specialists and consultations involved.[143] It is sometimes helpful to have the healthcare team discuss openly together some of these special difficulties and to develop an approach that is both caring and informative to the family and child.

Infective endocarditis does not appear to be a particular hazard in Down syndrome, although meticulous dental care is indicated,[36,211] and endocarditis prophylaxis is essential for those with congenital cardiac defects. The use of the usual childhood immunization protocols, together with periodic screening for hypothyroidism and vigorous treatment of upper respiratory infections, is part of the proactive approach, which continues to improve the quality of life of these children.[4] Cardiac surgical mortality figures in infancy for repair of AV septal defects are less than 10% and continue to improve. Nevertheless, Down syndrome is the cause of almost one tenth of severe congenital heart disease and remains a major source of childhood morbidity. Although a clear trend is not yet seen, prenatal detection methods could ultimately decrease the prevalence of this important syndrome.[78,86,148]

NOONAN SYNDROME OMIM 163950

Definition, Prevalence, and General Concepts

This constellation of anomalies,[146] also referred to as the Noonan-Ehmke syndrome,[145,147] is characterized by both cardiac and extracardiac defects (Fig. 46-2).[19,130,141,166] Familial Noonan syndrome is genetically heterogenic, but it can be caused by mutations in the gene *PTPN11* at chromosome 12q24.[113,199] Noonan syndrome has a prevalence of between 1/1000 to 1/2500 live births. Pulmonary valvar stenosis with valvar dysplasia is the most frequent cardiac anomaly, followed by hypertrophic cardiomyopathy. ASD is often associated with pulmonic stenosis, and a variety of other cardiovascular anomalies have been described.[3,5,130,178,216]

Originally the similarities between Noonan and Ullrich-Turner (XO) syndromes (neck webbing, lymphedema, short stature, and keloid formation) were emphasized in the literature.[145] The sex chromosomes are normal in Noonan syndrome, although a similar male phenotype has been rarely reported in 45X46XY mosaicism.[9] The syndrome may be sporadic but is familial in at least 40% of cases; an autosomal dominant mode of inheritance is usual,[19,141] but other genetic mechanisms have been described.[125] Additional defects of facial dysmorphism, kyphoscoliosis, vertebral anomalies, winged scapula, low-set ears, hypertelorism, male infertility, shield-shaped pectus sternal deformity, and coagulation factor deficits have been recorded. More recently, studies of

Noonan Syndrome
Autosomal Dominant Inheritance

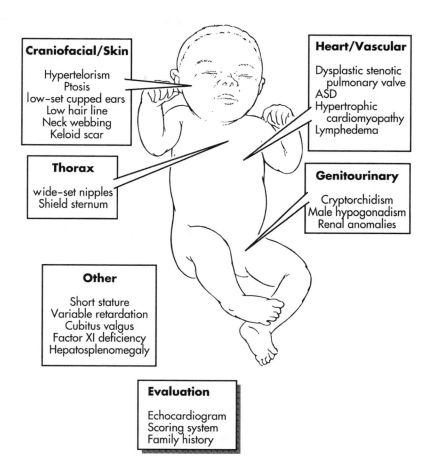

Craniofacial/Skin

Hypertelorism
Ptosis
low-set cupped ears
Low hair line
Neck webbing
Keloid scar

Thorax

wide-set nipples
Shield sternum

Heart/Vascular

Dysplastic stenotic
pulmonary valve
ASD
Hypertrophic
cardiomyopathy
Lymphedema

Genitourinary

Cryptorchidism
Male hypogonadism
Renal anomalies

Other

Short stature
Variable retardation
Cubitus valgus
Factor XI deficiency
Hepatosplenomegaly

Evaluation

Echocardiogram
Scoring system
Family history

FIGURE 46-2   Associated defects of Noonan syndrome.

families have focused on similarities between Noonan-Ehmke and cardiofaciocutaneous (CFC) syndrome.[67,68] Association with neurofibromatosis[183,194] and with basal cell nevus syndrome[77] has stimulated the hypothesis that an autosomal dominant mutation involving neural crest dysplasia cells may be the mechanism of the Noonan-Ehmke phenotype, a mechanism that differs from that proposed by Clark[31] for nondysplastic pulmonary valve stenosis. Gabrielli and associates,[69] in a study of magnetic resonance imaging, described Arnold Chiari malformation type I and a leptomeningeal cyst in one mildly retarded child with Noonan syndrome and recommended that more such studies might clarify the nature of the nervous system involvement.

Relevance of Noonan Syndrome in the Intensive Care Setting

This is a chronic disorder, and acute presentation with life-threatening illness is extremely rare. Nevertheless, several features make the syndrome of interest to the intensivist, who may be involved in perioperative management of cardiac or extracardiac anomalies. The relevant features are discussed under cardiac findings, anesthetic issues, postoperative sequelae, and diagnostic difficulties.

Cardiac Findings

Older reviews quote an incidence of congenital heart disease of from 50% to 66%, but in a recent study of 151 individuals with Noonan syndrome,[181] pulmonary stenosis was present in 62%, hypertrophic cardiomyopathy in 20%, and only 12.5% had a normal echocardiogram. Since the advent of pulmonary valvuloplasty,[98] most children and adults now have relief of pulmonary stenosis by valvuloplasty performed in the cardiac catheterization laboratory, and the great majority do not need overnight hospitalization or general anesthesia. However, in Noonan syndrome, the pulmonary valve is usually thickened and dysplastic (12 of 16 or 75% in Stanger's study)[192] and often responds poorly to valvuloplasty.[139,192] Surgery by partial valvectomy is sometimes necessary, and supravalvar patch is sometimes placed because of associated supravalvar stenosis. Such surgery is well tolerated, and despite postoperative pulmonary insufficiency, mortality and major cardiac morbidity are very rare.

Hypertrophic cardiomyopathy[161] was originally described as developing late in childhood but has now been recognized in infancy and even prenatally.[191] The presence of hypertrophic cardiomyopathy increases anesthetic and intraoperative risk. A recent echocardiogram should be available before anesthesia for cardiac or noncardiac surgery in infants or children with Noonan syndrome. A baseline preoperative electrocardiogram also is recommended, because an abnormal superior vector or low precordial lead voltage is frequent.

Perioperative and Anesthetic Issues

Some degree of psychomotor retardation is usual, even though almost 90% of children are able to attend regular school. Explanation and discussion of planned procedures is helped if the mental status has been evaluated earlier.

Severe bleeding seems to be a rare complication of surgery in patients with Noonan-Ehmke syndrome. Platelet-function deficit[62] and neonatal amegakaryocytic thrombocytopenia[54] have been described. Sharland and colleagues,[182] in a study of 72 affected individuals with a mean age of 11.4 years, found that 47 (65%) had a history of abnormal bruising or bleeding; 29 (40%) had a prolonged activated partial thromboplastin time. Specific abnormalities, including deficiencies of partial factor XI:C, XII:C, and VIII:C, were present in 36 (50%) patients, and 9 of the 36 had multiple deficiencies. This study suggests that preoperative assessment for coagulation-factor deficits may be warranted, despite the poor correlation reported by the authors between coagulation deficits and abnormal bleeding history.

A possible association of malignant hyperthermia with Noonan syndrome was postulated by Hunter and Pinsky,[89] based on a prior report of this complication in four boys with features suggestive of the Noonan phenotype. In a study of 27 patients, these authors found only one boy with mildly elevated creatine phosphokinase (CPK) levels and concluded that the association must be rare. Malignant hyperthermia was not mentioned in two large recent clinical series of Noonan syndrome,[166,181] including a total of almost 300 affected subjects. Appropriate screening may be warranted in a subset of patients with evidence of somatic myopathy.

Anesthetic management has been detailed in children with Noonan's cardiomyopathy.[23,179] Despite the facial dysmorphism, chest deformity, and high-arched palate, perioperative airway problems and sleep apnea are rare.

Postoperative Sequelae

Although anesthesia and surgery are well tolerated, it is helpful to the family to be aware that keloid scar formation is likely, and also that "catch-up growth" after relief of pulmonary stenosis is highly improbable.[141,166] The cause of the short stature and growth problem is not yet clarified, but Ahmed and coworkers[1] suggested a possible abnormality of the growth hormone/insulin-like growth factor (IGF)-I axis, with some response to treatment with human biosynthetic growth hormone.

Recurrent pleural effusion is a rare but troublesome postoperative complication. It appears to be due to a nonspecific effect of thoracotomy in exacerbating previously mild chronic low-grade pulmonary lymphangiectasia. Good response is generally obtained with a combination of thoracentesis, restriction from dietary long-chain fatty acids, fluid restriction, and/or diuretics. Although systemic lymphedema is well recognized,[12,125] pulmonary lymphangiectasia is rarer, but probably plays an important role in the pulmonary hypoplasia seen complicating the neonatal course of some infants with Noonan syndrome and nonimmune hydrops.[29]

Diagnostic Difficulties

Sharland and associates,[181] in an excellent report on the clinical profile of 151 affected individuals, found a mean age at diagnosis of 9.0 years, and others also commented on late diagnosis. Several factors contribute to this delay, which may lead to inadequate or inappropriate therapy and to lack of genetic counseling. These factors include the rarity of the syndrome, the phenotypic variability, the changes in facial pattern with growth,[2] and the multiplicity of healthcare providers who may see a child with ocular problems,[181] deafness,[38] dermatologic changes,[12,200] failure to thrive, undescended testes, and other manifestations or associations of the syndrome.[16,33]

Several reports exist of in utero diagnosis,[49,93] but after birth, the syndrome may have been overlooked by many observers because "the child looks just like his father (or mother)," who is also of short stature; the similar appearance may be because both parent and child are affected. Duncan and colleagues[51] has drawn up a valuable "score card" of anomalies, which is particularly helpful in the recognition of milder phenotypes. Hepatosplenomegaly was present in 50% of Sharland's series[181] but is often mild; when seen in a previously undiagnosed child or teenager with a heart murmur and lymphedema, an erroneous diagnosis of congestive heart failure has been made. Despite the diagnostic challenges, the pediatric intensivist confronted by a child with growth delay, pulmonary stenosis and/or cardiomyopathy, and cubitus valgus may be in a unique position to recognize the syndrome in the child and in a parent.

CHROMOSOME 22Q11.2 DELETION SYNDROMES: DIGEORGE (OMIM 188400), VELOCARDIOFACIAL (OMIM 192430), AND CONOTRUNCAL ANOMALY FACE (OMIM 217095) SYNDROMES

Definition, Prevalence, and General Concepts

The evolution in the description and understanding of these syndromes in the past few years can be attributed directly to advances in molecular diagnosis. Although initially described as separate syndromes, it now appears clear that these syndromes represent a spectrum of the same molecular disorder. An overlap also may exist with other disorders, and certainly some children may fit within the spectrum clinically who have an alternative genetic or teratogenic cause for their disorder. Historically, DiGeorge[48] described a syndrome with congenital absence of the thymus with associated immunodeficiency and congenital hypoparathyroidism with hypocalcemia. Although these infants did not have intracardiac defects, one was noted to have an aberrant right subclavian artery, and another, a right aortic arch. DiGeorge also referred to an infant described by Lobdell[116] with hypoparathyroidism and severe infectious complications who was noted at autopsy to have an aortic arch malformation, and an earlier letter by Harrington[80] reporting congenital absence of the thymus at autopsy of an 8-day-old who died of convulsions. DiGeorge noted that the association of thymic hypoplasia and hypoparathyroidism was not unexpected, in that both organs are derived from the third and fourth pharyngeal pouches, and commented that cardiac defects also might be expected.[48]

The velocardiofacial syndrome (VCFS) or Shprintzen syndrome was described by Shprintzen's group,[185,186] who reported on a group of patients with palatal abnormalities, typical facies, cardiac defects, most prominently VSDs, and learning disabilities. Other features noted include microcephaly, mental retardation, short stature, and slender hands and digits. Japanese investigators described the conotruncal anomaly face syndrome (CTAF) in a group of children with conotruncal defects.[184,198] This also has been given the eponym Takao syndrome. Wilson and coworkers[214] coined the term "CATCH22" to encompass the various manifestations of deletion in 22q11.2; however, this term was criticized for its negative connotations and has been withdrawn.[20]

These syndromes were brought together with the onset of widespread molecular diagnosis using fluorescent in situ hybridization (FISH) to probe for submicroscopic deletions in chromosome 22q11.2, based on the finding of more prominent deletions and translocations within 22q, first noted in patients with DiGeorge syndrome (DGS).[43] Studies have established that approximately 88% of infants with the clinical diagnosis of DGS have deletions, whereas 76% to 81% with the clinical diagnosis of VCFS have deletions detectable by DNA dosage analysis or FISH.[50,115] Similarly, 98% cases of CTAF have 22q11.2 deletions detectable by FISH.[124] The size of the deleted DNA segment itself cannot explain the variability in these clinical phenotypes; indeed, even when a deletion is inherited, variable phenotypes may be seen within a family.[112] These syndromes may be contiguous gene syndromes that are caused by allelic loss of multiple genes within the deleted region. However, recent evidence from mouse models indicates haploinsufficiency of the *TBX1* gene in the critical region may explain the cardiac defects in the syndromes.[131] Genetic heterogeneity also is present in DGS, cases of which also have been linked to deletions in 10p.[76,135]

DGS has been classified as a defect in a developmental field. A developmental field is an embryologic reactive unit in which the constituent cells and their primordia develop together. The malformation complex results when a perturbation causes this group of embryonic cells and primordia to develop abnormally together.[149] In DGS, the reactive unit consists of the third and fourth branchial arches, derived from a population of cephalic neural crest cells that have an important role in the development of the outflow tract of the heart as well as the thymus, parathyroid glands, and the facial aspects of the cranium.[104] Experimentally, premigratory extirpation of the cranial neural crest region in developing chicks produced conotruncal VSDs and thymic aplasia or hypoplasia.[105] Inherent in the concept of a developmental field defect is that either a genetic aberration affecting the reactive unit or exposure to an environmental agent that targets this unit may then result in a similar cluster of features. Indeed, DGS features have been associated with teratogen exposure in animal models.[15,150]

The prevalence of microdeletions in 22q11.2 is estimated to be approximately 1/4000.[215] Because up to 80% of children with 22q11.2 deletions are found to have congenital heart disease, it is likely that this is the second most frequent

Table 46-1 Cardiac Defects Associated with 22q11.2 Deletion

Defect	Percentage
No defect or clinically insignificant	22–25
Tetralogy of Fallot	17–20
Interrupted aortic arch	14–17
Ventricular septal defect (VSD)	14–16
Pulmonary atresia with VSD*	10
Truncus arteriosus	9
Aortic arch anormaly	5
Vascular ring	3
Pulmonary valve stenosis	2
Other significant defect	4–5

*Referred to as tetralogy of Fallot with pulmonary atresia in the chapter text.
From references 127 and 175.

genetic disorder seen by pediatric cardiovascular specialists. An index of suspicion is warranted because a confirmed or tentative diagnosis will influence management (for example, screening for hypocalcemia before and after surgical procedures and providing genetic counseling, because the deletion may be inherited in as many as 20% of cases). Certain rare cardiac defects should raise suspicion because of the high percentage of children with these lesions who are found to have 22q11.2 deletions (Table 46-1). These defects include interrupted aortic arch, tetralogy of Fallot with pulmonary atresia, tetralogy of Fallot with the so-called "absent" or "dysplastic" valve phenotype, truncus arteriosus, and unusual aortic arch variants such as aberrant subclavian artery or cervical arch. In addition, any child with a cardiac defect and family history of congenital heart disease should be assessed for features that might be suggestive of 22q11.2 deletion. Although it remains controversial, some would argue that the typical facies and dysmorphic features might be subtle or overlooked in the newborn with critical heart disease. Also controversial is whether all children with conotruncal lesions (for example, those with tetralogy of Fallot or conoventricular VSDs) should routinely be screened with FISH for this syndrome.[17,74,127] In tetralogy of Fallot without the variants discussed, the incidence is relatively low (~5%), and some argue a careful examination for dysmorphic features should guide whether to evaluate further.[96,175]

Diagnostic Criteria and Evaluation

The clinical presentations of these syndromes can be variable and are described in detail in clinical reviews.[127,175] Features of note in young infants include a nose with a broad nasal bridge; malar hypoplasia; narrow palpebral fissures; variable hypertelorism; ear anomalies with low-set posteriorly rotated ears, often circular in shape, with deficient upper helices; small and posteriorly displaced jaw (retrognathia) with a small mouth; and overt or more likely submucosal cleft palate (Box 46-1; Fig. 46-3). In older infants and children, notable features include a "hooded" effect of the eyes and velopalatal incompetence (VPI), which is present in high frequency if sought by experienced examiners.[126,223] More striking in older children is delayed expressive speech, hypernasal speech, and articulation problems, which may be improved after repair of VPI. Other features include short stature and long,

BOX 46-1 *Dysmorphic Features Associated with 22q11.2 Deletion Syndrome*

Narrow palpebral fissures
Hooded eyelids
Hypertelorism
Small, rounded protuberant ears
Broad nasal bridge
Bulbous nose tip
Hypoplastic alae nasae
Small mouth
Retrognathia/micrognathia
Palatal abnormalities
Long thin digits

Table 46-2   Evaluation for Patients with 22q11.2 Deletions[127,175]

Typical Subspecialty Evaluation
Genetics
Cardiology
Immunology
Otolaryngology
Plastic surgery
Speech and audiology
Neurodevelopmental

Additional Subspecialties as Necessary
Oral motor and swallowing
Endocrinology
Gastroenterology
Orthopedics
Urology
Pediatric surgery
Psychiatry

Laboratory Evaluation
FISH
Serum calcium
Complete blood count, T-cell studies, immunoglobulins
Echocardiography
Renal ultrasound

FISH, fluorescent in situ hybridization.

slender digits. Laboratory and imaging studies may reveal a variable degree of thymic hypoplasia or aplasia with associated T-cell defects, although profound clinically significant immunodeficiency is rare. Hypocalcemia may be found, particularly in young infants, and tends to resolve or respond to calcium supplementation. Another frequent finding is renal abnormalities detectable on ultrasound, including absent, dysplastic, or multicystic kidneys. Undescended testes are found in 8% of boys. Neurodevelopmental issues include motor and speech delay; learning disabilities are prominent, and structural brain lesions have been described.[109,117,132] Psychiatric disorders are reported in older individuals.[138,151]

The diversity of problems mandates evaluation by several specialty groups. The recommended specialties to evaluate these children are listed in Table 46-2. The specific evaluation should be dictated by the spectrum of problems in an individual.

Deletion of Chromosome 22q11.2 Syndrome

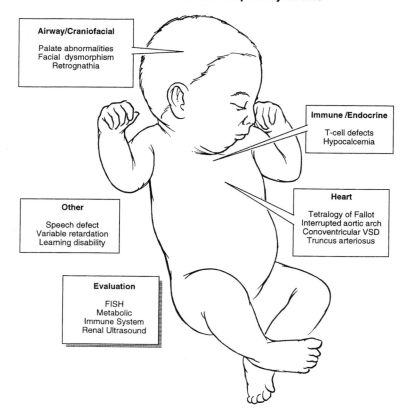

Airway/Craniofacial

Palate abnormalities
Facial dysmorphism
Retrognathia

Immune /Endocrine

T-cell defects
Hypocalcemia

Other

Speech defect
Variable retardation
Learning disability

Heart

Tetralogy of Fallot
Interrupted aortic arch
Conoventricular VSD
Truncus arteriosus

Evaluation

FISH
Metabolic
Immune System
Renal Ultrasound

FIGURE 46-3   Associated defects of 22q11.2 deletion syndromes.

Relevance in the Intensive Care Setting

Airway

The airway may be problematic in patients with 22q11.2 deletion syndrome (Box 46-2). Patients may have small mouths and posteriorly displaced jaws, which may complicate intubations and preclude easy visualization of the larynx during direct laryngoscopy. Depending on the severity of the anatomy, the equipment and personnel necessary to establish an alternative airway should be readily available before the administration of hypnotics and neuromuscular blocking agents.[61] A smaller subset of patients has laryngomalacia or structural laryngeal problems such as webs. Vascular rings may be present in this syndrome, and it is important to note that these frequently occur in patients without overt structural heart disease. Finally, infants with particularly complex cardiac defects may undergo prolonged and complex repairs, which may increase the risk of injury to the recurrent laryngeal or phrenic nerves. The resulting vocal cord or diaphragmatic paralyses should be rigorously excluded in infants for whom extubation fails or who require prolonged respiratory support.

Feeding Issues

Although overt or submucosal cleft palate occurs in approximately 25% of patients, confirmed or suspected VPI is even more prevalent. In the infant, feeding difficulties may occur in a third of patients.[127] These are seen as nasopharyngeal reflux, oral motor dysfunction, and gastroesophageal reflux and are not limited to the infants with congenital heart defects. Given the importance of adequate nutrition in the postoperative patient, early recognition of these issues will prompt investigation, with formal assessment of reflux and swallowing issues, and initiation of medical therapy, as described in Chapter 15. In some cases, tube feedings are necessary.

A caveat in the nutritional assessment of these patients: it is important to recognize that constitutional growth issues may be present. Approximately a third of older patients with or without heart disease have short stature.[127,175] Growth hormone deficiency has been found in a small percentage of these patients.

Immune Deficiency

Detailed studies of T-cell number and function, as well as evaluation of immunoglobulin levels, will reveal abnormalities in the majority of patients. These include decreased T-cell production in 67% of patients, as well as functional T-cell abnormalities in 18%.[196] Humoral abnormalities also are seen, in particular, IgA deficiency.[189,196] A large survey study of patients with 22q11.2 deletions found a clinical history of frequent infections in a small percentage of 218 patients in whom these data were recorded.[175] However, sufficient reason for concern exists about the risk of infectious complications and graft-versus-host disease from transfusion to warrant the use of cytomegalovirus-negative, irradiated blood products in the critically ill neonate and young infant requiring urgent heart surgery and in all infants and children who are known to have 22q11.2 deletions. Individual assessment of infants diagnosed with 22q11.2 deletion syndrome by an immunologist is warranted, with determination of need for antibiotic prophylaxis and need for avoidance of live viral vaccines.

> **BOX 46-2** *Critical Care Considerations in 22q11.2 Deletion Syndrome*
>
> Difficult intubation
> Laryngeal/tracheal abnormalities
> Hypocalcemia
> Hypocalcemic seizures
> Increased risk of infections
> Possibility of transfusion–related graft-versus-host disease
> Feeding diffculties

Hypocalcemia Hypocalcemia may result in seizures in infants with chromosome 22q11.2 deletion syndrome. Neonatal myocardial contraction is more dependent on transarcolemmal calcium entry than is mature muscle; thus hypocalcemia also may affect cardiac function, as well as contribute to abnormal cardiac rhythm and vasomotor tone.[27,73,95,221] Ryan and colleagues[175] reported that 60% of patients in whom calcium was measured were found to have hypocalcemia at some point in their course. In most cases, this was documented during the neonatal period and responded to calcium supplementation. The hypocalcemia generally resolves, although reports are found of late presentations with hypocalcemia.[40,41,71,197] Latent hypoparathyroidism also may be provoked to symptomatic hypocalcemia during periods of stress, such as surgery or systemic infections.

Long-term Management Issues

The severity of the cardiac defect is the major contributor to any early mortality in this syndrome. However, the majority of infants will have successful surgical therapy. Many infants and children will have ongoing issues of growth, speech delay, and ultimately some degree of learning disability or frank retardation. Psychiatric disorders may affect up to 30% of adults with this disorder[138] and may lead to problems in communication when a parent of a critically ill infant also is affected by a 22q11.2 deletion.

THE VISCERAL HETEROTAXY SYNDROMES (SPLENO-CARDIAC OR ISOMERISM SYNDROMES, IVEMARK SYNDROME, OMIM 208530, 306955)

Definition

The coexistence of cardiac malpositions, complex intracardiac architecture, and visceral heterotaxy (the abnormal position of the abdominal viscera) has been appreciated since the time of Aristotle.[155] Visceral heterotaxy (or situs ambiguous), with associated congenital anomalies of the spleen, is present in about one third of infants with cardiac malpositions. Fundamentally, instead of the normal asymmetry (a left-sided heart, stomach, and spleen and a right-sided major lobe of the liver), an abnormally symmetrical pattern of the lungs, liver, and vena cavae is found. The spleen either is absent (asplenia) or consists of a cluster of small splenuli (polysplenia) (Fig. 46-4).

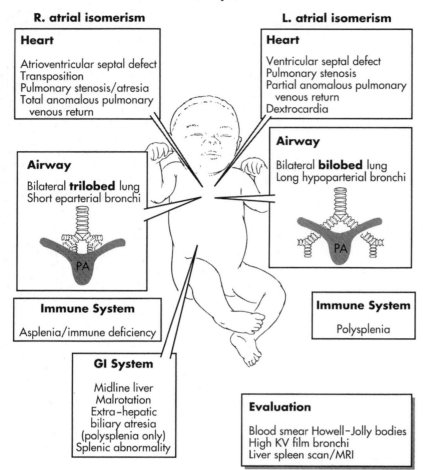

Ivemark Syndrome

R. atrial isomerism

Heart

Atrioventricular septal defect
Transposition
Pulmonary stenosis/atresia
Total anomalous pulmonary
    venous return

Airway

Bilateral **trilobed** lung
Short eparterial bronchi

Immune System

Asplenia/immune deficiency

GI System

Midline liver
Malrotation
Extra-hepatic
biliary atresia
(polysplenia only)
Splenic abnormality

L. atrial isomerism

Heart

Ventricular septal defect
Pulmonary stenosis
Partial anomalous pulmonary
    venous return
Dextrocardia

Airway

Bilateral **bilobed** lung
Long hypoparterial bronchi

Immune System

Polysplenia

Evaluation

Blood smear Howell-Jolly bodies
High KV film bronchi
Liver spleen scan/MRI

FIGURE 46-4   Associated defects of Heterotaxy/Ivemark syndrome.

Patients with asplenia characteristically have bilaterally trilobed lungs; the bronchi are bilaterally eparterial (i.e., posterior and superior to the right pulmonary artery). The term *bilateral right-sidedness* or *right atrial isomerism* is sometimes used as a mnemonic. By contrast, in polysplenia, both the right and left lungs are bilobed; both bronchi are hyparterial (i.e., anterior and inferior to the left pulmonary artery). The term *bilateral left-sidedness* or *left atrial isomerism* is often used.

In both asplenia and polysplenia, varying degrees of visceral heterotaxy may occur.[122,160,164] The normal visceral asymmetry is lacking; thus the liver frequently has two lobes of equal size, the stomach may be midline or on the opposite side of the body from the cardiac apex, and intestinal malrotation may occur. In 1954, Ivemark[158] tabulated the cardiac findings in 69 cases of congenital splenic anomalies, and many subsequent reviews have appeared.[204,206,209]

Prevalence and Etiologic Concepts

The heterotaxy syndromes account for between 2% and 3% of neonates first seen with critical heart disease. Although clinically most cases appear to be sporadic, familial clustering has long been recognized.[174] Recent human genetic studies and animal models[219] have implicated several genes in the development of normal laterality or asymmetry. Mutations and

submicroscopic deletions of *ZIC3*, an X-linked zinc-finger transcription factor, were found to cause laterality defects in both familial and sporadic cases.[72]

In the human embryo, the development of the spleen, growth of the endocardial cushions, lobation of the lungs, and connections between the left atrium and pulmonary venous plexus all occur between days 28 and 35 of gestation. In heterotaxy, all the defects arise early in development.[158] Opitz[149] suggested that the syndromes should be classified as the polyasplenia development field complex. Other etiologic mechanisms have been proposed.[24,90,164]

Pathology: The Nature of the Cardiac, Visceral and Vascular Anomalies in Heterotaxy Syndromes

Of 109 postmortem patients with visceral heterotaxy and congenital heart disease reported from the Boston Children's Hospital, 53% had asplenia, 42% had polysplenia, and 5% had an abnormally situated, morphologically normal spleen.[208] In the presence of heterotaxy, the best method of defining atrial situs has been the source of controversy. Many of these controversies are discussed and illustrated in Chapter 1 of this book.

Asplenia

Intracardiac defects are complex and severe,[158] including AV and ventriculoarterial relations. The most consistent finding is a complete AV canal defect with double-outlet right ventricle, transposition of the great arteries, pulmonary outflow atresia or severe stenosis, or a combination of these.

A complete AV canal defect with a common atrium occurs in 95% of patients. Severe malalignment of the AV valve often is associated with severe hypoplasia of the ventricle not receiving the AV valve. The ventriculoarterial relation is virtually always discordant.[204] Van Praagh and associates[209] noted the frequent association of unroofed coronary sinus with AV canal defects, adding to the "linkages" of intracardiac defects in asplenia noted by Ivemark. Bilateral sinus nodes and AV nodes are frequent, sometimes with a sling of conduction tissue between the two AV nodes.

Venous anomalies may affect both systemic and pulmonary veins. Bilateral superior venae cavae are the rule; when the persistent left superior vena cava drains into an unroofed coronary sinus, a posterior ASD is present, leading to a left-to-right atrial shunt. The inferior vena cava (IVC) usually drains normally into the primitive "right" atrium; however, in about one in four patients, the hepatic veins on the contralateral side drain directly into the atrium, often connecting to an unroofed coronary sinus.

Extracardiac obstructed total anomalous pulmonary venous drainage, either infradiaphragmatic or to a left vertical vein, is not infrequent and, in the past, was associated with a poor prognosis.

Visceral anomalies include a bilobed liver with equal-size lobes and often discordance between the situs of the stomach and the cardiac apex. The most common pulmonary pattern is that of bilaterally trilobed lungs with eparterial bronchi.

Polysplenia

The *intracardiac defects* in live-born infants tend to be less severe than those in asplenia. However, a recent study of heterotaxy detected in utero suggested that in fetal life, the cardiac anatomy is similar, perhaps indicating differences in fetal mortality in the two groups. In polysplenia, although one or both of the AV valves may be abnormal, the most frequent finding is a VSD with mild or moderate pulmonic stenosis. ASDs are frequent. In two thirds of infants, a concordant ventriculoarterial relation is found, with the remainder having a double-outlet right ventricle. With double-outlet right ventricle, frequently subpulmonary but no subaortic conus is noted. The sinus node is hypoplastic and abnormally located. With D-looped ventricles (70%), the AV node is solitary; in the inverted L-looped ventricle, often a pair of AV nodes is found.

Venous anomalies are frequent but differ from those in asplenia. The IVC is frequently (~80%) interrupted; a dilated azygous venous system provides a continuance of venous drainage from below the diaphragm to a superior vena cava.[156]

The drainage of the pulmonary veins is often ipsilateral, with those from the right lung entering the anatomic right atrium, whereas the two left pulmonary veins drain normally into the left atrium. This characteristic divided drainage has

Table 46-3 Anomalies in Heterotaxy Syndrome

Asplenia	Polysplenia
Common atrioventricular canal (85%) with double-outlet right ventricle, transposed great arteries, and pulmonic outflow atresia or extreme stenosis	Ventricular septal defect with pulmonic stenosis. Normal great arteries or DORV without subaortic conus
IVC intact: frequent anomalous drainage hepatic vein	IVC interruption with azygos drainage
SVC bilateral, unroofed coronary sinus	SVC may be bilateral
Pulmonary veins often drain into systemic vein, obstructed	Pulmonary venous drainage divided RPV to RA, LPV to LA
Lungs: bilateral trilobed	Lungs: bilateral bilobed
Liver: symmetrical	Liver: symmetrical or normally lobulated: risk of extrahepatic biliary atresia
Viscera: heterotaxy with risk of obstruction due to malrotation	Viscera: heterotaxy with risk of obstruction due to malrotation

This table summarizes the most frequently encountered anomalies, recognizing that a frequent overlap occurs in the cardiosplenic variants.[6]
DORV, double-outlet right ventricle; IVC and SVC, inferior and superior vena cavae; RPV and LPV, right and left pulmonary veins; RA and LA, right and left atria.

been attributed to hypoplasia or aplasia of the septum secundum, causing displacement of the septum primum.

Visceral anomalies affect the lungs and abdominal organs. Both lungs are characteristically bilobed and have hyparterial bronchi. Although less abdominal symmetry is seen than in asplenia (the major part of the liver is to one side, and the stomach is rarely in the midline), intestinal malrotation, absence of the gallbladder, and extrahepatic biliary atresia may be found. Splenic tissue is usually attached to the greater curvature of the stomach, often resembling the pattern of a cluster of small grapes.[156,172] Some of the characteristic findings in asplenia and polysplenia are summarized in Table 46-3.

Relevance of Heterotaxy Syndromes in the Intensive Care Setting

The complex nature of the cardiac defect[174,204] in many of these infants results in single-ventricle management and requires multiple operations. For example, an infant with asplenia, AV canal defect, pulmonary atresia, and total anomalous pulmonary venous drainage will require a neonatal operation to correct the pulmonary venous anomalies, and generally, placement of a systemic-to-pulmonary arterial shunt to provide pulmonary blood flow. Usually two subsequent procedures are needed, the last a Fontan operation variant.

Some infants with polysplenia can have a biventricular cardiac repair at one operation. However, those who have intestinal malrotation or extrahepatic biliary atresia will need both cardiac and extracardiac operations. Thus although heterotaxy is rare, the intensivist may see the syndrome disproportionately often.

Clinical Presentation

Patients with asplenia are predominantly male infants. They often have pulmonary outflow tract obstruction without significant aortopulmonary collaterals, and thus are cyanotic at presentation. If the obstruction is severe, pulmonary perfusion is ductal dependent. With the onset of ductal closure, profound cyanosis, metabolic acidosis, and ultimately cardiovascular collapse develop. With dextrocardia, the point of maximal impulse and site of best auscultation may be over the right hemithorax. A harsh systolic murmur is found in the setting of pulmonic stenosis; a continuous murmur is found in the setting of pulmonic atresia. A palpable midline liver may be appreciated.

The heart disease associated with the polysplenia is much more variable. In general, these infants initially are seen with a cardiac murmur, symptoms of congestive heart failure, or heart disease may be suspected because of visceral heterotaxy. Some children have no cardiac symptoms and may be first seen with associated gastrointestinal abnormalities.

Evaluation

Increasingly often, heterotaxy is recognized on fetal echocardiography, and delivery has been arranged in a center with optimal facilities for immediate cardiac diagnosis and therapy. Echocardiography is the essential tool for accurate evaluation, but roentgenography, the electrocardiogram, and other studies may provide some clues.

The radiographic manifestations of asplenia include a normal cardiac silhouette, oligemic lung fields, and an ectopic gastric bubble. Bilateral short bronchi suggest asplenia (right-sided isomerism). An overpenetrated frontal film may demonstrate bilateral eparterial bronchi,[44] but time spent in obtaining further radiographs is better used in skilled echocardiography. Cardiomegaly is suggestive of AV valve insufficiency. Pulmonary venous congestion is seen in the setting of obstructive pulmonary venous drainage. However, such congestion may not be appreciated on the radiograph, until prostaglandin therapy has reopened the ductus and increased the pulmonary blood flow.

The infant with polysplenia may have an absent IVC shadow on lateral chest radiographs; dilatation of the azygous vein, which accompanies redirection of venous return in the setting of interruption of the vena cava at the level of the liver, may occasionally be detected on the anteroposterior (AP) radiograph.[11,83] The bilateral hyparterial bronchi may be demonstrable on an overpenetrated chest radiograph.

The electrocardiogram in the infant with asplenia may show a P-wave axis of greater than 90 degrees if a single left-sided sinoatrial (SA) node is present[208]; occasionally bilateral sinus or AV nodes can be identified.[46,207] Normal sinus rhythm is usual, and congenital complete heart block, rare. Polysplenia is characterized by a displaced or hypoplastic sinus node and results in a P axis that is leftward and superior.[46,134] In contrast to asplenia, dysrhythmias are commonly seen in infants with polysplenia.[217] In Van Praagh's series,[209] complete heart block was seen in 22%, nodal rhythm in 9%, and coronary sinus rhythm in 7% of polysplenic patients. Fetal bradycardia due to complete heart block may be the presenting finding of polysplenia in the fetus.

Echocardiography can illustrate virtually all of the complex anatomic features that are associated with the heterotaxy syndromes. The abdominal venous anatomy is best seen with subxiphoid views, whereas the location of superior vena cavae on either side can be imaged by using suprasternal or high parasternal views.[87,88,190] The coronary sinus can be seen well in an apical four-chamber view. Pulmonary venous drainage can best be seen by using a suprasternal or high sternal border approach, enhanced by color Doppler flow mapping.[190] The atrial septum and atrial appendages can best be seen by using the subxiphoid and parasternal short-axis views.[13,187] The presence of outflow tract obstruction can be documented by using Doppler flow interrogation from the subxiphoid or apical views.[209]

Cardiac catheterization is usually unnecessary in the newborn, because echocardiography usually delineates the anatomy and physiology. Later, before a Glenn or Fontan procedure, a catheterization is needed, primarily to measure the pulmonary artery pressure and to exclude branch pulmonary artery stenosis.

Other laboratory tests may be useful to assess splenic function in heterotaxy patients. The presence of Howell-Jolly bodies on the peripheral blood smear is strongly suggestive of asplenia or a hypofunctioning spleen[159]; however, they are occasionally present in normal neonates in the first week of life.[21,160] The most widely accepted method for evaluating splenic function and demonstrating splenic malposition or asplenia is radionuclide scanning by using [^{99m}Tc]-sulfur colloid.[195] Radiocolloid scanning may not detect a small hypofunctioning spleen, or a large transverse liver may obscure its splenic image.[152] Current techniques in splenic imaging have recently been summarized.[6,153] Reliable quantitative splenic function may be assessed by using Fc receptor–mediated autologous erythrocyte clearance.[119,201]

Management

A majority of patients with asplenia have pulmonary outflow tract obstruction and are thus dependent on ductal flow to provide pulmonary perfusion. These infants' courses may be further complicated by abnormal and obstructed pulmonary venous drainage. Establishment of a normal and unobstructed pulmonary venous drainage should occur before or at the time of an aortopulmonary shunt procedure.[45] Further surgical management will depend on the exact nature of the congenital heart defects. Pulmonary arteriovenous or intrahepatic shunting may occur postoperatively after cavopulmonary anastomosis,[84] resulting in cyanosis, and requiring further intervention.

Children with congenital asplenia appear to have a greater risk for serious bacterial infections and fatal septicemia than do normal children, a risk that is analogous to that after surgical splenectomy. In a study of 59 children with asplenia, 16 instances of sepsis were documented.[212] Before age 6 months, Escherichia coli and Klebsiella organisms were most common, whereas pneumococcal and Haemophilus influenzae predominated in older children. Patients with polysplenia probably also have immune deficits.

As fatal septicemia may develop after trivial upper respiratory tract infections, these children require vigilant medical attention and aggressive treatment for suspected infections. Antibiotic prophylaxis with amoxicillin is appropriate.[165,212] In a study of eight children with the asplenia syndrome who had survived beyond the second year of life, all had normal serum complement activity, C3, and serum IgG and IgA levels.

However, their response to pneumococcal polysaccharide vaccination was profoundly abnormal. Of seven patients immunized, only three had a twofold increase in antibody response to pneumococcal antigen. Overall, the affected patients had only a 20% antibody response to antigen, as compared with a control group.[14] For this reason, bacterial vaccines should be administered, and antibody responses should be assessed.[14]

Another issue of concern is gastrointestinal malrotation, leading to an increased risk of developing acute obstruction due to volvulus. Prospective evaluation for malrotation with imaging studies is warranted in infants with heterotaxy. If malrotation were present, many would consider treatment with a Ladd procedure.

OTHER CARDIAC SYNDROMES

Prevalence

In some series, approximately one in four children born with a heart defect had some extracardiac anomaly.[57] Ferencz and colleagues[59] reported no noncardiac malformations in 3176 (72.3%) of 4390 of live-born infants with congenital heart defects registered in the Baltimore Washington Infant Study, 1981 to 1989. Chromosomal abnormalities were present in 522 (11.9%) of 4390, and Down syndrome in 385 of 522. Heritable named syndromes were identified in 327 (7.4%) of 4390. The most frequently encountered syndromes were Ivemark, 68; VACTERL, 37; DiGeorge, 30; Noonan, 15; Williams, 14; Goldenhaar, 8; and Holt-Oram, 7. The four relatively "common" syndromes, Down, Ivemark, VACTERL, and DiGeorge, were present in 520 (61%) of 849 of infants with chromosomal and heritable syndromes; the remaining 329 infants had, between them, 11 different chromosomal anomalies and a remarkable total of 50 other syndromes, ranging from Alagille to Werdnig Hoffman.[59]

Syndrome Load

A significant difference exists in the "syndrome load" of different cardiac defects, ranging from around 80% for AV septal defect to around 10% for transposition or pulmonary stenosis.[142] Natowicz and associates[140] found that 23 (28%) of 81 patients with hypoplastic left heart syndrome coming to autopsy over an 11-year period had a genetic disorder or major extracardiac anomaly or both. Thus heart defects can be considered to fall into three groups: (1) "isolated" defects (including complete transposition) with a statistically minor load of extracardiac anomalies; (2) the largest group of defects, including hypoplastic left heart or membranous VSD, with additional extracardiac anomalies present between 20% and 30% of the time; and (3) cardiac malformations such as the complete form of AV septal defect, which rarely occur in isolation, but more than 50% of the time form part of a major syndrome, such as Down or Ivemark syndrome.

The concept of syndromes is constantly changing with advances in understanding of pathogenetic mechanisms in cardiac development and with more sophisticated biochemical and genetic studies.[128] Some syndromes may be "hidden"; that is, the child may have no obvious dysmorphism or noncardiac problem, but have some biochemical marker indicative of a forme fruste of DiGeorge or other syndrome.[70] In the next few years, the classification of cardiac syndromes will be both expanded and simplified. The syndromes listed later include a number of that may be encountered in an intensive care setting. Although far from complete, it is intended to give a brief description of some of the more common associations. An excellent more detailed discussion is provided by Burn.[19]

Additional Cardiac Syndromes

ALAGILLE: OMIM 118450 (arteriohepatic dysplasia). Intrahepatic biliary cirrhosis, dysmorphic facies, and vertebral anomalies: *peripheral pulmonary stenosis.* Genetics: mutation of *JAG* gene located at chromosome 10p12. Often autosomal dominant (AD).[137]

BECKWITH WIEDEMANN: OMIM 130650 (Also EMG, *Exomphalos macroglossia gigantism*), hepatomegaly, hypoglycemia, risk of Wilms' tumor: *hypertrophic cardiomyopathy.* Genetics: mutation of *K1P2* gene located at chromosome 11p15.5. Complex inheritance, some AD with balanced translocation.

CHARGE: OMIM 214800. Eye anomaly (Coloboma), the Heart defect usually *VSD or tetralogy of Fallot,* (choanal Atresia), a kidney (Renal) Genital abnormality with cup-shaped Ear, and deafness. Cause unknown, approximately 8% familial.[42,128]

DIGEORGE: OMIM 188840 (DGS; see text under chromosome 22q11.2 deletion syndromes).

DOWN (TRISOMY 21): OMIM 190685 (see text). Genetics: trisomy of chromosome 21, including a specific cardiac region 21q22.

EHLERS DANLOS: OMIM (type I) 130000. A heritable disorder of connective tissue with hyperextensible skin and joints, and easy bruising. *Mitral valve prolapse* most usual. Genetics usually autosomal recessive (AR), but many variants.

ELLIS VAN CREVELD: OMIM 225500. Dwarfism with polydactyly, abnormal cartilage (chondroectodermal dysplasia). *Single atrium,* an incomplete form of AV septal defect. Genetics: mutation of gene located at chromosome 4p16. Usually AR: clusters noted among Amish communities. Growth remains impaired after cardiac repair.[118,173]

FETAL ALCOHOL: Facial dysmorphism, mental retardation, short fingers. A variety of heart defects with *VSDs and ASDs* being most common.[157]

FANCONI ANEMIA TYPE I: OMIM 227650. Rare hematologic syndrome, with difficulty in chromosome repair: hypoplastic thumbs, often a brownish discoloration of the skin: *patent ductus, VSD.* Genetics: a mutation of gene at chromosome 16q24.3.

GOLDENHAR: unilateral facial microsomia, microtia, preotic skin tag, and coloboma of the eye. Heart defects are present in one third of children and may include *tetralogy of Fallot.* Now included as one form of oculoauricular vertebral syndrome (OAV). Genetics probably AD, may be "sporadic."[170,171,176]

HOLT-ORAM: OMIM 142900. Although originally described as an AD syndrome with absent thumb and an ASD, considerable phenotypic heterogeneity exists, with "digitalized" (finger-like) thumb or rarely phocomelia. Cardiac defects variable, usually involve septation, *ASD most frequent.*[188] Genetics: mutation of the *TBX5* gene at chromosome 12q24, usually AD.[8]

HYPERTROPHIC CARDIOMYOPATHY: OMIM 192600 and other. When without extracardiac defects, genetics may be due to mutations in a number of sarcomeric genes[180] with AD inheritance. Infantile hypertrophic cardiomyopathy may have multiple etiologies, including Noonan, mitochondrial disorder with lactic acidosis,[32] and metabolic disease.

IVEMARK: OMIM 208530. See text under Heterotaxy Syndrome; a useful inclusive term for disorders of cardiac looping with visceral heterotaxy and congenital cardiosplenic anomalies. Genetics AR, AD, and X-linked, all with variable penetrance.

KARTAGENER: OMIM 244400, originally described as dextrocardia with situs inversus and bronchiectasis. Now used for syndrome of ciliary dyskinesia, with sinusitis and frequent male infertility. *Dextrocardia* of "mirror image" type, without other heart defects, frequent. Genetics AR, and both Ivemark and Kartagener have occurred in some families.

LEOPARD: *L*entigenes, *E*CG abnormalities, *O*cular change (hypertelorism), *P*ulmonary stenosis, *A*bnormal genital organs, *R*etardation, and *D*eafness. May be closely related to neurofibromatosis and may overlap with Noonan.

LONG-QT: OMIM 192500 and others. In the intensive care unit environment, prolonged QTc may be seen transiently in metabolic derangements or with neurologic damage. When persistent, it may be familial and associated with severe arrhythmias (*ventricular tachycardia* or fibrillation) on stress or exercise. Genetics: mutations in genes encoding cardiac potassium channels (chromosome 11 and chromosome 7), and a cardiac sodium channel (chromosome 3).[121]

MARFAN: see Chapter 47, "Heritable Heart Disease as Part of Multisystem Illness"

MUCOPOLYSACCHARIDOSIS: see Chapter 47

MUSCULAR DYSTROPHY: OMIM 310200 Duchenne type. Progressive muscular weakness often complicated by *cardiomyopathy.*[22,63] Genetics: mutation in the dystrophin gene located at chromosome Xq22. Sex-linked recessive.

NOONAN-EHMKE: OMIM 163950, see text.

OCULOAURICULAR VERTEBRAL (OAV): see Goldenhar.

OSTEOGENESIS IMPERFECTA: OMIM 166210 type I. Multiple fractures: *mitral prolapse*, aortic root dilatation with *aortic insufficiency*. Several genetic types, type I with blue sclerae, AD.[85]

POMPE: OMIM 232300. Most severe of the many forms of glycogen storage disease due to inherited deficiency in acid 1,4 glucosidase (acid maltase). *Cardiomyopathy with short PR interval.* Genetics, AR.[92]

RUBELLA: Congenital deafness, cataracts, and sometimes mental retardation and microcephaly may follow maternal rubella in early pregnancy. Cardiac sequelae usually *patent ductus and pulmonary arterial stenosis.* An example of a preventable "environmental" syndrome.[157]

SCIMITAR: Varying degrees of hypoplasia of the right lung and pulmonary artery: most or all of the right pulmonary veins drain into IVC, forming a "scimitar"-shaped shadow on chest radiograph. In severe infant form, right lung has systemic arterial supply from descending aorta. Occasionally familial.[52,144]

SHPRINTZEN: OMIM 192430. Velocardiofacial syndrome (VCFS): see text under chromosome 22q11.2 deletion syndromes.

SMITH-LEMLI-OPITZ: OMIM 270400. Mental retardation, microcephaly, skeletal anomalies, varying cardiac defects including *atrial and ventricular defects and tetralogy.* Genetics: mutation in the sterol delta7-reductase gene at chromosome at 11q12-q13 with AR inheritance.[101,213]

TAR (*thrombocytopenia absent radius*): OMIM 274000. Varying severity of limb defect and platelet deficiency. *ASD or tetralogy of Fallot.* Genetics, AR.[79]

TRISOMY 13 (*Patau*): Polydactyly, cleft lip and palate, holoprosencephaly. *ASD, VSD, cardiac positional anomalies.* Chromosomal anomaly, approximately 1 in 7000 births.[19,169]

TRISOMY 18 (*Edwards*): Multiple anomalies including clenched fists, rocker-bottom feet, micrognathia, severe retardation. *VSD, specific polyvalvar thickening.*[19]

TURNER (45XO): Ovarian agenesis, neck webbing, short stature. Cardiac defects in about 20%, usually left heart flow, varying from *hypoplastic left heart syndrome, coarctation, and/or bicommissural aortic valve.*[140]

VACTERL: OMIM 276950. *V*ertebral *A*nal *C*ardiac *T*racheo-esophageal *R*enal and *L*imb abnormalities. Heart defect varies, usually *VSD*, sometimes *tetralogy of Fallot.* Sporadic, sometimes seen with maternal diabetes. Attributed to disruption of blastogenesis.[37,102]

WILLIAMS: OMIM 194050. Irritability and slow growth in infancy, with elfin facies and sometimes documented hypercalcemia; older children show thicker features, varying mental retardation, abnormal dentition; *supravalvar aortic and pulmonary stenosis.* Genetics: A contiguous gene syndrome with hemizygosity at chromosome 7q11.2 including the elastin locus. Nonsyndromic familial supravalvar aortic stenosis also involves deletion of one elastin allele.[55,56]

ETHICAL CONSIDERATIONS

Child-Parent-Healthcare Team Triad

Ethics and cardiology are inseparable. When an infant or child with a heart problem needs intensive care, decisions involving life and death or possible long-term morbidity are made on a daily, even hourly basis. By necessity, these decisions are being made by surrogates, the family (or legal guardian) and the healthcare team, not by the child. We have referred elsewhere to this triangular relationship of child, family, and healthcare team as the "triangle of understanding."[143] Ethical issues are involved when a decision is made regarding the best site for care in a child with a complex heart problem: should care be local and convenient for the family, or does transfer to a regional center with specialized experience in that particular defect offer significant benefit to the child, always the apex of the triangle of understanding? It is an error to infer that ethical issues arise for discussion only when a disorder is in its terminal stages, or when a syndrome is present. Ethical considerations are always with us, as in Fost's memorable phrase "Ethics, ethics everywhere,"[65] even though less often discussed by cardiac teams than could be wished.

In this brief section, we describe an infant recently encountered in our pediatric ICU (PICU) setting and review some of the ethical considerations. These considerations are affected, not only by the rapid advances in technology, making previously lethal conditions treatable, but also by new genetic information and by rapid societal change.[10,28,39,220]

Illustrative Case

A young married woman, Mrs. M., had routine obstetrical ultrasound imaging at 18 weeks. Previous obstetrical history was significant for two previous uncomplicated pregnancies.

The prenatal sonogram documented multiple congenital anomalies, including microcephaly and hydrocephalus, bilateral shortened arms, and congenital heart disease. The couple declined amniocentesis. Despite the high potential for in utero fetal death, they wished to maintain the pregnancy. The next several sonograms showed poor fetal growth.

Mrs. M. arrived at the labor and delivery suite at 39 weeks for elective induction and delivery. A viable baby girl weighing 1.6 kg was delivered without difficulty: The Apgar scores were 6 and 8. The infant was transferred to the NICU for further evaluation. After multiple consultations, it was confirmed that she had complex congenital heart disease with microcephaly, hydrocephalus, imperforate anus, limb and vertebral anomalies, diffuse tracheomalacia, and renal anomalies. Chromosomes were 46 XX. A diagnosis of VACTERL syndrome was made. On the first day of life, the infant required intubation and mechanical ventilation.

Family meetings were arranged to review and discuss the infant's status. Based on examination and magnetic resonance imaging (MRI) scans, pediatric neurology anticipated that Baby M would be severely impaired, cognitively and physically, and partially blind and deaf. Bronchoscopic findings of severe diffuse tracheomalacia led pediatric pulmonologists to conclude that long-term mechanical ventilation would most likely be needed. Pediatric cardiologists predicted that surgery to repair the infant's complex heart defect was possible, but the current weight of 1.6 kg was a complicating factor. Pediatric orthopedic specialists, after reviewing the arm anomalies, concluded that future surgical intervention might be able to make the arms functional. Despite the poor overall prognosis and recommendations of the medical team not to intervene, the family wished to proceed with the multiple palliative and corrective surgeries.

Current Concepts

This infant presented a dilemma, which allows a chance to review some of the concepts now being brought to bear on pediatric ethical dilemmas in general. Landwirth,[111] in discussing pediatric and neonatal resuscitation, emphasized the unique nature of pediatrics, including the standing of the parents as surrogate decision makers. Others have stressed that in caring for the critically ill infant, three long-term issues must be considered: benefit to the child, the parents, and society as a whole. Some of the concepts currently under active discussion are those of beneficence, societal good, quality of life years, and patient autonomy. How can these concepts be applied to the difficult problem of Baby M? If the family and healthcare team disagree, what help is available to bring about consensus?

Although each of us tries to bring both reason and moral thinking to these discussions, we are each influenced by our prior experiences, whether of an infant once deemed unsalvageable who grew to give happiness to all his family, or of some child who, after many years of care and support, died tragically after prolonged suffering.

Beneficence

Beneficence, and its corollary, lack of maleficence, is clearly a paramount concept. In simple terms, the infant should receive treatment focused on ensuring or restoring an active happy life, with the minimum of pain and distress involved in the treatment.[26,210] The pediatrician, in considering beneficence, has to imagine how he or she would wish to be treated if in the infant's place.[35] Achieving such a goal is very difficult in an infant like Baby M with a complex cardiac problem and many extracardiac anomalies. For example, often lack of knowledge of the true prognosis exists; less often, controversy occurs over the certainty and accuracy of the various diagnoses.

Most physicians would not find it beneficent to submit an infant to several cardiac operations, multiple invasive procedures, and 6 months in intensive care on ventilator support, if the outcome for that particular condition were known to be uniformly fatal by age 1 year. However, in the real world, the knowledge database is very rarely that conclusive. For example, although most infants with trisomy 18 and heart disease die very early, between 5% and 10% live for more than a year, and no certain way is known at present of identifying the potential survivors.[25] Some parents of such an infant, even when informed of the poor prognosis for intellectual development, do not feel justified in withholding cardiac or other surgical care. Room exists for much honest disagreement on the optimal course to pursue, but it is essential that the parents and healthcare team have the best available facts and be able to participate knowledgeably in the decision.

Societal Good

Societal good is clearly achieved by the restoration to health of a child with coarctation of the aorta or tetralogy of Fallot, who can be expected to reach adult life and become a full member of society; indeed, although this is often not mentioned, society benefits in uncounted ways from the joy and activity of a healthy growing child. However, when an infant such as Baby M has severe multisystem involvement with anticipated mental retardation of uncertain degree, the picture is intuitively less clear. A wide philosophic gulf stretches between those who think societal good means raising a child who will be a wage earner and those who think society benefits from seeing and helping the handicapped. Sometimes, as may have happened with Baby M, the family's religious or ethical beliefs hold that the sanctity of individual life transcends all other considerations. The healthcare team always must consider societal good, but in a broad context.

Quality of Life Years (QALYs)

Quality of Life Years (QALYs) is a concept now discussed in medical ethics and also increasingly in medical economics. For the critically ill infant with successfully repaired coarctation of the aorta and no other anomalies, it is reasonable to estimate a future normal life expectancy of more than 70 years with an excellent quality of life. (The World Health Organization [WHO] program of vitamin A supplementation in the prevention of childhood blindness provides an even more dramatic example of low-cost QALY gained, with an estimated cost of 20 cents for each year of life with normal sight.) Any calculations of this kind are precarious in Baby M, because of uncertainties surrounding the duration of time on ventilator support and the ultimate neurologic and cognitive outcome. Again, individual philosophic variations exist as to the definition of quality of life. Individual lives vary in intensity, duration, and beauty, and each can have its own essential value. Some authors use the term "slippery slope" to express the dangers of being judgmental and derogatory about the quality of life of others.

Autonomy

Autonomy implies the importance of the individual in making his or her own life decisions. Respect for individual autonomy, implying the need for truly informed consent, is a concept increasingly accepted for both adults and children. Vicarious decisions must necessarily be made for infants such as Baby M, who are not yet autonomous, but are completely dependent on others for care, love, and decisions. In intensive care settings, the triangle of understanding may become complex, particularly if care is prolonged. Instead of one physician, a healthcare team is present, whose chief may change on a weekly or other timed basis; the ICU nurse and cardiac nurse specialist often provide most of the vital sense of continuity. Instead of two involved parents, there may be a single teenage mother, often accompanied by varying family members with differing philosophies; or the parents may already be separated or divorced, each accompanied by a new partner. When confronted with the question of whose autonomy should be most considered, that of the healthcare team or the family, it can be helpful to remember that the family will be the long-term caregivers.

Informed Consent

Informed consent is integral to respect for the patient's or family's autonomy: in the absence of good knowledge of the medical facts and the probable prognosis, they cannot act autonomously. Some of the recent public discussions of informed consent have involved gene therapy and other major advances involving the revolutionary upsurge in genetic knowledge.[64,75]

Other concepts discussed in the fast-growing literature on medical ethics concern futility and wrongful life. The *concept of futility* implies that treatment may be discontinued or withheld if efforts to prolong life will be futile or result in a meaningless existence. Decisions involving this concept are made almost daily in active intensive care settings in the presence of irreversible brain damage from various causes. Like most ethical concepts, this one is easier in the more extreme situations. Now generally accepted objective criteria are known

for a diagnosis of brain death. The presence of profound irreversible brain injury may be more difficult to determine with certainty. When doubt exists as to how long life may be prolonged, or the implications of a cardiac syndrome for a "meaningful" life, unanimity may be hard to achieve.

Bringing Ethical Concepts to the Bedside, or How Can These Concepts Be Applied to Baby M and Others with Severe Syndromes?

First, the healthcare team, in helping the child and family, must avoid being overly directive. Although the team has an obligation to share with the family their medical and scientific knowledge of the child's status and prognosis, they must separate the facts from their own individual feelings and beliefs. Some of us believe that it also is important to share at least some of one's uncertainties: For example, with Baby M, the degree of sight and hearing loss can probably be established with accuracy, but the cognitive function and needs for ventilator support are less predictable.

The forceful projection of medical beliefs on others is often described as "paternalism," although little evidence exists that the pattern is entirely confined to male physicians. Conversely, it is almost impossible, if even supposing it to be desirable, to counsel without conveying some sense of one's own stance. Each member of the healthcare team must know and examine his or her own ethical and moral viewpoint. This helps in the control of bias and provides assurance in the decision-making process. The increasing use of formal teaching on ethics and moral reasoning in medical and nursing schools is a major advance, one that will help future generations caring for the critically ill cardiac child.[47] Every physician, nurse, and healthcare team member involved in critical care knows how difficult the concept of beneficence can be in practice.

Second, if possible, the healthcare team should develop a consensus, so that the family's great and overwhelming sense of grief, loss, and uncertainty should not be further exacerbated by conflicting opinions and prognoses. Divisions among the healthcare team tend to arise most often in three critical situations: (1) the medical *facts* are unknown or in dispute; a consensus can be built only on what all know to be the truth; (2) the concept of *meaningful life* cannot be agreed on for the individual child; and (3) the moral, ethical, and philosophic *viewpoints* of the team and family either are unknown, at variance, or have not yet been properly discussed. After the medical facts are known with clarity, a consensus must be established. This involves much time and empathy. Discussion with an ethics committee[218] may clarify the facts and cool some of the heated dialogue. All the team members may be helped to realize that pediatrics, usually such a joyful field, may sometimes present severe ethical dilemmas.

It is very helpful to have seen older children and even adults who have survived long and arduous times in intensive care and are now leading healthy lives. The perspective of future possibilities is daily involved in the ethics of critical care. The child is and must remain the focus, the apex of the triangle of understanding.

Some of the ethical dilemmas faced today arise from technologic advances; some have always existed. The ethical challenge in an intensive care setting lies in providing skilled, compassionate, thoughtful, and well-informed care and information to the critically ill child and family. In most infants with heart defects and syndromes, societal good and many excellent individual QALYs can be achieved if the concepts of beneficence and autonomy accompany skilled and loving care. Even on the rare occasions when the goal of treatment and the assurance of a normal life fail, skilled care accompanied by compassion, love, and grace still avails much. The suffering of the child, the family, and the caregivers is, to some degree, allayed by ethical treatment. Each person reading this chapter should consider how he or she would have advised the family of Baby M, or how an ethics committee consultation could bring light and consensus. Caring for the heart of a child remains forever inseparable from ethics.

References

1. Ahmed ML, Foot AB, Edge JA, et al: Noonan's syndrome: Abnormalities of the growth hormone/IGF-I axis and the response to treatment with human biosynthetic growth hormone. *Acta Paediatr Scand* 80:446–450, 1991.
2. Allanson JE, Hall JG, Hughes HE, et al: Noonan syndrome: The changing phenotype. *Am J Med Genet* 21:507–514, 1995.
3. Amann G, Sherman FS: Myocardial dysgenesis with persistent sinusoids in a neonate with Noonan's phenotype. *Pediatr Pathol* 12:83–92, 1992.
4. American Academy of pediatrics Committee on Genetics: Health supervision for children with Down syndrome. *Pediatrics* 93:855–859, 1994.
5. Antonelli D, Antonelli J, Rosenfeld T: Noonan's syndrome associated with hypoplastic left heart. *Cardiology* 77:62–65, 1990.
6. Applegate KE, Goske MJ, Pierce G, Murphy D: Situs revisited: Imaging of the heterotaxy syndrome. *Radiographics* 19:837–852; discussion 853–854, 1990.
7. Arenson EB Jr, Forde MD: Bone marrow transplantation for acute leukemia and Down syndrome: Report of a successful case and results of a national survey. *J Pediatr* 114:69–72, 1989.
8. Basson CT, Bachinsky DR, Lin RC, et al: Mutations in human TBX5 cause limb and cardiac malformation in Holt-Oram syndrome. *Nat Genet* 15:30–35, 1997.
9. Batstone PJ, Faed MJ, Jung RT, Gosden J: 45,X/46,X dic (Y) mosaicism in a phenotypic male. *Arch Dis Child* 66:252–253, 1991.
10. Beller FK, Zlatnik GP: The beginning of human life: Medical observations and ethical reflections. *Clin Obstet Gynecol* 35:720–728, 1992.
11. Berdon WE, Baker DH: Plain film findings in azygos continuation of the inferior vena cava. *AJR Am J Roentgenol Radium Ther Nucl Med* 104:452–457, 1968.
12. Bernier-Buzzanga J, Su WP: Noonan's syndrome with extensive verrucae. *Cutis* 46:242–246, 1990.
13. Bierman FZ, Williams RG: Subxiphoid two-dimensional imaging of the interatrial septum in infants and neonates with congenital heart disease. *Circulation* 60:80–90, 1979.
14. Biggar WD, Ramirez RA, Rose V: Congenital asplenia: Immunologic assessment and a clinical review of eight surviving patients. *Pediatrics* 67:548–551, 1981.
15. Binder M: The teratogenic effects of a bis-dichloroacetyl-diamine on hamster embryos: Aortic arch anomalies and the pathogenesis of the DiGeorge syndrome. *Am J Pathol* 118:179–193, 1985.
16. Brewster SF, Kennedy RH, Smith PJ: A male pseudohermaphrodite with Noonan's syndrome. *Br J Urol* 69:96–97, 1992.
17. Bristow JD, Bernstein HS: Counseling families with chromosome 22q11 deletions: The catch in CATCH-22. *J Am Coll Cardiol* 32:499–501, 1998.
18. Brown PM, Lewis GT, Parker AJ, Maw AR: The skull base and nasopharynx in Down's syndrome in relation to hearing impairment. *Clin Otolaryngol* 14:241–246, 1989.
19. Burn J: The aetiology of congenital heart disease. In Anderson RH, Macartney FJ, Shinebourne EA, et al (eds): *Paediatric Cardiology.* Edinburgh, Churchill Livingstone, 1987, pp 15–63.
20. Burn J: Closing time for CATCH-22. *J Med Genet* 36:737–738, 1999.
21. Bush JA, Ainger LE: Congenital absence of spleen with congenital heart disease: Report of a case with antemortem diagnosis on the basis of hematologic morphology. *Pediatrics* 15:93, 1955.
22. Bushby KM: Recent advances in understanding muscular dystrophy. *Arch Dis Child* 67:1310–1312, 1992.
23. Campbell AM, Bousfield JD: Anaesthesia in a patient with Noonan's syndrome and cardiomyopathy. *Anaesthesia* 47:131–133, 1992.
24. Campbell M, Deuchar DC: Absent inferior vena cava, symmetrical liver, splenic agenesis, and situs inversus, and their embryology. *Br Heart J* 29:268–275, 1967.
25. Carey JC: Health supervision and anticipatory guidance for children with genetic disorders (including specific recommendations for trisomy 21, trisomy 18, and neurofibromatosis I). *Pediatr Clin North Am* 39:25–53, 1992.
26. Cassidy R, Fleishman A: *Pediatric Ethics: From Principles to Practice.* Amsterdam, Harwood, 1996.
27. Chaimovitz C, Abinader E, Benderly A, Better OS: Hypocalcemic hypotension. *JAMA* 222:86–87, 1972.
28. Chang AC: Pediatric cardiac intensive care: Current state of the art and beyond the millennium. *Curr Opin Pediatr* 12:238–246, 2000.
29. Chen SC, deMello D: Growth and development of lungs in siblings with nonimmune hydrops. *Chest* 97:1255–1257, 1990.
30. Clapp S, Perry BL, Farooki ZQ, et al: Down's syndrome, complete atrioventricular canal, and pulmonary vascular obstructive disease. *J Thorac Cardiovasc Surg* 100:115–121, 1990.
31. Clark EB, Takao A: Overview: A focus for research in cardiovascular development. In Clark EB, Takao A (eds): *Developmental Cardiology: Morphogenesis and Function.* New York, Futura, 1990, pp 3–12.
32. Clarke LA: Mitochondrial disorders in pediatrics: Clinical, biochemical, and genetic implications. *Pediatr Clin North Am* 39:319–334, 1992.
33. Cohen MM Jr, Gorlin RJ: Noonan-like/multiple giant cell lesion syndrome. *Am J Med Genet* 40:159–166, 1991.
34. Cohen WI: Atlantoaxial instability: What's next? *Arch Pediatr Adolesc Med* 152:119–122, 1998.
35. Cooke RE: Ethics in pediatric research. *Pediatr Res* 47:542, 2000.
36. Cooley WC, Graham JM Jr: Down syndrome: An update and review for the primary pediatrician. *Clin Pediatr (Phila)* 30:233–253, 1991.
37. Corsello G, Maresi E, Corrao AM, et al: VATER/VACTERL association: Clinical variability and expanding phenotype including laryngeal stenosis. *Am J Med Genet* 44:813–815, 1992.
38. Cremers CW, van der Burgt CJ: Hearing loss in Noonan syndrome. *Int J Pediatr Otorhinolaryngol* 23:81–84, 1992.
39. Cullen S, Sharland GK, Allan LD, Sullivan ID: Potential impact of population screening for prenatal diagnosis of congenital heart disease. *Arch Dis Child* 67:775–778, 1992.
40. Cuneo BF, Driscoll DA, Gidding SS, Langman CB: Evolution of latent hypoparathyroidism in familial 22q11 deletion syndrome. *Am J Med Genet* 69:50–55, 1997.
41. Cuneo BF, Langman CB, Ilbawi MN, et al: Latent hypoparathyroidism in children with conotruncal cardiac defects. *Circulation* 93:1702–1708, 1996.
42. Cyran SE, Martinez R, Daniels S, et al: Spectrum of congenital heart disease in CHARGE association. *J Pediatr* 110:576–578, 1987.
43. de la Chapelle A, Herva R, Koivisto M, Aula P: A deletion in chromosome 22 can cause DiGeorge syndrome. *Hum Genet* 57:253–256, 1981.
44. Deanfield JE, Leanage R, Stroobant J, et al: Use of high kilovoltage filtered beam radiographs for detection of bronchial situs in infants and young children. *Br Heart J* 44:577–583, 1980.
45. DeLeon SY, Gidding SS, Ilbawi MN, et al: Surgical management of infants with complex cardiac anomalies associated with reduced pulmonary blood flow and total anomalous pulmonary venous drainage. *Ann Thorac Surg* 43:207–211, 1987.
46. Dickinson DF, Wilkinson JL, Anderson KR, et al: The cardiac conduction system in situs ambiguus. *Circulation* 59:879–885, 1979.
47. Diekema DS, Shugerman RP: An ethics curriculum for the pediatric residency program: Confronting barriers to implementation. *Arch Pediatr Adolesc Med* 151:609–614, 1997.
48. DiGeorge A: Congenital absence of the thymus and its immunologic consequences: Concurrence with congenital hypoparathyroidism. In Bersma D (ed): *Immunologic Deficiency Diseases in Man.* Vol IV. White Plains, NY, March of Dimes-Birth Defects Foundation, 1968, pp 116–121.
49. Donnenfeld AE, Nazir MA, Sindoni F, Librizzi RJ: Prenatal sonographic documentation of cystic hygroma regression in Noonan syndrome. *Am J Med Genet* 39:461–465, 1991.
50. Driscoll DA, Salvin J, Sellinger B, et al: Prevalence of 22q11 microdeletions in DiGeorge and velocardiofacial syndromes: Implications for genetic counselling and prenatal diagnosis. *J Med Genet* 30:813–817, 1993.

51. Duncan WJ, Fowler RS, Farkas LG, et al: A comprehensive scoring system for evaluating Noonan syndrome. *Am J Med Genet* 10:37–50, 1981.

52. Dupuis C, Charaf LA, Breviere GM, Abou P: "Infantile" form of the scimitar syndrome with pulmonary hypertension. *Am J Cardiol* 71:1326–1330, 1993.

53. Epstein CJ: Down syndrome (trisomy 21). In Scriver CR, Beaudet AL, Sly WS, et al (eds): *The Metabolic and Molecular Bases of Inherited Disease.* New York, McGraw-Hill, 2001, pp 1223–1256.

54. Evans DG, Lonsdale RN, Patton MA: Cutaneous lymphangioma and amegakaryocytic thrombocytopenia in Noonan syndrome. *Clin Genet* 39:228–232, 1991.

55. Ewart AK, Jin W, Atkinson D, et al: Supravalvular aortic stenosis associated with a deletion disrupting the elastin gene. *J Clin Invest* 93:1071–1077, 1994.

56. Ewart AK, Morris CA, Atkinson D, et al: Hemizygosity at the elastin locus in a developmental disorder: Williams syndrome. *Nat Genet* 5:11–16, 1993.

57. Ferencz C, Neill CA: Cardiovascular malformations: Prevalence at live birth. In Freedom RM, Benson LN, Smallhorn JR (eds): *Neonatal Heart Disease.* New York, Springer Verlag, 1992, pp 19–29.

58. Ferencz C, Neill CA, Boughman JA, et al: Congenital cardiovascular malformations associated with chromosome abnormalities: An epidemiologic study. *J Pediatr* 114:79–86, 1989.

59. Ferencz C, Rubin JD, Loffredo CA, Magee CA: *Epidemiology of congenital heart disease: The Baltimore-Washington Infant Study 1981-1989.* Mount Kisco, NY, Futura Publishing, 1993.

60. Ferencz C, Rubin JD, McCarter RJ, et al: Cardiac and noncardiac malformations: Observations in a population-based study. *Teratology* 35:367–378, 1987.

61. Flashburg MH, Dunbar BS, August G, Watson D: Anesthesia for surgery in an infant with DiGeorge syndrome. *Anesthesiology* 58:479–481, 1983.

62. Flick JT, Singh AK, Kizer J, Lazarchick J: Platelet dysfunction in Noonan's syndrome: A case with a platelet cyclooxygenase-like deficiency and chronic idiopathic thrombocytopenic purpura. *Am J Clin Pathol* 95:739–742, 1991.

63. Forrest SM, Smith TJ, Cross GS, et al: Effective strategy for prenatal prediction of Duchenne and Becker muscular dystrophy. *Lancet* 2:1294–1297, 1987.

64. Fost N: Ethical issues in genetics. *Pediatr Clin North Am* 39:79-89, 1992.

65. Fost N: Introduction: Ethics, ethics everywhere. *Curr Probl Pediatr* 22:422–423, 1992.

66. Freeman SB, Taft LF, Dooley KJ, et al: Population-based study of congenital heart defects in Down syndrome. *Am J Med Genet* 80:213–217, 1998.

67. Fryer AE, Holt PJ, Hughes HE: The cardio-facio-cutaneous (CFC) syndrome and Noonan syndrome: Are they the same? *Am J Med Genet* 38:548–551, 1991.

68. Fryns JP, Volcke P, Van den Berghe H: The cardio-facio-cutaneous (CFC) syndrome: Autosomal dominant inheritance in a large family. *Genet Couns* 3:19–24, 1992.

69. Gabrielli O, Salvolini U, Coppa GV, et al: Magnetic resonance imaging in the malformative syndromes with mental retardation. *Pediatr Radiol* 21:16–19, 1990.

70. Gamallo C, Garcia M, Palacios J, Rodriguez JI: Decrease in calcitonin-containing cells in truncus arteriosus. *Am J Med Genet* 46:149–153, 1993.

71. Garabedian M: Hypocalcemia and chromosome 22q11 microdeletion. *Genet Couns* 10:389–394, 1999.

72. Gebbia M, Ferrero GB, Pilia G, et al: X-linked situs abnormalities result from mutations in ZIC3. *Nat Genet* 17:305–308, 1997.

73. Giles TD, Iteld BJ, Rives KL: The cardiomyopathy of hypoparathyroidism: Another reversible form of heart muscle disease. *Chest* 79:225–229, 1981.

74. Goldmuntz E, Clark BJ, Mitchell LE, et al: Frequency of 22q11 deletions in patients with conotruncal defects. *J Am Coll Cardiol* 32:492–498, 1998.

75. Green MJ, Fost N: Who should provide genetic education prior to gene testing? Computers and other methods for improving patient understanding. *Genet Test* 1:131–136, 1997.

76. Greenberg F, Elder FF, Haffner P, et al: Cytogenetic findings in a prospective series of patients with DiGeorge anomaly. *Am J Hum Genet* 43:605–611, 1988.

77. Grubben C, Fryns JP, Smeets E, Van den Berghe H: Noonan phenotype in the basal cell nevus syndrome. *Genet Couns* 2:47–54, 1991.

78. Haddow JE, Palomaki GE, Knight GJ, et al: Prenatal screening for Down's syndrome with use of maternal serum markers [see comments]. *N Engl J Med* 327:588–593, 1992.

79. Hall JG, Levin J, Kuhn JP, et al: Thrombocytopenia with absent radius (TAR). *Medicine (Baltimore)* 48:411–439, 1969.

80. Harrington H: Absence of the thymus gland. *Lond Med Gaz* 3:314, 1829.

81. Hattori M, Fujiyama A, Taylor TD, et al: The DNA sequence of human chromosome 21: The chromosome 21 mapping and sequencing consortium. *Nature* 405:311–319, 2000.

82. Hayes A, Batshaw ML: Down syndrome. *Pediatr Clin North Am* 40:523–535, 1993.

83. Heller RM, Dorst JP, James AE Jr, Rowe RD: A useful sign in the recognition of azygos continuation of the inferior vena cava. *Radiology* 101:519–522, 1971.

84. Hishitani T, Ogawa K, Hoshino K, Nakamura Y: Surgical ligation of anomalous hepatic vein in a case of heterotaxy syndrome with massive intrahepatic shunting after modified Fontan operation. *Pediatr Cardiol* 20:428–430, 1999.

85. Hortop J, Tsipouras P, Hanley JA, et al: Cardiovascular involvement in osteogenesis imperfecta. *Circulation* 73:54–61, 1986.

86. Huether CA, Haroldson K, Ellis PM, Ramsay CN: Impact of prenatal diagnosis on revised livebirth prevalence estimates of Down syndrome in the Lothian region of Scotland, 1978-1992. *Genet Epidemiol* 13:367–375, 1996.

87. Huhta JC, Smallhorn JF, Macartney FJ: Two dimensional echocardiographic diagnosis of situs. *Br Heart J* 48:97–108, 1982.

88. Huhta JC, Smallhorn JF, Macartney FJ, et al: Cross-sectional echocardiographic diagnosis of systemic venous return. *Br Heart J* 48:388–403, 1982.

89. Hunter A, Pinsky L: An evaluation of the possible association of malignant hyperpyrexia with the Noonan syndrome using serum creatine phosphokinase levels. *J Pediatr* 86:412–415, 1975.

90. Hutchins GM, Moore GW, Lipford EH, et al: Asplenia and polysplenia malformation complexes explained by abnormal embryonic body curvature. *Pathol Res Pract* 177:60–76, 1983.

91. Hyman BT: Down syndrome and Alzheimer disease. *Prog Clin Biol Res* 379:123–142, 1992.

92. Isaacs H, Savage N, Badenhorst M, Whistler T: Acid maltase deficiency: A case study and review of the pathophysiological changes and proposed therapeutic measures. *J Neurol Neurosurg Psychiatry* 49:1011–1018, 1986.

93. Izquierdo L, Kushnir O, Sanchez D, et al: Prenatal diagnosis of Noonan's syndrome in a female infant with spontaneous resolution of cystic hygroma and hydrops. *West J Med* 152:418–421, 1990.

94. Jacobs IN, Gray RF, Todd NW: Upper airway obstruction in children with Down syndrome. *Arch Otolaryngol Head Neck Surg* 122:945–950, 1996.

95. Johnson JD, Jennings R: Hypocalcemia and cardiac arrhythmias. *Am J Dis Child* 115:373–376, 1968.

96. Johnson MC, Strauss AW, Dowton SB, et al: Deletion within chromosome 22 is common in patients with absent pulmonary valve syndrome. *Am J Cardiol* 76:66–69, 1995.

97. Kalwinsky DK, Raimondi SC, Bunin NJ, et al: Clinical and biological characteristics of acute lymphocytic leukemia in children with Down syndrome. *Am J Med Genet Suppl* 7:267–271, 1990.

98. Kan JS, White RI Jr, Mitchell SE, Gardner TJ: Percutaneous balloon valvuloplasty: A new method for treating congenital pulmonary-valve stenosis. *N Engl J Med* 307:540–542, 1982.

99. Karr SS, Brenner JI, Loffredo C, et al: Tetralogy of Fallot: The spectrum of severity in a regional study, 1981-1985. *Am J Dis Child* 146:121–124, 1992.

100. Katz S, Kravetz S: Facial plastic surgery for persons with Down syndrome: Research findings and their professional and social implications. *Am J Ment Retard* 94:101–110; discussion 111–120, 1989.

101. Kelley RI, Hennekam RC: The Smith-Lemli-Opitz syndrome. *J Med Genet* 37:321–335, 2000.

102. Khoury MJ, Cordero JF, Greenberg F, et al: A population study of the VACTERL association: Evidence for its etiologic heterogeneity. *Pediatrics* 71:815–820, 1983.

103. Kidd L: Cardiorespiratory problems in children with Down syndrome. In Lott IT, McCoy EE (eds): *Down Syndrome: Advances in Medical Care.* New York, Wiley-Liss, 1992, pp 61–69.

104. Kirby ML, Gale TF, Stewart DE: Neural crest cells contribute to normal aorticopulmonary septation. *Science* 220:1059–1061, 1983.

105. Kirby ML, Turnage KL, Hays BM: Characterization of conotruncal malformations following ablation of "cardiac" neural crest. *Anat Rec* 213:87–93, 1985.

106. Korenberg JR, Chen XN, Schipper R, et al: Down syndrome phenotypes: The consequences of chromosomal imbalance. *Proc Natl Acad Sci U S A* 91:4997–5001, 1994.

107. Korenberg JR, Kawashima H, Pulst SM, et al: Molecular definition of a region of chromosome 21 that causes features of the Down syndrome phenotype. *Am J Hum Genet* 47:236–246, 1990.

108. Korenberg JR, Pulst SM, Gerwehr S: Advances in the understanding of chromosome 21 and Down syndrome. In Lott IT, McCoy EE (eds): *Down Syndrome: Advances in Medical Care.* New York, Wiley-Liss, 1992, pp 3–12.

109. Kraynack NC, Hostoffer RW, Robin NH: Agenesis of the corpus callosum associated with DiGeorge-velocardiofacial syndrome: A case report and review of the literature. *J Child Neurol* 14:754–756, 1999.

110. Kurnit DM, Aldridge JF, Matsuoka R, Matthysse S: Increased adhesiveness of trisomy 21 cells and atrioventricular canal malformations in Down syndrome: A stochastic model. *Am J Med Genet* 20:385–399, 1985.

111. Landwirth J: Ethical issues in pediatric and neonatal resuscitation. *Ann Emerg Med* 22:502–507, 1993.

112. Leana-Cox J, Pangkanon S, Eanet KR, et al: Familial DiGeorge/velocardiofacial syndrome with deletions of chromosome area 22q11.2: Report of five families with a review of the literature. *Am J Med Genet* 65:309–316, 1996.

113. Legius E, Schollen E, Matthijs G, Fryns JP: Fine mapping of Noonan/cardio-facio cutaneous syndrome in a large family. *Eur J Hum Genet* 6:32–37, 1998.

114. Levy J: The gastrointestinal tract in Down syndrome. *Prog Clin Biol Res* 373:245–256, 1991.

115. Lindsay EA, Goldberg R, Jurecic V, et al: Velo-cardio-facial syndrome: Frequency and extent of 22q11 deletions. *Am J Med Genet* 57:514–522, 1995.

116. Lobdell D: Congenital absence of the parathyroid glands. *Arch Pathol* 67:412–415, 1959.

117. Lynch DR, McDonald-McGinn DM, Zackai EH, et al: Cerebellar atrophy in a patient with velocardiofacial syndrome [see comments]. *J Med Genet* 32:561–563, 1995.

118. Mahoney MJ, Hobbins JC: Prenatal diagnosis of chondroectodermal dysplasia (Ellis-van Creveld syndrome) with fetoscopy and ultrasound. *N Engl J Med* 297:258–260, 1977.

119. Mantzouranis EC, Rosen FS, Colten HR: Reticuloendothelial clearance in cystic fibrosis and other inflammatory lung diseases. *N Engl J Med* 319:338–343, 1988.

120. Marino B, Papa M, Guccione P, et al: Ventricular septal defect in Down syndrome. Anatomic types and associated malformations. *Am J Dis Child* 144:544–545, 1990.

121. Maron BJ, Moller JH, Seidman CE, et al: Impact of laboratory molecular diagnosis on contemporary diagnostic criteria for genetically transmitted cardiovascular diseases: Hypertrophic cardiomyopathy, long-QT syndrome, and Marfan syndrome: A statement for healthcare professionals from the Councils on Clinical Cardiology, Cardiovascular Disease in the Young, and Basic Science, American Heart Association. *Circulation* 98:1460–1471, 1998.

122. Martin G: Observations on d'une anomalie dans la situation dans la configuration du coeur et des vaisseaux qui en partnet ou qui s'y redent. *Bulletin Soc Anat Paris* 3:39–43, 1826.

123. Mathew P, Moodie D, Sterba R, et al: Long-term follow-up of children with Down syndrome with cardiac lesions. *Clin Pediatr (Phila)* 29:569–574, 1990.

124. Matsuoka R, Kimura M, Scambler PJ, et al: Molecular and clinical study of 183 patients with conotruncal anomaly face syndrome. *Hum Genet* 103:70–80, 1998.

125. Maximilian C, Ioan DM, Fryns JP: A syndrome of mental retardation, short stature, craniofacial anomalies with palpebral ptosis, and pulmonary stenosis in three siblings with normal parents: An example of autosomal recessive inheritance of the Noonan phenotype? *Genet Couns* 3:115–118, 1992.

126. McDonald-McGinn DM, Driscoll DA, et al: Detection of a 22q11.2 deletion in cardiac patients suggests a risk for velopharyngeal incompetence. *Pediatrics* 99:E9, 1997.

127. McDonald-McGinn DM, LaRossa D, Goldmuntz E, et al: The 22q11.2 deletion: Screening, diagnostic workup, and outcome of results: Report on 181 patients. *Genet Test* 1:99–108, 1997.

128. McKusick VA: *Mendelian Inheritance in Man. A Catalog of Human Genes and Genetic Disorders.* Baltimore, Johns Hopkins University Press, 1998, p 3.

129. McKusick VA: *Online Mendelian Inheritance in Man.* Baltimore, Johns Hopkins University, 2000.

130. Mendez HM, Opitz JM: Noonan syndrome: A review. *Am J Med Genet* 21:493–506, 1985.

131. Merscher S, Funke B, Epstein JA, et al: TBX1 is responsible for cardiovascular defects in velo-cardio-facial/DiGeorge syndrome. *Cell* 104:619–629, 2001.

132. Mitnick RJ, Bello JA, Shprintzen RJ: Brain anomalies in velo-cardio-facial syndrome. *Am J Med Genet* 54:100–106, 1994.

133. Miyabara S: Cardiovascular malformations of mouse trisomy 21. In Clark EB, Takao A, (eds): *Developmental Cardiology: Morphogenesis and Function.* New York, Futura Publishing, 1990, pp 409–430.

134. Momma K, Linde LM: Abnormal P wave axis in congenital heart disease associated with asplenia and polysplenia. *J Electrocardiol* 2:395–402, 1969.

135. Monaco G, Pignata C, Rossi E, et al: DiGeorge anomaly associated with 10p deletion. *Am J Med Genet* 39:215–216, 1991.

136. Morris CD, Magilke D, Reller M: Down's syndrome affects results of surgical correction of complete atrioventricular canal. *Pediatr Cardiol* 13:80–84, 1992.

137. Mueller RF: The Alagille syndrome (arteriohepatic dysplasia). *J Med Genet* 24:621–626, 1987.

138. Murphy KC, Jones LA, Owen MJ: High rates of schizophrenia in adults with velo-cardio-facial syndrome. *Arch Gen Psychiatry* 56:940–945, 1999.

139. Nair M, Kaul UA, Prasad R, et al: Successful percutaneous pulmonary balloon valvuloplasty in Noonan's syndrome: A case report. *Indian Heart J* 42:123–125, 1990.

140. Natowicz M, Chatten J, Clancy R, et al: Genetic disorders and major extracardiac anomalies associated with the hypoplastic left heart syndrome. *Pediatrics* 82:698–706, 1988.

141. Neill CA: Congenital cardiac malformations and syndromes. In Pierpont ME, Moller JH (eds): *Genetics of Cardiovascular Disease.* Boston, Martinus-Nijhoff, 1986, pp 95–112.

142. Neill CA: Genetics and recurrence risks of congenital heart disease. In Long WA (ed): *Fetal and Neonatal Cardiology.* Philadelphia, WB Saunders, 1989, pp 125–133.

143. Neill CA, Clark EB, Clark C: *The Heart of a Child.* Baltimore, Johns Hopkins University Press, 2001.

144. Neill CA, Ferencz C, Sabiston DC, Sheldon H: The familial occurrence of hypoplastic right lung with systemic arterial supply and venous drainage "Scimitar Syndrome." *Bull Johns Hopkins Hosp* 107:1–21, 1960.

145. Noonan JA: Hypertelorism with Turner phenotype: A new syndrome with associated congenital heart disease. *Am J Dis Child* 116:373–380, 1968.

146. Noonan JA: Noonan syndrome revisited. *J Pediatr* 135:667–668, 1999.

147. Noonan JA, Ehmke DA: Associated noncardiac malformations in children with congenital heart disease. *J Pediatr* 63:468–470, 1963.

148. Olsen CL, Cross PK, Gensburg LJ, Hughes JP: The effects of prenatal diagnosis, population ageing, and changing fertility rates on the live birth prevalence of Down syndrome in New York State, 1983-1992. *Prenat Diagn* 16:991–1002, 1996.

149. Opitz JM: The developmental field concept. *Am J Med Genet* 21:1–11, 1985.

150. Oster G, Kilburn KH, Siegal FP: Chemically induced congenital thymic dysgenesis in the rat: A model of the DiGeorge syndrome. *Clin Immunol Immunopathol* 28:128–134, 1983.

151. Papolos DF, Faedda GL, Veit S, et al: Bipolar spectrum disorders in patients diagnosed with velo-cardio-facial syndrome: Does a hemizygous deletion of chromosome 22q11 result in bipolar affective disorder? *Am J Psychiatry* 153:1541–1547, 1996.

152. Pastakia B, Lieberman LM, Moodie D, Levy J: 99mTechnetium pyridoxylidene glutamate imaging in visceral heterotaxy (Ivemark's syndrome). *Gastroenterology* 77:1105–1108, 1979.

153. Paterson A, Frush DP, Donnelly LF, et al: A pattern-oriented approach to splenic imaging in infants and children. *Radiographics* 19:1465–1485, 1999.

154. Payne RM, Johnson MC, Grant JW, Strauss AW: Toward a molecular understanding of congenital heart disease. *Circulation* 91:494–504, 1995.

155. Peck AL: *Aristotle: Historica Animalium. Book II.* Cambridge, Harvard University Press, 1965, pp 132.

156. Peoples WM, Moller JH, Edwards JE: Polysplenia: A review of 146 cases. *Pediatr Cardiol* 4:129–137, 1983.

157. Pexieder T: Teratogens. In Pierpont ME, Moller JE (eds): *The Genetics of Cardiovascular Disease.* Boston, Martinus-Nijhoff, 1986, pp 25–68.

158. Phoon CK, Neill CA: Asplenia syndrome: Insight into embryology through an analysis of cardiac and extracardiac anomalies. *Am J Cardiol* 73:581–587, 1994.

159. Polhemus D, Schafer WB: Congenital absence of the spleen: Syndrome, with atrioventricularis and situs inversus. *Pediatrics* 9:696–708, 1952.

160. Polhemus DW, Schafer W: Absent spleen syndrome: Hematologic findings as aid to diagnosis. *Pediatrics* 24:254, 1959.

161. Pongratz G, Friedrich M, Unverdorben M, et al: Hypertrophic obstructive cardiomyopathy as a manifestation of a cardiocutaneous syndrome (Noonan syndrome). *Klin Wochenschr* 69:932–936, 1991.

162. Pueschel SM: Should children with Down syndrome be screened for atlantoaxial instability? *Arch Pediatr Adolesc Med* 152:123–125, 1998.

163. Pueschel SM, Scola FH, Tupper TB, Pezzullo JC: Skeletal anomalies of the upper cervical spine in children with Down syndrome. *J Pediatr Orthop* 10:607–611, 1990.

164. Putschar WGJ, Manion WC: Congenital absence of the spleen and associated anomalies. *Am J Clin Pathol* 26:429–470, 1952.

165. Radford DJ, Thong YH: The association between immunodeficiency and congenital heart disease. *Pediatr Cardiol* 9:103–108, 1988.

166. Ranke MB, Heidemann P, Knupfer C, et al: Noonan syndrome: Growth and clinical manifestations in 144 cases. *Eur J Pediatr* 148:220–227, 1988.

167. Reeves RH, Irving NG, Moran TH, et al: A mouse model for Down syndrome exhibits learning and behaviour deficits [see comments]. *Nat Genet* 11:177–184, 1995.

168. Reller MD, Morris CD: Is Down syndrome a risk factor for poor outcome after repair of congenital heart defects? *J Pediatr* 132:738–741, 1998.

169. Roberts DJ, Genest D: Cardiac histologic pathology characteristic of trisomies 13 and 21. *Hum Pathol* 23:1130–1140, 1992.

170. Rollnick BR: Oculoauriculovertebral anomaly: Variability and causal heterogeneity. *Am J Med Genet Suppl* 4:41–53, 1988.

171. Rollnick BR, Kaye CI: Hemifacial microstomia and variants: Pedigree data. *Am J Med Genet* 15:233–253, 1983.

172. Rose V, Izukawa T, Moes CA: Syndromes of asplenia and polysplenia: A review of cardiac and non-cardiac malformations in 60 cases with special reference to diagnosis and prognosis. *Br Heart J* 37:840–852, 1975.

173. Rosemberg S, Carneiro PC, Zerbini MC, Gonzalez CH: Brief clinical report: Chondroectodermal dysplasia (Ellis-van Creveld) with anomalies of CNS and urinary tract. *Am J Med Genet* 15:291–295, 1983.

174. Ruscazio M, Van Praagh S, Marrass AR, et al: Interrupted inferior vena cava in asplenia syndrome and a review of the hereditary patterns of visceral situs abnormalities. *Am J Cardiol* 81:111–116, 1998.

175. Ryan AK, Goodship JA, Wilson DI, et al: Spectrum of clinical features associated with interstitial chromosome 22q11 deletions: A European collaborative study. *J Med Genet* 34:798–804, 1997.

176. Ryan CA, Finer NN, Ives E: Discordance of signs in monozygotic twins concordant for the Goldenhaar anomaly. *Am J Med Genet* 29:755–761, 1988.

177. Schneider DS, Zahka KG, Clark EB, Neill CA: Patterns of cardiac care in infants with Down syndrome. *Am J Dis Child* 143:363–365, 1989.

178. Schon F, Bowler J, Baraitser M: Cerebral arteriovenous malformation in Noonan's syndrome. *Postgrad Med J* 68:37–40, 1992.

179. Schwartz N, Eisenkraft JB: Anesthetic management of a child with Noonan's syndrome and idiopathic hypertrophic subaortic stenosis. *Anesth Analg* 74:464–646, 1992.

180. Seidman CE, Seidman JG: Molecular genetic studies of familial hypertrophic cardiomyopathy. *Basic Res Cardiol* 93:13–16, 1998.

181. Sharland M, Burch M, McKenna WM, Patton MA: A clinical study of Noonan syndrome. *Arch Dis Child* 67:178–183, 1992.

182. Sharland M, Patton MA, Talbot S, et al: Coagulation-factor deficiencies and abnormal bleeding in Noonan's syndrome. *Lancet* 339:19–21, 1992.

183. Sharland M, Taylor R, Patton MA, Jeffery S: Absence of linkage of Noonan syndrome to the neurofibromatosis type 1 locus. *J Med Genet* 29:188–190, 1992.

184. Shimizu T, Takao A, Ando M, Hirayama A: Conotruncal anomaly face syndrome: Its heterogeneity and association with thymus involution. In Nora JJ, Takao A (eds): *Congenital Heart Diseases: Causes and Processes.* New York, Futura, 1984, pp 29–41.

185. Shprintzen RJ, Goldberg RB, Lewin ML, et al: A new syndrome involving cleft palate, cardiac anomalies, typical facies, and learning disabilities: Velo-cardio-facial syndrome. *Cleft Palate J* 15:56–62, 1978.

186. Shprintzen RJ, Goldberg RB, Young D, Wolford L: The velo-cardio-facial syndrome: A clinical and genetic analysis. *Pediatrics* 67:167–172, 1981.

187. Shub C, Dimopoulos IN, Seward JB, et al: Sensitivity of two-dimensional echocardiography in the direct visualization of atrial septal defect utilizing the subcostal approach: Experience with 154 patients. *J Am Coll Cardiol* 2:127–135, 1983.

188. Smith AT, Sack GH Jr, Taylor GJ: Holt-Oram syndrome. *J Pediatr* 95:538–543, 1979.

189. Smith CA, Driscoll DA, Emanuel BS, et al: Increased prevalence of immunoglobulin A deficiency in patients with the chromosome 22q11.2 deletion syndrome (DiGeorge syndrome/velocardiofacial syndrome). *Clin Diagn Lab Immunol* 5:415–417, 1998.

190. Snider AR, Silverman NH: Suprasternal notch echocardiography: A two-dimensional technique for evaluating congenital heart disease. *Circulation* 63:165–173, 1981.

191. Sonesson SE, Fouron JC, Lessard M: Intrauterine diagnosis and evolution of a cardiomyopathy in a fetus with Noonan's syndrome. *Acta Paediatr* 81:368–370, 1992.

192. Stanger P, Cassidy SC, Girod DA, et al: Balloon pulmonary valvuloplasty: Results of the Valvuloplasty and Angioplasty of Congenital Anomalies Registry. *Am J Cardiol* 65:775–783, 1990.

193. Stebbens VA, Dennis J, Samuels MP, et al: Sleep related upper airway obstruction in a cohort with Down's syndrome. *Arch Dis Child* 66:1333–1338, 1991.

194. Stern HJ, Saal HM, Lee JS, et al: Clinical variability of type 1 neurofibromatosis: Is there a neurofibromatosis-Noonan syndrome? *J Med Genet* 29:184–187, 1992.

195. Sty JR, Conway JJ: The spleen: Development and functional evaluation. *Semin Nucl Med* 15:276–298, 1985.

196. Sullivan KE, Jawad AF, Randall P, et al: Lack of correlation between impaired T cell production, immunodeficiency, and other phenotypic features in chromosome 22q11.2 deletion syndromes. *Clin Immunol Immunopathol* 86:141–146, 1998.

197. Sykes KS, Bachrach LK, Siegel-Bartelt J, et al: Velocardiofacial syndrome presenting as hypocalcemia in early adolescence. *Arch Pediatr Adolesc Med* 151:745–747, 1997.

198. Takao A, Ando M, Cho K, et al: Etiologic categorization of common congenital heart disease. In Van Praagh R, Takao A (eds): *Etiology and Morphogenesis of Congenital Heart Disease.* New York, Futura, 1980, pp 253–269.

199. Tartaglia M, Mehler EL, Goldberg R, et al: Mutations in *PTPN11*, encoding the protein tyrosine phosphatase SHP-2, cause Noonan syndrome. *Nat Genet* 29:465–468, 2001.

200. Tosti A, Misciali C, Borrello P, et al: A loose anagen hair in a child with Noonan's syndrome. *Dermatologica* 182:247–249, 1991.

201. Traub A, Giebink GS, Smith C, et al: Splenic reticuloendothelial function after splenectomy, spleen repair, and spleen autotransplantation. *N Engl J Med* 317:1559–1564, 1987.

202. Tredwell SJ, Newman DE, Lockitch G: Instability of the upper cervical spine in Down syndrome. *J Pediatr Orthop* 10:602–606, 1990.

203. Tubman TR, Shields MD, Craig BG, et al: Congenital heart disease in Down's syndrome: Two year prospective early screening study. *BMJ* 302:1425–1427, 1991.

204. Uemura H, Ho SY, Anderson RH, Yagihara T: Ventricular morphology and coronary arterial anatomy in hearts with isometric atrial appendages. *Ann Thorac Surg* 67:1403–1411, 1999.

205. Ugazio AG, Maccario R, Notarangelo LD, Burgio GR: Immunology of Down syndrome: A review. *Am J Med Genet Suppl* 7:204–212, 1990.

206. Van Mierop L, Gessner IH, Schiebler GL: Asplenia and polysplenia syndrome. *Birth Defect: Original Article Series* 5:36–44, 1972.

207. Van Mierop LHS, Wigelsworth FW: Isomerism of congenital asplenia with isomerism of the cardiac atria and sinoatrial nodes. *Am J Cardiol* 13:407, 1964.

208. Van Praagh S, Kreutzer J, Alday L, Van Praagh R: Systemic and pulmonary venous connections in visceral heterotaxy, with emphasis on the diagnosis of the atrial situs: A study of 109 postmortem cases. In Clark EB, Takao A (eds): *Developmental Cardiology: Morphogenesis and Function.* Mount Kisco, NY, Futura, 1990, pp 671–727.

209. Van Praagh S, Santini F, Sanders SP: Cardiac malpositions with special emphasis on visceral heterotaxy (asplenia and polysplenia syndromes). In Fyler DC (ed): *Nadas' Pediatric Cardiology.* Baltimore, Mosby-Year Book, 1992, pp 589–608.

210. Veatch R: *Medical Ethics.* Boston, Jones & Bartlett, 1997.

211. Vigild M: Dental caries experience among children with Down's syndrome. *J Ment Defic Res* 30:271–276, 1986.

212. Waldman JD, Rosenthal A, Smith AL, et al: Sepsis and congenital asplenia. *J Pediatr* 90:555–559, 1977.

213. Wassif CA, Maslen C, Kachilele-Linjewile S, et al: Mutations in the human sterol delta7-reductase gene at 11q12-13 cause Smith-Lemli-Opitz syndrome. *Am J Hum Genet* 63:55–62, 1988.

214. Wilson DI, Burn J, Scambler P, Goodship J: DiGeorge syndrome: Part of CATCH-22. *J Med Genet* 30:852–856, 1993.

215. Wilson DI, Cross IE, Wren C: Minimum prevalence of chromosome 22q11 deletions. *Am J Hum Genet* 55:A169, 1994.
216. Wong CK, Cheng CH, Lau CP, Leung WH: Congenital coronary artery anomalies in Noonan's syndrome. *Am Heart J* 119:396–400, 1990.
217. Wren C, Macartney FJ, Deanfield JE: Cardiac rhythm in atrial isomerism. *Am J Cardiol* 59:1156–1158, 1987.
218. Yen BM, Schneiderman LJ: Impact of pediatric ethics consultations on patients, families, social workers, and physicians. *J Perinatol* 19:373–378, 1999.
219. Yost HJ: The genetics of midline and cardiac laterality defects. *Curr Opin Cardiol* 13:185–189, 1998.
220. Zahka KG, Spector M, Hanisch D: Hypoplastic left-heart syndrome: Norwood operation, transplantation, or compassionate care. *Clin Perinatol* 20:145–154, 1993.
221. Zaloga GP: Hypocalcemia in critically ill patients. *Crit Care Med* 20:251–262, 1992.
222. Zipursky A, Poon A, Doyle J: Hematologic and oncologic disorders in Down syndrome. In Lott IT, McCoy EE (eds): *Down Syndrome: Advances in Medical Care.* New York, Wiley-Liss, 1992, pp 3–12.
223. Zori RT, Boyar FZ, Williams WN, et al. Prevalence of 22q11 region deletions in patients with velopharyngeal insufficiency. *Am J Med Genet* 77:8–11, 1998.

Chapter 47

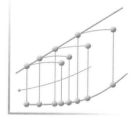

Heritable Heart Disease as Part of Multisystem Illness

DAVID G. NICHOLS, MD, MBA

INTRODUCTION

In a sense, all heart disease has a heritable component. However, this chapter focuses on patients who have a four-chambered heart, but have abnormal heart muscle or valve structure as part of an inherited multisystem disorder. These diseases often do not have cardiac dysfunction as the presenting manifestation, although cardiac disease may become the most life-threatening manifestation in due course. The major manifestation is usually in one or more noncardiac organ systems such as connective tissue, abdominal viscera, or the neuromuscular system. This chapter describes the presentation and management of heritable cardiovascular disease in the context of primary disease manifestations in other (noncardiac) organ systems. Cardiomyopathies with primary myocardial presentation are discussed in Chapter 48. Cardiomyopathies presenting as part of metabolic disease (e.g., carnitine deficiency) are discussed in Chapter 15 on *Nutrition and Metabolism*. The classically recognizable phenotypic syndromes associated with complex congenital heart disease (e.g., Down syndrome) are discussed in Chapter 46.

CONNECTIVE TISSUE DISEASES

Marfan Syndrome

Overview

Marfan syndrome is an inherited disease of connective tissue usually caused by a mutation in the fibrillin-1 or fibrillin-2 gene on chromosome 15. These genes code for fibrillin, a large glycoprotein constituent of elastin-associated microfibrils. The disease is autosomal dominant with high penetrance. Sporadic mutations appear in 10% to 20% of cases.

Classic Phenotype

Although the manifestations of Marfan syndrome may be variable, the habitus of the typical patient is readily recognizable. The musculoskeletal, ocular, and cardiovascular systems point to the disease. These patients are tall and thin with extremity length out of proportion to trunk length. Other skeletal deformities are frequently seen, including arachnodactyly, kyphoscoliosis, pectus excavatum, and hyperextensible joints. (Patients with the fibrillin-2 mutation may have joint contractures.) The ocular manifestations include subluxation of the lens, myopia, and occasionally retinal detachment. Because the molecular defect in Marfan syndrome involves microfibrils in elastin, the critical manifestations of the disease involve cardiac valves and blood vessels, which are discussed later.

Neonatal Phenotype

Recognition of the Marfan phenotype in the newborn signifies a particularly severe, usually lethal form of the disease. Neonatal Marfan syndrome exhibits arachnodactyly, small-joint laxity, and contractures of elbows, knees, and ankles. Dilated cardiomyopathy and valvular dysplasia lead to rapid onset of congestive heart failure.[18] In addition to pulmonary edema, these patients often have emphysema and chronic lung disease.

Cardiovascular Manifestations

Aortic Aneurysm and Dissection The patient with Marfan syndrome may develop a specific form of aortic aneurysm involving *dilation of the aortic root*. The age at onset of aortic root dilatation is unpredictable, but carries a particularly ominous prognosis if detected in the newborn. Unless corrected surgically, aortic dilatation is likely to lead to dissection and rupture of the aorta. The timing of surgical correction is critical, because patients first seen in shock or with a neurologic deficit after aortic dissection have a very high mortality rate.[24]

A variety of indications have been used to time the elective, prophylactic repair of a dilated aorta. Common indications include an ascending aortic diameter of more than 5 to 6 cm or an ascending aortic diameter more than twice the diameter of the descending aorta. In our experience, the average child with Marfan syndrome and aortic aneurysm undergoes operation at around age 10 years, at which time the aortic aneurysm was approximately 6 cm in diameter.[14] Dissection is very uncommon with careful monitoring and prophylactic operation. Therefore serial echocardiographic examination of aortic diameter at the sinus of valsalva is required in this population.

The standard surgical approach has been replacement of the entire aortic root and valve with a composite valve and graft prosthesis, with reimplantation of the coronary arteries.[15] This procedure, originally introduced by Bentall in 1968, has evolved to a low-risk standardized procedure.[2] Its major drawback is the need for lifelong anticoagulation for the mechanical valve prosthesis. For patients in whom lifelong anticoagulation is contraindicated or undesirable, there are two other options. The first entails replacement of the aortic root and valve with the biologic valve, either cryopreserved homograft or allograft valve (porcine or bovine pericardial) with a Dacron tube graft. The second option is a valve-sparing aortic root replacement, either the "Yacoub remodeling procedure" or the "David reimplantation procedure".[8,32] The reimplantation approach appears to be more reliable in patients with Marfan syndrome and is associated with a lower incidence of late aortic regurgitation.[22] Long-term follow-up studies have yet to clarify whether the composite valve graft or valve sparing aortic root replacement is preferable in patients with Marfan syndrome.

Mitral Valve Prolapse and Regurgitation The abnormalities in collagen and elastin associated with Marfan syndrome lead to redundant and elongated valve tissue. The defect may extend to the chordae and mitral annulus. Therefore symptomatic mitral regurgitation may result from the dilated annulus, infective endocarditis, or ruptured chordae, in addition to the more common leaflet prolapse. Patients with mitral valve prolapse may appear with syncope, dyspnea, palpitations, fatigue, or chest pain.

If evidence of mitral valve degeneration is present, early mitral valve repair should be considered to avoid later mitral valve replacement with the associated requirement of indefinite anticoagulation. Left ventricular dilatation, independent of symptoms, is generally considered an indication for surgery. The results of mitral valve repair have shown low mortality rate and generally absent or mild postoperative mitral regurgitation.[13]

Dysrhythmias Patients with Marfan syndrome who have mitral valve prolapse are at high risk for dysrhythmias. One third of such patients have been found to have premature ventricular contractions or ventricular tachycardia.[4] Delayed repolarization manifested by a prolonged QT interval is an additional risk factor for ventricular dysrhythmias in the Marfan patient. Caffeine, nicotine, or exercise may precipitate dysrhythmias. The presentations range from palpitations to sudden death.

Supraventricular dysrhythmias also are common in the Marfan patient with mitral valve prolapse, including premature atrial contractions and reentrant atrioventricular (AV) nodal tachycardia. The severity or frequency of the dysrhythmias generally does not bear any relation to the extent of mitral regurgitation. However, patients with chronic mitral regurgitation and left atrial distention may be seen initially with atrial fibrillation.

Preventive Management The ever-present risk of aortic dissection or dysrhythmias can be managed with good preventive cardiovascular care. Because elevated adrenergic tone appears to increase the risk, stimulant drugs such as caffeine and nicotine should be avoided. Exercise and sports must be carefully monitored. The National Marfan Foundation professional advisory board advises against contact sports. Pregnancy greatly increases the risk of the aortic dissection among women with Marfan syndrome and an enlarged aortic root.

Beta blockade slows the rate of growth of the aortic aneurysm in adult patients with Marfan syndrome.[27] For patients with asthma or other contraindications to beta blockade, calcium channel blockade is an alternative to decrease aortic stress. Similar data documenting benefit of beta blockade do not exist in children. However, many pediatricians believe that beta blockade is indicated in children with Marfan syndrome either prophylactically or at the first sign of aortic enlargement.

Osteogenesis Imperfecta

Overview

Osteogenesis imperfecta is an inherited disease characterized by decreased bone mass, which results in pathologic fractures. At least seven separate forms have been described by using a classification originally developed by Sillence and colleagues.[29]

However, for clinical purposes, the distinctions of mild, moderate (or variable), and severe forms based on bone fragility generally suffice. The most severe forms can be diagnosed in utero or shortly after birth. The most common genetic defect in osteogenesis imperfecta involves mutations in one of two genes encoding procollagen type I.

In addition to bone fragility, several other manifestations are noteworthy. Most types of osteogenesis imperfecta have blue sclerae, either permanently or at birth. Hearing loss is present in most patients with osteogenesis imperfecta, whereas abnormal dentition is found in some. Vertebral fractures may lead to kyphoscoliosis, restrictive lung disease, and pulmonary hypertension. The combination of these findings in the patient with pathologic fractures and a family history of the disease will make the diagnosis of osteogenesis imperfecta.

Cardiac Disease

Approximately 10% of children with osteogenesis imperfecta will have some form of structural heart disease.[32] The most common cardiac diagnoses are aortic stenosis and mitral valve prolapse. Children with the severe presentation may have aortic root dilatation in up to one third of cases and left ventricular wall thickening in two thirds of cases. Valve-replacement surgery carries a high mortality rate in this population. However, a successful double valve replacement has been reported.[5]

The more common clinical problem involves the perioperative management of these patients for noncardiac surgery, particularly orthopedic surgery, such as intramedullary rod placement. All patients with osteogenesis imperfecta should receive a cardiac evaluation before surgery. Endocarditis prophylaxis should be given in patients with valvular disease. If vasoactive infusions are used, tachycardia and systemic afterload reduction should be avoided in the aortic stenosis patient. Conversely, patients with mitral regurgitation may benefit from afterload reduction.

Significant extracardiac disease may complicate the management. *Postoperative bleeding* may be severe, despite a normal coagulation profile, because of extreme tissue friability. One case report suggests that recombinant factor VIIa (40 mcg/kg) may be effective in controlling postoperative hemorrhage.[20]

Dystrophic Epidermolysis Bullosa

Overview

Children with epidermolysis bullosa (EB) have a genetic disorder in which skin and other squamous epithelia (oropharynx, esophagus, and anus) fail to adhere to the subjacent connective tissue properly. A wide spectrum of the disease exists, with the recessive dystrophic variety being the most severe. Immunomapping of skin from biopsy can distinguish the recessive dystrophic EB from the other two major forms: EB simplex and junctional EB. The variation in the dystrophic disease is explained by the many different mutations of the gene for type VII collagen (COL7A1), which is important in attaching the epidermis to the basement membrane.

Dystrophic EB is a multisystem disease affecting the skin, gastrointestinal tract, the blood, and the heart. The diagnosis is usually made in the newborn period, when babies manifest severe blistering, erosions, and atrophic scarring of the skin. Painful blistering occurs throughout the entire gastrointestinal tract, from the mouth to the anus. The immediate consequences include dysphagia, gastroesophageal reflux, intestinal bleeding, and constipation. Patients with longer-term medical needs may experience severe nutritional deficiencies, which may contribute to mortality. Early gastrostomy tube placement allows full nutritional support and avoids of micronutrient deficiencies such as carnitine or selenium deficiency.

Cardiac Disease

Recent data suggest that approximately 10% of children with the recessive form of dystrophic EB develop a dilated cardiomyopathy (DCM).[28] Hence children with dystrophic EB should undergo regular cardiac evaluations. The precise etiology of DCM in this population is unclear. Candidate causes such as carnitine or selenium deficiency, anemia, iron overload, infections, or the effects of the underlying disease could not be identified in the EB patients with DCM. Although most children with dystrophic EB who receive good general care can survive into adulthood, 50% of children with DCM die soon after onset of heart disease.[28] No specific therapy exists for EB patients with DCM other than the usual supportive care for any patient with DCM (see Chapter 48).

STORAGE DISEASES

Mucopolysaccharidoses

Overview

Mucopolysaccharidoses (MPSs) are a family of heritable diseases that result from deficiencies of lysosomal enzymes responsible for the breakdown of complex carbohydrates known as glycosaminoglycans (GAGs). GAGs form protein-carbohydrate complexes in connective tissue. Based on the particular enzyme deficiency and resultant GAG accumulation, MPS can be divided into seven subtypes (Table 47-1). MPSs are first seen with the spectrum of phenotypic abnormalities including growth retardation, mental retardation, skeletal abnormalities, organomegaly, airway obstruction, and corneal opacities. All forms of MPS may include structural heart disease. The specific MPS is rarely diagnosable on clinical grounds alone and requires enzyme assay or DNA mutation analysis.

A multidisciplinary approach to management is required. This may include corneal transplantation (MPS I, II, IV, VI, and VII), range-of-motion therapy for stiff joints, and cervical fusion (MPS IV). MPS accumulation may obstruct the upper airway in MPS I (Hurler syndrome) and II (Hunter syndrome), necessitating noninvasive ventilation or tracheostomy. Bone marrow transplantation or specific enzyme replacement has been investigated and shows promising results.[19]

Cardiac Disease

Cardiac involvement based on echocardiographic abnormalities occurs commonly in all forms of MPSs, although children with Sanfilippo disease (MPS III) appear least affected.[7] Endocardial or endovascular accumulation of GAGs accounts for the abnormalities. The clinical presentation generally

Table 47-1 Mucopolysaccharidoses (MPS)

Type	Inheritance	Enzyme Deficiency	Storage Material	Onset	Major Noncardiac Features	Cardiac Features
MPS I (Hurler)	Autosomal recessive	α-L-Iduronidase	Dermatan sulfate; heparan sulfate	Infancy	MR, OM, SD, CO	CAD; valve thickening; aortic or renal artery narrowing; hypertension
MPS I (Scheie)	Autosomal recessive	α-L-Iduronidase	Dermatan sulfate; heparan sulfate	Adult	MR, OM, SD, CO	CAD; valve thickening; aortic or renal artery narrowing; hypertension
MPS II (Hunter)	X-linked	Iduronate sulfatase	Dermatan sulfate; heparan sulfate	Infancy to childhood	MR, OM, SD	CAD; valve thickening
MPS III A,B,C,D (Sanfilippo A-D)	Autosomal recessive	Various	Heparan sulfate	Late infancy	MR (severe)	Rare
MPS IV (Morquio)	Autosomal recessive	Various	Heparan sulfate	Childhood	SD (severe), CO	Aortic valve thickening
MPS VI (Maroteaux-Lamy)	Autosomal recessive	Arylsulfatase B	Dermatan sulfate	Late infancy	MR, SD (severe), CO	Valve thickening
MPS VII	Autosomal recessive	β-Glucuronidase	Dermatan sulfate; heparan sulfate	Newborn to adult	OM, SD, CO	CAD, vascular narrowing, cardiomyopathy, complete heart block

MR, Mental retardation; OM, organomegaly (liver and spleen); SD, skeletal dysplasia; CO, corneal opacities; CAD, coronary artery disease.

involves mitral stenosis or regurgitation secondary to thickening of the valve leaflets. Aortic valve thickening leading to aortic regurgitation, asymmetric septal hypertrophy, or hypertrophic cardiomyopathy occurs less commonly. Cardiovascular disease in MPSs is always progressive. Hence serial evaluations including echocardiography are indicated even if the first evaluation is negative. Increasing age, MPS I, and decreasing ejection fraction represent the cardiovascular risk factors for death in MPS.[26] Mitral or aortic valve lesions, by themselves, do not increase the risk of mortality in MPS.

Certain potentially fatal cardiac problems have been attributed to specific forms of MPSs. Severe diffuse *coronary artery disease* may arise during the first few years of life in children with MPS I (Hurler). The deposition of the GAGs dermatan sulfate and heparan sulfate in the intima of coronary arteries may produce fatal ischemic heart disease.[1] Coronary angiography may underestimate the extent of GAG infiltration in the coronary vessels. The deposition is progressive and usually fatal by age 10 years in the absence of treatment with bone marrow transplantation.

Hypertension is a complication of GAG accumulation in the intima of the aorta or renal artery in MPS I.[30] Aortic accumulation may be diffuse or localized. A localized accumulation in the thoracic aorta appears as coarctation of the aorta in imaging studies.

Complete heart block has occurred in patients with MPS during anesthesia or during right heart catheterization.[9,31] These patients had no obvious conduction system abnormality before the onset of complete heart block. The etiology of heart block is multifactorial, resulting from a combination of GAG infiltration around the conduction system, coronary ischemia, or direct trauma from the guide wire. The patients have been managed successfully with transvenous pacing.

Glycogen Storage Diseases

Glycogen storage diseases are inherited disorders marked by accumulation of normal or abnormal glycogen in excess quantities. The liver, skeletal muscle, and cardiac muscle are most commonly affected because these organs contain the most glycogen. The classic example of cardiomyopathy in glycogen storage disease is Pompe disease (lysosomal acid α-1,4-glucosidase deficiency). However, other glycogen storage diseases occasionally show cardiac involvement, including types IIIa (debrancher deficiency), IV (amylopectinosis), and IX (liver phosphorylase kinase deficiency).

Glycogen storage disease type II (Pompe disease) stands out among the glycogen storage diseases because of its prominent cardiac involvement in the infantile form of the disease. A deficiency of lysosomal acid α-1,4-glucosidase (acid maltase) leads to accumulation of glycogen in lysosomes in contrast to other glycogen storage diseases, in which the accumulation occurs in the cytoplasm. The inheritance is autosomal recessive.

The manifestations of the disease vary with the age. The severe infantile form exhibits hepatomegaly, severe cardiomegaly, macroglossia, and hypotonia. The electrocardiogram (ECG) shows very large QRS complexes and a shortened PR interval. Histologic examination shows glycogen accumulation in skin, liver, heart, and brain. Laboratory tests reveal an elevated serum creatine kinase, aspartate transaminase, and lactate dehydrogenase. A deficiency in acid glucosidase obtained

from cultured fibroblasts establishes the definitive diagnosis. No specific therapy is known, and these children die by early childhood.

Milder forms of Pompe disease begin in late childhood or even adulthood. These patients do not have cardiac involvement but have weakness and respiratory insufficiency.

NEUROMUSCULAR DISEASES

The Muscular Dystrophies (Dystrophinopathies)

Introduction

The muscular dystrophies comprise a heterogeneous group of diseases involving skeletal or cardiac muscle or both. Among muscular dystrophies, cardiac involvement is seen particularly with the so-called dystrophinopathies, which are x-linked disorders affecting the dystrophin gene. This group includes Duchenne muscular dystrophy (DMD), Becker muscular dystrophy (BMD), and x-linked dilated cardiomyopathy (XLDCM).

Manifestations

DMD manifests itself during the first decade of life, usually with delayed and clumsy (waddling) gait. To arise from the prone position, these children perform the *Gowers* maneuver, in which they first get on their hands and knees and then use their hands to push themselves up onto their legs to the erect position. The physical examination reveals pseudohypertrophy of the calves, proximal muscle weakness, and ultimately loss of the deep tendon reflexes. All patients are confined to a wheelchair by the teenage years. Severe kyphoscoliosis and respiratory muscle weakness often lead to respiratory failure and the need for ventilatory support. The laboratory examination shows very elevated creatine phosphokinase levels in the serum and small potentials of short duration on electromyography. Immunohistochemistry stain with anti-dystrophin antibodies yields no stain in the DMD patient. Conversely, a normal biopsy specimen will show the dystrophin stain in the sarcolemma of muscle tissue. The widespread use of assisted ventilation in this population has increased the survival rate to approximately 50% by age 25 years.[11] The manifestations of *BMD* are identical to those seen in DMD, but the onset is later in childhood, and the course is milder. Patients with BMD generally survive into their 50s.

XLDCM manifests itself solely as cardiomyopathy. No evidence of skeletal muscle weakness is seen, although the serum creatine kinase may be elevated.

Genetics and Molecular Biology

It is convenient to group the dystrophinopathies because they have identical genetic transmission, involve mutations within the same gene, and are associated with DCM to variable degrees. All three dystrophinopathies are x-linked. Therefore the full-blown manifestations of the disease appear in male patients. Female patients are said to be carriers. However, recent reports suggest that up to 10% of female carriers of dystrophin mutations for DMD or BMD may develop cardiomyopathy with or without (mild) skeletal muscle involvement.[16]

The dystrophin gene is one of the largest genes (2.5 million base pairs) in the human genome. The gene is located on the short arm of the X chromosome at Xp21. The gene product, dystrophin, is a sarcolemmal protein, which is part of a protein complex ("dystrophin-associated protein complex") that spans the cell membrane. This complex is believed to maintain the integrity of the sarcolemma during extreme exercise. Dystrophin deficiency leads to disruption of the dystrophin-associated protein complex and to disintegration of the sarcolemma. The muscle fiber undergoes necrosis and is replaced by connective tissue or fat. Various types of mutations in the dystrophin gene can account for the dystrophinopathy phenotypes. Approximately 65% of patients with DMD or BMD have deletions within the gene. The size of the deletion bears no relation to the severity of the phenotype. The remaining patients have duplications or mutations in the dystrophin gene.

Cardiac Involvement in Duchenne Muscular Dystrophy or Becker Muscular Dystrophy

The myocardial process in DMD and BMD involves the left ventricle selectively. The right side of the heart is spared. In particular, the left ventricular posterior basal and lateral walls undergo the most extensive replacement with connective tissue or fat. Degeneration of the conduction system may occur as an end-stage phenomenon when the entire left ventricle is involved.

The manifestations of cardiac involvement early in the course of the disease involve a characteristic ECG pattern, with tall R waves in the right precordial leads and a deep Q wave in the limb leads and the lateral precordial leads. Echocardiography reveals left ventricular dysfunction, the severity of which correlates with mortality risk.[6] As myocardial necrosis progresses, the symptoms are typical of congestive left heart failure in DCM. Because these children are immobile by the time cardiac involvement is manifest, the symptoms of dyspnea, orthopnea, and paroxysmal nocturnal dyspnea predominate. If the patient is already ventilator dependent, increased inspired oxygen concentrations or positive end-expiratory pressure (PEEP) may be necessary. For reasons that are unclear, patients may manifest sudden congestive heart failure after having appeared clinically stable for long periods. Conduction-system involvement during the late stages of the disease leads to ventricular tachydysrhythmias. If myocardial necrosis progresses, systolic dysfunction becomes pronounced, leading to hypotension and ultimately cardiac arrest. Although cardiac involvement can be demonstrated by clinical or ECG criteria in 90% of patients with DMD/BMD, it is the cause of death in only 20% of DMD and 50% of BMD patients.

Cardiac Involvement in X-Linked Dilated Cardiomyopathy

Teenagers with XLDCM appear entirely asymptomatic until exercise intolerance, fatigue, and dyspnea are noted. As noted earlier, these patients have a mutation in the dystrophin gene but no signs of skeletal muscle weakness. The symptoms of heart failure rapidly become intractable. Death often occurs within 1 to 2 years after diagnosis.

Cardiac Management of Patients with Dystrophinopathies

Guidelines on the evaluation and management of patients with dystrophinopathies have been published.[3] Children with DMD should have serial ECG and echocardiogram performed at the time of diagnosis and then every 2 years until age 10 years. After age 10 years, the cardiac evaluation should occur annually. After a full cardiac evaluation on diagnosis of BMD, it should be repeated at least every 5 years. If the patient has an abnormal ECG or cardiac symptoms, an elevated serum troponin I can be used to diagnose myocardial necrosis.[12] Neither total creatine kinase nor the MB fraction is useful for diagnosis of acute myocardial necrosis, because they may be elevated chronically. Boys with XLDCM by definition have cardiac symptoms on presentation. They should remain under close observation of a cardiologist with frequent reevaluation so that a prompt decision about the option of cardiac transplantation can be made.

Female carriers of the dystrophin mutations may develop heart failure in up to 10% of cases. However, cardiac involvement in female carriers is not seen until the mid-teenage years. Therefore a cardiac evaluation is indicated at least every 5 years after age 16 years.[3]

Initial treatment of the patients with a dystrophinopathy and an abnormal echocardiogram should begin with angiotensin-converting enzyme inhibitors. Case reports suggest that the addition of β-blockers may be helpful.[10] Because the cardiac failure is often exacerbated by obstructive sleep apnea or respiratory failure, these patients benefit from noninvasive ventilation either at night or around the clock. If the condition continues to deteriorate despite medical management, heart transplantation should be considered in BMD and XLDCM. The generalized muscle weakness and immobility is too severe in patients with DMD to contemplate heart transplantation. Successful heart transplantation has been reported both in BMD and XLDCM.[17,22]

Disorders of Trinucleotide Repeats (Friedreich Ataxia)

Several inherited neurologic diseases are associated with increased numbers of trinucleotide repeat sequences, generally in the intron of the gene. Among these disorders, myotonic dystrophy and Friedreich ataxia are associated with cardiomyopathy, but only Friedreich ataxia produces symptomatic heart disease in childhood.

Friedreich ataxia is an autosomal recessive disorder caused by GAA repeat expansion in the first intron of the gene for frataxin on chromosome 9. Frataxin is a protein involved in mitochondrial iron homeostasis. Frataxin deficiency is associated with abnormal oxidative phosphorylation. Patients are initially seen with ataxia, dysarthria, areflexia, loss of vibratory sensation, and weakness in the lower limbs. Associated skeletal abnormalities include pes cavus and scoliosis. The incidence of the disease is one in 50,000.

In most patients, hypertrophic cardiomyopathy, particularly septal hypertrophy, develops later in the disease. Although apparently extremely rare, hypertrophic cardiomyopathy has been reported as the presenting sign of Friedreich ataxia.[21] The medical management of the cardiomyopathy in this setting is the same as that described for other cardiomyopathies (see Chapter 48). Isolated case reports and a small clinical trial indicate that treatment with the free radical scavenger idebenone was associated with a reduction in septal thickness among Friedreich ataxia patients.[25]

References

1. Belani KG, Krivit W, Carpenter BL, et al: Children with mucopolysaccharidosis: Perioperative care, morbidity, mortality, and new findings. *J Pediatr Surg* 28:403–408, 1993.

2. Bentall H, De Bono A: Technique for complete replacement of the ascending aorta. *Thorax* 23:338–339, 1968.

3. Bushby K, Muntoni F, Bourke JP: 107th ENMC international workshop: The management of cardiac involvement in muscular dystrophy and myotonic dystrophy, 7th-9th June 2002. Naarden, the Netherlands. *Neuromuscul Disord* 13:166–172, 2003.

4. Chen S, Fagan LF, Nouri S, Donahoe JL: Ventricular dysrhythmias in children with Marfan's syndrome. *Am J Dis Child* 139:273–276, 1985.

5. Chrysant GS, Cassivi SD, Carey CF, Sundt TM: Double valve replacement in a patient with osteogenesis imperfecta. *J Heart Valve Dis* 11:751–754, 2002.

6. Corrado G, Lissoni A, Beretta S, et al: Prognostic value of electrocardiograms, ventricular late potentials, ventricular arrhythmias, and left ventricular systolic dysfunction in patients with Duchenne muscular dystrophy. *Am J Cardiol* 89:838–841, 2002.

7. Dangel JH: Cardiovascular changes in children with mucopolysaccharide storage diseases and related disorders: Clinical and echocardiographic findings in 64 patients. *Eur J Pediatr* 157:534–538, 1998.

8. David TE, Feindel CM: An aortic valve-sparing operation for patients with aortic incompetence and aneurysm of the ascending aorta. *J Thorac Cardiovasc Surg* 103:617–621, 1992.

9. Dilber E, Celiker A, Karagoz T, Kalkanoglu HS: Permanent transfemoral pacemaker implantation in a child with Maroteaux Lamy syndrome. *Pacing Clin Electrophysiol* 25:1784–1785, 2002.

10. Doing AH, Renlund DG, Smith RA: Becker muscular dystrophy-related cardiomyopathy: A favorable response to medical therapy. *J Heart Lung Transplant* 21:496–498, 2002.

11. Eagle M, Baudouin SV, Chandler C, et al: Survival in Duchenne muscular dystrophy: Improvements in life expectancy since 1967 and the impact of home nocturnal ventilation. *Neuromuscul Disord* 12:926–929, 2002.

12. Fiocchi R, Vernocchi A, Gariboldi F, et al: Troponin I as a specific marker for heart damage after heart transplantation in a patient with Becker type muscular dystrophy. *J Heart Lung Transplant* 16:969–973, 1997.

13. Fuzellier JF, Chauvaud SM, Fornes P, et al: Surgical management of mitral regurgitation associated with Marfan's syndrome. *Ann Thorac Surg* 66:68–72, 1998.

14. Gillinov AM, Zehr KJ, Redmond JM, et al: Cardiac operations in children with Marfan's syndrome: Indications and results. *Ann Thorac Surg* 64:1140–1144, 1997.

15. Gott VL, Greene PS, Alejo DE, et al: Replacement of the aortic root in patients with Marfan's syndrome. *N Engl J Med* 340:1307–1313, 1999.

16. Grain L, Cortina-Borja M, Forfar C, et al: Cardiac abnormalities and skeletal muscle weakness in carriers of Duchenne and Becker muscular dystrophies and controls. *Neuromuscul Disord* 11:186–191, 2001.

17. Grande AM, Rinaldi M, Pasquino S, et al: Heart transplantation in X-linked dilated cardiomyopathy. *Ital Heart J* 3:476–478, 2002.

18. Jacobs AM, Toudjarska I, Racine A, et al: A recurring *FBN1* gene mutation in neonatal Marfan syndrome. *Arch Pediatr Adolesc Med* 156:1081–1085, 2002.

19. Kakkis ED, Muenzer J, Tiller GE, et al: Enzyme-replacement therapy in mucopolysaccharidosis I. *N Engl J Med* 344:182–188, 2001.

20. Kastrup M, von Heymann C, Hotz H, et al: Recombinant factor VIIa after aortic valve replacement in a patient with osteogenesis imperfecta. *Ann Thorac Surg* 74:910–912, 2002.

21. Leonard H, Forsyth R: Friedreich's ataxia presenting after cardiac transplantation. *Arch Dis Child* 84:167–168, 2001.

22. Leprince P, Heloire F, Eymard B, et al: Successful bridge to transplantation in a patient with Becker muscular dystrophy-associated cardiomyopathy. *J Heart Lung Transplant* 21:822–824, 2002.

23. Leyh RG, Fischer S, Kallenbach K, et al: High failure rate after valve-sparing aortic root replacement using the "remodeling technique" in acute type A aortic dissection. *Circulation* 106:I229–I233, 2002.

24. Long SM, Tribble CG, Raymond DP, et al: Preoperative shock determines outcome for acute type A aortic dissection. *Ann Thorac Surg* 75:520–524, 2003.

25. Mariotti C, Solari A, Torta D, et al: Idebenone treatment in Friedreich patients: One-year-long randomized placebo-controlled trial. *Neurology* 60:1676–1679, 2003.

26. Mohan UR, Hay AA, Cleary MA, et al: Cardiovascular changes in children with mucopolysaccharide disorders. *Acta Paediatr* 91:799–804, 2002.

27. Shores J, Berger KR, Murphy EA, Pyeritz RE: Progression of aortic dilatation and the benefit of long-term beta-adrenergic blockade in Marfan's syndrome. *N Engl J Med* 330:1335–1341, 1994.

28. Sidwell RU, Yates R, Atherton D: Dilated cardiomyopathy in dystrophic epidermolysis bullosa. *Arch Dis Child* 83:59–63, 2000.

29. Sillence DO, Senn A, Danks DM: Genetic heterogeneity in osteogenesis imperfecta. *J Med Genet* 16:101–116, 1979.

30. Taylor DB, Blaser SI, Burrows PE, et al: Arteriopathy and coarctation of the abdominal aorta in children with mucopolysaccharidosis: Imaging findings. *AJR Am J Roentgenol* 157:819–823, 1991.

31. Toda Y, Takeuchi M, Morita K, et al: Complete heart block during anesthetic management in a patient with mucopolysaccharidosis type VII. *Anesthesiology* 95:1035–1037, 2001.

32. Vetter U, Maierhofer B, Muller M, et al: Osteogenesis imperfecta in childhood: Cardiac and renal manifestations. *Eur J Pediatr* 149:184–187, 1989.

33. Yacoub M, Fagan A, Stassano P, Radley-Smith R: Results of valve conserving operations for aortic regurgitation. *Circulation* 68:III321, 1983.

Chapter 48

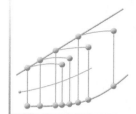

Cardiomyopathy

KATHERINE BIAGAS, MD, and DAPHNE T. HSU, MD

INTRODUCTION

Cardiomyopathies have been defined as diseases of the myocardium associated with cardiac dysfunction. The World Health Organization has identified three major classifications of primary cardiomyopathy based on morphology and dominant pathophysiology: dilated cardiomyopathy, hypertrophic cardiomyopathy, and restrictive cardiomyopathy.[61] Each class of cardiomyopathy has distinct modes of presentation and differs in short- and long-term management. Echocardiography has been the gold standard for empirical classification; however, cardiomyopathies are increasingly being defined by their metabolic and genetic basis.[68]

DEFINITIONS OF CARDIOMYOPATHY

Morphologic Classification of Cardiomyopathy

Dilated Cardiomyopathy

Dilated cardiomyopathy typically affects the left ventricle but may be bilateral and is characterized by ventricular dilation and impaired systolic function. The ventricular mass-to-volume ratio is reduced, although absolute ventricular mass may be normal or increased. Mitral insufficiency may be present secondary

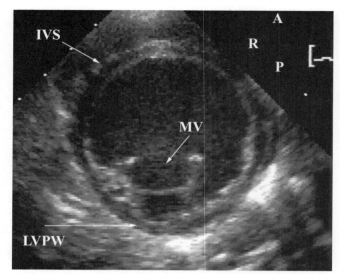

FIGURE 48-1   Dilated cardiomyopathy. Parasternal short axis echocardiographic view of the markedly dilated, thin-walled left ventricle. IVS, interventricular septum; LVPW, left ventricular posterior wall; MV, mitral valve.

to dilation of the valve annulus. Figure 48-1 depicts the echocardiographic appearance of dilated cardiomyopathy.

Hypertrophic Cardiomyopathy

Hypertrophic cardiomyopathy is characterized by left or right ventricular hypertrophy, or both, with normal to decreased ventricular volume. Hypertrophy is usually asymmetrical, with the interventricular septal thickness greater than the free wall; however, it may be concentric. Systolic ventricular function is normal or hyperdynamic until later phases of the

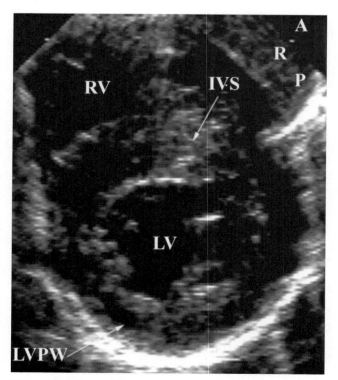

FIGURE 48-2   Hypertrophic cardiomyopathy with asymetric septal hypertrophy. Parasternal short axis echocardiographic view. IVS, interventricular septum; LV, left ventricle; LVPW, left ventricular posterior wall; MV, mitral valve; RV, right ventricle.

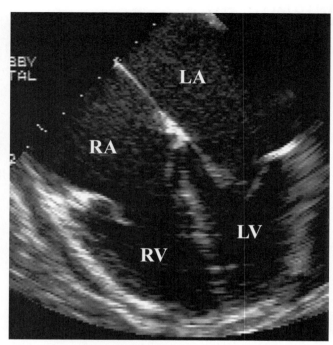

FIGURE 48-3   Restrictive cardiomyopathy. Apical four chamber echocardiographic view demonstrating biatrial enlargement with relative preservation of ventricular size. LA, left atrium; LV, left ventricle; RA, right atrium; RV, right ventricle.

disease. Obstruction to left or right ventricular outflow is common because of septal hypertrophy. Figure 48-2 depicts the typical echocardiographic appearance of hypertrophic cardiomyopathy.

Restrictive Cardiomyopathy

Restrictive cardiomyopathy is characterized by normal or reduced ventricular volume and by primarily diastolic dysfunction. Ventricular wall thickness is normal. Systolic function is normal until the later phases of the disease. Atrial enlargement is often present along with elevated atrial and ventricular end-diastolic pressures. Figure 48-3 depicts the typical echocardiographic appearance of restrictive cardiomyopathy.

Etiologic Classification of Cardiomyopathies

The etiology rather than the morphology can be used to classify cardiomyopathy (Table 48-1). Cardiomyopathy may affect primarily the heart or be a secondary complication of a more generalized systemic disease. In many patients with cardiomyopathy, no specific cause can be identified. As knowledge regarding the genetic and molecular basis of cardiac disease increases, the distinction between primary and secondary cardiomyopathies is less clear.

DILATED CARDIOMYOPATHY

Clinical Presentation

Infants and children with dilated cardiomyopathy most often are initially seen with signs of biventricular congestive heart failure. Manifestations of heart failure in infants include respiratory distress with tachypnea, retractions, and grunting.

Table 48-1   Etiologic Classification of Cardiomyopathy

Cardiac

Ischemic: anomalous left coronary artery, coronary calcinosis, Kawasaki disease, hyperlipidemia
Valvular: left ventricular outflow tract obstruction
Arrhythmia
Hypertensive

Inflammatory

Myocarditis in association with cardiac dysfunction

Infectious

Viral, Chagas's disease

Autoimmune

Systemic lupus erythematosus, polyarthritis nodosa, rheumatoid arthritis, scleroderma, dermatomyositis

Metabolic

Endocrine: thyrotoxicosis, hypothyroidism, adrenal cortical insufficiency, pheochromocytoma, acromegaly, diabetes
Infiltrative or toxic: iron, Wilson's disease
Dietary deficiency: carnitine, selenium

Inborn Errors of Metabolism

Amino acid metabolism: homocystinuria, alkaptonuria, oxalosis, hyperglycinemia
Mitochondrial disorders: respiratory chain diseases, cytochrome-*c* enzymes, MELAS, MERRF, mitochondrial myopathies
Storage diseases: glycogen storage, mucopolysaccharidoses, mucolipidoses, gangliosidoses, lipid storage, Gaucher's disease, Fabry's disease, neuronal ceroid lipofuscinosis

Amyloid

Neuromuscular Diseases

Duchenne and Becker muscular dystrophies, Nemaline myopathy, Friedreich ataxia, Kugelberg-Welander syndrome

Toxic Reactions

Anthracyclines, irradiation, alcohol

Peripartum

MELAS, mitochondrial myopathy, encephalopathy, lactacidosis, and stroke; MERRF, myclonic epilepsy associated with ragged red fibers.

Poor feeding and failure to thrive by weight criteria with relative preservation of length often occurs. The Ross Classification of heart failure in infants[65] is useful in quantifying heart failure in this young age group (Table 48-2). In the older child, clinical signs of pulmonary edema are often present. In addition, low cardiac output can be manifested by poor exercise tolerance and gastrointestinal distress. The New York Heart Association Classification can be used to quantify heart failure in the older child and adolescent (Table 48-3).

Cardiomyopathy associated with an inborn error of metabolism can appear as congestive heart failure as metabolic demand outstrips supply or as toxic metabolites accumulate (see Table 48-1). Infants with these disorders can have hypoglycemia, metabolic acidosis, encephalopathy, or a combination of these.

Table 48-2   Ross Classification of Heart Failure in Infants

Class I:	No limitations of symptoms
Class II:	Mild tachypnea and/or diaphoresis with feeds in infants; dyspnea on exercise in older children. No growth failure
Class III:	Marked tachypnea and/or diaphoresis with feeds or exertion and prolonged feeding time with growth failure
Class IV:	Symptomatic at rest with tachypnea, diaphoresis, or grunting

Physical Examination

On physical examination, signs of congestive heart failure include pulmonary edema, hepatomegaly, and poor peripheral perfusion. Cardiac findings include tachycardia, pulsus alternans, distant heart tones, an S_3 gallop, and often a murmur of mitral regurgitation. Jugular venous distention is uncommonly observed in the infant but is a useful indicator of central venous hypertension in the older child. Failure to thrive is common in patients with long-standing cardiomyopathy. Neurologic abnormalities, including hypotonia and generalized muscle weakness, are important findings leading to the diagnosis of cardiomyopathy associated with inborn errors of metabolism.

Cardiac Evaluation

Electrocardiography may demonstrate myocardial ischemia associated with coronary artery obstruction or due to congenital anatomic diseases such as anomalous left coronary artery. It also is essential to determine the predominant rhythm. Tachyarrhythmias, such as permanent junctional reciprocating tachycardia, ectopic atrial tachycardia, or junctional tachycardia, may result in ventricular dysfunction. Typically, increased left ventricular forces, flattening or inversion of the ST-T waves, atrial enlargement, or a combination of these characterize dilated cardiomyopathy. Low-voltage R waves and elevated ST-T segments are more characteristic of myocarditis.

Holter monitoring also is useful in diagnosing dysrhythmias, including ventricular premature beats or tachycardia, and in assessing the risk for malignant arrhythmias in patients with severely compromised function. As noted earlier, the arrhythmia may be the primary cause of dysfunction or may occur as a secondary complication in any cardiomyopathy in which severe ventricular dysfunction is found.

Chest radiography often shows pulmonary venous congestion and cardiomegaly. Congestive heart failure can be exacerbated by infectious respiratory disease, and the chest radiograph is essential in diagnosing these processes, including pneumonia. Pleural effusion and atelectasis, particularly of the left lower lobe, are commonly seen in severe cardiomyopathy.

Table 48-3   New York Heart Association Functional Classification of Heart Failure

Class I:	Patients with cardiac disease, but without resulting limitation of physical activity. Ordinary physical activity does not cause undue fatigue, palpitation, dyspnea, or angina
Class II:	Patients with cardiac disease resulting in slight limitation of physical activity. They are comfortable at rest. Ordinary physical activity results in fatigue, palpitation, and dyspnea or angina
Class III:	Patients with cardiac disease resulting in marked limitation of physical activity. They are comfortable at rest. Less than ordinary physical activity causes fatigue, palpitation, dyspnea, or angina
Class IV:	Patients with cardiac disease resulting in inability to carry on any physical activity without discomfort. Symptoms of heart failure or of angina may be present at rest. If any physical activity is undertaken, discomfort is increased

Echocardiography allows the quantitative determination of ventricular volume and function, both systolic and diastolic. It is essential to rule out anatomic causes of ventricular dysfunction, such as left ventricular outflow tract obstruction, coarctation, primary valvular disease, or coronary artery anomalies. The severity of atrioventricular valve regurgitation can be determined by using color flow Doppler. If tricuspid regurgitation is present, continuous-wave Doppler of the jet allows estimation of pulmonary artery pressure. Thrombi secondary to low cardiac flow may be seen most commonly in the left ventricular apex and in the left atrial appendage.

Other Noninvasive Studies for Determining Ventricular Volume and Function

Cardiac magnetic resonance imaging is useful in quantifying ventricular volumes and ejection fraction, especially in cases in which regional wall-motion abnormalities are present or when the echocardiogram is technically limited. Radionuclide ventriculography also can be used to determine ventricular ejection fraction.

Exercise stress testing with determination of maximal oxygen consumption has been shown to be useful in the prediction of 1-year survival in adult patients with dilated cardiomyopathy.[54] An oxygen consumption of less than 15 mL/kg/min is associated with a poorer 1-year survival. Although these data are not for children, exercise testing should be performed in the older child with stable cardiomyopathy.

Cardiac catheterization is not routinely performed to establish the diagnosis of cardiomyopathy. If anatomic abnormalities such as anomalous left coronary artery or aortic coarctation cannot be reliably excluded with noninvasive imaging, coronary angiography and aortography should be performed. Hemodynamic measurements such as cardiac output, ventricular filling pressures, and pulmonary vascular resistance may be helpful in determining both the effectiveness of therapy and the long-term prognosis. When significant ventricular outflow tract obstruction or valvular insufficiency is found, hemodynamic measurements may help to determine the relative contribution of the associated lesions to the heart failure syndrome. Endomyocardial biopsy may show distinctive histologic or ultrastructural findings that may be helpful in diagnosing myocarditis or certain metabolic diseases. However, myocardial biopsy may have only 60% sensitivity in detecting myocarditis, even when multiple biopsy specimens are obtained, because of the focal nature of myocardial involvement. Demonstration of myocardial fibrosis may indicate a worse prognosis.

Medical Therapy for Dilated Cardiomyopathy

The goals of medical therapy in dilated cardiomyopathy are threefold: control of the symptoms of congestive heart failure, promotion of measures to potentiate favorable ventricular remodeling, and prevention or treatment of complications including thromboembolism or arrhythmias. Decisions regarding specific therapies are tailored to the level of ventricular dysfunction and degree of heart failure as well as whether the patient is being treated immediately, such as in the intensive care unit, or over the long term, such as at home.

Short-term Management of Dilated Cardiomyopathy

Short-term management is directed toward the physiologic goals of improving ventricular function and contractility, optimizing preload, and reducing afterload. Continuous infusion of a selective β-adrenergic agonist such as dobutamine is often used to increase contractility and to reduce afterload, although low doses of dopamine will achieve the same effect (Table 48-4). Higher doses of dopamine should be avoided, as they cause α-adrenergic stimulation, resulting in peripheral vasoconstriction and increased afterload. It should be noted that both dobutamine and dopamine increase myocardial oxygen consumption and are proarrhythmic, both undesirable effects in the failing heart. Long-term use of β-agonists also may adversely affect prognosis. Reduction in right and left ventricular end-diastolic pressures is accomplished by diuresis. Loop diuretics, such as furosemide and bumetanide, are often used. In patients with very poor cardiac function, care should be taken to avoid rapid diuresis that may decrease preload and further reduce cardiac output. Continuous infusion of furosemide may be particularly effective in providing sustained diuresis with smaller swings in filling pressures.

Often these measures are sufficient to improve cardiac output. If not, additional afterload reduction may be required. The phosphodiesterase inhibitors, amrinone (no longer available in the U.S.) and milrinone, can be administered continuously for this purpose (see Table 48-4). Systemic hypotension can occur with either agent. Milrinone has the advantage of having a shorter half-life; thus it requires no loading bolus and can be more easily weaned if hypotension is present. Infusion of nitroprusside, a potent vasodilator, also may be used to decrease afterload (see Table 48-4).

Table 48-4 Intravenous Inotropic, Vasopressor, and Afterload Reducing Medications*

Medication	Dose Range†
Dopamine	
Dopaminergic‡	1–5 mcg/kg/min
β-adrenergic	2–10 mcg/kg/min
Alpha adrenergic‡	15–20 mcg/kg/min
Dobutamine	1–20 mcg/kg/min
Epinephrine	
β-adrenergic	0.01–0.2 mcg/kg/min
Alpha adrenergic‡	0.2–5 mcg/kg/min
Adult dose	1–4 mcg/min
Vasopressin	
Adult dose	0.0003–0.002 U/kg/min
Amrinone	
Loading	1–3 mcg/kg/dose
Maintenance	5–10 mcg/kg/min
Milrinone	
Loading	25–50 mcg/kg over 20–60 min
Maintenance	0.375–1 mcg/kg/min
Nitroprusside	0.05–4 mcg/kg/min

*Note adult dose
†All medications are administered by continuous infusion.
‡Doses of medications causing dopaminergic and/or α-adrenergic stimulation provided for information.

Careful titration of nitroprusside, starting at very low doses, is recommended to avoid hypotension.

Endotracheal intubation and positive-pressure ventilation may be beneficial. By decreasing ventricular transmural pressure, positive-pressure ventilation may improve cardiac mechanics. In addition, systemic oxygen demand is reduced as oxygen consumption associated with the work of breathing is reduced. Moreover, patients must be sedated to tolerate mechanical ventilation, and this may further reduce systemic oxygen requirements.

Patients with end-stage cardiac dysfunction or vasodilatory shock from multiple organ system failure or sepsis will have systemic hypotension. The management of these patients is particularly challenging and requires infusions of vasopressors to maintain systemic blood pressure. In such situations, judicious use of α-adrenergic agents, such as epinephrine or dopamine, may be required (see Table 48-4). One recent investigation reported the use of arginine-vasopressin, in addition to the use of α-adrenergic agents, in 10 patients with congenital heart disease and one patient with dilated cardiomyopathy (see Table 48-4).[64] Increased systemic blood pressure was found in patients with systemic hypotension from vasodilatory or severe cardiogenic shock. Additional beneficial effects may be derived as well. In an experimental model of ventricular dysfunction, infusion of arginine-vasopressin increased cardiac and urinary output, with improvement in overall hemodynamics.[49]

Critically ill patients must be monitored closely. Measurement of hourly urine output is essential to determine the adequacy of end-organ perfusion and the success of diuretic therapy. Monitoring of central venous and arterial blood pressure, by using indwelling lines, is usually indicated. In the older child or adolescent, management of cardiac output may be maximized by using a pulmonary artery (Swan-Ganz) catheter to determine optimal filling pressures and the effects of therapeutic interventions.

Long-term Management of Dilated Cardiomyopathy

Long-term therapy for dilated cardiomyopathy has many goals: afterload reduction, inhibition of the renin-angiotensin system, facilitation of factors likely to result in favorable ventricular remodeling, and optimization of preload with the use of diuretics.[75] All measures are intended to allow improvement in ventricular function and contractility.

It is becoming clear that the natural history of dilated cardiomyopathy also is positively affected by β-blockade,[70,72,73] administration of antagonists of aldosterone,[58] and angiotensin II receptor blockade. Angiotensin II receptor blockade has been demonstrated to affect positively the natural history of dilated cardiomyopathy and may have an additive effect beyond that achieved by angiotensin-converting enzyme inhibitors (see Chapter 4).[30] Recommended doses of common anticongestive medications are shown in Table 48-5.

The indications for treatment are based on the degree of heart failure and the level of ventricular dysfunction. In the child with class II to IV heart failure, standard therapy includes digoxin, diuretics, and angiotensin-converting enzyme inhibition. The latter are important because of a beneficial effect on both mortality and some measures of morbidity. Diuretic use is instituted in the presence of volume

Table 48-5 Oral Anticongestive Medications*

Medication	Dose	Dosing Interval
Digoxin		
Loading range†		
Infant	Total 20–30 mcg/kg IV	in 3 doses, ÷ q8h
Child	Total 25–35 mcg/kg IV	in 3 doses, ÷ q8h
>10 yrs	Total 8–10 mcg/kg IV	in 3 doses, ÷ q8h
Maintenance		
Infant/child	8–12 mcg/kg/day PO	÷ q12h
5–10 years	5–10 mcg/kg/day	÷ q12h
>10 years	2.5–5 mcg/kg/day	÷ q12h
Adult	0.125–0.5 mcg/kg/day	qd
Furosemide	1–6 mg/kg/day PO/IV	÷ q6–q24h
	Max adult dose 600 mg/day	
Spironolactone	1–3 mg/kg/day PO	÷ q8–q12h
	Adult dose, 25–100 mg	qd or bid
Captopril	1–4 mg/kg/day PO	÷ q12h
	Start dose, 0.1–0.3 mg/kg/dose	
	Adult dose, 12.5–50 mg	tid
	Max adult dose, 150 mg	tid
Enalapril	0.2–0.8 mg/kg/day PO	÷ q12h
	Adult dose, 10–40 mg	qd

*Not to exceed adult dose.
†IV doses are 80% of PO doses.

overload. Increasingly, aldosterone and β-blockade are used as well.

General Management

Anticoagulation Anticoagulation is recommended in patients with severe ventricular dysfunction because of the risk for thromboembolic disease, including pulmonary embolism and cerebrovascular accidents.[31] Warfarin is the drug of choice for long-term therapy; heparin should be used in the acute care setting. If the use of warfarin is contraindicated, antiplatelet therapy should be instituted.

Antiarrhythmic Therapy Antiarrhythmic therapy may be necessary because ventricular and supraventricular arrhythmias are common in patients with dilated cardiomyopathy. Supraventricular arrhythmias have been associated with worse outcome, although sudden death is rare in children with dilated cardiomyopathy. Antiarrhythmic therapy must be tailored to the type of arrhythmia. Ventricular arrhythmias are most commonly treated immediately with amiodarone infusion and over the long term with amiodarone or an automatic implantable defibrillator or both.

Biventricular Pacing Biventricular pacing has been reported, in adults with heart failure and interventricular conduction delay, to improve exercise tolerance significantly and to reduce the need for hospitalizations.[16] Comparable data have not yet been published for children. Biventricular pacing improves left ventricular function by synchronizing right and left ventricular contraction and septal wall motion.

Surgical Therapy Including Heart Transplantation

Close observation of the patient with congestive heart failure and severe ventricular dysfunction is essential because rapid deterioration can occur.[1] Mechanical ventricular-assist devices can be used in the acute rescue of intractable heart failure as a bridge to heart transplantation (see Chapter 21).[6] The indications for heart transplantation in dilated cardiomyopathy include heart failure refractory to medical therapy, severe failure to thrive, intractable arrhythmias, and severe limitations to activity. Pulmonary hypertension due to passive pulmonary venous congestion is a risk factor for poor outcome after transplantation; thus in the presence of elevated pulmonary vascular resistance, transplantation is considered, even in a relatively asymptomatic patient.[31,32] Results after heart transplantation for dilated cardiomyopathy in children indicate a 5-year survival of 72%.[11]

Prognosis

One-year survival after the diagnosis of dilated cardiomyopathy in children is reported to range between 50% and 75%, with 5-year survivals of 40% to 50%.[3,5,18,27,39,76,90] Factors that have been associated with worse outcome include older age,[5] lower shortening fraction, familial cardiomyopathy, endocardial fibroelastosis,[5,18] and elevated left ventricular end-diastolic pressure (>25 mm Hg).[39]

HYPERTROPHIC CARDIOMYOPATHY

The incidence of hypertrophic cardiomyopathy is 1 in 500 in the general population.[87] Tremendous heterogeneity exists in morphology, natural history, and the functional course of hypertrophic cardiomyopathy. Hypertrophic cardiomyopathy may involve either ventricle alone or together. The most common form of hypertrophy is asymmetrical, involving the interventricular septum; however, concentric hypertrophy also occurs. Midventricular and apical hypertrophy or isolated hypertrophy of the papillary muscles and apex alone are rare in children. Disease severity and symptoms, in particular, obstruction to ventricular outflow and myocardial ischemia, are related, although not consistently, to the extent and location of the hypertrophy.

Septal hypertrophy and systolic anterior motion of the mitral valve contribute to the mechanism of left ventricular outflow tract obstruction. The anterior mitral leaflet is pulled anteriorly by the Venturi effect during early systole, making contact with the septum and exacerbating subaortic obstruction. Repeated contact between the anterior leaflet and the septum may result in extensive leaflet fibrosis and further dysfunction.

Failure of proper coaptation of the mitral valve leaflets results in an interleaflet gap with mitral regurgitation directed posteriorly. The extent of mitral regurgitation is proportional to the duration that the interleaflet gap remains open. Thus the sequence of events that occurs is initial ejection with rapid filling of the aorta, then early systolic obstruction to flow through the outflow tract, followed by mid- to late-systolic mitral regurgitation. The degree of mitral leaflet dysfunction and septal wall contact determines the pathophysiologic features of hypertrophic cardiomyopathy. The magnitude of the pressure gradient across the outflow tract is a function of the extent of leaflet dysfunction and of the duration of leaflet–septal wall contact. The duration of mitral leaflet–septal wall contact also determines the degree of prolongation of left ventricular ejection time that is often seen in patients with hypertrophic cardiomyopathy. Last, the extent of mitral regurgitation can limit the volume of blood ejected from the left ventricle.

Clinical Presentation

Hypertrophic cardiomyopathy is seen in all phases of life, from the newborn infant to the elderly. The presentation often is a murmur related to turbulent flow in an outflow tract. Older children with obstructive hypertrophic cardiomyopathy typically complain of dyspnea, angina, presyncope, syncope on exertion, or a combination of these. Clinical symptoms in infants can be more difficult to detect but may be appreciated as increased work of breathing, failure to thrive, or significant diaphoresis. In infants, the pain of angina often appears as crying or agitation with feedings. Sometimes infants are mildly desaturated related to right-to-left shunting at the foramen ovale. Right ventricular outflow tract obstruction is more common in children. Patients with nonobstructive hypertrophic cardiomyopathy are first seen with milder symptoms.

Additional symptoms may occur in those with more severely obstructive hypertrophic cardiomyopathy or in patients with severe diastolic dysfunction or atrial fibrillation. Abnormalities in mitral valve morphology or function, such as anomalous papillary muscle attachments, calcification of the mitral annulus, marked anterior leaflet fibrosis, mitral valve prolapse, or a combination of these, may result in worsening symptoms from mitral regurgitation. Angina may be the presenting complaint for patients with hypertrophy in regions other than the septum because of infarction of hypertrophied papillary muscles or the apex. Malignant ventricular arrhythmias with near sudden death or syncope or both can be presenting signs. These patients may have been asymptomatic, with no signs of diastolic dysfunction or outflow tract obstruction.

The degree of systolic dysfunction in hypertrophic cardiomyopathy can be progressive. Left ventricular systolic function is usually normal or even hyperdynamic early in the disease. Later in the disease, myocardial fibrosis, ischemia, or infarction can result in impaired systolic function.

Diastolic dysfunction in hypertrophic cardiomyopathy results from impaired relaxation. Compliance in the right or left ventricle or both is decreased by an increased wall tone, decreased chamber volume, and myocardial fibrosis. Diastolic ventricular pressure is increased, and the volume of filling is reduced. The result is increased atrial pressure and venous congestion with pulmonary edema from left ventricular diastolic dysfunction and systemic venous congestion with hepatomegaly and peripheral edema from right ventricular diastolic dysfunction.

Physical Examination

Left ventricular involvement with hypertrophic cardiomyopathy is detected by a displaced and forceful left ventricular impulse. Diastolic dysfunction may be appreciated on auscultation with detection of loud fourth and third heart sounds, resulting from increased atrial systolic filling and restriction to ventricular filling, respectively. Patients with no obstruction to outflow will have no murmur or faint systolic murmurs appreciated at the apex. Patients with latent obstruction have a grade I or II/VI systolic apical murmur that increases to grade III/VI with provocation (Valsalva maneuver, assuming the upright posture, systemic hypotension, etc.) Patients with obstruction at rest will have a grade III to IV/VI murmur that radiates to the left sternal border and the axilla, reflecting the obstruction to flow and mitral regurgitation. Careful examination of patients with severe obstruction may reveal reverse splitting of the second heart sound, a mitral diastolic murmur, or an extra sound associated with mitral leaflet–septal contact.

Right ventricular involvement in hypertrophic cardiomyopathy may be difficult to detect, especially in the infant or young child. In the older child, a prominent A wave in the jugular venous pulse may be found. Rarely, a right-sided heart sound, reflecting diastolic dysfunction, or a right ventricular systolic ejection murmur may be appreciated.

Cardiac Evaluation

Electrocardiography is helpful, with the most common finding being that of left ventricular hypertrophy with or without a strain pattern. Signs of right ventricular hypertrophy may be appreciated in patients with prominent right ventricular or septal involvement. The QRS axis may be abnormal. Abnormal Q waves mimicking myocardial infarction are sometimes present. These reflect the increased forces of the hypertrophied septum. Signs of true myocardial ischemia may be seen under conditions of provocation. Patients with apical hypertrophy may have so-called giant negative T waves.

Holter monitoring is used routinely to determine the presence of associated dysrhythmias and to assess the risk for malignant arrhythmias. The presence of sustained ventricular tachycardia is an important predictor of the risk of sudden death, although in children, the absence of ventricular arrhythmias is not indicative of a low risk of sudden death.[46]

Chest radiography is often normal. Radiographic findings can include left ventricular, left atrial, or right atrial enlargement. Additional findings may include pulmonary vascular congestion and a bulge along the left heart border, reflecting anterior extension of septal hypertrophy.

Transthoracic echocardiography and Doppler study are the most informative laboratory investigation tools. The echocardiogram can determine the extent and location of the hypertrophy, the pressure gradient across the outflow tracts, and the degree of systolic and diastolic dysfunction. In addition, the severity and direction of mitral regurgitation can be estimated, and associated mitral valve abnormalities can be detected. Intraoperative and postoperative echocardiography is essential in guiding the surgery and assessing the outcome.

Other noninvasive modalities may be useful in assessing subtle or dynamic problems with hypertrophic cardiomyopathy and are used when the echocardiogram fails to explain fully the patient's symptoms. For example, magnetic resonance imaging is particularly useful in describing the extent of hypertrophy in unusual cases, such as patients with apical hypertrophy. Nuclear angiography may be used to assess systolic and diastolic function in patients with unexplained symptoms. Stress thallium or positron emission tomography can be sensitive techniques for diagnosing myocardial ischemia or infarction.

Cardiac Catheterization and Invasive Studies

The diagnostic accuracy of echocardiography and the other noninvasive studies has obviated the use of cardiac catheterization as a diagnostic tool. Cardiac catheterization is indicated in selected cases to evaluate the degree of ventricular outflow obstruction. Catheterization also is performed in a therapeutic intervention such as alcohol septal ablation or for the investigation of end-stage disease as part of the evaluation for cardiac transplantation. Invasive electrophysiologic studies have been used to provoke malignant arrhythmias and to guide antiarrhythmic therapy.

Medical and Surgical Treatment of Hypertrophic Cardiomyopathy

The management of hypertrophic cardiomyopathy is crafted to address the symptoms and hemodynamic problems unique to each patient. The manifestations of hypertrophic cardiomyopathy may vary considerably between patients, and therefore, so may the management.

Management of Ventricular Obstruction

Negative intropic agents like β-blockers and calcium channel blockers have, in some patients, brought relief of ventricular outflow tract obstruction and improvement of symptoms, particularly angina. Standard doses to achieve β-blockade are summarized in Table 48-6; however, much higher doses have been reported by some to produce a fivefold to10-fold reduction in the risk of disease-related death in children with hypertrophic cardiomyopathy.[55] β-Blockade has the additional advantage of reducing heart rate, allowing more time for cardiac filling in those patients with diastolic dysfunction As a general principle, these drugs should be sorted at their lowest doses and titrated upward as tolerated.

Calcium channel blockers also are used, particularly in patients with moderate or severe obstruction. Verapamil is the agent of choice, given its negative inotropic properties and relatively fewer vasodilator properties. It may be used in the long-term management of patients with hypertrophic cardiomyopathy. Care must be taken when administering this agent intravenously and in the acute setting, as hypotension can occur.[89] If used introvenously, preparations must be made for the immediate administration of intravenous calcium and

Table 48-6 β-Blockade Medications*

Medication	Dose	Dosing Interval
Propranolol		
Loading	0.01–0.1 mg/kg IV	Slow push
Infant	1–3 mg/kg/day PO	÷ q6–8h
Child	2–12 mg/kg/day PO	÷ q8h
Adult/adolescent	80–240 mg/dose	bid (sustained release)
Labetolol	0.4–1 mg/kg/hr IV	By infusion
	Adult, 1–2 mg/min	By infusion
Esmolol	0.2–1 mg/kg/min IV	By infusion
	Adult, 150–300 µg/kg/min	By infusion
Carvedilol	0.1 to 0.8 mg/kg/day PO	÷ q12h
	Adult, 6.25–50 mg/dose	bid
Metoprolol	0.5–12 mg/kg/day PO	÷ q12h
	Adult, 50–200 mg/dose	bid

*Not to exceed adult dose.

for full resuscitation of the patient. The combined use of verapamil and β-blockers is contraindicated because of the risk of hypotension.

Use of the oral type 1A antiarrhythmic agent, disopyramide, has been advocated by some for the prolonged management of obstructive hypertrophic cardiomyopathy. This agent has negative inotropic effects and has been used effectively in adults in combination with β-blockade for outpatient management.[89]

Dual-Chamber Pacing Dual-chamber (DDD) pacing has been used extensively in adults with obstructive hypertrophic cardiomyopathy to decrease obstruction to outflow. A 40% to 50% reduction in the pressure gradient across the outflow tract has been reported in selected patients.[24,44] DDD pacing decreases motion of the septum, decreases left ventricular contractility, and restores synchronous atrioventricular contraction and relaxation, especially in patients with arrhythmia. Optimal settings of the pacemaker involve slight prolongation of atrioventricular conduction, allowing complete ventricular capture. In the management of the older child or adult, dual-chamber pacing has been especially effective when combined with slowing of the heart rate by β-blockade. Until recently, use of these devices in the infant or small child presented technical difficulties, as the devices were rather bulky. Moreover, the growing infant or young child requires a large range of heart rates to meet changing levels of activity. However, recent adaptations in the device electronics have allowed at least single-chamber pacing of the infant or small child.

Surgical Relief of LVOTO Surgical relief of left ventricular outflow tract obstruction was described more than 25 years ago.[48] A transaortic myotomy or myectomy or both may be performed, with the goals of enlarging the ventricular outflow tract and thereby relieving obstruction. An additional benefit may be a reduction in mitral regurgitation by relief of mitral–septal wall contact. In patients with severe mitral disease, concomitant mitral valvuloplasty or mitral valve replacement may be required. Ideal surgical candidates are older children with obstructive hypertrophic cardiomyopathy for whom medical management fails. Other indications are significant mitral regurgitation and left atrial enlargement with arrhythmia. Some have advocated the use of myotomy-myectomy as primary therapy for selected adults (those with unexplained syncope or arrest).[89]

Management of Poor Diastolic Dysfunction

Calcium channel blockers have been demonstrated to improve diastolic filling immediately, and some have suggested using them over the long term as means of addressing the diastolic dysfunction frequently present in hypertrophic cardiomyopathy. Improvement in global left ventricular filling was noted in an observational study of 12 children with hypertrophic cardiomyopathy treated with verapamil.[56] Pretreatment with verapamil improved left ventricular filling in patients challenged with α- and β-adrenergic stimulation.[21] As stated earlier, calcium channel blockers are negative inotropes, and careful monitoring is required.

Diuretic therapy may be useful in later stages of the illness when venous congestion results in systemic or pulmonary edema. Clinical symptoms of coughing, dyspnea, orthopnea, abdominal pain, or a combination of these may be improved.

As discussed earlier, loop diuretics such as furosemide and bumetanide are effective, as are thiazide diuretics (see Table 48-5).

Management of Poor Systolic Dysfunction

Systolic function generally remains normal until the later stages of hypertrophic cardiomyopathy. Diastolic dysfunction usually occurs well before systolic dysfunction. Once systolic dysfunction is present, therapy resembles that used in dilated cardiomyopathy; however, use of inotropic and afterload-reducing agents is complicated by the potential for increasing outflow obstruction and the need to maintain preload in the setting of diastolic dysfunction. Given the chronotropic properties of most β-adrenergic agents, symptoms of diastolic dysfunction may be aggravated as well. Management of severe systolic dysfunction may be accomplished with intravenous dobutamine and diuresis and with the addition of a phosphodiesterase inhibitor as needed (see Table 48-4). Chronic systolic dysfunction is managed with oral medications, as described in Table 48-5.

Management of Arrhythmias

Treatment of malignant ventricular arrhythmias includes prolonged amiodarone therapy and placement of an automatic implantable defibrillator. Current recommendations for placement of an automatic implantable defibrillator include the presence of sustained ventricular tachycardia, near sudden death, or a family history of sudden death. Debate continues regarding the use of an automatic implantable defibrillator in the child with no evidence of ventricular arrhythmias and a negative family history.

Cardiac Transplantation

Cardiac transplantation is reserved for patients with end-stage cardiac function (see Chapter 16). Indications and contraindications for the procedure are essentially the same as those described for dilated cardiomyopathy. In general, patients who require transplantation have extensive disease. Pathologic specimens obtained from explanted hearts of adult and pediatric patients with hypertrophic cardiomyopathy show that 90% have ventricular scarring.[83] One- and two-year survival after cardiac transplantation in pediatric patients with congenital defects and cardiomyopathies is approximately 80%[71]; however, children who require transplantation for hypertrophic cardiomyopathy may be in a subgroup of patients with poorer prognosis.[52]

Prognosis

The clinical course of hypertrophic cardiomyopathy is highly variable, with some patients remaining asymptomatic until sudden death,[15,25] others developing progressive cardiac dysfunction, and still others having relatively benign disease.[15,25,42] The annual mortality rate reported by tertiary referral centers caring for children with hypertrophic cardiomyopathy is 3% to 6%.[2,45] However, studies in adults suggest that the risk of mortality may be much lower (<1% yearly) in the general population.[15] Sudden death composes up to 50% of the deaths in children with hypertrophic cardiomyopathy, with the risk increasing in patients with evidence of sustained ventricular tachycardia and those with a family history of sudden death.[55] Increased risk of mortality also is found in patients with a worse New York Heart Association Classification grade on presentation, evidence of myocardial infarction, need for anticongestive therapy, the severity of septal hypertrophy,[74] and the presence of atrial fibrillation.[15]

RESTRICTIVE CARDIOMYOPATHY

Restrictive cardiomyopathy is a rare form of myocardial disease characterized by diastolic ventricular dysfunction in the face of relatively preserved systolic function and normal wall thickness. Markedly elevated diastolic filling pressures and low cardiac output are the hemodynamic hallmarks of the disease. The majority of cases are sporadic; however, a primary restrictive cardiomyopathy associated with atrioventricular block and mild to subclinical myopathy has been associated with abnormal deposition of desmin in cardiac myocytes.[4,34]

The differential diagnosis of restrictive physiology includes secondary causes of diastolic dysfunction, such as constrictive pericarditis, myocarditis with associated myocardial fibrosis, coronary artery disease, and conditions increasing increased left ventricular mass such as left ventricular outflow tract obstruction or systemic hypertension. Systemic diseases or treatments can cause a restrictive cardiac physiology because of infiltration or injury. These include amyloid heart disease, scleroderma, doxorubicin (Adriamycin) or radiation, infiltrating neoplasms, and hemochromatosis.

Clinical Presentation

The clinical presentation of the patient with restrictive cardiomyopathy is often subtle because of the indolent nature of diastolic dysfunction. In small children, low cardiac output is manifested by growth failure or exercise intolerance. Acute pulmonary edema is rare; however, evidence of chronic systemic or pulmonary venous congestion is common. Systemic venous hypertension leads to ascites, peripheral edema, and hepatomegaly. Resting tachypnea and dyspnea on exertion also are common; in addition, a dry cough may be described in older children. Syncope also may be a presenting sign and carries a higher risk of mortality than do other presenting signs and symptoms.[20]

Arrhythmias are a common presenting sign of restrictive cardiomyopathy. Marked atrial dilation occurs in association with the elevated ventricular filling pressures and can lead to atrial flutter or fibrillation or supraventricular tachycardia. Complete heart block has been described in patients with desmin cardiomyopathy. Ventricular arrhythmias are less common but may occur, especially in the setting of depressed ventricular function. Restrictive cardiomyopathy also can appear as a thromboembolic event. Atrial thrombi form secondary to atrial dilation or atrial arrhythmias or both.

Physical Examination

Findings on physical examination include generalized growth failure; often with short stature, in conjunction with poor weight gain. Evidence of "right heart failure" is common, including hepatomegaly, jugular venous distention, and ascites. Borderline systemic hypotension can be present in

advanced disease. The cardiac examination can be unremarkable. An S_3 or S_4 may be audible; the P_2 may be accentuated in the setting of significant pulmonary hypertension. A murmur of tricuspid insufficiency may be present. A prominent apical impulse can be felt.

Cardiac Evaluation

Electrocardiography is characterized by bi-atrial enlargement. Nonspecific ST-T wave changes may be noted. In the setting of pulmonary hypertension, right ventricular enlargement may be present. The electrocardiogram (ECG) is essential to make the diagnosis of atrial arrhythmias or heart block associated with restrictive cardiomyopathy.

Echocardiography reveals prominent atrial enlargement with normal or even mildly reduced ventricular dimensions. The atrial four-chamber view is distinctive, and the appearance analogous to a "mushroom," with the ventricle reassembling the stalk, and the atrium, the cap. The hepatic veins and inferior vena cava are frequently quite dilated, reflecting elevated venous pressures. Pericardial effusion may be seen. Systolic ventricular function is normal or mildly reduced, but atrioventricular inflow patterns are frequently abnormal, reflecting diastolic dysfunction and elevated filling pressures. Pulmonary artery hypertension may be found.

Chest radiography can be normal, although careful inspection often reveals the presence of atrial enlargement. Pulmonary venous congestion may be present.

Holter monitoring is important in the clinical management to evaluate for the presence of tachyarrhythmias or bradycardia.

Cardiac magnetic resonance imaging may help to distinguish constrictive pericarditis from restrictive cardiomyopathy. Definitive diagnosis is made by direct inspection of the pericardium and pericardial biopsy; however, the risks of sternotomy are high in patients with low cardiac output secondary to restrictive cardiomyopathy. Magnetic resonance imaging can reliably evaluate the pericardial thickness and can lead to the diagnosis of constrictive pericarditis, allowing prompt surgical intervention.

Cardiac catheterization also may help in differentiating constrictive from restrictive processes. In restrictive cardiomyopathy, markedly elevated ventricular diastolic pressures are present, and in contrast to constrictive pericarditis, the end-diastolic pressure on the left is often higher than that on the right. In constrictive pericarditis, equalization of ventricular end-diastolic, atrial, and pulmonary artery end-diastolic pressures may be found. Maneuvers such as volume infusion may be necessary to bring out differences in ventricular filling pressures.

Cardiac catheterization also may yield important information in the prognosis of patients with restrictive cardiomyopathy. Pulmonary vascular resistance may be elevated at the time of diagnosis, secondary to left atrial hypertension. Low cardiac output or high pulmonary vascular resistance or both are important predictors of poor outcome and herald the need for cardiac transplantation.

Treatment of Restrictive Cardiomyopathy

Medical therapy has not proven effective in reversing the diastolic dysfunction found in restrictive cardiomyopathy. Symptomatic treatment includes the cautious use of diuretics to relieve systemic and pulmonary venous congestion, with careful attention to maintaining adequate intravascular volume to optimize cardiac output. In the terminal stages of disease, inotropic support may improve cardiac output (see Table 48-4).

Anticoagulation is recommended in patients with restrictive cardiomyopathy to prevent the thromboembolic complications. Antiarrhythmic therapy is important to treat atrial fibrillation or flutter, as a loss of atrioventricular synchrony will compromise cardiac output. In patients with malignant ventricular arrhythmias, placement of an automatic implantable defibrillator may be indicated. Mechanical pacing may be needed in cases of complete heart block.

Cardiac Transplantation

Cardiac transplantation may be the only therapeutic option available to patients with restrictive cardiomyopathy and low cardiac output. Pulmonary vascular resistance is elevated more commonly in patients with restrictive cardiomyopathy compared with that in children with other cardiomyopathies[32]; thus careful monitoring of patients for evidence pulmonary hypertension is essential in determining the optimal time for transplantation.

Prognosis

The prognosis of restrictive cardiomyopathy in children is grave, with reports of 44% to 50% 2-year actuarial survival after presentation.[17,38] Sudden death can occur. In one series of children, a 28% incidence of sudden death was reported, with female patients and those with signs and symptoms of ischemia, such as chest pain and syncope, being at greatest risk.[63] Patients also may die of worsening heart failure and congestion.

GENETICS OF CARDIOMYOPATHY

Original descriptions of the cardiomyopathies were generally made on entirely a clinical basis. Specific etiologies were rarely discovered. Although most primary cardiomyopathies were thought to arise sporadically, individual cases were noted to have familial associations. In recent years, increased understanding of molecular biology has resulted in elucidating specific genetic causes of certain cardiomyopathies. Statements from the World Health Organization recognize the evolving science and underscore this, stressing the importance of describing cardiomyopathies according to specific causes, including genetic defects.[29]

The heritable nature of hypertrophic cardiomyopathy was probably the first to be recognized. Extensive family pedigrees with autosomal dominant patterns of inheritance were identified. Early reports mapped a genetic defect to chromosome 6 in affected members.[35,43] However, linkage analysis of other affected patients demonstrated that considerable genetic heterogeneity is present. Rather than a few defective genes causing the heritable cases, the picture seems quite complex, with multiple diverse genes involved. Some have proposed a "final common pathway" hypothesis, which describes correlates between genotype and phenotype as functionally similar disruptions in a common pathway.[13] This hypothesis states that genetic heterogeneity for the same disease is observed because proteins with key functions exist within a common pathway. Mutations in the genes that encode these proteins disrupt the function of that pathway. A single phenotype is recognized from any of these mutations, because the result of dysfunction within the common pathway is the same clinically identifiable disease. Understood in this way, the cardiomyopathies can be classified according to the common pathways affected by the various mutations. Although this hypothesis does not fully describe the genetic basis for all the various forms of cardiomyopathy, it is a helpful unifying concept.

The remaining discussion focuses on the genetics of the two forms of cardiomyopathy now well studied: hypertrophic cardiomyopathy, which can be understood as a disease of the sarcomere, and dilated cardiomyopathy, which is a disease of the cytoskeleton. The genetics of restrictive cardiomyopathy are less well understood, although a dominant pattern of inheritance has been described.[4,34] Some of the specific cardiomyopathies, especially those associated with myopathy or neuropathy, are diseases of the mitochondria[82] or of carnitine metabolism.[57]

Molecular genetic studies have identified seven different genes encoding proteins of the myofibrillar apparatus of the sarcomere and associated with familial hypertrophic cardiomyopathy: β-myosin heavy chain,[28,33,59] cardiac troponin T,[87] cardiac myosin binding protein C,[77,85] α-tropomyosin,[78,87] ventricular myosin essential light chain,[7,66] ventricular myosin regulatory light chain,[67] and cardiac troponin I.[36,78,86] An estimated 70% of individuals thought to have familial hypertrophic cardiomyopathy have mutations in the first six of these.[69] Additional evidence implicates mutations in an eighth gene, which encodes for the atrial myosin light-chain protein, disturbing normal regulation of contractility.[62] In most cases, inheritance follows autosomal dominant patterns with variable penetrance.

Differences in phenotypic expression of the disease may be the result of a primary induced state or a compensatory response. The first option (i.e., primary production of hypercontractile, hypertrophied myocytes) is not thought to be the usual mechanism. Rather, it is the production of abnormal sarcomeric proteins that function as "poison peptides" and exert a dominant-negative effect on myocyte function. Specifically, incorporation of an abnormal protein in the sarcomeric structure alters the function of the sarcomere and myocyte sufficiently to cause a compensatory hypertrophy of cardiac muscle in an effort to preserve function.[10,41]

Differences in phenotypic expression also may be the result of mutational burden. Richard and colleagues[60] described a family pedigree with two sarcomeric mutations (mutations in genes encoding for the β-myosin heavy chain and cardiac myosin-binding protein C proteins). Patients with cosegregation of both mutations were more affected than their family members with a single defect.

In addition, differences in phenotypic expression can be explained by allelic variation. More than 100 different mutations have been identified in the sarcomeric genes listed earlier, but the impact of these mutations differs. Low disease prevalence has been seen in missense mutations causing one amino acid substitution in the β-myosin heavy chain, whereas nearly 100% disease penetrance has been seen with a different missense mutation in the same gene.[23,25,88] Allelic variation also may account for differences in disease severity and course. Certain mutations seem to have a profound effect on prognosis. Data on survival and incidence of sudden death in groups of unrelated individuals with the same mutations demonstrate significantly different prognosis. Groups with certain mutations have a high incidence of sudden death and shorter survival times, whereas groups with other mutations in the same genes have a better prognosis and nearly normal life span.[25,84] In the future, improved prediction of outcomes may be possible with this type of genotypic-phenotypic correlation.

As with hypertrophic cardiomyopathy, familial forms of dilated cardiomyopathy have been recognized. An estimated 20% to 30% of idiopathic dilated cardiomyopathy is familial.[47,51,79] Inheritance patterns are autosomal dominant, autosomal recessive, or X-linked. Over the past decade, linkage analysis, again conducted in families with affected individuals, has mapped loci on chromosomes 1q32,[22] 9q13-q22,[37] 10q21-q23,[12] Xq28,[9] and Xp21.[80] X-linked disease may be idiopathic,[8] recognized as Barth's syndrome (infantile-onset disease associated with the Xq28 locus), or arise in patients with Duchenne muscular dystrophy (associated with the Xp21 locus).

Further work has identified the autosomal genes as encoding for the proteins: actin,[53] desmin,[40] lamin A/C,[14,26] and possibly δ-sarcoglycan.[81] Linkage analyses suggest that several additional autosomal genes have not been identified to date. The X-chromosome genes encode for dystrophin[50,51,80,81] and tafazzin.[19] Mutations in the dystrophin gene account for the association of X-linked dilated cardiomyopathy with Duchenne muscular dystrophy (see Chapter 47). As stated earlier, the genetically recognized forms of dilated cardiomyopathy suggest that the disease is caused by dysfunction of cellular cytoarchitecture. These proteins are components of the cytoskeleton, such as lamin, or are elements associated with the skeletal architecture, such as dystrophin and sarcoglycan. Again, considerable phenotypic heterogeneity suggests numerous pathogenic mechanisms[47]; however, genetic explanations for some of the observed heterogeneity have not been explored to the extent that they have in hypertrophic cardiomyopathy.

SUMMARY

The cardiomyopathies are a group of diseases marked by myocardial dysfunction. Depending on the type of cardiomyopathy, clinical presentations in children vary markedly, as patients may have predominantly systolic dysfunction, diastolic dysfunction, arrhythmias, obstruction to ventricular outflow, or any combination of these. Short- and long-term management focuses on relief of the primary pathologic process(es), with some patients requiring surgical intervention, including cardiac transplantation. Recent advancements in genetic research have yielded information about the causes of some forms of cardiomyopathy. Improved understanding of the genetics of cardiomyopathy may generate better understanding of specific pathophysiology, guide therapy, or enhance prediction of outcomes.

References

1. Addonizio LJ, Hsu DT, Fuzesi L, et al: Optimal timing of pediatric heart transplantation. *Circulation* 80:III84–III89, 1989.
2. Ailman AG, Wigle ED, Ranganathan N, et al: The clinical course in muscular subaortic stenosis: A retrospective and prospective study of 60 hemodynamically proved cases. *Ann Intern Med* 77:515–525, 1972.
3. Akagi T, Benson LN, Lightfoot NE, et al: Natural history of dilated cardiomyopathy in children. *Am Heart J* 121:1502–1506, 1991.
4. Arbustini E, Morbini P, Grasso M, et al: Restrictive cardiomyopathy, atrioventricular block and mild to subclinical myopathy in patients with desmin-immunoreactive material deposits. *J Am Coll Cardiol* 31:645–653, 1998.
5. Arola A, Tuominen J, Ruuskanen O, Jokinen E: Idiopathic dilated cardiomyopathy in children: Prognostic indicators and outcome. *Pediatrics* 101:369–376, 1998.
6. Ashton RC Jr, Oz MC, Michler RE, et al: Left ventricular assist device options in pediatric patients. *Asaio J* 41:M277–M280, 1995.
7. Barton PJ, Cohen A, Robert B, et al: The myosin alkali light chains of mouse ventricular and slow skeletal muscle are indistinguishable and are encoded by the same gene. *J Biol Chem* 260:8578–8584, 1985.
8. Berko BA, Swift M: X-linked dilated cardiomyopathy. *N Engl J Med* 316:1186–1191, 1987.
9. Bolhuis PA, Hensels GW, Hulsebos TJ, et al: Mapping of the locus for X-linked cardioskeletal myopathy with neutropenia and abnormal mitochondria (Barth syndrome) to Xq28. *Am J Hum Genet* 48:481–485, 1991.
10. Bonne G, Carrier L, Richard P, et al: Familial hypertrophic cardiomyopathy: From mutations to functional defects. *Circ Res* 83:580–593, 1998.
11. Boucek MM, Faro A, Novick RJ, et al: The Registry of the International Society for Heart and Lung Transplantation: Fourth official pediatric report-2000. *J Heart Lung Transplant* 20:39–52, 2001.
12. Bowles KR, Abraham SE, Brugada R, et al: Construction of a high-resolution physical map of the chromosome 10q22-q23 dilated cardiomyopathy locus and analysis of candidate genes. *Genomics* 67:109–127, 2000.
13. Bowles NE, Bowles KR, Towbin JA: The "final common pathway" hypothesis and inherited cardiovascular disease: The role of cytoskeletal proteins in dilated cardiomyopathy. *Herz* 25:168–175, 2000.
14. Brodsky GL, Muntoni F, Miocic S, et al: Lamin A/C gene mutation associated with dilated cardiomyopathy with variable skeletal muscle involvement. *Circulation* 101:473–476, 2000.
15. Cannan CR, Reeder GS, Bailey KR, et al: Natural history of hypertrophic cardiomyopathy: A population-based study, 1976 through 1990. *Circulation* 92:2488–2495, 1995.
16. Cazeau S, Leclercq C, Lavergne T, et al: Effects of multisite biventricular pacing in patients with heart failure and intraventricular conduction delay. *N Engl J Med* 344:873–880, 2001.
17. Chen SC, Balfour IC, Jureidini S: Clinical spectrum of restrictive cardiomyopathy in children. *J Heart Lung Transplant* 20:90–92, 2001.
18. Chen SC, Nouri S, Balfour I, et al: Clinical profile of congestive cardiomyopathy in children. *J Am Coll Cardiol* 15:189–193, 1990.
19. D'Adamo P, Fassone L, Gedeon A, et al: The X-linked gene G4.5 is responsible for different infantile dilated cardiomyopathies. *Am J Hum Genet* 61:862–867, 1997.
20. Denfield SW, Rosenthal G, Gajarski RJ, et al: Restrictive cardiomyopathies in childhood: Etiologies and natural history. *Tx Heart Inst J* 24:38–44, 1997.
21. Dimitrow PP, Surdacki A, Dubiel JS: Verapamil normalizes the response of left ventricular early diastolic filling to cold pressor test in asymptomatic and mildly symptomatic patients with hypertrophic cardiomyopathy. *Cardiovasc Drugs Ther* 11:741–746, 1997.
22. Durand JB, Bachinski LL, Bieling LC, et al: Localization of a gene responsible for familial dilated cardiomyopathy to chromosome 1q32. *Circulation* 92:3387–3389, 1995.
23. Epstein ND, Cohn GM, Cyran F, Fananapazir L: Differences in clinical expression of hypertrophic cardiomyopathy associated with two distinct mutations in the beta-myosin heavy chain gene: A 908Leu----Val mutation and a 403Arg----Gln mutation. *Circulation* 86:345–352, 1992.
24. Fananapazir L, Cannon RO III, Tripodi D, Panza JA: Impact of dual-chamber permanent pacing in patients with obstructive hypertrophic cardiomyopathy with symptoms refractory to verapamil and beta-adrenergic blocker therapy. *Circulation* 85:2149–2161, 1992.

25. Fananapazir L, Epstein ND: Genotype-phenotype correlations in hypertrophic cardiomyopathy: Insights provided by comparisons of kindreds with distinct and identical beta-myosin heavy chain gene mutations. *Circulation* 89:22–32, 1994.

26. Fatkin D, MacRae C, Sasaki T, et al: Missense mutations in the rod domain of the lamin A/C gene as causes of dilated cardiomyopathy and conduction-system disease. *N Engl J Med* 341:1715–1724, 1999.

27. Friedman RA, Moak JP, Garson A Jr: Clinical course of idiopathic dilated cardiomyopathy in children. *J Am Coll Cardiol* 18:152–156, 1991.

28. Geisterfer-Lowrance AA, Kass S, Tanigawa G, et al: A molecular basis for familial hypertrophic cardiomyopathy: A beta cardiac myosin heavy chain gene missense mutation. *Cell* 62:999–1006, 1990.

29. Giles TD: New WHO/ISFC classification of cardiomyopathies: A task not completed. *Circulation* 96:2081–2082, 1997.

30. Hamroff G, Katz SD, Mancini D, et al: Addition of angiotensin II receptor blockade to maximal angiotensin-converting enzyme inhibition improves exercise capacity in patients with severe congestive heart failure. *Circulation* 99:990–992, 1999.

31. Hsu DT, Addonizio LJ, Hordof AJ, Gersony WM: Acute pulmonary embolism in pediatric patients awaiting heart transplantation. *J Am Coll Cardiol* 17:1621–1625, 1991.

32. Hughes ML, Kleinert S, Keogh A, et al: Pulmonary vascular resistance and reactivity in children with end-stage cardiomyopathy. *J Heart Lung Transplant* 19:701–704, 2000.

33. Jarcho JA, McKenna W, Pare JA, et al: Mapping a gene for familial hypertrophic cardiomyopathy to chromosome 14q1. *N Engl J Med* 321:1372–1378, 1989.

34. Katritsis D, Wilmshurst PT, Wendon JA, et al: Primary restrictive cardiomyopathy: Clinical and pathologic characteristics. *J Am Coll Cardiol* 18:1230–1235, 1991.

35. Kishimoto C, Kaburagi T, Takayama S, et al: Two forms of hypertrophic cardiomyopathy distinguished by inheritance of HLA haplotypes and left ventricular outflow tract obstruction. *Am Heart J* 105:988–994, 1983.

36. Kokado H, Shimizu M, Yoshio H, et al: Clinical features of hypertrophic cardiomyopathy caused by a Lys183 deletion mutation in the cardiac troponin I gene. *Circulation* 102:663–669, 2000.

37. Krajinovic M, Pinamonti B, Sinagra G, et al: Linkage of familial dilated cardiomyopathy to chromosome 9: Heart Muscle Disease Study Group. *Am J Hum Genet* 57:846–852, 1995.

38. Lewis AB: Clinical profile and outcome of restrictive cardiomyopathy in children. *Am Heart J* 123:1589–1593, 1992.

39. Lewis AB, Chabot M: Outcome of infants and children with dilated cardiomyopathy. *Am J Cardiol* 68:365–369, 1991.

40. Li D, Tapscoft T, Gonzalez O, et al: Desmin mutation responsible for idiopathic dilated cardiomyopathy. *Circulation* 100:461–464, 1999.

41. Marian AJ, Roberts R: Familial hypertrophic cardiomyopathy: A paradigm of the cardiac hypertrophic response to injury. *Ann Med* 30(suppl 1):24–32, 1998.

42. Maron BJ, Gardin JM, Flack JM, et al: Prevalence of hypertrophic cardiomyopathy in a general population of young adults: Echocardiographic analysis of 4,111 subjects in the CARDIA Study: Coronary Artery Risk Development in (Young) Adults. *Circulation* 92:785–789, 1995.

43. Matsumori A, Kawai C, Wakabayashi A, et al: HLA-DRW4 antigen linkage in patients with hypertrophic obstructive cardiomyopathy. *Am Heart J* 101:14–16, 1981.

44. McDonald KM, Maurer B: Permanent pacing as treatment for hypertrophic cardiomyopathy. *Am J Cardiol* 68:108–110, 1991.

45. McKenna WJ, Camm AJ: Sudden death in hypertrophic cardiomyopathy: Assessment of patients at high risk. *Circulation* 80:1489–1492, 1989.

46. McKenna WJ, Franklin RC, Nihoyannopoulos P, et al: Arrhythmia and prognosis in infants, children, and adolescents with hypertrophic cardiomyopathy. *J Am Coll Cardiol* 11:147–153, 1988.

47. Mestroni L, Rocco C, Vatta M, et al: Advances in molecular genetics of dilated cardiomyopathy: The Heart Muscle Disease Study Group. *Cardiol Clin* 16:611–621, vii, 1998.

48. Morrow AG, Reitz BA, Epstein SE, et al: Operative treatment in hypertrophic subaortic stenosis: Techniques, and the results of pre and postoperative assessments in 83 patients. *Circulation* 52:88–102, 1975.

49. Mulinari RA, Gavras I, Wang YX, et al: Effects of a vasopressin antagonist with combined antipressor and antiantidiuretic activities in rats with left ventricular dysfunction. *Circulation* 81:308–311, 1990.

50. Muntoni F, Cau M, Ganau A, et al: Brief report: Deletion of the dystrophin muscle-promoter region associated with X-linked dilated cardiomyopathy. *N Engl J Med* 329:921–925, 1993.

51. Muntoni F, Wilson L, Marrosu G, et al: A mutation in the dystrophin gene selectively affecting dystrophin expression in the heart. *J Clin Invest* 96:693–699, 1995.

52. Nunoda S, Kurosawa R, Kogashi K, et al: Points to note from indications for heart transplantation to post-heart transplant care: From the care of patients with refractory heart failure and overseas heart transplantation. *Heart Vessels Suppl* 12:37–40, 1997.

53. Olson TM, Michels VV, Thibodeau SN, et al: Actin mutations in dilated cardiomyopathy, a heritable form of heart failure. *Science* 280:750–752, 1998.

54. Osada N, Chaitman BR, Miller LW, et al: Cardiopulmonary exercise testing identifies low risk patients with heart failure and severely impaired exercise capacity considered for heart transplantation. *J Am Coll Cardiol* 31:577–582, 1998.

55. Ostman-Smith I, Wettrell G, Riesenfeld T: A cohort study of childhood hypertrophic cardiomyopathy: Improved survival following high-dose beta-adrenoceptor antagonist treatment. *J Am Coll Cardiol* 34:1813–1822, 1999.

56. Pacileo G, De Cristofaro M, Russo MG, et al: Hypertrophic cardiomyopathy in pediatric patients: Effect of verapamil on regional and global left ventricular diastolic function. *Can J Cardiol* 16:146–152, 2000.

57. Pierpont ME, Breningstall GN, Stanley CA, Singh A: Familial carnitine transporter defect: A treatable cause of cardiomyopathy in children. *Am Heart J* 139:S96–S106, 2000.

58. Pitt B, Zannad F, Remme WJ, et al: The effect of spironolactone on morbidity and mortality in patients with severe heart failure: Randomized Aldactone Evaluation Study Investigators. *N Engl J Med* 341:709–717, 1999.

59. Richard P, Charron P, Leclercq C, et al: Homozygotes for a R869G mutation in the beta-myosin heavy chain gene have a severe form of familial hypertrophic cardiomyopathy. *J Mol Cell Cardiol* 32:1575–1583, 2000.

60. Richard P, Isnard R, Carrier L, et al: Double heterozygosity for mutations in the beta-myosin heavy chain and in the cardiac myosin binding protein C genes in a family with hypertrophic cardiomyopathy. *J Med Genet* 36:542–545, 1999.

61. Richardson P, McKenna W, Bristow M, et al: Report of the 1995 World Health Organization/International Society and Federation of Cardiology Task Force on the definition and classification of cardiomyopathies. *Circulation* 93:841–842, 1996.

62. Ritter O, Luther HP, Haase H, et al: Expression of atrial myosin light chains but not alpha-myosin heavy chains is correlated in vivo with increased ventricular function in patients with hypertrophic obstructive cardiomyopathy. *J Mol Med* 77:677–685, 1999.

63. Rivenes SM, Kearney DL, Smith EO, et al: Sudden death and cardiovascular collapse in children with restrictive cardiomyopathy. *Circulation* 102:876–882, 2000.

64. Rosenzweig EB, Starc TJ, Chen JM, et al: Intravenous arginine-vasopressin in children with vasodilatory shock after cardiac surgery. *Circulation* 100:19(suppl): II182–II186, 1999.

65. Ross RD, Daniels SR, Schwartz DC, et al: Plasma norepinephrine levels in infants and children with congestive heart failure. *Am J Cardiol* 59:911–914, 1987.

66. Sanbe A, Nelson D, Gulick J, et al: In vivo analysis of an essential myosin light chain mutation linked to familial hypertrophic cardiomyopathy. *Circ Res* 87:296–302, 2000.

67. Sarkar S, Sreter FA, Gergely J: Light chains of myosins from white, red, and cardiac muscles. *Proc Natl Acad Sci U S A* 68:946–950, 1971.

68. Schwartz ML, Cox GF, Lin AE, et al: Clinical approach to genetic cardiomyopathy in children. *Circulation* 94:2021–2038, 1996.

69. Seidman CE, Seidman JG: Molecular genetic studies of familial hypertrophic cardiomyopathy. *Basic Res Cardiol* 93(suppl 3):13–16, 1998.

70. Shaddy RE: Beta-blocker therapy in young children with congestive heart failure under consideration for heart transplantation. *Am Heart J* 136:19–21, 1998.

71. Shaddy RE, Naftel DC, Kirklin JK, et al: Outcome of cardiac transplantation in children: Survival in a contemporary multi-institutional experience: Pediatric Heart Transplant Study. *Circulation* 94:II69–II73, 1996.

72. Shaddy RE, Olsen SL, Bristow MR, et al: Efficacy and safety of metoprolol in the treatment of doxorubicin-induced cardiomyopathy in pediatric patients. *Am Heart J* 129:197–199, 1995.

73. Shaddy RE, Tani LY, Gidding SS, et al: Beta-blocker treatment of dilated cardiomyopathy with congestive heart failure in children: A multi-institutional experience. *J Heart Lung Transplant* 18:269–274, 1999.
74. Spirito P, Bellone P, Harris KM, et al: Magnitude of left ventricular hypertrophy and risk of sudden death in hypertrophic cardiomyopathy. *N Engl J Med* 342:1778–1785, 2000.
75. Stern H, Weil J, Genz T, et al: Captopril in children with dilated cardiomyopathy: Acute and long-term effects in a prospective study of hemodynamic and hormonal effects. *Pediatr Cardiol* 11:22–28, 1990.
76. Taliercio CP, Seward JB, Driscoll DJ, et al: Idiopathic dilated cardiomyopathy in the young: clinical profile and natural history. *J Am Coll Cardiol* 6:1126–1131, 1985.
77. Thierfelder L, MacRae C, Watkins H, et al: A familial hypertrophic cardiomyopathy locus maps to chromosome 15q2. *Proc Natl Acad Sci U S A* 90:6270–6274, 1993.
78. Thierfelder L, Watkins H, MacRae C, et al: Alpha-tropomyosin and cardiac troponin T mutations cause familial hypertrophic cardiomyopathy: A disease of the sarcomere. *Cell* 77:701–712, 1994.
79. Towbin JA: The role of cytoskeletal proteins in cardiomyopathies. *Curr Opin Cell Biol* 10:131–139, 1998.
80. Towbin JA, Hejtmancik JF, Brink P, et al: X-linked dilated cardiomyopathy: Molecular genetic evidence of linkage to the Duchenne muscular dystrophy (dystrophin) gene at the Xp21 locus. *Circulation* 87:1854–1865, 1993.
81. Tsubata S, Bowles KR, Vatta M, et al: Mutations in the human delta-sarcoglycan gene in familial and sporadic dilated cardiomyopathy. *J Clin Invest* 106:655–662, 2000.
82. Wallace DC: Mitochondrial defects in cardiomyopathy and neuromuscular disease. *Am Heart J* 139:S70–S85, 2000.
83. Waller TA, Hiser WL, Capehart JE, Roberts WC: Comparison of clinical and morphologic cardiac findings in patients having cardiac transplantation for ischemic cardiomyopathy, idiopathic dilated cardiomyopathy, and dilated hypertrophic cardiomyopathy. *Am J Cardiol* 81:884–894, 1998.
84. Watkins H: Multiple disease genes cause hypertrophic cardiomyopathy. *Br Heart J* 72(6 suppl):S4–S9, 1994.
85. Watkins H, Conner D, Thierfelder L, et al: Mutations in the cardiac myosin binding protein-C gene on chromosome 11 cause familial hypertrophic cardiomyopathy. *Nat Genet* 11:434–437, 1995.
86. Watkins H, MacRae C, Thierfelder L, et al: A disease locus for familial hypertrophic cardiomyopathy maps to chromosome 1q3. *Nat Genet* 3:333–337, 1993.
87. Watkins H, McKenna WJ, Thierfelder L, et al: Mutations in the genes for cardiac troponin T and alpha-tropomyosin in hypertrophic cardiomyopathy. *N Engl J Med* 332:1058–1064, 1995.
88. Watkins H, Rosenzweig A, Hwang DS, et al: Characteristics and prognostic implications of myosin missense mutations in familial hypertrophic cardiomyopathy. *N Engl J Med* 326:1108–1114, 1992.
89. Wigle ED, Rakowski H, Kimball BP, Williams WG: Hypertrophic cardiomyopathy: Clinical spectrum and treatment. *Circulation* 92:1680–1692, 1995.
90. Wiles HB, McArthur PD, Taylor AB, et al: Prognostic features of children with idiopathic dilated cardiomyopathy. *Am J Cardiol* 68:1372–1376, 1991.

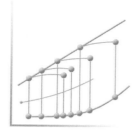

Index

Note: Page numbers followed by *b* indicate boxed material; those followed by *f* indicate figures; those followed by *t* indicate tables.